OXFORD TEXTBOOK OF PALLIATIVE MEDICINE

SECOND EDITION

Edited by
Derek Doyle
Geoffrey W. C. Hanks
and Neil MacDonald

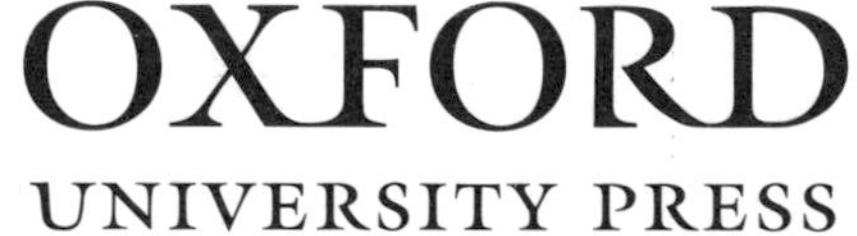

OXFORD
UNIVERSITY PRESS

Great Clarendon Street, Oxford OX2 6DP

Oxford University Press is a department of the University of Oxford.
It furthers the University's objective of excellence in research, scholarship,
and education by publishing worldwide in

Oxford New York

Athens Auckland Bangkok Bogotá Buenos Aires Calcutta
Cape Town Chennai Dar es Salaam Delhi Florence Hong Kong Istanbul
Karachi Kuala Lumpur Madrid Melbourne Mexico City Mumbai
Nairobi Paris São Paulo Singapore Taipei Tokyo Toronto Warsaw
with associated companies in Berlin Ibadan

Oxford is a registered trade mark of Oxford University Press
in the UK and in certain other countries

Published in the United States
by Oxford University Press Inc., New York

First edition published 1993
First published in paperback 1995
Second edition published 1998
Reprinted 1998
First published in paperback 1999
Reprinted 1999

A catalogue record for this book is available from the British Library

Library of Congress Cataloging in Publication Data
(Data available)

ISBN 0 19 263057 1 (Pbk)
ISBN 0 19 262566 7 (Hbk)

Printed in Great Britain
on acid-free paper by
Butler & Tanner Ltd., Frome and London

Foreword

Cicely Saunders

But I have promises to keep, and miles to go before I sleep.

Robert Frost

The time has come for this textbook, and demand has led to this second edition. It is the result of the past few decades of concentrated practice and a considerable body of research. It fills a gap, and the historical development as summarized by Wall in 1986 shows how it has been both necessary and possible. As he wrote:

> Up to the 19th century, most medical care related to the amelioration of symptoms while the natural history of the disease took its course toward recovery or death. By 1900, doctors and patients alike had turned to a search for root cause and ultimate cure. In the course of this new direction, symptoms were placed on one side as sign posts along a highway which was being driven toward the intended destination. Therapy directed at the sign posts was denigrated and dismissed as merely symptomatic. By the second half of this century, a reaction set in as seen by such remarkable developments as the hospice movement. The immediate origins of misery and suffering need immediate attention while the long-term search for basic cure proceeds. The old methods of care and caring had to be rediscovered and the best of modern medicine had to be turned to the task of new study and therapy specifically directed at pain.[1]

This volume has a wider perspective, however broadly pain may be interpreted to denote a whole spectrum of suffering. The challenge is as Wall has indicated.

Approaches to death and dying reveal much of the attitude of society as a whole to the individuals who compose it. The development of ideas of what constitutes a good death can even be traced to prehistory. Funeral rites can be dated back 50 000 years, and from this time show how early men laid down their dead in grief and in some hope of a continued existence.[2] Gentles traces the way funeral rites have become less and less elaborate and comparatively less costly over the millennia in proportion to the wealth of society.[3] But there seems to be more to it than that. The fantastic wealth of Egyptian funerals and the expenditure of time and human effort on such memorials as the pyramids were concentrated on the Pharaohs who in some sense personified the longings for immortality of the rest of the populace. Attitudes to death reflect attitudes to religion.

Aries reviewed western attitudes towards death from the Middle Ages to the present.[4] At the beginning of the period he describes 'tamed death', when the dying person was sure of his role in preparing for the end according to ritual or custom (Aries, pp. 2–9).[4] He was himself the centre of the stage, hopeful, if all was done in order, of a safe passage to the next world. Aries compares this with Solzhenitsyn's description of the death of the simple people of the country who 'departed easily, as if they were just moving into a new house'.[5] Similarly, Aries points out, the cemeteries of the early Middle Ages were open and public places and 'the living were as familiar with the dead as they were familiarised with the idea of their own death' (Aries, p. 25).[4]

Gradually during the Middle Ages subtle modifications gave a dramatic and personal meaning to this traditional familiarity. An increasing emphasis on the Last Judgement and the displacing of this to the end of each life with all its concentration on feelings of sin and failure, together with a macabre interest in physical decomposition, gave a more personal, threatening focus. One's own death, and an urge somehow to maintain identity despite the loss of all material attachments, took the place of the familiar resignation to the collective destiny of the species (Aries, pp. 27–52).[4] The individual has his particular place in the Christian Gospel (e.g. the search for the one lost sheep to join the ninety and nine safe in the fold) but the emphasis grew more urgent with the Renaissance: 'The discovery of the individual was made in early fifteenth century Florence. Nothing can alter that fact'.[6]

Aries traces in the exaggeration of mourning that developed in the nineteenth century a new fear, not so much of the death of the self as the death of another—the origin of the cult of tombs and cemeteries as we know them. This development was sharply brought to an end in many places in the twentieth century by a process far more abrupt than any so far summarized, surely related to the carnage of the War of 1914. From now on we see a process by which death becomes, as Aries puts it, 'shameful and forbidden', something to be hidden from those around. Death had become a taboo.[7]

The increasing tendency not to tell the dying person the truth of his condition, the likelihood of dying in hospital, often alone, rather than at home, and the inability of society to allow any display of emotions in public all made death an outlaw, a forbidden subject. We have not found our way to come to terms with our mortality, and each person, each family, with little help from ritual or tradition or from those around, has somehow to find a way to come to terms with and grow from loss. The old acceptance of destiny has gone, and a new sense of outrage that modern advances cannot finally halt the inevitable makes care of the dying and their families demanding and often difficult, but perhaps all the more rewarding.

The present volume, looking at the whole field of the multidisciplinary specialty of palliative medicine, addresses aspects of this problem and, importantly, shows how appropriate treatment before a patient can rightly be termed 'dying' can make a radical difference to his life and death.

The early hospices

A considerable part of this new and positive attitude to a whole new range of possibilities stems from the attitudes and skills of the modern hospice. An ancient word, although not originally concerned with dying, it has some connotations that introduce interesting comparisons with the aims of a modern hospice team. The Latin word *hospes* first meant 'stranger'. By late classical times, the word had changed and denoted a host, while *hospitalis* meant friendly, the welcome to the stranger. From it derived hospitality and thence many words used today; hospital, hostel, hostelry, hotel—and hospice. Another noun was derived—*hospitium*, originally the warm feeling between host and guest, and later the place where this feeling was experienced. The Greek version was *xenodochium* and by the fourth century came the first of many Christian institutions under both names, arising first in the Byzantine area[8] and later spreading to Rome and finally throughout Europe as hospice or hospital.[9] They were based on the Christian command 'As you did it to one of the least of these my brethren, you did it to me' (Matt. 25, v.40).[10] This was a radically different approach from the Hippocratic tradition, in which a doctor did not treat the incurably sick or terminally ill. It was thought unethical to treat a patient with a deadly disease, for in so doing the doctor risked paying the penalty awaiting those mortals who challenged nature and the gods.[11]

These hospices welcomed pilgrims, often very battered and perhaps dying, and gradually came the connotation of sickness, as Christians set out not only to welcome strangers and give food and drink but also to care for the sick.[12] As hospices developed along the pilgrim routes, local people in need undoubtedly came for help and were not sent away. Hospices lasted throughout the Middle Ages, but most came to a rather abrupt end with the Reformation. The state of the incurable and dying, no longer the honoured guests but often consigned to Poor Law or equivalent institutions, could be desperate. An example of how the Church's concern for the sick and poor was missed is illustrated by a petition to Henry VIII from the Lord Mayor and citizens of London. They implored the King to refound the priory of St Bartholomew in Smithfield and that of St Thomas across London Bridge in Southwark 'for the ayde and comfort of the poore sikke, blynde, aged and impotent persones, beying not able to helpe themselffs, nor hauyning any place certeyn whereyn they may be lodged, cherysshed and refressed tyll they be cured and holpen of theyre dyseases and syckesse'.[13]

The modern hospice movement

A family tree of the modern hospice movement was presented by Twycross at the Royal Society of Medicine in 1980 (Fig. 1).[14]

As has been pointed out, the medieval hospice was not primarily associated with dying people, and over the centuries it had come to welcome an impossible mix of patients along with travellers and pilgrims, orphans, and the destitute with varying degrees of segregation. Such cure as could be attained was a primary aim, but with comparatively little to offer many must have died, being cared for to the end with much emphasis on spiritual comfort.

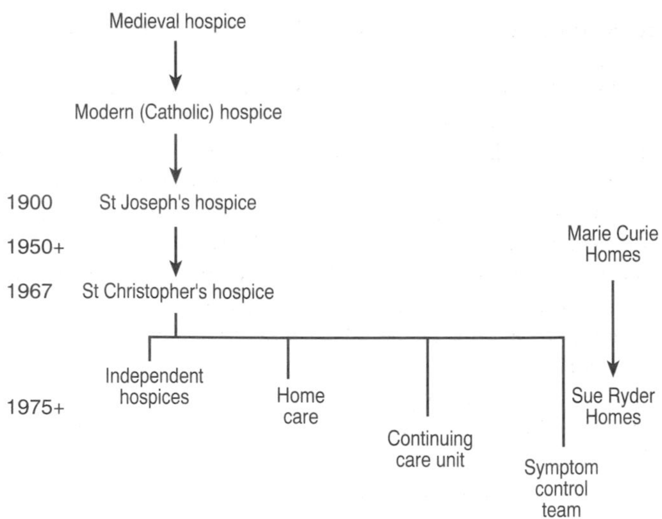

Fig. 1 Hospice development.

The first use so far discovered of the word 'hospice' solely for care of the dying was by Mme Jeanne Garnier in Lyons, France, in 1842, who founded several such hospices or *Calvaires*. There was no connection with the Irish Sisters of Charity who opened Our Lady's Hospice in Dublin in 1879 and St Joseph's Hospice in East London in 1905, both for incurable and dying patients, but Calvary Hospital in New York (1899) drew its inspiration from this source. Three Protestant Homes had been opened in London by the time St Joseph's welcomed patients. These were the Friedensheim Home of Rest (later St Columba's Hospital) in 1885, the Hostel of God (later Trinity Hospice) in 1891, and St Luke's Home for the Dying Poor in 1893. The author's seven years from 1948 as a volunteer nurse in St Luke's, by now named Hospital, and the reading of its many full and lively annual reports by Dr Howard Barrett, its founder, were a major influence in the early planning of St Christopher's Hospice.

These reports are full of individual stories of carefully observed people. Here we are not meeting 'the dying' but people, part of often destitute families. In 1909 Dr Barrett wrote:

> We do not think or speak of our inmates as 'cases'. We realize that each one is a human microcosm, with its own characteristics, its own aggregate of joys and sorrows, hopes and fears, its own life history, intensely interesting to itself and some small surrounding circle. Very often it is confided to some of us.

There was also much to learn from the Marie Curie Memorial Foundation. In 1952, it published a report detailing a great deal of suffering among patients dying of cancer at home.[15] Their response in supplying home nurses, and in opening a series of cancer care homes, marked another important milestone in terminal care. But above all, the author's seven years in clinical care at St Joseph's listening to patients, introducing records, and monitoring the results of the development of pain and symptom control (first seen in St Luke's as the regular administration of oral opioids) were crucial. Patients' comments and conditions revealed the need for appropriate treatments, for care in their own homes to supplement the existing community services, and for family support both before and after bereavement. Above all, the need for research and education in what was eventually to become a new specialty was revealed through much reading and many interviews during those years.

The Twycross tree (Fig. 1) summarizes the development of special units and teams to meet these new challenges. As he shows, the opening of St Christopher's led to several different systems of offering care in what began to be termed the Hospice Movement in North America, where the patterns other than free-standing inpatient units were first developed. The same systems arose not long afterwards in the United Kingdom. In 1974, The Connecticut Hospice began offering home care with a medical and professional team leading many volunteers but without its own backup beds. In New York, a consulting team began working throughout St Luke's Hospital during the same year. In early 1975, Mount opened the Palliative Care Service in The Royal Victoria Hospital, Montreal. The founders of all these teams had spent sabbatical periods of study and experience at St Christopher's Hospice. These developments demonstrated that hospice care did not have to be limited to a separate building, but that the new attitudes and skills could be practised in a variety of settings.

The Montreal Unit was not the first such use of the word palliative, although apparently there was no connection with an earlier use. In 1890, Dr Herbert Snow, Surgeon to the Cancer Hospital, Brompton, London, published a book on *The Palliative Treatment of Incurable Cancer, with an Appendix on the use of the Opium Pipe*.[16] He also published an article in the *British Medical Journal* on 'Opium and cocaine in the treatment of cancerous disease'.[17] The Cancer Hospital (now the Royal Marsden Hospital) was next door to the Brompton Hospital for Diseases of the Chest. Perhaps the pharmacists were in touch when the latter hospital produced the Brompton Cocktail in the early 1930s, with its main ingredients of morphine and/or diamorphine and cocaine. Its regular, four-hourly use in St Luke's Hospital, London can be traced back to 1935, through the memories of a former Matron (L. Pipkin, personal communication, 1948). The Cancer Hospital was committed to patients with advanced disease. In 1909, a Dr Horder was allocated 19 beds for such patients and in 1964 a ward was reopened with 16 beds in Dr Horder's name. I can find no record of what happened in the interim period.

New tools for relief

All the new teams set out first to establish control of the distress that had led to their patients' referral. For this they had many new tools on which to depend from the discoveries of the 1950s, including the new psychotropic drugs, the phenothiazines, antidepressants and anxiolytics, the synthetic steroids, and the non-steroidal anti-inflammatory drugs. New analgesics were also available, although none has so far replaced the well-tried opioids. Rather, it has been a continuing challenge to understand their actions, and to compare and test different routines and methods of administration. At the same time reports came from the new pain clinics, and work concerning better understanding of family dynamics and bereavement was undertaken at the Tavistock Centre for Human Relations. Developments in both cancer chemotherapy and intensive care units also had their impact, in both contrast and continuity, with the work of the new teams. The detailed study of 102 matched patients by Hinton[18] on the 'Physical and mental distress of the dying' documented the need to address problems largely ignored by the main thrust of medical development in general hospitals at that time.

Table 1

Hospice experience
Advances in clinical pharmacology
Clinical research in pain
Surveys and reports
Developments in palliative radiotherapy and oncology
Pain clinics
Potentials in home care
Tavistock Centre work on loss
Theology and death

During the 1960s Kubler-Ross began her series of interviews with patients talking about dying in a large general hospital in Chicago. Her book *On Death and Dying*[19] had a major impact on the public and on many professionals, and undoubtedly prepared the ground for the growth of hospice home-care teams in the United States. It also had an impact in other countries, although the original impetus, summarized above, came from more traditional sources.

At much the same time Parkes began publishing his studies of bereavement. His approach to the whole family had a major influence on the planning and early development of St Christopher's and, from there on, the whole movement. He was to carry out much of the early evaluation of hospice work.[20]

The influences that came together are summarized in Table 1, but, like the historical tree, it compresses many barely remembered influences. Most important is the impact of the many hundreds of patients whose notes were summarized, whose conversations were tape-recorded, and whose memories remain. They were the real founders of the hospice movement. Workers in clinical pain research such as Beecher,[21] Dundee,[22] Lasagna,[23] and LeShan,[24] were encountered and studied in researching the hospice foundation. Contacts with pain clinics were also developed.

There are, of course, other sources of the whole spectrum of palliative medicine as it is brought together in this book. The most important element that links the early teams and the present, widely developing branch of medicine is an awareness of the many needs of a person and his family as they grapple with all the demands and challenges introduced by the inexorable progress of a disease that has outstripped the possibilities of cure. Although the early foundations took such subtitles as 'for the dying', the new teams had early on established as their main objective the quality of life until death. The message was: 'You matter because you are you, and you matter until the last moment of your life. We will do all we can, not only to help you die peacefully, but also to live until you die'. These words together with the concept of total pain—a combination of physical, psychological, social, and spiritual elements—were built into St Christopher's and from thence into the modern hospice movement.

Table 2 lists the elements that St Christopher's Hospice brought together to set up this work, to demonstrate and evaluate its practice, and to encourage others to consider similar work in their different ways and settings. This had all been discussed in detail

Table 2

Beds integrated in local community
Development and monitoring of symptom control
Family support
Bereavement service
Home care
Research and evaluation
Education and training

with the Ministry of Health, and in 1966 a research and development grant was awarded to set up a home-care service (established in 1969), a comparative study of oral morphine and diamorphine (begun the same year), and an evaluation of local services and the effect that the presence of the Hospice would have upon them (from 1967). Research and rigour in developing clinical practice and education were built in from the beginning.

It was important to emphasize that what was being developed was not a soft option that would only be termed 'care', but a more appropriate treatment for people with advanced disease and their families. The main focus on malignant disease enabled the workers to concentrate on a limited range of symptoms and social and emotional problems and to produce a number of studies and publications, first from St Christopher's and soon from other centres such as Montreal and later Oxford, Southampton, and elsewhere. The present volume makes clear how widely these challenges are now recognized and tackled.

If there had not been a great amount of distress, documented among others by the Marie Curie Memorial Foundation (now called Marie Curie Cancer Care) in the home and by Hinton in hospital and felt deeply by all who could remember a sadly unrelieved death in their family or among their acquaintances, there would not have been the spread of interest and action first in the United Kingdom and then in North America, Europe, Australia, Southern Africa, and many countries throughout the world. If there had not been continued contact with both fundamental scientists and clinicians occupied in research in pain and with many workers in other specialties, there would have been no sound basis of practice to share and to become one of the roots of the whole development of the spectrum of palliative medicine as presented in this textbook with all the updating and many additions of this new edition.

Challenges and principles

A chapter on 'Terminal care' in the *Oxford Textbook of Medicine*[25] was reviewed as 'a characteristic mixture of tough clinical science and compassion'.[26] All the work of the professional team—the increasingly skilled symptom control, the supportive nursing, the social and pastoral work, the home care, and the mobilization of community resources—are to enable the dying person to live until he dies, at his own maximum potential, performing to the limit of his physical activity and mental capacity with control and independence wherever possible. If he is recognized as the unique person he is and helped to live as part of his family and in other relationships, he can still reach out to his hopes and expectations and to what has deepest meaning for him and end his life with a sense of completion.

Awareness of what 'quality of life' means to him now demands full consideration of both the nature of his suffering and the appropriateness of various possible treatments and settings in his particular circumstances. Alertness to any remission of his disease or disability should accompany the effective control of all the manifestations of an inexorable advance.

Patients should end their lives in the place most appropriate to them and their families, and where possible have choices in the matter. Some insight into the serious nature of his disease by the patient will help towards realistic decisions. Continuity of care can be maintained in the midst of change if there is effective communication and easy movement between different settings.

When a person is dying his family find themselves in a crisis situation with the joys and regrets of the past, the demands of the present, and the fears of the future all brought into stark focus.[27] Help may be needed to deal with guilt, depression, and family discord and in this time of crisis there is the possibility of resolving old problems and finding reconciliations that greatly strengthen the family.

If this time is to be fully used, there needs to be some degree of shared awareness of the true situation. Truth needs to be available (though not pressured) so that the family can travel together. In general, sharing is more creative than deception. The often surprising potential for personal and family growth at this stage is one of the strongest objections most hospice workers feel for the legalization of a deliberately hastened death or for an automatic policy of 'shielding' a patient from the truth. No one should have information forced upon them, but any continuing communication with a patient is likely to open up the subject sooner or later. The doctor who overcomes his own fears of the subject will learn how and when and what to tell.

At times the work will cause pain and bewilderment to all members of the staff. If they do not have the opportunity of sharing their strain and questions, they are likely to leave this field or find a method of hiding behind a professional mask. Those who commit themselves to remaining near the suffering of dependence and parting find that they are impelled to develop a basic philosophy, part individual and part corporate. This grows out of the work undertaken together as members find that they each have to search, often painfully, for some meaning in the most adverse circumstances and gain enough freedom from their own anxieties to listen to another's questions of distress.

Most of the early homes and hospices were Christian in origin, their workers believing that if they continued faithfully with the work to which they felt called, help would reach their patients from the God who had Himself died and risen again. Some of the traditional ways of expressing this faith are being interpreted afresh today, but there are also many people entering this field who do not have such a commitment, or who belong to other faiths or none.

Now that palliative care is spreading world-wide it has still, as in the World Health Organization definition,[28] kept a concern for the spiritual needs of its patients and their families. The whole approach has been based on the understanding that a person is an indivisible entity, a physical and a spiritual being. 'The only proper response to a person is respect: a way of seeing and listening to each one in the whole context of their culture and relationships, thereby giving each his or her intrinsic value' (M. Mayne, personal communication, 1996). The search for meaning, for something in which to trust, may be expressed in many ways, direct and indirect, in metaphor or silence, in gesture or symbol, or, perhaps most of all, in art and the unexpected potential for creativity. Those who work in palliative care may have to realize that they, too, are being challenged to face this dimension for themselves. Many, both helper and patient, live in a secularized society and have no religious language. Some will, of course, still be in touch with their roots in this area and find a familiar practice, liturgy, or sacrament to help their need. Others, however, will not and insensitive suggestions in this field will be unwelcome. However, if we can come not only in our professional capacity but in our common, vulnerable humanity, there may be no need of words on our part, only of concerned listening. For those who do not wish to share their deepest concerns, the way care is given can reach the most hidden places. Feelings of fear and guilt may seem inconsolable but many of us have sensed that an inner journey has taken place and that a person nearing the end of their life has found peace. Important relationships may be developed or reconciled at this time and a new sense of self worth developed.

A human as well as a professional basis has a fundamental bearing on the way that the work is done, and everyone meeting these patients and their families is challenged to have some awareness of this dimension. Their search for meaning can create a climate in which patients and families can reach out in trust towards what they see as true and find acceptance of what is happening to them.

'In a world in which technology threatens to undermine our sense of worth and meaning, hospice has appeared with the promise of not only easing the course for those who must die, but also of restoring the fundamental familial and religious ideals that have nourished our civilisation.'[29]

The values which the hospice movement tried to establish, alongside its commitment to excellence in practice, have shown that there are ways of seeking for the 'good death' today. Its 'holistic' approach has been built into the whole spectrum of palliative medicine and is presented anew by the contributors to this textbook.

References

1. Wall PD. Editorial—25 volumes of pain. *Pain,* 1986; **25**: 1–4.
2. Eisley L. *The Firmament of Time.* London: Gollancz, 1961: 113.
3. Gentles I. *Care for the Dying and the Bereaved.* Toronto: Anglican Book Centre, 1982: 121–32.
4. Aries P. *Western Attitudes towards Death from the Middle Ages to the Present.* London: Open Forum Series, Marion Boyars, 1976.
5. Solzhenitsyn A. *Cancer Ward.* London: Bodley Head, 1968: 115.
6. Clark K. *Civilisation.* London: BBC Publications, 1969: 108.
7. Gorer G. *Death, Grief and Mourning in Contemporary Britain.* London: Cresset Press, 1965: 9.
8. Miller TS. *The Birth of the Hospital in the Byzantine Empire.* Baltimore: Johns Hopkins University Press, 1988.
9. Phipps WE. The origin of hospices/hospitals. *Death Studies,* 1988: **12**: 91–9.
10. Goldin G, Thompson JD. *The Hospital: A Social and Architectural History.* New Haven, CT: Yale University Press, 1975: 6.
11. Lord Walton. *Method in Medicine. The Harveian Oration of 1990.* London: Royal College of Physicians, 1994.
12. Golding G. A protohospice at the turn of the century: St. Luke's House, London from 1893 to 1921. *Journal of the History of Medicine and Allied Sciences,* 1981; **36**: 383–415.
13. Clark-Kennedy AE. *London Pride: The Story of a Voluntary Hospital.* London: Hutchinson Benham, 1979: 11.
14. Twycross RG. Hospice care—redressing the balance in medicine. *Journal of the Royal Society of Medicine,* 1980; **73**: 475–81.
15. Marie Curie Memorial Foundation. *Report on a National Survey Concerning Patients Nursed at Home.* London: Marie Curie Memorial Foundation, 1952.
16. Snow H. *The Palliative Treatment of Incurable Cancer, with an Appendix on the Use of the Opium-Pipe.* London: J. and A. Churchill, 1890.
17. Snow H. Opium and cocaine in the treatment of cancerous disease. *The British Medical Journal,* 1896; **2**: 718–19.
18. Hinton JM. The physical and mental distress of the dying. *Quarterly Journal of Medicine,* 1963: **32**: 1–21.
19. Kubler-Ross E. *On Death and Dying.* Toronto: Macmillan, 1969.
20. Seale CH. What happens in hospices: a review of research evidence. *Social Science and Medicine,* 1989; **28**: 551–9.
21. Beecher HK. Non-specific forces surrounding disease and the treatment of disease. *Journal of the American Medical Association,* 1962; **179**: 437–40.
22. Dundee JW. Adjuvants in the relief of chronic pain. *Anaesthesia,* 1957; **12**: 330–44.
23. Lasagna L. The clinical evaluation of morphine and its substitutes as analgesics. *Pharmacology Review,* 1964; **16**: 47–83.
24. LeShan LL. The world of the patient in severe pain of long duration. *Journal of Chronic Diseases,* 1964; **17**: 119–26.
25. Saunders CMS. Terminal care. In: Weatherall DJ, Ledingham JGG, Warrell DA, eds. *Oxford Textbook of Medicine.* Oxford: Oxford University Press, 1983: 28.1–28.13.
26. Launer J. Overcoming prejudice. *British Medical Journal,* 1983; **286**: 1029.
27. Earnshaw Smith E. Dealing with dying patients and their relatives. *British Medical Journal,* 1981; **282**: 1779.
28. World Health Organization. *Cancer Pain Relief and Palliative Care,* 1990: 11–12.
29. Fulton R, Owen G. Hospice in America. In: Saunders CM, Summers DH, Teller N, eds. *Hospice: The Living Idea.* London: Edward Arnold, 1981: 11.

Preface to the Second Edition

When the first edition of this textbook was published in 1993 we were honoured to receive many appreciative reviews: several of them raised points to consider in a second edition and offered most constructive suggestions. We have been able to add comments from colleagues all over the world, to all of whom we express our appreciation. Our publishers have persuaded us to produce a new edition into which we can incorporate the many points raised.

Several people commented that the textbook appeared to be exclusively for doctors, yet palliative care, as is so frequently stated in the text, is team caring, interprofessional in fact rather than multiprofessional. We make no apology for it being a *medical textbook* for that is exactly what we intended and explained in the Preface to the first edition. We continue to see a need for a medical reference book whilst fully respecting and appreciating the roles of colleagues in other professions. In the same way we feel the title is right in referring to *palliative medicine* rather than palliative care or hospice care but readers will notice that throughout the text, wherever team collaboration is mentioned, the word used is *care* rather than *medicine*, and the much-loved word *hospice* is used when that is the title of a particular unit or service.

Another important comment was that the first edition appeared to focus on malignant disease although the principles of palliative medicine are said to apply to all diseases. In particular, some colleagues asked why a section had not been devoted exclusively to palliation in the geriatric population. The first comment has been addressed in this new edition by requesting all our contributors to demonstrate the relevance of palliative medicine across the clinical spectrum, where necessary highlighting special areas and issues for attention. We sought the opinion of specialist geriatricians and in the light of their comments have decided not to devote a special chapter to their patients.

What we *have* done is to introduce completely new chapters and make the book bigger and even more comprehensive. The increasingly important contribution of interventional radiology has been recognized with a full chapter, as have the subjects of audit and the economics of palliative medicine, and AIDS in children. A new chapter is devoted to pruritus and sweating, another to pain assessment, and yet another to pharmacological aspects of palliative medicine.

The section on cultural issues was appreciated by many readers and in this new edition it has been expanded with the additions of chapters on the cultures of sub-Saharan Africa, China and Japan, and Australian indigenous peoples, reflecting the worldwide spread and appropriateness of palliative medicine. A new team of authors has written the ethics section and, in recognition of the ethical issues in caring for children, a new chapter has been introduced on ethical issues in paediatric palliative medicine. Even when chapter titles have not been changed readers will find that many alterations have been made in the text, much new material added, and many new references cited, reflecting the considerable advances in this specialty in a very few years.

We pay tribute to those contributors to the first edition who so graciously agreed to stand down and hand over the baton to other authorities, and welcome our many new colleagues. To them all we express very sincere thanks for all the time, work, and endless patience they have so generously shared with us.

We have enjoyed working with our friends in Oxford University Press and make no apology for singling out Dr Irene Butcher whose skills, patience, and wisdom seem to us to be limitless. Finally, but with great sincerity, we acknowledge our immeasureable debt to our assistants, secretaries, and colleagues who in diverse ways made this new edition possible.

Derek Doyle
Geoffrey W.C. Hanks
Neil MacDonald
October 1997

Preface to the First Edition

We offer this new textbook as our contribution to modern palliative medicine. Our readers deserve some explanation about its contents and our fellow contributors our *unqualified* appreciation and respect.

Until quite recently terminal care, as it used to be called, consisted of little more than 'tender loving care' married to pain and symptom control using basic drugs skilfully prescribed. Some argued that there was little else to it and certainly not sufficient to merit a major textbook. We felt differently as, clearly, do many others who have made the subject their life's work. We were conscious of how much can be done, how much there is to learn, and how little we ourselves knew. Equally we were aware of how much our colleagues in related disciplines and specialties could share with us, how much valuable research had been done and how much remains to be done. Hence this textbook. Our aim has been to produce as comprehensive a book as possible, with a body of knowledge based on sound research as well as extensive clinical experience. To some extent we believe we have succeeded. Readers will note differing opinions, each firmly held by those with that level of experience and authority. We have made no attempt to reconcile all such differences for they are important. They demonstrate where dogmatism may be inappropriate and where further studies are still needed. Having said that, we have been impressed with the unanimity demonstrated in most areas and the professional open-mindedness and humility displayed by our contributors.

On many more occasions than might have been expected, we have been reminded what a strong scientific base palliative medicine is built on. Little of what has been written is merely anecdotal, valuable as that can be. Much has been studied and researched, forming the basis of this textbook.

Inevitably some will criticize the book as too much related to, and reflecting, 'Westernized' medical practice without due attention to the needs of the 'palliative care Third World'. Throughout, we have never ignored the needs of those having to work with limited resources but have tried to demonstrate not only what can be done in the medically-sophisticated world but also by colleagues less fortunate than ourselves. Treatment regimens include basic principles as well as sophisticated techniques, always emphasizing the totality of care, and the roles and needs not only of other professionals but also the relatives. We are deeply conscious that, while for a few, palliative medicine is the final stage of years of sophisticated therapeutic management, for millions of others all they can ever hope for is that its benefits will eventually become available to them and their families.

Clearly it would be impossible to detail each drug, each with as many different proprietary names, for every country where this book may be read. Rather we have chosen to use generic names.

Palliative medicine impinges on and frequently overlaps with many other medical specialties. Gone are the days when a patient receiving palliative care never again had further investigations or benefited from the advice of surgeons and oncologists. We have tried to demonstrate the contributions of other specialists by inviting them to share their knowledge and their contributions with us and have been honoured by their unstinting willingness to do so. Technical details of their work would have been out of place in such a textbook but readers will appreciate how they too can contribute to the complex kaleidoscope which confronts us and challenges us in palliative medicine.

In the same way in which we have encouraged these coauthors to share their wisdom in their own way, so too have we not attempted to impose a consistency of style on their writing but left them to express their thoughts and share their deeply-held feelings in their own inimitable way. We believe that this has enriched the book.

To our contributors we offer our profound thanks and respect. Few have worked alone; most have been assisted by many others, perhaps unnamed in this book, and by clinician colleagues who have acted for them when their writing took up days and weeks of precious time. To them all, named and unnamed, we extend our appreciation. They have all borne with our demands and our criticisms with unfailing patience making us appreciate what sensitive, understanding clinicians they must be.

Traditionally all authors and editors close with a grateful tribute to their publishers. In our case we would go further. We could never have dared to expect such patience with our shortcomings, such guidance when we so often called for it, and such genuine interest in, and enthusiasm for, our subject and this book. We are deeply grateful. We feel particularly privileged to have worked with Dr Irene Butcher who was an unfailing source of encouragement, support, and advice. No editors could have been better served.

Our secretaries deserve a special mention. Irene Turnbull (Edinburgh), Felicity Fleetwood (London), and Sheila Parr and Patricia McDonald (Edmonton) have given unstintingly of their skills, time, and loyalty, and to each we offer our unqualified thanks.

We dedicate this textbook to the colleagues with whom we work, those who have taught and inspired us and, most of all, to those we serve, our patients and their families.

Derek Doyle
Geoffrey W.C. Hanks
Neil MacDonald
1993

Contents

Contributors

A. ADAM
Professor of Interventional Radiology, United Medical and Dental Schools, Guy's and St Thomas' Hospitals, London, UK
8 Interventional radiology

SAM AHMEDZAI
Professor of Palliative Medicine, Royal Hallamshire Hospital, Sheffield, UK
9.5 Palliation of respiratory symptoms

DAVID A. ALEXANDER
Professor of Mental Health, Medical School, University of Aberdeen, UK
5.4 Psychosocial research in palliative care

H. RICHARD ALEXANDER, JR
Head, Surgical Metabolism Section, Surgery Branch, National Cancer Institute, Bethesda, Maryland, USA
9.3.5 The pathophysiology of cancer cachexia

T.G. ALLEN-MERSH
Reader in Surgery and Consultant Surgeon, Charing Cross and Westminster Medical School, Chelsea and Westminster Hospital, London, UK
9.1.3 Surgical palliation

EHUD ARBIT
Professor of Surgery (Neurosurgery), Cornell University Medical College; Director, Neurosurgical Oncology, Staten Island University Hospital, New York, USA
9.2.7 Neurosurgical approaches in palliative care

CAROLINE BADGER
Nurse Consultant in Chronic Oedema, Oxford, UK
9.7 Lymphoedema

VINCENT G. BAIN
Associate Professor of Medicine, University of Alberta, Edmonton, Canada
9.3.7 Jaundice, ascites, and hepatic encephalopathy

MARY J. BAINES
Consultant Physician, St Christopher's Hospice, London, UK
9.3.4 The pathophysiology and management of malignant intestinal obstruction

ADRIAN B.S. BALL
Consultant Surgeon and Surgical Oncologist, Crawley and Horsham NHS Trust, Sussex; formerly Lecturer in Surgery, Institute of Cancer Research, Royal Marsden Hospital, London, UK
9.1.3 Surgical palliation

M. BAUM
Professor of Surgery, University College London; Consultant Surgeon, UCL Hospitals Trust, London, UK
9.1.3 Surgical palliation

J. ANDREW BILLINGS
Director, Palliative Care Service, Massachusetts General Hospital and Assistant Clinical Professor, Harvard Medical School, Boston, Massachusetts, USA
21.2 Palliative medicine education

MARK H. BILSKY
Assistant Attending of Neurosurgery, Memorial Sloan Kettering Cancer Center; Assistant Professor of Neurosurgery, New York Hospital – Cornell University Medical Center, New York, USA
9.2.7 Neurosurgical approaches in palliative care

NIKKI BLACKWELL
Director of Accident and Emergency, Mount Isa Base Hospital, Queensland, Australia
10.5 Cultural issues in indigenous Australian peoples

MARK BOWER
Senior Registrar, Medical Oncology Unit, Charing Cross Hospital, London, UK
9.11 Endocrine and metabolic complications of advanced cancer

LUCY BRAZIL
Senior Registrar in Palliative Care, Royal Marsden Hospital, London, UK
9.11 Endocrine and metabolic complications of advanced cancer

NICHOLAS M. BREACH
Consultant Surgeon, Royal Marsden Hospital, London, UK
9.1.3 Surgical palliation

BRIGID BRECKMAN
Freelance Lecturer (Counselling and Communication), Hornchurch, Essex, UK
12.4 Stoma management

WILLIAM BREITBART
Associate Attending Psychiatrist, Memorial Sloan-Kettering Cancer Center, and Faculty Scholar, Open Society Institute, Project on Death in America, New York, USA
9.2.9 Psychological and psychiatric interventions in pain control
15 Psychiatric aspects of palliative care

R.P. BRETTLE
Reader and Consultant Physician, City Hospital, Edinburgh, UK
20.1 AIDS: aspects in adults

EDUARDO BRUERA
Professor of Oncology, Alberta Cancer Foundation Chair in Palliative Medicine, University of Alberta, Edmonton, Canada
5.3 Research into symptoms other than pain
9.3.6 Clinical management of cachexia and anorexia
9.4 Asthenia

ROBERT BUCKMAN
Medical Oncologist, Toronto-Sunnybrook Regional Cancer Centre, Toronto, Canada
4 Communication in palliative care: a practical guide

SIR KENNETH CALMAN
Chief Medical Officer, Department of Health, Whitehall, London, UK
5.1 Clinical and health services research

AUGUSTO CARACENI
Attending Neurologist, Pain Therapy and Palliative Care Division, National Cancer Institute of Milan, Italy
9.12 Neurological problems

MICHELE A. CARTER
Assistant Professor and Clinical Ethicist, Institute for the Medical Humanities, Galveston, Texas, USA
19.8 Child-centred care in terminal illness: an ethical framework

K.S. CHAN
Consultant Physician and Chief of Service, Hospice, Palliative Care Unit and Pulmonary Unit, Haven of Hope Hospital, Hong Kong
10.3 Chinese patients with terminal cancer

NATHAN CHERNY
Department of Medical Oncology, Shaare Zedek Medical Centre, Jerusalem, Israel
9.2.3 Opioid analgesic therapy

HARVEY MAX CHOCHINOV
Soros Faculty Scholar, Project on Death in America and Associate Professor, Department of Psychiatry, University of Manitoba, Manitoba Cancer Treatment and Research Foundation, Winnipeg, Canada
15 Psychiatric aspects of palliative care

ROXCO P.K. CHUN
Senior Lecturer, Department of Applied Social Studies, Hong Kong Polytechnic University, Hong Kong
10.3 Chinese patients with terminal cancer

SUSAN D. CLARK
Head Speech Therapist, Royal Victoria Infirmary, Newcastle upon Tyne, UK
12.5 Speech therapy

JENNIFER J. CLINCH
WHO Collaborating Centre for Quality of Life in Cancer Care, Winnipeg, Manitoba, Canada
2.7 Quality of life assessment in palliative care

R.C. COOMBES
Professor of Medical Oncology, Charing Cross and Westminster Medical School, London, UK
9.11 Endocrine and metabolic complications of advanced cancer

CHARLES A. CORR
Professor, Southern Illinois University at Edwardsville, USA
2.3 Death in modern society

MICHAEL J. COUSINS
Professor and Head, Department of Anaesthesia and Pain Management, Royal North Shore Hospital, University of Sydney, Australia
9.2.6 Anaesthetic techniques for pain control

INA CUMMINGS
Director, Palliative Care Program, Queen Elizabeth II Health Sciences Centre, Halifax, Nova Scotia, Canada
2.2 The interdisciplinary team
21.6 Training of volunteers

DAVID L.K. DAI
Consultant Physician, Hospice, Haven of Hope Hospital, Hong Kong
10.3 Chinese patients with terminal cancer

BETTY DAVIES
Professor, School of Nursing, University of British Columbia; Investigator, British Columbia Research Institute for Child and Family Health, Vancouver, Canada
19.5 Special services for children
19.6 Special issues in bereavement and staff support
19.7.1 The development of paediatric palliative care: introduction
19.7.3 Development in Canada

FRANCO DE CONNO
Director, Pain Therapy and Palliative Care Division, National Cancer Institute, Milan, Italy
9.10 Mouth care
21.2 Palliative medicine education

FRANCES DOMINICA
Founder and Honorary Director, Helen House, Children's Hospice, Oxford, UK
19.7.2 Development in the United Kingdom

DEREK DOYLE
Formerly Medical Director/Consultant in Palliative Medicine, St Columba's Hospice, Edinburgh, UK
1 Introduction
2.4 The provision of palliative care
12.1 Rehabilitation in palliative care: introduction
16 Domiciliary palliative care

DEBORAH DUDGEON
Associate Professor of Medicine, University of Manitoba and Director of Palliative Care, St Boniface General Hospital, Winnipeg, Canada
2.7 Quality of life assessment in palliative care

RHONA ELSE
Senior Physiotherapist, St Columba's Hospice, Edinburgh, UK
12.2 Physiotherapy

BRENDA ENG
Founding Director and Clinical Nurse Specialist, Canuck Place – A Hospice for Children, Vancouver, British Columbia, Canada
19.6 Special issues in bereavement and staff support

R.L. FAINSINGER
Assistant Professor, Division of Palliative Medicine, University of Alberta, Edmonton, Canada
9.3.6 Clinical management of cachexia and anorexia

KATHLEEN W. FAULKNER
Medical Director, Hospice Care, Inc., Stoneham, Massachusetts, USA
19.7.5 Development in the United States

BETTY R. FERRELL
Associate Research Scientist, City of Hope National Medical Center, Duarte, California, USA
14.2 The family

JACQUELINE FILSHIE
Consultant Anaesthetist, The Royal Marsden NHS Trust, London, UK
9.2.8 Transcutaneous electrical nerve stimulation (TENS) and acupuncture

KATHLEEN M. FOLEY
Co-Chief, Pain and Palliative Care Service, Memorial Sloan Kettering Cancer Center; Professor of Neurology, Neuroscience and Clinical Pharmacology, Cornell University Medical College, New York, USA
9.2.2 Pain assessment and cancer pain syndromes

KAREN FORBES
Macmillan Consultant Senior Lecturer in Palliative Medicine, University of Bristol, Bristol Oncology Centre, UK
9.2.10 Difficult pain problems

GILLIAN FORD
Medical Director, Marie Curie Cancer Care, London, UK
21.1 Multiprofessional education

DAVID R. FRAMPTON
Consultant Physician in Palliative Medicine, Mid-Essex Hospitals Trust and Medical Director, Farleigh Hospice, Chelmsford, Essex, UK
12.7 Creative arts and literature

COLETTE L. FULTON
Lecturer in Physiotherapy, Queen Margaret College, Edinburgh, UK
12.2 Physiotherapy

CHARLES S.B. GALASKO
Professor of Orthopaedic Surgery, University of Manchester; Consultant Orthopaedic Surgeon, Salford Royal Hospitals and Manchester Children's Hospitals NHS Trusts, UK
9.2.11 Orthopaedic principles and management

ANN GOLDMAN
CLIC Consultant in Paediatric Palliative Care, Great Ormond Street Hospital for Children, London, UK
19.2 Life threatening illnesses and symptom control in children

PETER GOLDSTRAW
Consultant Thoracic Surgeon and Director of Surgery, The Royal Brompton Hospital, London, UK
9.1.3 Surgical palliation

GILBERT R. GONZALES
Department of Neurology, Mayo Clinic Scottsdale, Scottsdale, Arizona, USA
9.2.1 Pathophysiology of pain in cancer and other terminal diseases

STEPHEN D.R. GREEN
Consultant Paediatrician, St Luke's Hospital, Bradford, UK
20.2 AIDS: aspects in children

JOSEPH G. HALL
Emeritus Professor of Immunology in the University of London; Formerly Chairman of the Section of Tumour Immunology at the Institute of Cancer Research and Honorary Consultant Pathologist, Royal Marsden Hospital, London, UK
9.7 Lymphoedema

GEOFFREY HANKS
Macmillan Professor of Palliative Medicine, University of Bristol, UK
1 Introduction
5.1 Clinical and health services research
7 The principles of drug use in palliative medicine
9.2.3 Opioid analgesic therapy
9.2.10 Difficult pain problems

ANNE P. HEMINGWAY
Professor and Chief of Service (Specialist Imaging), Hammersmith Hospitals NHS Trust and Royal Postgraduate Medical School, London, UK
8 Interventional radiology

IRENE HIGGINSON
Professor of Palliative Care and Policy, King's College School of Medicine and Dentistry, London, UK
2.6 Clinical and organizational audit in palliative care

P.J. HOSKIN
Consultant Clinical Oncologist, Mount Vernon Hospital, Northwood, Middlesex, UK
9.1.2 Radiotherapy in symptom management

DORIS HOWELL
UCSD Hospital, University of California, San Diego, USA
19.5 Special services for children

JANE INGHAM
Director, Palliative Care Program, Lombardi Cancer Center; Assistant Professor of Medicine, Georgetown University Medical Center, Washington, DC, USA
6 The measurement of pain and other symptoms

NORA T. JASKOWIAK
Clinical Associate, Surgery Branch, National Cancer Institute, Bethesda, Maryland, USA
9.3.5 The pathophysiology of cancer cachexia

NORA JODRELL
Macmillan Lecturer in Cancer Nursing, Department of Nursing Studies, University of Edinburgh, UK
21.3 Nurse education

TETSUO KASHIWAGI
Professor, Faculty of Human Sciences, Osaka University, Japan
10.4 Palliative care in Japan

SARAH KEIR
Senior Registrar, Medicine and Care of the Elderly, Bristol Royal Infirmary, Bristol, UK
7 The principles of drug use in palliative medicine

ZARINA C.L. LAM
Chairperson and Lecturer, Health, Disease, and Disability, Department of Applied Social Studies, Faculty of Health and Social Studies, Hong Kong Polytechnic University, Hong Kong
10.3 Chinese patients with terminal cancer

ANTHONY C.T. LEUNG
Hospital Chief Executive and Honorary Senior Consultant Physician, Haven of Hope Hospital, Kowloon, Hong Kong
10.3 Chinese patients with terminal cancer

MARCIA LEVETOWN
Clinical Assistant Professor, Pediatrics and Internal Medicine, University of Texas Medical Branch at Galveston and Pediatric Medical Director, Hospice of Galveston County and Houston Hospice, USA
19.8 Child-centred care in terminal illness: an ethical framework

IVAN LICHTER
Palliative Care Consultant, Te Omanga Hospice, Lower Hutt, New Zealand
17 The terminal phase

J. NORELLE LICKISS
Director of Palliative Care and Sydney Institute of Palliative Medicine, Royal Prince Alfred Hospital, Sydney, Australia
21.2 Palliative medicine education

CHARLES L. LOPRINZI
Professor of Oncology and Chair, Medical Oncology, Mayo Clinic, Rochester, Minnesota, USA
9.6.2 Pruritus and sweating

NEIL MACDONALD
Director, Cancer Ethics Program, Center for Bioethics, Clinical Research Institute of Montreal; Professor of Oncology, McGill University, Canada
1 Introduction
2.1 The interface between oncology and palliative medicine
3 Ethical issues in palliative care
9.1.1 Principles governing the use of cancer chemotherapy in palliative care
9.2.10 Difficult pain problems
21.2 Palliative medicine education

R.H. MACDOUGALL
Clinical Director, Clinical Oncology and Haematology, Western General Hospitals NHS Trust, Edinburgh, UK
9.9 Palliation in head and neck cancer

KATHRYN A. MANNIX
Honorary Palliative Physician, Newcastle City Health Trust, UK
9.3.1 Palliation of nausea and vomiting

CINZIA MARTINI
Associate Researcher Oncologist, Pain Therapy and Palliative Care Division, National Cancer Institute of Milan, Italy
9.12 Neurological problems

MITCHELL B. MAX
Chief, Clinical Trials Unit, Neurobiology and Anesthesiology Branch, National Institute of Dental Research, National Institutes of Health, Bethesda, Maryland, USA
5.2 Pain research: designing clinical trials in palliative care

PATRICIA A. MCGRATH
Director, Paediatric Pain Program, Child Health Research Institute and Professor of Paediatrics, University of Western Ontario, London, Canada
19.1 Pain control

J. MEIRION THOMAS
Consultant Surgeon, Sarcoma and Melanoma Unit, Royal Marsden Hospital, London, UK
9.1.3 Surgical palliation

CATHERINE MILLER
Group Nurse, Cancer and Related Services, London, UK
9.6.3 Skin problems: nursing aspects

BARBARA MONROE
Director of Social Work, St Christopher's Hospice, London, UK
13 Social work in palliative care

P.S. MORTIMER
Consultant Skin Physician and Reader in Dermatology, St George's Hospital and Royal Marsden Hospital, London, UK
9.6.1 Skin problems: medical aspects
9.7 Lymphoedema

BALFOUR M. MOUNT
Eric M. Flanders Professor of Palliative Medicine, McGill University, Montreal, Canada
21.2 Palliative medicine education

A.J. MUNRO
Professor of Radiation Oncology, University of Dundee, UK
9.9 Palliation in head and neck cancer

DEREK B. MURRAY
Principal Chaplain, St Columba's Hospice, and Lecturer in New College, Edinburgh, UK
21.5 Education and training of clergy

JULIA NEUBERGER
Chairman, Camden and Islington Community Health Service NHS Trust, London, UK
10.1 Cultural issues in palliative care: introduction

HANS NEUENSCHWANDER
Consultant Physician for Palliative Medicine, Department of Oncology, and Medical Director, Hospice Lugano, Bellinzona-Ticino, Switzerland
9.4 Asthenia

RICHARD W. NORMAN
Professor of Urology, Dalhousie University, Halifax, Nova Scotia, Canada
9.8 Genitourinary disorders

CHARLES L.M. OLWENY
Professor, University of Manitoba and Co-director, WHO Collaborating Centre for Quality of Life in Cancer Care, St Boniface General Hospital, Winnipeg, Canada
10.2 Cultural issues in sub-Saharan Africa

DAVID OSOBA
Director, Quality of Life Programme, British Columbia Cancer Agency; Professor, University of British Columbia, Canada
9.1.1 Principles governing the use of cancer chemotherapy in palliative care

SANDRO PAMPALLONA
Technical Officer, Cancer and Palliative Care Unit, World Health Organization, Geneva, Switzerland
22 Palliative medicine – a global perspective

COLIN MURRAY PARKES
Consultant Psychiatrist to St Christopher's Hospice, Sydenham and St Joseph's Hospice, Hackney, UK
18 Bereavement

STEVEN PASSIK
Clinical Assistant Attending Psychologist, Memorial-Sloan Kettering Cancer Center, New York, USA
9.2.9 Psychological and psychiatric interventions in pain control
15 Psychiatric aspects of palliative care

UGO PASTORINO
Consultant Thoracic Surgeon, Royal Brompton Hospital, London, UK
9.1.3 Surgical palliation

RICHARD PAYNE
Chief, Pain and Symptom Management Section; Associate Professor of Medicine (Neurology), University of Texas MD Anderson Cancer Center, Houston, USA
9.2.1 Pathophysiology of pain in cancer and other terminal diseases

DAVID PAYNE
Department of Psychiatry, Memorial-Sloan Kettering Cancer Center, New York, USA
9.2.9 Psychological and psychiatric interventions in pain control

MARK R. PITTELKOW
Associate Professor of Dermatology, Mayo Clinic, Rochester, Minnesota, USA
9.6.2 Pruritus and sweating

BRIAN POLLARD
Director (now retired), Palliative Care, Concord Hospital, Sydney, Australia
19.7.4 Development in Australia

SUSAN PORCHET-MUNRO
Music Therapist, Healthcare Educator, Zurich, Switzerland
12.6 Music therapy

RUSSELL K. PORTENOY
Associate Professor of Neurology, Cornell University Medical College and Associate Attending Neurologist, Memorial-Sloan Kettering Cancer Center, New York, USA
5.2 Pain research: designing clinical trials in palliative care
6 The measurement of pain and other symptoms
9.2.5 Adjuvant analgesics in pain management
9.2.10 Difficult pain problems

M.D. RAWLINS
Professor of Clinical Pharmacology, University of Newcastle upon Tyne, UK
9.2.4 Non-opioid analgesics

CLAUD REGNARD
Medical Director, St Oswald's Hospice; Honorary Consultant in Palliative Medicine, Royal Victoria Hospital; Honorary Lecturer in Pharmacological Sciences, Newcastle University, Newcastle upon Tyne, UK
9.3.2 Dysphagia, dyspepsia, and hiccup

ALISON RICHARDSON
Macmillan Lecturer in Cancer Nursing and Palliative Care, King's College London, UK
5.5 Nursing research
20.1 AIDS: aspects in adults

CARLA RIPAMONTI
Vice Director, Pain Therapy and Palliative Care Division, National Cancer Institute, Milan, Italy and Adjunct Professor of Oncology, Alberta University, Canada
9.10 Mouth care

M.A. ROBBINS
Lecturer in Social Policy, School of Social Sciences, University of Bath, UK
2.5 The economics of palliative care

CLIVE J.C. ROBERTS
Consultant Senior Lecturer, in Clinical Pharmacology, Bristol Royal Infirmary, UK
7 The principles of drug use in palliative medicine

DAVID J. ROY
Director, Center for Bioethics, Clinical Research Institute of Montreal; Research Professor, Faculty of Medicine, Université de Montreal: Director-Coordinator, Quebec Health Research Foundation (FRSQ) Network for Research in Clinical Ethics, Canada
3 Ethical issues in palliative care

LUIGI SAITA
National Cancer Institute, Milan, Italy
21.2 Palliative medicine education

MICHAEL J. SATEIA
Director, Sleep Disorders Center; Associate Professor of Psychiatry, Dartmouth Medical School, Lebanon, New Hampshire, USA
9.13 Sleep

CICELY SAUNDERS
Chairman, St Christopher's Hospice, London, UK
Foreword

ALBERTO SBANOTTO
Consultant in Palliative Care, European Institute of Oncology, Milan, Italy
9.10 Mouth care

HARVEY SCHIPPER
WHO Collaborating Centre for Quality of Life in Cancer Care, Winnipeg, Manitoba, Canada
2.7 Quality of life assessment in palliative care

JOHN F. SCOTT
Director, University of Ottawa Institute of Palliative Care, Canada
21.2 Palliative medicine education

R.J. SHEARER
Consultant Urologist and Medical Director, Royal Marsden Hospital, London, UK
9.1.3 Surgical palliation

F.M. SHELDON
Macmillan Lecturer in Psychosocial Palliative Care, Department of Social Work Studies, University of Southampton, UK
21.4 Education for social workers

JOHN H. SHEPHERD
Consultant Gynaecological Surgical Oncologist, St Bartholomew's Hospital and Royal Marsden Hospital, London, UK
9.1.3 Surgical palliation

PETER M. SILBERFARB
Raymond Sobel Professor of Psychiatry and Professor of Medicine; Chairman, Department of Psychiatry, Dartmouth Medical School and the Norris Cotton Cancer Center, Hanover, New Hampshire, USA
9.13 Sleep

ANTHONY M. SMITH
Medical Director, Pilgrims Hospices in East Kent, Canterbury, UK
21.2 Palliative medicine education

PETER SPECK
Chaplaincy Team Leader, Southampton University Hospitals NHS Trust, UK
11 Spiritual issues in palliative care

MICHAEL M. STEVENS
Senior Staff Specialist and Head, Oncology Unit, The New Children's Hospital at Westmead, Sydney, Australia
19.3 Psychological adaptation of the dying child
19.4 Care of the dying child and adolescent: family adjustment and support
19.7.4 Development in Australia

JAN STJERNSWÄRD
Medical Director, Global Cancer Concern, London, UK
22 Palliative medicine – a global perspective

ROBERT A. SWARM
Director of Pain Management and Instructor in Anesthesiology, Washington University School of Medicine, St Louis, Missouri, USA
9.2.6 Anaesthetic techniques for pain control

NIGEL P. SYKES
Consultant Physician, St Christopher's Hospice, London, UK
9.3.3 Constipation and diarrhoea

JOHN W. THOMPSON
Honorary Physician and Honorary Consultant in Medical Studies, St Oswald's Hospice; Emeritus Professor of Pharmacology, University of Newcastle upon Tyne; Emeritus Consultant Clinical Pharmacologist, Newcastle Health Authority, UK
9.2.8 Transcutaneous electrical nerve stimulation (TENS) and acupuncture

KENT NELSON TIGGES
Professor of Occupational Therapy, State University of New York at Buffalo, USA
12.3 Occupational therapy

A. ROBERT TURNER
Professor of Medicine (Hematology and Medicial Oncology), University of Alberta, Edmonton, Canada
9.14 Haematological aspects

ROBERT TWYCROSS
Macmillan Clinical Reader in Palliative Medicine, Oxford University; Consultant Physician, Sir Michael Sobell House, Churchill Hospital, Oxford, UK
9.3.2 Dysphagia, dyspepsia, and hiccup
17 The terminal phase

MARY L.S. VACHON
Consultant in Psychosocial Oncology/Coordinator of Palliative Care, Sunnybrook Health Science Centre/Toronto-Sunnybrook Regional Cancer Centre; Associate Professor, Department of Psychiatry and Behavioural Science, University of Toronto, Canada
14.1 The emotional problems of the patient
14.3 The stress of professional caregivers

VITTORIO VENTAFRIDDA
Director, WHO Collaborating Centre for Cancer Pain Relief, Milan, Italy
9.10 Mouth care

PHILIP D. WELSBY
Consultant Physician in Communicable Diseases, City Hospital, Edinburgh, UK
20.1 AIDS: aspects in adults

JANET A. WILSON
Professor of Otolaryngology, Head and Neck Surgery, University of Newcastle upon Tyne, UK
9.9 Palliation in head and neck cancer

JENIFER WILSON-BARNETT
Professor and Head of Division and Department, Division of Nursing and Midwifery-Department of Nursing Studies, School of Life, Basic Medical and Health Sciences, King's College London, UK
5.5 Nursing research

1

Introduction

1 Introduction

Derek Doyle, Geoffrey Hanks, and Neil MacDonald

It is customary for Editors to open with an explanation of why they have produced their book and who they hope may read and benefit from it. It must be rare for them to have to define their subject, but that is exactly the position in which we find ourselves.

What is 'palliative medicine'?

A useful definition with which to start is that prepared and adopted in Great Britain in 1987 when palliative medicine was recognized as a medical specialty. It states that 'Palliative medicine is the study and management of patients with active, progressive, far-advanced disease for whom the prognosis is limited and the focus of care is the quality of life'.

This definition is for palliative medicine; that is to say, the specialty practised by doctors. When describing the care offered by a team of doctors, nurses, therapists, social workers, clergy, and volunteers it is more correct to refer to palliative care, a useful definition of which has been suggested by the World Health Organization:[1]

> 'The active total care of patients whose disease is not responsive to curative treatment. Control of pain, of other symptoms, and of psychological, social and spiritual problems, is paramount. The goal of palliative care is achievement of the best quality of life for patients and their families. Many aspects of palliative care are also applicable earlier in the course of the illness in conjunction with anticancer treatment.'

By way of expanding and explaining the definition, the World Health Organization goes on:

> 'Palliative care: . . . affirms life and regards dying as a normal process, . . . neither hastens nor postpones death, . . . provides relief from pain and other distressing symptoms, . . . integrates the psychological and the spiritual aspects of care, . . . offers a support system to help patients live as actively as possible until death, . . . offers a support system to help the family cope during the patient's illness and in their own bereavement.'

Palliative care unquestionably grew out of hospice care, which some might claim was an euphemistic name for terminal care or care of the dying. Why then did we not entitle our book 'A Textbook of Hospice Medicine' or 'A Textbook of Terminal Care'?

The problem with the word terminal' in this context is one of definition. Does it refer to the last hours, days, weeks, or even months of life? Could it possibly be applied to the time when the goals changed from cure to care? Should it refer to the time when the patient, rather than his doctor, senses that death is approaching? The vagueness—the ambiguity—of the phrase 'terminal care' is obvious and is one of our reasons for not using it.

Much more important than the ambiguity is the implied negativism and passivity. 'Terminal' suggests that all is finished, that there is neither the time nor the opportunity to do more, and that active treatment is unjustified and might well be undignified. The essence of palliative care is a challenge to any such assumption. Even in the final days of life, care, whether undertaken by nurses or doctors, relatives or clergy, can always be positive, planned, and purposeful. It is not simply a matter of sitting by the bedside, grief-stricken and professionally helpless.

'Terminal care' suggests a preoccupation with dying and death, grief, loss, and sadness and, although we do not wish to create a sanitizing definition, the care outlined in this book affirms life rather than death.

Why not 'hospice medicine'? It is a term understood, respected, and used widely in many parts of the world. It remains the name for which most lay people best describe what is now called 'palliative medicine'. Why not use the word 'hospice'?

In Britain, where the 'hospice movement' might rightly be said to have begun its development (though the first hospice for the dying was established in France in 1842), most people would know what a hospice is for and could probably direct the enquirer to the nearest one and speak warmly of its reputation. They would know it was for the dying but might not realize that many patients were discharged home, nor that it ran a home care service for such patients. They might not appreciate that 'hospice care' is available in general hospitals. In the United States, people speak of 'hospice' as a philosophy, a concept of care, rather than a 'bricks and mortar' building, and unfortunately some hospices are viewed with suspicion and scepticism by doctors who see them as offering a 'soft' product without a scientific base. In some European countries, 'hospice' denotes a home for the destitute rather than a modern health-care centre. In short, the word so loved and understood by many and, in particular, the pioneers of palliative medicine, is itself difficult to define, used in widely differing ways, and is not as truly descriptive of this work as is needed.

However, the problem of nomenclature and definition does not stop if we adopt the term 'palliative medicine'. According to the *Oxford English Dictionary* to 'palliate' means, amongst other things, to mitigate, to alleviate, to lessen pain, to give temporary relief. We must ask, 'Do the limits of palliative care encompass all ultimately fatal illnesses?' To date, palliative care programmes have primarily addressed the needs of dying cancer patients and their families. More recently, programmes assisting AIDS patients are in place, and some palliative care groups also enrol patients with motor neurone disease and allied degenerative neurological disorders. All these disorders are characterized by constantly changing physical symptoms, increased risk of psychosocial distress, societal misunderstanding, and a relatively short period of final illness.

They lend themselves to special programme development. It remains unlikely that palliative care programmes will enrol many patients with other chronic illnesses, but the principles of palliative care can be applied with benefit throughout the medical care system.

We are now in a position to return to our original definition and to study it more clearly. Palliative medicine is, as befits a medical discipline, both about patient care and the study of that care. It is dedicated to those with an established diagnosis and also clinical evidence of the disease being active, progressive, and at an advanced stage such that death is inevitable within the foreseeable future.

The origins of palliative medicine

Presumably, man has attempted to relieve the suffering of his fellow creatures since he first appeared on earth. The history of hospices is well documented from the Middle Ages through their modern developments towards the end of the nineteenth century up to the final decades of this century, with their worldwide proliferation. The origins of palliative medicine as a discipline worthy of practising, study, and research are more recent, and to trace them we have only to look back about 25 years.

At the turn of the century and in the first decades of the twentieth century, what else could a doctor do but palliate? Much as he must have wanted to be able to do so, there were few conditions he could cure. Even today, with the exception of conditions amenable to curative surgery, the majority of curable conditions are infections. Our forefathers had no antibiotics, and so, even there, every skill they possessed was channelled into alleviating, palliating. Palliation was the norm, the description of all medical practice.

Then things began to change. Anaesthetic advances made more adventurous, radical surgery possible. Antibiotics came on the scene to combat the most common infections and, to a large extent, certainly in the Western World, reduced their threat as killers. Unfortunately, this is not the case in most other parts of the world. Advances, discoveries, and developments came in every field of medicine—radiology, nuclear medicine, immunology, radiotherapy, cancer chemotherapy . . . the list seems endless. New generations of doctors left medical school knowing that they would never see deaths from diphtheria, smallpox, and poliomyelitis, would easily cope with serious infections in patients' homes, and could confidently expect many of their cancer patients to be cured.

We have every reason to be proud of the medical discoveries and advances made in the second half of this century. We have at our disposal investigative procedures never dreamed of 50 years ago, a comprehensive pharmacopoeia with only a handful of drugs used then, and a cluster of new medical specialties reflecting these advances. While all this was happening, subtle changes were taking place in medical thinking and attitudes and in medical education.

Almost unnoticed doctors began to change their goal from palliative caring to absolute curing. No one taught them or told them to do so but, looking back, the change in attitude and approach began around the beginning of the antibiotic era. For the first time, cure seemed attainable in conditions with a hitherto high mortality. Increasingly sophisticated and technological investigations not only brought a much needed precision to our diagnoses but vastly increased our knowledge of the natural course of some conditions and led us to hope, quite justifiably, that earlier diagnosis—particularly in cancer—might increase the chance of cure. The increasingly 'scientific' basis of modern medicine appealed to a profession which, rightly or wrongly, regarded itself as scientific.

Insidiously, imperceptibly, doctors saw themselves primarily as diagnosticians and therapists (whether surgical, pharmacological, or radiation). Hospitals were seen as being for investigations, treatment, and early discharge home. Those who could not be cured, or at least put into a remission state, were often made to feel less welcome and less deserving of expensive, highly educated medical input. Those who were dying were given the lowest medical priority, and death itself became not the fact of life it had always been but a medical defeat or, worse still, a statistical embarrassment.

It would be outrageous to cast all blame on the clinicians and not look at the parallel changes in medical education. Once again the changes were subtle, and for a long time did not appear significant. The already packed curriculum was pruned here and added to there to accommodate details of the advances we have spoken of and ever-increasing scientific details and data. 'Softer' subjects, such as communication skills, ethics, psychological aspects of medicine, etc., were given less time, relegated to low priority slots, or omitted completely.

Until the last few years young doctors were leaving medical school with a comprehensive knowledge base, almost unattainably high professional expectations about what they would be able to do and offer, and a frightening paucity in the skills and attitudes essential for humane medical practice. Things are changing.

How clear so many changes seem when looked at in retrospect! Whilst this was happening—and let us never deny the importance and the impact of real medical developments—an uneasiness about the changes was being experienced by many in different walks of life, for this 'medical' problem was only part of a larger social upheaval. Some doctors became unhappy and sought to try to bring about changes. Nurses, who for a time seemed scarcely to notice that they were now copartners in increasingly scientific and technological care regimens and quite welcomed what was actually a changed role, also began to be troubled. Remarkably reluctant as most patients are to complain, or even hesitatingly to report on the quality of care they receive, some now confessed that they felt that one particular group of patients, the dying, were given less than optimal care. Formal studies of consumer experiences and views confirmed that pain control was inadequate, symptoms were often left uneased, fears were not answered, spiritual needs were left unrecognized, and doctors' home visits were becoming fewer. Study after study in hospital and community in many different countries produced the same type of report—the dying are a neglected and disadvantaged group in modern health-care systems.

Those best able to bring about change were the doctors, already aware and troubled and now conscious of nursing unease and consumer dissatisfaction. Doctors saw clearly that better care for the mortally ill did not mean a return to the 'old days', nor any rejection of scientific medical advances, but rather a healthy marrying of them both. If they had used their medical jargon they would probably have said 'Science and compassion are not antagonistic—they are symbiotic'. So 'hospice care' was begun for the terminally ill—care which was always patient (rather than pathology) centred, was holistic whilst remaining scientific. The years have passed and with them has come the realization that these patients need and deserve this quality of care not only at the end but from the minute that they, and their doctors and relatives, sadly recognize that time is short. Thus, palliative medicine was born.

The development of palliative medicine

The first modern hospice (for we must distinguish them from the 'homes for the dying' which had existed for some time, though few knew much of their work) began to appear in the late 1960s and 1970s, inspired by the pioneering work of St Christopher's in London. They were inpatient units, often with an associated home care service for those still able to be cared for at home. From the outset they recognized the need for comprehensive record-keeping and data collection, and for education of fellow professionals of the many disciplines with contributory roles in holistic care.

In recognition of the needs of patients in general hospitals, symptom relief or support teams were founded, staffed by medical specialists, and specially trained nurses, and with social workers, therapists, and chaplains on call. It was soon apparent that they could both improve the quality of life of those dying in general hospitals and enable more to go home under the care of general practitioners and home care services than might previously have been thought possible. Nevertheless, obvious as the benefits of such support teams now appear, there seemed less enthusiasm to develop them than inpatient units which, in the late 1970s and the 1980s, proliferated in Britain and, to a much lesser extent, in North America and beyond.

Hospices, or palliative care units, are to be found today in almost every country of the Western World, with similar practice in most countries but modified appropriately to meet local needs and patterns of health care provision. In Britain about one-fifth are run by the National Health Service, whilst the bulk are run by independent local bodies, funded by charities but assisted in many ways by the National Health Service. In Canada, where one of the pioneering services originated in a major Montreal teaching hospital, there are to be found other such designated in-hospital units, a few free-standing services, and others working alongside community nursing agencies, whilst in the United States the emphasis remains on home care but with notable initiatives in some of the major teaching hospitals. In many centres in Australia and New Zealand, there are now comprehensive palliative care programmes, many associated with medical and nursing colleges, and increasingly integrated with oncology services. At the time of writing, the first hospices have opened in Russia, others are planned in other Eastern European countries, Poland has several services initiated and developed against great odds even before the fall of communism, and each European country has groups seeking means to develop services appropriate for their needs.

Palliative care has developed most rapidly in the affluent countries of the world—Western Europe, North America, Australasia, and Japan—countries with well-developed and well-funded health care systems. The question must be asked: 'Does it have relevance worldwide?'.

Millions of people are suffering and dying in the Third World countries. Some have access to modern diagnostic and therapy facilities but the vast majority have not. Some are in countries without adequate food and water supplies, some are in countries where the uneven distribution of resources offers reasonable health care to some and none whatsoever to others, and many are in countries where ignorance or ill-informed legislation deprive those who most need them of access to opioid analgesics and other essential drugs.

In the West, palliative care is coming to be seen as a basic human right when curative care is no longer appropriate. Is it not equally appropriate for those who have never had the benefits of modern medicine with its possibility of early diagnosis, surgery, radiotherapy, antibiotics, and chemotherapy? Clearly, for vast numbers in the less developed countries, 'palliation' is all they can hope for, yet most will never receive it. For them it represents not the 'final luxury' but a basic human right which should be made available to them now even before their country's economies and politics develop and mature to provide technological services.

Clearly, the problem is not simply medical. It is political and economical, and as such might seem to be not the business of outsiders, yet perhaps we in the affluent West have a contribution to make. We can continue to demonstrate the benefits of palliative care, continue to evaluate and publish the merits and safety of such simple measures as the World Health Organization pain ladder, support the balanced WHO cancer care plan, and so encourage legislation which will at least make essential drugs available to millions more than have access to them at present.

We can enable medical and nursing colleagues from those countries to spend a few months working and studying in the palliative care centres of the West so that they can return home with confidence and the skill to relieve suffering even whilst they continue to press for the colleagues, the equipment, and the resources for better overall care. Most importantly, we should assist colleagues in developing countries to develop their own palliative care training centres of excellence.

Education and training in palliative medicine

Inevitably we have returned to the problem of education and training—the acquisition of skills, the changing of attitudes, the use of resources.

Following the many studies on patient/consumer views which have been alluded to, there inevitably came others on the attitudes of doctors, the training they had received, and their perceived needs for improved professional education in this field. Informal questioning in medical schools had already elicited the view of many teachers that everything which needed to be taught was already being taught throughout the undergraduate years. The recollections of newly qualified doctors belied that statement! Some recalled not having been taught anything about the special problems of the dying patient, and almost without exception they, and many more senior and experienced colleagues, expressed the need for more formal training, so incompetent and lacking in confidence did they feel when confronted by death. Their feelings were exactly mirrored by nurses, clergy, and others, as demonstrated in other studies. The time was ripe for developing teaching modules for undergraduates and postgraduates, and the challenge was eagerly taken up by those now involved in palliative medicine.

Certain subjects were clearly important and central to this work: pain and symptom control, emotional and social needs, and spiritual care. In 1990, every medical school in Britain had included them in the curriculum to a greater or lesser extent, but by 1992 on average less than 13 hours were devoted to them in a 5-year course. Similar changes were being reported from North America, Australia, and other countries. Soon, trainee family doctors and trainee oncologists were asking for help and courses were being devised for them, paralleled by similar courses extending over many weeks for nurses. Today, in Britain alone nearly 50 special courses are open to nurses in addition to several degree courses, with others rapidly being developed in Europe, North America, and elsewhere.

One has only to work in a palliative care service for a short time to appreciate that at the heart of all good care is good communication. Many of the emotional problems and anguish encountered in patients with advanced disease and their families stem from poor communications at an earlier stage—communications between doctors and patients, between patients and relatives, and between the professionals themselves. Very few of these problems are unique to palliative care, except in so far as they focus on loss and death, but are basic to all care. The dearth of good research in communication was slowly addressed by clinicians and psychologists in several centres, but much of the educational input by palliative medicine specialists came to focus on this issue and it was recognized that it should have been addressed long before as part of general professional training. Many have remarked that 'Palliative medicine is not new but a rediscovery'. To a large extent the same might be said of palliative medicine education; what was clearly needed, and now being offered to their colleagues by palliative medicine specialists, was what should have been taught much earlier in their training programmes. Chronic pain is not unique to advanced cancer. Fear, apprehension, and loneliness affect many more than the dying. Grief and loss are human experiences at all stages in life. Skilled empathetic communication is as necessary in acute medicine as in advanced cancer care. It is good that so many have accepted this challenge and are now deeply involved in, and committed to, improved education, but they must never lose sight of the fact that they are largely repairing the damage and making good the deficiencies of earlier years. What is still needed is an infusion of the principles of palliative medicine into all courses—a rediscovery of that undeniable fact we have stated, that the principles of palliative medicine are the principles of all good medical care. More widespread 'rediscovery' appears to be needed, but we shall show that means are being found to make this possible.

Three things have happened which give cause for some satisfaction and pride. The first is that so many doctors of high standing have chosen palliative medicine as their career. They very quickly began to change the attitude of otherwise sceptical colleagues to palliative medicine, particularly when their research was published and excellent books appeared. No longer was it possible to think of palliative medicine as a soft option for the less able, a quieter life for the less energetic, or an easier subject for those academically mediocre.

The second was the recognition in Britain of palliative medicine as a full specialty with its own clearly laid-down career training programme. In other countries the debate still continues as to whether this is the right course, but in Britain it has visibly raised the standing and the profile of palliative medicine and helped to make it creditable and respectable. The quality of young recruits, choosing palliative medicine as the career of choice, has enhanced it even further.

The third factor has been the development of academic palliative medicine with two Chairs in the subject occupied by coeditors of this textbook, seven Chairs in the United Kingdom, four in Australia, and several in other countries.

The scope and aims of this textbook

Palliative medicine is total care—of body, mind, and spirit. This is undeniable and unavoidable. So often in medical practice this is acknowledged and a claim made that it is always practised, but this is transparently not so. Often preoccupied with the technological aspects of care, many doctors find themselves focusing almost exclusively on physical problems. When so-called 'social problems' are encountered, they are passed to the social worker who may never meet the others involved in that patient's care. If 'spiritual problems' are uncovered, they are more likely to be met by embarrassed silence, trite platitudes, or a reluctant invitation to an overworked chaplain than to be addressed by a doctor or nurse directly involved in the care. Emotional problems are often encountered but are either described as psychological factors accounting for functional features or dealt with in a perfunctory manner as if a few minutes explanation and reassurance will cure all ills.

In palliative medicine, where the doctor is but one important member of a closely-knit, skilfully integrated and interdependent team, each patient is recognized as having physical, emotional, social, and spiritual needs as well as problems, and each need is given full and equal attention. No man can be rendered pain free whilst he still wrestles with his faith. No man can come to terms with his God when every waking moment is taken up with pain or vomiting.

If palliative medicine is total care, it is also team care with each member a specialist in his or her own right, each an equal member, and no one a prima donna. Let no one imagine that this is easy to achieve or easy to practise. It makes sense to work as a mutually supportive team because there is so much work to do, so many complex issues to occupy us, and so much at stake. It also makes sense for the needs of the individual team members themselves so that they can share the responsibility and therefore the burden, share the decisions as well as the strains, share the rewards as well as the pains.

These two key features of palliative medicine will feature many times in the pages which follow and will be implicit even in the sections and chapters which, at first sight, appear to be the technical prerogative of doctors only.

Palliative medicine is planned care, not crisis intervention.

There will always be unexpected emergencies and crises, but experience teaches us that many can be avoided by team-sharing and planning. The greater our knowledge of each condition and every nuance of management, the easier will we find it to reassure our patients through our improved professional skills.

This is a medical textbook, written for doctors whether generalist or specialist, written in the full recognition that doctors have a wealth of new knowledge to acquire and need a single book in which to find it. We do not apologize that it is not a 'Textbook of Palliative Care', but we certainly hope that it will be of equal value for nurses, social workers, therapists, and pastoral care workers. They have their own books to which doctors might also usefully refer, in the same way that our colleagues might hopefully dip into this textbook to their advantage.

Palliative medicine recognizes the skilled input of specialists from many disciplines—hence the range of sections that we have commissioned from acknowledged authorities from many countries. Some may feel that we have moved too far backwards in the care of our patients—backwards from those final weeks we used to equate with 'terminal care'—but we have done so within the limits of definitions which opened this chapter. We see laser therapy for bronchial obstructions as palliative if it will relieve dyspnoea. We embrace the contribution of surgical colleagues who can insert stents if, by so doing, they relieve biliary or ureteric obstruction. We see a role for the oncologist if his chemotherapy can reduce tumour bulk which is causing symptoms, for the radiotherapist who (amongst so many contributions) can ease the pain of bone secondaries or the asphyxiating sensation of the patient with superior vena caval obstruction. If pleurodesis prevents reaccumulation of a pleural effusion, or a pericardial window that of a pericardial effusion, that is palliation because it has the potential to relieve suffering and improve the quality of remaining life without in any way attempting either to extend or abbreviate it.

Palliative medicine has much to learn from other specialties. We believe that it has much to offer other specialties.

Distinction between palliative medicine approach and standard approach to topics

Many of the chapters in this textbook have identical titles to those encountered in other books. For example, we consider constipation, a topic also to be found in internal medicine or gastroenterology texts.

Apart from the convenience of locating subjects critical to palliative medicine within one binding, we believe that a different philosophical projection influences our discussion of physical or psychosocial problems. Again, considering the mundane but highly distressing symptom of constipation, we emphasize its special features in those with advanced illness and the need to adopt a consistently applied regimen to prevent it. The causative factors highly prevalent in palliative patients, such as the use of opioid and anticholinergic drugs, are stressed, and associated features such as voiding problems or confusion are emphasized.

Co-operation with nursing staff and use of family teaching programmes are essential features of a palliative medicine approach to symptom control. Our colleagues, throughout their discussions on constipation, or sleep disturbances, or the myriad other problems of the dying patient, place emphasis on the unique aspects of palliative care management. Recommendations on team approaches and family involvement simply represent good management, but we contend that they are not sufficiently emphasized.

Increasing need for palliative medicine

Advances in cancer and AIDS research may ultimately result in universally applicable curative therapy. For many years to come, however, most patients with these disorders will encounter pain, physical limitation, and emotional and spiritual distress, and ultimately will die of their disease. The incidence of cancer continues to increase throughout the world, particularly in those areas where tobacco is vigorously marketed. Even though North America may be spared the epidemic of cancer deaths secondary to promotion of tobacco in Europe and Third World countries, an increase in cancer mortality is anticipated. The cancers on the rise (most notably lung cancer) are, in the main, curable in only a small proportion of cases. Most of these cancers will occur in older patients. There is a tendency to assign a lower value to a loss of life in older age groups in relation to death from cancer in young populations. This is reasonable in terms of years of life, enjoyment, and productivity lost. However, a death at 35 and a death at 70 may both be associated with similar degrees of suffering.

Palliative medicine will increasingly involve AIDS patients and their loved ones. This disorder primarily affects the young—tragically, even infants and young children. While the disorder, at least in its current manifestation, may be near its peak in the Western World, mounting devastation and suffering will be the lot of many Third World countries where infection rates exceed 20 per cent of the population.

Major changes in the cure rates for cancer and AIDS patients are not expected to occur within the next 10 years. Research in molecular and tumour biology may result in widely accessible curative treatment, but this remains to be determined. Many of the new therapies, such as bone marrow transplants for metastatic cancer or monoclonal targeted therapy, may never be applied to impoverished countries. In the field of AIDS, until a vaccine or a simple curative agent becomes universally available, access to excellent palliative care must be the mainstay of AIDS therapy.

The fact that many conditions which cannot yet be cured may produce much unnecessary suffering has already been alluded to. Most such patients will, for the foreseeable future, be cared for in general hospitals or in their own homes. Indeed, we would never want to see everyone die in specialist palliative care units. As has been shown, we are very conscious of those millions who do not even have hospitals or healthy homes in which to live or die. The principles of palliative medicine, to which this textbook is devoted, apply wherever men and women suffer and die. We would want these principles of pain and symptom control, support and empathy, spiritual awareness, and team-caring to become the norm everywhere. Palliative medicine is appropriate for the practice of all doctors everywhere, whatever their specialty, whatever their culture and religious beliefs. The relief of unnecessary suffering, whatever its cause, is the concern of us all—the reason we entered this profession. It is indeed a rediscovery of age-old truths.

Research in palliative care

Even though most cancer patients will die of their disease, symptom and psychosocial research have been assigned a low priority in most cancer centres. The thrust of clinical research has been directed towards assessing survival and tumour regression. When symptom control is considered, one symptom, chemotherapy-related nausea and vomiting, has tended to receive most attention almost to the exclusion of everything else.

The major granting bodies provide very little funding for palliative care issues. While it may be argued that the palliative care submissions that grants panels receive do not meet the same standards established by the molecular biologists, it may be equally stated that the policies of most research bodies have not encouraged studies in palliative medicine. For example, until very recently, little encouragement was provided for the development of interinstitutional research, in contrast with the extensive network of chemotherapy clinical trials groups.

Apart from targeted support from cancer centres and research agencies, there are other reasons why palliative care research has not flourished. Clinical research is difficult to conduct at the end of life. Moreover, concern with patient and family care, rather than research interests, characterize the attraction of palliative care to most workers in this area. They have recognized the imbalance between cure and care in modern medical systems, and their religious and ethical convictions, rather than intellectual curiosity, draw them to palliative care. In contrast with laboratory research, it is extremely difficult, for ethical and medical reasons, to control variables over a prolonged period of time. Research is essential, and yet palliative care research presents the most difficult background for the conduct of a rigorous scientific investigation, while most people involved in palliative care do not have the research training of the basic research worker or the clinical pharmacologist working in the field of cancer chemotherapy.

However, in contrast with other fields of cancer research, immediate patient benefits may ensue from palliative care research and new knowledge can more readily be used to modify and improve clinical practice. For example studies of the use of oral morphine initially conducted by palliative care units have revolutionized cancer pain management. Subsequently, studies of the subcutaneous use of opioids and other medications have immediate application to patient care with consequent improvement in patient suffering, facilitation of home care, and resultant decreases in health costs.

Integrated research projects involving basic scientists, clinicians, and other health disciplines are unusual in palliative care. Where they exist, research has flowered. The happy constellation of common interest involving neurophysiologists, neuropharmacologists, academic neurologists, anaesthetists, palliative care physicians, and nurses has produced a compendium of knowledge which has revolutionized pain management.

Similar associations could enable us to understand more readily symptoms such as the cachexia–anorexia syndrome and the various poorly characterized forms of asthenia which bedevil cancer patients. The components of tumour biology, which result in some patients and not others developing pain and give rise to profound weight loss and weakness, have not been identified. Tumour biologists have not linked tumour growth and host response to symptom outcome. The encouragement of integrated basic science–clinical study groups is an essential feature needed to advance the field of palliative medicine and may profoundly influence research on other aspects of cancer and AIDS. Certainly it is reasonable to integrate palliative medicine with the care of cancer and AIDS patients early in their trajectory of illness with anticipated improvement in patient well-being and facilitation of palliative care research.

Today, palliative medicine is the care given to patients at the end of life when much else has been tried, often over many years, and now their need is for comfort, dignity, a sense of usefulness, a respect for their personhood, and a reaffirmation of life rather than a preparation for dying.

Tomorrow, the principles of palliative medicine should be the norm worldwide. It is our hope that this textbook may become a means of achieving this.

Reference

1. *Cancer Pain Relief and Palliative Care*. Technical Report Series 804. Geneva: World Health Organization, 1990.

2

The challenge of palliative medicine

2.1 The interface between oncology and palliative medicine

Neil MacDonald

A sixteenth century aphorism, penned by an anonymous author, defines the role of a physician:

To Cure Sometimes

To Relieve Often

To Comfort Always

Cure was achieved on few occasions by physicians at that time. Indeed, the odds of a patient encountering a physician and benefiting from the experience only evened toward the latter part of the nineteenth century. The introduction of anaesthesia and safe surgery, antibiotics, hormone and other biological replacement therapies, obstetric advances, and reductions in infant mortality now enable physicians to cure disease or to prolong the course of many chronic illnesses.

As in other areas of medicine and surgery, the scientific advances of the nineteenth and twentieth centuries led oncologists to adopt a biological model of disease. Cancer came to be regarded as a disease of organ dysfunction rather than an illness—an illness with psychological and spiritual dimensions embracing both the patient and the patient's family and community.

The public never fully accepted the biological model of cancer. To most non-physicians in every culture, cancer is regarded as an illness with panoramic social and psychological ramifications rather than as an organ-based disease. The community reaction to the biological model of cancer provides a continuing strong impetus for the palliative care movement.

Progress in the surgical management of cancer was rapid in the first half of the twentieth century. In the 1950s, the availability of megavoltage radiotherapy units increased the capacity for cure of localized cancers. Following the synthesis of alkylating agents and the first antimetabolite, amethopterin in 1945 to 50, progress in cancer chemotherapy led to the organization of a third cancer treatment specialty, medical oncology.

Cancer therapy was initially based on the concept that tumours were homogenous entities which proceeded in orderly fashion from local growth to lymph node involvement and subsequent haematological dissemination. Cancer was thought to consist of aberrant tissue that acted like a foreign invader and thus could be repulsed like other external threats such as bacteria. Indeed, the treatment of cancer is often expressed in military terms. A 'war' on cancer was declared and patients 'battled' with cancer. The 'war' however, resembled the First World War, with initial rapid change followed by a pattern reminiscent of the trench warfare of 1914 to 18. Similar to the optimism of Marshall Haig and his colleagues, oncologists hoped that a few more drugs or forms of radiation energy would bring about the cure of advanced cancer.

Unfortunately, current research on cell and molecular biology discounts this possibility. In 1997, cancer is recognized as a disorder involving near-normal cells with genetic errors which enable the cells to escape normal control systems and rapidly to develop cytotoxic drug resistance. Because of the propensity for cancer cells to alter their genetic apparatus, cancer tissue is soon composed of multiple populations of cells with different responses to growth factors and anticancer therapy.

Cancer cure rates now approach 40 to 50 per cent in the industrialized countries, but in developing countries cure remains an uncommon event. Success has been achieved through the early detection and treatment of localized cancers with surgery and/or radiation therapy, the use of adjuvant therapy in certain settings, and through the cure of germ cell tumours, childhood cancers, and certain haematological malignancies with chemotherapy. Current research involving immune modulation, transplantation, and increasingly complex chemotherapy regimens have modestly improved overall cancer mortality, while their costs burden the health-care system and limit their application in developing countries.

Our understanding of cancer continues to improve, allowing the introduction of more rational biological therapies. Research on tumour angiogenesis, differentiating agents, and molecular biology may ultimately result in uniformly available curative treatment, but this remains to be determined. In any event, the tortuous process of moving from the laboratory to the bedside and providing cost-effective therapies is likely, in the best of circumstances, to evolve over several years.

Because of success in preventing deaths from infectious diseases and, in the industrialized world, from degenerative cardiovascular disease, a rising incidence of cancer is anticipated. Contributing to the increased number of cases is the tobacco epidemic. At the present time in many Asiatic countries, the smoking rates exceed 60 per cent in males, and the habit is becoming more fashionable amongst females. Tobacco-induced cancers are notoriously difficult to diagnose and to cure. A rising incidence of certain other cancers, including cancer of the breast, prostate cancer, melanoma, and non-

Hodgkin's lymphomas, has recently been noted in the United States and other Western countries.[1] Therefore, we may expect a steady rise in the numbers of cancer patients who require palliative care.

When AIDS is considered, a similar situation is noted. As stated in the introduction to this textbook, while the rising incidence of this disorder, at least in its current manifestation, may be near its peak in the Western world, mounting social disruption and suffering may be anticipated in many Third World countries, where HIV infection rates of 20 per cent in certain urban populations are reported. Current World Health Organization estimates predict that 15 to 20 per cent of the African work-force could die of AIDS and there may be 10 000 000 African orphans at the turn of the century.[2]

Prevention programmes may begin to arrest the AIDS epidemic, while advances in vaccine research and the advent of new drugs may eventually control the disorder. For years to come, however, millions of AIDS patients will need palliative care in balance with disease modifying therapy. These principles are discussed in Section 20. The remainder of this chapter will concentrate on cancer care.

With the probability that in excess of 7 000 000 people will die each year from cancer, artificial lines drawn between disease modifying therapy and palliative care are inappropriate. More importantly, the role of surgery, radiation, and chemotherapy as agents enhancing quality of life requires more attention. This concept, at least as it applies to chemotherapy, is relatively new. This chapter will consider the principles governing the acceptance of palliative medicine as an integral component of cancer control.

Relations between cancer centres and palliative care programmes

There are four phases of cancer prevention:

(1) prevention of the disease (public education and policy);

(2) prevention of advanced disease (early diagnostic programmes);

(3) prevention of death (anticancer treatment);

(4) prevention of suffering.[3]

The four phases are often not co-ordinated within a seamless cancer-control programme. Until recently cancer centres have concentrated on the first three phases, which stimulated the development of the palliative care movement to deal with the fourth phase.

History—cancer centre interest in palliative medicine

Although most cancer patients will die of their disease, studies on the aetiology and treatment of their symptoms have not received a high priority within cancer centres. Research studies accurately assess survival and objective tumour response, but the effect of cancer therapies on pain, other physical symptoms, and on psychosocial parameters is seldom reported. For example the *Journal of Clinical Oncology* during 1986 and 1987 published 24 phase II–phase III studies of the chemotherapeutic response of advanced carcinoma of the oesophagus, stomach, colon, and pancreas, and non-small-cell lung cancer. These tumours tend to be poorly responsive to chemotherapy and, even in responders, prolongation of life is modest.

Because major changes in cure rates or survival could not be expected for patients with these poor response tumours, it is logical to expect that investigators would have concentrated on the impact of chemotherapy on the symptoms of these patients. Each article provided an assessment of tumour response and drug toxicity; not one of them reported on the effect of chemotherapy on pain.[4]

While psychologists and quality of life committees have become associated with a number of the major co-operative chemotherapy groups, the pattern is changing slowly. Information on quality of life and symptom control was not contained in the eight comparable reports to the 1986 to 1987 survey published in the *Journal of Clinical Oncology* between January and June, 1995. Nor was it offered in 13 of 15 abstracts of phase II or phase III chemotherapy studies on advanced non-small-cell lung cancer selected for presentation at the 1996 meeting of the American Society of Clinical Oncology.

Palliative medicine reaction—anticancer therapy

Because of the failure of disease modifying therapy to cure advanced cancer patients in many instances, palliative medicine physicians and nurses may deride the use of these therapies in situations where they may be helpful. The aim of palliative medicine to provide comfort for patients and families may cause an overestimation of the toxicities associated with chemotherapy and generate a viewpoint whereby oncologists may be regarded as automatons, enslaved by the icon of tumour response, without reference to the usefulness of a response for the patient. Conversely, oncology colleagues may sometimes think that palliative care workers are easing their patients' path to an earlier death than is necessary. A state of 'two solitudes' may come into existence wherein both groups fail to consult each other adequately .

Reluctance to encourage integration of palliative care with other aspects of cancer care is encountered from leaders in both spheres. As discussed in the *Canadian Brief on Palliative Care*,[5] both groups may feel that linkage will result in distortion of objectives and dilution of resources. Oncologists may say that we already look after all the needs of cancer patients (although we have not measured their degree of suffering as rigorously as we have measured the size of their tumour nodules). Alternatively, palliative medicine physicians may state that the oncologists, while mastering symptom control techniques (and that is all to the good), may miss the heart of the matter and fail to introduce the 'warm envelope' of care that characterizes palliative care at its best. Moreover, they believe that the complexity of the problem is such that, with the best of will, those whose primary interest lies in screening, tumour biology, or pharmacology will never have the time and energy to address the needs of dying patients and their families.[5] Although over 80 per cent of their patients have cancer, palliative medicine physicians may also be concerned that too close a tie with cancer programmes will blunt their efforts to provide palliative care for other dying patients. These concerns may confuse the community, as patients and families should reasonably expect continuity of care throughout their illness and are puzzled when jurisdictional priorities and barriers require them to take a zigzag path to obtain appropriate care. When this exists, patients and families caught in the centre will suffer.

The message is clear; the two solitudes state is unfair to patients. Palliative medicine physicians must be familiar with advances in oncology and maintain close ties with local oncologists and cancer centres. They must, together with other therapeutic options, consider the benefits of anticancer treatments for their patients, if only, once considered, to make a rational decision to eschew further anticancer treatment.

Integration of palliative medicine in a cancer control programme

Palliative care has traditionally concentrated on the last days of life; a time when pain, other symptoms, and psychosocial distress are often prominent and difficult to control. Would the task be easier if patients had received good palliative care throughout their trajectory of illness? The World Health Organization believes so. Their expanded definition of palliative care states that: 'many aspects of palliative care are also applicable earlier in the course of the illness in conjunction with anticancer treatment'.[6]

Tangible evidence of the wisdom of this philosophy exists for both cancer pain and the psychosocial problems of patients and families. Vachon and others report that poorly handled transfer of information and recognition of anxiety at the time of diagnosis translates into increased problems later in the course of illness. The pain literature is replete with studies demonstrating the plasticity of afferent sensory pain pathways when exposed to unrelieved chronic stimulation.[7] Pain thresholds are lowered, previously uninvolved neuronal systems transmit pain messages, and the relief of pain requires larger doses of analgesics and coanalgesics. More evidence to this point emerges from recent studies on confusional states at the end of life. Dr Bruera and his colleagues correlate a reduction in delirium with the introduction of preventive measures, including routine assessments, maintenance of hydration, and opioid rotation (see Chapter 9.2.10).[8]

Prevention is the cornerstone of medical practice. It is reasonable to assume that cancer centres imbued with the philosophy of palliative care, will be more likely to prevent long-term patient distress by integrating excellent palliative care and antitumour therapy earlier in the course of illness. They are more likely to achieve this end if the cancer centre has established close contact with a palliative care group or has included a palliative care division or department within their own organization. Most cancer centres throughout the world have not acted on this logical proposition. It is gratifying to note, however, that the *Policy Framework for Commissioning Cancer Services*[9] (United Kingdom, 1994) recommends both the formation of palliative care programmes within cancer centres and their co-ordination with community palliative care. The report strongly endorses the concept of palliative care as a preventive exercise —'Palliative care is required for many patients early in the course of their disease, sometimes from the time of diagnosis. It should not be associated only with terminal care. The palliative care team should integrate in a seamless way with all cancer treatment services to provide the best possible quality of life for the patient and their family.'

Palliative medicine—interface with oncology

Cancer centres and palliative care units can learn from each other to their mutual benefit and that of the people they serve.[10] Cancer centres will recognize more clearly that:

1. Continuity of care is important. Patients should not be exposed to constantly changing flotillas of doctors and nurses. A specific physician–nursing team should be recognized by the patient and family as their primary source of support within the centre.

In some jurisdictions, the patient may not have contact with a family practitioner skilled in palliative medicine. The cancer centre should not discharge the patient into a void for palliative care by the family doctor without assurance that community resources are in place to assist the patient and family. Oncologists, palliative care groups, and family practice programmes must establish these interfaces.

2. Pain and other symptoms can be assessed in a formal manner. Assessment dictates that we ask about the presence of problems. When asked, patients and families will bring forward information which otherwise could be passed over in a busy clinic.

There is current evidence that oncologists may underestimate their patients' pain and home–family concerns. Slevin *et al.*[11] compared quality-of-life assessments, finding a wide variation. Even Karnofsky ratings (a measure of physical status) showed low correlations between patient–physician pairs. In another study on prostate cancer,[12] one-quarter of severely disabled patients were judged by their physicians to be either asymptomatic or only slightly limited. Obtaining information on pain, other symptoms, and psychosocial distress is assisted through the use of patient-oriented assessment forms and assessments by other health professionals (see Chapter 9.2.2 and Section 6).

3. Pain and other symptoms can be relieved but, as in other areas of oncology, rigorous attention to detail, including protocols for patient–family teaching, are required.

4. Hierarchy of problems. At any time, the hierarchy of problems may vary considerably, between family, patient, and medical attendants.[13] The last may be most concerned with drug toxicity or drug doses; the family may have financial concerns uppermost, including the loss of income caused by prolonged waiting in an outpatient department, while the patient may be primarily upset by unrelieved pain and anxiety. A palliative care approach will elicit patient–family concerns and recognize their primacy.

5. Home care. The home is the focal point for palliative care and therapies are designed to be suitable for home use. Palliative care teams have established special techniques to allow previously hospital-bound patients to return home. Examples are the use of pump-delivered subcutaneous medications, epidural analgesic regimens, and, most importantly, regular assessment and follow-up by palliative care nurses in the home. Close integration between cancer centres and palliative care home-care teams, keeps people at home, enhances the patients' lives, and improves the efficient operation of the cancer centre (see Section 16).

6. Joint clinics. Patients constantly report that waiting in impersonal hospital clinics to see yet another new consultant is a most enervating experience. A cancer centre with a palliative care group can co-ordinate patient visits so that the antitumour therapy decisions are reached in concert with plans for home-care management of pain and other symptoms. The patient will appreciate the obvious evidence of a team approach to problems.

In turn, palliative care groups will learn from their close contact with cancer centres. Lessons to be learned include:

1. Self-criticism. The messianic aspects of palliative care should be complemented by critical review of existing dogma. Cancer centres will question unsubstantiated claims of therapeutic success and subject their therapies to tests of efficacy. Adoption of their approach will strengthen both the academic base and the resource base of palliative care. Recently, a *British Medical Journal* editorial stated 'evidence based medicine is a phrase that is currently familiar to only a few doctors, but we will all know it by the millennium'.[14] *Management of Cancer Pain*, a 1994 publication of the Agency for Health Care Policy and Research,[15] contains an analysis of the evidence supporting current pain management practice. While sound studies support current approaches using opioids and non-steroidal anti-inflammatory drugs, adjuvant drug therapy and non-pharmaceutical pain interventions are commonly based on modest evidence. One's recent encounters with health administrators and pharmacy committees indicate that hard data are needed to address their bottom-line financial concerns (see below). Evidence-based studies will not only improve clinical care but will influence and guide policy makers responsible for setting health-care priorities.

2. Emphasis on quality research. Cancer centres thrive on clinical trials and oncologists have established common classification systems and multi-institutional groups, enabling them to carry out first-rate clinical research. The cancer centres include basic science workers whose presence can result in a flow of research ideas from laboratory to the clinics.

The oncology co-operative model for conducting multicentre research could be copied with profit by palliative care groups. In contrast to oncology, internationally established criteria for definition and assessment of symptoms do not exist. Therefore, most palliative care research studies enrol small numbers of patients whose characteristics may not be clear to other investigators. If tumour biologists can be involved in symptom control research, they will produce needed information on the pathophysiology of currently uncontrolled symptoms, such as asthenia. Tumour biologists are located in cancer centres and may become interested in problems of importance to palliative medicine through regular contact with palliative medicine physicians.

3. Resources. Cancer centres tend to be relatively well supported by their communities and government institutions (a crass but important concept).

4. Enhanced access to palliative anticancer therapy. The need for quick and easy access to palliative radiotherapy is unpredictable and is facilitated if palliative care physicians work together with oncologists on a day-to-day basis. Moreover, the technical resources and consultant base of a cancer centre are often needed to resolve difficult symptom problems. A clinical example follows:

Mrs L., with metastatic breast cancer and leptomeningeal involvement, was receiving excellent care in her home community. She was on regular opioids which controlled her pain and allowed her to continue her life as a mother and community leader. The pain in her left hip became severe and her family physician steadily increased her dose of opioids, to the point where she was still in severe pain but stuporous. Radiographs of her bones did not suggest that she had any recent damage. Nothing else acute seemed to have happened. She was afebrile and her white blood cell count had not changed nor had her haemoglobin dropped. This lady needed the services of an acute care hospital and, when she was transferred to such a hospital, computed tomography scans and ultrasounds of her pelvis revealed that she had a pelvic abscess. She had been on steroids, which may have dampened the usual signs of infection. The abscess cavity was drained, the patient was placed on antibiotics, and she returned home in good pain control, alert on her previous dose of opioids.[16]

Mrs L. illustrates the benefits arising from continued interaction between community-based palliative care and a sophisticated cancer centre. On occasion 'high tech' approaches are required to alleviate suffering.

During the next decade, cancer centres will increasingly recognize their responsibility for balancing the phases of cancer prevention and should welcome the incorporation of palliative medicine within their organizations. They have recognized the need for subspecialty development in various fields of oncology, and it is reasonable that they should also develop programmes designed to address the palliative needs of cancer patients and their families and to conduct research and teaching in this special field.

Ethical considerations at the interface

Do cancer centres have a moral responsibility to ensure that cancer patients in the region they serve have access to impeccable palliative care? Institutions, like the professionals who staff them, have ethical duties.[17] These considerations must influence their role in a community, in concert with all the other factors which shape an institution's mission. It is common practice for cancer centres to publish formally their mission and goals and, in so doing, to state clearly the areas of cancer care for which they will accept responsibility. Centres, however, often have a mandated role to serve as a focal point for comprehensive cancer care in a region. Even in the absence of a formal mandate, their presence strongly influences overall arrangements for cancer care.

Commonly, a cancer centre may define itself as a centre for tertiary patient care, focusing on the application of complex technological approaches to treatment, and on the organization and conduct of clinical trials. Indeed, most cancer centres have a strong academic component and the physicians working in these centres are expected to carry out clinical research.

A cancer centre may define its mission in a manner which does not call upon it to assume responsibilities for all four phases of a comprehensive cancer control programme. If so, the centre must reconcile its role as an institution with specific priorities addressing the needs of a measured number of patients in its catchment area, and its role as a component of a comprehensive cancer programme within which all patients are entitled to equal consideration. Wearing the latter mantle, the centre has a responsibility to guarantee continuity of care for cancer patients. The onus is on the cancer centre to either develop a comprehensive palliative care service or to use its influence and resources to ensure that a fully co-ordinated, autonomous community programme is in place.

For example the emphasis in cancer centres in clinical trials must not damage the prospects of those patients who, for whatever reason, do not enter a trial or who subsequently discontinue participation in research protocols. Often, poor performance status will disenfranchise a patient for consideration in a trial or advancing disease will cause them to be dropped from continued care within a clinical trial setting. In some countries, the limited time of the clinicians within a cancer centre may be primarily taken up with clinical trial activities; if so, could a clinical trial impact negatively on the care of those patients not enrolled in the trial? This scenario could develop in centres where arrangements for formal interaction with community palliative care services are not in place, with consequent discharge of patients into a void.

The financial stringencies observed in every land can have a deleterious effect on cancer centre–palliative care interactions. Reimbursement increasingly relates to dictated norms; financial penalties are associated with deviations from these parameters. Dying often does not adhere to administrative fiats. As a result, patients with advanced disease who, nevertheless, need the technical skills of a cancer centre, may not be welcome. Factors diminishing the access of dying patients to hospitals may particularly affect the poor, who are less likely to afford home care[18] and who may have greater levels of distress.[19]

A single-minded emphasis on 'the bottom line' may not only be ethically problematic, but may also prove to be a bad business decision. A recent *Harvard Business Review* study illustrated the perils associated with cost cutting (in industries outside the health field) without due regard to maintenance of ethical standards.[20] The study provided examples of companies with an exclusive focus on cost cutting, with resultant drop in staff morale, customer satisfaction, and further financial losses, in contrast to other companies who thrived through balancing resource allocation with ethical reflection.

Callahan has stated 'No moral impulse seems more deeply embedded than the need to relieve suffering . . . it has become a foundation stone for the practice of medicine, and it is at the core of the social and welfare programmes of all civilized nations.'[21] If this tenet is applied to the organization of cancer control programmes, palliative care will thrive in a state of equipoise with other aspects of cancer care.

Will this newly-recognized responsibility of cancer centres damage the existing palliative care movement; a movement which has recruited thousands of theologians, social workers, trained volunteers, family practitioners, and others who have no ties with cancer programmes? The inclusion of palliative medicine as just another part of a large hospital programme would be a mistake, leading to a loss of the platform of community interest which has nourished palliative care. When the question is asked, the community gives the needs of dying patients a high priority.[22,23] Community support can be harnessed through creating parallel structures, such as palliative care community councils, with volunteer community members who will monitor the development of palliative care in a town or region and foster community–government education exercises. In some jurisdictions, these councils could assume funding and supervisory responsibilities. The advancement of palliative medicine at the community hospital level will extend the arm of palliative care towards people with other chronic, ultimately fatal, disorders, while the skills of palliative care physicians can be employed, in concert with others, to assist people with chronic non-fatal illnesses, such as those with post-traumatic pain syndromes.

An essential tenet of palliative care organizations is the establishment of broad community understanding and support. If this is present, then a programme web with strong filaments connecting cancer centre palliative care groups, community hospitals (where palliative inpatient units may be located), community volunteer groups, and dedicated home-care programmes servicing all hospitals can be developed. As in all areas of human endeavour, ultimately the success of an integrated community programme depends on the maturity and goodwill of the participants. If they are willing to lower institutional barriers and cherish co-operative activity rather than insularity, palliative care will thrive in all parts of the community, including the cancer centre.

The use of disease-modifying therapy in palliative medicine

Timing is all important when considering the use of palliative disease-modifying treatment. Surgical opportunities are limited, radiation therapy less effective, drug resistance develops, and drug access is more problematic as tumours increase in size. The patient's ability to tolerate therapy decreases in proportion to the extent of tumour progression.

Localized cancer

Localized cancers are potentially amenable to cure either with radiotherapy or surgery. Modern surgical techniques, together with improved radiotherapy equipment and technical skills, have improved the possibilities of local control and cure.

Certain localized cancers, such as anorectal tumours, can be cured, even in an advanced stage, by the combination of chemotherapy with surgery or radiation.[24]

The use of neoadjuvant (i.e. chemotherapy given before or at the same time as surgery or radiotherapy) chemotherapy may improve the operability and curability of other cancers such as cancers of the head and neck, stomach, oesophagus, and gynaecological cancers.

Guideline

Unless the patient has far advanced disease and a very poor performance status, the diagnosis of a localized cancer dictates an oncology consultation and/or consideration of anticancer therapy.

Metastatic cancer

Potentially curable metastatic cancer

Palliative physicians may see referred patients, diagnosed with an incurable disseminated malignancy, who may nevertheless benefit from curative anticancer therapy or other treatment measures. This may occur because:

1. Some referring physicians may still harbour excessively negative views about cancer and may fail to recognize curative situations.

2. The patient has been misdiagnosed. Occasionally patients with a past history of cancer may have all subsequent problems

Table 1 Guidelines for consideration of disease-modifying therapy

1. Review the patient's pathology
   Is a diagnosis of cancer established?
   Is the type of cancer established?
   Could illness be caused by a non-malignant correctable disorder?
   Is the patient's type of cancer usually amenable to curative or palliative anticancer therapy?
2. Review the patient's past therapy

Surgery	type and complications	
Radiotherapy	site(s)	
		dose, curative vs. palliative
		complications, acute; long term
Chemotherapy	Type	
		Hormonal
		Cytotoxic
		Biological
	Purpose	
		Curative
		Adjuvant
		Palliative drugs used
	Adequacy of therapy	
		Yes
		No
	Results	
		Effective
		Ineffective
	Toxicity	
		Life-threatening
		Major symptomatic
		Minor symptomatic

3. Review patient–family understanding
   (a) Are they properly informed of the purpose of past therapy and its outcome?
   (b) Was potentially helpful therapy withheld at family request?
   (c) Do they harbour bitterness and/or misunderstandings about past diagnostic and therapeutic exercises?
   (d) Do they hold views, realistic or unrealistic, about future interventional therapy?
4. Review the objectives of the patient's care
   (a) Are there well-localized symptom problems that could be controlled by surgery, radiotherapy, or chemotherapy?
   (b) Does the profile of past response to therapy suggest that interventional therapy may help?
   (c) Does the patient have a cancer normally amenable to interventional therapy?
   (d) If a slim chance for cure or long-term control is present but the risk of an adverse outcome is substantial, is the patient–family understanding clear and 'trade-off' position known?

Guidelines for the specific use of surgery, radiotherapy, and chemotherapy are contained in other chapters in this textbook.

assigned to the previous malignancy. Certain infectious processes closely mimic cancer (e.g. tuberculosis), other chronic disorders can produce cachexia (advanced pulmonary or cardiac disease, Addison's disease), or cause a pain syndrome difficult to distinguish from a malignant recurrence (vertebral body collapse secondary to osteoporosis or infection).

3. Even when 'proof' of cancer is present, the pathologic diagnosis may occasionally be in error. Some inflammatory states such as chronic pancreatitis can mimic cancer when only a sliver of tissue is available for analysis.

Guidelines

It is imperative that potentially curable disseminated tumours, such as germ cell cancers or lymphomas, are recognized. The situation most commonly arises when an unknown primary carcinoma is diagnosed. Patients with this diagnosis require investigation to rule out curable or highly responsive neoplasms. Occasionally, a therapeutic trial is justified.[25]

Verification of the presence of a malignancy is sometimes justified.

Incurable tumours

Chemotherapy

High-dose chemotherapy may cause more harm than benefit in patients with far advanced disease. Some cancers, however, are very sensitive to chemotherapy while, in some circumstances, chemotherapy and hormonal therapy may offer symptom relief with acceptable patient cost. In a palliative setting, the goal is to identify those patients who either wish to, or should, consider aggressive chemotherapy or whose symptoms could be alleviated by systemic anticancer therapy.

A global standard of anticancer assessment is the objective shrinkage of a tumour to 50 per cent of its previous size. The importance of this standard has been overemphasized, as the temporary shrinkage of a tumour does nothing to prolong life in most patients with far advanced solid tumours. The growth rate of tumours slow as they enlarge—the tumour appears to act as an integrated organ with growth influenced by growth regulatory factors. When the system is perturbed, by partially removing the tumour, the remaining tumour may be stimulated into a rapid growth phase.[26,27] The chemotherapy literature is replete with studies showing that 'responders' live longer than 'non-responders'—but in adult, advanced, solid tumour patients (equivalent to patients with a Karnofsky rating of <70) the survival of the total population will not usually be altered in comparison to an untreated population. Presumably the responsive population lived longer not as a result of therapy but because they would live longer in any event.[28,29]

The value of a partial remission achieved with chemotherapy is not decried. This standard of success, however, must be assessed in relation to changes in quality of life and alleviation of pain and other symptoms. Highly toxic regimens have no place in the care of cancer patients in the last days of life. There may be a place for low-dose, reduced toxicity regimens whose objective is to control symptoms and increase life enjoyment.

Radiotherapy

A recent Australian survey demonstrated that recent medical graduates infrequently thought of radiation therapy as a treatment for cancer pain.[30] Radiotherapy must be considered for all patients with tumour-induced, localized pain. Success can often be achieved with minimal disruption of the patient's life and comfort.

Radiotherapy also has a place in the palliation of selected other symptoms such as tumour-induced dysphagia, bronchial closing, haemoptysis, etc. Details on the palliative use of radiotherapy are discussed in Chapter 9.1.2.

Surgery

On occasion, the contribution of the surgeon is forgotten after the initial definitive therapy. Surgeons, however, should be consulted for many problems confronting the advanced cancer patient. The range of palliative surgical management is discussed elsewhere in this textbook (see, for example, Chapter 9.1.3) .

Table 1 summarizes the questions which must be answered by a palliative medicine physician on referral of a cancer patient. The resultant profile will assist the physician to assess whether oncological consultation is necessary.

References

1. Devesa SS, Blot WJ, Stone BJ, Miller BA, *et al.* Recent cancer trends in the United States. *Journal of the National Cancer Institute*, 1995; **87**: 175–82.
2. Palca J. The sobering geography of AIDS. *Science*, 1991; **252**: 372–3.
3. MacDonald N. Palliative care—the fourth phase of cancer prevention. *Cancer Detection and Prevention*, 1991; **15**: 253–5.
4. MacDonald N. The role of medical oncology in cancer pain control. In: Hill CS Jr and Fields WS, eds. *Advances in Pain Research and Therapy*, Vol 11. New York: Raven Press, 1989.
5. Scott J. *Canadian Brief on Palliative Care.* Presented to Cancer 2000 on behalf of the Canadian Palliative Care Association, 1990.
6. World Health Organization. *Cancer Pain Relief and Palliative Care: Report of a WHO Expert Committee.* Technical Bulletin 804. Geneva: WHO, 1990: 11.
7. Coderre TJ, Katz J, Vaccarino A, *et al.* Contribution of central neuroplasticity to pathological pain: review of clinical and experimental evidence. *Pain*, 1993; **52**: 259–85.
8. Bruera E, Franco JJ, Maltoni M, Watanabe S, *et al.* Changing pattern of agitated impaired mental status in patients with advanced cancer: association with cognitive monitoring, hydration and opioid rotation. *Journal of Pain and Symptom Management*, 1995; **10**: 287–91.
9. *A Policy Framework for Commissioning Cancer Services.* Calman Report/ Recommendations for Cancer Services. Consultative Document. London: Her Majesty's Stationery Office, 1994.
10. MacDonald N. Cure and care: interaction between cancer centres and palliative care units. In: Senn HJ and Glaus A, eds. *Recent Results in Cancer Research*, Vol 121. Berlin-Heidelberg: Springer-Verlag, 1991.
11. Slevin ML, Plant H, Lynch D, Drinkwater J, Gregory WM. Who should measure quality of life, the doctor or the patient? *British Journal of Cancer*, 1988; **57**: 109–12.
12. Fossa SD, Aaronson NK, Newling D, *et al.*, Quality of life and treatment of hormone resistant prostatic cancer. *European Journal of Cancer*, 1990; **26**: 1133–6.
13. Grobe ME, Ahmann DL, Ilstrup DN. Assessment of needs of terminal cancer patients. *Oncology Nursing Forum*, 1982; **9**: 26–30.
14. Morrison I, Smith R. The future of medicine. *British Medical Journal*, 1994; **309**: 1099–100.
15. *Management of Cancer Pain.* Clinical Practice Guideline Number 9. US Department of Health and Human Services, Public Health Service, Agency for Health Care Policy and Research, 1994: 221–5.
16. Mackey JR, Birchell I, MacDonald N. Occult infection as a cause of hip pain in a patient with metastatic breast cancer. *Journal of Pain and Symptom Management*, 1995; **10**: 1–4.
17. Reiser SJ. The ethical life of health care organizations. *Hastings Center Report*, 1994; **24**: 28–35.
18. Higginson I, Webb D, Lessof L. Reducing hospital beds for patients with advanced cancer. *Lancet* (letter), 1994; **344**: 409.
19. Cleeland CS, Gonin R, Hatfield AK, *et al.* Pain and its treatment in outpatients with metastatic cancer. *New England Journal of Medicine*, 1994; **330**: 392–6.
20. Paine LS. Managing for organizational integrity. *Harvard Business Review*, 1994; March–April: 106–17.
21. Callahan D. *The Troubled Dream of Life: In Search of a Peaceful Death.* New York: Simon and Schuster, 1993: 94.
22. Hadorn DC. The Oregon priority-setting exercise: quality of life and public policy. *Hastings Center Report*, 1991; May-June (suppl.): **21**: 11–16.
23. MacDonald N. *Evidence. Proceedings of the Senate Special Committee on Euthanasia and Assisted Suicide.* Issue No. 22. Ottawa: Canada Communication Group, 1994: 21–42.
24. Vokes EE, Weichselbaum RR. Concomitant chemoradiotherapy: rationale in clinical experience in patients with solid tumors. *Journal of Clinical Oncology*, 1990; **8**: 911–34.
25. Greco FA, Vaughn K, Hainsworth JD. Advanced poorly differentiated cancer of unknown primary site: recognition of a treatable syndrome. *Annals of International Medicine*, 1986; **104**: 547–53.
26. Prehn RT. The inhibition of tumor growth by tumor mass. *Cancer Research*, 1991; **55**: 2–4.
27. McMillan TJ, Hart IR. Can cancer chemotherapy enhance the malignant behaviour of tumours? *Cancer and Metastasis Reviews*, 1987; **6**: 503–20.
28. Anderson JR, Cain KC, Gelber RD. Analysis of survival by tumor response. *Journal of Clinical Oncology*, 1983; **1**: 710–19.
29. Joensuu H. Association between chemotherapy response and rate of disease progression in disseminated melanoma. *British Journal of Cancer*, 1991; **63**: 154–6.
30. Smith WT, Tattersall MHN, Irwin LM, Langshanks AD. Undergraduate education about cancer. *European Journal of Cancer*, 1991; **27**: 1448–53.

2.2 The interdisciplinary team

Ina Cummings

Introduction

The myriad of issues faced by a patient with a life-threatening illness, and a family who must adapt to the illness and eventual death of one of its members, exceeds the expertise of any one caregiver. Palliative care seeks to diminish suffering. As Cassel[1] points out, suffering occurs when any aspect of our personhood is threatened—our physical body, our role in the family, our perceived future, our ability to transcend ourselves. To understand adequately, to be able to intervene in each of these physical, psychosocial, and spiritual domains requires a range of skills. Patients are highly individual in those with whom they relate easily, and the availability of different team members provides opportunity for support from a number of sources. The interdisciplinary team, bringing together individuals with a diversity of training, who share the goal of improving the quality of life of the patient, is best equipped to provide a nurturing environment for patient and family. Many of the principles outlined in this chapter are relevant to, and could be practised in, most care settings.

Definition

In simple terms, a team is a group of individuals with a common purpose working together. Each individual will have a particular expertise and training, and will be responsible for making individual decisions within his area of responsibility. The common purpose will be understood by the individual members coming together to share knowledge and information, and out of this discussion will come plans for future action. To achieve the common purpose, the individual team members will be willing to subordinate their personal agendas for the good of the whole, and will be open to accept the contributions of other team members.

The interdisciplinary team differs in several important aspects from the traditional multidisciplinary team known in most medical settings. In the traditional team, individuals are known first by their professional identities and only secondarily by their team affiliation. They share information using the vehicle of the medical record, and the leader is the highest ranking member. As the team is not the primary vehicle for action, the interaction process is not of primary importance. Compare that to the interdisciplinary team. Here the identity of the team supersedes individual personal identities. Members share information and work interdependently together to develop goals. Leadership is shared among team members depending on the task at hand.

Because the team is the vehicle of action, the interaction process is vital to success.[2]

Palliative care teams can be defined at a number of levels. At a community level, if there is to be co-ordinated care between the primary care sector, the hospital sector, and the hospice services, there is a need for a district or regional planning team.[3,4] Each programme or service will develop its own team of health-care workers and volunteers. Traditionally, such teams often worked on hospice or palliative care units. Now an increasing number of supportive care teams work in acute care settings.[5,6,7] These facility-based teams will link with those providing care in the community.[8,9,10]

Traditional models have often been inadequate in the setting of HIV/AIDS. Many of these patients have been estranged from biological family, and live alone or with a partner. Home care has been provided by a network of friends, working in liaison with community services and health professionals. If one speaks of team from the perspective of the individual patient, it is necessary to review all those individuals who go to making up the team for that particular patient.[11]

Members of the team

The composition of an interdisciplinary team will vary depending on the stage of development of the programme, the objectives of the programme, or the particular needs of a given patient. Most programmes will include, as core personnel, physician, nurse, social worker, chaplain, and volunteers. Other disciplines tend to be brought in as needed, and may be available only for consultation. For each patient, there may be a core team, composed of those individuals who have regular contact with the patient, and the extended team, who have less regular or 'as needed' contact. The core team will need to communicate regularly to continually adapt the plan of care as the illness evolves, while the extended team members may only need to be kept informed.

The patient and family

The patient and family are central members of the palliative care team.[12,13] Their information about their unique life experience and response to illness is essential to the development of a care plan, and they should actively participate in its development.[14] If the patient and family are to be team members, then the patient must be informed of what is happening, and be able to talk with someone who will listen and attempt to understand; the patient and family must participate in decisions; and the patient must be able to express feelings without fearing judgement. It is the patient who is best able to report which problem is of greatest significance to him at the moment (often not the problem identified as primary by the health-care team), and it is patient and family who can tell what role they are able to play in ongoing care. It has been said that patients are our best teachers, if we but listen.

Making the patient and family team members requires acceptance—not an action but an attitude that is open to receive those of any background, culture, or world view—and empathy, such that we feel and understand the anguish of the patient, while at the same time remaining sufficiently detached to be effective. Visiting the patient at home, surrounded by personal effects gathered over the years, with any close family at hand, allows an immediate sense of this patient as a unique person. Much has been written about the depersonalization of the patient in today's health care institutions,[15] and about approaches that seek to restore the personal interaction.[16] The staff of the inpatient unit or supportive care team will need to exert extra effort to include the patient and family into the team in an effective way when they have not known the patient outside these settings.

Physicians

When uncontrolled pain and physical symptoms are present, all else is secondary. Relief of physical symptoms must be the foundation on which rests all other aspects of palliative medicine. It follows, then, that the physician plays a central role in the interdisciplinary palliative care team, whether in specialist palliative care or palliative care provision anywhere.

Physicians working in palliative medicine must be competent in general medicine, must have familiarity with the principles and practice of hospice care, and have an understanding of malignant disease and other diseases of the patient population. Training programmes for hospice physicians are now formalized in the United Kingdom, but North America is only beginning to move in this direction. Physicians may be attracted to palliative medicine from a wide variety of specialist backgrounds: surgery, anaesthesia, family medicine, oncology, psychiatry, internal medicine. The common denominator is a commitment to improving the quality of life for terminally ill patients and a philosophy of medicine that sees the patient as a total person. Physicians are called to be healers with their whole person and, thus, in addition to their professional competence, will need the personal qualities of compassion, patience, maturity, and confidence.[17]

Hospice physicians may play a variety of roles. Some will be the attending physician for hospice patients, either in the community or inpatient setting, and be responsible for assessment, supervision, and many of the difficult treatment dilemmas. There will be an additional responsibility to the interdisciplinary team for training and support. Other physicians working on symptom control teams may play a consultant role only. These physicians have an important educational role as they discuss medical management decisions with the primary team, for it is the interaction between the hospice physician and the primary physician that will maintain the balance between overlooking treatable disease and treating when there is no possibility of response.[18]

Nurses

The qualities that draw many people into nursing–intimacy, equality, nurturing, conscience[18]—are those which draw nurses to the field of palliative care. The nurse is the team member who will have greatest contact with the patient and family, whether at home or in the institution. This prolonged, close contact gives the nurse a unique opportunity to get to know the person who is the patient, and to observe what brings discomfort and what brings relief. It is the nurse's primary responsibility to assist the patient to cope with the effects of advancing disease.[19] This begins with attention to the details of physical care: bathing, control of odour, pressure areas, mouth care, bladder care, bowel care, diet, fluids.[20] The nurse can help organize the patient's environment to minimize loss of control. Other nursing strategies will assist the patient psychologically to reduce perceived symptoms.[21] The demonstrated interest and time spent often have a great placebo effect, enhancing the effectiveness of other therapies.

Specialized nurses may work as members of the team, or as resource personnel. Examples include stomae therapist, breast care nurses, clinical nurse specialists with particular knowledge of lymphoedema[22] or relaxation techniques, and family therapists. The day-to-day co-ordination of care will usually be done by the primary nurse,[23] ward sister, or patient care co-ordinator—an important role, for as Baines[24] reminds us, three staff members trying to have a meaningful discussion on the same day are doomed to failure.

Social worker

The goal of social work is to help the patient and family deal with the personal and social problems of illness, disability, and impending death. A social work assessment will cover: the patient's understanding of diagnosis, prognosis, and present expectations; the family's understanding of the same factors; the strengths and resources available to the family; the problems precipitated by the terminal illness; the past experiences of loss and how they were handled; particular cultural, social factors that are unique to this patient and family; and expectations and plans for the future. The social worker can be particularly helpful to the team when there is dysfunction within the family, financial difficulties, or problems with future planning. Social work interventions are of two types: instrumental services, including referral to needed community resources, discharge planning, and liaison with community; and emotional support, including individual counselling with patient or family members, family counselling, and bereavement counselling.

It is interesting to note that members of other professional groups do not expect social workers to play a role in counselling but look to them for concrete services, while social workers view that aspect of the role as less important than the counselling role.[25] Social workers, in particular, need to negotiate their role with other team members.

Chaplain

A sympathetic chaplain who is a skilled listener and able to meet patients without judgement is a key team member. His presence provides a focus and a stimulus for the airing of questions of meaning that are invariably present for these patients and their families. Sometimes there will be guilt for past events,[26] a sense of meaninglessness, a sense of life as unjust and unfair.[27] Faith that previously seemed secure may be questioned. If these issues can be identified, brought to the surface and resolved in some measure, it may well mean an improvement in total well being.[28] The role of chaplaincy is one of listening, facilitating past recollection, dealing with regrets, giving thanks for what has brought love and meaning, and growing in readiness for what lies ahead.[29]

The chaplain must be mature in his own religious faith, while at the same time being flexible to the needs of those from every other world view. For those with a past tradition, religious rituals and sacraments can be very meaningful. A liaison with community clergy will encourage continuity of relationships that have been meaningful. In addition to spiritual counselling, the chaplain will often be used as a confidant and source of support and encouragement, so counselling skills are particularly helpful. A chaplain may be involved in discussion of ethical questions, or may be a facilitator to the team during times of stress or conflict.

Physiotherapist

Rather than attempting to improve function, the goal of the palliative care physiotherapist is to help plan activity aimed at maximizing the patient's diminishing resources.[30,31] For the paralyzed or bedridden patient, an active or passive range of motion exercises will prevent painful contractures and improve circulation. Massage can be very relaxing for aching muscles, as well as providing an opportunity for talking. Other team members will benefit from instruction in transfers or positioning. The role is fundamentally different from the role of a therapist as a member of a rehabilitation team, and calls for much more time spent listening, problem solving, and providing emotional support.

Occupational therapist

Occupational therapy stresses a balance between work, self-care, and play/leisure.[32,33] Self-care needs are basic to a person's sense of integrity, and include such things as grooming, feeding, dressing, and moving about. The occupational therapist can assess which functions the patient needs assistance with, and which he is still capable of doing independently. Adaptive equipment or functional splints may increase independence. Particularly for patients at home, adapting household routines, simplifying meal preparation, providing adaptive self-help equipment for bathing and dressing can change a life of dependence to one of productive living. In the inpatient setting the focus of the occupational therapist on play and leisure can help restore a sense of normal living in what easily becomes a very medically oriented milieu.

Music therapist

Music can communicate across all language and cultural barriers. Frequently music is associated with significant life events, and facilitates a life review. It provides diversion and relaxation. Used in a very deliberate way, selected music can be invaluable in reducing anxiety, relaxing muscle tension, and thus in relieving dyspnoea or reducing pain. While any staff member or volunteer can provide musical selections for a patient, the use of music for a particular therapeutic goal requires a trained therapist.[34]

Art therapist

The use of art provides one more language with which patients can express themselves. Art or poetry will allow the expression of emotions often difficult to express in conversation.

Dietitian

The dietitian will seek to provide small, attractive portions of food or supplements according to the taste preferences of the patient. Quality of life, rather than nutrition *per se*, becomes the goal.

Pharmacist

Clinical pharmacists are establishing a role beyond the provision of medication. Their knowledge of pharmacology allows them to advise on potential drug interactions, side-effects, and suggest the best formulations.

Dentist

Many terminally ill patients have oral problems resulting from anti-cancer therapy and/or poor oral care during lengthy illnesses. By incorporating dentistry into the palliative care team, the dental needs of the dying patient will be managed more effectively.[35]

Volunteer

Volunteers are included in the palliative care team with the goal of assisting the health-care professionals to provide the optimum quality of life for the patient and family. Volunteers may come for all sectors of the community, including health-care professionals, business men and women, blue collar workers, home-makers, retired senior citizens, and students. Frequently the volunteer group will more closely match the social and cultural diversity of the community than will the health-care team. It is this potential diversity, this rich mix of skills and experience, that enlarges the scope of the palliative care programme. Fortuitously, expanding the possibilities of the team in this way also enables costs to be kept to a minimum.

Volunteers bridge the gulf between institution or health-care programme and the community served, bringing a dimension of community support and reminding the health-care professionals of the particular needs of the community. Volunteers will concentrate on the quality of life aspects of care, and bring a focus of normal living to a situation where all else seems to underline a medical crisis.

Volunteer needs assessment

If the function of the volunteer is to expand the potential of the palliative care programme, then the first task is to establish what the goals of the programme are and what resources are already in place. The first person needed is a volunteer co-ordinator, someone who can oversee the recruitment, screening, training, and supervision of volunteers within the programme. This individual should have a background in voluntary work, administration, and some knowledge of how health-care teams function. The volunteer co-ordinator with the programme staff can develop a list of functions and skills that will help to achieve programme goals, and recruit volunteers accordingly. Some functions will be ongoing and others related to particular projects.

Recruitment

Much will depend on the particular community. In some cultures there is a strong tradition of voluntarism, and the challenge is one of adapting previous practices to the needs of a palliative care programme. If the programme has received much publicity, there may be no need for initial recruitment. In other settings without a tradition of voluntarism, it may be difficult to stimulate interest in the community at large. Volunteer agencies often can give helpful advice on most effective local recruitment practices. Helpful strategies include speaking to community and service clubs, working through local volunteer bureaux, radio and television public service announcements, and announcements in bulletins of local places of worship.

Factors influencing the volunteer role

Several factors affect the roles that volunteers may be asked to consider. The traditional role of volunteers in a particular community may be important. In most of North America, there are minimal hierarchical structures in health care, and volunteers regardless of sex or age are welcomed in a wide variety of roles. In much of Europe, all roles are more structured and clearly defined. Health-care professionals may be much less familiar with the volunteer as a potential team member.

The developmental stage of the programme and the availability of other team members will be important. Programmes in the planning or early stages of development often have few professional staff and look to volunteers for functions of all kinds. As programmes become larger and more established, the increasing professionalism will mean changing roles for some volunteers.

In areas where there are strong professional and non-professional unions that define roles, there may be much less flexibility in adapting roles to volunteers. If it is clear that the role of the volunteer is to supplement but not to replace the role of the health-care worker, and if union representatives are informed of palliative care philosophy and goals and are involved in joint problem solving, any potential confrontation can usually be avoided.

Roles of the volunteer

Palliative care volunteers may be used in one of several capacities.[36]

Direct service to patient and family

While specific duties may vary depending on whether the patient is at home or in an institution, the focus is on improving the quality of life, providing a supportive presence that may facilitate communication, and assisting with the normal activities of daily living. Patients can dismiss or 'hire' volunteers, thus maintaining control.[37] In one survey of a community programme, the services judged most useful by the patients were companionship, shopping, home-making, visiting after the death of a loved one, letter writing, and relieving family members of care giving responsibilities.[38] Volunteers will frequently be able to provide feedback to the interdisciplinary team on patient/family needs and concerns.

Administrative support

Volunteers may help with a wide variety of administrative tasks, including acting as receptionists, typing, filing, handling mailings, supervision of a library. For the many programmes that depend on community support, volunteers play a large role in fund raising.

Public relations and community education

Trained volunteers can also share the load with professional staff in a wide variety of community educational services.

Special interest volunteers

Volunteers with particular expertise may focus on a relevant aspect of palliative care. Examples would be volunteers who work as pastoral assistants, in music or art therapy, or in bereavement counselling.

Volunteers as consultants

Some hospices may also have a pool of professionals who volunteer their services as consultants for particular projects or needs. Lawyers, accountants, computer specialists, fund raisers, and gardeners may be included. Such volunteers may need little more palliative care training than an understanding of the philosophy. Success requires clear definition of mutual expectations, tasks, and accountability.

Selection criteria for volunteers

As in any staff selection, best results are achieved when the skills and interests of the applicant match the needs and expectations of the programme. An in-depth interview with the volunteer co-ordinator is usually the first step in evaluating the potential volunteer. Volunteers being asked to do a specific administrative or professional task must obviously have the skills needed for that function. Working in a team setting, and with patients and families, requires a number of personal qualities.[39,40] These include:

(1) personal warmth, compassion, and empathy;

(2) non-judgemental attitude, open to a variety of life-styles and world views;

(3) ease in communication, good listening skills;

(4) flexibility;

(5) ability to work as a team member;

(6) emotional maturity;

(7) discretion and respect for confidentiality;

(8) commitment to the philosophy and goals of palliative care.

Other factors that will need to be reviewed in the screening process are listed below:

1. Particular areas of interest, skills, and hobbies.
2. Willingness to make a commitment. Many programmes require a regular weekly commitment of several hours.
3. Health status. Has the applicant presently or in the past had any life-threatening illness, and how has this altered his/her perception?
4. Bereavement or significant loss experience. Such life experiences that have been worked through can enhance the empathy and understanding of the potential volunteer. Applicants who are still feeling the pain of personal life experiences may be considered for administrative but not for direct care functions, lest the needs of the volunteer be imposed on a vulnerable patient.
5. Motivation. Why does the prospective volunteer want to work

Table 1 Characteristics of effective teams[41-43]

1. A team is organic, a whole that is greater than the sum of the individual component parts
2. A team is interdependent, all members succeeding or failing together
3. A team is stimulating, and spurs individual members to greater achievement
4. A team is fun, with members enjoying a sense of belonging and camaraderie
5. A team is civilized, structured, with members submerging their individual aspirations in a larger objective as they learn to share and interact. Roles are clearly defined
6. Teams demand a certain conformity, but not uniformity
7. Team members must share their vulnerabilities as well as their strengths
8. Difficult conversations are best conducted face to face
9. Effective teams are able to deal with disagreement and anger in a constructive manner
10. Palliative care teams must work with existing health care teams, and must not overstep their advisory role
11. Confident teams allow flexible professional roles
12. Difficult decisions need to be shared
13. Personal exchange can lead to professional growth
14. Formal review improves future performance

in this area, and why now? Those with a strong personal agenda, such as promotion of a religious view, should be declined.

6. Level of social support. The presence of a supportive family and/or social network is necessary if the volunteer's personal needs are to be met outside the workplace.

Team development

To understand the functioning of the interdisciplinary team in the palliative care setting, it is worth reviewing some of the principles of team development.

Characteristics of effective teams

Effective teams are defined by certain characteristics (Table 1). Such teams have been compared to competitive sports teams, but there are some significant differences. Health-care teams find that objective outcomes are often poorly defined, success is hard to measure, and credit is often lacking or attributed solely to the head of the team.

Obstacles to effective team functioning

The team may find itself frustrated and diverting excessive energy away from the goal of improved patient care for a number of reasons. There may, initially, be little trust between different disciplines represented on the team. Professional training provides little information about the resources of other disciplines, so team members may find their assumptions about the role of another discipline vary greatly from what they see in practice. Some disciplines are well established and secure, while others are emerging and aspiring to greater status. Art therapists, music therapists, and volunteers find themselves side by side in the palliative care team with physicians, nurses, and social workers. Even in the well established disciplines, roles are changing and evolving. The physician, accustomed to the traditional role of leader, may be threatened by the hospice nurse, who sees in hospice work the opportunity to experience the expanded role of nursing. Overlapping roles and issues of overlapping specialties will need to be addressed. Many teams, particularly small support teams, include staff who have part-time commitments to other services. Conflicting loyalty to two areas of responsibility often results. The palliative care team may be resentful that the staff member never seems to be available when needed, while the staff person who is juggling responsibilities feels resentful at being misunderstood and not appreciated. A team member who feels a greater loyalty toward the line manager of their discipline than toward the team is involved but not committed, and will rarely give the team goals first priority. In turn, the team will resent being used by the individual pursuing discipline goals.

Hazards inherent in interdisciplinary teamwork

The very diversity that gives the interdisciplinary team its potential for effectiveness makes the team vulnerable if there is ineffective co-ordination.[44] Co-ordination requires effective communication and leadership, both of which can lead to difficulties. Communication requires that team members have opportunities to meet, to exchange information, and plan interventions. Meetings can multiply and expand until there is little time left for patient care. Talking can be excessive, while true communication is minimal, and waiting until everyone has had an opportunity to make a contribution may lead to excessively delayed decision making. The notion of shared responsibility may mean that no one individual fully accepts responsibility or feels accountable.[45] Attention to process is important but excessive amounts of time can be consumed in introspection. Unrealistic expectations that the team cannot meet are frequently raised.

Life-cycle model of team development

Just as individuals and families have a predictable life-cycle, with each phase bringing its own issues and challenges, so various authors have described the life-cycle of team development.[46,47] Understanding this organizational life-cycle can be extremely helpful in interpreting problems as they arise in the team, and in planning for the future.

In the first stage, hospice team development brings together a few idealistic individuals, many of them volunteers, highly motivated to initiate a new programme, and often playing many roles simultaneously. Interaction is polite, but often superficial; listening is intense but there is little sharing; and as the expression of feelings is avoided, there is minimal conflict. To be successful in achieving the public recognition that gains community support, leadership must be dynamic and often charismatic. Leader competence is usually technical and clinical rather than administrative. The enthusiasm and commitment to an ideal often over-rides the need for self-care among team members, and personal limits are not acknowledged.

The next stage brings increased formalization of the programme, with increasing definition of roles, a need for strengthening of the management component, and a need to develop a sound financial base. The tension between immediate patient and family needs and the need for future oriented planning, between idealism and pragmatism, and between delegation of responsibility and 'ownership', frequently leads to frustration, confrontation, poor team morale, and an expenditure of organizational energy that slows momentum. Staff who must care for an increasing number of patients face increased accountability and documentation requirements, and frequently feel unappreciated as everyone tries to meet the demands. The potential for conflict is high. Successful leadership must be less autocratic and more sensitive to staff concerns, less based on personal attributes and more on administrative expertise.

If these transitional issues are successfully negotiated, the team moves into a further phase in which roles are better understood and delineated. Decision making is based on individual expertise with open communication, and the internal structure of the programme becomes more complex through the addition of staff and services. The idealistic pioneers may not have the skills, personality, or desire to fulfil the new management roles, and some may leave. The programme finds a new equilibrium balancing idealistic, humanistic concerns with a pragmatic response to legal and financial pressures from the environment.

How effective is the team?

As palliative medicine becomes better defined and developed, there is increasing consensus on reasonable outcomes of interventions. Standards of practice are undergoing a 'paradigm shift' to focus on patient well-being and outcomes rather than on the process of care delivery. Restricted resource availability requires us to ensure efficient practice. In response to these trends, teams are starting to define outcome criteria, and measure their performance against these criteria.[48,49,50] This trend will continue as we look to the future.

Components of interdisciplinary team work

How a team functions depends on several components. Successful interdisciplinary team management requires attention to each of these.[51]

Roles within the team

In some medical settings, roles are very clear. In the operating theatre, for example, surgeon, anaesthetist, scrub nurse, and orderly each know what is expected of him, and each knows whether he is performing appropriately. When time is critical it is not the moment to sit down to negotiate whether some aspect of the task would be best done by someone else.

In the palliative care setting, the task is more variable and open to interpretation. What does improved quality of life mean for an individual patient? What needs to be done to achieve that goal? Who is best equipped to help with the task? Who would the patient prefer to be helped by? What is the role of any individual staff person in working toward this goal?

Palliative care seeks to approach the patient as a total person, to recognize the multiplicity of needs, and to integrate the care; roles cannot be sharply defined. The team member who is present at the time will do his best to relieve the immediate situation. It may be the nurse who counsels a distraught family, or the chaplain who helps a patient find a comfortable position. Unfortunately this blurring of traditional role boundaries can also lead to confusion and conflict.

Role expectations

A professional, while training in a particular discipline, learns a certain subject content and assumes a value system that determines how the professional role is understood. This professional identity, together with personal values such as honesty, determines how an individual views himself as a professional, and his expectations for a particular clinical role. The type of organization, the size of team, and the professions of the other team members will all influence a set of external expectations of any role. Internal and external expectations of a role may not always be congruent. A nurse who sees herself as a nurturing supporting individual may seek out hospice as an environment where she will be able to focus on emotional support, only to find that the case load and the physical care requirements of her patients leave little time to sit and talk.

Role ambiguity

Traditional roles in a non-traditional setting, or non-traditional roles are often poorly defined. Individuals themselves may have difficulty knowing how they should focus their efforts. A physiotherapist trained to help others regain function must redefine the aspects of that training which apply to patients with diminishing function. When outcomes are unpredictable, success is hard to measure. Some staff adapt well to this ambiguity, while others feel lost without greater structure, repeatedly turning to others for assistance and questioning their own competence.

Role conflict

Lack of congruence of expectations leads to potential conflict. Ideally, each staff person's input and opinion is considered equally and is complementary to those of other staff, and all are integrated in the best approach to care. In practice it may seem quite different. Each discipline will evaluate the problem from their frame of reference, and each may interpret the same information to arrive at quite different assessments. If the patient reports back pain, the physician may immediately suspect spinal metastases and begin investigation, the social worker may note that pain is only reported when family is present and conclude that a family conference is a priority, and the music therapist, noting taut muscles and a strained expression suggests that relaxation training may be most effective. Conflict arises when each team member feels that their contribution should have priority, or is consistently overlooked by other staff. This kind of tunnel vision that comes from discipline-specific training often prevents optimum team function.

Many patients, by virtue of poor education, illness, or reticence, have difficulty making their wishes and preferences known in a medical world, and several disciplines, including medicine,[52] nursing,[19] pharmacy,[53] and social work would see themselves as being the advocate for the patient. If each views his relationship with the patient as being more insightful that the others, the stage is set for conflict.

Each discipline has an area of training that gives it an exclusive role in meeting particular needs, while many other needs can be met by several different disciplines. If team members are to work together without undue conflict, they must be mature within their discipline, confident of their ability, and able to educate other team members about the skills they have to offer in their exclusive role. At the same time they must be flexible, and ready to let other team members invade their specialty in their inclusive role without becoming threatened. Role conflicts can be negotiated and overcome if the patient is kept central in discussion, and there is mutual, strong commitment to the well-being of the patient. Because the role is so dependent on what the individual brings to it, a team that has been functioning smoothly will face a new phase of negotiation whenever there is any change in key team members.

Role overload

Role overload exists when either a team or one of its members carries too large a role or too many roles to accomplish the assigned work. New programmes consisting of only a few individuals are anxious to establish their credibility and will strive to meet all demands. Such programmes are also usually changing rapidly—another source of strain. Team members can attempt to achieve the impossible by meeting all demands with inadequate resources, or set priorities and delay some of the demands.

Decision making

In the traditional, hierarchical work group, decisions are made by the leader; other members of the group who have no part in the decision have no particular investment in carrying it out except as required. What happens in the interdisciplinary team? Nurses have often felt that they are not included in decisions where they have relevant information.[54] If all disciplines are considered to have equally important input, does that mean that they are all involved in all decisions? Such a process would be so cumbersome little would be achieved. Sorting out how decisions should be made within the team requires certain questions to be asked.

1. Who has the information necessary to make the decision? Before a decision can be made to send an immobile, oxygen-dependent patient home for a week-end, it is necessary to know if transport will be possible, if there are stairs that must be negotiated, how to arrange oxygen in the community, who will be able to stay with the patient, and who will be available should things not work out. It is unlikely the chaplain or dietitian, for example, would need to be involved in such a decision.

2. Who needs to be consulted before the decision is made? Using the above example, this decision requires consultation between the patient, his family, the physician, the nurse, and possibly the social worker and the community nurse. Failing to consult all those who will be implicated in carrying out the decision may mean that some important information is overlooked.

3. Who needs to be informed of a decision after it is made? In this example some of those needing to be informed might be the dietitian (no meals on the unit for the week-end), administration (statistics, census), and community liaison (arranging ambulance transportation).

It follows that some levels of decision are made by individual team members alone, some by individuals in conjunction with others (usually the core team for day-to-day decisions), and still others require the team as a group (developing a care plan, or deciding on policy). Poor decisions will result from failure to include team members with important information, but inefficiency results from including members who are not implicated in a particular decision.

Table 2 Qualities of team centred leaders

1. Can be a visionary about what people can achieve as a team. Can share vision and act accordingly.
2. Proactive in most relationships. Stimulates excitement and action. Inspires teamwork and mutual support.
3. Gets people involved and committed. Allows people to perform. Makes it easy to see opportunities for teamwork.
4. Seeks out people who can work constructively with others.
5. Considers problem solving to be the responsibility of team members.
6. Communicates fully, openly, welcoming questions.
7. Mediates conflict before it becomes destructive.
8. Makes an effort to see that both individual and team accomplishments are recognized at the right time in an appropriate manner.
9. Keeps commitments and expects the same in return.

Leadership

A team without a captain lacks focus and direction. Historically in health care, it is the physician who has been accorded the highest status and he is looked to as leader of the health-care team. In palliative care programmes, the physician still bears ultimate medico-legal responsibility for the patient, but other disciplines increasingly share in this responsibility. The functional co-ordination of the programme is often the responsibility of the patient care co-ordinator, who may have a nursing administration background, while the executive director of the programme will increasingly come from an administrative background. The size of the programme and local policies will determine who are officially named leaders.

The functions of a leader are well known: to motivate the team to the highest possible standard (to persuade the team members that they want to go in the direction in which you are pushing them), and to take responsibility for planning and problem solving.[55] A new group with inexperienced members and much to achieve in a short time will be best served by a leader who is quite directive. This same style will be counterproductive with a group of experienced team members who individually have much to contribute (Table 2). The most effective leader will be the one who can adapt his style to the circumstances, and who can maintain the best balance between pressure to get the job done, and need to nurture and motivate the team members.[56]

Within the palliative care team leadership can be quite flexible and based on expertise, depending on the problem under consideration. The social worker may be the best leader in working with a dysfunctional family, while the physician will take leadership in sorting out the cause and best approach to control vomiting. The formal team leader then can act as co-ordinator, ensuring that there is follow through and regular re-evaluation.

Communication

Communication is the thread that runs through interdisciplinary team work, bringing all the pieces together into a coherent whole. Having accepted that all team members may have valuable information, the challenge is how to achieve information exchange in the most concise, efficient way possible. Communication can take two forms—reporting and problem solving.

In the former approach, one team member has information that needs to be conveyed to other members, and which will be lost unless there is a written record. The medical record serves as the vehicle for clinical reporting, whether physical symptoms or a family meeting. Such information may be reported on verbally at 'change of shift' reports or at team meetings. Organizational information can be conveyed in memorandum form and kept in a readily available 'information book' available to all staff.

An example of problem-solving communication is the formulation of a care plan. This requires the team to meet together, usually weekly. The facilitator of such a meeting has the task of making sure that all team members have a chance to contribute, that no member dominates the meeting, that extraneous anecdotal discussion is kept to a minimum, and that a clear plan evolves with members knowing their area of responsibility. Such team meetings will also provide opportunities for continuing education and team support.

Programme goals

Each programme will define a purpose or mission, which must be congruent with that of any parent institution or body. Such external goals are not usually negotiable, but within this global purpose, the team must set its own more limited or short-term goals. For example a palliative care programme in a university hospital may be expected to have a teaching programme. The team may decide that it will accept students on a regular rotational basis, with nurses acting as preceptors. Since each team member has his own personal goal, the nurse whose goal is to spend as much time as possible with her patients may resent the time spent with a student and the delay to the routine of the day. To consider programme goals, then, is to consider a series of questions.

1. How are goals defined, who sets the goals, and how well are they understood by the whole team?
2. How much fit is there between individual, team, and organizational goals?
3. How much consensus is there about the programme goals?
4. How much commitment is there to the goals?
5. How are the goals reviewed and up-dated?
6. How is goal achievement measured, what does success look like, and how does it benefit individual team members?

Norms

These are the unwritten rules that govern behaviour in the team, and will determine the topics discussed, how conflict is dealt with, formality of dress and speech, etc. New members of the team will need to become accustomed to and adopt the norms if they are to be fully integrated.

Conflict management

Conflict occurs when two or more people, or ideas, or activities, attempt to occupy the same space at the same time. Conflict is intrinsically neither good nor bad: different ideas and different perspectives can lead to the kind of creative brain storming that produces a better idea than any of the participants had at the beginning. A lack of conflict would result in the uniformity of approach that would stifle growth. However, staff may expend significant energy in intrapersonal and interprofessional conflict management[57] and, if the conflict becomes personal and bitter, it has the potential to be very destructive. Either option is always present. The manner in which the interdisciplinary team works makes conflict inevitable, so the challenge becomes not how to avoid conflict, but how to manage it so that it enriches the programme.

Levels of conflict

Conflict can take place at three levels, intrapersonal, interpersonal, and interorganizational, and each influences the other. The intrapersonal conflict is always present between those aspects of our personality that reflect in behaviour that is overbearing and critical, overprotective and smothering, or the helpless victim, or conversely, behaviour that is supportive, nurturing, and problem-solving. This will be reflected in our personal style of interaction. 'You should know I can't get all my patients done by noon' (victim) tends to provoke a different response than 'I'm running late–can we talk after lunch?(problem-solving). Any team member who finds themselves repeatedly in conflict would do well to look at their personal style. Interpersonal conflict will be discussed below. Interorganizational conflict is outside the control of the team, but may result in external pressures on team members that can exacerbate team conflict.

Antecedents to conflict in the interdisciplinary team

Many of the factors previously discussed will lead to conflict from time to time:

(1) ambiguous role boundaries, roles that are changing, protective territorialism of role area;

(2) interdisciplinary professional rivalry;

(3) communication barriers; small problems that are not dealt with because of time becoming larger problems;

(4) leadership style that is not congruent with the needs of the team;

(5) decision making that does not include individuals involved;

(6) team members with different goals, expectations;

(7) prior conflicts, displaced hostility;

(8) differing personality styles;

(9) continuing change, change threatening the existence of individual roles or the programme, change which affects team members unequally;[58]

(10) scarcity of resources.

Variables affecting the course of conflict

Several factors will influence the way a conflict will develop:

1. The characteristics of the individuals involved: their motivations, values, resources, aspirations.
2. The prior relationship of the individuals to one another. If the relationship has been one of trust, then conflict is more likely to lead to creative problem-solving than if the relationship has a history of difficulty.
3. The nature of the problem giving rise to the conflict. If the

problem is relatively minor, then it is unlikely that either party will have much invested in pursuing their point of view. On the other hand, if the problem involves a value that is important to one individual, then the significance is much greater.

4. The social environment. Is the team fatigued and stressed, or does either party stand to lose self-esteem?
5. Interested audience. Is this a problem limited to two individuals, or is there a split in the team?
6. Tactics employed by the individuals in conflict. Is the conflict focused on issues, or has it become personal? Are promises, threats, coercion part of the communication?
7. What will be the consequences of the conflict—gains or losses, precedents set, influences on relationships?

Understanding these factors may help to avoid destructive interactions, and favour problem-solving.

Managing interpersonal conflict

Conflict cannot be resolved unless it is acknowledged, and suppressing or avoiding conflict only postpones the inevitable. Smoothing things over with diplomatic platitudes also fails to deal with the real issues. Discuss the problem directly with the individual(s) concerned and involve third parties only if resolution cannot be achieved between the directly involved parties. A problem-solving approach to confrontation[59] will involve the following factors:

1. Timing. Deal with an issue as soon as possible after it arises, but not until emotions have cooled. Make an appointment for tomorrow rather than confront a colleague when the heat of emotion over-rules rational thinking.
2. Location. Use a private, quiet area where you will not be interrupted.
3. Describe what has happened—'Are you aware that I was not informed of the meeting to plan Mrs. K's discharge?'
4. Describe the consequences of the actions of the other person in personal terms—'I was very frustrated because I had spent a lot of time looking into Mrs. K's situation.'
5. Protect the self-respect of the other individual. What is at issue is behaviour, and not the credibility or integrity of the other.
6. Specify what you would like to see happen, and how you can help. 'I believe the primary nurse should be involved in all meetings concerning her patients.'
7. Describe the consequences for the other person if they were to change their behaviour—'. . . that way there will be less duplication of effort and better co-ordination.'
8. Together generate all possible solutions to the problem.
9. Choose the best solution. Agree that after trying it for a given period of time you will review the question again.

Managers and leaders within the programme will have to evaluate conflicts as they arise to determine if they are significant. If several team members are involved, and the effectiveness of the team is threatened, then intervention is indicated (Fig. 1).

Facilitating conflict resolution

If conflicts cannot be resolved by the individuals involved, then it is useful to bring the matter to a group, preferably with an objective third party outside the authority structure to act as facilitator.[60,61,62]

The facilitator should take the following steps:

1. Welcome the existence of the conflict, bring it into the open, and use it as potential for change.
2. Listen with understanding and not evaluation.
3. Clarify the nature of the problem as seen by both parties. Is this the real problem? Suppose the nurse is complaining that the doctor is not prescribing sufficient doses of analgesic for a patient, and isn't listening to her. The doctor is upset that the nurse is telling him what to do when the patient seems very comfortable. The real problem may be that the nurse has not learned to perform a systematic pain assessment, or how to report the evidence to back up her statement to the doctor—not primarily a problem of analgesia but of communication! 'Scapegoating' is a common response to a problem, but the removal of the person who is being blamed for a situation seldom solves the problem. Scapegoating is a convenient way of attributing blame away from self, and should always trigger a further assessment of the issues.
4. Reduce the area of conflict. Both parties should individually list the specific problems and agree to work only with those problems listed by both parties. This reduces the number of issues, and starts with establishing an initial agreement.
5. Suggest the procedures and ground rules. It is important that someone should be in charge, and that the process is 'safe' for all concerned.
6. Identify the goals. Short-term and long-term goals should be assessed and the question of whether they are compatible should be considered. Winning at the cost of the quality of the relationship is self-defeating.
7. Identify the variables keeping the individuals in conflict. Organizational conflicts are felt at the lowest level of the system, but can only be resolved at the level at which they originate. For example, if a conflict between nurses and physicians arises because nurses cannot take verbal orders, the only way of resolving the conflict is to take it to the level of nursing administration that set the policy.
8. Create and evaluate as many solutions as possible, looking for a solution that preserves everyone's self-esteem.
9. Agree on one solution, record it, and ensure that both parties agree on the meaning as it is written.
10. Plan implementation and subsequent re-evaluation after a defined period.

Staff selection

Professional competence is the first consideration as in any health-care team. As palliative medicine becomes more common as a

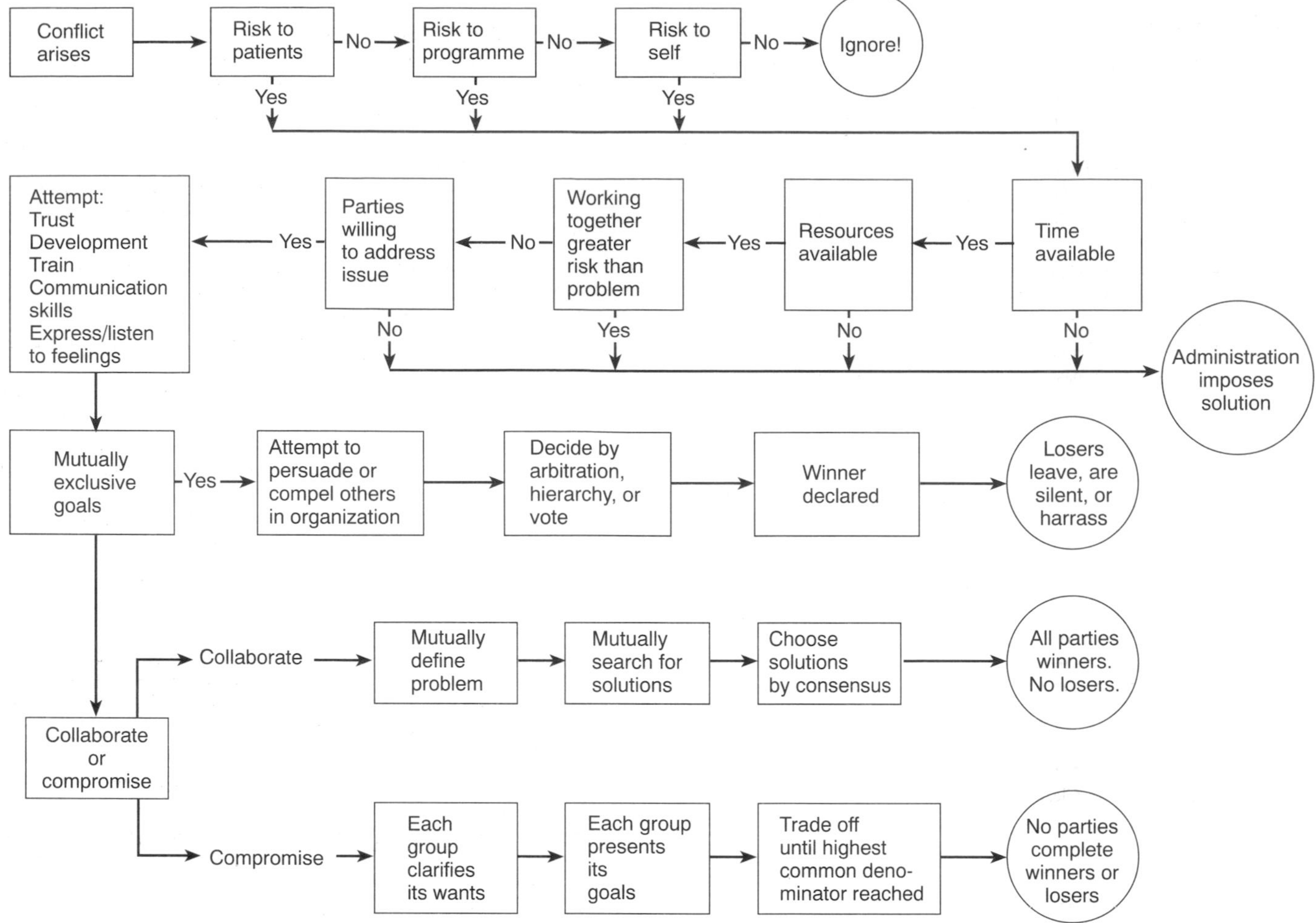

Fig. 1 Interdisciplinary team conflict management flow chart.

career path, and training programmes become more available, a standard may be established for staff who would like to work in the field. Pending that evolution, it falls to each programme to determine the skills that will be required to perform any particular role, and to ensure that potential staff have those skills or are able to acquire them.

Potential staff members need to be mature and secure within their discipline. It follows that staff should have some work experience prior to joining an interdisciplinary team. Working within an interdisciplinary team can be very rewarding, but is not easy, and is not for everyone. Personal characteristics that are required include a willingness and ability to trust others; flexibility, openness and tolerance for ambiguity; respect for others and their contributions; patience; sensitivity; a willingness and ability to support colleagues; and an ability not to take oneself too seriously—a sense of humour is invaluable.

Team members who are 'loners' will effectively sabotage team interaction. While physicians are often guilty in this respect, it can be a problem for any team member. Since many potential staff members will have had a personal life experience that leads them to this field, so any history of personal losses should be explored. This background often results in an increased sensitivity and commitment, but can also lead to over involvement and 'burnout'. Above all, potential staff members need to have personal maturity—the ability to accept one's self, to acknowledge one's feelings without being overcome by them, to take responsibility for one's actions and behaviour, and to set personal limits.

The most effective way to avoid many of the pitfalls of this type of team functioning is to select staff who are best suited. Mount[63] provides helpful guidelines to a selection process. One of the keys is to match the idiosyncrasies of the applicant to the idiosyncrasies of the job; thus a good job description is an important starting point.

Stress and support in the interdisciplinary team

The palliative care team faces particular stresses as a result of their work including the stress of continually forming relationships with dying patients and simultaneously preparing for the termination of these relationships, and the stress related to the work group and work place.[64,42] Approaches that are reported to diminish stress include attention to informal staff support, staff support meetings with a facilitator, and continuing education aimed at increasing skills.[65] A full discussion of these issues is found elsewhere in this volume.

References

1. Cassel EJ. The nature of suffering and the goals of medicine. *New England Journal of Medicine*, 1982; **305**: 635–45.
2. Lowe JI, Herranen M. Interdisciplinary Team. In: *Hospice Education Program for Nurses.* Washington: US Department of Health and Human Services Publication No. HRA 81–27, 1981: 1047–8.
3. Bennett M, Corcoran G. The impact on community palliative care services of a hospital palliative care team. *Palliative Medicine*, 1994; **8**: 237–44.
4. Thorne CP, Seamark DA, Lawrence C, Gray DJ. The influence of general practitioner community hospitals on the place of death of cancer patients. *Palliative Medicine*, 1994; **8**: 122–8.
5. Campbell ML, Field BE. Management of the patient with do not resuscitate status: compassion and cost containment. *Heart-Lung*, 1991; **20**: 345–8.
6. Cohen IL. Establishing and justifying specialized teams in intensive care units for nutrition, ventilator management and palliative care. *Critical Care Clinics*, 1993; **9**: 511–20.
7. Dunlop RJ, Hockley JM. *Terminal Care Support Teams; the hospital-hospice interface.* Oxford: Oxford Medical Publishers, 1990.
8. McWhinney IR, Steward MA. Home care of dying patients. Family physicians' experience with a palliative care support team. *Canadian Family Physician*, 1994; **40**: 240–6.
9. Dunne C, Falkenhagen M. Palliative care in the community: a specialized approach. *Journal of Palliative Care*, 1998; **4**: 47–8.
10. Chekryn J, Pfaff GA. Generalist team with specialist consultants is preferable. *Journal of Palliative Care*, 1988; **4**: 44–6
11. Johnson A. *Living with dying, dying at home: an AIDS care team resource manual.* Toronto: AIDS Committee of Toronto (ACT) and Le projet Accès, National AIDS Clearing House, 1994.
12. Hull R, Ellis M, Sargent V. *Teamwork in Palliative Care.* Oxford: Radcliffe Medical Press, 1989.
13. Wilson DC, Ajemian I, Mount BM. The Royal Victoria Hospital palliative care service. In: Davidson GW, ed. *The Hospice: Development and Administration.* Washington: Hemisphere Publishing Corporation, 1978: 14–15.
14. Joint Commission on Accreditation of Hospitals. *Hospice Standards Manual.* Chicago: JCAH, 1983.
15. Duff RS, Holingshead AB. *Sickness and Society.* New York: Harper, 1968.
16. Mount BM. Caring in today's health care system. *Canadian Medical Association Journal,* 1978: **26**: 303–4.
17. Swanson RW. Role of the family physician in treatment of cancer. *Canadian Family Physician,* 1990; **36**: 839.
18. Fagin C, Diers D. Nursing as metaphor. *New England Journal of Medicine,* 1983; **309**: 116–17.
19. Dicks B. The contribution of nursing to palliative care. *Palliative Medicine,* 1990; **4**: 197–203.
20. Cockburn M. Nursing care of dying persons and their families. In: Corr CA, Corr DM, eds. *Hospice Care: Principles and Practice.* New York: Springer Publishing Company, 1983: 119–134.
21. McCaffery M, Beebe A. *Pain, Clinical Manual for Nursing Practice.* St. Louis: Mosby, 1989.
22. Badger C. Lymphoedema: management of patients with advanced cancer. *The Professional Nurse,* 1987; **January**: 100–2.
23. Athlin E, Furaker C, Jansson L, Norberg A. Application of primary nursing within a team setting in the hospice care of cancer patients. *Cancer Nursing,* 1993; **16**: 388–97.
24. Baines M. Tackling total pain. In: Saunders C, ed. *Hospice and Palliative Care: An Interdisciplinary Approach.* London: Edward Arnold, 1990: 34.
25. Kulys R, Davis MA. Nurses and social workers: rivals in the provision of social services? *Health and Social Work,* 1987; **12**: 101–12.
26. Clark R. Forgiveness in the hospice setting. *Palliative Medicine,* 1990; **4**: 305–10.
27. Kemp C. Spiritual care in terminal illness. *The American Journal of Hospice and Palliative Care,* 1994; **11**: 31–6.
28. Doyle D. Have we looked beyond the physical and psychosocial? *Journal of Pain and Symptom Management,* 1992; **7**: 302–11.
29. Hoy T. Hospice chaplaincy in the caregiving team. In: Corr CA, Corr DM, eds. *Hospice Care: Principles and Practice.* New York: Springer Publishing Company, 1983: 195.
30. Doutre D, Stillwell DM, Ajemian I. Physiotherapy in palliative care. In: Ajemian I, Mount BM, eds. *The R.V.H. Manual on Palliative/Hospice Care.* New York: Arno Press, 1980: 216–22.
31. Ebel S, Langer K. The role of the physical therapist in hospice care. *American Journal of Hospice/Palliative Care,* 1993; **10**: 32–5.
32. Tigges KN. Occupation therapy in hospice. In: Corr CA, Corr DM, eds. *Hospice Care: Principles and Practice,* New York: Springer Publishing Company, 1983: 160–76.
33. Dawson S. The role of occupational therapy groups in an Australian hospice. *American Journal of Hospice and Palliative Care,* 1993; **10**: 13–7.
34. Munro S, Mount BM. Music therapy in palliative care. *Canadian Medical Association Journal,* 1978; **119**:1029–34.
35. Lapeer GL. The dentist as a member of the palliative care team. *Journal of the Canadian Dental Association,* 1990; **56**: 205–7.
36. Bates IJ, Brandt KE, eds. *Volunteer Training Curriculum: Recommended by the National Hospice Organization.* Arlington: National Hospice Organization,1990: 43–4.
37. Moore MK. Dying at home: a way of maintaining control for the person with ALS/MND. *Palliative Medicine,* 1993; **7** supplement (4): 65–8.
38. McGill A, Wares C, Huchcroft S. Patients' perceptions of a community volunteer support program. *The American Journal of Hospice and Palliative Care,* 1990; **7**: 43–6.
39. Kilburn LH. *Hospice Operations Manual.* Arlington: National Hospice Organization,1988: 127–8.
40. Markey K. Volunteers in palliative care. In: Ajemian I, Mount BM, eds. *The R.V.H. Manual of Palliative/Hospice Care.* New York: Arno Press, 1980: 522–38.
41. Teamwork in Business. *Royal Bank Letter,* 1982; **63**: 1–4.
42. Vachon MLS. Staff stress in hospice/palliative care: a review. *Palliative Medicine,*1995; **9**: 91–113.
43. Dellepoort WTA. Teamwork and collaboration. *Canadian Oncology Nursing Journal,* 1994; **4**: Supplement 2: 65–7.
44. Zimmerman JM. *Hospice: complete care for the terminally ill.* 2nd edn. Baltimore: Urban and Schwarzenberg, 1986.
45. Rae-Grant Q, Maruse D. The hazards of teamwork. *American Journal of Orthopsychiatry,* 1968; **38**: 4–8.
46. Tuckman BW, Jensen MAC. Stages of small-group development revisited. *Groups and Organization Studies,* 1977; **2**: 419–42.
47. Lowe JI, Herranen M. Conflict in teamwork: understanding roles and relationships. *Social Work in Health Care,* 1978; **3**: 323–30.
48. Ellershaw JE. Assessing the effectiveness of a hospital palliative care team. *Palliative Medicine,* 1995; **9**: 145–52.
49. Higginson I, Wade A, McCarthy M. Effectiveness of two palliative support teams. *Journal of Public Health Medicine,* 1991; **14**: 50–6.
50. McCarthy M, Higginson I. Clinical audit by a palliative care team. *Palliative Medicine,*1991; **5**: 215–21.
51. Branon B, Bohnet NL, Amenta MR. The interdisciplinary team. In: Amenta, MR, Bohnet NL, *Nursing Care of the Terminally Ill.* Boston; Little Brown and Company,1986: 273–89.
52. Latimer EJ. When a patient is dying...the physician's responsibilities and rewards. *Pain Management Newsletter,* 1988; **1**: 1–2.
53. Schulz RM, Brushwood DB. The pharmacists role in patient care. *Hastings Center Report,* 1991; **21**: 12–17.
54. Rodney P. A nursing perspective on life-prolonging treatment. *Journal of Palliative Care,* 1994; **10**: 40–4.
55. Jackson L. Team building. In: Saunders C, ed. *Hospice and Palliative Care: an Interdisciplinary Approach.* London: Edward Arnold, 1990: 21–3.

56. Maddux RB. *Team Building: an Exercise in Leadership* (revised edition). Menlo Park, California: Crisp Publications Inc.,1992: 5–11.
57. McWilliam CL, Burdock J, Wamsley J. The challenging experience of palliative care support team nursing.*Oncology Nursing Forum,* 1993; **20**: 779–85.
58. Perlman D, Takacs GJ. The 10 stages of change. *Nursing Management,*1990; **21**: 33–8.
59. White TA. Nose to nose conflict. *Nursing Life,* 1985; **March/April**: 49–51.
60. Wallace JA. The death of a child: the use of a group for conflict resolution. *American Journal of Hospice Care,*1989; **6**: 43–6.
61. Lemieux-Charles L. Physicians in health care management: managing conflict through negotiation. *Canadian Medical Association Journal,* 1994; **151**: 1129–32.
62. Tagliere DA. *How to Meet, Think and Work to Consensus.* San Diego: Pfeiffer and Company, 1992: 34–5.
63. Mount BM. Personnel selection: applying the McMurray principles in palliative care. In Ajemian I, Mount BM. eds. *The R.V.H. Manual on Palliative/Hospice Care.* New York: Arno Press, 1980: 431–47.
64. Vachon MLS. *Occupational Stress in the Care of the Critically Ill, the Dying and the Bereaved.* Washington: Hemisphere Publishing Corporation, 1987.
65. Harris RD, Bond MJ, Turnbull R. Nursing stress and stress reduction in palliative care. *Palliative Medicine,* 1990; **4**: 191–6.

2.3 Death in modern society

Charles A. Corr

Introduction

With respect to death, there is a sense in which each of us is like all other persons who are now alive in the world and who have been or will be alive at some time. There is another sense in which each of us is only like some other persons who have been, are, or will be alive. There is yet another sense in which each of us is like no other person who has ever been, is now, or will at some future time be alive. In the first of these senses, for example, for every human being death means that this life is over once and for all. Barring the possibility of miracles, death is the end of life for each person in the world. At the same time, each person's experience of death—when it occurs, how and where it takes place, and how he or she feels about it—is unique and individual. My death is my own. No one else can experience it for me.

The ways in which death is experienced by some human beings in the particular set of historical, temporal, and societal circumstances which represent modern society are addressed in this chapter. The principal aim of this analysis is to outline the main features whereby contemporary human beings find themselves to be living with the changing face of death near the end of the twentieth century. These features constitute the proximate context within which palliative care will or will not be found to be desirable and/or feasible.

The main emphasis in this discussion is on the developed countries of Western Europe and North America. Nevertheless, it is useful to introduce selected contrasts with other patterns of death-related experiences at different times in history. Also, several examples of distinctive sets of societal experiences with death from other countries around the globe are introduced towards the end of the chapter.

Death-related experiences

Two principal dimensions can be distinguished in order to understand how human beings experience death. These two dimensions are encounters which represent the ways in which human beings confront or meet death and attitudes which encompass the dispositions or stances that humans develop towards their encounters with death.[1] Encounters and attitudes are not independent components of human experience, but are distinguished here for purposes of discussion. As individuals live out their lives, encounters and attitudes intertwine and interact as the warp and weft of death-related experiences. Different types of death-related encounters are likely to engender different sorts of attitudes, just as differing attitudes are likely to encourage or to inhibit death-related encounters.

In the following analysis we first discuss changing encounters with death and then changing attitudes towards death. We begin with death-related encounters and attitudes in the developed countries of Western Europe and North America, and then turn to selected examples drawn from other societies around the world. The account is introduced through a consideration of Goldscheider's model of 'uncontrolled' and 'controlled' mortality,[2] a set of ideal types around which comparisons and contrasts can usefully be organized.

'Uncontrolled' versus 'controlled' mortality

In Goldscheider's model the Industrial Revolution is selected as the point of division between two contrasting patterns of human experiences with mortality. Therefore his analysis is based upon broad historical trends in human society. However, historical evidence can only be depicted in a general way, particularly as one moves backwards in time from modern societies and their complex systems for recording demographic data. Thus the main value of Goldscheider's analysis lies in the ways in which its contrasting typologies stimulate thinking and self-understanding. There is no pure historical example of 'uncontrolled' mortality, because all human beings throughout history have striven to influence their relationships with death. Similarly, there is no pure historical example of 'controlled' mortality, since no human beings throughout history have been able to control their relationships with death completely.

According to Goldscheider, there are three important features of the experience with death in preindustrial societies, which he takes as the model of uncontrolled mortality. He points out that 'mortality was high, fluctuated over short periods, and varied widely at any point in time between areas and subpopulations' (ref. 2, p. 106), i.e. in most societies prior to the Industrial Revolution and in many societies which remain largely in a preindustrial state today, human beings experienced very high death rates and correspondingly low average life expectancies. Some individuals in such societies lived to an old age, but most died at what would now be regarded as a relatively young age. High mortality rates, particularly among infants, children, and women during pregnancy and childbirth, or shortly thereafter, would reduce average life expectancy to what many now think of as the prime of life.

Widowers would probably be relatively young or middle-aged adult males whose wives had died giving birth to the latest of what would now be considered to be a large number of children.

Mortality rates fluctuate significantly from time to time as a result of famine, epidemics, and wars, and also vary in important ways from place to place when, for example, infection is carried along principal routes of travel, ignoring isolated towns and small villages located away from the main routes of commerce, only to strike hardest in cities along those routes or in the large metropolitan communities which are their nodules. Early transmission of the AIDS virus in some countries resembled this pattern quite closely.

When one does not understand the underlying causes of these temporal fluctuations and spatial variations, death is a capricious and puzzling phenomenon, an event shrouded in mystery. Even so, defensive tactics such as the use of quarantine can often be effective in preventing infection from entering or leaving the boundaries of an isolated community.

In a context of more or less controlled mortality, death rates are much lower, and both temporal fluctuations and spatial variations are much less significant, if not almost non-existent in any substantive sense. Because average life expectancy is inversely related to mortality rates, Goldscheider is able to illustrate changes associated with increasing control or influence over mortality patterns in the following way: 'By 1840, the population in the most advanced European countries had a life expectancy of over forty years slowly increasing to forty-five years by 1880, to fifty-one years by the turn of the twentieth century, to over sixty years by 1930, and to over seventy years by the 1950s' (ref. 2, p. 110).

In the model of controlled mortality, the large fluctuations and variations which characterized encounters with death in the pre-industrial world have been virtually eliminated. Mortality rates have declined steadily, eventually reaching low levels that have no known precedent in human history. In such societies, average life expectancy has for the first time achieved the biblical promise of 'three-score years and ten'.

An important feature of this shift from one model of mortality experiences to another is that it started and was far advanced prior to the advent of modern medicine. Alterations in mortality patterns began as a result of changes in social systems and in standards of living. These changes included better housing and working conditions, developments in agriculture, advances in communications and transportation, and improvements in public health and sanitation measures. The influence of antibiotics, beginning in the 1930s, and more recent cure-oriented interventions augmented and extended these changes. However, such interventions are relatively new, and modern medical technology simply augments the effects of a very broad base of improvement in societal living standards and preventative measures.

Therefore changes in a society and in its health care system can have a direct impact upon its experiences with death; similarly, changes in the specific features of the mortality patterns in a particular society will influence the larger society in one way or another. The former point can be illustrated by current and projected changes in demographic patterns in those societies in which the proportion of elderly members in the population is increasing. The latter point is apparent in the ways in which the influence of AIDS is spreading throughout society, far beyond those who are carriers of the human immunodeficiency virus. How death is experienced is in part a function of the society in which that experience takes place; what society is like is in part a function of its encounters with and attitudes towards death.

Table 1 Mortality rates per 1000 population by age and gender, United States, 1900 and 1994

Age (years)	1900			1994		
	Both sexes	Males	Females	Both sexes	Males	Females
All ages	17.2	17.9	16.5	8.8	9.2	8.4
Under 1	162.4	179.1	145.4	8.1	9.0	7.2
1–4	19.8	20.5	19.1	0.4	0.5	0.4
5–14	3.9	3.8	3.9	0.2	0.3	0.2
15–24	5.9	5.9	5.8	1.0	1.5	0.5
25–34	8.2	8.2	8.2	1.4	2.1	0.8
35–44	10.2	10.7	9.8	2.4	3.4	1.4
45–54	15.0	15.7	14.2	4.5	5.8	3.3
55–64	27.2	28.7	25.8	11.4	14.7	8.4
65–74	56.4	59.3	53.6	25.9	33.5	19.9
75–84	123.3	128.3	118.8	59.1	74.9	49.2
85 and over	260.9	268.8	255.2	153.1	179.4	143.0

Source: refs. 3 and 4.

Encounters with death in modern developed societies

In modern societies encounters with death are characterized by a number of factors, including mortality rates, temporal fluctuations, spatial variations, average life expectancy, causes of death, dying trajectories, professionalization, specialization, and institutionalization.

Mortality rates have declined dramatically (Table 1). For example, in the United States the mortality rate for the total population in 1900 was 17.2 deaths per 1000; in 1994 that rate had dropped to 8.4 per 1000.[3,4] This unprecedented reduction of more than 50 per cent in less than a century has been paralleled in nearly every other developed country in Western Europe and North America.

Within these impressive declines in overall mortality rates, reductions in infant mortality rates have been even more significant. For example, infant mortality rates in the United States were more than 20 times higher in 1900 than in 1994. This has important implications for children, for parents (particularly mothers), and for society as a whole in such matters as family planning and in the design of programmes in paediatrics and child care.

There are also gender, ethnic, and class differences within overall mortality rates. For example, the mortality rate for males in the United States declined from 17.9 per 1000 in 1900 to 9.2 per 1000 in 1994, and that for females declined from 16.5 to 8.4. In terms of ethnic, class, and other social groupings, as a general rule those who are socially disadvantaged experience higher mortality rates. This should not be surprising, since low socio-economic standing, poverty, and inadequate access to health care have immediate and unhappy implications for death rates. One study exemplified this sad disparity by showing that black males living in

Table 2 The 10 leading causes of death, by rank, in the United States, 1900 and 1994

Rank	Cause of death	Deaths per 100 000 population	Percentage of all deaths (%)
1900			
All causes		1719.1	100.0
1	Influenza and pneumonia	202.2	11.8
2	Tuberculosis (all forms)	194.4	11.3
3	Gastritis, duodenitis, enteritis, etc.	142.7	8.3
4	Diseases of the heart	137.4	8.0
5	Vascular lesions affecting the central nervous system	106.9	6.2
6	Chronic nephritis	81.0	4.7
7	All accidents	72.3	4.2
8	Malignant neoplasms (cancer)	64.0	3.7
9	Certain diseases of early infancy	62.6	3.6
10	Diphtheria	40.3	2.3
1994			
All causes		876.9	100.0
1	Diseases of the heart	281.6	32.1
2	Malignant neoplasms (cancer)	206.0	23.5
3	Cerebrovascular diseases	59.2	6.8
4	Chronic obstructive pulmonary diseases and allied conditions	39.1	4.5
5	Accidents and adverse effects	34.6	3.9
6	Pneumonia and influenza	31.5	3.6
7	Diabetes mellitus	21.2	2.4
8	HIV infection	16.1	1.8
9	Suicide	12.4	1.4
10	Chronic liver disease and cirrhosis	9.9	1.1

Source: refs. 3, 4.

the New York City neighbourhood of Harlem are less likely to reach the age of 65 than men living in Bangladesh, one of the poorest countries in the world today.[5]

Rates of decline in nearly all mortality rates in developed societies appear to have levelled off in recent years, suggesting that changes have been brought about in many of the factors that are most obviously or directly linked to death. Further reductions in mortality rates in such societies may be much harder to achieve.

As has been suggested earlier, declines in overall mortality rates in modern societies are accompanied by decreases in temporal fluctuations and spatial variations, as well as increases in average life expectancy. Fluctuations and variations in mortality rates and differences in average life expectancies do exist within various developed societies, but these are demographically far less significant than those encountered in preindustrial societies.

This has led one knowledgeable scholar (ref. 6, p. 85) to speak of a 'death-free generation', i.e. one that is born, lives through infancy, childhood, and adolescence, enters into adulthood, marries, and has children, all without experiencing the death of a significant close family relative. Perhaps it is something of an exaggeration to say that recent generations are wholly free of death-related encounters. However, it is certainly true that one frequently meets young parents who are able to describe their lives in this way. If this is the pattern of their confrontations with death, perhaps it is not surprising that death seems to be a stranger or an alien figure which has no natural or appropriate place in their lives.

Other features which characterize encounters with death in modern society have to do with the causes of death and the ways in which we die. Around 1900 most deaths were due to communicable diseases such as influenza, cholera, scarlet fever, measles, smallpox, and tuberculosis (Table 2). Such diseases are often accompanied by symptoms such as diarrhoea, nausea, vomiting, headache, fever, and muscle ache, and therefore they were relatively easy to identify. However, it was not until Pasteur's discovery in the late nineteenth century that communicable diseases are caused by microbial agents, and the subsequent development of antimicrobial drugs in the 1930s, that caregivers were able to do much more than respond to the symptoms rather than overcome their underlying causes.

In developed societies death is mainly the result of degenerative diseases which are largely the result of the wearing out of bodily organs, a deterioration associated with lifestyle, environment, and ageing. The three leading causes of death in modern society are all degenerative diseases: diseases of the heart, malignant neoplasms (cancer), and cerebrovascular diseases.

In order to contrast ways in which people die from communicable versus degenerative diseases, it is helpful to consider the notion of dying trajectories.[7] Dying trajectories or patterns of dying are primarily distinguished by duration (the time taken between the onset of dying and the arrival of death) and shape (the course of the dying process, and particularly whether one can predict how it will advance, and whether or not death is expected or unexpected). Some dying trajectories involve a swift or almost instantaneous onset of death, while others last for a long period of time; some can be anticipated, others are ambiguous or unclear (perhaps involving a series of remissions and relapses), and still others give no advance warning at all.

As a general rule, communicable diseases are characterized by a relatively brief dying trajectory, usually resolving in either death or recovery in a period of hours, days, or a few weeks. Although some degenerative diseases (such as heart attacks, strokes, embolisms, and aneurysms) may cause rapid unanticipated death, the more typical dying trajectory associated with a degenerative disease is one of gradual and increasing debilitation.

In modern societies, degenerative diseases can often be identified and treated with surgery, chemotherapy, and/or radiation. If this can be done, quantity and quality of life may be restored; if not, intervention may only have the effect of prolonging the dying trajectory. In any event, the interval between the onset of a degenerative disease and death—the so-called 'living/dying interval'[8,9]—is characteristically measured in terms of months or even years. There are also some degenerative diseases for which significant cure-oriented interventions are not available; in other cases, the disease may not be identified until the stage has passed where cure-oriented interventions are likely to be fruitful. Thus there are a number of situations in modern society in which palliative or symptom-oriented care is particularly relevant to the ways in which people die.

Partly as a result of changes in society and in its health care systems, and partly as a result of changes in the ways in which people die, care of the dying in modern society has been increasingly marked by professionalization and specialization. Many of the causes of death which in former times would have produced patterns of dying for which care would have been relatively easy have been eradicated or minimized. These have to do with dying trajectories which are of short duration and for which interventions are relatively few in number or simple in nature.

Dying in modern society is likely to take more time than in previous years and to be more complex. As a result, care of the dying has increasingly involved professional caregivers with specialized skills. This has also come about, in part, because the demands for such care are likely to be more closely interwoven with cure-oriented interventions and to be more burdensome over a longer period of time for family caregivers.

This increasing professionalization and specialization in care of the dying has been associated with increasing institutionalization. In the United States and many other developed societies, a significant majority of all deaths now take place in a public institution such as a hospital or long-term care facility.[1] About 100 years ago, roughly the same proportion of all deaths would have taken place in the home. Most people in modern society die in a strange place, in a strange bed, surrounded mostly by sights, sounds, smells, and people who are strange to them. In many of these institutions, family members (particularly children) are excluded or are only permitted to be present and to participate in limited ways. It is not a condemnation of health care institutions or their staff to say that this is a significant alteration in the way in which death is encountered in modern society.

Because dying is most likely to take place outside the home in modern societies, family members are often not present at the moment of death; they will probably learn about a death through a telephone call from an institution. Cleaning, dressing, and preparation of the body, actions that were once regarded as final gestures of love and respect, are now likely to be performed by nurses, nurses' aids, and funeral directors. The body will probably be removed from the place where death occurred to a funeral home and may reappear in a different form at a wake, or it may be cremated and/or buried without the presence of family members.

In short, direct encounters with all facets of death have been diminished in many modern societies. Care for the dying and care of the dead has been moved away from the family and out of the home. Death is increasingly distanced from the mainstream of life's events and has become a less familiar feature of life and a more alien event.

Attitudes towards death

Attitudes are our dispositions, the patterns of feeling which enter into and often become habitual in our ways of thinking about the world. Social attitudes toward death have changed with time and have typified certain societies and periods in history. The French cultural historian Philippe Ariès has examined attitudes toward death in Western societies from the early Middle Ages to the present.[10,11] His analysis led him to identify five basic patterns in such attitudes, and he gave them the following descriptive titles arising from their most distinctive features: tame death ('all people die'), death of the self, remote and imminent death, death of the other, and forbidden death. We need not consider each of these five patterns here, but it may help to focus on a contrast between the first and the last (with some additional comments on the second and fourth) in order, once again, to understand our own situation better.

Tame death

Tame death is the most basic attitudinal pattern relating to death in the sense that it is the oldest, the most pervasive or widespread, and the most persistent. Death is said to be 'tame' in this pattern because it was familiar; those who shared this attitude were not surprised when death occurred. Encounters with death were common in their lives, much as present-day encounters with a household pet are familiar and common. When this attitude was dominant, most dying persons knew that they were dying and did not attempt to evade it. Rather than perceiving death as something that could be avoided, they calmly accepted the inevitable.

Dying persons could wait quietly for death because they did not expect their experience in dying to be long, drawn-out, or painful. One might regret that one's life was coming to an end, but the experience itself was often very much like going to sleep. In fact, most people in Christian Europe during the early Middle Ages, when this attitude was most prominent, believed death to be a kind of sleep that would last until the Second Coming of Christ. At that time, the saints would enter their celestial home, while those who were not saints would remain forever asleep. In each case, death is perceived as peaceful and non-threatening—calm, simple, and without menace.

Death was also tame because it was a public event which occurred within the community of family, friends, and neighbours. Indeed, it was the community that was most important, not the individual. It was important not to die suddenly or alone, without the comfort of one's companions, and without time to collect oneself, ask forgiveness for offences, and commend both one's friends and oneself to God.

Tame death also encompasses an attitude towards the dead themselves and their bodies. Many ancient and primitive peoples have feared proximity to a corpse because they thought of the dead as impure, polluting, or potentially harmful to the living. When that view prevailed, the living might relocate after a death and cemeteries were located outside towns. This does not describe the attitude of tame death as Christianity became the dominant religious belief during the early Middle Ages. In the Christian context of that time, people wanted to be buried near the bodies of martyrs, presumably because they were holy people who could intercede for and protect other human beings. Cemeteries and other grave sites were located near churches, inside their grounds, or even below the floor of the actual church buildings. Bodies were buried on top of each other in large unmarked common graves. Such grave sites were reused periodically; the bones were relocated to open attics (charnels) around the cemeteries and were replaced by new bodies. These bones provided moral lessons for the living, while the cemeteries themselves were centres of social life in which marketing, judicial proceedings, and social gatherings took place.

The twelfth and thirteenth centuries saw a change in these death-related attitudes from tame death to death of the self. This was associated with a shift in emphasis within religious belief from the Second Coming of Christ to the Last Judgement, when the just are to be separated from the damned. If the saints did not include all believers who had died, then one could no longer be assured of one's own salvation. Death was no longer perceived as merely neutral but held the potential for everlasting suffering, and individuals began to feel anxiety about what would happen to them after death and to wonder what they might do to influence that outcome.

This emphasis on personal salvation was associated with a strong sense of self: life, history, and biography became important, not just for themselves, but in terms of what they would mean for the salvation of the soul. The ordeal to be faced was gradually perceived to be the moment of death, a time at which there would be a struggle between a patron saint and the devil for the soul and when judgement would be rendered. This dramatic moment could decide the meaning of an entire life. Facing this moment by 'dying well' became of utmost importance, and the art of dying (*ars moriendi*) developed. This was an elaborate ritual of prayer and action which was to be carried out just before death in order to influence the judgement in which it would culminate.

We need not pursue this shift from tame death to death of the self any further. Significant differences are obvious and they reveal a number of elements which differ in each case. Each pattern fits its own modes of encounters with death, in part shaping and in part being shaped by those encounters. No pattern of death-related attitudes is simply given or inevitable, no matter how unstudied or ingrained it may seem to be. Is this also true of the typical pattern of attitudes toward death in our century?

Forbidden death

In the nineteenth century, the emphasis in attitudes was largely on death of the other, on relationships which were broken by death. There was much stress on lamenting the separation brought about by death and upon reunion with loved ones in the next life. In this romanticized view of death, mourning, not dying, became the central art. Vertical headstones now came to bear epigraphs and sometimes effigies. Death was seen as happiness, a release into the immensity of the beyond. The dead were thought of as disembodied spirits whose separation from the living was intolerable. Harsh realities of death were concealed and new cults of the dead developed, including interest in communicating with the spirits of the dead.

All of this depends upon sharp contrasts between the living and the dead who are seen as 'other'. In the twentieth century, this distancing of self from other has been enhanced. Death is now perceived as socially unacceptable or forbidden. Death is dirty and indecent, an unfair violation of life which should be preventable. It is somehow offensive to die in public. We are now told that dying persons would prefer to be left alone. Who previously would have made that claim and whose interests does it serve?

Attention has now shifted away from those who are dying and towards the feelings and sensibilities of those who are around the dying person. It is their discomfort which takes precedence. This is not a shift to caring for those who are soon to be survivors or for the already bereaved; their association with death is also a source of social discomfort. The shift is towards attitudes which give priority to that which is acceptable to the society as a whole. Death is to be removed or hidden from social view. Dying is displaced from the home to institutions. Bodies are transported almost invisibly and their disposal may not involve much ritual. Funeral activities are strictly limited both in duration and in terms of those who are expected to participate. Mourning is restrained and often almost perfunctory.

The pornography of death

In a short essay which has been widely circulated and reprinted (and which influenced some of Ariès' thinking), Gorer[12,13] suggested that modern societies have developed attitudes which amount to the pornography of death. He drew a contrast between obscenity, which he linked to universal rules of seemliness (that sort of appearance which is pleasing or fitting to the situation), whose violation in fact or in anecdote provokes social laughter, and pornography, which he linked to prudery (particularly in literate societies) and which is enjoyed primarily in private fantasies. For Gorer, 'prudery is defined by subject; some aspect of human experience is treated as inherently shameful or abhorrent, so that it can never be discussed or referred to openly, and experience of it tends to be clandestine and accompanied by feelings of guilt and unworthiness' (ref. 13, p. 194).

In Gorer's view, during much of the nineteenth century copulation and birth were the great unmentionables, while death was a common topic of discussion. This view has been supported by other research, such as that of Stannard concerning the Puritans in New England.[14,15] People encountered death frequently, the cemetery was at the centre of most villages, and the execution of criminals was both a public holiday and a public warning. Children, in particular, were encouraged to think about their own deaths, and the deaths of others were portrayed to children either as edifying or as cautionary examples for moral behaviour.

According to Gorer, in the twentieth century 'death has become more and more "unmentionable" as a natural process' (ref. 13, p. 195). We are now commonly told that the natural processes of corruption and decay are disgusting, and that preoccupation with such processes is morbid and unhealthy. Encounters with death in modern society have diminished, even as 'violent death increased in a manner unparalleled in human history' (ref. 13, p. 197). Thus our century has witnessed an unparalleled degree of human-induced death in wars and concentration camps,[16] a new set of encounters with death by way of automobile accidents, and a significant rise in the role that violent death plays in the fantasies offered to mass audiences. In this last form, the newly arisen pornography of death appears to be a substitute gratification for increased distancing from death as a natural reality.

The language of death

Prominent illustrations of ways in which death is forbidden in much of modern society include the language of ordinary social discourse, professional speech, and communications about dying. It is important to pay attention to these linguistic practices because naming helps to define and to determine reality. How we speak says a good deal about who we are and the attitudes that we hold.

In ordinary conversation, modern society teaches us to go to great lengths to avoid saying the words 'dead' or 'dying' when discussing the realities to which those words refer. Instead, we employ euphemisms or ways of speaking that seem to many to be more pleasing or less distasteful. In the past, many euphemisms originated in a rich soil of experiential contact with death. Thus Homer spoke of those who 'bit the dust', the Bible spoke of 'giving up the ghost' and 'going the way of all flesh', and Shakespeare spoke of 'shuffling off this mortal coil'. However, when contacts with natural human death are more attenuated, language tends to objectify and trivialize death-related events. The result both discloses and contributes to a kind of distancing from important and fundamental events of life itself.

In modern society, euphemisms tend to shy away from honest and straightforward speech by covering death with a linguistic shroud. People do not die; they 'pass away'. Euphemisms of all sorts need not be condemned. Their weakness is in the unspoken assumption that direct speech cannot be sensitive and caring. Their danger arises when they tend to supplant direct speech entirely and when they themselves are emptied of content and become unfeeling clichés.

Professional speech is euphemistic when it tells us that 'we lost Mrs Jones last night' or that she 'expired'. Surely, she has not simply vanished or gone missing. Perhaps the suggestion is that caregivers accustomed to think in metaphors of the conflict against illness ('the fight against cancer') see death as loss or failure in battle? Similarly, in an etymological sense 'to expire' is for the spirit or last breath to go out of the person. However, it is not likely that those who use this language today are drawing upon this sort of historical linguistic meaning. More typically, they are simply unwilling to speak directly. Once entered upon this path, one easily ends up in bureaucratic hyperbole which redefines death as 'negative patient care outcome'.

Consider the state to which we have come in trying to express in ordinary language what veterinary surgeons do to very sick, old, or infirm cats and dogs. They 'put them to sleep', 'put them out of their misery', or 'put them down'. Can one describe these actions in some other non-euphemistic and non-metaphorical language that would be both recognizable and effective? Would we say that such animals are simply 'killed' or 'euthanized', which is, of course, true? What is an enquiring child to make of these events and their descriptions when he is told that his pet was put to sleep and then is admonished to go away now, lie down, and take a nap?

Note that the evident unwillingness of many to employ death-related language only applies when death and dying are being directly discussed in their own right. When the subject of discussion concerns events that do not have to do with the realities of death and dying, most people are quite willing to use death-related language.[1] One would be 'dead wrong' to imagine that death-related language has simply been banished from most ordinary speech. Rather, death language is commonly used to convey intensity or absoluteness in matters that do not relate to death, as when one is 'dead certain' or 'dying to meet someone'.

When Glaser and Strauss[17] studied patterns of communication with the dying, they found four basic types of what they called 'awareness contexts' or social interactions between those who are dying and those around the dying.

1. 'Closed awareness' means that the person who is dying does not know or suspect that fact, and for various reasons medical staff, perhaps acting in concert with family members, who do know the truth do not convey it.

2. 'Suspected awareness' arises when the person who is ill has begun to suspect (for a variety of possible reasons) that more is going on than is being said.

3. 'Mutual pretence' represents a kind of shared drama in which everyone realizes the truth but acts out roles that are intended to suggest that things are not as they know them to be. Without explicit acknowledgement, the social pretence may even be conducted so as to cover over embarrassing moments when the strategy of dissembling temporarily fails or risks revealing the true situation.

4. 'Open awareness' is distinguished by the fact that everyone involved knows the condition of the person who is ill, and everyone is willing to talk about it.

This description of awareness contexts should not be misconstrued as an outline of a linear process; rather, it sets forth a typology of different patterns of interaction which represent alternative possibilities which may change, as human relationships always do. The important point about these awareness contexts is what they reveal about options for communication within the small groups that are engaged in coping with dying.

Many people consider it desirable not to convey to the dying person full and accurate information about his or her diagnosis and prognosis. Some professional caregivers have also argued that such information should not be given to family members of the dying person. In defence of this strategy, it has been argued that candour could undercut the will of dying persons to live or even encourage them to end their own lives. When Oken[18] conducted a survey about communicating accurate information to patients with a terminal illness, physicians indicated a strong preference for not providing this information to patients, a desire to be given accurate information if they themselves were such patients, and an unwillingness to provide such information even to patients who were also physicians. In a later study,[19] exactly the opposite results were reported. Have attitudes of American physicians towards telling dying patients the truth changed so dramatically in a brief period of time? If so, is that change based upon a reliable scientific or clinical foundation, or does it represent the influence of changing societal attitudes and other factors not directly related to optimal care for dying persons?

An unwillingness to be candid, particularly with dying persons, can be found among professional caregivers and lay persons in many parts of the contemporary world.[20] Why are such attitudes so widespread? On the basis of very little objective empirical support, it has been claimed that providing such information can be detrimental to the dying person. Thus 'clinical experience' was cited by nearly all the respondents (those with many years of practice, as well as those who were newly qualified) in both of the research studies cited above, despite their opposing results.

In fact, there is no reliable evidence that honest communication has detrimental effects, at least not when that communication is responsive to the needs of the dying person and is carried out in a thoughtful and caring way. In fact, the content of the communication may not be as important as the ways in which it is expressed and understood. One can brutalize a vulnerable person with the truth, just as one can harm with falsity.

It also seems evident that untrue, misleading, or incomplete communications can have detrimental effects. One might argue, for example, that most dying persons have some awareness of their own situation, and this seems to have been confirmed in the literature.[21] Most of us are aware when unusual things are happening within our own bodies, although we may not understand precisely what is going on and may not be able to describe it in technical language. Patients in modern societies also obtain information about their conditions from a variety of sources. If this is the case, will not such 'middle knowledge'[22] result in undermining trust in the patient–caregiver relationship when it is not addressed by reliable communication?

Waechter[23] demonstrated that children who were terminally ill exhibited far more anxiety than children who were healthy and children who had an acute or a chronic illness, even though the terminally ill children had not been told the truth about their diagnoses. If this is the case, do not such children and other dying persons have a broad general right to access to information about their own condition that may be in the possession of professionals who are providing care for them? How else can such persons cope effectively with their fears and anxieties, or determine how to live out the balance of their lives?

All interpersonal contexts of awareness and communication bring with them potential benefits and hazards; the point is to determine which serve the best interests of those involved. Barring certain situations involving mental illness or a clearly established (not merely imputed) danger of direct harm, the role of such communications should be to serve the interests of dying persons as they themselves perceive them.

Those who share a context of open awareness may or may not actually spend much time discussing the fact that the person is dying. As has aptly been said, no one is dying 24 hours a day. The ability to discuss the facts honestly and fully often frees dying persons to set that issue aside and to concentrate upon making the best use of the time that is available for living. Others should not try to dictate the course of that living. Instead, they should foster responsible autonomy which permits dying persons to live their own lives, 'sing their own songs', and die their own deaths.[24]

Societal death systems

Many of the central elements in this discussion can be drawn together in the concept of a societal death system.[25] Kastenbaum defined a death system as the 'sociophysical network by which we mediate and express our relationship to mortality' (ref. 25, p. 310). By this, he meant that every society works out, more or less formally and explicitly, a system which it interposes between death and its citizens. Systems of this sort intervene to help a society and its citizens deal with death and its implications, and to interpret death to the members of the society in socially approved ways.

Any societal death system includes the following elements.

1. People—individuals who can be defined by their more or less permanent or stable roles in the death system, such as physicians and nurses, funeral directors, florists, life insurance agents, and lawyers.
2. Places—specific locations which have assumed or taken on a death-related character, such as cemeteries, funeral homes, health care institutions, and the 'hallowed ground' of a battlefield or death-related disaster.
3. Times—occasions which are associated in some special way with death, such as Memorial Day in the United States (originally Armistice Day, but now a remembrance of all those members of the military who have died in the service of their country), the Day of the Dead in Mexico, Good Friday in the Christian world, or the anniversary of a death.
4. Objects—things whose character is somehow linked to death, such as death certificates, hearses, obituaries and death notices in the newspaper, weapons, tombstones, a gallows, a guillotine, or an electric chair.
5. Symbols—things which have come to signify or represent death, such as a flag at half mast or a black armband signifying bereavement, a pirate's skull and crossbones flag, warning symbols on containers of poison, certain solemn organ music, and selected words or phrases.

The following are functions of a death system.

1. To give warnings and predictions, as in the role of civil defence sirens or forecasts of violent storms.
2. To prevent death, as in the efforts of emergency medical care and resuscitation procedures.
3. To care for the dying, as in the work of modern hospice or palliative care programmes.
4. To dispose of the dead, as in the activities of funeral directors and those who work at crematoria or cemeteries, or procedures for burial at sea.
5. To work toward social consolidation after death, as in the aims of funeral ritual or self-help groups for the bereaved.
6. To help make sense of death, as in the examples provided by many religious or philosophical systems.
7. To bring about socially sanctioned killing, as in some aspects of police work, training for war, procedures for capital punishment, or the killing of some animals and other living things to provide food for humans.

Aspects of societal death systems in selected countries

A death system will be found in some form in every society; it may be formal, explicit, and widely acknowledged in some of its aspects, or largely hidden and often unspoken in other aspects. This can be illustrated by considering how one very specific cause of death is regarded in different settings, and by considering some of the larger similarities and differences between death-related experiences that have been described above as typical of Western Europe and North America and those in Colombia, Eastern Europe, China, India, and Japan.

The phenomenon of sudden infant death syndrome has attracted varying attention and responses in different societies during recent years. In Western Europe, North America, and many other modern developed societies, it is of significant social concern as the leading cause of death for infants between the ages of 1 month and 1 year.[26] As the cause of one to two deaths per 1000 live births in many of these societies, sudden infant death syndrome has been recognized as an approved diagnostic category by the World Health Organization, but its diagnosis depends upon a sophisticated post-mortem examination, investigation of the death scene, and review of the case history.[27]

In contrast, societies with high infant mortality rates and low average life expectancy may have to deal with far more basic problems in health care and living conditions. Reversible conditions, such as malnutrition and diarrhoea, and communicable diseases are likely to be leading causes of death in these societies. Lack of sanitary facilities and unsafe water sources contribute to illness and death. With a high rate of infant mortality in general, such societies rarely possess the investigational and record-keeping systems that would permit them to identify and undertake research on sudden infant death syndrome. Relatively sudden and unexpected deaths in early childhood will be familiar to such societies, and the allocation of major resources to a phenomenon such as sudden infant death syndrome may not be possible or desirable in such societal contexts.

Therefore the dominant patterns of encounters with death which have been described in this chapter for Western Europe and North America are not typical of all contemporary societies. In many undeveloped or developing societies around the world, and in some subgroups within developed societies, encounters with death take on a quite different form.

In Colombia, for example, and in many other societies in Central and South America, a strong familial and societal network of support is provided to the dying and their relatives.[28, 29] Extended families, which provide company for the dying and the bereaved, are common in such societies. Thus isolation and loneliness in dying are neither as common nor as feared as they are in supposedly more developed and more sophisticated societies.

However, societies with strong family networks may also struggle with poverty, inadequate living conditions, and professional authoritarianism. Management of distressing symptoms may not always be practicable or well understood, decision-making may be the sole province of the physician, open communication may not be practised, and there may be wide discrepancies between the health care that is available to a wealthy few and that available to a much larger, but less advantaged, segment of the population. Inpatient facilities may be inadequate and home care may be ineffective or non-existent. In the case of Colombia, in particular, there are special problems arising from an underground economy of drug processing and distribution, and the presence of well-organized guerrilla armed forces; more deaths arise from homicide and violence than from cancer.

Despite the very great differences between the death systems in Eastern Europe and in China, there are some interesting similarities. For example, during the 1980s Poland witnessed the rise of a diverse and vital hospice movement,[30] which has no parallel as yet in China. Nevertheless, in Poland, as in other East European countries and China, death remains a taboo subject in many ways. Candour is not well understood or widely practised as a value in communications with those who are coping with dying.[20] In China, for example, this may lead to an unwillingness to discuss their illness with children who have potentially fatal conditions, an unspoken message to ill children that parental frustrations and irritations are the responsibility of the children, and even decisions by parents not to attend funeral services for their children or not to mark their children's graves.[31] Resources for the management of distressing symptoms associated with terminal illness may be limited in both Eastern Europe and China, although in the latter society non-Western forms of traditional care may compensate in part.

In India, the most notable feature of a very large and diverse society is the extensive discussion of death in a variety of scriptural writings (the Vedas, the Upanishads, and the Gita) and in diverse religious viewpoints. Particularly prominent in the Indian subcontinent are accounts of the life of the soul after death and issues related to reincarnation,[32,33] associated with lengthy discussions as to how one should understand and cope with suffering.[34] However, as one knowledgeable commentator has written, ' "scientific" enquiry into issues related to death and dying is only just beginning in India, and is limited to a handful of us who work with patients suffering from an incurable illness'.[35] In other words, a detailed analysis of the Indian death system of the kind presented earlier for other societies is yet to be performed.

In contrast, there are many ways in which the situation in Japan is similar to that prevalent in Western Europe and North America a few years ago. For example, in Japan it is common to avoid using the number 4 for room and floor numbers, much as Americans do not use the number 13, because the Japanese word for 'four' is similar in pronunciation to the word for 'death'.[36] Also, most Japanese physicians do not tell patients the truth about their illnesses (although that information may be communicated to the families), emotional isolation often develops around dying persons, last thoughts may go unexpressed, and there may be a legacy of guilt, sadness, and regret for bereaved survivors.

Leading causes of death in Japan are similar to those in other developed countries, but other factors have hindered a humanitarian approach to patient-centred care of the dying. These include an influential medical ethics textbook which warns against the dangers of suicide when patients are told of an incurable disease, cultural associations between cancer, pain, and death, negative images and taboos surrounding death, lack of confidence on the part of physicians in their ability to reveal bad news and effectively support patients afterwards, little respect for the self-reliance of individual patients, and the lack of both modern death education and an established system of terminal care.[37] Modern terminal care in Japan dates from a palliative care team that was founded in Osaka in 1973, but the Japanese government did not approve a distinct medical insurance benefit for four programmes of terminal care until April 1990.[38]

Death systems in modern societies

In many of the modern societies in Western Europe and North America, the death system seems to function in numerous powerful ways to keep death at a distance from the mainstream of life and to gloss over many of its harsher aspects. This may also be true, although perhaps in quite different ways, in societies such as those of Colombia, Eastern Europe, China, India, and Japan. In yet other societies, the death system may work in some ways to make death a prominent social reality around which major cultural events and a large part of private living are organized. The important point is that no society is without some system for coping with the fundamental realities that death, dying, and bereavement present to human existence. In contrast, one interesting aspect of every society is its views on death, the nature of its death system, and the ways in which that system functions.[39,40]

Some commentators[41] have concluded that many modern societies in Western Europe and North America (particularly the United States) are best described as 'death denying'. This appears to imply that death has largely been exiled from such societies as a social or public presence. This conclusion has been challenged by Dumont and Foss,[42] who have asked whether the broad societal view of death in the United States need be one of either acceptance or denial; rather, it could include elements of both postures simultaneously.

Kastenbaum's notion of a societal death system,[25] together with most of what we know about the complexity of individual encounters and attitudes that relate to death, seems to fit best with a multidimensional account of death-related experiences and death systems in modern societies. Despite common themes, it seems likely that the nature of that account will be different for each modern society as the societies differ in their own ways from each other.

Conclusion

Two central points emerge from this discussion. The first is suggested by a statement from Craven and Wald (ref. 43, p. 1816): 'What people need most when they are dying is relief from distressing symptoms of disease, the security of a caring environment, sustained expert care, and assurance that they and their families will not be abandoned.' Adequate responses to such needs are primarily dependent, not upon certain sorts of facilities or a particular system of care, but upon the development of a comprehensive philosophy of hospice or palliative care.[44] Such a philosophy transcends buildings or programmes. It reflects the efforts of societies to develop within their death systems new modes of caring communities which can then be applied not only to elderly cancer patients, but also to other contexts such as situations involving children.[45-47]

Second, Kashiwagi[48] has written the following:

> Regardless of the differences in the concept of death, socio-economic and religious backgrounds, and medical and nursing situations, a common hope of people all over the world is to die peacefully. . . . Therefore the need for palliative care services in every part of the world is a consideration that reaches beyond the boundaries of country and nationality.

This means that our discussion of death in modern society is not confined to a particular community or geographical area. Nevertheless, the actual implications of dying, death, and bereavement must be lived out and coped with in the concrete circumstances of societal conditions and individual situations. Therefore sensitivity to the character of death-related experiences in any particular circumstances is essential to providing effective care and maximizing quality in living.

References

1. Corr CA, Nabe CM, Corr DM. *Death and Dying, Life and Living*. 2nd edn. Pacific Grove, CA: Brooks Cole, 1997.
2. Goldscheider C. *Population, Modernization, and Social Structure*. Boston, MA: Little, Brown, 1971.
3. United States Bureau of the Census. *Historical Statistics of the United States, Colonial Ttimes to 1970, Bicentennial Edition* (2 parts). Washington, DC: US Government Printing Office, 1975.
4. Singh GK, Mathews TJ, Yannicos T, Smith BL. Annual summary of births, marriages, divorces, and deaths: United States, 1994. *Monthly Vital Statistics Report*, 1995; **43**. Hyattsville, MD: National Center for Health Statistics.
5. McCord C, Freeman HP. Excess mortality in Harlem. *New England Journal of Medicine*, 1990; **322**:173–7.
6. Fulton, R. *Death and Identity*. Revised edn. Bowie, MD: Charles Press, 1976.
7. Glaser B, Strauss A. *Time for Dying*. Chicago, IL: Aldine, 1968.
8. Pattison EM. *The Experience of Dying*. Englewood Cliffs, NJ: Prentice-Hall, 1977.
9. Pattison EM. The living–dying process. In: Garfield CA, ed. *Psychosocial Care of the Dying Patient*. New York: McGraw-Hill, 1978: 133–68.
10. Ariès P. *Western Attitudes Toward Death: From the Middle Ages to the Present*. Transl. P. Ranum. Baltimore, MD: Johns Hopkins University Press, 1974.
11. Ariès P. *The Hour of Our Death*. Transl. H. Weaver. New York: Knopf, 1981.
12. Gorer G. The pornography of death. In: G. Gorer, ed. *Death, Grief, and Mourning*. Garden City, NY: Doubleday, 1965: 192–9.
13. Gorer G. The pornography of death. *Encounter*, 1955; **5**:49–52.
14. Stannard DE. Death and the Puritan child. In: DE Stannard, ed. *Death in America*. Philadelphia, PA: University of Pennsylvania Press, 1974: 9–29.
15. Stannard DE. *The Puritan Way of Death:A Study in Religion, Culture, and Social Change*. New York: Oxford University Press, 1977.
16. Elliot G. *The Twentieth Century Book of the Dead*. New York: Random House, 1972.
17. Glaser B, Strauss A. *Awareness of Dying*. Chicago: Aldine, 1965.
18. Oken D. What to tell cancer patients: a study of medical attitudes. *Journal of the American Medical Association*, 1961; **175**:1120–8.
19. Novack DH, Plumer R, Smith RL, Ochitill H, Morrow GR, Bennett JM. Changes in physicians' attitudes toward telling the cancer patient. *Journal of the American Medical Association*, 1979; **241**:897–900.
20. Corr CA. Some impressions from a hospice-related visit to Poland. *Journal of Palliative Care*, 1991; **7**(1):53–7.
21. Hinton J. The physical and mental distress of the dying. *Quarterly Journal of Medicine*, 1963; **32**:1–21.
22. Weisman AD. *On Dying and Denying: A Psychiatric Study of Terminality*. New York: Behavioral Publications, 1972.
23. Waechter EH. Children's awareness of fatal illness. *American Journal of Nursing*, 1971; **71**:1168–72.
24. Brady EM. Telling the story: ethics and dying. *Hospital Progress*, 1979; **60**:57–62.

25. Kastenbaum R. On the future of death: some images and options. *Omega, Journal of Death and Dying*, 1972; **3**:306–18.
26. Corr CA, Fuller H, Barnickol CA, Corr DM, eds. *Sudden Infant Death Syndrome: Who Can Help and How*. New York: Springer, 1991.
27. Jones AM, Weston JT. The examination of the sudden infant death syndrome infant: investigative and autopsy protocols. *Journal of Forensic Sciences*, 1976; **21**:833–41.
28. de Jaramillo I. Some notes on death and dying in Colombia, South America. Paper presented to the Meeting of the International Work Group on Death, Dying, and Bereavement, Asilomar, CA, 2 January 1989.
29. de Jaramillo I. Personal communication, 30 January 1991.
30. Sikorska E. The hospice movement in Poland. *Death Studies*, 1991; **15**:309–16.
31. Lee PWH, Lieh-Mak F, Hung BKM, Luk SL. Death anxiety in leukemic Chinese children. *International Journal of Psychiatry in Medicine*, 1984; **13**:281–9.
32. Abhedananda S. *Life Beyond Death: A Critical Study of Spiritualism*,7th edn. Calcutta: Ramakrishna Vedanta Math, 1984.
33. Sivananda S. *What Becomes of the Soul After Death*, 11th edn. Shivanandanagar, India: Divine Life Trust Society, 1989.
34. Central Chinmaya Mission Trust. *Beyond Sorrow*. Bombay: Central Chinmaya Mission Trust, 1988.
35. Chakravorty SG. Personal communication, 16 March 1991.
36. Saito T. Dealing with attitudes about death and aging in Japan. *Japan Christian Quarterly*, 1986; **52**:225–8.
37. Okayasu M. Presenting a diagnosis of cancer to patients in Japan. *Nihon University Journal of Medicine*, 1988; **30**:259–67.
38. Kashiwagi T. Hospice care in Japan. *Postgraduate Medical Journal*, 1991; **67**(Supplement 2):S95–9.
39. Berger A, Badham P, Kutscher AH, Berger J, Perry J, Beloff J., eds. *Perspectives on Death and Dying: Cross-cultural and Multi-disciplinary Views*. Philadelphia, PA: Charles Press, 1989.
40. Irish DP, Lundquist KF, Nelson VJ, eds. *Ethnic Variations in Dying, Death, and Grief: Diversity in Universality*. Washington, DC: Taylor and Francis, 1993.
41. Kübler-Ross E. *On Death and Dying*. New York: Macmillan, 1969.
42. Dumont R, Foss D. *The American View of Death: Acceptance or Denial?* Cambridge, MA: Schenkman, 1972.
43. Craven J, Wald FS. Hospice care for dying patients. *American Journal of Nursing*, 1975; **75**:1816–22.
44. Corr CA, Corr DM, eds. *Hospice Care: Principles and Practice*. New York: Springer, 1983.
45. Corr, CA, Corr DM, eds. *Hospice Approaches to Pediatric Care*. New York: Springer, 1985.
46. Corr CA, Corr DM. Situations involving children: a challenge for the hospice movement. *Hospice Journal*, 1985; **1**:63–77.
47. Corr CA, Corr DM. Pediatric hospice care. *Pediatrics*, 1985; **76**:774–80.
48. Kashiwagi T. Palliative care in Japan. *Palliative Medicine*, 1991; **5**:165–71.

2.4 The provision of palliative care

Derek Doyle

The history of palliative care

It is tempting to think of palliative care as something new, one of the many medical innovations of the second half of the twentieth century, when in fact it is as old as medicine itself. Long before doctors ever realistically dreamed of being able to cure any patient, they saw their task as the relief of suffering. Much of the professional lives of doctors before the middle of the twentieth century was spent in easing pain with opium preparations, the lowering of temperature with tepid sponging and various potions, the bringing of comfort to those dyspnoeic with dropsy or chest infections, and allaying the fears and loneliness of the dying by sitting at their bedside. This was palliative care but no one glorified it with such a descriptive name. In those days, medical practice and palliative care were synonymous. This simple, unsophisticated relief of suffering was all that was possible, a noble objective, and certainly not one to be despised.

On to the scene came modern surgery, largely made possible by developments in anaesthesia and the ability to control infection with newly-discovered antibiotics. There followed radiotherapy, anticancer chemotherapy, the new sciences of immunology, endocrinology, radiology, isotope and computer scanning, organ replacement and transplantation surgery—and, as a result, a real possibility of cure for some and life prolongation or long-term disease remission for most others. Almost imperceptibly the goal of medicine shifted from symptom relief to cure and with it came the unintentional downgrading of the former. Soon, and ever increasingly, one came to hear what sounded like a sinister sentence. . . . 'We can only palliate . . .', made to sound, as in fact it was obviously felt, like a nihilistic admission of failure expressed as bitter disappointment. The implication was clear. The primary aim was always to cure and anything less—'just palliative care'—was seen not as a continuing responsibility of the modern doctor but as something which could be left to nurses and the less scientifically-minded members of the medical profession whose ambitions were perhaps more modest.

Definitions and descriptions

Cynical as this brief historical description may sound, it serves to remind us of certain indisputable facts which must be recognized and understood if we are to look at the provision of modern palliative care. The relief of suffering when cure is impossible ('palliation') has always been at the heart of all good medical practice, even before it was called palliative care. It was, and surely still is, what every patient hopes for—and has a right to expect—whatever his condition. It has never been, nor should ever be, regarded as a luxury, an optional extra available to the privileged few. Not only does every person have a right to expect it—every health-care professional has a responsibility to provide it—wherever he or she is, whatever their discipline or specialty. To few of us is given the chance to cure but to all is given the challenge and the chance to relieve the suffering of our fellow men and women. This is palliative care or, as the National Council for Hospice and Specialist Palliative Care Services describes it, 'employing the palliative approach'.

To the question, 'Who should provide palliative care?', the answer must be every doctor and nurse. To the question, 'Where should they provide palliative care?', the answer must be where they work day-in, day-out. If some are able to cure a few patients as part of their surgical, medical, oncological, or family practice, all credit to them but the ambition to cure must never obscure the imperative to care through the relief of suffering. The development of palliative care as a new medical and nursing specialty in the last two decades of the twentieth century is not, as some would suggest, evidence of a newly-created subject but rather a renewed emphasis on the hallowed principles and precepts of traditional medicine, principles which are increasingly being rediscovered and put into practice in many branches of medicine.

It is worth remembering that many valuable procedures carried out by surgeons are palliative—the formation of ostomies, the insertion of biliary, ureteric, oesophageal, and tracheal stents. None will lead to cure but each will materially alleviate symptoms, hence they can rightly be described as palliative procedures. The physician who drains a pleural effusion or performs a paracentesis abdominis is employing palliative procedures as surely as the anaesthetist who inserts a spinal cannula for opioids, the neurosurgeon who operates to relieve spinal cord compression or sets out to debulk a cerebral tumour, or the radiation oncologist who irradiates to ease bone pain. The general practitioner who employs his psychotherapeutic skills or his ability to bring together a dysfunctional grieving family is employing palliative techniques though he, like the surgeon and the physician, is not likely to define them as such.

We see, therefore, that in this chapter we have already used two different terms—'palliative care' meaning a philosophy of care, an approach, and 'palliative techniques and procedures' used as part of the therapeutic armamentarium of many specialists who are not, nor would they wish to be called, palliative medicine specialists.

This textbook, and this chapter in particular, recognizes that every doctor wants to care better and offers guidelines to assist them in doing so as part of their everyday work. What follows in this chapter is a description of the provision of specialist palliative care, that new discipline defined and developed in the past two decades primarily to ensure: that all who need it can be guaranteed that their care will be as appropriate, skilled, and comprehensive in the later stage of a mortal illness as it was when it was first diagnosed; that such care can be made available to them whether they are at home or in a hospital; that all who care for them—professional carers, relatives, and friends—will themselves be supported and their particular needs addressed. This is a tall order, made more difficult by the fact that medical care and resources differ in so many respects, not only from country to country but even from town to town.

Definitions of palliative care have been given in Section 1. They are important not least because they do not confine the need for the provision of palliative care to any one pathology, most emphatically not to any social, religious, or ethnic group, nor to the medically affluent, advanced West.

Two particular features of the definitions need to be highlighted. The first is the reference to . . . 'a limited prognosis. . .'. No time limit is set or intended (though certain health-care funding bodies have themselves set arbitrary limits). The implication is that such care is primarily for those with a terminal illness. Inevitably this has caused confusion and much heated debate. Including such a clause in the universally-accepted definition does not deny the imperative to provide palliative care when one cannot cure in all manner of chronic, disabling conditions from which patients may suffer for years and years before they could ever be described as 'terminal'. It does not deny the obligation of all doctors and nurses to ease suffering whenever, wherever, they encounter it—that is, to provide palliative care—nor does it seek to diminish the importance of the palliative procedures and techniques just described. It does, however, unequivocally describe and define specialist palliative care as that required for, and essential to provide for, the terminally ill.

The second feature to be recognized and honoured in the definitions is the focus of all such specialist palliative care on the quality of life. This indisputably makes such care patient-centred rather than pathology-centred; affirms patient autonomy and emphasizes that the patient is, in effect, a partner in decision making; emphasizes that the aim of all such care is neither prolongation nor abbreviation of life but quality of life as defined by the patient rather than by the professional carers.

It has often been asked, and indeed continues to be asked in many countries, why there needs to be a specialty if palliation is the responsibility of all professional carers.

The country which first recognized it as a medical specialty (and indeed a nursing specialty) was the United Kingdom. By this was meant not that some doctors had chosen to work exclusively in this area and made it a career choice, but that the official, professional bodies who define and approve training programmes leading to professional accreditation deem the subject worthy of being regarded as a specialty. Before such recognition was granted, proof had to be furnished that there was a substantial body of knowledge built up on the subject, that other specialties were expressing a need for professional guidance and advice from the practitioners of the subject, that research was taking place, the results of which were to be found in peer-reviewed scientific journals, that there was a professional association representing its practitioners, that there was a significant number of doctors wanting to make it their exclusive work and, finally, that there was a substantial bibliography building up on the subject. Such criteria may appear to some as obvious and reasonable as the need for specialist recognition, but many have been offended by the emergence of a specialty many of whose principles and therapeutic regimens are already known to and commonly practised by doctors. There are, however, analogies in other areas of medicine. Though many doctors care for patients with cardiac conditions, they do not question the need for cardiologists to advise on the most difficult cases, nor the need for cardiac intensive care units for a significant minority of patients whose needs call for high levels of medical and nursing expertise. The same could be said for respiratory medicine, communicable diseases such as AIDS, and many more. Whether we approve of it or not in Western medicine, we live in an age of specialization—specialization which recognizes and generates a new body of knowledge and expertise, without in any way denying or diminishing the skills to be found in other medical disciplines caring for the same groups of patients. Indeed, it should be hoped that creating such a body of knowledge, expertise, and experience will actually enhance the skills of those working in other disciplines, particularly if all its specialists acknowledge their responsibility to share their knowledge and skills through education and training.

We can take the United Kingdom as an example and ask why specialization was needed there. Why should a few hundred doctors and a few thousand nurses undertake years of further study and training? Why should special units and services be developed, staffed by these experts, for a relatively small but significant number of needy patients? Why should such an august body as the Royal College of Physicians encourage it? Why does the government encourage it and include it in strategic health-care planning?

Deficiencies in care

Many studies revealed that, no matter how good was the care of other patients, those in the terminal phase were suffering unnecessary pain and other symptoms even when the necessary drugs were readily available to them.[1] The situation was the same in patients' homes, in general hospitals, and in cancer centres. Toscani[2] and Terzoli[3] studied the quality of care in hospitals, oncology centres, and homes in Italy and noted the same gross inadequacies. A study of care in Sicily, comparing 1988 and 1990, found fewer patients being visited at home and only 19 per cent of doctors prescribing essential opioids.[4–6] Major studies in the United States revealed high levels of pain in cancer patients, inadequate analgesia, poor understanding of opioids, and a need for much better education and training.[7–9] Walsh,[10] reviewing continuing care in a major United States medical centre, asserts that any centre claiming to care from diagnosis to death, as most oncology units do, should have a palliative care service; something also described by Magno[11] and supported by an overview of the challenges faced in providing oncology care in rural North America.[12–14] A United Kingdom recommendation now states that each regional oncology centre should have specialist palliative care input.[15]

Many reports confirm that the elderly patient is disadvantaged. Cartwright,[16] looking at the role of the family doctor in caring for people in their last year of life, confirmed that there were fewer home visits not only for the elderly but particularly for those with an illness other than cancer, even though the elderly have more needs than the younger patients. Another United Kingdom study of family doctor care of patients discharged from hospital found 'apathy, neglect. . .'.[17] Not only is there a dearth of information on pain and in particular opioid therapy in the elderly, sometimes old people are excluded from research trials and studies.

There is certainly inequality in care provision. Higginson[18] confirmed that the percentage who die at home is proportional to socio-economic status, 5 per cent of the underprivileged and 46 per cent of the more privileged, but these figures must be taken alongside Hinton's.[19,20] He found that the declared preference for home care fell from 100 per cent to 54 per cent for these terminally ill patients and 45 per cent for relatives as the mortal illness advanced, and most relatives eventually approved of where the patient had been treated and died. The longer care continued the more likely that hospital admission would be needed and, perhaps not surprisingly, the reasons for admission to a palliative care unit so far as relatives were concerned were their fatigue, anxiety, and depression.

One of the most comprehensive studies of what patients and carers suffer and the care they receive remains that by Cartwright (1973)[21] but her subsequent study in 1991[22,23] still reported inadequate pain control. This was confirmed a year later by Sykes[24] who found 65 per cent of carers citing inadequate control of suffering, 58 per cent not being told of benefits available to them, and more than 50 per cent offered no bereavement support. A sensitive study of general practitioner care in a semirural area found that, '. . . expert advice would have helped'.[25] No matter how many differences in care in different settings are described, overall 'consumer' satisfaction appears to be highest with home palliative care.[26]

As is graphically described in Section 22, the situation is often even worse in many countries where such essential drugs as opioids are not available for one reason or another. There, too, the problems are compounded by a lack of personnel trained in the basics of palliative care.

Deficiencies in experience and expertise

As more and more people are taken into hospital when terminally ill—a pattern seen not only in the United Kingdom but wherever medical care becomes more sophisticated—so inevitably the necessary experience and expertise of the general practitioner/family doctor diminish in this area of medicine. This is not a reflection of palliative medicine becoming a specialty but of a changing social pattern. This is not a value judgement. It is widely attested to by the doctors and nurses themselves,[27,28]—some trainee family doctors allegedly never seeing a terminally ill patient in their trainee year working in the community.[29]

One study of a two-man partnership responsible for 3800 patients had 31 deaths in the year but only six occurred at home.[30] This would suggest that the average family doctor will encounter remarkably few terminally ill patients who tax all his skills of palliation, in any one year, even though that doctor and his colleagues will care for many such patients.

In another review of 85 dying patients cared for by a group of five doctors, 50 deaths were expected (25 from malignant and 25 from non-malignant disease). In eight cases the doctors themselves were dissatisfied with communications and what they regarded as poor pain and symptom control.[28] This makes it all the more surprising to learn of apparent reluctance of younger doctors to refer patients to a palliative care service.

A Scottish study[31] of 80 family doctors and 84 consultants found that 76 per cent and 69 per cent respectively felt they needed further training in pain control, 55 per cent and 52 per cent on symptom control, and similar percentages wanted further training in communication skills. More than 50 per cent felt it would be worthwhile spending 4 weeks in a specialist palliative care unit to develop their skills. These figures are very similar to those from a study of 300 registered nurses questioned about their sense of competence and confidence in nursing the dying.[32] Many studies confirm that family doctors appreciate specialist help with pain control and emotional support. A Canadian study found only two-thirds feeling comfortable, competent, and in control and, interestingly, the same proportion happy with the quick response, support, and communications of a palliative care team.[33] A Spanish study noted that general practitioners were highly motivated but the motivation exceeded competence.[34]

Public dissatisfaction

Reluctant as many patients may be to report deficiencies in care, there has been an increasing number of reports of relatives' dissatisfaction with care received by the patient or themselves.

Many had felt that patients at home were not visited frequently enough and often rated the quality of domiciliary care in terms of the doctor's visiting pattern rather than his skills in symptom relief.[35] In particular, the elderly and those with non-malignant conditions appeared to be disadvantaged.[16,17,23,36,37] Another study reported 6 per cent of those at home and 19 per cent in hospital even before the terminal phase, having severe unrelieved pain. Forty per cent of patients at home had pain severe enough to justify transfer to hospital but even there 20 per cent were left in unrelieved pain.[38] Yet another study of carers' views reported 65 per cent of patients having inadequate symptom control, whilst another study from Sheffield, United Kingdom, found 34 per cent critical of general practitioner care.[24]

Not all reports related to pain and other symptoms.[39,40] Many complained that nurses were called in too late[41] and family support was felt to be inadequate,[42] yet in one study only 26 per cent of general practitioners felt that family care (as distinct from patient care) was a very important part of their work, another 25 per cent actually declaring that it was relatively unimportant.[23]

Nurses' frustration

We have seen how nurses also feel less than adequately trained to provide good palliative care but they are also very critical of their medical colleagues, particularly in domiciliary care from where most of the studies have emanated.[43,44] They call for a less controlling role for general practitioners/family doctors, better and earlier invitations to become involved in care (citing instances where 20 per cent of patients were faecally incontinent yet no nurse had been called in), and proposing self-help teaching of patients. They are particularly conscious of the strains imposed on relatives, noting that in 74 per cent of cases it was the emotional strain on them and avoidable suffering of the patients which led to admission into hospital.[12,23,45] The situation may not be improving. A comparative study of 1969 and 1987 found the problem of late referrals to nurses in the community worsening rather than improving. Another study found 33 per cent of community nurses unclear who had overall responsibility and 28 per cent feeling they were underrated.[46]

Inadequate professional training

This has been alluded to above but recognition of the deficiencies led not to more medical school and nursing college faculty addressing the problem but greater reliance on palliative care workers (and units where they were based) taking on the responsibility for teaching and training. Today, every British medical school includes aspects of palliative medicine in its curriculum but in almost all the principal teachers are local consultants/specialists from specialist palliative care services with, on average, 50 per cent of such units contributing to the training of medical students, trainee general practitioners, and local general practice principals, in addition to scores of nursing courses and degrees. Hunt, looking at community care in Australia, found that quality was directly proportional to the general experience and training of the family doctors.[47]

By late 1987, when medical specialization in palliative medicine was officially recognized, there was overwhelming evidence of unmet needs and every reason to believe that only by creating a new specialty would palliative medicine come to have the place it needed and its practitioners the credibility and authority necessary to bring about change. The succeeding years have seen a sustained growth in the specialty, a proliferation of specialist palliative care services, and discernible improvements in the provision of palliative care across the board, some of which are attributable to the presence and influence of the specialist services.

Specialist palliative care services

Specialist palliative care can be provided in inpatient units and in the patient's home. These services will now be described in detail.

Inpatient services

Specialist unit

A unit dedicated to specialist palliative care may be:

(1) a ward within a general/specialist hospital;

(2) a separate, free-standing unit within a hospital complex;

(3) a free-standing unit geographically separate from any other hospital.

The benefits of the first two include ready access to on-site diagnostic and specialist consultation services, availability of junior medical staff to provide out-of-hours cover, and convenience for patient transfer and visiting by relatives. An important advantage is the potential for providing palliative care advice for patients in non-cancer wards and the considerable educational potential for non-palliative care doctors, nurses, and others to learn from, and be inspired by, the palliative skills evidenced in the specialist unit so close at hand. Contrary to what some expect, provided the unit's ethos is one of palliation and rehabilitation rather than 'death row', patients readily accept or even request transfer to the specialist unit knowing full well what it stands for.

In theory, it should be of benefit for student nurses to be rotated through the specialist unit but unless there is a high quality of preparation, support, and in-service supervision for these young nurses, they may find it particularly stressful at this early stage in a nursing career. For this reason most such units do not use student nurses but rely on registered nurses and nursing auxiliaries, in this way striving to maintain the necessarily high nurse:patient ratio which good palliative care requires, provided management accepts the inevitable cost implications.

A free-standing specialist palliative care unit, geographically independent of a larger hospital, whether it is run by a national health service or is independent (wholly or partly funded by charity) can benefit from unshackled management and all the possibilities of small unit flexibility but is not likely to have on-site diagnostic facilities (except possibly simple radiology) nor the ready availability of consultants in other specialties. In the United Kingdom, 80 per cent of units are free-standing (independent) and 20 per cent are run by the National Health Service; the independent ones include most of the traditional hospices, the forerunners of modern specialist palliative care.

The staffing of any such unit is of the utmost importance. It is essential that all senior medical and nursing staff should be appropriately qualified in palliative care, having had the necessary training and been officially accredited as specialists by the appropriate professional body. Similarly, such staff as physiotherapists, occupational therapists, chaplains, and clinical pharmacists should have had considerable experience in palliative care even though the subject may not yet be officially recognized as a specialty by their peers. No matter how committed the general practitioner/family doctor may be, a unit where his input is the only medical contribution, inevitably not full time, cannot expect to be regarded as a specialist palliative care unit.

No recommended staffing ratios are available but most aim to have one nurse to 1.5 patients around-the-clock and one consultant physician for 10 to 15 beds, partly depending on whether or not the physician is also employed to see out patients, do domiciliary and hospital consultations, play a major role in an educational outreach, carry out research, and contribute to clinical and organizational audit.

As an example, looking at the United Kingdom, the average unit has 15 beds, (most common sizes 10, 12, 25, and 6 beds), a throughput per bed per annum of 18 to 20, and a discharge rate of three in every seven patients admitted.

Symptom relief team (hospital or palliative care team)

One of the most interesting and important developments in the provision of specialist palliative care in recent years has been the emergence of these teams.[48]

They are usually composed of a consultant in palliative medicine (or a specialist registrar/trainee consultant working under the supervision of an accredited specialist), at least one clinical nurse specialist, and part-time social workers and pastoral care workers, all supported by adequate clerical and record staff.

Such a team usually has no dedicated beds of its own (though a few may have access to them in different wards) but responds to invitations from any and every department in a major hospital of 500 plus beds, advising on every aspect of palliative care. Prescribing and arranging investigations remain the responsibilities of the ward staff caring for these patients, under the guidance of the team, unless otherwise authorized by clinical managers.

The benefits of such an advisory team can scarcely be overstated. The costs are almost entirely salaries. The patients can remain in familiar wards under doctors and nurses they have come to trust, close to all the therapeutic and diagnostic facilities they may need. Junior doctors and nurses gain valuable experience in the provision of palliative care under expert guidance and learn both to plan, prescribe and monitor within the context of general medical care, an educational experience probably much more relevant and valuable than any gained in more formal tutorials and lectures. Within the world-wide economic constraints which characterize health-care services, this seems to be a nearly ideal way of providing specialist care and, at the same time, encouraging and training the doctors and nurses of the future.

Experience, however, suggests that as in specialist inpatient units with their own beds, the majority of referrals are still of patients with malignancies. For reasons as yet undefined and seldom researched, many non-oncology specialist units within the general hospital do not regularly take advantage of the expertise of the hospital's peripatetic team which could offer so much for patients with far-advanced cardiac, respiratory, neurological, and endocrine problems. Is this because clinicians find it difficult to recognize 'end-stage disease' and approaching death, or regard it as a medical failure when someone cannot be kept alive? Is it simply that they feel expert enough in palliative care and do not see the need for any outside specialist advice? Is it that the 'terminal phase' of most malignant conditions is longer and better defined? This subject needs to be researched.

In the United Kingdom, the number of such teams has risen from 5 to 240 in the space of less than 20 years and they are now actively encouraged by the Department of Health, which no longer encourages the creation of more independent/charity-funded specialist palliative care units.[49]

Domiciliary services

In most countries where specialist palliative care is developing, there are well developed primary health-care facilities usually provided by general practitioners/family doctors with or without associated community nurses, either working as part of a team with the doctors or serving a defined geographical area.

Reference has already been made to the changing pattern of place of death and the consequent reduction in experience and expertise for general practitioners. What must be remembered, however, is that 90 per cent of the last year of life is spent at home[50] where, inevitably, most of their care problems and complications arise. Clearly, what is needed is for specialist palliative care expertise to be made available for patients in their own homes, enabling primary care teams to care as comprehensively and efficiently as they would like to, or have the specialist palliative care team itself provide total comprehensive care.

Two types of specialist domiciliary palliative care services have developed:

(1) a team consisting of a palliative medicine specialist and as many clinical nurse specialists as are required for the population served;[51]

(2) an all-nurse team, each member specially trained and accredited in palliative nursing care.

Such teams may be based in, and work from, a specialist palliative care unit with its own inpatient beds or be based entirely in the community managed by, and accountable to, its own clinical managers. At first sight there seems to be little to choose between them except the lesser cost of the all-nurse team without the high cost of medical salaries, but experience suggests that multiprofessional teams can better influence doctors' prescribing habits and the proactive planning of palliative care, and can better demonstrate an indisputable feature of all palliative care—namely, the interdisciplinary/multidisciplinary approach which should, in theory, produce the best care. No matter how experienced and skilled a doctor or nurse is, neither can have the skills and the insights they need to provide or advise on comprehensive palliative care without the other.

By far the majority of such domiciliary teams ('Home Care Services') in the United Kingdom are multiprofessional and advisory and have as their aims the provision of:

(1) a complementary, advisory, and supportive service for primary health-care teams;

(2) advice on all palliation for the patient (physical, psychological, social, and spiritual);

(3) advice on, and provision of additional support for, the caring relatives;

(4) liaison with other medical and nursing specialists involved in palliative care;

(5) support for the members of the primary health-care team.

Many domiciliary services operate 24 hours, around-the-clock, others a '9 to 5' service, largely dependent on the quality of local primary care and its resources.[52,53]

The availability or otherwise of back-up beds seems to be important. One study demonstrated that if a service was independent of a unit with palliative care beds, even if beds were available in a nearby general hospital, patients would elect to be cared for at home and up to 67 per cent died there. On the other hand, if back-up beds were available in a palliative care unit from which the service operated, most patients preferred to die there, the percentage dying at home falling to 31 per cent.[54] Another study demonstrated that a comprehensive domiciliary service did not increase the number dying at home but demonstrably enabled more patients to remain at home longer, eventually spending only a few days in the special unit.[53] Evidence on this subject is, however, conflicting.[55] Some reports suggest that a good specialist domiciliary service helps more to achieve their aim to remain and die at home.[56] This may be related to the comprehensiveness and staffing of the service as demonstrated by the Motala (Sweden) model[57,58] which has a significant medical component, offering all the nursing care the patient needs over 24 hours, and the necessary equipment for such care. Whichever the model, there is always found a need both for more equipment (beds, commodes, feeding equipment, etc.)

and up to 117 per cent increase in home visiting by other community nurses providing 'hands-on' care.[59]

That totally comprehensive care can be provided at home is beyond question.[60] Reports have been published of patients able to receive intravenous chemotherapy at home, having blood transfusions,[61] and benefiting from spinal opioids managed at home.[62] In the United Kingdom, such comprehensive domiciliary care is increasingly being sought by, and provided for, AIDS patients, as is the case for 90 per cent of AIDS patients in California.

Much depends on the wishes of the patients, the readiness of well-supported relatives to co-operate in providing care, the views and skills of each member of the primary care team (if in fact one exists), and the composition and resources of the specialist domiciliary team. It can fail completely if there is not genuine team caring and mutual support, and a high level of interprofessional communication.

In the United Kingdom, where specialist domiciliary palliative care services are now an established feature, all the nurses employed have had training in palliative care in addition to advanced training in community care, and many also possess qualifications in counselling, oncology, and other specialties.

The question must be asked whether these services are found acceptable and useful not just by the patients and their relatives but also by general practitioners and their community nurse colleagues. Without any doubt many were suspicious of them at the outset, seeing them as a threat, an indictment of their previous caring, particularly if inadequacies of care had not been recognized by them, as was often the case. The longer these services are operational, the better they are accepted, until the time comes when many community workers wonder how they coped without them. Others state that they would not now accept back into their care on discharge from hospital some terminally ill patients if there was not a specialist domiciliary palliative care service available to assist them.

It is a timely reminder of the principles described at the beginning of this chapter. Every doctor and nurse provides palliative care, often of a high standard, but every now and again a problem arises which needs specialist input. It is then that the specialist palliative care team becomes invaluable, supporting but hopefully never supplanting the primary health-care team. Each needs the other.[63–66]

Very recently two new types of domiciliary service have been developed in the United Kingdom to deal with well recognised problems encountered in the communiy, problems which can easily lead to unnecessary hospital admission: rapid response teams and respite care teams.

Rapid response teams

This is, in effect, an emergency 'crisis intervention' service. When a crisis develops at home such that urgent admission would normally be called for, the family doctor can call out this team composed of a medical specialist in palliative medicine, and palliative nursing specialists. They respond within an hour or so, deal with whatever problems they encounter and then the nurse may remain in the house, relieved by colleagues, for a day or so until the situation has settled. Crises include sudden inexplicable pain, acute confusional states or paranoia, the need for urgent suprapubic catheterization, and status epilepticus.

Respite care teams

It is now well recognized that the strain on caring relatives can often be the final trigger leading to hospital admission. Often the offer of a short respite admission for the patient has been declined early in the illness because relatives felt they should be able to cope. The Respite Care Team differs from an ordinary domiciliary team in that palliative care nursing specialists remain with the patient for several hours each day, offering all the care the patient needs, so that relatives can take time off, the better to cope with the few weeks or days that remain. They are in addition to the specialist night-sitting services (Marie Curie Cancer Care) which have been a feature of the United Kingdom for many years.

Both these types of service are currently being evaluated.

Day care (day hospices)

In several countries there are now growing numbers of day care units (in the United Kingdom, usually termed 'day hospices') for patients under domiciliary care.

Most of the 216 in the United Kingdom are based in specialist palliative care units, operate on weekdays and cater for 10 to 15 patients each day, often augmented by patients fit enough to attend from the inpatient unit. Those attending from home are brought by car or ambulance at 10 a.m. and taken home between 3 and 4 p.m.

Each day unit, staffed by nurses, physiotherapists, occupational therapists, and volunteers, is committed to maximizing the quality of life of its patients through social activities, crafts, and creative arts, skilfully tailored to meet the individual needs of patients. The atmosphere is relaxed and informal, more like a home than a hospital, with decor, furnishings, and ambience specially created for this group of people. Creative arts and activities range from modelling, ceramics, painting, and confectionery, to music, travel talks, poetry readings, and indoor gardening, recognizing the untapped potential of so many patients and the undoubted benefits of bringing together people with similar problems and needs. In spite of the presence of nurses and the availability of doctors near at hand to help these patients, every effort is made to create a deliberately low key clinical environment. Contrary to what might be thought, these activities are not diversional but a means of emphasizing personal worth and usefulness, of helping patients look back to happy days and relationships.

Few studies have been done on day care but the important subjective views of patients suggest that they do much to reaffirm living rather than dying, often shown by patients going into long-term remissions. What is equally important is the respite accorded to the caring relatives who can resume some normal home activities during the hours the patient is out of the house, confident that the patient is in safe hands because they, the relatives, have been given the opportunity to visit the day hospice and experience for themselves its unique atmosphere and philosophy.

Outpatient (ambulatory) consultation services

When palliative care is deemed appropriate for patients still able to attend the specialist palliative care unit, there is much value in offering an outpatient consultation service. This enables general practitioners/family doctors to obtain specialist advice on any or every aspect of a patient's needs whilst still maintaining care at home, exactly as would be done at any other time of life.

Such a facility should not be regarded as an alternative to, or a substitute for, a domiciliary service where the patient is visited at home by the team. It enables patients to be given specialist advice before they are seriously incapacitated but it does not enable the team to see and assess the home situation nor to meet many of the caring relatives and address their needs. As any experienced family doctor will attest, a patient seen as an outpatient often gives a different picture from the one seen at home on his own territory, where the doctor and nurse are the patient's guests.

Obstacles to the provision of specialist palliative care

When palliative medicine and specialist palliative care services are developing so rapidly in many innovative ways in different countries and cultures, it may seen unnecessary or churlish to look at obstacles to their development but progress has often been slow and many hurdles are encountered. These will now be reviewed.

Misunderstandings about palliative care

Much was said on the subject of definitions and descriptions at the start of this chapter because of widespread misunderstandings. There remain some doctors, but fewer nurses, who cannot accept the need for specialists in this subject, believing, in spite of the evidence to the contrary, that they are currently providing the necessary quality of care as part of their daily work. Many still regard palliative care as 'terminal care', the care of those with only days to live. Others see it as exclusively a nursing responsibility (a claim sometimes made by those nurses who have undertaken additional training in palliative care nursing and see no need for medical input) or primarily psychosocial, requiring not medical input but companionship, emotional support, and pastoral care ('tender loving care'—TLC). Mistakenly they believe that all that is needed by such patients is time spent with them, something they feel they cannot give but which is available in abundance in a special unit, overlooking the fact that it is quality of time, not quantity, which these patients need.

Paradoxically, the many new pharmacological therapies and skills developed by palliative medicine for the relief of symptoms have brought their own problems as more doctors have learned these therapies and themselves become better 'symptomatologists', choosing to ignore the ever present, often greater, challenges of emotional and spiritual problems and the myriad needs of relatives. They manage to control a person's pain and feel that in so doing they have practised comprehensive modern palliative care. They forget that a patient freed from pain may still be, and often is, frightened, lonely, and shorn of dignity.

Palliative care is not exclusively for cancer patients. Specialist palliative care grew out of cancer care and has developed in parallel with oncology; however, it is not a branch of oncology but of all medical care irrespective of a person's life-threatening pathology. To see it as a subdivision of oncology is to limit its application and to deprive thousands of patients of appropriate care. As is repeatedly stressed in this textbook, there is no reason why these specialist services should not be used for cardiac, neurological, and other patients, but health-care planners and managers need to be reminded of this. Too few studies have been done on the advanced care of these patients. Particularly when needs assessments are being done, health-care planners fail to take into account the many non-malignant disease patients who could benefit from palliative care.

Low priorities in professional education

This is dealt with in Section 21. Basically, the problem is that different component parts of medical care are identified and included in professional training curricula but not the subject as a comprehensive, cohesive whole. Thus, pain control is taught, often very minimally, but not the palliation of other symptoms, emotional needs, pastoral care, and the interdisciplinary approach. Communications and ethical issues are often alluded to but not taught in any detail and are often divorced from other aspects of palliative care, confined to 'breaking bad news' and euthanasia. Almost universally there is little co-ordination or cohesion, with aspects of palliative care being mentioned at many different stages in the curriculum but not taught as a package, resulting in doctors and nurses failing to learn its relevance and its potential benefits for so many of their patients, and never learning how to plan integrated care.

Low priority in resource allocation

In an age when every health-care service seems to be based on a market economy, it is perhaps inevitable that in some countries specialist palliative care is often accorded lower priority than the provision of high-profile specialties, each characterized by sophisticated technology, easily defined outcome measures, and considerable expense, the provision of which is thought to enhance the standing of some ambitious politicians.

Again there is the problem of understanding and appreciation of what specialist palliative care is and can achieve on the part of health-care economists and strategic planners. The situation is not helped by the generosity of the public in the United Kingdom, United States, and many other countries who often founded, funded, and continue to meet close on 60 per cent of the revenue needs of many of the specialist palliative care services in their country. Without them there would not be such services but the longer the public are willing to support them so magnanimously, the less incentive is there for governments to face up to their obligations.[67]

Some blame lies with the specialty itself which has until recently signally failed to research its work to ensure it is truly 'evidence-based medicine', define outcome measures, measure its effectiveness, and prove/disprove the claims made by its practitioners. That the public, the patients ('consumers'), appreciate and value specialist palliative care is beyond question but this carries little weight in any competition for limited financial resources. Even more is this the case when some health-care planners are unclear what specialist palliative care is and how it fits into the jigsaw of service provision. Even some palliative care practitioners have tended to be content with consumer/patient satisfaction and plaudits, and have not been prepared themselves to negotiate with the purchasers of care in a cut-throat market economy.

The place of specialist palliative care in a health service

Clearly this will depend on many factors—the national pattern of health-care provision, local and national resources, the sophistication or otherwise of a country's health service, the politics and priorities of health care, and the knowledge and understanding of specialist palliative care and what it has to offer.[68,69]

These factors are so obvious that little space need be devoted to the study of them. At one extreme we may have an economically poor and underdeveloped country with the most rudimentary health service. Though it can be argued that the greatest need in such a country is for palliative care because the vast majority of its peoples will not, for many years, have the resources and equipment necessary if there is to be any hope of ever curing anyone, often poor countries develop health services for non-infectious diseases from the top and work downwards. They develop specialist expensive, high technology, prestigious medical centres with no palliative care facilities, before they look to providing basic care for the bulk of the population, often to be found in rural areas. At the other end of the spectrum are some of the most affluent and scientifically-advanced countries who give priority to superspecialties that aim to cure and they too need to be reminded of the needs of those whose condition is incurable and fatal. This subject is dealt with in detail in Section 22.

In most countries hospital medical care is, and always has been, better resourced than domiciliary and community care. One sequel is that general practice is less attractive than hospital practice, less respected and valued, and may consequently be of poorer quality from the viewpoint of palliative care. In others, private health care is the norm with state health care a poor relation in all respects. Specialist palliative care is rarely, if ever, a part of private medicine and may consequently be looked down upon by private practitioners or, more commonly, seen as a financial threat to them.

In only a few countries is specialist palliative care slowly being integrated into mainstream health care, notably in the United Kingdom, Canada,[70] Australia, and New Zealand. Notable as its practitioners are, and great their example and commitment, even in the United States[11] such services are often outside mainstream care, and to a large extent the responsibility of charitable bodies and thousands of voluntary workers. In many European countries, Hong Kong,[71] Israel,[72,73] Singapore, and South Africa, the picture resembles that in the United Kingdom some years ago—a few medical and nursing pioneers setting an example within their own units and practices, striving to establish palliative care as the norm for everyone rather than a luxury for a few, with much effort having to go into persuading governments and colleagues of its value[74] because these efforts are being made to integrate palliative care into the full spectrum of health care provision.

The United Kingdom picture may be of interest (Figs 1 and 2). The developing pattern of provision reflects the definition which opened this chapter. Primary health care is the responsibility of the family doctor caring for patients at home and in nursing homes, and he or she is responsible for offering palliative care whenever it is required. The assistance of medical and nursing specialists in palliative care is available to him on request (see Section 16). If the patient goes into a hospital, whether general or specialist, once again the services of specialists are available to complement the skills of all the other specialists in that hospital—an example of a hospital palliative care team at work. Should it be thought appropriate for a patient to be transferred to a specialist palliative care unit for terminal care, palliative care, or rehabilitation before returning home, the responsibility shifts to the specialist palliative service which becomes totally responsible for the patient; all the professional carers then, for the first time, being specially trained in palliative care.

This evolving pattern acknowledges the skills of family doctors and community nurses, the palliative skills of many hospital staff, and the additional and sometimes unique skills of the specialist team, ensuring that wherever the patient requires care, wherever they move to, expertise is available without any encroachment into colleague's territory or any threat to patients' or professionals' autonomy. Such a pattern ensures that palliative care follows the patient rather than the patient having to seek out palliative care.

Evaluating specialist palliative care

Clinical and organizational audit are dealt with in Chapter 2.6. Here we focus on reports and impressions from published studies of palliative care provision worldwide.

Children's hospices are the subject of Chapter 19.5 and 19.7; a study from the world's first such unit in Oxford, United Kingdom,[75] not only demonstrated improved care but found how parents want such improved care for their dying children, want better mobilization of resources, and want to be listened to and acknowledged as experts in their care. With close on 14 children's hospices operational or planned, it is interesting to note how they are regarded as respite, rehabilitation, or palliation units rather than the places where children go to die.

A detailed clinical and financial assessment of patients with advanced Alzheimer's disease[76] found that they fared better when offered palliative care in a specialist unit than when catered for in a traditional long-term unit. The impact of a specialist unit on local care standards has been reported in several studies. One from the United Kingdom looking at palliative care at home, in hospitals, and in special units over a 5 year period, found not only more doctors prescribing opioids better but an overall improvement in care.[77] Another study of family doctors and local consultants a year after the establishment of a local specialist unit, found high levels of professional acceptance and appreciation, a high take-up of its resources, and an acknowledgement that the specialist unit raised standards of care in the hospitals, a view shared by family doctors and specialists alike.[78,79] The same raising of care standards was observed in London by Parkes, the notable exception being in the care of relatives.

Somewhat similar reports come from Spain,[80] Finland,[81] Japan,[82] Hong Kong,[71] Australia, New Zealand,[83] Russia,[84] Israel,[72,73] and Italy.[3] In 1990, the Japanese government authorized medical incentives for hospice care, the first such unit having opened in 1987, followed by five others in the next 9 years. The concept is now widely accepted with plans to develop home care.[82]

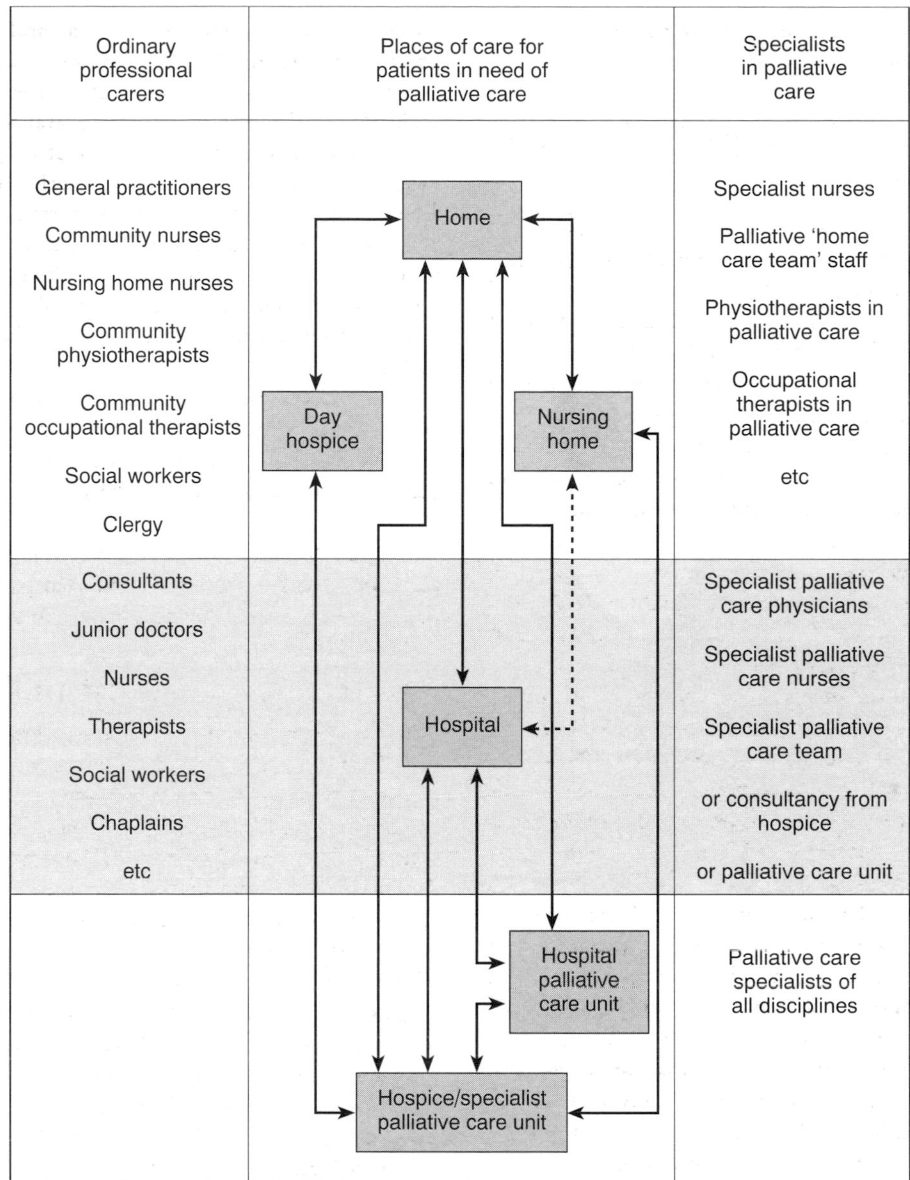

Fig. 1 'Palliative care follows the patient'. When the patient is at home the ordinary day-to-day professional carers are the general practitioner (family physician), community nurses, and therapists. The patient may move between his home, a nursing home, and a Day Centre, but always these are his carers, assisted if needs be by the specialists in the right column. If the patient goes to hospital the ordinary staff there also have palliative care specialists to help and advise them, in touch with those who assisted in the community. If admission to a specialist palliative care unit is needed, even if the patient leaves there to return to hospital, home, or nursing home, still there are palliative care specialists on hand.

Specialist palliative care is now recognized in Hong Kong[71] with several units serving its dense population and active plans taking shape to develop home care staffed by nurses similar to the specialist palliative care ('Macmillan') nurses so familiar in the United Kingdom. Argentina now has several services and in 1994 there was the first report of developments in Colombia.[85] In the United States there are over 2000 services, a small number of which have inpatient beds. Most are home-care services, but in many of the larger medical centres, including some of the world's most famous centres, there are now specialist palliative care teams.

Australia[86] now recognizes palliative medicine as a specialty, has 4 academic chairs, and provides a full range of services in areas as different as settlements in the Northern Territories and all the major cities; places such as Sydney are served not only by inpatient units with 100 beds but also by consultant-led teams in major hospitals.

So acceptable has specialist palliative care become in Catalonia, Spain, that centres have been established throughout the whole province and a 5-year strategic plan has been devised to involve primary care doctors to take it wherever it is needed.[87] Canada has long been a pioneer in this work, with one of the world's first specialist units within a major hospital (Royal Victoria, Montreal), but even she does not yet have comprehensive or fully co-ordinated services in every city, nor is palliative medicine yet accorded specialist recognition.

New Zealand[83] has, at the time of writing, 23 services, some consultant-led, serving all the main cities and many rural areas. In the past few years, palliative care services have been developed in

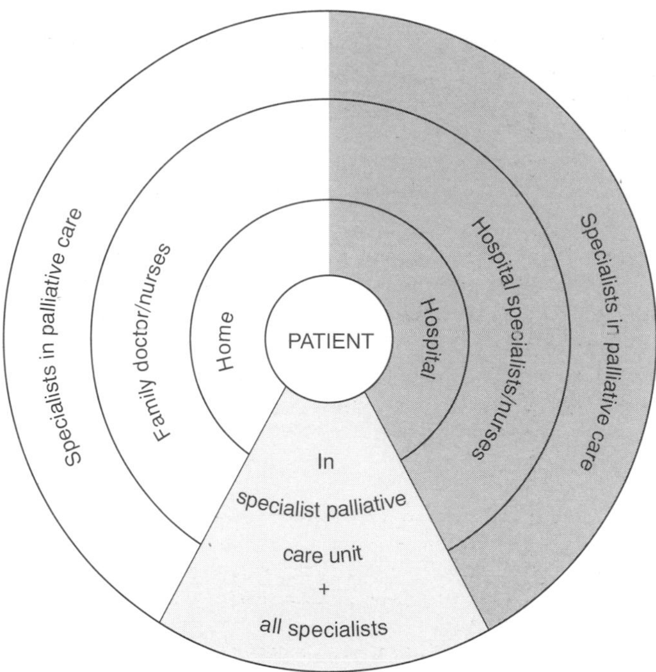

Fig. 2 'Palliative care follows the patient'. As any patient moves between home, hospital, and specialist palliative care unit he or she always has access to specialist palliative care. All that is needed is for the general practitioner or hospital physician/surgeon to call in the specialist in palliative care, whether that be a nurse or a doctor.

St. Petersburg and Moscow,[84] with others planned, and high hopes of others starting in Romania and Bulgaria. Poland has many services and a vigorous education and training programme. In Western Europe, there is now no country which does not have such services, some still embryonic, others highly developed and usually recognized by statutory health authorities.

The majority of reports emanate from primary care (Section 16) many describing major deficiencies of care for the home-based patient, that are improved with the availability of specialist domiciliary services.[88] Workers in Israel[72] speak of 29 per cent of the terminally ill dying at home, 40 per cent in general hospitals, and 31 per cent in chronic care institutions, but claim that with better palliative care services two-thirds could have been managed at home. A similar report from Norway[89] shows how rewarding relatives found it to care for their loved ones at home, provided specialist skills and supports were available for them. Other reports and evaluations have been published from Sicily,[4,5] Italy,[2] Australia,[90] France,[74] Finland,[81] Spain,[80] Denmark,[56] and Portugal.

Few question that if home care is impossible, the next best is for the patient to be cared for by the family doctor in a general practitioner hospital or a hospital in which the doctor has admitting rights, provided that he also has the necessary skills and access to specialists.[91,92] The alternative is to take all the benefits of a specialist service into the patient's home or, as in Sweden[57,58] and in some parts of Canada, to provide totally comprehensive care there without the involvement of the family doctor. It has to be noted, however, that a few family doctors can feel threatened by a specialist service, as has been alluded to above.[93]

The most comprehensive details of palliative care services, particularly domiciliary services, in the United Kingdom and Ireland are to be found in reports by Smith *et al.*[94] and Hinton;[19,20] one of the best comparative-cost studies is that by Gray *et al.*[95]

Planning the provision of services

No health care service can, or should, be planned or provided without:[96–99]

(1) a scientific needs assessment by purchasers and providers;

(2) a review of existing services and their efficacy and potential;

(3) a review of resources available and those likely to be needed;

(4) plans for audit and regular reviews;

(5) consideration of the type(s) of service most likely to meet identified needs.

It must be admitted that few of the existing specialist palliative care services in the world were established after this process. In most cases need was identified but not measured. It was simply recognized that care was inadequate, improvement was demonstrably possible, and a start was made. Public support was often overwhelming, with professional and governmental interest and backing lagging behind. This led to problems and continues to do so in many places. Because there has usually been such consumer pressure and satisfaction, the temptation has been to take it for granted that the most appropriate model had been selected. The same insatiable public demand has led to indiscriminate proliferation of units with little if any needs assessment or re-evaluation being carried out, or the establishment of home-care services without consultation with planners, family doctors, or even existing palliative care services.

The definitions and descriptions so frequently referred to in this chapter cannot be ignored. Whatever type of service is decided upon—if in fact one is demonstrated as necessary—it must never be forgotten that most doctors and nurses can be enabled to provide better palliative care through improved education, training, and sympathetic encouragement. Any specialist service—an inpatient unit, a hospital team, or a home-care service—MUST have an built-in educational component from its conception and MUST be designed to meet clearly identified local needs rather than being developed as a clone, a mirror image, of some long-established famous unit elsewhere. One community may need only a day hospice, another a few beds to be under general practitioner care, whilst nearby the local district hospital perhaps needs a palliative care team.

Needs assessment

Needs assessment in this field is difficult but not impossible.[98,100] It must take into account:

(1) geographical location and population;

(2) demography profile;

(3) health profile (looking separately at malignant and non-malignant conditions);

(4) existing provision of services.

For long it has been said, without any hard data to support it, that 50 beds set apart for specialist palliative care are required per million of population. However, this figures does not take into account the changing pattern of place of death (with diminishing numbers at home and more in hospital), nor the effects of improved resources put into the community (including types of home care service), nor the increasing ability of a specialist palliative care service to rehabilitate, nor the almost completely unmet needs of those with non-malignant conditions, nor the world-wide shortage of adequately trained staff for such services, nor the financial implications.

Recent guidlines published in the United Kingdom [105] suggest the *minimum* provision of adequate specialist palliative care services for a population of 500 000 are:

- 2 WTE consultants/specialists in palliative medicine (to provide service in both hospital and community settings)
- 25 specialist palliative care inpatient beds
- 10 WTE *community* clinical nurse specialists in palliative care
- at least 2 WTE *hospital* clinical nurse specialists in each cancer unit or district general hospital (the latter usually having 350-500 beds)
- 200 specialist palliative day care patient places per week.

Evaluation and outcome measures

Anecdotes abound but objective evaluations are few.[52,79,101] How should the effectiveness of services be measured? What should be the acceptable outcome measures? The traditional ones of cure, mortality, infection control, etc., are inappropriate.

Many have studied symptom relief and pain control, both measurable in a multitude of ways. Others have recorded consumer views of needs and to what extent they have been met. Others have looked at anxiety and depression in patients and carers, subsequent bereavement, and staff stress.

Predictably, health-care purchasers want high quality care at the lowest cost but how does one cost a home-care service or a hospital palliative care team and with what other services are they to be compared in financial terms? Many services make much use of trained volunteers but how is their contribution to be costed or in any other way evaluated? Indeed, it might be argued that any saving as a result of using them may be offset by the cost of training, organizing, and supervising them.

Is a specialist service justified merely because the public approve of it and support it in so many ways or is its worth related to its taking patients from a hospital and so releasing for those who need them 'precious' beds in a high-technology unit? At a more basic but arguably important level, is an 'efficient' palliative care unit one with high throughput as would be said of a general hospital or one where patients could feel there was no pressure on them to return home, something rarely acceptable in hospital practice.

Much work on all these diverse and difficult questions continues to be done by the National Council for Hospice and Specialist Palliative Care Services (England, Wales, and Northern Ireland) and its 'Occasional Papers' dealing with contracting from purchasers, quality standards, audit, definitions, ethnic minorities, research, and education. These are all commended to the reader provided it is remembered that they come from a country with a reasonably well-financed National Health Service, a long and notable tradition of general practice, and the longest history of specialist palliative care provision in the world—not necessarily of relevance therefore for planners in the medical third world.[96,99,102–109]

It is important to continue not only appropriate planning and provision of specialist palliative care services, but to be responsible and bold enough to look into the future, asking such questions as who will need such care, what will the family doctor of the future want to do, what services will be both effective and economically efficient, and—everywhere—how much specialization is needed? Perhaps, in time, one mark of a caring community will be its willingness to look at 'the future of palliative care' as eagerly as it looks at other health-care issues.

References

1. Thorpe G. Enabling more dying people to remain at home. *British Medical Journal*, 1993; **397**: 915–8.
2. Toscani F, Mancini C. Inadequacies of care in far-advanced cancer patients: a comparison between home and hospital in Italy. *Palliative Medicine*, 1989; **4**: 31–6.
3. Terzoli E, *et al.* Medical oncology and home care in Italy. *Tumori*, 1993; **79**: 30–3.
4. Mercadente S. Family doctor and palliative care team: 1988 versus 1990. *Journal of Palliative Care*, 1991; **7**: 38–9.
5. Mercadente S, *et al.* Home palliative care: results of 1991 versus 1988. *Journal of Pain and Symptom Management*, 1992; **7**: 414–8.
6. Mercadente S. Prevalence, causes and mechanisms of pain in home-care patients with advanced cancer. *Pain Clinic*, 1994; **7**: 131–6.
7. Portenoy RK, *et al.* Pain in ambulatory patients with lung and colon cancer. *Cancer*, 1992; **70**: 1616–24.
8. Cleeland CS, *et al.* Pain and its treatment in outpatients with metastatic cancer. *New England Journal of Medicine*, 1994; **330**: 592–6.
9. Von Roenn JH, *et al.* Physician attitudes and practice in cancer pain management: a survey from the Eastern Co-operative Oncology Group. *Annals of Internal Medicine*, 1993; **119**: 121–6.
10. Walsh TD. Continuing care in a medical center: the Cleveland Clinic Foundation Palliative Care Service. *Journal of Pain and Symptom Management*, 1990; **5**: 273–8.
11. Magno J. USA Hospice care in the 1990s. *Palliative Medicine*, 1992; **6**: 158–65.
12. Hileman JW, Lackey NR, Hassanein RS. Identifying the needs of home caregivers of patients with cancer. *Oncology Nursing Forum*, 1992; **19**: 771–7.
13. Hileman JW, Lackey NR. Self-identified needs of patients with cancer at home and their caregivers: a descriptive study. *Oncology Nursing* Forum, 1990: **17**: 907–13.
14. Curtiss CP. Trends and issues for cancer care in rural communities. *Nursing Clinics of North America*, 1993; **28**: 241–51.
15. 'A Policy Framework for Commisioning Cancer Services.' *Expert Advisory Group on Cancer's report to the Chief Medical Officers*, HMSO, London, 1995.
16. Cartwright A. The role of the general practitioner in caring for people in the last year of their lives. *King Edward's Hospital Fund Report*, 1990.
17. Williams EL, Fitton F. General practitioner response to elderly patients discharged from hospital. *British Medical Journal*, 1990; **300**: 159–61.
18. Higginson I, Webb D, Lessor L. Reducing hospital beds for patients with advanced cancer. *Lancet*, 1994; **344**: 409.
19. Hinton J. Can home care maintain an acceptable quality of life for patients with terminal cancer and their relatives? *Palliative Medicine*, 1994; **8**: 183–96.
20. Hinton J. Which patients with terminal cancer are admitted from home care? *Palliative Medicine*, 1994; **8**: 197–210.
21. Cartwright A, Hockey L, Anderson R. *Life Before Death*. Kegan Paul, London. 1973.

22. Cartwright A. Balance of care for the dying between hospital and the community: perceptions of general practitioners, hospital consultants, community nurses and relatives. *British Journal of General Practice*, 1991; **41**: 271–4.
23. Cartwright A. Changes in life and care in the year before death. *Journal of Public Health Medicine*, 1981: **13**: 81–7.
24. Sykes NP, Pearson SE, Chell S. Quality of care of the terminally ill: the carer's perspective. *Palliative Medicine*, 1992; **6**: 227–36.
25. Herd EB. Terminal care in a semi-rural area. *Journal of the Royal College of General Practitioners*, 1990; **40**: 248–51.
26. Haines A, Booroff A. Terminal care at home: perspective from general practice. *British Medical Journal*, 1986; **292**: 1051–3.
27. Boyd KJ. Palliative care in the community: views of general practitioners and district nurses in East London. *Journal of Palliative Care*, 1993; **9**: 33–7.
28. Blyth AC. Audit of terminal care in a general practice. *British Medical Journal*, 1991; **330**: 983–6.
29. Copperman H. Hospice home care services (letter). *Palliative Medicine*, 1992; **6**: 260.
30. Barritt PW. Care of the dying in one practice. *Journal of the Royal College of General Practitioners*, 1984; **34**: 446–8.
31. Doyle D. Education in palliative medicine and pain therapy: an overview. In: Twycross RG, ed. *The Edinburgh Symposium on Pain Control and Medical Education*. Royal Society of Medicine International Congress and Symposium Series Number 149. London, 1989.
32. Doyle D. Nurse Education in Terminal Care. *Nurse Education Today*, 1982; **2**: 4–6.
33. Lubin S. Palliative care—could your patient have been managed at home? *Journal of Palliative Care*, 1992; **8**: 18–22.
34. Lopez de Maturana A, *et al.* Attitudes of general practitioners in Bizkaia, Spain, towards the terminally ill patient. *Palliative Medicine*, 1993; **7**: 39–45.
35. Reddall C. People with cancer have the right to expect the best possible treatment and care. *European Journal of Cancer Care*, 1994; **3**: 39–43.
36. Bradshaw PJ. Characteristics of clients referred to home, hospice and hospital palliative care services in Australia. *Palliative Medicine*, 1993; **7**: 101–7.
37. Cartwright A. Dying when you're old. *Age Ageing*, 1993; **22**: 425–30.
38. Parkes CM. Home or hospital? Terminal care as seen by surviving spouses. *Journal of the Royal College of General Practitioners*, 1978; **28**: 19–30.
39. Brivio E, Gamba A. Home care for advanced cancer patients: the efficacy of domiciliary assistance. *European Journal of Cancer Care*, 1992; **1**: 24–8.
40. Smith N. The impact of terminal illness on the family. *Palliative Medicine*, 1990; **4**: 127–35.
41. Seale C. Community nurses and the care of the dying. *Social Science and Medicine*, 1992; **34**: 375–82.
42. Jones RV, Hansford J, Fiske J. Death from cancer at home: the carer's perspective. *British Medical Journal*, 1993; **306**: 249–51.
43. Dunphy KP, Amesbury BDW. A comparison of hospice and home care patients: patterns of referral, patient characteristics and predictors of place of death. *Palliative Medicine*, 1990; **4**: 105–11.
44. Reilly PM, Patten MP. Terminal care in the home. *Journal of the Royal College of General Practitioners*, 1981; **31**: 531–7.
45. Grieco AJ, Kowalski W. The 'care partner'. In: Bernstein LH, Grieco AJ, Dete MK, eds. *Primary Care in the Home*. Philadelphia: J.B. Lippincott, 1987: 71–82.
46. Seamark DA, *et al.* Knowledge and perceptions of a domiciliary hospice service among general practitioners and community nurses. *British Journal of General Practice*, 1993; **43**: 57–9.
47. Hunt RW, *et al.* The community care of terminally ill patients. *Australian Family Physician*, 1990; **19**: 1835–41.
48. Dunlop R, Hockley J. *Terminal Care Support Teams: The Hospital–Hospice Interface.* Oxford: Oxford University Press, 1990.
49. Wilkes E. *Standing Medical Advisory Committee on Terminal Care. Report of a Working Party.* London: HMSO, 1980.
50. Levy B, Selare AB. Fatal illness in general practice. *Journal of the Royal College of General Practitioners*, 1976; **26**: 303–7.
51. Kindlen M. Hospice home care services: a Scottish perspective. *Palliative Medicine*, 1988; **2**: 115–21.
52. Hockey L. St. Columba's Hospice Home Care Service: an evaluation study. *Palliative Medicine*, 1991; **5**: 315–22.
53. Doyle D. A home care service for terminally-ill patients in Edinburgh. *Health Bulletin* (Edinburgh), 1991; **49**: 14–23.
54. Ward AWM. *Home Care Services for the Terminally Ill.* Sheffield: Medical Care Research Unit, University of Sheffield, 1985.
55. Maltoni M, *et al.* Description of a home care service for cancer patients through quantitative indexes of evaluation. *Tumori*, 1991; **77**: 453–9.
56. Palleson AE. Care for the dying in Denmark. *Danish Medical Bulletin*, 1992; **39**: 265–8.
57. Beck-Friis B, Strang P. The organization of hospital-based home care for terminally ill cancer patients; the Motala model. *Palliative Medicine*, 1993; **7**: 93–100.
58. Beck-Friis B, Strang P. The family in hospital-based home care with special reference to terminally-ill cancer patients. *Journal of Palliative Care*, 1993; **9**: 5–13.
59. Doyle D. Domiciliary terminal care—demands on statutory services. *Journal of the Royal College of General Practitioners*, 1982; **32**: 285–91.
60. Spencer J. Caring for a terminally ill person with pain at home: an Australian perspective. *Cancer Nursing*, 1991; **14**: 55–8.
61. Sciortino AD, *et al.* The efficacy of administering blood transfusions at home to terminally ill cancer patients. *Journal of Palliative Care*, 1993; **9**: 14–17.
62. Mercadente S. Intrathecal morphine and bupivacaine in advanced cancer patients implanted at home. *Journal of Pain and Symptom Management*, 1994; **9**: 201–7.
63. Jones R. Primary health care: what should we do for people dying at home with cancer? *European Journal of Cancer Care*, 1992; **1**: 9–11.
64. McWhinney IR, Stewart MA. Home care of dying patients: Family physicians' experience with a palliative care team. *Canadian Family Physician*, 1994; **40**: 240–6.
65. McWhinney, IR. *A Textbook of Family Medicine.* Oxford: Oxford University Press, 1989.
66. Robinson L, Stacy R. Palliative care in the community: setting practice guidelines for primary care teams. *British Journal of General Practice*, 1994; **44**: 461–4.
67. Vainio A. Palliative care in Finland. *Palliative Medicine*, 1990: **4**: 225–7.
68. Constantine M, *et al.* Palliative home care and place of death among cancer patients: a population-based study. *Palliative Medicine*, 1993; **7**: 323–31.
69. Saunders J, Rosenthal S. Improving domiciliary terminal care. *Nursing Times*, 1992; **88**: 32–4.
70. Roe DJ. Palliative care 2000—home care. *Journal of Palliative Care*, 1992; **8**: 28–32.
71. Tsao SY, Leung A. Palliative care in Hong Kong. *Palliative Medicine*, 1991; **5**: 262–6.
72. Loven D, *et al.* Place of death of cancer patients in Israel; the experience of a home care programme. *Palliative Medicine*, 1990; **4**: 299–304.
73. Margarit D. The first two years of a palliative home care programme—Jerusalem. *European Journal of Cancer*, 1993; **29A** (Suppl): S268.
74. Gomas JM. Palliative care at home: a reality or 'mission impossible'? *Palliative Medicine*, 1993; **7** (Suppl): 45–59.
75. Burne R. The dying child at home. *Journal of the Royal College of General Practitioners*, 1987; **37**: 291.
76. Volicer L, *et al.* Impact of special care unit for patients with advanced Alzheimer's disease on patients' discomforts and costs. *Journal of the American Geriatric Society*, 1994; **42**: 597–603.
77. Rees WD. Changes in prescribing for terminal care patients in general practice, hospital and hospice over a 5 year period. *Journal of the Royal College of General Practitioners*, 1987; **37**: 504–6.
78. Macdonald ET, Macdonald JB. How do local doctors react to a hospice? *Health Bulletin*, 1992; **50**: 351–5.
79. McIllmurray MB, Warren MR. Evaluation of a new hospice: the relief of

symptoms in cancer patients in the first year. *Palliative Medicine*, 1989; **3**: 135–40.

80. Sanz-Oriz J, Llamazares Gonzales A. Home care in a palliative care unit. *Medicina Clinica* (Barcelona) 1993; **101**: 446–9.
81. Nikkonen M, Siikanen E. Home care nurses' support of the relative caregiver of the patient dying at home. *Sairaanhoitaja*, 1993; **8**: 14–15.
82. Kashiwagi T. Hospice care in Japan. *Postgraduate Medical Journal*, 1991; **67** (suppl): S95–9.
83. Lichter I. Palliative care services in New Zealand. *Palliative Medicine*, 1990; **4**: 219–23.
84. Karajaeva E. Out of Russia. *Hospital Bulletin*, 1994; **22**: 8–9.
85. De Lima L, Bruera E. Palliative care in Columbia: programme in 'La Viga'. *Journal of Palliative Care*, 1994; **10**: 42–3.
86. MacAdam DB. A review of 715 terminal patients cared for at home by a hospice palliative care service. *Cancer Forum*, 1985; **9**: 101–4.
87. Gomez-Batiste X. Catalonia's five year plan: basic principles. *European Journal of Palliative Care*, 1994; **1**: 45–9.
88. Dawson NJ. Need satisfaction in terminal care settings. *Social Science and Medicine*, 1991; **32**: 83–7.
89. Norum J, Wist E. When a cancer patient dies at home: experience of the relatives. *Kreftavdelingen Recionsykehuset; Tromso Tidsskrift for den Norske Laegeforening*, 1993; **113**: 1107–9.
90. Cavenagh JD, Gunz FW. Palliative Hospice Care in Australia. *Palliative Medicine*, 1988; **2**: 51–7.
91. Lyon A, Love DR. Terminal care: The role of the general practitioner hospital. *Journal of the Royal College of General Practitioners*, 1984; **34**: 331–3.
92. Thorn CP, *et al.* The influence of general practitioner community hospitals on the place of death of cancer patients. *Palliative Medicine*, 1994; **8**: 122–8.
93. Aldridge D. A team approach to terminal care: personal implications for general practitioners. *Journal of the Royal College of General Practitioners*, 1987; **37**: 364.
94. Smith AM, Eve A, Sykes NP. Palliative Care survey in Britain and Ireland 1990—an overview. *Palliative Medicine*, 1992; **6**: 277–91.
95. Gray D, MacAdam, Boldy D. A comparative cost analysis of terminal cancer care in home hospice patients and controls. *Journal of Chronic Diseases*, 1987; **40**: 807–10.
96. National Council for Hospice and Specialist Palliative Care Services. *Guidelines for Voluntary Hospices Contracting with the National Health Service*. Occasional Paper No. 1, June 1992.
97. National Council for Hospice and Specialist Palliative Care Services. *Quality, Standards, Organizational and Clinical Audit for Hospice and Palliative Care Services*. Occasional Paper No. 2, Nov. 1992.
98. National Council for Hospice and Specialist Palliative Care Services. *Needs Assessment for Hospice and Specialist Palliative Care Services: From Philosophy to Contracts*. Occasional Paper No. 4, Dec. 1993.
99. National Council for Hospice and Specialist Palliative Care Services. *Opening Doors*. Occasional Paper No. 6, 1995.
100. *Palliative Care Guidelines*. Palliative Care Services. Health Services and Promotion Branch, Department of Health and Welfare, Canada. 1989
101. Parkes CM. Terminal care: evaluation of an advisory domiciliary service at St. Christopher's Hospice. *Postgraduate Medical Journal*, 1980; **56**: 685–9.
102. National Council for Hospice and Specialist Palliative Care Services. *Education in Palliative Care*. Occasional Paper No. 9, 1996.
103. National Council for Hospice and Specialist Palliative Care Services. *Key Ethical Issues in Palliative Care: Evidence to House of Lords Select Committee on Medical Ethics*. Occasional Paper No. 3, July 1993.
104. National Council for Hospice and Specialist Palliative Care Services. *Research in Palliative Care: the Pursuit of Reliable Knowledge*. Occasional Paper No. 5, April 1994.
105. *Palliative Care for Adults with Cancer in the West Midlands: A Framework for Good Practice*. A Report of a Multidisciplinary Working Party. September 1995. NHS Executive, West Midlands, Birmingham, UK.
106. National Council for Hospice and Specialist Palliative Care Services. *Dilemmas and Directions: The Future of Palliative Care*. Occasional Paper No. 11, 1996.
107. National Council for Hospice and Specialist Palliative Care Services. *Palliative Care in the Hospital Setting 1996*. Occasional Paper No. 10, 1997.
108. National Council for Hospice and Specialist Palliative Care Services. *Feeling Better: Psychosocial Care in Specialist Palliative Care*. Occasional Paper No. 13, 1997.
109. National Council for Hospice and Specialist Palliative Care Services. *Making Palliative Care Better: Quality Improvement, Multiprofessional Audit and Standards*. Occasional Paper No. 12, 1997.

2.5 The economics of palliative care

M.A. Robbins

Introduction

There are three questions which are increasingly being asked of every health-care intervention: Does it really work? Is it value for money? How should it be organized in the future? Searching for the answers to these interconnected questions has become an important health services research task as politicians and policy-makers emphasize that health budgets are finite. Faced with increasingly expensive health technologies, ageing populations, and rising public expectations of health care, cost-containment policies focus attention on minimal levels of health care which are effective, cost effective, and acceptable, and which meet assessed population needs. Similar questions about rationing and priority setting in health care are being asked across the world, but particularly in Europe, North America, and Australasia.[1]

Palliative care services have developed in a rapid and relatively uncoordinated manner over the past 25 years. As a popular concept and philosophy of care, the 'hospice' was taken up and developed at local levels, albeit supported by national charities, cancer foundations, and religious orders, rather than being developed within general health service frameworks. Current patterns of palliative care provision reflect this bottom-up approach. Groups of committed individuals have been able to mobilize significant amounts of voluntary and charitable support to subsidize or replace the mainstream or conventional care offered to terminally ill and dying patients. Inevitably, substantial variation in the range and type of palliative care provision has arisen between localities and regions, and the extent to which national funding has been secured has reflected variable appreciation of the need for this specialized sector of care.

However, more general acceptance of the principles of palliative care and the increasing integration of the voluntary hospice–palliative care sector into the mainstream has produced a range of questions concerning the model (or combination of models) of palliative care that offers the best quality care for dying patients and their relatives, and that will be financially sustainable in the future. These questions are not straightforward, because the choices and trajectories of dying are infinitely varied leading to practical problems in assessing the need for palliative care, and they are also conceptually linked to societal values concerning best practice in the management of terminal illness, dying, and death.

We begin this chapter by describing funding policies for palliative care services in a range of health care systems, principally in Europe and North America, and then move on to a consideration of more formal methods of cost analysis in palliative care. The demands that economic evaluation places on robust and repeatable research methodology are reviewed. Finally, attention is directed to the processes of priority setting and health policy as they relate to palliative care services.

National funding policies for palliative care

Overview

In this chapter we are principally concerned with the economics of palliative care services in the richer countries of the world. In many less developed countries, there have been efforts to establish palliative care services and to draw attention to the problem of cancer pain. However, where per capita expenditures on health care are minimal and general health care services are underdeveloped, the economics of palliative care represent a largely peripheral and academic debate. However, rising health-care costs in the richer countries have forced a move towards cost-effective purchasing and, in relation to palliative care, fundamental questions concerning the balance between voluntary and statutory funding, and the priority given to palliative care funding within the total demands on health care budgets.

United Kingdom

The specialist palliative care sector in the United Kingdom largely grew out of the hospice movement which gathered momentum in the early 1970s. The opening of St Christopher's Hospice in 1967 has been credited with initiating a world-wide hospice movement, much of which has followed the United Kingdom example by depending on charitable funding for its establishment. There is now a complex web of financial support for the specialist palliative care sector in the United Kingdom. Independent hospices receive a mixture of funding; a considerable amount comes from local fund-raising, and some is received in the form of grants and contracts from public funds, directed through purchasing authorities. Palliative care services located within the National Health Service are additionally supported (and 'pump-primed') by the charitable foundations as well as by local hospices. Nurses, doctors, and other therapists move between all sectors, taking their skills, developed and paid for in one sector, into another sector and sometimes back again.

Formal statutory support of the independent hospice sector was established in 1987, with the allocation of limited 'ring-fenced' vouchsafed funds administered through district health authorities. This was accompanied by the requirement that health authorities should review their palliative care services and plan future developments in partnership with the voluntary sector, with the recommendation that health authority support for hospices should approach the 50 per cent level,[2] which has generally not been achieved. The government's special allocation to hospices came to an end in the financial year 1993–1994, with the expectation that the contracting process of the newly reorganized National Health Service would provide the machinery for the long-term funding of hospices and other specialist palliative care services.[3]

At present, many independent hospices have entered into contracts with their local purchasers (which may be single health authorities or a number of authorities which have formed joint commissioning agencies) to supply specified volumes and types of palliative care to district residents. The revenue supplied by such contracts may amount to 30 or 40 per cent (or more) of the running costs of such hospices, with the remainder being raised through donations, legacies, and fund-raising (for example, the charity shops of some hospices are able to raise 10 to 20 per cent of total income[4]). As well as providing inpatient beds, many hospices provide day-care facilities, outpatient clinics, domiciliary medical support, bereavement follow-up, and home care nursing (ranging from advisory only to 24-h hands-on nursing). Differing combinations and volumes of all these types of activities may be specified in contracts with local purchasers.

Other forms of palliative care provision which are subsidized by the voluntary sector include hospital and primary care advisory palliative care nurses. Some of these posts have been funded initially by Cancer Relief Macmillan Fund on the understanding that the health care trust (and ultimately the health authority purchaser) will contribute long-term funding (for example, after 3 years). To acknowledge the source of the initial funding, such nurses may be called Macmillan nurses. Full-time and sessional medical posts have also been funded by the charities to expand the hospital-based provision of palliative care. Community nursing support is subsidized by Marie Curie Cancer Care which provides 50 per cent of the costs of home nurses (called Marie Curie nurses) who offer principally night nursing services to terminally ill patients who are being principally cared for at home by the primary health care team. The remaining 50 per cent of the costs are met by the National Health Service health care trust which manages the community nursing service. While the Marie Curie service has traditionally been limited to patients with terminal cancer, since 1994 Marie Curie nurses have been available to help in the home care of patients with any terminal illness, although all the costs then have to be borne by the health care trust.

As well as being a major provider of palliative care, the United Kingdom voluntary palliative care sector has also taken a major lead in education and training. The cancer charities (for example, Cancer Relief Macmillan Fund, Marie Curie Cancer Care, Help the Hospices, and Europe Against Cancer) have funded research and teaching posts in United Kingdom universities and hospitals as well as supporting conferences, training events, and the development of teaching material. Many of the independent hospices have developed educational centres and now offer courses to a wide range of health care professionals, including nursing home staff.

Although the charitable and voluntary sector has played a large part in the development and expansion of specialist palliative care services, hospice care funded by the National Health Service has also been a feature of the United Kingdom specialist palliative care sector. Currently, 533 hospice beds are provided in 46 National Health Service hospice units, which represents about 20 per cent of overall hospice provision.[5] In addition to the National Health Service specialist palliative care sector (which also includes hospital-based palliative care teams) there is the provision of non-specialist palliative care which is far more difficult to quantify. Palliative care services can be 'generalist' when they are provided by a range of clinicians in the primary and secondary care sectors during the course of routine medical and nursing care. Many of these clinicians have specialist qualifications in palliative care but do not work as specialists, although they bring their skills and experience to each patient encounter. This may be particularly noteworthy in community nursing teams operating in the primary care setting where many nurses will have completed training in care of the dying or bereavement counselling, and where they feel that the differences between themselves and the specialist palliative care providers lie in the availability of time and resources rather than expertise and approach.

One of the main features of the National Health Service reforms of 1990 was the new purchasing role of district health authorities. This brought the question of costs and funding policies into sharper focus. District authority purchasers are now responsible for assessing the health care needs of their populations and buying the range of services which meet these needs, increasingly in collaboration with social service purchasers and general practitioner fund-holders. Thus health purchasing, as this process is termed, involves 'buying the best value for money services to achieve the maximum health gain for those most in need'.[6] Over the years since the reforms, understanding of the commissioning, purchasing, and contracting aspects of the internal market has developed and expanded. Early contracts were based on previous patterns of activity, and by necessity had to be 'block' contracts in the absence of detailed purchasing information. Future contracts are likely to be more sophisticated, to reflect strategy, and also to be less provider-driven, with a greater understanding of the cost-effectiveness of services.

The implications of these changes for palliative care services are significant, particularly in relation to needs assessment. While different approaches to needs assessment have been identified (for example, the comparative and corporate approaches[3]), the Department of Health approach emphasizes the population-based assessment of need and uses the term 'epidemiologically based needs assessment'.[7] This rests on a triadic model, with measures of prevalence and incidence at one corner, evidence concerning effectiveness and cost-effectiveness at the second, and knowledge of existing services at the third. It is asserted that these three components form the basis of 'triangulation' whereby 'purchasers can determine the policy directions they wish to pursue'.[7]

The broad-based nature of palliative care is a source of difficulty to health authorities in their attempts to assess service needs. Not only does the palliative care sector overlap with other care sectors (e.g. care of the elderly), but there is also confusion over the boundaries between specialist and non-specialist palliative care. Traditionally, specialist palliative care has been offered to people who are terminally ill with cancer. However, not all terminally ill people with cancer require such services, and it is asserted that other patients who are terminally ill with non-malignant disease would benefit from specialist palliative care input.[8] It has also been suggested that the specialist palliative care approach can also benefit patients who are not imminently terminally ill.[9] The triadic model of needs assessment also requires information relating to service provision, incidence and prevalence figures, and evidence of effectiveness and cost-effectiveness. However, health authorities face considerable difficulty in amassing this kind of intelligence since most descriptions of specialist palliative care services emphasize the variation between different localities. It is also very difficult to estimate from routine statistics the proportion of the population likely to benefit from different types and amounts of specialist palliative care input, since the need for palliative care is related to symptomatology (and often social circumstances) rather than the disease categories which are used for classification. Finally, evidence relating to the effectiveness of palliative care as a personal service as opposed to the effectiveness of different components of the service (e.g. methods of pain relief) is lacking, particularly in the form of evidence from randomized controlled trials.

Evidence is increasing that the contractual (or service agreement) arrangements with specialist palliative care providers reflect a picture of uncertainty over this care sector. Guidance from the National Health Service Executive exhorts health authorities to enter into 3-year contracts for hospice care where possible 'in order to ensure stability of funding and service provision'.[10] One recent study of district health authority contracts reveals that over half the contracts examined (63 per cent) were limited to 1 year, with wide variation between health authorities in their requirements for clinical audit, statistical returns, and service specifications.[11] Some districts appear to be considerably more proactive and supportive of specialist palliative care service than others.

There is now no national funding policy for palliative care services in the United Kingdom. Although national guidance is offered (for example the *Policy Framework for Commissioning Cancer Services* which includes core palliative care services[12]), health purchasers are given 'free-ish' rein to develop local health strategies and priorities. The creation and dissemination of nationally applicable guidelines and recommendations is now more likely to derive from the major cancer charities and non-governmental organizations such as the National Council for Hospice and Specialist Palliative Care Services.

United States of America

The first hospice programme in the United States was established in 1974 and was funded by the National Cancer Institute. The hospice philosophy and approach became popular, and the number of programmes had risen to 516 by 1983 and to 1700 by 1989.[13] Owing to the funding structure of the American health care system (insurance-based rather than centrally funded from public taxation), costs have always been higher up the policy agenda. When insurance companies took on the funding of palliative care services, more attention was paid to the prediction and containment of costs as well as value for money.

During the late 1970s and early 1980s, the principles and practice of hospice care became more widely known at the same time as it was realized that high-technology acute-hospital-based care of the dying could well be inappropriate and needlessly expensive. In the United States, more than in the United Kingdom at this time, hospice care was quickly seen as a way of reducing the costs of terminal illness. It was believed that the emphasis on less aggressive and less interventionist care that was not based in an acute hospital would reduce costs. Partly on this assumption, in 1983 Medicare (insurance coverage for those aged over 65) extended its cover to include care provided by hospice programmes. Hospice programmes were required to become certified to become eligible for Medicare funding, and the care packages that they were subsequently able to offer terminally ill patients and their families were quite closely circumscribed. For example, Medicare will reimburse inpatient hospice care only when it does not exceed 20 per cent of the total amount of care offered to a patient.

A number of advantages and disadvantages of the Medicare hospice benefit have been identified over the years since its introduction. Because it is calculated as a *per diem* total cost which does not always cover the costs of care in the final period (when they are highest), there is a tendency to introduce hospice care earlier in the course of terminal illness (when the actual costs are likely to be lower than the daily rate) in order to compensate for the later costs.[14,15] In addition, the close financial management and control required for licensing have been viewed as a disincentive to innovation and experiment; processes which might be regarded as part of the hospice philosophy of helping each patient to find his or her own path through terminal illness. When the Medicare Hospice Benefit was introduced in 1983, only half the existing hospice programmes applied for Medicare certification, although by 1990 this had increased to two out of every three hospice programmes (996 out of 1500),[13] implying that Medicare reimbursement was important to the running of many hospice programmes across the United States.

Although, like their British counterparts, American hospice programmes developed inpatient units in the early 1970s and 1980s, by 1990 many of these had been closed. The emphasis shifted more clearly onto home care, which is regarded as possible in about 95 per cent of cases.[13] Day hospice facilities are also increasing, and attention is being focused on the incorporation of hospice-style care into care of the elderly, particularly nursing home care. A feature of hospice programmes in the United States has been the comparative absence of significant medical (physician) input in their running and service delivery. As Walsh puts it, 'many patients referred to hospice programs are never again seen by a physician during the remainder of their illness'.[14] The reasons for this are varied, but it is interesting to note in the context of this chapter that the development of hospital-based palliative care teams is viewed as a way of increasing physician involvement as well as integrating palliative care into medical speciality care. In Cleveland, Ohio, the hospital palliative care service is part of medical oncology, and financial viability is assured by billing for services as medical oncology consultations.[14]

Although starting with a common approach, hospice programmes in the United States and the United Kingdom have developed differently. Cost containment and financial viability have been stronger pressures on the models of care in the United States, with a resulting stronger emphasis on nurse-led home care services.

The increasing integration of the principles of palliative care into the discipline of oncology may bring significant alternative funding streams to the palliative care sector in the future.

Other countries

A review of national funding policies for palliative care in every country in the world that has adopted the principles and practice of the hospice movement is outside the scope of this chapter. Instead, a number of issues influencing funding policies that have emerged in different countries can be outlined. As mentioned in the Introduction, societal values concerning best practice in the management of terminal illness and death will affect the expansion of palliative care services as well as the availability of financial resources. Without public understanding, sympathy, and support, the hospice approach may not be valued as a help during terminal illness nor benefit from the voluntary support that has accompanied its expansion elsewhere. Denial of cancer diagnosis and stoicism in the face of terminal illness can limit the extent to which doctors and nurses can intervene, and where health resources are perceived to be scarce, expenditure on people with incurable illness may not be socially sanctioned. In the past World Health Organization policies on the availability of analgesics for cancer pain have faced such social and institutional barriers as fear of opioid dependence and the priority given to curative treatment.[16]

In many countries, however, the hospice approach has been quickly embraced and resources invested in the development of palliative care teams. Hospices were established in the 1970s in New Zealand, Australia, and Canada, and palliative care teams developed in many of the European countries as well as the Far East during the 1980s. The 1990s have seen limited palliative care services developing in South American countries, India, and in some African countries (South Africa established palliative care services earlier). In most countries the funding of specialist palliative care services reflects a mixture of charitable, private, and state support. However, the creation of an additional network of care for the dying, as has occurred in the United Kingdom, is not a model that all countries wish to follow. It is planned that hospice principles should be adopted by the public health systems in the Scandinavian countries, and in Finland the running costs of the few inpatient hospice units are met by the communes and the state.[17]

The capital investment needed to build inpatient hospice units has focused attention on alternative ways of providing provision. The conversion of convalescent wards in existing hospitals has proved to be one way of redeploying health care resources to the care of the terminally ill.[18] Using existing hospital provision as well as reorganizing oncology services so that they embrace the principles of palliative care are ways in which integration with mainstream health care can contribute to the financial viability of palliative care initiatives, although this approach inevitably brings dilemmas in the management, philosophy, control, and direction of such services.

Cost analysis in palliative care

Health economics

Cost-effective health care purchasing in the United Kingdom, the United States, and other countries has become more important over the past few decades as rising health technology costs are forcing choices to be made between competing types of health care provision. The evaluation of health care interventions has become necessary in order to inform any rationing decisions that have to be made. It has commonly been observed that many current health care interventions have not been assessed for their effectiveness and efficiency, and that other services of proven effectiveness could be expanded if the waste inherent in current practice could be eradicated.[1]

Health care evaluation is approached from a number of angles and uses a range of outcome indicators. Clinical effectiveness can be assessed according to criteria of disease abatement, reduction of symptoms, objective tumour response, survival, post-treatment complications, and so on. A social evaluation may involve an assessment of the impact of an intervention on quality of life including social functioning, resumption of employment or usual activities, and a range of psychological indicators, as well as patient and carer preferences and satisfaction. Increasingly, however, economic evaluation is regarded as an important dimension of assessing the effectiveness of health care. In this section of the chapter we first discuss the different kinds of economic evaluation that can be performed, and then review some of the ways in which cost analysis has been carried out in relation to palliative care.

In essence, economic evaluation involves a comparison of the costs (resources) and benefits (outcomes or outputs) of alternative treatment options, and theoretically can provide useful information to purchasers about which interventions represent best value for money. A number of concepts are important to the health economist: scarcity, opportunity cost, and margin. Resource allocation always starts with the assumption that resources are scarce and will never be sufficient to meet all demands. Opportunity cost is the benefit that a resource (cost) could have generated if it had been used in the best alternative manner. Margin relates to the idea that alternatives in health care generally concern service additions or reductions, rather than an all-or-nothing situation. Underlying these concepts is a concern with utilitarian ethics.

The principles of economic evaluation are clearly and extensively described elsewhere.[19-25] In brief there are four main types of evaluation, all of which involve comparing the costs (resource inputs) and consequences (outcomes) of alternative interventions. Thus all economic evaluation is based on comparison and on seeking to put a value on the opportunity cost of one intervention in relation to alternative (even dissimilar) ones. A full economic evaluation should take the view of society in general when considering costs and benefits, no matter to whom they accrue, thus accounting for direct, indirect, and intangible costs. For the purposes of health care purchasing this wider-based perspective may be replaced with the perspective of the agency responsible for funding. Purchasers may decide to include only direct treatment costs and ignore non-medical costs, the indirect costs to patients and their families, and intangible costs (iatrogenic effects).

Cost-minimization analysis

Cost-minimization analysis is considered to be the simplest form of economic evaluation where the direct costs of interventions are compared, assuming that the outcomes or consequences are equal. The intervention which costs least is taken to be the most efficient. The direct costs of two kinds of palliative care delivery can be compared using this kind of analysis only if the outcomes can reasonably be assumed to be similar. Methodologically, as discussed below, outcome measurement is complex because of the interacting and multilayered nature of multidisciplinary palliative care. This in turn requires multidimensional measurement from different perspectives.[26,27] Cost-minimization analysis cannot be performed without prior evidence of equivalence of such multidimensional outcomes.

Cost–effectiveness analysis

A way of valuing the health care resources used in alternative interventions when outcomes are known to differ is to reduce the outcomes to some kind of natural unit, for example a pain-free day or a life saved or a life-year gained. Such units can then be compared in relation to the resource costs. Simple cost–effectiveness analyses use one dimension of outcome for ease of comparison, but it is also possible to consider multiple outcomes and present a range of dimensions (e.g. clinical effectiveness after a period of follow-up, incidence of postintervention complications, patient satisfaction).

Cost–utility analysis

Cost–utility analysis goes one step further than cost–effectiveness analysis by comparing the costs of different procedures with their outcome measures in utility-based rather than natural units. The derivation of utility-based units involves a subjective evaluation on the part of the subject as to the quality of their health status or well being, i.e. their quality of life. This goes beyond cost effectiveness by attaching a value to the life-year gained or the pain-free day. The most widely used utility-based measure in cost–utility analysis is the quality-adjusted life-year (QALY), although other measures have been developed such as the Euroqol, healthy year equivalents, and saved young life equivalent.[28]

Cost–benefit analysis

Cost–benefit analyses have a longer history than the other types of economic evaluation, as they have been used in public sector investment planning for many years.[23] Efficiency is measured in monetary terms at both the input and the output (outcome) stage. In this type of analysis it is assumed that every aspect of a health intervention can be valued using a monetary unit, i.e. that a cost in pounds or dollars can be attached to an inpatient stay or a community nursing visit. Cost–benefit analysis has been a popular approach because of its potential for comparison across different forms of health care and returns on investments in other areas of the economy. However, the emphasis on monetary evaluation has led to reservations about the flexibility, scope, and ethics of this approach.

Inputs and outputs

All four types of economic evaluation described above begin with an analysis of resource costs, and indeed many cost analyses go no further than the estimation of these as they do not have the effectiveness (outcomes) evidence to perform an evaluation. The calculation of direct inputs is itself a major task, and it becomes more complex when non-medical, societal, and psychological costs are calculated additionally.

Direct costs can be divided into those which are medical (or treatment-related) and those which are non-medical 'out-of-pocket' expenses. Direct medical costs include medical, nursing, pharmacy, hotel, capital, and marginal costs which are common to all forms of health care. The types of non-medical costs that should be considered are those borne by the patient and family, and include travel costs, extra fuel consumption for heating, air conditioning, lighting, and appliances, special foods and drinks, laundry, bedding, and cleaning costs, special furniture, aids, and equipment that are purchased rather than borrowed, private nursing costs, and so on. Indirect costs are those associated with the loss of productive time incurred by either the patient or the family as a result of the treatment, while intangible costs relate to the pain and suffering caused by the treatment.

In order to undertake economic evaluation, information is required on the consequences of the interventions being compared. As described above, outcomes can be measured in different kinds of units—natural units such as pain-free days, utility units such as perceived states of health, or actual monetary units. Therefore the choice of outcome indicators and units of measurement is of fundamental importance. Many cost comparisons are carried out on the assumption that outcomes are equivalent. However, without evidence of outcome measurement, such cost analyses are of dubious worth, relying as they do on assertion, prejudice, and rhetoric to justify the costs. Economic evaluation allows the comparison of costs according to clearly defined outcome indicators.

Comparisons of palliative care services

An economic evaluation of palliative care may seek to compare any of the following alternative models of delivery.

1. Comparisons within a specialist palliative care service, for example inpatient hospice care compared with home care services (ranging from advisory nursing services to 'hospice at home').

2. Comparisons between specialist palliative care services, for example one independent hospice service compared with another, or a hospital palliative care team (as part of oncology services) compared with an independent hospice service.

3. Comparisons between specialist palliative care services and conventional (mainstream) services, for example a hospital palliative care team compared with general hospital care, hospice services (both inpatient and home-based) compared with hospital services, and community-based hospice services compared with community-based conventional care.

Which kind of economic analysis is carried out (cost minimization, effectiveness, utility, or benefit) will depend on the particular question being posed, by whom, and for what purpose.

A review of the literature on economic analyses of palliative care services reveals that very few economic evaluations have actually been performed. Tables 1 and 2 present summaries of a number of studies which have attempted to compare costs for different specialist palliative care services, and for specialist palliative care services and conventional services. Very few have collected outcomes data in addition to direct costs data (generally medical costs) to enable cost-effectiveness, cost–utility or cost–benefit analyses to be carried out. These studies reveal a series of methodological and theoretical problems which face cost analyses in palliative care.

Table 1 Comparisons of specialist palliative care services

Type of care examined	Type of study	Sample size	Country	Derivations of costs measured	Outcomes measured?	Reference	Main conclusions
Inpatient hospice units	Survey	20 hospices in 1984 40 hospices in 1989	UK	Financial costs relative to inpatient care Capital costs excluded	No	4, 29.	Cost per bed per week higher in units with lower numbers of beds. Costs rise with units having over 30 beds. Unable to comment on whether hospice care is cheaper than hospital care, nor whether NHS hospice care is cheaper than independent hospice care owing to incompatible and unavailable data
Home care service and hospital care of advanced cancer patients (both groups receiving palliative care)	Quasi-experimental study	30 hospital patients with input from palliative care team 30 patients cared for by home palliative care service	Italy	Medical, nursing, institutional, and family expenses	Yes	30	Clinical outcomes similar in the home care group compared with the hospital group, but better scores on psychosocial parameters. Costs of a day's home care was \$37.4 (1987) compared with \$261.4 mean daily cost for inpatient care
Hospice services	Survey	11 hospices	Scotland	Volunteer input, admissions, services, staffing details (divided total cost of running the unit from annual financial statement, by measure of activity — crude average cost per case)	No	31	No sound conclusions can be made from the data — accounting policies vary between hospices (a feature of the charitable sector). Better to build up episodic costs for patients in each hospice
Hospice services	In-depth case study	1 independent hospice 1 NHS hospice	Scotland	Calculated costs involved in caring for individual patients. Direct and indirect costs, fixed overhead costs	Yes	32	Overall costs between the two hospices not found to be substantially different. However medical overheads were higher in the NHS hospice, whereas administrative costs per patient were four times higher in the independent hospice. More time was spent by staff in the independent hospice in direct patient care. Great variability in *per capita* costs within and between units.

Measuring costs

In relation to calculating the direct costs of palliative care, the costs of volunteer input have proved a point of contention.[38] The ratio of paid staff to volunteer staff in hospice programmes in the United States has been noted to range from 1:1 to 1:5,[39] possibly reflecting the specification of Medicare reimbursement that 5 per cent of hospice programme services must be provided by volunteers. A number of studies have examined the volunteer role in detail[40,41] and have identified four types of volunteer: administrative workers, direct carers, counsellors, and ancillary workers engaging in domestic, reception, gardening, building maintenance and driving roles. Field and Johnson[40] found that 30 per cent of the 276 volunteers that they contacted who worked for one hospice in the United Kingdom also carried out voluntary work for other charities, and were predominantly relatively affluent older women. Influences on becoming a hospice volunteer included experiencing the death of a close relative or friend.

Two observations relating to the costing of volunteer input can be made. One, which is also made by Whynes,[38] is that hospices that can substitute volunteer labour for paid labour will lower their nominal care costs per patient. However, given the variation between hospices with respect to their volunteer lists and patterns of utilization, comparisons between hospice programmes in terms of their nominal care costs will have an almost unquantifiable inexactness. This observation has been supported by others.[4,31] The second point is that, although the concept of opportunity cost is conventionally applied to volunteer input (i.e. if volunteers do not work for one charity or cause then they are likely to donate their time and resources to another), it may be a different case when applied to volunteers in hospice programmes. It is conceivable that

Table 2 Comparisons of specialist palliative care services and conventional care

Type of care examined	Type of study	Sample size	Country	Derivations of costs measured	Outcomes measured?	Reference	Main conclusions
Hospice compared with conventional care	Randomized controlled trial	137 hospice patients 110 control patients	USA	Hospital billing estimates, hospital utilization data, inpatient charts	Yes	33	Hospice care not cheaper than conventional care. Only difference in satisfaction — implies that hospice patients and their carers appreciated the qualitative difference in hospice care. Only one hospice studied
Hospice home care compared with conventional care	Retrospective population-based survey	152 hospice patients 1397 conventional care patients	USA	Medicare Part A and Blue Cross hospital insurance claims	No	34	When dying patients are shifted from conventional care to hospice care, hospital use decreased by 50%, home visits increased 10-fold. Savings of about 40% over conventional care. Unclear whether this was patient selection or hospice effect
Hospice home care compared with conventional care	Retrospective case–control	98 who died with hospice service 98 who died without	Australia	Bed day costs, services procedures, and investigations	No	35	Bed day costs account for greatest proportion of total costs. No significant difference in costs between home hospice and non-home hospice patients. Results only generalizable to patients dying of cancers which have relatively short survival times. Hospice care is labour intensive and will never be cheap for that reason
Demonstration home and hospital hospice care compared with non-demonstration hospice care and conventional care	Quasi-experimental	1754 total 833 home care 624 hospital-based 297 conventional care	USA	Health service utilization data obtained from the primary care person. Medicare and other reimbursement records, hospice inpatient and home care unit cost coefficients. Medicare hospital reporting data	Yes	36	Hospice home care patients less costly to care for than conventional care patients in last year of life. Hospital-based hospice patients also but to lesser extent. Because of patient selection unable to establish the effect of hospice care
Hospice care compared with conventional care	Quasi-experimental	65 hospice patients 55 conventional care patients	Australia	Marginal costs of direct patient care (as well as hotel and administrative costs)	Yes	37	Some improvements in some measures of patient care. No reduction in cost to community. Equivalence between hospice care and best traditional care

people are attracted to volunteering for hospice work because of a specific set of beliefs and motivations which might not necessarily apply to other charitable work. In addition, since many of the volunteers have themselves been bereaved, there may be a therapeutic dimension to working in the hospice programme, i.e. personal gains to the volunteers, which implies further complexity in the calculation of benefits.

It is important to take the non-medical direct costs of palliative care into account, particularly when the impact of home care programmes is being assessed. The cost savings believed to accrue to certain types of home care when compared with inpatient care derive from the transfer of the hotel, capital, and caring costs (of hospital care) to the patient and his or her household.

In insurance-based health systems, the payment of both inadequately covered medical costs and out-of-pocket expenses can cause major family anxiety. An American study carried out by Lansky *et al.* in 1979[42] examined the non-medical costs of childhood cancer and reported that for half of the families surveyed the total expenses plus loss of pay amounted to more than 25 per cent of the weekly income. A similar study conducted amongst adult American cancer patients receiving outpatient chemotherapy found that 14 per cent of the patients were estimated to be spending more than 50 per cent of their weekly incomes on non-medical expenses, and these patients were found to be in the lower-income categories.[43] Similar expenditure of high proportions of weekly income on out-of-pocket expenses was found by a British study of the families of children referred to the regional oncology centre at Birmingham Children's Hospital.[44]

Work still needs to be done on the calculation of non-medical costs during terminal illness and how these are affected by the different models of palliative care delivery. Keeping diaries which itemize household costs can be an additional burden for carers at a time of stress, and may be subject to a low and selective compliance rate. However, without estimations of such costs, the real impact of transferring substantial amounts of care into the community will remain hidden.

Although indirect costs are generally defined as the costs associated with the loss of productive time when caring roles are taken on by members of the household (e.g. taking time away from salaried work), the cost of leisure time forgone may also come into this category, although this is more difficult to quantify and classify. Attention has been drawn to the opportunity costs of cancer treatment which have otherwise been neglected, i.e. the opportunity costs of time spent on treatment (receiving chemotherapy, attending outpatient appointments, and so on).[45]

By their nature, intangible costs (meaning the pain and suffering associated with medical treatment) are difficult to measure and translate into monetary units. In the transition from aggressive curative treatment to active palliative treatment, and from there to less interventionist supportive care, it is important to assess the impact of continuing medical interventions, even when the expected time of survival is short. Scheithauer *et al.*[46] conducted a randomized comparison of combination chemotherapy plus supportive care with supportive care alone in patients with metastatic colorectal cancer, using the Functional Living Index—Cancer (FLIC) to assess quality of life. Although only a small number of patients (40) were studied, preliminary findings indicated that there was increased survival in the chemotherapy group and that the overall quality of life for asymptomatic patients was at least as good as that for patients receiving supportive care, and was better in symptomatic patients. It is precisely in this area, where conventional wisdom may assume that the toxicity associated with invasive (and expensive) therapy is likely to be associated with a decline in quality of life and to bring unacceptable iatrogenic costs, that more sophisticated evaluation needs to be performed and placed in a wider policy context. This area where continuing treatment can be perceived as overtreatment, but where patient choice also has to be respected, has been explored in a collection of papers on cost versus benefit in cancer care.[47]

Measuring outcomes

There are two related questions in the setting of appropriate outcome indicators. First, what outcome indicator(s) arbitrate(s) between good and unacceptable quality? Second, how can such indicator(s) be measured in a reliable and valid fashion? Cure- and recovery-related indicators are clearly inappropriate in palliative care, and the practical and ethical difficulties of researching terminally ill patients have been well rehearsed.[48] Such problems have contributed to the current scarcity of experimental evaluations of palliative care, and the consequent lack of data on effectiveness. It has been more common to undertake observational and descriptive studies which, while illuminating and disclosing, have not been able to address the more rigorous hypotheses questioning the value of specialist palliative care, hospice care, and other psychosocial interventions in relation to each other and to conventional or mainstream care.

There are increasing numbers of texts describing the range of health status and quality-of-life instruments which can be used in outcome measurement.[28,49–52] Such accounts discuss the psychometric qualities of disease-specific measures, measures of functional status, and generic quality-of-life indices and scales. Those of interest in relation to palliative care include specific measures for assessing symptom levels (including pain), measures to assess psychological morbidity, functional dependency scales, and scales that attempt to assess overall quality of life. Other domains which relate to quality of life are social functioning and satisfaction (e.g. location of care, adequacy of information and advice, and the care given by professionals), as well as spiritual comfort.

Outcome measures are generally patient based, although both professional and lay carers can be used as surrogates when patients are too incapacitated to answer for themselves. The validity of measurement by proxy has been discussed by Higginson *et al.*[53] in relation to one study using the Support Team Assessment Schedule. The study found that ratings by the palliative care team were usually closer to those of the patients than to those of the family member, although all parties demonstrated differences in their perceptions of problems. However, patient-derived scores may not constitute the only measure of effectiveness; staff perceptions of the quality of care (in terms of both its process and outcome) may also be utilized, as well as the perceptions of patients' lay carers (an approach used in surveys of bereaved carers[54]). Thus the question of whose perspective is used in the evaluation of palliative care is fundamental when setting parameters of effectiveness.

Specialist and conventional care

Many types of palliative care seek not to replace mainstream (or conventional) services with a completely alternative system of care, but to augment, complement, and fill in gaps present in mainstream care. In this sense, many palliative care services (e.g. advisory home-care nursing services and hospital symptom control teams) aim to work alongside the mainstream health-care professionals, and to offer specialist expertise, extra time, and resources. Working with other health professionals has also been an objective in the wider dissemination of palliative care principles and practice. Even when some palliative care services appear to take over the complete care of terminally ill patients, they do so against the backdrop and context of the wider health-care system.

Therefore the 'pure' effect of palliative care input may be very difficult to distinguish at both the structural and the patient level. Under palliative care, the individual requirements of each patient are met through a unique package of care that is reassessed as the illness progresses. Part of the difficulty of evaluating a 'service' is that it is made up of different components which are offered in different ways and volumes to meet personal circumstances and personal preferences. In addition to service variability, there is the fact of patient variability and the possibility that patients who choose or accept hospice care are systematically different from those who do not.

Several studies have noted the lower costs of hospice home care compared with conventional care,[34,36] but were not able to conclude that it was the hospice effect that was responsible for the lowered costs. Instead, it was plausible that the patients enrolled in the hospice programmes were generally low utilizers of health care services anyway. The randomized controlled trial methodology theoretically circumvents these problems, but is not easy to apply in this field. There has been one randomized controlled trial of hospice care in the United States,[33] performed in the early 1980s, which failed to show major cost differentials between hospice and conventional care. However, it was limited to only one hospice service. More recently, a randomized controlled trial of a palliative home care service in Canada was attempted, but failed to reach its sample size.[55] The problems faced by those designing randomized controlled trials lie primarily in recruitment and obtaining consent. Referrals to palliative care services come from other clinicians who may exercise judgement over who is referred, and patients can also be self-selecting in that some will not want all the services on offer from a palliative care team. The resulting sample of patients who are randomized into receiving or not receiving palliative care may already be unrepresentative of the general population of terminally ill patients, making cost comparisons more difficult to perform. The problem of patient selectivity remains a methodological challenge to palliative care researchers.

Philosophy of palliative care

The assumption that palliative care should cost less than conventional care in order to be seen as effective is questionable. Much of the concern with the costs of health care in the last year of life, which has been a feature of the American literature, has over-emphasized the correlation of high costs with the inappropriate use of medical technologies. It was assumed that as hospice care advocated less aggressive care it would therefore be cheaper care. As Emanuel and Emanuel[56] state, 'the persistent interest in saving money at the end of life through the use of advance directives and hospice care makes it imperative to assess how much money might realistically be saved'. However, it has become clear that the greatest cost component during terminal illness is hospital bed occupancy and nursing time, and even the introduction of advance directives (which in general instruct against the use of heroic interventions to postpone death) has not had a significant effect on the cost of the hospital care of terminally-ill patients.[57] The practice of palliative care generally involves increased levels of nursing, medical, and psychosocial assessment, and inpatient hospice care is characterized by high staff-to-patient ratios. The costs of increased patient contact are offset by the use of volunteer labour, but it is clear that the very elements of care that have been found to account for the major costs of terminal illness are those which palliative care services seek to maximize.

Economic evaluation in palliative care should seek to investigate whether the quality of care is such that for each pound or dollar spent on a particular service, considerably more 'health gain' is derived than for each pound or dollar spent on an alternative one. Theoretically, higher service charges which result in very high valuations of service quality could be more cost effective than a service with lower costs which obtained lower valuations. In turn, it then becomes a matter of priority setting as to how much can be spent on palliative care, understanding the kinds of returns that are likely to accrue. At present, however, there has been no research of a sufficiently rigorous nature to enable economic evaluations of the different types of palliative care to be performed.

Health policy in palliative care

Priority setting

Priority setting is not a new activity in the allocation of health care resources; what is new is that health planners are now emphasizing that it should be explicit. To this end, a great deal of interest is now focused on how priorities can be decided, and how to integrate the variety of perspectives and interests that are involved. This process is struggling to reconcile competing pressures on the health services, i.e. that budgets will always be finite, that patients have increasing expectations of health care and their own rights in relation to health care delivery systems, that health technology research continues to develop new and expensive forms of diagnostic tests and treatments, that it is increasingly untenable to expect health care professionals to ration access to treatment without a wider supporting policy structure, and that theories of ethical resource distribution are socially and politically driven.

Internationally, there have been a series of exercises attempting to set explicit priorities in health care. One of the best known is the Oregon Health Plan, which was conceived to replace the system of rationing based on excluding part of the population (the uninsured) with a system based on excluding medical treatments deemed to be low priority (the resource wasters). The plan came into effect in 1994 after extensive research, ranking procedures, and public consultation. The exercise has drawn attention to a range of methodological and practical difficulties,[58] and also demonstrates how such processes cannot take place in the absence of good-quality information on health needs, outcomes data, and costs of services, or without effective methods of involving the public.[59] Attempts have also been made in The Netherlands and New Zealand to define a minimum package of health care that should be universally accessible, but these have also encountered a dearth of research evidence relating to the effectiveness and cost effectiveness of interventions. As Maynard[58] observes, the lack of information on effectiveness means that 'it is difficult to rank interventions and all prioritisation exercises will inevitably be crude and subject to fundamental criticism'.

Thus there is considerable debate at the international level about the methods through which priority setting might be achieved, and also what research is required to provide the necessary evidence. In the United Kingdom, the process of priority setting has recently been investigated by the House of Commons Health Committee, which reported in 1995.[59] The report reiterates the need for an 'honest and realistic set of explicit, well-understood ethical principles at national level to guide the NHS into the next century', building on the basic principles of equity, public choice, and the effective use of health service resources. The report concludes with a manifesto for research rather than a template for priority setting at the national and local level, but emphasizes again that transparency in decision-making, taking full account of the views of all interested parties, is the preferred way forward.

Policy directions in palliative care

The debate on national priority setting reinforces the need for methodological development in palliative care research. As a complicated package of care that crosses boundaries between social and health care, and between primary and secondary care, and where utility measures based on quality of survival time are clearly inappropriate, the methodological challenges of research in palliative care are particularly pressing. The future development of services should clearly be based on the principles of equity, patient choice, and effective use of resources as outlined above in relation to health services in general.

Equity

The accusation that specialist palliative care services have focused on the needs of one group of terminally ill patients (those with malignant disease) to the detriment of others has been taken up in a number of recent publications,[8,60–62] and in response many palliative care services have widened their remit. Needs assessment carried out on the basis of symptomatology and nursing need, domestic circumstances, and psychosocial need may represent a more egalitarian method of targeting resources, particularly home care nursing support. Thus developing and refining methods of needs assessment which are able to model the time-dependent nature of the changing requirements of the terminally ill population is a priority for a palliative care research programme.

Patient choice

The tremendous charitable support for the voluntary hospice sector has been taken as *de facto* evidence of the public's demand and support for this kind of care. As Clark[61] observes of the hospice movement, 'By championing holism and the reform of the dominant system, it attracted massive popular support and colonised a new field of moral concern'. However, if this is the kind of care which the public desire, this is a very strong argument for hospice care becoming a core component of the publicly funded health service. Does willingness to subsidise palliative care through charitable giving and donations not in fact allow national health services to renege on the provision of adequate palliative care for the majority population? It can be argued in these terms that the quicker that palliative care services are integrated into mainstream services, the more likely public choice is to be represented at the macrolevel.

It remains to be investigated just how much public understanding there is of palliative care as a distinct set of caring activities, and what expectations are held of the capacity of the national health services to deliver that care. In the United Kingdom, for example, there has been long acceptance of the pioneering and gap-filling role of voluntary organizations *vis à vis* statutory services,[63] but how far the public accept the increasingly mixed economy of health care, in particular the substitution of a substantial amount of national health service care by the voluntary hospice sector, is unknown.

Effective use of resources

Issues in the measurement of effectiveness and cost effectiveness have already been discussed in this chapter, and it is clear that major research activity should focus on the development of valid and reliable outcome measures in palliative care. The need to develop palliative care research has been recognized for many years in the face of the rapid expansion of services,[64–67] and much has already been achieved. However, the next few years will see increasing pressure for the palliative care sector to justify its 'anecdotal success and emotional appeal',[64] and to demonstrate that 'if one hospice program is good, 1400 are better'.[66]

Conclusion

In the first section of this chapter we discussed national funding policies for palliative care and implied that the importance of public and professional support had been instrumental in the relatively recent development of this sector. However, because of the emphasis on cost containment (particularly in the United States) and cost-effective purchasing, it has become increasingly strategic to evaluate the effectiveness of services to demonstrate that health care resources are not being wasted. In the second section on cost analysis we introduced the principles of economic evaluation and examined how far such methods had been used in palliative care research. A range of methodological problems relating to the calculation of costs were noted, as was the lack of development in multidimensional outcome indicators. In the final section we briefly discussed general issues in priority setting and how these might be applied to palliative care. It would be a mistake to finish this chapter with the impression that palliative care services have been exceptionally underevaluated compared with other interventions. The type of cost-effectiveness data which have proved difficult to derive for palliative care services have also been difficult to derive for many other forms of health care. The challenge ahead is to address the methodological and theoretical barriers to service evaluation.

References

1. Maynard A. The significance of cost-effective purchasing. In: Drummond MF, Maynard A, eds. *Purchasing and Providing Cost-effective Health Care*. Edinburgh: Churchill Livingstone, 1993: 3–15.
2. Contracting with the National Health Service: revised guidelines for voluntary hospices. National Council for Hospice and Specialist Palliative Care Services. Occasional Paper 6. 1994.
3. Neale B, Clark D, Heather P. Purchasing palliative care: a review of the policy and research literature. Occasional Paper 11. Sheffield: Trent Palliative Care Centre. 1993.
4. Hill F, Oliver C. Hospice—an update on the cost of patient care. *Palliative Medicine*, 1989; **3**:119–24.
5. Hospice Information Service. *1995 Directory of Hospice and Palliative Care Services*. London: St Christopher's Hospice, 1995.
6. Øvretveit J. *Purchasing for Health*. Buckingham: Open University Press, 1995.
7. Stevens A, Raftery J. Introduction. In: Stevens A, Raftery J, eds. *Health Care Needs Assessment: The Epidemiologically Based Needs Assessment Reviews*. Oxford: Radcliffe Medical Press, 1994: 11–30.
8. Standing Medical Advisory Committee and Standing Nursing and Midwifery Advisory Committee. *The Principles and Provision of Palliative Care*. London: HMSO, 1993.
9. Davis C, Hardy JR. Palliative care. *British Medical Journal*, 1994; **308**:1359–62.
10. National Health Service Management Executive. *Contracting for Specialist Palliative Care Services*. EL(94)14. London: Department of Health, 1994.
11. Robbins M, Frankel S. Palliative care services: what needs assessment? *Palliative Medicine*, 1995; **9**: 287–94.
12. Expert Advisory group on Cancer. *A Policy Framework for Commissioning Cancer Services*. London: Department of Health, 1994.
13. Magno JB. USA hospice care in the 1990s. *Palliative Medicine*, 1992; **6**:158–65.
14. Walsh TD. Continuing care in a medical center: the Cleveland Clinic Foundation Palliative Care Service. *Journal of Pain and Symptom Management*, 1990; **5**:273–8.
15. Baker M. Cost-effective management of the hospital-based hospice program. *Journal of Nursing Administration*, 1992; **22**:40–5.
16. World Health Organization Expert Committee. *Cancer Pain Relief and Palliative Care*. Geneva: World Health Organization, 1990. (WHO Technical Report Series 804.)
17. Vainio A. Palliative care in Finland. *Palliative Medicine*, 1990; **4**:225–7.
18. Tsao SY. Palliative care in Hong Kong. *Palliative Medicine*, 1991; **5**:262–6.
19. Robinson R. Economic evaluation and health care: what does it mean? *British Medical Journal*, 1993; **307**:670–3.

20. Robinson R. Economic evaluation and health care: costs and cost-minimisation analysis. *British Medical Journal*, 1993; **307**:726–8.
21. Robinson R. Economic evaluation and health care: cost-effectiveness analysis. *British Medical Journal*, 1993; **307**:793–5.
22. Robinson R. Economic evaluation and health care: cost-utility analysis? *British Medical Journal*, 1993; **307**:859–62.
23. Robinson R. Economic evaluation and health care: cost-benefit analysis. *British Medical Journal*, 1993; **307**:924–6.
24. Drummond MF. The contribution of health economics to cost-effective health-care delivery. In: Drummond MF, Maynard A, eds. *Purchasing and Providing Cost-effective Health Care*. Edinburgh: Churchill Livingstone, 1993: 16–27.
25. Coyle D, Davies L. How to assess cost-effectiveness: elements of a sound economic evaluation. In: Drummond MF, Maynard A, eds. *Purchasing and Providing Cost-effective Health Care*. Edinburgh: Churchill Livingstone, 1993: 66–79.
26. Goddard M. The role of economics in the evaluation of hospice care. *Health Policy*, 1989; **13**:19–34.
27. Goddard M. The importance of assessing the effectiveness of care: the case of hospices . *Journal of Social Policy*, 1993; **22**:1–17.
28. Brooks RG. *Health Status Measurement: A Perspective on Change*. Basingstoke: Macmillan, 1995.
29. Hill F, Oliver C. Hospice—the cost of in-patient care. *Health Trends*, 1984; **16**:9–11.
30. Ventafridda V, De Conno F, ViganÒ A, Ripamonti C, Gallucci M, Gamba A. Comparison of home and hospital care of advanced cancer patients. *Tumori*, 1989; **75**:619–25.
31. King M, Lapsley I, Llewellyn S, Tierney A, Anderson J, Sladden S. Purchasing palliative care: availability and cost implications. *Health Bulletin*, 1993; **51**:370–84.
32. Tierney AJ, Sladden S, Anderson J, King M, Lapsley I, Llewellyn S. Measuring the costs and quality of palliative care: a discussion paper. *Palliative Medicine*, 1994; **8**:273–81.
33. Kane RL, Wales J, Berstein L, Leibowitz A, Kaplan S. A randomised controlled trial of hospice care. *Lancet*, 1984; **April 21**:890–4.
34. Brooks CH, Smyth-Staruch K. Hospice home care cost-savings to third-party insurers. *Medical Care*, 1984; **22**:691–703.
35. Gray D, MacAdam D, Boldy D. A comparative cost analysis of terminal cancer care in home hospice patients and controls. *Journal of Chronic Disease*, 1987; **40**:801–10.
36. Kidder D. The impact of hospices on the health-care costs of terminal cancer patients. In: Mor V, Greer DS, Kastenbaum R, eds. *The Hospice Experiment*. Baltimore, MD: Johns Hopkins University Press, 1988: 48–68.
37. Dunt DR, Cantwell AM, Temple-Smith MJ. The cost-effectiveness of the Citymission Hospice Programme, Melbourne. *Palliative Medicine*, 1989; **3**:125–34.
38. Whynes DK. Counting the true costs of palliative care. *Progress in Palliative Care*, 1993; **1**:47–50.
39. Harris MD. Volunteers—a priceless treasure. *Home Healthcare Nurse*, 1990; **8**:7–8.
40. Field D, Johnson I. Satisfaction and change: a survey of volunteers in a hospice organisation. *Social Science and Medicine*, 1993; **36**:1625–33.
41. Hoad P. Volunteers in the independent hospice movement. *Sociology of Health and Illness*, 1991; **13**:231–48.
42. Lansky SB, Cairns NU, Clark GM, Lowman J, Miller L, Trueworthy R. Childhood cancer: nonmedical costs of the illness. *Cancer*, 1979; **43**:403–8.
43. Houts PS *et al.* Nonmedical costs to patients and their families associated with outpatient chemotherapy. *Cancer*, 1984; **53**:2388–92.
44. Bodkin CM, Pigott TJ, Mann JR. Financial burden of childhood cancer. *British Medical Journal*, 1982; **284**:1542–4.
45. Munro AJ, Ebag-Montefiore D. Opportunity cost—a neglected aspect of cancer treatment. *British Journal of Cancer*, 1992; **65**:309–10.
46. Scheithauer W, Rosen H, Kornek GV, Sebesta C, Depisch D. Randomised comparison of combination chemotherapy plus supportive care with supportive care alone in patients with metastatic colorectal cancer. *British Medical Journal*, 1993; **306**:752–5.
47. Stoll BA. Saying no is difficult in cancer. In: Stoll BA, ed. *Cost Versus Benefit in Cancer Care*. Baltimore, MD: Johns Hopkins University Press, 1988: 97–111.
48. Cassileth BR, Lusk EJ. Methodologic issues in palliative care psychosocial research. *Journal of Palliative Care*, 1989; **5**:5–11.
49. McDowell A, Newell C. *Measuring Health: A Guide to Rating Scales and Questionnaires*. Oxford University Press, 1987.
50. Bowling A. *Measuring Health*. Buckingham: Open University Press, 1991.
51. Bowling A. *Measuring Disease*. Buckingham: Open University Press, 1995.
52. Wilkin D, Hallam L, Doggett MA. *Measures of Need and Outcome for Primary Health Care*. Oxford University Press, 1992.
53. Higginson IJ, McCarthy M. Validity of the support team assessment schedule: do staffs' ratings reflect those made by patients or their families? *Palliative Medicine*, 1993; **7**:219–28.
54. Addington-Hall J, McCarthy M. Regional Study of Care for the Dying: methods and sample characteristics. *Palliative Medicine*, 1995; **9**:27–35.
55. McWhinney IR, Bass MJ, Donner A. Evaluation of a palliative care service: problems and pitfalls. *British Medical Journal*, 1994; **309**:1340–2.
56. Emanuel EJ, Emanuel LL. The economics of dying: the illusion of cost-savings at the end of life. *New England Journal of Medicine*, 1994; **330**:540–4.
57. Schneiderman LJ, Kronick R, Kaplan RM, Anderson JP, Langer RD. Effects of offering advance directives on medical treatments and costs. *Annals of Internal Medicine*, 1992; **117**:599–606.
58. Maynard A. Future directions for health care reform. In: Drummond MF, Maynard A, eds. *Purchasing and Providing Cost-effective Health Care*. Edinburgh: Churchill Livingstone, 1993: 242–54.
59. House of Commons Health Committee. *Priority Setting in the NHS: Purchasing*. London: HMSO, 1995.
60. Harris L. The disadvantaged dying. *Nursing Times*, 1990; **86**:26–9.
61. Clark D. Whither the hospices?. In: Clark D, ed. *The Future for Palliative Care*. Buckingham: Open University Press, 1993: 165–77.
62. Wilson IM, Bunting JS, Curnow RN, Knock J. The need for inpatient palliative care facilities for noncancer patients in the Thames Valley. *Palliative Medicine*, 1995; **9**:13–18.
63. Lewis J. Voluntary organizations in 'New Partnership' with local authorities: the anatomy of a contract. *Social Policy and Administration*, 1994; **28**:206–20.
64. Lunt B, Hillier R. Terminal care: present services and future priorities. *British Medical Journal*, 1981; **283**:595–8.
65. Mount BM, Scott JF. Whither hospice evaluation? *Journal of Chronic Disease*, 1983; **36**:731–6.
66. Torrens PR. Hospice care: What have we learned? *Annual Review Public Health*, 1985; **6**:65–83.
67. Higginson I, McCarthy M. Evaluation of palliative care: steps to quality assurance. *Palliative Medicine*, 1989; **3**:267–74.

2.6 Clinical and organizational audit in palliative care

Irene Higginson

Quality of care: a worldwide crusade?

Throughout the world there is a growing concern to ensure quality and thereby value for money in health care. Higher public expectations and the move towards quality service in many public and private companies have all heightened the desire to introduce quality assurance, audit, and evaluation into clinical care.[1] In response, clinicians, managers, and governments have sought to standardize clinical practice to that which is the 'best' possible or which is proven to be the most effective and efficient.[1] Although many terms in the quality dictionary are new, many of the ideas, such as clinical review, are not. In 1518 the Charter of the Royal College of Physicians of London included the statement: 'to uphold the standards of medicine both for their own honour and public benefit'.[2] Florence Nightingale was one of the first clinicians to insist on measuring the outcome of care for her patients, i.e. to evaluate treatment.[3] Ward rounds, postgraduate lectures, and clinical presentations already contribute to the review of medical and nursing performance. However, the new emphasis on audit and quality assurance has resulted in four main differences:[2]

- explicit criteria for good practice should be applied by all clinicians rather than those in exemplary centres;
- all patients in care should be included in quality monitoring rather than a few 'interesting' cases;
- patients and their families should be able to seek empowerment;
- funding or accreditation may be withheld from those units which do not comply with quality standards or which are found to be ineffective or inefficient.

References to quality assurance and clinical audit in the medical and nursing literature began in the late 1970s and they continue to rise (Fig. 1).

What is audit?

Audit aims to improve care for patients and families by assessing whether we are doing the right thing well. Therefore, to audit, first we have to know what we are trying to achieve, second we must have a way of observing practice to assess whether we achieve the goals or standards, and third we must change practice to improve care. Effective audit is a cycle. Standards for the delivery of care are agreed. Then practice is observed and compared with the standards. This often demonstrates successes, but also failings and a need for change. The results are then fed back and examined so that new or modified standards can be set. The audit cycle is then repeated anew.[2,4–7] The cycle can be entered at any point; for example it is possible to begin by observing practice and acting on the results, and then proceed to setting standards.[1,2,8]

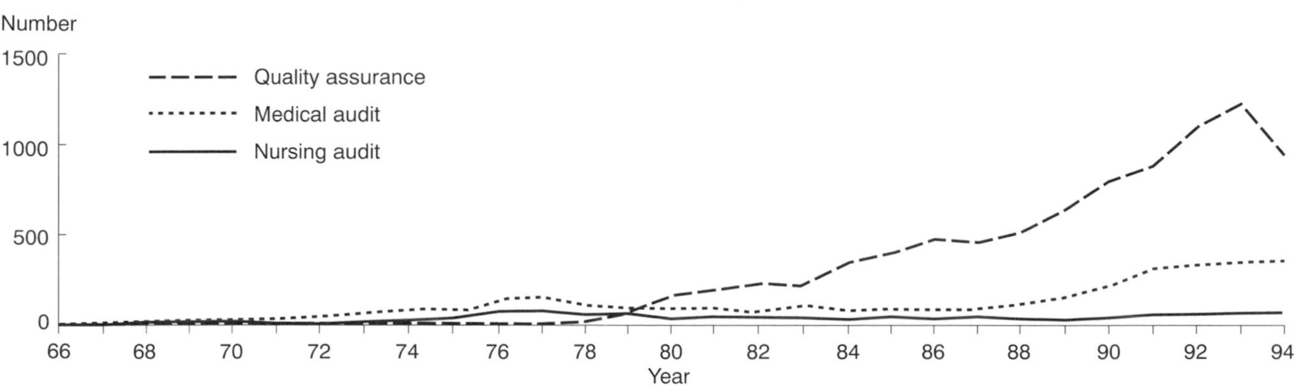

Fig. 1 Number of Medline references per year (1966–1994).

Why audit palliative care: benefits and costs?

Palliative care arose out of a desire to improve the quality of care for patients with advancing disease and their families. The newness of the specialty coupled with scepticism or reluctance to support this form of care often resulted in many of the early evaluations of palliative services which compared hospice, home, and hospital care.[9-12] Therefore palliative care often led the way in developing methods of examining the quality of care and sought to influence those working in oncology and other professions.[12] However, there is no room for complacency as these evaluations were limited to a few exemplary centres.[12] Palliative practice varies from one part of the country to another, even in simple aspects such as staffing levels and mix within a hospice or home care team, the catchment populations, the operational policies, and the throughput.[13-15] We need to know which models of care work best and for which types of problems palliative care is most effective. Those providing and those purchasing palliative services will need to know which interventions and which combinations work best, for what kinds of patients and families, and in which types of locality.

Hospices and palliative services provide novel therapies, such as new treatments for symptoms, support and counselling services, or complementary therapies.[12] However, new therapies and approaches must be evaluated and audited to determine if and to whom these are useful. Otherwise, hospice resources and patients' time will be wasted. There is a great danger of concentrating on current concerns without reviewing previous failings and using those findings to plan improved care in the future.

Antipathy to audit is based on various arguments such as the following.

- There is no problem since palliative care is of a high quality and is self-auditing.
- The outcomes of palliative care cannot be measured.
- Resources, information, and time for auditing are not available.
- Audit looks back at practice which has gone, not at the problems which lie ahead.

None of these arguments are supported by evidence. Audits of palliative care can help to improve care in the following ways.[16,17]

1. Review of the quality of work and identification of ways of improving it should mean that future patients and families will not suffer the same failings.
2. Identification of areas where care is effective and where it is not could allow services to be better targeted and will mean that patients and families receive the most up-to-date care.
3. Prospective audits with systematic assessments of patients and families during care can help to ensure the following:
   (a) aspects of care are less likely to be overlooked;
   (b) there is a more holistic approach to care;
   (c) new staff have a clearer understanding of what they should assess.
4. Audit can help most patients and families receiving palliative care because it looks at routine practice rather than a few 'special' cases. Quite apart from mistakes, suboptimal care may be due to professional or administrative problems which tend to escape anecdotal case reviews.[2]

Audit is important for education and training, because the structured review allows analysis, comparison, and evaluation of individual performance; it also promotes adherence to local clinical policies and offers opportunity for publication of results.[1] Educational programmes can be constructed to meet the demonstrated needs of individuals or groups.

In the future, audit may also be required for the recognition of training posts. Royal Colleges and faculties increasingly seek evidence of formally organized review and could withdraw recognition from departments that do not provide this.[1]

Audit is important for purchasers of health care[18] because it provides tangible evidence that the service is seeking the most effective use of existing clinical resources and aims to improve the quality of care. This is increasingly important in competition for health-care contracts.[18] Requirements for audit and the implementation of research findings may well be included in such contracts.[19]

The costs of not auditing are as important as the benefits of auditing.[16,17] These include the following.

- Extra inappropriate treatment which wastes patients' and families' time and resources as well as wasting staff time and resources. Such resources could be used elsewhere where they may be more effective.
- Uncontrolled symptoms may result in admission to hospice or hospital or delay discharge. Most significantly this causes suffering to the patient, family, and staff.
- There may be extra inappropriate services, for example unnecessary outpatient attendances.

However, audit takes time and resources. These should not be underestimated and can include the following.

- Time from all staff to prepare for audit, to agree the standards or topics, and to review the findings.
- Time from some staff to carry out the audit and to analyse its results and document the findings and any recommendations.
- Commitment from all staff (managers, nurses, doctors, etc.) to consider the results and act upon them.
- Resources to pay for the staff time involved plus any other analytical or computing support needed.

The costs of audit mean that it is important to ensure that the audit itself is as effective as possible. What is the purpose of collecting audit data if the changes recommended are not acted on? Mechanisms to review the audit and to ensure that it is effective are discussed in a later section.

Computers are not necessary for audit. They can help if they are used to streamline the information collected and if they include standard programs to make the analysis easy.[20,21] However, if the

Box 1 Audit by any other name

Medical	Care	Evaluation
Health	Standards	Assessment
Clinical	Activity	Assurance
Professional	Review	Audit
Total	Quality	Management
	Monitoring	

Adapted and updated from refs. 2 and 4.

audit is small or in its early stages, too rigid a use of computers by inexperienced staff can be a hindrance, because the need to update the computer delays the evolution of the audit.

Approaches to audit and assessing quality: their relevance to palliative care

There are various other terms for audit (Box 1). Some of the widely accepted definitions of audit are shown in Table 1.

The different approaches to audit and the assessment of quality can be categorized according to two axes: first, who carries out the audit (the local clinicians, managers, or an external organization), and second, whether the audit considered the care of an individual or a few patients, or the whole organization or population. Common forms of audit identified according to these two axes (internal versus external and individual versus organization/population) are shown in Fig. 2. The appropriate type of audit is determined by the setting. It is extremely difficult for those purchasing the services or external bodies to assess the clinical quality of care. Instead, they are more likely to rely on organizational or environmental standards or, when determining whether the professionals are employing proven high-quality treatments, to examine staff mix and whether a clinical audit programme is in place.

Clinical audit

Clinical audit is the systematic critical analysis of the quality of clinical care including the procedures used for diagnosis and treatment, the use of resources, and the resulting outcome and quality of life for the patient.[5]

Early forms of audit involved only single professions, for example medical or nursing audit (Table 1). However, it is now widely accepted that audit in palliative care should be multiprofessional, to reflect the multiprofessional nature of care. Clinical audit is like medical and nursing audit but involves all professionals and volunteers, rather than only doctors or nurses.

The audit can be prospective, where the standards and measures are agreed at the start and are recorded for patients and families

Table 1 Common definitions: audit and quality assurance

Term	Definition
Medical audit	The systematic critical analysis of the quality of medical care including the procedures used for diagnosis and treatment, the use of resources, and the resulting outcome and quality of life of the patient[5]
Clinical audit	The systematic critical analysis of the quality of clinical care including the procedures used for diagnosis and treatment, the use of resources, and the resulting outcome and quality of life of the patient
	Clinical audit is like medical audit but involves all professionals and volunteers rather than only doctors
Nursing audit	The methods by which nurses compare their actual practice against pre-agreed guidelines and identify areas for improving their care
Prospective audit	The standards and measures are recorded on patients and their families during their care
Retrospective audit	This looks back at the care of patients who have been discharged or have died, and the standards are applied to the information available from case notes or by asking families about the care after the patient has died
Quality assurance	The definition of standards, the measurement of their achievement and the mechanisms to improve performance[2]
	The quality assurance cycle is as for medical audit or clinical audit. However, quality assurance implies a planned programme involving the whole unit or health services. Clinical or medical audit is usually described as one part of a quality assurance programme

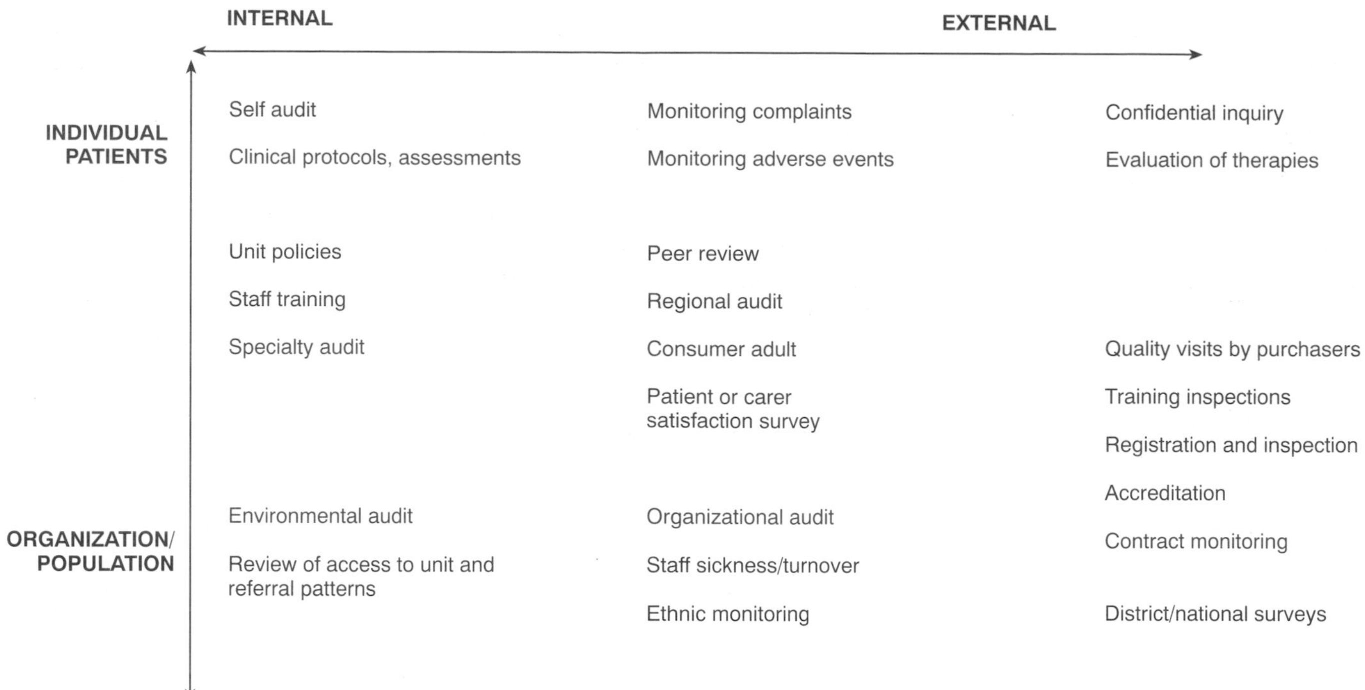

Fig. 2 Alternatives in monitoring quality and audit.

during their care, or retrospective, where the care of patients is reviewed either by extracting the information from the clinical notes or by asking families.

Organizational audit

The King's Fund Centre, London, described organizational audit as a developmental and voluntary stage towards accreditation.[22] Accreditation schemes exist in many countries and usually operate nationally. For example, medical Royal Colleges inspect training posts and agree where doctors can be trained. In the United Kingdom there are two main country-wide systems of organization audit. The King's Fund Centre, London, developed a project, initially called 'Accreditation UK' and later 'Organizational Audit',[22] which worked voluntarily with the National Health Service and private hospitals to agree a lengthy document of standards. In the first 3 years of the programme (to the end of 1992) over 130 acute general hospitals were assessed against published standards. Standards for primary care[1] are now being piloted, and a palliative care organization audit has been developed following this system (see examples later in this chapter). The Hospital Accreditation Programme was established at the Clinical Audit Unit in the South Western Region in Bristol, and was designed to assess smaller hospitals or community-based services.[23] In its first 3 years as a pilot scheme limited to general practitioner hospitals in one region, the Hospital Accreditation Programme completed 61 surveys on 70 per cent of eligible hospitals and accredited 75 per cent against standards based on action research.[24] This programme became available nationally in April 1993 for community hospitals, generally smaller than those eligible for the King's Fund hospital programme.[1]

Organizational standards were developed because of evidence of organizational variation, which limits the quality of care. This included administrative delays, uncoordinated care, poor environment or sign-posting, poor staff training, etc.[22,23,25] Organizational standards need to be sufficiently straightforward to be monitored by an external surveyor.[23]

Organizational audit and accreditation are usually developed in three stages.[22]

1. Developing organizational standards of the systems and process of care.

2. Implementation of the standards by the hospices, hospitals, or units included.

3. Evaluation of compliance with the standards, usually by external surveyors or auditors.

The first stage of developing standards can often be quite lengthy, because the standards need to be agreed and written in clear non-ambiguous language, and then tested to determine if they can distinguish between good and suboptimal practice. If only the poorest level of practice is detected, then standards could be reduced to just above this level because units will not need to strive higher. Units with higher standards, which were undetected, may appear to have higher costs for the same level of practice as units with just acceptable standards.

The following alternative definition of quality assurance has been provided by those working in organizational audit at the Cancer Relief Macmillan Fund, United Kingdom (personal communication):

> an independent and voluntary audit of a entire organisation or team infrastructures that promote consistency in care and service. Such examination promotes multi-disciplinary working and teamwork to assist co-ordination of care and service by examining the inter-relationships between departments and

the differing roles of clinicians (very important as role blurring is a key feature of palliative care).

Quality assurance and total quality management programmes

Although there are various definitions of quality assurance, one which is widely accepted is the 'definition of standards, the measurement of their achievement and the mechanisms to improve performance'.[2] Thus the cycle is the same as for clinical audit. Clinical audit lies within the frame of quality assurance: it is the review of the quality of local clinical practice on a regular basis, for example through internal 'peer review' by practising clinicians.

Quality in health care can be assessed from various angles: equity and accessibility (the provision and availability of services to everyone in need), effectiveness (achieving the intended benefits within a population), acceptability and humanity (to the consumer and the provider), and efficiency (the avoidance of waste).[2,26] Simple general definitions of quality are available; for example, that quality is meeting the customer requirements, or meeting people's health care requirements.[27] Of course, quality includes these criteria, but the more comprehensive definitions provide a broad way of looking at quality. The danger of using the simple definitions is that a service may assert that it has high quality based on a satisfaction survey of patients, but have overlooked problems in another area, for example the service may be inequitable or have a poor clinical effectiveness.

Total quality management is a term which has recently become part of the jargon of quality in health care and its definition is included for completeness. It has been defined as a strategy to ensure that an organization is working to its maximum effectiveness and efficiency.[27] It has been facilitated by closer working relationships been clinicians and managers[1] and builds on the other definitions, but switches the focus from quality practised by professionals to quality within the whole organization. Thus clinical audit would be part of a total quality management programme. It also introduces the concept of managing the quality process, such as cataloguing reports of local quality initiatives[1] and using managers to ensure that improvements in quality occur.

Applying audit to palliative care

Know what we are trying to achieve: goals or standards

The definitions of palliative care and palliative medicine (see Chapter 2.4) provide guidance on the goals of palliative care which might be measured in audit. These include aspects of pain and symptom control, improving the patient's quality of life, relieving fears and anxiety, and caring for the family members or carers. Therefore, in analysing the goals or standards of care, many have audited their effectiveness in controlling symptoms such as pain or dyspnoea, their effect on a patient's quality of life or psychological well being, or the patient's or families' satisfaction with care.[28-37]

There are other aspects which might be included. Weisman[38] defined 'appropriate death' as 'an absence of suffering, preservation of important relationships, an interval for anticipatory grief, relief of remaining conflicts, belief in timeliness, exercise of feasible option in activities, and consistency with physical limitations, all within the scope of one's ego ideal'. Kellehear[39] described the features of a modern 'good death' as 'awareness of dying, social adjustments and personal preparations, public preparations (legal, financial, religious, funeral, medical), work or activities reduced, and farewells'. These two definitions suggest audit of aspects of patient and family awareness of the illness or their planning of personal and public preparations.

In many countries the role of palliative care in supporting, advising, and educating other professions is stressed[40-42] (see also other chapters). Family practitioners have identified needs for education in symptom control and patient and family support.[43,44] Therefore another form of audit could examine the educational and supportive role of palliative care services.

Poor communication is a frequent cause of stress for patients and families.[45-47] Doctors and nurses need to communicate well with patients and their families rather than withdrawing or appearing hurried or abrupt in their manner. Communication is needed between professional staff caring for the patient and family members, to ensure liaison and to prevent duplication or delay. These aspects are also goals suitable for audit.

Total pain has been described as including physical, emotional, social, and spiritual components.[48] Although the earlier discussions have covered the emotional and physical aspects of palliative care, it is also important to consider the audit of spiritual and social aspects. Spiritual audit might consider whether patients are able to raise spiritual concerns and to find a mechanism to relieve problems or whether patients are in any form of spiritual crisis.[49] Social aspects might include whether the patient and family have sufficient practical and financial support to remain at home.[8,49]

How can these goals be turned into standards? Any goal or standard which is set must be measurable and sufficiently challenging, but achievable. It would be unrealistic to set freedom from pain for all patients as a goal or standard, but it would be reasonable to set a goal of what proportion of patients' pain might be controlled and in what circumstances pain might be uncontrolled. A baseline could be established from current practice. Standards of action when pain is uncontrolled could be audited.

Have a way of assessing and reassessing whether we achieve the goals or standards

The goals or standards of health services can usually be assessed in terms of the following.[2,16,25,50]

- Structure and/or inputs: resources in terms of manpower, equipment, and money.
- Process: how the resources are used (e.g. domiciliary visits, beds, clinics, drugs or treatments given).
- Output: productivity or throughput (e.g. rates of clinic attendance or discharge, throughput).
- Outcome: change in health status or quality of life that can be attributed to health care.

Structural aspects influence the process of care so that its quality can be either diminished or enhanced. Similarly, changes in the process of care, including variations in its quality, will influence the output and in turn the effect of care on health status and outcomes. Thus we have the following functional relationship:[50]

structure → process → output → outcome.

Structure is easiest to measure because its elements are the most stable and identifiable. However, it is an indirect measure of the quality of care and its value depends on the nature of its influence on care.[50] Structure is relevant to quality in that it increases or decreases the probability of a good performance. Process and output are closer to changes in the health status of individuals. Their advantage is that they measure the most immediately discernible attributes of care activities. However, they are only valuable as a measure once the elements of process are known to have a clear relationship with the desired changes in health status.[50] Outcome reflects the true change in health status, and thus is the most relevant for patients and society. However, it is difficult to eliminate other causes for change, such as prior care or external events. A useful approach is to focus on the difference between the desired outcome and the actual outcome.[4] Services can then identify whether or not their goals are being achieved and investigate any failings.[2] Organizational audits usually assess the structure and process of care, whereas clinical audits often measure the process and outcome of care. Although structure is easiest to measure, it is furthest from influencing change in the patient and family. Outcome is most difficult to measure but is of direct relevance to the patient and family. Standards of structure or process are most useful when these are of proven effectiveness, or if there is an overwhelming consensus that these are desirable. Structure, process, and outcome measures which have been either used or advocated to assess palliative care are shown in Table 2.

Change practice to ensure that any deficiencies are corrected

This stage closes the audit loop in the cycle.[4,16] Any weaknesses in practice need to be considered and discussed with the whole team to determine what changes might be appropriate. This may involve a review of the literature or consulting with other individuals to determine whether they have solutions to particular problems. For example, in London we identified that our control of dyspnoea in the last weeks of life was not reaching our targets; this was the most severe symptom in patients.[31] To decide what change was needed we consulted chest physicians, physiotherapists, and other colleagues about what treatment might be appropriate in the home, reviewed the literature on effective treatment, and examined the possible causes of dyspnoea. This led us to make substantial changes in our practice and has probably also led to further research into the management of dyspnoea.

Difficulties in implementing changes have been described in larger specialist palliative care services. These include the following.

1. Inadequate cascading of the information from those present at the audit meetings to other staff.
2. Difficulties in ensuring that those who have hands-on patient contact but are at the end of the cascade, such as auxiliary nurses, feel ownership of any changes and therefore are willing to accept them.
3. Difficulties if the main communicator is a resistor to change. Many health care professionals have an innate conservatism and resist changes of long-cherished beliefs. This may be partly from fear of their deficiencies being revealed.[29]

Continuing education is important if change is to be achieved.[19,51] It can be targeted to ensure that those being educated feel part of the teaching or learning process. In one mechanism, which has been described by Finlay[29], the full team of nurses is asked to evolve policy themselves with the tutor as facilitator.

Types of audit: an appraisal of their use in palliative care

Once the standards or goals are agreed, a method of audit must be chosen. This is analogous to choosing a research method in a study once the research question or hypothesis is decided. Two methods—key indicators and topic review—have been commonly used in palliative care.

Key indicators

These can be based on the structure or process of care, as in organizational audit, or can be based on clinical indicators, such as in clinical audit. In organizational audit the indicators are reviewed by inspection; in clinical audit they are reviewed by the clinical team (see Fig. 1).

Routinely collected data, such as throughput, visits, or readmission rates, can be used in some areas of health care, but these may not be appropriate in palliative care. The clinical record may have to be amended to include relevant items. In clinical audit a few key indicators are chosen and recorded prospectively, and are examined after a period of care. In organizational audit the survey team asks for information about the indicators and then seeks evidence of these. Examples in palliative care include the organizational audit of the Cancer Relief Macmillan Fund,[52] and in clinical audit the Support Team Assessment Schedule,[49,53] the Edmonton Symptom Assessment System,[28] and the Palliative Care Core Standards.[32]

Topic review

A topic is chosen and reviewed prospectively or retrospectively. Although the latter often reveals inadequacies in the clinical records, it can be valuable in providing a baseline for later comparison. Examples of topics are medical records and letters,[54] referral or admission procedures, control of a particular symptom, prescribing practice, or the diagnostic procedures used. This technique has also been used successfully in palliative care.[29,54]

Random case review

Here notes are selected at random and critically reviewed by doctors who are not involved in the care of that particular patient. This method may lose direction if the aims and criteria for quality are not clear. One way to focus the audit is to develop a previously agreed checklist for use in the critical review. The method can be linked with key indicators—a random sample of notes is examined for the key indicators.

Patient or family satisfaction

The simplest method is to analyse patient and family complaints. However, in palliative care patients may die before they are able to

Table 2 Example of potential measures of structure, process, or outcome in palliative care

Type of measure	Examples
Structure	Values or aims of the service Financial resources Home care/hospital/hospice services Day hospice places Number of staff or services per cancer patient in the population Staffing mix, grades Number of staff per patient Drugs and equipment available Building design Physical environment (e.g. safety, pleasantness of surroundings)
Process	Number of visits Number of admissions Procedures followed Documentation Time taken in a visit Polices and procedures for staff training and working Mechanism for handling complaints and the documentation of this Adherence to ethical and legal codes Staff support given
Output	Rate of discharge Number of completed consultant episodes Throughput Rate of equipment given out Drugs correctly given Well-coordinated care (telephone communication etc.) Supply of medicines after discharge Completed patient management plans Early arrival of discharge information to general practitioner Satisfaction of professionals referring to the service
Outcome	Reduction in distressing symptoms Improved mental health of patient and carer Patient and carer satisfaction Satisfied with place of care Open and honest communication as the patient wishes Resolved communication, fears, grief, anger Resolved need to plan future events (e.g. funeral or meetings) Good use of remaining time Any spiritual problems resolved or fulfilment Reduced carer strain Improved carer health Resolved grief after death (if appropriate)

complain. Surveys of patients' or families' views may be included in the overall quality improvement plan of a hospice or hospital. Care has also been examined via a national survey of families' views after the death.[35] However, detailed surveys tend to be beyond the resources of single units.

Adverse patient events

Events during a patient's treatment which may indicate some lapse in the quality of care are systematically identified. Patients' clinical records are reviewed retrospectively by a health professional or a ward clerk for examples of agreed adverse events. This method is of value in specialities such as surgery, where adverse events (e.g death or postoperative infection) are usually recorded in the patients' records. However, it is unsatisfactory in palliative care because adverse palliative events are more difficult to identify routinely and may not be included in the patient's records unless these are standardized.

Examples of audits in palliative care

Organizational audit

The Cancer Relief Macmillan Fund has developed an organizational audit for specialist care services with and following the King's Fund organizational audit programme[52] A working group consisting of six regional coordinators for palliative care, five of whom were nurses, and a representative from Cancer Relief

Macmillan Fund developed an initial draft of standards. These were piloted in several palliative care units in the United Kingdom and then modified. The organizational audit aims to take a macroview of the organization, identifying how internal quality mechanisms are used to promote good practice and examining the structures in place to facilitate improvements.[52] The 11 standards and their purposes are as follows.[52,55]

1. Service values: a statement of service values and objectives related to the palliative care service guides the organization and delivery of high-quality care.
2. Organization and management: the palliative care service or organization is managed efficiently to ensure that patients and families receive suitable and effective multidisciplinary care.
3. Organizational and operational policy: organizational and operational policies reflect current knowledge and principles, and are consistent with the requirements of statutory bodies, purchasing authorities, and service objectives.
4. Physical environment for care: the physical environment is safe and accommodates individual and shared needs.
5. Self-determination and climate for care: the caring environment for patients and families is conducive to independence, self-esteem, and participation in daily life.
6. Direct patient and family care: professional staff manage to ensure that patient and family needs are assessed, planned, implemented, and evaluated on an individual basis.
7. Multidisciplinary working and team work: a range of skills is available to meet service goals, and specific contributions are identified and integrated.
8. Staffing and skill mix: good employment practices are in place and staffing levels are systematically determined in order to meet service needs.
9. Education, training, and staff development: staff have access to education and training programmes, which reflect the different levels of activity and practice necessary to meet service goals, provide appropriate care, and respond to change.
10. Staff support: staff support systems are in place as an integral part of the organization, and a healthy working environment is promoted which recognizes the possible physical and emotional effects of work on staff.
11. Ethics and law: there is guidance and support for staff to comply with statutory requirements and use a systematic approach to decision-making where ethical and legal status issues are involved.

Each of these 11 standards has a rationale followed by criteria which are used by a team of external surveyors to determine the extent to which each standard is achieved. Guidance is provided on the questions to ask when assessing a criterion.[55] As an example, the criteria for standard 7 are shown in Box 2, and the questions used to assess these criteria in Box 3.

The validity, reliability, practicality, and sensitivity of the questions are unreported. The audit is in the relatively early stage; an independent evaluation or one similar to that undertaken for the Hospital Accreditation Programme would help to assess its utility and problems.[24] There is a charge for carrying out the audit; fee structures are available from Cancer Relief Macmillan Fund. In 1995, fees were in the region of £6500, depending upon the circumstances of the unit. Units could pay over a 2-year period (personal communication).

An example of the Cancer Relief Macmillan Fund organizational audit in practice and its use, as reported by an inspection team member, is given below (personal communication).

> Upon noticing that a patient bathtub and equipment was exceptionally dirty in one organization, I asked whose responsibility it was to clean it. I was told by the nursing staff that it was the domestic's responsibility. The domestic told me that it was the nursing staff's responsibility. As this issue had not been discussed or agreed, no one cleaned the tub and the patients had to use a tub that was unhygienic and that was clearly unacceptable. Having a hygienic environment is an essential part of the comfort and good care of patients, but it clearly falls outside the ambit of clinical audit. Issues such as those would never be addressed as a part of a clinical audit programme. Organizational audit puts those issues into another context and encourages different departments to talk to each other to plan and coordinate their efforts.

Box 2 The criteria from standard 7 of the Cancer Relief Macmillan Fund organizational audit[56]

Interdisciplinary working and teamwork

Criteria

1. Systems exist for referral to the therapy professions, social workers, and ministers of religion
2. Mechanisms exist for liaison within and between disciplines, including volunteers, to ensure continuity of care
3. Staff demonstrate awareness of differing roles, relationships, and responsibilities
4. Mechanisms exist for monitoring the performance of the multidisciplinary team
5. There are systems to inform patients and families of the range of skills and services available
6. There are arrangements for liaison and co-operation between patients and families and health care agencies

Box 3 Evidence to be considered from standard 7 of the Cancer Relief Macmillan Fund organizational audit[56]

Interdisciplinary working and teamwork

For Criterion 1—Do systems exist for referral to the therapy professions, social workers/counsellors, ministers of religion, complementary therapists, dietitians, interpreters, and other specialist medical or nursing services (i.e. ostomy nurse, psychiatrist)?

Documents
Referral forms
Response time statistics

Discussion
How is liaison maintained?
How are referrals made?
How quickly are referrals met?
Do these staff have post-qualification specialist training?

Observation
Observe referrals and team relationship

Clinical audits

Although palliative care cannot be audited by the usual measures of mortality and morbidity, an array of measures suitable for clinical audit are now available. These cover aspects of process, such as documentation standards and procedures followed,[54] and aspects of output and outcome, such as symptom control, co-ordination, communication, and psychosocial problems.[28–37,53]

The range of measures available should provide most clinicians with a choice for their own practice. The setting of standards and the development of instruments can be a lengthy process, and it is probably better to adapt those measures which are available or are being tested, if this is possible. Common published measures for audit are described in the next section, together with examples of the results where these are available. Although some of the measures were designed for use in audits of key indicators, some aspects of them could be used for topic audits.

The measures described are at very different stages of use and development. Three—the Support Team Assessment Schedule (STAS),[53] the Trent Documentation Standards,[54] and the Regional Study of Care of the Dying[35]—have been used in a wide variety of settings or in different regions of the United Kingdom. Items in the STAS have also undergone testing for validity and reliability,[56–58] and such testing is under way for the Edmonton Symptom Assessment System[28,59] and the Palliative Care Core Standards.[32] At the other end of the spectrum, the *Guidelines for Good Practice and Audit Measures,*[60] developed by the Royal College of Physicians, London, several years ago, has never yet been used (to the knowledge of the author and the co-ordinator of this audit (personal communication)).

Examples of measures used in palliative care audit

The Support Team Assessment Schedule[48,53,56–58]

This schedule includes 17 items covering pain and symptoms (two), patient anxiety and insight and spiritual support (three), family anxiety and insight (two), planning affairs (two), communication (three), home services (three), and support of other professionals (two). It assesses outcomes, intermediate outcomes, and outputs. The items included are shown in Box 4, and details of the rating for one item, pain control, are shown in Box 5. It was developed by means of collaboration with five support teams, and revised in light of presentations at professional meetings, observation of palliative care, and interviews with patients and families. It is now used in a variety of settings.

The STAS is used widely. There are over 100 registered users, including home, hospital, and hospice settings, in nine different countries (to the knowledge of the author). The time to complete ratings for one patient averages 2 min. It is validated to ensure that professional ratings reasonably reflect patient views,[57] and it is acceptably reliable.[56] Reliance on assessments by professionals may be a problem,[57] but where possible the schedule is tested with some patients completing some items, such as pain, directly for comparison with the team assessments. The symptom assessment has been expanded,[33] items for day care[61] and primary care[62] are being tested, and a database has been developed in collaboration with the Irish Cancer Society.[63] A study funded by the NHS Executive (UK) is seeking to develop a smaller core audit. The audit has two components, a patient completion form and a trained staff schedule based on STAS. The study has a nationally representative steering group, including hospital, hospice, community and primary care staff. The project aims to develop a core measure which can be used beyond specialist palliative care settings.

There is no charge for using the STAS, but users must register and sign an agreement to state that they will not sell it.

Results have been useful in demonstrating how patients' problems change during care. Figure 3 and Box 6 show examples of findings in a group of patients.

Box 4 Items in the STAS[48,53]

Patient and family items
Pain control
Symptom control
Patient anxiety
Family anxiety
Patient insight
Family insight
Spiritual
Planning
Predictability
Communication between patient and family

Service items
Practical aid
Financial
Wasted time
Communication from professionals to patient and family
Communication between professionals
Professional anxiety
Advising professionals

Edmonton Symptom Assessment System[28,59]

This measure includes nine visual analogue scales (Fig. 4): pain, activity, nausea, depression, anxiety, drowsiness, appetite, well being, and shortness of breath. Assessments are usually completed by the patient; if this is not possible, the family member or nursing staff complete the ratings. It assesses outcome and can be used to track individual patients during care (Fig. 5), and the results for groups of patients can also demonstrate successes and failures.

Box 5 Definition and ratings of the STAS item 'pain control'

Rating definition

Pain control = effect of his/her pain on the patient

0 None

1 Occasional or grumbling single pain; patient is not anxious to be rid of symptom

2 Moderate distress, occasional bad days, pain limits some activity possible within extent of disease

3 Severe pain present often; activities and concentration markedly affected by pain

4 Severe and continuous overwhelming pain; unable to think of other matters

WEEK OF CARE	**0**	1	2	3	4	5	**6**
Nine core STAS items							
Pain control	4	2	0	0	0	0	0
Symptom control	3	3	2	2	2	2	2
Patient anxiety	3	2	2	2	3	1	1
Family anxiety	3	1	1	1	3	1	1
Patient insight	3	3	2	2	1	1	1
Family insight	0	0	0	0	0	0	0
Communication between patient and family	4	4	4	2	2	1	1
Communication between professionals	1	1	1	1	1	0	0
Communication professionals to patient and family	3	3	2	2	0	0	0
Total nine STAS items	24	19	14	12	12	6	6
Other STAS items							
Practical aid	2	2	0	0	0	1	1
Financial	3	2	2	2	2	2	2
Wasted time	1	0	0	0	0	0	0
Spiritual	?	?	?	?	1	1	1
Professional anxiety	2	2	1	1	1	1	1
Advising professionals	3	2	2	1	3	0	0
Planning	3	3	2	2	2	0	0
Predictability	2	2	1	1	1	1	1
Main other symptom: Dyspnoea throughout							
Days at home		6	7	7	7	7	7
Days in hospital	7	1					
Days in a hospice							

Fig. 3 STAS scores for one patient, showing control of pain and anxieties during care and later improved patient insight, but difficulties in controlling dyspnoea and alleviating financial problems.

This measure was developed by members of a hospice service and is intended for in-patient hospice use. It is also being used widely in many countries and is being validated. It is particularly useful where patients' assessments are needed. A study to compare the Support Team Assessment Schedule and the Edmonton Symptom Assessment System is planned. There is no charge for the use of the Edmonton Symptom Assessment System.

Box 6 Some of the main findings from palliative care audit using STAS

- Family needs are not assessed by some hospital-based teams
- Shortness of breath is not improved
- Late referrals had more problems and needed much work in short time
- Spiritual assessments often missed by some teams
- STAS is useful as clinical tool

Palliative Care Core Standards[32,34]

This measure includes six standard statements and 56 process and outcome items: collaboration with other agencies (eight items); symptom control (six items); patient and carer information (nine items); emotional support (11 items); bereavement care and support (13 items); specialist education and training for staff (nine items). It assesses structure, process, and outcomes so that the relationship between these elements can be examined. This may be very useful in identifying where failings occur. Development was by the regional collaboration of hospice and home care units, and in-patient hospice and community teams.

A pilot audit is underway to evaluate the Core Standards and

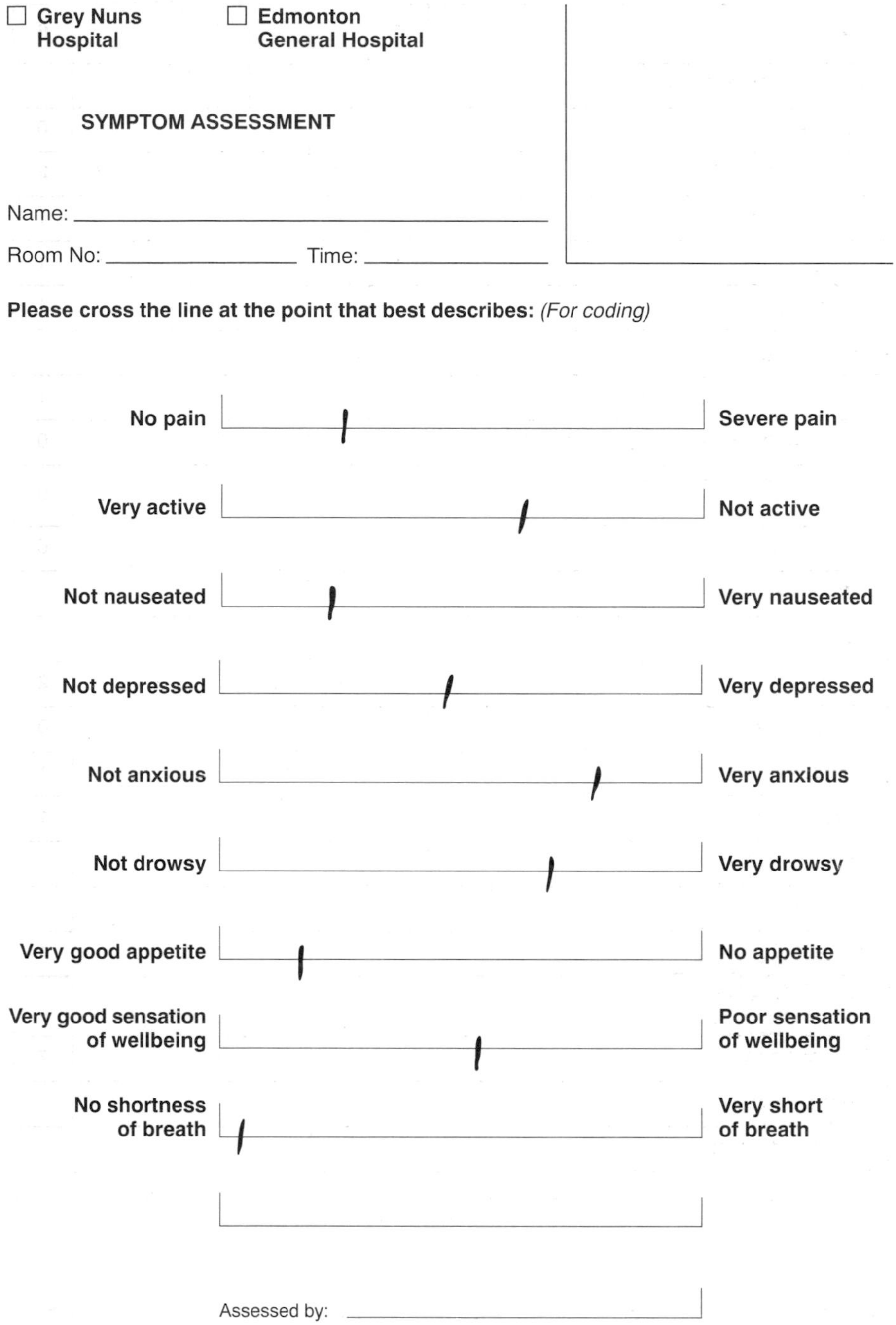

☐ Grey Nuns Hospital ☐ Edmonton General Hospital

SYMPTOM ASSESSMENT

Name: ______

Room No: ______ Time: ______

Please cross the line at the point that best describes: *(For coding)*

No pain	______	**Severe pain**
Very active	______	**Not active**
Not nauseated	______	**Very nauseated**
Not depressed	______	**Very depressed**
Not anxious	______	**Very anxious**
Not drowsy	______	**Very drowsy**
Very good appetite	______	**No appetite**
Very good sensation of wellbeing	______	**Poor sensation of wellbeing**
No shortness of breath	______	**Very short of breath**
	______	

Assessed by: ______

Fig. 4 Edmonton Symptom Assessment System: visual analogue scales.

their validity and reliability and to determine the criteria for the standard's usage.

Regional Study of Care of the Dying[35]

This audit uses a questionnaire administered to the person who knew most about the patient approximately 7 months after his or her death. It assesses process and outcomes including services received, symptoms during the last year of life, communication, satisfaction with care, and mental status of the carer. The questionnaire was developed and adapted from studies by Cartwright and co-workers[46,64].

The work builds on information collected 20 years ago and 5 years ago, so that patterns of care and symptoms can be compared. In the new study the carers of 3500 people who died in 20 districts in England were interviewed. Such an enterprise is not suitable for frequent audit; it is a valuable way of obtaining information about all patients who die, by identifying their carers through the death registration, rather than only those receiving services. Districts were able to buy into the 1992 study, and another national picture may be needed in 5 years time.

Documentation standards[54]

This measure, which assesses processes, includes 62 documentation standards covering general topics (four), referral details (23), admission assessment and progress (26), after death (five), and after discharge (four). It was developed with the help of six medical

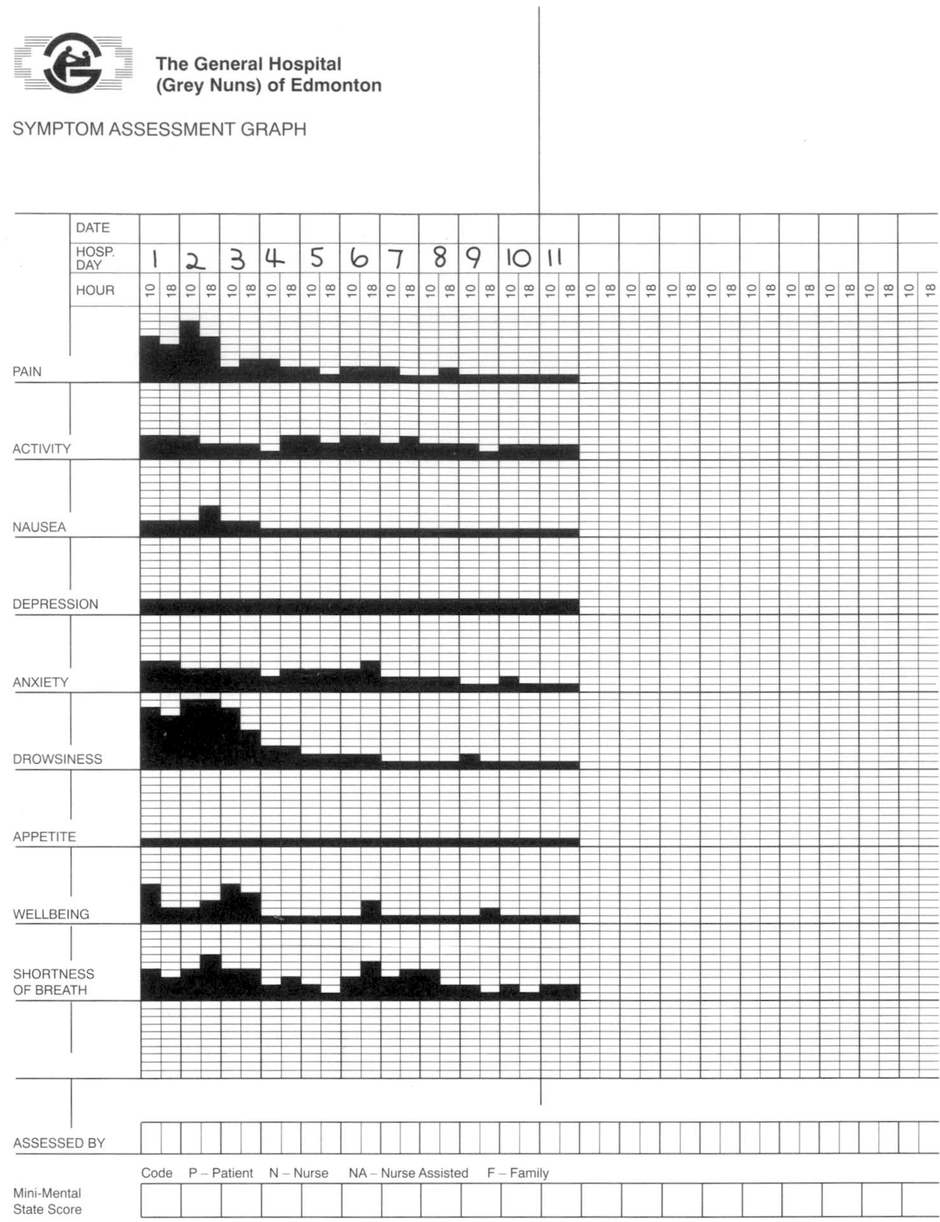

Fig. 5 Edmonton Symptom Assessment System: demonstrating symptom control for a patient during care.

directors and an in-patient hospice. The standards went through three rounds of testing, improvement, and revision, and have been used to audit care in six units.

Topic audits[29]

This measure, which assesses process and outcome, consists of topic audits including blood transfusion, drug chart recording, restlessness, pressure sores, and communication. It was developed by members of a hospice service and an in-patient hospice.

Other measures which have been proposed for auditing palliative care

Some other measures which have been proposed, although rarely used at present, and their potential for palliative care audit are described in this section.

Palliative care: guidelines for good practice and audit measures[60]

This measure, which assesses the structure and process of care, includes 29 items covering admission policy (five), clinical management (six), support of patient and family (five), communication (four), and documentation and administration (nine). It was developed by a working group of the Royal College of Physicians of London, which included many representatives from palliative care including the Association for Palliative Medicine of Great Britain and Ireland. The group met to consider key papers and then corresponded. The intended settings are inpatient hospices.

The audit items are listed but have not been tested in practice. There are a number of anecdotal reports of attempts to use this instrument which have failed because the questions used to assess care are too broad. There is also some criticism that the criteria are insufficiently challenging (personal communication from various hospices).

Care of people with a terminal illness[65]

This document, which assesses structure and process, includes 10 standards for contracts covering policies, provision, consumer participation, education, direct care, attitude, skills, and mix of staff, and 10 areas with numbers of standards for care in nursing homes. It was developed by an advisory group. Although standards are published, measures of the standards are not.

Standards of care for palliative nursing[66]

This includes seven topics: symptom control, spiritual support, family care, bereavement care, multiprofessional team, ethical practice and staff support, each with structure, process and outcome criteria. It was developed by a working group of the Royal College of Nursing, which included five senior nurses for various settings. Standards follow the principles of the Dynamic Standard Setting System. It was designed for a wide range of settings and is the second revision of an earlier document. Standards can be adapted for local use. Like the Palliative Care Core Standards, outcome criteria are given but ways of measuring these are not. Such measures need to be developed.

Rotterdam symptom checklist[67]

This measure includes 34 physical and psychosocial problems for the patient. It was developed on the basis of items identified from three studies: cancer patients undergoing chemotherapy or follow-up with early disease, cancer patients undergoing chemotherapy for advanced ovarian cancer, and cancer patients who were disease free. This measure is used widely in research, and different formats are available. It has been shown to be valid and reliable. Assessments are self-rated—there is evidence of missing data in half or more completed by patients close to death.[68]

Hebrew Rehabilitation Centre for Ageing—Quality-of-Life index (HRCA-QL)[69]

This includes five items: health, support, outlook, daily living, and mobility. It was developed and adapted from a quality-of-life index developed by Spitzer,[70] with the item 'mobility' replacing one called 'activity'. Items were identified by consensus of patients, the general public, and professionals, and were designed to apply to cancer patients at all stages of disease.[70] It was used in the largest evaluation of hospice care in the United States—the US National Hospice Study.[71] It is designed for completion by professionals, although it has been completed by patients.[69] The original index developed by Spitzer was validated, but the adapted index was not revalidated. It has been criticized for a lack of responsiveness in patients with advanced disease.[72]

European Organization for Research and Treatment of Cancer QLQ-C30[73]

This measure includes 30 items, both multi-items and single scales. It was developed by an international collaboration of professionals to devise items and scales. It has been tested before and during chemotherapy in lung cancer patients in different countries, and is now being tested widely in settings other than where originally developed. Patients take 11 min to complete it. It has been shown to distinguish between patients at different stages of disease, and is valid and reliable in those settings for which it was originally developed.[73]

Short Form-36 (SF-36)[74,75]

This measure includes 36 items assessing bodily pain, self-reported general health, mental health, limitations, energy, social functioning, and change in health in the previous year (this last item is not a core domain and the time period can vary). It is one of several health status questionnaires developed in the United States by the Medical Outcomes Study. It is a 36-item short form of a longer questionnaire and has been developed to assess the outcomes of hospital care in the United States. It is designed for patients at all stages of disease—from those who are completely well to those with symptoms. It is becoming very widely used. An English (not American) version is available. It is very quick and takes just a few minutes to complete. This is its main advantage over other general (generic) measures such as the Nottingham Health Profile. Its validity, reliability, and responsiveness are often well regarded, but the measure is undergoing further testing. It has been tested in elderly patients, although not in patients with advanced disease, and seems to be of most use in assessing populations. Caution is urged when trying to assess therapies or services.[74,75]

Hospital Anxiety and Depression Scale (HAD)[76]

This measure includes 14 items divided into two subscales: seven items to assess anxiety and seven to assess depression. It was developed for patient completion in sick populations and has been translated into several languages. It has been validated against other scales and has been described as quick and easy to use. It is used widely in cancer patients, but its application in palliative care is still being tested.

McGill pain questionnaire[77]

This assesses pain according to description (e.g. throbbing) and severity. It was developed for completion by patients. At least five versions of the index are available, ranging from the short form (15 descriptors) to the longest version (128 descriptors). It only assesses pain. Self-completion and verbal versions are available, although the originator recommended the verbal form. It has good test–retest reliability.[78]

Conclusions

Audit approaches and methods are now well advanced in palliative care, particularly in clinical audit. There is a choice of tried and tested methods and measures which can be adapted for specific needs, rather than having to develop new procedures. Practical measures for clinical audit include the Support Team Assessment Schedule and the Edmonton Symptom Assessment Scale (both of which have either been validated or are being tested) and Finlay's topic audits. Clinical audits which use satisfaction surveys or surveys after bereavement are probably more costly, but are still possible. These may prove useful for national audits of palliative care. Again, measures are available. Apart from completing the audit cycle, clinical audit can look to developing clinical protocols for treatment or algorithms to predict patient problems and the need for specialized care. Organizational audit is less well advanced, and we need research to determine what patient benefit results from the advocated structures of care. The question of who should be the 'experts' who decide what constitutes an ideal structure remains unanswered. Nevertheless, one system of organizational audit for palliative care has been developed in the United Kingdom and its results are likely to provide some very useful data to assist this debate.

Audit is here to stay, and is now widely accepted. However, it requires resources, and so it must be sure to benefit patients and families, be kept as simple and efficient as possible, and have a strong educational component. Further work is needed to evaluate the impact of different audit approaches and methods on improving care so that we know which approach is most cost-effective. If palliative approaches extend backwards to include patients earlier in care, rather than only those near to death, audit could become a means for clinical dialogue and education between specialties. Practitioners of palliative medicine could take the lead in encouraging this, promoting methods among their medical and surgical colleagues and presenting their own results.

References

1. Shaw CD. Quality assurance in the United Kingdom. *Quality Assurance in Health Care*, 1993; **5**(2):107–18
2. Shaw CD. *Medical Audit. A Hospital Handbook*. London: King's Fund Centre, 1989.
3. Rosser RM. A history of the development of health indices. In: Smith GT, ed. *Measuring the Social Benefits of Medicine*. London: Office of Health Economics, 1985.
4. Shaw CD. Aspect of audit. 1. The background. *British Medical Journal*, 1980; **280**:1256–8.
5. Department of Health. *Working for Patients. Medical Audit Working Paper 6*. London: HMSO, 1989.
6. Department of Health. *Medical Audit in the Hospital and Community Health Services*. Draft Health Circular. London: Department of Health, 1990.
7. Department of Health. *Medical Audit in the Hospital and Community Health Services*. HC(91)2. London: Department of Health, 1991.
8. Butters E, Higginson I, George R, Smits A, McCarthy M. Assessing the symptoms, anxiety and practical needs of HIV/AIDS patients receiving palliative care. *Quality of Life Research*, 1992; **1**(1):47–51.
9. Parkes CM. Terminal care: evaluation of in-patient service at St Christopher's Hospice. Part I. Views of surviving spouse on effects of the service on the patient. *Postgraduate Medical Journal*, 1979; **55**:517–22.
10. Parkes CM. Terminal care: home, hospital, or hospice? *Lancet*, 1985; **i**:155–7.
11. Hinton J. A comparison of places and policies for terminal care. *Lancet*, 1979; **i**:29–32.
12. Higginson I. Palliative care: a review of past changes and future trends. *Journal of Public Health Medicine*, 1993; **15**(1):3–8.
13. Johnson I, Rogers C, Biswas B, Ahmedzai S. What do hospices do? A survey of hospices in the United Kingdom and Republic of Ireland. *British Medical Journal*, 1990; **300**:791–3.
14. Kirkham S, Davis M. Bed occupancy, patient throughput and size of independent hospice units in the UK. *Palliative Medicine*, 1992; **6**:47–53.
15. Eve A, Smith AM. Palliative care services in Britain and Ireland—update 1991. *Palliative Medicine*, 1994; **8**(1):19–27.
16. Higginson I. Clinical audit: getting started, keeping going. In: Higginson I, ed. *Clinical Audit in Palliative Care*. Oxford: Radcliffe Medical Press, 1993.
17. Higginson I. *Quality, Standards, Clinical and Organisational Audit for Palliative Care*. London: National Council for Hospice and Specialist Palliative Care Services, 1992.
18. Clark D, Neale B, Heather P. Contacting for palliative care. *Social Science and Medicine*, 1995; **40**(9):1193–1202.
19. Haines A, Jones R. Implementing findings of research. *British Medical Journal* 1994; **308**: 1488–92
20. Butters E, Higginson I, Murphy F, McDonnell M. Audit experience: using a data base to audit care. In: Higginson I, ed. *Clinical Audit in Palliative Care*. Oxford: Radcliffe Medical Press, 1993:156–67.
21. Dale RF. The Cambridge Audit System in a service hospital. *Journal of the Royal Naval Medical Service*, 1990; **76**(3):147–54.
22. King's Fund Centre. *Organisational Audit (Accreditation UK): Standards for an Acute Hospital*. London: King's Fund Centre, 1990.
23. Shaw CD, Brooks TE. Health service accreditation in the United Kingdom. *Quality Assurance in Health Care*, 1991; **3**(3):133–40.
24. Hayes J, Scrivens E. *An Evaluation of the Accrediation Programme for Community Hospitals 1990–93*. Bristol: Hospital Accreditation Programme, 1993.
25. Shaw CD. *Speciality Medical Audit*. London: King's Fund Centre, 1992.
26. Black N. Quality assurance of medical care. *Journal of Public Health Medicine* 1990; **12**(2):97–104.
27. NHS Management Executive. *The Quality Journey. A Guide to Total Quality Management in the NHS*. Leeds: NHS Management Executive, 1993.
28. Bruera E, MacDonald S. Audit methods: The Edmonton Symptom Assessment system. In: Higginson I, ed. *Clinical Audit in Palliative Care*. Oxford: Radcliffe Medical Press, 1993.
29. Finlay I. Audit experience: views of a hospice director. In: Higginson I, ed. *Clinical Audit in Palliative Care*. Oxford: Radcliffe Medical Press, 1993.
30. Hayes A. Audit experience: assessing staff's views. In: Higginson I, ed. *Clinical Audit in Palliative Care*. Oxford: Radcliffe Medical Press, 1993.
31. Higginson I, McCarthy M. Measuring symptoms in terminal cancer:are pain dyspnoea controlled? *Journal of the Royal Society of Medicine*, 1989; **82**:264–7.
32. Hunt J. Audit methods: palliative care core standards. In: Higginson I, ed. *Clinical Audit in Palliative Care*. Oxford: Radcliffe Medical Press, 1993.
33. McKee E. Audit experience: a nurse manager in home care. In: Higginson I, ed. *Clinical Audit in Palliative Care*. Oxford: Radcliffe Medical Press, 1993.
34. Trent Hospice Audit Group. *Palliative Care Core Standards: A Multidisciplinary Approach*. Trinity Street, Derby: Nightingale Macmillan Continuing Care Unit, 1992.
35. Addington-Hall J, McCarthy M. Audit methods: views of the family after the death. In: Higginson I, ed. *Clinical Audit in Palliative Care*. Oxford: Radcliffe Medical Press, 1993.
36. Keay TJ, Fredman L, Taler GA, Datta S, Levenson SA. Indicators of quality medical care for the terminally ill in nursing homes. *Journal of the American Geriatric Society*, 1994; **42**(8):853–60.
37. Boys L, Peat SJ, Hanna MH, Burn K. Audit of neural blockade for palliative care patients in an acute unit. *Palliative Medicine*, 1993; **7**(3):205–11
38. Weisman AD. The psychiatrist and the inexorable. In Feifel JC, ed. *New Meanings of Death*. New York: McGraw-Hill, 1977.
39. Kellehear A. *Dying of Cancer. The Final Year of Life*. London: Harwood, 1990.
40. James N. A family and a team. In Gilmore A, Gilmore S, ed. *A Safer Death: Multidisciplinary Aspects of Terminal Care*. New York: Plenum, 1988.
41. Working Group on Terminal Care (Wilkes E, chairman). National terminal care policy. *Journal of the Royal College of General Practitioners*, 1980; **30**:466–71.
42. Ford G, for Working Group on Clinical Guidelines of the National Council for Hospice and Specialist Palliative Care Services. *Guidelines for Specialist Palliative Care Services*. London: National Council for Hospice and Specialist Palliative Care Services, 1995.
43. Haines A, Booroff A. Terminal care at home: perspective from general practice. *British Medical Journal*, 1986; **292**:1051–3.
44. Charlton RC. Attitudes towards care of the dying: a questionnaire survey of general practice attenders. *Family Practitioner*, 1991; **8**(4):356–9.
45. Higginson I, Wade A, McCarthy M. Palliative care: views of patients and their families. *British Medical Journal* 1990; **301**:277–81.
46. Cartwright A, Hockey L, Anderson JL. *Life before Death*. London: Routledge and Kegan Paul, 1973.

47. Addington-Hall J, MacDonald L, Anderson H, Freeling P. Dying from cancer:the view of bereaved family and the friends about the experiences of terminally ill patients. *Palliative Medicine*, 1991; **5**:207–14.
48. Saunders C, Sykes N. *The Management of Terminal Malignant Disease.* 3rd edn. London: Edward Arnold, 1993.
49. Higginson I, Wade A, McCarthy M. Effectiveness of two palliative support teams. *Journal of Public Health Medicine*, 1992; **1**:50–6.
50. Donabedian A. The definition of quality and approaches to its assessment. In *Explorations in Quality Assessment and Monitoring*, Vol. 1. Michigan: Health Administration Press, 1980.
51. Coles C. Making audit truly educational. *Postgraduate Medical Journal*, 1990; **66**(Supplement 3):S32–6.
52. Prouse M. Organisational audit for palliative care services. *European Journal of Palliative Care*, 1994; **1**(4):184–6.
53. Higginson I. Audit methods: a community schedule. In Higginson I, ed. *Clinical Audit in Palliative Care.* Oxford: Radcliffe Medical Press, 1993.
54. Catterall RA. Audit methods: regional documentation standards. In Higginson I, ed. *Clinical Audit in Palliative Care.* Oxford: Radcliffe Medical Press, 1993.
55. Cancer Relief Macmillan Fund. *Organisational Audit for Specialist Palliative Care Services.* London: Cancer Relief Macmillan Fund, 1994.
56. Higginson I. Audit methods: validation and in-patient use. In Higginson I, ed. *Clinical Audit in Palliative Care.* Oxford: Radcliffe Medical Press, 1993.
57. Higginson I, McCarthy M. Validity of the support team assessment schedule: do staffs' ratings reflect those made by patients or their families? *Palliative Medicine*, 1993; **7**:219–28.
58. Higginson I, McCarthy M. Validity of a measure of palliative care—comparison with a quality of life index. *Palliative Medicine*, 1994; **8**(4):282–90.
59. Bruera E, Kuehn N, Miller M, Selmser P, MacMillan K. The Edmonton Symptom Assessment System (ESAS): a simple method for the assessment of palliative care patients. *Journal of Palliative Care*, 1991; **7**(2):6–9.
60. Working Group of the Research Unit, Royal College of Physicians. *Palliative Care—Guidelines for Good Practice and Audit Measures.* London: Royal College of Physicians of London, 1991.
61. McDaid P. New STAS items: sadness/grief and confidence/self worth. In Webb D, ed. *STAS Newsletter.* London: Palliative Care Research Group, 1994:6–7.
62. Higginson I. Clinical teams, general practice, audit and outcomes. In *Outcomes into Clinical Practice.* London: British Medical Association Books, 1994.
63. Butters E, *et al. The Palliative Care Management System—Users Manual and Package.* Dublin: Irish Cancer Society, 1995.
64. Cartwright A. Changes in life and care in the year before death 1969–1987. *Journal of Public Health Medicine*, 1991; **13**(2):81–7.
65. National Association of Health Authorities and Trusts. *Care of People with a Terminal Illness.* Birmingham: National Association of Health Authorities and Trusts.
66. RCN Dynamic Quality Improvement Programme. *Standards of Care for Palliative Nursing.* London: Royal College of Nursing, 1993.
67. de Haes JCJM, van Knippenbery FCE, Neijt JP. Measuring psychological and physical distress in cancer patients: structure and application of the Rotterdam Symptom Checklist. *British Journal of Cancer*, 1990; **62**:1034–8.
68. Hopwood P, Howell A, Maguire P. Psychiatric morbidity in patients with advanced cancer of the breast: prevalence measured by two self-rating questionnaires. *British Journal of Cancer*, 1991; **62**(2):349–52.
69. Greer DS, Mor V, Morris JN, Sherwood S, Kidder D, Birnbaum H. An alternative in terminal care: results of the National Hospice Study. *Journal of Chronic Disease*, 1986; **39**:9–26.
70. Spitzer WO, *et al.* Measuring the quality of life of cancer patients: a concise QL index for use by physicians. *Journal of Chronic Disease*, 1981; **34**:585–97.
71. Mor V, Greer DS, Kastenbaum R. *The Hospice Experiment.* Baltimore, MD: Johns Hopkins University Press, 1988.
72. Mount BM, Scott JF. Whither hospice evaluation? *Journal of Chronic Disease*, 1983; **36**:731–6.
73. Aaronson NK, *et al.* The European Organisation for Research and Treatment of Cancer QLQ-C30: a quality of life instrument for use in international clinical trials in oncology. *Journal of the National Cancer Institute*, 1993; **85**(5):365–75.
74. Dixon P, Heaton J, Long A, Warburton A. Reviewing and applying the SF-36. *Outcomes Briefing (UK Clearing House on Health Outcomes)*, 1994; **4**:3–25.
75. Hill S, Harris U. Assessing the outcome of health care for the older person in community settings: should we use the SF-36? *Outcomes Briefing (UK Clearing House on Health Outcomes)*, 1994; **4**:26–7.
76. Zigmond AS, Snaith RP. The Hospital Anxiety and Depression Scale. *Acta Psychiatrica Scandinavica*, 1983; **67**:361–70.
77. Melzack R. The McGill pain questionnaire: major properties and scoring methods. *Pain*, 1975; **1**:277–99.
78. Wilkin D, Hallam L, Doggett MA. *Measures of Need and Outcome for Primary Health Care.* Oxford University Press, 1992.

Recommended reading

National Council for Hospice and Specialist Palliative Care Services, London. *Making palliative care better: quality improvement, multiprofessional audit and standards.* Occasional paper no. 12, March 1997.

2.7 Quality of life assessment in palliative care

Jennifer J. Clinch, Deborah Dudgeon, and Harvey Schipper

Measurement of quality of life provides a broad biopsychosocial paradigm for the evaluation of medical therapy. In addition to the physiological parameters to which we are accustomed, the quality-of-life paradigm adds the psychological and sociological dimension, as well as specific representation of symptoms of both disease and treatment. This broadened base of evaluation is well suited to palliative medicine.

Contemporary palliative care takes its root in the comprehensive care of people whose medical illness is progressive and not amenable to curative therapies. Most frequently this is toward the end of life, when the illness is manifest and symptomatic. However, palliation can be viewed from a broader perspective, as extending from diagnosis of an incurable disease onward. Attempts to control symptoms and alter the fundamental biology of an illness are not necessarily incompatible. If one considers cancer control as a spectrum, beginning with prevention and proceeding through early detection, diagnosis, and treatment and finally the management of advanced incurable illness, each point in the continuum is characterized by a requirement for both biological and symptomatic understanding of the process. The patient receiving adjuvant chemotherapy, though not strictly 'palliative', also has symptom control and quality-of-life concerns. These are analogous to those experienced by patients with early incurable disease or advanced recurrence. At each point along the spectrum, the overall therapeutic strategy may differ, but the expanded horizon offered by an analysis based on quality of life is consistent. The measures of success of our interventions may be multiple (e.g. in a prevention setting, diminished incidence of disease and the various consequences of the intervention), and they will differ along the spectrum. Measures of tumour response are important in curative therapies, but of less consequence at the end of life, where treatment is more symptom driven. In each instance a focus on therapeutic goals leads to the selection and balancing of measures of efficacy. This expanded concept of palliation provides an opportunity for knowledge gained in the care of the dying to be applied to the suffering of those fortunate to face a better prognosis. What follows is an overview of the concept and its attendant technology. The intent is to facilitate its use as an evaluative tool and to help shape a humane, mainstream palliative medicine.

Towards a definition of quality of life

Framing the concept

A number of different models have been proposed to define the quality of life construct. Many have unique perspectives which have important implications for how the construct is turned into something measurable. A few of these different views are presented below.

Calman's gap: patient's expectations

Calman described quality of life in inverse relationship to the size of the gap between an individual's expectations and the reality of the situation;[1] the smaller the gap, the better the quality of life. The gap principle is also implicitly present in most quality-of-life questionnaires, where it is assumed that the individual automatically assesses his/her function based upon what is normal for him/her. Thus, the score on a question does not reflect some absolute level of quality of life but is relative to the individual's expectations. According to this model, a person's quality of life can be influenced either by change in his/her actual condition or by a change in his/her expectations. In the palliative care setting, it is important to keep this in mind as the person's expectations are often adjusted as acceptance of functional limitations, secondary to disease progression, occurs. As such, in addition to assessing the actual condition, a measure of expectations needs to be developed in order to use this model properly.

The utility concept: trade-offs now and later

Relative quality of life can also be defined in terms of its utility or value compared to normal function. Utilities are on a scale of zero to one, with normal function having a value of one and death a value of zero. If some level of function is assigned a value of 0.5, then 1 year of life at the lower functional level is considered equivalent to only half a year at the normal level. This is the essence of the concept of quality-adjusted life-years (QALYs) of survival. The TWiST model, developed by Gelber and Goldhirsch, has attempted to apply this concept to breast cancer patients.[2] **TWiST** stands for time without symptoms and toxicity of either disease or therapy. The patient can thus assign a lower utility value for time with symptoms and time with toxicity. This narrow physiological analysis has recently been broadened to encompass other dimensions, more closely approximating the quality-of-life construct.[3,4]

Another method of assessing utility is the time trade-off approach. This was exemplified by McNeil *et al.* in a study of healthy individuals faced with the hypothetical question of a choice between surgery and radiation for treatment of laryngeal cancer, that is, a choice between possibly longer survival with loss of speech or shorter survival while retaining speech.[5] The survival time that individuals were willing to trade off, in order to retain their ability

Table 1 Commonly identified dimensions of quality of life

Physical concerns (symptoms; pain)	Treatment satisfaction (including financial concerns)
Functional ability (activity)	Future orientation (planning; hope)
Family well-being	Sexuality/intimacy (including body image)
Emotional well-being	Occupational functioning
Spirituality	
Social functioning	

to communicate, depended upon their chosen profession and the importance of speech to that work. Executives were willing to trade off more years of life to keep their voice than firefighters. This emphasizes the very individual and personal nature of what constitutes quality of life.

Although not impacting on survival, an analogous situation in patients with chronic pain might be one person's choice for complete analgesia regardless of the level of sedation, while another might accept more pain to achieve greater wakefulness.

A recent study by Cassileth *et al.* provides prospective quality-of-life data in men with previously untreated stage D prostate cancer who chose as treatment either orchiectomy or the leuteinizing hormone releasing hormone agonist goserelin acetate. Six months later the hormonally treated group showed a maintained improvement in overall quality of life and mood while the initial improvement at 3 months had declined to baseline in the orchiectomy group. Sexual function, as expected, declined in both groups but marital relationship improved in the hormonal group and declined in the orchiectomy group.[6] In this case the trade-off was the cost and inconvenience of monthly subcutaneous injections as compared to an inexpensive one-time procedure.

Reintegration: the effort to return to function

Wood-Dauphinee and Williams have proposed the concept of reintegration to normal living as a proxy for quality of life.[7] This is defined as the reorganization of an individual's physical, psychological, and social characteristics into a harmonious whole, so that well-adjusted living can be resumed after an incapacitating illness or trauma. Essentially, this is a rehabilitation concept, and it is important because it focuses upon the recovery side of illness or toxic treatment. Related to this is the competency-based model of coping with cancer. There are three components to this model: problem specification, response enumeration, and response evaluation. An instrument for assessing the first component has been developed by Schag and Heinrich and is known as the cancer rehabilitation evaluation system (CARES).[8] The focus of this instrument is on assessing the specific components of behaviour affected by cancer. It is a deliberate move away from an assessment of cancer's impact in terms of emotional distress. This component, and symptom distress, were also deliberately omitted from the reintegration concept. Although both these models lack components usually included in quality-of-life assessment, the questionnaires generated from each have been found to correlate well with quality-of-life measures. Further, such instruments are not particularly appropriate to the palliative care setting, the basic concept of reintegration has definite application. An individual whose chronic pain has prevented him/her from performance of his/her usual roles at work or in the family setting can usually resume those roles, albeit temporarily, when the pain is adequately controlled.

Patient-centred or community-centred quality of life

Most conceptual definitions of health-related quality of life are patient-centred and do not go much beyond the immediate impact on the patient. However, Ware views quality of life in the broader context of a patient's immediate and more distant environment.[9] The impact of a disease on quality of life is structured much like the concentric surface ripples seen after dropping a stone in water. Initially, the effect is on the patient's physiology; this then spreads to physical functioning, psychological functioning, general health perception, and, finally, social role functioning. The outermost ripple also affects the community at large. The causal directions implicit in this model have not been tested but questionnaires have been developed to measure these various components of the impact of disease.

Quality of life and the meaning of illness

Kleinman, a medical anthropologist and psychiatrist, believes that quality of life in a medical context is an attempt to measure the illness side of the illness/disease construct.[10] Quality of life is the measurement of the perception of the impact of the disease and is, therefore, both subjective and culturally bound.

In any serious illness, but particularly in the case of terminal illness, an individual may experience a spiritual crisis and ask questions such as 'why me?' and 'why now?'.[11] Attempts to answer such questions represent efforts to attribute meaning to the illness and to cope with it. Support for such emotional work should be available to patients from their physicians and/or other health-care professionals. Measures of spiritual well-being represent some of the earliest attempts to measure quality of life,[12] but with few exceptions these seem to have been largely ignored in later developments of the paradigm.[13-15]

Over the past few years, a number of similar quality-of-life questionnaires have been developed. After reviewing the different names (now more than 30) for quality-of-life dimensions listed by various authors, Cella and Tulsky thought that 10 were distinct enough to warrant separate listing (Table 1).[16]

Many of the dimensions in the right hand column of Table 1 could possibly be subsumed under one of the dimensions on the left. However, there is no real consensus regarding whether the additional areas do indeed represent a real expansion of the quality-of-life construct. This question needs to be tested empirically.

It is also possible that several of the areas in the list may be much more relevant for one type of illness than another. In order to resolve this problem Aaronson proposed the 'core-plus-module' model that has been used for development of a quality-of-life questionnaire by the European Organization for Research and Treatment of Cancer (EORTC).[17] This model proposes that there are core items for quality of life applicable to all types of cancer. In addition, they propose to develop a set of disease-specific modules that include questions relevant only to one form of cancer. Several modules have now been developed.[18-20] A module does not necessarily add new information but is designed to expand on certain disease-specific issues in order to improve sensitivity. There is little data as yet relating to the added precision, sensitivity, or predictive validity that such an approach provides in the clinical setting.

Most quality-of-life instruments were developed for use in patients in the earlier stages of their disease where cure or long-term control was considered possible. The 'core-plus-module' model could possibly be used to capture changes in quality of life along the spectrum of the disease trajectory. A module specific to the advanced patient could be developed and added to an established instrument for earlier stages of disease. One such study is under way using the Functional Living Index–Cancer (FLIC).[21]

Taken across the spectrum of disease there seems to be general agreement upon some of the component parts of quality of life, or at least those parts that it is relevant to measure in ill people.[16,22] These areas of agreement are:

(1) physical function

(2) emotional or psychological function

(3) social function

(4) symptoms of disease or its treatment.

There is no consensus on a full definition of these components or how they relate to each other or to other areas not always included in the quality-of-life construct. Areas still debated include the financial impact of disease,[23] sexual function,[24] body image concerns, [25] and spirituality.[26]

A full conceptual model of quality of life in disease states should also incorporate an explanation of the inter-relationships of the elements of the composite construct throughout the stages of a disease and its treatment. Such models could be very useful for generating hypotheses to investigate the links among the variables studied and specific quality-of-life outcomes. Of 11 conceptual models characterized by Hollen *et al.*, only two have delineated interdependent dimensions with directional relationships amenable to testing.[27] Also, all of the measurement issues that have been implied by the various models must be addressed before the construct can be made fully operational.

In the absence of a full theoretical model for quality of life, the tendency is to allow the construct to be defined by the operations used to measure it. For a conceptual definition to be practically useful, a method of measurement must be developed for the construct. This process often falls short of fully representing the original concept due to the difficulties encountered in developing an objective measure of an abstract concept. One very good example of this problem is that nobody has ever succeeded in developing a measure of creativity, despite the fact that everyone has an intuitive knowledge of what the term means. Thus, of necessity, the quality-of-life questionnaire comes to define quality of life.

Asking the question and weighing the answer

Whatever the model, the relative impact of the various components on overall quality of life is an issue to consider. The importance of these components varies not only between individuals but from time to time in the same person over the course of an illness. Should a set of items, representing a specific component of quality of life, be summed and weighted in such a way as to reflect the importance of that component to the patient? This would seem to be the only meaningful method of defining intra- and inter-individual variation in overall quality of life. In the functional assessment of cancer therapy (FACT) index, Cella *et al.* attempt to address this issue.[28] An experimental item at the end of each subscale in this questionnaire allows explicit appraisal of the effect each dimension has on overall quality of life.

The notion of weighting scores has been extended to the individual items on a quality-of-life questionnaire by Ferrans and Powers;[29] however, this method of weighting ignores the issue of how many questions represent each quality-of-life component. If a total score for the whole questionnaire is used to represent overall quality of life, then a whole dimension could be over- or under-emphasized simply by having more or fewer questions than the other dimensions. When neither items nor scales are weighted according to importance, a total score obtained by adding all the item scores is implicitly weighted by the number of questions representing each component.

Another general conceptual issue is how questions are put to the patient. It is not the mere presence or absence of symptoms that is important but rather the extent to which symptoms affect the patient's overall well-being. Again, to emphasize the differences between individuals, this impact may vary considerably from patient to patient for the same degree of impairment as judged by an observer.[30] Thus, questions asking 'Are you bothered by . . .' symptom X are included as well as 'Do you have . . .' symptom X.

The issue of culture

Cultural sensitivity may be more important in palliative care than in other areas of medicine and oncology. The focus is less physiological, and more holistic with matters of family, world view, and spirit coming to the forefront, especially toward the end of life. Quality of life is important in most places, and it is likely that current tools and procedures can form the basis of good research. However, the process requires understanding of the principles of cross-cultural research. This area of inquiry examines differences in culture, and provides a framework for describing these in cultural perspective, potentially enabling ideas derived from one setting to be applied in another. Moving tools across languages and cultures requires more than literal translation. Equivalent concepts may be expressed in totally different ways.

Palliation is a distinctly Western notion in the sense we understand it, meaning 'The active total care of patients whose disease is not responsive to curative treatment'.[31] In some cultures disease is not considered as much of a departure from the normal life process as we perceive it to be in the West. Symptoms or 'suffering' may have a different connotation. The conundrum was eloquently put by a former Minister of Health of Cameroon, Dr Victor Ngu, who described suffering as '. . .what is left after you take the pain away.' He went on to explain that illness and death are part of life, and in his community where material expectations were less, and the North American death aversion culture less evident, the impending end of life drew families together in a manner that seemed different from his experience of European society. Clearly those differences in cultural expression will affect formal measurement of quality of life.

Apart from its contextual meaning, the translational meaning of pain may also be different. The Christian theological concept of pain as a purifying force is even contested within the Judaeo-Christian religious community. Goh relates the remarkable story of a man from Singapore with advanced cancer whose pain seemed inexplicably out of control, despite careful assessment and appropriate medication administered by an attentive family (personal communication). After a considerable period of anguish and confusion it became clear this man's pain was spiritual. A life-long Buddhist, he had recently converted to Christianity in the expectation that this would ease and speed his transition to the next life, as it seemed to have done for a friend. When the desired result was not obtained after a few weeks, the man's despondency became anguish which was translated as 'pain' and treated with morphine, not surprisingly without success. Thus, from a cultural perspective the first step in quality-of-life assessment, whether for a clinical trial or the individual patient, is to learn enough about the culture to ensure that the entire direction of inquiry makes sense.

Given the preceding caution, there is an emerging body of evidence that the quality-of-life concept has cross-culturally robust constructs.[32,33] In part, this is due to the limited, function-oriented nature of the tools. Physical, psychological, and social function, noxious symptoms and sensations, and family hardship appear broadly relevant. There is, however, scant literature describing the relative importance of these or similar factors in different cultures.

Instrument development

We have devised some general guidelines for the development of both general and disease-specific indices of quality of life.[21] Obviously the first step in any such undertaking is to explore the relevant literature for any previous work in the area and for information on the symptoms and concerns displayed by individuals suffering from the disease in question. Once this background information is available a panel is convened, composed of individuals who may have insight into the problems experienced by the patient which are associated with the illness. This panel should include present and former patients, their spouses and other relatives, and health professionals who regularly provide therapy for the condition. The last group will probably include physicians (from a number of specialties), nurses, social workers, psychologists, and rehabilitation therapists.

At the first meeting of the panel the general areas of patient concern are discussed and consensus reached upon the domains that should be represented in the questionnaire. In preparation for the next panel meeting, each member is asked to develop several questions to cover all the domains equally. Individuals are requested to contribute beyond their usual area of concern because they may bring a different perspective. At this early stage it is important to make sure that the domains have been adequately sampled thus ensuring good content validity for the questionnaire.

After the first batch of questions has been generated, they are collated and obvious duplications are removed. If some domains are not covered adequately or equally after removing duplicates, the panel members will then be asked to generate more questions in specific areas. Once there is a sufficient pool of questions, the panel meets again to consider issues of question comprehensibility. These include making sure that each question contains only one idea, that the language is sufficiently simple for it to be understood by most people, and that assumptions have not been made that would preclude some individuals from answering the question. At this stage the questionnaire is ready for pilot testing.

A few patients of the appropriate type are approached to complete the questionnaire plus a debriefing form that asks about any difficulties experienced when answering questions and any additional areas of concern to the patient. Adjustments are made to the questionnaire based on these responses. The modified questionnaire is then administered to a large group of patients so that the responses can undergo factor analysis, in an attempt to reduce the overall number of questions.[34] Factor analysis determines the number and nature of the dimensions required to account for the total variance in the answers to the questionnaire. A rule of thumb to determine the required sample size is that there should be 10 patients per question. This is unlikely to be possible if the number of questions is too large. A compromise must usually be made between the number of questions and the number of patients tested.

After completing the factor analysis, factor loadings (correlations between questions and factors) are examined to determine the nature of the underlying element of quality of life that the factor represents. If the original work of defining the questions was done well there should be a good match between the hypothetical domains of quality of life and the factors. Reduction of the number of questions is accomplished by selecting the highest loading questions for each domain until the questionnaire is the desired overall length.

There will often be questions that load fairly highly on more than one factor, indicating that they are not pure measures of any one domain. These questions should be eliminated from the final questionnaire but should be studied carefully to determine the reason for their multidimensionality. This procedure should enable better question design if more questions are needed.

Another difficulty that may occur is that some factors do not have a sufficient number of high loading questions to provide a proper representation of that facet of quality of life. If subscales are desired, and they usually will be, then it is important to have enough questions for each subscale.

Some quality-of-life questionnaires have been criticized because they provide an overall score rather than several subscale scores. The reason for this criticism is that an overall score from a multidimensional scale can be arrived at in a variety of ways. One person may have poor physical function but good psychological function and another person the reverse, yet both may have the same overall score. An overall score does not provide much insight if the quality-of-life assessment is to be used to direct clinical practice. Therefore, if the first factor analysis reveals a poor representation of one quality-of-life domain, additional questions must be prepared and the new version of the questionnaire administered to a new sample of patients.

The final version of the questionnaire should be administered to at least two groups of subjects to ensure that the factor structure is stable. This is particularly important if only a few patients were tested in relation to the number of items on the questionnaire. At the same time additional tests relating to the various subscales should be administered to establish concurrent validity. Construct validation is a cumulative process and is best assessed by the behaviour of the questionnaire scores under various conditions. Every time a clinical trial demonstrates a hypothesized between-group difference in scores on a quality-of-life dimension this adds to the weight of evidence for construct validity. Since the validity of an instrument is limited by its reliability, that is the extent to which scores are consistent over time, it is also important to assess reliability.

Internal consistency is one measure of reliability but it is only reasonable to expect consistency within subscales and not between them. Cronbach's alpha should be calculated for each subscale separately. Since quality of life is variable over time it may not be reasonable to expect high values for test–retest reliability if the time interval between the two administrations of the test is large. For short time intervals, such as one day, the correlation coefficients should be in the acceptable range of 0.8 or higher.

For the clinician contemplating quality-of-life assessment in a different culture, shaping a culturally appropriate question is the starting point. Thereafter comes the decision about instrumentation. Provided rigorous techniques are used, a locale-specific instrument might be developed. The problem then becomes the relationship between data collected with the new instrument and that from more established measures. A logical alternative is to adapt an existing tool. It is now generally accepted that simple language translation and back-translation is not sufficient. A certain amount of careful patient interviewing and analysis must be undertaken to determine the contextual meaning of questions, a matter significantly more nuanced than verbatim translation. For example, a question relating to physical function, and perhaps scaled, might use the ability to climb stairs as the measure. It will not work in a setting where there are no stairs. Our experience in Asia offers another example. A household activities question on the FLIC could not be answered by most men and many middle to upper class women because these roles were totally foreign to the local culture.[32] The verbatim translation was understandable but it had no meaning, an observation only made during a carefully designed testing and de-briefing process. The debriefing and translation/back-translation are iterative and one informs the other. Often disparities uncovered in the back-translation lead to a subtler understanding of fundamental concepts and differences.

It is tempting to transpose quality-of-life methodologies from Western society because there are important questions to ask. There may be a highly prevalent disease in Africa (HIV-related Kaposi's sarcoma for example), or an opportunity for intellectual collaboration. In the West, the methodologies have been well established, and it seems efficient to 'use what we know'. In working in another culture, there are three seminal questions to ask:

1. Are the concepts being explored compatible and is the question of value or relevance to the subject?
2. Is the study feasible, given the cultural and physical setting?
3. Can a valid and understandable textual translation of measurement tools be made?

The design and validation of a quality-of-life assessment tool is clearly a substantial undertaking: the foregoing gives some impression of the process required. It makes sense to use established tools wherever possible, reserving the major design effort for situations for which appropriate instruments do not exist.

These design and conceptual issues reflect an important balance in quality-of-life research. The field is populated by two overlapping and synergistic groups of investigators—those who devise instruments and those who use them to answer clinical and policy questions. In this whole exercise it is important for both groups to understand each other's perspectives and goals.

Clinical use of the quality-of-life paradigm

How does one use the quality-of-life paradigm in clinical research? Its major strength is that it represents a patient-centred measure of success that reflects all aspects of the medical and social intervention. None of the quality-of-life tools measure physiological parameters *per se*; they measure the effect of physiological change. In the broadest sense, quality-of-life measures depict what happens to patients on a day-to-day basis. How are they able to function, what is their level of social interaction, what is their psychological state, and what is the impact of any of the range of noxious somatic stimuli? Clearly the pattern can be applied to individual patients, as well as in the more formal, clinical experiment. Thus, while the following discussion focuses on the clinical trial, it can in principle be extrapolated to the management of individuals. At the present time the available instruments do not have subscales of sufficient reliability to allow clinical decisions to be made with confidence on the basis of individual patient scores.

The conduct of a clinical trial can be divided into four components:

(1) the design of the trial (or the definition of the question);

(2) the selection of measures of success;

(3) the implementation of the experiment;

(4) the analysis and interpretation of the data.

There are a number of texts and articles which explore this process in considerable detail.[35-37] A short summary of the general approach as applied to quality-of-life trials follows.

Asking the question

The first and most difficult step in any experiment is framing the question. Marshall McLuhan commented that 90 per cent of the success of an experiment is asking a question which will lead to an interesting answer. The palliative care setting offers a wealth of opportunities for altering the quality of life of patients by intervening not only physiologically, but also psychologically, sociologically, and environmentally. The application of the quality-of-life paradigm provides a final common pathway for the analysis of all of these interventions, from the viewpoint of the patient.

A few specific examples may further clarify the issue. One might improve quality of life by relieving pain. This is a widely held expectation, though relatively few trials have compared different approaches to the management of pain for their overall quality-of-life impact. In a study conducted by Tannock *et al.*,[38] 14 of 37 men with symptomatic bone metastases from cancer of the prostate treated with prednisone had improvement in all indices of pain. The McGill pain questionnaire and a series of 17 linear analogue self-assessment (LASA) scales measuring pain and various aspects of quality of life assessed the response to treatment. At the time of maximum improvement in pain, 46 per cent of the quality-of-life scales had improved, 11 per cent deteriorated, and 43 per cent were unchanged. This study clearly shows that pain control is not the sole determinant of quality of life.

The venue of care can also be explored. The American national hospice study was a fairly early quality-of-life study which sought to document the natural history of patients in their last days.[39] The hope was that clear evidence could be found in support of the principle that care within a hospice met the needs of the dying patient better than that administered within the active treatment hospital. The focus on analgesia, supportive rather than interventive measures, and the aggregation of social resources were postulated to provide for a better quality of life. This early quality-of-life study was inhibited by the relative inadequacy of quality-of-life-measurement tools and techniques compared with those available today. In an attempt to capture better the impact of hospice care, a secondary analysis of the data from the national hospice study was conducted using a new measure 'quality of death'. An analysis of covariance showed that quality of death was lower for patients who received conventional care than those who received home-base or hospital-based hospice care.[40] Even simple venue issues may provide provocative outcomes leading to changes in the pattern of health-care delivery. The social isolation which comes with institutional care may carry its own substantial price in terms of quality of life.

From the outset we are aware that many malignancies are not curable and many therapeutic interventions are essentially palliative in nature. Treatment of any of the advanced epithelial malignancies falls into this category.[41] With the emerging data that intensity of chemotherapy does not materially alter survival of patients with advanced epithelial tumours, the setting is ripe for serious quality-of-life oriented trials, measuring dose of therapy against quality-of-life response. The study of chemotherapy for advanced breast cancer undertaken by Coates *et al.* is one of a number of such trials which have been reported.[42] In this particular study, a comparison was made between continuous and intermittent chemotherapy for women with metastatic breast cancer. Another study, currently taking place in Zimbabwe, extends the logic one step further. It compares four essentially palliative treatments for advanced Kaposi's sarcoma; hemibody radiotherapy, combination chemotherapy, single agent oral chemotherapy with etoposide (all in combination with best supportive care), and best supportive care alone.[43] There is no evidence that treating the tumour with radiotherapy or chemotherapy will improve quality of life to any greater extent than simply providing best supportive care alone. However, in conducting such studies, the investigator must be prepared for the situation in which the physiological response (tumour shrinkage) appears to diverge from the quality-of-life response.

Finally, the quality-of-life paradigm makes it possible to compare medical and non-medical interventions. Studies which compare physiological interventions against psychological or sociological interventions might be considered, particularly where there is no clear evidence of either primary drug efficacy or an increase in the duration of physiological responses observed. As an example in the Kaposi's sarcoma study outlined above, the patients on etoposide do not require inpatient treatment whereas those on combination chemotherapy do. This difference in the locale for treatment might have different effects on both compliance and quality of life, assuming an equal effect on the disease itself.

All of these are examples to illustrate a fundamental experimental design point—the quality-of-life paradigm permits the evaluation of physiological and non-physiological interventions. Questions must be designed in which clinically significant differences in effect may be anticipated. It probably makes little sense to assume the cost and burden of quality-of-life outcome measurement in clinical trials which compare the relative efficacy and toxicity of rather similar chemotherapy and/or radiation treatment regimens. While many of these trials are currently being conducted and some are mandated by government regulatory agencies, it is unlikely that differences in outcome will be substantial enough to be detected reliably by the instrumentation, or important enough to form the basis of broad changes in therapeutic approach.

There are five general situations where quality of life is a predominant, though not necessarily exclusive, measure of success. The first two settings are particularly relevant to palliative care:

1. A clinical trial comparing therapies where only a slight survival difference is anticipated. The more dissimilar the therapies being compared, the more likely the experiment will yield worthwhile information.
2. Trials in which survival is not a consequential outcome criterion.
3. Disease states for which there are multiple, clinically effective therapies with potentially different quality-of-life outcomes.
4. Treatments which reduce mortality but at significant toxic cost.
5. Where treatment is lifelong, the complication rate relatively low, and patients asymptomatic; hypertension is an example.

Choosing the tools

The selection of an appropriate quality-of-life instrument depends upon definition of the experimental question. The evaluation of outcome is critically dependent on the selection of both measurement technique and measurement timing.

Since quality of life is a patient-centred subjective parameter, the measurement devices must represent the patients' perceptions of their day-to-day performance in each of the dimensions of quality of life. Further, the ability to determine the success of the intervention or experiment depends on the match between the clinical situation and the chosen instrument.

Whether one is assessing quality of life in an experimental study or during programme evaluation, the first issue to be determined is whether quality of life is being measured as an entry prognostic variable, a final outcome variable, or is evaluated repetitively in the course of treatment, or all of these. In general, the more frequently quality of life is measured, the more compact the measurement instrument should be. A necessary corollary is that as an instrument becomes more compact, the information derived from it becomes less detailed and reliable. Thus, if all that is required is an initial detailed quality-of-life assessment, measures such as the McMaster general health questionnaire or the Nottingham health profile might be appropriate.[44,45] However, since quality of life is a phenomenon which varies with time, it is our view that more emphasis should be placed on the selection of well-validated instruments that are compact and designed for repeated use. What may be lost in resolution will be gained in insight into the natural course of the disease. The core-plus module approach, as outlined by Aaronson and discussed earlier, represents a reasonable compromise.

No ideal quality-of-life measure currently exists. Nonetheless, a number of quality-of-life instruments have been devised, both for general application in cancer and for specific disease sites.[8,18,21,44,46–48] In principle, the best clue to the value of an index is its long-term acceptance by the professional community. However, there are some specific criteria which are helpful to the clinician seeking to select particular instruments. Originally set out in the early 1980s, they seem to have withstood a reasonable test of time.[49]

Selection of indices

A quality-of-life measure should satisfy the following criteria:

1. The quality-of-life measure should be specific enough to the disease population to detect differences in functional state between patients. Unlike broad-based medical quality-of-life indices designed to measure the medical functional state of free living populations, these tests should take into account that patients have already been diagnosed as having an incurable illness and therefore should concentrate on distinguishing functional states within this population.

2. The index should address day-to-day living issues that represent the global construct of quality of life.

3. Most quality-of-life indices are self-administered. However, in the palliative care population alternative response formats may be considered. For example, instead of recording on a linear analogue scale, patients could respond verbally on a scale of 1 to 10 to questions asked verbally by an interviewer. Such changes in the method of administration and response for existing questionnaires require testing for equivalency to the original, since it is well known that both presence of interviewers and method of response alter scores.

4. The questions should be designed with general applicability, ease, and consistency of interpretation in mind. The number of questions should be sufficiently low to permit high compliance despite repeated administration.

5. The questionnaire should be designed for repeated use, to allow a patient's score to be followed over a period of time, permitting trends, both within patients and between groups, to be evaluated.

6. It should be sensitive across the range of clinical practice to distinguish degrees of dysfunction between patients with varying extent of disease and intensity of therapeutic intervention.

7. The instrument should have demonstrated adequate reliability and validity.

8. Where an instrument is intended for use in a culture different from the one in which it was designed and validated, cross-cultural validation needs to be addressed.

9. The instrument should have published rules of administration, scoring, and interpretation to ensure that its application is consistent and evaluable.

Many established quality-of-life measures were developed for patients undergoing curative or life-prolonging treatment and hence focus on symptoms and functional ability. It may be that questions designed for this population are less appropriate for patients in palliative or terminal care settings. In addition, even relatively short questionnaires may be burdensome.[50] While control of symptoms and maintenance of functional ability are important areas for palliative care, it has been suggested that persons retain a need and capacity for personal growth at the end of life and that quality-of-life questionnaires designed for this population should reflect this positive aspect also. Byock *et al.* have developed an 31-item instrument with five dimensions: symptoms, functional status, interpersonal relations, emotional well-being, and transcendence.[14] The fifth dimension is what distinguishes this instrument from most others and provides a means of assessing the psychosocial interventions of palliative care. At present, the instrument is undergoing testing of its psychometric properties but results are expected by late 1995 (I. Byock, personal communication).

An instrument developed by Cohen *et al.*,[51,52] the McGill quality of life questionnaire (**MQOL**), is also designed specifically for the palliative care population. The most current version of the instrument has four subscales representing physical, psychological, existential, and support domains, all having Cronbach's alphas above 0.84. When the subscale scores were used in a multiple regression to predict a single-item overall quality-of life-assessment, the existential subscale was weighted much more heavily by patients with local or metastatic disease than by those with no evidence of disease. This attests to the importance of the existential domain in determining and assessing quality of life in palliative care.

Although assessment of physical status must be part of any quality-of-life assessment, inclusion of long lists of symptoms makes measures lengthy and creates noise in the data because only a few symptoms impact on any one individual. The MQOL deals with this problem by allowing patients to state their three most troublesome symptoms when responding to the physical domain items.

The newly developed hospice quality of life index (**HQLI**)[53] includes four conceptual domains of physical, psychological/spiritual, social, and financial well-being. These domains have not been confirmed by factor analysis and no subscale scores are available. In addition to answering items on a visual analogue scale, patients are asked to rate the importance of each item on a 0 to 3 scale. Items ranked most important were relationship with God, physical care received, and support from the hospice team, from family, and friends. These items also were among those having the highest scores on the visual analogue scales, supporting the notion that a better quality of life can be achieved through the attention given to these areas in the palliative care setting.

Despite the potential problems of using standard quality of life instruments in the palliative care population, we have used the FLIC in a pilot study of a palliative care population in conjunction with a needs assessment form (NAF).[54] In the ongoing study, we are assessing needs and quality of life of patients over time from admission to palliative care to death. Selected items from the purpose-in-life test[55] have been added to the evaluation and hence we will be able to determine the importance of the existential domain over time.

Conducting the trial

Perhaps the greatest point of departure for quality-of-life trials from more conventional pharmacological or survival trials is in the day-to-day conduct of the experiment. Two critical properties of the quality-of-life paradigm must be kept in mind.

First, quality of life itself is multifactorial and varies with time. Unlike survival or disease-free survival data, quality-of-life data are not recoverable once lost. It is therefore essential that the timing of data collection is carefully considered so that it is symmetrical across treatment arms. Once measurement points are determined, every effort must be made to collect all of the data, on each subject, at each data point.

Second, quality-of-life measurement uses patients as their own internal controls. Normative results are generally not available. The point of first data collection is thus critical, as it serves as the anchor against which individual patient responses are subsequently judged.

These two general principles lead directly to some operational guidelines for the conduct of quality-of-life studies.

1. *In calculating patient numbers for clinical trials*, the quality-of-life trial is unlikely to require more patients than a similar trial whose only outcome parameters are response, duration of response, and survival. This is because each patient is assessed on multiple occasions. In contrast, survival and disease-free survival data only provide a single data point for each experimental subject.

2. *The careful timing of entry level quality-of-life measures* cannot be overemphasized. This is a problem which is not amenable to trivial solutions. The logical entry point for a clinical trial frequently occurs when a patient's condition is both emotionally and physically volatile. The data suggest that the first few weeks after the diagnosis of any malignancy is a time of considerable emotional upheaval perhaps even more so on admission to palliative care with its tacit connotation of a not too distant death. Anxiety and depression almost universally accompany such a diagnosis yet, for most patients at least, partial recovery takes place. Further major medical interventions begin during that same period. Finally, depending on the pace of evolution of the individual tumour, the patient's overall condition may change markedly, independent of any specific medical intervention.

In selecting the initial data point, the experimenter must carefully consider all of these dynamic variables so that the window for initial evaluation meets the pragmatic compromise between the stability of individual quality-of-life parameters and the logistics of therapy. In the palliative care setting, the heterogeneity of the patient population may impose yet another constraint on this important timing issue.

3. *Frequency of measurement* is a third important design issue. The operational properties of the quality-of-life paradigm impose no limitations on the frequency of measurement or on the duration of follow-up. However, it is generally assumed that too frequent assessment may become burdensome for the patient with limited energy. On the other hand, there is consensus that the period of recall of a quality-of-life measure is relatively short—2 to 4 weeks. Thus, quality of life assessment asking for recall further back than 2 weeks may introduce distortion into the data.

As a general principle, it is advisable to measure quality of life at times of anticipated change in patient status. A general strategy to employ would be to measure quality of life at regular intervals, and add extra times of measurement to capture the effect of interventions. It is important to evaluate all patients at similar intervals in each treatment arm.

4. *Cognitive function* is of particular concern toward the end of life. Apart from the observed clear shifting of interests and concerns, the ability to focus diminishes and the burden of even simple tasks increases. This is an area of active exploration in palliative care, and one where the issue of surrogate assessment is being reconsidered—a direction at variance with the majority of quality-of-life research but potentially appropriate in this circumstance.

5. *Data collection personnel* play a critical role in quality-of-life studies. Since the assessment is patient-centred and subjective, care must be taken to ensure that the intervention of the researcher does not distort the data. Roles of the data collection staff must be precisely defined in terms of the method of presentation of the instrument, their role in assisting in its completion, and their role in facilitating completion of missing or delinquent forms. There is evidence in the literature that quality-of-life estimates made by nurses and physicians may differ from each other and from the patient's self-estimate.[30,56,57] The data collection process clearly has to be carefully standardized in order that these important distortions are avoided.

6. *Guidelines for follow-up.* As yet, no clear guidelines regarding duration of follow-up for quality-of-life trials have been established. The major considerations are the duration of impact of the intervention being considered and its side-effects, and also and the natural history of the disease.

7. *Quality of life.* The palliative care setting is one where quality of life may be the sole measure of success in a trial. In some circumstances it might be appropriate to measure outcomes in addition to quality of life. This may allow one to understand the mechanism for any changes in quality of life.

Analysing the data

The goal of the statistical design and analysis process is to ensure that the data derived from the experiment provide an answer to the test question. We want to have confidence that the observed differences in the sample, or lack thereof, represent the true state in the population under study. Understanding the relationship between the statistic and the process is particularly relevant in the analysis of quality-of-life data. The multidimensional and time variable nature of quality-of-life data means that, in our analyses, we are seeking to describe differences in curves and shapes. However, this ignores both the time variability of weightings of quality-of-life components, and the relative utility of present versus delayed benefit. Similarly single point comparisons for time variable data are probably of limited value.

Currently, no statistic is ideal. In the following discussion of specific methodologies it is wise to remember that one has to practice the art of the possible rather than the ideal. This only serves to emphasize the need to evolve a more representative statistical process. In particular, extension of the TWiST methodology to the quality-of-life parameter should be explored.

Quality-of-life information is usually only one part of the data collected during a study. Account must be taken of the other data sources in designing the study and planning the data analysis. Cancer clinical trials have customarily used such outcome measures as tumour response, survival, disease-free survival, and treatment toxicity. Any or all of these may be used in a specific study. The two aspects of quality-of-life data which make them quite different from other kinds of outcome measures are that measurement may be repeated at many points in time and that a single assessment is multidimensional. This means that a large number of comparisons may be made both between different points in time and between different aspects of quality of life or any number of combinations of the two.

If one is interested in any difference in trend in the overall quality-of-life score over time between two groups then this question can be analysed by a repeated measures analysis of variance.[37] However, this type of analysis requires that rather restrictive statistical assumptions about the data be met. An alternative type of analysis is a multivariate analysis of variance which allows differences between groups to be assessed on several variables simultaneously. In this case the values to be analysed are the differences between two consecutive measurement times. These could be differences between overall quality-of-life scores or differences between quality-of-life component scores. At its simplest this method of analysis could look at a difference in overall quality of life from diagnosis to the end of treatment.

One of the problems with multiple times of assessment using multi-item questionnaires is that of missing data. Many computer programmes for the multivariate and repeated measures analyses referred to above require that no data are missing on an individual; otherwise that person is deleted from the analysis. When individual items have not been answered in questionnaires it is usually possible to develop rules for estimating overall scores. However, the problem is much more severe when trying to estimate an entire set of scores because a time of measurement is missed. Stringent follow-up procedures should be in place to ensure that patients complete questionnaires at the times required by the research protocol.

Multivariate techniques are generally conservative statistical methods and they will therefore have lower power than comparable univariate analyses. This raises the issue of the two types of experimental errors: Type I error—the probability that the null hypothesis has been rejected erroneously, and Type II error—the probability that the null hypothesis has been accepted erroneously.

If very simple quality-of-life questions are asked, such as whether two forms of pain management differ in their impact on quality of life, this could be assessed by as few as two times of measurement, if those times were carefully chosen. In this case only one statistical comparison might be made; that of comparing the time one to time two difference in overall quality-of-life scores for the two groups. This comparison might be tested at the usual 0.05 level of significance. However, as the question asked develops more facets, such as comparing the time one to time two difference for each quality-of-life component, then the probability of committing a Type I experimental error increases almost additively as the number of subquestions increases. That is, five subquestions each tested at the 0.05 level of significance give an overall probability of Type I error of 0.25. If one rejected the null hypothesis for one of the subquestions it would be virtually impossible to tell if this were a false-positive or true-positive result. The usual way to resolve this problem is to divide the significance level between the various hypotheses. If there were five subquestions then the level of significance at which each would be tested would be 0.01. This procedure greatly reduces power, as does the multivariate method of assessing all five questions simultaneously.

The resolution of this dilemma is to keep the number of hypotheses small and to make sure that the sample size is adequate to give a reasonable power—say 0.80. It is important to have a few very carefully specified hypotheses that have a definite priority in relation to each other. There is no reason why the overall Type I error rate, say 0.05, cannot be divided unequally between the various hypotheses with the more important hypotheses receiving a larger share of the overall 0.05.[37]

If there are few missing data then multivariate and/or repeated measures analyses can proceed but if there is a considerable quantity of data missing then alternative analyses should be performed on those portions of the data that are available. This may bias the results, depending upon the reason for missing data, and it is important to be aware of these potential sources of confounding of the results. If data are missing for any reason associated with the conditions of the experiment, this is referred to as informative censoring. For example if only patients who are feeling very unwell at the time of data collection do not complete questionnaires, the data will yield an overestimate of actual quality of life. Potential sources of bias should be considered and indicated in the reporting of the results. In other cases where the source of bias is unclear, initial quality-of-life scores can be compared for those who do and those who do not complete a questionnaire at a later point in time. In cases where data is missing intermittently for reasons unrelated to the experimental treatment there are various methods for imputing missing values.

In palliative care drop-out due to death is a major data analytic problem which may preclude the use of multivariate and repeated measures analyses. Some means of combining quality and quantity of life, appropriate to this population needs to be developed. The quality adjusted life year has been used in other populations. Quality in this context means the utility associated with precisely described health states derived from a utility index. The utilities associated with these health states have been determined by methods such as the standard gamble on normal population samples. The problem with applying this methodology to the palliative care population is that the broad ranging health states applicable to the general population will not have the sensitivity to discriminate in the palliative care setting. Additionally, techniques for establishing health state utilities are very time-consuming and difficult for subjects to understand. The nature of the palliative care patient population would preclude their participation in such an exercise. Utilities for palliative care health states could be obtained on other populations and proponents assure us that there would be little difference in utility assignments since groups with and without a particular condition assign similar utilities to that health state. The attractiveness of utilities is that they are on a ratio scale of measurement with a true zero. No existing quality of life measure has this feature and attempts to transform scores to conform to this requirement have been unsuccessful.

When planning the data collection and analysis it is as well to anticipate the possibility of missing data and decide *a priori* on a back-up procedure for the preferred form of data analysis. This planning phase should always include an individual with statistical expertise who will be able to advise on the required sample size and the correct data analytic procedure for various data collection difficulties.

Recently Matthews *et al.* suggested a two-stage method of analysing serial measurements in medical research.[58] In the first stage the aim is to select and calculate a single measure that summarizes all the serial measurements taken over time on a single individual. The type of summary measure chosen will be dictated by the particular type of serial data and the research questions that are to be answered. Examples of summary measures in a longitudinal series of quality-of-life measures might include the area under the curve, time to achieve a peak or nadir, or duration of a quality-of-life response. In the second stage of analysis the summary measures can be analysed using the simplest of statistical techniques because there is now only one measure for each person. This method also has the advantage that, unlike multivariate methods, a summary measure can often be calculated even if a few times of measurements are omitted.

Interpretation of results

Quality of life is patient-centred and subjective. It is multifactorial. It is also time variable. These properties distinguish this paradigm from many other outcome measures to which we are accustomed and add complexity to the interpretation of experimental results.

A number of interpretive examples follow, each making the assumptions that the experiment was properly designed and conducted, the measurement tools reliable and valid for the study, and the statistical analysis process appropriate.

Example 1: the concordant result

The situation in which all experimental data point toward the same solution is an outcome which is both desired and straightforward in its interpretation. A comparative study of two treatments in which one offers both better survival and improved quality of life leads directly to affirmation and further exploitation of the superior therapy.

However, the data will be rich in clues to the reasons for the quality-of-life difference and the natural history from a bio-psychosocial perspective. There is more than survival or response data to examine. Each component of the quality-of-life measure is influenced by the illness and the treatment. For example could the superior therapy be further improved by a psychological or sociological manipulation without compromising the physiological effect? Not to be forgotten, could the inferior treatment be improved by a similar modification of its quality-of-life impact?

Example 2: the dissonant outcome

In this case, all of the physiological data and a preponderance of quality-of-life data favour one therapy. However, one or more quality-of-life component is significantly contradistinct. A study conducted by Ferrell *et al.*[59] demonstrates this phenomenon. They compared the effectiveness of controlled-release analgesia to short acting analgesia. The City of Hope Medical Centre quality-of-life survey and the present pain intensity scale of the McGill pain questionnaire were used as two of the primary instruments. The results showed not only a greater improvement in pain intensity and distress scores with controlled-release analgesia than with short acting analgesia, but also a greater improvement in adjustment to disease, attainment of affection, strength, and overall quality of life. However, patients receiving the controlled-release analgesia had significantly more problems with constipation and nausea than those receiving the short acting preparations. The data of Sugarbaker *et al.*,[60] demonstrating sexual impairment as a consequence of limb-sparing therapy for sarcomas, is another example. When encountered, the response should be a concerted effort to address the specific deficiency. The quality-of-life paradigm is the tool by which such outcome disparities may be more systematically identified.

Example 3: partial equivalence

Imagine a two-arm trial. In the end both are equivalent in either quality of life or survival, not both. At first examination one is tempted to take equivalent arms as equal and choose the therapy superior by virtue of the non-equivalent outcome measure. However, this assumes that the value, to the patient, of both measures of success are the same. This may not be the case. It becomes important in this case to attempt to assess the marginal change in quality-of-life outcome which results from altering therapy so as to improve survival. Equally, the argument can be made from the opposite perspective, namely marginal change in survival resulting from efforts to improve quality of life.

Example 4: complete discordance: the hung jury

Perhaps most vexing is the situation in which one treatment has a demonstrable and substantial survival advantage, but with an equally marked inferior quality-of-life outcome. This is the logical extreme of example 2, the dissonant outcome. In seeking to resolve the conundrum it helps to recall that measuring quality of life has not in itself created the dilemma. This procedure simply offered the mechanism by which the paradox could be identified and partially quantified. Clearly, one must dissect the disparity in all its dimensions in order to devise a new approach to therapy that provides less paradoxical outcomes. Such results may reflect the distinction between third-party (read health professional) preference and first party (read patient) preference. The quality-of-life paradigm provides the information for informed decision making.

Extrapolation beyond outcome: the next generation of questions

Considerable quantities of data are now available which support quality of life as an independent prognostic factor in a number of clinical cancer settings, including advanced non-small-cell lung cancer,[61,62] and advanced breast cancer.[63,64] There is also a long anecdotal history of changes in life quality, much more broadly described, influencing physiological outcome.

Suggestions are beginning to emerge that altering quality of life, as defined in the current context, may influence physiology and perhaps survival. A new interface area, psychoneuroimmunology, examines these issues specifically in the relationship between the brain and immunity.[65,66] As we gain confidence in the robustness of the construct and the rigour of its application we can begin to explore manipulation of quality of life as a primary therapeutic manoeuvre.

The palliative care setting is perhaps an ideal place to begin. The tenet of palliative care is that cure is unattainable. Hence the physician-scientist in palliative care is unlikely to be faced with the hung jury. At the very least, survival is not the overwhelming measure of success. Studies with low-dose chemotherapy for metastatic breast cancer can be interpreted as tentative steps in this direction.

The preceding discussion has focused on the quality-of-life trial. Managing an individual patient is, in effect, a trial of one, but even such a trial can be a rigorously controlled experiment.[67,68] Commonly, however, it represents our day-to-day management approach, a setting in which the quality-of-life paradigm has particular relevance for palliative care. Recognizing that 'quality-of-life' has meaning for both patient and physician is the starting point. Beginning to think about the component parts of quality of life—physical/occupational function, psychological/emotional, social function, and symptoms of disease and treatment—opens a range of potential therapeutic approaches that can be employed daily.

The needs of each patient must be assessed at the physiological level and from the broadened perspective which has come to be defined as 'quality of life'. There are potential interventions of benefit along each axis. At a given moment a sociological 'therapy' may be of more consequence than any other. At each point in the disease trajectory the balance is shifting, at no time more so than towards the end of life. To be aware of the range and to be sensitive to the balance is the heart of the matter. It is not new science. It is good old medicine.

References

1. Calman KC. Quality of life in cancer patients–an hypothesis. *Journal of Medical Ethics*, 1984; **10**: 124–7.
2. Gelber RD, Goldhirsch A. A new endpoint for the assessment of adjuvant therapy in postmenopausal women with operable breast cancer. *Journal of Clinical Oncology*, 1986; **4**: 1772–9.
3. Gelber RD, Goldhirsch A, Cavalli F. Quality-of-life-adjusted evaluation of adjuvant therapies for operable breast cancer. The International Breast Cancer Study Group. *Annals of Internal Medicine*, 1991; **114**: 621–28.
4. Gelber RD, Goldhirsch A, Cole BF. Evaluation of effectiveness: Q-TWiST. The International Breast Cancer Study Group. *Cancer Treatment Reviews*, 1993; **19** Suppl A: 73–84.
5. McNeil BJ, Weichselbaum R, Pauker SG. Speech and survival: tradeoffs between quality and quantity of life in laryngeal cancer. *New England Journal of Medicine*, 1981; **305**: 982–7.
6. Cassileth BR, Soloway MS, Vogelzang NJ, *et al.* Quality of life and psychosocial status in stage D prostate cancer. Zoladex Prostate Cancer Study Group. *Quality of Life Research*, 1992; **1**: 323–9.
7. Wood-Dauphinee S, Williams JI. Reintegration to normal living as a proxy to quality of life. *Journal of Chronic Diseases*, 1987; **40**: 491–9.
8. Schag CC, Heinrich RL. Development of a comprehensive quality of life measurement tool: CARES. *Oncology*, 1990; **4**: 135–8.
9. Ware JE, Jr. Conceptualizing disease impact and treatment outcomes. *Cancer*, 1984; **53**: 2316–23.
10. Kleinman A. *The Illness Narratives: Suffering, Healing and the Human Condition*. New York: Basic Books, 1988.
11. Hiatt JF. Spirituality, medicine, and healing. *Southern Medical Journal*, 1986; **79**: 736–43.
12. Paloutzian RF, Ellison CW. Loneliness, spiritual well-being and the quality of life. In: Peplau LA, Perlman D, eds. *Loneliness: A Sourcebook of Current Theory, Research and Therapy*. New York: John Wiley & Sons, 1982: 224–37.
13. Warner SC, Williams JI. The meaning in life scale: determining the reliability and validity of a measure. *Journal of Chronic Diseases*, 1987; **40**: 503–12.
14. Byock I, Kinzbrunner B, Pratt M. Assessing quality of life in the terminally ill: A developmental approach. *Journal of Palliative Care*, 1994; **10**(3)127 (Abstract).
15. McGill JS, Paul PB. Functional status and hope in elderly people with and without cancer. *Oncology Nursing Forum*, 1993; **20**: 1207–13.
16. Cella DF, Tulsky DS. Measuring quality of life today: methodological aspects. *Oncology*, 1990; **4**: 29–38.
17. Aaronson NK, Bullinger M, Ahmedzai S. A modular approach to quality-of-life assessment in cancer clinical trials. *Recent Results in Cancer Research*, 1988; **111**: 231–49.
18. Aaronson NK, Ahmedzai S, Bullinger M, *et al.* The EORTC core quality-of-life questionnaire: interim results of an international field study. In: Osoba D, ed. *Effect of Cancer on Quality of Life*. Boca Raton, Florida: CRC Press, 1991: 185–203.
19. Bergman B, Aaronson NK, Ahmedzai S, Kaasa S, Sullivan M. The EORTC QLQ-LC13: A modular supplement to the EORTC core quality of life questionnaire (QLQ-C30) for use in lung cancer clinical trials. *European Journal of Cancer* Part A, 1994; **30A**: 635–42.
20. Bjordal K, Ahlner-Elmqvist M, Tollesson E, *et al.* Development of a European Organization for Research and Treatment of Cancer (EORTC) questionnaire module to be used in quality of life assessments in head and neck cancer patients. *Acta Oncologica*, 1994; **33**: 879–85.
21. Schipper H, Clinch J, McMurray A, Levitt M. Measuring the quality of life of cancer patients: the functional living index-cancer: development and validation. *Journal of Clinical Oncology*, 1984; **2**: 472–83.
22. Schipper H, Clinch J, Powell V. Definitions and conceptual issues. In: Spilker B, ed. *Quality of Life Assessments in Clinical Trials*. New York: Raven Press, 1990: 11–24.
23. Padilla GV, Presant C, Grant MM, Metter G, Lipsett J, Heide F. Quality of life index for patients with cancer. *Research in Nursing and Health*, 1983; **6**: 117–26.
24. Wolberg WH, Romsaas EP, Tanner MA, Malec JF. Psychosexual Adaptation to Breast Cancer Surgery. *Cancer*, 1989; **63**: 1645–55.
25. Lasry JM, Margolese RG, Poisson R. Depression and body image following mastectomy and lumpectomy. *Journal of Chronic Diseases*, 1987; **40**: 529–34.
26. Ellison CW. Spiritual well-being: conceptualization and measurement. *Journal of Psychology and Theology*, 1983; **11**: 330–40.
27. Hollen PJ, Gralla RJ, Kris MG, Cox C. Quality of life during clinical trials: conceptual model for the Lung Cancer Symptom Scale. *Support Care Cancer*, 1994; **2**: 213–22.
28. Cella DF, Tulsky DS, Gray G, *et al.* The functional assessment of cancer therapy scale: development and validation of the general measure. *Journal of Clinical Oncology*, 1993; **11**: 570–9.
29. Ferrans CE, Powers MJ. Quality of life index: development and psychometric properties. *Advances in Nursing Science*, 1985; **8**: 15–24.
30. Slevin ML, Plant H, Lynch D, Drinkwater J, Gregory WM. Who should measure quality of life, the doctor or the patient? *British Journal of Cancer*, 1988; **57**: 109–12.

31. *Cancer Pain Relief and Palliative Care*. Technical Report Series 804. Geneva: World Health Organization, 1990.
32. Goh CR, Lee KS, Tan TC, *et al.* Measuring quality of life in different cultures: translation of the Functional Living Index for Cancer (FLIC) into Chinese and Malay in Singapore. *Annals of Academic Medicine of Singapore*, 1996; **25**: 323–4.
33. Borok M, Gudzal I, Kiire C, Levy L, Otim-Oyet D. Fulminant epidemic Kaposi's sarcoma (EKS): hallmark of AIDS in Zimbabwe. *Proceedings of the Annual Meeting of the American Society of Clinical Oncologists*, 1996, Abstract.
34. Harman HH. *Modern Factor Analysis*. 3rd edn. Chicago: University of Chicago Press, 1976.
35. Spilker B. *Guide to Clinical Studies and Developing Protocols*. New York: Raven Press Books, 1984.
36. Teeling-Smith G, ed. *Measuring Health: A Practical Approach*. Chichester: John Wiley & Sons, 1988.
37. Kirk RE. *Experimental Design: Procedures for the Behavioral Sciences*. Belmont, California: Brooks/Cole, 1968.
38. Tannock I, Gospodarowicz M, Meakin W, Panzarella T, Stewart L, Rider W. Treatment of metastatic prostate cancer with low dose prednisone: evaluation of pain and quality of life as pragmatic indices of response. *Journal of Clinical Oncology*, 1989; **7**: 590–7.
39. Greer DS, Mor V. An overview of national hospice study findings. *Journal of Chronic Diseases*, 1986; **39**: 5–7.
40. Wallston KA, Burger C, Smith RA, Baugher RJ. Comparing the quality of death for hospice and non-hospice cancer patients. *Medical Care*, 1988; **26**: 177–82.
41. De Vita VT, Hellman S, Rosenberg SA, eds. *Cancer: Principles and Practice of Oncology*. 3rd edn. Philadelphia, PA: J.B. Lippincott, 1989: 2.
42. Coates A, Gebski V, Bishop JF, *et al.* Improving the quality of life during chemotherapy for advanced breast cancer. A comparison of intermittent and continuous treatment strategies. *New England Journal of Medicine*, 1987; **317**: 1490–5.
43. Olweny CLM, Clinch J, Schipper H, *et al.* Quality of Life (QOL) in epidemic Kaposi's sarcoma (EKS) in Zimbabwe. *Proceedings of the Annual Meeting of the American Association for Cancer Research*, 1995; **14**: 510 (Abstract).
44. Chambers LW, MacDonald LA, Tugwell P, Buchanan WW, Kraag G. The McMaster health index questionnaire as a measure of quality of life for patients with rheumatoid disease. *Journal of Rheumatology*, 1982; **9**: 780–4.
45. Hunt SM, McKenna SP, McEwen J, Williams J, Papp E. The Nottingham health profile: subjective health status and medical consultations. *Social Science and Medicine*, 1981; **15A**: 221–9.
46. Coates A, Dillenbeck CF, McNeil DR, *et al.* On the receiving end–II. linear analogue self-assessment (LASA) in evaluation of aspects of the quality of life of cancer patients receiving therapy. *European Journal of Cancer and Clinical Oncology*, 1983; **19**: 1633–7.
47. Levine MN, Guyatt GH, Gent M, *et al.* Quality of life in stage II breast cancer: an instrument for clinical trials. *Journal of Clinical Oncology*, 1988; **6**: 1798–810.
48. Priestman TJ, Baum M. Evaluation of quality of life in patients receiving treatment for advanced breast cancer. *Lancet*, 1976; **1**: 899–901.
49. Schipper H, Levitt M. Measuring quality of life: risks and benefits. *Cancer Treatment Reports*, 1985; **69**: 1115–25.
50. Donnelly S, Walsh D. Quality of life assessment in advanced cancer. *Palliative Medicine*, 1996; **10**: 275–83.
51. Cohen SR, Mount BM, Strobel MG, Bui F. The McGill Quality of Life Questionnaire: a measure of quality of life appropriate for people with advanced disease. A preliminary study of validity and acceptability. *Palliative Medicine*, 1995; **9**: 207–19.
52. Cohen SR, Mount BM, Tamas JJ, Mount LF. Existential well-being is an important determinant of quality of life. Evidence from the McGill Quality of Life Questionnaire. *Cancer*, 1996; **77**: 576–86.
53. McMillan SC, Mahon M. Measuring quality of life in hospice patients using a newly developed hospice quality of life index. *Quality of Life Research*, 1994; **3**: 437–47.
54. Dudgeon D, Clinch J. A longitudinal study of needs and quality of life (QOL) in advanced cancer patients. *Proceedings of the Annual Meeting of the American Society for Clinical Oncology*, 1994; **13**: 437 (Abstract).
55. Crumbaugh JC. Cross-validation of the purpose-in-life test based on Frankl's concepts. *Journal of Individual Psychology*, 1968; **24**: 74–81.
56. Degner LF, Henteleff PD, Ringer C. The relationship between theory and measurement in evaluations of palliative care services. *Journal of Palliative Care*, 1987; **3**: 8–13.
57. Spitzer WO, Dobson AJ, Hall J, *et al.* Measuring the quality of life of cancer patients: A concise Q/L index for use by physicians. *Journal of Chronic Diseases*, 1981; **34**: 585–97.
58. Matthews JNS, Altman DG, Campbell MJ, Royston P. Analysis of serial measurements in medical research. *British Medical Journal*, 1990; **300**: 230–5.
59. Ferrell B, Wisdom C, Wenzl C, Brown J. Effects of controlled-released morphine on quality of life for cancer pain. *Oncological Nursing Forum*, 1989; **16**: 521–6.
60. Sugarbaker PH, Barofsky I, Rosenberg SA, Gianola FJ. Quality of life assessment of patients in extremity sarcoma clinical trials. *Surgery*, 1982; **91**: 17–23.
61. Ganz PA, Lee JJ, Siau J. Quality of life assessment. An independent prognostic variable for survival in lung cancer. *Cancer*, 1991; **67**: 3131–5.
62. Ruckdeschel JC, Piantadosi S. Assessment of quality of life (ql) by the functional living index-cancer (FLIC) is superior to performance status for prediction of survival in patients with lung cancer. *Proceedings of the Annual Meeting of the American Society for Clinical Oncology*, 1989; **8**: 311.
63. Winer EP, Gold DT, Lees J, Affronti ML, Westlund R, Ross M, *et al.* Quality of life following high dose chemotherapy with autologous bone marrow support in patients with metastatic breast cancer. *Proceedings of the Annual Meeting of the American Society for Clinical Oncology*, 1991; **10**: 62 (Abstract).
64. Ganz PA, Schag CA, Cheng HL. Assessing the quality of life–a study in newly-diagnosed breast cancer patients. *Journal of Clinical Epidemiology*, 1990; **43**: 75–86.
65. Schleifer SJ, Keller SE, Stein M. Central nervous system mechanisms and immunity: implications for tumor response. In: Levy SM, ed. *Behavior and Cancer*. San Francisco,CA: Jossey-Bass, 1985: 120–33.
66. Ader R, ed. *Psychoneuroimmunology*. Orlando, FL: Academic Press, 1981.
67. Guyatt G, Sackett D, Taylor DW, Chong J, Roberts R, Pugsley S. Determining optimal therapy–randomized trials in individual patients. *New England Journal of Medicine*, 1986; **314**: 889–92.
68. Keller JL, Guyatt GH, Roberts RS, Adachi JD, Rosenbloom D. An N of 1 service: applying the scientific method in clinical practice. *Scandinavian Journal of Gastroenterology*, 1988; **147** (suppl.): 22–9.

3

Ethical issues in palliative care

3 Ethical issues in palliative care

David J. Roy and Neil MacDonald

Introduction

Simply stated, ethical issues in palliative care centre around decisions which will enable us to satisfy the criteria for a peaceful death, dignified and assisted by a helpful society.[1] A qualification, however, must be added. While the origins of palliative care stem from a recognition of the needs of dying patients, it is now clearly recognized that suffering at the end of life often relates to problems earlier in the trajectory of illness. Moreover, the attitudes, skills, and knowledge engendered in a palliative care programme can alleviate suffering encountered by patients with a prolonged course of illness or who may be cured of their disorder.

The need to match technical and scientific aspects of care with a moral component is not unique to palliative care. Ethical considerations arising at the end of life, however, have always received a special priority from the world's great religions and philosophies. More recently, secular agencies such as the press, the legal profession, and medical bodies have highlighted a number of issues.

When morality was clearly the purview of religion, and one followed the dictates of a well-defined and inflexible culture, what was right and good was easily identified and few decision-making dilemmas would occur. Currently, we live in constantly changing societies where absolutism no longer rules, and where religious expression ranges from dogmatic interpretation to liberality in thought and deed. Strong secular pressures lead many to question previously absolute tenets of morality. Cultural change heavily influences bioethics, but the most profound perturbations arise secondary to the explosive growth of information presenting us with an extraordinary range of options where previously few existed. Thus, moral decisions may seem less secure as new perspectives on biology and disease appear, and new options for interfering with the life cycle come forward.

Table 1 categorizes the principal palliative care ethical issues.[2] This chapter will not address each of them, as many topics are discussed in other chapters of this textbook. We have selected seven issues for detailed consideration because they are not considered elsewhere in this book and are of paramount importance in our field. The seven issues are:

(1) clinical ethics

(2) confidentiality

(3) competence

(4) research

(5) resource allocation

(6) withholding or withdrawing therapy

(7) euthanasia.

Our approach is primarily not that of philosopher, although we trust that reason and logic characterize our account. Rather, we are emphasizing what may be termed 'muscular ethics'—the practical application of ethical decision making at the bedside. In so doing, we do not negate the contemplative aspects of ethics which are thoughtfully expressed by our colleagues in theology, law, and philosophy. The products of their intellectual pursuit grace practical applications of right and wrong which occur in the crucible of our institutions and in the homes of our patients.

Clinical ethics

Ethical issues bearing upon the rights and wrongs of human behaviour arise when the answers proposed to any given question are uncertain or conflicting. We hold conflicting beliefs about how human beings should live and die; about the values individuals and groups should uphold; about which values may be sacrificed when all values in a specific situation cannot be honoured and maintained.[3] These are ethical issues in palliative medicine and palliative care because they occur at the bedsides of seriously ill and dying people; because they centre on what should and should not be done, as well as upon clinical acts that may be tolerable, if not ideal, in the care of patients afflicted with advanced or terminal disease.

Ethics, as understood in this chapter, is a function of and an exercise of human intelligence. As such, ethics shares a common cognitive goal with science: to distinguish mere appearances from reality. Scientific research, using measurement as its cardinal procedure, seeks to express the actual relationships between phenomena. Uncritical reliance on initial observations, potentially distorted by bias, can lead to a systematic divergence from truth.[4]

Ethics, a process of interdisciplinary critical reflection, acts against a tendency to diverge systematically from what is right. Just as initial observations may fail to reveal true correlations between phenomena, so also may it happen that spontaneous desires or compulsions may not correspond to what is truly good and to what we really ought to do. What appears to be good in a limited perspective may contradict a greater and more commanding value.

Table 1 The care of patients with advanced chronic illness—ethical issues

Competence

1. Access to skilled control of pain and other symptoms may be regarded by some as a fundamental patient–family right. However, the competence of health professionals in pain and symptom control varies. How important is it to ensure that patients have access to the most competent care? Is competent relief of relievable suffering a fundamental right?
2. Are patients and families sufficiently aware that there are relative levels of health care competence? Should they have such information in a form that will help them to make decisions to seek appropriate medical care?

Communication with health professionals

1. Medical information is complex and constantly developing. Do patients and their families with advanced chronic illness have the necessary information in order to assist them in making logical choices?
2. Should it be a priority to develop information systems that provide as even access as possible to information for patients and familes?

Confidentiality

We recognize that, in order to assist patients and families with all aspects of their illness, we need to involve physicians, nurses, other health professionals, and, on occasion, volunteers as members of a team. How do we exchange sensitive information within the team, while preserving patient–family rights to confidentiality and preservation of dignity?

Cultural sensitivity

We encounter many patients who speak neither French nor English and whose cultural backgrounds influence decision making. Truth-telling is only one example of cultural differences in the management of patients with advanced chronic illnesses such as cancer or AIDS. In some cultures, the family may know the diagnosis, but they prefer that the patient not know the nature of illness or prognosis.

And yet, we regard patient autonomy—i.e., the right to have information on which they will make decisions—to be an important ethical issue. How do we respect cultures, yet maintain a consistent ethical approach?

Dual ethical standards

The promotion of many legal products greatly increases the incidence of suffering in members of the community. For example tobacco manufacturers may promote their products, company lawyers may protect their ability to promote their products, and merchants may promote the sale of tobacco products.

Promoting ill health for personal gain would not be judged as ethically acceptable by health professionals.

Is it acceptable that business people adhere to a lower standard of ethical behaviour than health professionals?

Education of health professionals

The principles of palliative care (encompassing pain and symptom control) may be regarded by some as essential components of medical practice. Does our current health professional educational system recognize and reflect this view?

Euthanasia and physician-assisted suicide

The policy of The Netherlands, the actions of Dr Kevorkian in the United States, the death of Sue Rodriguez, and the decision of people in Oregon to support a legal option for physician-assisted suicide and euthanasia, have all served to bring this issue to public attention.

1. Autonomy is highly valued—should patient autonomy extend to allow them to choose their options?
2. Should a society consider legalizing euthanasia and physician-assisted suicide if patients who may consider this option do not have impeccable access to excellent palliative care and symptom control?

Life-prolonging therapy

1. In the care of many patients with advanced chronic illnesses, aggressive therapies may be considered in situations where the risk of adverse effects is high and beneficial outcome low. Many of these therapies have a high cost, both in money and in investment of health professional time and effort, family resources, and public funds. How do we balance the relative benefit to few people against the personal and societal costs?
2. Nurses and other health profesisonals have responsibility for assisting patients who may be undergoing aggressive treatments, but they do not have the authority to decide when therapy should proceed, or for how long therapy should be applied. Does this create ethical dilemmas for them?

Research

Many patients with advanced chronic illness are asked to participate in a research study. Aside from immediate benefit which may accrue to the patient, many patients believe that participation in research studies enchances the meaning of their existence, as they are making a positive contribution to the public good. However, a number of ethical dilemmas arise in the course of enrolling patients and family members in research studies.

1. Are some studies, by their very natures, unethical to be conducted in a fragile population of patients and familes?
2. In situations where a loss of clear thinking ability (cognitive failure) is common, must we ensure that patients are, indeed, competent to give informed consent?
3. Do physicians, other health professionals, the patient, and the family share a mutual understanding of their responsibilities?
4. Sponsorship of research—much private research, notably in the pharmaceutical area, is supported by private pharmaceutical firms. Does the availability of funds from private industry drive the public research agenda, and subsequently influence resource allocation, fuelling futile efforts, with increased costs in suffering and waste of resources?
5. In a time of limited hospital and professional resources, does ineligibility for a trial or refusal to participate in a trial adversely affect a patient's future medial care?

Responsibilities of health professionals

In the past it was clearly a health professional's ethical responsibility to treat the needs of the patient as the highest priority, with other responsibilities secondary to this demand. In today's complex society, what are the responsibilities of health professionals to:

1. the patient?
2. the patient and family?
3. the institutions in which they work?
4. society at large as reflected in government actions to restrict costs and to obtain patient information in certain settings?
5. the health professional's family—in an age when others have increased leisure time, and we are generally advised to place our responsibilities to our families above all others, does this create unresolvable tensions for physicians and other health professionals?

Resource allocation

1. Is there evidence that the increasing reduction of resources may force health professionals and institutions to select health care options which compromise patient care?
2. Institutions are reducing their bed availability. Is this move matched by a satisfactory increase in resources for home care?
3. It is clear that there is a steady increase in the numbers of patients with advanced incurable cancer, AIDS, and a number of chronic conditions affecting the elderly. This increase is projected well into the next century. Is this immutable fact mirrored in decisions on the training of health professionals, in their availability in different settings, or in the resources to meet this demand?

Standards of care

Should hospitals and other health care institutions be expected to demonstrate that they maintain an acceptable standard of care and competence?

Withholding or withdrawing of therapy

Therapies which may sustain life for a period of time may be available to patients with a poor quality of life, comatose patients, and those who will not recover from their illness to any extent, and where every day of life adds a day of suffering.

Under these circumstances, it may be wise to either withdraw futile therapy, or to make the decision not to offer futile therapy in the first instance.

1. Do we and our patients and families understand the difference between these acts and physician-assisted suicide or euthanasia?
2. Are physicians and other health professionals programmed to offer futile therapy inappropriately?
3. Do patients and families exert pressure for the use of these therapies which are not to their benefit, and which increase health costs?
4. Are there legal strictures which lead patients or families to carry on futile therapies?

Unorthodox therapies

1. In a society which cherishes free speech and free will, are there ethical limits of tolerance extended to charatans who exploit patient ignorance and fear for personal advantage?
2. The search for unorthodox therapies reflects, in part, a desire for continued survival, but also for autonomy and free choice. May health professionals ethically support the use of certain unorthodox therapies which their patients wish to use?

Value judgements, like judgements of fact and of truth, are governed by concurrence with sufficient evidence, not by submission to custom, convention, authority, sheer brilliance, or any overpowering attraction.

People in western societies today clash profoundly on two levels: on the level of their cultural beliefs, within which people define the goals of life and the meaning of death; and on their hierarchies of value against which people decide which values may be sacrificed and which values must be maintained at all costs. In this context, ethics requires a shift from a divergent to a convergent method and mode of thought. The required shift is from the task of constructing arguments to the work of constructing practical judgements about what must be done, what should be prohibited, and what can be tolerated. The shift from theoretical to practical reasoning in ethics is needed to reach the decisions that often have to be made quite rapidly at the bedside of the sick and the dying. This is the shift required to extricate clinical ethics and the ethics of palliative care from the deadlock of interminable discourse about matters upon which people are likely never to agree.[5]

Ethics in palliative care is a matter of practical reasoning about individual patients, specific cases, and unique situations. Attention to this unique nature, and respect for it, may lead to decisions that we cannot always show to be consistent with either widely accepted principles or decisions taken earlier in similar situations. The starting point of clinical ethics, as also of clinical practice, is the consideration of a patient as a person like any other, what Charles Fried has called the principle of personal care.[6]

The patient's body and biography—his or her clinical course, life plans, relationships, strengths, weaknesses, and personal history—constitutes the most proximate norm governing the decisions to be made at the bedside. This bedside norm, of course, operates within a society that incorporates the principles of its religious, philosophical, moral, and medical traditions. But clinical ethics works with patients' clinical and personal biographies to interpret the meaning of these principles; that is, to determine what these principles command, permit, tolerate, or prohibit at the bedside of this particular patient. As such, clinical ethics is a particular kind of inductive ethics, for we do not know what our philosophical and moral traditions mean until we test them on a range of particular cases. We cannot simply pass each individual case through a grid of philosophical and religious moral principles to reach a clinical ethical conclusion. We simultaneously have to pass these principles through the grid of individual cases to arrive inductively at a reconstruction of these traditions—a reconstruction mediated through a range of personal histories confronting the suffering of multiple loss, as well as the threat of personal disintegration and death.

Clinical ethics, then, is not applied philosophy or theology. It is an original, distinctive intellectual activity, not a derivative one. Clinical ethics is an integral part of a clinician's work. Ethical dilemmas at the bedside will be misconstrued if the clinical situation is not understood in all its subtle medical and human complexity. The thesis that clinical ethics is a doctor's work does not imply that the doctor resolves issues by deciding in solitary eminence what is best for patients. Quite the contrary. A clinician must seek and orchestrate the contributions of team members, patients, and families. Ethical competence presupposes the skill and the sensitivity to carry out this task so as to understand the patient and what constitutes the patient's best interests. This is particularly necessary when patients cannot speak for themselves.

The complete physician holds together two seemingly incompatible excellences; sensitivity to signals of the patient's body and receptivity to the messages of a life in crisis—at the crossroads or at the terminus of a personal history. Competence in palliative medicine is an ethical condition of adequate professional response to the signals of a dying person's body and mind.

Confidentiality

What I may see or hear in the course of the treatment or even outside of the treatment in regard to the life of men, which on no account one must spread abroad, I will keep to myself holding such things shameful to be spoken about.

Oath of Hippocrates

Not all of the dictums in the ancient oath of Hippocrates have stood the test of time. He was an antiabortionist who would restrict medical practice to 'brothers in male lineage'. The concept of risk versus benefit for patients was not familiar to him, as Hippocrates abjures the use of any 'deadly' drug in treatment, and he may have been unduly paternalistic in his approach to patients—the oath says nothing about providing patients with information or respecting patient autonomy.

Amongst the Hippocratic principles, the statement on confidentiality remains fresh and topical. One cannot visualize that modern societal mores could or should challenge the bedrock principles of a physician's individual responsibility for a patient, including respect for 'what I may see or hear in the course of treatment or even outside of treatment in regard to the life of men'. In more prosaic language, current codes of medical practice include the unalloyed physician's guarantee to respect patient confidentiality as a fundamental tenet. For example the Code of Ethics of the Canadian Medical Association states 'An ethical physician will keep in confidence information derived from his patient, or from a colleague, regarding a patient, and divulge it only with the permission of the patient, except when the law requires him to do so'.

Some codes outline the conditions under which disclosure by a physician to others of information that should normally be kept secret is justified. For example the Code of Medical Ethics of the College of Physicians of Quebec states 'The physician must keep in confidence what he has learned in the practice of his profession. However, he may divulge those facts he knows personally, when the patient so authorizes him, when the law permits, when there are imperative and justifiable motives relating to the health of his patient or of the community or in the case of a commanding higher objective'.

The views of society are consonant with these codes. Physicians should refrain from disclosure of patient information, even after the death of a patient. Exceptions are permitted:

(1) with patient consent;

(2) for legal demand;

(3) when judged to be in the patient's interest—that is, family discussions on occasion;

(4) for registration of illnesses;

(5) to protect society.

Although subject to case by case variation throughout the Western legal world, the law echoes societal views and anticipates that patients regard their communications with physicians as privileged, and expect that these communications will not be revealed to others without consent. The physician may breach this contract only if it is clearly to the patient's benefit (generally, in situations where the patient may not be competent), where the duties to protect society outweigh patient privilege (for example where a psychiatrist may know about forthcoming events whereby the patient may harm others[7]), or where the law demands that a physician breach the vow of confidentiality. In general, physicians do not enjoy the same level of respect for privileged communication enjoyed by their legal brethren.[8,9] Absolute privilege is an aspect of lawyer–client interaction, as the law believes that it could not properly function if this rule were not in place. Arguably, the significance of trust in medical communications can be viewed in a similar light, but it is clearly not regarded by the law as absolute; the protection for patient–physician discourse varies from place to place.

Modern medical ethical principles and western trends of thought value highly the principle of autonomy. Central to a respect for personal autonomy, is the concept that the privacy of individuals must be respected.

Fidelity and trust are essential characteristics of a physician's covenant with sick and vulnerable people seeking treatment, care, and healing. For this relationship to work, doctors need information from patients as much as patients seek information from doctors. There is a difference though. To give their professional advice and counsel, and to guide their treatment prescriptions, doctors often require kinds of information about the body and biography of sick people, information patients would normally not be willing to share with anyone else.

The duty to protect confidentiality binds not only the physician primarily in charge of a patient's treatment and care. That duty extends to all other members of a clinical team who need access to a patient's medical chart if they are to make their special contribution to the patient's care. It is misguided to consider their access to a patient's medical records as a break of confidentiality. It may happen, however, that patients may entrust to a doctor or nurse confidences of a particularly personal nature that should not be written down in the medical record. Decisions in this matter call for sound judgement and open discussion with patients.

Confidentiality in research

Participants in research may be harmed psychologically, socially, or even financially if their privacy is invaded or if information about them, including their participation in certain kinds of research, is not kept confidential. There is now heightened sensitivity to the critical importance of safeguards for privacy and confidentiality, particularly in surveillance studies and in research on conditions that are socially stigmatizing and likely to render people susceptible to various kinds of discrimination. The HIV epidemic, for instance, has occasioned the development of detailed guidelines and of ingenious coding methods for electronic data storage to protect privacy and confidentiality in the research setting.

Information sheets accompanying consent forms for participants in clinical research should routinely state that rights to privacy and to confidentiality of information will be respected in clinical trials. The World Medical Association Declaration of Helsinki states that every precaution should be taken to respect the privacy of research subjects. The Code of Federal Regulations of the United States requires, for Institutional Review Board approval of research with human subjects, that there are adequate provisions to protect the privacy of subjects and to maintain the confidentiality of data.

The requirements for adequate protection of privacy and confidentiality will vary in keeping with the nature of the research, the disease or condition under study, and the laws of each country. Some countries provide legal shields to protect the confidentiality of research data against civil, criminal, administrative, or other proceedings to compel disclosure. Where such shields do not exist in law, researchers may be restricted with regard to the extent of protection of confidentiality they can guarantee research subjects. Clinical studies involving follow-up of patients after closure of the study require that particular attention be given to protection of privacy. Research subjects should be alerted to the possibility of future contact and they should give free and informed consent to any follow-up plan.[10]

Moreover, it is reasonable for purposes of medical audit and epidemiological surveys that records be accessed by responsible colleagues. Ordinarily, specific patient consent for this type of work is not required, although an official custodian of the records must review requests and provide access only if scientific standards and strict confidentiality are assured.

Perhaps the public's greatest concern relevant to the privacy of health information relates to 'macroissues' such as the intrusion of modern techniques of communication into the health field, with the potential for broad access to individual health data by a wide range of agencies and individuals. The participation by many professionals and volunteers in the therapy of patients, the demands by a host of agencies for patient information, and the ready electronic recording and transfer of this information challenge the maintenance of the ancient dictum of strict confidentiality.

It is now possible to embed all of our health information on a plastic 'smart card'. This advance is helpful as our health profiles will follow us as we make our way through increasingly complex health care systems. The risks are obvious—this information could be available to people with less-than-charitable interest in us. Access to information about us by alien agencies is a clear and evident risk which has been discussed in a number of publications and editorials on both sides of the Atlantic.[11-15]

Common issues in confidentiality

In the rest of this section we will consider immediate ethical issues in confidentiality which palliative care colleagues may encounter on a daily basis. We will limit further discussion to the problem of balancing the interpretation of psychosocial information for patient good and the casual distribution of privileged patient information with consequent loss of respect and dignity. Three scenarios, based on actual experiences, with details changed to preserve confidentiality, will illustrate the issues which arise.

Case 1 (Fig. 1) is an account where information about a family, of a nature which any of us would regard as privileged, is disclosed by a medical consultant. Several issues arise:

Medical consultation

To : Psychiatry

REASON FOR REQUEST : 'Drug addiction' (patient has metastatic chondrosarcoma with severe chronic pain syndrome secondary to invasion of a knee joint.)

Consultative note: male, 35 years old, with metastatic chondrosarcoma. In pain and using up to 100 codeine plus paracetamol (acetaminophen) tablets a week. Wife feels he is addicted—sleeps most of the day, no ambition. Patient doesn't think his medications are a concern, but he is worried about things—bills are piling up, he has a family to support, fights constantly with his wife. The pain in his knee is severe (average 8/10 on pain scale). Any movement makes it worse; the patient cannot weight-bear. He is severely anhedonic—no appetite for food or zest for life. He can't concentrate on any task and can't 'get it together' to do anything. No interest in sex x months according to his wife. He knows he is depressed, but denies suicidal thoughts. However, he told his wife he might shoot self if things got worse.

Social history: unhappy childhood; history of dysphoric family with spousal abuse. Wife states still in love, but she can't cope with his physical problems and moods. She feels like leaving him sometimes (he doesn't know this). On social assistance—financially strapped. (Physical examination and recommendations re pain management, family counselling, and antidepressants follow.)

Fig. 1 Case 1.

1. When we are provided with private information about a patient, can we share information with others while withholding it from the patient?
2. A medical chart is a public record. Does not our duty to protect patient privacy require us to preclude the publication of implicitly private matters in a public record?
3. Information changes the way we think about a patient. As information may be inaccurate and cause us to adopt attitudes or policies inimical to a patient, questions of dignity aside, is it not our duty to reconcile our information with the patient's account?

Public record

An institutional medical chart may be read by scores of people. Seigler, describing the chart access of a woman entering hospital for a routine cholecystectomy, notes that in excess of 80 people (physicians, students, volunteers, administrators, maintenance staff, and other health professionals) may read the record.[16] A colleague who has worked in hospitals for thirty years has stated 'If I must be hospitalized, I'll react like a military prisoner and give them only my name, occupation, and Medicare number!' His circumspect view may be extreme, albeit based on disturbing observations over time. However, maintaining due respect for the public nature of a medical record should temper both the nature of matters discussed and the language chosen to relate those matters.

Hearsay information

This consult note (Fig. 1) discusses the patient's mental state, family problems, and sexuality. When private information on a patient is received from others, the burden is on the physician to justify withholding this material from a patient. However, this general moral principle must be wisely interpreted in the individual situation—will feedback to the patient cause alienation and family strife, as it almost certainly would in this case?[17] Physicians traditionally are repositories of patients' secrets, both those relayed by patients and by friends and family. We may conclude that, while openness remains the ideal, we are free to use this information as we deem appropriate to further the patient's good, including remaining silent.

Team discussion

Working as a team requires periodic meetings to discuss patients' problems. Nevertheless, the salutary goal of working together to assist patients and families may adversely affect privacy and patient–family dignity. It is a privilege to share a family's most intimate secrets. If we are to help a family to the fullest extent, it is sometimes necessary that we are able to share this information with colleagues in our interdisciplinary team. Team discussions of patient–family problems, however, have a potentially serious negative component. Hearsay information on marital infidelities, spousal abuse, sexual performance, and other subjects usually regarded as inherently of a confidential nature, may be bandied about, sometimes in a humorous vein. Transmission of information on our Case 2 (Fig. 2) patient without her specific permission violates universally held principles of timeless importance. Revelations of this nature before a group represent a fundamental attack on patient–family dignity, while unsubstantiated information may influence the reaction of hospital staff to a patient or family member.

Are we so professional that accounts of peccadilloes and moral failings will not influence unfavourably our degree of involvement and patient concern? The saintly amongst us may not be unduly swayed; for the rest, it is best that the physicians not test the charity and understanding of health-care colleagues sharing patient responsibilities through unhelpful revelations.

While communication of patient information with hospital teams is essential for patient well being, physicians and nurses should remember that when we pass on information, we are acting

You have been asked to see Mrs C.H., a 38-year-old woman with advanced metastatic breast cancer, primarily to bone, with consequent generalized pain. Her pain control, previously good, is now inadequate, despite therapy with regularly increasing doses of opioids, corticosteroids, spot radiation therapy, and a recent trial of a bisphosphonate. The ward nurses report increasing mood swings, with periods of obvious sadness and weeping. After a period of hesitant conversation in which Mrs C.H. appears reluctant to discuss psychosocial issues which may contribute to her suffering, she suddenly states 'You would have pain, too, if your husband was playing around with your best friend'. She then reports that she had previously partnered her husband in a small business. As she was no longer able to work with him, she encouraged a friend to take her place. The staff had previously noted that Mrs C.H. was often visited by her husband, accompanied by this friend. Following further discussion, it seems to you that the depth of anguish created for Mrs. C.H. by this situation is indeed a major contributor to her deteriorating physical and psychological status. Shortly after this interview, you are participating in the weekly palliative care team review of all patients on the unit. How should you contribute to the discussion on Mrs C.H.?

Fig. 2 Case 2.

as if we have implied consent from the patient. We should get the patient's specific permission to pass on to specifically designated members of a health-care team material which an ordinary person would judge to be sensitive.

In Case 2 (Fig. 2), it may be important for certain members of the palliative care team to know about Mrs C.H.'s suspicions, as they are contributing to her suffering and may be incorrect. Counselling will help. Quite certainly, Mrs C.H.'s permission to share this information should be sought. She may give that permission willingly, and she may want and need to speak to certain members of the team about her sadness and distress. She may also have her own personal reasons for restricting disclosure only to certain team members in whom she has a particularly high degree of trust. As the case evolved, Mr C.H. was probably not unfaithful. The staff concluded that corticosteroids may have contributed to Mrs C.H.'s paranoia.

Probably all of us have violated the tenets of confidentiality in a scene similar to Case 3 (Fig. 3). Discussion of patient information in public elevators and cafeterias is an obvious avoidable problem. However, few hospitals are built with adequate provisions for private space. A particular problem still emerges from the 'grand ward round', wherein senior staff, residents, students, and nursing colleagues parade around from bed to bed, discussing patient issues. This scenario has been associated with offences to patient dignity in a variety of guises. The patient may be referred to in the third person as people hover around the bed, while personal information is bandied about amongst both the members of the ward walk and the patients and visitors currently in the room at that time.

Efficiency of operation does not take precedence over the fundamental ethical responsibilities of physicians to honour patient privacy. The ward walk must be tailored to demonstrate that the common violations which were the product of our training are not accepted as a standard which will be followed by future generations of physicians.

Competence

It is axiomatic that patients and families expect that their physicians will competently address the various components of human suffering. However, using cancer pain as an index problem, recent surveys on three continents demonstrate defects in physicians' basic pain knowledge, education, and patient treatment.[18–23] Paradoxically, evidence of poor practice stands in contrast to the availability of simple management strategies.[24–26] Relief of suffering is not simply an item for faculty debate on the time assigned to garnering experience in palliative care *vis-à-vis*, for instance, spending more time in the operating room on a surgical clerkship. Such debates are not always based on ethical principles and may hinge on the current power base of the competing faculty departments or programmes.

The competence of physicians in relieving suffering is an ethical issue. It is morally untenable for those responsible for medical education to fail to offer support for the introduction to the principles of palliative medicine by retreating behind a facade of balancing competing faculty initiatives. Palliative medicine is not just another subdivision of medical practice simply clamouring for its rights and privileges. Its principles constitute an essential foundation for all medical instruction.[27,28] Changes in physicians' attitudes, wrought through an understanding of these principles, will not burden health-care systems. Rather, impeccable pain and symptom management may prevent otherwise tragic and expensive manifestations of human suffering.

You are standing within the confines of the ward station, discussing with a colleague the behaviour of a delirious patient. Your eye is drawn to the nearby elevator where a startled visitor, not associated with the patient in question, has obviously overheard your discussions. He appears shocked, and you wonder if the visitor may believe that you were discussing his loved one. With a sense of remorse, you once again resolve not to discuss patient information in other than a fully secure environment.

Fig. 3 Case 3.

Once the ethical dimension of palliative care education is accepted, relatively simple organizational and educational approaches can result in a tangible expression of an ethics-based educational process. These include:[29,30]

1. A formal place for palliative medicine in medical faculties. 'The education of a physician requires a positive exemplar.'[31] Palliative medicine divisions and/or chairs in palliative medicine are focal points for academic leadership.

2. The introduction of palliative care consult teams into teaching institutions. In the course of consultations, opportunities arise for 'real-time', case-based teaching. Palliative care consultants may wish to enhance this opportunity through framing their consultations as teaching instruments. For example their use of assessment techniques may further their general use throughout an institution.

3. Publication of practice guidelines for the management of pain and other symptoms. Experience with guidelines demonstrates that they do not work unless they are backed up by authoritative agencies and credible individuals in a community who put their principles into action.[32] They do provide a benchmark for acceptable practice and are readily constructed.

4. Use of patient-based assessment techniques on the clinical record. Symptom assessment measures should be given the same priority as assessment of tumour anatomy or drug toxicity. Patient-based, readily completed assessment scales should be included on the clinical record of all patients with advanced cancer or other chronic illnesses in which distressing symptoms are anticipated (see Chapter 9.2.2).

5. A palliative care curriculum should be endorsed by a faculty. It is not necessary for each faculty to develop its own curriculum. Numerous models currently exist (see Section 21). The principles enunciated by the palliative care curriculum should be integrated throughout the medical programme.

6. Obtain formal community input on faculty educational committees. The importance of including non-professional representatives on research review committees has long been recognized by medical faculties. This concept should be extended to the educational sphere. The presence of members of the community on medical school curriculum committees will add balance and community wisdom to what has often been an isolated professional arrangement.

7. Ultimately, the content of professional examinations influences the priorities of our trainees. The rites of passage within our medical faculties and professional licensing bodies should reflect the importance of the principles of palliative medicine.

8. In addition to their role in policing the profession and protecting the community, licensing authorities should use their data bases for educational purposes. Computer-generated information on practices which are important in palliative care, such as the prescription of opioids, were designed for after-the-fact control, rather than for the ongoing education of physicians.[33] However, the data obtained on opioid use may positively influence practice if it is fed back with informed commentary to practitioners.[32]

9. The accreditation of educational facilities should recognize the responsibility of these facilities to include relief of suffering in their stated missions and goals. In the process of accrediting facilities, the interest and success of an institution in matching their mission and goals with tangible achievement may be readily assessed.

The above considerations cannot be viewed in isolation from other topics in this chapter, including euthanasia and physician-assisted suicide. One cannot, in a moral society, consider terminating a fellow citizen's life if that citizen is suffering because of a lack of access to informed medical care. Surely as a first principle of any society, impeccable care for dying citizens must be ensured.

Research

More than a quarter of a century after the birth of the modern palliative care movement, research on dying patients continues to generate ethical debate. The same issues which touch upon the moral conduct of research studies at other times in the trajectory of an illness are pertinent to the involvement of end of life patients in research trials. There are, however, specific factors which amplify the ethical issues posed by research on dying patients.

Ethical distinctiveness of research in palliative care

Among the factors that complicate the ethical conduct of research on the dying, the following deserve particular mention.

1. Purpose—patients enrolled in a palliative care programme may be offered the opportunity to participate in research. In this setting, the trial objectives may be to improve the patient's quality of life or to determine factors which impact on patient–family well being. As such, the trial interventions generally have a low risk of causing harm, while the benefit of participating in a successful trial could be rapidly realized, particularly in studies focusing on improving quality of life and of care.

A patient with far advanced illness may also be asked to participate in a Phase I drug trial, where the chance of benefit is small.[34,35] Indeed, the major objective of such a trial is to determine the tolerable human dose of an agent. This scenario is replete with ethical concerns, as evidence to date suggests that patients (and sometimes their physicians) often do not fully understand the rationale of a Phase I trial.[36,37]

2. Vulnerability—dying patients and their families represent a highly vulnerable group. They may be more desperate than others, with a sense that options have collapsed around them. They may be particularly dependent upon health workers, and could be unduly influenced by them. The patients are ill, exhausted, often depressed, and, because of these factors, possibly more susceptible to proposals that are not in their best interests. Their sense of trust in physicians is often strong; to lose this sense of trust would be intolerable in their circumstances. They may have variable degrees of cognitive failure, as will be discussed below. The inherent degree of vulnerability of the dying magnifies the requirement for their protection.[38]

3. Competence—patients engaged in research must understand their options after receiving relevant information, and must be able

A.T., a 70-year-old business woman with three adult children, is referred to the palliative care unit of a teaching hospital with breast carcinoma widely metastatic to bone and brain. Several of her presenting symptoms, including multiple bone pains, nausea, and constipation, are rapidly controlled. Neuropathic pain involving her chest wall, however, responds poorly to the opioid and non-steroidal anti-inflammatory drug she has been given. The addition of carbamazepine and amitriptyline to her medication regimen has resulted in some improvement but she is left with a residual burning pain that measures 4 to 6 out of 10 on the daily visual analogue scales carried out on the ward, with occasional spikes, usually late in the day, reaching 7 to 9 out of 10. A.T. requires assistance for even limited ambulation because of generalized weakness. She is judged to be mentally competent on the basis of her admission history and physical examination, during which she was found to be drowsy but pleasant, co-operative, and oriented as to time, place, and person.

A.T. is a candidate for two current research studies: a randomized, double-blind, placebo-controlled trial of mexiletine in the management of neuropathic pain; and a qualitative study of music therapy employing semistructured interview techniques. She gives informed consent for participation in both studies. Several members of the palliative care team, including nurses and a physician, do not agree with palliative care research of any type.

Fig. 4 Case 4.

both to use that information to reach a decision and to clearly communicate that decision.[39] The competence of patients to give informed consent is a particular concern at the end of life. The incidence of dementia and delirium is increased[40,41] while, without formal testing, defects in cognitive function may be masked.[42] Bruera reports that 13 of 67 patients otherwise judged eligible to participate in a research study were found to have Folstein Mini-Mental Status examinations of less than 24 out of 30; these patients appeared to be mentally competent in clinical assessments, were able to read and sign a consent form, but probably could not offer valid, informed consent.

4. Personal goals—at any time, the uniqueness of individuals and the need to ensure that their goals are consonant with those of the investigators is important. Using cancer as an example, earlier in the trajectory of illness it is more likely that these goals will be fully shared—that is, both parties may be primarily interested in curing the illness or in a meaningful prolongation of life. Towards the end of life, when a curative therapeutic trial is no longer possible, the aims of investigators, patients, and families may be quite different or, indeed, in conflict. These differences may affect a variety of research processes, including mutual agreement on research objectives, obtaining informed consent, trial design (for example parallel versus cross-over designs), changes in design as the study proceeds, and trial termination.

5. Clinical instability—patients with advanced illness are subject to a barrage of constantly changing physical and psychosocial problems. At any time, patients may average 8 to 11 symptoms, occurring against a background of comorbidity from other chronic illnesses.[43] Each problem may demand its own therapeutic approach and many of the drugs employed will result in the addition of other agents to balance the adverse effects of the first drugs. For example, opioid use is often accompanied (wisely) by laxatives and, less commonly, central nervous system stimulants. Non-steroidal anti-inflammatory drugs are often associated (sometimes unwisely) with agents added to obviate gastrointestinal toxicity. As a result, polypharmacy may reign and a patient with constantly changing patterns of illness may also suffer from iatrogenic problems, further compounding the patient's fragile status. Aside from the impact of the patient's unstable condition on research results, the patient may not be able to complete the research trial. In any event, more than in any other research setting, informed consent will constantly need to be renegotiated and termination of a trial may, more commonly, be judged to be in the patient's best interests.

6. Age—aged patients are often excluded from participation in clinical trials.[44] Aside from AIDS patients, the majority of patients dying with advanced chronic illness are elderly. The role of an older person in a research trial is compounded by all of the issues raised in the above sections. Nevertheless, many research programmes are particularly germane to the needs of the aged.

7. Performance status—investigators either preclude enrolment of patients with limited performance status or choose not to approach them.[45] As one consequence, information on the effects of anticancer therapy on symptom status is limited. While the risk of inducing harm out of proportion to benefit primarily influences decisions to exclude some patients, a misguided application of this principle could reduce interest in designing trials of gentler therapy particularly germane to the problems of patients with more advanced illness.

Issues which can arise in the conduct of research in dying patients, illustrated by Case 4 (Fig. 4), include: Can quantitative studies such as the mexiletine study be justified in this patient population? Can qualitative studies be justified? Do current methods for obtaining informed consent reliably indicate mental competence and adequately protect patients in studies such as these?

Questioning research in palliative care

The physician and nurses in the above scenario might express the following concerns to justify their antiresearch stance:[46]

1. Clinical researchers, whether using quantitative or qualitative strategies, risk treating subjects merely as a means to the research end, thus contravening the central palliative care tenet that considers the patient and family member and their needs as ends in themselves. Palliative care physicians and nurses state that they aim to support the goals and aspirations of patient and family, rather than enlisting their support in fulfilling the researchers' goals.

2. In safeguarding the well-being of the research subject, the depersonalization implicit in the impersonal nature of the experimental method may introduce unavoidable role conflict as the

investigator acts as agent for both patient well-being and study completion.

3. Informed consent is problematic because the stability and duration of consent are uncertain and may be influenced by events emerging in the course of the study. Thus 'informed consent' at the outset can, at best, be simply consent to commence; benefit to participants from the study cannot be predicted and consent must be repeatedly negotiated as the study progresses.

4. Participant observation in palliative care research may be burdened by an intrinsic power differential between researcher and subject. Typically when we speak of consent to research participation, we assume that physician and patient are on a 'level playing field'; information is exchanged, risks are described, and the patient can decide for herself whether to participate (investigators often invoke this claim when dealing with institutional review boards). But, of course, sick people, particularly terminally ill people, are not on a level playing field with physicians. Cassell helpfully described illness as a state of 'diminished autonomy', and a purpose of therapy as being to restore autonomy.[47]

5. Palliative care patients may be particularly vulnerable to the close attention of the researcher in qualitative studies and to a deepening relationship with the researcher as the study progresses. Role blurring may become an additional problem which may interfere with withdrawal from the study. Is the researcher perceived to be a friend, nurse, or researcher? The researcher must be adequately trained and supervised to identify and manage the transference and counter-transference that are likely to occur. Are adequate safeguards built into the termination of the relationship?

6. The whole research process remains value laden by virtue of the selective availability of research funding which supports issues dictated by cultural or economic preoccupations.

One commentator, articulating many of these concerns, states 'To research at all into the needs and experiences of this client group could be said to be an affront to the dignity of those people who are terminally ill and an expression of profound disrespect for the emotional and physical state of such patients'.[47] This author goes on to say 'one wonders whether they (research questions) should ever be asked by the living to the dying'.

In support of palliative care research

In rebuttal, to this article, a group of physicians engaged in palliative care research state 'We disagree with this distinction.[48] The terminally ill are living. Furthermore, the suggestion that others have the right to deprive them of making their own decisions regarding whether they wish to participate in clinical research is paternalistic, demeaning and disrespectful. The frailty of the very ill does not preclude autonomous decision-making, participating in society, giving to others or finding purpose and meaning. The personhood, integrity and sanctity of all individuals must be equally respected'. The place of research in palliative care emerges from the following considerations.

Acceptability in principle

Research wherein the patient is the 'means to the end' is not, *prima facie*, unethical. If this were the case, a moral imperative against all clinical research would exist. Moreover, the 'means–end' language may misrepresent the real relationship existing between researchers and participant patients. The collaboration requires a unique contribution of each to the research venture. In that collaboration, it is difficult to say that either the researcher or the participating patient is a means to the attainment of the other's end. Both should strive towards the same end. This breaks down when researchers manipulate patients, fail to respect their dignity, and reduce them to 'means'.

Independent of benefit to patients, research may advance the pool of human knowledge and the investigator's prestige and career. These research outcomes are not inherently odious; they only become so if they represent the prime purpose of research with participatory patient interests as secondary goals.

Purpose is a key issue in ethical discussions. While the investigator's main purpose may be to produce generalizable knowledge, secondary benefits potentially accruing to the patient, to other patients, or to the investigator are ethically acceptable ends. The above point is reasonably straightforward. What if the patient is unlikely to benefit from the research?

Informed consent

Truly informed consent, if freely offered, may resolve ethical issues arising in this situation—the concept of patient autonomy supports the potential involvement of patients in research that may not be of immediate benefit to themselves. It remains a noble gesture to 'shake one's fist at the inevitable' and to make a contribution to the common good. The sense of purpose, sometimes lost in the course of suffering from a chronic illness, may be enhanced even from one's bed if a continuing contribution to the community may be offered. The noble nature of man is demeaned if research is simply conceived as a utilitarian effort.

However, analyses of patients participating in some Phase I trials tells us that many patients participate in these studies primarily in the hope of personal benefit.[35] Did they not understand the study explanation? Was it properly carried out? Did they choose to see only what they wished to see? We don't know but their responses raise the concern that 'informed consent' may be reduced to a medical oxymoron,[49] as will be discussed below. In the final analysis, the patient's protection must lie in the physician's observation of the Helsinki dictum—'the interest of science and society should never take precedence over the well being of the subject'.

This issue represents a tangible application of the cardinal principles of medical ethics. These principles are sterile if not applied within a compassionate environment by wise, charitable, and moral investigators.

Placebo use in research

Placebo use is regarded by some as controversial in palliative care research. Recent guidelines on research in palliative care[50] state 'Giving a placebo is not just if there is a therapy known to be more effective than a placebo. Therefore, placebo-controlled, double-blind trials are unlikely to be ethical.' This view presupposes that a treatment is known to be effective before study. If this is so, then a placebo trial is obviously unethical, regardless of the phase in the trajectory of the patient's illness in which it is conducted. Placebo trials are ethical at all stages of illness providing that placebos do not replace standard efficacious therapy and providing that patients know and understand that they may be receiving a placebo.

Participation in a clinical trial can never be justified if it results in less than optimal care. However, many 'standard' approaches in palliative care may not have proven efficacy, may not confer patient benefit, and, under certain circumstances, may be harmful. For example progestational agents, in certain doses at certain stages of illness, appear to be helpful in increasing appetite, patient weight, and possibly even energy levels with low risk of toxicity. However, at higher doses in conjunction with chemotherapy, toxicity may be a problem.[274] A blind assumption from early trials that corticosteroids or progestational agents are helpful in all circumstances would result in erroneous and harmful practice.

There is a consensus that at the beginning of a random clinical trial (RCT) comparing two or more treatments, an honest null hypothesis must exist.[51] In other words, uncertainty must exist as to the relative merits of the treatments being tested in the trial.[6] Some authors have argued that this means the treatments in a trial must be precisely balanced—referred to as 'theoretical equipoise'—that is, no empirical grounding for a preference for one treatment over another in a trial can exist.[52] As Freedman has pointed out, this understanding of equipoise is all too fragile; the fate of a single patient in a RCT could throw the balance in favour of one treatment or the other, thus requiring that the trial be stopped.[53] Freedman has persuasively argued for a different understanding of equipoise termed 'clinical equipoise'. Clinical equipoise exists when there is 'an honest, professional disagreement among expert clinicians about the preferred treatment'.[53]

At the start of the trial, there must be a state of clinical equipoise regarding the merits of the regimens to be tested, and the trial must be designed in such a way as to make it reasonable to expect that, if it is successfully concluded, clinical equipoise will be disturbed. In other words, the results of a successful trial should be convincing enough to resolve the dispute among clinicians.[53]

The question hinges on the analysis of equipoise. If, in the physician's opinion, equipoise is not absolute, this view should be shared with the patient. Even if equipoise does exist, patients must receive an explanation of what this means. If there is no scientifically relevant difference between two treatments under study, there may be a personally relevant difference for the patient. Subsequent decisions in practice will depend on other factors such as cost and drug access.

Must a patient always have the right to the active agent? This issue has surfaced in many AIDS trials, albeit primarily with respect to therapies used in early or mid-disease trajectory.

This issue is negated in research trials involving 'n of 1' or short-span, cross-over designs. These are particularly useful approaches for palliative care research, although inherent design problems such as carry-over effects and the constantly changing clinical setting may limit study interpretation. Moreover, regulatory agencies prefer randomized placebo studies.[54]

Aside from ethical issues, research involving dying patients presents formidable logistic, demographic, and academic barriers (outlined in Table 2).[28] Consequently, few investigators are currently attracted to this area of endeavour.

However, we know from other settings that, aside from the direct benefits of a trial, participation in research and access to the research milieu is often beneficial for patients (Weijer C, Freedman B, Fuks A, Robbins J, Shapiro S, Skrutkowska M, in press).[55] Is it therefore possible that the care of patients with advanced illness is unfairly jeopardized by the devaluing of palliative care research by funding agencies? As a result, dying patients may have less access to the 'best and brightest', as these physicians and nurses concentrate on issues more readily resolved and more likely to satisfy their academic mentors.

Table 2 Limiting factors in palliative care research[a]

Logistic – demographic

- Small population base—individual programmes
- Lack of training in research techniques
- Balance of workload versus research opportunities
- Problems in control of variables in rapidly changing patient populations

Academic priority

- Lack of association with academic units
- Where association exists, lower priority in comparison with oncology and other disciplines
- Lower priority of granting agencies
- Unrealistic expectations leading to excessive targeting and funding of certain fields, such as cancer chemotherapy trials

Developmental

- Lack of internationally recognized classification and assessment systems
- Absence of multi-institutional groups
- Lack of tie-in of basic science and palliative care
- Absence of support from large pharmaceutical firms
- Semantics—What is palliative therapy?

[a] From MacDonald, N. Priorities in education and research in palliative care. *Palliative Medicine* 1993;7(suppl 1):65–76.

Double agents?

Yes, a physician or nurse conducting clinical research is acting as a double agent. While this situation can induce an ethical dilemma, it does not, *de facto*, place one in an unethical stance. Increasingly, we are called upon to act as double agents, with responsibilities not only to our patients but to their families, our colleagues, departments and institutions, medical faculties, and, most problematic of all, the state (or, in the United States, private insurance agencies or health management organizations). Moreover, in our private lives we must constantly address the balance between responsibilities to our own families and the patients we serve.

While one must often accept double agency status, the ethical problems arising therein may be resolved if priorities are set so that, as has been the tradition in medical practice throughout the ages, patient well-being is maintained as a physician's top priority.

This problem is not unique to research settings. Indeed, although not receiving proportionate attention, it may be of greater concern in the non-research setting.[56,57] Currently, clinical research protocols must be accompanied by carefully constructed informed consent documents which should, prior to their introduction, be reviewed by uninvolved physicians, scientists, and members of the lay community. While comprehension by patients of these forms and the purposes of research is often poor,[58] this may reflect a more general ethical problem in communicating with patients. If a patient's understanding of their illness and the purpose of the clinical research trial is often not clear, what happens in the course of day to day care outside a research setting?

The data on cognitive impairment at the end of life are sufficient in the authors' opinion to dictate the use of a screening tool, such as the Folstein Mini-Mental Status test, on participants in palliative care research where the risk of masked incompetence is present. While not an absolute litmus test, an abnormal test result should raise serious questions about a patient's capability to provide informed consent.

As in other research areas, informed consent may need to be repeatedly renegotiated during the course of a study. It is not a blanket permit. This is necessary to provide patients with updated information which may alter study equipoise. It is of particular importance in palliative care research, since patient cognition, health status, and degree of vulnerability may change, with consequent resetting of the terms for informed consent.

The community as partners in research

Clemenceau, noting the singularly unimaginative approach of his military to First World War battle strategy, stated 'War is too important to be left in the hands of the generals'. A similar sentiment may apply to the dearth of research interest in the problems of dying patients. The 1996 American Society of Clinical Oncology abstracts contain 10 times as many studies on one chemotherapeutic agent, paclitaxel, as there are on cancer pain.

Even though this agent is neurotoxic and could have a beneficial or harmful effect on pain, this issue does not appear to interest oncologists. In order to make clinical trials at the end of life more responsive to the needs of patients, greater involvement of patients and their families in the design and conduct of cancer research is clearly needed.[59] Clinical science inevitably involves value-laden decisions. Currently these decisions appear to be weighted heavily towards seemingly repetitive interventional trials, with consequently reduced emphasis on psychosocial and symptom control issues. The balance will be heavily influenced by the traditional interests of academic oncology, buttressed by the availability of support from the pharmaceutical industry. Is this balance logical and does it reflect the expectations of the community? Possibly not—the answer will be more clearly apparent when we involve patients and patient communities, not only in the ethical review of trials (a practice now well established) but also in the planning and conduct of research. The AIDS community has achieved this aim, to a certain extent. With respect to cancer, the concerned community may be less clearly defined. However, as cancer affects between one in three and one in four members of the community, there is an abundance of thoughtful, well-informed people whose families have been touched by cancer and who could be drawn upon to help in this process.

Towards resolving the case dilemma

The following steps are suggested to resolve dilemmas generated when the imperative for academic palliative care units to conduct clinical research is seemingly challenged by their primary responsibility to ensure the well-being of their patients.

1. Patients have a right to participate in research which may add meaning to their lives and may offer imediate relief from suffering. However, the compentence of the patient must be ensured. Use a mental status examination when competence is in question.
2. Even if competence is assured, participation in two research trials at one time may produce an undue burden. The nurses, physicians, family members, and patients involved should candidly discuss these issues. These discussions should be rational rather than emotive, using reasoned rather than theoretical language. They need to address clearly the following questions.
   (a) Improving the well-being of the patient is clearly the first priority — will participation in research compromise this objective?
   (b) May research participation provide a reasonable chance, with little downside risk, to improve the patient's lot?
   (c) Is the research programme so structured that the patients may view themselves as partners in the process, rather than simply as subjects?
   (d) If participation in a research trial is associated with appreciable risks such as development of adverse drug effects, even in the face of assured patient competence, are processes in place to identify adverse events at the earliest possible moment, and are processes in place which ensure the opportunity for patient renegotiation of participation throughout the study? Always, is patient risk commensurate with patient benefit?
3. Units considering participation in research should commence their activities with a workshop on ethical issues in palliative care research. Apart from identification of important principles, a workshop enables colleagues to discuss a series of situations which may arise in a forum which encourages reasoned discourse. This should facilitate decision making when similar problems are encountered in 'real time'.

Resource allocation

No moral impulse seems more deeply embedded than the need to relieve suffering...it has become a foundation stone for the practice of medicine, and it is at the core of the social and welfare programmes of all civilized nations.

Daniel Callahan

Few readers of this textbook would argue with Dr Callahan.[60] Government commissions on euthanasia and physician-assisted suicide in three countries (United Kingdom, Canada, and New York State in the United States) concluded, after public hearings, that their communities should give a priority to palliative care. The citizens of Oregon, when asked, also gave a high priority to pain relief and control of suffering.[61]

Why then does the allocation of resources fail to match basic moral principles and expressed community expectations? Some possible reasons are:

1. Substantial funds are already spent on dying patients.

Indeed, this is the case. The costs for treating patients are heavily concentrated towards the last year of life, with much of the expenditure devoted to institutional care.[62] Good value for money, however, may not be received, as a financial outlay in some cases purchases predictably futile therapy, while in other instances quality of care does not appear to correlate with the money spent on care. Numerous studies quoted in other parts of this textbook describe the inadequate attention to symptom control and quality of life which is still a characteristic of many of our institutions.

2. In a time of fiscal restraint funds cannot be allocated for major new programmes.

Many harried administrators, physicians, and educators may regard palliative care as yet another special interest advocacy initiative. If thought of in this light, it becomes an easy task to assign it to a lower order of fiscal need. What may be a common view is stated in a letter received from an Associate Dean in a Canadian medical school. In response to a request by the Canadian Palliative Care Education Group, suggesting that a film, *The Edge of Being*, be made available to Canadian medical students, he replied :

'I receive proposals such as yours regularly throughout the year. Each proposal is important and worthy. In the past six months they have included violence towards women, assaults on children and abuse of the elderly. As you know the concern of medical educators is that the curriculum is already overloaded leading to too little time for students to learn. You must also know that post-graduate training is at least two years, and is usually longer than the other undergraduate programmes.

I'm therefore surprised that proposals such as yours don't seem to consider that the education you propose be fitted into the post-graduate programme. I question whether undergraduates are ready to learn 'how to do palliative care.'

The group Chairman replied:

'I was struck by your comparison of palliative care to such topics as abuse of the elderly. I sense that you regard palliative care as yet another single issue advocacy initiative. If you think of palliative care in this light, it becomes an easy task to assign it to a lower order of educational priority. I also note that you believe that palliative care is not a suitable topic for undergraduate education. I think we are still teaching respiratory medicine, cardiology, haematology, etc., in the undergraduate programme. Why should palliative care that encompasses the skilled application of a wide range of medical techniques to assist patients and their families with advanced chronic illness, not be a suitable topic for undergraduate teaching? Indeed, palliative care education should inform all clinical teaching in medicine, surgery, gynaecology, paediatrics, etc., which we expect our students to master in their undergraduate programme.

Perhaps therein lies the reason for our misunderstanding. Palliative care is not a single issue topic, but rather presents to undergraduate students a method of whole patient care that will certainly benefit the students in specific technical areas such as the proper use of analgesics but, more importantly, should influence their overall approach to medical care.'

An attitudinal change, wherein decision makers come to respect palliative care as a method of whole patient care, rather than yet another advocacy initiative, could result in sensible fiscal redistribution of funds already expended on dying patients and their families.

3. Proof is lacking that palliative care will save money.

The task of supporting palliative care programmes would be eased if one could prove that they reduce costs while improving patient–family welfare.[63] Hospital administrators may point out that inpatient palliative care is labour intensive and that costs for personnel will balance savings in medications and procedures. However, lower hospital admissions for care of chronic diseases correlates with access to good community health care. Palliative care programmes foster measures that enable patients to be maintained in a home setting who otherwise would require hospitalization. The introduction of subcutaneous medication techniques,[64,65] together with regular home visiting services, stand as examples. Based on an analysis of total health care costs, rather than simply concentrating on the institutional component, some regional health authorities have now introduced comprehensive community palliative care programmes in order to save money as well as improve patient care (the Capitol Regional Palliative Care Programme, E. Bruera, personal communication). While further studies in this complex area are required, if total health care costs were taken into consideration, palliative care programmes may not necessarily increase societal costs and might result in overall savings.

4. Money should only be expended when expenditures are clearly balanced with defined needs.

Lack of support for comprehensive palliative care exists not because of ethical shortcomings of health planners and medical leaders but, in large part, because the basic needs of those who suffer have not been clearly identified and defined. Therefore it is not surprising that needs were not balanced by resource allocation. A paradox, however, is apparent. Granting agencies and clinical researchers may already have their hands full with studies on other issues of interest to the medical establishment of the day or on research programmes which are influenced by external, well-endowed sources. For example studies may demonstrate a 'need' for the community to have access to a lookalike chemotherapeutic agent because of the forceful support of pharmaceutical firms and a research establishment which thrives on drug studies. The needs of a community may be reflected in the public press through the lobbying efforts of well-organized, disease-specific constituencies. There is no 'National Society of the Dying' to drive the public agenda in most countries. Therefore, detailed information on the needs of those suffering with chronic illness remains *terra incognita* in most jurisdictions. Recently, a series of studies in Canada has addressed this issue (see Chapter 14.1). Moreover, the landmark work of Dr Cleeland and his group in the United States and other countries, complemented by recent surveys by Portenoy and the Canadian Pain Management Group, consistently demonstrate that the need of cancer patients for skilled pain control is not sufficiently addressed. As illustrated by Kristianson *et al.*, research methodology is now in place for identifying patient–family needs and views on care.[66]

5. Health care costs must be reduced. Everyone must share the burden.

Many countries are revising their health systems. Often, the organizing feature of this effort is reduction in cost, with other features of health care subservient to this principle. This single-minded approach is thought to mimic hard-nosed, effective business practice. It is ironic that some non-health industries now regard a dogged, soulless emphasis on money making as not only greedy but often also as bad business. As recently described in the *Harvard Business Review*, the business world is finding that using an ethical base for decision making can make business sense.[67] Businesses with their eyes only on expenditures compounded their financial problems as their employees cut corners, with consequent customer dissatisfaction. Conversely, other model companies which redeveloped their business strategy on a framework marrying ethics and sound finance enjoyed increasing success in a highly competitive market area. Bottom line, short-term decisions may turn out to be rash, expensive, and inefficient.

Assuming general acceptance of Dr Callahan's statement at the beginning of this section, it should also be accepted as an ethical base for policy decisions. For practice to match principle, additional funds are probably not required; rather, a change in attitude, with a concomitant adjustment in allocation of resources.

Ethical issues related to home care resource allocation

A man's castle is his daughter's work house and his wife's prison
George Bernard Shaw

An increased emphasis on home care presents a number of ethical dilemmas.[68] Clearly, one is acting in the patient's best interests if he or she can return home with adequate provision of medical care. Discharge from an institution enhances patient autonomy and maintenance of dignity. However, the home caregiver can be harmed in a number of ways. The freedom of time and activities of that individual will be further limited. Existing funding arrangements in many countries offend the tenet of distributive justice, as expenses incurred in the home which might have been covered, in whole or in part, by the state or an insurance agency if the patient had been hospitalized are now the responsibility of the family.

Whether the costs to health-care systems are lower or not, it is clear that the costs of home care to the family are higher. Aside from direct financial costs (drugs and other home therapies), caregivers may incur indirect costs as they may be required to take time off from work. Sometimes, remodelling of the home to accommodate a sick family member is necessary.

In addition to economic costs, there is an emotional price to pay for the lost sleep and constant association with a loved one's suffering. The patient's illness creates a new duty for the caregiver, with sharp limitation of that caregiver's freedom. For some this can become very wearing and can create a sense of onerous duty.

Should there not be limits on this imposed duty? How do we balance the moral duty to care for a family member with other ethical issues, such as combating a culturally reinforced expectation of women who all too readily have embraced self sacrifice and a selfless life—in practice, most family caregivers are women.[69] It is easily assumed that families should look after loved ones. However, the exceptional dedication of home caregivers should not be taken for granted. As Callahan states, if we are to ask families to undertake a heroic sacrifice then it becomes imperative that we find out how we might sustain them.

Patients in many cultures still enjoy the privileges which come with membership of a large extended family. However, in the Western world, families are smaller, often fragmented, and without access to previously supportive community institutions such as churches and fraternal organizations. Family members often live at a distance, with alternate responsibilities which cannot be easily discharged.

Home caregivers will soon be bereaved. It cannot always be assumed that the heroism of a caregiver who has looked after a loved one for a long time in a home setting will assist the bereavement process as this individual looks back with satisfaction upon a job well done. Balancing this positive scenario, the caregiver may be exhausted and an ambivalent relationship between the caregiver and the dying patient may be established, which will rebound into a poor bereavement reaction. Among the critical markers of a pathological bereavement reaction are the absence of close social contacts and an ambivalent reaction towards the deceased (see Section 18). Prolonged home-care responsibilities can intensify all of these factors.

Therefore, as we shift care from institution to home, we have an ethical responsibility to look after not only the patient but also the home caregiver. Policy on palliative care in the home should be dictated by ethical considerations in addition to clinical and financial concerns. Specific programme elements may include :

1. If the state is shifting cost to individual patients and families, the state has a duty to shift resources to provide support for those bearing the burden of care which would otherwise fall upon state institutions. Some jurisdictions are addressing this issue by providing financial support to family members who give up employment to care for dying loved ones at home.

2. Programmes to sustain home caregivers should receive a high priority. These include:

   (a) educational programmes specially designed for lay caregivers;

   (b) ready availability of respite beds and day-care centres;

   (c) establishment of a clear line of contact with professional help at all hours;

   (d) identification of caregivers who will require specific bereavement assistance.

Ethical issues related to society-generated costs

Most countries either direct public money to practices which increase suffering or support such practices through low taxation policies and over-tolerant legislation. Any ethical consideration of resource allocation must take these egregious practices into consideration. For example in every country toleration of dual ethical standards in society leads to much of the suffering which is encountered in palliative care practice. The standard of ethical behaviour allowable to tobacco executives, and the sporting figures, cultural leaders, lawyers, and advertising agencies who support their reprehensible practices, gives evidence that often the term 'business ethics' is an oxymoron. Rich rewards would ensue if the same moral standards quite properly applied to medicine and nursing were expected of our political colleagues and those who engage in the commerce of hazardous products. The term 'beneficence' would take on new universal meaning.

If society continues to tolerate and support major sources of suffering, such as the tobacco industry, it surely must balance the ill-gotten resources which ensue with added resources allocated to the tragic aftermath of this tolerance. Practical resolutions of this ethical dilemma could include:

(1) abolition of tobacco advertising;

(2) increase in tobacco taxation;

Dr X is a renowned physician with an impeccable standing amongst his peers. He served as Chief of Staff of his home hospital and head of a medical division prior to leaving his home Canadian province to take up a senior academic position at another Canadian university.

Shortly after his departure, the provincial health authorities, through an agreement with the province's specialists and family practitioners, agreed to provide each medical group with a global budget. This enables the government to predict more clearly their medical expenditure while, as reasoned by the physician groups, the authority to influence the distribution of funds to individual physicians, albeit within a limited budget, remains with physicians.

Dr X completes, with further distinction, his work at a university in the adjacent province. In the course of his work, he developed an interest in palliative medicine. The palliative medicine division in the home hospital attempts to recruit him. In this locale, as in every Canadian province, palliative care physicians with demonstrated skills in teaching and research, are in very short supply. Clearly, Dr X represents an extraordinary resource for the palliative care division, and the patients and families it serves.

Dr X applies to his medical specialty association, who refuse to provide him with the authorization which will enable him to receive recompense for his work in palliative medicine. He will not be practising his medical specialty, as it is usually construed and they do not wish to allow a colleague, no matter how distinguished, to dilute the income pool. Dr X joins a palliative care programme in another part of Canada.

Fig. 5 Case 5.

(3) government–community transfer of the current support of sporting and cultural events by tobacco companies, with assignment of these funds to a public trust, which could fund our ballets and symphonies without odious expressions of 'thanks' to tobacco firms;

(4) direct allocation of tobacco revenues to palliative care programme-support. Tobacco victims probably do not add health care costs as so many of them die early after a few months of illness.[70] However, their suffering can be alleviated if they have access to impeccable palliative care. In a sense, they have already paid for it.

Ethical issues related to health system redesign

The physician as a double agent

In a previous day, the moral responsibility of a physician was primarily to the individual patient and only secondarily to others, be it the patient's family or to agencies and the state. In this historic setting, the physician's ethical hierarchy was straightforward.[71] Most countries are now introducing innovative, organizational arrangements designed to control costs and, possibly, improve the health of their societies. Many of these macroadministrative processes have unexpected, detrimental effects on palliative care patients. Case 5 (Fig. 5) illustrates an ethical problem arising when physicians function as double agents.

Placing physicians in situations where decisions affecting their financial rewards within a private, for-profit health system or publicly funded system are in conflict with patient care has major ethical connotations.[72–74] The above scenario illustrates the double-agent role which physicians are increasingly forced to accept. While this scenario is particularly germane to the health-care system in Canada, similar dilemmas affect other systems. For example a related dilemma may be noted in an American health maintenance organization whose physicians earn a higher income for both the organization and themselves if the medical care costs of their patients are truncated.[75] Dying patients generate costs; many plans may attempt to exclude 'costly' patients. Where are these patients to turn?

The legal and moral codas of most countries demand that physicians accept a fiduciary responsibility to put an individual patient's interest first, regardless of cost to himself, rather than a purely contractual arrangement, wherein each side bargains, presumably on an equal basis, to obtain favourable arrangements with the limitations of the contract clearly listed and limited. This is so as the physician's power and knowledge *vis-à-vis* the patient precludes establishing a fair business contract.[76]

In the scenario outlined, the medical group acted as agents both for the state and for their fellow members but consequently with probable harm to the individual patients who would be served by the palliative care group. They would not recognize any of these patients individually as their responsibility and, as such, would argue that they have not breached their responsibility to any specific patient.

Be it in war or in medicine, the harm which one inflicts upon faceless groups is more readily carried out with good conscience. Even if it is accepted that they did not harm any of their patients, do they not have an obligation to serve as not only an agency of the state and their organization (where they have a self-serving role), but also to the broader society of suffering patients who would benefit from access to first-rate palliative care physicians?

The issue of physician fidelity to patients when the doctor is forced into double agency is surfacing in American health care. Millions of American patients, and thousands of their physicians, are pressured into 'co-operating' with for-profit, managed care organizations. Amongst the many ethical abuses therein entailed, one notes that some of these organizations had required the agreement of participating physicians to withhold information from their patients about alternate treatments or opportunities for referral outside the managed care network to which the physician and patient belong.[76] Physicians may also be instructed not to pass on information on the nature of their financial arrangements with managed care operations; the patient, as a result, will not be aware that limitation of their rights for referrals or medical procedures will enrich both the physician and the commercial firm with which he is enrolled. As in research, patients must be aware of their full rights and conflicts of interest which may influence the judgements, on their behalf, of their physicians.

The moral dilemma of the physician double agent could be partially resolved if the physician regarded himself as an agent, not only for his patient, but for all patients. One can wear two hats. 'When I am dealing with a patient, he is my priority. But when I am not, I am a knowledgeable citizen and free to advise the collectivity (state, hospital, etc.) on how to use their limited resources' (M. McGregor, personal communication). Physicians should support a fair distribution of resources not only to their patients but all dying patients, and should regard this objective as a higher calling than adherence to professional organizations, institutions, or the state.

Does the high moral stance suggested in the previous paragraph indicate that physicians must never serve a gatekeeper function? Of course, physicians have always acted as gatekeepers, for only through them could patients have access to the various components of medical care.[72] Physicians have also always rationed care, as they have always rationed their initiative on behalf of a particular patient according to the time available, the resources at hand, and patient's characteristics. These characteristics may include those which suggest to the physician that he could intervene effectively. Unfortunately, using cancer care as a marker, the rationing process may also be influenced by the patient's age, gender, race, and economic status. Physicians are products of their society and, while ethically troublesome, it is not surprising that social characteristics would influence physicians' decisions.

If one accepts the thesis that a physician cannot avoid serving as a gatekeeper but that decisions in this role should be based fairly on the needs of the individual patient, then what guidelines may be considered for that allocation of resources which is influenced by physicians? These include:

1. Transparency—physicians should inform their patients of rationing decisions and who is involved in these decisions should be open to public scrutiny and debate.

2. Respect for the hierarchy of responsibility—the conduct of affairs in a democracy involves creative tensions between groups with possibly disparate perspectives and responsibilities. Physicians must recognize state imperatives but, in the care of their patients, this recognition does not change their primary ethical focus. While government and institutional functionaries will adequately address the priorities of the organizations they represent, physicians must balance the equation through patient representation. They cannot serve the state, their hospitals, or professional groups if this service jeopardizes their primary responsibility to patient interests.

3. Physicians can improve the sensible application of resources through recommending less costly therapies if there is no evidence that more expensive options are superior, improving administrative efficiency, discontinuing futile or ineffectual therapies, and participating in defining guideline development. They may also shed their white coats and provide expert advice to governments and agencies on societal issues where their training and experience provide unique, valuable perspectives.

The above ethical progression may sound naïve and unlikely to be perfectly realized in a complex society. However, as stated by Randall and Downie '... so much of life seems to be about the struggle to achieve goals which in the end are rarely attained, such as the struggle for justice in law, for international peace, and for fulfilling relationships. We value these ends and so value the struggle to attain them, possibly because the striving affirms our commitment to them as well as enabling us to inch forward slowly towards them'.[77]

Resource allocation—the aged

In 1996, the United States Court of Appeals for New York State ruled that the existing ban on physician-assisted suicide in that state is unconstitutional. Their judgement, commented upon elsewhere in this chapter, contained a chilling sentence 'Surely the state's interest lessens as the potential for life diminishes'. The court's views are echoed in the priorities that seem to be assigned by physicians to the care of elderly patients with advanced chronic illnesses. For example, where studied, an age bias was demonstrated in the opportunity for the elderly to receive anticancer therapy. Studies to date, primarily from the United States, indicate that :

(1) elderly patients are less likely to receive aggressive therapy;

(2) they are less likely to have alternate therapies presented to them;

(3) they are less likely to receive adjuvant therapy.[78,79]

These perceived behaviours of physicians stand in contrast to the treatment preferences of elderly patients. Suzanne Yellen and colleagues presented cancer patients at Rush-Presbyterian Hospital in Chicago with a series of clinical vignettes of people with the same diagnosis as the patient. Patients were asked to make hypothetical decisions about treatments; their decisions reflecting their acceptance of chemotherapy and their willingness to trade survival for toxicity and harm. While elderly patients were averse to taking major toxic risks, the study demonstrates that they were as willing to choose chemotherapy as younger patients.[80]

The management of pain and other symptoms may be particularly problematic in an older population. There is no evidence to suggest that older patients suffer less than younger cohorts. Indeed, the average number of symptoms which older patients may have is higher, while the symptoms of cancer are often expressed against a background of comorbid disease and related suffering. Wherever studied, cancer pain appears to be under-diagnosed and under-treated throughout the world. The consequences of this mistreatment may fall most heavily upon the elderly, particularly if they are female and poor. The Rush-Presbyterian study enrolled a small number of patients but, even within this limited group, there was wide variability in preference.

The assigning of stereotypic characteristics of a group to an individual is absolutely decried by society, at least for race, sex, ethnicity, or sexual preference. However, the elderly are still subject to stereotyping. In our pop culture, the doddering old fool remains the socially accepted butt of jokes. In our hospitals, these adverse attitudes are still reflected in occasional conversations on our wards—for example the young student or physician, who could be the grandchild of an elderly patient, addressing him or her by a first name, as 'George' or 'Ethel'. The stereotyping is never logical but it is particularly ironic when applied to elderly people. The elderly probably represent a more heterogeneous group than younger cohorts but their unique characteristics may be ignored by medical attendants who usually are much younger than their elderly patients.

The quote which began this section and the above observations suggest that, at a time of financial stringency, decisions on resource allocation may be made to the particular disadvantage of the elderly. They may be the only large publicly-targeted group singled out for restrictive funding.

The shift from institutional to home care will have the greatest impact upon older citizens. As recently expressed by the National Advisory Council on Ageing in Canada, rhetoric is not matched by reality—the shift of funds from institutions to the community sector is not yet proportionate to the shift of patients. The patient with advanced cancer at home usually presents a very complex set of problems. The studies of Cartwright remind us of the multiple symptoms that the aged encounter as they die, both those with cancer and otherwise. Most symptoms are common in incidence and severity to patients dying at an earlier age but a few vary with age.[81,82] Some of these symptoms, notably mental confusion and bladder and bowel control, put particular pressure upon caregivers in their efforts to both control the symptoms and to maintain the dignity of their aged parent or spouse.

Ignorance or anxiety on the part of the patient or the caregiver is the principle cause for problems in a home-care programme. Few individuals in the older age group have more than the most rudimentary knowledge of science and biology and are frightened by the need to involve themselves in such things as injections and medication adjustments.

If attitudes are adopted which assign a priority to care of elderly patients, programmes of the type outlined in the section on 'Home care' can succeed. Of greatest importance to the elderly, the following issues must be considered in an ethical context:

1. If rationing is necessary, it should be carried out using medical benefit criteria rather than group criteria.[72]
2. Funding arrangements setting up an arbitrary distinction between institutional care which is paid for, and home care which is not, must be reconsidered.
3. Short-term respite admissions, which provide relief for care-givers, must be more readily available.
4. Day care facilities allowing careful monitoring of elderly patients on a frequent basis, while providing respite for care-givers, should be introduced.
5. The availability of educational material and nurse instructors to provide instruction and follow-up advice is essential.

Conclusion

Ultimately, the availability of resources for the dying depends on societies' views on their rights versus competing rights. A 'right' is defined in the *Concise Oxford Dictionary* as 'that which one may legally or morally claim. . .'. Rights are assigned by law or by community consensus. Rights recognize a perceived 'need' which may be characterized as a 'requirement' or a 'want'. We cannot obtain everything we 'want' but most of us would concur that the basic requirement of a person to find respite for treatable suffering frames a morally assigned societal right. To what extent does this moral claim translate into a legal–financial claim? This must vary from country to country, as some may have over $2000 per capita to spend on health, and others less than $2. However, if the address of suffering is granted the status of a 'right', then each country is ethically required to endorse a basic palliative care programme, commensurate with their resources. The basic elements of a programme are not expensive, as they include simple educational initiatives, changes affecting drug availability, and access to trained health professionals (the level of training dependent upon a country's health system). Adoption of this proposal can balance the equation between sensible analysis of 'need' and assignment of a corresponding 'right'.

Withholding or withdrawing therapy

A contemporary consensus

Dying with dignity has become a slogan of opposition to aggressive, technologically aided attempts to prolong life when a sick person's organism, though still minimally functional, no longer supports or permits the exercising of control over life's events. To treat a person as a mere object is an appalling degradation of human dignity, and the rejection of such treatment of human beings is a moral basis of our dealings with one another in all phases of life. The expression, dying with dignity, appeals to doctors, nurses, families, and others involved with the care of the sick to respect this moral foundation in their relationship to those who are gravely ill or dying.

Blaise Pascal once said that a human being, even if subject to the laws of nature that dictate descent into death, remains superior to the entire universe. This is so because human beings can know that they must die and why, while the universe knows nothing about what it does. This is only part of the truth. The balancing truth is that human dignity does not reside in the power for thought and knowledge alone. Dignity also comes to mature expression in the power to act knowledgeably and sensibly and to command respect for one's considered and cherished intentions.[83]

People may wonder about 'the worth of being superior to the universe' when they see themselves or their sick loved ones as inferior to today's life-extending technology; inferior because of their own inability and powerlessness to command if, when, and for how long that technology will be used. Patients surviving on intensive, life-support technology and care have not always been able to act in accordance with their considered and cherished intentions, particularly so when they have wanted to refuse life-prolonging care and to be left free to die as peacefully and as quickly as possible. These patients would have needed help so to act, and they were often unable to command attention, under-standing, and respect from others for a choice that seemingly contradicted a constitutive goal of medicine—the saving of life.

Although saving lives always has been, and will ever remain, a primary goal of clinical practice, the initiation and continuation of intensive, life-prolonging procedures may result in little more than a stretching out of the dying curve or the extension of an unbearable and unrelentingly miserable life. Over the last twenty years or so, patients, families, nurses, doctors, and people from all walks of life have been asking whether extension of life to the bitter, biological end is the right thing to do, particularly when the sick and the dying find the physical, emotional, and personal costs of such treatment to be hardly bearable. A trend has developed over two decades, and its direction is away from an ethic of prolonging life at all costs towards an ethic emphasizing the quality of life and of dying over the duration of life taken as an absolute value.

This trend demonstrates a much clearer understanding than was detectable in the early days of intensive-care high technology, that the availability of medical technologies is not of itself an ethical command that these technologies be used. For many years, treatments were characterized as ordinary or extraordinary (terms now abandoned for reasons to be discussed below) as though the ethical indications for use were built into the treatments or technologies as such. The contemporary clinical ethical consensus about withholding and discontinuing life-prolonging treatments emerges from the realization that treatments are a means, and their use is not an end independent of the clinical goals that a patient accepts and clinicians can achieve. It is these clinical goals that govern, or should govern, decisions about initiating or discontinuing treatments, recalling all the while that these goals vary along the course of a disease; that these also vary from patient to patient even when they have similar clinical conditions.

The clinical goals to be pursued for each patient, and the requirements of clinical care, inevitably change along the continuum of disease. While diseases vary considerably both as to rate and as to continuity of evolution, the evolution of disease is also always unique to each individual patient. It is the nature of a patient's response to treatment plans that indicate when the time arrives to down regulate intensive life-prolonging care and to up regulate palliative care. The shift is rarely abrupt or of the on–off, binary kind of change. Moreover, certain interventions, such as radiotherapy or surgery, may serve curative clinical goals for some patients and palliative goals for others. Along this continuum of evolving disease and correspondingly changing clinical goals, moments are reached when it is clinically, ethically, and legally justifiable to withhold or to discontinue clinical treatments, such as resuscitation procedures, respiratory support, dialysis, antibiotics, chemotherapy, surgery, and assisted hydration and nutrition; the discontinuance of this last mentioned intervention being still very controversial.

Some people, including physicians, nurses, and other health-care professionals, may still be quite unaware of this trend and consensus; and others may think this direction is simply wrong. Moreover, some particular cases, perhaps even many, will inevitably provoke agonizing discussions, intricate deliberations, and difficult decisions, if for no other reason than that persons, both in their bodies and biographies, are simply too complex to be reduced to principles. Nevertheless, the trend, as evidenced in a line of court cases and in a voluminous literature in medicine, nursing, ethics, and law, is against the tethering of people with advanced, irreversible illness to life-prolonging treatments and technologies, particularly when the underlying disease is progressing and cannot be halted and when the life extended is only marginally bearable or definitely miserable.[84–88]

However, there is a gap, and it varies in width from place to place, between clinical–ethical practice as reflected in the literature and clinical practice in reality. The contemporary clinical–ethical consensus about withholding or discontinuing life-prolonging treatments may simply fail to operate when: there is no continuing communication between doctors, nurses, patients, and families; when doctors and nurses are not educated to attend both to the body and the biography of patients; and when the organization of care in hospitals promotes the unreflective use of technology rather than the careful mastery of technology in the service of the patients' goals and aspirations.[89] When these failures occur, a technologically and bureaucratically dominated system tends to take charge, and that system may not know when or how to stop life-extending treatments, in great part because that system is not in intimate contact with the sick and dying people it is meant to serve.[90]

The path to consensus

The attainment of a now widely-shared, but not universally implemented, understanding about when allowing people to die is the right thing to do has resulted from a slow, long, and complex process. This consensus has not flowed from the pens of any single group of particularly clairvoyant thinkers. It has, rather, come about from multiple interactions over many years between patients and families, clinicians, nurses, judges, lawyers, and people from various disciplines and professions working on solutions to the clinical, ethical, and legal problems encountered so frequently in the care of incurably ill or dying persons. In another sense, the process has been complex because it has involved cycles of interaction between changes in clinical practice, changes in the normative concepts used in clinical ethics and legal doctrine, and changes in the standards and arguments of jurisprudence. Numerous court cases, often called 'right-to-die' case, over twenty years, and the many ensuing commentaries illustrate these changes and the interactions between them.[91–97]

Socially high-profile discussions, at times intense debates, about life-prolonging decisions have centred on a relatively few cases that have gone both to trial courts and appeal courts. The estimate in the United States is that about 13 million deaths over the period 1976 to 1991 involved prior decisions to discontinue or to forego life-sustaining treatments. Only 2900 to 7000 of these cases ever went to trial courts, and of these, only 50 to 75 went into appeal.[98,99] Clearly the high-profile cases—such as the Karen Ann Quinlan and Nancy Cruzan cases in the United States, the Nancy B case in Québec,[100,101] and the Anthony Bland case in the United Kingdom[102,103]—have occurred against a background of increasing social and clinical adjustment, over the last twenty years, to the idea that persistence in the use of life-sustaining treatment is often not the right thing to do.

Milestones on the path to consensus

The space of a chapter does not favour a detailed tracking of the many interactions involved in this twenty-year long clinical, ethical, legal, and social dialogue. Certain milestones, however, have been passed and they could well be marked here as likely points of no return.

1. Decisions about withholding or discontinuing life-sustaining treatments cannot be made adequately simply on the basis of a predetermination that some treatments are extraordinary and others are ordinary. The distinction between extraordinary and ordinary means has a long history and has provoked extensive

discussion and controversy.[104,105] However, medical science and technology has developed in ways so varied and complex that the distinction between ordinary and extraordinary means, once useful in clinically simpler times, has, for over a decade, been recognized as quite useless as a criterion for clinical decisions and public policy.[86] Even the Roman Catholic Church, within which this distinction was once widely used in statements on matters of medical ethics, suggested over fifteen years ago that this distinction should be abandoned in favour of the more meaningful distinction between proportionate and non-proportionate treatments.[106] The real clinical–ethical issue is whether any treatment, be it technically simple or complex, be it an instrument of basic or of advanced life support, is in keeping with the current clinical goals of each individual patient.

2. The implication of the proportionate–non-proportionate distinction is the now widely-held view that there are no intrinsic moral or ethical imperatives attached to different categories of treatment, such as cardiopulmonary resuscitation, ventilatory support, dialysis, medication (such as vasopressors, antibiotics, and insulin), and the provision of assisted nutrition and hydration. Decisions to use, to forego, or to discontinue any of these and other kinds of treatment should be taken as a function of, and not in isolation from, the clinical goals of the total treatment plan for each patient.

3. Binary thinking that would set sacredness of life in opposition to quality of life, so that respect of the one would require abandonment of the other, is not the way to reach ethically sound, clinical decisions.

Quality-of-life decisions are inescapable in clinical practice because physicians and clinical teams are ethically and professionally obligated to gauge the consequences of their work on the bodies and lives of the people they are professionally presuming to help. Yet, the quality of human life varies from person to person, and, indeed, varies for each person across the ages of the life cycle. The ethical danger in 'quality of life' decisions is that some lives maybe judged as not worth living because they will never match up to some single inflexible notion or scale, inevitably culturally conditioned, of what worthwhile human living means. Thinking of quality of life in absolute rather than relative terms risks the mistake of ignoring that a meaningful human life is possible even far out from the centres of biological, psychological, and intellectual normality. The doctor forgot this when he refused, on a quality-of-life basis, to remove an operable lung tumour from a man afflicted with Korsakoff's syndrome. The doctor judged that this man's brain impairment combined with his need to live out his life in a long-term care institution amounted to an intolerable quality of life.

An ethical danger also lurks within any absolute emphasis on the sacredness of life. It is the particular danger of subjugating sick and dying persons to life-preserving interventions that are really intended to serve a sick person's life plans, not to substitute for them. Since the introduction of powerful life-prolonging technologies into hospitals, people have often feared dying more than death. They have feared being technologically tethered to the biologically living relic of the persons they once were, and can never be again. They have feared being clinically forced into the extension of a life now irreversibly damaged by disease, depleted of energy, and intolerant of enjoyment. In such and similar circumstances, it is now widely recognized as being ethically erroneous to read the sacredness-of-life principle as compelling absolute persistence in extending life by all means and at all costs, right up to the moment when a patient's biology has utterly lost all capacity to respond. Allowing a gravely ill person to die on time, on his or her chosen time, is quite perfectly consonant with the sacredness-of-life principle. To insist on the contrary would be equivalent to insisting that a sick person's biology is more sacred than her person.

4. The wide attention given over the last twenty years in professional medical and ethics journals, and in the media, to a series of court cases involving decisions about life-prolonging treatments may obscure a cardinal point in the contemporary consensus about where these decisions should be made and who should make them. The law generally follows standard, or widely accepted, clinical practice in these matters. This means that these decisions, generally, should be made in the clinical setting, at the bedside, and not before the bench. Today this does not mean, as was often clinical practice in the past, that the doctors alone decide if and when life-prolonging treatment is to be started or stopped. The emphasis in the contemporary consensus, at least within the countries and culture of the West, is on shared decision-making between physician and patient, with the patient holding primary of power to decide. This emphasis comes to expression, to cite one example, in an amendment to the Criminal Code of Canada, proposed some years ago by the then existing, and now disbanded, Law Reform Commission of Canada. The amendment was designed to prohibit any relevant paragraph of the code from being interpreted as requiring a physician 'to continue to administer or to undertake medical treatment against the expressed wishes of the person for whom such treatment is intended'.[107]

The trend towards according primacy of decisional power to the patient rather than to the doctor in matters of life-prolonging treatments would be misread if it were interpreted to mean that doctors are now expected to act against their personal and professional consciences. Although a readiness to respect a patient's will, wishes, and decision should occupy primacy of place in a clinician's professional conscience, some patients' choices or refusals of treatment may elicit reasoned opposition from a doctor or other health-care professional. There is no consensus without its complexities and conflicts. These conflicts are inescapable and they will continue to challenge the courts on an episodic basis and clinical ethics on a daily basis.

5. The self-determination of patients has moved from an earlier periphery to central place in contemporary consensus about how decisions concerning withdrawing or withholding life-prolonging treatments should be made. Legal provisions have been made in many jurisdictions to allow for, and to recognize, living wills, advanced directives, or assignment of power of attorney to a person of one's choice, each of these being one of several strategies to assure that sick persons' wishes about life-extending treatments will be respected when they are no longer conscious or able to participate in the decisions that have to be made.[108–111]

There is a continuing uncertainty and reticence about not initiating or discontinuing life-extending interventions for gravely ill persons who are no longer capable of expressing their wishes and who never did, or never could do so, before their disease progressed to its current advanced state. Some courts that have recognized the justification of withdrawing life-support treatments in the cases of persons who could no longer express their will have explicitly sought evidence that these now unconscious patients had at some earlier time in their lives expressed a desire not to have their lives prolonged if, for example, they ever lapsed into a state of permanent unawareness.[112,113]

It would be mistaken to read the contemporary emphasis on self-determination as implying that there is no place in the contemporary consensus for withholding or discontinuing life-prolonging treatment when patients can no longer express their will and never expressed any thought about these matters before falling gravely ill. There is general agreement that incompetent patients have the same rights as competent patients.[114,115] There is also general agreement that doctors and clinical teams should not be bound by law to administer treatments that are therapeutically useless and not in the patient's best interests.[107,116] There is debate and uncertainty regarding the ways of determining what a person's best interests are when they can no longer speak for themselves. However, just as patients themselves, in consort with physicians and members of the clinical team, can usually come to decide reasonably about which treatments are in their best interests and which are not, so also, the proximity principle suggests, are family members and loved ones usually able to reach reasonable decisions in a similar way about what is or is not in the best interests of an unconscious or incompetent person who is in a state of advanced and irreversible disease.

Physicians, clinical teams, and family members do not, of course, always agree on what is right or wrong to do for irreversibly ill or dying persons. Moreover, the proximity principle may not be in operation in certain families. Some family members may not have the best interests of a dying person as their decisive priority when speaking with doctors about discontinuing life-prolonging treatments. These situations, as will be considered below, may provoke intensely difficult scenes at the bedside and, if these conflicts cannot be resolved, then ultimately judicial proceedings may follow.

The consensus in practice: principles and cases

The kinds of decisions that have to be taken for and with gravely ill and dying persons are not purely technical. These decisions become an intrinsic component of the event of dying. Depending on the content of these decisions, and on the way they are made, some people will have the chance to die well, masters of their dying, not alone and not lonely. Others may die before their time, without a chance to live their dying through. Others may die too late, reduced to biological systems that have to be tended. Some may die uninformed and unenlightened, caught trying to play 'scene two' when life's drama is in fact about to close. Still others may die who could have lived.

Decisions having such consequences demand that comprehensive attention be given to patients in their full particularity; that attention is focused on the unique biology, clinical condition, needs, desires, life plans, hopes, sufferings, strengths, vulnerabilities, and limitations of this particular person now. Decisions of this kind, and they are the primary outcome of clinical ethics in palliative medicine, cannot be deduced from any one principle or set of principles. These decisions result rather from a process of highly practical reasoning. The method of clinical ethics in palliative medicine is inductive. It works by passing the existing principles of the philosophical and religious moral traditions through the grid of particular personal and clinical histories to learn gradually what these principles command, prohibit, or tolerate. This knowledge is not all worked out in advance, completed, and waiting to be applied. The clinical ethical order within these principles is, to use an expression of David Bohm, an implicate order.[117] An implicate order cannot be made explicit as a whole. It is manifested slowly and only partially as it is worked out in the case-by-case practical judgements reached at the bedsides of unique persons as their disease advances and their biographies come to a close.

This method of clinical ethics in palliative medicine will now be exemplified in a series of considerations of when and why it is ethically justified to withhold or to discontinue life-extending therapy. These considerations refer to the principles most frequently invoked when decisions about treatment have to be made with or for the dying. Specific, real cases, greatly modified to protect confidentiality, are described to illustrate how principles have to be interpreted in the light of individual patient histories if they are to offer any practical guidance at the bedside. It is in the following situations that withholding or discontinuing life-prolonging treatment is most often considered and ethically justifiable.

When patients refuse treatment

If confusion, the undue influence of other persons, and pathological depression can be excluded, many hold to the principle that 'the will of the patient, not the health of the patient, should be the supreme law' governing decisions about initiating or discontinuing life-prolongation measures.[118] A classic expression of the principle of self determination is Justice Benjamin Cardozo's 1914 statement 'Every human being of adult years and sound mind has a right to determine what shall be done with his own body.'[119] In the same vein, the Law Reform Commission of Canada has proposed an amendment to the Criminal Code of Canada to prohibit any relevant paragraph of the code from being interpreted as requiring a physician 'to continue to administer or to undertake medical treatment against the expressed wishes of the person for whom such treatment is intended.'[107]

This clear and reasonable principle may conflict sharply with strongly held clinical perceptions and certain dominant values in our culture. People increasingly give public support to patient autonomy and to the value of self-determination against the potential abuse of medical technology. However, it is not always easy to live according to the same categories in which we think. People can generally agree on the justification of abandoning life-prolonging procedures when a patient's loss of consciousness is irreversible. Many, however, experience a strong visceral opposition to discontinuing or withholding life-prolongation treatment—whether this be respiratory support, chemotherapy, or total parenteral nutrition—from an intelligent, conscious, and lucid patient.

This spontaneous opposition may be reinforced by bonds to the patient forged during the earlier fight for life. Decisive and distressed family members may also intensify the difficulty of respecting a patient's refusal of life support. Moreover, although the principle of autonomy or of self-determination may be easy to state, it is often very difficult to ascertain whether some patients who are speaking coherently are not perhaps so dominated by a particular state of mind, such as a depression, that they really are unable to make decisions on their own behalf.

Several years ago, a 27-year-old woman entered hospital with leukaemia. She had been abandoned by her parents shortly after her birth and subsequently lived in one foster home after another. Through adolescence she lived a wild sex and drug life and came to despise herself at the age of 19. At this time she met a couple who had never had children and they offered her a room in their home. She gradually became their own child in fact, if not in law, and this young woman, highly intelligent, went on to finish her schooling, her university undergraduate studies, and had dreams of becoming an architect.

Her leukaemia was diagnosed at this point in her life. A young physician was very supportive, assuring this young woman that effective treatments were available, and that she had every chance of pursuing her professional dream. When he outlined the treatment plan, the young woman agreed to everything except the blood transfusions. She could not accept transfusions she said, because her new parents' Jehovah's Witness faith had become her own. She didn't want to die but could not accept a treatment that for her was tantamount to betrayal of her faith, and to a betrayal of the parents and extended family who had given her a new life.

The physician opposed her refusal, insisted that she was not going to enter the cemetery because of some silly belief, and that she was totally wrong in refusing a treatment when that refusal was, in his view, equal to a choice of death. When he threatened to force treatment on the young woman the relationship broke down and another, older physician entered the scene. He spoke to the younger physician, reminding him of their shared religious beliefs, some of which were looked upon as bizarre and even foolish by some of their very bright and competent colleagues. The older physician said 'It's not for us to judge her faith but to make sure she is really speaking her own mind and is not being pressured by others'.

It became quite clear over several considerations that this young woman was quite thoroughly independent, was not being pressured by family or friends, and held the Jehovah's Witness belief as her very own. Her refusal of transfusions was then respected by the entire clinical team, with the young physician maintaining a very reluctant silence.

After the young woman's death and funeral, that reluctant silence exploded in rage directed against the older physician who had orchestrated respect for the young woman's decision. The young physician's accusation? 'If it were not for you and your ethics, doctor, she'd be at the university now, and probably dancing on Saturday. Now she's dead and you seduced me into betraying my basic mission as a doctor, which is to save life. I could have saved hers.' The older physician's response? 'Do you think it is your mission to save life at all costs? Even at the costs of crushing a patient's liberty? If you do, you're wrong. At times liberty is a value higher than health or even life.'

This one case illustrates how difficult it can be at times to respect an instance of human freedom that is highly conscious of itself, superbly capable of self-expression, and articulating itself in a choice that affronts a dominant value or moral persuasion. This case also illustrates how the whole biography of this young patient, not only her clinical condition and the treatments available, entered into the deliberation required to reach a clinical decision. Many, but not all, would argue that the decision reached in this case matched the full particularity of this young woman. For that reason, it was the right decision. However, if principles can be generalized, specific clinical–ethical decisions cannot.

The clinical circumstances of the following case are quite different from those of the young woman with leukaemia, just discussed.

A woman, 53 years old, entered hospital in a state of renal failure. She was accompanied by her husband and her adult daughter. The physician explained to the woman that she would have to start dialysis, but she refused, stating that it was time for her 'to go into the arms of God'. Over lengthy conversations that afternoon, the woman's refusal of dialysis was persistent and her refusal was strongly supported by her husband and daughter. She appeared lucid and coherent but fatigued and withdrawn. She insisted on leaving hospital and returning to her village many miles away, to be cared for by her doctor there, and basically to let nature take its course.

Her son, however, arrived at the hospital late in the afternoon, before her departure, and explained that his mother had been depressed over the last ten years and had never, in his opinion, been adequately diagnosed or treated. Supported by her son, and against her protests and those of her husband and daughter, the doctor had the woman admitted to hospital and dialysis was started. The woman also received psychiatric attention. Over months she improved and changed her mind thoroughly about the dialysis, with which she collaborated enthusiastically, and about wanting to live. As she gradually rediscovered her former better self, she took up activities and re-established friendships she had long abandoned. Her husband and daughter changed too, recognizing in her the woman they had once loved but who, over years of depression, had become for them a constant source of stress and even a symbol of death.

It was not immediately obvious to the doctor, even after lengthy conversation that afternoon, that this woman's depression, not her genuine self, was refusing treatment and seeking death. This case illustrates one situation in which respect for a patient's self determination requires clinical opposition to a patient's and to her family's refusal of treatment.

When burdens are not proportionate to benefits

The principle of proportionality, succinctly stated, affirms that life-prolonging treatments are contraindicated when they cause more suffering than benefit.[118] This principle also comes to expression in the Canadian Law Reform Commission's recommendation that the Criminal Code should not bind physicians to administer therapeutically useless treatments or treatments that conflict with a patient's best interests.[107] Other position papers have also cited this principle or its equivalent.[87,115] The Vatican Declaration on Euthanasia proposes that it is ethically justifiable to discontinue the use of life-prolonging techniques 'where the results fall short of expectations'. Direct appeal is made to the principle of proportionality when this document observes that patient, family, and staff may judge that 'the techniques applied impose on the patient strain or suffering out of proportion with the benefits which he or she may gain from such techniques'.[106]

It was on the basis of a proportionality judgement that the court supported a mother's and grandmother's refusal of additional chemotherapy treatment for Carole Couture-Jacquet's saccrococcygeal teratoma. This little girl, under 5 years old, had already suffered greatly from the side-effects of previous chemotherapeutic regimens. The suffering included constant nausea, loss of at least 50 per cent of kidney function, and a significant diminishment of hearing function. Physicians estimated that a renewed chemotherapy regimen had a 10 to 20 per cent chance of arresting the advance of Carole's cancer. The Quebec Court of Appeal did not find the mother's and grandmother's refusal of additional chemotherapy for Carole to be unreasonable. That refusal, rather, was seen as based on reasonable proportionality judgement that the low probability of success did not justify submitting Carole to more of the intolerable suffering she had already endured.[120]

A 42-year-old man, severely handicapped intellectually, and with multiple metastases to the brain presented his two sisters and a clinical team with a choice found, initially, by all involved to be most difficult. The treatments available at the time would probably prolong this man's life for a period of 6 months to a year beyond the time he could be expected to live without treatment. Yet these treatments required the patient's collaboration, and he could not collaborate. He didn't understand what doctors and nurses and hospitals were, and had no concept whatsoever of disease, treatment, or side-effects. He was a powerfully built person and still capable of quite devastating resistance to anyone he thought threatening or harmful. He also had lovely hair, and prized this personal characteristic above everything. He would spend hours grooming himself and admiring himself in the mirror, and would glow when complimented about his hair.

How, his sisters and physician asked, would he react to the hair loss and other side-effects of his treatment? Would he resist treatment if he made the connection between his hair loss and what doctors were doing to him? Would it not be better for our brother, the sisters asked, if he could have a relatively comfortable 8 months of life rather than 11 months or so of life filled with losses, complications of daily living, and misery he could never understand? This is how the sisters and the clinical team came to understand the choice they had to make for this man; they judged aggressive antitumour treatment as being out of keeping with what this patient could tolerate as it was likely to cause this man harm out of all proportion to the good it would bring him.

When treatments are bound to fail

There is general agreement today that patients are not obliged to undergo, and physicians are not obliged to offer, begin, or maintain, treatments that are futile.[84,85] It is nearly a tautology to say that those patients may be allowed to die for whom life-prolonging treatment is futile. However, this statement is not tautologous because there is confusion and controversy about the meaning of futility.[121,122]

The futility of an intervention is to be judged in terms of the clinical goals for each individual patient. The central question is—will the intervention benefit the patient as a whole? Antibiotics will clear up a pneumonia in a patient locked into a persistent state of unawareness. That effect can be achieved. Because this effect can be achieved, some physicians believe antibiotic therapy in this situation is not futile and hence it is obligatory. However, what is the goal of treatment for a patient who will never regain consciousness? If the clinical goal of this treatment is to return the patient to even a minimum of intellectual and relational capacity, then this treatment for patients in this state is indeed futile and non-obligatory, for those patients will never return to consciousness and awareness.

It is essential to distinguish and even separate two components in the concept of futility—the component of physiological effect and the component of benefit.[123] Some treatments are futile because they cannot produce a desired physiological effect for a particular patient or a particular category of patients. For example the probability of chemotherapeutically halting a metastatic process may, on the basis of clinical trial results or on the basis of accumulated clinical experience, be nil or so low as to constitute the rare and unpredictable exception.

Other treatments may be futile because they are useless in attaining the clinical goals of care, even if they can have the effect of prolonging biological life. If the goal of clinical treatment is to restore a patient to a measure of independent life, then treatments are futile if they only prolong a dying process, or preserve the patient in a permanent state of unconsciousness, or tether the patient indefinitely to life-support machines in an intensive care unit.[123]

Consideration of each individual patient in his or her body and biography—the total patient—is the key to proper use of futility as a criterion for withholding or discontinuing advanced or even basic life support. Prolonging a dying process may be justifiable if the patient and family need that extra time to achieve important personal goals.

One man in an irreversible and advanced stage of leukaemia returned to hospital time and again for blood transfusions. Some members of the clinical team accused others of excessive agressivity in their treatment of this man. They came to think differently, though, on the day the man returned to hospital one last time, this time to die. He explained that, though he knew the treatments would never cure him, they at least gave him the time to complete the porch he was building around the house for his wife.

In a quite different situation, a physician aggressively maintained life support for a severely brain damaged teenager so that the mother and father could synchronize their schedules of grief. The father, unrealistically expecting his son's return to conscious life, was accusing his more realistic wife of abandoning hope, of abandoning their son. The marriage and the equilibrium of the surviving 9-year-old brother were in danger. The physician, a neurologist, worked carefully and sensitively with the father who, 5 months later, came to hospital with his wife and son. He apologized to his wife in the presence of the doctor and both husband and wife requested that no further efforts whatsoever be continued to prolong the biological shell of their child. Efforts to prolong the life of a non-salvageable child can be justified, within reasonable limits, if they contribute to the healing of an endangered family life.

Treatments of the most varied sorts are means to ends and the futility of treatments in clinical practice should be judged in terms of how likely it is that any given treatment will obtain the current clinical goals for this patient, now.

What, in general, are the clinical goals of care for patients with advanced cancer, for patients who are now receiving palliative care, or who should be receiving such care? What place does cardiopulmonary resuscitation have as a means to the attainment of these goals? When people dying from advanced cancer suffer cardiopulmonary arrest, surely resuscitation will have very little effect in helping these patients die in peace, free from pain and suffering. If such a death is generally inevitable and quite imminent for patients in palliative care, then resuscitation is generally futile.[124] There may be exceptions, but these will be adequately assessed only if the clinical team knows the patient well.

The sources of clinical problems linked to cardiopulmonary resuscitation of patients in advanced states of cancer may well go beyond any particular clinician's lack of sensitivity. When the law requires the writing of no resuscitation orders, physicians may be reluctant to do so because they know that such an order in a given hospital will be equivalent to abandonment of the patient. When dying patients have to court the risk of futile resuscitation so that they can receive the very basics of the palliative care they require, the ethical problem at the bedside mirrors a more pervasive ethical problem at the level of how care is organized and delivered in a hospital. A system of care that is out of touch with the specific and changing needs of dying patients is likely to favour the proliferation of futile treatments.[125-127]

When being alive is no longer meaningful

There is general agreement that survival in a state of persistent unawareness is not meaningful human existence and may indeed be a fate worse than death.[128] Useful studies and reviews[129–132] discuss the clinical characteristics of persistent vegetative state and the basis for its diagnosis. Our concern in this section is to discuss how far physicians may ethically go in allowing patients in states of persistent unawareness to die. Is there an ethically defensible distinction between advanced life-support measures that may be discontinued and basic support measures, such as assisted nutrition and hydration, that ethically must be continued?

As mentioned earlier in this section (and it bears repeating) medical, ethical, and even legal consensus[133–136] is growing in support of the view that there are no intrinsic moral differences between categories of treatment, such as cardiopulmonary resuscitation, ventilatory support, medications, and the provision of nutrition and hydration by artificial means. Decisions to start or discontinue assisted nutrition and hydration, as for all other treatment decisions, should be taken as a function of, and not in isolation from, the goals of the total treatment plan for each patient.[137] This question, however, remains controversial.[138]

The ethically critical question regarding assisted nutrition and hydration of children and adults in persistent vegetative state is not 'Are we justified in discontinuing such treatment?' but rather 'What justification is there for continuing this treatment?' This latter question is based upon the assumption that every medical and surgical intervention into the body of a patient has to be justified. A range of invasive procedures in emergency and intensive care units are normally justified by the likelihood of curing the patient, stabilizing the patient, or restoring the patient to a level of meaningful life.

When physicians reliably diagnose that a patient is in a state of persistent unawareness and that the patient's emergence from that state is impossible or overwhelmingly unlikely, there is little justification for continuing assisted nutrition and hydration. These procedures, as one mother expressed it, are only preventing my son from completing his death.

The role of intravenous or subcutaneous hydration in the palliative care of persons dying from advanced cancer remains controversial. The statement that dehydration in the terminally ill is beneficial for all dying patients is probably an unwarranted generalization. Some dying patients experience symptoms, such as confusion or opioid toxicity, that may well be relieved by parenteral hydration.[139]

If assisted nutrition and hydration may be essential measures in the palliative care of some dying patients, this is rarely the case for patients, adults or children, in deep and irreversible coma.[140] Relatives, and some physicians and nurses, may be very opposed to discontinuing assisted hydration and nutrition for a patient in a state of persistent unawareness because they believe and fear that the patient will suffer the pain and discomforts of hunger and thirst. This is unlikely if the diagnosis of persistent vegetative state is correct. A person in this state is, by definition, unable to perceive a wide range of stimuli, and the brain functions required to permit self-perceived affective response to stimuli have been destroyed.[141] At least one other working group agrees that the neurological mechanisms needed for the experience of pain and suffering are no longer operating in vegetative state patients, and that feeding does not benefit these patients.[142] If decisions have been taken to discontinue assisted hydration and nutrition, good nursing care and oral hygiene will assure the patient's bodily dignity until death occurs.

When the evolution of the disease is uncertain

The evolution of the patient's clinical course usually indicates when the time has arrived to discontinue life-sustaining treatment and to allow a patient to die. However, time is not always on the physician's or the patient's side. The conscious, alert, and ventilator-dependent patient certainly presents one of the greatest and most difficult challenges to clinicians and family in deciding when to stop support that could prolong life indefinitely in an intensive care unit.[143] The term 'entrapment' has been used to describe this situation that may occur more frequently in spinal cord injury and neuromuscular disease than in other clinical conditions.[144] Entrapment may also occur outside the context of respiratory support, for example in clinical situations marked by a slowly cascading series of organ failures and infections.

There is no single ethical protocol that can cover these situations. The following considerations, however, offer a direction for difficult decisions.

1. There is no clinical or moral obligation for physicians and family to adhere to a treadmill of increasing therapy and diminishing returns for a patient who will, in all probability, never be freed from a regimen of intensive care.
2. There is no ethical difference, and it is also increasingly recognized that there is no legal difference, between not starting and stopping life-prolonging treatment.[145,146]
3. The purpose of resuscitation, respiratory support, and other emergency and intensive care measures is to return a person in acute collapse to some reasonable measure of normal human life. Intensive care treatment has reached its limits when its only result is to entrap a patient into permanent bondage and residency in an intensive care unit. Intensive care has reached its limits, and may be stopped, when it can do little more than totally tie the patient's time and energy to the procedures of survival.[123,147]
4. It is not always possible, but it sometimes happens, that patients are able to understand their predicament and are able also to help family and physicians with the difficult decisions that have to be made.

One 10-year-old boy, neurologically damaged but cognitively unimpaired after an automobile accident, had already suffered several episodes of respiratory failure and would continue to do so indefinitely. This little boy, while still on a respirator after his last respiratory arrest, clearly told his parents and doctor that he wanted to go home and was altogether too fatigued by the whole process to ever want to be resuscitated again.

Nancy B., a 25-year-old woman in Québec, afflicted with extensive muscular atrophy resulting from Guillain–Barré syndrome, initiated the discussion and deliberation that eventually elicited Superior Court agreement with her request to stop the respirator on which she would be dependent for breath for the rest of her life.[148,149]

When families clash with physicians

Decisions about life-prolonging treatments involve a complex interplay of clinical facts and probabilities and personal values. They are not purely medical in nature. Physicians, on the basis of their knowledge and experience, carry prime responsibility for ascertaining a patient's condition and prognosis, and for assessing the clinical efficacy, benefits, and risks of alternative treatments. Patients and families, on the other hand, have a need and a right to receive from physicians clear and comprehensive clinical information so that they can decide which of alternative available treatments, or whether only palliative treatment, is in their own or their family member's best interests.

When patients are unconscious, confused, or otherwise unable to participate in decisions about their care, physicians inevitably have to share these decisions with parents, close family members, with close friends of the patient, or with the patient's guardian, as the case may be. The principle of proximity states that loved ones who have lived years with a gravely ill and dying person are normally best situated to interpret what is in that patient's best interests and to defend those interests. To act responsibly on behalf of a dying loved one, family members need the same clinical information that the patient herself would require.

Information alone, however, is rarely enough. A physician's leadership may and should include the giving of clinical advice. Indeed, it is rare that family members would expect a physician simply to provide a range of clinical facts and options and to leave them without any guidance as to which of several alternatives is best for their gravely ill loved one.[150] Identification of possible treatments, the balancing of benefits and burdens, and the formulation of therapeutic recommendations are an integral part of a physician's responsibilities.[151]

When shared decision-making works well, neither physician nor family members take the 'final' decision alone. They carry responsibility for that decision together. Yet some family members may be intellectually or emotionally unable, or culturally unprepared, to assume their central role in decisions for their loved ones. In these situations, physicians will have to exercise an even greater degree of leadership in guiding the family towards the decision that is best for the patient. Experienced nurses can often be of great service in these circumstances in helping physicians guide parents or family members towards necessary and highly distressing decisions. This is particularly true when nurses, perhaps over many weeks of contact, have acquired the trust of family members and an intimate knowledge of a family's strengths, weaknesses, uncertainties, and anxieties.

Shared decision-making may, on occasion, break down totally. The causes of such breakdowns are usually complex and may, in some situations, be due to a physician's insensitivity to, and lack of understanding of, a particular patient and family. Some physicians may also be relatively uncommunicative or may be seeking to impose their moral views on the patient or family. Since case descriptions of breakdowns in shared decision-making would require at least a chapter, attention may be best focused here on situations where families are trying, as it were, to play doctor.

The impending death of a central figure in a family can provoke multiple shifts in the relationship of the family members, one to all and all to each. The relationship of power and leadership among family members may undergo rapid change right at the bedside, and precisely on the issue of what is to be done for a dying relative.

A large family led by one of the sons demanded that all antibiotics and all other supportive treatments be stopped so that their mother could die in peace. Extensive discussions between the clinical team and four consultants had the greatest difficulty in bringing the family to understand that the patient was going through a normal postoperative course after repair of an abdominal aorta. The patient's situation was indeed most grave, and prognosis was most guarded, but it was still too early, 10 days after the operation, to say that this woman would not recover and was dying. The family finally opposed the dominant and dominating son and agreed to the continuation of all treatments so that their mother's body would have time to 'have its say'.

This family, however, was most unstable. Within 3 days of the clinical discussion that ended with the family's acceptance of life-supporting treatment, the family arrived in full numbers, led by the son, and demanded of the physician in charge that all treatments be stopped. The physician was overwhelmed and complied. They thought their mother would die within a few hours. When their mother was still alive 2 days later, the family panicked and asked that treatment of the postoperative infections be started again. It was too late, though. Septicaemia had spread and a woman died who might have lived.

Families who try to play doctor need to be gently and firmly opposed, while all efforts continue to achieve common understanding between the family and clinical team. This opposition may be particularly important when family members are insisting on maximal aggression treatment of a dying patient. Physicians and hospitals, unfortunately, can be fearful—fearful of bad publicity, fearful of legal entanglements, and they can fail for these reasons to oppose unreasonable family demands that are damaging to dying patients.

Such an event occurred when a niece demanded on behalf of her 82-year-old aunt, who was in the terminal phase of advanced cancer, that dialyses be started when her aunt's kidneys failed. The niece also threatened legal proceedings if she suspected her aunt died more rapidly than expected due to heavy administration of analgesics. This elderly patient's dying was prolonged because of hospital and physician acquiescence to the niece's demands, and this patient's pain was inadequately medicated because of the niece's threats.

When advance directives cause ethical dilemmas

Advance care planning is a strategy to ensure that the norm of consent is still operative and respected when sick persons are no longer able to discuss their treatment options with physicians and thereby exercise control over the course of their care. Planning in advance may typically include written directives indicating who a person would want to make treatment decisions on his or her behalf, and also specifying what kinds of treatment one would or would not want in certain states of illness (Singer PA, Robertson G, Roy DJ, in press).

The preparation of advance directives may favour improved communication between physicians and patients and these directives may reduce anxiety and uncertainty on the part of both clinicians and family members when the time eventually comes for difficult decisions about care, particularly if the patient is unable to participate in the making of these decisions.

It is illusory, however, to think that advanced directives or living wills will prevent all clinical-ethical uncertainties and conflicts. People themselves may change, and may change their minds and attitudes towards certain states of illness, between the time they write their advance directives and the occasion arrives for their implementation. Proxy decision makers, appointed in advance, may be uncertain as to whether the sick person, now unconscious or otherwise incompetent, really is in the clinical situation described in the advance directives as requiring non-initiation or discontinuance of certain kinds of treatment. It may also happen that people, in their advanced directives, have requested life-prolonging interventions that now, in their current specific clinical condition, are totally unrealistic.

Quite different situations can occur within which advance directives create an ethical dilemma for clinicians, and possibly also for family members.

Such an event occurred in an emergency unit when a woman arrived in ambulance accompanied by the ambulance physician and her two sons. This 67-year-old woman had a long history of rheumatoid arthritis and had taken an overdose of barbiturates. Finding their mother unconscious, the sons called the ambulance. However, they also arrived with two documents, signed by their mother and stating clearly that she intended to end her life when her arthritis reached a stage that no longer permitted her to live independently and in her own apartment. One document was a living will or advance directives text, signed 6 months earlier, and naming her sister as the person who should speak and decide for her when she was no longer able to do so herself. The second document was signed the day before the woman took the overdose. That document specified that the woman intended to end her life, that no resuscitation should be attempted, and that she would sue in the event that she were to be successfully resuscitated.

The physician in the emergency service telephoned the sister and she, along with the woman's two sons, insisted that this woman should not be resuscitated.

This woman did not have a medical record in the hospital where she was brought by ambulance and the physician felt extremely uneasy about not resuscitating a suicide victim about whom he has so little medical information. Should this woman, despite her clear advance directives, be resuscitated, only to be left in the situation of having to try suicide all over again? Was this woman suffering from a treatable depression? Had this woman really received optimal treatment for her arthritis? In the face of all these unknowns, and with only minutes to spare, the emergency room physician decided not to attempt resuscitation, and the woman died shortly after that decision was taken.

This situation provoked intense controversy within the hospital and it was impossible to achieve consensus in several discussions that followed upon this event.[152]

When anguish or pain are overwhelming

Whether heavy sedation of patients prior to their deaths is ever ethically justifiable remains controversial. The controversy, in part, is about what happens to people who are dying from advanced cancer. Some claim and others deny that there is a crescendo of pain and suffering in the final days of dying from cancer, a crescendo admitting of relief only through heavy sedation and the induction of sleep prior to death.[153-155] This controversy is about events and numbers and it can only be resolved by additional research.

The use of heavy sedation to control pain and other causes of suffering is ethically controversial not least because one class of sedatives, the barbiturates, are frequently used to administer capital punishment, for euthanasia, and for suicide.[156-158] Some who can ethically accept the use of heavy sedation to manage refractory pain and refractory symptoms such as dyspnoea and agitated delirium may be ethically very uncertain about the use of sedation to control severe and persistent anxiety, depression, and existential distress.[159,160]

Pain and symptoms are said to be refractory when they 'cannot be adequately controlled despite aggressive efforts to identify a tolerable therapy that does not compromise consciousness.'[161] The ethical evaluation of heavy sedation, including the use of barbiturates for the control of refractory symptoms, largely depends on the clinical goals and intentions of both patients, families, and clinicians. There should be no ethical objection to the use of heavy sedation when this is the only effective measure available to bring patients relief from agonies that torment their bodies and minds. The choice of which sedative to use, in what doses, and by which route of administration, remains a matter of clinical assessment and clinical judgement in palliative medicine. Attention should be given to the fact that clinical strategies for managing refractory existential suffering and severe anxiety in the dying are perhaps less well established than for the management of pain and physical symptoms.[161] Moreover, existential suffering and anxiety may not be constant and may wax and wane over time.

The determination that suffering of the mind is refractory requires 'repeated assessment by a knowledgeable clinician who has established a relationship with the patient and his or her family.' If anxiety, depression, and existential suffering resist all consciousness-preserving methods of control, then the use of heavy sedation may be ethically justifiable.[156,162,163] Relief from crushing agonies is for some, and perhaps for many, dying patients a higher value than the maintenance of consciousness.

These general considerations cannot be expected to silence the multiple uncertainties that will occur in particular situations. The case of a man in his late fifties, receiving palliative care 14 months after diagnosis of a left parietal glioblastoma multiforme illustrates some of the uncertainty attaching to the use of sedation when anguish is overwhelming.

This patient had been receiving parenteral steroids and midazolam for a period of 41 days when the decision was taken, because of the patient's continuing and intense anguish, to increase the midazolam and diminish the dexamethasone gradually over 6 days ending with cessation of steroidal treatment. The patient died on day 45, 4 days after initiation of this treatment plan.[164]

Although the palliative care team and family members were of one accord in accepting this treatment plan, the physician and nurse reporting on this case have asked whether condoning sedation for psychological distress is not entering onto a slippery slope.[164] Two commentaries in this case report queried whether the administration of dexamethasone for over 40 days resulted in an unnecessary and avoidable prolongation of this man's dying and agony.[165,166] Although she agreed that sedation, in addition to antianxiety and antidepressant drugs is a part of the management of end-stage symptoms, one commentator on this case considered that induction of continuous sleep was the equivalent of euthanasia.

Although some may find the difference between euthanasia and induction of deep sleep or heavy drowsiness to be thin and logically uncompelling, the distinction, despite this perception, is clinically, ethically, and legally real and essential. Some people do need to sleep before they die, and conflicts of perception regarding the ethereality versus the reality of the distinction between sedation and euthanasia should never be allowed to frustrate fulfilment of that need.

Towards a discussion of euthanasia

A widely shared consensus has crystallized gradually over the past two decades, in both clinical ethics and law, about the conditions that justify foregoing or discontinuing various kinds of life-sustaining treatments. However, clinical practice may be very much out of phase with the current state of discussion and reflection in the professional literature of medicine, ethics, and law. If the established ethical consensus on withholding and discontinuing life-sustaining treatments, and on the requirements of palliative medicine, were widely implemented in clinical practice, we would probably not now be in the midst of the renewed, intense debate that has been running on for over five years at least.

Yet, as already mentioned above, patients are all too frequently still treated in ways that fail miserably to honour the particular needs of the dying. At times, it is almost as though a technologically well-equipped hospital system is operating on its own, without patient-sensitive clinical guidance; a system programmed to prolong life to its bitter biological end, come what may. Terrible omissions occur, when the governing focus of those caring for persons with advanced illness is on biology and not on the total person. These omissions regard adequacy of pain relief and symptom management, and they are almost systematic in some places and hospitals. They contribute mightily to intensifying the agony of the dying and to enflaming the demands for euthanasia and for its legalization. Demands for euthanasia, it is also true, may be most acute when life-prolonging treatments and inadequate palliative care have little or nothing to do with the agony of dying and the delay of a desired death. It is some person's own stubborn biology that is keeping body and brain alive when the mind is prepared for death and the person is wanting so intensely to die. Some of the dying today do demand death, and they do so unambiguously and unambivalently.

It is precisely because demands for euthanasia do occur, and also because current discussions frequently enough confuse both withdrawal of treatment as well as the palliative control of pain and symptoms with euthanasia, that this chapter turns in the following section to a survey of the main points to be made regarding euthanasia within the ethics of palliative medicine.

Euthanasia

A hundred and seventy years ago, on 29 July 1826, Dr Carl Friedrich Heinrich Marx, on the occasion of his installation as assistant professor of medicine at the University of Goettingen, delivered an address, published that same year by Dieterich, on medical euthanasia, *De Euthanasia Medica*.[167] A little over fifty years later, Rohlfs, in his *History of German Medicine*, lauded Marx's treatise as 'a medical classic, worthy to be on the bookshelf of the educated physician for many a century to come'.[168]

What Dr Marx called 'medical euthanasia', we would today call palliative medicine. He spoke of euthanasia as that science 'which checks oppressing features of illness, relieves pain, and renders the supreme and inescapable hour a most peaceful one'.[167] If the sacred duty of physicians is 'to lay to peaceful rest a life they can no longer save', then physicians will use medicines to eliminate or curb anxiety, pain, torment, spasm, convulsion, restlessness, and long-drawn-out sleepless nights. Indeed, a point may come in the evolution of disease when the dying have a right, so Marx would advise, 'to be deprived of all consciousness',[167] an issue discussed in a preceding section of this chapter when the use of sedation was considered for the relief of overwhelming anguish or pain.

Does Marx's treatise on medical euthanasia set any limits on the means physicians may use to discharge their sacred duty of laying to peaceful rest a life they can no longer save? There is at least this limit—least of all, should a physician 'be permitted, prompted either by other people's requests or by his own sense of mercy, to end the patient's pitiful condition by purposely and deliberately hastening death. How can it be permitted that he who is by law required to preserve life be the originator of, or partner in, its destruction?'[167]

Dr Marx's treatise on medical euthanasia is in fact an early nineteenth-century treatise on palliative medicine, capturing in its essentials the dominant contemporary consensus to date about how palliative medicine should be practised. Aside from the advances in palliative medicine available today, as compared with the palliative medical knowledge of a hundred-and-seventy years ago, the major difference between Marx's palliative medicine and palliative medicine today centres on the meaning and use of the term euthanasia.

The demand for euthanasia today

If one refers to the Greek origin of the word, euthanasia, etymologically means a good death, a gentle easy death. Dr Marx cites Suetonius[169] and Francis Bacon[170] as using the word in that same sense; laying peacefully to rest a life one can no longer save is what Marx meant by euthanasia. That is not what euthanasia, as debated before the courts and as discussed in countless publications, means today. Today euthanasia means exactly what Marx excluded from his use of the term, namely, the administration of death to the dying—the hastening or advancing of death.

A gentle, peaceful, easy death—this is the way Solzhenitsyn describes the dying of older folk in *The Cancer Ward*. People did not fight against death. They did not pretend they were not going to die. They prepared themselves quietly and they departed easily 'as if they were just moving into a new house.'[171] A central contemporary problem in Canada, the United States, the United Kingdom, The Netherlands, and other parts of Europe and the world is that people fear they will not be able to die in this gentle easy way. They fear they will have little or no control over their dying. They fear, as a recent editorial in *Nature* states, 'a twilight life tethered to feeding tubes or respirators'.[172] As they have been doing for over twenty years, people are now still, and with increasing intensity, echoing Montaigne's statement, 'It is dying, not death, that I fear'.

The euthanasia we are now debating in the media, in the courts, in countless symposia and publications is linked to the fact that so many people today do not die 'as if they were just moving into a new home'. People used to die at home, in the midst of their families, surrounded by all the objects, furniture, photos, and memories that kept a life history alive and present to the dying during their last days, hours, and moments. Most of the time today, people do not die at home at all. They die in institutions, in strange and sterile places, places that bear no mark or memory of where one has lived, of those with whom one has lived.

People often die today in places that are equipped with complex technology capable of supporting and prolonging life, often only biological life, when a cure and return to health, vitality, and normal living are no longer possible. Terminally ill and dying patients may be technologically bound to biological existence long beyond the time when they could have died consciously and in mastery of their ultimate moments of life.

However, enslavement to life-prolonging technology is not the primary driving force behind contemporary discussions of euthanasia and current debates over its legalization. The fear of some patients, a fear backed by fact, is not that they will die tethered to life-prolonging technology, but that they will die tethered to unrelieved pain and symptoms. Others fear exactly what they think palliative care has to offer, a release from pain at the cost of their being plunged into a lingering state of semiconsciousness, of being doped into stupor, while all around sit and await one's death. Some find the prospect of this particular kind of loss of control to be quite unbearable.

But there is another quite different experience of loss of control. It comes from heightened consciousness of one's condition, not from an analgesic induced dimming of awareness. Demands for euthanasia often are most acute when life-prolonging technology has nothing to do with death's delay, and when pain is not the main factor in the agony of the dying. We live in a fragmented world, in a world in which language, to a large extent, no longer conveys the shared vision of humanity and the shared hopes within which we could once talk to one another about the terrible uncertainties towards which our own intelligence, if given free rein, would thrust us when we face death. To face those uncertainties, and to confront them openly in fragile conversation with others, would drag us all towards a darkness where no data, no concepts, no hypotheses, and no proof can silence or calm the dread, and possibly the rage with which an awakened human spirit can shake, when contemplating the apparently all-too-real and inevitable fate of personal extinction.

To enter this darkness is to lose control, and that loss is what we, at the end of this century, seem increasingly to dread above all. That dimension of suffering—the sense of a loss of control over our own existence, the sense that we are not absolute masters of our destiny, just as we are not our own creators—seems to be increasingly intolerable to many today as they face their own death.

To be conscious is indeed to suffer, and heightened consciousness opens the mind onto frontiers of the deepest existential uncertainty. What do we then do when we cannot find a language within which we can suffer these uncertainties together? One option is to flee into autonomy, into an act of seemingly ultimate control; the act of ending one's life, of destroying that consciousness within which one senses one's own essential isolation, as well as one's profound dependency.

Current debates about euthanasia are not only about inadequate management of pain and symptoms; not only about insensitive misuse of life-prolonging technology. The demands for rapid, painless death, and the debates these demands provoke, are a signal that we all, at the end of this century, have entered a very deep crisis about how we understand, experience, and should bear the human condition.

Sometimes a dying person's request or demand for death is ambiguous and ambivalent. The requests leave space for manoeuvring. Doctors, nurses, family members then have pathways they can explore. They can decode the request for death, uncover the other requests the death demand is masking, and then set about achieving what the dying person 'really' wants.

Some will dogmatically claim, and others will desperately hope, that all demands of the dying for death are ambiguous and ambivalent. That would be comforting. It would confirm a world view within which we never have to face our limits, suffer our finiteness, acknowledge our helplessness. But that does not seem to be the way the world today actually works. Some demands of the dying for death are quite definitive, unambiguous, and unambivalent. Death now is what they want and what they are demanding.

There is the case of a young man in the terminal stages of AIDS. This young man had a head full of projects and wanted to live. Yet, knowing he would inevitably die soon from AIDS, he asked for sufficient drugs and instructions on how to use them so that he could time his death to occur before he wasted away and lost his mental competence. And that is what he did. There is a similar story in the recent medical literature, the story of Diane, a young married woman with a husband, a college-age son, a business, and her artistic work. Diane, diagnosed as having a form of leukaemia, rejected the chemotherapy option. The side-effects and the roughly 25 per cent chance of long-term survival were not for her. What Diane feared most, according to Dr Quill, her physician, was increasing discomfort, dependence, and hard choices between pain and sedation. Diane made it clear to her family and to Dr Quill that when the time came, she wanted to advance her death in the least painful way possible. Dr Quill thought this made sense, aware as he was of Diane's desire for independence and of her wish to stay in control. He consequently referred her to the Hemlock Society for information about suicide and made sure Diane knew how to use the barbiturates for sleep as well as the amount needed to bring about her own death. This is what Diane did—she advanced her own death when bone pain, weakness, fatigue, and fevers began to assume control of her life.[173]

These two brief case descriptions are presented to illustrate that euthanasia now means administering death to the dying or assisting the dying to administer death to themselves. The contemporary debate centres on the question of whether euthanasia, or assisting euthanasia, should be decriminalized, legalized, or, as in The Netherlands today, excused under some regulatory scheme while upholding legal prohibition. This issue has returned periodically into public discussion throughout this century in the countries of the western world.

The reasons and arguments advanced today for and against the ethical acceptability, and for and against the legalization, of euthanasia are often substantially the same as those presented in earlier debates over the last hundred years. A defining characteristic of a complex question is that it will and it must be taken up again and again by each successive generation. This does not mean that any given generation cannot learn from the mistakes and from the wisdom of people in earlier times. Yet, it would be naïve and intellectually misguided to think that we could simply lift euthanasia proposals and arguments out of their historical contexts to compare and apply them today, as though the social, political, and medical particularities of each period had no influence at all on euthanasia reasoning and practice.

People in any generation have to think through for themselves those questions that most deeply affect their own lives and destinies. Ancestors cannot do that, once and for all for their descendants. Each generation in each society and culture, that regularly differ so profoundly one from another, has to seek, often through intense and even acrimonious discussion, what it stands for, what it stands against, and what it can tolerate. Not all questions are so pressing or decisive for individuals and societies seeking to discover who they really are, but euthanasia certainly is one of these questions for us today, as it has been throughout the moral history of the Western world.

Limits and purpose of the discussion

There are several excellent surveys, covering the period from the 1870s to the present, of how people have thought, acted, and legislated regarding euthanasia.[174–178] Physicians of various medical specialties, nurses, and the general public have been polled over the last several years to ascertain their attitudes towards euthanasia.[179–185] Various associations and working groups have issued positions on the matter[186–192] and philosophers, theologians, ethicists, lawyers, physicians, and nurses have, over the last decade, analysed, defended, and criticized the many reasons and arguments put forth to justify or reject the legalization of euthanasia or its ethical acceptability.[193–198]

A comprehensive review of this voluminous reflection would far exceed the space of a chapter, let alone a subsection of a chapter, on ethics in palliative medicine, and might even distract from the purpose of this chapter's discussion of euthanasia. That purpose is to stimulate those involved in the practice of palliative medicine to formulate reasoned responses to two crucial questions; crucial because they affect in a major way how palliative medicine will be understood, practised, and supported. The first question is whether euthanasia can ever be ethically acceptable or tolerable within palliative medicine. The second question is whether euthanasia should be decriminalized, legalized, or declared to be an excusable exception, under some regulatory scheme or other, to homicide laws.

These two questions are quite distinct,[199,200] although there is a tendency to collapse the second question about the status of euthanasia in law to the status of euthanasia in the clinical ethics of palliative medicine. Some would propose that if euthanasia can reasonably be thought to be ethically acceptable, or at least ethically tolerable as the lesser evil in some circumstances, then euthanasia should be permitted in law. The central argument of this chapter is that euthanasia, even if it is ethically tolerable in some circumstances, should not be decriminalized, nor legalized, nor legally excused under some regulatory scheme of conditions that would uphold the legal prohibition of euthanasia in principle.

Euthanasia: a definition and distinctions

Discussions of euthanasia often become extremely entangled because people use the same term, euthanasia, but understand it in very different, and even diametrically opposed, ways.

Definitions of euthanasia are frequently shaped, often inadvertently, by the moral stances people have already adopted on the issue. Those in favour of euthanasia may, in defining the term, speak of it as a 'deliverance', or as 'helping people to die a peaceful, dignified death', or as 'aid-in-dying', and who could possibly be against that? Those against euthanasia may, in defining the term, speak of it as 'killing' or as 'destruction of life', and who could possibly be in favour of that? These kinds of definitions signal a moral stance and are really opening moves in a moral debate. They do not contribute much to the logical task of distinguishing euthanasia from other acts, from which it is both conceptually and clinically different.

Moreover, people involved in the controversy are often really constructing quite different kinds of definitions. Some want to include under 'euthanasia' acts that they believe to be morally equivalent, even if they are conceptually and clinically different. For example some see no moral distinction between withholding life-prolonging treatment, discontinuing such treatment, and administering death. So, they speak of passive and active euthanasia. Moreover, there is a lingering confusion in society, and at times even within professional circles, about the purposes and methods of palliative medicine. People who do not know very much about how pain can be and is controlled in advanced disease still think that doctors have to hasten death to relieve pain and to control distressing symptoms. Those afflicted with this confusion see no difference between using medication to relieve pain and to bring about death. So they use the term euthanasia to cover two acts that are clinically, ethically, and legally totally different.

Agreement on the meaning of euthanasia is also difficult, because the term is not historically neutral. Those who believe that euthanasia is ethically justifiable and should be legalized want the understanding of the term, as used today, to be freed from any connection to the programme of the Nazi doctors. Some who oppose euthanasia believe that decoupling euthanasia today from euthanasia as practised under Hitler's Reich may well lead to uncivilized abuses, similar to those committed by some doctors in the Nazi period.

To facilitate discussion of the two central questions of this chapter's discussion of euthanasia, we first propose a working definition of euthanasia and then distinguish euthanasia, so defined, from acts of foregoing or discontinuing life-prolonging treatments as well as from the use of various analgesics or sedatives to relieve the dying from pain, symptoms, or overwhelming distress.

A definition

People have been thinking, writing, and proposing legislation about euthanasia for a long time but the discussion, as noted above, is bedevilled by the many different and conflicting understandings of what euthanasia means. If what is said is not what is meant, then many things that should be done may remain undone, and what should not be done may be championed as the only right thing to do.

A large measure of confusion could be removed from discussions about the ethical acceptability of euthanasia or about its legalization, if the term were taken to mean: the deliberate and painless termination of life of a person afflicted with an incurable and progressive disease leading inexorably to death. Euthanasia in this chapter means the administration of death to the dying.

This definition assumes:

(1) that the termination of life in this way, of a sick person in these circumstances, will be motivated by compassion (however, since motivation is often difficult to ascertain reliably, 'merciful' or 'compassion-motivated' is not included in the above definition);

(2) that termination of life will be of persons afflicted with a condition or disease that is inexorably drawing them towards death, even if that death may not be imminent;

(3) that painless termination of life will usually be achieved by parenteral or oral administration of a lethal dose of a drug or of a combination of drugs;

(4) that euthanasia may be either self administered or administered by someone else, usually a physician;

(5) that euthanasia is voluntary or non-voluntary depending on whether the sick person has or has not requested and given full consent (informed, comprehending, and voluntary) to the termination of his or her life;

(6) that assisted euthanasia would occur when a sick person desiring to advance his or her death would require help from others, usually physicians or health-care professionals, to obtain lethal dosage of drugs and instructions on how to use these effectively.

Euthanasia should not be confused with cessation of treatment or with relief from pain, symptoms, or distress

Central to the controversy on euthanasia is the fact that some people acknowledge, and others deny, that there is a distinction between euthanasia and withholding or discontinuing life-prolonging treatment.[201,202]

Our position is that the distinction between euthanasia, as defined above, and withholding or discontinuing life-prolonging treatment, as well as the distinction between euthanasia and adequate control of pain, are both clinically, ethically, and legally essential and logically defensible.[203–206] The defence of these distinctions, and their meaning, rest upon three assumptions.

The first assumption is about the goals and mandates of palliative medicine. These may be summarized as the professional and humanitarian responsibility:

(1) to help those, who need not die now, to live as fully as they possibly can;

(2) to help those, who can no longer live, to die on time, not too early and not too late;

(3) to help those, who now must die, and who are dying, to die in peace and with dignity.

The second assumption is that doctors do not possess unlimited authority to intervene in the bodies and lives of sick people. Each intervention has to be justified, and that justification derives from the clinical goals that come to predominate as a disease progresses. When treatments, including life-sustaining treatments, have been started, as justified by an earlier governing clinical goal, and are now doing more harm than good, the ethically critical question is not 'Are doctors justified in discontinuing these treatments?' but rather 'Is there any justification for continuing the treatment?' The burden of justification shifts from discontinuance to continuance of treatment when clinical goals have changed with the evolution of the disease. Treatments do not carry their own in-built ethical imperative. It is when doctors lose sight of the clinical goals they should be pursuing for a particular patient at a particular time that patients risk being enslaved to technologies doctors mistakenly believe they ethically must employ.

A point arrives in the course of a progressive disease when it is no longer possible to restore health, function, or consciousness, when it is also no longer possible to reverse a dying process. Treatments designed to do these things are then futile, and may even be harmful. In these situations, it is correct to speak of allowing a person to die.

Allowing a dying person to die differs from euthanasia in intent, in act, and in professional mandate. The intent in euthanasia, even when the doctor's motivation is compassion, is to cause death immediately. The intent in discontinuing life-prolonging treatments of the dying, even if the patient's death is desired by the doctors, families, and the patients themselves, is to cease hindering an inevitable process from reaching its timely end. In fact, death often does not immediately follow upon discontinuance of such treatments.

It is in part because dying patients often do not die immediately after discontinuance of life-sustaining treatments that euthanasia is put forward by some as the ultimate act of compassion that the dying have a right to request and expect of doctors. If euthanasia differs from discontinuance of treatment, in intent, act, and results, the difference between both as regards professional mandate also merits emphasis. With the act of euthanasia a doctor assumes, however temporarily, a mandate of total dominion over a human life *in extremis*. The act of discontinuing life-sustaining treatments from patients who are in the advanced stages of disease implies that the mandate of doctors over a human life *in extremis* is limited to accompanying and serving a dying patient with all the scientific and compassionate skills of comforting a life that cannot be saved. Acceptance or rejection of this limit marks the difference between palliative medicine and euthanasia.

It is because of these differences between euthanasia and discontinuance of life-prolonging treatments that people all over the world are now engaged in intense debate over the legalization of euthanasia, and are being pressed to rethink fundamental assumptions about the moral limits of dominion people should have over their own lives, and about the limits of dominion doctors should be authorized to exercise over the dying.

The third assumption derives directly from the third of the three clinical goals and mandates of palliative medicine, as identified above. One of the essential elements of dying with dignity is freedom from pain, and the various kinds of bodily and mental fatigue and distress, that can dominate consciousness and leave free no psychic space for the personally important things people want to think, say, and do before they die. Constant, racking, and mind-twisting pain separates dying persons from themselves and from their loved ones. That pain combined with other kinds of relentless biological and psychic stress can drive the dying from coping, control, and integration to chaos and hopelessness.[207,208]

Patients have a right to request, and doctors have an obligation of fidelity to the dying to employ, every proportionate means available to relieve the suffering and agony provoked by relentless pain and symptom distress. Administering medications in combinations, dosages, and frequencies needed to relieve effectively the suffering of the dying is logically, clinically, and ethically totally different from the act of administering death. These two acts differ both as to end and as to means. The goal of palliative medicine is emancipation, the freeing of the dying person's consciousness from the domination of pain. The goal of euthanasia is death.

It is in part because of a failure to grasp the essential distinction between euthanasia and the palliative control of pain and symptoms that some doctors, unreasonably fearful of legal liability for hastening death, have gone just so far, and not far enough, in their use of medications to give patients the relief they need and request. Patients should never have to beg for relief because of doctors' unenlightened fears. And it is indeed foolish to deny patients relief from suffering because of unsubstantiatable fears and concerns that effective relief of pain will shorten life.[209,210] A dying patient receiving frequent medication for pain and symptom control will eventually die after receiving a dosage of medication. It is a fallacy to conclude that the medication and not the last surge of the underlying disease caused the patient's death.

The Law Reform Commission of Canada demonstrated remarkable clinical perspicacity when it proposed that the possible effect of analgesics on a dying person's length of life is no basis whatsoever for holding physicians criminally liable when they (competently) administer pain and symptom relief.[107] When the clinical goal is to maintain dying patients in a state of conscious tranquillity, the effect on length of life of the medications required to achieve this is relatively irrelevant. It would be cruel and inhumane to argue that analgesics should not be given because they probably lengthen the time of life and dying, and patients should therefore be allowed to die rapidly, even if pain is the price to pay. It is equally inhumane and foolish to withhold adequate combinations and dosages of palliative medication because of concerns that these medications may have the secondary effect of shortening the dying process. Legal and other lay colleagues may not fully appreciate the relative risks of using opioids. Tolerance to respiratory depression readily occurs in patients on chronic opioid therapy. In such patients, increasing opioid use to ensure pain relief, and sometimes sedation in concert with other drugs, is rarely the direct cause of a patient's demise.

The distinction between the administration of death, which is what euthanasia is, and the administration of relief from suffering, which is what palliative medicine is, should serve as a directive for law, ethics, medical education, and health-care planning. Doctors must not be barred by any law of the state or by any dictate of morality from freeing the dying, as best their knowledge and skills allow, from the agonies of advanced and terminal stages of disease. If laws are outdated or obscure on palliative medicine, they should be changed or clarified. If doctors are unclear about their mandate to relieve suffering, they should be educated rapidly and expertly. Where competent palliative medicine and care are not available, health-care planners should set the organization and equitable delivery of such care as a top priority of a civilized health-care system. To court and defend the idea of euthanasia when resources and programmes have not been mobilized to make palliative medicine available to all is equivalent to employing the short sightedness, apathy, and ignorance of health-care planners and medical educators as major premises in an argument favouring the legalization of the administration of death.

The distinction between active and passive euthanasia leads to confusion

Many articles and books on euthanasia distinguish active from passive euthanasia.[201,211,212] Equivalent distinctions, such as direct and indirect euthanasia or euthanasia by act and euthanasia by omission, are also used to create two categories of euthanasia.

The distinction between active and passive euthanasia leads to confusion and distracts attention from the current, central ethical and legal controversy about the acceptability of administering death.

This distinction leads to confusion because the category of passive euthanasia (or indirect euthanasia or euthanasia by omission) encompasses two kinds of decisions and acts that are logically and clinically different—acts of withholding or discontinuing treatments that can reverse a disease process leading to death (for example withholding surgery from infants afflicted with an intestinal blockage); and acts of withholding or discontinuing treatments that cannot reverse a disease process leading to death but can only prolong the dying process.

The kinds of acts encompassed by the category of withholding or discontinuing life-prolonging treatment have been at the centre of a particular kind of ethical and legal controversy that has been underway within hospitals and the courts for at least two decades. A high degree of ethical and legal consensus has been attained on this controversy, as discussed in the preceding section of this chapter. We should not confuse that controversy with the current, renewed conflict of views about whether administering death should be legalized or is ever ethically justifiable.

The term euthanasia should be reserved for the painless termination of life of persons afflicted with diseases or conditions that are drawing them inexorably to death, even if death is not imminent. When euthanasia is used in this sense there is no doubt that the administration of death is what is intended and attempted. Whether euthanasia in this sense should ever be acceptable in ethics or in law is precisely what is at issue in the current controversy.

One point, however, needs emphasis. Rejection of the distinction between active and passive euthanasia, and reservation of the term euthanasia for the act of administering death, does not mean that all acts of withholding or discontinuing life-prolonging treatments are ethically and legally justifiable acts of allowing the dying to die. Euthanasia, it is argued here, is the painless administration of death to the dying. Withholding life-saving treatments from those who need not die, but who will die without such treatment, is not euthanasia. Decisions to withhold or discontinue such treatments may be ethically justifiable in some circumstances and ethically, as well as legally, reprehensible in others. Decisions and acts of withholding or discontinuing life-sustaining treatments should be ethically evaluated on their own merits and should not be confused with euthanasia.

The legalization of euthanasia: recent events

In the 1990s the practice of euthanasia is still illegal in most countries. One exception, widely known and discussed, is The Netherlands. Although euthanasia is still a criminal offence, as stated in Article 293 of the Penal Code of The Netherlands, the Dutch Supreme Court in 1984 declared that euthanasia would be legally excusable if physicians found themselves in a conflict of duties consisting of the dilemma: respect the Penal Code's prohibition of euthanasia or respect a patient's request for euthanasia as a release from suffering. The Supreme Court recognized the defence of necessity or of *force majeure* when physicians found themselves in such a dilemma.[213]

The Royal Dutch Medical Association has formulated five requirements that have to be fulfilled for euthanasia to be acceptable or legally excusable. The combination of the third and fourth requirements specify the meaning of *force majeure*. The five requirements are:

(1) there is voluntary, competent, and durable request on the part of the patient;

(2) the request is based on full information;

(3) the patient is in a situation of intolerable and hopeless suffering (either physical or mental);

(4) there are no acceptable alternatives to euthanasia;

(5) the physician has consulted another physician before performing euthanasia.[213,214]

A notification procedure was adopted in 1990, requiring of physicians practising euthanasia that they do not issue a declaration of natural death but that they inform the local medical examiner of the act of euthanasia by filling out an extensive questionnaire. The medical examiner then reports the euthanasia to the public prosecutor and the prosecutor decides if prosecution is required.[215] A new law, accepted in 1993 and effective on 1 June 1994, gave formal legal status to the notification procedure. However, this law extends the notification procedure to cover cases involving euthanasia without the patient's explicit request.[213]

In North America, pressure is growing to legalize assisted euthanasia. In November 1991, voters in Washington State took part in a referendum on death with dignity, which included a provision to legalize euthanasia. Despite public opinion polls that showed a two-thirds majority in favour of voluntary euthanasia, the proposal was defeated by 54 per cent of voters. A similar proposal was defeated by California voters in November 1992, by an almost identical margin.

Two years later, on 8 November 1994, Oregon voters approved the Death with Dignity Act. That act allows terminally ill adult patients to request in writing a prescription for medication to end their life. This law specifically prohibits physicians from performing euthanasia but allows them to assist patients by prescribing medications patients can then use to advance their own deaths.[216]

In Canada, the Supreme Court, in September 1993, ruled against a British Columbia woman's request for physician-assisted euthanasia. Sue Rodriguez was dying of amyotrophic lateral sclerosis, a motor neurone disease. The Supreme Court judges were split five to four in their ruling that the Criminal Code's prohibition of assisted suicide or euthanasia does not violate the Canadian Charter of Rights and Freedoms.

Australia's Northern Territory legalized voluntary euthanasia when it passed its Rights of the Terminally Ill Act on 25 May 1995. Physicians are specifically prohibited from administering or assisting euthanasia if there are effective palliative care options available for the relief of a patient's pain and suffering.[217] This Act was reversed by the Australian Federal Parliament in March 1997.

Recently, two United States Appeal Courts have ruled against the ban of physician-assisted death by certain states. On 6 March 1996, the Ninth Circuit Court of Appeals, exercising jurisdiction over the State of Washington and eight other states, ruled that terminally ill patients have the right to seek a doctor's aid to hasten death. The ruling applies to terminally ill adults, who have 'a strong liberty interest in choosing a dignified and humane death rather than being reduced at the end'.[218] On 2 April 1996, the Second Circuit Court of Appeals, which covers the states of New York, Vermont, and Connecticut, ruled that the state of New York's ban on physician-assisted suicide or euthanasia was unconstitutional. The Court expressed the view that 'Physicians do not fulfil the role of 'killer' by prescribing drugs to hasten death any more than they do by disconnecting life-support systems'.[219] Moreover, prohibitions of physician-assisted euthanasia or suicide, in the view of this Court, 'are not rationally related to any legitimate state interest'. That interest, the Court stated, 'lessens as the potential for life diminishes. And what business is it of the state to require the continuation of agony when the result is imminent and inevitable?'[219]

Legalize euthanasia? The controversy

The film *Breaker Morant* demonstrated the thesis that in war, situations occur which fall outside all existing rules. Similar situations seem to arise from time to time in caring for the terminally ill. If decisions to stop all life-prolonging treatments and to allow 'nature to take its course' are morally and legally justifiable, should not society, as Dr John Freeman asked twenty-five years ago, allow physicians to help nature take its course—quickly?[220]

How is such a question to be answered? By measuring the proportion of benefits to harms? The focus then would be on the patient. If the patient is bound to die, given the irreversibility of a lethal disease and the rightness of a decision not to intervene to prolong life, of what good to the patient, family, or to anyone is an interim period of slow decline into death? Why should patients, families, and caregivers be bound passively to await death? But should the focus be only on the patient when the balance of benefits to harms is considered?

Do we answer the question (about helping nature to take its course quickly) by considering community consequences? Here the focus would be on the medical profession and society. Should a society give such power to doctors, or to any profession? There are many kinds of suffering and there are sufferers of all ages. If we justify euthanasia for some patients on the grounds of mercy, is it possible to establish generally acceptable and non-arbitrary limits to the putative medical mandate to shorten 'useless dying curves' by administering death? Do we try this as an experiment and closely monitor what happens? Or do we, in the fear that 'things might get out of hand', arbitrarily decree that no one, doctors included, is ever morally justified in terminating a patient's life?

Some, many perhaps, would argue that such a decree is not arbitrary at all. It is simply the expression of the most basic of all principles—that no human being has dominion over the life of another. Judges, philosophers, and religious leaders have reiterated this principle in various ways over the ages.

That fact, however, does not silence the questions. How do we know that this principle should hold, and should hold without exception? Even if one accepts that no human being has dominion over the life of another, do human beings not have dominion over their own lives? How can the constraint of the dominion principle be justified, when the act it prohibits, euthanasia, appears, in some circumstances, desirable from every empirical point of view and is, in fact, desired by everyone involved in a particular case? Is the authority of reason able to resolve this most important of our ethical questions, or does the prohibition of euthanasia rest rather on belief?

Reasoning in favour of legalizing euthanasia

The strongest arguments advanced to support the legalization of euthanasia are usually complex combinations of statements of fact, of principle, of logic, and of belief.

As to statements of fact, those requesting that euthanasia be decriminalized, legalized, or legally excused under some regulatory scheme emphasize the current limits of palliative medicine. Euthanasia, it is claimed, is often the only effective means of relieving dying patients from intense suffering. Although palliative medicine and palliative care have, over the last three decades, make remarkable progress, it is still quite true, as a *Lancet* editorial on the Dr Nigel Cox case observed, that there is a long way to go before it becomes possible to promise that no terminal state is so bad that it cannot be palliatively controlled, with dignity maintained by the co-ordinated administration of medications and other forms of treatment and care.[221] Moreover, it is also a matter of fact, documented in a number of studies, that current, effective methods of palliative medicine are so frequently neither mastered nor used by clinical teams that patients continue to die miserably.[127,222,223] It is also quite true that access to expert palliative medicine and care remains extremely limited in most countries of the world.[224–227]

At this point statements of principle lock into the argument. There is the principle of compassion. Over twenty-five years ago, A.B. Downing, in advocating the legalization of euthanasia, emphasized that we shall probably never be able to eliminate totally from human experience the suffering that is both hard to bear and hard to behold. He buttressed this observation with the words of the former Dean of St Paul's Cathedral, the Very Reverend W.R. Matthews, who stated 'It seems to be an incontrovertible proposition that, when we are confronted with suffering that is wholly destructive in its consequences and, so far as we can see, could have no beneficial result, there is a *prima facie* duty to bring it to an end.'[228] Because palliative medicine and care are neither universally effective nor universally available, and probably never will be, compassion requires that euthanasia be legally available to patients when no other effective means of relief are at hand.

A second statement of principle in the prolegalization argument would limit the administration of legalized euthanasia to those who are suffering consciously and who voluntarily request the hastening of their deaths. Only those should receive euthanasia, who, with full knowledge of their condition, stably request death, unpressured by others and unconstrained by depression. This is an appeal to the principle of autonomy and self determination. The combination of the principle of compassion with the principle of self determination leads to the ethical conclusion that it would be wrong not to honour patients' informed, lucid, free, and stable requests for rapid and painless death, as their chosen way of release from suffering they find unbearable. Physicians should be authorized to administer euthanasia to suffering patients, who want to advance their death but cannot do so themselves for lack of knowledge, ability, or both. Given the primacy of individual liberty among the values Western societies hold dear, the burden of proof should be on those who would legally restrict the liberty of competent adults to request and receive euthanasia.

The prolegalization argument evolves with an appeal to statements of logic. If we ethically and legally allow doctors to withhold or to discontinue life-prolonging treatments, fully aware that patients will die as a result, then there is no logically compelling reason to treat voluntary euthanasia differently. There is no compelling ethical reason to reject the legalization of euthanasia, since discontinuance of life-sustaining treatments are already widely accepted, clinically, ethically, and legally, and there is no ethical difference between death resulting from the withdrawal of life-prolonging treatment and death resulting from euthanasia. In fact, so the logic presses, it would be more compassionate to deliver death rapidly and painlessly to those who request it than to force them, by our euthanasia inaction, to stumble through a perhaps lengthy dying until they collapse, exhausted, into death. The United States Federal Second Circuit Court of Appeal's ruling, on 2 April 1996, that the State of New York's ban on doctor-assisted suicide should be struck down, invoked the logic of 'no difference' when the court stated 'Physicians do not fulfil the role of 'killer' by prescribing drugs to hasten death any more than they do by disconnecting life-support systems.'[219]

Nearly all proposals for the legalization of euthanasia admit the necessity of procedures and safeguards to prevent potential abuses of euthanasia. If not legalized, euthanasia, it is believed, will be practised clandestinely, and without adequate legal supervision and control, abuses are likely to occur. However, it is also believed, practicable, effective, and enforceable safeguards which will not bureaucratically complicate that last days of those asking for euthanasia, are designable. Moreover, it is also believed, these safeguards will prevent most categories of abuse, if not every possible instance of abuse within any given category.

What would constitute an abuse of euthanasia? The most frequently cited examples refer to various categories of non-voluntary euthanasia: the administration of euthanasia to patients who have been submitted to pressure and manipulation; to persons who have not consented, or who cannot consent, to the advancing of their deaths.

At this point a decisive statement of belief enters into the prolegalization argument. One may grant, for the sake of argument, that safeguards and regulations may be effective in preventing abuse but they will be so only so long as certain acts of euthanasia continue to be seen as an abuse. The statement of belief is that a society, our society, will never come to perceive euthanasia as an act of compassion for the comatose, for those in persistent vegetative state, for those in prolonged states of senile dementia, for persons afflicted with persistent, difficult-to-treat depression, or for persons afflicted with other forms of chronic mental or physical disability.

A proposal for regulating physician-assisted death, published in the *New England Journal of Medicine* in 1994, reflects much of the argument, just sketched above. The proposal defends a policy 'of legalized physician-assisted death restricted to competent patients suffering from terminal illness or incurable–debilitating disease who voluntarily request to end their lives'.[229] The policy includes a regulatory framework with safeguards, judged as adequate to protect the professional integrity of physicians and to reserve euthanasia as a measure of last resort. The moral goals of respect for patient self-determination and compassion in the relief of suffering are the basis for the proposal.

This policy promotes comfort care or palliative care as standard treatment for dying patients and physician-assisted death is presented as permissible non-standard care of suffering persons, who voluntary and repeatedly request to die. This policy would not limit physician-assisted death to terminally ill patients. Certified palliative care consultants would play the central safeguard role in this policy's regulatory framework, for these consultants 'would have the authority to override agreements by patients and physicians to undertake physician-assisted death'.[229]

This proposal has been challenged on at least the following grounds:

1. The proposed regulations and safeguards are a charade because physicians, under this regulation scheme, would have to submit themselves voluntarily to the control of palliative care consultants.[230]

2. If the practice of physician-assisted death is not to be frustrated from the very start, it would clearly not do to have persons opposed to euthanasia as the palliative care consultants. These persons would have to be screened out in favour of persons who are neutral or impartial.[230] But who is impartial on this matter of euthanasia?

3. If palliative care services are now far from adequately available, how possible would it be to prepare a sufficient number of competent and impartial palliative care consultants for this regulatory safeguard function? Should the emphasis be on mobilizing these cadres of consultants or on mobilizing adequate palliative medicine and palliative care services?[231,232] If the latter is neglected, the former, as overseers of euthanasia, may come to be seen as just as necessary as euthanasia.

4. This policy's emphasis on the self-determination of patients requesting euthanasia is practically silent on the need to assess the autonomy-constricting influence of depression on patients afflicted with terminal disease or with incurable, handicapping, or progressive conditions.[233]

5. This proposal's emphasis on palliative care consultants as arbiters of requests for physician-administered euthanasia subverts the philosophy, the values, and the ethics of palliative care as practised since its inception in the middle of this century.

As in many other proposals for legalizing euthanasia, this proposal also emphasizes clear criteria for selection of those patients whose request for death will be honoured; rigorous procedures to assure that physicians will be publicly accountable; and safeguards to prevent abuse.[234] Unfortunately, what seems straightforward and simple, particularly in the delivery of death, has to have been simplified.[235] The Cartesian assumption that clarity, order, and pre-established procedure will govern the practice of euthanasia, and will do so successfully, floats in abstraction above the real world in which euthanasia will be practised. This is a world of infinitely complex interactions, across society as a whole, between patients, doctors, nurses, families, hospital managers, health-care budget planners, politicians, and conflicting moral groups who, so is the human condition, so often fall far short of the ideal agents these euthanasia proposals would require.

One can never prove, in advance of history, that the legalization of euthanasia will lead to abuse and possibly to moral disaster in a society. But one must admit the possibility and the risk, once the delivery of death has begun, that interlocking chains of consequence and change may emerge, and break away from civilized oversight, to extend the delivery of death far beyond the borders thought sacred by the original planners and legislators.

Should a society accept this risk and legalize euthanasia? The answer to this question does not result from an argument ending with a QED (*quod erat demonstrandum*) that would command the assent of anyone capable of following the reasoning. The taking of a stand for or against the legalization of euthanasia calls for judgement, and enlightened people of good will may well differ on matters of judgement. In our judgement, as will be explained below, euthanasia should neither be legalized nor given advance legal immunity under any regulatory scheme.

Why euthanasia should not be legalized

There is a valid distinction between ethically justifying or tolerating an individual act of euthanasia and ethically defending a regulatory policy or law authorizing a wide range of acts of euthanasia.[199] We accept this distinction and now turn to a summary of the reasons why euthanasia should not be legalized.

As already noted above, some who advocate the legalization of voluntary euthanasia take it as a starting point that the voluntary request for euthanasia is a liberty that does not have to be justified. Legal restrictions on this liberty are what require justification. Those who think this way ask why should criminal law restrain the liberty of a patient and physician by prohibiting them from doing what they want and choose to do when suffering is in ascendance at the end of life.

We take it as a starting point that any legal restriction on the liberty to request or perform euthanasia should not, in pluralistic societies, be equivalent to the imposition of the religious and moral beliefs of some people on others, who hold quite different beliefs. The justification of the legal restriction on euthanasia would have to demonstrate that the restriction is a necessary protection of the common good and of the individual good and rights of people who may not desire or who cannot consent to euthanasia.

When a society accords physicians a mandate to eliminate suffering by eliminating the sufferer, it wanders far beyond the perimeters of responsibility and liberty traditionally given to the medical profession in Western civilized thought. Such a profound change indeed requires reasoned, credible justification. A simple appeal to the liberty and autonomy of conscious patients desiring euthanasia will not suffice. Those who favour legalization of voluntary euthanasia emphasize that doctors are not assuming the authority to terminate a patient's life. That authority is rather bestowed upon a doctor by a conscious and free patient seeking release from intolerable suffering, and society, it is said, should not interfere with this exercise of liberty and autonomy. However, the principles of liberty and autonomy are not absolute. Societal checks and balances on the exercise of liberty and autonomy are justified, and have been traditionally imposed, when the exercise of some liberties imperils the liberties and needs of others and imperils the common good.

Opposition to the legalization of euthanasia is not only a matter of theoretical reasoning and argument. In its most decisive phase, that opposition is also a matter of practical judgement. A change in the law prohibiting euthanasia would represent a profound societal change, and a most significant departure from the accumulated wisdom of generations of human beings, who have thought it essential to circumscribe the administration of death with clear and stable restrictions. In our judgement it is the cumulative impact of the high questionability, if not illusions, of so many of the assumptions of those favouring legalization of euthanasia that militates decisively against any legal change that would grant doctors, or any other persons, authority to administer death to the dying. The questionable or illusory assumptions are as follows.

Regarding voluntariness

It is highly questionable that any society will be able to uphold the voluntary character of euthanasia once euthanasia becomes a legally and socially acceptable option. Voluntary means freedom from coercion, pressure, undue inducement, and psychological and emotional manipulation. There is no law permitting voluntary euthanasia that could, even if implemented via complex procedures, protect conscious and vulnerable people against subtle manipulation to request socially acceptable administered death when they would rather live and be cherished.

Attention should be given to the fears many have of being a burden on others when they are very old or very sick and dependent. This fear was cited as one of the two most common reasons people in the United States put forth in support of legalizing euthanasia, the other reason being a fear of dying a painful death.[199,236] The decision of two United States Federal appeal courts to lift bans on euthanasia has provoked the observation 'People who are sick already feel that they are a financial and emotional burden to their families and to society. ... Now society is telling them "You have an option. You have the right to die." For them, this translates easily into an obligation to die'.[237]

The position in favour of legalizing voluntary euthanasia rests upon an assumption of ideal hospitals, doctors, nurses, and families. But we do not live in an ideal world. The assumption of idealism is often illusory, and when it is in fact an illusion the voluntariness of euthanasia is in peril.

Regarding extension of euthanasia to those who cannot consent

Those who propose legalization of euthanasia usually, but not always, claim that only voluntary euthanasia should be legally permitted. The assumption is that after legalization of voluntary euthanasia, societies in the Western world would be enduringly willing and able to withstand pressure for an extension of euthanasia to those who never were able, or to those who have irreversibly lost the ability, to request or to consent to the termination of their lives.

There are good reasons to believe this assumption is illusory. There are many persons in hospitals, chronic care wards, and nursing homes across the land whose lives, by standards external to themselves and in the eyes of others, are hardly worth living. Many of these persons retain little more than the ability to sense and experience biological pain and comfort, gentleness of care, pleasing sound, human presence and warmth. Some can hardly experience even these things, but their relatively strong bodies still cling to life.

It is naïve to imagine that social barriers against non-voluntary euthanasia would not crumble in a society that legalizes voluntary euthanasia on the basis of compassion. Should compassion not also extend to those who, in the eyes of others, are suffering the indignity of profound mental and physical handicaps, even if they are suffering no pain, but who cannot request euthanasia?

This naïvety is reinforced when one adverts to the fact that insistence on voluntary euthanasia is for some proponents of euthanasia in The Netherlands little more than a strategic move towards a much more expanded administration of euthanasia.[238] The 1985 report of The Netherlands State Commission on Euthanasia accepted euthanasia for comatose patients upon family request when such patients continued to live despite discontinuance of life-prolonging treatments. Moreover, the most recent Dutch law on notification procedures for euthanasia includes a notification procedure for euthanasia when persons, such as handicapped new-born children or comatose patients, cannot request or consent to the termination of their lives.[213] Some physicians in The Netherlands do not even consider such terminations of life to be euthanasia because they consider that euthanasia, by definition, has to be voluntary. Some would consider the rapid and painless termination of life in these circumstances to be little more than normal medical practice.[239]

Regarding the necessity of euthanasia

The case for legalizing euthanasia appeals to compassion. Euthanasia, it is claimed, should be legalized because it is inhumane to allow people to continue suffering when they request release by the painless termination of life. The assumptions behind this claim are: that patients frequently suffer agony from pain that is uncontrollable; and that administration of death is the only effective release from suffering that arises, not from unmanageable pain, but from the human condition.

The illusion in this assumption is not that patients do not frequently suffer agony from improperly controlled pain and symptoms. They do, as studies have documented. The illusion is in the idea that measures to control adequately pain and symptoms do not exist. But they do exist.

It is simply wrong to assume that pain can be frequently managed only by administering death to the patient. The binary logic—dying with pain or euthanasia—may have held true in earlier periods prior to the development of modern methods of palliative medicine and palliative care. That logic need not hold true anywhere in the world today. For example the World Health Organization guidelines for the relief of cancer pain have been shown to be effective in controlling pain adequately up to the time of death.[240] These guidelines propose both the sequential use and the skilful combination of non-opioid and opioid pain medication.

The second component to this illusion is the notion that doctors and nurses have generally mastered the state-of-the-art knowledge and skills that bring about an adequate management of pain and symptoms. But they have not. Where the binary logic—dying with pain or euthanasia—still holds true, the most reasonable solution would require widespread education of doctors and nurses in the methods of palliative medicine and palliative care. Legalization of euthanasia is an unjustifiable substitute for such education.

Suffering, as is widely recognized, involves more than the experience of pain. Each person is distinctive, individuated, and profoundly different from everyone else. So also is each person's suffering. Memories, lost opportunities, guilts, dated moments of hurt and betrayal, the fragility of loves and joys, loneliness, and unfulfilled dreams are all as unique as the days, times, places and persons to which they are bound. Suffering of this existential sort is universally part of the human condition and it can be unbearable for anyone isolated in loneliness. Euthanasia is no adequate answer to this kind of suffering. If such suffering cannot be borne alone, then the solution rests with mobilizing a community of caring persons around those who suffer deeply. Legalization of euthanasia is no civilized substitute for the formation of such communities of care.

Regarding the ability of doctors to communicate with the dying

It is illusory to think that doctors are generally masters of the sensitive arts of communication with the dying. Some are and others are not. It would be very unwise to give doctors legal authorization to administer death when they do not know how to talk to their dying patients and are untrained in the principles and methods of palliative medicine. There should be no move to decriminalize or to legalize euthanasia until we have mounted a credible and sustained effort to train doctors in the skills required for the care of the dying.

Regarding the protection of doctors against prosecution

Some have argued that legalization of euthanasia is needed to protect well-meaning doctors against prosecution when they administer euthanasia to suffering persons who, on their own initiative, truly request rapid termination of their lives.

The illusion here is in the assumption that a law can be devised, so clear in its conditions and implementation procedures, that professionals and family survivors will generally conclude that a euthanasia-administering doctor honoured the patient's true desires and abided by all the conditions and procedures of the law. But that honouring and abiding are matters of fact. These are matters that are brought before courts of law, particularly by well-meaning, or even ill-meaning, persons who suspect a physician of insensitivity or negligence, or by families torn by dissension over the fact that death was administered to their relative.

Some believe, citing The Netherlands as an example, that a law permitting voluntary euthanasia would reduce the likelihood or frequency of doctors appearing before the courts to defend their administration of euthanasia. That may be so in countries where euthanasia is widely accepted or tolerated. In other countries, where such acceptance or tolerance of euthanasia does not exist, and where there is a particularly litigious atmosphere, the more frequent these acts of euthanasia would become, the more likely it is that a law permitting voluntary euthanasia would be used as a legal opportunity for the pursuit of doctors by those who do not morally accept the law; or by those who doubt the law was respected in a particular case; or by some grieving family members who believe other family members were all too eager in supporting a loved one's request for euthanasia.

Regarding the stability of societal compassion

The illusion to be mentioned here, the most dangerous of all, docks in the bay of well-meaning simplicity, the simplicity of assuming that a society permitting voluntary euthanasia and tolerating non-voluntary euthanasia could remain committed to high standards of care for vulnerable, poor, and marginalized people. The simplicity, and the naïvety, consists in the narrow focus on the particular situation in which one person, a physician, wants to do good for another person, a patient requesting release from unbearable suffering. It is naïve to imagine that a policy and a law permitting euthanasia will not lead to insensitive, inhumane, and intolerable abuse simply because those who designed the law were governed by pure motives and noble purposes.[241]

This narrow and naïve focus of attention is blind to what Loren Graham, writing about eugenics and genetics in Russia and Germany during the 1920s, has called 'second-order' links between changing values and the uses a society can make of a science or a policy. Second-order links are difficult to see. They depend upon existing, and changing, political and social situations and upon the persuasiveness of current, and emerging, philosophies and ideologies, however flawed these may be.[242] The abuses which a law permitting euthanasia could come to serve depend upon second-order links between such a law and currently latent, or later emergent, ideologies of human insensitivity.

Regarding the costs of care

It is illusory to imagine that second-order links are not now being forged between social–economic stresses and a future law that would permit voluntary euthanasia and possibly tolerate non-voluntary euthanasia. The constraints and strains on our health-care budgets, and our much vaunted universal health-care systems, are growing in intensity. As many have observed, medical and hospital costs rise steeply with increasing age. In these circumstances, could socially and legally acceptable euthanasia not come to seem altogether too socially convenient? Could euthanasia then not come to be seen as a tolerable substitute for spending limited resources to develop and expand programmes of palliative care tailored for patients with cancer, HIV disease, amyotrophic lateral sclerosis, and other destructive and mortal diseases?

The danger in economically tough times is that we may easily slip into a triage mentality and adopt for everyday life the principles of exception that are tolerable only in extreme emergency situations. In such situations, where resources are just not immediately at hand to treat all who are sick or injured, treatment begins with those who are most severely ill or injured but who are salvageable, then moves on to those who are in lesser danger of dying, and finally is given last of all to those who cannot be saved, to the dying. This approach becomes particularly threatening to the humanitarian values and ethic of a society when it is put forth as necessary not only in crises of short duration, but as a matter of course. That the dying should come last when resources are distributed is reflected in the statement from the United States Court of Appeals in its decision to strike down the New York State ban on euthanasia. The Court said 'Surely the state's interest lessens as the potential for life diminishes'.[219] Those who believe that palliative care should be one of the first of the services to be cut when health care and hospital budgets are drastically slashed should stop and reflect upon the consequences of extending to everyday life these principles of exception. Charles Fried has warned 'It is when emergencies become usual that we are threatened with moral disintegration, dehumanization'.[243]

There is reason for concern that legalized euthanasia could come to be an expression of a moral disintegration and of a dehumanization of which we would never have thought ourselves capable.

Caution in reasoning against the legalization of euthanasia

In this chapter, opposition to the legalization of euthanasia is presented as a matter of practical and prudential judgement. Each of the reasons advanced in the preceding subsection against changing laws currently prohibiting the administration of death to the dying is open to question, and has been questioned in one publication or another written by those who believe and argue that healers should be legally authorized to administer euthanasia in response to voluntary requests of competent patients suffering from a terminal illness.[244-246] In our judgement, the reasons put forward to promote 'a carefully designed social experiment with legalized, voluntary euthanasia'[246] are, both when taken individually and when taken together as an argument, too naïve and too insensitive to the complexities and to the extremes of moral views in pluralistic modern societies to justify such a radical departure, as euthanasia would be, from long-standing legal interdictions on the administration of death.

The practical and prudential judgement of this chapter that euthanasia should not be legalized does not depend upon a theologically or philosophically buttressed position that voluntary euthanasia is unethical in any and all circumstances. The following and closing section of the chapter accepts that voluntary euthanasia may, in some circumstances, be at least ethically tolerable. Our central concern is this: the crystal clear rationality of those proposing careful design, precise conditions, and detailed safeguards to prevent any slippage from voluntary to non-voluntary, and to only partially voluntary, euthanasia may well fracture along unpredictable fault lines when it enters the highly varied and variable moral world in which euthanasia will be practised. Those who, with pure motives and clearly defined purposes, initiate actions of profound human significance in complex situations often find that the action, with time, can become evermore separated from the initial agents and their rational designs.[247] It is indeed naïve to imagine that a policy authorizing voluntary euthanasia 'would not be abused simply because those who were present at its conception and birth had pure motives and well spelled out purposes.'[241]

The judgement of this chapter that legalizing euthanasia would be to court an unjustifiable risk of abuse definitely involves a slippery-slope concern and slippery-slope reasoning, if not a formal slippery-slope argument. This chapter's judgement would be very weak, however, if its concern and reasoning were based upon an historically and socially questionable analogy between euthanasia in pre-Nazi and Nazi Germany and euthanasia in societies today. Some have appealed to such an analogy in their opposition to the legalization of euthanasia[248,249] but this chapter does not do so, because we share the view that 'comparisons with Nazi killing operations do not illuminate today's discussion' of euthanasia;[250] this is for the following reasons.

First, euthanasia, as proposed for legalization today, generally means the painless administration of death to persons suffering from incurable and advanced disease. That is not what euthanasia meant when proposed in 1920 by Alfred Hoche and Karl Binding in their book, *Die Freigabe der Vernichtung lebensunverten Lebens* (Authorization for the Destruction of Life Unworthy of Life). Alfred Hoche, a psychiatrist and specialist in neuropathology, was then a professor at Freiburg University and Klaus Binding was a retired legal scholar who had taught at the University of Leipzig. This book is only incidentally concerned with euthanasia for persons suffering from terminal illness. The authors' main preoccupation is for the legalized administration of euthanasia to those who are unworthy of life. This expression embraces the feebleminded, those with incurable mental retardation, and more generally, to those persons whose lives are of no worth to themselves or to society. The euthanasia defended in this book was primarily for human beings therein described as 'Ballastexistenzen' (beings who are nothing but ballast and can be jettisoned) and 'leeren Menschenhülson' (empty human shells).[251,252] Many of the people targeted in this book for euthanasia were capable of living on for years without pain or suffering, persons, however, whose care represented, in the authors' estimate, a gross misappropriation of human resources.[253,254]

Second, euthanasia under Nazi rule was really a euphemism for a racially and eugenically motivated secret government programme to rid the German people of all those who were defective and inferior, and included were persons with mental illness, mental retardation, as well as the blind, the deaf, the epileptic, and persons with other kinds of physical or mental disability or both.[255]

Third, the Nazi euthanasia programme, it has been strongly argued, was not just a step down the slope to genocide, but rather a euphemism for the mass murder of human beings because they belonged to biologically defined groups.[256,257] It was genocide from the beginning.

Slippery-slope reasoning and arguments have been reasonably criticized for their frequent vagueness and lack of detail.[258-260] The sketchiness of the reasoning often afflicts the descriptions of the forces that would supposedly propel a society away from socially and legally acceptable forms of euthanasia and down the slope to morally and socially intolerable abuses. What is required, it is said, for strong and convincing slippery-slope reasoning is detailed empirical evidence about the conditions and causes of communal moral deterioration, and that 'detailed empirical evidence is conspicuously lacking.'[258] We agree with this assessment and critique, and we are far from prepared to argue against the value of methodologically sound studies in social psychology, political sociology, and social history for any reasoning about euthanasia.[258] However, if evidence is currently lacking to buttress slippery-slope reasoning against the legalization of euthanasia, it is equally lacking to support the beliefs of those who think that legalizing euthanasia will not lead to abuse. The judgement of this chapter is that it is reasonable to maintain the legal prohibition of euthanasia until sufficient evidence were to accumulate, through whatever studies now underway or still to be undertaken, that a given society is with great probability able to prevent abuses of legalized euthanasia.

The slippery-slope reasoning in this chapter's opposition to the legalization of euthanasia recognizes the difference between reasonable and effective distinctions.[261] The distinctions between voluntary euthanasia on the one hand and non-voluntary or pressured euthanasia on the other are intellectually clear and ethically significant. Our concern and practical judgement is that it will probably be very difficult effectively to maintain these distinctions in practice. Will societal attitudes towards non-voluntary euthanasia change and become more benign as people become more and more accustomed to various extensions and modifications of voluntary euthanasia?

An event in the world of art may suggest what could happen in the world of ethics. Bernard Williams cites Nelson Goodman's explanation of how increasingly incompetent forgeries by van Meegeren came to be accepted as genuine Vermeers.[261,262] What process was at work that could so distort the faculties of aesthetic perception and judgement? It was a process of incremental adaptation to incrementally poor forgeries. Only when the latest and poorest of the forgeries were compared, not to preceding and somewhat better forgeries, but to the original Vermeers did the poverty of the fakery become strikingly clear.

The chapter's judgement that voluntary euthanasia as a compassionate release from suffering should not be legalized includes the concern that a process similar to that at work with the van Meegeren forgeries may come to distort ethical perceptions and evaluations of extensions of euthanasia to those who are neither dying nor able to consent. This concern is not purely speculative. The tolerance, if not the desire, for non-voluntary euthanasia in The Netherlands,[263] the 1994 legal authorization of a notification procedure for non-voluntary euthanasia in The Netherlands, and the Dutch Supreme Court's decision in June 1995 not to penalize psychiatrist Dr Boudewijn Chabot for assisting the suicide of a woman suffering from grief and depression[264] are all events that give justifiable cause to pause and to wonder how far enlightened societies in the late 1990s will be prepared to go in extending the putative benefits of compassionate euthanasia.

Can euthanasia ever be ethically tolerable?

Some clinical situations are exceptional in that commonly respected rules do not apply. What should one do when the wife and adult children ask, in front of her husband and their father dying from throat cancer, and with his nodding agreement, that the doctor put him 'to sleep' on Thursday or Friday, the days when everyone expected him to die. His pain was bearable, but the periodic choking episodes were terrifying to this man. He wanted to die in peace and tranquillity. He did not want his last moments of consciousness to be the consciousness of panic and terror. The doctor believed that euthanasia was the only route open to him to give this man and his family what they so deeply and reasonably desired. But the doctor could not walk that route. The man did die on the Friday and in a choking episode.

After the funeral, the wife and children were crushed by guilt, and so were the staff who had cared for this man. What should have been done? Everything necessary should have been done to ensure that this man died, not in choking anxiety, but in tranquillity. It was wrong to let him die in terror.

This man was dying. His death was inevitable and imminent. His life was already out of the doctor's hands, and anyone else's hands for that matter. Only the timing of his death was still in the doctor's control and he, upon the man's silent request and upon the explicit request of his family, would have been quite justified ethically in timing that death for a moment of tranquillity.

Some physicians will reject euthanasia in all circumstances because they believe such an act is against the fundamental meaning and purpose of medicine. It would be a fundamental contradiction for a healer and saver of life to administer death. In M. Mead's interpretation it is the Hippocratic Oath and its prohibition of killing that permitted patients to trust physicians without reservation and permitted physicians to practise the art and science of healing without being conscripted to administer death for social purposes.[265,266]

However, care and compassion motivate some physicians to administer euthanasia when all other available means seem powerless to relieve intensely suffering patients. Thus did Dr Nigel Cox in England inject two ampoules of potassium chloride into a 70-year-old woman who had suffered for over twenty years from acute rheumatoid arthritis. Mrs Lilian Boyes' pain was so intense that she could not bear to be touched. She refused all treatment other than painkillers and when these were no longer having their desired effect, Mrs Boyes asked Dr Cox for a fatal injection. He at first refused, then later complied when Mrs Boyes did not appear about to die rapidly on her own but was likely to continue to live perhaps for days or longer in intense pain. His act provoked considerable debate and led to a conviction of attempted murder.[267–270] Dr Cox, it may be noted, could have explored the option of sedating Mrs Boyes to give her relief without giving her death. Physicians should be respected, not accused of hypocrisy, in showing great hesitancy to assume the terrible power of giving death.

It is quite difficult, if not impossible, to assert in any absolute way that situations never do and never will occur in clinical practice where advancing death seems to be the only way to give patients relief from certain kinds and intensities of suffering. However, if euthanasia or advancing death may at times be clinically and ethically justifiable, or at least ethically tolerable as the lesser of two evils, should euthanasia for that reason be legalized or decriminalized?

This chapter distinguishes the ethical justifiability or tolerability of individual acts of euthanasia in certain circumstances from the ethical justifiability of legalizing euthanasia. This distinction rests upon the view that the 'existence of a justified act does not necessarily justify a policy condoning such an act, and an act that is an exception to a policy does not necessarily invalidate the policy'.[199]

The pressing need today is not to change legal prohibitions of euthanasia to guarantee doctors immunity from prosecution if and when they and their patients decide that euthanasia is the only practicable release from intolerable suffering. The most pressing need is to perfect and expand programmes of palliative medicine and palliative care that will reduce, even if they will never totally eliminate, requests for euthanasia. If and when a request for euthanasia has to be honoured, the need is for enhanced communication between patients, families, doctors, and clinical staff, so that, when such circumstances occur, all together will know and come to agree on what is the right thing to do.

It is not inconsistent to judge certain acts of hastening death to be ethically acceptable or tolerable and yet simultaneously to hold that laws should not be modified to grant doctors or anyone else legal authorization in advance to carry them out.

Position statement

At the end of this century, the signs in Western societies of overt discrimination, of latent racism, of utilitarian insensitivity to vulnerable people, and of tendencies to devalue human beings[271] are too prominent to justify insouciant attitudes regarding the legalization of euthanasia. The law prohibiting euthanasia, even voluntary euthanasia, should be maintained.

Those who favour legalization of voluntary euthanasia believe it to be utterly unproved and quite unlikely that legalization of euthanasia will provoke a societal slide down the slippery slope to intolerable abuses. Admittedly, such a slide is not certain. The issue is whether we should try this social experiment. This chapter argues that we should not.

Of course, there is no law, not even a law prohibiting euthanasia, that can cover the infinite variety of human situations or the infinite variety of unique human suffering. Maintaining a law against euthanasia will require of all of us the kind of common sense that knows when such a law should not be applied, or not applied in all its force.

Conclusion

At the close of this chapter we draw attention to the important distinction between ethics within palliative care and the ethic within which palliative care operates.

This chapter has been about ethics within palliative care. The bedside of the dying has centred the chapter's discussions about resolving value conflicts and uncertainties, about how to make and justify the myriad decisions required of the dying, of families, and of doctors, nurses, and other professionals on behalf of the dying. The clinical goal of palliative medicine underlying the discussion of ethical issues encompasses the co-ordination of knowledge, skills, reflection, and compassion to allow us, at the end of our days, to die as Philip Aries outlines:

> Death must simply become the discreet but dignified exit of a peaceful person from a helpful society. A death without pain or suffering, and ultimately without fear.[1]

But what of those who do not find their way into this ideal place? Who die alone, abandoned in their final plight? Any answer to this question confronts the ethic within which palliative care operates. That ethic encompasses a vision and the reach of humanity beyond the bedside. That ethic calls for society discourse, conflict resolution, and decision on how we value and respect life at the moment that life is ending. It is an ethic of action.

In his novel *The Death of Virgil,* Hermann Brock has the poet considering a decision to destroy his manuscript of the Aeneid.[272] Why? Because Brock sees Virgil coming to realize that the beauty and truth of language are inadequate to cope with human suffering. A poetry more immediate that that of words is needed—a poetry of action.[273]

Like such a poetry, the ethic within which palliative care operates needs to be an ethic of action, an ethic that mobilizes and links governments, institutions, programmes, services, persons, and resources to form a tissue of effective bonds of compassion, a vision that no one is a stranger to us among those who anguish and suffer as they face loss and death.

References

1. Ariès P. *L'Homme Devant la Mort*. Paris: Éditions du Seuil, 1977: 608.
2. MacDonald N. From the front lines. *Journal of Palliative Care*, 1994; **10**: 44–7. (Adapted with permission.)
3. Roy DJ, Williams JR, Dickens BM. *Bioethics in Canada*. Scarborough, Ontario: Prentice-Hall Canada, 1994: 27.
4. Sackett DL. Bias in analytic research. *Journal of Chronic Diseases*, 1979; **32**: 51–63.
5. Toulmin S. The tyranny of principles. *Hastings Center Report*, 1981; **11**: 31–9.
6. Fried C. *Medical Experimentation, Personal Integrity and Social Policy*. Amsterdam, Oxford: North-Holland Publishing Company, 1974: 101–5.
7. Quinn KM. The impact of Tarasoff on clinical practice. *Behavioral Sciences and the Law*, 1984; **2**: 319–29.
8. Hoffman B. Disclosure of medical information without consent: the patient's right to confidentiality. *Health Law in Canada*, 1992; **13**: 156–9.
9. Marshall M. Case comment: R. v. Gruenke. *Health Law in Canada*, 1992; **12**: 112–4.
10. Tri-Council Working Group. *Code of Conduct for Research Involving Humans*. (Draft document.) Ottawa: Minister of Supply and Services Canada, 1996.
11. Marr P. Maintaining patient confidentiality in an electronic world. *International Journal of Bio-Medical Computing*, 1994; **35** (Suppl.1): 213–17.
12. Gostin LO, Turek-Brezina J, Powers M, *et al.* Privacy and security of personal information in a new health care system. *Journal of the American Medical Association*, 1993; **270**: 2487–93.
13. Anderson R. NHS-wide networking and patient confidentiality. *British Medical Journal*, 1995; **311**: 5–6.
14. Editorial. The selling of patients' data. *Lancet*, 1989; **ii**: 1078.
15. Black D. Personal health records. *Journal of Medical Ethics*, 1992; **18**: 5–6.
16. Siegler M. Confidentiality in medicine—a decrepit concept. *New England Journal of Medicine*, 1982; **307**: 1518–21.
17. Burnum JF. Secrets about patients. *New England Journal of Medicine*, 1991; **324**: 1130–3.
18. Von Roenn JH, Cleeland CS, Gonin R, *et al.* Physician attitudes and practice in cancer pain management. A survey from the Eastern Cooperative Oncology Group. *Annals of Internal Medicine*, 1993; **119**: 121–6.
19. Cleeland CS, Gonin R, Hatfield AK, *et al.* Pain and its treatment in outpatients with metastatic cancer. *New England Journal of Medicine*, 1994; **330**: 592–6.
20. Portenoy RK, Miransky J, Thaler HT, *et al.* Pain in ambulatory patients with lung or colon cancer. *Cancer*, 1992; **70**: 1616–24.
21. Larue F, Colleau S, Brasseur L, Cleeland CS. A multicentre study of cancer pain and its treatment in France. *British Medical Journal*, 1995; **310**: 1034–7.
22. Vainio A. Treatment of terminal cancer pain in France: a questionnaire study. *Pain*, 1995; **62**: 155–62.
23. Vachon M. The emotional problems of the patient in palliative medicine. In: Doyle D, Hanks GW, MacDonald N (eds). *Oxford Textbook of Palliative Medicine*. 1st edn. Oxford: Oxford University Press, 1993: 575–605.
24. Jacox A, Carr DB, Payne R. New clinical practice guidelines for the management of pain in patients with cancer. *New England Journal of Medicine*, 1994; **330**: 651–5.
25. World Health Organization. *Cancer Pain Relief.* 2nd edn. Geneva: World Health Organization, 1996.
26. MacDonald N. Topic 4. Pain management for breast cancer patients. In: *Clinical Practical Guidelines for the Care and Treatment of Breast Cancer.* Canadian Breast Cancer Initiative, 1996.
27. MacDonald N. Evidence/Témoignages. *Proceedings of the Senate Special Committee on Euthanasia and Assisted Suicide/Délibérations du Comité Sénatorial Spécial sur l'Euthanasie et le Suicide Assisté*. Issue/Fascicule No. 22. Ottawa: Canada Communication Group/Groupe Communication Canada, 1994: 21–42.
28. MacDonald N. Priorities in education and research in palliative care. *Palliative Medicine*, 1993; **7**(Suppl.1): 65–76.

29. MacDonald N. Teaching palliative care: a structural overview. In : MacLeod RD, James C (eds). *Teaching Palliative Care: Issues and Implications.* Newmill, Penzance: Patten Press, 1994.
30. MacDonald N. A proposed matrix for organisational changes to improve quality of life in oncology. *European Journal of Cancer*, 1995; **31A** (Suppl. 6): S18–21.
31. Calman KC. New methods of teaching and the evaluation of teaching. In: Twycross RG (ed.). *The Edinburgh Symposium on Pain Control and Medical Education.* Royal Society of Medicine, 1989: 175–80.
32. Hagen N, Young J, MacDonald N. Diffusion of standards of care for cancer pain. *Canadian Medical Association Journal*, 1995; **152**: 1205–9.
33. Andersen JF, McEwan EL, Hrudey WP. Effectiveness of notification and group regulation in modifying prescribing of regulated analgesics. *Canadian Medical Association Journal*, 1996; **154**: 31–9.
34. Decoster G, Stein G, Holdener E. Responses and toxic deaths in Phase I clinical trials. *Annals of Oncology*, 1990; **2**:175–81.
35. Kodish E, Stocking C, Ratain MJ, Kohrman A, Siegler M. Ethical issues in Phase I oncology research: a comparison of investigators and institutional review board chairpersons. *Journal of Clinical Oncology*, 1992; **10**: 1810–16.
36. Daugherty C, Ratain MJ, Grochowski E, Stocking C, Kodish E, Mick R, Siegler M. Perceptions of cancer patients and their physicians involved in Phase I trials. *Journal of Clinical Oncology*, 1995; **13**: 1062–72.
37. Daugherty C, Lyman K, Mick R, Siegler M, Ratain MJ. Differences in perception of goals, expectations and level of informed consent between oncologists (oncs) and patients (pts) involved in Phase I clinical trials. *Proceedings of ASCO* (Abstract Number 1713), 1996: 530.
38. Lipsett MB. On the nature and ethics of Phase I clinical trials of cancer chemotherapies. *The Journal of the American Medical Association*, 1982; **248**: 941–2.
39. Appelbaum PS, Grisso T. Assessing patients' capacities to consent to treatment. *New England Journal of Medicine*, 1988; **319**: 1635–88.
40. Bruera E, Franco JJ, Maltoni M, Watanabe S, Suarez-Almazor M. Changing pattern of agitated impaired mental status in patients with advanced cancer: association with cognitive monitoring, hydration, and opiate rotation. *Journal of Pain and Symptom Management*, 1995; **10**: 287–91.
41. Massie MJ, Holland JC, Glass E. Delirium in terminally ill cancer patients. *American Journal of Psychiatry*, 1983; **140**: 1048–50.
42. Bruera E, Spachynski K, MacEachern T, Hanson J. Cognitive failure in cancer patients in clinical trials (Letter). *The Lancet*, 1993; **341**: 247–8.
43. Portenoy RK, Thaler HT, Kornblith AB, *et al.* Symptom prevalence, characteristics and distress in a cancer population. *Quality of Life Research*, 1994; **3**:183–9.
44. Kennedy BJ. Needed: clinical trials for older patients. *Journal of Clinical Oncology*, 1991; **9**: 718–20.
45. MacDonald N. Principles governing the use of cancer chemotherapy in palliative medicine. In: Doyle D, Hanks GW, MacDonald N (eds). *Oxford Textbook of Palliative Medicine.* 1st edn. Oxford: Oxford University Press, 1993: 105–17.
46. de Raeve L. Ethical issues in palliative care research. *Palliative Medicine*, 1994; **8**: 298–305.
47. Cassell EJ. *The Nature of Suffering and the Goals of Medicine.* Oxford: Oxford University Press, 1991: 27.
48. Mount BM, Cohen R, MacDonald N, Bruera E, Dudgeon E. Ethical issues in palliative care research revisited. *Palliative Medicine*, 1995; **9**: 165–70.
49. Raghavan D. Clinician surrogates and equipoise: an analogy to lawyers who represent themselves? *European Journal of Cancer*, 1991; **27**: 1072–4.
50. The National Council for Hospice and Specialist Palliative Care Services. *Guidelines on Research in Palliative Care.* London: The National Council for Hospice and Specialist Palliative Care Services, 1995.
51. Levine RJ. *Ethics and Regulation of Clinical Research.* New Haven: Yale University Press, 1988: 187–90.
52. Shaw LW, Chalmers TC. Ethics in cooperative clinical trials. *Annals of the New York Academy of Sciences*, 1970; **169**: 487–95.
53. Freedman B. Equipoise and the ethics of clinical research. *New England Journal of Medicine*, 1987; **317**: 141–5.
54. Elliott C, Weijer C. Cruel and unusual treatment. *Saturday Night*, December 1995: 31-4.
55. MacDonald N. Suffering and dying in cancer patients: research frontiers in controlling confusion, cachexia, and dyspnea. *Western Journal of Medicine*, (Caring for patients at the end of life. Special Issue), 1995; **163**: 278–86.
56. Annas GJ. Informed consent, cancer, and truth in prognosis. *New England Journal of Medicine*, 1994; **330**: 223–5.
57. MacDonald N. Quality of life in clinical and research ethics. *Journal of Palliative Care*, 1992; **8**: 46–51.
58. Williams CJ, Zwitter M. Informed consent in European multicentre randomised clinical trials—Are patients really informed? *European Journal of Cancer*, 1994; **30A**: 907–10.
59. Weijer C. Our bodies, our science. *The Sciences*, 1995; **May/June**: 41–5.
60. Callahan D. *The Troubled Dream of Life: In Search of a Peaceful Death.* New York: Simon and Schuster, 1993: 94.
61. Hadorn DC. The Oregon priority-setting exercise: quality of life and public policy. *Hastings Center Report*, 1991; **May-June**: 11–16.
62. Lubitz JD, Riley GF. Trends in medicare payments in the last year of life. *New England Journal of Medicine*, 1993; **328**: 1092–6.
63. Emanuel EJ. Cost savings at the end of life. What do the data show? *Journal of the American Medical Association*, 1996; **275**: 1907–14.
64. Bruera E, Brenneis C, Michaud M, *et al.* Use of the subcutaneous route for administration of narcotics in patients with cancer. *Cancer*, 1988; **62**: 407–11.
65. Ferris FD, Wodinsky HB, Kerr IG, *et al.* A cost-minimization study of cancer patients requiring a narcotic infusion in hospital and at home. *Journal of Clinical Epidemiology*, 1991; **44**: 313–27.
66. Kristjanson LJ. Validity and reliability testing of the Famcare Scale: measuring family satisfaction with advanced cancer care. *Social Science Medicine*, 1993; **36**: 693–701.
67. Paine LS. Managing for organizational integrity. *Harvard Business Review*, 1994; **March-April**: 106–17.
68. Arras JD. The technological tether. An introduction to ethical and social issues in high-tech home care. *Hastings Center Report*, 1994; **September-October** (Special Supplement): S1–2.
69. Callahan D. Families as caregivers: the limits of morality. *Archives of Physical Medicine and Rehabilitation*, 1988; **69**: 323–8.
70. Kluger R. A peace plan for the cigarette wars. *New York Times Magazine*, 1996; **April 7**: 28–35, 50, 54.
71. Angell M. The doctor as double agent. *Kennedy Institute of Ethics Journal*, 1993; **3**: 279–86.
72. Sulmasy DP. Physicians, cost control and ethics. *Annals of Internal Medicine*, 1992; **116**: 920–6.
73. Emanuel EJ, Dubler NN. Preserving the physician-patient relationship in the era of managed care. *Journal of the American Medical Association*, 1995; **273**: 323–9.
74. Miles SH, Weber EP, Koepp R. End-of-life treatment in managed care. The potential and the peril. *Western Journal of Medicine*, 1995; **163**: 302–5.
75. Woolhandler S, Himmelstein DU. Editorial. Extreme risk - The new corporate proposition for physicians. *New England Journal of Medicine*, 1995; **333**: 1706–7.
76. Mehlman MJ, Massey SR. The patient-physician relationship and the allocation of scarce resources: a law and economics approach. *Kennedy Institute of Ethics Journal*, 1994; **4/4**: 291–308.
77. Randall F, Downie R. *Palliative Care Ethics. A Good Companion.* New York: Oxford University Press, 1996.
78. Newcomb PA, Carbone PP. Cancer treatment and age: patient perspectives. *Journal of the National Cancer Institute*, 1993; **85**: 1580–4.
79. Newschaffer CJ, Penberthy L, Desch CE, *et al.* The effect of age and comorbidity in the treatment of elderly women with nonmetastatic breast cancer. *Archives of Internal Medicine*, 1996; **156**: 85–90.
80. Yellen S, Cella DF, Leslie WT. Age and clinical decision making in

oncology outpatients. *Journal of the National Cancer Institute*, 1994; **86**: 1743–4.

81. Cartwright A. The role of hospitals in caring for people in the last year of their lives. *Age and Ageing*, 1991; **20**: 271–4.
82. Cartwright A. Dying when you're old. *Age and Ageing*, 1993; **22**: 425–30.
83. Roy DJ. Living on dialysis and dying with dignity. *Renal Family*, 1986; **8**: 17–22.
84. The Hastings Center. *Guidelines on the Termination of Life-Sustaining Treatment and the Care of the Dying*. Briarcliff Manor, New York: The Hastings Center, 1987.
85. Stanley JM (ed.). The Appleton International Conference. Developing guidelines for decisions to forego life-prolonging medical treatment. *Journal of Medical Ethics*, 1992; **18** (Suppl): 3–23.
86. President's Commission for the Study of Ethical Problems in Medicine and Biomedical and Behavioral Research. *Deciding to Forego Life-Sustaining Treatment. Ethical, Medical, and Legal Issues in Treatment Decisions*. Washington, D.C.: U.S. Government Printing Office, 1983.
87. National Council for Hospice and Specialist Palliative Care Services. *Key Ethical Issues in Palliative Care: Evidence to House of Lords Select Committee on Medical Ethics*. Occasional Paper 3, July 1993.
88. Council on Ethical and Judicial Affairs, American Medical Association. Decisions near the end of life. *Journal of the American Medical Association*, 1992; **267**: 2229–33.
89. Feinstein AR. An additional basic science for clinical medicine: IV. The development of clinimetrics. *Annals of Internal Medicine*, 1983; **99**: 848.
90. Lo B. Improving care near the end of life. Why is it so hard? *Journal of the American Medical Association*, 1995; **274**: 1634–6.
91. Sherlock R. For everything there is a season; the right to die in the United States. *Brigham Young University Law Review*, 1982; **3**: 545–616.
92. Gostin L. A right to choose death: the judicial trilogy of Brophy, Bouvia, and Conroy. *Law, Medicine and Health Care*, 1986; **14**: 198–202.
93. Meisel A. *The Right to Die*. New York: John Wiley and Sons, 1989.
94. Ruark JE, Raffin TA, Stanford University Medical Center Committee on Ethics. Initiating and withdrawing life support. *New England Journal of Medicine*, 1988; **318**: 25–30.
95. Buchanan AE, Brock D. *Deciding for Others: The Ethics of Surrogate Decisionmaking*. Cambridge University Press, 1989.
96. Wanzer S *et al.* The physician's responsibility toward hopelessly ill patients: a second look. *New England Journal of Medicine*, 1989; **244**: 1846–53.
97. Solomon MZ *et al.* Decisions near the end of life: professional views on life-sustaining treatments. *American Journal of Public Health*, 1993; **83**: 14–23.
98. Meisel A. The legal consensus about forgoing life-sustaining treatment: its status and its prospects. *Kennedy Institute of Ethics Journal*, 1993; **2**: 309–45.
99. Hafemeister TL, Keilitz I, Banks S. The judicial role in life-sustaining medical treatment decisions. *Issues in Law and Medicine*, 1991; **7**: 53–72.
100. Annas GJ. Sounding board. Nancy Cruzan and the right to die. *New England Journal of Medicine*, 1990; **323**: 670–3.
101. Roy DJ. Refus des traitements de prolongation de vie dans le cas de patients dont la mort n'est pas imminente: éthique clinique et jurisprudence récente au Québec. *Médecine/Sciences*, 1992; **8/7**: 747–9.
102. Brahams D. Medicine and the law. Persistent vegetative state. *The Lancet*, 1992; **340**: 1534–5.
103. Brahams D. Medicine and the law. Persistent vegetative state. *The Lancet*, 1993; **341**: 428.
104. McCartney JT. The development of the doctrine of ordinary and extraordinary means of preserving life in Catholic moral theology before the Karen Quinlan case. *Linacre Quarterly*, 1980; **47**: 215–24.
105. McCormick RA. *How Brave a New World? Dilemmas in Bioethics*. New York: Doubleday and Company, 1981.
106. Sacred Congregation for the Doctrine of the Faith. *Declaration on Euthanasia*. Rome, 1980: 4–10.
107. Law Reform Commission of Canada. *Euthanasia, Aiding Suicide and Cessation of Treatment*. Report 20. Ottawa: Minister of Supply and Services Canada, 1983.
108. Emanuel LL, Emanuel EJ. The medical directive: a new comprehensive advance care document. *Journal of the American Medical Association*, 1989; **261**: 3288–93.
109. Hackler C, Moseley R, Vawter D. *Advance Directives in Medicine*. New York: Praeger, 1989.
110. Singer PA *et al.* Advance directives: are they an advance? *Canadian Medical Association Journal*, 1992; **146**: 127–34.
111. Silverman HJ, Vinicky JK, Gasner MR. Advance directives: implications for critical care. *Critical Care Medicine*, 1992; **20**: 1027–31.
112. Annas GJ *et al.* Bioethicists' statement on the U.S. Supreme Court's Cruzan decision. *New England Journal of Medicine*, 1990; **323**: 686–7.
113. Weir RF, Gostin L. Decisions to abate life-sustaining treatment for nonautonomous patients. Ethical standards and legal liability for physicians after Cruzan. *Journal of the American Medical Association*, 1990; **264**: 1846–53.
114. Meisel A. The legal consensus about forgoing life-sustaining treatment: its status and prospects. *Kennedy Institute of Ethics Journal*, 1993; **2**: 309–45.
115. Paris J, Reardon FE. Moral, ethical, and legal issues in the intensive care unit. *Journal of Intensive Care Medicine*, 1991; **6**: 175–95.
116. Task Force on Ethics of the Society of Critical Care Medicine. Consensus report on the ethics of foregoing life-sustaining treatments in the critically ill. *Critical Care Medicine*, 1990; **18**: 1435–9.
117. Bohm D. *Wholeness and the Implicate Order*. London: Routledge and Kegan Paul, 1980.
118. Cassem N. When illness is judged irreversible: imperative and elective treatments. *Man and Medicine*, 1980; **5**: 154–66.
119. Faden R, Beauchamp TL, King NMP. *A History and Theory of Informed Consent*. Oxford: Oxford University Press, 1986: 123.
120. Carole Couture-Jacquet c. The Montreal Children's Hospital [1986]. *R.J.Q.* 1221–8 (Cour d'Appel). 1986.
121. Veatch RM, Spicer CM. Medically futile care: the role of the physician in setting limits. *American Journal of Law and Medicine*, 1992; **18**:15–36.
122. Truog RD, Brett AS, Frader J. The problem with futility. *New England Journal of Medicine*, 1992; **326**: 1560–4.
123. Schneiderman LJ *et al.* Medical futility: its meaning and ethical implications. *Annals of Internal Medicine*, 1990; **112**: 949–54.
124. Faber-Lagendoen K. Resuscitation of patients with metastatic cancer: is transient benefit still futile? *Archives of Internal Medicine*, 1991; **151**: 235–9.
125. Green M. Cardiopulmonary resuscitation and the dying patient with cancer: a resuscitator's response. *Archives of Internal Medicine*, 1992; **152**: 1529–30.
126. Haines IE *et al.* Not-for-resuscitation orders in cancer patients—principles of decision-making. *Medical Journal of Australia*, 1990; **153**: 225–9.
127. The SUPPORT Principal Investigators. A controlled trial to improve care for seriously ill hospitalized patients. The study to understand prognosis and preferences for outcomes and risks of treatments (SUPPORT). *Journal of the American Medical Association*, 1995; **274**: 1591–8.
128. Feinberg WM, Ferry PC. A fate worse than death. The persistent vegetative state in childhood. *American Journal of Diseases of Children*, 1984; **138**: 128–30.
129. Munstat TL *et al.* Guidelines on the vegetative state: commentary on the American Academy of Neurology statement. *Neurology*, 1989; **39**: 123–4.
130. American Neurological Association Committee on Ethical Affairs. Persistent vegetative state: report of the American Neurological Association Committee on Ethical Affairs. *Annals of Neurology*, 1993; **33**: 386–90.
131. Tresch DD *et al.* Clinical characteristics of patients in the persistent vegetative state. *Archives of Internal Medicine*, 1991; **151**: 930–2.
132. Working Group, Royal College of Physicians. The permanent vegetative state. Review by a Working Group convened by the Royal College of Physicians and endorsed by the Conference of Medical Royal Colleges and

their Faculties of the United Kingdom. *Journal of the Royal College of Physicians of London*, 1996; **30**: 119–21.

133. Steinbrook R, Lo B. Artificial feeding—solid ground, not a slippery slope. *New England Journal of Medicine*, 1988; **318**: 286–90.
134. Cantor NL. The permanently unconscious patient, non-feeding and euthanasia. *American Journal of Law and Medicine*, 1989; **15**: 381–437.
135. Lynn J (ed.). *By No Extraordinary Means*. Bloomington: Indiana University Press, 1986.
136. Pollock. Life and death decisions; who makes them and by what standards? *Rutgers Law Review*, 1989; **41**: 505.
137. Bernat JL *et al.* Patient refusal of hydration and nutrition. *Archives of Internal Medicine*, 1993; **153**: 2723–7.
138. Kamisar Y. Dilemma over the night that ends all nights; right to die, or license to kill? *New Jersey Law Journal*, 1989; **124/21**: 7.
139. MacDonald N, Fainsinger R. Indications and ethical considerations in the hydration of patients with advanced cancer. In: Bruera E (ed.). *Cachexia-Anorexia Syndrome in Cancer Patients*. Oxford: Oxford University Press, 1996.
140. Lynn J, Childress JF. Must patients always be given food and water? *Hastings Center Report*, 1983; **13**: 17–21.
141. Council of Scientific Affairs and Council on Ethical and Judicial Affairs. Persistent vegetative state and the decision to withdraw or withhold life support. *Journal of the American Medical Association*, 1990; **263**: 426–30.
142. Institute of Medical Ethics Working Party on the Ethics of Prolonging Life and Assisting Death. Withdrawal of life-support from patients in a persistent vegetative state. *The Lancet*, 1991; **337**: 96–8.
143. Gillis J *et al.* Ventilator-dependent children. *Medical Journal of Australia*, 1989; **150**: 10–14.
144. Gillis J, Kilham H. Entrapment. *Critical Care Medicine*, 1990; **18**: 897.
145. Smedera N *et al.* Withholding and withdrawal of life support from the critically ill. *New England Journal of Medicine*, 1990; **322**: 309–15.
146. NIH Workshop. Withholding and withdrawing mechanical ventilation. *American Review of Respiratory Disease*, 1986; **134**: 1327–30.
147. McCormick RA. A proposal for "quality of life" criteria for sustaining life. *Hospital Progress*, 1975; **56**: 76–9.
148. Roy DJ. Decision offers Nancy B. a measure of dignity. Life-support technology not sole solution. *Financial Post*, 1992; **January 8**: 10.
149. Roy DJ. Respecter le désir et la dignité de Nancy B. *Le Devoir*, 1991; **December 2**: 1, 4.
150. Wanzer SH *et al.* The physician's responsibility toward hopelessly ill patients. *New England Journal of Medicine*, 1984; **310**: 955–9.
151. Paris JJ, Crone RK, Reardon F. Physicians' refusal of requested treatment. The case of Baby L. *New England Journal of Medicine*, 1990; **322**: 1012–5.
152. Désaulniers P. L'éthique clinique à l'urgence: réfléchir contre la montre. In: Roy DJ, Rapin C-H, Morissette MR (eds). *Collection Panétius - Archives de l'éthique Clinique. 1. Au Chevet du Malade: Analyse de Cas à Travers les Spécialités Médicales*. Montréal: Centre de Bioéthique, Institut de Recherches Cliniques de Montréal, 1994: 99–101.
153. Ventafridda V *et al.* Symptom prevalence and control during cancer patients' last days of life. *Journal of Palliative Care*, 1990; **6**: 7–11.
154. Mount B. A final crescendo of pain? *Journal of Palliative Care*, 1990; **6**: 5–6.
155. Roy DJ. Need they sleep before they die? *Journal of Palliative Care*, 1990; **6**: 3–4.
156. Truog RD, Berde CB, Mitchell C, Grier HE. Barbiturates in the care of the terminally ill. *New England Journal of Medicine*, 1992; **327**: 1678–81.
157. Bedau HA (ed.). *The Death Penalty in America*. 3rd edn. New York: Oxford University Press, 1982: 17–8.
158. Quill TE. Death and dignity: a case of individualized decision-making. *New England Journal of Medicine*, 1991; **324**: 691–4.
159. Sholl JG. Barbiturates in the care of the terminally ill (Letter). *New England Journal of Medicine*, 1993; **328**: 1350.
160. Donnelly S, Nelson K, Walsh TD. Barbiturates in the care of the terminally ill (Letter). *New England Journal of Medicine*, 1993; **328**: 1350–1.
161. Cherny NI, Portenoy RK. Sedation in the management of refractory symptoms; guidelines for evaluation and treatment. *Journal of Palliative Care*, 1994; **10**: 31–8.
162. Cherny N., Coyle N, Foley KM. The treatment of suffering when patients request elective death. *Journal of Palliative Care*, 1994; **10**: 71–9.
163. Saunders C. Pain and impending death. In: Wall P, Melzack R (eds). *Textbook of Pain*. New York: Churchill Livingstone, 1984: 477–8.
164. Mount B, Hamilton P. When palliative care fails to control suffering. *Journal of Palliative Care*, 1994; **10**: 24–6.
165. Scott M. Commentaries. When palliative care fails to control suffering. *Journal of Palliative Care*, 1994; **10**: 30.
166. Cooper MD. Commentaries. When palliative care fails to control suffering. *Journal of Palliative Care*, 1994; **10**: 27–8.
167. Cane W. Medical euthanasia. *Journal of the History of Medicine and Allied Sciences*, 1952; **VII**: 401–16.
168. Rohlfs. *Geschichte der Deutschen Medizin*. Stuttgart, 1880. Cited here from the article by Walter Cane. Medical euthanasia. *Journal of the History of Medicine and Allied Sciences*, 1952; **VII**: 401–16.
169. Suetonius Tranquillus C. *The Lives of the Twelve Caesars*. London: George Bell, 1890:145.
170. Bacon F. *The Advancement of Learning*. London: J.M. Dent, 1958: 114–15.
171. Solzhenitsyn A. *The Cancer Ward*, (Bethell N, Burg D, trans.). New York: Farrar, Straus and Giroux, 1969: 97.
172. Anon. Final exit: euthanasia guide sells out. *Nature*, 1991; **352**: 553.
173. Quill TE. Death and dignity. A case of individualized decision making. *New England Journal of Medicine*, 1991; **324**: 691–4.
174. Emanuel EJ. Euthanasia. Historical, ethical, and empirical perspectives. *Archives of Internal Medicine*, 1994; **154**: 1890–1901.
175. Van Der Sluis I. The movement for euthanasia 1875–1975. *Janus*, 1979; **66**: 131–71.
176. Gruman GJ. An historical introduction to ideas about voluntary euthanasia; with a bibliographic survey and guide for interdisciplinary studies. *OMEGA*, 1973; **4**: 87–138.
177. Silving H. Euthanasia: a study in comparative criminal law. *University of Pennsylvania Law Review*, 1954; **103**: 350–89.
178. Portnoy RK (ed.). Special issue on medical ethics: physician-assisted suicide and euthanasia. *Journal of Pain and Symptom Management*, 1991; **6**: 279–339.
179. Davis AJ *et al.* An international perspective of active euthanasia: attitudes of nurses in seven countries. *International Journal of Nursing Studies*, 1993; **30**: 301–10.
180. Ward BJ, Tate PA. Attitudes among NHS doctors to requests for euthanasia. *British Medical Journal*, 1994; **308**: 1332–4.
181. Shapiro RS *et al.* Willingness to perform euthanasia. A survey of physician attitudes. *Archives of Internal Medicine*, 1994; **154**: 575–84.
182. Paume P, O'Malley E. Euthanasia: attitudes and practices of medical practitioners. *Medical Journal of Austria*, 1994; **161**: 137–44.
183. Kinsella TD, Verhoef MJ. Alberta euthanasia survey: 1. Physicians' opinions about the morality and legalization of active euthanasia. *Canadian Medical Association Journal*, 1993; **148**: 1921–6.
184. Verhoef MJ, Kinsella TD. Alberta euthanasia survey: 2. Physicians' opinions about the acceptance of active euthanasia as a medical act and the reporting of such practice. *Canadian Medical Association Journal*, 1993; **148**: 1929–33.
185. Stevens CA, Hassan R. Management of death, dying and euthanasia: attitudes and practices of medical practitioners in South Australia. *Journal of Medical Ethics*, 1994; **20**: 41–6.
186. British Medical Association. *Euthanasia*. London: British Medical Association, 1988.
187. American Geriatrics Society Ethics Committee. Physician-assisted suicide and voluntary active euthanasia. *Journal of the American Geriatrics Society*, 1995; **43**: 579–80.
188. Institute of Medical Ethics Working Party on the Ethics of Prolonging Life and Assisting Death. Assisted death. *The Lancet*, 1990; **336**: 610–3.
189. House of Lords Select Committee on Medical Ethics. *Report*. London: HM Stationery Office, 1994.

190. Canadian Medical Association. Canadian Medical Association policy summary. Physician-assisted death. *Canadian Medical Association Journal*, 1995; **152**: 248A–B.
191. The Senate of Canada, Special Senate Committee on Euthanasia and Assisted Suicide. *Of Life and Death. Report of the Special Senate Committee on Euthanasia and Assisted Suicide.* Ottawa: Minister of Supply and Services Canada, 1995.
192. Académie Suisse des Sciences Médicales. Directives médico-éthiques sur l'accompagnement médical des patients en fin de vie ou souffrant de troubles cérébraux extrêmes. *Bulletin des Médecins Suisses*, 1995; **29/30**: 1226–8.
193. Gillett G. Euthanasia, letting die and the pause. *Journal of Medical Ethics*, 1988; **14**: 61–8.
194. Brock DW. Voluntary active euthanasia. *Hastings Center Report*, 1992; **22**: 10–22.
195. Callahan D. When self-determination runs amok. *Hastings Center Report*, 1992; **22**: 52–5.
196. Miller FG, Fletcher JC. The case for legalized euthanasia. *Perspectives in Biology and Medicine*, 1993; **36**: 159–76.
197. Kamisar Y. Against assisted suicide—even a very limited form. *University of Detroit Mercy Law Review*, 1995; **72**: 735–69.
198. Keown T (ed.). *Euthanasia Examined. Ethical, Clinical and Legal Perspectives.* Cambridge University Press, 1995.
199. Truog RD, Berde CB. Pain, euthanasia, and anesthesiologists. *Anesthesiology*, 1993; **78**: 353–60.
200. Brock DW. Euthanasia. *The Yale Journal of Biology and Medicine*, 1992; **65**: 121–9.
201. Rachels J. Active and passive euthanasia. *New England Journal of Medicine*, 1995; **292**: 78–80.
202. Gillon R. Euthanasia, withholding life-prolonging treatment, and moral differences between killing and letting die. *Journal of Medical Ethics*, 1988; **14**: 115–17.
203. Callahan D. Can we return death to disease? (Suppl. Mercy, Murder and Morality: Perspectives on Euthanasia). *Hastings Center Report*, 1989; **19/1**: 4–6.
204. The New York State Task Force on Life and the Law. *When Death is Sought: Assisted Suicide and Euthanasia in the Medical Context.* New York, 1994.
205. Larson EJ. Seeking compassion in dying: the Washington State law against assisted suicide. *Seattle University Law Review*, 1995; **18**: 509, 517.
206. Scofield GR. Exposing some myths about physician-assisted suicide. *Seattle University Law Review*, 1995; **18**: 473, 481.
207. Chapman CR, Gavrin J. Suffering and its relationship to pain. *Journal of Palliative Care*, 1993; **9**: 5–13.
208. Liebeskind JC. (Editorial) Pain can kill. *Pain*, 1991; **44**: 3–4.
209. Trowell H. *The Unfinished Debate on Euthanasia*. London: SCM Press, 1973: 83.
210. Smith RS. Ethical issues surrounding cancer pain. In: Chapman CR, Foley KM (eds). *Current and Emerging Issues in Cancer Pain: Research and Practice.* New York: Raven Press, 1993: 385–92.
211. Loewy EH. Healing and killing, harming and not harming: physician participation in euthanasia and capital punishment. *The Journal of Clinical Ethics*, 1992; **3**: 29–34.
212. Sawyer DM, Williams JR, Lowy F. Canadian physicians and euthanasia: 2. Definitions and distinctions. *Canadian Medical Association Journal*, 1993; **148**: 1463–6.
213. Schwartz RL. Euthanasia and assisted suicide in the Netherlands. *Cambridge Quarterly of Health Care Ethics*, 1995; **4**: 111–21.
214. Royal Dutch Medical Association. *Vision on Euthanasia*. Utrecht: Royal Dutch Medical Association, 1984.
215. Dillmann RJM, Legemaate T. Euthanasia in the Netherlands: the state of the legal debate. *European Journal of Health Law*, 1994; **1**: 81–7.
216. Annas GJ. Death by prescription. The Oregon initiative. *New England Journal of Medicine*, 1994; **331**: 1240–3.
217. Ryan CJ, Kaye M. Euthanasia in Australia—The Northern Territory rights of the terminally ill act. *New England Journal of Medicine*, 1996; **334**: 326–8.
218. *United States Court of Appeals for the Ninth Circuit, Compassion in Dying, a Washington non-profit corporation; Jane Roe; John Doe; James Poe; Harold Gluchsberg, M.D., v. State of Washington; Christine Gregoire, Attorney General of Washington.* March 6, 1996: 14.
219. *United States Court of Appeals for the Second Circuit, Timothy Quill, M.D., Samuel C. Klagskrun, M.D., and Howard A. Grossman, M.D. v. Denaris C. Vacco, Attorney General of the State of New York, George E. Palaki, Governor of the State of New York, Robert M. Morgenthau, District Attorney of New York County.* April 2, 1996: 12.
220. Freeman J. Is there a right to die—quickly? *Journal of Paediatrics*, 1972; **80**: 905.
221. Editorial. The final autonomy. *The Lancet*, 1992; **340**: 757–8.
222. Cleeland CS, *et al.* Pain and its treatment in outpatients with metastatic cancer. *New England Journal of Medicine*, 1994; **330**: 592–6.
223. Foley KM. The relationship of pain and symptom management to patient requests for physician-assisted suicide. *Journal of Pain and Symptom Management*, 1991; **6**: 289–97.
224. Stjernsward J *et al.* Opioid availability in Latin America: the Declaration of Florianoloplis. *Journal of Palliative Care*, 1994; **10**: 11–14.
225. Vainio A. Treatment of terminal cancer pain in France: a questionnaire study. *Pain*, 1995; **62**: 155–62.
226. Rhymes J. Hospice care in America. *Journal of the American Medical Association*, 1990; **264**: 369–72.
227. Wank R, *et al.* Country Reports: status of cancer pain and palliative care in Argentina, Australia, Canada, China, Columbia, Costa Rica, Egypt, France, Germany, Greece, Hungary, India, Indonesia, Japan, Papua New Guina, Philippines, Singapore, Thailand, United States, and Vietnam. *Journal of Pain and Symptom Management*, 1993; **8/6**: 385–442.
228. Downing AB (ed.). *Euthanasia and the Right to Death.* London: Peter Owen, 1969: 23.
229. Miller FG *et al.* Regulating physician-assisted death. *New England Journal of Medicine*, 1994; **331**: 119–121.
230. Callahan D. Regulating physician-assisted death: to the Editor. *New England Journal of Medicine*, 1994; **331**: 1656.
231. Lynn J. Regulating physician-assisted death: to the Editor. *New England Journal of Medicine*, 1994; **331**: 1657.
232. Finlay IG, Gilbert J, Randall F. Regulating physician-assisted death: to the Editor. *New England Journal of Medicine,* 1994; **331**: 1657–8.
233. Billings JA, Block SD. Regulating physician-assisted death: to the Editor. *New England Journal of Medicine*, 1994; **331**: 1657.
234. Benrubi GI. Euthanasia—The need for procedural safeguards. *New England Journal of Medicine*, 1992; **326**: 197–9.
235. Morin E. *La Méthode. 1. La Nature de la Nature.* Paris: Éditions du Seuil, 1977: 365.
236. Blondin RJ, Szalay US, Knox RA. Should physicians aid their patients in dying? *Journal of the American Medical Association*, 1992; **267**: 2658–62.
237. Fein EB. Will the right to suicide become an obligation? *New York Times*, 1996; **April 7**: 24.
238. de Watcher MAM. Euthanasia in the Netherlands. *Hastings Center Report*, 1992; **22**: 29.
239. ten Have HAMJ, Welie JVM. Euthanasia: normal medical practice? *Hastings Center Report*, 1992; **22**: 34–8.
240. Grond S *et al.* Validation of World Health Organization guidelines for cancer pain relief during the last days and hours of life. *Journal of Pain and Symptom Management*, 1991; **6**: 411–22.
241. Fairbairn GJ. Kuhse, Singer and slippery slopes. *Journal of Medical Ethics*, 1988; **14**: 132–4.
242. Graham LR. Political ideology and genetic theory: Russia and Germany in the 1920's. *Hastings Center Report*, 1977; **7**: 30–9.
243. Fried C. Rights and health care—Beyond equity and efficiency. *New England Journal of Medicine*, 1975; **293**: 245.
244. Quill TE, Cassel CK, Meier D. Care of the hopelessly ill. Proposed criteria for physician assisted suicide. *New England Journal of Medicine*, 1992; **327**: 1380–4.
245. Brody H. Assisted death—A compassionate response to a medical failure. *New England Journal of Medicine*, 1992; **327**: 1384–8.

246. Miller TG, Fletcher JC. The case for legalized euthanasia. *Perspectives in Biology and Medicine*, 1993; **36**: 159–76.
247. Morin E. *La Méthode. 2. La Vie de la Vie.* Paris: Éditions du Seuil, 1980: 82.
248. Reichel W, Dyek AJ. Euthanasia: a contemporary moral quandary. *The Lancet*, 1989; **2**: 1321–3.
249. Lamb D. *Down the Slippery Slope: Arguing in Applied Ethics.* London: Croom Helm, 1988.
250. Friedlander H. *The Origins of Nazi Genocide. From Euthanasia to the Final Solution.* Chapel Hill, North Carolina and London: The University of North Carolina Press, 1995: xxii.
251. Binding K, Hoche A. *Die Freigabe der Vernichtung lebensunwerten Lebens: Ihr Mass und ihre Form.* Leipzig: F. Meiner, 1920. (Translation in: Permitting the destruction of unworthy life. *Issues in Law and Medicine*, 1992; **8**: 231–65).
252. Reference 251, pp. 54–5.
253. Friedlander H. *The Origins of Nazi Genocide. From Euthanasia to the Final Solution.* Chapel Hill, North Carolina and London: The University of North Carolina Press, 1995: 15.
254. Reference 251, pp. 29–32.
255. Reference 253, p. xi.
256. Müller-Hill B. *Murderous Science: Elimination by Scientific Selection of Jews, Gypsies, and Others, Germany, 1933–1945.* (Fraser GR, trans.). Oxford: Oxford University Press, 1988.
257. Lifton RJ. *The Nazi Doctors. Medical Killing and the Psychology of Genocide.* New York: Basic Books, 1986.
258. Burgess JA. The great slippery-slope argument. *Journal of Medical Ethics*, 1993; **19**: 169–74.
259. Govier T. What's wrong with slippery slope arguments? *Canadian Journal of Philosophy*, 1982; **12**: 303–16.
260. Van der Burg W. The slippery slope argument. *Ethics*, 1991; **102**: 42–65.
261. Williams B. Which slopes are slippery? In: Lockwood M. *Moral Dilemmas in Modern Medicine.* Oxford: Oxford University Press, 1985: 126–37.
262. Goodman N. *Languages of Art—An Approach to a Theory of Symbols.* Indianapolis: Hackett, 1976: 110–1.
263. Hendin H. Seduced by death: doctors, patients, and the Dutch care. *Issues in Law and Medicine*, 1994; **10**: 123–68.
264. CQ Interview. Arlene Judith Kotzko and Dr. Boudewijn Chabot discuss assisted suicide in the absence of somatic illness. *Cambridge Quarterly of Health Care Ethics*, 1995; **4**: 239–49.
265. Mead M. The right to die. *Nursing Outlook*, 1968; **16/10**: 20–2.
266. Mead M. Population: the need for an ethic. *Journal of Medical Education*, 1969; **44/11** (suppl. 2): 30–5.
267. Brahams D. Euthanasia: doctor convicted of attempted murder. *Lancet*, 1992; **340**: 782–3.
268. Lewis J. Doctor convicted of mercy killing. *Manchester Guardian Weekly*, 1992; **September 27**: 3.
269. Radcliffe Richards J. Excuses and euthanasia. *Manchester Guardian Weekly*, 1992; **September 27**: 3.
270. Lackland P, Widdrington C. Letters to the Editor: the conviction of Dr. Cox. *Manchester Guardian Weekly*, 1992; **October 4**: 2.
271. Woollacot M. Paying the price for insecurity. *Manchester Guardian Weekly*, 1994; **August 28**: 25.
272. Broch H. *The Death of Virgil.* San Francisco: North Point Press, 1983.
273. Steiner G. The hollow miracle. In: Steiner G. *Language and Silence. Essays on Language, Literature, and the Inhuman.* New York: Atheneum, 1982: 103.
274. Rowland KM, Jett JR, Jung SH, Loprinzi CL, Washburn JH, Shaw EG. Phase III randomized double-blind placebo-controlled trial of cisplatin and etoposide plus megestrol acetate/placebo in extensive stage small cell lung cancer: a North Central Cancer Treatment Group Study. *Proceedings of ASCO*, 1994; **13**:330.

4

Communication in palliative care: a practical guide

4 Communication in palliative care: a practical guide

Robert Buckman

Introduction: objectives of this chapter

Effective symptom control is impossible without effective communication. The most powerful analgesics will be of little value if health-care professionals do not have an accurate understanding of the patient's pain, and this can be obtained only by effective communication. Despite its cumbersome form, 'health-care professionals' is the only acceptable phrase that encompasses members of all health disciplines: doctors, nurses, social workers, psychologists, psychiatrists, chaplains, or any other. The words 'professional' and 'practitioner' are used interchangeably in this chapter to refer to this group. Almost invariably, the act of communication is an important part of the therapy: occasionally it is the only constituent. It usually requires greater thought and planning than a drug prescription, and unfortunately it is commonly administered in subtherapeutic doses.

There is no lack of published literature concerning the emotional and psychosocial needs of the dying patient[1-7] and the importance of communication as a major component of the delivery of all medical, and particularly palliative, care.[8-16] There is also some published work on the obstacles to, and the deficiencies in, communication between the dying patient and the health-care professional.[17-19] However, there is very little in the general medical literature that provides detailed practical assistance for the palliative care practitioner in improving his or her communication skills. The major objective herein is to remedy that omission, and to provide an intelligible and coherent approach to communication in a palliative care setting between professionals and their patients. Much of this material may be known to experienced professionals, but very little of it has previously been published or documented. The objectives of this chapter are, therefore, practical and pragmatic, and its somewhat unusual structure and style reflect that emphasis.

The details of communication can be considered under three headings.

1. **Basic listening skills;**
2. **The specific communication tasks of palliative care:**
   (a) breaking bad news;
   (b) therapeutic dialogue;
3. **Communicating with the family and with other professionals.**

However, before considering the details of doctor–patient communication, it is worthwhile undertaking a brief survey of the major obstacles to good communication with the dying patient. It is an undeniable fact that in our society any conversation about death and dying is awkward and difficult, and even more so when it occurs between doctor and patient. Some of that awkwardness is social and has its origins in the way society currently views death, some of it originates with the individual patient, and some originates with the professional, since our own professional training, while it prepares us to treat sick people, paradoxically leads us to lose touch with our own human skills when the medical treatment of the disease process fails.

In addition, there is no adequate working concept of the process of dying. Currently accepted systems do not provide a good working model of the transition from living to dying. Without such a conceptual framework or model to guide us, communication will always be suboptimal because we will be unable to understand or interpret what we are hearing, and will be unable to anticipate what may happen next, or to place the patient's feelings within the broader context of the dying process or of that individual's life and experience.

Therefore, the following two sections of this chapter will provide an overview of these issues, starting with a summary of the main areas of difficulty in discussing death and dying, and moving on to put forward a new three-stage concept of the process of dying which, it is hoped, will be of practical value to all practitioners in palliative care.

Sources of difficulty in communication with dying patients

Whatever the experience—or lack of it—of the health-care professional, a conversation with a dying patient almost always causes some degree of discomfort or awkwardness. It is important to recognize the fact that this discomfort is universal and is not the product of any personal fault or deficiency of the health-care professional. The major causes of this sense of unease originate long before the individual patient and the individual doctor begin the conversation. Therefore, a brief overview of the causes of that discomfort may have some value in relieving the sense of awkwardness, personal inadequacy, or even guilt which so commonly hinders communication in palliative care.

The sources of difficulty can be divided into three groups: first, those related to society (the social causes), second those related to the individual patients, and third those related to the health-care professional, arising from the professional's own social background and also from the professional's training—in medical school or nursing college for example.

The social denial of death

Contemporary society is going through a phase of virtual denial of death.[20] Such attitudes are probably cyclical, and we may now be seeing this denial phase beginning to fade. However, the price of the current attitude of denial or avoidance is paid by the person whose life is threatened and who has to face death, and by those who look after and support the patient—the family and the professionals. The major social roots of the contemporary fear of dying are discussed below.

Lack of experience of death in the family

Nowadays, most adults have not witnessed the death of a family member at home when they themselves were young and still forming their overall view of life. Whereas a century ago approximately 90 per cent of deaths occurred in the home, for the last few decades over 65 per cent (varying with regional demographics) occur in hospitals or institutions. This is associated with a change in family structure as the norm has changed from the extended family to the nuclear family. Thus, elderly people are less likely to be living with their grandchildren and are usually without young, fit relatives to support them at the time of their last illness. By the same token, a normal childhood and adolescence in contemporary society does not include a personal experience of death in the family occurring in the home.

Another factor in determining the place of most deaths is the rise and range of modern health services and the increase in facilities and treatments on offer. While these services undoubtedly offer advantages in medical and nursing care for the person dying in an institution, it means that there is disruption of family support for the patient as well as a lack of experience and understanding of the dying process for the surviving relatives.

This is not to imply that witnessing a death at home in the past was always a serene or tranquil experience. But even if a death at home was not a pleasant event, a child growing up in such a home would be imprinted with a sense of the continuity of life, the process of ageing and the natural inevitability of death ('when you are older you look like dad, when you are much older you look like grandad, when you are very very old you die'). As the extended family has disappeared, so dying has become the province of the health-care professional and/or institution; most people have lost that sense of continuity and now regard the process of dying as intrinsically alien and divorced from the business of living.

High expectations of health and life

Advances in medical sciences are often over-reported in the media and hailed as major breakthroughs. The constant bombardment of the public with news of apparently miraculous advances in the fight against disease subconsciously raises expectations of health and even offers tantalizing hopes of immortality. It, thus, becomes even harder for an individual to face the fact that he or she will not be cured despite the many miracles seen on television or in the papers.

Materialism

It is beyond the scope of a textbook to assess the materialist values of the modern world, except to point out that our society routinely evaluates a person's worth in terms of material and tangible values. This is our current social system of values and is neither good nor bad. However, it is universally accepted in our society that dying means being parted from material possessions. Hence, a society that places a high and almost exclusive value on material possessions implicitly increases the penalty of dying for its members.

The changing role of religion

The role of religion has changed, and the previously near-universal view of a single exterior anthropomorphic God is now fragmented and individualized. Religion is currently much more of an individual philosophical stance than it was in the last century, and it is no longer possible to assume that everyone shares the same idea of a God or of an after-life. Whereas a Victorian physician might have said to a patient 'Your soul will be with your Maker by the ebb-tide' and may have meant it genuinely as a statement of fact and of consolation, we cannot nowadays assume that such a statement will bring relief to all, or even most, patients.

For all these reasons, then, our society is passing through a phase of development during which the process of dying is perceived as alien and fearsome, and during which the dying person is separated and divided from the living. This increases the discomfort that surrounds any conversation about dying.

Patients' fears of dying

The fear of dying is not a single emotion. It can be composed of any or all of many individual fears, and it is probably true to say that every human being will have a different and unique combination of fears and concerns in facing the prospect of dying. An illustration of some of these is shown in Table 1. This concept of the patient's fear of dying has important implications for communication in palliative care. First, recognizing that fear of dying is not a single monolithic emotion should prompt the professional into eliciting from the patient the particular aspects of terminal illness that are uppermost in his or her mind. Thus, a patient's statement that he or she is afraid of dying should become the beginning of a dialogue, not the end of one.[21] Second, being aware that there are so many different aspects of dying that may cause fear will help the professional recognize some triggers of the patient's feelings. This recognition and the ensuing familiarity with the causes of fear often enhances the professional's ability to empathize with the patient and thus increases the value of his or her support.

Factors originating in the health care professional

As professionals in any health-care discipline we are subject to several sources of pressure that add to the discomfort caused by talking about dying. Some of these factors arise simply because we are human beings (albeit professionals whose behaviour has been ostensibly modified by training) and are in the presence of another person, the patient, who is in distress. Other factors arise from, or

Table 1 Common fears about dying

Fears about physical illness e.g. physical symptoms (such as pain, nausea), disability (paralysis, loss of mobility)
Fears about psychological effects e.g. not coping, 'breakdown', losing mind/dementia
Fears about dying e.g. existential fears, religious concerns
Fears about treatment e.g. fear of side-effects (baldness, pain), fears of surgery (pain, mutilation), fears about altered body image (surgery, colostomy, mastectomy)
Fears about family and friends e.g. loss of sexual attraction or sexual function, being a burden, loss of family role
Fears about finances, social status and job e.g. loss of job (breadwinner), possible loss of medical insurance with job, expenses of treatment, being 'out of the mainstream'

are amplified by, the same professional training that purports to prepare us for the death of our patients, but which usually has not. The following is a brief survey of the factors operating on the health-care professional (fuller discussions have been published elsewhere).[19,22]

Sympathetic pain

We are likely to experience considerable discomfort simply by being in the same room as a person who is going through the distress of facing death. This sympathetic pain may seem so patently obvious that it does not need to be stated, but it is often the case that professionals feel distressed by a painful interview and markedly underestimate the intensity of feeling that has originated from the patient. Commonly, and particularly with trainees and junior staff, a consideration of the intensity of the patient's distress leads to the realization that this was indeed the major source of the professional's stress. Until this is openly acknowledged, the professional may feel personally inadequate or guilty—another factor blocking good communication.

Fear of being blamed

As professionals we have a fear of being blamed that is partly justified. There are two main components of this fear.

First, if we are bearing bad news we are likely to be blamed for the news itself ('blaming the messenger for the message'). This is probably a basic human reaction to bad news and one with which we are all familiar in daily life (for instance, blaming a traffic-warden for writing out a parking ticket). We, thus, justifiably expect it when it is our role to bring bad news. Furthermore, many of the trappings of our profession (such as uniforms, jargon, ward rounds) help support the concept that we are in control of the situation. This may be valuable when the patient's condition is improving, but the same trappings increase the likelihood that we will become targets for blame when the patient's clinical condition begins to deteriorate.

Second, there is the concept imbued into us during our training that when a patient deteriorates or dies there must be somebody at fault. This attitude is strongly reinforced by medicolegal practice in which monetary sums are attached to deteriorations in health. For physicians, training in medical school inadvertently reinforces this feeling. Medical school education prepares doctors (appropriately) to deal with the myriad of reversible or treatable conditions (whether they are common or rare). However, there is usually little or no teaching on the subject of what to do when the disease cannot be reversed (hence, the need for this textbook). Most medical schools do not teach palliative medicine in the undergraduate curriculum and as a result most medical students evolve into physicians who are keen to treat the curable conditions and who have little training in what to do with chronic, irreversible diseases. This omission makes it even more difficult for the physician to deal with his or her own sense of therapeutic failure when communicating with the dying patient.[23]

Fear of the untaught

We also fear talking to a dying patient if we do not know how to do it properly. In all professional training, trainees are rewarded for doing a particular task 'properly'. In essence this means 'by following conventional procedures' and avoiding deviations from standard practice. While this is the accepted and justifiable norm for any procedure for which there are established guidelines, if it happens that there are no guidelines—as is the case with communicating with the dying—then the professional will naturally feel ill at ease and will show a tendency to avoid the area entirely.[24]

Fear of eliciting a reaction

In the same way in which, as professionals, we dislike doing tasks for which we have not been trained, we also avoid the side-effects or reactions caused by any intervention unless we have been taught how to cope with them.[25] It is an axiom of medical practice that we 'don't do anything unless you know what to do if it goes wrong'. If there has been no effective training in this form of interview,[26] there will also have been no training in dealing with complications or side-effects of these interviews (such as the patient becoming angry or bursting into tears). Not knowing how to cope with these reactions to the interview will further increase the aversion of an untrained person to communicating with a dying patient.[27]

Furthermore, interviews in which patients show emotional reactions may earn discouraging responses from other professionals. Although it is now less common than a few years ago, there are still senior physicians and senior nurses who think it is a bad thing to 'get the patient all upset'. It should be an obvious fact (but it is often ignored) that if you have had an interview about a patient's grave prognosis and if the patient, for example, bursts into tears, it is not the interview that has caused the tears but the medical situation.

Fear of saying 'I don't know'

No matter what discipline we are trained in, health-care professionals are never rewarded for saying 'I don't know'. In all training, and particularly in examinations, we expect our standing to be diminished if we confess that we do not know all the answers. In everyday clinical practice, by contrast, any honesty shown by the professional strengthens the relationship, increases trust, and encourages honesty from the patient in return. Conversely, attempts to 'flannel' or 'snow' the patient, or attempts to disguise ignorance or to pretend greater knowledge or experience weaken the bond between the patient and the doctor or nurse and discourage honest dialogue. Thus, our fears of displaying our ignorance—appropriate in examinations but not in clinical practice—make communication increasingly difficult when the answers are unknown and, often, unknowable.

Fear of expressing emotions

We are also encouraged and trained to hide and suppress our own emotions (more true of medical students than of nursing students or trainees in other disciplines). It is, of course, essential for truly professional behaviour that we do not show such emotions as irritation or panic (or that we try not to show them). However, while we are being trained not to show panic or rage, inadvertently we are being encouraged to envisage the ideal doctor as one who never shows any emotions and is consistently calm and brave. While that is not necessarily a bad paradigm for a doctor dealing with emergencies or reversible crises, it is unhelpful in the palliative care setting. When a patient is facing death, a professional who expresses no emotions is likely to be perceived as cold or insensitive.

Ambiguity of the phrase 'I'm sorry'

Even if we want to show some human sympathy, the moment we begin there are some linguistic problems that threaten to create further difficulties. Most of us do not realize that the word 'sorry' has two quite distinct meanings. It can be a form of sympathy ('I am sorry for you') and can also be a form of apology accepting responsibility for an action ('I am sorry that I did this'). Unfortunately both are customarily abbreviated to 'I am sorry'. This reflex abbreviation can commonly lead to misunderstanding, for example:

A. . . . and then my mother was brought into hospital.

B. Oh, I am sorry.

A. You've got nothing to be sorry for.

The first speaker is so used to hearing the word 'sorry' as an apology, that she or he responds with a reflex reply to an apology before realizing that it was not an apology that was being offered, but an expression of sympathy. This has relevance to all of us as professionals. Not only is it difficult for us to overcome some of our trained responses in order to express our own emotions of sympathy and empathy, but the moment we try to do so, we fall foul of a linguistic slip and appear to be accepting responsibility (with the associated medicolegal implications) instead of offering support. (The solution to this ambiguity lies in paying careful attention to your own speech patterns: make sure that if you want to say 'I am sorry' you use the specific words 'I am sorry for you'.)

Own fears of illness/death

Most of us have some degree of fear about our own deaths—perhaps more so than the general population.[28] In fact, some psychologists would suggest that the desire to deny one's own mortality and vulnerability to illness is a component of every health-care professional's desire to be a doctor or nurse. This is sometimes called counter-phobic behaviour, and means in real terms that each time we go into an encounter with a sick person and emerge from the encounter unharmed we are reinforcing our own illusions of immortality and invulnerability. If this is indeed a major constituent of the desire to be a health-care professional, then it might lead to avoidance of those situations in which those illusions are challenged.[29] Hence the professional's own fear of dying will lead to avoidance or block of any communication with the dying patient.

Fear of the medical hierarchy

Finally, there is the discomforting fact that not all professionals think of these issues as important, perhaps because of their own fears of illness and death, or fears of the untaught and so on. A junior member of a medical team may, thus, be under pressure from a senior staff member when trying to hold conversations with patients about dying. In more old-fashioned hierarchical systems (in the United Kingdom in the 1960s for instance) it was quite possible for a senior physician to state 'no patient of mine is ever to be told that they have cancer'. Nowadays that stance is less tenable for ethical and legal reasons, but there are still occasional instances of this attitude which then make it difficult to respond to the patient's desire for information and support. (Fortunately, this problem has a solution since in any circumstances, however adverse, the health-care professional can always perform advocacy and transmit the patient's questions and reactions and knowledge or suspicions upwards to the senior person concerned.)

The stages of dying—a new conceptual framework

An appraisal of the five-stage model of the process of dying

The Kubler-Ross staging system of dying—which divides the process of dying into five consecutive stages termed denial, anger, bargaining, depression, and acceptance—has achieved considerable professional and public attention and is widely thought to be the only appropriate model of dying.[30] Within the community of palliative care practitioners, however, this staging system is often regarded as a model with many flaws and deficiencies,[31] requiring some modification, and alternatives have been put forward (for an overview see Rando[32]). Without demeaning the considerable achievement of Kubler-Ross in devising the system, and in considering the process of dying as a transition in the first place, it does seem that an alternative framework can be put forward which more accurately reflects the dying patient's progress and which will allow the professional greater power of analysis and prediction.

The major flaws in the Kubler-Ross five-stage system can be considered under two headings—first, deficiencies in the overall concept itself, and second, several reactions to dying which are seen commonly in clinical practice but are not included in the five-stage schema.

Some deficiencies of the five-stage system

In the very concept of stages numbered 'first' through to 'fifth' (even with the caveat that patients do not behave in sequence and may dart back and forth) there is a central flaw. It seems closer to reality to conceive human emotions not as serial and universal, but as idiosyncratic (characteristic of the individual) and simultaneous. When confronted with any serious threat, particularly the prospect of dying, each individual exhibits reactions that are characteristic of that person and of the way in which that person has reacted to difficulties in the past, not of the stage in the process or the diagnosis.

We all develop our own in-built repertoire of emotions as we grow up (subject presumably to our experiences in childhood and other factors). Thus, some individuals are easily roused to anger and others are not. Some greet every reverse or trouble by turning their backs and shutting it out—others face it directly and wish to know the worst possible outcome as early as they can. Each of us, therefore, carries with us our personal internal palette of emotions from which we pick our own emotional reactions. These are not in fact stages of a universal process but are the essential components of the emotional side of that person's character. It is more useful, then, to view the emotions or responses exhibited by the patient facing death as sources of insight into that individual and not indicators of the stage that he or she is passing through.

Further, those emotions are usually exhibited simultaneously, not serially. A common example of simultaneous responses to stress is what happens when a parent loses a child temporarily in a supermarket and then finds the child again. At the moment of reunion, the parent experiences relief, guilt, happiness, anger (at both child and self), fear (at what might have happened), and regret. These emotions, some of which are conflicting, occur simultaneously and are not consecutive stages. This is a useful analogy to what happens to a person facing the prospect of dying. Denial and anger, for example, are often experienced at the same time. A patient may easily be angry with the disease but may express the anger as resentment at the doctor while simultaneously exhibiting denial (in, for instance, accusing the doctor of making a mistake in the diagnosis). Intellectually, these emotions are incompatible (how can one be angry at something whose very existence is being denied?) but in the reality of human emotions they frequently coexist.

It is, therefore, more useful to view the patient's emotions as a mosaic, comprising different personal emotions often expressed simultaneously, but in a pattern that is a feature of that individual. By contrast, in the Kubler-Ross staging system, the patient is seen as a chameleon, changing from one emotion to another as he or she progresses through the stages (albeit with the caveats stated in the original work about the sequence and inconsistency of individual patient's reactions).

Thus the first, second, and fourth stages of dying (denial, anger, and depression) can be more usefully considered as reactions to dying experienced by some patients, but not all, and which are exhibited (in those patients who experience them) not serially but simultaneously. It is also likely that the third stage in the five-stage system (bargaining) is a false entity. Bargaining is more usefully viewed as an attempt by the patient to construct a rational link between a hope and a fear. ('I hope that my disease will respond to chemotherapy, I fear that it will not respond—therefore if I promise to perform actions X and Y, perhaps what I hope for will occur.') Bargaining is more usefully considered, then, as an individual strategy for coping and not as a universal or even common stage in the dying process.

Emotions and responses missing from the five-stage system

While there are paradigmatic problems with the five stages of the Kubler-Ross system there are also several responses to dying which are seen commonly in palliative care practice and which the system does not include. The most obvious omission is fear. Fear of dying is so universal[20] that if a particular patient does not exhibit it, the professional's first thought should be 'has this patient understood the situation?'. There are the rare individuals who are so comfortable and well-balanced in their lives that they can face the end of life with perfect equanimity and without any fear at any stage of the process. Such instances are extremely uncommon and any attempt to describe the process of dying should include some mention of fear within the model.

Second, there is guilt which is seen commonly, and is quite often expressed with great force and with considerable influence on the patient's state. Guilt is not universal, but it is undoubtedly common enough to be accommodated in any practical framework that relates to the clinical picture.

Third, it is a common occurrence in palliative care that a patient experiences hope and despair as alternating emotions, replacing each other on a cyclical basis. It is as if hope and despair were mutually exclusive emotional reactions to the same data. Thus, if a patient's condition has a 40 per cent chance of responding to therapy, on one day the patient might hope and feel that she or he is in that fortunate 40 per cent and will improve. The following day, the same patient may feel that she or he is in the unlucky 60 per cent. The facts have not changed, but the patient's emotional response to those facts has altered. Unless one sees hope and despair as mutually displacing emotional reactions, there will be great difficulty in tracking the patient's progress.

Another response that is seen very commonly but which is missing from the five-stage system is humour. Humour is commonly used by some patients to maintain a sense of perspective in the face of potentially overwhelming news. It is an individual coping strategy that, like denial defends the ego and reinforces the central personality of the patient when external forces threaten it. Humour during grave illness is usually only used by those who have habitually used it as a coping strategy in their past, but it is certainly important enough to warrant consideration in any conceptual system of the dying process.

A three-stage model of the process of dying

A better approximation of common clinical experience can be obtained with a different staging system. The three-stage system (detailed at greater length elsewhere[22,33]) is based on two central principles.

1. Patients facing death exhibit a mixture of reactions and response which are characteristic of the patient, not of the diagnosis or the stage of the dying process.

2. Progress through the dying process is marked, not by a change in the type or nature of emotions, but by resolution of the resolvable elements of those emotions.

The system proposed here divides the process of dying into three stages—the initial stage, the chronic stage, and the final stage.

The initial stage is defined as starting when the patient first faces the possibility of dying from his or her disease, not as an abstract concept but as a concrete reality. At that stage, popularly termed 'facing the threat', the patient may show a combination of

Table 2 The three-stage model of the dying process

Initial stage ('facing the threat')	Chronic stage ('being ill')	Final stage ('acceptance')
A mixture of reactions which are characteristic of the individual and which may include any, or all, of: Fear Anxiety Shock Disbelief Anger Denial Guilt Humour Hope/despair Bargaining	1. Resolution of those elements of the initial response which are resolvable 2. Diminution of intensity of all emotions ('monochrome state') 3. Depression is very common	1. Defined by the patient's acceptance of death 2. Not an essential state provided that the patient is not distressed, is communicating normally, and is making decisions normally

emotional responses which represents that person's individual recipe of coping strategies and reactions. For instance, individuals who have met every stress with anger will exhibit anger now and patients who have always used denial will use denial at this stage. That mixture may be selected from any of the emotions listed in Table 2.

The middle or chronic stage ('being ill') follows the initial stage as the patient resolves those elements of the initial reactions that are resolvable (with or without assistance). It is the process of resolution that identifies the second stage, not a change in the emotions themselves. A few patients do not achieve any resolution of their emotions and remain with unmodified reactions until the end of their lives. In such patients, the chronic stage does not exist and the total absence of any form of resolution should prompt the professional to seek help for that patient. For the patients that do achieve some resolution, the intensity of their emotional responses diminishes but the nature of those feelings usually does not. This phase is, therefore, marked by the beginnings of what will later develop, in many patients, into acceptance.

An important characteristic of the second stage is depression. Often the patient may be functioning with high emotional intensity in the first stage and may be surrounded by friends and relatives who have equally intense responses (both helpful and unhelpful). As the dying process continues and as the most intense emotions diminish, the patient and family often experience an almost anticlimactic sense of depression. This was most perceptively identified by one patient 'as if my life was now being photographed in monochrome'. At this time, the patient is aware that he or she is going to die from this disease, but that death is not imminent. The patient is likely to become withdrawn and may appear apathetic and depressed. It is during this period that the patient may require more support from the professional (as well as from relatives and friends).

The third stage is defined (as in the five-stage system) by acceptance. It should be noted that many practitioners in palliative care believe that acceptance is helpful but not an absolute necessity.[34] A few patients die without ever overtly acknowledging the imminence of their death, and if they are not distressed by this, if they are communicating normally with friends and family, and are able to function and to make decisions normally (for example concerning their treatment or social arrangements) then there seems to be no rationale for intervening and forcing acceptance on them.

The potential value of this model

It is, of course, impossible to prove definitively that the system set out here is a closer approximation to the dying process or is a more useful framework than the five-stage system. There are no objective data available to support either and it is virtually impossible to envisage any studies that could achieve this. The only criterion by which a staging system can be assessed is its pragmatic utility. If the three-stage system helps the professional to understand what she or he is hearing from the patient, to respond with greater sensitivity, to provide more effective support, and to predict what is most likely to occur next, then it will have proved its worth.

A practical guide to communication in palliative care

This section will provide a series of practical steps that can be taken by any health care professional to make her or his communication more effective. First there is a summary of general listening skills which are essential for all professional–patient interviews, not just those in palliative care. Next, the two most common tasks of palliative care—breaking bad news and therapeutic (or supportive) dialogue—are discussed. The criteria by which the patient's response can be assessed, together with some suggestions for resolving conflict are considered. Finally some guidelines for improving communication between health-care professionals and family, and between different health care disciplines are offered.

Basic listening skills for palliative care

All medical interviews, and particularly those with a dying patient, contain the potential for going wrong. Often the seeds of failure are sown in the first few minutes. Even though readers of this textbook may already be familiar with the rules of effective listening it is worth stressing them again since under the pressure of a difficult interview it is often the simplest omissions that cause the biggest problems.[35] Furthermore, patients are more likely to disclose their understanding of their medical situation to those staff who demonstrate that they are prepared to listen and discuss.[36]

The basic listening skills that are most crucial in palliative care may be considered under the headings of physical context, facilitation techniques, and the empathic response. (For a general review of interviewing skills see Lipkin *et al.*[37])

Physical context

The physical context of an interview sends important signals to the patient even before verbal communication begins.[38] It is, therefore, extremely important to observe with particular care the usual rules of good interviewing. A few seconds spent establishing the physical context may save many minutes of frustration (for both the professional and the patient). The rules are not complex but are often omitted in the heat of the moment.[39] Although privacy is difficult to obtain in institutions, consider the patient's dignity and ensure that trenchant conversations of great import are carried out in a private setting if at all possible.

Introductions

Ensure that the patient knows who you are and what you do. Many practitioners, including the author, make a point of shaking the patient's hand but this is a matter of personal preference. Often the handshake tells you something about the family dynamics as well as about the patient. Frequently the patient's spouse will also extend his (or her) hand. It is worthwhile making sure that you shake the patient's hand before that of the spouse (even if the spouse is nearer) in order to demonstrate that the patient comes first, and the spouse (although an important member of the team) comes second.

Sit down

This is an almost inviolable rule. It is virtually impossible to assure a patient that she or he has your undivided attention and that you intend to listen seriously if you remain standing up. Only if it is absolutely impossible to sit should you try and hold a medical interview while standing. Occasionally, in hospitals or hospices, the only available seat is a commode. If so, it is worth asking permission to sit and then saying that you are aware of what you are sitting on to reduce embarrassment. Whatever you sit on, the result will be better than if you remain standing.

Clinical impressions (B. Mount, personal communication) suggest that when the doctor sits down, the patient perceives the period of time spent at the bedside as longer than if the doctor remains standing. Thus, not only does the act of sitting down indicate to the patient that he or she has control and that you are there to listen, but it also saves time and increases efficiency.

Next, get the patient organized if necessary. If you have just finished examining the patient, allow or help him or her to dress and to restore the sense of personal modesty.

Then, get any physical objects out of the way. Move any bedside tables, trays, or other impedimenta out of the line between you and the patient. Ask for any televisions or radios to be turned off for a few minutes. If you are in an office or room, move your chair so that you are adjacent to the patient not across the desk. If you find the action embarrassing, state what you are doing ('It may be easier for us to talk if I move the table/if you turn the television off for a moment').

Your body language

It is important to be seated at a comfortable distance from the patient. This distance (sometimes called the 'body buffer zone') seems to vary from culture to culture, but a distance of 50 to 90 cm will usually serve the purpose for intimate and personal conversation.[40] This is another reason why the doctor who remains standing at the end of the bed ('six feet away and three feet up' known colloquially as 'the British position') seems remote and aloof.

The height at which you sit can also be important; normally your eyes should be approximately level with the patient's. If the patient is already upset or angry, a useful technique is to sit so that you are below the patient, with your eyes at a lower level. This often decreases the anger. It is best to try and look relaxed, particularly if that is not the way you feel. To achieve an air of relaxation, sit down comfortably with both your feet flat on the floor. Let your shoulders relax and drop. Undo your coat or jacket if you are wearing one, and rest your hands on your knees.

Touching the patient

Most of us have not been taught specific details of clinical touch at any time in our training.[41] We are, therefore, likely to be ill at ease with touching as an interview technique until we have had some practice. Nevertheless there is considerable evidence (although the data are somewhat 'soft') that touching the patient (particularly above the patient's waist to avoid misinterpretation) is of benefit during a medical interview, even though patients may not expect to be touched the first time that they meet the physician.[42] It seems likely that touching is a significant action in the context of palliative care and should be encouraged, with the proviso that the professional should be very sensitive to the patient's reaction. If the patient is comforted by the contact, continue: if the patient is uncomfortable, stop. Touch can be misinterpreted (as lasciviousness, aggression, or dominance for example) so be aware that touching is an interviewing skill that requires extra self-regulation.

Facilitation techniques

As dialogue begins, the professional should show that she or he is in 'listening mode'. This is the fundamental interviewing skill known as facilitating. The most important guidelines to good facilitation are listed below.

Let the patient speak

If the patient is speaking, don't talk over him or her. Wait for the patient to stop speaking before you start your next sentence. This, the simplest rule of all, is that most often ignored, and is most likely to give the patient the impression that the doctor is not listening.[43]

Encourage the patient to talk

You can use any or all of the following gestures: nodding, pauses, smiling, saying 'Yes', 'Mmm hmm', 'Tell me more', or anything similar. Maintain eye contact for most of the time while the patient is talking (sometimes if things are very intense it may be helpful to the patient for you to look away briefly).

Tolerate short silences

Silences are important and revealing.[44] Usually, a patient will fall silent when he or she has feelings that are too intense to express in words. A silence, therefore, means that the patient is thinking or feeling something important, not that he or she has stopped thinking. If you can tolerate a pause or silence, the patient may well express the thought in words a moment later. If you have to break the silence, the ideal way to do so is to say 'What were you thinking about just then?' or 'What is it that's making you pause?', or something to that effect.[45]

Having encouraged the patient to speak, it is necessary to prove that you are hearing what is being said. The following techniques enhance your ability to demonstrate this.

Repetition and reiteration

Repetition is probably the single most important technique of all interviewing skills (apart from sitting down). To show that you are really hearing what the patient is saying, use one or two key words from the patient's last sentence in your own first one. Reiteration means repeating what the patient has told you but in your words, not hers or his. If the patient says 'Since I started those new tablets, I've been feeling sleepy' a response such as 'You seem to be getting some drowsiness from the tablets' is reiterative (using the word 'drowsiness' where the patient said 'sleepy') and confirms to the patient that she or he has been heard.

Reflection

Reflection, the restating of the patient's statement in terms of what it means to the listener, takes the act of listening one step further, and shows that you have heard and have interpreted what the patient said. (For example 'If I understand you correctly, you're telling me that you lose control of your waking and sleeping when you're on these tablets . . .'.)

The empathic response

The empathic response is an extremely useful technique in an emotionally-charged interview, and yet is frequently misunderstood by students and trainees. There are three essential components of the empathic response.

(a) identifying the emotion that the patient is experiencing;

(b) identifying the origin and root cause of that emotion;

(c) responding in a way that tells the patient that you have made the connection between (a) and (b).

Often the most effective empathic responses follow the format of 'You seem to be . . .' or 'It must be . . .'; for example 'It must be very distressing for you to know that all that therapy didn't give you a long remission'. The objective of the empathic response is to demonstrate that you have identified and acknowledged the emotion that the patient is experiencing, and by doing so you are giving it legitimacy as an item on the patient's agenda. In fact, if the patient is experiencing a strong emotion (rage or crying, for example) you must acknowledge the existence of that emotion or all further attempts at communication will fail. If strong emotions are not acknowledged in some way, you will be perceived as insensitive and this will render the rest of the interaction useless.

In making an empathic response, however, you do not necessarily have to feel the emotion yourself—you do not have to 'cry and bleed for every patient'. In fact, if you experience the same emotion as the patient, your feelings are termed sympathetic rather than empathic (see under sympathetic pain above). It is therefore possible to formulate an empathic response for all your patients, provided that you identify and acknowledge the feelings that they are describing.

Table 3 Six-step protocol for breaking bad news

1. Getting the physical context right
2. Finding out how much the patient knows
3. Finding out how much the patient wants to know
4. Sharing information (aligning and educating)
5. Responding to the patient's feelings
6. Planning and following through

Two specific tasks of communication in palliative care

Communication in palliative care is important from the moment that the patient first meets a palliative care professional until the last moment of life. Most significant conversations in palliative care comprise two major elements: one in which medical information is transmitted to the patient ('bearing the news'), and the other in which the dialogue centres around the patient's feelings and emotions and in which the dialogue itself is a therapeutic action ('therapeutic or supportive dialogue'). In practice most conversations are a mixture of the two, although commonly there is more medical information transmitted in the early conversations shortly after starting palliative care, and there is usually a greater need for therapeutic dialogue in the later stages.

For the purposes of clarity, the two components will be considered separately.

Breaking bad news

In palliative care, there are many occasions when new medical information needs to be discussed. This is almost universal when the patient is first assessed in palliative care, and is quite common later on. Hence it is essential to have a logical and systematic approach to the sharing of medical information.[46] The following protocol has been detailed at greater length elsewhere.[22] In practice, it has been found to be useful in all interviews concerning bad news, whether the patient and the professional know each other well or not. However, formal studies of this protocol (or any other) have not been carried out, and even the design of such investigations pose major difficulties.[47] It consists of six steps or phases, which are summarized in Table 3.

Physical context

The physical context of the interview has already been reviewed. It is of even greater importance for the interview in which bad news is shared than for any other.

Finding out how much the patient knows or suspects

It is always important to obtain directly from the patient an impression of what he or she already knows about the seriousness of the medical condition and about its effect on the future before providing further information. In fact, sharing information may be awkward, superfluous, or even impossible without first knowing what the patient already knows.[48] In all cases, you should be trying to establish what the patient knows about the impact of the illness on his or her future, not about the fine details of basic pathology or nomenclature of the diagnosis. There are many ways in which this information can be gathered. Some of the phrases that may be useful include:

'What have you made of the illness so far?'

'What did the previous doctors tell you about the illness/operation etc?'

'Have you been worried about yourself?'

'When you first had symptom X, what did you think it might be?'

'What did Dr X tell you when he sent you here?'

'Did you think something serious was going on when . . .?'

As the patient replies, analyse the response. Important information can be obtained from three major features of the reply.

The factual content of the patient's statements

It must be established how much the patient has understood, and how close to the medical reality is the impression. Some patients may at this point say that they have been told nothing at all. This may or may not be true, but even if you know it to be false, accept the patient's statement as a symptom of denial and do not confront it immediately. First, the patient may be about to request information from you, and may, in part deliberately, deny previous information to see if you tell the same story. Second, if the patient has previously been given information, you are unlikely to appear supportive to a patient in denial by immediate confrontation.

In fact, a patient denying previous information quite often precipitates anger or resentment on the professional's part ('My goodness, doesn't Dr Smythe tell his patients what he found at the operation!'). If you find yourself feeling this, pause and think. You may be seeing a patient in denial and this may be causing you to suffer from the professional syndrome known as the 'nobody-ever-tells-their-patients-anything-until-I-do' syndrome. It is very common when patients are sick and the emotional atmosphere is highly charged.

The style of the patient's statements

Much can be gleaned from the patient's emotional state, educational level, and articulational ability by the manner in which she or he is speaking. Listen to the vocabulary, the kind of words being said, and the kind of words being avoided. Note the style so that when you come to speak, you can start at the right level.

You should, however, ignore the patient's profession in making this assessment, particularly if he or she happens to be a member of a health-care profession. Far too often you will find yourself making assumptions. Even physicians when they are patients may not be experts in their own disease and may not understand something like 'It's only a Stage II but I don't like the mitotic index' when they hear it as a patient.

Emotional content of the patient's statements

There are two major sources of these—verbal and non-verbal. Both may yield information about the patient's state, and discordance between the two (for instance, apparent calm in the speech, but major anxiety in the body language) may give valuable signals regarding state and motivation.

Finding out how much the patient wants to know

This is the single most crucial step in any information-giving discussion. It is far easier to proceed with giving the news if there is a clear invitation from the patient to do so. Conversely, although it is universally acknowledged that in contemporary society patients have a right to truth and information,[49,50] it is often impossible to predict which patients will not want to hear the truth[51] (for fuller reviews see Billings and Reiser[52,53]). The exact proportion of patients who do want full disclosure varies from study to study, but current figures range from 50 to 98.5 per cent depending on patient demographics and the diagnosis suspected[51,54–57] (for a detailed review see McIntosh[58]). Since no characteristics predict whether a patient desires disclosure,[54] it seems logical simply to ask him or her.[59] The way in which this important and sensitive question is phrased is largely a matter of personal style. Some examples are given below.

Are you the kind of person who likes to know exactly what's going on?

Would you like me to tell you the full details of the diagnosis?

Are you the kind of person who likes the full details of what's wrong—or would you prefer just to hear about the treatment plan?

Do you like to know exactly what's going on or would you prefer me to give you the outline only?

Would you like me to tell you the full details of your condition—or is there somebody else that you'd like me to talk to?

Note that in all of these, if the patient does not want to hear about the full details you have not cut off all lines of communication. You are saying overtly that you will maintain contact and communication (for example about the treatment plan) but not about the details of the disease. If the patient does not want to hear the information, you should add that if, at any time in the future, the patient changes her or his mind and wants further information, you will provide it. The phrase '. . . the sort of person who' is particularly valuable because it suggests to the patient that there are many patients like him or her, and that if he or she prefers not to discuss the information, this is neither unique, nor a sign of extraordinary feebleness or lack of courage.

Sharing medical information

The process by which medical information is transmitted can be thought of as consisting of two crucial steps.

Aligning

At this point in the interview, you have already heard how much the patient knows about the situation, and something of the vocabulary used to express it. This is the starting point for sharing the information. Reinforce those parts which are correct (using the patient's words if possible) and proceed from there. It gives the patient a great deal of confidence in himself or herself (as well as in you) to realize that his or her view of the situation has been listened to and is being taken seriously (even if it is being modified or corrected).

This process has been called 'aligning';[46,60] a useful term to describe the process by which you line up the information you wish to impart on the baseline of the patient's current knowledge. (Maynard uses the word 'aligning' to describe one particular style of doctor–patient communication.[60] The meaning has been extended in this schema to describe the first part of the information-sharing process.)

Educating
In the next phase of the interview, having started from the patient's starting point (i.e. having aligned your information on the patient's original position) you now have to bring his or her perception of the situation closer to the medical facts as you know them.

There is no word in current usage that fully describes this part of the interview, but perhaps 'educating' is the closest. The process of sharing information should be a gradual one in which the patient's perception is steadily shifted until it is in close approximation to the medical reality. This part of the interview can usefully be compared to steering an oil tanker. You cannot make sudden lurches and expect the patient's perception to change instantly. You have to apply a slow and steady guidance over the direction of the interview, observing the responses as you do so. In the process, you build upon those responses from the patient that are bringing him or her closer to the facts, and emphasize the relevant medical information if it becomes apparent that the patient is moving away from an accurate perception of the situation. The key ingredients are steady observation and continued gentle guidance of the direction of the interview rather than sudden lurches.

Give information in small amounts: the warning shot
Medical information is hard for patients to digest and more so if it concerns a grave prognosis or threat of death. Recall of information is poor at the best of times and likely to be very poor if medical facts are grim ('The moment you said 'cancer', doctor, . . . I couldn't remember a thing from that moment on . . .'). The rule is, therefore, give the information in small amounts.

One of the most useful principles is the idea of 'the warning shot'. If there is clearly a large gap between the patient's expectations and the reality of the situation, you can facilitate understanding by giving a warning that things are more serious than they appear ('well, the situation was more serious than that . . .') and then grading the information, gradually introducing the more serious prognostic points, waiting for the patient to respond at each stage.[61,62]

Use English
Technical jargon ('medspeak') is an efficient language for transmitting codified information in a short time. Since it takes many years to learn, it is also comforting to the professional. However, the patients have not learned to speak it and cannot express their emotions in it; hence it reinforces the barrier between patient and professional, and is most likely to make the former feel angry, belittled, and isolated. We should avoid jargon if we are trying to support the patient at a difficult time.

Check reception frequently
Check that your message is being received—and check frequently.[63] You can use any phrase that feels comfortable—anything to break the monologue. Examples are:

Am I making sense?

Do you follow what I'm saying?

Does this all seem sensible to you?

This must be a bit bewildering, but do you follow roughly what I'm saying?

Do you see what I mean?

These interjections serve several important functions: (a) they demonstrate that it matters to you if the patient doesn't understand what you are saying; (b) they allow the patient to speak (many patients feel so bewildered or shocked that their voices seem to seize up, and they need encouragement and prompting to speak); (c) they allow the patient to feel an element of control over the interview; (d) they validate the patient's feelings and make them legitimate subjects for discussion between you.

You should also check that you are transmitting the information at the same intellectual level as the patient is receiving it, by ensuring that your vocabulary and that of the patient are similar.

Reinforce the information frequently
There are several ways in which you can reinforce what you are telling the patient.

1. Get the patient to repeat the general drift of what you have been saying.

2. Repeat important points yourself: because it is difficult to retain information, particularly if the news is serious, and even more so if denial is operating, you may have to repeat crucial points several times. Accept this as a fact of life when looking after seriously ill patients (you can cover this with a phrase such as 'I know it's difficult to remember all this stuff at one go . . .').

3. Use diagrams and written messages. A few simple scribbles on the back of an envelope or a scrap of paper may serve as a useful *aide-memoire*.

Blend your agenda with that of the patient
While transmitting information to the patient, it is important to elicit his or her agenda or 'shopping list' of concerns and anxieties, so that further information can be tailored to answer major problems. The following are useful guidelines.

Elicit the 'shopping list' Quite often the patient's major concerns are not the same as those of the professional. For instance, patients may be more worried about severe pain or loss of mental functioning, than about the primary disease itself (see above). You do not necessarily have to deal with the items at that particular moment, but you should indicate that you understand what the patient is talking about and will return to it in a moment. ('I know you're very worried about drowsiness, and I'll come to that in a moment, but can I first cover the reasons that we recommend increasing the painkillers in the first place?').

Listen for the buried question Deep personal worries may not emerge easily. Sometimes the patient asks questions while you are talking. These questions ('buried questions') are often highly significant to the patient. When the patient does this, finish your own sentence and then ask the patient what he or she was saying. Be prepared to follow that train of thought from the patient—it is quite likely to be important.

Be prepared to be led Quite often you may draw an interview to a close and then find that the patient wants to start part of it again.

This is not simply contrary behaviour. It often stems from fear and insecurity; by restarting the interview the patient is exerting some measure of control.

Responding to the patient's feelings

In many respects the patient's reactions to his or her medical condition, and the professional's response to those reactions, define their relationship and determine whether or not it offers support for the patient. Hence, the professional's ability to understand and respond sensitively to the emotions expressed by the patient are central to all communication in palliative care. In essence, this part of the communication becomes therapeutic (or supportive) dialogue.

In the short space of this chapter it is not possible to illustrate the wide range of patients' reactions to dying or to bad news in general. However, a detailed analysis has been published elsewhere,[22] together with several options available to the professional in each situation. The central components of the professional's response are (a) assessment of the response and (b) empathic responses from the professional. For the sake of convenience, these two topics are discussed under the heading of therapeutic dialogue below.

Organizing and planning

The sixth and final step in the breaking bad news protocol is the stage at which the professional summarizes the situation and makes an operational plan and a contract for the future. This process is of great importance to the patient, and is a process that should conclude every interview with a palliative care patient, not just an interview in which bad news is discussed.

Frequently, after hearing news that is new or distressing, the patient may feel bewildered, dispirited, and disorganized. While the professional should be sensitive to those emotions and be capable of empathy, our responsibilities consist of more than simply reflecting the patient's emotions. The patient is looking to us to make sense of any confusion and to offer plans for the future. At this point in the interview, therefore, it is important to try to put together what is known of the patient's agenda, the medical scenario, the plan of management, and a contract for the future. This process can be logically divided into six tasks.

Demonstrate an understanding of the patient's problem list

If the interview has been effective so far, this is what you have been achieving since the beginning. From the outset, you have been demonstrating that you have been hearing what bothers the patient most, and a brief 'headline' reference to the major concerns of the patient reinforces the fact that you have been listening.

Indicate that you can distinguish the 'fixable' from the 'unfixable'

With both medical problems and psychosocial problems, some are 'fixable' and some are not. We shall be discussing this further in relation to the patient's responses in the next section but it is a pragmatic step without which your support will appear to be less effective. If the interview gets stuck or bogged down as the patient explores her or his problems, it is often helpful to try to enumerate the problems as a list, getting the patient to arrange them in order of priority. You can then begin to set your own agenda—stating the problems you are going to try and tackle first. This leads logically to the next step.

Make a plan or strategy and explain it

When making a plan for the future, it is quite permissible for that plan to include many uncertainties, 'don't knows', and choices ('if the dizziness doesn't get better, then we'll . . .'), acknowledging that uncertainty is often a painful and difficult state to cope with.[64] What you are actually doing is presenting a decision-tree or algorithm. Patients need to know that you have some plan in mind—even if it consists of little more than 'we'll deal with each problem as it arises'—which, at least, implies that you will not abandon the patient. The act of making a plan and explaining it to the patient is part of what the patient sees as support—it defines the immediate future of your relationship with this particular patient and reinforces the individuality of this person and what you are going to do for him or her.

Identify coping strategies of the patient and reinforce them

There is a lot of emphasis in our training on what we do to patients or for patients. Obviously in acute emergencies the professionals have to do all of the work. However, this attitude of 'we will do it all for you' may influence the professional's approach to all patients in every situation, particularly if the patient is feeling overwhelmed and helpless in the face of bad news. This may be bad for the patient, and also bad for us as we may later become overwhelmed by the sense of our responsibilities. At this point in the interview, then, it is important to look at the resources available to the patient, both internally and externally.[65] We cannot, and should not, live the patient's life for him or her. Hence, as the problem list and the plan begin to take shape the professional should begin helping the patient to evaluate what he or she can do for himself or herself. This part of the process involves helping the patient to identify his or her own coping strategies and is a continuous process, not usually completed in one interview. It also leads logically on to the next component.

Identify other sources of support for the patient and incorporate them

Not only do we tend to forget that the patient has capabilities of his or her own, we also tend to forget that there is anyone outside the professional–patient relationship who can assist. Most people have at least one or two friends or relatives who are close in some way and can add support. For those patients who have no social supports of their own, it will be necessary to enrol and co-ordinate the other services available.

Summary and conclusion

The final part of the interview is the summary and contract for the future. The summary—which also requires a great deal of thought—should show the patient that you have been listening and that you have picked up the main concerns and issues. It is not a particularly easy task but you should try to give an overview of the two agendas (yours and the patient's). It need not be a long statement, and often consists of no more than one or two sentences.

Having summarized the main points, you should then ask 'Are there any (other) questions that you'd like to ask me now?'. Sometimes the patient has been bottling up concerns over some issue that simply has not arisen, or one aspect of the treatment or the disease that you have merely touched on. This part is as important as the question period after a lecture—it is the time when any unresolved issues can be discussed.

Finally, you should make a contract for the future. Even though this may be very simple ('I'll see you at the next visit in two weeks' or 'We'll try the new antisickness medicine and I'll see you tomorrow on the ward-round') patients may otherwise be left at the conclusion of the interview with the feeling that there is no future and may be glad to hear that there is one.

Therapeutic (or supportive) dialogue

Many physicians under-rate the value of therapeutic dialogue because it is not included in the curricula of most medical schools, and they are thus unfamiliar with its use. Supportive communication is obviously central to psychiatric and psychotherapeutic practice, but is generally not taught to medical or nursing students outside those disciplines.[66] Hence, it often seems an alien idea that a doctor or nurse can achieve anything by simply listening to the patient and acknowledging the existence of that individual's emotions.

Nevertheless, supportive dialogue, during any stage of palliative care, is an exceptionally valuable resource and may be the most important (and sometimes the only) ingredient in a patient's care. The central principle of effective therapeutic dialogue is that the patient should perceive that his or her emotions have been heard by the professional and acknowledged. It may then become apparent that there are problems that can be solved, emotions that can be resolved, and needs that can be met, but even if there are no solutions, the simple act of supportive dialogue can reduce distress.

For the main objective of acknowledging the patient's emotions, the empathic response is of prime importance, although it cannot be the only component of the professional's side of the dialogue. Obviously a single technique cannot create an entire relationship; nevertheless, many professionals are unfairly perceived as being insensitive or unsupportive, simply because they do not know how to demonstrate their abilities as listeners. The empathic response is one of the most reliable methods of demonstrating effective listening. In addition to responding in this way, the professional should also attempt to assess the nature and value of the patient's responses in coping with the situation, to disentangle the emotions that have been raised by the discussion, and to try to resolve any conflicts that may have arisen.

Assessment of the patient's responses

Even though we have not, in this chapter, detailed all the possible reactions that a patient might experience it is possible to offer some brief guidelines for assessing those emotions, so that the professional may know which emotions are best reinforced and which require intervention. In essence, there are three criteria by which patients' responses may be assessed.

Acceptability

First, a patient's reactions must meet the broadest definitions of socially acceptable behaviour. These definitions vary from culture to culture (and some of the gravest misunderstandings arise from misinterpretation—behaviour that is normal in one culture being seen as aberrant in another). In the context of palliative care, however, interpretation of 'socially acceptable' should be very wide. The professional should err on the side of generosity and only if extreme behaviour is a genuine danger to the patient, staff, other patients, or family members should assistance be called in. For all but these very rare cases, you should accept the behaviour even if you do not like it, and assess it on the other two criteria—does it help the patient, and (if it does not) can it be improved by intervention?

Table 4 Some adaptive and maladaptive responses

Adaptive	Maladaptive
Humour	Guilt
Denial	Pathological denial
Abstract anger	
Anger against disease	Anger against helpers
Crying	Collapse
Fear	Anxiety
Fulfilling an ambition	The impossible 'quest'
Realistic hope	Unrealistic hope
Sexual drive	Despair
Bargaining	Manipulation

Distinguishing the adaptive from the maladaptive

Second, facing the end of life usually induces major stress and distress: an individual's response to that distress may either help the person to reduce it (an adaptive response) or may increase it (a maladaptive response). Frequently, it is difficult to distinguish one from the other at the first interview and it may require several interviews over a longer period to decide whether a patient is adapting to the medical circumstances.

It is not easy to be dogmatic about which responses are always maladaptive but some guidelines are shown in Table 4. There seems to be a consensus opinion that, for example, a feeling of guilt is always maladaptive and cannot help a patient. It may be somewhat more controversial, but still helpful, to regard denial in the early stages as an adaptive response, allowing the patient to adjust to the situation in small 'bites' when otherwise the threat would be overwhelming. It is also important to note that some responses will buy the patient an immediate short-term decrease in distress, but will accumulate trouble later on. For instance, denial that is prolonged and which prevents a patient from making decisions with which he or she is comfortable ('We won't even think about that . . . ') may later increase distress. Only the professional's clinical experience and the passage of time can define the situation in some cases.

Distinguishing the 'fixable' from the 'unfixable'

The third criterion by which responses may be assessed is what might be termed 'fixability'. If there is a problem that is increasing the patient's distress or obstructing adaptation, can it be remedied? This is largely a matter of clinical experience, and depends on the professional's confidence and competence in addressing psychosocial problems.[67] Two points, however, are worth stressing. First, the chance of damage is higher when the professional feels that he or she can fix a problem, and then perseveres without seeking help, than when a professional knows his or her own limitations. Second, it is even more important that, if there appears to be a problem that is not 'fixable', a second opinion is sought—preferably from a psychologist or psychiatrist. In problems that appear to the medical

Table 5 In the event of conflict

1. Try to take a step back
2. Identify your own emotions and try to describe them, not display them
3. Try to define the area of conflict that is unresolved
4. Try to obtain agreement on that area of difference, even if it cannot be resolved
5. Find a colleague and talk about it

team to be 'unfixable', some improvement can be achieved by psychologists in up to two-thirds of cases.[68]

Distinguish your emotions from those of the patient

Another task that often has to be undertaken during therapeutic dialogue is the disentangling of the emotions experienced during the interview by both the patient and the professional. We have already seen that strong emotions cannot be ignored without jeopardizing all communication. We should also try to be aware of our own emotions in dealing with an individual person who is dying. We may experience strong emotions because of our own previous experience (counter-transference) or we may be moved, attracted, or irritated and intolerant as a result of the patient's behaviour patterns. In any event, whenever emotions arise it is essential to try to take a step back and ask yourself what you are feeling and where that feeling comes from. If the professional can recognize a strong emotion in himself or herself, the recognition itself partly negates the effect of the emotion on judgement and communication. If the emotion goes unrecognized, it is far more likely to produce damage.

Dealing with conflict

We all want to do our best for the patient, but we all have our limits. Sometimes we simply cannot ease a patient's distress, sometimes the patients do not wish to be relieved, and sometimes they appear to have a need for antagonism or conflict in order to give themselves definition or some other gain.

Despite pretences to the contrary, all of us at some time feel exhausted, frustrated, and intolerant. This is unavoidable. There are, however, a few guidelines that may reduce the impact of those feelings in our professional life.[69] The most useful are shown in Table 5.

In summary, the single most useful tool of therapeutic dialogue is the empathic response which indicates to the patient that the emotional content of his or her reaction is being heard and is legitimized. In addition, the professional should attempt to assess the patient's response, disentangle his or her emotions from those of the patient, and try to resolve conflict.

These, then, are some of the most important aspects of communicating with the dying patient. However, there are almost always other parties involved, and in the next section we shall deal with communication issues concerning the family and those that may arise between health-care disciplines.

Communication with other people

All efforts in palliative care are directed to ameliorating the situation of the patient. However, there are other parties to be considered who may assist or hinder efforts at effective communication (for a major review of communication issues with cancer patients, their families, and professionals see Northouse and Northouse.[70]). Only a few broad guidelines can be offered in this limited space, but attention to even these simple issues can improve quality of care noticeably.

Communication with friends and family

The responses of friends and family to the imminent death of the patient may be as varied as those of the patient himself. Similarly, they may assist the patient and be of support, or they may be counter-productive and form part of the patient's problem rather than part of the solution. They may be similar in nature to the patient's responses or they may be qualitatively different. Even when they are the same as those of the patient, they may be asynchronous with the patient's responses; for example the patient may have resolved his or her anger and may have come to accept his or her death, while the family are still angry or in denial. In the same way, therefore, as the patient's responses may be considered adaptive or maladaptive, so the family's responses may also serve to decrease or increase the patient's distress and increase or decrease support.

When a patient's treatment is palliative, some effort should always be made to identify leading members of his or her support systems (friends and family). However, in communicating with the family, there are two principles which may at first seem mutually exclusive.

The patient has primacy

A mentally competent patient has the right (ethical and legal) to determine who shall be informed about his or her medical condition. All rights of friends or family are subsidiary to this. If a patient decides not to share information with anyone else, although that may be an aggressive and vengeful action, it cannot be countermanded by the professional at the family's request. Similarly, however well intentioned, a relative stating that 'the patient is not to be told' does not have primacy over the patient's wishes if the patient wishes full disclosure.

The family's feelings have validity

Despite the secondary rank of the family's feelings, those feelings have validity and must be acknowledged even if their wishes or instructions cannot be acceded to. Often a family's wishes arise from a desire to show that they are good and caring sons or daughters (rationalizing their own feelings as 'If I cannot stop mother becoming ill, I can at least stop her finding out too much about it.') It is important for the professional to identify the family's emotions and to acknowledge them; for this purpose, the empathic response is of great value.

Communication between physicians

Doctors are notoriously bad at communicating with each other. We do not do it frequently enough, and more importantly, when we do communicate with each other, we are often disorganized and unfocused in our communication. Perhaps the most dangerous gaps in doctor–doctor communication occur when a patient moves from one care setting to another—for example into a palliative care unit or from a hospital to home.

It is difficult to give useful guidelines about something as ill-defined as interspecialty communication, but perhaps the key principles are that all communication should be task-orientated and should clearly define frontiers of responsibility. This means that communications should be related to those aspects of the patient's situation that may have an impact on the care. Much of what is discussed between doctors is found to be, on analysis, simply opinion or conjecture. Although there is nothing wrong with this in itself, it often gives us the feeling that we have thoroughly discussed the case, when in fact vital management issues have not been discussed at all.

The five-point checklist that follows may be of some value when considering a letter or telephone call to another physician about a palliative care patient.

1. Am I addressing the right person? (For instance, does the patient know the family practitioner well? Have I asked the patient whom he or she wished me to contact?)
2. What do I know about this patient that the other person should know? (and/or what do I want to know from the other person?).
3. What does this mean for the patient's future care?
4. Who is going to do what? Who is now 'the doctor' for this patient?
5. How shall we communicate again if things are not going well?

Even if communications are limited to these five points, they will be more effective than many of the current communications between doctors—not because we are negligent or malevolent, but because we are often too polite and too afraid of stepping on each other's toes in making suggestions for the patient's benefit.

Communication between physicians and nurses

By definition, professionals belong to different teams because they have special expertise and training that identifies them with that discipline. This is essential for good patient care. However, there is a side-effect—namely that we each speak a different language and we all tend to believe that our particular language is the only one truly relevant to the patient's care. As a result, different aspects of the patient's problems are often poorly integrated and there are often large gaps in communication between the teams. The most common gaps—because of the way the jobs inter-relate—occur between doctors and nurses.

One of the greatest paradoxes (and perhaps one of the greatest losses) in the recent evolution of the nursing profession has been the diminishing of the ward-round as the standard method for exchanging information between patient, doctor, and nurse. Although this idea that the ward-round is essential in patient care is a controversial one, it is a view that is now receiving increasing support from all disciplines and from patients and families. The days of the three-hour ward-round during which four patients are reviewed are over—nursing time is at a premium and nursing tasks have increased greatly in number and complexity. However, without the 'trinity' of patient–doctor–nurse present in the same place at the same time, inpatient care is rendered unnecessarily complex and incomplete. In hospitals or hospices where time is limited, it is often possible to agree on time-limits (for example an average of 10 min per patient can accomplish almost all of the necessary exchanges).

In our own unit, we ensure that the three following points are addressed during the minimum 10-min period allotted to each patient for discussion.

1. The medical game-plan: what is known about the patient's medical status, what measures are planned or being considered. What is the prognosis?
2. Nursing concerns: what are the main difficulties in the day-to-day care of the patient?
3. What does the patient know and what are the patient's major concerns? For instance, does the patient have strong views about the type of therapy or where she or he would like to be looked after?

It is surprising how efficient communication can be if all concerned are aware that time is limited and that these three main areas must be covered in the discussion.

Conclusion

In palliative care, everything starts with the patient—including every aspect of symptom relief and every aspect of communication. There is no doubt that we all want to do our best, but often the major challenges in palliative care arise because we do not know how to approach the problem. Nowhere is this more true than in communication—a professional who feels ill-equipped and inept at communication will become part of the problem instead of part of the solution. The act of following relatively straightforward guidelines, however simplistic they may appear, will at least give us a feeling of competence and enhance our ability to learn as we practise.

An expert in palliative care is not a person who gets it right all the time: an expert is someone who gets it wrong less often—and is better at concealing or coping with his or her fluster and embarrassment. We are, after all, only human beings.

References

1. Houts PS, *et al.* Unmet needs of persons with cancer in Pennsylvania during the period of terminal care. *Cancer*, 1988; **62**: 627–34.
2. Saunders JM, McCorkle R. Models of care for persons with progressive cancer. *Nursing Clinics of North America*, 1985; **20**: 365–77.
3. Wilkes E. Dying now. *Lancet*, 1984; **ii**: 950–2.
4. Hockley JM, Dunlop R, Davies RJ. Survey of distressing symptoms in dying patients and their families in hospital and the response to a symptom control team. *British Medical Journal*, 1988; **296**: 1715–17.
5. Schulz R. *The Psychology of Death, Dying and Bereavement*. Reading, MA: Addison Wesley, 1978.
6. Stoll BA. Quality of life as an objective in cancer treatment. In Stoll BA, ed. *Cancer Treatment: End-point Evaluation*. Chichester: Wiley, 1983: 113–38.
7. Stedeford A. *Facing Death: Patients, Families and Professionals*. London : Heinemann, 1984.
8. Cousins N. How patients appraise physicians. *New England Journal of Medicine*, 1985; **313**: 1422–4.
9. Klein SJ. Hospice care. In: Higby DJ, ed. *Issues in Supportive Care of Cancer Patients*. Boston: Martinus Nijhoff, 1986.
10. Ley P. *Communicating with Patients*, London: Croom Helm, 1988.

11. Kristjanson LJ. Quality of terminal care: salient indicators identified by families. *Journal of Palliative Care*, 1989; **5**: 21–8.
12. Lichter I, Davidson GP. Caring for the dying. *New Zealand Medical Journal*, 1981; **93**: 15–18.
13. Linn MW, Linn BS. Caring for the terminal patient. In: Stoll BA, ed. *Coping with Cancer Stress.* Lancaster: Martinus Nijhoff, 1986: 155–61.
14. Twycross RG, Lack SA. *Therapeutics in Terminal Cancer.* London: Churchill Livingstone, 1990: 209–15.
15. Fallowfield L. *The Quality of Life: the Missing Measurement in Health Care.* London: Souvenir Press, 1990: 186–203.
16. Kaplan SH, Greenfield S, Ware JE. Impact of the doctor-patient relationship on the outcomes of chronic disease. In: Stewart M, Roter D, eds. *Communicating with Medical Patients.* Newbury Park: Sage Publications, 1989: 228–45.
17. Stedeford A. Couples facing death. II Unsatisfactory communication. *British Medical Journal*, 1981; **283**: 1098–101.
18. Maguire P. Barriers to psychological care of the dying. *British Medical Journal*, 1985; **291**: 1711–13.
19. Buckman R. Breaking bad news: why is it still so difficult? *British Medical Journal*, 1984; **288**: 1597–9.
20. Becker E. *The Denial of Death.* New York: Free Press, 1973.
21. Saunders CM, Baines M. *Living with Dying.* Oxford: University Press, 1983: 10.
22. Buckman R. *How to Break Bad News—a Guide for Health Care Professionals.* London: Macmillan Medical, 1993.
23. Scravalli EP. The dying patient, the physician and the fear of death. *New England Journal of Medicine*, 1988; **319**: 1728–30.
24. Maguire P, Faulkner A. How to do it: improve the counselling skills of doctors and nurses in cancer care. *British Medical Journal*, 1988; **297**: 847–9.
25. Gorlin R, Zucker HD. Physicians' reactions to patients. *New England Journal of Medicine*, 1983; **308**: 1059–63.
26. Perez EL, Gosselin JY, Gagnon A. Education on death and dying: a survey of Canadian medical schools. *Journal of Medical Education*, 1980; **55**: 788–9.
27. Michaels E. Deliver bad news tactfully. *Canadian Medical Association Journal*, 1983; **129**: 1307–8.
28. Streim JE, Marshall F. The dying elderly patient. *American Family Practitioner*, 1988; **38**: 175–83.
29. Radovsky SS. Bearing the news. *New England Journal of Medicine*, 1985; **513**: 586–8.
30. Kubler-Ross E. *On Death and Dying.* London: Tavistock Publications, 1970.
31. Parkes CM. Psychological aspects. In: Saunders CM, ed. *The Management of Terminal Diseases.* London: Edward Arnold, 1978: 50–2.
32. Rando TA. Death and the dying patient. In: *Grief Dying and Death.* Chicago: Research Press Company, 1984: 199–223.
33. Buckman R. *I Don't Know What to Say—How to Help and Support Someone Who is Dying.* London; Macmillan, 1988.
34. Taylor SE. Adjustment to threatening events: a theory of cognitive adaptation. *American Psychologist*, 1983; **38**: 1161–73.
35. DiMatteo MR, Prince LM, Taranta AJ. Patients' preceptions of physicians' behaviour: determinants of patient commitment to the therapeutic relationship. *Community Health*, 1979; **4**: 280–90.
36. Hinton J. Whom do dying patients tell? *British Medical Journal*, 1980; **281**: 1328–30.
37. Lipkin M, Quill TE, Napodano RJ. The medical interview: a core curriculum for residencies in internal medicine. *Annals of Internal Medicine*, 1984; **100**: 277–84.
38. DiMatteo MR, Taranta A, Friedman HS, Prince LM. Predicting patient satisfaction from physicians' non-verbal communication skills. *Medical Care*, 1980; **18**: 376–87.
39. Maguire P. Communication skills. In: *Patient Care Health Care and Human Behaviour*, London: Academic Press, 1984:153–73.
40. Hall ET. *The Silent Language.* New York: Doubleday, 1959 (reprinted Anchor, 1981).
41. Older J. Teaching touch at medical school. *Journal of the American Medical Association*, 1984; **252**: 931–3.
42. Larsen KM, Smith CK. Assessment of nonverbal communication in the patient–physician interview. *Journal of Family Practice*, 1981; **12**: 481–8.
43. Blau N. Time to let the patient speak. *British Medical Journal*, 1989; **298**: 39.
44. Frankel RM, Beckman HB. The pause that refreshes. *Hospital Practice*, 1988; **Sept 30**: 64–7.
45. Bendix T. *The Anxious Patient.* London: Livingstone, 1982.
46. Maynard D. On clinicians co-implicating recipients' perspectives in the delivery of diagnostic news. In: Drew P, Heritage J, eds. *Talk at Work: Social Interaction in Institutional Settings.* Cambridge: University Press, 1990.
47. Waitzkin H, Stoeckle JD. The communication of information about illness. *Advances in Psychosomatic Medicine*, 1987; **8**:180–215.
48. Maynard D. Notes on the delivery and reception of diagnostic news regarding mental disabilities. In: Helm DT, Anderson WT, Meehan AJ, eds. *The Interactional Order: New Directions in the Study of Social Order.* New York: Irvington Publishers, 1989: 54–67.
49. Lichter I. Rights of the individual patient. In: Stoll BA, ed. *Ethical Dilemmas in Cancer Care.* London: Macmillan, 1989: 7–16.
50. Goldie L. The ethics of telling the patient. *Journal of Medical Ethics*, 1982; **8**: 128–33.
51. Jones JS. Telling the right patient. *British Medical Journal*, 1981; **283**: 291–2.
52. Billings A. Sharing bad news. In: Billings A. *Out-patient Management of Advanced Malignancy.* Philadelphia: Lippincott, 1985: 236–59.
53. Reiser SJ. Words as scalpels: transmitting evidence in the clinical dialogue. *Annals of Internal Medicine*, 1980; **92**: 837–42.
54. Cassileth BR, Zupkis RV, Sutton-Smith MS, March V. Information and participation preferences among cancer patients. *Annals of Internal Medicine*, 1980; **92**: 832–6.
55. Henriques B, Stadil F, Baden H. Patient information about cancer. *Acta Chirurgia Scandinavica*, 1980; **146**: 309–11.
56. McIntosh J. Patients' awareness and desire for information about diagnosed but undisclosed malignant disease. *Lancet*, 1976; **ii**: 300–3.
57. Kelly WD, Friesen SR. Do cancer patients want to be told? *Surgery*, 1950; **27**: 822–6.
58. McIntosh J. Processes of communication, information seeking and control associated with cancer: a selective review of the literature. *Social Science and Medicine*, 1974; **8**: 167–87.
59. Reynolds PM, Sanson-Fisher RW, Poole AD, Harker J, Byrne M. Cancer and communication: information giving in an oncology clinic. *British Medical Journal*, 1981; **282**: 1449–51.
60. Maynard D. Breaking bad news in clinical settings. In: Dervin, B, ed. *Progress in Communication Sciences*, Norwood NJ: Ablex Publishing Co, 1989: 161–3.
61. Maguire P, Faulkner A. How to do it: communicate with cancer patients. 1 Handling bad news and difficult questions. *British Medical Journal*, 1988; **297**: 907–9.
62. Premi J. Communicating bad news to patients. *Canadian Family Physician*, 1981; **27**: 837–41.
63. Rando TA. Caring for the dying patient. In: *Grief, Dying and Death.* Chicago: Research Press Company, 1984: 278–83.
64. Maguire P, Faulkner A. How to do it: communicate with cancer patients. 2 Handling uncertainty, collusion and denial. *British Medical Journal*, 1988; **297**: 972–4.
65. Manuel GM, Roth S, Keefe FJ, Brantley BA. Coping with cancer. *Journal of Human Stress*, 1987:149–58.
66. Fallowfield L. Counselling for patients with cancer. *British Medical Journal*, 1988; **297**: 727–8.
67. Skinner JB, Erskine A, Pearce S, Rubenstein I, Taylor M, Foster C. The evaluation of a cognitive behavioural treatment programme in outpatients with chronic pain. *Journal of Psychosomatic Research*, 1990; **34**: 13–19.

68. Buckman R, Doan B. Enhancing communication with the cancer patient: referrals to the psychologist—who and when? In: Ginsburg D, Laidlaw J, eds. *Cancer in Ontario 1991*. Toronto: Ontario Cancer Treatment and Research Foundation, 1991: 78–86.
69. Lazare A, Eisenthal S, Frank A. In: Lazare A, ed. *Outpatient Psychiatry: Diagnosis and Treatment*. 2nd edn. Baltimore: Williams and Wilkins, 1989: 157–71.
70. Northouse PG, Northouse LL. Communication and cancer: issues confronting patients, health professionals and family members. *Journal of Psychosocial Oncology*, 1987; 5:17–45.

Further reading

Becker E. *The Denial of Death*. New York: Free Press, 1973.
Rando TA. *Grief, Dying and Death*. Chicago: Research Press Company, 1984.
Buckman R. *How to Break Bad News—a Guide for Healthcare Professionals*. London: Macmillan Medical, 1993.

5

Research in palliative care

5.1 Clinical and health services research

Sir Kenneth Calman and Geoffrey Hanks

'Ignorance has risks, but they are largely unseen and unnoticed. Gaining knowledge has risks which are noticed, but largely unpredictable, and it is very costly (though less so than prolonged ignorance). It focuses blame, whereas ignorance dispels it. So, maintaining ignorance often seems more attractive than gaining knowledge'. Duncan Vere.[1]

Modern palliative care has its origins in the opening of St Christopher's Hospice in London just over 30 years ago. St Christopher's was different from other long-established hospices and homes for the terminally ill because its aim was to integrate 'a scientific programme concerned with the discriminating use of drugs with the tender loving care' provided within these other institutions.[2] From the outset, research was a priority and the studies in pain control by Twycross[3] and in the evaluation of hospice care by Murray-Parkes[4] had a considerable impact on the development of the specialty and widespread influence outside it. Since that time, much has been achieved and there have been many advances which are described throughout this book. However, that initial urgency and enthusiasm properly to evaluate the care that was provided and the methods that were being used has not grown and matured as it should have done. As the specialty has developed research has tended to take a back seat. Indeed, there is a view that scientifically rigorous clinical research is incompatible with the basic tenets of palliative care and the emotive accusation of experimenting on the dying has been an ever-present deterrent to some.

In palliative care, the issues of the primacy of the individual and whole person care versus the 'greatest happiness of the greatest number'[5] are brought sharply into focus. The physician's obligation to keep the interests of his patient as paramount is a fundamental precept of medical practice and is given great emphasis in palliative care. However, the physician has another obligation, which is to promote the acquisition of scientific knowledge. These obligations constitute a real conflict and raise difficult ethical dilemmas.

The purpose of this section of the book is to highlight the importance of research to the future of palliative care, to review the ethical and practical difficulties which may be encountered, and to indicate the scope of what has been done and what needs to be done.

Why carry out research in palliative care?

To many readers of this book this will be an unnecessary question: medical progress, in whatever field, must be based on research and, in a clinical discipline, this means research involving patients. There is a view also (which some might find controversial) that everyone who uses health care has an obligation to participate in the research necessary to permit progress.[6] Thus, if there are to be developments and improvements in palliative care, research is essential. However, two cogent arguments have been aired to discourage clinical research in palliative care. First, that the patient population involved is too ill and too vulnerable to allow meaningful scientific research and that, in such a situation, advances in knowledge must rely on clinical experience and empiricism. Second, that there is not much more to find out—that the problems of pain and symptom control have been well worked out and that the accumulated wisdom on the management of psychological and social issues leaves no great hiatus in present knowledge. Neither argument holds water but both require a thoughtful response rather than a facile rejection. The first argument concerns ethics and the second the scope of research in palliative care.

The ethics of research in palliative care (see also Section 3)

Much progress in medicine is achieved through advances in basic science, but it also depends on clinical research which, by definition, means research involving patients. Serendipity continues to play a role in advancing knowledge as does astute clinical observation. But neither of these mechanisms can be relied on to ensure progress; human experimentation based on the scientific method is essential for medicine to continue to advance. This argument applies to palliative care as it does to any other area of medicine.

The Declaration of Helsinki, drawn up by the World Medical Association in 1964 (and amended in 1975 and 1983) was a response to the need for a code of ethics on human experimentation which would be applicable to all countries and all situations where human subjects were involved in research.[7] The code acknowledges the need for guidance for physician investigators caught in the conflict between the patient's own best interests and the necessity to advance knowledge for the benefit of society as a whole.

The Declaration of Helsinki is generally accepted as an ethical code of practice for clinical research and its principles are applicable to palliative medicine. It is important that clinical research is seen to conform to these principles and that all research projects are scrutinized by independent assessors to ensure that this is the case. This function is usually undertaken by a local Research Ethics Committee. In the United Kingdom, there is a comprehensive network of local research ethics committees whose constitution and function generally follows the guidelines set out in a report of the Royal College of Physicians (originally published in 1984 and revised in 1990).[8] The Department of Health has also issued its own guidelines.[9] There are similar provisions in other westernized societies. Research projects in palliative care should undergo ethical committee assessment and approval in the same way as any other clinical research.

Controlled clinical trials and informed consent in palliative medicine

Austin Bradford Hill set out the ethical precepts for randomized controlled trials in his Marc Daniels Lecture at the Royal College of Physicians in 1963.[10] In the United States, Henry Beecher had a similar influence on the development of ethical guidelines for clinical research,[11,12] and the subject has been debated in many places since.[1,13-18] It is not appropriate to discuss this subject in detail here but the reader is referred to these reviews which make two important points. The first is that the prospective randomized controlled trial is the most efficient, scientific way of evaluating a new treatment or of comparing alternative treatments, but the second is that it is not the only way of ensuring the advance of reliable knowledge.

Controlled clinical trials are necessary in palliative medicine, and the usual guidelines and ethical principles will apply. Some points need particular emphasis in the palliative care setting. Patients are invariably at a low ebb physically and many are elderly and frail; most have a multitude of physical and emotional and perhaps social and spiritual problems. When they come to the palliative care unit or team many of these problems will be dealt with, and some, particularly the psychosocial issues, may receive attention for the first time. The supportive environment in palliative care may make patients particularly keen to give something back to the carers, to show their gratitude for the care they are receiving. All of these factors make patients particularly vulnerable when they are asked to participate in any sort of research project, for many will feel almost an obligation to accede to such a request.

Researchers in palliative care must be on their guard not to take advantage of this situation. It is generally good practice always to involve a family member when the patient is first approached about a study, together with a member of the nursing staff involved in the care of the patient. Explanation must be as thorough and meticulous but also as simple as possible and should be backed up by some written material which can be left for the patient and family to read at leisure. The Helsinki Declaration requires that 'the potential subject must be adequately informed of the aims, anticipated benefits and potential hazards of the study', and this should apply to the family member as well.

In palliative care, confusion is a problem encountered in many patients; when this is obvious they will be excluded from consideration for entry to a study. However, often the confusion is mild or variable. Such patients need careful assessment, and, wherever there is any doubt that the patient is able to understand what is being asked of him, he or she should not be considered for inclusion.

There is a fine balance that needs to be achieved here. The special vulnerability of patients receiving palliative care dictates the need for special handling in obtaining the consent to participate in research but at the same time the researcher must not go out of his or her way to talk the patient out of wanting to take part. Patients should be given time to discuss the project with their families and of course must understand that they can decline or change their minds without needing to give any reason. Once they are sure and have agreed to participate, consent should be obtained in writing.

The scope of research in palliative care

Since the first edition of this textbook there have been significant developments relating specifically to palliative care research and to the general area of evidence-based medicine.

Palliative care research

One of the barriers to palliative care research has been a lack of funding from traditional research-funding sources, both statutory and voluntary. To some extent this reflected a widely-held view that palliative care is not a well-defined scientific discipline but rather a model of humane health-care delivery. This view has changed and the need for science-based research in palliative care has been recognized in several important initiatives. In the United Kingdom, the National Health Service has embarked on a major research and development programme in which priority areas are first established and research then commissioned specifically to improve knowledge and practice in those areas.[19] The overriding consideration in developing these priorities is to address issues directly related to the burden of disease on the National Health Service. Palliative care research figures prominently in the cancer research and development programme,[20] encompassing both clinical topics ('optimal treatment strategies for unrelieved symptoms') and health services research ('cost-effective models of service delivery and provision of palliative care services'). Outside the United Kingdom, the European Union launched its BIOMED 2 programme (Biomedicine and Health Research) in 1994 and again palliative care was identified as a priority area both within the cancer programme and in the area of biomedical ethics.[21]

The two major cancer care charities in the United Kingdom have also developed research activities in palliative care as an integral part of their overall strategy. The Cancer Relief Macmillan Fund supports palliative care research through the establishment of academic posts in nursing, medicine, and social work. Marie Curie Cancer Care has allocated specific funds to palliative care research supported by a number of educational activities to improve understanding of research concepts, organization, and methodology. In order to identify areas of particular need the Cancer Relief Macmillan Fund undertook a study to identify the perceived research priorities amongst practitioners of various disciplines working in the field.[22] Social workers, occupational therapists, physiotherapists, chaplains, doctors, and two groups of nurses were surveyed to determine priorities for clinical research in palliative care. A large number of topics were identified by 1304 participants, and two priority areas picked out by several of the professional groups were multiprofessional teamwork and symptom management.

These developments indicate a significant shift in attitudes both within and outside palliative care. The culture within the specialty has evolved to one where it is recognized that maintaining high standards of care depends on advances in knowledge and that in order to achieve this there is an obligation to contribute to those advances.

Evidence-based palliative care

Evidence-based medicine is a term of recent provenance which has rapidly become part of the jargon not just of professional researchers but of politicians and health service managers. It will take a little longer to be taken up generally by clinicians, but there is little doubt that the philosophy underlying it will have a major impact in all areas of health care. Evidence-based medicine 'is the conscientious, explicit, and judicious use of current best evidence in making decisions about the care of individual patients. The practice of evidence-based medicine means integrating individual clinical expertise with the best available external clinical evidence from systematic research'.[23]

Evidence-based medicine is not a new idea. It has always been implicit that clinical practice should be based on the best possible evidence. However, what is relatively new is the widespread recognition that this is not happening. In one often-cited study Antman and his colleagues compared the evidence from randomized trials and systematic reviews of treatments for myocardial infarction with recommendations in current medical textbooks.[24] They found that 6 years after the first meta-analysis confirmed the efficacy of thrombolytic therapy, most texts failed to recommend it.

There is a problem in applying the evidence from randomized trials and other clinical investigations to day-to-day clinical practice. Part of this problem is the huge amount of data available. It is estimated that the total number of randomized trials currently is between 250 000 and 1 million.[25] Evidence-based medicine is about finding ways in which to bridge the gap between the available data and clinical practice, and encompasses a number of strategies. One of these strategies has been the development of scientific methods (systematic reviews and meta-analyses) to combine data from a number of different randomized studies of the same or similar treatments in any particular condition. Systematic reviews differ from other types of review in that they adhere to a strict scientific design in order to make them more comprehensive, to minimise the chance of bias, and so ensure their reliability.

Taken at face value, it seems reasonable to assume that the data from several studies which have been combined according to agreed scientific methodology should be more meaningful than the evidence from single studies. This is not universally accepted[26,27] and there is no doubt that the methodology and application of these techniques must continue to be looked at critically. However, systematic reviews are a powerful tool in aggregating and evaluating large amounts of data.

This has been recognized by a growing international group who form the Cochrane Collaboration.[28] Cochrane had highlighted the fact that there was no ready access to reviews of reliable evidence from randomized controlled trials. He wrote in 1979 that 'it is surely a great criticism of our profession that we have not organized a critical survey, by specialty or subspecialty, updated periodically, of all relevant randomized controlled trials'.[29] The Cochrane Collaboration has developed in response to this hiatus and aims 'to create a register of all completed and continuing randomized controlled trials; to combine the results of trials that meet set standards of quality; to produce regularly updated systematic reviews or meta-analyses; and to make these reviews widely available in journals, on CD-ROM, and eventually on line through the Internet'.[28] These developments have implications for all areas of health care, including palliative medicine. There are many areas within palliative medicine which would be amenable to systematic reviews. For example in the field of pain relief there is already considerable activity with recent published reviews of the WHO analgesic ladder,[30] anticonvulsant drugs,[31] and pre-emptive analgesia.[32] Other groups are putting together databases which focus on topics in psychosocial care, complementary therapies, and a number of other areas within the broad field of palliative care.

Systematic reviews and meta-analyses will become an important area of research activity in palliative medicine over the next few years. However, this approach will highlight even more the continuing need for high quality clinical research.

Evidence-based medicine and the future of palliative care

Evidence-based medicine is not merely a new piece of jargon. Rather it represents a philosophy which will have a major impact on the development of health care in a time of ever increasing demands but limited resources. It is likely that resource allocation will increasingly be based on evidence not just of efficacy but of cost effectiveness. Where proof of efficacy is lacking, funds will not be provided by government or other health-care agencies. This has particular implications for palliative care because it is an area where such research-based evidence is sparse. There are many activities within palliative care which are not amenable to investigation by randomized controlled studies. But, as noted above, the randomized controlled trial is not the only valid method of ensuring advances in knowledge. The recent focus on evidence-based medicine makes all the more urgent the development of palliative care research as an integral part of palliative care services.

Clinical research in palliative care

There are particular difficulties associated with clinical research in palliative care, in addition to the ethical constraints described above. The patient population from which potential trial candidates are taken is characterized by old age, multisystem disease, generally severe illness with many symptoms, a progressive clinical condition, and limited survival time. In addition, polypharmacy is the rule, and environmental and psychological factors have a variable but potentially very great influence on physical well-being. Prospective randomized controlled studies of drug treatments in symptom control are thus particularly difficult to carry out.

The choice of trial design for prospective studies will be much influenced by these characteristics of the patient population. Endpoints or outcomes are also difficult to define. Outcome measures are not based on hard data such as biochemical indices or survival, which are relatively easy to quantify, but on changes in symptoms and quality of life which are much more difficult to measure. The choice of trial design and measurements will be influenced also by the need to ensure that all procedures are designed to place the least possible additional burden on patients.

Practical considerations

The nature of palliative medicine practice means that the number of patients who may be suitable for entry to a particular study will be small. A common miscalculation of those beginning research in this area is to assume that they will have many suitable subjects and this will lead to wildly over-optimistic estimates of the time required to complete a project. This is a well-known aspect of any clinical research[33,34] but is particularly true of palliative medicine. Most drug studies will involve inpatient observation, at least in the early phase of the study. In palliative medicine practice, patients who are stable enough to be considered for such studies will rarely want to remain as inpatients in the palliative care unit or hospice. Conversely most patients receiving inpatient care will be too ill or unstable to be suitable subjects.

It is discouraging and disheartening for researchers to embark on a study and experience very slow patient recruitment. The availability of suitable patients must receive careful consideration at the outset. Few individual units will have access to sufficient patients to complete a study single-handed in a reasonable period of time. Thus, we are moving into an era where multicentre studies will be the most efficient way of successfully completing clinical research in palliative medicine. There are problems associated with multicentre studies[33] but the benefits in this area of medicine outweigh them.

Multicentre studies will also solve the problems faced by many palliative care units, particularly those in the voluntary sector or those not associated with a larger institution. Practitioners in many units will have no experience of clinical research or clinical trial methodology, or its scientific basis. They may not have easy access to advice about such matters or access to a statistician or perhaps to an ethics committee. They may, however, be keen to be involved in research and will of course have access to patients. Co-operation between such units and centres experienced in research will reap benefits for both and ultimately will facilitate research in palliative medicine. Such collaboration is being encouraged and endorsed by a number of organizations in the field, including the World Health Organization, the European Association for Palliative Care, and individual national associations of palliative care.

These are the difficulties encountered in carrying out research in palliative care; there are solutions. In the following chapters the main areas of clinical research in palliative care are discussed in detail by researchers who have successfully completed studies in this area. They are able to describe the theoretical considerations which need to be taken into account but also pass on much practical advice. They highlight problems in methodology and design, review past experience, and indicate some directions for future research.

Health services research in palliative care

Health services research involves the examination of some aspect of health care in a structured and systematic way. Health services research has been defined as 'strategic and applied research concerned with the needs of the community as a whole, including the provision of health services to meet those needs'.[35] It emphasizes the importance of research based information for planning and policy development to allow clinical staff and managers to deal with complex issues and dilemmas concerning the equity, effectiveness, and efficiency of health care. Many of the current issues surrounding the delivery and effectiveness of palliative care are complex and need careful consideration, backed by reliable data, before they can be resolved. In practice, those involved in the specialty are more likely to understand these complexities, yet paradoxically may be least likely to see the benefits of this type of research. Yet it is vital if palliative care is to continue to be of high quality.

The basic measure of health services research is that of outcome, the result of one or more episodes of care. In some clinical situations this can be related to a particular event such as mortality, the development of the recurrence of the disease, a complication, or a clearly measurable change in an objective finding such as a radiograph or blood test. These may be considered to be 'hard data', available in some clinical settings and providing a great deal of valuable information. In palliative care such outcomes are often more difficult to define, as discussed above, and are associated with 'softer' issues such as quality of life, symptom relief, comfort, and patient and family satisfaction. The fact that the majority of patients, by definition, die means that in palliative care terms the 'good death' becomes the preferred outcome, even though this may be more difficult to evaluate. Health services research is often, therefore, concerned with clinical trials and psychological and sociological research rather than basic medical research, though they may well overlap.

Health services research, therefore, concentrates on outcomes, delivery of care, option appraisal, and economic measurement. Its overall purpose is to improve care and its delivery, and the methods used are those of the appropriate discipline (such as medicine, psychology, nursing, sociology). Clinical audit would be one such tool. Like all research the key to its usefulness is the implementation of the research findings. Indeed, one of the important areas of health services research is to study the diffusion of new ideas and techniques into general clinical practice. Inevitably the economic and resource allocation aspects of health services research raise ethical issues which must then be tackled.

Health services research covers a very wide area of clinical and non-clinical practice. In palliative care the following areas would be an appropriate focus for investigation.

Organization and planning of services

In addition to providing a service to the local population or community, it is also necessary to consider the wider regional and national planning of palliative care. By virtue of its development many of the current services have grown up around specific individuals, organizations, or groups with a special interest in the subject. This may well mean that services are haphazard in their distribution and provision. For this reason regional and national bodies have a responsibility to ensure that the wider public are considered and that there is equity in the provision of care. Each of the models of care described should be considered and where possible a range of services provided to meet individual patients' needs. This should cover a range of cultural and religious backgrounds. Co-ordination of the services is required together with the restricted development of special services (e.g. specialized pain services, radiotherapy, nutritional techniques). Such planning should ensure the appropriate distribution of resources and expertise.

Information requirements

The planning of any health-care facility depends on an accurate database and a knowledge of the population to be served. Too often little attention is paid to this fundamental assessment of the need for a palliative care service. For example the population structure, age and sex distribution, and socio-economic status of the population should be available to the planners of the service. In addition, there is a need to know about the incidence, prevalence, and type of major illnesses to be managed by the service. Thus, if the hospice is to deal only with cancer patients there should be some knowledge of the major types of cancer in the population and an assessment of the range of facilities already available for such patients. If the service is to widen its remit to cover AIDS, chronic neurological conditions, or other illnesses then a similar requirement for data collection is necessary.

The purpose of collecting these data is twofold. The first is to establish a patient population on which to base a service. The second is to monitor the actual throughput of the service compared to the overall population. This can be a very salutary exercise, when it is recognized that not all patients who might be eligible are referred to the service, and that those who are referred may constitute a skewed sample. Following the changes in referral over the years will give some indication of the way in which the service is developing. In addition, it might provide appropriate information for use in developing new services and the generation of resources.

Associated with the collection of population information is the need for data on the service itself. The collection of routine data may not seem exciting, but can provide valuable information on the activities of the unit. Without such data it becomes impossible to compare activity with other similar units and to assess the value of the service in the wider context of health care. As will be discussed later, such basic data does allow clinical audit to be carried out and an assessment made of the value of the care provided.

In almost all health care systems in the world there is an increasing emphasis on 'value for money'. Palliative care services cannot be exempt from this if they are to compete for national or private resources. The starting point of this is a database of population and service information. This can be obtained manually or using computer-based systems; the only important point is that the data are collected and analysed. This inevitably means committing resources to acquiring such a database which may not seem to have a high priority with those whose particular skills and talents are for patient care. Nevertheless, palliative care services will need to give increasing effort to setting out their forward plans to establish their role in the overall health care system of the country.

Models of care

In the development of a palliative care service consideration should be given to the type of service to be provided, or the 'model of care' to be used. This will depend on several factors including the resources available, the skill mix of staff, the physical facilities, and the needs and culture of the community. Before deciding on the type of service to be provided there is a need to assess the size of the problem and the range of care to be delivered. This is covered in Chapter 2.4. During the development of the service over a period of years it is useful to review, at intervals, the current service provision and the possibility of extending or modifying the range of care available. It is also important to emphasize that a diversity of models will be required in different settings, and that the translation of one model to another setting may not always be appropriate. What is crucial is that the model of care is adequately evaluated and that the findings are made available to a wider audience.

Within one service the way in which care is provided, the skill mix, special services available, community outreach, patient participation groups etc., would all be open to investigation. New ways of handling and maintaining medical records, the value of computers, resource management initiatives all might be studied. Inevitably an economic appraisal of the work of the palliative care team, in whole or in part, could be carried out. This aspect is likely to be of increasing importance as economic pressures, and a need to control health care spending, becomes more pressing.

It is perhaps worth pointing out that palliative care services as relatively 'new' developments in health care are facing many of the same issues as other services have in the past—lack of recognition of their special skills, lack of resources, opposition or cynicism, and a blurring of traditional boundaries. On a positive note it is worth recalling that orthopaedics, cardiology, urology, neurosurgery, and many other specialties have been through the same process, which concerns the specialization of health care. Those involved in palliative care can learn a great deal from those who have gone before.

Staffing issues

Staffing issues are crucial if the palliative care service is to work to its full potential. In most services the great bulk of recurrent funding is required for staff and it is therefore essential that careful thought is given to the skill mix required, their career development, and continuing education.

The first issue to be considered is the skill mix of staff required. This needs to cover the number and training of the medical staff, and their relationship to other doctors working in the public or private sector. Attention to this early on may assist in better integration of the service. Nursing staff provide the backbone of the service in many places. Consideration needs to be given to the mix of highly specialized nurses, trained nurses, or health-care assistants. This decision will affect not only the quality and type of care provided, but also the funding required to sustain the service. These are fundamental decisions and need very careful thought. Those unfamiliar with the issues would be well advised to seek outside help in this matter. Other professional groups, such as physiotherapists, dietitians, or occupational therapists, all provide essential input. What is needed, however, is a plan which will provide these services to meet patient needs within available resources. Finally, there is the role of volunteers, a group which in many palliative care services provides an essential input. There is a need here to consider training issues and the selection of volunteers.

Many palliative care services throughout the world have been established outside the traditional or national health-care setting. For this reason there is a special need for those concerned with staff issues to ensure that there are programmes of continuing education and that individual professionals are able to retain links with professional colleagues. Such educational programmes can be arranged within the service or in association with outside groups. However, if the palliative care service is to maintain its quality of service the investment in education and training must have some priority.

The importance of selection of volunteers has already been mentioned but the importance of selection applies equally to all staff. In general, the palliative care service will have been established with a particular philosophy, culture, or religious background in mind. In addition, it will fit into the prevailing ethos of the country in which it is based. A service should consider producing a clear statement of its purpose and philosophy in order that those involved can be clear about its objectives and that those entering the service understand its basis. Such a 'mission statement' can help to clarify issues and avoid problems.

Guidelines, standards, and clinical audit

In most health-care settings throughout the world there is a move to set standards of care and to produce guidelines of 'best practice'. This is often associated with the development of clinical audit, a method of systematically examining and evaluating clinical practice. Each of these inter-related developments puts the onus on the provider of care to ensure that standards are met and maintained. Palliative care services are no exception to this.

Clinical audit provides a tool for the evaluation of the efficiency and effectiveness of clinical services. It requires the systematic review of clinical practice based on existing data, and its purpose is critically to examine the quality of care in order continually to improve it. It is therefore not a 'once and for all' exercise but an ongoing review of the results of care. It may be concerned with structure (the organization of a service), process (how that service is delivered), and outcome (the overall result of an episode or episodes of care). It is, therefore, wide-ranging in its application and can be concerned with one professional group, or more usually in the palliative care setting, a variety of different staff groups. Patients and relatives will naturally be part of this process.

The methodology involved is generally straightforward and may not need sophisticated data collection. In general, it begins with the assessment of a topic, with data collection and analysis. This is followed by planning the service and then implementing some new or existing strategy. Finally there is an evaluation of the change and a new and improved service is planned. This 'audit cycle' is equivalent to other cycles of planning and improving services. Audit is discussed in detail in Chapter 2.6.

From clinical audit and other activities, standards of care can be developed. These are well advanced in many clinical areas and are established as key aspects of the delivery of care. Again the international health care scene is demanding more explicit standards of care and the palliative care sector will be required to be part of this. The providers of care will need to spend effort and resources defining what they can provide and to what level. Simply to say that a high quality service is delivered without considering the implications of that statement will not be sufficient in many places in the future.

In palliative care there is a complicating factor in terms of defining specialist and non-specialist care.[36] Purchasers of health care will want to know the 'added value' of a specialist nurse or doctor or multidisciplinary service. There is, thus, also a need to define standards at different levels of care.

Alongside the setting of standards is the development of guidelines or treatment protocols. In this case patients are managed according to an agreed protocol depending on the illness or symptom. It is possible that such guidelines could remove clinical freedom or the right of the patient to direct a care programme. This is not the intention. Rather it is to set out appropriate care plans which can be reviewed (by the process of medical or clinical audit) and an assessment made of the value of the care provided. Those involved in palliative care may consider that by virtue of being in the specialty, they are bound to provide a high quality of care. This is not always the case and the palliative care unit has a duty, as do other clinical specialities, to record and evaluate the care provided.

There have been relatively few attempts to evaluate palliative care services—the most ambitious being the national hospice study in the United States.[37] The finding that 'there appear to be few robust patient quality of life advantages associated with hospice' was not the conclusion expected but highlights the need for such studies. Other investigations have demonstrated benefits in terms of pain control, mobility, and psychosocial care within palliative care programmes.[38]

The importance of clinical audit has been generally recognized in the United Kingdom and has been given added stimulus by the changes within the National Health Service which require that all clinical services institute an audit programme. Clinical standard setting and guidelines for good practice are being developed as a basis for multidisciplinary clinical audit in palliative care.[39,40]

Thus, there are a number of areas which would be amenable to investigation under the broad heading of health services research. Its purpose is to improve patient care, and it is important that those involved in palliative care can see its value and be proactive in carrying out research in this fascinating field.

References

1. Vere D. Controlled clinical trials: the current ethical debate. *Journal of the Royal Society of Medicine*, 1981; **74**: 85–7.
2. Saunders C. Hospice care. *American Journal of Medicine*, 1978; **65**: 726–8.
3. Twycross RG. Choice of strong analgesic in terminal cancer: diamorphine or morphine? *Pain*, 1977; **3**: 93–104.
4. Murray Parkes C. Terminal care: home, hospital or hospice? *Lancet*, 1985; **i**: 155–7.
5. Anonymous. Emotion and empiricism. *British Medical Journal*, 1979; **i**: 288–9.
6. Caplan AC. Is there an obligation to participate in biomedical research? In: Spicker SF, Alon I, de Vries A, Engelhardt HT, eds. *The Use of Human Beings in Research*. Dordrecht: Kluwer, 1988: 229–48.

7. Anonymous. Human experimentation: code of ethics of the World Medical Association. *British Medical Journal*, 1964; **2**: 177.
8. Royal College of Physicians. *Guidelines on the Practice of Ethics Committees in Medical Research Involving Human Subjects*. 2nd edn. London: Royal College of Physicians, 1990.
9. Department of Health. *Local Research Ethics Committees*. London: Department of Health, 1991.
10. Bradford Hill A. Medical ethics and controlled trials. *British Medical Journal*, 1963; **ii**: 1043–9.
11. Beecher HK. Ethics and clinical research. *New England Journal of Medicine*, 1966; **274**: 1354–60.
12. Beecher HK. *Research and the Individual*. Boston: Little Brown, 1970.
13. Burkhardt K, Keinle G. Controlled clinical trials and medical ethics. *Lancet*, 1978; **ii**: 1356–9.
14. Anonymous. Controlled trials: planned deception? *Lancet*, 1979; **i**: 534–5.
15. Relman AS. The ethics of randomized clinical trials: two perspectives. *New England Journal of Medicine*, 1979; **300**: 1272–5.
16. Schafer A. The ethics of the randomized clinical trial. *New England Journal of Medicine*, 1982; **307**: 719–24.
17. Cancer Research Campaign Working Party in Breast Conservation. Informed consent: ethical, legal, and medical implications for doctors and patients who participate in randomized clinical trials. *British Medical Journal*, 1983; **286**: 117–21.
18. Dudley HAF. The controlled clinical trial and the advance of reliable knowledge: an outsider looks in. *British Medical Journal*, 1983; **287**: 957–60.
19. Research and Development Division, Department of Health. *Research for Health*. London: Department of Health, 1993.
20. Department of Health. *R and D Priorities in Cancer. Report to the NHS Central Research and Development Committee*. London: Department of Health, 1994.
21. European Commission. *Biomedicine and Health Research (BIOMED 2) 1994–1998 Workprogramme*. Brussels: European Commission, 1994.
22. Cawley N, Webber J. Research priorities in pallaitive care. *International Journal of Palliative Nursing*, 1995; **1**: 101–13.
23. Sackett DL, Rosenberg WMC, Gray JAM, Haynes RB, Richardson WS. Evidence-based medicine: what it is and what it isn't. *British Medical Journal*, 1996; **312**: 71–2.
24. Antman EM, Lau J, Kupelnick B, Mosteller F, Chalmers TC. A comparison of results of meta-analyses of randomized controlled trials and recommendations of clinical experts. *Journal of the American Medical Association*, 1992; **268**: 240–8.
25. Sackett DL, Rosenberg WMC. The need for evidence-based medicine. *Journal of the Royal Society of Medicine*, 1995; **88**: 620–4.
26. Eysenck HJ. Meta-analysis and its problems. *British Medical Journal*, 1994; **309**: 789–92.
27. Grahame-Smith D. Evidence-based medicine: Socratic dissent. *British Medical Journal*, 1995; **310**: 1126–7.
28. Godlee F. The Cochrane collaboration. *British Medical Journal*, 1994; **309**: 969–70.
29. Cochrane AL. 1931–1971: a critical review, with particular reference to the medical profession. In: *Medicines for the Year 2000*. London: Office of Health Economics, 1979: 1–11.
30. Jadad AR, Browman GP. The WHO analgesic ladder for cancer pain management. Stepping up the quality of its evaluation. *Journal of the American Medical Association*, 1995; **274**: 1870–3.
31. McQuay H, Carroll D, Jadad AR, Wiffen P, Moore A. Anticonvulsant drugs for management of pain: a systematic review. *British Medical Journal*, 1995; **311** 1047–52.
32. McQuay HJ. Preemptive analgesia: a systematic review of clinical studies. *Annals of Medicine*, 1995; **27**: 249–56.
33. Friedman LM, Furberg CD, DeMets DL. *Fundamentals of Clinical Trials*. Littleton: PSG Publishing, 1985.
34. MacIntyre IMC. Tribulations for clinical trials. Poor recruitment is hampering research. *British Medical Journal*, 1991; **302**: 1099–100.
35. Anonymous. *Priorities in Medical Research*. The Third Report of the House of Lords Select Committee on Science and Technology HL54 1987/88. London: Her Majesty's Stationery Office, 1988.
36. National Council for Hospice and Specialist Palliative Care Services. *Specialist Palliative Care: a Statement of Definitions*. Occasional paper 8. London: National Council for Hospice and Specialist Palliative Care Services, 1995.
37. Greer DS, Mor V. An overview of national hospice study findings. *Journal of Chronic Diseases*, 1986; **39**: 5–7.
38. Mount BM, Scott JF. Whither hospice evaluation? *Journal of Chronic Diseases*, 1983; **36**: 731–6.
39. Report of a working group of the research unit, Royal College of Physicians. Palliative care: guidelines for good practice and audit measures. *Journal of the Royal College of Physicians of London*, 1991; **25**: 325–8.
40. South West Thames Regional Health Authority. *A Framework for the Care of the Terminally Ill*. London: South West Thames Regional Health Authority, 1991.

5.2 Pain research: designing clinical trials in palliative care

Mitchell B. Max and Russell K. Portenoy

Introduction

The development of a scientific basis for symptom treatment is an imperative for the field of palliative care. Several historical circumstances make pain research an area of particular promise. First, a range of new treatments have been made possible by advances in both neuroscience and therapeutic technology. Examples include the development of selective agonists and antagonists of neural receptors mediating pain and analgesia, and the development of novel methods of analgesic administration, such as spinal, transdermal, or patient-controlled analgesic infusions. Second, the scientific foundation for research into pain therapy has already been established. Thousands of clinical trials have shown that simple measures of pain relief can reliably quantify analgesic efficacy. Third, there are great opportunities for methodological innovation, including multidose drug comparisons, assessment of treatment toxicity and quality of life, and controlled studies of spinal opioid infusions or neurolytic procedures.

This chapter is written for the palliative care clinician who plans to conduct controlled clinical trials of treatments for pain. In this brief review, no attempt will be made to be comprehensive; for example biostatistical issues, such as sample size calculation, sequential analysis methods, and specific statistical tests, are left to other works. Rather, several of the key issues in designing a clinical analgesic trial will be discussed in some depth: formulating the research question, choosing treatments and controls in a way that will maximize the chance for a meaningful positive or negative result, and tailoring the most efficient study procedures for a particular situation (e.g. patient selection, the choice between parallel or crossover design, and the choice of outcome measures). To complement this chapter, the novice investigator may wish to refer to longer works on analgesic study design,[1-3] monographs on clinical trials methods in general,[4-6] pain assessment,[7-9] and biostatistics.[10,11]

Clarifying the question to be studied

Clinical trials in palliative medicine might examine any of a wide variety of pain relief interventions, including treatments aimed at the lesion causing pain, new analgesic drugs or routes of drug administration, neuroablative procedures, cognitive treatments for pain, and efforts to improve physicians' prescribing practices. Each type of investigation requires numerous design choices. For most of these interventions, there have been few or no clinical trials, and it is not possible to give specific rules for their design. Nonetheless, there are several general questions common to all studies that may help the investigator to focus limited resources on the crucial issues.

What shortcomings of conventional treatments is the proposed treatment intended to correct?

The outcome measures and overall design of the study should focus on the components of this particular clinical dilemma. For example the most common dose-limiting side-effects of opioids are sedation and nausea. In studies of adjuvant drugs intended to specifically augment opioid analgesia, these side-effects must be carefully quantified, and the treatments, controls, and outcome measures must be sufficient to prove that the addition of the adjuvant not only increases analgesia but causes less sedation and nausea than an equianalgesic dose of the opioid alone. Such data are lacking on adjuvants in current use (Chapter 9.2.5 and Max[12]).

Is the study primarily intended to elucidate a biological principle, or to guide the clinician's empirical choice of treatment in that particular patient population?

Schwartz and Lellouch[13,14] distinguish between two different purposes of clinical trials, which they call 'explanatory' and 'pragmatic.' An 'explanatory' approach seeks to elucidate a biological principle. The study population is considered to be a model from which one may learn principles of analgesic pharmacology or pain physiology—principles that are likely to shed light on a variety of clinical problems. For example the 'analgesic equivalency tables' that guide opioid prescribing in a variety of conditions are largely based on studies in cancer patients.[1,2] A 'pragmatic' approach, in contrast, focuses on the question, 'What is the better treatment in the particular clinical circumstances of the patients in the study?

As an illustration of how these approaches to design differ, consider a hypothetical analgesic that animal studies had shown to be effective in models of visceral pain. Looking first at patient selection, a palliative care researcher oriented towards the explanatory approach might select only a small subset of cancer patients in whom there was unequivocal radiological proof of hollow viscera involvement, while the pragmatic clinical researcher might open the study to patients with ill-defined abdominal pain. An explanatory approach would try to maximize the therapeutic response by selecting a high dose and monitoring patients frequently; the pragmatically-oriented investigator might choose an intermediate dose and provide the looser supervision common in clinical practice. An explanatory approach will usually mandate a placebo, because even small amounts of pain relief over the placebo response may provide information about the mechanisms of visceral pain transmission and relief. A pragmatic approach, in contrast, generally compares the new treatment to the best treatment in clinical use. Placebo comparisons may still be desirable in such studies, particularly when there is no significant difference between the study drug and standard control (see below), but detection of a small therapeutic effect is of less interest.

The dichotomous explanatory/pragmatic schema is an oversimplification, of course. The investigator usually wishes to address both theoretical and practical concerns. This distinction may, however, offer a useful perspective for making design choices in complex cases.

How can previous clinical experience with the proposed treatment guide the design of a controlled trial?

Retrospective or prospective surveys of clinical experience can provide insights into the nature and variety of therapeutic and adverse effects produced by a treatment, and thereby help determine the methods for future controlled studies. Among other factors, surveys can suggest the major sources of variability in the response to an intervention. For example a survey of approximately 700 cancer patients treated with non-steroidal anti-inflammatory drugs suggested that pain relief was greater in patients with bony or other somatic lesions than in those with nerve lesions.[15]

Surveys may also enable the investigator to estimate the time-course of response. In a controlled trial, treatment periods should be long enough so that patients will approach maximal response, unless a significant incidence of dropouts or spontaneous change in the disease over that length of time mandates a compromise on study duration. This will help to maximize the power of the study to detect treatment differences. In some cases, survey data must be supplemented by prospective open-label pilot studies. For analgesic drug treatments, survey data or prospective dose-ranging studies will suggest a maximum safe dose for initial studies and may suggest a range of doses or blood levels that will produce analgesia.[16] Such pilot studies can also provide variance estimates for the major outcome measures, which are needed to choose the sample size.[4] The use of surveys and non-randomized controlled trials are discussed further in other articles.[17,18]

Choice of treatments and controls

A clear-cut positive or negative result of a clinical trial is often useful to other researchers and, ultimately, to patients. Unfortunately, many clinical studies turn out to be inconclusive (and often unpublishable) because of poor selection of control groups. During the 40-year history of analgesic clinical trials, a distinct logic has evolved regarding the choice of controls and the interpretation of clinical trials. This framework, illustrated in Fig. 1(a-h), is now widely applied in determining the validity of single-dose analgesic trials.[19,20]

Interpreting analgesic studies: test drug, placebo, and positive control

Although the simplest of the classic designs consists of two treatments—the test medication and a placebo—most modern single-dose trials also include a standard analgesic 'positive control.' In single-dose trials, common positive controls include morphine, aspirin, or ibuprofen.

To demonstrate the value of these controls, consider a hypothetical study comparing the putative analgesic drug X to a morphine 'positive control' and a placebo (Fig. 1(a)). Using summed pain relief scores as the measure of analgesia, drug X tended to be slightly but not statistically significantly more effective than morphine, and both drug X and morphine were statistically superior to placebo. The conclusions are straightforward; drug X is an effective analgesic and the study methods were sufficiently sensitive to distinguish morphine from placebo.

The omission of a positive control does not fatally flaw the study if drug X is superior to placebo (Fig. 1(b)), although one cannot be certain about the strength of the effect. The positive control serves as a yardstick against which to compare the magnitude of the analgesia produced by drug X. In pain syndromes for which there is no accepted positive control—for example some types of neuropathic pain—the comparison of test drug to placebo must suffice. Should drug X fail to produce more analgesia than the placebo, however, the omission of the positive control will render the study uninterpretable (Fig. 1(c)). One cannot reliably conclude that drug X is ineffective in this condition. Perhaps the drug is truly analgesic in patients with this condition, but the study methods were too insensitive to observe this effect. This could happen because patients were too stressed by the clinical setting to respond to medication, the pain questionnaires were insensitive, the procedures of the nurse-observer were variable or confusing, or merely because of random variation. If a morphine positive control were included and shown superior to both placebo and drug X (Fig. 1(d)), this would validate the study methodology and indicate that drug X was not analgesic in this population. Alternatively, if morphine produced no more analgesia than drug X and the placebo (Fig. 1(e)), one could conclude that the study methods were inadequate to show the effects of even a strong analgesic.

What are the consequences of omitting the placebo and comparing drug X only to a standard analgesic? As in the previous case, this omission is less damaging when the assay shows a difference between the two treatments. The data in Fig. 1(f) suggest that drug X is an effective analgesic in this population, although the proportion of analgesia attributable to the placebo effect cannot be determined for either drug X or morphine. If the responses to drug X and standard analgesic were similar, however (Fig. 1(g)), interpretation would be troublesome. The data might reflect either that drug X and morphine were both effective analgesics, or that neither were effective and there was a large placebo effect.[21]

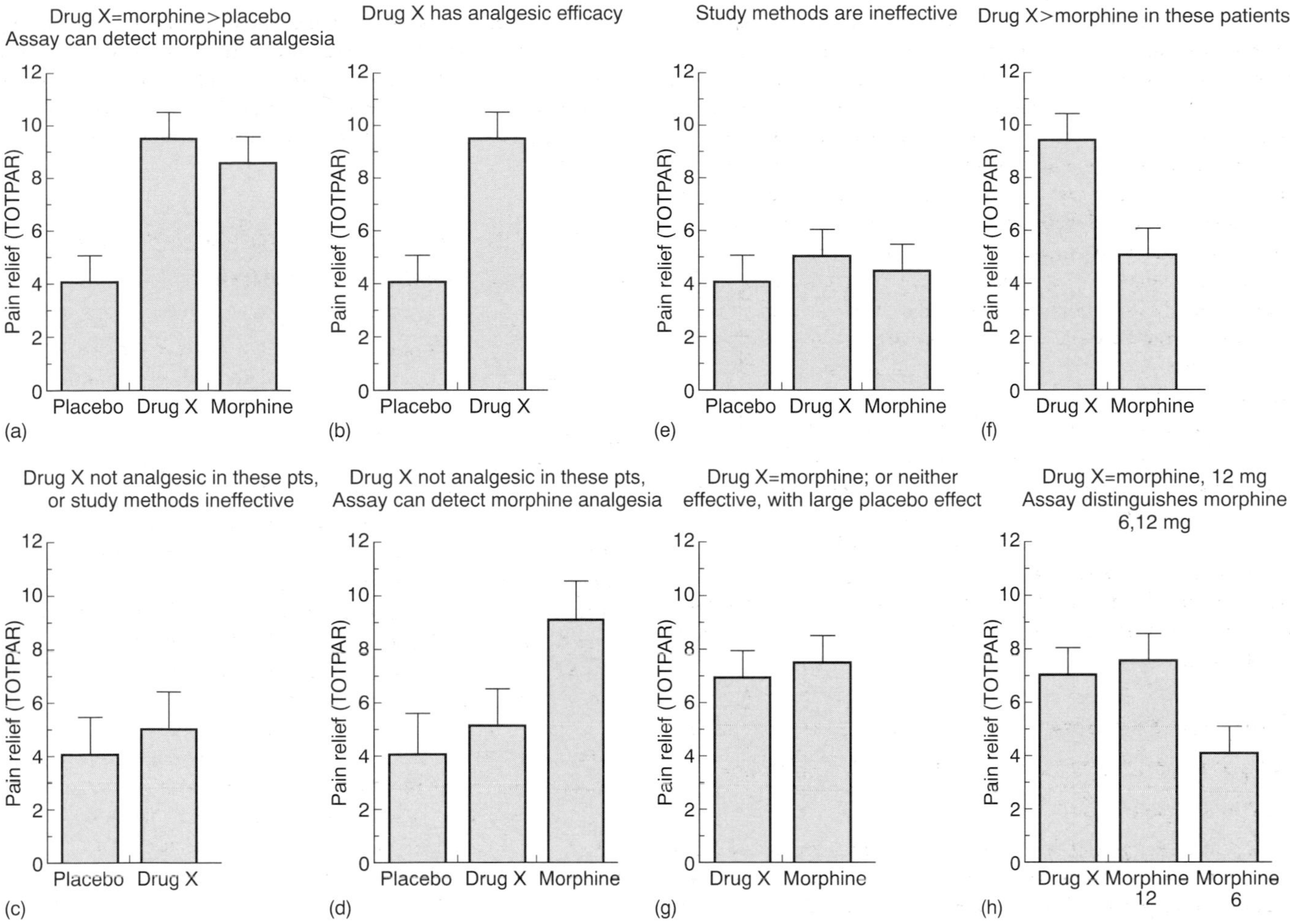

Fig. 1 (a)-(h)Placebo and standard analgesic in the interpretation of analgesic trials (see text). Explanation of symbols: >, statistically significantly greater than; =, not significantly different from. TOTPAR = 'total of pain relief scores' during the study period. (Reproduced from Max and Laska,[19] with permission.)

If the use of a placebo group is difficult, an alternative approach is to use a second dose level of the standard analgesic. Fig. 1(h) shows that morphine 12 mg surpassed morphine 6 mg, demonstrating the sensitivity of the study methods, and implying that the effects of both drug X and morphine 12 mg were not merely placebo effects.

In addition to doses of a test drug, a standard analgesic, and a placebo, most analgesic studies include additional treatment groups or controls that are chosen to further elucidate the major research question. For example when evaluating a range of doses of test analgesic, one might add additional doses of standard analgesic spanning that analgesic range, both to serve as a comparative yardstick and to verify that the study methods can separate high from moderate analgesic doses. (For further discussion of this point see Max *et al.* pp.77–8.[3]) To test the soundness of proposed designs, the investigator may wish to graph the possible outcomes as in Fig. 1(a-h). If the conclusion given a particular outcome is ambiguous, it may be wise to consider additional treatment groups that would distinguish among the alternative explanations. The addition of treatment or control groups is costly, however. One must either recruit more patients or reduce the size of each treatment group, lessening the statistical power of the comparisons. In many cases, particularly where negative results will not be of great interest, researchers may choose to omit controls whose main value is to clarify the interpretation of the negative result.

Placebo and positive controls in chronic palliative care studies

In single-dose analgesic studies in cancer pain, there are rarely ethical objections to the use of placebos, because patients understand that they can terminate the study and take additional analgesic at any time. In actual practice, many patients experience some placebo analgesia, and most tolerate the study for the 1 to 2 h needed to evaluate the response to the placebo.

Chronic studies are a different matter, however. Although a placebo control has been considered to be appropriate in studies of pain syndromes that have no reliable treatment, such as some painful neuropathies, chronic administration of a placebo cannot be justified in pain syndromes that generally respond to therapy, such as most cancer pain syndromes. Moreover, attrition rates under such circumstances are likely to be high; for example in a placebo-controlled drug trial in cancer patients,[22] 90 per cent of the placebo group withdrew in the first day. The same problem exists for

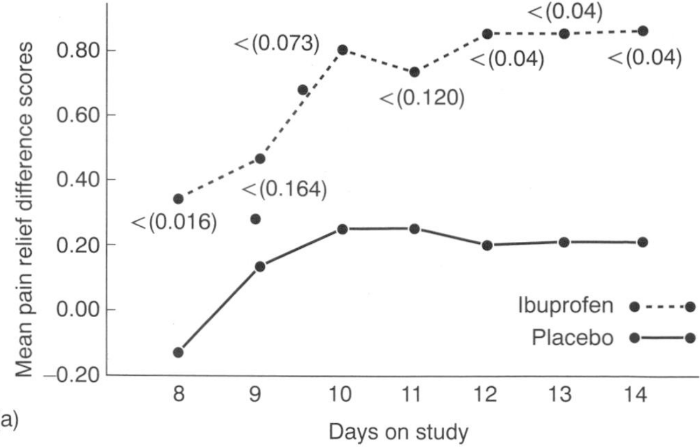

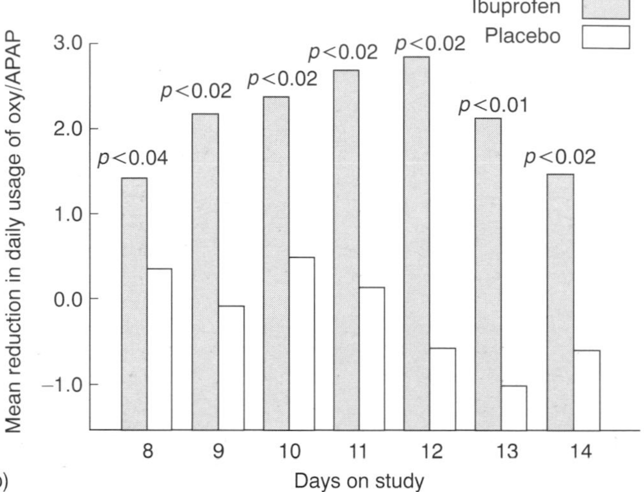

Fig. 2 (a) Comparison of mean pain relief differences of ibuprofen, 600 mg four times/day and placebo, both in combination with oxycodone/paracetamol (oxy/APAP) as needed. Positive values represent greater pain relief. Values in parentheses represent *p* values of ibuprofen v. placebo. Day 8 was the first day ibuprofen or placebo were added, after 7 days of baseline observations of pain and oxy/APAP consumption. (b) Alterations of oxy/APAP use after the addition of ibuprofen or placebo. Mean reduction scores were determined by comparing oxy/APAP use on days 6 and 7 with means for each of days 8 through 14. For each day, oxy/APAP use was reduced by the addition of ibuprofen. (Reproduced from Stambaugh and Drew,[23] with permission.)

studies of discrete interventions, for example coeliac block, that require a prolonged observation period after the treatment.

In these situations, therefore, the only feasible way to conduct placebo-controlled studies may be to give both placebo and active treatment groups access to a standard analgesic 'rescue' dose. An example of a chronic placebo-controlled study of ibuprofen for metastatic bone pain is shown in Fig. 2. Stambaugh *et al*[23] enrolled a group of inpatients whose bone pain required at least four daily doses of an oxycodone/paracetamol combination. Strong parenteral opioids were also given for severe breakthrough pain, but patients requiring more than one injection daily were dropped from the study. For the first 7 days of the study, no intervention took place; the daily dose of oxycodone/paracetamol was monitored, and patients assessed pain intensity and relief once a day. On days 8 to 14, half the patients received ibuprofen 600 mg orally four times daily, and the other half received placebo. Figure 2 shows that pain relief was better with ibuprofen than placebo, and that the ibuprofen-treated group reduced their oxycodone/acetaminophen consumption relative to the placebo group. This example illustrates how use of the background or rescue analgesic becomes another important outcome measure. Similar strategies have been used to study the analgesic effects of sustained-release morphine in cancer patients[24-26] and many types of interventions in postoperative pain.[27,28]

In these designs, the rescue analgesic may be given by any of a variety of routes, including oral, intramuscular, or intravenous (commonly by patient-controlled analgesia devices). Both pain report and rescue analgesic consumption should be examined as primary outcome measures. Although some investigators have used the amount of rescue drug consumed as the only outcome measure, many patients may not change their analgesic demands enough to completely offset any change in pain (as in Fig. 2 and Portenoy *et al.* and Lehmann[26,27]). In addition, the reduction of analgesic consumption alone is not a compelling clinical advantage, unless pain or analgesic side-effects can also be shown to be reduced. An analytic method has been proposed that integrates pain score and rescue analgesic consumption into a single summary variable.[29]

In repeated dose studies just as in single-dose studies, positive controls or multiple levels of the test drug may also be used to answer the research question.[30,31] As with the placebo-controlled studies discussed above, provisions must generally be made for a rescue analgesic treatment of some sort. In addition, the protocol should allow for lowering doses of the test drug or standard analgesic should drug toxicity occur.

Designing the appropriate control interventions may also be a challenge for non-pharmacological treatments. Control or sham interventions are possible with diverse treatments such as cognitive pain control techniques or acupuncture but they are often open to criticism.[32] With more invasive methods such as neuroablative procedures, placebo or sham procedures are generally considered inappropriate.

Comments on several specialized design problems

Dose-ranging studies

Knowledge of a drug's dose–response curve guides its use in clinical practice. This relationship is clarified through studies that compare the effects produced by a range of doses. The dose range to be examined in these trials may be chosen on the basis of phase I toxicity studies, which indicate an upper limit, or by prior clinical experience. Methods for examining the dose–response relationship is an area of current research interest,[33-35] although there has been little work with chronic analgesic therapies.

A few general points can be made about dose-ranging. First, doses should be chosen over a wide range of levels. For dose ranges that may be of clinical interest, several levels of a standard analgesic control are also often desirable, allowing a direct comparison of adverse effects for the test and standard treatment at levels producing equal analgesia. Second, efforts to estimate the optimal therapeutic range are often assisted by the analysis of blood levels of drug or active metabolites, particularly in the case of drugs whose pharmacokinetics have great variability.[16] Third, to draw firm conclusions about dose–response curves, it is important that several different dosing schemes be specified prospectively; these

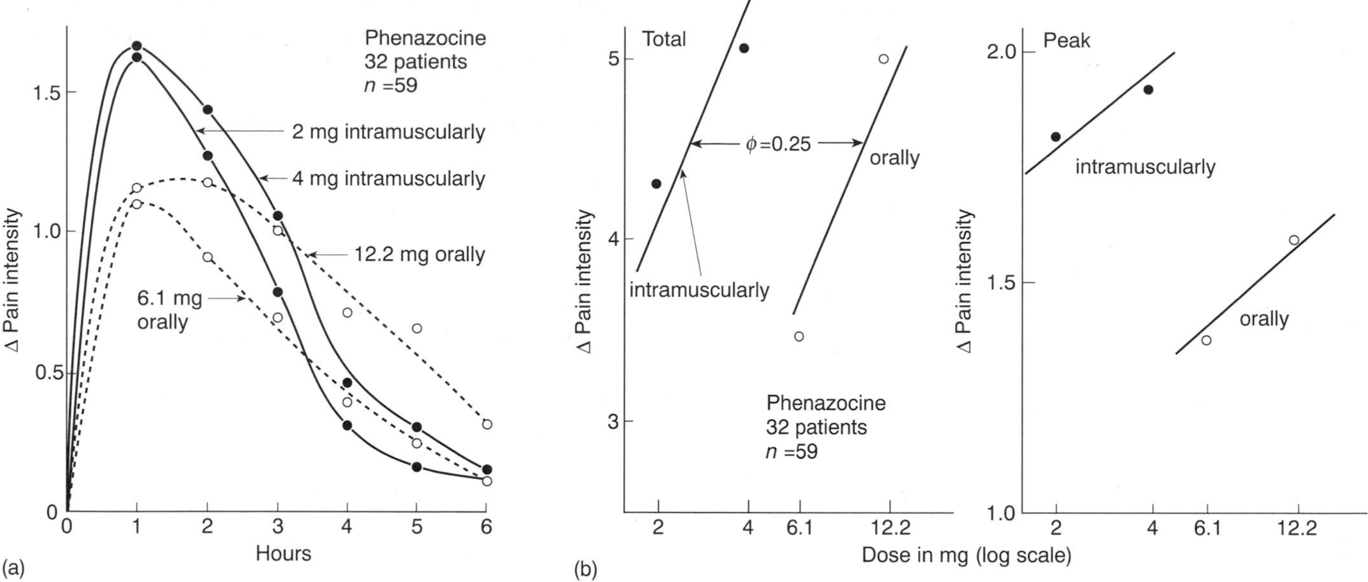

Fig. 3 Four-point relative potency study comparing intramuscular (filled circles) and oral (open circles) phenazocine. (a) Pain intensity difference (category scale) is plotted against time. Note the difference between the time course of analgesia for the two routes. (b) Total (left) or peak (right) changes in pain intensity are plotted against dose. For total scores, oral phenazocine is one-fourth as potent as the intramuscular drug. For peak scores, no relative potency can be calculated because there was no overlap between the levels of response seen with the two routes. Because the time course of response differs between the routes, note that the relative potency calculated for total scores will change according to the length of the study; for example if only the first 3 h were considered, the intramuscular/oral disparity would have appeared even greater. (Reproduced from Beaver *et al.*,[38] with permission.)

may include parallel group designs, crossover studies[33] (see below), or studies using several different ascending dose-titration schedules.[36]

Relative potency studies

One of the most useful tools in guiding the dosing of opioid analgesics has been the class of designs called relative potency bioassays.[37] Relative potency bioassays consist of a comparison of two or more doses of a test drug with two or more doses of a standard (Fig. 3). A placebo may not be necessary in such trials because the demonstration of a statistically significant positive slope for the dose–response curves establishes assay sensitivity. A placebo is necessary, however, if one wishes to estimate the lowest dose at which analgesic efficacy might be detected.

There are several advantages in expressing the outcome of a study or group of studies[38,39] in terms of relative potency. First, such estimates allow clinicians to tailor the dosing of a new drug to the individual patient, based on the specific dose of the standard usually used by that patient. Secondly, this method eliminates the problem of expressing a drug's effect in units on an arbitrary analgesic scale, measurements whose absolute size may vary with the patient population, study methods, and placebo effect. Finally, relative potency studies allow one to test whether a new analgesic or drug combination is superior to the standard in terms of toxicity as well as efficacy; the relative intensity of adverse effects can be estimated for the two treatments at doses providing the same analgesia.[12,40]

There are also pitfalls in interpreting relative potency assays. If the dose–response curves of the test and standard drugs are not linear and parallel, or the doses chosen are not in the same analgesic range, the calculated relative potency may be incorrect or meaningless. In addition, if the drugs to be compared have different kinetics, the relative potency may vary greatly depending upon whether the peak pain relief or the summed scores over time are used. For example using summed scores over time will favour a drug with longer duration (Fig. 3(b)).

In addition, relative potency estimates derived from single-dose studies may not be sufficient to predict chronic dosing requirements, particularly when the pharmacokinetics of the treatments and their active metabolites differ. For example the slowly-metabolized analgesic methadone is equipotent to morphine as a single parenteral dose but many times more potent in chronic treatment. The relative potency design could potentially be used with chronic dosing regimens—for example comparing two different levels of chronic epidural morphine infusion to two levels of parenteral infusion, but the previously discussed requirement for rescue analgesics or dose reductions would present challenges in analysis.

Studies to assess whether two treatments are equivalent

A common error in study design is to assume that the demonstration of no significant difference between two analgesics proves that they are equivalent.[41] The error in this reasoning is illustrated by the following example. In a controlled trial, cancer patients received either intramuscular morphine, 10 mg, or intramuscular morphine, 5 mg, plus a peptide shown to potentiate opioid analgesia in animals. In the clinical trial, similar pain relief scores were observed for the two treatments and the investigator concluded that the peptide doubled the analgesic effects of morphine. The data do not support this; without controls such as morphine 5 mg alone or placebo, there was no demonstration that the study methods would have been sensitive enough to detect a true difference between analgesics (Fig. 1(g)). Even if both 10 mg morphine and 5 mg morphine+peptide had surpassed a control group, a convincing demonstration of equivalence would require demonstrating that the 95 per cent confidence interval for the difference between the two treatments was also small.[42–44] This generally requires a much larger sample size than is needed to distinguish an active treatment from placebo.[41]

Drug combinations

Many advances in pain treatment are likely to involve drug combinations and controlled clinical trials of such combinations present particular challenges.[45] If a test drug is simply added to a standard regimen whose optimal dose is well known, the need for dose-ranging is limited to the test drug.[46] Should uncertainty exist about the dose of each component, however, a rather complex study may be needed.[47] For example one might determine dose–response curves for each component alone and for several dose-ratios of the combination. Reviews of current work are given in the reference list.[12,19,45,48–50]

Parallel versus crossover designs

In a parallel group (also termed 'completely randomized') design, each patient receives a single treatment. In a crossover design, each patient receives some (incomplete block) or all (complete block) of the treatments being studied.

There are several obvious advantages to crossover designs. Analgesic studies often require large sample sizes because detection of a drug effect must compete with so many other causes of variation in pain report; the subject's painful lesion, tolerance to opioid medications, psychological make-up, previous pain experience, age, race, weight, interaction with the study personnel, etc. Much of this between patient variation can be eliminated by using a crossover design, in which treatment comparisons are largely or entirely within the same patient.[51–56] Because of this reduction in variance, and because each patient is used several times, crossover studies usually have greater statistical power for a given sample size than parallel group designs.[45] This is an important practical advantage, particularly when studies are performed in a single centre. Crossover designs have been used frequently in studies of cancer pain.[1,57]

Such advantages notwithstanding, there may be problems with the use of crossover designs in palliative care settings. First, change in the painful lesions over time may introduce great variability into patient responses, thereby undermining the major potential advantage of the crossover design. This necessitates that the total duration of the crossover study be short enough to ensure such within-patient variation will be less than the variation already existing between the patients enrolled. The changes in the underlying disease, as well as logistical factors and voluntary withdrawals, usually cause a higher dropout rate in crossover than in parallel group studies. Although the greater power of the crossover approach may compensate for a higher dropout rate, reviewers may doubt the general applicability of the results of a study completed by a minority of the patients entered.

Another major concern with crossover studies is the possibility of bias produced by unequal 'carryover effects'. Carryover effects are changes in the efficacy of treatments resulting from treatments given in earlier periods; they may be mediated by persistence of drug or metabolites, changes in brain or peripheral tissues caused by the treatment, or behavioural or psychological factors. The major problem with carryover effects occurs with the two-treatment, two-period design ('2 × 2'; Table 1, left). Results may be difficult to interpret whenever the treatment effect differs for the two periods. In this event, one cannot distinguish with any certainty whether this is due to a carryover effect (persistence of a pharmacological or psychological effect of the first treatment into the second period), a 'treatment × period interaction' (the passage of time affects the relative efficacy of the treatments; for example by the second period, patients who initially received placebo might be too discouraged to respond to any subsequent treatment), or a difference between the groups of patients assigned the two different orders of treatment. For this reason, regulatory agencies have been particularly reluctant to rely upon data from such designs.

Table 1 Some alternative designs for two-treatment crossover studies

Standard 2 x 2	Alternative 1	Alternative 2	Alternative 3
A–B	A–B	A–B–B	A–B–B
B–A	B–A	B–A–A	B–A–A
	A–A		A–B–A
	B–B		B–A–B

Fortunately, these statistical difficulties are largely limited to the 2 × 2 case. If the investigator adds several other treatment sequences (Table 1, alternative 1) or a third treatment period (alternatives 2 and 3) unbiased estimates of treatment effects are possible even in the presence of various types of carryover effects.[54–56,58] For studies involving three or more treatments, there are a variety of designs that allow these effects to be distinguished.[54,59] Thus, although the relative brevity and simplicity of the 2 × 2 design may make it attractive for single-centre pilot studies and for situations in which previous experience suggests that there is no significant carryover effect, the need to estimate treatment effects with greater certainty will usually recommend the use of alternative designs.

A variant of the crossover design, the 'enriched enrolment' design, may be useful in studying treatments to which only a minority of patients respond.[60] If the results are not statistically significant in a conventional clinical trial, one cannot retrospectively point at the responders and claim that the treatment accounted for their relief. One can, however, enter them into a second prospective trial, or a series of comparisons between treatment and placebo. If the results of the second trial considered alone are statistically significant, this suggests that the patients' initial response was not just due to chance. While statistically defensible, enriched enrolment designs are open to the criticism that prior exposure to the treatment defeat the double-blind procedure (particularly with treatments that have distinctive side-effects) and sometimes result in spurious positive results.

Parallel study designs are preferable when there are strong concerns about carryover effects or when the natural history of the pain syndrome makes disease-related changes in pain likely during the period required for a crossover study. Between-patient variability is the major problem posed by parallel group designs and several approaches have been suggested to mitigate its impact.[61] For

Table 2 Factors that contribute to the heterogeneity of the population suffering from cancer pain

Pain-related factors	Pain characteristics
	intensity and duration of chronic pain
	pain intensity at study onset
	quality
	temporal pattern
	precipitants
	Pain mechanisms and site of lesion
	Prior therapy
	duration and extent of prior analgesic use
	efficacy of previous analgesics
	prior adverse effects from analgesics
Patient-related factors	Demographics
	Psychological factors
	affective disorder
	other psychiatric disorders
	behavioural disturbances
	cognitions, expectations, and fears
	intellectual capacity
	degree of placebo response
	Other historical factors
	history of chronic pain
	history of substance abuse
	history of psychiatric disorder
Disease-related factors	Related to neoplasm
	type of tumour
	extent of disease
	previous antineoplastic therapy
	ongoing antineoplastic therapy
	Other pathological processes
	major organ dysfunction
	number and severity of other symptoms
	Other treatments
	concurrent use of centrally acting drugs
	use of drugs that may be coanalgesic

example baseline pain scores may be subtracted from the treatment scores to yield pain intensity difference scores, or they may be treated as a covariate. This often eliminates a large part of the variance, thereby increasing the power of treatment comparisons. In single-dose analgesic drug trials, the baseline has generally been determined under 'no treatment conditions' but, as discussed above, a standard pain treatment regimen will generally be needed in palliative care contexts.

The investigator should also make an effort to balance the treatment groups for variables that predict response whenever these predictors are known or suspected.[62] If one wishes to examine response in specific subgroups, assignments must also be balanced appropriately. Groups can be balanced using stratification or various techniques of adaptive randomization.[4,6] In studies with sample sizes typical of single centre trials (20-40 patients per group) these methods can significantly increase the power of a study if the prognostic variables are well chosen and the statistical methods take the balancing method into account.[61] If stratification is not feasible, *post hoc* covariate analyses or other statistical techniques may be an acceptable substitute if the variables in question are distributed fairly evenly among the treatment groups.

Selecting the patient sample

Many characteristics of the patients may influence the outcome of analgesic studies (Table 2). Depending upon the purpose of the study (see above), investigators may either choose to define the population narrowly for a number of factors, or may open the study to a broad group of patients. Narrow criteria bring certain benefits—potentially lower variance in outcome measures and, as discussed above, more solid grounding for 'explanatory' conclusions. On the other hand, multiple rigorous entry criteria may slow patient accrual or introduce selection biases that may limit the generalizability of the results. For example the decision to exclude elderly cancer patients from a trial may reduce the risk of adverse effects but will also limit the value of the efficacy and safety data for treating older patients.

Factors related to the pain

In selecting patients for cancer pain studies, particular attention should be paid to pain mechanisms, temporal characteristics, baseline pain intensity, and prior opioid intake.[63]

It is reasonable to assume that pain mechanisms may not be uniform among pains arising from different tissues, and that these differences may affect responses to particular treatments. Although pain mechanisms may sometimes be directly assessed using techniques such as stimulation or blockade of particular nerve fibre populations, this will rarely be practical in palliative care clinical trials. Pain mechanisms may be imputed from knowledge of the involved tissues, and from the patient's pain report. Therefore, it is important that researchers characterize patients by the site of pain-producing lesions during enrolment into the study, and by the quality and temporal characteristics of the pain. Current studies at Memorial Sloan-Kettering Cancer Center use the following categories.

1. Somatic pain denotes pain arising from bone, joint, muscle, skin, or connective tissue, which is usually aching or throbbing in quality and well-localized. For some purposes, investigators may wish to consider particular subclasses, such as bone pain.
2. Visceral pain can be subdivided into a relatively well-localized and aching pain associated with tumour involvement of organ capsules and the poorly localized, usually intermittent cramping associated with obstruction of a hollow viscus. These two subtypes should be distinguished in analgesic studies.
3. Neuropathic pain is most commonly burning or stabbing in quality, is often associated with a sense of distortion of the body part or light-touch evoked discomfort, and is accompanied by evidence of appropriately localized injury to the peripheral or central nervous system.

Although many pains in patients with cancer are relatively steady, some patients have intermittent transient pains, such as the so-called 'incident pains' that are triggered by movement. The analgesic efficacy of any therapeutic modality may be difficult to assess when these pains are frequent and severe. In some studies, it may be reasonable for the investigator to exclude patients in whom they are particularly prominent, whereas in other studies it may be useful to consider quantifying the frequency and intensity of these pains as an additional outcome measure.

Baseline pain intensity and consumption of analgesic drugs prior to the study (including type and dose of drug, duration of treatment, and time of last dose) must also be recorded as potentially important covariates.[64,65] In the case of opioids, the latter factor may operate, at least in part, through the influence of tolerance. Variability in prior opioid consumption may greatly increase the variation in response to the test doses of the experimental opioids. This possibility is usually addressed during the study through the use of appropriate selection criteria (e.g. a designated range of prior opioid consumption) or by stratification by previous drug intake. Alternatively, variable degrees of tolerance within the study sample can potentially be managed by flexibility in the test doses used during the study; if the relative potency of the test drug and baseline drug is known, doses of the study drug can be determined as a proportion of the patient's prior opioid exposure, rather than as a fixed milligram amount.

Factors related to the patient

A large number of patient characteristics (Table 2) must also be considered in the selection of appropriate candidates for study. In those patients who participate in the study, these characteristics may become important covariates to evaluate *vis-à-vis* the analgesic response.

Factors related to the disease

The medical condition of the patient must be carefully considered in the selection process. Major organ failure, including pulmonary or renal insufficiency, cardiac or liver disease, or encephalopathy, may increase the risks to the patient of participation in the study, potentially undermine data collection, or bias patients towards rating treatments as unacceptable even if they relieve pain. Mild degrees of delirium or dementia are common in cancer patients[66] and may impair the patient's ability to discriminate effects.

Outcome measures

Pain and pain relief

Most of the clinical analgesic trials in the literature have used category scales and visual analogue scales, such as those shown in Table 3. In single-dose analgesic comparisons, patients are asked to complete these scales at regular intervals and derived measures such as peak relief (or reduction in pain intensity score) and summed relief scores are used as outcome measures.[19] In these studies, relief category scales and visual analogue scales for pain intensity and relief appear somewhat more sensitive than pain category scales in detecting drug treatment effects.[68,69]

In chronic studies, researchers have generally used category scales, visual analogue scales, or the McGill Pain Questionnaire[70] to assess pain. A measure developed specifically for the cancer patient, the Brief Pain Inventory combines a 0 to 10 rating of pain intensity with assessments of mood, common daily activities, and sleep.[71] Studies to compare these tools in palliative care settings are needed.[72]

Many investigators prefer to use pain intensity rather than pain relief scales in chronic studies because they allow the patient to directly estimate the pain. Any assessment of pain relief, in contrast, requires a comparison with the memory of baseline pain, which may be difficult in studies of long duration. Although single-dose studies have suggested that the pain intensity visual analogue scales may be more sensitive than the pain intensity category scale,[68] the visual analogue scales may be confusing to some elderly patients and those with a poor grasp of English. A study in which only written instructions were given found that 11 per cent of chronic pain patients failed to complete the visual analogue scales, while all used the category scale correctly.[73] Some of these failures can be prevented by careful instruction of the patient.[74,75]

The McGill Pain Questionnaire has been extensively validated as a multidimensional pain scale for acute and chronic pain conditions.[76] Its disadvantages are that it takes about 5 minutes to complete (compared to seconds for visual analogue scales and category scales), requires a rich vocabulary, and confuses some patients.[71,77] In a study of cancer patients, an Italian version of the McGill Pain Questionnaire was shown to reflect only one dimension, which appeared to be most closely related to pain intensity.[78] If this finding generalizes within the cancer population, it would suggest that the potential value of multidimensional assessment is not realized in cancer pain. A pain intensity rating is more simply acquired using a briefer scale, such as the visual analogue scales.

Table 3 Examples of standard category and visual analogue scales used to assess pain and pain relief in analgesic studies (adapted from ref. 67, with permission).

Pain intensity category scale (4-point)		Pain relief category scale (5-point)	
Severe	3	Complete	4
Moderate	2	Lots	3
Mild	1	Moderate	2
None	0	Slight	1
		None	0

LEAST possible pain	Visual analogue scale, pain intensity	WORST possible pain
NO relief of pain	Visual analogue scale, pain relief	COMPLETE relief of pain

An important issue in the conduct of analgesic trials is the frequency of pain assessment. Many chronic studies have used single ratings before and after treatments, even though many types of cancer-related pain fluctuate over hours or days. Because single retrospective ratings covering a long period may be strongly affected by the pain level over the past day or two, treatment effects determined using the mean of frequent ratings over a long period (e.g. daily or several times daily) may be more robust;[79] there will still be random fluctuations but they will tend to average out over the study period. Although the possibility of missing data is compounded by the request for frequent pain measurement, the successful completion of studies that incorporated nightly[80] or multiple daily pain measures[26] suggests that this degree of patient burden is not excessive for most ambulatory populations. Frequent and prospective pain evaluation is particularly important if separate pains (e.g. steady pain and incident pains) or various characteristics of the pain are to be assessed independently. This type of evaluation can yield data that may be relevant to pain mechanisms or to the clinical utility of an intervention.

Analgesic use

As discussed above, most chronic studies of cancer pain require the use of a background analgesic regimen and/or the provision of rescue doses, the need for which can be used as an ancillary measure of analgesic efficacy. Before the study begins, it is often advisable to revise patients' analgesic regimen to a standard set of treatments—for example an aspirin-like agent and an appropriate dose of morphine. This may make the population more homogeneous and enhance the sensitivity of the study. Whatever the method for adjusting analgesic maintenance or rescue doses, it is important that procedures for making decisions are as uniform as is practical, particularly between clinicians or study sites. As discussed above, the efficacy of a standard opioid rescue dose may vary with the degree of prior opioid tolerance.

A recent controlled study[80] evaluated the analgesic outcome associated with a new chemotherapy for pancreas cancer using change in pain and analgesic consumption as two of the primary outcome measures. To accomplish this, a standardized opioid regimen was implemented during a 'run-in' period. This regimen incorporated a baseline opioid and a rescue dose. During the study period that followed, patients were randomly assigned to receive one of two chemotherapeutic drugs. Each patient received multiple treatment cycles over a period of many months. The treating oncologist made whatever adjustments in the opioid regimen that were needed to retain optimal pain control during this lengthy period. At the end of the study, both pain scores and analgesic consumption differed significantly between the two study groups. The standardization of the analgesic regimen in this design presumably reduced the within-group variability, and may have increased the likelihood that these significant group differences would be found.

Drug side-effects

Numerous checklists have been devised to survey adverse effects during drug trials.[81] The more extensive of these[82,83] assess a variety of characteristics for each adverse event, including severity, relationship to the drug, temporal characteristics (timing after a dose, duration and pattern during the day), contributing factors, course, and action taken to counteract the effect. Symptoms can be listed a priori or can be recorded as observed by the investigator. Each characteristic can be quantified with scales of various complexity. For example the likelihood of a relationship between the adverse event and the study drug in clinical drug trials has been recorded on a categorical scale (none, remote, possible, probable, definite) according to the presence or absence of specific features;[84] these may include a reasonable temporal relationship, foreknowledge that such an event may occur with the specific drug, improvement following discontinuation of the drug, and reappearance of the effect following repeated exposure. If appropriate, specific instruments can be used to assess one or more side-effects, such as nausea[85] or cognitive impairment.[86] A simpler approach assesses the intensity of a symptom on a visual analogue scale adapted for the purpose; this has been accomplished successfully with sedation, for example.[87]

The detailed assessment of adverse events can add considerably to the time and effort required for the evaluation of the study intervention. The degree to which the various characteristics are pursued should be determined by the overall goals of the study. The evaluation of a new type of analgesic drug, for example, may warrant this effort, whereas such detail may be appropriately neglected in lieu of other assessments in studies of accepted opioids for which the side-effect spectrum is well appreciated.

In studies comparing a placebo to a putative therapeutic drug that also produces side-effects, patients' perception of side-effects may increase their expectation of benefit, and lead to a false positive result.[88,89] While there is no consensus about how to deal with this potential bias, suggestions have included the use of 'active placebos' that mimic the side-effects of the test drug, use of questionnaires to assess whether patients and staff can see through the blind,[90] or simpler measures such as the careful recording of side-effects or the use of multiple dose levels of the test drug. In the latter case, the finding of a positive dose–response relationship above the level where side-effects begin suggests a specific analgesic effect.

Mood, function, and global assessments

The effects of pain treatment on mood, function, and other dimensions of the quality of life are essential measures for chronic pain studies in palliative care settings. Measurement of these outcomes is discussed in Chapters 2.7, 9.2.9, and Section 15 of this volume.

Because a treatment may relieve pain, but produce side-effects or worsen symptoms associated with the underlying disease, it is valuable to have the patient make an overall rating of treatment acceptability. In parallel designs, a category scale can be used (e.g., 'How satisfied have you been with the treatment you received during the study? Not at all, slightly, moderately, a great deal, completely'). In crossover trials, patients may be asked to compare one intervention to the other ('Did you prefer treatment A, treatment B, or have no preference?'). All studies can incorporate a query about the future use of a treatment ('Would you be willing to continue treatment with this intervention?').

Conclusion

This brief chapter has sought to identify key issues in designing controlled trials of pain relief in palliative care settings. Practical difficulties of research in this patient group are great, but aided by patience, frequent consultations with a statistician and other pain researchers, and a familiarity with the principles of pain research outlined here, palliative care clinicians have the opportunity to shape a new research tradition.

References

1. Houde RW, Wallenstein SL, Beaver WT. Evaluation of analgesics in patients with cancer pain. In: Lasagna L, ed. *Clinical Pharmacology. Section 6. International Encyclopedia of Pharmacology and Therapeutics.* New York: Pergamon Press, 1966: 59–97.
2. Houde RW, Wallenstein SL, Beaver WT. Clinical measurement of pain. In: de Stevens G, ed. *Analgesics.* New York: Academic Press, 1965, 75–122.
3. Max MB, Portenoy RK, Laska EM, eds. *The Design of Analgesic Clinical Trials.* New York: Raven Press, 1991.
4. Friedman LM, Furberg CD, DeMets DL. *Fundamentals of Clinical Trials*, 2nd edn. Littleton, Massachusetts: PSG Publishing Company, 1985.
5. Pocock SJ. *Clinical Trials: a Practical Approach.* Chichester, UK: John Wiley and Sons, 1983.
6. Meinert CL. *Clinical Trials: Design, Conduct, and Analysis.* New York: Oxford University Press, 1986: 71–89.
7. Chapman CR, Loeser JD, eds. *Issues in Pain Measurement.* New York: Raven Press, 1989.
8. Price DD. *Psychological and Neural Mechanisms of Pain.* New York: Raven Press, 1988: 28–38.
9. Turk DC, Melzack R, eds. *Handbook of Pain Assessment.* New York: Guilford Press, 1992.
10. Bailar JC III, Mosteller F. *Medical Uses of Statistics.* Waltham, Massachusetts: New England Journal of Medicine Books, 1986.
11. Pocock SJ. Group sequential methods in the design and analysis of clinical trials. *Biometrika,* 1977; **64**: 191–9.
12. Max MB. Challenges in the design of clinical trials of drug combinations. In: Gebhart GF, Hammond DL, Jensen TS, eds. *Proceedings of the VII World Congress on Pain.* Seattle: IASP Publications, 1994: 569–86.
13. Schwartz D, Lellouch J. Explanatory and pragmatic attitudes in therapeutic trials. *Journal of Chronic Diseases*, 1967; **20**: 637–48.
14. Schwartz D, Flamant R, Lellouch J. *Clinical Trials* (trans. Healy MJR). London: Academic Press, 1980.
15. Ventafridda V, Fochi C, De Conno F, Sganzerla E. Use of nonsteroidal anti-inflammatory drugs in the treatment of pain in cancer. *British Journal of Clinical Pharmacology*, 1980; **10**: S343–6.
16. Inturrisi CE, Colburn WA. Application of pharmacokinetic-pharmacodynamic modeling to analgesia. In: Foley KM, Inturrisi CE, eds. *Opioid Analgesics in the Management of Clinical Trials.* New York: Raven Press, 1986: 441–52.
17. Feinstein AR. An additional basic science for clinical medicine: II. The limitations of randomized trials. *Annals of Internal Medicine*, 1983; **99**: 544–50.
18. Portenoy RK. Cancer pain: general design issues. In: Max MB, Portenoy RK, Laska EM, eds. *The Design of Analgesic Clinical Trials.* New York: Raven Press, 1991: 233–66.
19. Max MB, Laska EM. Single-dose analgesic comparisons. In: Max MB, Portenoy RK, Laska EM, eds. *The Design of Analgesic Clinical Trials.* New York: Raven Press, 1991: 55–95.
20. Food and Drug Administration. *Guideline for the Clinical Evaluation of Analgesic Drugs.* Rockville, Maryland: U.S. Department of Health and Human Services, 1992.
21. Turner JA, Deyo RA, Loeser JD, Von Korff M, Fordyce WE. The importance of placebo effects in pain treatment and research. *Journal of the American Medical Association*, 1994; **271**: 1609–14.
22. Stambaugh JE, McAdams J. Comparison of intramuscular dezocine with butorphanol and placebo in chronic cancer pain: a method to evaluate analgesia after both single and repeated doses. *Clinical Pharmacology and Therapeutics*, 1987; **42**: 210–9.
23. Stambaugh JE, Drew J. The combination of ibuprofen and oxycodone/acetaminophen in the management of chronic cancer pain. *Clinical Pharmacology and Therapeutics*, 1988; **44**: 665–9.
24. Savarese JJ, Thomas GB, Homesley H, Hill CS. Rescue factor: a design for evaluating long-acting analgesics. *Clinical Pharmacology and Therapeutics*, 1988; **43**: 376–80.
25. Cundiff D, *et al.* Evaluation of a cancer pain model for the testing of long-acting analgesics. *Cancer*, 1989; **63**: 2355–9.
26. Portenoy RK, Maldonado M, Fitzmartin R, Kaiko R, Kanner R. Controlled-release morphine sulfate: analgesic efficacy and side effects of a 100 mg tablet in cancer pain patients. *Cancer*, 1989; **63**: 2284–8.
27. Lehmann KA. Patient-controlled intravenous analgesia for postoperative pain relief. In: Max MB, Portenoy RK, Laska EM, eds. *The Design of Analgesic Clinical Trials.* New York: Raven Press, 1991: 481–506.
28. VadeBoncouer TR, Riegier FX, Gautt RS, Weinberg GL. A randomized double-blind comparison of the efficacy of interpleural bupivicaine and saline on morphine requirements and pulmonary function after cholecystectomy. *Anesthesiology*, 1989; **71**: 339–43.

29. Silverman DG, O'Connor TZ, Brull SJ. Integrated assessment of pain scores and rescue morphine use during studies of analgesic efficacy. *Anesthesia and Analgesia*, 1993; **77**: 168–70.
30. Max MB. Divergent traditions in analgesic clinical trials. *Clinical Pharmacology and Therapeutics*, 1994; **56**: 237–41.
31. Jadad AR, Carroll D, Glynn CJ, Moore RA, McQuay HJ. Morphine responsiveness of chronic pain: double-blind randomized crossover study with patient-controlled analgesia. *Lancet*, 1992; **339**: 1367–71.
32. Chapman CR, Donaldson GW. Issues in designing trials of nonpharmacological treatments for pain. In: Max MB, Portenoy RK, Laska EM, eds. *The Design of Analgesic Clinical Trials.* New York: Raven Press, 1991: 699–711.
33. McQuay HJ, Carroll D, Glynn CJ. Dose-response for analgesic effect of amitriptyline in chronic pain. *Anaesthesia*, 1993; **48**: 281–5.
34. Sheiner LB, Beal SL, Sambol NC. Study designs for dose-ranging. *Clinical Pharmacology and Therapeutics*, 1989; **46**: 63–77.
35. Temple R. Dose-response and registration of new drugs. In: Lasagna L, Erill S, Naranjo CA, eds. *Dose-Response Relationships in Clinical Pharmacology.* Amsterdam: Elsevier, 1989: 145–70.
36. Bolognese JA. A Monte Carlo comparison of three up-and-down designs for dose ranging. *Controlled Clinical Trials*, 1983; **4**: 187–96.
37. Laska EM, Meisner MJ. Statistical methods and applications of bioassay. *Annual Review of Pharmacology and Toxicology*, 1987; **27**: 385–97.
38. Beaver WT, Wallenstein SL, Houde RW, Rogers A. A clinical comparison of the effects of oral and intramuscular administration of analgesics: pentazocine and phenazocine. *Clinical Pharmacology and Therapeutics*, 1968; **9**: 582–97.
39. Laska EM, Sunshine A, Mueller F, Elvers WB, Siegel C, Rubin A. Caffeine as an analgesic adjuvant. *Journal of the American Medical Association*, 1984; **251**: 1711–18.
40. Belville JW, Forrest WH, Elashoff J, Laska E. Evaluating side effects of analgesics in a coooperative clinical study. *Clinical Pharmacology and Therapeutics*, 1968; **9**: 303–13.
41. Temple R. Government viewpoint of clinical trials. *Drug Information Journal*, 1982; **16**: 10–17.
42. Detsky AS, Sackett DL. When was a 'negative' clinical trial big enough? How many patients you needed depends on what you found. *Archives of Internal Medicine*, 1985; **145**: 709–12.
43. Makuch RW, Johnson MF. Some issues in the design and interpretation of 'negative' clinical studies. *Archives of Internal Medicine*, 1986; **146**: 986–9.
44. Makuch R, Johnson M. Issues in planning and interpreting active control equivalence studies. *Journal of Clinical Epidemiology*, 1989; **42**: 503–11.
45. Beaver WT. Combination analgesics. *American Journal of Medicine*, 1984; **77** (suppl. 3A): 38–53.
46. Lavigne GJ, Hargreaves KM, Schmidt EA, Dionne RA. Proglumide potentiates morphine analgesia for acute surgical pain. *Clinical Pharmacology and Therapeutics*, 1989; **45**: 666–73.
47. Levine JD, Gordon NC. Synergism between the analgesic actions of morphine and pentazocine. *Pain*, 1988; **33**: 369–72.
48. Carter WH Jr, Carchman RA. Mathematical and biostatistical methods for designing and analyzing complex chemical interactions. *Fundamentals of Applied Toxicology*, 1988; **10**: 590–5.
49. Plummer JL, Short TG. Statistical modelling of the effects of drug combinations. *Journal of Pharmacological Methods*, 1990; **23**: 297–309.
50. Brunden MN, Vidmar TJ, McKean JW. *Drug Interactions and Lethality Analysis.* Boca Raton, FL: CRC Press, 1988.
51. James KE, Forrest WH, Rose RL. Crossover and noncrossover designs in four-point parallel line analgesic assays. *Clinical Pharmacology and Therapeutics*, 1985; **37**: 242–52.
52. Louis TA, Lavori PW, Bailar JC, Polansky M. Crossover and self-controlled designs in clinical research. *New England Journal of Medicine*, 1984; **310**: 24–31.
53. Brown BW Jr. The crossover experiment for clinical trials. *Biometrics*, 1980; **36**: 69–79.
54. Jones B, Kenward MG. *Design and Analysis of Cross-over Trials.* London: Chapman and Hall, 1989.
55. Ratkowsky Da, Evans MA, Alldredge JR. *Cross-Over Experiments: Design, Analysis, and Application.* New York: Marcel Dekker, 1993.
56. Senn S. *Cross-Over Trials in Clinical Research.* Chichester: John Wiley, 1993.
57. Bruera E. Cancer pain: chronic studies of adjuvants to opioid analgesics. In: Max MB, Portenoy RK, Laska EM, eds. *The Design of Analgesic Clinical Trials.* New York: Raven Press, 1991: 267–81.
58. Laska EM, Meisner M, Kushner HB. Optimal crossover designs in the presence of carryover effects. *Biometrics*, 1983; **39**: 1087–91.
59. Cochran WG, Cox GM. *Experimental Designs*, 2nd edn. New York, NY: John Wiley and Sons, 1957.
60. Byas-Smith MG, Max MB, Muir J, Kingman A. Transdermal clonidine compared to placebo in painful diabetic neuropathy using a two-stage 'enriched enrollment' design. *Pain*, 1995; **60**: 267–74.
61. Lavori PW, Louis TA, Bailar JC, Polansky M. Designs for experiments—parallel comparisons of treatment. *New England Journal of Medicine*, 1983; **309**: 1291–8.
62. Kaiko RF, Wallenstein SL, Rogers AG, Houde RW. Sources of variation in analgesic responses in cancer patients with chronic pain receiving morphine. *Pain*, 1983; **15**: 191–200.
63. Bruera E, MacMillan K, Hanson J, MacDonald RN. The Edmonton staging system for cancer pain: preliminary report. *Pain*, 1989; **37**: 203–10.
64. Thaler HT. Outcome measures and the effect of covariates. In: Max MB, Portenoy RK, Laska EM, eds. *The Design of Analgesic Clinical Trials.* New York: Raven Press, 1991: 106–11.
65. Wallenstein SL, *et al.* Clinical analgesic assay of repeated and single doses of heroin and hydromorphone. *Pain*, 1990; **41**: 5–14.
66. Silberfarb PM, Oxman TE. The effects of cancer therapies on the central nervous system. In: Goldberg, RJ, ed. *Psychiatric Aspects of Cancer.* Basel: Karger, 1988: 13–25.
67. Fishman B, Pasternak S, Wallenstein SL, Houde RW, Holland J, Foley KM. The Memorial pain assessment card: a valid instrument for the evaluation of cancer pain. *Cancer*, 1987; **60**: 1151–8.
68. Littman GS, Walker BR, Schneider BE. Reassessment of verbal and visual analog ratings in analgesic studies. *Clinical Pharmacology and Therapeutics*, 1985; **38**: 16–23.
69. Sriwatanakul K, Lasagna L, Cox C. Evaluation of current clinical trial methodology in analgesimetry based on experts' opinions and analysis of several analgesic studies. *Clinical Pharmacology and Therapeutics*, 1983; **34**: 277–83.
70. Melzack R. The McGill Pain Questionnaire: major properties and scoring methods. *Pain*, 1975; **1**: 277–99.
71. Daut RL, Cleeland CS, Flannery RC. Development of the Wisconsin Brief Pain Questionnaire to assess pain in cancer and other diseases. *Pain*, 1983; **17**: 197–210.
72. Bradley LA, Lindblom U. Do different types of chronic pain require different measurement technologies? In: Chapman CR, Loeser JD, eds. *Issues in Pain Measurement.* New York: Raven Press, 1989: 445–54.
73. Kremer E, Atkinson JH, Ignelzi RJ. Measurement of pain: patient preference does not confound pain measurement. *Pain*, 1981; **10**: 241–8.
74. Scott J, Huskisson EC. Graphic representation of pain. *Pain*, 1976; **2**: 175–84.
75. Sriwatanakul K, Kelvie W, Lasagna L, Calimlim JF, Weis OF, Mehta G. Studies with different types of visual analog scales for measurement of pain. *Clinical Pharmacology and Therapeutics*, 1983; **34**: 234–9.
76. Melzack R, Katz J, Jeans ME. The role of compensation in chronic pain: analysis using a new method of scoring the McGill Pain Questionnaire. *Pain*, 1985; **23**: 101–12.
77. Chapman CR, Casey KL, Dubner R, Foley KM, Gracely RH, Reading AE. Pain measurement: an overview. *Pain*, 1985; **22**: 1–32.
78. De Conno F, Caraceni A, Gamba A, *et al.* Pain measurement in cancer patients: a comparison of six methods. *Pain*, 1994; **57**: 161–6.
79. Jensen MP, McFarland CA. Increasing the reliability and validity of pain intensity measurement in chronic pain patients. *Pain*, 1993; **55**: 195–203.

80. Moore M, Anderson J, Burris H, *et al.* A randomized trial of gemcitabiline (GEM) versus 5FU as first-line therapy in advanced pancreatic cancer (abstract). *Proceedings of ASCO*, 1995; **14**: 199
81. Koeppen D, Mohr R, Streichenwien W. Assessment of adverse drug events during the clinical investigation of a new drug. *Pharmacopsychiatry*, 1989; **22**: 93–8.
82. Guy W, ed. *ECDEU Assessment Manual for Psychopharmacology (DOTES: Dosage Record and Treatment Emergent Symptom Scale)*. Rockville, Maryland: National Institute of Mental Health, 1976: 223–44.
83. Levine J, Schooler N, eds. *Systematic Assessment for Treatment Emergent Events (SAFTEE-GI)*. Rockville, Maryland: National Institute of Mental Health, 1983.
84. Karch FE, Lasagna L. Adverse drug reactions. *Journal of the American Medical Association*, 1975; **234**: 1236–41.
85. Morrow GR. The assessment of nausea and vomiting. *Cancer*, 1984; **53**: 2267–80.
86. Bruera E, Macmillan K, Hanson J, MacDonald RN. The cognitive effects of the administration of narcotic analgesics in patients with cancer pain. *Pain*, 1989; **39**: 13–16.
87. Inturrisi CE, Portenoy RK, Max MB, Colburn WA, Foley KM. Pharmacokinetic-pharmacodynamic relationships of methadone infusions in patients with cancer pain. *Clinical Pharmacology and Therapeutics*, 1990; **47**: 565–77.
88. Greenberg RP, Fisher S. Seeing through the double-masked design: a commentary. *Controlled Clinical Trials*, 1994; **15**: 244–6.
89. Max MB. Neuropathic pain. In: Max MB, Portenoy RK, Laska EM, eds. *The Design of Analgesic Clinical Trials.* New York: Raven Press, 1991: 193–220.
90. Moscucci M, Byrne L, Weintraub M, Cox C. Blinding, unblinding, and the placebo effect an analysis of patients' guesses of treatment assignment in a double-blind trial. *Clinical Pharmacology and Therapeutics*, 1987; **41**: 259–65.

5.3 Research into symptoms other than pain

Eduardo Bruera

Introduction

Adequate management of physical and psychosocial distress are the main purposes of palliative medicine. Most palliative medicine programmes treat a large percentage of patients with terminal cancer. In these patients, pain is a highly prevalent and devastating symptom that significantly affects patients quality of life. However, terminally ill patients frequently present with a large variety of severe physical and psychosocial symptoms in addition to pain. Table 1 summarizes the prevalence of a number of symptoms in a series of 275 consecutive patients with terminal cancer seen by our service. Similar results have been reported by other groups.[1,2] It is not infrequent that a terminally ill cancer patient may have severe pain in addition to profound anorexia, asthenia, chronic nausea, confusion, and mood changes such as anxiety or depression.

Because of the severity of illness, the presence of several coexisting symptoms, polypharmacy, and other logistic and administrative factors, very little research has taken place in this patient population.

Research in pain has been discussed in a previous chapter. In the following paragraphs some of the administrative issues related to research on symptoms other than pain and some guidelines for research in this area are discussed. Finally, some areas where future research in this field should focus will be discussed.

Administrative issues related to research on symptoms other than pain

Although the areas of service and education in palliative medicine have improved considerably during the last 10 years, there is very limited evidence for any improvement in their research efforts. A comprehensive review of the literature in the second half of 1988 suggested that there was an extremely low number of research trials performed each year in the management of symptoms other than pain, and that most of these trials had not been performed by palliative care units or in the setting of palliative care programmes.[3] An update of the review by our group during 1994 suggested no significant improvement in this situation. Some issues related to the absence of an adequate number and quality of research studies and possible approaches to the problem will be discussed in the following paragraphs.

Table 1 Symptom prevalence in 275 consecutive patients with advanced cancer

Symptom	Prevalence (%)	95% confidence interval
Asthenia	90	81 – 100
Anorexia	85	78 – 92
Pain	76	62 – 85
Nausea	68	61 – 75
Constipation	65	40 – 80
Sedation–confusion	60	40 – 75
Dyspnoea	12	8 – 16

Funding

Palliative medicine requires the generation of a solid body of knowledge. This can only be obtained with adequate funding. At the present time, research on issues related to the control of symptoms other than pain and the psychosocial issues associated with the dying patients or their families have had extremely low priority among the traditional cancer and medical scientific granting agencies. Many of the outcome measures that are regarded as the most important by palliative medicine research are seen by many scientists as 'soft' and deserving low priority for funding as compared to more 'objective' research. Less than 1 per cent of the budget of the National Cancer Institute of Canada went to all areas of supportive care and psychosocial support during 1994. One way in which funding can be made available is by including in the different granting agencies individuals who understand and can promote the importance of funding research in this area. Most granting agencies assess research proposals by allocating them to judgement panels. Proposals with the highest scores are then taken by the panel chair to the agency governing committee to compete for funding with successful proposals from other panels. Panels with limited or mixed expertise (as is usually the case with palliative care) are less likely to rank proposals with top marks, thereby limiting their chance of successful funding. Another way of increasing funding is to generate independent granting agencies for palliative medicine research, as has been done recently in the UK and European Community.

University recognition

Because of the fact that most of the original palliative care groups developed outside mainstream academic medicine, the process of gaining university recognition and generation of faculty has been extremely slow. The generation of adequate faculty is crucial to the

Table 2 Number of abstracts published at the Annual Meeting of the American Society of Clinical Oncology

	1983	1984	1985	1986	1987	1988
Number of abstracts published	952	1058	1082	1086	1082	1160
Number of abstracts in the Supportive Care, Infection, and Nutrition Session[a]	58(6)	85(8)	73(7)	76(7)	57(5)	80(7)

[a] Percentages in parentheses.

future of any national palliative care effort. In some countries, such as the United Kingdom or Australia, postgraduate training programmes have developed. Unfortunately, in the rest of the world, the absence of consensus among palliative care physicians on the future of our discipline has certainly delayed the process of forcing recognition of palliative medicine departments or palliative medicine divisions in different universities.

Adequate forms for the dissemination of research

There is clearly inadequate space for dissemination of palliative care research. Table 2 summarizes a review of the space allocation for research in supportive care and symptom control within the Annual Meeting of the American Society of Clinical Oncology. This society is recognized as the main forum in the world for the dissemination of cancer-related knowledge. Although the total allocation of space was approximately 7 per cent, Table 3 shows that approximately 70 per cent of the space was allocated for chemotherapy-induced nausea trials. That left less than 1/3 of that 7 per cent space for the discussion of all the subjects related to palliative medicine. A similar allocation of space is common in the World Cancer Congress, the European Congress in Clinical Oncology, and other major congresses. Pain research can be reported in congresses or journals that mostly deal with pain. On the other hand, research on symptoms other than pain is almost ignored in major congresses and journals.

There is also a clear lack of space in the major internal medicine or cancer journals for the dissemination of palliative care research.

As in the case of funding, the generation of adequate space for the dissemination of knowledge can take place by either creating a space along with the currently available scientific meetings or journals, or by the creation of meetings and journals that will specifically address research issues in palliative medicine.

Table 3 Main subject of the abstracts presented at the session on supportive care, infection and nutrition

Subject	1985	1986	1987	1988
Chemotherapy-induced emesis (%)	65	71	65	70
Blood products—infection (%)	7	6	7	9
Pain (%)	3	2	3	3
Nutrition (%)	2	1	1	2
Terminal care (%)	0	0	0	0
Other (%)	23	20	29	16

Integration of service with research

Relevant research on symptoms other than pain can only take place upon proper observation of the problems related to the care of terminally ill patients. Therefore, adequate research can only take place in areas where excellent care is provided. It is important for researchers with an interest in palliative care to have access to clinical facilities where there is an adequate concentration of patients in order to interact closely with the clinicians.

Co-ordination between different centres with an interest in palliative care research

Because of the lack of resources, it would be ideal to co-ordinate the effort of the different centres with an interest in developing palliative medicine research as a co-operative national or international group, or as research centres. Such an effort has proven to be extremely successful in oncology. The disadvantage of using some of the already established medical research networks for palliative care research is that many centres that provide excellent palliative care are not represented within those organizations.

Guidelines for research in symptoms other than pain

Clinical research on symptoms other than pain presents the investigator with a series of unique obstacles related to the characteristics of the drug or intervention under investigation, the patient population, and the nature of the effects which will be measured. The major considerations are summarized in the following paragraphs.

Patient population

Clinical trials should be performed in a population that resembles, as much as possible, the population that will clinically benefit from the use of the drug on a daily basis. Advanced cancer patients are often elderly, malnourished, and suffer multisystem failure. In addition, this population is in a dynamic state in which the nature and intensity of symptoms and the response to treatment are changing continuously. This means that the baseline for any studies is rarely stable. Unfortunately, in an effort to better characterize the biological effects of certain agents and to simplify clinical trials, investigators frequently study patients who are more stable than those who would ultimately benefit from the new treatment. One example of this problem is the development of long-acting morphine preparations. Most of the studies on these new agents were done on a population of very stable patients requiring an overall low dose of opioid analgesics.[4–6] The results from these trials cannot be automatically applied to populations of patients with severe pain, who require much higher doses of opioids and have significant impairment of gastrointestinal motility. Many of the studies of psychoactive drugs have also been performed in a population of patients who are younger and in better health than terminally ill cancer patients.[7,8]

Sometimes, the characteristics of the drug preclude evaluation in the population that would most likely employ it. If this is the case, the investigators should report this fact in the 'Patients and Methods' section and discuss the possible impact of the patient population on the final results of the study.

The patient population should be properly characterized using all known prognostic parameters. In the case of a crossover trial, this will help other investigators and clinicians to understand the population in which the trial was performed. In the case of a parallel-group trial, this information is even more important. Patients should either be stratified according to the most important prognostic factors before randomization takes place, or multivariate analysis should take place in order to determine the influence of different prognostic factors on the overall outcome. Unfortunately, the natural history of the most frequent symptoms present in terminally ill patients is not well known. Therefore, adequate staging systems are lacking. Staging systems have been crucial in the development of clinical research and cancer medicine.[9,10] These systems have allowed for adequate comparison of different treatment interventions on similar patient populations, and have allowed for the development of a common language for identification of patients for service and research purposes. Staging systems have been designed and are currently being tested for cancer pain.[11,12]. It is imperative that similar staging systems be developed for the adequate assessment of patients with nausea, dyspnoea, asthenia, anorexia, cognitive failure, and mood changes such as anxiety or depression.

It is important to consider how many potentially eligible patients can be entered in the trial within a reasonable period of time. The assistance of a biostatistician is invaluable at this stage of the planning of the trial. By postulating what would be considered a clinically relevant difference between the study drug and a control, the number of cases needed to significantly reject a type II error (the possibility that a real symptomatic benefit exists even if the study design does not find it) can be estimated. The probability that the study will be able to reject this type II error is defined as the 'power' of the study. As will be discussed later, study power is relatively less with a parallel-group design than a crossover design.

In some studies, large numbers of patients are required to answer some fundamental questions concerning the effects of different drugs. Even the largest individual palliative medicine centre may not be able to perform such trials. In cancer medicine, this problem has been overcome very successfully by the creation of co-operative groups. These groups are able to design a significant number of clinical trials, and all member institutions co-operate by entering patients. Unfortunately, no such group exists for palliative medicine research.

If the problem under study occurs very rarely and the patient remains stable for long periods of time, the 'N-of-1' design can be used.[13]

Trial design

Choice of study

Retrospective studies are unlikely to be particularly useful in symptom research unless they are conducted in institutions that regularly assess and document the intensity and prevalence of different symptoms.[14] These trials have been useful in assessing patterns of treatment of symptoms[15] or symptom prevalence.[16] However, results of different symptom prevalence trials are difficult to compare because of the absence of uniformly accepted techniques for the assessment of the presence and severity of different symptoms.

In the assessment of therapeutic interventions prospective studies are almost mandatory. Because of the subjective nature of the study end-points, these trials should be double-blind whenever possible.

During recent years, oncologists have compared chemotherapy versus 'best supportive care' or chemotherapy versus corticosteroids.[17] These studies are not blinded, although the main outcomes are symptom control or quality of life. The high potential for bias makes it difficult to interpret the data from this research. Occasionally, open pilot studies could provide some useful information on the nature of therapeutic or toxic effects of a certain drug that might help in the design of a more expensive, blinded trial.

Parallel versus crossover designs

For drugs with a long latency to maximal effects, such as tricyclic antidepressants, patients need to receive the drug or placebo for several days before an assessment can take place. If a crossover design is tried in these conditions, the status of the patient's symptoms may change significantly before the completion of the trial. This change may relate to the development of tolerance to some of the drugs the patient may be receiving such as opioids or amphetamines, or to the development of new complications of the disease such as confusion or bowel obstruction. In trials performed in advanced cancer patients, the number of non-evaluable patients at the end of the study may be large enough to invalidate the results. For these reasons, some investigators[18] have chosen a parallel-group design for the evaluation of the effects of the experimental drug. There are problems associated with this choice:

1. The statistical power of the trial decays very significantly, and therefore, a larger number of patients will be required for completion of the study.

2. Cognitive failure or sedation in the patient population receiving the study drug may not be readily perceived.

3. The final choice of the patient and investigator as an overall assessment of satisfaction is lost.

Finally, it is important to consider that the long latency may not necessarily be proof for all the effects of the drug. For example, although the antidepressant effect of tricyclics takes place approximately 2 to 3 weeks after starting the treatment, analgesic effects in postherpetic neuralgia are evident between 48 and 72 h after they are started.[19] Similarly, although the maximal effect of the non-steroidal anti-inflammatory drug in the treatment of rheumatic conditions usually takes several weeks, its effect on cancer pain can usually be measured after just a couple of days.[20]

Before embarking on a long and expensive controlled trial of a new agent, it is extremely useful to perform a pilot, uncontrolled trial in a small number of patients. This study can determine the onset of action and duration of different effects of the new drug. During this pilot trial, it is also possible to test different doses of the drug under study. Comparing the results of this trial with historical controls provides information very useful in planning the controlled trial. The main drawback of a pilot trial is the absence of a systematic evaluation of the placebo effect.

In the case of short acting drugs, the design is much more simple. A double-blind, crossover trial is very useful for the assessment of the symptomatic effects of these drugs.

The statistical power of this design is much higher than that of the parallel design, and it allows for a blinded choice by patients and investigators. The blinded choice provides an overall estimation of the satisfaction with the new agent. Advanced cancer patients suffer from a variety of extremely complex symptoms that have strong interaction with each other and are also frequently treated with a number of drugs that interact with each other and probably with the new experimental agent. Therefore, the introduction of a new symptomatic agent could have a large number of very complex effects that are best assessed by comparing the effect of the experimental drug with a placebo in the same patient.

Some drugs should not be tested in a double-blind, crossover trial, despite having a short effect. Drugs with sedating effects may not be evaluated well this way, since the patient and the investigator are much more likely to discriminate the effects or side-effects of drugs in a crossover trial. Therefore, drugs with a significant number of side-effects may need to be given in a very low dose or be tested in a parallel-group design, in which the patient is not given the opportunity to compare the study drug with placebo. Other drugs that may not be used in a short-term crossover trial are those that have a rapid onset of action but a long-lasting effect. For example, studies on the effects of antibiotics on different symptoms associated with ulcerated tumours, such as pain or odour, could not be designed as a crossover trial because of the significant effect that 3 or 4 days of antibiotic therapy could have on the natural history of the local infection.

'N-of-1' studies

A number of symptoms such as dyspnoea, pruritus, or hiccups have been suggested to improve significantly with a number of therapeutic interventions. However, the majority of those interventions have not been tested in controlled clinical trials. For example, in the case of dyspnoea, some authors have found that the administration of oxygen could bring significant symptomatic relief[21] while other authors have found no significant effects.[22] At the present time, the decision to administer oxygen to patients with terminal cancer dyspnoea is usually made on an individual basis. A similar situation occurs with a number of other therapeutic interventions.

The N-of-1 trial consists of doing a number of crossovers between a certain therapeutic agent and a placebo, or between two different therapeutic agents in the same patient. These crossovers should take place on a double-blind basis, and outcome measurements such as visual analogue scales and patient choices should be assessed after each crossover. The results at the end of the multiple crossovers can be analysed statistically using both parametric and non-parametric tests for crossover trials.

The N-of-1 might be a very useful clinical trial in order to help increase the patient's and clinician's confidence in a given symptomatic treatment. Some of the criteria for applying the N-of-1 are the presence of doubt on the effectiveness of a certain treatment, the fact that the treatment, if effective, should be continued for a long period, the patient's willingness to collaborate in the trial, and the fact that the treatment should have a rapid onset and termination of action.[13] A recent report has used the N-of-1 trial for the assessment of the effects of oxygen on terminal cancer dyspnoea.[23]

Table 4 Adjuvant drugs used for symptom control in patients with advanced cancer*

Drug	Percentage
Phenothiazines	87
Corticosteroids	57
Night sedation	54
Antiemetics*	44
Daytime sedatives	35
Non-steroidal anti-inflammatory drugs	32
Antidepressants	19
Anticonvulsants	8

* Excluding phenothiazines

From: Walsh TD. Chronic studies of adjuvants to opiate analgesics. *Advances in Pain Research and Therapy*, 1991; **18**: 283–6.

The drug

A certain experimental drug administered for the management of a given symptom has specific effects on the given symptom, but is also likely to interact with some of the multiple syndromes that the patient is likely to have (Table 1) or with some of the multiple medications that terminally ill patients are likely to be receiving (Table 4). An almost constant characteristic of these trials is that the patients are polysymptomatic and are already receiving other drugs, mainly opioids.

The interaction between the new drug and the variety of symptoms and other drugs is, therefore, a critical aspect of these studies. The new drug may have effects on the bioavailability of opioids—as suggested in a recent report demonstrating that orally administered imipramine can increase the bioavailability of morphine, possibly by reducing its rate of elimination.[24] A study of an antiemetic that can increase gastric emptying could also show a change in the rate of absorption of orally administered opioids.[25]

One of the most sensitive effects of a new experimental drug would be that of increased sedation or confusion. These could be the effects of the new drug or be caused by interaction with some other drug the patient is already receiving. An increased level of obtundation or confusion may make a symptomatic assessment difficult and may result in false positive findings of symptomatic relief, particularly when the symptom assessment and the administration of the drugs are done by a third person. If the experimental drug has possible side-effects of sedation or confusion (for example benzodiazepines and phenothiazines, antihistamines), it is important to assess prospectively the cognitive status and the level of sedation of the patient during the administration of the study drug and control. If the symptomatic effect, or the 'blinded' choice by the patient and investigator are accompanied by a significant cognitive deterioration or increased sedation, it cannot be ruled out that the effects are just a consequence of the increased central toxicity caused by the experimental drug.

If the experimental drug is likely to potentiate sedation induced by other drugs such as opioids, patients should be asked at the end of the trial if they believe they received the active drug or placebo, and why, in order to assess the effectiveness of the blinding. One double-blind, placebo-controlled crossover study of cyproheptadine by our group was cancelled after 13 consecutive patients easily recognized the drug phase because of somnolence. This failure might have been avoided by doing a pilot study in a small number of patients. Some studies on dyspnoea have masked the sedating effects by controlling the results of the experimental drug not only with the placebo, but also with other drugs with sedative effects.[26,27] This is likely to improve the blinding, but is also likely to make the trial longer and more complicated.

Some other characteristics of the drugs that might affect the choice of trial design have been discussed previously in this chapter.

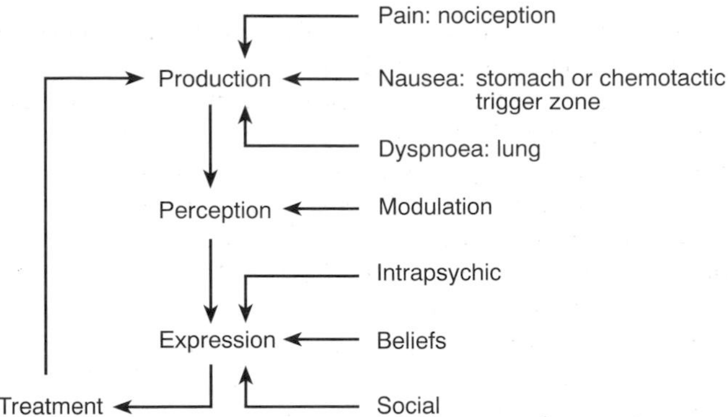

Fig. 1. Mechanisms of symptoms in cancer patients.

End-points of the study

An experimental drug given to a patient who is experiencing a variety of severe symptoms and who is already receiving a number of drugs can change the effects of some of the drugs the patient is receiving (e.g., analgesics, antinauseants, sedatives, laxatives) or have therapeutic effects and side-effects of its own (in the case of the tricyclic antidepressants; for example, antidepressant effects occur with autonomic effects, dry mouth, hypotension, and arrhythmias). For these reasons, the effect of the experimental drug can be extremely complex. Moreover, different effects can have a varying latency (in the case of tricyclic antidepressants, dry mouth and sedation can occur immediately, whereas analgesia requires 3 or 4 days, and mood effects can take weeks), duration, and intensity.

From this, it is evident that no single study is able to fully characterize the symptomatic effects of a given drug. Short term, intensive crossover trials will provide ample information on the acute effects of a given drug, but miss some of the important long-term effects. Less intensive, long-term studies will determine long-term effectiveness and side-effects, but potentially miss early effects. Research on amphetamines provides a useful example of these problems. Forrest *et al.*[28] proved in an elegant double-blind study that a single dose of dextroamphetamine was able to potentiate morphine-induced analgesia and decrease sedation. However, it is not possible to conclude from this study that repeated doses of amphetamines are useful for patients with terminal cancer. Our group found that in two short-term crossover trials amphetamines could decrease opioid-induced sedation in cancer patients and potentiate analgesia,[29,30] but significant toxicity and a rapid development of tolerance were detected. The results of our studies suggest that amphetamines can be useful adjuvant drugs, at least for the short-term, and in some patients with pain due to advanced cancer. However, from our studies, it cannot be assumed that amphetamines will be useful during long-term administration.

The finding of a significant improvement in one or more isolated variables does not necessarily mean that an experimental drug will be clinically useful. For example, at the end of our double-blind, crossover trial of mazindol, the patients had significantly better pain control and lower analgesic consumption on mazindol as compared to placebo,[29] but their overall preferences were equally distributed between 'drug', 'placebo', and 'no choice'. In the case of mazindol, the low level of patient satisfaction with the drug is probably due to the significant anxiety and anorexia it caused.[29] These facts could only be determined because we were measuring several other variables in addition to pain. However, even the simultaneous measurement of several variables would not always provide an explanation for the observed global satisfaction or dissatisfaction. It is always possible that deterioration occurs in a variable that is not measured or that the patient's choice reflects improvement, or the deterioration, of several variables combined, each of which does not independently reach statistical significance. A recent trial of clonidine in the treatment of anticipatory nausea in patients receiving chemotherapy is illustrative: although clonidine was able to decrease anticipatory nausea, patients preferred not to receive it in subsequent courses of chemotherapy and the reasons for this remains unclear.[31] In both parallel and crossover studies a global rating of response with statements ranging from 'no difference' may allow the patient to express his/her overall satisfaction with the new intervention.

Although it is useful to combine objective variables (daily dose of antiemetics, number of rescue doses for nausea or dyspnoea, the need for administration of enemas, etc.) and subjective variables (nausea, somnolence, confusion, etc.) in these trials, it must be clear that the clinical usefulness of an adjuvant drug will depend on it's ability to modify the subjective parameter.

The assessment of symptoms

Different chapters in this book make reference to the adequate assessment of symptoms. Figure 1 summarizes the process of production, perception, and expression of the symptoms. It is important to bear in mind that research oriented towards symptom control will be dealing with the patient's expression of the different symptoms more than with an assessment of the mechanism of production or perception of those symptoms. The actual expression of many of the symptoms can bear very limited relationship to the clinical manifestations of production of such symptoms. For example, it is well known that the intensity of cancer pain does not necessarily bear a clear relationship with the location or size of the tumour.[32] It is also known that the severity of subjective dyspnoea may not bear a close relationship to the level of deterioration of ventilatory function.[17-19,26,33] Other factors such as the patient's cognitive status, mood, and beliefs can have more impact on the expression of symptom distress than the actual severity of the disorder at the source of production of the symptom. Symptom control research lacks a 'gold standard' for the assessment of different symptoms as can be commonly seen in internal medicine trials (e.g. serum glucose for diabetic trials, arterial blood pressure for antihypertensive trials). Therefore, it is advisable to use a variety of different techniques such as numerical scales, verbal scales, and visual analogues, in order to assess the intensity of different symptoms.

Future areas of research

The development of staging systems for the most common symptoms in palliative medicine patients should be one of the main research priorities. These staging systems should be based on adequate determination of the natural history of those different symptoms and on identification of different prognostic factors for good or poor response of every given symptom. Adequate staging systems for nausea, dyspnoea, cognitive failure, mood disorders, asthenia, and anorexia will allow for the development of a common language to be used in therapeutic interventions.

Because of the presence of several different severe symptoms in one patient, these symptoms are likely to have a complex and important interaction between each other. The nature of the interaction between pain, nutritional status, confusional state, dyspnoea, and mood, has been very poorly established. The effects that different therapeutic interventions aimed at a specific symptom might have on the other symptoms have also been poorly characterized. The relative importance of different symptoms for a given patient and his or her family and the relative importance of the different side-effects associated with symptomatic treatment should also be the target of future research trials.

Novel pharmacological agents and novel routes for the administration of the currently existing pharmacological agents should be defined. In the area of pharmacological interventions, particular emphasis should be made on properly establishing the interaction between different experimental agents and the drugs the patients are usually receiving, such as opioid analgesics, antiemetics, etc. It is hoped that a better understanding of the interaction between these different agents should result in a better utilization of these agents and might prompt the development of newer agents.

Finally, we need to develop better understanding of the pathophysiology of different symptoms. In the future, we should be able to establish why some patients with severe lung dysfunction do not suffer considerable dyspnoea, while other patients with minimal dysfunction suffer profound symptom distress. The same is valid for the presence of nausea, anorexia, and confusional syndromes. This pathophysiological research may require us to interact closely with basic researchers in order to be able to develop animal experimental models of the most frequent symptoms of terminal disease.

References

1. Coyle N, *et al.* Character of terminal illness in the advanced cancer patient: pain and other symptoms during the last 4 weeks of life. *Journal of Pain and Symptom Management*, 1990; **5**: 83–93.
2. Doyle D. Symptom relief in terminal illness. *Medicine in Practice*, 1983; **1**: 694–8.
3. Bruera E. Current research in symptom control. Presented *at 6th International Congress on Care of the Terminally Ill*. Montreal, Quebec, October 1988.
4. Hanks G, Twycross R, Bliss J. Controlled release morphine tablets: a double-blind trial in patients with advanced cancer. *Anaesthesia*, 1987; **42**: 840–4.
5. Walsh TD. Clinical evaluation of slow release morphine tablets. *Proceedings of the American Society of Clinical Oncology*, 1985; **4**: 266.
6. MacDonald RN, Bruera E, Brenneis C, *et al.* Long acting morphine in the treatment of cancer pain: a double-blind, crossover trial. *Proceedings of the American Society of Clinical Oncology*, 1987; **6**: 1054.
7. Greenblatt D, Harmatz J, Shapiro L, *et al.* Sensitivity to triazolam in the elderly. *New England Journal of Medicine*, 1991; **324**: 1691–8.
8. Gillin C. The long and the short of sleeping pills. *New England Journal of Medicine*, 1991; **324**: 1735–6.
9. American Joint Committee for Cancer Staging and End Result Reporting. *Manual for Staging of Cancer*. Chicago, Il: American Joint Committee, 1977.
10. Paterson AHG. Clinical staging and its prognostic significance. In: B. Stall B, ed. *Pointers to Cancer Prognosis*. Dordrecht: Martinus Nijhoff, 1988: 37–48.
11. Stiefel F, Bruera E. On symptom control when death is near. *Journal of Palliative Care*, 1991; **7**: 39–41.
12. Bruera E, Macmillan K, Hanson J, MacDonald RN. The Edmonton staging system for cancer pain: preliminary report. *Pain*, 1989; **37**: 203–9.
13. Guyatt GH, Keller JL, Jaeschke R, Rosenbloom D, *et al.* The N-of-1 randomized controlled trial: clinical usefulness. Our three-year experience. *Annals of Internal Medicine*, 1990; **112**: 392–9.
14. Bruera E, Kuehn N, Miller MJ, Selmser P, Macmillan K. The Edmonton Symptom Assessment System (ESAS): A simple method for the assessment of palliative care patients. *Journal of Palliative Care*, 1991; **7**: 6–9.
15. Bruera E, Fox R, Chadwick S, Brenneis C, MacDonald RN. Changing pattern in the treatment of pain and other symptoms in advanced cancer patients. *Journal of Pain and Symptom Management*, 1987; **2**: 139–45.
16. Bruera E. Symptom control in patients with cancer. *Journal of Psychosocial Oncology*, 1990; **8**: 47–73.
17. Tannock I, Osoba D, Ernst S, *et al.* Chemotherapy with mitoxantrone (M) and prednisone (P) palliates patients with hormone-resistant prostate cancer (HRPC). Results of a randomized Canadian trial. *Proceedings of the American Society of Clinical Oncology*, 1995; **14**: 245.
18. Walsh TD. Controlled study of imipramine and morphine in chronic pain due to cancer. *Proceedings of the American Society of Clinical Oncology*, 1986; **5**: 327.
19. Watson C, Evans R, Reed K, *et al.* Amitryptiline versus placebo in postherpetic neuralgia. *Neurology*, 1982; **32**: 671–73.
20. Ferrer-Brechner T, Ganz P. Combination therapy with ibuprofen and methadone for chronic cancer pain. *American Journal of Medicine*, 1984; **77**: 78–83.
21. Swinburn CR, Mould H, Stone TN, *et al.* Symptomatic benefit of supplemental oxygen in hypoxemic patients with chronic lung disease. *American Review of Respiratory Disease*, 1991; **143**: 913–5.
22. Ashutosh K, Mead G, Dunsky M. Early effects of oxygen administration and prognosis in chronic obstructive pulmonary disease and cor pulmonale. *American Review of Respiratory Disease*, 1983; **127**: 399–404.
23. Bruera E, Schoeller T, MacEachern T. Symptomatic benefit of supplemental oxygen in hypoxemic patients with terminal cancer: the use of the N of 1 randomized controlled trial. *Journal of Pain and Symptom Management*, 1992; **76**: 365–8.
24. Feinman C. Pain relief by antidepressants: possible modes of action. *Pain*, 1985; **23**: 1–8.
25. Manara A, Shelly M, Quinn K, *et al.* The effect of metoclopramide on the absorption of oral controlled release morphine. *British Journal of Clinical Pharmacology*, 1988; **25**: 518–21.
26. Woodcock A, Gross E, Gellery A. A comparison of diazepam and promethazine in the treatment of breathlessness in patients with chronic obstructive lung disease. *British Medical Journal*, 1982; **1**: 96–9.
27. Woodcock A, Gross E, Gellery A, *et al.* Effects of dihydrocodeine, alcohol and caffeine on breathlessness and exercise tolerance in patients with

chronic obstructive lung disease. *New England Journal of Medicine*, 1981; **305**: 1611–18.

28. Forrest W, Brown B, Brown C, *et al.* Dextroamphetamine with morphine for the treatment of post-operative pain. *New England Journal of Medicine*, 1977; **296**: 712–15.
29. Bruera E, Carraro S, Roca E, Barugel M, Chacon R. Double-blind evaluation of the effects of mazindol on pain, depression, anxiety, appetite and activity in terminal cancer patients. *Cancer Treatment Reports*, 1986; **70**: 295–8.
30. Bruera E, Brenneis C, Chadwick S, Hanson J, MacDonald RN. Methylphenidate associated with narcotics for the treatment of cancer pain. *Cancer Treatment Reports*, 1987; **71**: 67–70.
31. Fetting J, Stefanek M, Sheidlen J, *et al.* Noradrenergic activity in anticipatory nausea. *Proceedings of the American Society of Clinical Oncology*, 1988; **7**: 284.
32. Bruera E. Continuing challenges in the management of cancer pain. *Oncology* (Special Supplement), 1989; 1101: 31–6.
33. Bruera E, Macmillan K, Pither J, MacDonald RN. The effects of morphine on the dyspnea of terminal cancer patients. *Journal of Pain and Symptom Management*, 1990; **5**: 341–4.

5.4 Psychosocial research in palliative care

David A. Alexander

Introduction

The early studies of the medical care of the dying exposed the limitations of the contemporary approaches which, at that time, reflected largely technological and paternalistic attitudes. Increasing lay and professional dissatisfaction culminated in the hospice movement which strongly asserted the need to address the psychosocial needs, not just of patients, but also of their families.

Initially, this new approach thrived on a diet of clinical observation, articles of faith, and anecdotes, but 'well-intentioned amateurism' had to be replaced by 'hard-headed professionalism'.[1] Moreover, practitioners of a behavioural approach to palliative care criticized the reliance on a priori assumptions and on clinical prescriptions lacking empirical justification.[2]

In this chapter we focus on research developments relevant to psychosocial issues from the standpoint of the patient, the family, and the palliative care staff. In addition, we address methodological problems associated with such research, and highlight future research objectives.

Psychosocial issues

The patient

A seminal contribution to our understanding of patients' psychosocial needs was made by Kubler-Ross[3] when she identified how patients adapt progressively to a life-threatening illness by means of denial, anger, depression, and reconciliation. (Of course, these are descriptions; they should not be used prescriptively.) Other psychological reactions include despair, helplessness, hopelessness, and guilt, although the impact of cancer may vary with age because of the different roles and responsibilities associated with various stages of the lifecycle.[4] The stage of the illness *per se* is also a major determinant of patients' quality of life. In a survey of 26 American hospices the quality of life was noted to decline markedly for most patients in the last 2 weeks of life.[5]

Of course, patients faced with life-threatening illnesses are confronted not by a single event but by a series of consequences. These may provoke 'anticipatory grief' (i.e. a preparation for the loss to come), a reappraisal of achievements, and efforts to find some personally acceptable meaning in their illness and plight. Some investigators[6] have studied patients' attributions (i.e. to what they attribute their illness). Their results suggest that what patients blame has little bearing on how well they adjust; indeed, there is some evidence that not making any causal links and accepting their plight as something which could happen to anybody may be more adaptive than blaming, for example, themselves or God. Self-blame may even interfere with adaptation and leave the individual feeling guilty and rejected. Denial is perhaps one of the most commonly recognized reactions to a life-threatening illness. There are various uses of this concept,[7] but essentially it refers to a person's inability to accept the implications of some anxiety-provoking item of news or circumstance. As a defence, denial may be adaptive or maladaptive; therefore it should not be challenged without justification, or at times when the patient has no opportunity to find alternative ways of coping.[8] However, staff must not inappropriately foster denial by, for example, masking the reality of death. A recent study[9] demonstrated the positive value of hospice patients witnessing the peaceful death of a fellow patient. The authors claim further that shielding the patients from the reality of such events would have been more distressing.

Different methods of responding to psychosocial problems have been considered.[10] It has been argued that effective intervention should include accurate information and an understanding of how patients cope in order that these methods can be incorporated into the overall management plan. Several investigators have also emphasized the need to encourage self-determination in patients and to allow them to be actively involved in their own management.[11] However, the extent to which some principles can be effectively implemented is likely to depend, at least to some degree, on the nature of staff–patient relationships. These may vary considerably, as has been shown in participant–observer studies (studies in which the investigator plays an active role, e.g. as a patient or member of staff, while observing what takes place). In one such study[12] it was noted that efforts to implement a hospice philosophy may be thwarted by pressures on staff to conform to the more paternalistic and traditional medical model operating in the neighbouring hospital. Also, surgical staff have been observed to spend less time with the dying than is the case with their hospice counterparts, even when the numbers of staff–patient contacts are similar.[13] A detailed conceptual analysis of general practitioners' communications has also revealed the different strategies and tactics used to cope with the difficult issues which arise with the terminally ill.[14]

The psychosocial needs of dying children have been less thoroughly researched, but there have been some helpful efforts.[15] These have highlighted the fact that younger patients pose particular problems because of their limited ability to verbally express their feelings and needs. Another study, comparing two paediatric hospitals, also emphasized the special problems of dependence and overprotection with children, and showed that staff spend more time with those children whose deaths were uncertain.[16]

In conclusion, attention to patients' psychosocial needs is an essential feature of palliative care. Patients use different psychological defences which need to be understood, respected, and upheld, unless they interfere with other aspects of their care. However, researching patients' psychosocial needs (especially among children) is not easy, particularly because of the lack of adequate measures and techniques.

The family

Traditionally, hospitals have not displayed great enthusiasm for attending to the needs of families or for involving them in patient care. Too often it is assumed that they will cope, but there is ample evidence that dealing with a seriously ill patient makes enormous demands on the rest of the family,[17,18] particularly when a child is dying.[19] Looking after a patient at home can disrupt the patterns of relationship, and it is often the breakdown of these which leads to the patient's admission.

If the family is truly the unit of care, it is essential to understand how the members cope. The concept of 'anticipatory grief' has already been raised above in relation to patients, but it is also relevant to families. They also show a number of reactions typical of grief in advance of the patient's death, as a way of preparing themselves for the ultimate loss. A revision of roles and responsibilities may be required: husbands may have to assume unfamiliar domestic duties, and wives may have to become the primary breadwinners. The development of children may also be disrupted by the presence of a terminally ill relative. Other researchers[2] point to changes in the way that families respond to each other emotionally. For instance, it may become difficult to express negative feelings (e.g. resentment, anger, and impatience) when there is a dying family member involved. To avoid uncomfortable feelings, families may distance themselves from the dying and avoid any closeness or intimacy. An unwillingness to acknowledge their own distress is displayed by families' use of denial. This defence may appear in many guises but, characteristically, it disrupts the way that the family members usually communicate with the patient or among themselves. The dying may not be told the facts pertaining to their illness, or the family may never talk openly about the sick relative. Such disturbed communication patterns are likely to create anxiety, isolation, and suspicion in the dying patient.

Identifying what families find helpful is an important challenge for researchers. In one study,[20] families who were asked to rate the actions of palliative care nurses placed 20 out of the 25 most helpful actions in the 'psychosocial' category. In particular, it was apparent that families preferred patients to be allowed to participate in their own management and to maintain a degree of independence. From interviews with bereaved relatives, general practitioners were seen to be most helpful when they visited regularly (often without a request to do so), offered their home telephone numbers, and considered the effectiveness of the patients' medication before providing repeat prescriptions.[21] Families also like information about help available outside the health service.[22] In a recent longitudinal study using the technique of 'methodological triangulation' (i.e. an interview, a measure of hope in the family caregiver, and biographical data), the need for families to be helped to maintain a sense of hope was emphasized.[23]

An interesting approach to the psychosocial needs of families has been made by considering them in terms of a systems model.[24] A systems approach reminds us that a setting determines what happens inside it, and that the parts can only be understood in relation to the whole. Thus the behaviour of one family member has to be understood in relation to others who constitute the family unit. This approach also emphasizes the need to identify the family's requirements and problems at different stages of the disease process. Those families which have a number of flexible ways of coping and which can function as a cohesive unit appear to cope better.

To conclude this section it is necessary to restate the cardinal importance of the psychosocial needs and defences of families when dealing with their dying relatives. Generally, families prefer to be actively involved, and they benefit from good communications with staff. Families defend against the distress created by a dying relative in a variety of ways, including denial and distancing, and sometimes these methods may be detrimental to the patient.

The staff

It has been claimed that the 'physician who chooses to fully participate in the psychosocial support of the cancer patient and family may experience rich personal and professional rewards that counterbalance any psychologic risks involved in participating in the profound challenges associated with living and dying'.[10]

Palliative care staff find their work rewarding,[25] as do general practitioners who deal with the dying,[26] but it is equally true that palliative care makes many demands on staff. In one study it was reported that 22 per cent of hospice nurses admitted that dealing with the dying was a major stressor,[27] and other investigators[28] have established that, in addition to intractable pain, psychiatric symptoms in patients and dealing with relatives were the major sources of stress; this was irrespective of whether the nurses were full-time or part-time, trained or auxiliary, or on day or night shift. It is possible that palliative care staff have unrealistically high expectations in terms of what they believe that they should be able to offer patients and their families, but the findings from the last study, as well as those from a survey of staff working with terminally ill children,[29] suggest that they commonly experience a sense of therapeutic impotence and helplessness which engenders anxiety and distress. In the extensive National Hospice Study[17] it was noted that those staff experiencing burnout were younger and better educated, and worked full time in direct contact with patients.

Other studies have compared the psychological impact of palliative care with that of other kinds of nursing.[25,30] Although hospice staff and intensive care staff may be more troubled by issues involving death than colleagues in other medical and surgical units, there is no evidence that hospice staff are more stressed. However, palliative care staff may have a wider repertoire of methods of coping with stress.[25]

It has been shown from audio and video recordings that, in the face of psychological and interpersonal stressors, staff distance themselves from their patients.[31] Also, some staff rationalize their lack of response to patients' psychological and emotional needs on the grounds that patients are expected to be upset by their plight. In one participant–observer study[13] the author masqueraded as a terminally ill patient and found that in the surgical unit he had only brief contact with doctors, who were usually accompanied by other staff. In the hospice, however, the staff were more likely to make contact with him on their own and initiate communication about personal matters. Two distinctive patterns of communication are displayed by doctors who find it difficult to deal with their own psychological reactions: they become either increasingly vague or inappropriately abrupt and frank.[10]

A longitudinal study has also shown the presence of gender differences between doctors in the way that they cope with the terminally ill and their families.[32] For instance, 10 years after graduation female physicians are more likely than their male colleagues to avoid telling patients directly about their terminal prognosis.

Why should there be apparent resistance to dealing with patients and relatives at a psychosocial level? It may be a lack of training,[28] or perhaps staff fear that, if they encourage patients and relatives too much, they will trigger reactions and emotions with which they will not be able to cope. Alternatively, they may believe that such matters are the responsibility of other staff, such as social workers.

Factors, such as personal qualities, which might mitigate the impact of palliative care on staff have been the subject of considerable research. For instance, it has been reported that hospice nurses are more assertive, more independent, and more imaginative than other nursing colleagues.[33] A claim has also been made that successful hospice nurses are emotionally more mature and derive support from their own firmly established philosophy of life.[6] 'Satisfactory' volunteers have also been found to be less anxious about death and to display more flexibility and tolerance than 'unsatisfactory' volunteers.[34]

Other bulwarks against stress and burnout appear to be the use of cognitive-behavioural methods (e.g. distraction techniques and graded exposure).[35] Organizational factors such as the creation of a home-like atmosphere, a redistribution of workload, not being involved exclusively with dying patients, and a team approach have all been proposed as ways of preventing occupational stress and burnout.

The psychoprophylactic value of training has been emphasized by a number of investigators.[28,31] One group of investigators assessed the effects of 14 courses on the attitudes of 122 staff and compared the results with those from 43 controls who underwent no training. Whilst there were positive changes in attitudes to palliative care, these did not seem to be very durable when reassessed 1 year after the courses had finished.[36]

Psychosocial care of the dying is only as good as the ability of the staff to care for themselves.[10] The value of support groups in dealing with the staff's own psychological needs has been proclaimed, but the aims and methods of such groups need to be carefully considered and their outcome evaluated because there is nothing intrinsically and inevitably healing about individuals organizing themselves into groups.[37] The contribution of family support has also been highly rated by hospice staff as a means of reducing the deleterious impact of palliative care on those who provide it.[28,38]

In conclusion, the observations discussed in this section have confirmed that, whilst palliative care creates an opportunity for job satisfaction, it also makes many psychological demands on those who provide it (even although their overall levels of stress may be no higher than those of other staff in specialist fields). Some protection against and relief from these psychological pressures may be afforded by certain personality traits and coping methods, by peer and family support, and by training and sensitive organization.

Methodological challenges

Palliative care poses significant challenges to the researcher. It is only possible to consider them briefly here; those readers with a particular interest in these matters are referred to other texts.[39–41]

Reliability and validity are not issues specific to palliative care, but they are so important that they merit attention here. A reliable instrument is one which measures consistently whatever it measures. A valid instrument is one which measures that which it claims to measure. Attempts to assess quality of life and denial, for example, have been bedevilled by the lack of reliable and valid measures. It should be noted that a measure may be valid in one setting but not in another. Certain scales for assessing depression may be valid when used on psychiatric patient samples but invalid when used with terminally ill patients because the scales are sensitive to changes in biological functions (such as sleeping, eating, and activity levels) which are often markedly impaired by physical illness and its treatment. Validation also requires a standard for the phenomenon being measured. This can be very difficult, as has been shown in assessments of the quality of life.[39–42]

The clinical state of the patient is an important determinant of which research procedures can be used. The psychosocial assessment of very ill patients may be contaminated by the disease itself, by cerebral metastases and confusion, or by medication and other forms of treatment. Because of this, informants such as relatives may be used, but there is always the risk of bias—conscious and/or unconscious—in the reports that they offer.[43] Trained observers and participant observers are alternatives, but even they may not be totally free from bias and their training is often costly and lengthy.

The use of control groups or comparison groups frequently helps to put research findings in perspective, as was shown by those studies[25,30] which used comparison groups to determine whether palliative care staff have higher levels of psychological difficulties and different problems compared with nurses in other areas of work. Similarly, any attempt to investigate the value of different psychosocial interventions will benefit from random allocation (with or without stratification) to different groups.[44] One could use a matched design as an alternative to random allocation, provided that one is clear as to the relevant variables on which the groups should be matched. Another option for outcome studies, which resolves some problems (e.g. small sample size) is the multicentre randomized controlled trial.[45]

Researchers have to decide whether to use a longitudinal or a cross-sectional design. In the former, subjects are followed up at different intervals to obtain an index of change. However, this is a time-consuming method which may result in a high drop-out rate when dealing with very sick patients or troubled patients and staff. The 'practice effect', which occurs as patients become familiar with the measures used, may also be a problem. The cross-sectional method (perhaps involving the assessment of different groups of patients at different stages of their illness) may lack the rigour of the longitudinal approach (because subjects do not act as their own controls), but it is a useful way of assessing large numbers of subjects in a short period of time.

The choice of a retrospective as opposed to a prospective approach also has to be made. The former is a relatively quick and easy method for establishing, for example, the quality of care by interviewing bereaved relatives, but it is subject to distortion owing to fallible recall and the impact of intervening events and experiences. In the prospective approach a particular cohort of subjects (e.g. relatives of dying patients) are followed up and their psychosocial welfare is assessed at prescribed intervals.

The possible influence of bias always has to be considered. For instance, there is the 'ceiling effect' due to the generally high levels of satisfaction expressed by patients. Patients and relatives usually want to give favourable reports on those who care for them; therefore criticism may be difficult to elicit. Conversely, staff may find it difficult to express their own psychosocial problems because they may fear that they will be seen as 'weak' and unsuited for the job or for promotion.

Just as the Heisenberg Uncertainty Principle or the 'observer effect' is acknowledged in the natural sciences, so it has to be accepted in the psychosocial field that measurements and observations of a particular phenomenon will affect that phenomenon.

In conclusion, psychosocial research in palliative care is not easy, and it is challenged by a number of issues. Some relate to the physical vulnerability of the patients (which circumscribes the duration, nature, and frequency of assessments) and others relate to the limitations of some of the measures used in this field. Researchers often have to display sensitivity and ingenuity in their selection of research instruments and procedures.

Future research objectives

In the previous sections we have shown that psychosocial issues provide a valuable and exciting research focus in palliative care. However, such research activity remains something of a cottage industry when contrasted with the energy, time, and resources invested in palliative care itself. Some possible research objectives are identified in this final section.

There is a need for more refined methodologies and measuring instruments, the reliability and validity of which have been demonstrated specifically within palliative care and which have not been merely purloined from other areas. In terms of identifying what is helpful to families and patients, efforts must continue to be made to devise rigorous evaluation strategies and procedures. Within the field of psychotherapy research there is a challenging question, yet to be fully answered, about the relative impact of special features of specific therapies as opposed to that of 'non-specific factors' (such as hope and a persuasive rationale for the illness and its treatment). Their contribution in palliative care also has to be systematically assessed. The use of random allocation and control and comparison groups to evaluate the impact of psychosocial interventions has to be encouraged.

Longitudinal studies are also needed to identify how the psychosocial needs of families and patients change over time. In particular, it would be helpful to conduct a prospective study of families who are assessed before the diagnosis of a terminal illness is made and who could be followed up through the demise of the patient and for a period thereafter. Not only are we unable to identify how psychosocial needs change over time, but it is not clear what determines why, when, and from whom families will seek help. Families should also be assessed in terms of those individuals who are actively involved in the welfare of a sick member of the family and those who are not. Are there different losses and rewards for these two groups, and do they have different needs?

The concept of 'anticipatory grief' is often used in this field but without much rigour; it is a more complicated concept than its simple name might imply.[46] What is the evidence that relatives do grieve in advance of the patient's death and that this is beneficial? Are there times when it is unhelpful—perhaps even to the patient who is subjected to unintentional isolation and separation? The whole question of the relationship between effective palliative care and successful grieving has yet to be answered.

Whom we study and when we do so are important considerations. There is a risk that researchers are exposed only to the individuals who are not coping, whether they be staff, patients, or relatives. However, there is much to be gained from identifying and studying those who are coping effectively. What is different, for instance, about the small groups of patients who have been observed to maintain a good quality of life even in the last 14 days[5] compared with those patients who commit suicide?[47]

The role of individual differences is itself a fascinating topic. Little is known about successful methods of coping, or the range of coping methods called upon at different times or in response to different demands. Also, the extent to which we can teach, foster, or develop successful ways of coping has yet to be determined, although this possibility has been considered.[48]

For a number of reasons patients with malignant disease have been the most commonly studied, but there are other conditions, such as AIDS[49] or motor neurone disease, which are worthy of more detailed investigation in terms of the psychosocial issues that they raise for staff and families as well as for those who suffer from them. Children and adolescents have also been a neglected group.[50]

The literature on occupational stress among staff is developing,[25,51] but rarely is any knowledge achieved about whether the stressors are chronic or transient. Similarly, little effort has been made to identify the relationship between, on the one hand, stress and functioning at work and, on the other hand, psychosocial pressures outside the workplace. How to select staff who will cope with the demands of their work in a way which also ensures excellent care for patients needs further consideration. We should also study successful 'copers', not only among the groups who traditionally have been the target for research, namely nurses and doctors, but also among the ranks of ancillary staff such as porters and cleaners. Many professional staff must have observed, with no little envy and respect, those staff who 'just have a way' with patients. Research into training is still embryonic in terms of identifying what particular psychosocial attitudes, skills, and knowledge have to be taught, and how they can be taught in a way which ensures a long-term link between training and effective palliative care.

In conclusion, psychosocial issues in palliative care offer a rich source of challenging but important research questions. However, it is imperative that findings from the research domain continue to be translated into action and guidelines,[52–54] particularly in relation to effective psychosocial interventions.[55]

Bibliography

Brege JA. Terminal care: a bibliography of the psychosocial literature. *Hospice Journal*, 1985; **1**:51–79.

Broadfield L. Evaluation of palliative care: current status and future directions. *Journal of Palliative Care*, 1988; **4**:21–8.

Clarke D. *The Future of Palliative Care.* Buckingham: Open University Press, 1993.

Stedeford A. *Facing Death*. Oxford: Sobell, 1994.

References

1. Anonymous. Problems of hospices (editorial). *British Medical Journal*, 1984; **288**:1178–9.
2. Sobel HJ. Toward a behavioral thanatology in clinical care. In: Sobel HJ, ed. *Behavior Therapy in Terminal Care*. Cambridge: Ballinger, 1981.
3. Kubler-Ross E. *On Death and Dying.* New York: Macmillan, 1969.
4. Cain J, Stacy L, Jusenius K ,Figge D. The quality of dying: financial, psychological and ethical dilemmas. *Obstetrics and Gynaecology*, 1990; **76**:149–52.
5. Turk DC, Salovey P. Toward an understanding of life with cancer: personal meanings, psychosocial problems, and coping resources. *Hospice Journal*, 1985; **1**:73 84.
6. Gotay CC. Why me? Attributions and adjustment by cancer patients and their mates at two stages in the disease process. *Social Science and Medicine*, 1985; **20**:825–31.
7. Connor SR. Measurement of denial in the terminally ill: a critical review. *Hospice Journal*, 1986; **2**:51–68.
8. Connor SR. Denial in terminal illness: to intervene or not to intervene. *Hospice Journal*, 1992; **8**:1–15.
9. Honeybun J, Johnston M, Tookman, A. The impact of a death on fellow hospice patients. *British Journal of Medical Psychology*, 1992; **65**:67–72.
10. Herman F. Psychosocial support: interventions for the physician. *Seminars in Oncology*, 1985; **12**:466–71.
11. Geyman JP. Toward increased patient autonomy and choice of terminal care options. *Journal of Family Practice* 1986; **22**:399–400.
12. James V. Care and work in nursing the dying: a participant study of a continuing care unit. PhD Thesis. University of Aberdeen, 1986.
13. Buckingham RW. Living with the dying: use of the technique of participant observation. *Canadian Medical Association Journal*, 1976; **115**:1211–15.
14. Todd C, Still A. General practitioners' strategies and tactics of communication with the terminally ill. *Family Practice*, 1993, **10**:268–76.
15. Le Baron S, Zeltzer LK. The role of imagery in the treatment of dying children and adolescents. *Developmental and Behavioral Pediatrics*, 1985; **10**:252–8.
16. Doka KJ. The social organization of terminal care in two pediatric hospitals. *Omega*, 1981–2; **12**:345–54.
17. Greer DS, Mor V. An overview of National Hospice Study findings. *Journal of Chronic Diseases*, 1986; **39**: 5–7.
18. Gomas JM. Palliative care at home: a reality or 'mission impossible'? *Palliative Medicine*, 1993; **7**(Supplement 1):45–49.
19. Jefidoff A, Gasner R. Helping the parents of the dying child: an Israeli experience. *Journal of Pediatric Nursing*, 1993; **8**:413–15.
20. McGinnis SS. How can nurses improve the quality of life of the hospice client and family? An explanatory study. *Hospice Journal*, 1986; **2**:23–36.
21. Wilkes E. Terminal care: how can we do better? *Journal of the Royal College of Physicians of London*, 1986; **29**:216–18.
22. Jones RVH. Death from cancer at home: the carers' perspective. *British Medical Journal*, 1993; **306**: 249–51.
23. Herth K. Hope in the family caregiver of terminally ill people. *Journal of Advanced Nursing*, 1993; **18**:538–48.
24. Levitt JM. The conceptualization and assessment of family dynamics in terminal care. *Hospice Journal*, 1986; **2**:1–19.
25. Vachon M. *Occupational Stress in the Care of the Critically Ill, the Dying and the Bereaved.* Washington, DC: Hemisphere, 1987.
26. Still AW, Todd CJ. Role ambiguity in general practice: the care of patients dying at home. *Social Science and Medicine*, 1986; **23**:519–25.
27. Turnipseed DL. Burnout among hospice nurses: an empirical assessment. *Hospice Journal*, 1987; **3**:105–19.
28. Alexander DA, Ritchie E. 'Stressors' and difficulties in dealing with the terminal patient. *Journal of Palliative Care*. 1990; **6**:28–33.
29. Woolley H, Stein A, Forrest GC, Baum JD. Staff stress and job satisfaction at a children's hospice. *Archives of Disease in Childhood*, 1989; **64**:114–18.
30. Foxall MJ, Zimmerman L, Standley R, Captain BB. A comparison of frequency and sources of nursing job stress perceived by intensive care, hospice and medical–surgical nurses. *Journal of Advanced Nursing*, 1990; **15**:577–84.
31. Maguire P. Barriers to psychological care of the dying. *British Medical Journal*, 1988; **291**:1711–13.
32. Dickinson GE, Tournier RE. A longitudinal study of sex differences in how physicians relate to dying patients. *Journal of the American Medical Women's Association*, 1993; **48**:19–22.
33. Amenta MM. Traits of hospice nurses compared with those who work in traditional settings. *Journal of Clinical Psychology*, 1984; **40**:414–20.
34. Layer B. Predicting performance and persistence in hospice volunteers. *Psychological Reports*, 1989; **65**:467–72.
35. Jones K, Johnston M, Speck P. Despair felt by the patient and the professional carer: a case study of the use of cognitive behavioural methods. *Palliative Medicine*, 1989; **3**:39–46.
36. Razavi D, Delvaux N, Farvacques C, Robaye E. Brief psychological training for health care professionals dealing with cancer patients: a one-year assessment. *General Hospital Psychiatry*, 1991; **13**:253–60.
37. Alexander DA. Staff support groups: do they support and are they even groups? *Palliative Medicine*, 1993; **7**:127–32.
38. Chiriboga DA, Jennings G, Bailey J. Stress and coping among hospice nurses: test of an analytic model. *Nursing Research*, 1983; **32**:294–9.
39. Mor V. Assessing patient outcomes in hospice: what to measure? *Hospice Journal*, 1986; **2**:17–35.
40. Dobkin PL, Morrow GR. Biopsychosocial assessment of cancer patients: methods and suggestions. *Hospice Journal*, 1986; **2**:37–59.
41. Cassileth BR. Methodologic issues in palliative care psychosocial research. *Journal of Palliative Care*, 1989; **5**:5–11.
42. Rathbone GV, Horsley S, Goacher J. A self-evaluated assessment suitable for seriously ill hospice patients. *Palliative Medicine*, 1994; **8**:29–34.
43. Spiller JA, Alexander DA. Domiciliary care: a comparison of the views of terminally ill patients and their family caregivers. *Palliative Medicine*, 1993; **7**:109–15.
44. McCorkle R, Packard N, Landenburger K. Subject accrual and attrition: problems and solutions. *Journal of Psychosocial Oncology*, 1985; **2**:137–46.
45. McQuay H, Moore A. Need for rigorous assessment of palliative care. *British Medical Journal*, 1994; **309**:1315–16.
46. Rando TA. Anticipatory grief: the term is a misnomer but the phenomenon exists. *Journal of Palliative Care*, 1988; **4**:70–3.
47. Hietanen P, Lönnqvist J, Henriksson M, Jallinoja P. Do cancer suicides differ from others? *Psycho-Oncology*, 1994; **3**:189–95.
48. Smith DC, Maher MF. Achieving a healthy death: the dying person's attitudinal contributions. *Hospice Journal*, 1993; **9**: 21–32.
49. Butters E, Higginson I, George R, McCarthy M. Palliative care for people with HIV/AIDS: views of patients, carers and providers. *AIDS Care*, 1993; **5**:105–16.
50. Christ GH, *et al.* Impact of parental terminal cancer on latency-age children. *American Journal of Orthopsychiatry*, 1993; **63**:417–25.
51. Alexander DA, MacLeod M. Stress among palliative care matrons: a major problem for a minority group. *Palliative Medicine*, 1992; **6**:111–24.

52. Robinson L, Stacy R. Palliative care in the community: setting practice guidelines for primary care teams. *British Journal of General Practice*, 1994; **44**:461–4.
53. Smith N, Regnard C. Managing family problems in advanced disease—a flow diagram. *Palliative Medicine*, 1993; 7:47–58.
54. Faulkner A, Maguire P, Regnard C. Dealing with anger in a patient or relative: a flow diagram. *Palliative Medicine*, 1994; 8:51–7.
55. Fawzy IF, Fawzy NW, Arndt LA, Pasnau O. Critical review of psychosocial interventions in cancer care. *Archives of General Psychiatry*, 1995; **52**:100–13.

5.5 Nursing research

Jenifer Wilson-Barnett and Alison Richardson

Nursing is a broad-based discipline which requires knowledge from many subject areas. As the main focus for nursing is the 'whole person', his or her needs and responses to health or illness, and the care received, research by nurses is wide ranging. It covers the social context of care, as well as psychosocial and spiritual needs. It also includes work which explores the relationship between psychological and physical phenomena and ways in which nurses can intervene to improve the welfare of patients and their carers. This breadth of relevant topics is represented in the new core curriculum for courses in palliative nursing care described by Tiffany.[1] An impressive range of subjects is integrated into a core of study to prepare specialist nurses in palliative care.

Just as the topics of nursing enquiry are varied, so are the research approaches and methods used. A combination of basic disciplines and research paradigms serves to increase nurses' understanding of how people feel, what they require and appreciate, and how practitioners can assist them. Therefore in this chapter we cover the areas most pertinent to nursing and review work which straddles many issues in palliative nursing internationally. Several recently published studies are included in this edition of the textbook, although there do not appear to have been any major shifts in direction or substantial findings since the publication of the first edition.

Authors of other chapters in this book have addressed similar topics in more depth and from a different perspective. In this chapter we indicate current progress in relevant nursing research and provide access to other sources of literature. We commence with an overview of research progress in the speciality, touching on the different settings for care and how these affect patients. Family care is then discussed briefly before we deal more specifically with psychological and physical care. In the final section we discuss the overall contribution of nurses and nursing research to this speciality. Throughout, we highlight areas where additional research is necessary to inform practice.

Overview of nursing research

The majority of studies in the 1970s, 1980s, and early 1990s have concentrated on the attitudes and experiences of nurses in caring for the dying and on communication patterns within the ward team and with patients and relatives. Both areas have been found to present disappointing pictures, in that nurses (in the general setting) feel anxious and ill-prepared to care for the dying and their families and therefore tend not to engage in open communication which may be more supportive and helpful for all involved.[2,3]

Recently, there have been more systematic attempts to identify the needs of patients and their relatives and also to quantify and measure symptoms and quality of life for patients.[4,5] There have also been a few studies of psychological intervention, particularly for the bereaved,[6] and practice-based innovations and evaluations using research findings which have identified needs of relatives.[7] Progress has been made by building on these findings and attempting to explore more specific nursing approaches to problems.

A great diversity of research methods has been recognized by other reviewers in this area,[8] who have also noted how complex and difficult it is to test 'best nursing treatments' by experimental methods. Clearly, it is extremely important to establish appropriate research methods in order to address specific questions. It is not always appropriate or desirable to conduct randomized trials, and in a new research area, such as nursing, great insight may be gained from case studies and other in-depth systematic descriptive methods. A combination of qualitative and quantitative methods also has advantages in this particular field.[9] A recent review of palliative care research[10] also reflects this diversity of approach and acknowledges the great advances which can be made through a multidisciplinary approach. This report also provides an excellent analysis of the particular ethical considerations necessary in this specialty.

The settings for palliative care

It is evident that a majority of individuals in the Western world still die in hospital. Although many may die rather rapidly after emergency admission from a coronary thrombosis or cerebrovascular accident, others die after serious illnesses for which they receive protracted treatments in the medical or surgical wards of a general hospital. Research indicates that the care received by those who are dying in this setting is far from ideal. A recent editorial in the *Journal of Advanced Nursing*[11] asserted that a holistic philosophy, privacy, and supportive staff relationships should be developed wherever care is given. Evidence suggests that this is more difficult in the acute setting with its obvious and pressing competing demands. When the care of 50 dying patients was observed in hospital wards,[12] the research team concluded that care was poor, basic interventions to maintain comfort were not often provided, and hygiene, thirst, and nutritional needs were often not attended to: 'Contact between nurses and the dying patients was minimal; distancing and isolation of patients by most medical and nursing staff were evident; this isolation increased as death approached' (ref. 12, p. 583). Field[13] also found poor communication, leading to inadequate support for relatives and staff. This has been verified by interviews with staff who feel inadequately prepared and rather upset and ashamed at what they recognize to be a failure in the system.[14] In this last study, a modest educational workshop lasting for 3 days was found to help nurses to feel more confident in their ability to comfort patients and their families. Their realization that as newly registered nurses they were responsible for such care motivated them to explore their own feelings and consider ways in which they could help to improve the general ward climate. As these studies were undertaken several years ago, it is now appropriate that they should be repeated in order to establish the extent of change in practice and the effect of, for example, palliative care teams within the acute hospital setting.

Recent work[15] has confirmed that trained nursing staff use several blocking techniques when communicating with cancer patients, whether they are working in the general or specialized setting. This is particularly worrying since, in the specialist setting, a number of nurses had received advanced education.

In addition, a qualitative study[16] of hospital nurses found the same problems with disclosure of prognosis that had been identified over 20 years ago. Despite a policy that nurses should be present during such interviews with patients and relatives, they often felt excluded and ill-informed. This was interpreted as undervaluing their potential and, more specifically, their ability to offer continued support.

Despite general acceptance of what good practice should be in hospital—that nurses should spend time with and be available for the patient and relatives, and that the multidisciplinary team should discuss and plan for care—priorities do not seem to have shifted away from acute curative medical care. Policy guidelines for general hospitals, advising on management and administrative procedures concerned with family follow-up and support, are widely available. However, general staff do not seem to cope well with dying patients or prevent unnecessarily distressing events. Hence specialist teams have been established to link hospital and home care, provide continuity, and identify and help with particular problems. Evaluation of these teams[17] shows that they can have a direct effect in improving care and also help to educate other staff in the general wards.

Contrasts in philosophy and practice across sectors are also highlighted by evidence that different problems are identified by nurses in different settings when caring for those who are dying.[18] While nutrition and pain were found to be the problems occurring most frequently across all settings, weakness and confusion were found to be the most difficult to manage in the community, while pain persisted as the most difficult to manage in acute care. More nurses in community care mentioned physical problems, although this could reflect either their client group or their more sensitive assessment of such problems. Team problems were also perceived as greatest in acute care; and this probably influenced opinions that the support offered to nursing staff was inadequate. Adaptation by patients to their dying status was seen as a difficult and frequent problem for nurses in all sectors.

There appears to be general acceptance that most people would prefer to die at home,[19] although support from community and, in particular, nursing care teams is a vital component of this choice. Services in the United Kingdom have been extended in the form of community teams which include specialist nurses. These seem to provide a higher standard of care than other arrangements based on either hospitals or general practitioners.[20] However, further work is required to evaluate the particular roles that specialist nurses should play and their relationship to the rest of the community team.[19] Such roles and services should be evaluated through quality assurance programmes and action research. Recently, a small qualitative interview study[21] with a mixed sample of patients, relatives, and community staff, exploring the role of Macmillan nurses, demonstrated that they are highly valued for their knowledge and contribution, and that they can also work harmoniously with members of the caring team. It is suggested that their work should be structured flexibly within teams, so that, for instance Macmillan nurses and district nurses should work together, not necessarily adhering to rigid predefined roles.

As the developed world's population becomes older, with fewer able carers, and family units become smaller, it is likely that demand for palliative care will increase for all age groups. For example, short-stay and day care are increasingly seen as appropriate for some palliative treatments. It could be said that nursing partially compensates for lack of family support, as hospice nursing has been characterized as intensive care, collaborative sharing, continuous knowing or counselling, and giving.[22] Clearly, the philosophy of providing constant care and emotional support satisfies a need for the dying person and also helps to support family members who may become isolated and unable to cope.

However, the enormous challenge of attempting to provide perfect care or role models must be recognized. A more philosophical analysis of these issues[23] has revealed that nurse specialists often feel that they have impossible goals, because holistic care has been reinterpreted as a perfect comprehensive and ideal package which they should be able to deliver.

In summary, nursing research which examines hospice care tends to describe the service, organization, costs, and attitudes, while practice-based or direct patient care research is 'sadly lacking'.[24] More collaborative studies between educationalists and practitioners are needed to ensure work of relevance to the welfare of patients.

Family care

To date, research identifying the needs of family members and evaluating the nursing care required to meet these seems to be more plentiful and consistent than that focused directly on patient care. Descriptions of these needs have been based on interview studies such as that by Dracup and Brue.[7] These showed that the primary requirement of all relatives was reliable information about the patient's present condition and prognosis. Relatives caring for the patient at home were particularly appreciative of instructions on aspects of patient care or treatment procedures. Nurses were seen to be in an ideal position to provide this information. Relatives have also consistently reported that they feel more secure if they can be near the patient, visiting whenever they wish or contacted at home by staff. However, they considered that nurses should spend time comforting the patient and seeing to his or her needs, rather than attempting to provide certain types of counselling for themselves and other relatives.[25]

Research with families has often asked members to identify helpful or supportive behaviours of nurses. Honest information about all aspects of care was most important to families. Adequate pain control and assurance that their relatives were receiving competent nursing care were also major concerns.[26–28] Families did not want attention focused on themselves and consistently identified as least supportive behaviours that encouraged them to ventilate their feelings.[29]

Thus families should be recognized as experts in generating information about specific behaviours that communicate caring. With this in mind, a qualitative study[30] was conducted which examined the caring behaviours of hospice nurses as perceived by family caregivers. Four areas of caring were identified: 24-h accessibility, effective communication, a non-judgemental attitude, and clinical competence. A discrepancy in the findings with respect to previous research was highlighted. This was concerned with whether families wanted to share their feelings. The researcher suggests that if families need to maintain control of their emotions, yet nurses encourage them to express their feelings, this is distressing and unsupportive. In contrast, if families want to discuss problems and share feelings, the nurses' ability to explore these feelings is perceived as caring. Obviously, sensitivity is required in taking cues from families as to what is comfortable. Future research should address this aspect of communication, with specific approaches to psychological care being correlated with families' satisfaction and bereavement outcomes.

Interesting work on the changing pattern of the family's needs as the patient's condition changes or deteriorates has been reported.[31] It was found that as the disease (cancer) progressed, relatives expected less attention for themselves from nurses. At the same time, families expected to be more involved in care and requested more explanation and teaching from nurses. It has also been found that with lengthening periods of terminal illness, the main informal carers become the channel of communication with the hospice team and other relatives.[32] Findings show that relatives generally wish to maintain a close relationship with the dying person and do not find long periods of sustained contact difficult, except when the patient manifests signs of distress and confusion.

Although this body of research has provided guidelines for practice and one specific study has used these to evaluate improvements,[7] reviews of research in the area have criticized the lack of a theoretical basis and consequently the absence of ideas to explain findings. For instance, Hull[25] explores the need for interpretation in which attempts are made to relate findings to other work on coping and separation. Need for further clarification of the concepts of 'support' and 'emotional isolation' is also required to avoid confusion when advising on nursing practice. Despite this, Hull advocates that these findings should form the basis of further correlational research and recommends that nurses provide more opportunities to give information and discuss concerns with family members.

The context of care and death has been seen to influence the degree of family support and level of bereavement care received by relatives, particularly the spouse. A study performed in the United Kingdom[33] highlighted the difference between hospital and hospice in this regard. Hospital staff tended to be rushed and failed to give relatives sufficient time to say goodbye to their loved one (a similar finding was reported in the United States). Staff's inability or perceived unwillingness to talk and comfort the grieving relatives was reported by some relatives. Cowley's[34] research in one district, interviewing widows some months after the death of their spouse, supports this general finding and produced several examples where relatives had to wait to see staff or were inappropriately informed on aspects of prognosis or deterioration. This seemed to have a lasting and deleterious impression on their own grieving process.

Much advice on supportive care at the time of death and subsequently is available in the literature. Yet again it has not been evaluated as a package of nursing care which has demonstrable benefits. Difficulties in designing and carrying out such a study are legion, but ward-based evaluative research might help by involving all staff as participants.

In contrast with the lack of supportive care received by relatives of patients in hospital, hospice staff have initiated active programmes to support families over time. The nature of such support varies, but a Canadian study[35] stands out as an attempt to identify the essential component of such care. Samples of 11 hospice nurses and 12 families were selected in order to explore what was described as the spiritual relationship between nurses and families through in-depth unstructured interviews. Families described the openness and ready availability of the nurses as fundamental; their knowledge and faith in themselves and their ability to give were seen as valuable and helpful for their adjustment. Somehow their capacity to share, listen, and grieve with the relatives made the experience more worthwhile for them all, and subsequently the specialist nurse role became encapsulated in the term 'the shining stranger'.[36] Nurses themselves felt vulnerable at times but realized that there was a quality in their relationships with relatives which helped them to grow and continue to give of themselves. This type of work can illuminate palliative nursing and seems to exemplify what can be achieved and what is highly valued.

Psychological aspects of nursing care

In the main, models for good psychological care have arisen from specialist practice. In contrast, other general staff seem to fail to assess and plan psychological care systematically.[37] However, there is a growing body of research-based knowledge on which assessments and interventions could be based. For instance, Weisman[38] suggests that one can identify stressful aspects of the 'dying situation' which can be ameliorated through careful support. Successful copers tend to confront problems, seek information, and discuss their fears and worries. Others may need much more time to establish trust and build a relationship with a primary nurse before facing particular problems. Recognition of the stages involved in 'fading away' was also clarified in work with relatives.[39] These qualitative accounts were used to design a practical framework for psychological care at different terminal stages. Growing evidence that successful coping is associated with fewer physical discomforts and symptoms[40] demonstrates the importance of this area.

Psychological intervention which can be tailored to individual needs is needed to help adjustment.[41] The three tasks of adjustment are seen as searching for meaning, regaining mastery, and enhancing self esteem. Relevant interventions may induce effective communication, participation in care, group support, and stress reduction techniques. Research assessing the efforts of group support and stress reduction techniques is perhaps more plentiful than that in the other areas identified. For instance, the experience of nurse-run groups in the United States[42] showed that such groups were well appreciated and helped to raise the self-esteem of participants. Stress reduction techniques for patients have also been employed by nurses[43] with reported beneficial results. Muscle relaxation and massage have been shown to reduce anxiety, to reduce 'congestion' by aiding circulation, and to improve general well being.

Sims[44] contends that the purposeful use of touch has significance for all patients, and that it has particular significance for patients with far advanced disease. Touch should be valued as a therapeutic intervention. It is a powerful way to facilitate communication; it enhances verbal communication and facilitates social interaction, information giving, and expression of feeling. Touch may also form an integral part of comfort care with the possibility of enhancing both physical and psychological comfort. It would appear beneficial to explore further the systematic forms of touch such as gentle massage, exploring the benefits that they may have for patients in a more rigorous research evaluation.[45]

Central to all effective psychological care is the nature of close relationships for those who are vulnerable. Interviews with hospice patients[46] revealed that an empathic relationship with a nurse was felt to influence improved and maintained physical and emotional well being.

Likewise, Hunt[47] identified ease of communication, in which nurses were valued for being friendly and informal. From these data it appeared that 'chatting' (about topics not related to illness) was crucial for the development of this type of easy relationship.

Nurse researchers have also focused on the concept of 'hope' as a positive and motivating response which can give meaning to and energize those who are dying. Fostering hope is seen to improve the quality of life and help patients to achieve goals,[48] although little practical guidance is available for nurses on how to do this. Herth's study[48] aimed to elicit aspects of patients' experiences which encouraged or discouraged hope. This interview study revealed that seven key strategies were seen as facilitating hope:

(1) the presence of a meaningful relationship;

(2) the ability to feel light-hearted;

(3) personal attributes of determination, courage, and serenity;

(4) clear aims;

(5) spiritual beliefs;

(6) ability to recall positive moments;

(7) having one's individuality accepted and respected.

Negative effects on hope were identified as follows:

(1) physical and emotional loss of others;

(2) uncontrolled pain and discomfort;

(3) being treated in a 'devaluing' manner.

Herth[49] also proposed that an understanding of 'hope' from the viewpoint of family caregivers was essential for their support. She found enduring levels of what was conceived as an 'inner strength'. However, physical problems of a long-term nature for patients were found particularly to hinder hope among this sample.

Clearly, all these features help to provide a framework on which to base psychological care. This work has shown that nurses can provide an enduring and caring relationship which fosters hope. As this is so important to the well being of patients and their families, care should always be organized to enable this.

Discussion on how this can be sustained by staff is important; some maladaptive reactions to multiple deaths and poorly managed deaths cause distress and health problems. Experience derived from extensive work in this field and from workshops with staff has been used to provide guidelines for managing grief,[50] in which emphasis on understanding personal signs of distress and poor coping is combined with various policy recommendations for managers. Another recent study also demonstrates that nurses in palliative care teams need to expend substantial energy on role adaptation and coping with conflict among the team in order to sustain their own personal integrity.[51] Only when this is an active element of their work can they prevent signs of distress associated with patient care.

Physical problems and nursing care

There is abundant evidence that resistant symptoms cause patients to suffer at the end of their lives.[52] Advances and success in analgesia are not matched by the palliation of many other common problems such as dyspnoea, fatigue and nausea.[53] It is impossible and inappropriate to discuss these in detail here as they are well covered elsewhere. However, some nursing research is useful in identifying the specific role of the nurse and those aspects of nursing care which are particularly helpful for patients and relatives.

As previously mentioned, measurement of symptoms and their effect on the quality of life has received concentrated attention from researchers such as McCorkle and Young[5] and Sutcliffe and Holmes.[4] The importance of producing reliable tools to monitor and assess the effects of nursing interventions is clear. Progress in testing interventions has been slow, partly because of the absence of measuring tools and partly because of the methodological challenges related to controlling other influential variables.

Work identifying the prevalence of symptoms and problems is also progressing with more general nursing assessment tools available, and the range of interventions span the physical and psychological realms of practice. The following six major research areas of palliation have emerged from the literature on the whole spectrum of problems: ambulation, bowel management, comfort, diet, pain care, and wound and skin care.[54] These areas demonstrate a reasonable selection of nursing support functions but overlook the general aim of maximizing the patient's own coping strategies and other more specific actions which might be employed.

There are still several problems which are seemingly difficult to alleviate such as dyspnoea, a prevalent and distressing problem shown to be a predictor of imminent death among hospice admissions.[55] This and other problems, such as malodour, incontinence, and general malaise, tend to tax all staff. Little research by nurses has been done in these areas.

Nutrition and mobilization are generally important in maintaining health but may become progressively more difficult. Helping to sustain choice and the comfort of a sociable environment is generally advised, and nurses are encouraged to recognize the symbolic importance of nutrition as life sustaining.[56] Staff in one hospice demonstrated the positive benefits of arranging food to suit patients, with smaller plates and a peaceful attractive setting in which to eat.[57] This encouraged a better dietary intake for many patients.

In continuing to realize that psychosocial factors influence physical discomfort, recent nursing studies of side-effects and symptoms have attempted to identify and modify such factors where appropriate. Patients' own coping strategies and resources clearly need to be maximized and their participation in care is essential. Information-giving and exchange and individualized teaching can frequently facilitate patients' efforts. For example, Payne[58] demonstrated that women undergoing palliative chemotherapy for breast cancer inevitably seemed to suffer from nausea. Their coping strategies were of varying success, but the 'positive fighters' had a greater sense of control and a wider repertoire of strategies including diversion, minimization, humour, and making new special friends. A recent review[59] of self-care strategies for alleviating side-effects of chemotherapy echoes many of these findings. Prerequisites for self-care are seen as essential knowledge, skills, and responsibility, sufficient motivation and energy, a need to place a high value on health, and a perception that new health behaviours will reduce vulnerability to further illness.[60] Greater social support and better economic status of patients have a positive influence on their use of self-care strategies.[61] However, other symptoms such as tiredness and weakness have been found to have an adverse effect on attempts to cope actively and to use self-care strategies.[62] Dodd [63,64] has produced a number of reports on the utilization of self-care strategies in response to the side-effects of cancer therapies. It may be beneficial to focus attention on the utility of self-care in the relief of symptoms associated with the disease process, complications of the disease, and medications such as opioid analgesics. It has been suggested[62] that individuals with symptoms attributed to illness make attempts to modify their behaviour in attempts to maintain normal function. There are fewer expectations of self-care when symptoms are associated with treatment strategies. The relationships between perception of the cause of a symptom and the likelihood of performance of self-care need to be clarified. Self-care could usefully be employed as a means of more successful symptom control and as a way of handing over control of a situation to the patient.

Responses to chemotherapy and radiotherapy (whether at the treatment stage or used as palliative strategies) include fatigue and weakness. This is well recognized across disciplines, and nurse researchers are now starting to study these conditions. Dodd[64] has explored self-care for all the side-effects of treatment and the measuring instruments should be useful for future research. Despite disappointing results (which indicated that self-care behaviours were not associated with less distress), she found that anxiety was reduced as a consequence of self-care at one stage of treatment.

Hart *et al.*[65] discussed the variables associated with fatigue and made the following recommendations, which we support, to assist nurses to help patients:

(1) to increase awareness of levels of fatigue and the factors which make this worse;

(2) to recognize when rest and restoration is needed;

(3) to identify and use an activity–rest programme that results in the restoration of energy;

(4) to accept assistance from a support network;

(5) to develop a lifestyle that stimulates and involves physical activity..

Although these recommendations appear sensible, the practicalities of encouraging those who feel deeply fatigued and unwell could be extremely difficult. These strategies clearly need to be appropriately applied and evaluated.

There are many causes of fatigue, and those who are dying may well manifest several related not only to treatments for alleviation of pain or obstruction from tumour growth, but also to malnutrition, anaemia, infections, and cancer. Pathologies other than cancer can also lead to fatigue and generalized weakness, known as asthenia, but as many as 75 per cent of patients with cancer may complain of this.[66] Any obvious physical and medical intervention needs to be applied where possible, but complementary approaches to care may also be helpful. Sim[44] has reviewed alternative therapies which can be applied by nurses and may be particularly useful in alleviating these more general symptoms. Massage and relaxation might well be included in programmes of care and evaluated carefully through research using the adapted symptom distress scales mentioned previously (see Chapter 9.4).[4]

Accurate descriptions of problems need to proceed in tandem with identification of appropriate supportive interventions. For instance, the sensations of people experiencing dyspnoea who suffer from obstructive, restrictive, and vascular lung disease have been investigated.[67] Physical sensations were clustered into the categories of suffocation, tightness, and congestion. Further work with lung cancer patients[68] provided descriptions of the sensations of dyspnoea and identified coping and adaptive strategies utilized by this group. The subjects suffered significant dyspnoea, felt extreme fatigue, and experienced loss of concentration, memory, and appetite when short of breath. Many useful strategies of either a short-term or a long-term nature were identified. Short-term strategies included actions to manage acute episodes of breathlessness such as changes in position and activity. Long-term strategies focused upon adaptive lifestyle changes such as advanced planning of activities and alterations in attitude. Rather worryingly, it was revealed that no patients identified any useful strategies that had been taught by nurses; any strategies that had been learnt had been self-taught.

Further efforts to quantify and explore the significance of this problem of dyspnoea is recommended, as there is evidence that it is underdetected by staff and unreported by patients.[69] The measurement tools used could be usefully employed in the clinical setting to aid the detection of the level of dyspnoea that a patient may be experiencing. The information obtained could lead to appropriate planning for change with nursing interventions evaluated against a reliable measurement of the subjective symptoms of dyspnoea.

From the evidence obtained so far[70] patients provide a wealth of information on how to manage dyspnoea. In future, nurse researchers could usefully investigate the provision of information concerned with combinations of these strategies in different subgroups of patients experiencing different degrees of dyspnoea.

There are two other specific physical problems which concern nurses a great deal and have been the object of nursing research. Wound care is important to patients; discomfort and low morale may be caused by resistance to healing or by fungating and ulcerating malignant lesions. According to Ivetic and Lyne[71] there is little published work dealing specifically with such lesions, but this topic is considered in detail in Chapter 9.6.3. The second specific physical problem, which affects patients after treatment for cancer and those suffering from advanced disease, is lymphoedema. A heavy oedematous limb is a distressing condition, leading to restriction of movement and discomfort, and it has a significant effect on the patient's quality of life, particularly when associated with terminal cancer.[72] One study[73] reports an incidence of 38 per cent in women with breast cancer, depending on treatment. Radiotherapy was isolated as being one of the most important risk factors, but this contrasts with the findings of a smaller study.[74] A simple mastectomy or radiotherapy required as a palliative measure may often be complicated by lymphoedema. Selection of a short effective treatment programme would seem prudent in people with a limited life expectancy. The management of lymphoedema is discussed in detail in Chapter 9.7.

The range of physical problems requiring palliation is extensive. Research indicates careful monitoring and specific care for most of these, but it is also clear that nurse researchers are attempting to employ complementary strategies which strengthen the patient's coping style and behaviour. Self-caring and family participation in care seem to be particularly satisfying strategies for providing comfort and support. However, much more evidence is required to demonstrate how these may be perfected and evaluated.

Palliative nursing and further directions for research

The most recent research-based papers in these areas show that work is building on previous findings and greater clarity is emerging. More guidelines for practice and theoretical analyses are presented from data which increasingly reflects the consumers' views. In most areas specialists continue to receive praise and positive evaluation from consumers, whereas generalists are seen to require much more confidence and skill to give that extra dimension of care that dying patients and their families need. When attempting to identify what that special dimension might be, Davies and Oberle[75] conducted in-depth interviews with one expert nurse based on 10 cases. Using an inductive interperative approach, these researchers derived themes from these data which described the features and role of the specialist. These included the following:

(1) 'valuing' others and the patient as an individual;

(2) 'connecting' or establishing and continuing a good relationship with the family;

(3) 'empowering' and facilitating strengths within the family by encouraging and defusing;

(4) 'doing for' the patient as necessary by controlling pain and resolving problems;

(5) 'finding meaning' by focusing on living and acknowledging death;

(6) 'preserving own integrity' by valuing oneself as a nurse and being aware of one's own needs and attachments.

This small study crystallized the value and special nature of the role. It encompassed several dimensions, but the skill of providing comprehensive family care was seen to be based on knowledge, wisdom, and personal strengths. Not all nurses caring for the dying may be able to give so much of themselves, but the ideal picture may give insights into what is valued and sometimes expected.

Further study by McWilliam *et al.*[51] has confirmed the importance of this framework. Nurses' effort was conceptualized as primary (or direct care) and secondary, in which barriers were overcome. The work environment is still likely to produce most stress. As always, better team work and recognition of an individual's need for support are highlighted.

Nursing research is increasing in volume, value, and diversity. In 1983 Quint Benoliel[3] concluded her review by identifying three areas of established evidence from nursing research as follows:

(1) planned support which can enhance adjustment after bereavement;

(2) focused education which can improve nurses' attitudes and knowledge about death and grief;

(3) innovations in practice which can be introduced into the complex environment of care.

A more recent review[2] of research in areas of social and psychological care, coping, and comfort care found evidence that more knowledge existed in the areas of psychosocial care than in the field of physical and comfort care. To some extent this is still the case, but an encouraging trend for researchers to tackle the more resistant and abstract problems of fatigue and malaise has emerged. No doubt greater understanding will be gained from really imaginative qualitative exploration as well as from carefully controlled comparative or quasi-experimental evaluations. This eclectic approach which is now encouraged across disciplines[10] would seem to suit the wide-ranging issues and dimensions of palliative nursing.

The quantity, degree of focus, and quality of research have all improved in the last 3 years. The confidence of researchers to tackle important yet 'difficult to study' areas is impressive. Recognition of the sensitivities involved as well as the pluralistic influence on the quality of consumers' experience is evident across this literature. Sadly, however, the need to improve hospital care and staff support is enduring.

References

1. Tiffany R. A core curriculum for a postbasic course in palliative nursing care. *Palliative Medicine*, 1990; **4**:261–70.
2. Wilson-Barnett J and Raiman J. *Nursing Issues and Research in Terminal Care*. Chichester: Wiley, 1988.
3. Quint Benoliel J. Nursing research on death, dying and terminal illness: development, present state and prospects. *Annual Review of Nursing Research*, 1983; **1**:101–30.
4. Sutcliffe J, Holmes S. Quality of life: verification and use of a self-assessment scale in two patient populations. *Journal of Advanced Nursing*, 1991; **16**:490–98.
5. McCorkle R and Young K. Development of a symptom distress scale. *Cancer Nursing*, 1978; **1**:373–8.
6. Vachon MLSV, Lyall WAL, Rogers J, Freeman-Letofsky K, Freeman SJJ.

A controlled study of self-help intervention for widows. *American Journal of Psychiatry*, 1980; **137**:1380–4.
7. Dracup K, Brue CS. Using nursing research findings to meet the needs of grieving spouses. *Nursing Research*, 1978; **27**:212–16.
8. Cassileth BR, Lusk SJ. Methodologic issues in palliative care: psychosocial research. *Journal of Palliative Care*, 1989; **5**:5–11.
9. Corner J. In search of more complete answers to research questions: quantitative versus qualitative research methods: is there a way forward? *Journal of Advanced Nursing*, 1991; **10**:718–27.
10. Twycross RG, Dunn V. *Research in Palliative Care: The Pursuit of Reliable Knowledge*. London: National Council for Hospice and Specialist Palliative Care Services, 1994.
11. Bircumshaw D. Guest editorial: Palliative care in the acute hospital setting. *Journal of Advanced Nursing*, 1993; **18**:1665–6.
12. Mills M, Davies HTO, Macrae WA. Care of dying patients in hospital. *British Medical Journal*; 1994; **309**:583–6.
13. Field D. *Nursing the Dying*. London: Tavistock/Routledge, 1989.
14. Corner J. The newly registered nurse and the cancer patient. PhD Thesis, King's College London, 1990.
15. Wilkinson S. Factors which influence how nurses communicate with cancer patients. *Journal of Advanced Nursing*, 1991; **16**:677–88.
16. May C. Disclosure of terminal prognoses in a general hospital: the nurse's view. *Journal of Advanced Nursing*, 1993; **18**:1362–8.
17. Hockley J, Dunlop R, Danes R. Survey of distressing symptoms in dying patients and their families in hospital and the response to a symptom control team. *British Medical Journal*, 1988; **296**:1715–17.
18. Copp G, Dunn V. Frequent and difficult problems perceived by nurses caring for the dying in community, hospice and acute care settings. *Palliative Medicine*, 1993; **7**:19–25.
19. Bergen A. Nurses caring for the terminally ill in the community: a review of the literature. *Journal of Advanced Nursing*, 1991; **28**(1):89–101.
20. Ward A. Home care services: an alternative to hospices. *Community Medicine*, 1987; **9**:47–54.
21. Cox K, Bergen A. Exploring consumer views of care provided by the Macmillan nurse using the critical incident technique. *Journal of Advanced Nursing*, 1993; **18**:408–15.
22. Dobratz MC. Hospice nursing: present perspectives and future directions. *Cancer Nursing*, 1990; **13**:116–22.
23. Cribb A, Bignold S, Ball S. Linking the parts : an exemplar of philosophical and practical issues in holistic nursing. *Journal of Advanced Nursing*, 1994; **20**:233–8.
24. Petrosino BM. Nursing research in hospice care. *Hospice Journal*, 1988; **4**:29–45.
25. Hull MM. Family needs and supportive nursing behaviours during terminal cancer: a review. *Oncology Nursing Forum*, 1989; **16**:787–92.
26. Hampe S. Needs of the grieving spouse in a hospital setting. *Oncology Nursing Forum*,1975; **24**:113–19.
27. Wright K, Dyck S. Expressed concerns of adult cancer patients' family members. *Cancer Nursing*, 1984; **7**:371–4.
28. Skorupka P, Bohnet N. Primary caregivers' perceptions of nursing behaviours that best meet their needs in a home care hospice setting. *Cancer Nursing*, 1982; **5**:371–4.
29. Freihofer P, Felton G. Nursing behaviours in bereavement: an explanatory study. *Nursing Research*, 1976; **25**:332–7.
30. Hull M. Hospice nurses, caring support for caregiving families. *Cancer Nursing*, 1991; **14**:63–70.
31. Dyck S, Wright K. Family perceptions: the role of the nurse throughout an adult's cancer experience. *Oncology Nursing Forum*, 1985; **12**:53–6.
32. Yang C-T, Kirschling JM. Exploration of factors related to direct care and outcomes of care giving: caregivers of terminally ill older persons. *Cancer Nursing*, 1992; **15**(3):173–81.
33. Lunt B. *A Comparison of Hospice and Hospital Care for Terminally Ill Cancer Patients and their Families*. London: Cancer Relief Macmillan Fund, 1985. (Research Report.)
34. Cowley S. Supporting dying people. *Nursing Times*, 1993; **89**:42, 52–5. (Occasional Paper.)
35. Stiles MK. The shining stranger: nurse–family spiritual relationship. *Cancer Nursing*, 1990; **13**:235–45.
36. Stiles MK. The shining stranger : application of the phenomenological method in the investigation of the nurse–family spiritual relationship. *Cancer Nursing*, 1994; **17**(1):18–26.
37. Knight M, Field D. A silent conspiracy: coping with dying cancer patients on an acute surgical ward. *Journal of Advanced Nursing*, 1981; **6**:221–9.
38. Weisman A. *Coping with Cancer*. New York: McGraw-Hill, 1979.
39. Reimer JC, Davies B. Palliative care: the nurse's role in helping families through the transition of 'fading away'. *Cancer Nursing*, 1991; **14**(6):321–7.
40. Carr A. In Hall J, ed. *Psychology for Nurses and Health Visitors*. London: Macmillan, 1982: 217–36.
41. Taylor S. Adjustment to threatening events: a theory of cognitive adaptation. *American Psychologist*, 1983; **November**:1161–73.
42. Fredette S, Beattie H. Living with cancer: a patient education programme. *Cancer Nursing*, 1986; **9**:308–15.
43. Sims S. Slow stroke back massage for cancer patients. *Nursing Times*, 1986; **82**:47–50. (Occasional Paper.)
44. Sims S. The significance of touch in palliative care. *Palliative Medicine*, 1988; **2**:58–61.
45. Sims S. Complementary therapies as nursing interventions. In: Wilson-Barnett J, Raiman J, eds. *Nursing Issues and Research in Terminal Care*. Chichester: Wiley, 1988: 163–82.
46. Raudonis BM. The meaning and impact of empathic relationships in hospice nursing. *Cancer Nursing*, 1993; **16**(4):304–9.
47. Hunt M. Being friendly and informal. reflected in nurses', terminally ill patients' and relatives' conversations at home. *Journal of Advanced Nursing*, 1991; **16**:929–38.
48. Herth K. Fostering hope in terminally-ill people. *Journal of Advanced Nursing*, 1990; **15**:1250–9.
49. Herth K. Hope in the family caregiver of terminally ill people. *Journal of Advanced Nursing*, 1993; **18**:538–48.
50. Saunders JM, Valente, SM. Nurses' grief. *Cancer Nursing*, 1994; **17**(4):318–25.
51. McWilliam CL, Burdock J, Namsley J. The challenging experience of palliative care support-team nursing. *Oncology Nursing Forum*, 1993; **20**(5):779–85.
52. Corless IB. Dying well : symptom control within hospice care. In: Fitzpatrick J, Stevenson J, eds. *Annual Review of Nursing Research*, 1994; **12**:125–46.
53. Thomas M.. Coping with distressing symptoms. In: Wilson-Barnett J, Raiman J, eds. *Nursing Issues and Research in Terminal Care*. Chichester: Wiley, 1988: 91–118.
54. Grobe M, Illstrup D, Ahman D. Skills needed by family members to maintain the care of an advanced cancer patient. *Cancer Nursing*, 1981; **4**:371–5.
55. Heyse-Moore LH, Ross V, Mullee MA. How much of a problem is dyspnoea in advanced cancer? *Palliative Medicine*, 1991; **5**:20–6.
56. Sandstead HM. A point of view: nutrition and care of terminally ill patients. *American Journal of Clinical Nutrition*, 1990; **52**:767–9.
57. Williams J, Copp G. Food presentation and the terminally ill. *Nursing Standard*, 1990; **51**:29–32.
58. Payne SA. Coping with palliative chemotherapy. *Journal of Advanced Nursing*, 1990; **15**:652–8.
59. Richardson A. Theories of self-care: their relevance to chemotherapy-induced nausea and vomiting. *Journal of Advanced Nursing*, 1991; **16**:671–6.
60. Orem D. *Nursing: Concepts of Practice*. 3rd edn. New York: McGraw-Hill, 1985.
61. Hanucharurnkul S. Predictors of self-care in cancer patients receiving radiotherapy. *Cancer Nursing*, 1989; **12**:21–7.
62. Rhodes V, Watson P, Hanson B. Patients' descriptions of the influence of tiredness and weakness on self-care abilities. *Cancer Nursing*, 1988; **11**:186–94.
63. Dodd M. Assessing patient self-care of side effects of cancer chemotherapy. *Cancer Nursing*, 1982; **5**:447–51.

64. Dodd M. Patterns of self-care in patients with breast cancer. *Western Journal of Nursing Research*, 1988; **10**:7–24.
65. Hart LK, Freel M, Milde KK. Fatigue. *Nursing Clinics of North America*, 1990; **25**:967–76.
66. Bruera E, MacDonald RN. Asthenia in patients with advanced cancer. *Journal of Pain and Symptom Management*, 1988; **3**:9–14.
67. Janson-Bjerklie S, Carrieri V, Hudes M. The sensations of pulmonary dyspnoea. *Nursing Research*, 1986; **35**:154–9.
68. Brown M, Carrieri V, Janson-Bjerklie S, Dodd M. Lung cancer and dyspnoea: the patient's perception. *Oncology Nursing Forum*, 1986; **13**:19–24.
69. Roberts DK, Thorne SE, Pearson L. The experience of dyspnoea in late-stage cancer: patients' and nurses' perspectives. *Cancer Nursing*, 1993; **16**(4):310–20.
70. Carrieri V, Janson-Bjerklie S. Strategies patients use to manage the sensation of dyspnoea. *Western Journal of Nursing Research*, 1986; **8**:284–305.
71. Ivetic O and Lyne PA. Fungating and ulcerating malignant lesions: a review of the literature. *Journal of Advanced Nursing*, 1990; **15**:83–8.
72. Gray B. Management of limb oedema in advanced cancer. *Nursing Times*, 1987; **83**:39–41.
73. Kissin M, Querci della Rovere G, Easton D, Westbury G. Risk of lymphoedema following the treatment of breast cancer. *British Journal of Surgery*, 1986; **73**:580–4.
74. Markby R, Baldwin E, Kerr P. Incidence of lymphoedema in women with breast cancer. *Professional Nurse*, 1991; **6**:502–8.
75. Davies B, Oberle K. Dimensions of the supportive role of the nurse in palliative care. *Oncology Nursing Forum*, 1990; **17**:87–94.

6

The measurement of pain and other symptoms

6 The measurement of pain and other symptoms

Jane Ingham and Russell K. Portenoy

Introduction

Medical intervention aims to eliminate disease, mitigate disease effect, and maximize quality of life. As clinicians endeavour to fulfil these goals, symptoms present both diagnostic clues and therapeutic challenges. For patients, the disease experience is inextricably linked to symptoms and the distress they produce. Distress, in turn, is influenced by diverse psychosocial and cultural factors. The assessment of symptoms and symptom distress is, therefore, a vital aspect of clinical care, particularly in advanced and incurable illnesses for which the primary goals of care may relate to comfort and quality of life.

Ideally, the management of symptoms should be guided by a comprehensive assessment that incorporates an understanding of the multidimensional nature of symptoms and quality of life. Symptom measurement is a part of symptom assessment and should similarly reflect the complexity of patient perceptions. This complexity can be addressed by reviewing:

(1) the principles of symptom assessment and measurement;

(2) the clinical and research applications of these principles;

(3) the measurement instruments for several common symptoms;

(4) the challenges in the application of symptom measures in the palliative care setting.

Principles of symptom assessment and measurement

Symptoms—a general definition

The study of symptoms has been hampered to some degree by a lack of consistency in terminology. Symptom has been defined as 'a physical or mental phenomenon, circumstance or change of condition arising from and accompanying a disorder and constituting evidence for it....specifically a subjective indicator perceptible to the patient and as opposed to an objective one (compare with sign)'.[1] Thus, symptoms are inherently subjective. They are perceptions, usually conveyed by language. Symptom measurement attempts to quantify aspects of these perceptions in a manner that is valid and reliable.

This definition highlights the distinction between symptoms and pathological processes or diagnoses. Usually, a disease process causes a spectrum of symptoms, each of which may clarify the disease process and diagnosis. Symptoms are subjective physical and psychological phenomena that arise from pathological states or disorders and should never be viewed as diagnoses. The existence of confusion, for example, should not be used synonymously with either the diagnosis of delirium or dementia, or with any of the specific disease processes with which these diagnoses may be associated.

Defining specific symptoms

Although languages are made rich by the many nuances that are applied to words that describe human perceptions, the measurement of these perceptions is made more challenging by these nuances. The complexity of measurement is compounded when the words used to label symptoms, such as 'pain' or 'fatigue', have a plethora of meanings for patients and a wide range of implications in the medical setting.

In contrast to the generally accepted definition for 'pain' and the development of a taxonomy for the study of this symptom,[2] no such definition or taxonomy has evolved to clarify other symptoms. For example the measurement of 'fatigue', 'confusion', and even 'breathlessness', is complicated by the absence of specific definitions and the range of implications associated with each. Fatigue may be interpreted by some patients as sleepiness and by others as muscle weakness. Confusion may refer to impaired concentration, disorganized thinking, forgetfulness, or even hallucinations. A study that investigated the descriptors used by patients with dyspnoea found that 8 per cent answered 'no' to the statement 'I feel breathless' despite answering 'yes' for numerous descriptors that are applied to dyspnea.[3] Another study explored quality of life in a population of cancer patients and found that there was instrument to instrument variation in the prevalence of identical symptoms (Table 1) (Chang and Hwang, unpublished data).[4-6] In addition, items that appeared to assess similar experiences, such as 'anxiety' and 'nervousness,' had differing prevalence rates. These data indicate that symptom assessment and measurement is dependent on the clarity of meanings attached to symptom descriptors. The variability of these meanings justifies the need for formal validation of symptom assessment instruments.

Subjectivity in assessment and measurement

Because symptoms are inherently subjective, patient self-report must be the primary source of information.[7-13] Numerous studies

Table 1 Prevalence of selected symptoms by instrument (n = 200)[a]

Symptom	ESAS[b] (%)	FACT[c] (%)	MSAS[d] (%)
Pain	55.4	47.7	46.0
Nausea	26.6	22.4	21.5
Depression	35.7	–	–
Sadness	–	41.3	27.5
Anxiety	61.3	–	–
Nervous feeling	–	46.0	35.5

[a] Chang VT, Hwang, SS, Unpublished data
[b] Edmonton symptom assessment scale[4]
[c] Functional assessment of cancer therapy scale[5]
[d] Memorial symptom assessment scale[6]

have demonstrated that observer and patient assessments are not highly correlated, and that the accuracy of a clinician's assessment cannot be assumed.[7-11] For example a recent study of pain perception demonstrated a low correlation between patients' visual analogue scores for pain and those of health-care providers.[7] Clinician accuracy was especially poor when assessing patients with the most severe pain, suggesting that inferences about subjective states may be most uncertain at a level of patient distress that is most clinically relevant. A study that concurrently assessed patients and their spouse caregivers found that, although the caregivers agreed with patients on objective measures with observable referents (e.g. ability to dress independently), they disagreed with subjective aspects of patient functioning (e.g. depression, fear of future, and confidence in treatment).[8] Another study revealed that retrospective assessments by bereaved family members did not accurately depict patient symptoms at the end of life.[9]

The optimal approach to symptom assessment and measurement must incorporate patient ratings of subjective experiences. In some cases, objective signs can be monitored to complement subjective data but this information cannot substitute for self-report. For example, dyspnoea measurement may be complemented by measurement of oxygen saturation or blood gases. Nausea measurement may be supplemented by assessment of the frequency of emesis, and pain measurement may be clarified by functional assessment.

In some populations, such as demented or obtunded patients or preverbal children, it may not be possible to obtain or interpret patient self-reports. Although family members and staff may be useful proxies for clinical and research purposes, these data must be interpreted cautiously. This approach to data collection has been effective in some studies of symptoms and quality of life towards the end of life.[14-19] To facilitate accurate interpretation of data, investigators should always acknowledge the source of the data and describe the self-report and proxy data separately, if both are acquired.[20]

Symptoms as measurable multidimensional experiences

Symptoms are multidimensional experiences that may be evaluated in terms of their specific characteristics and impact (Table 2). The impact of symptoms may be described in relation to spheres of functioning—any variety of family, social, financial, spiritual, and existential issues or various global constructs such as overall symptom distress or quality of life.[21-24]

Symptom characteristics

Although surveys of symptoms have often assessed prevalence, or prevalence and a single descriptor (usually severity), a more detailed assessment of the characteristics of specific symptoms is often valuable. This may appear to be self evident in the clinical setting, where history taking frequently incorporates the assessment of the frequency, severity, and distress associated with each symptom. Assessment of these characteristics has not, however, been extensively applied in the research setting.

The variability of symptom characteristics has been described repeatedly.[6,21-23,25] For example, a study of 215 patients with prostate, colon, breast, or ovarian cancer described variations in the frequency, severity, and distress (the degree to which they considered the symptom to be bothersome) associated with 32 physical and psychological symptoms.[21] Some of the symptoms were reported to be frequent or severe but not highly bothersome or distressing, suggesting that the mere report of a symptom does not imply that it is burdensome or in need of treatment.

Symptom impact

The impact of symptoms can be evaluated in terms of many other phenomena. In the setting of advanced medical disease, the presence of multiple symptoms and other adverse influences on quality of life can complicate efforts to define the impact of a particular symptom.

Pain provides a useful example of this complexity. Pain may induce depression, exacerbate anxiety, interfere with the ability to interact socially, impair physical performance, prevent the patient from working, and decrease family income. These secondary effects can be specifically measured. The Brief Pain Inventory, for example, contains a validated subscale that assesses pain-related interference with function, mood, and enjoyment of life.[26] Surveys in the cancer population have shown that the relationship between pain severity and interference with function is non-linear and characterized by a disproportionate impairment in function above a pain severity rating of four on a ten-point scale.[27,28] This finding was consistent across four cultures and may ultimately be useful in research to quantify target ranges of pain severity and better assess the effectiveness of pain treatment strategies.[28]

The complexity of symptom impact is reflected in the many options available to measure it. Depending on the goals of measurement, symptom impact may be illuminated by the evaluation of other physical or psychological symptoms, patient function, global symptom distress, or other domains of quality of life.

Symptoms and global constructs

Several studies have explored the utility of the construct 'global symptom distress' as an indicator of overall symptom burden in the cancer population.[6,24,29] Brief measures have been validated to measure this construct (see below).[6,24] The development of these brief measures demonstrates that unidimensional assessment of a small group of highly prevalent physical and psychological symptoms can validly indicate global symptom distress, which correlates with both a relatively poor quality of life and impairment of performance status.[6,21] Although multidimensional assessment probably has a greater potential for clarifying the impact of

Table 2 The measurable aspects of symptoms

Specific dimensions	Frequency Severity Distress
Symptom impact on specific factors	Other physical and psychological symptoms or diagnoses Function Family, social, financial, spiritual, and existential resources and concerns
Symptom impact on global constructs	Global symptom distress Health-related quality of life

symptoms on quality of life,[6] the use of a brief measure, requiring limited evaluation time, can provide clinically relevant information with minimal effort.

The multidimensional construct of quality of life reflects the broad influence of many positive and negative factors on perceived well being.[20,30–37] Physical and psychological symptoms contribute to quality of life, but are merely elements within a complex set of factors that increase or temper distress, or enhance well being. This complexity is particularly apparent in the setting of advanced medical disease, which is characterized by numerous physical and psychological symptoms[21,22,38–47] and a diverse range of physical, emotional, social, ethical, and spiritual phenomena. Each of the latter concerns has the potential independently to influence quality of life, and to augment or lessen the distress associated with specific symptoms.

Figure 1 illustrates the impact that a pathophysiological process and various modifying factors may have on the perception of symptom-associated distress and overall quality of life. Assessment of these complex interactions may be facilitated by the use of valid multidimensional measures of quality of life.

Multidimensional measurement of symptoms may provide the most information about the interactions between symptoms and quality of life. For example, a recent study of symptoms in patients with cancer provided empirical evidence that information relating to the impact of symptoms on quality of life was maximized by concurrent measurement of symptom distress and either frequency or intensity.[6] Of the three dimensions assessed, distress was the most informative. These data suggest that distress, or if possible distress and another dimension, should be assessed if the goal of the evaluation is to clarify the interaction between symptoms and quality of life.

Symptom assessment and measurement over time

Symptoms usually change over time. Characteristics may change or the symptom itself may remit or recur. Clinically, this observation is usually addressed through repeated assessments throughout the course of disease. In the research setting, and particularly in clinical trials, the challenge of symptom measurement is to capture relevant concerns as they evolve using measures that are simple and brief enough to limit patient burden and encourage compliance.

Numerous factors influence the changes in symptom prevalence and characteristics. Even problems that remain static, such as aphonia following laryngectomy, may be perceived differently as the disease, or the availability of treatment, changes or the consequences on function or psychosocial status evolve. Although such symptoms may continue to be described by the patient as severe, the associated distress and impact on quality of life may increase or decrease. These observations suggest that longitudinal measurement of multiple symptom dimensions may be essential to characterize accurately the long-term impact of symptoms, interventions, or disease-related processes on quality of life.

Clinical and research applications

Historically, symptom measurement has been used in clinical investigations to determine the positive and negative impact of disease-oriented therapies or palliative treatments. Although symptom measurement could potentially have clinical utility as a part of the routine monitoring of cancer patients in treatment settings,[7,13,48–51] it has rarely been applied in this way.

Symptom measurement in routine clinical management

The effective implementation of therapeutic strategies is contingent on comprehensive symptom assessment. The clinical approach, which has been well described in basic medical textbooks and in specialized reviews, requires a detailed evaluation of symptom characteristics, pathogenesis, and impact (Table 3).[52–55] Although rarely used, instruments for structured history taking and for assessment of patient needs have been developed.[56,57,58]

Symptom measurement is one aspect of comprehensive evaluation but the routine clinical application of symptom measures, particularly for symptoms other than pain, has not been systematically explored. This is unfortunate given the possibility of increased awareness of symptom-related distress and improved outcomes associated with careful, ongoing monitoring.[51] Systematic pain measurement may improve caregiver understanding of pain status in hospitalized patients.[59] In a cancer centre, regular measurement has been incorporated into a continuous quality

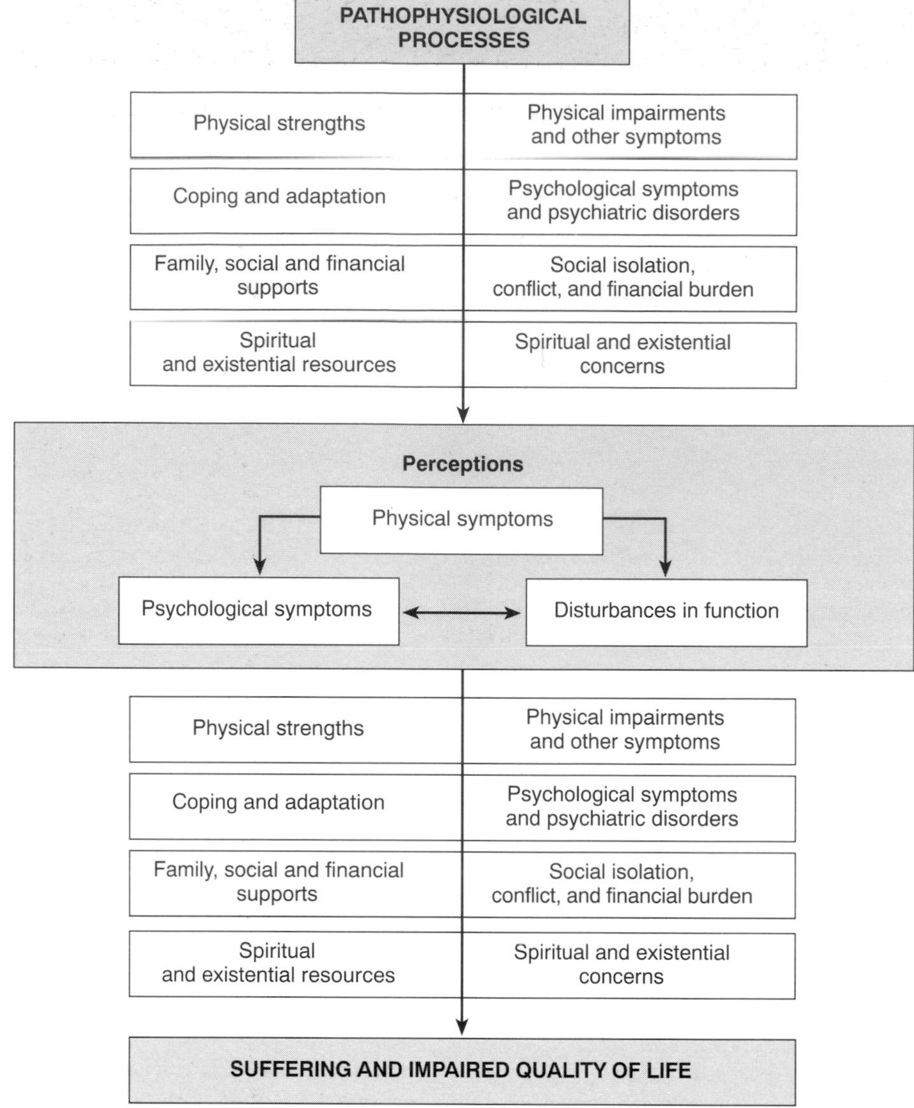

Fig. 1 Interactions between pain, symptoms, and quality of life

improvement strategy and preliminary data suggest that nurses' knowledge and attitudes about pain, and patient satisfaction with pain management, have improved subsequently (Bookbinder *et al.*, in press).[50] In the latter study, pain measurement was facilitated by the addition of a pain scale to the bedside chart (Fig. 2). Recent guidelines from the Agency for Health Care Policy and Research[13] and the American Pain Society[49] have recommended the regular use of pain rating scales to assess pain severity and relief in all patients who commence or change treatments. These recommendations also suggest that clinicians teach patients and families to use assessment tools in the home to promote continuity of pain management in all settings.

The experience with pain measurement in the clinical setting could be expanded to the measurement of other symptoms. Symptom checklists, which have been developed to explore the spectrum of common physical and psychological symptoms in particular disease states, may be useful in symptom detection. Unfortunately, these simple, face-valid instruments have notable limitations, which include the lack of adequate validation and the inability to address more than one symptom dimension.[4,60–63] Face validity, by which is meant the intuitive assumption of validity based on the appearance of the items, is less than adequate in the research setting. In the routine clinical setting, where the scale is complemented by a full clinical evaluation, extensive validation of an instrument may not be needed. Recent studies have yielded validated measures that supersede these simple checklists for research purposes (see below).[6,21,24,29,64,65] Although the application of the newer, more comprehensive measures has not been explored outside the research setting, some of the simple checklists have been used in routine clinical practice in palliative care units.[4,61] In addition to focusing staff attention on symptom assessment, such measures may be used as a means of reviewing the quality of patient care and ascertaining situation-specific barriers to symptom control.[4,44,66,67]

In the clinical setting, comprehensive symptom assessment should also query the impact of symptoms on global symptom distress and other quality of life concerns. Although instruments exist for the evaluation of global distress[6,21,24,29] and quality of

Table 3 Clinical symptom assessment

Medical history	**Psychosocial issues**	**Current medications**
Diagnosis	Family history	
Chronology	Social resources	
Therapeutic interventions including operative procedures, chemo- and radiotherapy	Impact of disease and symptoms on patient and family	
Patient's knowledge of current extent of disease		
Assessment	**Global symptom impact**	**Pathophysiology**
Review of systems For each symptom: chronology and frequency severity degree of distress impact on function other clinical characteristics impact of each symptom on other symptoms patient perception of aetiology prior treatment modalities and their efficacy other factors that alleviate or modulate distress associated with specific symptoms e.g. coping strategies and supports	Global symptom distress impact of overall symptom distress on quality of life Impact of symptoms on quality of life: physical condition psychological status social interactions Factors that modulate global symptom distress e.g. coping strategies and family supports	For each symptom: inferred pathophysiology relationship to other symptoms differing pathophysiologies same pathophysiology causal pathology induced by another symptom causal factor is treatment directed at another symptom
Physical examination	**Assess available laboratory and imaging data**	

Adapted from Ingham and Portenoy (1996).[54]

life,[5,37,68–71] the use of this type of instrument also has not been adopted in routine patient care.

Symptom measurement in clinical research

Systematic symptom assessment, when utilized in clinical trials, may clarify the toxicity or palliative potential of a treatment, or expose the need to alter clinical management at the time of its administration. In investigations of symptom epidemiology or quality of life, the use of validated instruments for symptom measurement may also be important. Numerous factors must be considered when planning methodology for symptom-related research (Table 4).

In most clinical trials, symptom measurement has been limited to standardized toxicity scales, such as those recommended by the World Health Organization and the National Cancer Institute.[60] These recommendations do not mandate the use of patient-rated scales for the grading of severity and data are frequently collected at relatively long intervals. Although recent modifications recommend documentation of side-effect duration,[72] conventional side-effect assessment remains limited and may not accurately assess the severity and distress associated with a symptom, particularly when a symptom is transitory.

Clinical trials now frequently incorporate a quality of life instrument. Validated multidimensional instruments that have been used for this purpose include the QLQ C30 of the European Organization for Research and Treatment of Cancer,[37] the Functional Living Index—Cancer,[68,69] the Functional Assessment of Cancer Therapy Scale,[5] the Cancer Rehabilitation Evaluation System,[70] and the SF-36 of the Medical Outcome Study.[71] Recent studies have also explored the application of modified versions of some of these and other instruments for quality of life assessment in populations with symptomatic HIV infection and other illnesses.[73–77]

All of these recently developed, validated, multidimensional measures of health-related quality of life assess a selected group of prevalent symptoms, including pain, fatigue, and anxiety.[5,37,68,70] Although this information may be clinically meaningful and sufficient for many purposes, these instruments cannot clarify the prevalence rates or characteristics of the diverse array of physical and psychological symptoms experienced by patients.

Although a detailed assessment of symptoms may not be required in some studies, large clinical trials or epidemiological surveys may benefit from measurement of a broad spectrum of physical or psychological symptoms. This can be accomplished by the concurrent use of a quality of life instrument and an instrument that measures symptoms. Alternatively, a more 'tailored' approach can be used in which a screening instrument is combined with

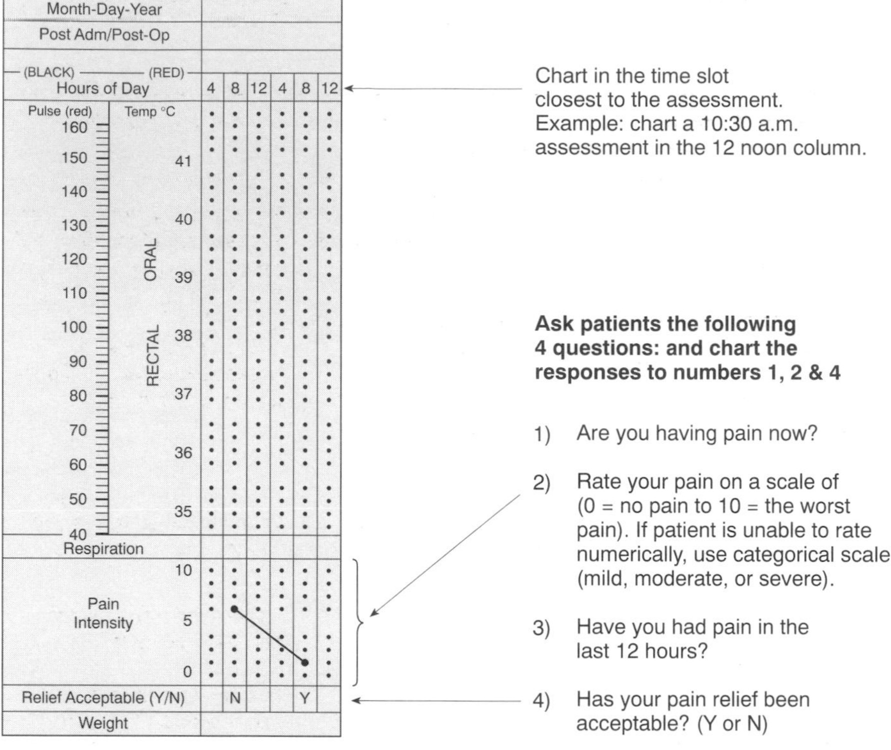

Fig. 2 Memorial Sloan-Kettering observation chart with patient-rated pain intensity and relief measures. Reproduced with permission from Bookbinder *et al.*, ref. 50.

some specific supplemental measures that capture information relevant to the disease or clinical setting. The recent development of multidimensional quality of life instruments with disease-specific or treatment-specific modules derives from this perspective.[5,31,32,37] Depending on the purpose of the assessment, the aims of the research, the anticipated outcomes and toxicities, and the resources of the investigator, tailoring can be focused on specific assessment of a single symptom or phenomenon, assessment of multiple symptoms, or assessment of related disease and treatment-specific issues (e.g. performance status or psychological function).[5,31,32,37,78]

The utility of this 'tailored' approach to symptom and quality of life assessment was demonstrated in a recent study which explored the importance of specific pain assessments during routine quality of life evaluation (Ingham *et al.*, in press). [78] In this phase II trial of paclitaxel and recombinant human granulocyte-colony stimulating factor for breast cancer, previously observed clinical observations had suggested that frequent, short-lived episodes of pain were likely to occur during this treatment regimen. To capture this information, supplemental pain measurements were included with quality of life measures. The assessment revealed a marked disparity between the pain data obtained during a routine quality of life assessment performed at intervals of 3 weeks and those acquired through the supplemental pain evaluation obtained twice weekly. In contrast to the interval assessment, which revealed a marked decline in median pain scores, the supplemental assessment demonstrated transient acute and severe pains in almost half the patients. Clearly, such a tailored approach to measurement may be important in clarifying the usefulness of a therapy in symptom palliation, altering clinical management at the time of treatment or determining the long-term effects of therapy on well being. This study also illustrates the need, in all settings, for careful consideration of the optimal timing of evaluations.

Validated instruments for symptom assessment

The selection of instruments for symptom measurement must be guided by an understanding of the goals of assessment and the practicality, applicability, and acceptability of the instrument, or instruments, in the particular patient population. Careful consideration must be given to the burden imposed on both patients and investigators by the use of each instrument. Measurement strategies that are simple and brief may limit patient burden and encourage compliance. The effort to achieve this, however, should not impede the necessary assessment to capture complex symptom-related concerns or quality of life. If the information is salient and would not be assessed otherwise, the increased burden may be warranted.

Table 4 Methodological considerations for symptom measurement in research settings

Patient-related factors	Factors related to investigator goals and resources	Instrument-related factors
Patient's ability to provide consent and comprehend instruments	**Study aims and method**	**Validity and reliability**
Age-related factors Cognitive state Cultural and language barriers Patient's descriptors for symptom Presence of other symptoms	Which symptoms and dimensions of symptoms need to be assessed? When should symptoms be assessed? What methodological controls are needed?	Validity of instrument for assessment of symptom in general and in particular population Ability of instrument to assess the dimensions and impact of symptom
Patient's willingness to participate in data collection	**Data management and statistical analysis**	**Clinical utility and appropriateness**
Patient reluctance to participate in investigation or to report specific symptom	Available resources for data collection and analysis	Capacity of instrument to assess hypothesis Instrument complexity and respondent burden

Instruments for the measurement of multiple symptoms

Historically, the spectrum of common physical and psychological symptoms has, most frequently, been explored using simple, face-valid measures, often in the form of symptom checklists.[4,44,60,61] One of these measures, the Edmonton Symptom Assessment System,[4] evaluates eight symptoms on visual analogue scores and has been extensively used in palliative care research. Although the validity and reliability of this instrument have not been clarified to date, its convenience, applicability in patients with far-advanced disease, and ease of use may prove to be advantageous.

As alluded to above, recent studies have resulted in the development of new, validated measures that may supersede these simple checklists, particularly in the assessment of multiple symptoms.

Memorial Symptom Assessment Scale[6,21]

The Memorial Symptom Assessment Scale (**MSAS**) is a validated, patient-rated measure that provides multidimensional information about a diverse group of common symptoms (Fig. 3). This instrument characterizes 32 physical and psychological symptoms in terms of intensity, frequency, and distress. The MSAS provides a Global Distress Index (MSAS-GDI), a ten item subscale that reflects global symptom distress, and separate subscales that measure physical (MSAS-PHYS) and psychological (MSAS-PSYCH) symptom distress, respectively. The MSAS may be a useful measure in a variety of research settings. Further studies are needed to establish its reliability and validity with repeated administration, assess its utility as an outcome measure in cancer clinical trials, and confirm its value in patients with various types of cancer and disease states.

Rotterdam Symptom Checklist[64,65]

The Rotterdam Symptom Checklist is a validated, patient-rated measure that evaluates a spectrum of common symptoms in terms of patient-rated distress. Thirty physical and psychological symptoms are included and an additional eight items specifically attempt to define the impact of symptoms on physical activity and function. The Rotterdam Symptom Checklist provides quantitative information about global symptom distress and subscales that distinguish physical and psychological symptom distress. The issue of multidimensional assessment is not addressed by this instrument and no information is provided about potentially relevant dimensions, such as intensity or frequency. Some symptoms that may be common in advanced disease, such as change in taste and appearance, are not evaluated. Although there are questions about pain in the head, back, abdomen, and mouth there is no general pain item.

Symptom Distress Scale[24,29]

The Symptom Distress Scale is a 13-item, patient-rated scale that evaluates 11 symptoms, nine physical and two psychological, in terms of either frequency, intensity, or distress. Responses are answered on a five-point Likert scale ranging from one (no distress) to five (extreme distress). Although the Symptom Distress Scale provides only limited information about specific symptoms, it is a

MEMORIAL SYMPTOM ASSESSMENT SCALE

NAME: DATE:

SECTION 1:

INSTRUCTIONS: We have listed 24 symptoms below. Read each one carefully. If you have had the symptom during this past week, let us know how OFTEN you had it, how SEVERE it was usually and how much it DISTRESSED OR BOTHERED you by circling the appropriate number. If you DID NOT HAVE the symptom, make an "X" in the box marked "DID NOT HAVE".

DURING THE PAST WEEK, Did you have any of the following symptoms?	DID NOT HAVE	IF YES, How OFTEN did you have it?				IF YES, How SEVERE was it usually?				IF YES, How much did it DISTRESS or BOTHER you?				
		Rarely	Occasionally	Frequently	Almost Constantly	Slight	Moderate	Severe	Very Severe	Not At All	A Little Bit	Somewhat	Quite A Bit	Very Much
Difficulty concentrating		1	2	3	4	1	2	3	4	0	1	2	3	4
Pain		1	2	3	4	1	2	3	4	0	1	2	3	4
Lack of energy		1	2	3	4	1	2	3	4	0	1	2	3	4
Cough		1	2	3	4	1	2	3	4	0	1	2	3	4
Feeling nervous		1	2	3	4	1	2	3	4	0	1	2	3	4
Dry mouth		1	2	3	4	1	2	3	4	0	1	2	3	4
Nausea		1	2	3	4	1	2	3	4	0	1	2	3	4
Feeling drowsy		1	2	3	4	1	2	3	4	0	1	2	3	4
Numbness/tingling in hands/feet		1	2	3	4	1	2	3	4	0	1	2	3	4
Difficulty sleeping		1	2	3	4	1	2	3	4	0	1	2	3	4
Feeling bloated		1	2	3	4	1	2	3	4	0	1	2	3	4
Problems with urination		1	2	3	4	1	2	3	4	0	1	2	3	4

Continued on other side..........

DURING THE PAST WEEK, Did you have any of the following symptoms?	DID NOT HAVE	IF YES, How OFTEN did you have it?				IF YES, How SEVERE was it usually?				IF YES, How much did it DISTRESS or BOTHER you?				
		Rarely	Occasionally	Frequently	Almost Constantly	Slight	Moderate	Severe	Very Severe	Not At All	A Little Bit	Somewhat	Quite A Bit	Very Much
Vomiting		1	2	3	4	1	2	3	4	0	1	2	3	4
Shortness of breath		1	2	3	4	1	2	3	4	0	1	2	3	4
Diarrhea		1	2	3	4	1	2	3	4	0	1	2	3	4
Feeling sad		1	2	3	4	1	2	3	4	0	1	2	3	4
Sweats		1	2	3	4	1	2	3	4	0	1	2	3	4
Worrying		1	2	3	4	1	2	3	4	0	1	2	3	4
Problems with sexual interest or activity		1	2	3	4	1	2	3	4	0	1	2	3	4
Itching		1	2	3	4	1	2	3	4	0	1	2	3	4
Lack of appetite		1	2	3	4	1	2	3	4	0	1	2	3	4
Dizziness		1	2	3	4	1	2	3	4	0	1	2	3	4
Difficulty swallowing		1	2	3	4	1	2	3	4	0	1	2	3	4
Feeling irritable		1	2	3	4	1	2	3	4	0	1	2	3	4

Continued on next page ....

SECTION 2:

INSTRUCTIONS: We have listed 8 symptoms below. Read each one carefully. If you have had the symptom during this past week, let us know how SEVERE it was usually and how much it DISTRESSED OR BOTHERED you by circling the appropriate number. If you DID NOT HAVE the symptom, make an "X" in the box marked "DID NOT HAVE".

DURING THE PAST WEEK, Did you have any of the following symptoms?	DID NOT HAVE	IF YES, How SEVERE was it usually?				IF YES, How much did it DISTRESS or BOTHER you?				
		Slight	Moderate	Severe	Very Severe	Not At All	A Little Bit	Somewhat	Quite A Bit	Very Much
Mouth sores		1	2	3	4	0	1	2	3	4
Change in the way food tastes		1	2	3	4	0	1	2	3	4
Weight loss		1	2	3	4	0	1	2	3	4
Hair loss		1	2	3	4	0	1	2	3	4
Constipation		1	2	3	4	0	1	2	3	4
Swelling of arms or legs		1	2	3	4	0	1	2	3	4
"I don't look like myself"		1	2	3	4	0	1	2	3	4
Changes in skin		1	2	3	4	0	1	2	3	4

** IF YOU HAD ANY OTHER SYMPTOMS DURING THE PAST WEEK, PLEASE LIST BELOW AND INDICATE HOW MUCH THE SYMPTOM HAS DISTRESSED OR BOTHERED YOU.

OTHER:	0	1	2	3	4
OTHER:	0	1	2	3	4
OTHER:	0	1	2	3	4

Fig. 3 Revised version of the Memorial Symptom Assessment Scale.[6] Copyright 1994, reprinted with permission from Elsevier Science Ltd, The Boulevard, Langford Lane, Kidlington OX5 1GB, UK.

valid and useful measure of global symptom distress. The potential utility of this score has been further demonstrated in a study of lung cancer patients in which the symptom distress score was a significant predictor of survival.[79]

Instruments for the measurement of specific symptoms

Although numerous instruments have been validated for the assessment of some symptoms, such as pain and depression, there is a paucity of similar instruments for other symptoms that are prevalent in advanced disease, such as anorexia, dry mouth, or change in appearance. Moreover, many symptom-specific instruments have been validated in specific populations and may not be valid in others. For example dyspnoea measurement has been developed in the disciplines of pulmonary medicine and cardiology,[80–84] and, there is little information specifically derived in the oncology setting.[85–87] To illustrate the range of options available and the practical issues that may be important in selecting an instrument, the following discussion focuses on measures for four common symptoms—pain, impaired cognition, dyspnoea, and fatigue.

Instruments for the assessment of pain

Unidimensional scales of intensity or relief (including visual analogue, numerical, and categorical scales) have been the traditional focus of pain measurement. Multidimensional instruments which provide a more comprehensive evaluation of pain and its impact, comprise the McGill Pain Questionnaire[88–90] and an instrument that has been extensively validated in the cancer population, the Brief Pain Inventory.[26]

The Memorial Pain Assessment Card[91] is a brief, validated measure that uses visual analogue scores to characterize pain intensity, pain relief and mood, and an eight-point verbal rating scale to characterize pain intensity further (Fig. 4). The mood scale correlates with measures of overall psychological distress, depression, and anxiety and is considered to be a valid measure of global psychological distress. Although this instrument provides limited information, its brevity, simplicity, and reliability are attractive and it has been used in many analgesic trials.

The Brief Pain Inventory[26] is a self administered, easily understood measure that provides information about pain history, intensity, location and quality (Fig. 5). Numeric scales (range one to ten) indicate the intensity of pain in general, at its worst, at its least, and right now. A percentage scale quantifies relief from current therapies. A body figure allows localization of the pain. Seven questions evaluate the degree to which pain interferes with function, mood, and enjoyment of life. The Brief Pain Inventory has now been translated into several languages.

The McGill Pain Questionnaire[88–90] is a self-administered questionnaire that evaluates the sensory, affective, and evaluative dimensions of pain and provides global scores and subscale scores for each of these dimensions. The scores are derived from the adjectival pain descriptors selected by the patient. A five-point verbal categorical scale characterizes the intensity of pain and a pain drawing localizes the pain. Additional information is collected about the impact of medications and other therapies. This instrument does not assess the impact of pain on function. To date, the predominant application of the McGill Pain Questionnaire has

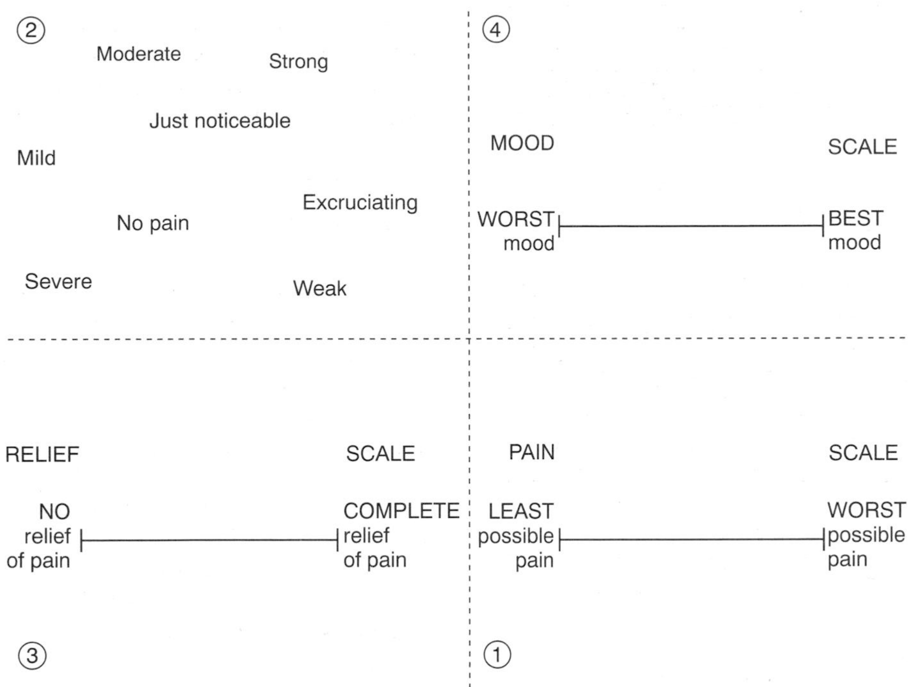

Fig. 4 The Memorial pain assessment card. (Reproduced with permission from reference 91)

been in the assessment of chronic, non-malignant pain and the utility of the subscale scores has not been demonstrated for cancer pain.[92]

Instruments for the assessment of impaired cognition

Instruments have been developed to identify cognitive impairment and determine the likelihood that the impairment can be ascribed to a specific diagnosis, such as delirium. Delirium is common in hospitalized cancer patients[46,47,67] and in the medically ill elderly.[93,94] It is also prevalent in those with chronic illness who are nearing the end of life.[67,95-97] The instruments for delirium assessment have recently been extensively reviewed.[98]

Screening tests for cognitive impairment include the Mini Mental Status Exam[99] and the Blessed Orientation-Memory-Concentration Test.[100] These tools are sensitive indicators of impairment,[67,101,102] but are not specific for the diagnosis of delirium. Further assessment with either a clinical interview or the administration of another validated instrument is necessary to clarify the diagnosis. Electroencephelography or brain imaging studies may supplement the clinical assessment and assist in clarifying the diagnosis.

The clinical psychiatric interview using the criteria outlined by the American Psychiatric Association in the Diagnostic and Statistical Manual (DSM) IV[103] remains the 'gold standard' for the diagnosis of delirium. Several instruments are available that can facilitate the diagnosis, including the Confusion Assessment Method,[104] the Delirium Symptom Interview,[105] and the Delirium Rating Scale.[106] These instruments, which were developed based on the earlier criteria outlined in the DSM III[107] or DSM III-R,[108] use an interview format to clarify the characteristics of the cognitive impairment. Either a score above a cut-off point or an algorithm documents the presence or absence of delirium. Although none of these measures have been adequately validated as a measure of delirium severity, they may be useful in providing a method for the monitoring of patients predisposed to delirium or receiving treatment for this condition.

Instruments for the assessment of fatigue

Fatigue is among the most prevalent symptoms reported by patients with advanced illness, including cancer. Despite this there is no generally accepted definition of fatigue. The experience is frequently characterized by a spectrum of disturbance that includes muscular weakness, lethargy, sleepiness, mood disturbance (particularly depression), cognitive disturbances (such as difficulty concentrating), and others. The measurement of fatigue attempts to capture this spectrum of disturbances.[109-112]

Although unidimensional scales have been used, the most meaningful assessment of fatigue evaluates the temporal dimensions of the symptom, its physical and psychological components, and its associated distress. Unidimensional fatigue scales include single items incorporated into symptom checklists and the fatigue subscale of the Profile of Mood States.[24,64,113] Scales developed in the industrial setting have also been applied to clinical assessment.[111,114-118] Another approach has involved the assessment of specific symptoms associated with fatigue. For example, in a series of studies evaluating psychostimulants in patients receiving opioids, investigators used a visual analogue score to assess 'drowsiness' and other scales to evaluate cognitive status.[119-122]

Several multidimensional scales have been validated in the medically ill. The 41-item Piper Fatigue Self Report Scale addresses the severity, distress, and impact of fatigue, and can be administered as either a series of visual analogue scores or as numerical scales.[123] This scale was developed to assess the multiple dimensions of fatigue in patients receiving radiation therapy and has demonstrated excellent reliability and moderate construct validity in this population.

The Visual Analogue Scale—Fatigue is an 18 item, multidimensional patient-rated instrument. It has been validated in a

Brief Pain Inventory

Date: __/__/__

Name: ____________ ____________ ____________
Last First Middle Initial

Phone: ( ) ____________ Sex: ☐ Female ☐ Male

Date of Birth: __/__/__

1) Marital Status (at present)
1. ☐ Single 3. ☐ Widowed
2. ☐ Married 4. ☐ Separated/Divorced

2) Education (Circle only the highest grade or degree completed)
Grade 0 1 2 3 4 5 6 7 8 9
10 11 12 13 14 15 16 M.A./M.S.
Professional degree (please specify) ____________

3) Current occupation ____________
(specify titles; if you are not working, tell us your previous occupation)

4) Spouse's Occupation ____________

5) Which of the following best describes your current job status?
☐ 1. Employed outside the home, full-time
☐ 2. Employed outside the home, part-time
☐ 3. Homemaker
☐ 4. Retired
☐ 5. Unemployed
☐ 6. Other

6) How long has it been since you first learned your diagnosis? ____ months

7) Have you ever had pain due to your present disease?
1. ☐ Yes 2. ☐ No 3. ☐ Uncertain

8) When you first received your diagnosis, was pain one of your symptoms?
1. ☐ Yes 2. ☐ No 3. ☐ Uncertain

9) Have you had surgery in the past month? 1. ☐ Yes 2. ☐ No

10) Throughout our lives, most of us have had pain from time to time (such as minor headaches, sprains, and toothaches). Have you had pain **other** than these everyday kinds of pain during the **last week?** 1. ☐ Yes 2. ☐ No

IF YOU ANSWERED YES TO THE LAST QUESTION, PLEASE GO ON TO QUESTION 11 AND FINISH THIS QUESTIONNAIRE. IF NO, YOU ARE FINISHED WITH THE QUESTIONNAIRE. THANK YOU.

11) On the diagram, shade in the areas where you feel pain. Put an X on the area that hurts the most.

Front Back
Right Left Left Right

12) Please rate your pain by circling the one number that best describes your pain at its **worst** in the last week.
0 1 2 3 4 5 6 7 8 9 10
No Pain — Pain as bad as you can imagine

13) Please rate your pain by circling the one number that best describes your pain at its **least** in the last week.
0 1 2 3 4 5 6 7 8 9 10
No Pain — Pain as bad as you can imagine

14) Please rate your pain by circling the one number that best describes your pain on the **average.**
0 1 2 3 4 5 6 7 8 9 10
No Pain — Pain as bad as you can imagine

15) Please rate your pain by circling the one number that tells how much pain you have **right now.**
0 1 2 3 4 5 6 7 8 9 10
No Pain — Pain as bad as you can imagine

16) What kinds of things make your pain feel better (for example, head, medicine, rest)?
____
____

17) What kinds of things make your pain worse (for example, walking, standing, lifting)?
____
____

18) What treatments or medications are you receiving for your pain?
____
____

19) In the last week, how much relief have pain treatments or medications provided? Please circle the one percentage that most shows how much relief you have received.
0% 10% 20% 30% 40% 50% 60% 70% 80% 90% 100%
No Relief — Complete Relief

20) If you take pain medication, how many hours does it take before the pain returns?
☐ 1. Pain medication doesn't help at all
☐ 2. One hour
☐ 3. Two hours
☐ 4. Three hours
☐ 5. Four hours
☐ 6. Five to twelve hours
☐ 7. More than twelve hours
☐ 8. I do not take pain medication

21) Circle the appropriate answer for each item.
I believe my pain is due to:
☐ Yes ☐ No 1. The effects of treatment (for example, medication, surgery, radiation, prosthetic device).
☐ Yes ☐ No 2. My primary disease (meaning the disease currently being treated and evaluated).
☐ Yes ☐ No 3. A medical condition unrelated to primary disease (for example, arthritis).

22) For each of the following words, check yes or no if that adjective applies to your pain.

Aching	☐ Yes	☐ No	Exhausting	☐ Yes	☐ No
Throbbing	☐ Yes	☐ No	Tiring	☐ Yes	☐ No
Shooting	☐ Yes	☐ No	Penetrating	☐ Yes	☐ No
Stabbing	☐ Yes	☐ No	Nagging	☐ Yes	☐ No
Gnawing	☐ Yes	☐ No	Numb	☐ Yes	☐ No
Sharp	☐ Yes	☐ No	Miserable	☐ Yes	☐ No
Tender	☐ Yes	☐ No	Unbearable	☐ Yes	☐ No
Burning	☐ Yes	☐ No			

23) Circle the one number that describes how, during the past week, **pain** has interfered with your:

A. General Activity
0 1 2 3 4 5 6 7 8 9 10
Does not Interfere — Completely interferes

B. Mood
0 1 2 3 4 5 6 7 8 9 10
Does not Interfere — Completely interferes

C. Walking ability
0 1 2 3 4 5 6 7 8 9 10
Does not Interfere — Completely interferes

D. Normal work (includes both work outside the home and housework)
0 1 2 3 4 5 6 7 8 9 10
Does not Interfere — Completely interferes

E. Relations with other people
0 1 2 3 4 5 6 7 8 9 10
Does not Interfere — Completely interferes

F. Sleep
0 1 2 3 4 5 6 7 8 9 10
Does not Interfere — Completely interferes

G. Enjoyment of life
0 1 2 3 4 5 6 7 8 9 10
Does not Interfere — Completely interferes

Pain Research Group, Department of Neurology, University of Wisconsin-Madison

Fig. 5 Brief pain inventory. Reproduced with permission from the Pain Research Group, University of Wisconsin, Madison Medical School.

population with sleep disorders and has demonstrated high internal consistency and significant correlations with the Profile of Mood States fatigue subscale and a sleepiness scale.[124] The Visual Analogue Scale—Fatigue has not been widely used in populations with advanced medical disease, but may prove useful because of its comparative brevity.

Fatigue itself may impose limitations on assessment. The length of the multidimensional fatigue assessment instruments may be problematic in populations with advanced disease and/or severe fatigue. In the initial validation study of the Piper Fatigue Self Report Scale, for example, 24 per cent of patients experienced difficulties in responding to the scales and almost half the patients approached for the study refused to participate.[123] This problem compounds the challenges posed by the lack of a widely accepted definition, the complexity of the dimensions that constitute the symptom, and the paucity of instruments that are both validated and accepted. Ongoing research will hopefully clarify some of these problems and guide the development of assessment instruments.

Instruments for the assessment of dyspnoea

The instruments for the measurement of dyspnoea have, for the most part, been developed in the setting of chronic pulmonary and cardiac conditions. Like other symptoms, numerous aspects and dimensions of dyspnoea can be assessed. These include: antecedents, or physiological and psychogenic factors, that precede the onset of the symptom; environmental or personal characteristics that mediate dyspnoea; subjective responses and reactions to dyspnoea; and consequences or outcomes of dyspnoea.[83] Instruments may assess one or more of these dimensions.

To clarify the appropriateness of the language employed in dyspnoea assessment, the descriptors used by patients have been explored using adjectival checklists.[3,125,126] These studies indicate that patients use a variety of descriptors for dyspnoea and that particular descriptors, or clusters of descriptors, vary in relation to specific lung pathologies. For example a study of patients with a spectrum of chronic lung diseases (including emphysema–bronchitis, asthma, restrictive lung disease, and vascular lung disease) demonstrated that although all groups of patients endorsed the descriptor 'I feel short of breath', those with asthma were more likely than others to describe 'chest tightness.'[125] Such disease-specific characteristics emphasize the importance of selecting instruments for dyspnoea measurement that have been validated in the appropriate disease population.

Visual analogue scales are the most commonly utilized measures for the assessment of dyspnoea in patients with advanced disease. Visual analogue scales generally have good within subject reproducibility, particularly when dyspnoea is assessed repeatedly in a single session using an exercise task to induce dyspnoea.[80,127] The visual analogue score has been found to be less reliable when the same exercise task is repeated at a longer intervals, such as 2 weeks.[128] In addition, considerable between subject variation has been demonstrated[129] and, in some individuals, visual analogue scores are insensitive and poorly reproducible.

Verbal categorical scales and numerical scales have also been used to assess dyspnoea.[81,82,126,130] The modified Borg scale is an example of a commonly used categorical scale.[131,132] This scale, which has been validated in healthy individuals and in patients with chronic non-malignant pulmonary disease, rates the patient's perception of their dyspnoea in relation to a perceived level of exertion. For example the dyspnoea is rated as equating with exertion that is 'very, very weak', 'very, very strong' and varying degrees in between.

The measurement of dyspnoea, unlike that of many other symptoms, frequently involves the administration of an instrument with a dyspnoea-producing task, usually standardized or graded exercise. Indeed, although the reliability and validity of the commonly used dyspnoea measures, such as visual analogue scores and the Borg scale,[131,132] have been documented in response to an exercise task, these measures have not been evaluated without such a stress for historical, one-time, or repeated administration. The reliability of assessment can be improved by the use standardized exercise task. One approach involves the assessment of each subject's ability to reproduce a dyspnoea score on the visual analogue scale in response to a standard degree of exertion.[127] Other investigators have attempted to use a standardized exercise to 'calibrate' the visual analogue score with respect to the each subjects quantity and quality of breathlessness.[81,82] In such a 'calibrated' scale, the upper end of the visual analogue score is 'anchored' to the dyspnoea associated with a specific strenuous exercise.[81] The dyspnoea at the moment that the exercise is terminated is defined as the maximum point on the visual analogue score.

In addition to enhancing the reliability of the assessment, an approach that incorporates an exercise task allows the assessment of therapeutic interventions that may have little impact on baseline dyspnoea but substantial effect on exercise-induced dyspnoea. For example, a standardized exercise task may be administered both before and after an intervention, and the level of dyspnoea induced by the task measured.

When assessing dyspnoea in a population with advanced disease, it is important to define a standardized exercise that is not limited by other symptoms or disabilities. For example the use of a short walk or treadmill exercise may be limited by pain or fatigue, whereas the use of repetitive arm or leg lifting exercises may be a feasible option.

Other instruments assess the consequences of dyspnoea in relation to limitations on function. Although useful in the patient suffering from breathlessness as a single symptom, these instruments (which include the Modified Medical Research Council Dyspnoea Scale,[133] the American Thoracic Society Five Level Scale of Breathlessness,[134] the Baseline Dyspnoea Index,[135] and the Transition Dyspnoea Index[135]) have obvious limitations when function is limited by other symptoms such as pain or fatigue.

Challenges in palliative medicine

There are significant challenges in bringing systematic symptom measurement to the palliative care population. These include both attitudinal and conceptual barriers to the use of such measures, practical barriers, and barriers that are specific to special populations.

Conceptual and attitudinal barriers to the use of symptom measures

Conceptual and attitudinal barriers to the use of health-status measures in patient care and clinical trials[136] are likely to be relevant in the palliative care setting. These include scepticism about the validity and importance of self-rated health measures, preferences for physiological outcomes or death rates, unfamiliarity of health-care providers with the scoring of measures, and a paucity of direct comparisons among instruments.

Education of health professionals about measurement techniques should be viewed as a priority in efforts aimed at eliminating barriers and improving symptom management. In a recent survey of physicians providing care for patients with cancer, 76 per cent stated that the single most important barrier to adequate pain management was poor pain assessment.[137] In another survey, fewer than one-half of patients with pain had a staff member ask about pain or note pain in their record during the 72 h period after their admission to the hospital.[138] The routine use of symptom assessment measures in clinical practice may be useful in approaching these difficulties.[51]

To improve clinicians' understanding of research involving subjective end-points, studies are needed to compare newer measures with traditional outcomes.[136] This issue has been explored, to some degree, in the recent studies that have assessed the impact of particular symptom scores, or ranges of scores, on function.[28,139]

Practical barriers that occur in patients with advanced disease

The absence of valid measures for the assessment of many common symptoms represents a major methodological barrier to improving symptom measurement. As a result, many studies have used checklists to measure symptom prevalence without reference to symptom distress and impact. New, validated measures that assess symptom characteristics are clearly preferable. Instruments are needed for the specific assessment of the less common symptoms.

Some symptoms are difficult to measure or, in themselves, compromise the assessment of subjective concerns. The high prevalence of delirium and fatigue in patients with advanced disease is a potential barrier to the completion of subjective measures. Studies have suggested that the prevalence of delirium in hospitalized medical and surgical patients is approximately 10 per cent.[94,140] A higher prevalence, ranging to 50 per cent in some studies, exists in some inpatient populations, including the elderly and patients in the postoperative period.[93,94] The prevalence of delirium in hospitalized cancer patients ranges from 8 to 40 per cent.[46,47,67] A consistently higher prevalence, up to 85 per cent, has been found in studies of cancer populations with very advanced disease, particularly those in the last week of life.[67,97]

Cognitive impairment may preclude accurate measurement of subjective data. The difficulty that some cognitively intact individuals experience in completing visual analogue scores[81,141–143] is likely to be increased among the cognitively impaired. It has been suggested that studies should incorporate a methodology for assessing an individual's ability to use measurement instruments consistently, such as the visual analogue score, and consideration should be given to eliminating patients who are unable reliably to use the instrument from studies designed to assess the specific interventions.[81]

Fatigue is also an extremely prevalent concern in patients with advanced disease. Fatigue is the most common symptom in populations with advanced cancer, occurring with a prevalence of 40 to 70 per cent[21,22,38–40,43,144] and, although the impact of fatigue on the ability of patients to complete assessment measures has not been empirically evaluated, it is an important theoretical concern.

A further methodological difficulty relates to the measurement of symptoms in patients experiencing multiple symptoms concurrently. In a study of patients with prostate, colon, breast, or ovarian cancer the median number of symptoms per patient was 11.5 and the range was 0 to 25.[21]. The development of instruments for the measurement of global symptom distress has provided a method by which the impact of multiple symptoms can be explored.[6,21,24,29]

The priorities of the patient and family may be another barrier to systematic symptom assessment in the palliative care setting. Patients may be unwilling to participate in clinical studies or provide information that requires the use of complex, time-consuming instruments. One survey demonstrated that patients in a palliative care unit gradually reduced their compliance with twice daily visual analogue score measures for pain, activity, nausea, drowsiness, appetite, sensation of well being, depression, and anxiety as their disease progressed.[44] In contrast to the day of admission, when 69 per cent of the visual analogue score were completed by the patient and 28 per cent by the nurse, only 8 per cent of the measures were completed by the patient on the day of death.

The willingness or ability of patients with advanced medical disease to participate in symptom studies has not been studied. Clearly, this willingness will vary with the characteristics of the patient, family, disease, and study methodology. Several surveys of symptoms and quality of life in patients with advanced medical illness suggest that relatively good compliance is possible. Of 1427 consecutive outpatients with recurrent or metastatic cancer who were asked to participate in a study using the Brief Pain Inventory, only 119 patients (8.3 per cent) did not participate; of these, 68 (4.7 per cent) refused, 34 (2.4 per cent) were too ill to participate, and 17 (1.2 per cent) were unable to comprehend or complete the forms.[145] In another study of 308 patients with advanced, symptomatic HIV disease, 67 per cent participated, 15 per cent refused and the remaining 18 per cent could not be enrolled for 'logistic' reasons.[146] The group who participated provided self-report data despite severe symptoms (mean symptom number 11) and a low performance status (41 per cent limited in self-care activities).

Concern about the response of medically ill patients to sensitive questions at a time when they are experiencing numerous physical, psychological, and emotional stressors has also not been addressed in the literature. Evidence exists, however, that sensitive areas of concern can be assessed. For example in a survey of patients with cancer who were expected to die within a year, patients were asked to participate in interviews at biweekly or monthly intervals to discuss issues regarding their preferred place of death.[147] Of 98 patients approached, 84 (86 per cent) agreed to be interviewed, of whom 70 (83 per cent) died during the study.

In summary, the concerns that cognitive impairment may interfere with subjective reporting, and that fatigue and/or symptom burden may limit patient ability or willingness to provide subjective data, have important implications for clinical practice and research methodology in the palliative care population. Clinically, these issues impact on the approach to assessing patient concerns. In the research setting, these issues emphasize the importance of selection criteria, documentation of cognitive status, and recording of reasons for refusal or inability to participate in data collection.

Special populations

Symptom measurement is particularly challenging in several subpopulations. These include the paediatric population, the imminently dying, and those patients whose language or culture differs from that of the health-care professionals involved in their care.

In the paediatric literature, symptom assessment has predominantly focused on postoperative and procedural pain.[148–151] In these settings, pain has been evaluated with self-report visual analogue scores and 'faces' scales,[152–157] and observational scales such as the Observational Scale of Behavioural Distress[158] and the Procedure Behaviour Checklist.[154] These measures have been used to quantify the occurrence, intensity, and range of a child's pain. Children over the ages of 6 to 7 years are thought to be able to indicate pain intensity using self-report measures. Although a behavioural observation scale for assessment of tumour-related pain in children aged 2 to 6 years has been developed,[159] the 17 items in the scale have not, as yet, been validated, lack operational definitions, and have demonstrated poor inter rater reliability. Other scales have been used for the assessment of chemotherapy-related nausea and vomiting,[160,161] including visual analogue scores and 'face' scales for frequency, severity, and distress, but these have not been extensively validated. To date, there has been little attention directed towards assessment issues relating to chronic pain or other symptoms that occur in the setting of chronic illness. Reviews of the current state of knowledge in this area are available in the paediatric literature.[162]

The difficulties encountered in the assessment of the imminently dying population have led both clinicians and investigators to rely on observer-rated data despite concerns about the validity of this approach. However, the prevalence of cognitive impairment varies by disease and general rules cannot be proffered. For example only 15 per cent of 16 000 decedents in the National Mortality Followback Survey had trouble understanding where he or she was during the 'last few hours or days'.[163] Although some surveys have described cancer patients with advanced disease as commonly being unable to communicate for significant periods of time towards the end of life,[44,95,100,164,165] a recent survey of 154 inpatient and homecare cancer deaths found that approximately 33 per cent of patients were able to interact 24 h prior to death; 25 per cent could interact 12 h before, and 8 per cent were communicative in the hour before death (Ingham *et al.*, unpublished data). This issue poses significant methodological challenges for the assessment of distress in the imminently dying.

Significant problems relating to symptom assessment and measurement also may be encountered in patients whose culture and language differ from the professionals involved in their care.[166] Without meticulous attention to skilled translation, the nuances of the language used to describe symptoms may obscure meaning across cultures. Only a few instruments have been shown to be reliable and valid across cultures and languages,[167,168] and translation and validation of other symptom measures is needed.

In the clinical setting, health-care professionals may need to develop simple, face-valid symptom measures to overcome language barriers. A discussion among the clinician, the patient, and an interpreter can facilitate the construction of a simple, two-language verbal rating scale to keep by the bedside. To assist the patient with communication of symptom-related issues, the symptoms on the rating scale should take into account the current concerns of the patient and anticipated concerns given the patient's clinical problems. To monitor the level of distress and impact of interventions, such scales should, at a minimum, address both symptom intensity and relief. This approach is important to ensure that symptom distress can be minimized at all times, particularly when interpreters are not freely available.

Conclusion

Systematic symptom assessment is a foundation of clinical practice and research. Instruments for the measurement of symptoms have been developed and may facilitate this process. Quantification of symptoms may be able to improve symptom management and further the goal of enhanced quality of life. Clinicians and investigators should become familiar with these instruments and develop methods for their use in routine clinical practice, the research environment, and the palliative care setting.

References

1. *The New Shorter Oxford English Dictionary.* Oxford: Clarendon Press, 1993.
2. IASP Subcommittee on Taxonomy. Pain terms: a list with definitions and notes on usage. *Pain,* 1980; **8**: 249–52.
3. Elliott MW, Adams L, Cockcroft A, MacRae KD, Murphy K, Guz A. The language of breathlessness. Use of verbal descriptors by patients with cardiopulmonary disease. *American Review of Respiratory Disease,* 1991; **144**: 826–32.
4. Bruera E, Kuehn N, Miller M, Selmser P, Macmillan K. Symptom Assessment System (ESAS): a simple method for the assessment of palliative care patients. *Journal of Palliative Care,* 1991; **7**: 6–9.
5. Cella DF, Tulsky DS, Gray G, Sarafian B, Linn E, Bonomi A, *et al.* The functional assessment of cancer therapy scale: development and validation of the general measure. *Journal of Clinical Oncology,* 1993; **11**: 570–9.
6. Portenoy RK, Thaler HT, Kornblith AB, Lepore JM, Friedlander KH, Kiyasu E, *et al.* The memorial symptom assessment scale: an instrument for the evaluation of symptom prevalence, characteristics and distress. *European Journal of Cancer,* 1994; **30A**: 1326–36.
7. Grossman SA, Sheidler VR, Swedeen K, Mucenski J, Piantadosi S. Correlation of patient and caregiver ratings of cancer pain. *Journal of Pain and Symptom Management,* 1991; **6**: 53–7.
8. Clipp EC, George LK. Patients with cancer and their spouse caregivers. Perceptions of the illness experience. *Cancer,* 1992; **69**: 1074–9.
9. Higginson I, Priest P, McCarthy M. Are bereaved family members a valid proxy for a patient's assessment of dying? *Social Science and Medicine,* 1994; **38**: 553–7.
10. Slevin ML, Plant H, Lynch D, *et al.* Who should measure quality of life, the doctor or the patient. *British Journal of Cancer,* 1988; **57**: 109.
11. Kahn SB, Houts PS, Harding SP. Quality of life and patients with cancer: a comparative study of patient versus physician perceptions and its implications for cancer education. *Journal of Cancer Education,* 1992; **7**: 241.
12. Osoba D. Lessons learned from measuring health-related quality of life in oncology. *Journal of Clinical Oncology,* 1994; **12**: 608.
13. Jacox A, Carr DB, Payne R, Berde CB, Brietbart W, Cain JM, *et al.* *Management of Cancer Pain. Clinical Practice Guideline. No. 9.* U.S. Department of Health and Human Services, Public Health Service, Agency for Health Care Policy and Research, 1994.

14. Greer DS, Mor V, Morris JN, Sherwood S, Kidder D, Birnbaum H. An alternative in terminal care: results of the National Hospice Study. *Journal of Chronic Diseases*, 1986; **39**: 9–26.
15. Morris JN, Suissa S, Sherwood S, Wright SM, Greer D. Last days: a study of the quality of life of terminally ill cancer patients. *Journal of Chronic Diseases*, 1986; **39**: 47–62.
16. Reuben DB, Mor V. Dyspnea in terminally ill cancer patients. *Chest*, 1986; **89**: 234–6.
17. Mor V. Cancer patients' quality of life over the disease course: lessons from the real world. *Journal of Chronic Diseases*, 1987; **40**: 535–44.
18. Mor V, Masterson-Allen S. A comparison of hospice vs conventional care of the terminally ill cancer patient. *Oncology*, 1990; **4**: 85–91.
19. Higginson IJ, McCarthy M. A comparison of two measures of quality of life: their sensitivity and validity for patients with advanced cancer. *Palliative Medicine*, 1994; **8**: 282–90.
20. Aaronson NK. Quality of life research in cancer clinical trials: a need for common rules and language. *Oncology*, 1990; **4**: 59–66.
21. Portenoy RK, Thaler HT, Kornblith AB, Lepore JM, Friedlander KH, Coyle N, *et al.* Symptom prevalence, characteristics and distress in a cancer population. *Quality of Life Research*, 1994; **3**: 183–9.
22. Dunlop GM. A study of the relative frequency and importance of gastrointestinal symptoms and weakness in patients with far advanced cancer. *Palliative Medicine*, 1989; **4**: 37–43.
23. Welch JM, Barlow D, Richardson PH. Symptoms of HIV disease. *Palliative Medicine*, 1991; **5**: 46–51.
24. McCorkle R, Young K. Development of a symptom distress scale. *Cancer Nursing*, 1978; **1**: 373–8.
25. Portenoy RK, Hagen NA. Breakthrough pain: definition, prevalence and characteristics. *Pain*, 1990; **41**: 273–81.
26. Daut RL, Cleeland CS, Flanery RC. Development of the Wisconsin Brief Pain Questionnaire to assess pain in cancer and other diseases. *Pain*, 1983; **17**: 197–210.
27. Daut RL, Cleeland CS. The prevalence and severity of pain in cancer. *Cancer*, 1982; **50**: 1913–18.
28. Serlin RC, Mendoza TR, Nakamura Y, Edwards KR, Cleeland CS. When is cancer pain mild, moderate or severe? Grading pain severity by its interference with function. *Pain*, 1995; **61**: 277–84.
29. McCorkle R, Quint-Benoliel J. Symptom distress, current concerns and mood disturbance after diagnosis of a life-threatening disease. *Social Science and Medicine*, 1983; **17**: 431–8.
30. Till JE, McNeil BJ, Bush RS. Measurements of multiple components of quality of life. *Cancer Treatment Symposium*, 1984; **1**: 177.
31. Aaronson NK, Bullinger M, Ahmedzai S. A modular approach to quality of life assessment in cancer clinical trials. In: Scheurlen H, Kay R, Baum M, eds. *Recent Results in Cancer Research*, Vol 111. Berlin: Springer-Verlag, 1988: 231.
32. Moinpour CM, Feigl P, Metch B, Hayden KA, Meyskens FJr, Crowley J. Quality of life endpoints in cancer clinical trials: review and recommendations. *Journal of the National Cancer Institute*, 1989; **81**: 485–95.
33. Moinpour CM, Hayden KA, Thompson IM, Feigl P, Metch B. Quality of life assessment in Southwest Oncology Group trials. *Oncology*, 1990; **4**: 79–84.
34. Cella DF, Tulsky DS. Measuring quality of life today: methodological aspects. *Oncology*, 1990; **4**: 29–38.
35. Aaronson NK. Methodologic issues in assessing the quality of life of cancer patients. *Cancer*, 1991; **67** (Suppl 3): 844–50.
36. Nayfield SG, Ganz PA, Moinpour CM, Cella DF, Hailey BJ. Report from a National Cancer Institute (USA) workshop on quality of life assessment in cancer clinical trials. *Quality of Life Research*, 1992; **1**: 203–10.
37. Aaronson NK, Ahmedzai S, Bergman B, Bullinger M, Cull A, Duez NJ, *et al.* The European Organization for Research and Treatment of Cancer QLQ-C30: a quality-of-life instrument for use in international clinical trials in oncology. *Journal of the National Cancer Institute*, 1993; **85**: 365–76.
38. Curtis EB, Krech R, Walsh TD. Common symptoms in patients with advanced cancer. *Journal of Palliative Care*, 1991; **7**: 25–9.
39. Coyle N, Adelhardt J, Foley KM, Portenoy RK. Character of terminal illness in the advanced cancer patient: pain and other symptoms during the last four weeks of life. *Journal of Pain and Symptom Management*, 1990; **5**: 83–93.
40. Dunphy KP, Amesbury BDW. A comparison of hospice and homecare patients: patterns of referral, patient characteristics and predictors on place of death. *Palliative Medicine*, 1990; **4**:105–111.
41. Brescia FJ, Adler D, Gray G, Ryan MA, Cimino J, Mamtani R. Hospitalized advanced cancer patients: a profile. *Journal of Pain and Symptom Management*, 1990; **5**: 221–7.
42. Grosvenor M, Bulcavage L, Chlebowski RT. Symptoms potentially influencing weight loss in a cancer population. Correlations with primary site, nutritional status, and chemotherapy administration. *Cancer*, 1989; **63**: 330–4.
43. Ventafridda V, DeConno F, Ripamonti C, Gamba A, Tamburini M. Quality-of-life assessment during a palliative care programme. *Annals of Oncology*, 1990; **1**: 415–20.
44. Fainsinger R, Miller MJ, Bruera E, Hanson J, MacEachern T. Symptom control during the last week of life on a palliative care unit. *Journal of Palliative Care*, 1991; **7**: 5–11.
45. Reuben DB, Mor V, Hiris J. Clinical symptoms and length of survival in patients with terminal cancer. *Archives of Internal Medicine*, 1988; **148**: 1586–91.
46. Levine PM, Silberfarb PM, Lipowski ZJ. Mental disorders in cancer patients: a study of 100 psychiatric referrals. *Cancer*, 1978; **42**: 1385–91.
47. Derogatis LR, Morrow GR, Fetting J, Penman D, Piasetsky S, Schmale AM, *et al.* The prevalence of psychiatric disorders among cancer patients. *Journal of the American Medical Association*, 1983; **249**: 751–7.
48. Jacox A, Carr DB, Payne R. New clinical-practice guidelines for the management of pain in patients with cancer. *New England Journal of Medicine*, 1994; **330**: 651–5.
49. Max M. American Pain Society quality assurance standards for relief of acute pain and cancer pain. In: Bond MR, Charlton JE, Woolf CJ, eds. *Proceedings VI World Congress on Pain*. Amsterdam: Elsevier, 1990: 185–9.
50. Bookbinder M, Kiss M, Coyle N, Brown MH, Gianella A, Thaler HT. Improving pain management practices. In: McGuire DB, Yarbo CH, Ferrell BR, eds. *Cancer Pain Management*, 2nd edn. Boston: Jones and Bartlett, 1995.
51. Foley KM. Pain relief into practice: Rhetoric without reform. *Journal of Clinical Oncology*, 1995; **13**: 2149–51.
52. Foley KM. Pain assessment and cancer pain syndromes. In: Doyle D, Hanks G, MacDonald N, eds. *Oxford Textbook of Palliative Medicine*; Oxford: Oxford University Press, 1993: 148–65.
53. Cherny NI, Portenoy RK. Cancer pain: principles of assessment and syndromes. In: Wall PD, Melzack R, eds. *Textbook of Pain*. Edinburgh: Churchill Livingstone, 1994: 787–823.
54. Ingham J, Portenoy R. Symptom assessment. In: Cherny NI, Foley KM. *Pain and Palliative Care—Hematology/Oncology Clinics of North America*, 1996; **10**: 21–39.
55. Sui AL, Reuben DB, Moore AA. Comprehensive geriatric assessment. In: Hazzard WR, Bierman EL, Blass JP, Ettinger WH, Halter JB, eds. *Principles of Geriatric Medicine and Gerontology*; 3rd edn. New York: McGraw-Hill, 1994: 203–11.
56. Pecoraro RE, Inui TS, Chen MS, Plorde DK, Heller JL. Validity and reliability of a self-administered health history questionnaire. *Public Health Reports*, 1979; **94**: 231–8.
57. Brodman K, Erdmann AJ, Lorge I, Wolff HG. The Cornell Medical Index, an adjunct to medical interview. *Journal of the American Medical Association*, 1949; **140**: 530–4.
58. Coyle N, Layman-Goldstein M, Passik S, Fishman B, Portenoy R. Development and validation of patient needs assessment tool (PNAT) for oncology clinicians. *Cancer Nursing*, 1996; **19**: 81–92.
59. Au E, Loprinzi CL, Dhodapkar M, Nelson T, Novotny P, Hammack J, *et al.* Regular use of a verbal pain scale improves the understanding of oncology inpatient intensity. *Journal of Clinical Oncology*, 1994; **12**: 2751–5.

60. Miller AB, Hoogstraten B, Staquet M, Winkler A. Reporting results of cancer treatment. *Cancer,* 1981; **47**: 207–14.
61. Donnelly S, Walsh D. The symptoms of advanced cancer. *Seminars in Oncology,* 1995; **22**(2), Suppl 3: 67–72.
62. Burgess AP, Irving G, Riccio M. The reliability and validity of a symptom checklist for use in HIV infection: A preliminary analysis. *International Journal of STD and AIDS,* 1993; **4**: 333–8.
63. Osoba D. Self-rating symptom checklists: a simple method for recording and evaluating symptom control in oncology. *Cancer Treatment Reviews,* 1993; **19**(Suppl A): 43–51.
64. de Haes JCJM, Raatgever JW, van der Burg MEL, Hamersma E, Neijt JP. Evaluation of the quality of life of patients with advanced ovarian cancer treated with combination chemotherapy. In: Aaronson NK, Beckman J, eds. *The Quality of Life of Cancer Patients.* New York: Raven Press, 1987: 217–25.
65. de Haes JCJM, van Kippenberg FCE, Neijt JP. Measuring psychological and physical distress in cancer patients: structure and application of the Rotterdam Symptom Checklist. *British Journal of Cancer,* 1990; **62**: 1034–8.
66. Bruera E, MacMillan K, Hanson J, MacDonald N. Palliative care in a cancer center: results in 1984 versus 1987. *Journal of Pain and Symptom Management,* 1990; **5**: 1–5.
67. Stiefel F, Fainsinger R, Bruera E. Acute confusional states in patients with advanced cancer. *Journal of Pain and Symptom Management,* 1992; **7**: 94–8.
68. Schipper H, Clinch J, McMurray A, Levitt M. Measuring the quality of life of cancer patients: The Functional Living Index-Cancer: Development and validation. *Journal of Clinical Oncology,* 1984; **2**: 472–83.
69. Morrow GR, Lindke J, Black P. Measurement of quality of life in patients: psychometric analyses of the Functional Living Index-Cancer (FLIC). *Quality of Life Research,* 1992; **1**: 287–96.
70. Ganz PA, Schag CA, *et al.* The CARES: a generic measure of health related quality of life for patients with cancer. *Quality of Life Research,* 1992; **1**: 19–29.
71. Stewart AL, Hays RD, Ware JE. The MOS short-form general health survey: reliability and validity in a patient population. *Medical Care,* 1988; **26**: 724–35.
72. Creekmore SP, Urba WJ, Longo DL. Principles of the clinical evaluation of biological agents. In: Devita VT, Hellmen S, Rosenberg SA, eds. *Biologic Therapy of Cancer*; 1st edn. Philadelphia, Pa: Lippincott, 1991: 67–86.
73. Kaplan RM, Anderson JP, Wu AW, Christopher WM, Kozin E, Orestein D. The Quality of Well-Being Scale: applications in AIDS, cystic fibrosis, and arthritis. *Medical Care,* 1989; **27**: 35–49.
74. Wu AW, Rubin HR, Mathews WC, Ware JE, Brysk LT, Hardy WD, *et al.* A health status questionnaire using 30 items from the Medical Outcomes Study. *Medical Care,* 1991; **29**: 786–98.
75. Wachtel T, Piette J, Mor V, Stein M, Fleishman J, Carpenter C. Quality of life in persons with human immunodeficiency virus infection: measurement by the Medical Outcomes Study instrument. *Annals of Internal Medicine,* 1992; **116**: 129–37.
76. Cleary PD, Fowler FJ, Weissman J, Massagli MP, Wilson I, Seage GR, *et al.* Health-related quality of life in persons with Acquired Immune Deficiency Syndrome. *Medical Care,* 1993; **31**: 569–80.
77. Bozzette SA, Hays RD, Berry SH, Kanouse DE. A Perceived Health Index for use in persons with advanced HIV disease: Derivation, reliability and validity. *Medical Care,* 1994; **32**: 716–31.
78. Ingham JM, Seidman A, Lepore J, Belletierri R, Yao TJ, Thaler H, *et al.* The importance of frequent pain measurement in quality of life assessment in cancer clinical trials. *Presented at the American Pain Society Meeting, Orlando, Florida. Nov 4,* 1993.
79. Kukull WA, McCorkle R, Driever M. Symptom distress, psychosocial variables and survival from lung cancer. *Journal of Psychosocial Oncology,* 1986; **4**: 91–104.
80. Stark RD, Gambles SA, Lewis JA. Methods to assess breathlessness in healthy subjects: a critical evaluation and application to analyse the acute effects of diazepam and promethazine on breathlessness induced by exercise or by exposure to raised levels of carbon dioxide. *Clinical Science,* 1981; **61**: 429–39.
81. Stark RD. Dyspnoea: assessment and pharmacological manipulation. *European Respiratory Journal,* 1988; **1**: 280–7.
82. Cockcroft A, Adams L, Guz A. Assessment of breathlessness. *Quarterly Journal of Medicine,* 1989; **72**: 669–76.
83. McCord M, Cronin SD. Operationalizing dyspnea: focus on measurement. *Heart Lung,* 1992; **21**: 167–79.
84. Eakin EG, Kaplan RM, Ries AL. Measurement of dyspnoea in chronic obstructive pulmonary disease. *Quality of Life Research,* 1993; **2**: 181–91.
85. Brown ML, Carrieri V, Janson-Bjerklie S, Dodd MJ. Lung cancer and dyspnea: the patient's perception. *Oncology Nursing Forum,* 1986; **13**: 19–23.
86. Bruera E, DeStoutz N, Velasco-Leiva A, Schoeller T, Hanson J. Effects of oxygen on dyspnoea in hypoxaemic terminal-cancer patients. *Lancet,* 1993; **342**: 13–14.
87. Roberts DK, Thorne SE, Pearson C. The experience of dyspnea in late-stage cancer. Patients' and nurses' perspectives. *Cancer Nursing,* 1993; **16**: 310–20.
88. Melzack R. The McGill pain questionnaire: Major properties and scoring methods. *Pain,* 1975; **1**: 277–99.
89. Graham C, Bond SS, Gerkovich MM, Cook MR. Use of the McGill Pain Questionnaire in the assessment of cancer pain: replicability and consistency. *Pain,* 1980; **8**: 377–87.
90. Melzack R. The short-form McGill Pain Questionnaire. *Pain,* 1987; **30**: 191–7.
91. Fishman B, Pasternak S, Wallenstein SL, Houde RW, Holland JC, Foley KM. The Memorial pain assessment card. A valid instrument for the evaluation of cancer pain. *Cancer,* 1987; **60**: 1151–8.
92. DeConno F, Caraceni A, Gamba A, Mariani L, Abbattista A, Brunelli C, *et al.* Pain measurement in cancer patients: a comparison of six methods. *Pain,* 1994; **57**: 161–6.
93. Lipowski ZJ. Delirium (acute confusional states). *Journal of the American Medical Association,* 1987; **258**: 1789–92.
94. Levkoff SE, Evans DA, Liptzin B, Cleary PD, Lipsitz LA, Wetle TT, *et al.* Delirium. The occurrence and persistence of symptoms among elderly hospitalized patients. *Archives of Internal Medicine,* 1992; **152**: 334–40.
95. Exton-Smith AN. Terminal illness in the aged. *Lancet,* 1961; **2**: 305–8.
96. Witzel L. Behavior of the dying patient. *British Medical Journal,* 1975; **2**: 81–2.
97. Massie MJ, Holland J, Glass E. Delirium in terminally ill cancer patients. *American Journal of Psychiatry,* 1983; **140**: 1048–50.
98. Smith MJ, Breitbart WS, Platt MM. A critique of instruments and methods to detect, diagnose, and rate delirium. *Journal of Pain and Symptom Management,* 1995; **10**: 35–77.
99. Folstein MF, Folstein SE, McHugh PR. Mini-mental state. *Journal of Psychiatric Research,* 1975; **12**: 189–98.
100. Katzman R, Brown T, Fuld P, Peck A, Schechter R, Schimmel H. Validation of a short orientation-memory-concentration test of cognitive impairment. *American Journal of Psychiatry,* 1983; **140**: 734–9.
101. Bruera E, Miller L, McCallion J, MacMillan K, Krefting L, Hanson J. Cognitive failure in patients with terminal cancer: a prospective study. *Journal of Pain and Symptom Management,* 1992; **7**: 192–5.
102. Fainsinger RL, Tapper M, Bruera E. A perspective on the management of delirium in terminally ill patients on a palliative care unit. *Journal of Palliative Care,* 1993; **9**: 4–8.
103. American Psychiatric Association. *Diagnostic and Statistical Manual of Mental Disorders,* 4th edn. Washington, D.C.: American Psychiatric Association, 1994.
104. Inouye SK, Van Dyck CH, Alessi CA, Balkin S, Siegal AP, Horwitz RI. Clarifying confusion: The confusion assessment method. *Annals of Internal Medicine,* 1990; **113**: 941–8.
105. Albert MS, Levkoff SE, Reilly C, Liptzin B, Pilgrim D, Cleary PD, *et al.* The delirium symptom interview: an interview for the detection of delirium symptoms in hospitalized patients. *Journal of Geriatric Psychiatry and Neurology,* 1992; **5**: 14–21.

106. Trzepacz PT, Baker RW, Greenhouse J. A symptom rating scale for delirium. *Psychiatry Research,* 1988; **23**: 89–97.
107. American Psychiatric Association. *Diagnostic and Statistical Manual of Mental Disorders,* 3rd edn. Washington, D.C.: American Psychiatric Association, 1980.
108. American Psychiatric Association. *Diagnostic and Statistical Manual of Mental Disorders* , 3rd rev. edn, Washington, D.C.: American Psychiatric Association, 1987.
109. Irvine DM, Vincent L, Bubela N, Thompson L, Graydon J. A critical appraisal of the literature investigating fatigue in the individual with cancer. *Cancer Nursing,* 1991; **14**: 188–99.
110. Smets EM, Garssen B, Schuster-Uitterhoeve AL, de Haes JC. Fatigue in cancer patients. *British Journal of Cancer,* 1993; **68**: 220–4.
111. Glaus A. Assessment of fatigue in cancer and non-cancer patients and in healthy individuals. *Support Care Cancer,* 1993; **1**: 305–15.
112. Winningham ML, Nail LM, Burke MB, Brophy L, Cimprich B, Jones LS, *et al.* Fatigue and the cancer experience: The state of the knowledge. *Oncology Nursing Forum,* 1994; **21**: 23–34.
113. McNair D, Lorr M, Deoppleman LF. *Profile of Mood States Manual.* San Deigo: Educational and Industrial Testing Service, 1971.
114. Pearson PG, Byars GE. *The Development and Validation of a Check List Measuring Subjective Fatigue.* School of Aviation, USAF, Randolf AFB, Texas, 1956.
115. Yoshitake H. Relations between the symptoms and feelings of fatigue. *Ergonomics,* 1971; **14**: 175–96.
116. Haylock PJ, Hart LK. Fatigue in patients receiving localized radiation. *Cancer Nursing,* 1979; **2**: 461–7.
117. Kogi K, Saito Y. Assessment criteria for mental fatigue. A factor-analytic study of phase discrimination in mental fatigue. *Ergonomics,* 1971; **14**: 119–27.
118. Kobashi-Schoot JAM, Hanewald GJFP, VanDam FSAM, Bruning PF. Assessment of malaise in cancer patients treated with radiotherapy. *Cancer Nursing,* 1985; **8**: 306–13.
119. Bruera E, Chadwick S, Brenneis C, Hanson J, MacDonald N. Methylphenidate associated with narcotics for the treatment of cancer pain. *Cancer Treatment Reports,* 1987; **71**: 67–70.
120. Bruera E, Brenneis C, Paterson AH, MacDonald N. Use of methylphenidate as an adjuvant to narcotic analgesics in patients with advanced cancer. *Journal of Pain and Symptom Management,* 1989; **4**: 3–6.
121. Bruera E, Fainsinger R, MacEachern T, Hanson J. The use of methylphenidate in patients with incident cancer pain receiving regular opiates. A preliminary report. *Pain,* 1992; **50**: 75–7.
122. Bruera E, Miller MJ, MacMillan K, Kuehn N. Neuropsychological effects of methylphenidate in patients receiving a continuous infusion of narcotics for cancer pain. *Pain,* 1992; **48**: 163–6.
123. Piper BF, Lindsey AM, Dodd MJ, Ferketich S, Paul SM, Weller S. The development of an instrument to measure the subjective dimension of fatigue. In: Funk SG, Tornquist EM, Champange MT, Copp LA, Wiese RA, eds. *Key Aspects of Comfort. Management of Pain, Fatigue and Nausea.* New York: Springer Publishing Company, 1989: 199–208.
124. Lee KA, Hicks G, Nino-Murcia G. Validity and reliability of a scale to assess fatigue. *Psychiatry Research,* 1991; **36**: 291–8.
125. Janson-Bjerklie S, Carrieri VK, Hudes M. The sensations of dyspnea. *Nursing Research,* 1985; **35**: 154–9.
126. Simon PM, Schwartzstein RM, Weiss JW, Lahive K, Fencl V, Teghtsoonian M, *et al.* Distinguishable sensations of breathlessness induced in normal volunteers. *American Review of Respiratory Diseases,* 1989; **140**: 1021–7.
127. O'Neill PA, Stretton TB, Stark RD, Ellis SH. The effect of indomethacin on breathlessness in patients with diffuse parenchymal disease of the lung. *British Journal of Diseases of the Chest,* 1986; **80**: 72–9.
128. Wilson RC, Jones PWA. Comparison of the visual analogue scale and modified Borg scale for the measurement of dyspnea during exercise. *Clinical Science,* 1989; **76**: 277–82.
129. Stark RD, Morton PB, Sharman P, Percival PG, Lewis JA. Effects of codeine on the respiratory responses to exercise in healthy subjects. *British Journal of Clinical Pharmacology,* 1983; **15**: 355–9.
130. Eakin EG, Kaplan RM, Ries AL. Measurement of dyspnea in chronic obstructive pulmonary disease. *Quality of Life Research,* 1993; **2**:181–91.
131. Borg G. Perceived exertion as an indicator of somatic stress. *Scandinavian Journal of Rehabilitation Medicine,* 1970; **2–3**: 92–8.
132. Borg G. Psychophysical bases of perceived exertion. *Medical Science and Sports Exercise,* 1982; **14**: 377–81
133. Research Council Committee on the Aetiology of Chronic Bronchitis. Standardized questionnaires on respiratory symptoms. *British Medical Journal,* 1960; **2**: 1665.
134. Thoracic Society. Recommended respiratory disease questionnaires for use with adults and children in epidemiological research. *American Review of Respiratory Diseases,* 1978; **118**: 7–53.
135. Mahler D, Weinberg D, Wells C, Feinstein A. The measurement of dyspnea: contents, interobserver agreement, and physiologic correlates of two new clinical indexes. *Chest,* 1984; **85**: 751–8.
136. Deyo RA, Patrick DL. Barriers to the use of health status measures in clinical investigation, patient care, and policy research. *Medical Care,* 1989; **27** suppl 3: S254–68.
137. VonRoenn JH, Cleeland CS, Gonin R, Hatfield AK, Pandya KJ. Physician attitudes and practice in cancer pain management: A survey from the Eastern Cooperative Oncology Group. *Annals of Internal Medicine,* 1993; **119**: 121–6.
138. Donovan M, Dillon P, McGuire L. The incidence and characteristics of pain in a sample of medical-surgical outpatients. *Pain,* 1987; **30**: 69–87.
139. Cleeland CS. The impact of pain on the patient with cancer. *Cancer,* 1984; **54**: 263–7.
140. Lipowski ZJ. *Delirium: Acute Confusional States.* New York: Oxford University Press, 1990.
141. Stark RD, Gambles SA, Chatterjee SS. An exercise test to assess clinical dyspnoea: estimation of reproducibility and sensitivity. *British Journal of Diseases of the Chest,* 1982; **76**: 269–78.
142. Ganz PA, Haskell CA, Figlin RA, *et al.* Estimating the quality of life in a clinical trial of patients with metastatic lung cancer using the Karnofsky Performance Status and the Functional Living Index-Cancer. *Cancer,* 1988; **61**: 849.
143. Selby P, Robertson B. Measurement of quality of life in patients with cancer. *Cancer Surveys,* 1987; **6**: 521–43.
144. McCarthy M. Hospice patients: a pilot study in 12 services. *Palliative Medicine,* 1990; **4**: 93–104.
145. Cleeland CS, Gonin R, Hatfield AK, Edmonson JH, Blum RH, Stewart JA, *et al.* Pain and its treatment in outpatients with metastatic cancer. *New England Journal of Medicine,* 1994; **330**: 592–6.
146. Cunningham WE, Bozzette SA, Hays RD, Kanouse DE, Shapiro MF. Comparison of health-related quality of life in clinical trial and nonclinical trial human immunodeficiency virus-infected cohorts. *Medical Care,* 1995; **33**: AS15–25.
147. Townsend J, Frank AO, Fermont D, Dyer S, Karran O, Walgrove A, *et al.* Terminal cancer care and patients' preference for place of death: a prospective study. *British Medical Journal,* 1990; **301**: 415–7.
148. Karoly P. Assessment of pediatric pain. In: Bush JP, Harkins SW, eds. *Children in Pain: Clinical and Research Issues from a Developmental Perspective.* New York: Springer-Verlag, 1991: 59–82.
149. Manne SL, Andersen BL. Pain and pain-related distess in children with cancer. In: Bush JP, Harkins SW, eds. *Children in Pain: Clinical and Research Issues from a Developmental Perspective.* New York: Springer-Verlag, 1991: 337–72.
150. Matthews JR, McGrath PJ, Pigeon H. Assessment and measurement of pain in children. In: Schechter NL, Berde CB, Yaster M, eds. *Pain in Infants, Children and Adolescents.* Baltimore: Williams and Wilkins, 1993.
151. Porter F. Pain assessment in children: Infants. In: Schechter NL, Berde CB, Yaster M, eds. *Pain in Infants, Children and Adolescents.* Baltimore: Williams and Wilkins, 1993.
152. Jay S, Elliot C, Katz E, Seigal S. Cognitive-behavioral and pharmacologic interventions for childrens' distress during painful medical procedures. *Journal of Consulting and Clinical Psychology,* 1987; **55**: 860–5.

153. Katz E, Kellerman J, Ellenberg L. Hypnosis in the reduction of acute pain and distress in children with cancer. *Journal of Pediatric Psychology*, 1987; **12**: 379–94.
154. LeBaron S, Zeltzer LK. Assessment of pain and anxiety in children and adolescents by self-reports, and a behavior checklist. *Journal of Consulting and Clinical Psychology*, 1984; **52**: 729–38.
155. Kuttner L, Bowman M, Teasdale M. Psychological treatment of distress, pain and anxiety for children with cancer. *Developmental and Behavioral Pediatrics*, 1988; **9**: 374–81.
156. Manne S, Redd WH, Jacobson P, Gorfinkle K, Schorr O, Rapkin B. Behavioral intervention to reduce child and parent distress during venipuncture. *Journal of Consulting and Clinical Psychology*, 1990; **58**: 565–72.
157. Jay S, Elliott C. Behavioral observation scales for measuring childrens' distress: The effects of increased methodological rigor. *Journal of Consulting and Clinical Psychology*, 1984; **52**: 1106–7.
158. Elliott C, Jay S, Woody P. An observational scale for measuring childrens' distress during medical procedures. *Journal of Pediatric Psychology*, 1987; **12**: 543–51.
159. Gauvain-Piquard A, Rodary C, Rezvani A, Lemerle J. Pain in children aged 2–6 years: a new observational rating scale elaborated in a pediatric oncology unit—a preliminary report. *Pain*, 1987; **31**: 177–88.
160. Zeltzer LK, LeBaron S, Richie DM, Reed D. Can children understand and use a rating scale to quantify somatic symptoms? Assessment of nausea and vomiting as a model. *Journal of Consulting and Clinical Psychology*, 1988; **56**: 567–72.
161. Tye VL, *et al*. Chemotherapy induce nausea and emesis in pediatric cancer patients: external validity of child and parent emesis ratings. *Developmental and Behavioral Pediatrics*, 1993; **14**: 236–41.
162. Schechter NI, Berde CB, Yaster M, eds. *Pain in Infants, Children and Adolescents*. Baltimore: Williams and Wilkins, 1993.
163. Seeman I. National Mortality Followback Survey: 1986 Summary, United States National Center for Health Statistics. *Vital and Health Statistics*, 1992; **20**: 19.
164. Saunders C. Pain and impending death. In: Wall P, Melzack R, eds. *Textbook of Pain*. Churchill Livingston: New York, 1984: 472–8.
165. Hinton JM. The physical and mental distress of the dying. *Quarterly Journal of Medicine*, 1963; **32**: 1–21.
166. Waxler-Morrison N, Anderson JM, Richardson E, eds. *Cross Cultural Caring: A handbook for Health Professionals in Western Canada*. Vancouver: University of B.C. Press, 1990.
167. Lipson JG, Dibble SL, Minarik PA, eds. *Culture and Nursing Care: A Pocket Guide*. San Francisco: UCSF Nursing Press, 1996.
168. Cleeland CS, Ryan KM. Pain assessment: global use of the Brief Pain Inventory. *Annals of Academic Medicine Singapore*, 1994; **23**: 129–38.
169. Cleeland CS, Ladinsky JL, Serlin RC, Nugyen CT. Multidimensional measurement of cancer pain: comparisons of US and Vietnamese patients. *Journal of Pain and Symptom Management*, 1988; **3**: 23–7.

7

The principles of drug use in palliative medicine

7 The principles of drug use in palliative medicine

Clive J. C. Roberts, Sarah Keir, and Geoffrey Hanks

The control of distressing symptoms is central to the practice of palliative medicine. It is the foundation of 'whole patient' care in that it is not possible to deal with psychological, social, or spiritual concerns if patients have uncontrolled physical symptoms. The management of these symptoms is largely based on drug treatment, which means that effective symptom control requires some understanding of clinical pharmacology. The purpose of this chapter is to describe those principles of clinical pharmacology that are relevant to day-to-day palliative medicine practice.

Symptom management is unfortunately not a simple exercise of targeting a particular symptom with a specific drug. Patients with advanced disease are a vulnerable population and it is necessary to recognize that environmental and psychological factors have a variable but potentially very great influence on physical well-being. The response to drug treatment may be sometimes unpredictable for these reasons.

There are other complicating factors in this patient population. The patients are predominantly elderly with many concurrent symptomatic problems and often with multisystem dysfunction. Polypharmacy is almost invariable and the potential for drug interactions and modified or abnormal responses to drugs is considerable. Iatrogenic problems are commonplace in that prescription of one symptomatic remedy—for example an opioid analgesic—will invariably cause other symptoms, in this case constipation, drowsiness, and possibly nausea and dry mouth. A laxative, antiemetic, psychostimulant, and artificial saliva may all be added to the treatment regimen as a result. The skill of the palliative medicine physician is to deal effectively with each symptom without imposing a greater burden on the patient because of intolerable, unwanted drug effects or too complex a drug regimen. The principles of effective symptom control need always to be kept in mind: make a diagnosis of the underlying mechanism or cause of each symptom, individualize the treatment, and keep it simple.

Clinical pharmacology

Clinical pharmacology may be broadly divided into pharmacokinetics ('what the body does to the drug') and pharmacodynamics ('what the drug does to the body'). It is often assumed that these are theoretical and rather esoteric disciplines that do not in fact have much direct 'clinical' relevance. As we shall demonstrate this assumption is wrong. For example palliative care patients commonly require parenteral administration of drugs at some stage of their illness, and disordered handling of drugs by the body as a result of disease is common. Drugs are often used in special formulations, either involving modified release of orally administered agents or novel forms designed for administration by other routes. These are everyday clinical situations which cannot be properly managed without some pharmacokinetic knowledge.

Pharmacodynamics is about drug action in man and, like pharmocokinetics, its measurement has become highly sophisticated; for example in the use of imaging techniques to monitor biochemical changes in target organs such as the brain. However, one of the challenges of drug use in palliative care is that outcome measures are often not easy to define and measure. In palliative care, drugs are not being used to cure disease but to improve comfort. Subjective symptoms such as pain, nausea, or depression are less easy to quantify than biochemical changes in the brain or even tumour size, serum calcium, or haemoglobin concentrations. Yet these are common targets for drug treatment in palliative medicine. Knowledge of the basic modes of action of drugs will underpin the logical selection and use of the most appropriate remedies for these symptoms.

Pharmacokinetics

Pharmacokinetics is often arbitrarily described under the headings of absorption, distribution, metabolism, and excretion of drugs. A number of other terms are used to describe the way in which the body handles drugs. These terms can be defined and modelled mathematically. However, the practising clinician should not be put off by the emphasis on mathematics which is often applied to the subject. A broad understanding of the physiological, pharmacological, and pathophysiological factors which influence the ultimate concentration of a drug in the blood stream is invaluable and does not need an understanding of complex mathematical models.

This section will define commonly used kinetic terms and identify, where possible, factors contributing to the variability of each. In order to illustrate the terminology, some pharmacokinetic parameters for frequently used drugs will be described at the end of each section.

Half-life ($t_{1/2}$)

This is perhaps the most well known and commonly used pharmacokinetic parameter. It is a measure of the rate at which a particular process takes place. For example the elimination half-life is a measure of the time taken for half the drug in the body to be removed. However, the process is often complex. For example the decay in drug concentration following intravenous administration may comprise several exponentials, representing movement of drug inwards and outwards of body compartments and also the elimination of the drug from the body. It is generally the elimination half-life which correlates most closely with the duration of action of the drug, though this is not always the case. Technical difficulties in defining a drug's half-life may account for variation in quoted figures.

The elimination half-life is a dependent variable—dependent on volume of distribution and clearance. In the simplest kinetic model, half-life ($t_{1/2}$) equals volume of distribution (Vd) multiplied by a constant (k) divided by clearance (Cl):

$$t_{1/2}=k\frac{\mathrm{Vd}}{\mathrm{Cl}}.$$

What this means is that half-life is prolonged as distribution volume increases and clearance reduces. These terms are defined below.

Drugs with a long half-life may accumulate over a prolonged period of time and build up to toxic levels. For example this may happen with methadone[1] which on regular dosing has a half-life of 20 to 40 h.

The elimination half-life of benzodiazepine hypnotics to some extent predicts the potential of each drug to cause residual or hangover effects the next day. Temazepam ($t_{1/2}$ 8–10 h) and triazolam ($t_{1/2}$ 2–3 h) are much less likely to cause daytime drowsiness than flurazepam (which has an active metabolite desalkylflurazepam with a $t_{1/2}$ of 2–4 days).

Apparent volume of distribution (Vd)

This term is defined as the volume into which all the drug in the body would need to be distributed to achieve the blood concentration. For drugs which are taken up into fat stores or muscle the volume may be many times body size. Thus, it is not a real volume which can be described in anatomical terms but a mathematical concept which is a convenient way of expressing how a drug is distributed in the body. This is why it is termed 'apparent'. Similarly a 'compartment' does not have an anatomical equivalent but is a theoretical space (often shown diagramatically as a box).

The volume of distribution is important as a determinant of half-life and is also of theoretical importance in the calculation of a loading dose where one is needed. Alteration in body composition and in the physicochemical environment of the body causes changes in distribution volume. Such changes for individual drugs in specific conditions may be quite difficult to predict. However, emaciation may reduce the distribution volume of many centrally acting agents and lead to an enhanced effect after single doses. If a drug is normally heavily plasma protein bound, distribution volume may increase when plasma proteins are reduced because more drug is available for tissue binding sites. However, because the proportion of active (unbound) drug is increased, a lower plasma concentration of drug will produce a given therapeutic effect. Thus, the net result is that the effects of these changes will tend to cancel each other out.

Digoxin is rapidly and extensively taken up by body tissues, particularly skeletal and cardiac muscle and in a 70 kg man has a volume of distribution of some 490 litres. In contrast, morphine, which is relatively hydrophilic and little taken up in tissue stores, has a volume of distribution of 140 litres. In both of these examples the 'apparent' volume of distribution is greater than the size of the body.

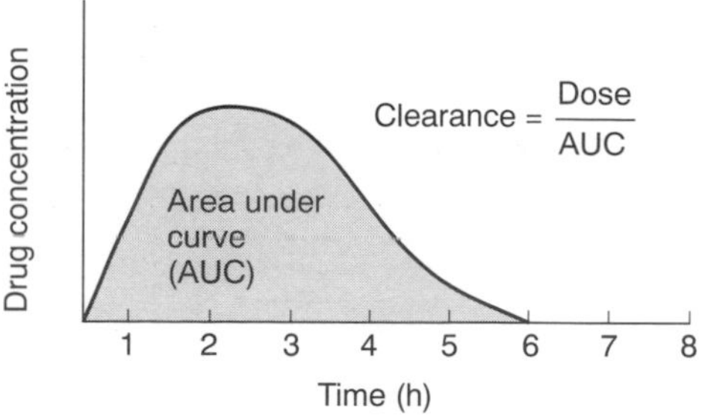

Fig. 1 Plasma concentrations of a typical drug after oral administration. The shaded area is the 'area under the curve' of plasma concentration versus time and can be calculated mathematically, and from this can be derived the clearance.

Clearance

This is the volume of blood which is completely cleared of the drug in a unit of time. It therefore most closely reflects the efficiency of the elimination process. It is a major determinant of half-life and of the steady state drug concentration. This is because at steady state the amount of blood being cleared in the interval between doses will contain an amount of drug equivalent to the dose (assuming 100 per cent bioavailability). The two major organs of elimination are the liver and the kidney, both of which are susceptible to pharmacological and pathophysiological sources of variability. Clearance can be measured experimentally by plotting blood concentrations of the drug after a dose has been administered. Clearance (Cl) can then be calculated as:

$$\mathrm{Cl} = \frac{\text{dose}}{\text{area under the plasma concentration/time curve}}$$

This is illustrated in Fig. 1.

Most drugs are cleared from the bloodstream either by metabolism in the liver or by excretion by the kidney or by a combination of both. Total blood clearance determines steady state concentration and is the sum of all clearance mechanisms. Whilst it is often claimed that if one organ of elimination is compromised by disease the other can compensate by allowing increased excretion of the drug, this does not prevent a rise in drug level in the body, which is determined by total clearance.

Steady state plasma concentration (C_{ss})

The aim of any dosing regimen in an individual patient is to achieve a concentration of drug in the blood which is not so high as to produce adverse effects but high enough to give the intended effect (Fig. 2). This concentration can never be completely steady as peaks will occur at the point of maximum drug absorption after administration and troughs occur immediately before each dose (Fig. 3). Steady state is said to have been achieved when all trough and all peak concentrations do not vary. The degree of swing between peak and trough is determined by the drug's elimination half-life and the frequency of drug administration. For instance where a drug has a short half-life and the difference between peak concentration and trough concentration is small, then dosing should be frequent. The actual steady state concentrations achieved in any patient are dependent on the dose administered, the

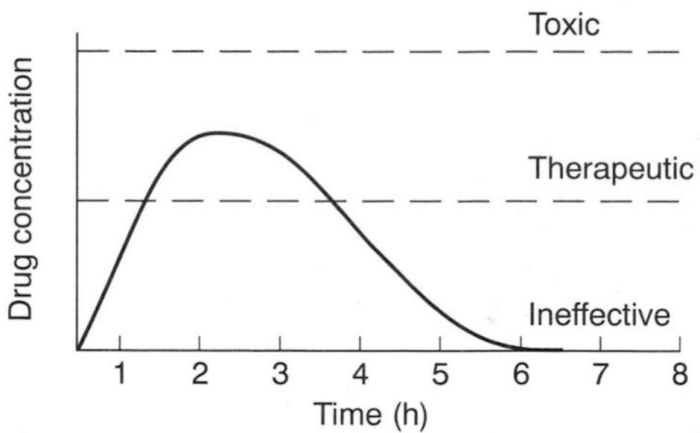

Fig. 2 Plasma concentrations of a typical drug after oral administration of a single dose. The aim in chronic dosing is to maintain plasma concentrations within the therapeutic range.

bioavailability of the drug in that patient, and the clearance of the drug from the blood in that patient.

It is a common misconception that steady state drug concentration is dependent on the size of the body. In fact the volume into which the drug is distributed plays no part. The reason why smaller people and children often require reduced doses is because they have smaller organs of elimination and therefore lower clearance rates. This is pertinent in the context of palliative care where it cannot be predicted that a patient whose body is wasted may need to be given a smaller dose. The elimination process itself may be unimpaired.

Time to reach steady state plasma concentration

Whilst the actual concentration of drug in the blood is independent of its half-life, the time it takes to reach that level is entirely and solely dependent on this parameter. As a rough guide, if a drug is given to a patient in constant dosage at a constant time interval it takes about four half-lives to reach 95 per cent of the steady state plasma concentration. This applies only to drugs whose elimination is governed by 'first order kinetics'. Fortunately this comprises the vast majority of drugs, with phenytoin being the notable exception. During a first order process a constant proportion of remaining drug is eliminated in a unit of time. Indeed that is why the term half-life can be applied—that is, half the drug in the body is removed in the half-life interval.

A first-order process is independent of the concentration of drug; the proportion eliminated is the same per unit of time whilst the actual amount of drug eliminated increases. A zero-order process is dependent on concentration and the amount eliminated per unit of time is fixed. Phenytoin is initially metabolized according to first-order kinetics but the enzyme system responsible has limited capacity. Once this system is 'saturated', metabolism of phenytoin continues as a zero-order process.

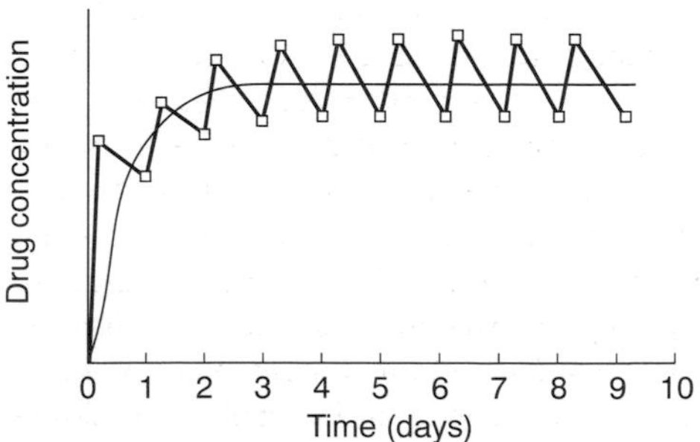

Fig. 3 Steady state plasma concentration of a short-acting drug showing peaks and troughs after each dose.

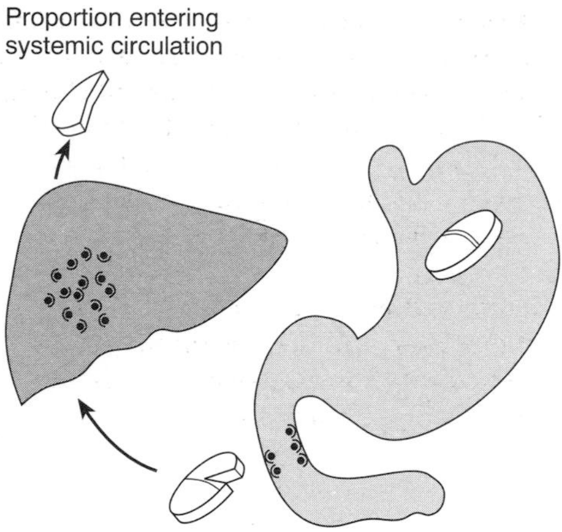

Fig. 4 'First pass' metabolism may take place in the liver (and sometimes also in the intestinal mucosa) before the absorbed drug enters the systemic circulation.

It is clear, therefore, that for a first-order process the amount of drug in the body must build up until the amount of drug being eliminated during the dose interval equates with the dose. Because the time to reach steady state depends on half-life, when this is very long it may be necessary to give a loading dose initially and then to follow with a reduced maintenance dose.

The elimination half-life ($t_{½}$) of morphine is 2 to 4 h. Thus, when morphine is administered at regular 4-hourly intervals steady state will be 95 per cent achieved after 16 h or so. In contrast, the half-life of digoxin is about 2 days so that it would take at least 8 to 10 days to achieve steady state. It is usual to give a loading dose of digoxin and then maintain patients on a single daily dose.

Bioavailability

This is the percentage of administered drug which gains access unchanged to the systemic circulation. It is of most clinical relevance after oral administration. It can be measured in individual patients by comparing the area under the plasma concentration time curves after oral and after parenteral administration allowing for any difference in the dose administered and assuming no change in the rate of elimination. Many factors may contribute to a reduction of bioavailability below 100 per cent. Variation in the pharmaceutical formulation of drugs such as digoxin and phenytoin may account for significant differences in bioavailability and the extent of drug absorption may be susceptible to changes in gastrointestinal function.

More important, however, is the extent of presystemic (or 'first pass') metabolism (Fig. 4). Once absorbed from the gastrointestinal tract, all drugs must pass via the portal venous system through the liver. If within that organ there is an avid system of enzymes for metabolizing the particular drug, then a percentage will be biotransformed before passing through the liver to the systemic circulation. For some drugs the amount extracted during one pass through the liver (extraction ratio) may be as high as 80 per cent, giving an oral bioavailability of only 20 per cent. The steady state blood concentration of such drugs after oral administration may exhibit high variability; minor changes in the extraction ratio will be reflected by large percentage changes in bioavailability. Thus, interactions with other drugs which induce or inhibit hepatic enzymes or changes in hepatic function due to disease may have a profound effect on such drug levels after oral administration but relatively little effect when the drug is given parenterally. In patients with chronic liver disease or hepatic metastases, there may develop shunts of blood from portal to systemic vessels. Drug may thus bypass hepatic enzymes, the presystemic metabolism will be reduced, and the bioavailability may be considerably increased. Consequently very much higher levels of drug may build up after oral administration if the enhanced bioavailability is not taken into account. The effect of presystemic metabolism on drug bioavailability must also be taken into account when calculating oral doses during conversion from parenteral regimens. The bioavailability of some drugs may also be reduced by intraluminal degradation in the gastrointestinal tract or metabolism by enzymes within the intestinal wall.

Drug absorption

In the main, the absorption of drugs is a passive process along a concentration gradient across a lipid cell membrane. As long as the drug is in solution and has a degree of lipid solubility, there is sufficient surface area for diffusion, and the drug remains in contact with the absorptive areas for long enough then problems should not arise.

Most drugs are absorbed where the greatest surface area is available; that is, in the small bowel. A reduced rate of absorption may therefore occur if there is a delay in emptying of the stomach. This might arise as part of a pathological process or result from pharmacological agents which slow gastric motility, such as drugs with anticholinergic effects or opioid analgesics.

Drugs must have the physicochemical characteristics to facilitate dissolution in the gut and once presented to the vast surface area of the small bowel their potential for full absorption should be easily achieved. Only the most severe of structural gastrointestinal disease will cause problems.

Many drugs are now formulated as controlled release preparations. For them to achieve their expected absorptive profile they may need to remain in the small bowel for a prolonged length of time. Such formulations have usually only been tested under ideal conditions in healthy volunteers. For the patient with gastrointestinal hurry who takes a controlled release drug there is a considerable risk that it will be propelled past the absorptive zone of the gut before all of the drug has been released and this will result in therapeutic failure.

Within the gut there is some potential for drug interaction which results in reduced bioavailability. Most examples are well known and involve loose chemical binding between two drugs within the gut lumen. For example cholestyramine binds many drugs, iron salts and tetracycline bind to each other, and sucralfate binds phenytoin. Other less obvious drug interactions may occur. Some broad-spectrum antibiotics decrease the effectiveness of the oral contraceptive and this may relate to increased gastrointestinal transit caused by the antibiotic and reduced absorption of the contraceptive.

Absorption and bioavailability are not the same. Morphine, for example, is more or less completely absorbed (i.e. 100 per cent). However, it undergoes extensive presystemic metabolism, mainly in the liver but also in the wall of the gastrointestinal tract. The bioavailability of morphine is thus about 20 to 30 per cent.

Drug metabolism

Drug biotransformation takes place mainly in the liver and contributes both to the rate of elimination of drug and to its bioavailability. The rate at which the metabolic process proceeds usually determines the clearance but where the removal is particularly avid (high extraction ratio) the rate of delivery of drug to the liver rather than the rate of metabolism may determine clearance (flow dependent kinetics). In these circumstances if liver blood flow is markedly reduced, drug accumulation will result.

The biochemical processes of drug metabolism are complex. The concept of two phases of metabolism involving initially oxidation or hydrolysis (phase I) followed by conjugation (phase II) is commonly used but can be misleading. All of the reactions involve the production of products which are more polar and therefore more water soluble and amenable to excretion by the kidney. So-called phase II reactions may take place in some circumstances without prior phase I. Phase I reactions involve oxidation, reduction, hydrolysis, hydration, dethioacetylation, and isomerization. Such reactions may prepare the drug molecule for a phase II reaction by producing or uncovering a chemically reactive group which then forms the substrate for a phase II reaction.

Of the phase I reactions, oxidation involving the 'mixed-function oxidase system' is the most important and its behaviour is best understood. This system of enzymes is based in hepatic microsomes and requires molecular oxygen, NADPH and cytochrome P450, and NADPH-cytochrome P450 reductase. Amongst the reactions catalysed by the mixed-function oxidase system are aromatic hydroxylation, aliphatic hydroxylation, epoxidation, *N*-dealkylation, *O*-dealkylation, oxidative deamination, *N*-oxidation, *S*-oxidation, and alcohol oxidation. Not all oxidative processes are carried out by this system; alcohol dehydrogenation is performed by a non-microsomally located enzyme which is responsible for the major pathway for alcohol detoxification (in non-enzyme induced subjects).

Phase II reactions mostly involve conjugation; glucuronidation, glycosylation, sulphation, methylation, and acetylation or conjugation with glutathione or with certain amino acids.

The intricacies of drug metabolism may appear irrelevant to clinicians but an appreciation of the complexity of the process is necessary in developing a scientific approach to dose management.

Pharmacodynamics

Drugs produce their effects on the body by combining with receptors, by modifying enzyme processes, or by a direct chemical or physical action.

Receptors, agonists, and antagonists

Receptors are specialized areas of the cell membrane which are highly specific for certain drug or hormone molecules. A drug which combines with a receptor to 'activate' it is called an agonist and this terminology initially derived from the actions of hormones and neurotransmitters. The term refers to a drug which binds to cell receptors to induce changes in the cell which stimulate

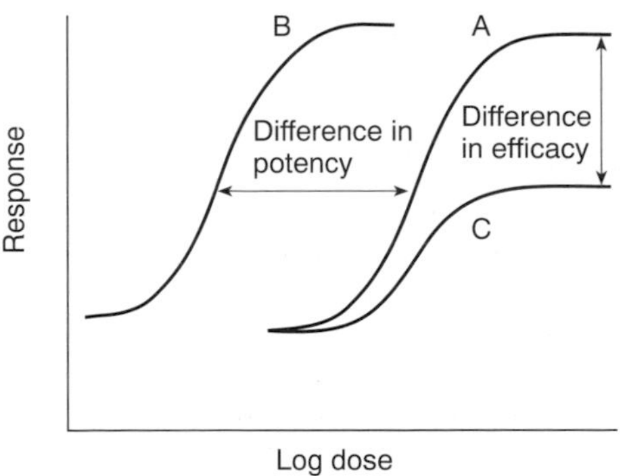

Fig. 5 Log dose–response curves for two full agonist drugs A and B, and a partial agonist C. Drug B is more potent than drug A but no more effective. Drug A is more effective than drug C but has similar potency.

physiological activity. Some drugs can combine with receptors without initiating any change in cell function. Such drugs are called antagonists because they interfere with the action of agonists by blocking the receptor sites ('competitive antagonists'). Non-competitive antagonists do not compete for the same receptor as the agonist but block the effect of the agonist in some other way.

A partial agonist is a drug with low intrinsic activity (efficacy) so that its dose response curve exhibits a ceiling effect at less than the maximal effect produced by a full agonist. The difference between a partial agonist and a full agonist is thus a difference in efficacy (Fig. 5). This should not be confused with potency which is a measure of the amount of drug required to produce a given effect, and is a measure also of affinity for receptors; the more potent a drug, the greater its affinity for receptors. Thus a drug may be a partial agonist (less effective) but still more potent than a full agonist. This is the case with buprenorphine which has limited efficacy compared with morphine but greater potency (0.3 mg intramuscular buprenorphine ≡ 10 mg intramuscular morphine).[2] However, because it is more potent it has greater affinity for μ opioid receptors and can displace morphine from them. In this way it can act as an 'antagonist' of morphine by reducing the overall μ opioid effect (see Chapter 9.2.3). Buprenorphine is therefore classified as an 'agonist antagonist'. Other opioid analgesics, such as pentazocine, are also classified as 'agonist antagonists' but have a different profile. These drugs have both agonist and antagonist effects at receptors, but at different receptors (see below).

There are similar examples in other therapeutic areas, and they are likely to increase as new receptors and receptor subtypes are identified. For example metoclopramide has been long regarded primarily as a dopamine receptor blocker, which it is at low doses. At high doses metoclopramide blocks (antagonizes) 5-HT_3 receptors and is a much more effective antiemetic. Metoclopramide also has a prokinetic effect on the upper gastrointestinal tract and this is mediated through an agonist effect at 5-HT_4 receptors, leading to an enhancement of the effects of acetylcholine release in the gut. Metoclopramide is thus both an agonist and an antagonist at different serotonin receptors.

Morphine is an agonist at μ opioid receptors. Buprenorphine is a partial agonist at μ receptors and can in certain circumstances reverse ('antagonize') the effects of morphine. Pentazocine is a weak competitive antagonist at μ receptors (so may also antagonize the effects of morphine but by a different mechanism) and is a partial agonist at a different type of opioid receptor, κ. Naloxone is an antagonist at the μ opioid receptor and will block the effects of μ agonists and partial agonists (but with varying efficiency).

Drugs which alter enzyme activity

Non-steroidal anti-inflammatory drugs block the effect of the enzyme cyclo-oxygenase and thereby interfere with the synthesis of prostaglandins; this is believed to be the basis for their anti-inflammatory activity. Monoamine oxidase inhibitor antidepressants interfere with the degradation of monoamine neurotransmitters thus enhancing their effect in central synapses; angiotensin-converting-enzyme inhibitors block the conversion of angiotensin I to angiotensin II by inhibiting the relevant enzyme and are effective in the treatment of hypertension and cardiac failure. Thus, drugs affecting enzyme processes may have diverse therapeutic applications but many of them share in common the fact that they are inhibitors of enzyme actions.

Drugs which have a direct chemical or physical action

Antacids are an example of drugs with a direct chemical action. They are bases which neutralize gastric acid. Drugs with a physical mode of action include the bulk laxatives such as ispaghula husk. While the mode of action of such drugs seems far less complex than that of drugs which interact with receptors, the same attention to detail in their use and individualized approach are necessary to maximize the benefits and reduce potential adverse effects.

Routes of administration of drugs in palliative care

If individuals need to take drugs, most prefer to take them by mouth and this is the commonest route of administration in palliative care. However, other routes are often either necessary or preferred. In one study of patients with advanced cancer almost a quarter required drug administration by three or more routes prior to death.[3] Analgesic drugs in particular may be delivered by several different routes and the following section should be read in conjunction with Chapter 9.2.3.

Oral

The oral route is non-invasive and the most convenient and most acceptable to patients. However, in many ways it is the most complicated because of the various processes which take place between ingestion of the medication and entry of the drug into the systemic circulation. The drug has to pass from the mouth into the stomach, and tablets or capsules need to disperse and dissolve before they can be absorbed. As described above, absorption takes place predominantly in the small bowel and the drug is then conveyed via the portal system to the liver, and hence to the systemic circulation. Numerous factors can affect absorption and bioavailability.

In spite of this complicated process, drugs may enter the systemic circulation rapidly. For example peak plasma concentrations (C_{max}) of immediate release morphine (solution or tablets) are achieved within 1 h after ingestion (t_{max}, the time to peak concentration) and sometimes within 15 to 30 min (Fig. 6). Patients

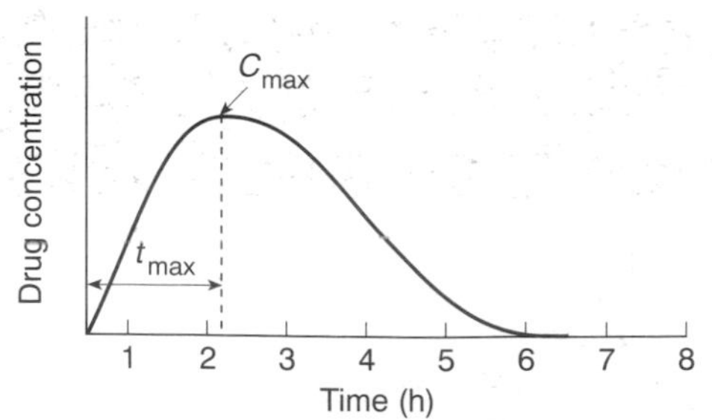

Fig. 6 Plasma concentrations of a typical drug after oral administration. C_{max} peak plasma concentration; t_{max} time to peak plasma concentration.

may therefore start to experience effects from such a drug within minutes of ingesting it.

Modified release formulations for oral administration

There are two theoretical benefits of sustained or controlled release oral preparations. They are either to prolong the absorption time and thereby extend the overall duration of action of a short-acting drug (Fig. 7) or to attenuate peak plasma concentrations of a drug where such peak concentrations could be associated with adverse effects. The commonest example in palliative medicine is controlled release morphine. Morphine is a short-acting drug with a duration of analgesia of about 4 h, so that in order to maintain control of chronic pain it has to be given six times a day. Controlled release morphine tablets have a 12- or 24-h duration of effect. Reduction in the frequency of dosing has important benefits in terms of patient acceptance and patient compliance. The theoretical reduction in adverse effects has not been demonstrated in practice with controlled release morphine.

Controlled release formulations are in general designed for maintenance treatment. The plasma concentration profile is different from that of an immediate or normal release preparation in that the time to peak plasma concentration is delayed and the peak is attenuated. This has implications for the use of such preparations. For example some drugs need to be rapidly absorbed and have a relatively short duration of action if they are to achieve their intended therapeutic effect without producing significant unwanted effects. This applies to analgesics used in the treatment of acute pain and it is inappropriate to use controlled release preparations in such situations.

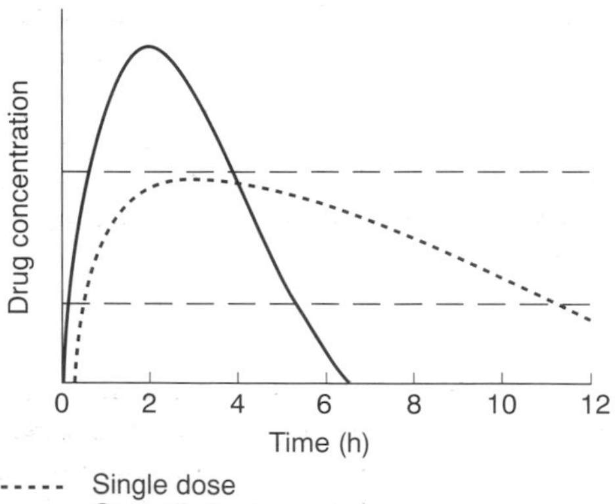

Fig. 7 Typical plasma concentration profile for an immediate release and controlled release formulation of the same drug.

Controlled release formulations prolong the absorption phase, but do not change the elimination process. For example the elimination half-life of morphine (2–4 h) is the same whether or not an immediate release or controlled release formulation is used.[4]

Subcutaneous and intramuscular

There are two main indications for parental administration of drugs in palliative medicine: when the oral route is unavailable or impractical, or when a rapid effect is required. If patients are unable to take oral medication, the alternative route most often used in palliative medicine is subcutaneous, and in general this mode of administration has replaced intramuscular injection.

In an historical context, this means that practice has come full circle in that the subcutaneous route was the first parenteral route to be adopted with the invention of the hypodermic syringe (hence the name) in the middle of the last century. The speed of absorption of drugs after subcutaneous and intramuscular injection is probably much the same and peak plasma concentrations are achieved within 15 to 30 min. The time to peak concentrations will be much influenced by blood flow to the site of injection. Blood flow through the skin is thought to be less than through the muscles, and this will certainly be the case in shocked patients with poor peripheral perfusion though in such circumstances blood flow through muscles is also reduced.

The disadvantages of subcutaneous injection compared with the intramuscular route are that there are limitations to the volume that may be injected because of the more superficial site, and drugs which are irritant may cause local pain and lead to the formation of sterile abscesses. The advantages of subcutaneous injection are that a smaller (and therefore less painful) needle is required, the chance of damage to nerves is less so that the site of injection is not so crucial, and the possibility of inadvertent intravenous injection is also less because veins can be seen more easily; subcutaneous injection is therefore simpler.

It is generally assumed that drugs administered by subcutaneous or intramuscular injection are completely absorbed into the systemic circulation (i.e. have a bioavailability near to 100 per cent) and this process may be very rapid. The absorption of many drugs may be complete within 30 min. In general intramuscular or subcutaneous injections will lead to a more rapid onset of drug action than oral administration but this does not always apply. Some drugs are not well absorbed after intramuscular injection and are likely to be even less well absorbed subcutaneously. Diazepam is a common example; oral administration of diazepam is more predictable and produces a more rapid effect than intramuscular injection.

Drugs administered by parenteral routes do not undergo presystemic ('first pass') metabolism. This needs to be taken into account when calculating equivalent doses if the route of administration is changed. Oral to parenteral relative potency ratios for opioid analgesics are discussed in Chapter 9.2.3.

Continuous subcutaneous infusions

The invention of portable, battery-operated, syringe drivers to administer a continuous, slow infusion of drugs was a major step forward from the cumbersome mains-operated syringe pumps which preceded them. They were first used widely to give desferrioxamine to patients with thalassaemia.[5] Many of the patients were children or adolescents and many were in developing countries and this use highlighted the relative cheapness, convenience, and acceptability of these devices. Other applications were soon reported including the continuous subcutaneous infusion of diamorphine to treat pain in patients with advanced cancer.[6] This technique is now very widely used in palliative medicine to administer a range of drugs using a variety of simple infusion devices and discussion of its application in specific indications will be found in other chapters (particularly Chapters 9.2.3, 9.3.4, and 17).

The main indications for a continuous subcutaneous infusion in palliative medicine are relatively few; persistent nausea and vomiting, inability to take oral medication in the final stages of illness before death, and, less commonly, severe dysphagia. However, there have been concerns almost from the time they were introduced into palliative care, that syringe drivers and similar devices are being inappropriately used to administer parenteral drugs to patients when there is no clear indication for them.[7] Anecdotal reports suggest that in some specialist palliative home-care services almost 100 per cent of patients had used a syringe driver at some stage of their final illness.

When properly indicated, continuous subcutaneous infusion of drugs is a simple and effective technique, which causes the minimum of discomfort to patients and facilitates nursing care particularly in the terminal stages. It is this simplicity and convenience which has sometimes led to its misuse in patients who could continue with oral medication. It is worth re-emphasizing (particularly with regard to opioid analgesics) that drugs given by the subcutaneous route (or any other parenteral route) are not inherently more effective than when given orally, a common misconception.

In the United Kingdom, diamorphine is the drug most commonly used in continuous subcutaneous infusions, but a recent survey found that 19 other drugs were being given by this means.[8] The most frequently used drug groups are opioid analgesics, antiemetics, anxiolytic sedatives, corticosteroids, non-steroidal anti-inflammatory drugs, and anticholinergic agents. Many of these drugs are used in combination with morphine or diamorphine, usually mixed in the same syringe or infusor. There have been concerns about chemical compatibility and stability of such mixtures[9] but relatively few specific investigations.[10,11] Some drugs are used in this way though the manufacturers do not have a licence for such use. However, there are sufficient data to support some specific guidelines for the most commonly used drugs.[12,13] Most of the published data on compatibility relates to drugs which can be mixed with diamorphine, which include cyclizine, dexamethasone, haloperidol, hyoscine butylbromide, hyoscine hydrobromide, methotrimeprazine, metoclopramide, and midazolam (Table 1).[13] Recently, data have been published on the compatibility of a variety of drugs likely to be used in palliative medicine with solutions of fentanyl citrate, hydromorphone hydrochloride, methadone hydrochloride, and morphine sulphate.[14] Outside of the United Kingdom, hydromorphone and morphine are the most widely used opioids for continuous infusions. Some of these mixtures may precipitate if high concentrations are used or if the drugs are not mixed at body temperature. If this occurs or if the solution becomes discoloured (particularly metoclopramide) the mixture should be discarded. The drugs listed above may also be mixed with morphine. In every case the infusion should be monitored to ensure that precipitation or discoloration has not occurred.

Table 1 Drugs which may be mixed with diamorphine in a syringe driver for continuous subcutaneous infusion:

Cyclizine[a]
Dexamethasone[b]
Haloperidol[c]
Hyoscine butylbromide
Hyoscine hydrobromide
Methotrimeprazine
Metoclopramide[d]
Midazolam

[a] Cyclizine may precipitate at concentrations above 10 mg/ml or in the presence of physiological saline or as the concentration of diamorphine relative to cyclizine increases; mixtures of diamorphine and cyclizine are also liable to precipitate after 24 h.

[b] Special care is needed to avoid precipitation of dexamethasone when preparing.

[c] Mixtures of haloperidol and diamorphine are liable to precipitate after 24 h if haloperidol concentration is above 2 mg/ml.

[d] Under some conditions metoclopramide may become discoloured; such solutions should be discarded.

Reproduced with permission from Anonymous. *Prescribing in Palliative Care. British National Formulary.* No. 31. London: British Medical Association and Royal Pharmaceutical Society of Great Britain, 1996.[13]

The use of two or three drugs concurrently in a continuous infusion raises questions about possible pharmacological interactions, quite apart from simple chemical reactions relating to the immiscibility or otherwise of drug solutions. For example diamorphine has been mixed together with haloperidol and midazolam[9] and other more exotic cocktails have been reported. It is important to promote a cautious approach to such mixtures. One of the major advances of modern palliative care has been the increasing sophistication of palliative therapeutics which is characterized by the effective use of the simplest available therapeutic tools. The increasing tendency to use drug cocktails by infusion is akin to the now outdated fashion for oral drug mixtures (the Brompton Cocktail, Mist Euphoriens, Cocktail Lytique) and is a step backwards to the dark ages of terminal care.

A number of drugs are too irritant to be given by continuous subcutaneous infusion. This applies to chlorpromazine and prochlorperazine, and diazepam. Some patients may also develop idiosyncratic local reactions to other drugs, including diamorphine given alone, which may lead to the formation of sterile abscesses.[15]

Continuous subcutaneous infusion of drugs has been an important development in palliative therapeutics and it is essential to ensure that it is seen neither as a panacea nor as an opportunity for therapeutic excesses.

Rectal

The rectal route was the traditional first choice for patients unable to take drugs by mouth. In palliative medicine it has tended to give way to subcutaneous infusions which are now generally more acceptable to patients, particularly if repeated rectal administration is required. However, this route may still be applicable if simple infusion devices are not available or in other situations where chronic administration is not planned and an alternative to oral dosing and injections is desirable.

The venous plexus surrounding the rectum and anal canal drains into the superior, middle, and inferior rectal veins. The superior rectal vein drains into the portal system whereas the others drain directly into the systemic circulation. Thus, it is possible that a proportion of any drug absorbed from the rectum will bypass the portal system and will not therefore be subject to first pass metabolism. This could result in greater bioavailability by the rectal route and an enhanced effect.

In practice, even drugs which undergo extensive presystemic metabolism often do not have a markedly increased bioavailability when given rectally. Morphine, for example, has similar bioavailability by oral and rectal routes. This probably reflects some of the limitations of rectal administration which will balance any enhancement that may result from avoiding first pass metabolism. These are the limited surface area for absorption, the presence of faeces which may prevent access to the rectal mucosa, interruption of absorption by defecation, and enzymatic degradation of the drug within the lumen and or the mucosal lining of the rectum.

The rectal route may in some circumstances provide a convenient mode of administration for dealing with emergency situations in palliative medicine. Rectal diazepam (in solution) achieves very rapid plasma concentrations and has been used in the management of status epilepticus in children. In palliative medicine respiratory panic attacks can be a difficult problem to cope with, particularly for patients being cared for at home who do not have immediate access to medical or nursing staff to administer drugs by injection. In such circumstances it is often possible to abort the attack by administering diazepam per rectum. This can be managed quite easily by relatives if the patient is at home, and diazepam is available in a liquid formulation designed for rectal administration.

A large number of drugs are available in suppository form for administration per rectum, in particular analgesics (opioid, non-opioid, and non-steroidal anti-inflammatory drugs), antiemetics, and anxiolytic sedatives.

Intravenous

This is the quickest way to achieve a drug effect, by introducing the drug directly into the systemic circulation. In palliative medicine this route is usually reserved for emergency situations, for example a patient with an excruciating exacerbation of pain or a patient with status epilepticus, where a rapid effect is necessary. Another indication for the intravenous route is for the administration of drugs to patients who have been unable to tolerate subcutaneous or intramuscular injection, or for children or adults who have an indwelling intravenous line. Irritant drugs such as cytotoxics are given intravenously and also drugs which need careful control of blood levels because of potential toxic effects (for example some antibiotics such as gentamicin).

There are several disadvantages to the intravenous route. The first is the need to gain venous access which may be a particular problem in some cancer patients who have received a lot of chemotherapy. In general terms the inability to remove a drug once it has been given, the higher incidence of anaphylaxis, and damage caused by extravasation of irritant substances are all potential problems. In long-term use of intravenous lines, infection may also be a problem.

Patients receiving drugs intravenously, particularly drugs with a narrow therapeutic index such as opioid analgesics, require close monitoring. Specific indications for using drugs intravenously in palliative medicine are relatively limited, so this route is generally avoided if there is a viable alternative.

Sublingual and buccal

Drugs may be placed under the tongue or between the cheek and gingiva for sublingual or buccal absorption. The putative advantages of these routes is that a very rapid effect may be obtained and drugs are absorbed directly into the systemic circulation, thus avoiding any first pass metabolism. Some drugs, for example glyceryl trinitrate, are absorbed extremely rapidly sublingually and glyceryl trinitrate produces relief of angina within minutes. Glyceryl trinitrate also undergoes extensive presystemic metabolism when given orally, so the sublingual route has major advantages for this drug. Unfortunately few other therapeutic agents are as effective by this route.

The number of drugs used by the sublingual and buccal routes in palliative medicine is limited. There have been anecdotal reports of the sublingual use of opioid analgesics, including morphine in solution, but pharmacokinetic studies have shown that absorption of these drugs by this route is generally poor and certainly unpredictable.[16] An exception is buprenorphine which is absorbed well by the sublingual route such that its analgesic potency by sublingual and intramuscular administration is more or less the same.[2] Sublingual lorazepam and buccal prochlorperazine are occasionally useful but many patients dislike the sensation of tablets or 'grittiness' under the tongue or in the buccal sulcus, and often the drug or excipients leave a bitter taste. In this patient population, in whom dry mouth is endemic, the potential for these preparations is very limited.

Dermal

A number of drugs are absorbed well through the skin and the amount of absorption and time course are sufficient to produce predictable systemic effects. The first drugs to be specifically formulated in skin patches were glyceryl trinitrate for the treatment of angina and hyoscine (scopolamine) for motion sickness. Several other transdermal preparations are now available: oestrogen for hormone replacement, clonidine for hypertension, nicotine for use in patients who are giving up smoking, and the potent opioid fentanyl for chronic pain.

There are several potential advantages of the transdermal route. It is a non-invasive parenteral route which may be particularly appropriate, for example, in patients who are nauseated or vomiting, or for drugs which undergo extensive presystemic metabolism (such as glyceryl trinitrate). Other patients in palliative medicine practice may benefit from this option, notably patients with severe dysphagia or with any other problem which restricts oral administration of drugs. Transdermal administration produces continuous plasma concentrations akin to subcutaneous or intravenous infusion, with less fluctuation than intermittent parenteral injections. The disadvantages are the delay in achieving therapeutic plasma concentrations and the delay in reaching steady state. There is a further complication with fentanyl in that a subcutaneous depot of the drug is formed so that absorption continues for a significant period following removal of the patch. The use of transdermal fentanyl is discussed in more detail in Chapter 9.2.3.

Transdermal hyoscine and fentanyl are both widely used in palliative medicine, though the latter is relatively recent and it is still finding its place in palliative therapeutics. Transdermal administration of both drugs may cause local irritation to the skin but the incidence of this adverse effect seems to be small.

Absorption of drugs through the skin may vary in different parts of the body, though this variation does not follow the same pattern with different drugs. Hyoscine patches are usually attached behind the ear; transdermal fentanyl to the lateral chest wall. Convenience and inconspicuousness are important considerations.

Inhalation

The alveoli of the lungs provide an enormous surface area for the absorption of drugs by inhalation. The most common use of this route is to provide general anaesthesia with volatile anaesthetic agents.

Drugs for inhalation can be administered either in the form of a liquid aerosol or as a dry powder. This route is in general designed to deliver drugs directly to the mucosal surfaces of the lungs in order to achieve a local effect. Bronchodilators and topical corticosteroids used in the treatment of reversible airways obstruction are common examples. These drugs are used in a conventional way to treat bronchospasm in palliative medicine.

The penetration of drug particles into the lungs depends on particle size. A particle size of 1 μm is required to get into the smallest bronchioles and alveoli, and in order to achieve this, an ultrasonic nebulizer is required. In palliative medicine there remains controversy about the efficacy of nebulized morphine for treating dyspnoea and in particular some debate as to whether any beneficial effect is mediated locally in the lungs or is a result of systemic absorption of morphine. This and the use of nebulized local anaesthetics for the relief of cough are described in Chapter 9.5.

Inhalation is not an efficient way to administer drugs topically to the alveolar membranes because a significant proportion is absorbed through the oropharyngeal mucosa or in the upper airways. Only about 10 to 20 per cent of each dose reaches the lungs. Large volume spacers improve this proportion by removing large particles on the wall of the spacer and reducing the speed of propulsion of the particles, allowing the propellant coating each particle to evaporate. Spacers also reduce the speed of impact of the particles on the oropharynx, reducing the amount of drug deposited there. Spacers are bulky and may be inconvenient to use but they significantly improve drug administration via aerosol inhalers, particularly in elderly patients.

Spinal

Spinal administration includes both epidural and intrathecal routes and is discussed in detail in Chapter 9.2.6.

In palliative medicine these routes will most often be used to administer analgesic drugs so that they are delivered directly to the relevant central nervous system receptors. The terminology can be confusing. 'Spinal' was a term originally synonymous with 'intrathecal injection' (which is the same as 'subarachnoid'), and 'extradural' is an alternative name for 'epidural'. In general, the convention that 'spinal' refers to both intrathecal and epidural administration is to be preferred.

Variability in drug response

Wide variability in the rates of drug metabolism occurs between individuals as a result of genetic factors, pathological processes, concurrent medication, and ageing and creates the major obstacle to matching dose to patients' requirements.

Both pharmacokinetic and pharmacodynamic factors may be responsible for therapeutic failure or adverse effects and the mechanism of each may relate to drug interaction, disease, genetics, or the effect of old age. The study of variability in drug response encompasses the whole of the science of clinical pharmacology. In this section we will merely highlight important principles and provide examples most relevant to palliative medicine.

Pharmacogenetics

Wide inter-individual variation in the rates of metabolism of drugs has been observed for many years and a combination of genetic and environmental factors is assumed to be responsible. Our understanding of the influence of genetic factors is increasing rapidly with the advent of modern molecular biological techniques. For example the rate of elimination of isoniazid within populations has been recognized to have a bimodal distribution.[17] This drug is N-acetylated and it is well known now that the rate of drug acetylation is under the control of two autosomal alleles, R for fast acetylation and r for slow (R being dominant and r recessive).[18] 'Fast acetylators' of isoniazid may be more susceptible to hepatic damage caused by the drug and at the same time may be at risk of under dosage with other agents which are acetylated.[19]

The high incidence of the recessive trait, which determines slow acetylation, may indicate a selective advantage for slow acetylators which is not related to drug metabolism. There is variation in the proportion of fast and slow acetylators in different populations and ethnic groups. In most European groups about 40 per cent are fast acetylators and in the United States 45 per cent, but 80 to 90 per cent of Asian populations and nearly 100 per cent of Canadian Eskimos are fast acetylators.[20] Numerous drugs are metabolized by acetylation and the effects of genetic polymorphism have not been studied for all. Hydralazine, some sulphonamides, and some benzodiazepines are worthy of mention but within the field of palliative medicine, where in general dose can be titrated to patients' needs, there do not appear to be significant clinical implications of this phenomenon.

A genetic component to drug oxidation was first documented when rates of metabolism of antipyrine were shown to have a greater degree of concordance in identical twins than in fraternal twins.[21] This was difficult to interpret because of the singular lack of any observed correlation in the rates of oxidation of different drugs between individuals. However, it was subsequently demonstrated that people who were slow oxidizers of debrisoquine were also slow metabolizers of other drugs such as sparteine, phenformin, phenytoin, metoprolol, nortriptyline, and others.[22] We now know that the enzyme system involved, cytochrome P450, can be classified into a number of subfamilies each of which is probably under genetic and environmental control. The most widely studied is the debrisoquine 4-hydroxylation phenotype which is under the control of cytochrome P450 2D6. About 90 per cent of the population are extensive metabolizers of debrisoquine and family studies have indicated that this is a dominant trait.[23,24] Using kinetic tests it has been shown that different racial groups exhibit different proportions of poor and extensive metabolizers. Egyptians show the lowest incidence of debrisoquine poor metabolizer status (about 1 per cent), whereas West Africans show the highest (about 13 per cent) and Caucasians have an intermediate incidence. There is evidence of genetic control in the metabolism of mephenytoin in which another isoform of cytochrome P450 is involved (2C9). About 3 per cent of Caucasians and 18 per cent of Japanese are poor metabolizers of mephenytoin.[25] The variation between poor and extensive metabolism is wide and it is important therefore that the doses of drugs linked to the debrisoquine or mephenytoin phenotype should be very carefully managed.

There are, of course, pharmacodynamic examples of genetic variation in drug response. These include resistance to the effects of warfarin due to increased sensitivity to vitamin K, haemolysis in patients with glucose 6-phosphate dehydrogenase deficiency in response to drugs such as sulphonamides or nitrofurantoin, and flushing in response to alcohol in patients taking chlorpropamide.[26]

Disease states

A myriad of conditions, both acute and chronic, can affect the response to drugs by both pharmacokinetic and pharmacodynamic mechanisms. From the pharmacokinetic viewpoint, diseases of the two most important organs of elimination, the kidney and the liver, are most important.

Excretion of drugs by the kidney depends either upon filtration of drug unbound to plasma protein at the glomerulus or upon the active transport systems which secrete drug at the renal tubule. In reality the reduction in the renal clearance of any drug closely follows renal function as measured by creatinine clearance. The consequences of renal disease therefore depend upon the extent to which renal clearance contributes to total drug clearance and how critical drug concentration is in terms of toxicity. Information about the need for dose adjustment in patients with renal impairment is usually readily available in prescribing information sources.

A more complex situation exists for hepatically metabolized drugs. The relevance to palliative medicine is much greater because centrally-active drugs tend to be those requiring metabolism simply because they are lipid soluble—a necessary property for penetration into the brain. The metabolic process converts them into more polar, water soluble metabolites. The liver is also much more commonly affected in malignant disease, not least because it is a common site for metastases.

In chronic liver disease there exist intrahepatic and extrahepatic anastomoses ('shunts') between the portal and systemic circulation. This means that drugs which normally have a low bioavailability because of presystemic metabolism in the liver can by-pass that metabolic process and may achieve a greatly increased oral bioavailability. This has been shown to occur with pentazocine, pethidine,[27] and chlormethiazole[28] (and many other drugs not used in palliative medicine) and may be expected to occur with methadone,[29] metoclopramide,[30] and others. Reduced metabolite formation of several drugs in the absence of a reduction in systemic clearance in patients with hepatic metastases suggests that such shunting can also take place within tumour deposits inside the liver.[31] This has great implications for oral dosing in malignant disease of drugs with normally low bioavailability.

In chronic liver disease the total mass of functioning hepatocytes is reduced. It is not surprising that drug metabolism is generally impaired. However, normal interindividual variation in drug metabolism rates is so wide that the effect of the disease may only be evident when severe. The level of serum albumin has been shown to correlate as closely as any parameter to the degree of pharmacokinetic disturbance.[32]

The situation is further complicated by an apparent differential effect on the enzyme system involved. Thus, glucuronidation seems to be relatively protected from the effects of liver disease compared to oxidation and demethylation and there is also evidence of a differential effect on the subfamilies of cytochrome P450.[31]

Hepatic drug metabolizing capacity is not just susceptible to local effects within that organ but widespread pathophysiological changes may affect drug clearance rates. Acute febrile illnesses and endocrine abnormalities may impair drug metabolism.

Some drugs rely on conversion within the liver to their active moiety, for example prednisone, methylprednisone, and many of the angiotensin converting enzyme inhibitors. This may render some drugs less effective than others in the presence of liver disease and influence the choice of drug in this situation.[31]

In malignant disease of the liver there appears to be no overall loss of functional hepatocytes so that systemic clearance is usually unimpaired.[33] Some more detailed studies of cytochrome P450 subfamilies are now emerging. It has been shown that CYP1A2 and CYP2E1 are decreased in cirrhosis but not in hepatocellular carcinoma[34] and there is evidence that P450s of the 2C subfamily may actually be upregulated (i.e. have increased activity) in patients with carcinoma.[35]

Not only renal and hepatic failure but also other organ failures can cause changes in distribution volume either through reducing plasma proteins to which drugs bind or through a qualitative change in the binding sites. Tissue binding may also be affected and the changes in body composition in relation to organ failure and cachexia may be expected to change a drug's distribution volume according to whether they are distributed mainly in water or in lipid tissue. Although poorly studied, the kinetic profile of many drugs is likely to be abnormal in the presence of advanced malignant disease.

In disease states pharmacodynamic mechanisms may cause altered response. Increased sensitivity to centrally acting agents and those acting on the cardiovascular system is common. Particular care is needed when both pharmacodynamic and pharmacokinetic changes are potentially occurring in the same patient, for example when using drugs with sedating properties in patients with hepatic impairment or respiratory insufficiency.

Ageing

Much of what has been said in respect of disease processes can be applied to the elderly, for after the age of about 65 years there is a gradual decline in renal and hepatic function. Body composition changes so that there is an increase in lipid in relation to total body weight and plasma albumin gradually declines. However, it should be emphasized that the changes in pharmacokinetics are quite small and are only detectable in group studies. The most notable change associated with ageing is an increase in variability so that no assumptions can be made about reduced doses being required and titration of dose to patients' requirements is just more difficult in the aged.

Well studied and of great interest is the effect of the ageing process on hepatic drug metabolism. Total hepatic mass decreases with age and much of the documented decline in drug metabolizing capacity can be attributed to the sheer reduction in total functional hepatocyte mass.[36] It appeared from studies with antipyrine and other agents that it was only microsomally-located enzyme systems which decline in activity with age but the results of studies are inconsistent[37] and it has been estimated that only 3 per cent of total variance in drug metabolic rate could be attributed to ageing.[38] A further source of debate is the response of the cytochrome P450 system to enzyme inhibitors and inducers with the obvious implications for drug interaction. There appears little doubt that cimetidine, and presumably other enzyme inhibitors, have a similar effect in the elderly compared to the young.[39] Earlier studies had suggested that microsomal enzymes in the elderly were incapable of being induced[40] (see below) but this suggestion is now completely refuted[37,41] and it is clear that elderly patients are at risk of drug interaction through these mechanisms in the same way as the young.

Reduced cardiovascular and other homeostatic mechanisms and reduced central nervous system function in the aged make this group susceptible to excessive effects from diuretics, blood pressure lowering agents, and central nervous system depressants. The prescription of prochlorperazine for the symptom of dizziness illustrates the potential hazards. The dizziness is usually due to age-related postural hypotension. However, the α-adrenergic blocking properties of the phenothiazine cause vasodilation and worsen the symptom, the dopamine receptor blocking effect precipitates parkinsonism, and the sedating effect causes intellectual impairment!

Drug interaction

Patients who develop terminal illnesses may already be receiving drugs for a variety of conditions. Some may still be required but others may not be necessary but may be continued because of the adverse impact of discontinuing them. If drugs to relieve symptoms are added, this creates an enormous potential for drug interaction. Interaction is adverse if it causes therapeutic failure or toxicity from any one drug. It may be regarded, therefore, as simply another source of variability in drug response. Remembering all the possible drug interactions is virtually impossible so frequent consultation with prescribing information is important. However, a knowledge of the underlying mechanisms of drug interaction can put the prescriber on guard.

In broad terms, drug interactions are either pharmacokinetic or pharmacodynamic. Kinetic interaction results in a change in the total body exposure to the drug reflected in a change in blood concentration. The effect is entirely predictable from that change. However, the existence of a pharmacokinetic interaction can not be easily predicted—every drug has to be studied before its potential for kinetic interaction can be recognized.

The site of pharmacodynamic interaction is the receptor and so it follows that the consequences of such interaction are common to pharmacological groupings of drugs and are therefore to some extent predictable from a working knowledge of each drug group.

Kinetic interaction arises through alteration in rate and extent of absorption, changes in metabolism (both presystemic and elimination), changes in distribution, and in renal excretion. Drugs such as metoclopramide, anticholinergics,[42] and opioid analgesics[43] which alter the rate of gastric emptying will affect the speed of absorption of other agents. Again, the resultant effects may not be easily predictable. It is of interest, for example, that food increases the bioavailability of morphine[44] and metoclopramide increases morphine's rate of absorption and sedative effects.[45] Some drugs bind others in the gastrointestinal tract and affect their bioavailability. Certain antacid preparations, iron salts, and cholestyramine are the worst offenders and care is necessary in the use of these drugs concurrently with others.

Of least importance are interactions through changes in distribution. This is because, as we have seen, volume of distribution is not a determinant of steady state concentration although an acute change could cause a temporary effect. In the past, much was made of interactions between drugs as a result of plasma protein binding displacement but this is actually rarely a problem. Even if a drug is very heavily bound to protein, displacement will result in only a temporary rise in the free (unbound) fraction because of immediate compensatory mechanisms. There will be wider distribution throughout the distribution volume and the first order nature of the elimination process results in increased removal of drug. Most clinically significant interactions previously ascribed to protein binding displacement have now been explained by enzyme inhibition.[46]

Drug interaction resulting from changes in the rate of metabolism by the liver will result in both changes in bioavailability (for those drugs with significant first pass effect) and decreased clearance. Steady state concentrations of drug may be profoundly affected. A number of drugs (particularly the barbiturates, carbamazepine, phenytoin, and rifampicin) are capable of inducing the mixed function oxidase and glucuronidase enzyme systems in the liver. The process involves hypertrophy of the endoplasmic reticulum and takes some weeks to be fully achieved. There is a myriad of substrates for this interaction, amongst them warfarin, corticosteroids, the oral contraceptive, and anticonvulsant drugs. Serum methadone levels can be reduced by the concurrent use of carbamazepine, phenobarbitone, and phenytoin[47] and by rifampicin.[48] The oestrogen component of the oral contraceptive has been shown to double the clearance of morphine by induction of glucuronyl transferase, suggesting the need for increased doses in patients on oestrogens.[49] Important to the care of patients with malignancy is the trebling in plasma clearance of dexamethasone which can occur in patients receiving concurrently phenytoin, phenobarbitone, or rifampicin, or presumably other enzyme inducers, leading to a reduced bioavailability and shortened half-life.[50]

Our understanding of the process of inhibition of the mixed function oxidase system by drugs has increased dramatically in recent years with the identification of the subfamilies of cytochrome P450. Previously, there was no explanation as to why one drug might reduce the clearance of a second but not that of a third. It is now clear that some drugs inhibit specific subfamilies whilst others, such as cimetidine, are capable of inhibiting all forms of cytochrome P450. That is why cimetidine causes interaction with so many other agents. Cimetidine has been reported to precipitate apnoea in patients taking methadone[51] and to have had a similar effect in a patient taking morphine[52] but others have found only a small and insignificant effect on morphine kinetics.[53] Other H_2 receptor blocking drugs have no enzyme inhibitory effect and the proton pump inhibitor omeprazole has a modest and rather unpredictable effect.

Clomipramine and amitriptyline increase the bioavailability and reduce the clearance of morphine and enhance the analgesic effect. The mechanism seems to be both kinetic, through enzyme inhibition, and pharmacodynamic, through the antidepressants' analgesic effects.[54] Enzyme inhibition tends to occur rapidly so that the full effect is seen after four or five of the newly prolonged half-lives. The list of drugs which cause interaction through enzyme inhibition is long but non-steroidal anti-inflammatory drugs, especially azapropazone,[55] and some of the opioid analgesics, such as dextropropoxyphene,[56] are implicated.

The most important drug interactions in the kidney involve competition between agents for active tubular secretion. This process is used by organic acids and the most frequent 'interactors' are the loop diuretics and some non-steroidal anti-inflammatory drugs. The renal excretion of methotrexate may be inhibited by some non-steroidal anti-inflammatory drugs through this mechanism.[57] Although renal excretion of some drugs is pH dependent, and this can be useful in the management of poisonings, it has in general minor implications in normal therapeutics. There are a few exceptions; for example methadone's renal clearance is considerably enhanced by concurrent use of urinary acidifiers such as acetazolamide.[58]

Of pharmacodynamic interactions, those of greatest import in palliative medicine involve intracerebral mechanisms. Drugs which cause sedation also have the potential to cause confusion. Not only can central nervous system depressants summate in their action but if the ionic or metabolic environment is deranged by other drugs such as diuretics the problem may be compounded. It is of interest that certain benzodiazepines have been shown to oppose the respiratory depressant action of some opioid analgesics[59] whilst increasing the drowsiness associated with others without affecting kinetics.[60] Phenothiazines increase the risk of respiratory depression, sedation, and hypotension.[61]

Polypharmacy

Polypharmacy is endemic in palliative medicine. A recent survey of 385 patients 3 weeks after referral to a palliative care service found that the median number of drugs per patient was five, with a maximum of 11.[62] These numbers are similar to those reported in other elderly patient populations, particularly those admitted to hospital with drug-induced illness.[63] There are several causes of polypharmacy[64] and in palliative medicine some justification. Patients with advanced cancer invariably suffer several symptoms, many of which will be amenable to drug therapy. This may justify the use of combinations of drugs but the overriding principle here must be to avoid unnecessary duplicate prescribing which may occur with significant frequency even in leading specialist centres[62] and to be aware of potential consequences of multiple drug use. Clearly, the more drugs employed at any one time the greater the likelihood of drug interaction. Sometimes such interaction will be unpredictable, but often adverse consequences of polypharmacy may be both predictable and avoidable. Increasingly, there is a move towards the production of clinical guidelines and drug formularies which should have the effect of improving prescribing habits and encouraging the use of the simplest effective remedies.

Apart from avoiding duplicate prescribing of similar drugs, there are other important principles of good practice which will reduce the tendency towards polypharmacy. The drug regimen should be regularly reviewed and potentially redundant treatments identified. It is always easier to continue treatments particularly if they are not causing any obvious problems, and often patients are reluctant to give up old friends. Both patient and physician need to be persuaded of the benefit of stopping drugs. Adverse effects of one symptomatic remedy may be self limiting, both in terms of severity and duration, so that any additional treatment introduced to deal with them may be continued unnecessarily. Nausea associated with morphine for example is usually an initiation side-effect, if it occurs at all, and may need specific treatment only for a few days; similarly drowsiness, which will usually not require any additional drug intervention. Trials of therapy for specific symptoms should be encouraged and the treatment changed if ineffective rather than continued in conjunction with a new drug.

Conclusions

The skilful use of drugs to palliate symptoms is essential to the practice of palliative medicine. Individualization of drug and dose and simplicity are the watchwords whatever type of treatment is being used. An understanding of the principles outlined in this chapter should facilitate day-to-day management of clinical problems, improve the risk–benefit ratio of drugs used in symptom control, and ultimately contribute to improving the quality of life of patients with advanced disease.

References

1. Ettinger DS, Vitale PJ, Trump DL. Important clinical pharmacologic considerations in the use of methadone in cancer patients. *Cancer Treatment Reports*, 1979; **63**: 457–9.
2. Bullingham RES, McQuay H, Dwyer D, Allen MC, Moore RA. Sublingual buprenorphine used post-operatively: clinical observations and preliminary pharmacokinetic analysis. *British Journal of Clinical Pharmacology*, 1981; **12**: 117–22.
3. Coyle N, Adelhardt J, Flowy KM, Portenoy RK. Character of terminal illness in the advanced cancer patient: pain and other symptoms during last four weeks of life. *Journal of Pain and Symptom Management*, 1990; **5**: 83–9.
4. Savarese J, Goldenheim PD, Thomas GB, Kaiko RF. Steady-state pharmacokinetics of controlled release oral morphine sulphate in healthy subjects. *Clinical Pharmacokinetics*, 1986; **11**: 505–10.
5. Wright B M, Callan K. Slow drug infusions using a portable syringe driver. *British Medical Journal*, 1979; **2**: 582.
6. Russell PSB. Analgesia in terminal malignant disease. *British Medical Journal*, 1979; **1**: 1561.
7. O'Neill WM. Subcutaneous infusions—a medical last rite. *Palliative Medicine*, 1994; **8**: 91–3.
8. Johnson I, Patterson S. Drugs used in combination in the syringe driver—a survey of hospice practice. *Palliative Medicine*, 1992; **6**: 125–30.
9. Regnard CFB, Mannix K. Subcutaneous drug compatibility in palliative care. *Lancet*, 1989; **iii**: 1044.

10. Allwood MC. Diamorphine mixed with anti-emetic drugs in plastic syringes. *British Journal of Pharmaceutical Practice,* 1984; **6**: 88–90.
11. Regnard C, Pashley S, Westrope F. Anti-emetic/diamorphine mixture compatibility in infusion pumps. *British Journal of Pharmacutical Practice,* 1986; **8**: 218–20.
12. Twycross RG. Alternative routes of administration. In: Twycross RG (ed). *Pain Relief in Advanced Cancer.* Edinburgh: Churchill Livingstone, 1994: 349–63.
13. Anonymous. Prescribing in palliative care. In: *British National Formulary, Number 32.* London: British Medical Association and the Royal Pharmaceutical Society of Great Britain, 1996: 12–15.
14. Chandler SW, Trissel LA, Weinstein SM. Combined adminstration of opioids with selected drugs to manage pain and other cancer symptoms: initial safety screening for compatibility. *Journal of Pain and Symptom Management,* 1996; **12**: 168–71.
15. Hoskin PJ, Hanks GW, White ID. Sterile abscess formation by continuous subcutaneous infusion of diamorphine. *British Medical Journal,* 1988; **296**: 1065.
16. Ripamonti C, Bruera E. Rectal, buccal and sublingual narcotics for the management of cancer pain. *Journal of Palliative Care,* 1991; **7**: 30–5.
17. Evans DAP, Manley KA, McKusick VA. Genetic control of isoniazid metabolism in man. *British Medical Journal,* 1960; **ii**: 485.
18. Sim E, Hickman D. Polymorphism in human N-acetyltransferase—the case for the missing allele. *Trends in Pharmacological Science,* 1991; **12**: 1211–13.
19. Ellard GA, Gammon PT. Acetylator phenotyping of tuberculosis patients using matrix isoniazid on sulphadimidine and its prognostic significance for treatment with several intermittent isoniazid-containing regimens. *British Journal of Clinical Pharmacology,* 1977; **4**: 5–14.
20. Lunde PKM, Frislid K, Hansteen V. Disease and acetylation polymorphism. *Clinical Pharmacokinetics,* 1977; **2**: 182.
21. Vesell ES. Pharmacogenetics. *Biochemical Pharmacology,* 1975; **24**: 445–50.
22. Steiner E, Iselius L, Alvan G, Lindstein J, Sjoqvist F. A family study of genetic and environmental factors determining polymorphic hydroxylation of debrisoquine in man. *Clinical Pharmacology and Therapeutics,* 1985; •**38**: 394–401.
23. Eichelbaum M, Gross AS. The genetic polymorphism of debrisoquine/sparteine metabolism—clinical aspects. *Clinical Pharmacology and Therapeutics,* 1990; **46**: 377–94.
24. Gonzalez FJ, Meyer UA. Molecular genetics of the debrisoquine/sparteine polymorphism. *Clinical Pharmacology and Therapeutics,* 1991; **50**: 233–8.
25. Gibson GG, Skett P. *Introduction to Drug Metabolism.* 2nd edn. Glasgow: Blackie Academic and Professional, 1994.
26. Sjoqvist F, Borga, Orme M. Fundamentals of clinical pharmacology. In: Speight TM (ed). *Avery's Drug Treatment.* Auckland: ADIS, 1987.
27. Pond SM, Tong T, Benowitz NL, Jacob P. Enhanced bioavailability of pethidine and pentazocine in patients with cirrhosis of the liver. *Australian and New Zealand Journal of Medicine,* 1980; **10**: 515.
28. Pentikainen PJ, Neuvonen PJ, Jostell KG. Pharmacokinetics of chlormethiazole in healthy volunteers and patients with cirrhosis of the liver. *European Journal of Pharmacology,* 1980; **17**: 275.
29. Inturrusi CE, Verebely K. Disposition of methadone in man after a single oral dose. *Clinical Pharmacology and Therapeutics,* 1972; **13**: 923–30.
30. Bateman DN. Clinical pharmacokinetics of metoclopramide. *Clinical Pharmacokinetics,* 1983; **8**: 523–9.
31. Morgan DJ, McLean AJ. Clinical pharmacokinetic and pharmacodynamic considerations in patients with liver disease. *Clinical Pharmacokinetics,* 1995; **29**: 370–91.
32. Homeida, M, Jackson L, Roberts CJC. Decreased first pass metabolism of labetalol in chronic liver disease. *British Medical Journal,* 1978; **2**: 1048.
33. Robertz-Vaupel GM, Lindecken KD, Edeki T, *et al.* Disposition of antipyrine inpatients with extensive metastatic liver disease. *European Journal of Clinical Pharmacology,* 1992; **42**: 465–9.
34. Guengerich FP, Turvy CG. Comparison of levels of several human microsomal cytochrome P450 enzymes and epoxide hydrolase in normal and disease states using immunochemical analysis of surgical liver samples. *Journal of Pharmacology and Experimental Therapeutics,* 1991; **256**: 1189–91.
35. Murray M. P450 enzymes: inhibition mechanisms, genetic regulation and effects of liver disease. *Clinical Pharmacokinetics,* 1992; **23**: 132–46.
36. Swift CG, Homeida M, Halliwell M, Roberts CJC. Antipyrine disposition and liver size in the elderly. *European Journal of Clinical Pharmacology,* 1985; **20**: 119–28.
37. Durnas C, Loi CM, Cusack BJ. Hepatic drug metabolism and aging. *Clinical Pharmacokinetics,* 1990; **19**: 359–89.
38. Vestal RE, Norris AH, Tobin JD, Cohen BH, Shock NW, *et al.* Antipyrine metabolism in man: influence of age, alcohol, caffeine and smoking. *Clinical Pharmacology and Therapeutics,* 1975; **18**: 425–32.
39. Feely J, Pareira I, Guy E, Hockings N. Factors affecting the response to inhibition of drug metabolism by cimetidine—dose response and sensitivity of elderly and induced subjects. *British Journal of Clinical Pharmacology,* 1984; **17**: 77–81.
40. Salem SAM, Rajjayabun P, Shepherd AMM, Stevenson IH. Reduced induction of drug metabolism in the elderly. *Age and Ageing,* 1978; **7**: 68–73.
41. Pearson MW, Roberts CJC. Drug induction of hepatic enzymes in the elderly. *Age and Ageing,* 1984; **13**: 313–16.
42. Nimmo J, Heading RC, Tothill P, Prescott LF. Pharmacological modification of gastric emptying: effects of propantheline and metoclopramide on paracetamol absorption. *British Medical Journal,* 1973; **1**: 587–9.
43. Nimmo WS, Heading RC, Wilson J, Tothill P, Prescott LF. Inhibition of gastric emptying and drug absorption by narcotic analgesics. *British Journal of Clinical Pharmacology,* 1975; **2**: 509–13.
44. Gourlay GK, Plummer JL, Cherry DA, Foate JA, Cousins MJ. Influence of a high fat meal on the absorption of morphine from oral solutions. *Clinical Pharmacology and Therapeutics,* 1989; **46**: 463–8.
45. Manara AR, Shelley MP, Quinn K, Park GR. The effect of metoclopramide on the absorption of oral controlled release morphine. *British Journal of Clinical Pharmacology,* 1988; **25**: 518–21.
46. Kristensen MB. Drug interaction and clinical pharmacokinetics. In: Gibaldi M, Prescott L (eds). *Handbook of Clinical Pharmacokinetics.* Auckland: ADIS Health Science Press, 1983.
47. Bell J, Seves V, Bowren P, Lewis J, Batey R. The use of serum methadone levels in patients receiving methadone maintenance. *Clinical Pharmacology and Therapeutics,* 1988; **43**: 623–9.
48. Bending MR, Skacel PO. Rifampicin and methadone withdrawal. *Lancet,* 1977; **i**: 1211.
49. Watson KJR, Ghabrial H, Mashford ML, Harman PJ, Breen KJ, Desmond PV. The oral contraceptive pill increases morphine clearance but does not increase hepatic blood flow. *Gastroenterology,* 1986; **90**: 1779.
50. Anonymous. Dexamethasone. In: Dollery C, Boobis AR, Burley D, *et al.* (eds.) *Therapeutic Drugs.* Edinburgh: Churchill Livingstone, 1991: D44–D50.
51. Dawson GW, Vestal RE. Cimetidine inhibits the *in vitro* N-demethylation of methadone. *Research Communications in Chemical Pathology and Pharmacology,* 1984; **46**: 301–4.
52. Fine A, Churchill DN. Potential lethal interaction of cimetidine and morphine. *Canadian Medical Association Journal,* 1981; **124**: 1434.
53. Lam AM, Clement JL. Effect of cimetidine pre-medication on morphine-induced ventilatory depression. *Canadian Anaesthetic Society Journal,* 1984; **31**: 36–43.
54. Ventafridda V, Ripamonti C, De Conno F, Bianchi M, Pazzuconi F, Panerai AE. Antidepressants increase bioavailability of morphine in cancer patients. *Lancet,* 1987; **i**: 1204.
55. Roberts CJC, Daneshmend TK, Macfarlane D, Dieppe PA. Anticonvulsant intoxication precipitated by azapropazone. *Postgraduate Medical Journal,* 1981; **57**: 191.

56. Orme M, Breckenridge A. Warfarin and distalgesic interaction. *British Medical Journal,* 1976; **i**: 200.
57. Daly HM, Scott GL, Boyle J, Roberts CJC. Methotrexate toxicity precipitated by azapropazone. *British Journal of Dermatology,* 1986; **114**: 733–5.
58. Bellward GD, Warren DM, Howald W, Axelson JE, Abbott PS. Methadone maintenance: effect of urinary pH on renal clearance in chronic high and low doses. *Clinical Pharmacology and Therapeutics,* 1977; **22**: 92–9.
59. McDonald CF, Thomson SA, Scott NC, Scott W, Grant IWB, Crompton GK. Benzodiazepine–opiate antagonism—a problem in intensive care therapy. *Intensive Care Medicine,* 1986; **12**: 39–42.
60. Pond SM, Benowitz NL, Jacob P, Rigod J. Lack of effect of diazepam on methadone metabolism in methadone-maintained addicts. *Clincial Pharmacology and Therapeutics,* 1982; **31**: 139–43.
61. Grothe DR, Ereshefsky L, Jann MW, Fidone GS. Clinical implication of the neuroleptic–opioid interaction. *Drug Intelligence in Clinical Pharmacology,* 1986; **20**: 75–7.
62. Twycross RG, Bergl S, John S, Lewis K. Monitoring drug use in palliative care. *Palliative Medicine,* 1994; **8**: 137–43.
63. Colt AG, Shapiro AP. Drug induced illness as a cause for admission to a community hospital. *Journal of the American Geriatric Society,* 1989; **37**: 323–6.
64. Kroenke K. Polypharmacy. Causes, consequences, and cure. *The American Journal of Medicine,* 1985; **79**: 149–52.

8

Interventional radiology

8 Interventional radiology

A. Adam and Anne P. Hemingway

One of the most significant medical discoveries was that of X-rays by Roentgen in 1895. Exactly a century later, the discipline of radiology would be unrecognizable to the early pioneers. Conventional radiography techniques have been joined by other modalities including computerized tomography, nuclear medicine, ultrasound, and magnetic resonance imaging. Added to all these diagnostic modalities has been the discipline of interventional radiology.[1,2] The emergence of this specialty has been made possible by the enormous technological advances in relation to catheter and instrument design and manufacture, imaging systems, and radiological expertise. Some of the procedures encompassed by interventional radiology have virtually replaced more invasive and hazardous surgical alternatives. Other interventional manoeuvres offer completely new therapeutic options. Invasive techniques are subdivided into diagnostic and therapeutic categories although in any one patient a diagnostic procedure is frequently followed by a therapeutic manoeuvre. For example percutaneous antegrade pyelography performed to delineate the site and nature of renal obstruction is usually followed immediately by the placement of a nephrostomy drainage catheter.[3] The purely diagnostic procedures (e.g. biopsy, etc.) will not be discussed in any detail as they are largely inappropriate for the patient with a known terminal or neoplastic process receiving palliative care.

All interventional procedures carry some risk which is interdependent on the underlying condition, the nature of the procedure, and the experience of the radiologist. Therefore, it is important in patients with advanced malignant disease receiving palliative care to contemplate only those procedures which will alleviate symptoms, improve the quality of life, and where the potential benefits outweigh the risks.

Interventional radiology can make a significant contribution to the palliation of patients with irresectable malignant tumours, as many of the procedures can relieve symptoms without the need for general anaesthesia, a prolonged stay in hospital, or the discomfort associated with recovery from a surgical operation. The vast majority of procedures are performed using local anaesthesia and mild sedation where necessary. The emphasis in this chapter is on the indications, contraindications, and likely success rate as opposed to detailed technical descriptions.

Therapeutic interventional radiological procedures

A summary of procedures which may be useful in patients undergoing palliative care is shown in Table 1.

Percutaneous puncture and drainage procedures

Utilizing fluoroscopy, ultrasound, or computerized tomography it is possible to image and drain obstructed renal and biliary systems, cysts, abscesses, and effusions.

Renal tract[4]

Antegrade pyelography and percutaneous nephrostomy are useful in the management of a variety of situations including malignant obstruction of the urinary tract, haemorrhagic cystitis secondary to chemotherapy where it is desirable to divert the urine to 'rest' the bladder, and in patients with pelvic malignancy where either the disease or the treatment has resulted in the development of fistulas between the bladder and rectum or vagina and hence incontinence. Diversion of urinary flow may assist in healing of the fistulas, ease nursing problems, and allow patients to become 'dry' (Fig. 1).

The pelvicalyceal system is initially punctured with a fine-gauge needle through which radiographic contrast medium is instilled to opacify the system and hence to determine the anatomy and level of obstruction. Percutaneous nephrostomy entails the insertion into the collecting system of a pigtail configuration catheter with multiple, large side ports. If drainage is to be of short duration, an

Table 1 Interventional radiological procedures

Procedure	Examples of indications
Drainage	Malignant obstruction of renal or biliary tract
Dilatation	Oesophageal obstruction, superior vena caval obstruction, etc
'Feeding'	Venous access—Hickman lines, percutaneous gastrostomy
Extraction	Retrieval or resiting of venous lines
Infusion	Regional, selective infusion of chemotherapeutic agents
Embolization	Hormone producing metastases, primary hepatomas, skeletal metastases, etc.

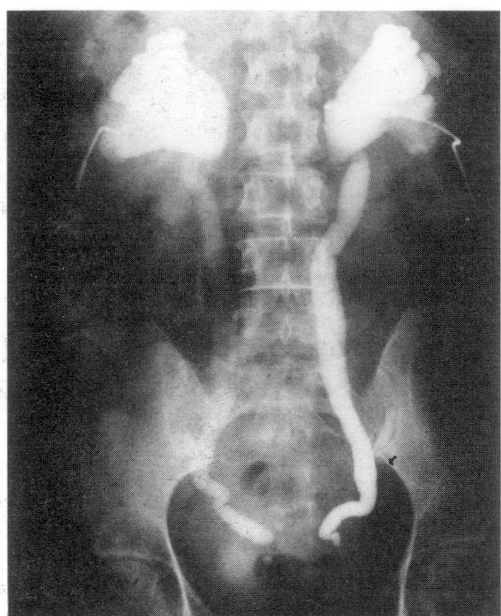

Fig. 1 Percutaneous renal drainage.

external bag may be satisfactory; however, if long-term drainage is required and if it is possible to cross the area of obstruction, an internal drain (e.g. double-ended pigtail catheter) or stent is preferred,[5] thus allowing the patient to be free of 'bags'. It is noteworthy that, in most cases, it is possible to manipulate a catheter across an area of apparently complete obstruction. Although a contrast study may indicate total obstruction, a hydrophilic guide wire can usually be advanced through the 'obstruction', as it finds the (very narrow) lumen and follows it. The balloon catheter can then be advanced over the guide wire to dilate the stricture and restore patency before a stent is inserted.

In patients with pelvic malignancy and fistulas to the perineum it may prove necessary to combine nephrostomy with ureteric embolization using steel coils or segments of gelatine sponge to prevent any urine reaching the skin of the perineum.[6] A catheter can be manipulated into the ureter and embolic materials, such as steel coils and sterile sponge, can be injected to occlude the ureter.

Biliary tract

Ultrasound is used to determine the site of malignant biliary tract obstruction, following which a percutaneous transhepatic cholangiogram is performed. An external drain is inserted into the dilated biliary system to allow decompression. If drainage is required for any significant length of time, and providing it is technically feasible, an internal–external drain or a completely indwelling stent (endoprosthesis) can be inserted (Fig. 2). An endoprosthesis is desirable in all patients with inoperable malignant obstructive jaundice as it is not associated with the physical and psychological problems that accompany external catheters. Endoprostheses may be inserted endoscopically for lesions affecting the low common bile duct or percutaneously in patients with lesions at the hilum of the liver. Self-expandable metallic stents can be inserted using a relatively small introducing catheter and yet these achieve a large internal diameter when released across the lesion.

The commonest form of occlusion of biliary endoprostheses is bile encrustation, the occurrence of which is inversely proportional to the calibre of the stent. As self-expandable metallic stents have a much larger internal lumen than plastic endoprostheses, they are much less prone to occlusion due to encrustation of bile. However, they can become blocked by tumour growing through the mesh of the stent or extending above or below the endoprosthesis. The overall failure rate of plastic stents is in the region of 30 to 40 per cent, whereas that of metallic stents is 10 to 15 per cent. The frequency of cholangitis is approximately 30 per cent in patients with plastic stents and approximately 10 per cent in patients with metallic endoprostheses. Haemorrhage is an unusual complication with both types of stent; it is seen in 2 to 4 per cent of patients. Occluded plastic stents can be replaced using a variety of endoscopic or percutaneous techniques. Occluded metallic endoprostheses cannot be removed but their patency can be restored by the introduction of a second device inserted coaxially within the first. Unless a patient with an occluded stent is considered to have a very short life expectancy, it is well worth considering restoring the patency of an occluded stent as this can greatly improve the patient's quality of life.[7,8]

Abscess drainage[9]

In appropriate situations, that is except where surgery is safer and more effective, percutaneous puncture of an abscess cavity under computerized tomography or ultrasound guidance and aspiration of contents for bacteriological analysis can be followed by insertion of a drainage catheter. It is possible to instil antibiotics into the cavity and percutaneous drainage may be effective either as the definitive treatment or as a temporary measure until the appropriate surgery can be contemplated.

Dilatation techniques[2]

The dilatation procedures are most commonly employed for the treatment of non-malignant conditions in the vascular tree (percutaneous transluminal angioplasty). These techniques can, however,

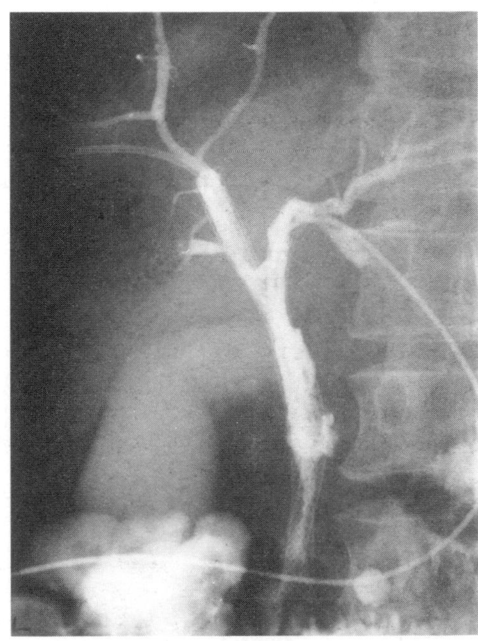

Fig. 2 Percutaneous biliary drainage.

also be applied to benign and malignant narrowings (or stenoses) and occlusions in other systems including the gastrointestinal tract, renal, and biliary systems.

Gastrointestinal tract

Within the gastrointestinal tract, oesophageal dilatation has proved to be a particularly useful technique. Dilatation alone is unlikely to be effective in malignant oesophageal strictures and should be followed by some form of stenting. Rigid plastic tubes inserted endoscopically or under fluoroscopic guidance have been used for several years. However, recently self-expandable metallic endoprostheses have become available;[10] some of these are covered with plastic in order to prevent ingrowth of tumour through the wall of the stent. These stents can be inserted using fluoroscopic guidance under light sedation, unlike rigid plastic tubes which are too large to be inserted without the use of general anaesthesia. A commonly used device, the Wallstent endoprosthesis (Schneider SA, Bulach, Switzerland), is inserted using an 18F or 22F introducing catheter and expands to a diameter of 20 mm or 25 mm. The procedure can be rapidly performed, on an outpatient basis if necessary. The quality of swallowing can be graded from 0 for normal swallowing to 4 for complete dysphagia. The mean dysphagia score of patients with oesophageal carcinoma treated with self-expandable metallic endoprostheses is 1 (Adam *et al.*, data submitted for publication). Most patients treated with rigid plastic tubes have a dysphagia score greater than 2, and the majority can manage only a liquid or semiliquid diet. We have recently carried out a prospective randomized comparison of self-expandable metallic stents with endoscopic laser treatment in patients with oesophageal carcinoma; this has shown that the mean reduction in dysphagia score was 2 points in patients treated with metallic stents and only 1 point in patients with laser treatment. In addition to greater improvement in the quality of swallowing, the rate of perforation of the oesophagus is negligible with metallic stents (there have been no perforations in our own series) whereas it is in the region of 10 to 15 per cent when using rigid plastic tubes and 5 to 10 per cent when using laser. A prospective randomized comparison has shown that although metallic stents are more expensive than rigid plastic tubes, they are cost-effective because they minimize the rate of complications and reduce the length of hospital stay.[11]

Plastic-covered stents are also very useful in the management of malignant oesophageal fistulas. They result in an immediate seal of the fistula and the patient can drink fluids a few hours after the procedure, resuming a normal diet on the following day[10] (Fig. 3).

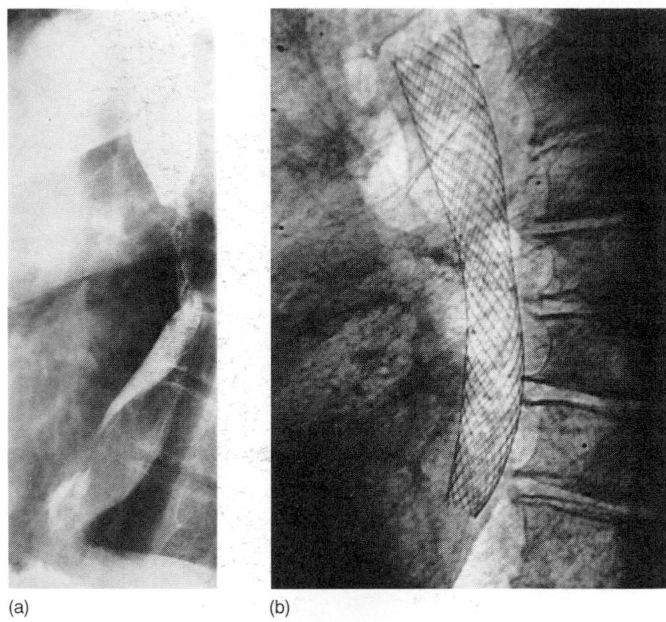

(a) (b)

Fig. 3 Oesophageal stenting.

Venous obstruction

The superior vena caval syndrome often represents a very distressing and unpleasant preterminal event in patients with thoracic malignancy. It is most commonly (approximately 90 per cent of cases) related to mediastinal neoplasia, particularly primary and secondary lung tumours and lymphoma. The obstruction, which can be partial or complete, can be caused by either caval compression and/or invasion by tumour and is frequently complicated by venous thrombosis.

Superior venacavography delineates the site and extent of the obstruction. If extensive thrombosis is present, selective intravenous thrombolysis with a catheter placed within the thrombus is undertaken under local anaesthesia. Percutaneous transfemoral dilatation of the narrowed superior vena cava is followed by the insertion of self-expandable metallic endoprostheses. Flow is restored immediately providing excellent and immediate palliation of symptoms[12] (Fig. 4). This procedure can be performed prior to, in conjunction with, or after therapy, including radiotherapy or chemotherapy (Fig. 5).

Malignant involvement of the inferior vena cava can be managed in a similar fashion. It is inappropriate for any patient to suffer the distress of superior vena cava obstruction without consideration for this relatively straight forward and successful procedure which can readily improve the quality of life.

Self-expandable metallic stents can be inserted in the trachea or main bronchi of patients with inoperable tracheobronchial malignancy to restore patency of the airways and prevent collapse and/or infection of the lung distal to a malignant stenosis. This procedure is best carried out, under general anaesthesia, as a combined effort between an interventional radiologist and a bronchoscopist. Bronchoscopic visualization is used to determine the position of the stricture, the limits of which are marked with a radio-opaque marker. The stricture is then dilated under fluoroscopic guidance. Following dilatation, a self-expandable metallic stent (such as a Wallstent endoprosthesis) is released across the stricture, again under fluoroscopic guidance. This can result in significant symptomatic improvement and prevent infection and abscess formation beyond an obstructing lesion.

Feeding techniques

Venous access

Central venous access may be essential in some patients with terminal disease for feeding and the delivery of drugs, particularly analgesia. In many centres, radiological techniques are now used to insert Hickman catheters under fluoroscopic control. The procedure is performed in the radiology department under local anaesthesia and strict asepsis. The advantage over the usual surgical method is that performing the procedure under fluoroscopic

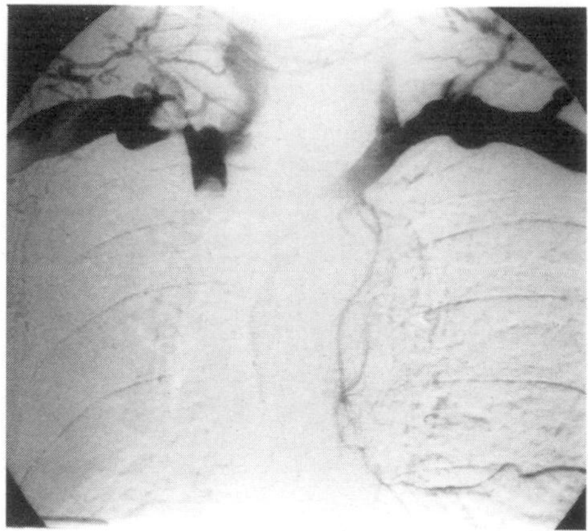

(a)

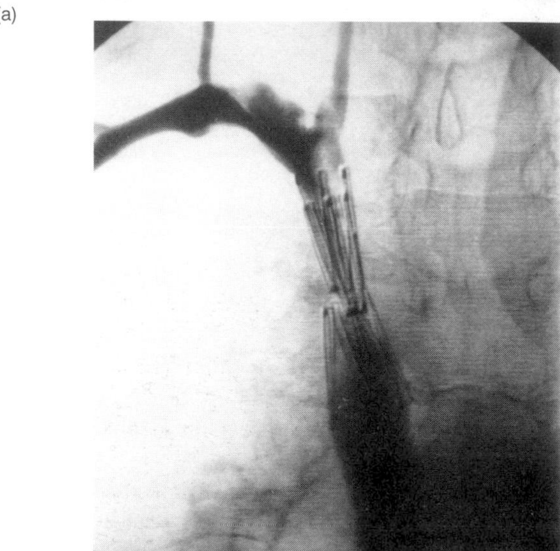

(b)

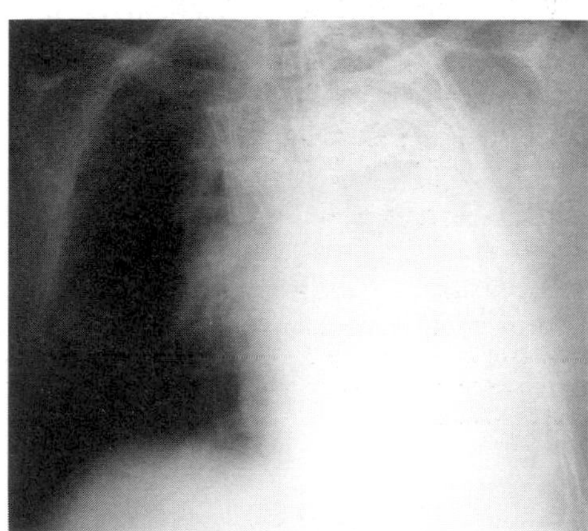

(c)

Fig. 4 Superior vena caval stenting. (a) Superior venacavogram reveals extensive thrombosis and narrowing of the superior vena cava by tumour. (b) Following selective thrombolysis, metallic stents have been placed across the compressed area which was initially dilated with a balloon. A repeat venogram confirms patency of the superior vena cava. (c) A chest radiograph shows the stents in place and the extensive tumour affecting the left hemithorax and mediastinum. The patient's symptoms showed immediate improvement and had completely resolved by 24 h.

control ensures that the tip of the catheter is always in the correct position and virtually eliminates the need for repositioning the catheter at a later date. The procedure is rapid, well tolerated by the patient, and associated with a high success and low complication rate.[13] In our experience, it is virtually always possible to gain venous access using intervention radiological methods. The rate of occurrence of pneumothorax when using a subclavian approach is approximately 1 per cent. This complication is very rare when access is gained via the internal jugular vein. The long-term complications of occlusion and infection of the catheter are not significantly different from those observed when a surgical method of venous access is used. The traditional surgical method of placement without imaging guidance is associated with a misplacement rate of approximately 6 per cent, whereas this complication does not occur when catheter placement is performed under imaging guidance.

Percutaneous gastrostomy

Patients with terminal disease of neoplastic and non-neoplastic origin may require intervention to assist with feeding and hydration.

The insertion of a feeding gastrostomy tube either under fluoroscopic or endoscopic guidance and local anaesthesia can significantly improve the patients well being and ease of management, often avoiding the need for uncomfortable and psychologically distressing nasogastric tubes and intravenous lines. A gastrostomy tube can be readily managed in the home environment by the patient's family and carers as well as by nursing staff.[14]

Extraction techniques[2,15]

Developments in intravenous feeding therapy and monitoring techniques have led to a vast increase in the number of indwelling venous cannulas and catheters. Unfortunately, these occasionally break or become disconnected and a part or all of the catheter is 'lost' within the venous system.[16] It is important to retrieve these

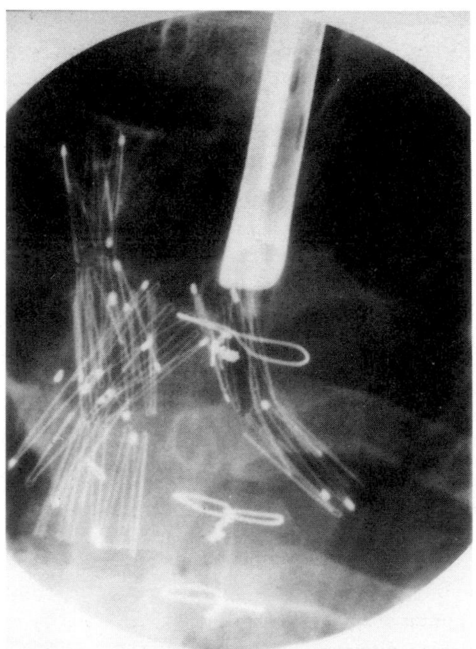

Fig. 5 Tracheal and superior vena cava stenting. Double bronchial stents and superior vena cava stents in a patient with myasthenia gravis with compression following surgery and radiotherapy. (Reproduced with kind permission from I.D. Irving and R. Dick.)

intravascular foreign bodies as they not only perforate vascular structures and cause dysrhythmias but also act as a seat of infection, particularly in immunosuppressed patients. Surgical retrieval of catheter fragments is hazardous (and sometimes impractical) necessitating a thoracotomy. It is almost invariably possible to retrieve these catheter fragments, which usually lodge within the right side of the heart or the pulmonary arteries, percutaneously under fluoroscopic guidance. Detailed descriptions of all the retrieval techniques available are beyond the scope of this chapter but any interventional radiologist offering a comprehensive vascular service is well advised to acquaint himself or herself with the various methods and have the necessary equipment available.[17]

The ability to snare or 'catch' the end of a catheter can also be of value in patients receiving intravenous cytotoxic chemotherapy in whom the tip of an indwelling central venous catheter has become displaced and lodged in the jugular vein as opposed to the superior vena cava. It is usually possible to 'pull' such a catheter back into its proper position using a percutaneous vascular approach under local anaesthetic.

Infusion

The ability to site vascular catheters in virtually any area of the body in either the venous or arterial system has enabled the radiologist/clinician to deliver a variety of chemotherapeutic agents directly to the site of disease. Cytotoxic agents, thrombolytic agents, and analgesics can be delivered safely and effectively by this method if required.

Vascular embolization[2]

This technique, that is the deliberate occlusion of arteries and/or veins by the injection of embolic agents through selectively placed catheters, is one of the major therapeutic applications of interventional radiology in the patient with neoplastic disease. The technique has been employed in the management of severe and disabling symptoms from a very wide variety of tumours throughout the body. Embolization, which is usually performed employing a percutaneous approach under local anaesthesia, offers an attractive alternative to surgery under general anaesthesia and, in some situations, offers the only therapeutic option available. A wide variety of embolic agents is available[18] and a detailed description is beyond the scope of this chapter. The broad categories of substances used include particulate emboli (Spongostan; polyvinyl alcohol—Ivalon), mechanical emboli (balloons, steel coils), and liquids (50 per cent dextrose, absolute alcohol, lipiodol). The appropriate agent or combination of agents depends on the lesion to be treated and its site (with particular reference to adjacent vulnerable vascular structures).

Embolization can be used definitively to treat benign conditions and preoperatively to assist effective, safe surgery, but in many cases it is used palliatively to alleviate distressing symptoms (Fig. 6).

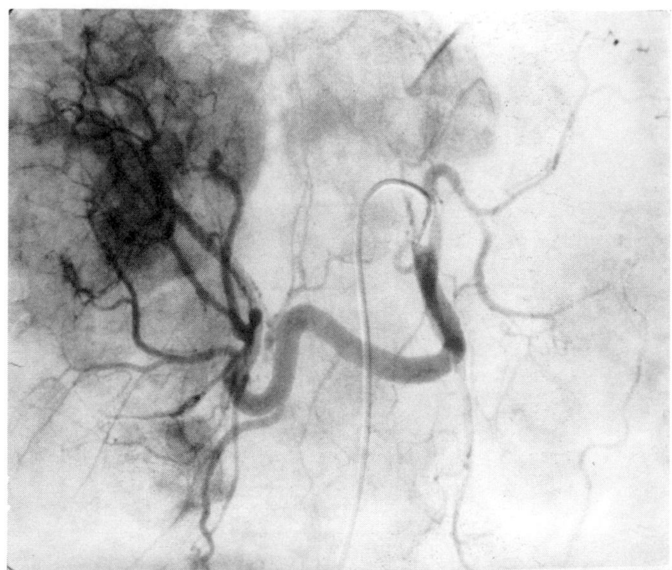

(a)

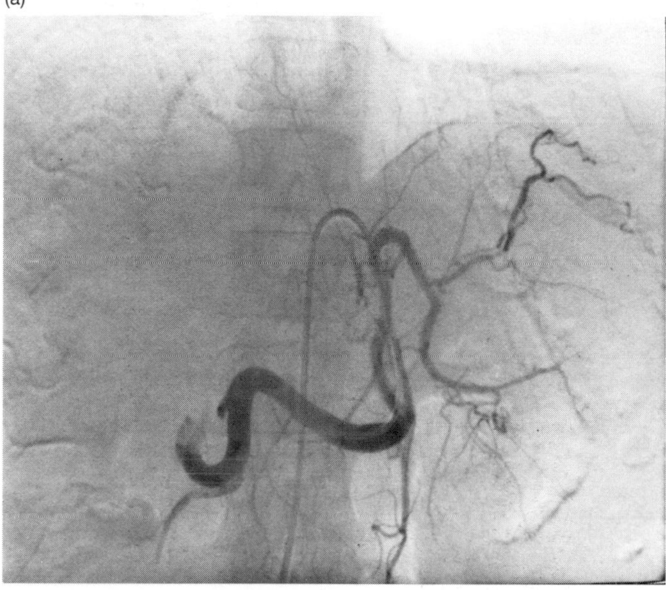

(b)

Fig. 6 Hepatic embolization for metastatic carcinoid tumour. (a) The arterial parenchymal phase shows hepatic enlargement and reveals multiple tumour deposits. (b) Postembolization arteriogram shows that the arterial supply has been obliterated. The patient's symptoms (flushing and diarrhoea) were dramatically alleviated by this procedure.

Palliative embolization

In patients receiving palliative care embolization can be used to control pain, haemorrhage, and hormone production as well as to reduce tumour bulk. The technique may be used as the primary mode of treatment in inoperable malignancy and embolization of metastatic deposits has, in some situations, been shown to extend survival times in advanced disease.[19] Tumours in all sites have been treated in this fashion (liver, kidney, bone, lung, soft tissues, nervous system, and gastrointestinal tract). Tumours which are secreting hormone (e.g. metastatic, carcinoid, and amine precursor uptake and decarboxylation cell tumours) show the greatest therapeutic response to arterial embolization. Appropriate pharmacological blockade is necessary during the embolization to avoid the effects of a dramatic outpouring of hormone as the tumour is deprived of its blood supply. The beneficial effects of embolization may become apparent within a matter of hours. In embolization procedures it is important that adequate premedication is given prior to the procedure, including broad spectrum antibiotics. In many situations, for example liver and bone, it is necessary to

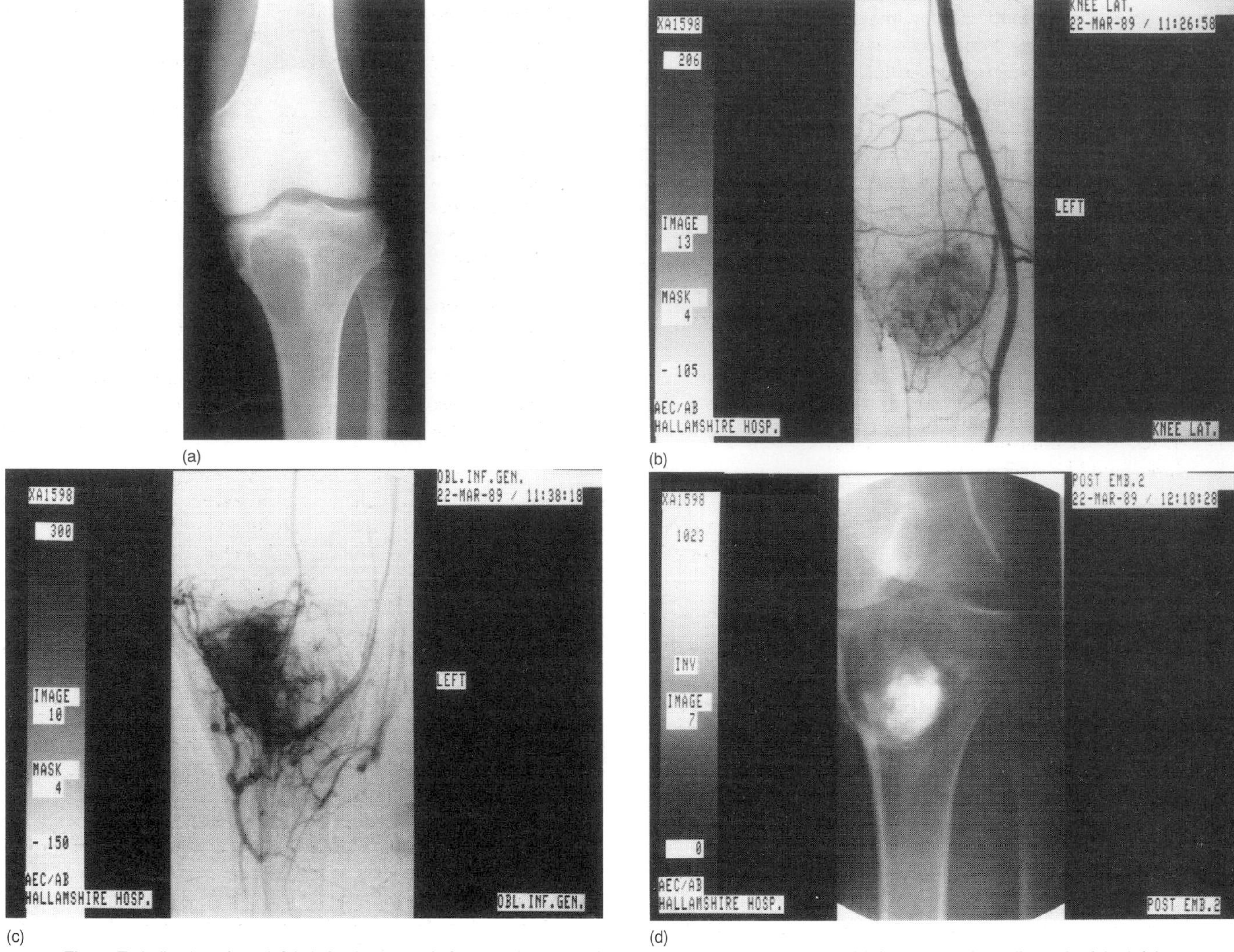

Fig. 7 Embolization of a painful skeletal metastasis from a primary renal carcinoma in a 55-year-old man. (a) Anteroposterior radiograph of the left knee shows a large lytic metastasis in the upper tibia in a patient with a known renal malignancy. (b) A femoral arteriogram (lateral) shows hypervascularity in the region of the metastasis. (c) The main vessel supplying this region was selectively catheterized. Fine particulate embolic material suspended in contrast medium and hypertonic dextrose was injected selectively into the vessels supplying tumour. (d) Postembolization radiograph shows stagnant contrast and embolic agent within the tumour. The patient experienced some increased pain for 24 h controlled by opioid analgesic. After this period his symptoms were significantly alleviated.

continue antibiotics for 10 days after the procedure to prevent sepsis developing in the devascularized tissue.

One of the more exciting recent developments in tumour embolization (especially liver) is the discovery that vascular tumours appear to have a particular affinity for lipiodol injected into the hepatic artery. The possibility of tagging cytotoxic agents or labelled monoclonal antibodies to the lipiodol is under investigation in many centres worldwide. Some preliminary results in, for example, in primary hepatoma, are very encouraging.[20,21]

In patients with cirrhosis of the liver complicated by hepatocellular carcinoma it is best to avoid arterial embolization because it may lead to further deterioration in liver function. In such patients percutaneous injection of alcohol into the tumour under ultrasound guidance has been shown to lead to a significant prolongation of life expectancy. Unfortunately, the results of this procedure in patients with multiple hepatic metastases are not as satisfactory as those obtained in hepatocellular carcinoma. This is because hepatocellular carcinoma is a very vascular tumour and alcohol diffuses throughout the mass, whereas most metastases are not very vascular resulting in uneven diffusion of alcohol with many cells surviving the injection. Percutaneous treatment with laser and radiofrequency probes is now being tried in metastatic disease, and the preliminary results are encouraging.

Skeletal metastases and primary malignant bone tumours are frequently very vascular. Therapeutic embolization (Fig. 7) can be useful in the following situations:

1. Prebiopsy, to reduce vascularity sufficiently to enable an adequate biopsy to be taken.

2. Preoperatively to reduce tumour bulk and vascularity prior to tumour resection. This technique has proved to be of value prior to limb preservation surgery for malignant or for potentially malignant lesions such as osteoclastoma and osteogenic sarcoma.

3. For palliation of inoperable neoplasms to reduce pain and tumour bulk. The commonest embolization materials are sterile absorbable gelatine sponge and steel coils. Occasionally, liquid emboli, such as absolute alcohol and iso-butyl-2-cyanocrylate, are used. The last-named substance sets quickly in contact with human tissue and, though its behaviour can be modified by mixing it with myodil and other substances, it can be difficult to handle. If it is used, great care must be taken not to embolize outside the target area and measures must be taken to avoid the adhesive incorporating the tip of the delivery catheter tip into the embolic plug. Various types of resins and polymers with more controllable setting characteristics are currently being developed.

Although embolization is effective, the treatment is invasive and can be associated with complications such as embolization of vascular territories uninvolved by malignancy. In view of this, this procedure should be reserved for patients who have not responded to more conventional therapy.

After embolization of large tumour masses, patients may experience some discomfort and pain and they may have a fever for a few days accompanied by a feeling of malaise and an elevated white cell count. This combination of signs and symptoms is indicative of the postembolization syndrome, an indicator of the presence of necrotic tissue and effectiveness of the procedure. A sustained pyrexia should alert the clinician to the possibility of abscess formation and blood cultures plus regional ultrasound should be performed. Serum C-reactive protein estimations can also provide a useful indication that infection may be present.[22]

Conclusions

This chapter was not intended to be an exhaustive list of every procedure that can be performed but to give an overall impression of the vast range of techniques available. The patient undergoing palliative care should not be subjected to any unnecessary procedure or instrumentation. However, there is a vast range of readily performed, well tolerated, and safe interventional procedures which can significantly alleviate distressing symptoms, improve the quality of remaining life, and ease the nursing burden. Further detailed information can be obtained from the many reviews, journals, and books on the subject, some of which are included in the reference list.

References

1. Athanasoulis CA, Pfister RC, Greene RE, Roberson GH. *Interventional Radiology*. Philadelphia: W.B. Saunders, 1981.
2. Allison DJ, Wallace S, Machan LS. Interventional radiology. In: Grainger RG, Allison DJ, eds. *Diagnostic Radiology: An Anglo-American Textbook of Organ Imaging*, 2nd edn. Edinburgh: Churchill Livingstone, 1992; 2329–88.
3. Wallace S, Charanangavej C. Interventional radiology in renal neoplasms. *Seminars in Roentgenology*, 1987; **22**: 303.
4. Pfister RC, Yoder IC, Newhouse JH. Percutaneous uroradiologic procedures. *Seminars in Roentgenology*, 1981; **16**: 62–71.
5. Pingoud EG, Bagley DH, Zeman RK, *et al*. Percutaneous antegrade bilateral ureteral dilation and stent placement for internal drainage. *Radiology*, 1980; **134**: 780.
6. Dick R, Adam A, Allison DJ. Interventional techniques in the hepatobiliary system. In: Grainger RG, Allison DJ, eds. *Diagnostic Radiology: An Anglo-American Textbook of Organ Imaging*, 2nd edn. Edinburgh: Churchill Livingstone, 1992; 1111–27.
7. Adam A, Chetty N, Roddie M, Yeung E, Benjamin IS. Self-expandable stainless steel endoprostheses for treatment of malignant bile duct obstruction. *American Journal of Roentgenology*, 1991; **156**: 321–5.
8. Davids PHP, Groen AK, Rauws EAJ, Tytgat GNJ, Huibregtse K. Randomized trial of self-expanding metal stents versus polyethylene stents for distal malignant biliary obstruction. *Lancet*, 1992; **340**: 1488–92.
9. Gerzof SG, Spira R, Robins AH. Percutaneous abscess drainage. *Seminars in Roentgenology*, 1981; **16**: 62–71.
10. Watkinson AF, Ellul J, Entwisle K, Maron RC, Adam A. Oesophageal carcinoma: initial results of palliative treatment with covered self-expanding endoprostheses. *Radiology*, 1995; **195**: 821–7.
11. Knyrim K, Wagner HJ, Bethge N, Keymling M, Vakil N. A controlled trial of an expansile metal stent for palliation of osophageal obstruction due to inoperable cancer. *New England Journal of Medicine*, 1993; **329**: 1302–3.
12. Irving JD, Dondelinger RF, Reidy JF, Schild J, Dick R, Adam A, Maynar M, Zollikofer CL. Gianturco self-expanding stents: Clinical experience in the vena cava and large veins. *Cardiovascular and Interventional Radiology*, 1992; **15**: 351–5.
13. Page AC, Evans RA, Kaczmarski R, Mufti GJ, Gishen P. The insertion of chronic indwelling central venous catheters (Hickman lines) in interventional radiology suites. *Clinical Radiology*, 1990; **10**: 105–9.
14. Bell SD, Carmody EA, Yeung EY, Thurston WA, Simons ME, Ho CS. Percutaneous gastrostomy and gastrojejunostomy: additional experience in 519 procedures. *Radiology*, 1995; **194**: 817–20.
15. Rossi P. Percutaneous removal of intravascular foreign bodies. In: Wilkins RA, Viamonte M, eds. *Interventional Radiology*. Oxford: Blackwell Scientific Publications, 1982: 359–69.
16. Gibson RN, Hennessy OF, Collier N, Hemingway AP. Major complications of central venous catheterization. A report of five cases and brief review of the literature. *Clinical Radiology*, 1985; **36**: 204–8.
17. Belli AM, Hemingway AP. Retrieval of intravascular foreign bodies. In: Belli AM, ed. *Interventional Radiology in the Peripheral Vascular System*. Edward Arnold. 1993; **4**: 88–92.
18. Hemingway AP. Materials for embolization. *Radiology Now*, 1986; 63–4.
19. Chuang VP, Wallace S. Hepatic artery embolisation in the treatment of hepatic neoplasms. *Radiology*, 1987; **140**: 51–8.
20. Takayasu K, Shima Y, Muramatsu Y, *et al*. Hepatocellular carcinoma: treatments with intra-arterial iodized oil with and without chemotherapeutic agents. *Radiology*, 1987; **162**: 345–51.
21. Kobayashi H, Inoue H, Shimada J, *et al*. Intra-arterial injection of adriamycin/mitomycin C lipiodol suspension in liver metastases. *Acta Radiologica*, 1987; **28**: 275–80.
22. Hemingway AP, Allison DJ. Complications of embolization: analysis of 410 procedures. *Radiology*, 1986; **166**: 669–72.

9

Symptom management

(continued)

9.1 Disease-modifying management

9.1.1 Principles governing the use of cancer chemotherapy in palliative care

David Osoba and Neil MacDonald

Introduction

Recently, the palliative benefits of cancer chemotherapy have been emphasized in numerous clinical trial reports. Cancer chemotherapy was once commonly regarded as an often futile and always dangerous type of therapy by both the public and by many palliative care physicians and nurses. Administrators viewed the rising costs of new aggressive protocols with alarm and all parties queried the risk versus benefit ratios of treatment. The best symptom control, however, will follow reduction of the cancer burden, control of neoplastic growth, or alteration of tumour biology and metabolic activity. Even when survival is not prolonged, the comfort of many patients can be enhanced following chemotherapy, provided that the toxic side-effects do not significantly impair health-related quality of life.

The object of this chapter is to provide a rational perspective for the palliative use of anticancer drugs. We intend to counteract some of the undue pessimism surrounding the employment of chemotherapy and to help readers ensure that those advanced cancer patients who may benefit are considered for anticancer treatment. The chapter will not provide specific details of management but will concentrate on general principles of treatment and will emphasize those situations where consultation with oncologists is in the patient's best interests.

The authors do not believe that the mixing and matching of combinations or dose forms of currently available chemotherapy drugs will appreciably alter the advice contained in this chapter. However, in the life of this textbook, new drugs will be developed and antimetastatic or differentiating agents now showing promise in the laboratory or in clinical trials may enter practice, while the slow progress noted in early trials of biologic modifiers may be improved upon. It is imperative that palliative care physicians are familiar with the clinical oncology literature and maintain or develop ongoing contacts with oncology groups in order to be aware of new therapies.

Chemotherapy as a symptom control agent

Pain, dyspnoea, and other symptoms will be improved following tumour shrinkage or removal. Even if life will not be prolonged, patients will benefit if reduction of a tumour mass opens a bronchus or an obstructed bowel, reduces pain, stabilizes hypercalcaemia or other metabolic abnormalities, or relieves pressure on vital organs.

However, more effort should be made to assess the effect of any intervention(s) on symptoms in an organized, systematic fashion. The use of simple symptom assessment methods, completed either by patients (when possible) or by significant others and professional care givers, such as the Edmonton symptom assessment scale,[1] or by a checklist approach, provides reliable and reproducible information. These methods can accurately describe changes in symptoms, but also form a basis for rational decisions to change interventions or to alter dosages or frequency of dosing of a pharmacological intervention. Greater detail on these approaches will be provided below.

Table 1[2] outlines a number of painful events common to cancer patients which may respond to chemotherapy intervention.

It is not clear whether symptom relief may occur in the absence of tumour regression. There are theoretical reasons why pain and other symptoms could be modified by chemotherapy independent of tumour response.

Potential analgesic effects of cancer chemotherapy

Corticosteroids are well-established coanalgesics. They may produce their effects by altering vascular permeability around a tumour, thus reducing 'tumour oedema', or by blocking the synthesis of cytokines, such as the eicosanoids, which contribute both to inflammation and nociception. They may also reduce cytokine production through their cytolytic effect on lymphoid cells.

Cytotoxic drugs also have a profound effect on granulocytes, lymphocytes, and monocytes. Populations of these cells are located in and around a tumour and contribute to tumour bulk.[3]

Cancer pain and other symptoms are not simply related to mechanical pressure effects. Nociceptive chemicals may be released by the tumour, host reactive cells, and the neovasculature. The presence of algesic chemicals probably accounts for the observation that pain produced by tumours is often disproportionate to their size or degree of bone involvement.

Figure 1 illustrates the 'chemical stew' which characterizes the tumour milieu. Many of the ingredients of the stew either sensitize

Table 1 Efficacy of chemotherapy in relieving pain

Primary cancer	Source or site of pain	Degree of pain relief[a]
Breast	Tumour ulceration } Chest wall infiltration }	+++
	Bone metastasis	++
	Lymphoedema of arm	+
Prostate	Bone metastasis	+++
Lymphomas	Para-aortic adenopathy > back pain	++++
	Superior vena cava obstruction	+++
	Spinal cord compression	+++
Leukaemia } Myeloma }	Periosteal irritation/invasion } Increased medullary pressure }	+++
Testicle	Para-aortic adenopathy > back pain	++
Oral/ Pharyngeal	Tumour ulceration } Invasion of nerves }	++
Lung	Pancoast's syndrome	+
Colorectal } Cervical } Bladder }	Low abdominal pain } Perineal pain } Low pain }	+
Intracranial tumours	Increased cerebral fluid pressure > severe headache	
	(a) with corticosteroids	+++
	(b) without corticosteroids	+

[a]++++ complete relief; +++ very good, but incomplete relief; ++ moderate relief; + little or no relief.
From Bonadonna G and Molinari R. Role and limits of anticancer drugs in the treatment of advanced cancer pain. In: *Advances in Pain Research and Therapy*, Vol. 2. Eds JJ Bonica and V Ventafridda. New York, Raven Press, 1979, pp. 131–44.

nociceptive nerves or directly stimulate them. One would anticipate that cytotoxic chemotherapy, through its effects on lymphocytes, granulocytes, and other rapidly growing normal reactive cell populations, could influence tumour-induced pain if the cytokines produced by these cells contribute to cancer pain.

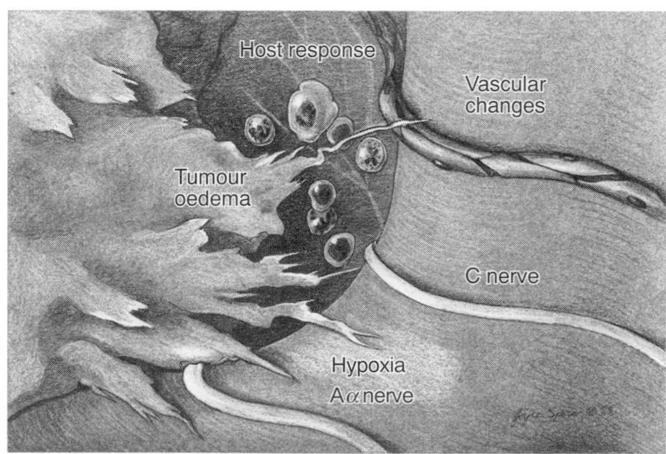

Fig. 1 Milieu surrounding a tumour (reproduced by courtesy of Joyce Spicer, Medical Artist, Cross Cancer Institute).

The independent analgesic effects of cytotoxic chemotherapy were not commonly studied.[4] Of interest, early studies on high-dose intra-arterial chemotherapy often contained an analysis in which the authors reported pain control in the absence of significant antitumour effects.[5–12] As with radiation therapy (Chapter 9.1.2), analgesia was often noticed immediately after therapy, before significant alteration in the size of the tumour could be expected.

As some cytotoxic drugs alter peripheral nerve function and can cross the blood–brain barrier, they could alter both peripheral and central neurotransmitter systems. Therefore, cytotoxic drug effects on neurones could influence pain and other symptoms, independent of tumour effect.

Chemotherapy—effect on symptoms

Cytotoxic chemotherapy as a symptom inducer

Cytotoxic chemotherapy has well-known, acute, self-limited, adverse effects. Involved physicians respect the severe bone marrow depression and secondary infections associated, sometimes unpredictably, with cytotoxic therapy. Patients may express more concern about chemotherapy-induced symptoms than about the ultimate effect of the cancer.[13,14] Nevertheless, when the effects of the symptoms associated with chemotherapy were assessed for their effects on quality of life in a randomized trial of 'intermittent' versus 'continuous' chemotherapy for metastatic breast cancer, chemotherapy-induced symptoms were less disruptive to quality of life than were the effects of the cancer itself.[15] The cancer was not controlled as effectively in the group receiving 'intermittent' chemotherapy as in the group receiving 'continuous' chemotherapy, and women in the former group had lower scores for well being as compared to the latter group. The only symptom that was worse in the 'continuous' chemotherapy group was nausea and vomiting. Therefore, it is important for health-care professionals and patients to understand that the major source of deterioration in quality of life in symptomatic cancer is likely to be the cancer itself rather than the chemotherapy for the cancer. However, it is still important to consider the symptom-inducing capacity of the chemotherapy that will be used and its dosing frequency. Chemotherapy with a high symptom-inducing capacity, given frequently, may do more harm than good.[16]

Nausea and vomiting

Palliative care physicians should be aware that nausea and vomiting can be alleviated with antiemetics, without major risk. The observation that metoclopromide could be used in this fashion marked a major change in the degree of comfort with which cancer patients could receive emesis-inducing chemotherapy.[17] Recently, the introduction of selective serotonin antagonists, the 5-hydroxytryptamine (**5-HT$_3$**) blockers, enables patients to have superior emesis control without risk of extrapyramidal side-effects.[18,19]

In addition, we are now beginning to appreciate the very important contribution of corticosteroids to the control of chemotherapy-induced emesis.[20] Dexamethasone, or other corticosteroids, add measurably to the control not only of emesis occurring in the first day after chemotherapy but are also a mainstay in the control of emesis during the week following chemotherapy. The quality of life of patients taking dexamethasone for several days after chemotherapy is demonstrably better than in patients not taking dexamethasone. The combined use of 5-HT_3-antagonist antiemetics and dexamethasone can completely abrogate chemotherapy-induced emesis in nearly half of patients, even after highly emetogenic chemotherapy such as high-dose cisplatin.

Finally, it should also be noted that chemotherapy-induced emesis may not be as disruptive on some quality of life domains as formerly suggested by early studies. When postchemotherapy quality of life scores for physical, role, cognitive, emotional, and social functioning, for global quality of life, and for symptoms such as fatigue, pain, and anorexia are controlled for prechemotherapy scores in the same domains, social functioning, global quality of life, fatigue, and anorexia are adversely affected by the emesis.[21] Other decrements in quality of life domains, such as in physical and role functioning and increased insomnia after chemotherapy, are probably attributable to other effects of chemotherapy.

Nausea and vomiting are normally short-term complications which are not known to influence the subsequent incidence of chronic nausea. The relationship between late-stage chronic nausea and earlier chemotherapy experiences has not been studied.

Bone marrow depression

Recovery from bone marrow depression after a cycle of chemotherapy usually occurs in 1 to 3 weeks, depending upon the nature and doses of the chemotherapeutic drugs used. However, repeated cycles may produce a cumulative effect in some patients. Occasionally, patients exposed to certain alkylating agents, such as busulphan, phenylalanine mustard, the nitrosoureas, and the antibiotic mitomycin C, may have profound, long-standing marrow depression.[22]

Haemopoetic growth factors can partially alleviate the degree and time at risk with severe granulocytopenia. At present, this therapy is expensive and is used in megadose chemotherapy protocols rather than for supplementary support in therapies which may be considered in palliative care patients.

Neurological problems

A variety of neuromuscular disorders are associated with cancer. Most commonly, severely cachectic patients may exhibit poorly characterized, mixed neuromyopathies; carcinomatous sensory neuropathies are, otherwise, the most common paraneoplastic syndrome, albeit unusual.[23] Frequently, however, the direct effects of cancer or its therapy produce nerve damage. Amongst chemotherapeutic drugs, cisplatin, procarbazine, the vinca alkaloids, and paclitaxel are particularly liable to induce a neuropathy. Uncommonly, cytosine, arabinoside, alkylating agents, etoposide, and a new agent, suramin, are implicated.

1. Cisplatin. This causes a dose-dependent sensory polyneuropathy, secondary to axonal degeneration. The neuropathy may progress for several weeks after completion of therapy and recovery may be slow and incomplete. Recently, prior cisplatin therapy has been reported to cause longer-term cognitive–attentional deficits.[24]

2. Vinca alkaloids. Sensorimotor peripheral neuropathies, secondary to alteration in axon transport, are commonly noted. Autonomic nerve toxicity, often manifested as constipation, is also common. Recovery from major neurological complications is usually complete, but absent reflexes and some degree of sensory neuropathy may persist.

3. Paclitaxel. Sensory neuropathies, rarely with a motor component, are commonly encountered at higher cumulative doses of paclitaxel.[25,26] When paclitaxel is added to other neurotoxic drugs, such as cisplatin, neuropathies may become the dose-limiting adverse event.[27]

4. Cytokines. These are associated with a wide range of neuropsychiatric effects.[28] While these usually reverse when therapy is stopped, occasionally long-term neurotoxicity is noted.[29] Most reports stem from clinical trials of interferon or interleukin-2; as other cytokines are used, more examples of neurotoxicity may be expected. It is not known whether prior neurotoxic therapy influences the patient's mental status in the last days of life.

Cancer patients often have tumour-related neurological defects, compounded by the presence of comorbid neuropathies in elderly diabetic or alcoholic patients. Against this background, the addition of higher doses of nerve-damaging drugs made possible by advances in bone marrow support may increase symptomatic neuromyopathies in palliative care patients. The incidence of this risk, which may be balanced by the use of neuroprotective agents,[30] is a reasonable topic for future research.

Dyspnoea

Pulmonary toxicity (interstitial pneumonitis followed by fibrosis) commonly occurs in patients treated with bleomycin.[31] There are no studies relating prior treatment with this agent to the onset of chronic dyspnoea in late-stage cancer patients. Interstitial pneumonitis with fibrosis is an unusual complication of melphalan, chlorambucil, cyclophosphamide, busulphan, and mitomycin C. Nitrosourea therapy causes dose-related lung fibrosis which can induce progressive pulmonary symptoms. Indeed, in one study of children with brain tumours treated with BCNU and radiation, 35 per cent of survivors died of lung fibrosis.[32] Certain chemotherapy combinations and chemotherapy–radiation joint therapy enhance the risk of long-term pulmonary complications.[33] A pneumonitis of uncertain aetiology, without sequelae, is uncommonly associated with methotrexate therapy.[34]

Cardiomyopathy

Permanent cardiac muscle damage with risk of chronic congestive failure is associated with anthracycline therapy. The risk is proportional to the cumulative dose of the anthracycline drugs, and probably also dose intensity. Cardiomyopathy is unusual in adults below total doses of 350 mg/m^2 of doxorubicin or 500 mg/m^2 of daunorubicin. Children may be at risk at lower doses.[35] Patients with cardiac disease and those who received multiagent chemotherapy (notably with actinomycin D or cyclophosphamide) are also more susceptible.[36]

Cardiac toxicity, usually as an acute effect, has occurred following high-dose cyclophosphamide therapy and in association with mitomycin C, mitoxantrone, and 5-fluorouracil. Acute cardiotoxicity, usually rapidly reversed after discontinuation of therapy, may occur with recombinant interleukin-2 and interferon as therapy.[37] Other biological response modifiers may prove to be cardiotoxic.

Germ cell failure

Permanent reduction in sperm production and ovarian failure are common sequelae of chemotherapy treatment, particularly if alkylating agents are used.[38] More relevant to palliative care patients, sexual interest and performance are often diminished while receiving therapy. It is not known whether reduced sexual activity later in the course of illness relates to prior chemotherapy.

Hair loss

Hair loss and other integumentary changes are commonly encountered following therapy with many (but not all) cytotoxic drugs. These changes are reversible over time. The amount of hair loss may be diminished in patients receiving drugs with a short half-life of the active compound by cooling the scalp or placing tourniquets around its margins.[39]

Genitourinary complications

Changes in excretory capacity increase the risk of adverse drug effects. Therefore, long-term nephrotoxicity secondary to chemotherapy may complicate the management of palliative care patients. Agents of particular note include:

1. Mitomycin C may induce thrombotic microangiopathy (causing a variant of the haemolytic–uraemic syndrome). This syndrome is also associated with vinblastine–bleomycin combinations.[40]
2. Nitrosoureas therapy may cause irreversible alterations in renal function.[41]
3. Cisplatin can produce dose-related tubule–interstitial damage, causing a permanent reduction in glomerular filtration rate.[42]
4. Methotrexate can cause dose-dependent tubular damage which is usually reversible.
5. Cyclophosphamide/ifosphamide both form the metabolite acrolein, which produces uroepithelial damage. While hydration and concomitant use of a sulfhydryl donor (mesna) are protective, patients with long-term ureter–bladder sequelae may be encountered. These patients may have bladder contraction, ureteric obstruction, and readily induced haematuria.[43]

Pain

Acute pain syndromes are often associated with cytotoxic therapy and, less commonly, with hormonal therapy. These include pain secondary to stomatitis (antimetabolites—notably methotrexate and 5-fluorouracil), headaches (intrathecal therapy), colicky abdominal pain (vinca alkaloids), peripheral neuropathy (vinca alkaloids, platinum compounds, cytosine arabinoside, taxanes), and jaw pain (vinca alkaloids). With the exception of peripheral neuropathy and some hormone-induced pain syndromes (see below) these painful episodes clear without sequelae. Many cytotoxic agents cause demyelination and axis cylinder fragmentation in animal experiments,[44] which correlate with their propensity to induce clinical neuropathies. The introduction of marrow-stimulating agents and autologous bone marrow transplantation allows dose escalation of drugs formerly limited by the risk of myelosuppression. As a result, an increase in neuropathies and other non-haematological, long-term adverse effects may occur.

Long-term side-effects of cytotoxic agents are summarized in Table 2.

Hormones as symptom inducers

In general, hormonal therapy is associated with fewer short-term adverse effects, but in the case of corticosteroids there is a greater risk of chronic adverse effects.

Corticosteroids

In the palliative care patient, aside from facilitation of infections, the principal adverse effects of corticosteroids are as follows.

Neuropsychiatric

High-dose corticosteroids induce psychiatric problems in many patients.[45] Paranoia, other delusions, hallucinations, delirium, and affective disorders (major depression and anxiety) may occur. Perhaps related to concomitant illness and drug therapy, organic brain disorders such as delirium are more common than affective disorders in corticosteroid-treated cancer patients. The risk of mental complications is dose related.[45]

Peptic ulcer

Controversy still ensues concerning the risk of peptic ulcers with corticosteroids. The risk is probably low, primarily affecting patients with a prior history of peptic ulcer on higher doses of steroids.[46] Peptic ulcer risk is sharply increased when patients use corticosteroids together with non-steroidal anti-inflammatory drugs. In this circumstance, the risk is estimated at 15 times that of patients not taking either drug.[47]

Steroid myopathy

Cancer patients become asthenic as their disease progresses. Muscle weakness limits the patient's independence, mobility, and choice of living arrangements. Patients on corticosteroids may develop a proximal myopathy whose symptoms meld into the general pattern of cancer asthenia. The legs are more severely affected and patients will complain that they cannot rise from a chair or have increasing trouble climbing stairs. Exercise probably reduces the effects of steroid myopathy. However, the admonition to use muscles lest we lose them is often not helpful in our palliative care population.

The appellation 'proximal' may be inexact as the muscle fibres principally effected by steroids are the Type IIB fast-twitch muscles, primarily dependent on non-oxidative glycolysis. These fibres are also abundant in respiratory muscles, notably the diaphragm, raising the possibility that long-term steroid use could contribute to dyspnoea in susceptible patients.[48] A clinical association remains to be established.

Hyperglycaemia

Corticosteroids provoke hyperglycaemia by inducing both insulin resistance and non-insulin dependent inhibition of muscle glucose transport.[49] Even in patients with no prior history of diabetes, dangerous serum glucose levels may occur[50] which result in glucosuria, dehydration, mental slowing, and, on occasion, frank hyperosmolar coma. Patients with steroid-induced diabetes usually have comorbid conditions which accentuate hyperglycaemic risk. For example an elderly patient with a brain tumour on dexamethasone may be poorly nourished, with decreased thirst appreciation. She may be on phenytoin and a diuretic, and then develop

Table 2 Potential long-term side-effects of cytotoxic agents

Cytotoxic agent	Long-term side-effects
Alkylating agents	
e.g. Busulphan	Bone marrow depression
Melphalan	Pulmonary fibrosis
Cyclophosphamide	Gynaecomastia
Chlorambucil	Leukaemia
Nitrosoureas	Germ cell failure
Ifosphamide	Inappropriate ADH secretion
	Cystitis (cyclophosphamide) (ifosphamide)
	Hepatitis
Antimetabolites	
Folic acid analogues (methotrexate)	Pulmonary fibrosis
	Renal failure (risk combined with non-steroidal anti-inflammatory drugs combined with hepatitis
	Encephalopathy (post-intrathecal use)
Pyrimidine analogues	
Cytarabine	Peripheral neuropathy
	Encephalopathy
	Hepatitis
5-Fluorouracil	Cerebellar atrophy
Vinca alkaloids	
Vincristine	Peripheral neuropathy
Vinblastine	Inappropriate ADH secretion
Tumour antibiotics	
Bleomycin	Pulmonary fibrosis
	Raynaud's syndrome
Mitomycin C	Pulmonary fibrosis
	Renal failure
	Germ cell failure
Doxorubicin	Cardiac failure
Duanorubicin	Cardiac arrhythmias
Epipodophyllotoxins	
Etoposide	Peripheral neuropathy
Teniposide	
Platinum compounds	Peripheral neuropathy
	Hearing loss
	Germ cell failure
	Renal failure
	Cognitive changes
Mitoxantrone	Renal failure
Taxanes	Peripheral neuropathy
Hormonal agents	
Corticosteroids	Delirium
	Affective disorders
	Osteoporosis
	Aseptic necrosis—femur
	Peptic ulcer
	Infections
	Myopathy
	Hyperglycaemia
Oestrogens	Gynaecomastia
	Fluid retention
	Thrombosis
Megesterol	Weight gain
	Fluid retention
	Thrombosis
Tamoxifen	Retinopathy
Antiandrogens	Gynaecomastia
	Hepatotoxicity

an acute infection which precipitates a severe hyperglycaemic crisis.

Regular screening of patients at risk should reduce hyperglycaemic complications.[51] Aside from specific antidiabetic therapy, maintenance of hydration, particularly in patients with glucosuria, is critically important.

Pain

Steroids enhance osteoporosis. Their contribution to metastatic bone pain through this mechanism is uncertain. They can also induce an aseptic necrosis of the femoral head associated with characteristic hip pain. Diffuse myalgias and arthralgias may occur after steroid withdrawal.

Addison's disease

This is a well known complication which may develop after steroid withdrawal following long-term use. The edict that corticosteroids must be tapered, and replacement therapy sometimes offered, is well known to physicians.

Patients at risk

Usually, patients receiving the equivalent of less than 20 mg/day of prednisolone have a reduced risk for any of the above complications. Patients taking 9-α-fluorinated glucocorticoids have a greater risk of developing a myopathy.[52,53] The commonest corticosteroids in this category which are used in palliative medicine are betamethasone, dexamethasone, and triamcinolone. If long-term, high-dose corticosteroid therapy is required, it is our practice to discontinue fluorinated corticosteroids and switch the patient to prednisolone. However, improvement may not occur unless steroid doses can be sharply decreased.

The above complications should be prevented by limiting long-term use, using alternate-day therapy if possible, and keeping the corticosteroid dose as low as possible.

Other hormonal complications

Other hormonal agents commonly used in oncology are listed in Table 2. Oestrogens, tamoxifen, and zoladex may cause a 'flare' of bone pain when first employed. Pain in this situation does not represent tumour stimulation and is not a reason for stopping therapy. Otherwise, with the exception of fluid retention and a variable increased risk of deep vein thrombosis, adverse effects interfering with patient comfort are not common. Subtle effects, such as their impact on sexuality, could be lost within a complex clinical presentation.

Summary

With the increased use of high-dose chemotherapy regimens, long-term adverse effects may increase. Protocols for assessment of these programmes should not solely concentrate on short-term toxicity, but should include provisions for assessing long-term, drug-induced adverse effects. Corticosteroids often have noteworthy effects when used long-term.

Guidelines for the use of chemotherapy in a palliative setting

Palliative medicine stresses the importance of maintaining patient control of his or her destiny and the importance of symptom

Table 3 Commonly-used general quality-of life questionnaire in patients with cancer

Acronym	Name	References
MQOL	McGill quality of life questionnaire	54
CARES-SF	Cancer rehabilitation evaluation system short form	55
EORTC QLQ-C-30	European Organization for the Research and Treatment of Cancer core quality of life questionnaire	56
FACT	Functional assessment of cancer therapy	57
FLIC	Functional living index—cancer	58
LASA	Linear analogue self-assessment scale	59
MOS SF-36	Medical outcomes study short form	60
QLI	Quality of life index	61
QL-Index	Quality of life index	62
RSCL	Rotterdam symptom checklist	63

control in achieving that objective. There is nothing inherently wrong in using any avenue of approach which will assist this process. Clearly, palliative radiotherapy has a role, as does palliative systemic anticancer therapy in many circumstances. The palliative care physician must be able to identify patients whose lives can be prolonged and, less clearly defined, situations where drug therapy can relieve symptoms and improve patients' well being even in the absence of prolongation of life.

Assessment

In the past, medical oncologists were remiss in not assessing the effects of their therapies on patient symptoms and psychosocial well being. Palliative care physicians are trained in the art of symptom control assessment and should set up an evaluation programme to complement the usual measurements of tumour size. Indeed, the latter measurements are less relevant in a palliative care setting, although tumour change should be assessed if assessment does not require arduous or dangerous technical procedures.

More importantly, a standard battery of simple symptom control and quality of life tests should be used when patients are receiving chemotherapy. Assessment must fit the resources of the unit and the patient's tolerance.

Recently developed assessment methods are important tools in evaluating levels of symptom relief and improvement in well being. For assessing symptom relief, the Edmonton symptom assessment scale,[1] developed for patients in a palliative care setting and completed by patients, relatives, and nursing or medical staff is an excellent tool that deserves wide use. A somewhat simpler approach is the use of symptom checklists which can be completed by most patients in both ambulatory care and inpatient settings.

Although symptom relief should result in an improvement in well being and in quality of life, it is not self-evident that this is always true. The control of some symptoms may lead to the emergence or expression of other previously hidden concerns that were of minor importance in the presence of an overwhelming symptom such as pain or dyspnoea. Also, when patients are preoccupied with a symptom they may not remember or think it important to raise other concerns. Thus, a method for making certain that such concerns are not missed would be a valuable addition to the usual means of eliciting symptoms. This is now possible to achieve, to a degree, by using self-report, health-related, quality-of-life questionnaires that have been designed to tap into a broad range of quality of life domains and symptoms which are of concern to most patients with cancer. The domains include one or more functions, such as physical, role, cognitive, emotional, and social function, as well as overall quality of life and a number of common symptoms such as fatigue, pain, nausea/vomiting, dyspnoea, insomnia, and appetite loss. The more popular of these questionnaires have been developed primarily for patients who are not in a palliative care setting and thus may not address all of the important concerns of such patients (e.g. existential issues), but they may be modifiable for hospice and palliative care wards. The current questionnaires, however, probably do address the concerns of patients who are receiving palliative anticancer therapy. Since not all tumour-specific or situation-specific concerns are covered, regardless of the setting, additional checklists and modules of questions can be designed and added to the general self-report, health-related, quality-of-life questionnaires.

Recently, a number of instruments, exemplified by the McGill quality-of-life questionnaire,[54] that address the unique concerns of palliative care patients have been developed. They consider existential domains in addition to traditional physical, social, and psychological domains. A listing of the most commonly available, general questionnaires is given in Table 3.[54–63]

It should also be remembered that patients with progressive or recurrent cancer are concerned not only with pain, suffering, and dying, but also with being a burden to their families, as well as other family concerns.[64] These concerns need to be addressed throughout the illness trajectory and particularly in the palliative care setting.

Table 4 Karnofsky performance status scale

Definition	%	Criteria
Able to carry on normal activity and to work; no special care needed	100	Normal; no complaints; no evidence of disease
	90	Able to carry on normal activity; minor signs or symptoms of disease
	80	Normal activity with effort; some signs or symptoms of disease
Unable to work; able to live at home and care for most personal needs; varying amount of assistance needed	70	Able to care for self; unable to carry on normal activity or to do active work
	50	Requires considerable assistance and frequent medical care
Unable to care for self; requires equivalent of institutional or hospital care; disease may be progressing rapidly	40	Disabled; requires special care and assistance
	30	Severely disabled; hospitalization is indicated, although death not imminent
	20	Very sick; hospitalization necessary; active supportive treatment necessary
	10	Moribund; fatal processes progressing rapidly
	0	Dead

Goals of therapy

In a palliative care setting, improvement in symptoms and quality of life are usually the principal aims of therapy. Patients and family may over-estimate the life-prolonging benefits of chemotherapy and relate its use to hopes for cure or prolonged survival. Physicians should ensure at the outset that patients and their families share an understanding of the reasons for inaugurating therapy.

Performance status

Chemotherapy trials commonly employ the Karnofsky performance scale (Table 4), the World Health Organization scale, or the similar Eastern Cooperative Oncology Group scale (Table 5) to describe the status of the enrolled patient. These scales are simple measures of patient function, as judged by a physician, which have a good correlation with tumour regression, length of response, and quality of response.

Analysis of performance status provides a major reason why clinical trials results may not be matched in the palliative care setting. A review of phase II–III trials in the 1990 *Journal of Clinical Oncology* on patients with advanced melanoma, colorectal cancer, renal cancer, or non-small-cell lung carcinoma reveals that over 80 per cent of enrolled patients were Karnofsky level 80+ or Eastern Cooperative Oncology Group status 0–1; similar findings are noted in a 1995 review. For example in a study by Poon *et al.*,[65] describing the palliative benefits of 5-fluorouracil–leucovorin in advanced colorectal cancer, 85 per cent of the patients enrolled had an Eastern Cooperative Oncology Group status of 0–1. The palliative response of the more advanced patients is not specified. These are not the patients usually seen in palliative care units; a survey of 12 British hospices stated that only 8 per cent of their patients were classified as Eastern Cooperative Oncology Group 0–1 at the time of hospice admission.[66] Patients with poor performance status fare badly in chemotherapy trials; response rates are reduced, the usefulness of a response is usually minimal in comparison to toxicity, and the length of response is reduced.[67]

This information is not surprising as the national hospice study reported that, in the absence of treatment, the Karnofsky performance scale was the best determinant of ultimate patient survival. Patients with a Karnofsky performance scale of 40 lived on the average less than 50 days, while those with a performance status of

Table 5 ECOG scale performance status

Grade	Definition
0	Fully active, able to carry on all predisease performance without restriction
1	Restricted in physically strenuous activity but ambulatory and able to carry out work of a light or sedentary nature (e.g. light housework, office work)
2	Ambulatory and capable of all self care but unable to carry out any work activities; up and about more than 50% of waking hours
3	Capable of only limited self care, confined to bed or chair more than 50% of waking hours
4	Completely disabled; cannot carry on any self care; totally confined to bed or chair

20 had only 10 to 20 days of life left.[68] Patients with poor performance status will not tolerate high doses of chemotherapy. Their tumours tend to be bulky, providing poor access for drugs, which in any event will encounter a heterologous population of tumour cells, many of which have genetically transformed to become chemotherapy resistant. Therefore, patients considered for chemotherapy with any tumour type should receive treatment before they are severely limited by disease.

Several recent studies indicate that quality-of-life status may be more strongly predictive of survival than is performance status. In patients with metastatic lung cancer, breast cancer, and malignant melanoma, scores for such attributes of quality of life as 'physical well being', 'quality of life index' and 'psychosocial well being' were found to be independently predictive of survival even after allowance for treatment group, performance status, and tumour response.[69,70,71,72] A Canadian study has confirmed these findings in a heterogeneous group of patients, the majority of whom had either lung, breast, or ovarian cancer, and also found that the predictive value of 'global quality of life' was present in patients with local or regional disease as well as in patients with metastatic disease (Dancey J, Zee B, Osoba D, *et al.* in press).

Age

For most cancers (excluding lymphomas and leukaemias), chemotherapy response rates probably do not change with advanced age, but toxicity may be enhanced.[73,74] In the past, many clinical trials excluded people over 70. Outside a research setting, older patients were less likely to be informed about or to receive chemotherapy.[75] Therefore, information on chemotherapy response in the elderly is not adequate. Many elderly patients will have reduced bone marrow reserve and renal function (probably the most common physiological changes associated with ageing).[73] The presence of other chronic illnesses will influence decisions to use chemotherapy. The risk of untoward drug interactions is also increased as many elderly patients are taking a variety of drugs.

Nevertheless, biological and chronological ages often differ because of genetic make-up and past life styles. Desch and Smith remind us that assigning negative characteristics of a group to an individual is a form of 'ageism', stereotypical reasoning otherwise decried by society.[76] Therefore, arbitrary age divisions for chemotherapy should not be employed. Rather, caution based on assessment of measurable parameters of organ function should be exercised when considering older patients for chemotherapy. Risk is proportional to the effects of chemotherapy on normal tissue, the pathways used to metabolize and excrete the drugs, and the current health of organs subject to damage or involved in drug removal. Personal costs and dependency (including travel and housing arrangements) related to chemotherapy are considerations for everyone but may be of particular importance to elderly patients. Older patients will welcome a full account of their options, although they may be less likely to accept the risks of a high-dose regimen than their younger counterparts, opting for gentler therapies.[77]

Patient preference

Patients and families vary considerably in acceptance of risk, as do physicians. Patients may be more willing than their physicians to accept toxic risks for minimal chance of gain.[78] Everyone wishes to die with dignity, but patients may translate the meaning of 'dignity' differently from their families or their doctors. For some it may mean a continuing valiant fight against the inevitable.

The patient has the right to be fully informed of all options, including chemotherapy. One cannot assume that previous physicians have covered all salient points with the patient or family. This situation may particularly apply to older patients (see above). Many doctors remain unaware of the indications for chemotherapy, while some radiation and surgical oncologists may be unduly pessimistic about the role of systemic therapy. Formalized models for assessing patient preference and degree of risk acceptance have been used in clinical trials but are not readily available for clinical use.[79]

Patient–family understanding of their situation is normally reviewed when patients enter a palliative care programme. An appreciation of their experience with anticancer therapy and their views on this topic should be part of the admission interview. The palliative cancer physician and nurse must have a reasonable knowledge of the state of the art of oncology therapy in order to hold up their part of their conversation.

Type of cancer

Table 6 outlines the relative sensitivities to systemic therapy of the major cancers. It must be highly unusual for patients with Group I tumours (a child, a leukaemia–lymphoma patient, or a young man or woman with a germ cell tumour) to be registered in a palliative care programme without prior oncological consultation and treatment. If this should happen, referral, even for patients with late stage disease, should be arranged. This dictum must be tempered with good sense if the patient is nearly moribund. Referral does not necessarily translate into therapy, but as a general rule consultation is advisable. Some patients may have missed prior referral because of primary physician error, cultural barriers, or a phobic fear of medical procedures. The palliative care setting may provide the first opportunity for detailed counselling; the opportunity should not be missed.

Cancers in Group II will not be cured by chemotherapy once disease is disseminated. Exceptions to this rule exist, such as a few patients with small cell lung carcinoma, ovarian carcinoma, and, possibly, post-bone marrow transplant breast cancer, chronic myelogenous leukaemia, and multiple myeloma patients. Many other Group II patients may experience prolongation of comfortable life for a measured period of time. As a general rule, one should consider the use of systemic therapy in this group of patients, the final decision being dependent on an analysis of patient preference and characteristics.

Group III contains a large group of tumours where the responses to systemic therapy are modest in percentage and substance. Patients with Group III tumours who have a good performance status should have the opportunity to consider participation in a clinical trial. This may offer some of them a chance for a few more months of quality life. As stated elsewhere, the evidence supporting improved quality of life is rarely obtained in chemotherapy trials but there is gathering evidence[80,81,82] that the well being of some patients may be enhanced by treatment with new clinical protocols. It is the authors' belief that submitting patients in Group III to 'one-off' clinical adventures, conducted by inexperienced physicians practising without access to a sophisti-

Table 6 Locally advanced or disseminated cancers response to chemotherapy

Group	
Group I	*Highly sensitive—chemotherapy must be considered*
	Germ cell tumours—Testicle
	Choriocarcinoma
	Acute lymphocytic leukaemia
	Acute myelogenous leukaemia
	Paediatric tumours—Ewing's sarcoma
	—Wilms' tumour
	—Rhabdomyosarcoma
	Lymphomas—Hodgkin's
	—non-Hodgkin's
Group II	*Sensitive—chemotherapy usually employed*
	Prostate cancer
	Breast cancer
	Small-cell lung cancer
	Chronic myelogenous leukaemia
	Ovarian cancer
	Bladder cancer
	Endometrial cancer (hormones)
	Neuroendocrine cancer
	Kaposi's sarcoma
	Multiple myeloma
	Neuroblastoma
	Adult sarcoma[a]
	Gastric carcinoma[a]
	Cervical carcinoma[a]
	Head and neck cancer[a]
	Non-small-cell lung cancer[a]
Group III	*Low sensitivity—poor response to chemotherapy*
	Oesophageal carcinoma
	(Melanoma) tumours often treated with biological response modifiers in combination with chemotherapy
	Renal cell cancer
	Pancreatic cancer (gemcitibine may change group III assignment)
	Hepatocellular cancer
	Osteogenic sarcoma (metastatic)
	Colorectal cancer

[a] Some would argue that these are group III tumours

cated follow-up and monitoring system, is not likely to benefit palliative care patients. Nowhere more than in Group III tumours is transfer from the research setting to the community fraught with greater opportunity for harm.

Prior chemotherapy

Patients in Groups II and III with poor performance status (Karnofsky <70) and a recent adequate trial of chemotherapy are not candidates for further systemic treatment. Patients with a remote trial of chemotherapy and a good performance status may be candidates. For example women with breast cancer who received adjuvant chemotherapy can still respond to systemic chemotherapy upon relapse.[83,84] The use of agents selected from new chemotherapy drug classes may help patients with a good performance status and more sensitive tumours (e.g. breast cancer),[85] although the opinions of oncologists remain mixed on this issue.[86] Hormonally-influenced tumours in Group II (notably breast and prostate cancer) may benefit from a trial of alternate hormone therapy. This is further discussed in the section on specific tumour therapy.

Hormone response

Patients with tumours subject to endocrine control may benefit for long periods of time from hormonal manipulation or blockade. Drugs in these classes are not highly toxic and their side-effects are either mild or readily controlled. It is imperative that the history of past hormonal therapy is elicited and specifically considered on the admission of a patient with cancer of the breast, prostate, or endometrium. At present, hormone therapy has a minimal role in advanced ovarian cancer; the literature reports occasional responses to tamoxifen or progestins.[87–89]

The cells of certain tumours, including melanomas, cancer of the pancreas, or lung cancer, which are ordinarily not thought to be under endocrine control, may have hormonal receptors. Attempts to influence the behaviour of these tumours with tamoxifen or other hormonal agents have resulted in trivial response rates.

While hormonal agents may not reduce tumour size, they can influence tumour production of peptides and other biologically active substances. The mechanism of the effect of corticosteroids on pain is unknown but may relate, in part, to interference with production of leukotrienes and cytokines. The inhibitory hormone somatostatin dramatically reduces production of gastrin and other gut peptides by neuroendocrine tumours. These are rare tumours but the observation is important as it suggests the possibility of hormonal inhibition of the tumour products of more common tumours. For example progestational agents do not have anti-tumour activity against tumours arising in non-sex-hormone influenced tissues, but have a profound effect on the cachexia-inducing properties of these tumours (see Chapter 9.3.6).

Length of therapy

Recommending a trial of sometimes arduous therapy in a situation where the outcome for an individual patient is problematic creates an ethical dilemma. Outcome figures for groups are published, but they may not apply to the individual patient. Chemotherapy trials for Group III patients still represent an exercise where many patients would be better off if they never received therapy—but which patients fall into this group? The clinician is obliged to assess meticulously patient costs versus benefits, and to stop therapy as early as possible if there is no evidence of response or patient improvement. It is unlikely that patients with Group II or III tumours will benefit from further chemotherapy if they have not stabilized or improved after two full courses of therapy (if given every 3 weeks) or after 6 weeks of therapy (administered daily or weekly). Objective response in certain sites (liver, bone) may be delayed for 3 to 4 months.[90] Changes in tumour size, however, should not be the major criterion for continuing therapy. Rather, therapy should be continued if the patient is stable, with improvement in symptoms and general sense of well being.

If the patient has improved, then treatment should continue as, at least for breast cancer, the quality of life is better in patients treated continuously than in those receiving intermittent therapy.[15] Careful reassessment after each subsequent treatment is required. The decision to continue therapy should be based on quality of life criteria not tumour size.

Palliative care units—use of chemotherapy

Depending upon the regimen, palliative chemotherapy can be administered within a palliative care unit. Palliative care physicians and nurses have a heightened sensitivity to whole patient assessment, comprehensive evaluation techniques are generally in place, and, in collaboration with oncology colleagues, the additional assessment procedures required for monitoring patients on chemotherapy can be introduced. The critical decision involves the use of palliative therapies rather than the site of therapy. Those patients who should be treated with high-dose toxic regimens should be transferred.

Evaluation of the literature

To both oncologist and palliative care physician alike, the cancer chemotherapy literature is a confusing mix of multidrug cocktails and outcomes of uncertain significance. Increases in survival, measured in weeks, are sometimes trumpeted, conflicting results are common, and the permutations and combinations of drug protocols appear limitless.

The history of modern systemic cancer therapy encompasses five decades. Today, as in the past, certain conclusions remain pertinent:

1. Small, non-randomized studies usually report better results than subsequent, large, randomized trials using the same study drugs.
2. Results from single institutions tend to be better than those reported from multi-institutional trials using the same protocol.
3. A common closing sentence in a single-arm, open trial is a variant of 'these results are encouraging and warrant further investigation'. It is often wise to await the results of 'the further investigation'.
4. Publication bias. Small, positive trials are more likely to be submitted for publication than negative trials.

Reflecting a therapeutic era where most advances are reminiscent of trench warfare rather than *blitzkrieg,* complex statistical calculations and mathematical models are employed to chart progress which otherwise may not be self-evident. Reports of '*p*' values yielding significance in various components of a clinical trial do not necessarily have clinical relevance. They are simply statements of the likelihood that a subset of activity within the artificial environment of a clinical trial could have occurred by chance. They relate only to that trial but the observation may lead the investigator to false or grandiose conclusions.

The author of a recent surgical journal review states: 'Authors who use '*p*' values to support their conclusions about the magnitude or importance of differences in group data are making the most serious and the most common error to be found in the clinical literature'.[91] For example an improved median survival of 6 weeks may reach statistical significance in a large trial, but is this finding helpful? Literature interpretation will be eased when investigators establish important quantitative goals for their studies and provide the readers with an account of their success in reaching these goals.

Likelihood of change

With the exception of the taxanes and topoisomerase inhibitors, few fundamentally new, useful chemotherapy agents have been introduced since cisplatin in the early 1970s. Since then, most new drugs are representative of existing classes with advantages in certain settings. The existing response range of cancer chemotherapy has changed only modestly in 20 years.

Recent advances in the use of chemotherapy are concentrated in the adjuvant setting. Chemotherapy in combination with surgery and/or radiotherapy in patients with limited colorectal cancer will improve patient survival.[92] Similar findings have been reported for patients with other tumours including breast cancer,[90] and subsets of small cell lung cancer.[93] Continued progress in the management of early cancer can be anticipated, but similar success with advanced cancer therapy is unlikely using the chemotherapeutic agents available today.

Two basic problems bedevil the future of systemic drug therapy; drug access within large tumours and drug resistance. Access will always limit drug efficacy in advanced cancer patients. Theoretically, once mechanisms of drug resistance are known, it may prove possible to alter this phenomenon.[94] The genetic instability and consequent heterologous nature of metastatic cancers, however, creates a dismaying prospect for success.

Success in cancer chemotherapy is usually judged to encompass both complete tumour remissions and partial remissions in excess of 50 per cent of the tumour volumes. Partial remissions demonstrate that a drug can kill a proportion of tumour cells. It is debatable whether this partial destruction has survival value for the patient. It has been postulated that partial tumour destruction may actually stimulate tumour growth,[95] a postulate recently demonstrated in a study of myeloma cells.[96] Could this explain, in part, the conundrum wherein therapies which clearly improve response rates do not always improve survival? Other factors, notably the effect of cross-over therapies upon failure of the primary approach, are often present. Enhanced tumour growth following failed chemotherapy, however, remains a theoretical possibility. Where only partial remission is anticipated, assessment of symptom relief and quality of life clearly become the most important features.

There is now renewed interest in enhancing or stimulating natural defences against cancer. Earlier attempts with non-specific immune stimulation therapies achieved limited success. In the 1990s, efforts to specifically enhance the numbers and effects of natural antitumour immune cells will continue. Early results are promising in limited tumour types but, like chemotherapy, response relates to patient performance status. Therapy with specific cytokines or with antitumour lymphocytes is both toxic and expensive. There is no current evidence that immune modulation will improve the quality of life of cancer patients in the last months of life.

The promise of targeting cancer cells with monoclonal antibodies, either alone or as carriers for anticancer drugs, remains unfulfilled. If and when success is achieved, monoclonal antibodies will probably be used primarily as tumour diagnostic agents or as therapy for patients with small tumour masses.

Other avenues of approach include reversing the abnormal genetic mechanism of the cancer cell, and blocking the phenotypic expression of oncogenes. There will be growing interest in compromising tumour nourishment by blocking tumour angiogenesis (the stimulation and production of new blood vessels in cancer).

In summary, improve understanding of the molecular biology of cancer cells and the relationship between these cells and their host environment is creating new directions for systemic cancer therapy. The new therapies promise to be expensive, highly sophisticated, and limited to research settings for some years to come. They will be most readily applied to patients with a small tumour burden; they do not auger a change in the lot of most far advanced cancer patients during the decade of the 90s.

Palliative chemotherapy—selected tumour types

In the following disease specific section, advice on restricting chemotherapy use to clinical research settings is sometimes included. The attention to detail and standards inherent in clinical research protocols is usually beneficial for all patients. However, location, costs, disease characteristics, and availability of skilled oncology colleagues may limit the access of patients to enrolment in a formal clinical trial. We have attempted to delineate those situations where the use of chemotherapy is indicated outside an established trial from those where the results of so-called 'standard' treatment (for example intermittent bolus therapy with 5-fluorouracil for advanced pancreatic cancer) are so bad and toxic results so harmful that occasional therapeutic adventures are to be discouraged.

The purpose of this exercise is primarily to help non-specialists to recognize palliative opportunities for anticancer therapy. A secondary benefit will stem from the recognition of the patient's right to be presented with all realistic options, including participation in clinical research.

Lung cancer

Small-cell lung cancer

It is important to distinguish between patients with small-cell lung cancers and those with non-small-cell lung cancers. The former have an excellent chance of responding to cancer chemotherapy and a small percentage of patients with limited-stage disease may even be cured. Small-cell lung cancer is normally disseminated at diagnosis but it will respond to chemotherapy in 65 to 80 per cent of cases with extensive disease.[97] In most cases, response periods are brief but complete responses are common, occurring in 15 to 30 per cent of patients. In favourable subsets (patients with clinically localized disease, a good performance status, and normal biochemical parameters) over 20 per cent disease free survival at 2 years has been reported.[93]

As most patients will have a clinically significant response, which for a few may continue for several years, all small-cell lung cancer patients should be referred to an oncology centre for treatment as early in their course of illness as possible. These patients may expect alleviation of distressing pulmonary symptoms, pain, and the superior vena cava syndrome. If the patients are elderly or in poor general health, single agent therapy with etoposide[98] may still provide symptomatic relief.

If disease progresses on therapy or if rapid relapse occurs, second line chemotherapy is unlikely to help.[99]

Non-small-cell lung cancer

Chemotherapy protocols in common use include a combination of etoposide and cisplatin, often with one or two additional agents. Tumour response and drug toxicity are closely linked to performance status.

In contrast to small cell lung cancers, chemotherapy response rates in this group of disseminated non-small-cell lung cancers are low, ranging from 10 to 40 per cent in large inter-institutional studies. Several new agents, including the taxanes, gemcitibine, topotecan, and vinorelbine, demonstrate activity against non-small-cell lung cancers, and are now factored into combination drug regimens.

Complete response of advanced disease is rarely achieved, but two recent meta-analyses concluded that chemotherapy reduced mortality during the first 6 months to 1 year.[100,101] While the newer protocols often bring about a modest survival advantage (a few months) in comparison with earlier regimens or 'best supportive care', it is unlikely that the agents at hand will substantially alter the grim prognosis of metastatic non-small-cell lung cancer. These discouraging results may lead one to conclude that the cost and side-effects of therapy do not justify the use of chemotherapy in non-small-cell lung cancer.

Indeed, until recently, some cancer centres abjured the use of chemotherapy for patients with advanced non-small-cell lung cancers. This is a reasonable decision if survival is the objective of therapy. Non-small-cell lung cancer, however, is a tumour where chemotherapy has been reported to improve symptoms, sometimes even in the absence of objective tumour response.[4,102-104]

In addition, in the National Cancer Institute Canada non-small-cell lung cancer trial, while reporting that chemotherapy statistically improved patient survival,[80] also showed that patients receiving chemotherapy required less hospitalization and fewer palliative radiotherapy treatments throughout their course of illness.[81] One of the chemotherapy regimens was associated with less overall costs than supportive care alone. In contrast to the Canadian report, a larger study using a similar treatment protocol achieved only trivial responses and concluded that 'combination chemotherapy with currently available drugs in advanced non-small cell lung cancers does not meaningfully improve survival'.[105] Unfortunately, this otherwise excellent trial does not contain any symptom control information.

Herein lies the problem. Surely, the major value of current chemotherapy in non-small-cell lung cancers must lie in its effect on symptoms and quality of life. Tantalizing data from small studies and retrospective data from one large study suggest that chemotherapy can enhance quality of life.[104] Nevertheless, most investigators to date have not been interested in assessing the symptom-control role of chemotherapy in non-small-cell lung cancers.[106] In the 1991 *Proceedings of the American Society for Clinical Oncology*, 51 abstracts on the use of chemotherapy in non-small-cell lung cancers were published. All gave an account of tumour response and toxicity; only two mention symptom control but without data. In 1995, again only two abstracts amongst the 25 studies on advanced non-small-cell lung cancers selected for slide or poster presentation reported symptom control information.

In summary, chemotherapy should not be dismissed out of hand in the management of non-small-cell lung cancer patients. It may improve survival when used together with radiotherapy in local disease. Chemotherapy may marginally improve survival, with enhanced symptom control and quality of life of patients with disseminated disease but this has not been prospectively demonstrated in large, controlled trials. Where possible, patients should be enrolled in clinical trials as the drugs employed require expertise in administration and toxicity management. What favourable data exist, relate to patients with good performance status. There is no support for the view that patients with a poor performance status will benefit from an encounter with chemotherapy for non-small-cell lung cancers as it now stands. As a combination of paclitaxel and cisplatin, with its inherent risk of neuropathy, is regarded as a combination of great promise, one hopes that future phase III studies on this regimen will contain impeccable quality-of-life information.

Metastatic colorectal cancer

Metastatic colorectal cancer tends to run an inexorable course towards death with a medium survival of 6 to 10 months.[107] The linchpin of chemotherapy for this disorder remains, as it was 30 years ago, 5-fluorouracil. Recently, a more specific thymidylate synthetase inhibitor is undergoing clinical trial.[108] To date, it appears to give equivalent results to 5-fluorouracil, possibly with fewer adverse effects. Symptom control information on this agent or on camptothecine (another group of drugs of study interest in colorectal cancer) is lacking.

In the adjuvant setting, combining 5-fluorouracil with various immunological or biochemical modulators can enhance the opportunity for cure. For example 5-fluorouracil in combination with the immune modulator, levamisole, has been shown to improve the curability of surgically treated patients with regional lymph node involvement.[92,109]

In contrast, the response rates of patients with metastatic disease to standard 5-fluorouracil therapy are in the range of 10 to 20 per cent without associated improvement in overall survival.[110] These figures have improved somewhat for patients who receive a continuous infusion of 5-fluorouracil, or 5-fluorouracil together with citrovorum factor. While response rates now lie in the 20 to 35 per cent range, the overall effect on survival remains modest.[110,111]

5-Fluorouracil is simply administered; it does not cause local skin irritation or severe nausea. Troubles start a week later when, sometimes not in proportion to dose, the patient's white count and platelet count plummets at the same time as the mucosa of the mouth and gastrointestinal tract begin to slough. Few oncologists have escaped caring for patients with the above constellation of findings. While they ruminate on their choice of dose, they gain increasing respect for the morbidity and mortality which 5-fluorouracil can cause.

A number of studies confirm that 5-fluorouracil in combination with leucovorin factor (which enhances the link between 5-fluorouracil and its target enzyme) brings about an improvement in symptoms and overall quality of life[65,112] equal to or in excess of the objective tumour response.[113] However, in Poon and Buroker's studies[65] 80 per cent of the patients had an Eastern Cooperative Oncology Group status score of one or better—this corresponds to a group of fully ambulatory patients. As stated earlier, the authors do not comment upon symptom relief in the few patients with poorer performance status.

Guidelines for therapy

1. 5-Fluorouracil will normally be combined with other chemotherapy drugs or biologic modifiers. It should be administered following rigorously controlled protocols by experienced oncologists. These protocols must include quality of life evaluation.

2. 5-Fluorouracil, alone or in combination, should not be employed in palliative care patients with poor performance status. It will not prolong life and there is no available evidence that the considerable risk of toxicity is balanced by improvement in symptom control. The same admonition holds for newer chemotherapeutic agents, pending evidence of reduced toxicity and symptom control.

3. Patients with recurrent colorectal cancer who have metastases restricted to their liver may be considered for local surgery or regional chemotherapy. A surgical option is sensible for patients with solitary or a few isolated metastases.[114] Interest is again developing in the use of percutaneous, locally ablative techniques, now using alcohol.[115] Intra-arterial chemotherapy administration requires installation of an infusion apparatus with consequent increased costs and risk. This remains a clinical research programme restricted to patients with early symptomatic metastases.[11,116,117]

Cancer of the pancreas

The prognosis of patients with exocrine ductal carcinoma of the pancreas has improved only slightly in 50 years. The occasional patient may present with a localized resectable tumour, particularly if it is located adjacent to the common bile duct, causing early jaundice. At present, overall cure rates lie in the range of 3 to 5 per cent, while less than 20 per cent of patients are alive 1 year after diagnosis.[118]

In the past, 5-fluorouracil or combinations of drugs with 5-fluorouracil have been the 'standard chemotherapy' for cancer of the pancreas. Results were dismal; 5-fluorouracil is ineffective and should not be regarded as the standard chemotherapy for patients with advanced cancer of the pancreas. While the combination of leucovorin factor with 5-fluorouracil appears to improve colorectal cancer response rates, it does not do so in pancreatic cancer.

As discussed in the section on abdominal pain, 5-fluorouracil has radiosensitizing properties and has been used in combination with radiation therapy in order to provide palliative relief of pancreatic cancer pain. Its role in this setting is not clear as the protocols using radiation and 5-fluorouracil were primarily designed to study tumour response and patient survival rather than symptom relief. One study reported a 30 per cent pain response, but the parameters for measuring pain relief were not defined.[119]

Aside from survival benefits, may chemotherapy improve the patient's symptoms? Evidence supporting 5-fluorouracil in this role does not exist. Recently, a new antimetabolite, gemcitabine, demonstrated alleviation of symptoms in 27 per cent (phase II trial) and 24 per cent (versus inactive 5-fluorouracil in a phase III trial) of patients with advanced pancreatic cancer.[120,121]

Sensibly, these two trials used pain, analgesic consumption, improvement in Karnofsky status, and, in one study, lean body mass as the principal criteria for assessment. One hopes that these studies will spawn others with similar, rational aims.

Some pancreatic tumours have oestrogen receptors, while a number of them also are subject to the stimulatory effects of gastrin and balanced inhibitory action of somatostatin. Recently, clinical trials with octreotide (a somatostatin analogue), sometimes in combination with tamoxifen, have been published. While objective remission rates are modest, improvements in symptom control are observed. To date, only a few small studies have appeared. Physicians will wish to follow this story closely.[122-125]

Also of interest, a study on a new angiogenesis inhibitor[126] shows that it has some impact on pancreatic cancer; data on pain and quality of life are awaited.

Guidelines for therapy

1. 5-Fluorouracil is not an appropriate treatment for patients with cancer in the pancreas. Gemcitibine has a role.
2. Radiation therapy may be used to control pain.
3. Participation of patients in clinical research protocols as a first line of treatment is appropriate in view of the lack of standard treatment options.
4. Early coeliac plexus block for patients should be considered in locales where there is access to experienced anaesthetic consultation. Studies using an integrated approach combining plexus block with palliative radiotherapy and/or gemcitibine are awaited.
5. Patients commonly are depressed. Evaluation and antidepressant therapy are recommended for those judged to be clinically depressed.

Metastatic prostate cancer

Eighty per cent of patients with metastatic prostate cancer report relief of pain after hormonal therapy interfering with androgen production or action at the cell level. Survival, and possibly pain relief, are diminished in patients who present with a combination of low testosterone levels, poor performance status, bone pain, and a high alkaline phosphatase.[127]

It is imperative that all prostate cancer patients in a palliative care setting should be reviewed to determine whether they have had an orchiectomy or an adequate trial of an androgen suppressant. If the disease relapsed following an adequate trial, second line hormone therapy generally is unsuccessful. Infrequent responses have been noted with high-dose oestrogens, antiandrogens, or corticosteroids. It is reasonable to treat relapsed patients with a trial of low-dose corticosteroids,[128-130] which may suppress residual androgen production arising from the adrenals and have a direct effect on eiconasoid production around bone tumours, thus reducing pain. Tannock and his colleagues noted a 30 per cent improvement in symptoms using prednisone in a dose of 5 mg twice daily as second line therapy.[130] This dose should not be associated with adverse corticosteroid effects and may be maintained for a long time, although the duration of symptomatic response is usually brief.

It is the custom of urologists and oncologists to treat relapsed prostate cancer with an antiandrogen on the thesis that this will suppress cancer cell populations still responsive to androgens.[131] In the interests of reducing costs, reducing polypharmacy and the possible side-effects of useless agents, the authors believe that it is reasonable to discontinue antiandrogen therapy when low-dose corticosteroids are started. As the issue is not proven, this decision should be reviewed if other androgen suppressants are discontinued and the patient experiences a flare-up of pain.

There is recent evidence suggesting that the addition of moderate doses of mitoxantrone to prednisone is better than prednisone alone in reducing pain and improving other aspects of quality of life.[132] This study illustrates that endpoints other than tumour response and survival can be measured and can provide useful information in the care of patients with metastatic disease. Other studies on cytotoxic therapy which include data on pain and quality of life are beginning to appear.[133]

Patients may obtain pain relief following therapy with an isotope, strontium 89,[134] or a bisphosphonate.[135,136] Of note, strontium therapy may reduce the need for multiple 'cherry picking' radiotherapy treatments.

Guidelines for therapy

1. Every patient must have had an adequate trial of androgen suppression.
2. Patients who have progressive disease following initial androgen-suppressive therapy should receive secondary treatment with low-dose corticosteroid therapy. The addition of mitoxantrone may improve quality of life.
3. Patients with pain should be considered for bisphosphonate or strontium 89 therapy when pain control with oral analgesics is problematic. The role of bisphosphonates in preventing adverse skeletal events is under study.
4. Selected patients with a good performance status, pain, and advancing disease, whose symptoms have failed to respond to androgen suppressive therapy and low-dose corticosteroids, may wish to consider participation in clinical trials of new cytotoxic agents.

Metastatic breast cancer

Patients with early breast cancer receiving adjuvant chemotherapy often record a decreased quality of life linked to the occurrence of side-effects.[137,138] Most patients will accept these adverse circumstances, trading off temporary illness against improved chances for long-term survival.

In contrast to the adjuvant studies, chemotherapy for metastatic breast cancer is commonly associated with symptom improvement and a better quality of life[1,5,139] even though life is not usually prolonged.[90] Patients will experience side-effects yet the evidence of tumour regression, the hope engendered by this event, and the abatement of symptoms counterbalances the toxicity of therapy.

The temptation is present to employ minimal doses of chemotherapy, hoping to avoid toxicity yet garner the reward of symptom control. Unfortunately, this simple premise is not usually successful in practice.[139] Too little therapy may waste the patient's time and resources to no avail. Very-high-dose regimens, including exercises in autologous marrow transplant, continue to be explored.

Hormone therapy must be used in women with disease factors associated with hormonal response (positive sex hormone receptors on the tumour, a long disease-free interval prior to recurrence, slowly progressive disease not involving brain or liver). A sensible regimen combines tamoxifen and low dose prednisone (less than 20 mg/day).[90] Progestins are alternate choices in women with anorexia or cachexia.

Standard chemotherapy regimens following failure of hormone therapy, or as first therapy in hormone-receptor-negative patients, should be considered for all women with metastatic breast cancer. A variety of 'standard' protocols exist—the most commonly studied treatment includes a combination of cyclophosphamide, 5-fluorouracil, and methotrexate.

Of interest, pain relief has been reported within days of initiation of therapy,[139] well before tumour regression has occurred. While this may be a placebo effect, it is possible that the chemotherapy interfered with chemical mediators of pain.

If the trajectory of illness is rapid, with liver involvement prominent, time may not allow a trial of hormone therapy. In these patients immediate use of chemotherapy should be considered. Therapy, if successful, should continue until relapse, if side-effects are tolerable.

Patients who have had prior chemotherapy may still benefit from another course of alternate treatment, particularly if rapid disease progression has not occurred while the patients were on therapy.[140] Response rates between 30 and 45 per cent have been reported with doxorubicin alone or in combination with other drugs in patients without prior exposure to this agent. Other regimens, including less toxic agents such as mitoxantrone, may prove to have equal palliative benefit.[141] Recently, the introduction of the taxanes together with cisplatin, offers new hope for the treatment of metastatic disease.[142,143]

There is one caveat—the database for the above recommendations consists of studies which predominantly enrolled women with a good performance status. One of these studies points out that the small subset of women with poor performance status (only 12 per cent of this study population) had reduced response rates which were short in duration.[15] Separate quality-of-life data are not available for this group.

Both the progression and symptoms of metastatic bone disease can be favourably influenced by bisphosphonates. Recent data strongly support their role in preventing adverse skeletal events (hypercalcaemia, pain, pathological fractures, number of metastases).[144-146] Strontium-89 may also have a role in bone pain management.[147]

Guidelines for therapy

1. Women with advanced breast cancer are candidates for systemic therapy. Usually, initial therapy will include tamoxifen.

2. Systemic chemotherapy may be subsequently employed with reasonable expectation that patient's quality of life will improve.

3. As symptom control and quality of existence are enhanced in many patients, therapy should start when symptoms occur and while the patient has a good performance status.

4. Women who have had prior adjuvant chemotherapy may respond to chemotherapy if they develop metastatic disease.

5. Salvage regimes should be considered when primary therapy fails.

6. Initial therapy, in the absence of clear evidence of progression, should continue if symptom relief is noted or if the disease is stable and side-effects are tolerable.

7. In women with prior failed chemotherapy and a poor performance status chemotherapy responses are unlikely and, if obtained, are of poor quality. In this group of patients, hormonal therapy continues to be a consideration.

Metastatic head and neck cancer

Most cancers in the head and neck region are squamous cell cancers arising in the mouth, nasopharynx, oropharynx, pharynx, or hypopharynx. Their initial treatment is by surgery for early stage disease when it is amenable to a surgical approach which does not involve the loss of a function important to quality of life, for example speech. Cancers of the nasopharynx and larynx are treated initially by radiation therapy and, when tumours are bulky, both approaches may be used in a combined modality approach. The primary cancers frequently metastasize to lymph nodes of the cervical chain and, thus, surgical neck dissection for excision of the lymph nodes on the affected side is a common procedure. Cure rates for stage I and II disease using these approaches vary from 65 to 95 per cent depending on the anatomical site, size of the primary tumour, and the ability to render the first echelon of nodes free of tumour by radiation or surgical extirpation. However, for bulkier tumours with fixed nodes or bilateral nodes, cure rates are less than 50 per cent. Unfortunately, a large proportion of patients present with advanced stage disease, partly because even relatively small tumours are 'anatomically large' given the close proximity of many complex structures in a relatively small anatomical area, and partly because one of the predisposing factors (high alcohol intake) may lead patients to disregard early symptoms and to delay seeking medical attention.

The poor cure rate in advanced stage disease means that a significant number of such patients will experience either progression or recurrence of the primary disease, or regional metastatic disease after initial treatment. Some, particularly those with nasopharyngeal carcinoma, will develop distant metastases in the lungs, liver, or bones as the first sites of recurrence. For other primary sites, recurrence at the primary site or in regional lymph nodes is the most common manifestation of incurable disease but some of these patients will present with more distant metastases, usually in the lungs. Furthermore, patients with head and neck cancer frequently present with a second primary tumour in the respiratory tract, since the main predisposing factor, tobacco smoke, affects the entire respiratory system and upper digestive tract.

When the disease has recurred at the primary site or in regional lymph nodes, the patient may often be treated surgically or with a course of radiation, even when the primary or regional metastases have previously been treated surgically or by radiation therapy. Unfortunately, the relief of symptoms from treatment of a local recurrence is often short and, upon further recurrence or the development of more distant metastases, the patient is referred to a medical oncologist for consideration of chemotherapy.

Before briefly reviewing chemotherapy for recurrent and distantly metastatic disease, it should be mentioned that chemotherapy has also been used in a neoadjuvant fashion, that is before the definitive treatment (surgery or radiation) or concomitantly with radiation therapy or as adjuvant or maintenance therapy after the definitive treatment.[148] To date, there is little to indicate that any chemotherapy used as neoadjuvant, adjuvant, or maintenance therapy has improved survival or improved short-term symptom control or quality of life. However, some studies indicate that when chemotherapy is used concomitantly with radiation therapy, there is some modest survival advantage. Further studies are in progress to determine the kind of chemotherapy that is best used in this fashion.

Chemotherapy for recurrent and metastatic disease has ranged from the use of single agents such as methotrexate, 5-fluorouracil, bleomycin, hydroxyurea, and others to complex three and four-drug combinations. One combination that seems to be in favour currently in many centres is high-dose cisplatin given as a single dose at the beginning of a four or five-day infusion of 5-fluorouracil. The popularity of this drug combination is curious, since it is not clear that it produces longer survival times than do standard doses of methotrexate alone in patients with recurrence or distant metastases.[149] Response rates for both approaches are 11 to 30 per cent and median response durations are 4 to 5 months. Both have the potential for producing significant and unexpected toxicity (mucositis and myelosuppression of nephrotoxicity). The combination of high-dose cisplatin and 5-fluorouracil requires the use of prehydration and mannitol infusion, most likely in an inpatient setting, and is far more expensive than the use of methotrexate in the ambulatory care setting. None of the chemotherapy trials with single or multiple agents has cured more than a few patients. Since symptom control and quality of life assessment are still uncommon in these patients, little can be said about whether such therapy benefits large numbers of patients, although it clearly has the potential for doing so. Clearly, further studies in this significant group of tumours are required.

Guidelines for therapy

1. Although high-dose cisplatin and 72 to 96 h 5-fluorouracil infusion is considered standard chemotherapy for recurrent and widely metastatic head and neck cancer, consideration should also be given to less expensive, single agent therapy with methotrexate. Tumour responses are accompanied by relief of symptoms in many patients.

2. Second and third-line chemotherapy should be considered primarily in formal clinical trials.

3. Patients with advanced and recurrent cancer localized to the primary site or to regional lymph nodes can benefit from supportive care such as nutritional supplements, dressings for ulcerated lesions, metronidazole to control offensive odours, and good pain control.

Emergency use of chemotherapy

Elsewhere in this textbook the management of the superior vena cava syndrome and spinal cord compression are detailed. Both accounts stress the role of corticosteroids and radiation therapy as the mainstays of medical management. This is appropriate, but there are situations where radiation therapy, or surgery in the case of spinal cord compression, is either unavailable or is contraindicated because of prior therapy or patient debility. In developing countries access to immediate radiation treatment may not be possible. Thus, there are emergency situations where chemotherapy may have a role.

Spinal cord compression

Aside from breast cancer, multiple myeloma, and small cell carcinoma of the lung, the tumours most commonly associated with epidural cord compression (non-small-cell lung, prostate and kidney cancer, and malignant melanoma) tend not to be sensitive to chemotherapy. Cord compression secondary to lymphomas is relatively less common, but these tumours usually respond to chemotherapy and may cause cord compression independent of structural damage to the vertebral column.

The literature contains several examples of excellent responses to chemotherapy alone in the treatment of lymphoma-induced spinal cord compression.[150,151] Good responses to chemotherapy alone have been reported in another haematological tumour, multiple myeloma.[152] Less information is available on the management of non-haematological cancer.

Cyclophosphamide, methotrexate, and 5-fluorouracil were successfully employed by Marshall and Langfitt in the management of two patients with epidural disease from breast cancer who refused radiation.[151] Germ cell tumours, the most sensitive of tumours to chemotherapy, have been treated with good effect.[153] Many paediatric cancers are also highly sensitive to chemotherapy. Neuroblastoma and Ewing sarcoma causing cord compression have been treated with cyclophosphamide and doxorubicin.[154] In Hayes' report all patients responded initially with eight out of nine demonstrating complete resolution of neurological abnormalities. An excellent response to the chemotherapeutic management of cord compression in a patient with nasopharyngeal carcinoma has been reported.[155]

Similar responses would not be expected in patients with epidural compression secondary to more resistant tumours such as melanoma and non-small-cell lung cancer. Nevertheless, in an emergent situation where no other options are available a trial of chemotherapy could be considered.

There is no clear evidence with respect to the ideal chemotherapy to be employed. In general, it appears wise to use chemotherapy which is known to be effective in the tumour to be treated. Cyclophosphamide, an alkylating agent, is commonly reported as a component of chemotherapy regimes used to treat cord compression. If one agent was to be employed in an emergency situation, a rapidly acting alkylating agent would probably be the drug of choice.

Superior vena cava syndrome

This syndrome should more properly be regarded as an 'urgent' rather than 'emergency' problem. However, it may be a marker for an associated acute problem, airway compromise. The distinction is important, as usually time is available to establish a tissue diagnosis with consequent definitive therapy. In most cancer patients this syndrome is secondary to lung cancer (75 per cent) or lymphoma (15–20 per cent). Patients with small-cell lung cancer and lymphomas have been treated with chemotherapy with reasonable results.[156,157] Other patients are usually treated with radiation therapy and high-dose corticosteroids. The addition of nitrogen mustard therapy does not appear to improve the outcome of patients with superior vena cava syndromes secondary to bronchogenic carcinoma.[158] In an emergency situation where access to excellent radiotherapy is not available, chemotherapy could be used—the regimen to be related to the probable cause of the obstruction.

Hypercalcaemia

Mithramycin is a third line agent in the management of tumour-related hypercalcaemia. Other chemotherapeutic agents may be useful in maintaining a tumour response after a return to a normal calcium level, but they should not be regarded as drugs for emergency management of this condition (see Chapter 9.11).

References

1. Bruera E, Kuehn N, Miller MJ, *et al.* The Edmonton symptom assessment system (ESAS): a simple method for the assessment of palliative care patients. *Journal of Palliative Care,* 1991; **7**: 6–9.
2. Bonadonna G, Molinari R. Role and limits of anticancer drugs in the treatment of advanced cancer pain. *Advances in Pain Research and Therapy,* 1979; **2**: 131–44.
3. Rosenberg SA *et al.* Use of tumor-infiltrating lymphocytes and interleukin-2 in the immunotherapy of patients with metastatic melanoma. *New England Journal of Medicine,* 1988; **319**: 1676–80.
4. Osoba D *et al.* Combination chemotherapy with bleomycin, etoposide, and cis-platin in metastatic non-small cell lung cancer. *Journal of Oncology,* 1985; **5**: 1470–85.
5. Estes NC *et al.* Intra-arterial chemotherapy and hyperthermia for pain control in patients with recurrent rectal cancer. *American Journal of Surgery,* 1986; **152**: 597–601.
6. Klopp CT *et al.* Fractionated intra-arterial cancer chemotherapy with methyl bis amine hydrochloride; a preliminary report. *Annals of Surgery,* 1950; **132**: 811–32.
7. Woodhall B *et al.* Effect of hyperthermia upon cancer chemotherapy; application to external cancers of head and face structures. *Annals of Surgery,* 1960; **151**: 750–9.
8. Bateman Jr, Hazen JB, Strolinsky DC, Steinfeld J. Advanced carcinoma of the cervix treated with intra-arterial methotrexate. *American Journal of Obstetrics and Gynecology,* 1966; **96**: 181–7.
9. Latbrop JC, Frates RE. Arterial infusion of nitrogen mustard in the treatment of intractable pelvic pain of malignant origin. *Cancer,* 1980; **45**: 432–8.
10. Laufe LE *et al.* Infusion through inferior gluteal artery for pelvic cancer. *Obstetrics and Gynecology,* 1966; **28**: 650–9.
11. Beyer JH *et al.* Intra-arterial perfusion therapy with 5-fluorouracil in patients with metastatic colo-rectal carcinoma and intractable pelvic pain. *Recent Results in Cancer Research,* 1983; **86**: 33–6.
12. Heim ME, Eberwein S, Georgi M. Palliative therapy of pelvic tumours by intra-arterial infusion of cytotoxic drugs. *Recent Results in Cancer Research,* 1983; **86**: 37–40.
13. Coates A, Abraham S, Kaye S, Sowerbutts T, Frewin C, Fox RM, Tattersall MHN. On the receiving end patient perception of the side-effects of cancer chemotherapy. *European Journal of Cancer and Clinical Oncology,* 1983; **1**: 203–8.
14. Sutherland HJ, Lockwood GA, Boyd NF. Ratings of the importance of quality of life variables: Therapeutic implications for patients with breast cancer. *Journal of Clinical Epidemiology,* 1990; **43**: 661–6.
15. Coates A, Gebski V, Bishop JF, *et al.* for the ANZ Breast Cancer Trials Group. Improving the quality of life during chemotherapy for advanced breast cancer. A comparison of intermittent and continuous treatment strategies. *New England Journal of Medicine,* 1987; **317**: 1490–5.
16. Richards MA, Hopwood P, Ramirez AJ, *et al.* Doxorubicin in advanced breast cancer: influence of schedule on response, survival and quality of life. *European Journal of Cancer,* 1992; **28A**: 1023–8.
17. Gralla RJ *et al.* Antiemetic efficacy of high-dose metoclopramide: randomized trials with placebo and prochlorperazine in patients with chemotherapy-induced nausea and vomiting. *New England Journal of Medicine,* 1981; **305**: 905–9.
18. Marty M *et al.* Comparison of the 5-hydroxytryptamine (serotonin) antagonist ondansetron (GR 38032F) with high-dose metoclopramide in the control of cisplatin-induced emesis. *New England Journal of Medicine,* 1990; **322**: 816–21.
19. Milne RJ, Heel RC. Ondansetron: therapeutic use as an antiemetic. *Drugs,* 1991; **41**: 574–95.
20. Johnston D, Latreille J, Laberge F, *et al.* Preventing nausea and vomiting during days 2–7 following high-dose cisplatin chemotherapy (HDCP). A study by the National Cancer Institute of Canada Clinical Trials Group (NCIC CTG) (abstract 1745). *Proceedings of the American Society of Clinical Oncology,* 1995; **14**: 529.
21. Osoba D, Warr D, *et al.* Quality of life studies in chemotherapy-induced emesis. *Oncology,* 1996; **53** (suppl. 2): 92–5.
22. Colvin M, Chabner BA. Alkylating agents. In: Chabner BA, Collins JM, eds. *Cancer Chemotherapy: Principles and Practice.* Philadelphia: J.B. Lippincott, 1990.
23. Stubgen JP. Neuromuscular disorders in systemic malignancy and its treatment. *Muscle and Nerve,* 1995; **18**: 636–48.
24. Troy LA *et al.* The impact of cisplatin-based therapy on attentional processes in patients with testicular cancer (abstract). *Psycho-Oncology,* 1996; **5** (suppl.): 23.
25. Rowinsky EK, Donehower RC. Paclitaxel (Taxol). *New England Journal of Medicine,* 1995; **332**: 1004–14.
26. Gelmon K. The taxoids: paclitaxel and docetaxel. *Lancet,* 1994; **344**: 1267–72.
27. Belli L, Le Chevalier T, Gottfried M, *et al.* Phase I-II Trial of Paclitaxel (Taxol ®) and Cisplatin in Previously Untreated Advanced Non-Small Cell Lung Cancer (NSCLC). *Proceedings of the American Society of Clinical Oncology,* 1995; **14**: 350.
28. Forman AD. Neurologic complications of cytokine therapy. *Oncology,* 1994; **8**: 105–17.
29. Meyers CA, Scheibel RS, Forman AD. Persistent neurotoxicity of systemically administered interferon-alpha. *Neurology,* 1994; **41**: 672–6.
30. Cascinu S, Cordella L, Del Ferro E, *et al.* Neuroprotective effect of reduced glutathione on cisplatin-based chemotherapy in advanced gastric cancer: a randomized double-blind placebo-controlled trial. *Journal of Clinical Pharmacology,* 1995; **13**: 26–32.
31. Chabner BA. Bleomycin. In: Chabner BA, Collins JM, eds. *Cancer Chemotherapy:Principles and Practice.* Philadelphia: J.B. Lippincott, 1990.
32. O'Driscoll BR, Hasleton PA, Taylor PM, *et al.* Active lung fibrosis up to 17 years after chemotherapy with carmustine (BCNU) in childhood. *New England Journal of Medicine,* 1990; **323**: 378–82.
33. McDonald S, Rubin P, Phillips TL, *et al.* Injury to the lung from cancer therapy: clinical syndromes, measurable endpoints, and potential scoring systems. *Journal of Radiation Oncology Biology Physics,* 1995; **31**: 1187–203.
34. Allegra CJ. Antifolates. In: Chabner BA, Collins JM, eds. *Cancer Chemotherapy: Principles and Practice.* Philadelphia: J.B. Lippincott, 1990.
35. Sorensen K, Levitt G, Sebag-Montefiore D, *et al.* Cardiac function in Wilms' tumor survivors. *Journal of Clinical Oncology,* 1995; **13**: 1546–56.
36. Watts RC. Severe and fatal anthracycline toxicity at cumulative doses below 400 mgm/m^2. Evidence for enhanced toxicity with multiagent chemotherapy. *American Journal of Hematology,* 1991; **3**: 337–42.
37. Schechter D, Nagler A. Recombinant interleukin-2 and recombinant interferon α immunotherapy cardiovascular toxicity. *American Heart Journal,* 1992; **123**: 1736–9.
38. Schilsky RL, Erlichman C. Infertility and carcinogenesis: late complications of chemotherapy. In: Chabner BA, Collins JM, eds. *Cancer Chemotherapy: Principles and Practice.* Philadelphia: J.B. Lippincott, 1990.
39. Seipp CA. Alopecia. In: Wittes RE, ed. *Manual of Oncologic Therapeutics 1991–92.* Philadelphia: J.B. Lippincott, 1991.

40. Jackson AM, Rose BD, Graff LG, *et al.* Thrombotic mieroangiopathy and renal failure associated with antineoplastic chemotherapy. *Annals of Internal Medicine,* 1984; **101**: 41–4.
41. Narins RB, Carley M, Bloom EJ, *et al.* The nephrotoxicity of chemotherapeutic agents. *Seminars in Nephrology,* 1990; **10**: 556–64.
42. Hamilton CR, Bliss JM, Horwich A. The late effects of cis-platinum on renal function. *European Journal of Cancer and Clinical Oncology,* 1989; **25**: 185–9.
43. Marks LB, Carroll PR, Dugan TC, *et al.* The response of the urinary bladder, urethra, and ureter to radiation and chemotherapy. *Internatonal Journal of Radiation Oncology Biology Physics,* 1995; **31**: 1257–80.
44. Woodhall V *et al.* Effect of chemotherapeutic agents upon peripheral nerves. *Journal of Surgical Research,* 1962; **2**: 373–81.
45. Stiefel FC, Breitbart WH, Holland JC. Corticosteroids in cancer: neuropsychiatric complications. *Cancer Investigation,* 1989; **7**: 479–91.
46. Effershaw S, Kelly MK. Corticosteroids and peptic ulceration. *Palliative Medicine,*1994; **8**: 313–19.
47. Piper JM, Ray WA, Dougherty JR, Griffin MR. Corticosteroid use and peptic ulcer disease: role of nonsteroidal anti-inflammatory drugs. *Annals of Internal Medicine,* 1991; **114**: 735–40.
48. Bowyer SL, LaMothe MP, Hollister JR. Steroid myopathy: incidence and detection in a population with asthma. *Journal of Allergy and Clinical Immunology,* 1985; **76**: 234–42.
49. Weinstein SP, Paquin T, Pritsker A, *et al.* Glucocorticoid-induced insulin resistance: dexamethasone inhibits the activation of glucose transport in rat skeletal muscle by both insulin- and non-insulin-related stimuli. *Diabetes,* 1995; **44**: 441–5.
50. Siperstein MD. Diabetic ketoacidosis and hyperosmolar coma. *Endocrine and Metabolic Clinics of North America,* 1992; **21**: 415–32.
51. Lorber D. Nonketotic hypertonicity in diabetes mellitus. *Medical Clinics of North America,* 1995; **79**: 39–52.
52. Braunstein PW Jr, deGirolami U. Experimental corticosteroid myopathy. *Acta Neuropathologica,* 1981; **55**: 167–72.
53. Falude G, Gotlieb J, Meyers J. Factors influencing the development of steroid-induced myopathies. *Annals of the New York Academy of Sciences,* 1966; **138**: 61–72.
54. Cohen SR, Mount BM, Tomas JJN, Mount LF. Existential well-being is an important determinant of quality of life. Evidence from the McGill Quality of Life Questionnaire. *Cancer,* 1996; **77**: 576–86.
55. Coscarelli Schag CA, Ganz PA, Heinrich RL. Cancer rehabilitation evaluation system—short form (CARES-SF). A cancer specific rehabilitation and quality-of-life instrument. *Cancer,* 1991; **68**: 1406–13.
56. Aaronson NK, Ahmedzai S, Bergman B, *et al.* The European Organization for Research and Treatment of Cancer QLQ C-30. A quality-of-life instrument for use in international trials in oncology. *Journal of the National Cancer Institute,* 1993; **85**: 365–76.
57. Cella DF, Tulsky DS, Gray G, *et al.* The functional assessment of cancer therapy scale: development and validation of the general measure. *Journal of Clinical Oncology,* 1993; **11**: 570–9.
58. Schipper H, Clinch J, McMurray A, *et al.* Measuring the quality of life of cancer patients: the functional living index—cancer development and validation. *Journal of Clinical Oncology,* 1984; **2**: 472–83.
59. Selby PJ, Chapman J-AW, Etazadi-Amoli J, *et al.* The development of a method for assessing quality of life of cancer patients. *British Journal of Cancer,* 1984; **50**: 13–22.
60. Ware JE, Sherbourne CD. The MOS 36-item Short Form Health Survey (SF-36): Conceptual framework and item selection. *MedCare,* 1992; **30**: 473–83.
61. Padilla GV, Presant C, Grant MM, *et al.* Quality-of-life index for patients with cancer. *Research Nursing Health,* 1983; **6**: 117–26.
62. Spitzer WO, Dobson AJ, Hall J, *et al.* Measuring the quality of life of cancer patients: A concise QL-index for use by physicians. *Journal of Chronic Diseases,* 1981; **34**: 585–97.
63. de Haes JCJM, Welvart K. Quality of life after breast cancer surgery. *Journal of Surgical Oncology,* 1985; **28**: 123–5.
64. Dudgeon DJ, Raubertas RF, Doerner K, O'Connor T, Tobin M, Rosenthal SN. When does palliative care begin? A needs assessment of cancer patients with recurrent disease. *Journal of Palliative Care,* 1995; **11**: 5–9.
65. Poon MA *et al.* Biochemical modulation of fluorouracil with leucoverin: confirmatory evidence of improved therapeutic efficacy inadvanced colorectal cancer. *Journal of Clinical Oncology,* 1991; **9**: 1967–72.
66. McCarthy M. Hospice patients: a pilot study in 12 services. *Palliative Medicine,* 1990; **4**: 93–104.
67. Miller RJ. The role of chemotherapy in the hospice patient. A problem of definition. *American Journal of Hospice Care,* 1989; 19–26.
68. Reuben DB, Mor V, Hiris J. Clinical symptoms and length of survival in patients with terminal cancer. *Archives of Internal Medicine,* 1988; **148**: 1586–91.
69. Ruckdeschel JC, Piantadosi S. Quality of life assessment. An independent prognostic variable for survival in lung cancer. *Journal of Theoretical Surgery,* 1991; **6**: 201–5.
70. Kaasa S *et al.* Prognostic factors for patients with inoperable non-small cell lung cancer, limited disease. *Radiotherapy Oncology,* 1989; **15**: 235–42.
71. Coates A, Gebski V, Signorini D, *et al.* Prognostic value of quality-of-life scores during chemotherapy for advanced breast cancer. *Journal of Clinical Oncology,* 1992; **10**: 1833–8.
72. Coates A, Thomson, D, McLeod GRM, *et al.* Prognostic value of quality of life scores in a trial of chemotherapy with or without interferon in patients with metastatic malignant melanoma. *European Journal of Cancer,* 1993; **29A**: 1731–4.
73. Kennedy BJ. Aging and cancer. *Journal of Clinical Oncology,* 1988; **6**: 1903–11.
74. Fentiman IS. Treatment of cancer in the elderly. *British Journal of Cancer,* 1991; **64**: 993–5.
75. Yellen SB, Cella DF, Leslie WT. Age and clinical decision making in oncology patients. *Journal of the National Cancer Institute,* 1994; **86**: 1766–70.
76. Desch CE, Smith TJ. Defining treatment aims and end-points in older patients with cancer. *Drugs and Aging,* 1995; **6**: 351–7.
77. Weeks JC. Preferences of older cancer patients: can you judge a book by its cover? *Journal of the National Cancer Institute,* 1994; **86**: 1743–4.
78. Slevin ML *et al.* Attitudes to chemotherapy: comparing views of patients with cancer with those of doctors, nurses, and general public. *British Medical Journal,* 1990; **300**: 1458–60.
79. O'Connor AMC *et al.* Eliciting preferences for alternative drug therapies in oncology: influence of treatment outcome description, elicitation technique and treatment experience on preferences. *Journal of Chronic Diseases,* 1987; **40**: 811–18.
80. Rapp E *et al.* Chemotherapy can prolong survival in patients with advanced non-small cell lung cancer. *Journal of Clinical Oncology,* 1988; **6**: 633–41.
81. Jaakkimainen L *et al.* Counting the costs of chemotherapy in a National Cancer Institute of Canada randomized trial in non-small cell lung cancer. *Journal of Clinical Oncology,* 1990; **8**: 1301–9.
82. Poon MA *et al.* Biochemical modulation of fluorouracil: evidence of significant improvement of survival and quality of life in patients with advanced colorectal cancer. *Journal of Clinical Oncology,* 1989; **7**: 1407–18.
83. Kardinal CG *et al.* Responses to chemotherapy or chemo-hormonal therapy in advanced breast cancer patients treated previously with adjuvant chemotherapy. *Cancer,* 1988; **61**: 415–19.
84. Valagussa P, Tancini G, Bonadonna G. Salvage treatment of patients suffering relapse after adjuvant chemotherapy. *Cancer,* 1986; **58**: 1411–17.
85. Hudis CA. Do we need a 'stopping rule' for breast cancer? *Cancer Investigation,* 1994; **12**: 543–4.
86. Benner SE, Fetting JH, Brenner MH. A stopping rule for standard chemotherapy for metastatic breast cancer: lessons from a survey of maryland medical oncologists. *Cancer Investigation,* 1994; **12**: 451–5.
87. Sikic BI *et al.* High-dose megestrol acetate therapy of ovarian carcinoma: a phase II study of the Northern California Oncology Group. *Seminars in Oncology,* 1986; **13**: 26–32.

88. Geisler HE. The use of high-dose megestrol acetate in the treatment of ovarian adenocarcinoma. *Seminars in Oncology,* 1985; **13**: 20–2.
89. Belinson JL, McClure M, Badger G. Randomized trial of megestrol acetate vs. megestrol acetateltamoxifen for the management of progressive or recurrent epithelial ovarian carcinoma. *Gynecologic Oncology,* 1987; **28**: 151–5.
90. Rubens RD. Corticosteroids. In: Powles TJ, Smith IE, eds. *Medical Management of Breast Cancer.* London: Martin Dunitz, 1991: 117–21.
91. Yancey JM. Ten rules for reading clinical research reports. *American Journal of Surgery,* 1990; **159**: 533–8.
92. NIH Consensus Conference on Adjuvant Therapy for Patients with Colon and Rectal Cancer. *Journal of the American Medical Association,* 1990; **264**: 1444–50.
93. Spiro SG. Management of lung cancer. *British Medical Journal,* 1990; **301**: 1287–8.
94. Goldie J, Ling V. The evolution of drug resistance in tumor. *Canadian Journal of Oncology,* 1991; **1**: 1–10.
95. Prehn RT. The inhibition of tumor growth by tumor mass. *Cancer Research,* 1991; **51**: 2–4.
96. Maidand JA *et al.* Evidence that multiple myeloma may be regulated by homeostatic control mechanisms: correlation of changes in the number of clonogenic myeloma cells *in vitro* with clinical response. *British Journal of Cancer,* 1990; **61**: 429–33.
97. Ihde DC. Chemotherapy of lung cancer. *New England Journal of Medicine,* 1992; **327**: 1434–41.
98. Catney DN *et al.* Single-agent oral etoposide for elderly small cell lung cancer patients. *Seminars in Oncology,* 1990; **17**: 49–53.
99. Ihde DC. Small cell lung cancer. In: Macdonald JS, Haller DG, Mayer RJ, eds. *Manual of Oncologic Therapeutics,* 3rd edn. Philadelphia: J.B. Lippincott, 1995: 148–52.
100. Souquet PJ, Chauvin F, Boissel JP, *et al.* Polychemotherapy in advanced non small cell lung cancer: a meta-analysis. *Lancet,* 1993; **342**: 19–21.
101. Non-small Cell Lung Cancer Collaborative Group. Chemotherapy in non-small cell lung cancer: a meta-analysis using updated data on individual patients from 52 randomised clinical trials. *British Medical Journal,* 1995; **311**: 899–909.
102. Gurney H *et al.* Ifosfamide and mitomycin in combination for the treatment of patients with progressive advanced non-small cell lung cancer. *European Journal of Cancer,* 1991; **27**: 565–8.
103. Hardy JR, Noble T, Smidh IE. Symptom relief with moderate dose chemotherapy (mitomycin-C vinblastin and cisplatin) in advanced non-small cell lung cancer. *British Journal of Cancer,* 1989; **60**: 764–6.
104. Fernandez C *et al.* Quality of life during chemotherapy in non-small cell lung cancer patients. *Acta Oncologica,* 1989; **28**: 29–33.
105. Luedke DW *et al.* Randomized comparișon of two combination regimens versus minimal chemotherapy in non small cell lung cancer: southeastern cancer study group. *Journal of Clinical Oncology,* 1990; **8**: 886–91.
106. McVie JG. Non-small cell lung cancer: meta-analysis of efficacy of chemotherapy. *Seminars in Oncology,* 1996; **23**: 12–14.
107. Grem JL. Current treatment approaches in colorectal cancer. *Seminars in Oncology,* 1991; **18**: 17–26.
108. Seitz JF *et al.* Final results and survival data of a large randomised trial of 'Tomudex' in advanced colorectal cancer (ACC) confirm comparable efficacy to 5-fluorouracil plus leucovorin (5FU+LV) (abstract). *Proceedings of the American Society for Clinical Oncology,* 1996; **15**: 201.
109. Moertel CG. Chemotherapy for colorectal cancer. *New England Journal of Medicine,* 1994; **330**: 1136–42.
110. MacDonald JS. Colorectal cancer. In: Wittes RE, ed. *Manual of Oncologic Therapeutics 1991–92.* Philadelphia: J.B. Lippincott, 1991.
111. Kemeny N. Chemotherapy for colorectal carcinoma: one small step forward, one step backward. *Journal of Clinical Oncology,* 1995; **13**: 1287–90.
112. Glimelius B *et al.* Quality of life during cytostatic therapy for advanced symptomatic colorectal carcinoma: a randomized comparison of two regimens. *European Journal of Cancer and Clinical Oncology,* 1989; **25**: 829–35.
113. Buroker TR, O'Connell MJ, Wie HS, *et al.* Randomized comparison of two schedules of fluorouracil and leucovorin in the treatment of advanced colorectal cancer. *Journal of Clinical Oncology,* 1994; **12**: 14–20.
114. Allen-Mersh TG Colorectal liver metastases: is 'no treatment' still best? *Journal of the Royal Society of Medicine,* 1989; **82**: 2–3.
115. Perrone S, Silva F, Sala A, *et al.* Treatment of liver metastases from colorectal neoplasia with percutaneous ethanol injection (PEI) under ultrasound (US) guidance (abstract). *Proceedings of the American Society for Clinical Oncology,* 1995; **14**: 203.
116. Kemeny N *et al.* Intra-hepatic or systemic infusion of fluorodioxyuridine in patients with liver metastases from colorectal carcinoma. *Annals of Internal Medicine,* 1987; **107**: 459–65.
117. Hohn DC *et al.* A randomized trial of continuous intravenous versus hepatic intra-arterial floxuridine in patients with colorectal cancer metastatic to the liver. *Journal of Clinical Oncology,* 1989; **7**: 1646–54.
118. Lillemoe KD. Current management of pancreatic cancer. *Annals of Surgery,* 1995; **221**: 133–48.
119. Moertal CE *et al.* Therapy of unresectable pancreatic carcinoma: a randomised comparison of high dose radiation alone, moderate dose radiation and high dose radiation plus 5-FU. *Cancer,* 1981; **48**: 1705–10.
120. Rothenberg ML, Burtis HA, Andersen JS, *et al.* Gescitabine: effective palliative therapy for pancreas cancer patients failing 5-FU (abstract). *Proceedings of the American Society for Clinical Oncology,* 1995; **14**: 198.
121. Moore M, Andersen J, Burris H, *et al.* A randomized trial of gemcitabine (GEM) versus 5FU as first-line therapy in advanced pancreatic cancer (abstract). *Proceedings of the American Society for Clinical Oncology,* 1995; **14**: 199.
122. Cascinu S, Del Ferro E, Catalano G. A randomized trial of octreolide vs best supportive care only in advanced gastrointestinal cancer patients refractory to chemotherapy. *British Journal of Cancer,* 1995; **71**: 97–101.
123. De Conno F, Saita L, Ripamonti C, *et al.* Suboutaneous octreotide in the treatment of pain in advanced cancer patients. *Journal of Pain and Symptom Management,* 1994; **9**: 34–8.
124. Rosenberg L, Barkun AN, Denis MH, *et al.* Low dose octreotide and tamoxifen in the treatment of adenocarcinoma of the pancreas. *Cancer,* 1995; **75**: 23–8.
125. Taylor OM, Benson EA, McMahon MJ, *et al.* Clinical trial of tamoxifen in patients with irresectable pancreatic adenocarcinoma. *British Journal of Surgery,* 1994; **80**: 384–6.
126. Rosemurgy A *et al.* Marimastat, a novel matrix metalloproteinase inhibitor in patients with advanced carcinoma of the pancreas (abstract). *Proceedings of the American Society for Clinical Oncology,* 1996; **15**: 207.
127. Chodak GW *et al.* Independent prognostic factors in patients with metastatic (stage D2) prostate cancer. *Journal of the American Medical Association,* 1991; **265**: 618–21.
128. Yagoda A. Genitourinary cancers. In Wittes RE, ed. *Manual of Oncologic Therapeutics 1991–92.* Philadelphia: J.B. Lippincott, 1992: 178–88.
129. Berry N, MacDonald N. Cisplatin, cyclophosphamide, and presdnisone therapy for state D prostatic cancer. *Cancer Chemotherapy Reports,* 1982; **66**: 1403–4.
130. Tannock I *et al.* Treatment of metastatic prostatic cancer with low-dose prednisone: evaluation of pain and quality of life as pragmatic indices of response. *Journal of Clinical Oncology,* 1989; **7**: 590–7.
131. Gittes RF. Carcinoma of the prostate. *New England Journal of Medicine,* 1991; **324**: 236–45.
132. Tannock I, Osoba D, Ernst S, *et al.* Chemotherapy with mitoxantrone plus prednisone or prednisone alone for symptomatic prostate cancer: A Canadian randomized trial with palliative endpoints. *Journal of Clinical Oncology,* 1996; **14**: 1756–69.
133. Maulard-Durdux C *et al.* Phase II study of the oral cyclophosphamide and oral etoposide combination in hormone-refractory prostate carcinoma patients. *Cancer,* 1996; **77**: 1144–8.
134. Hoefnagel CA. Radionuclide therapy revisited. *European Journal of Nuclear Medicine,* 1991; **18**: 408–31.
135. Fitton A, McTavish D. Pamidronate: a review of its pharmacological properties and therapeutic efficacy in resorptive bone disease. *Drugs,* 1991; **41**: 289–314.
136. Ernst DS, MacDonald N, Paterson AHG, Jensen J, Brasher P, Bruera E.

A double-blind, crossover trial of intravenous clodronate in metastatic bone pain. *Journal of Pain and Symptom Management*, 1992; **7**: 4–11.

137. Maguire GP *et al.* Psychiatric morbidity and physical toxicity associated with adjuvant chemotherapy after mastectomy. *British Medical Journal*, 1980; **281**: 1179–80.
138. Palmer BV, Walsh GA, McKinna JA, Greening WP. Adjuvant chemotherapy for breast cancer: side effects and quality of life. *British Medical Journal*, 1980; **281**: 1594–7.
139. Tannock IF *et al.* A randomized trial of two dose levels of cyclophosphamide, methotrexate, and fluorouracil chemotherapy for patients with metastatic breast cancer. *Journal of Clinical Oncology*, 1988; **6**: 1377–87.
140. Garber JE, Henderson IC. Use of chemotherapy in metastatic breast cancer. *Hematology and Oncology Clinics of North America*, 1989; **3**: 807–21.
141. Henderson IC *et al.* Randomized clinical trial comparing mitoxantrone with doxorubicin in previously treated patients with metastatic breast cancer. *Journal of Clinical Oncology*, 1989; **7**: 560–71.
142. Gelmon KA, O'Reilly S, Plenderleith IH, *et al.* Bi-weekly paclitaxel and cisplatin in the treatment of metastatic breast cancer (abstract 87). *Proceedings of the American Society for Clinical Oncology*, 1994; **13**: 71.
143. Gelmon K. The taxoids: paclitaxel and docetaxel. *Lancet* 1994; **344**: 1267–72.
144. Paterson AHG, McCloskey EV, Ashley S, Powles TJ, Kanis JA. Reduction of skeletal morbidity and prevention of bone metastases with oral clodronate in women with recurrent breast cancer in the absence of skeletal metastases (abstract). *Proceedings of the American Society for Clinical Oncology*, 1996; **15**: 104.
145. Theriault R, Lipton A, Gluck S, *et al.* Reduction of skeletal related complications in breast cancer patients with osteolytic bone metastases receiving hormone therapy, by monthly pamidronate sodium (Aredia) infusion (abstract). *Proceedings of the American Society for Clinical Oncology*, 1996; **15**: 122.
146. Conte PF, Latreille J, Mauriac F, *et al.* Delay in progression of bone metastases in breast cancer patients treated with intravenous pamidronate: results from a multinational randomized controlled trial. *Journal of Clinical Oncology*, 1996; **14**: 2552–9.
147. Robinson RG *et al.* Strontium 89 therapy for the palliation of pain due to osseous metastases. *Journal of the American Medical Association*, 1995; **274**: 420–4.
148. Tannock IF. General principles of chemotherapy. In: Million RR, Cassisi NJ, eds. *Management of Head and Neck Cancer: A Multidisciplinary Approach*, 2nd edn. Philadelphia: JB Lippincott, 1994: 143–56.
149. Forastiere A, Metch B, Schuller DE, *et al.* Randomized comparison of cisplatin plus fluorouracil versus carboplatin plus flourouracil versus methotrexate in advanced squamous-cell carcinoma of the head and neck. A Southwest Oncology Group study. *Journal of Clinical Oncology*, 1992; **10**: 1245–51.
150. Murphy WT, Bilge N. Compression of the spinal cord in patients with malignant lymphoma. *Radiology*, 1964; **82**: 495–500.
151. Marshall LF, Langfitt IW. Combined therapy of extradural tumors of the spine. *Cancer*, 1977; **40**: 2067–70.
152. Sinoff CL, Blumsohn A. Spinal cord compression in myelomatosis: response to chemotherapy alone. *European Journal of Cancer in Clinical Oncology*, 1989; **25**: 197–200.
153. Gale GB, O'Connor DN, Chu S. Successful chemotherapeutic decompression of epidural malignant germ cell. *Medical Pediatric Oncology*, 1986; 1497–9.
154. Hayes FA *et al.* Chemotherapy as an alternative to laminectomy and radiation in the management of epidural tumour. *Journal of Pediatrics*, 1984; **104**: 221–4.
155. Leung SF, Tsao SY, Shiu W. Treatment outcome of spinal cord compression by nasophryngeal carcinoma. *British Journal of Radiology*, 1990; **63**: 716–19.
156. Dombernowsky P, Hanson H. Combination chemotherapy in the management of superior vena caval obstruction in small cell anaplastic carcinoma of the lung. *Acta Medica Scandinavica*, 1978; **204**: 513–16.
157. Perez-Soler R *et al.* Clinical features and results of management of superior vena cava syndrome secondary to lymphoma. *Journal of Clinical Oncology*, 1984; **2**: 260–6.
158. Levitt SH, Jones GK, Kilpatrick SJ. Treatment of malignant superior vena caval obstruction. *Cancer*, 1969; **24**: 447–51.

9.1.2 Radiotherapy in symptom management

P. J. Hoskin

Introduction

Over 50 per cent of cancer patients will require radiation therapy at some time in the course of their disease, and over half of all radiation treatments are given with palliative intent for the control of local symptoms. Radiotherapy has a major role in controlling symptoms from a tumour at a specific site but will have no influence over the natural history of the tumour outside the irradiated area.

General principles of radiotherapy

Radiobiology

Radiotherapy is the process of treatment with ionizing radiation which results in damage to cellular DNA. X-rays and gamma rays are the forms of ionizing radiation used most frequently in clinical radiotherapy; similar effects result from the release of beta particle irradiation when radioisotopes are used. The results of radiation of this type passing through a living cell are to cause both direct and indirect damage to the reproductive material of the cell. Direct damage occurs in the form of base deletions and single and double strand breaks in the DNA chain. Indirect damage occurs by the interaction of radiation with water molecules in the cell releasing toxic free radicals. Considerable repair of the damage may be possible within the cell and normal tissues have a marked repair capacity allowing recovery from this 'sublethal' radiation damage. Differences in repair capacity between different types of cancer cell may partly account for the variation seen in radiosensitivity. It is also increasingly recognized that programmed cell death (termed apoptosis) is an important factor in the pathway resulting in cell death after irradiation.

The response of cells to radiation is affected by many factors including oxygenation (hypoxic cells are relatively radioresistant), the number of cells actively dividing (cells in certain phases of the cell cycle are more sensitive than others; non-cycling cells are relatively radioresistant), and the rate of repopulation within the tumour. These parameters of repair, reoxygenation, repopulation, and redistribution within the cell cycle form the basis of radiobiology. Application of these principles is used in clinical practice to maximize tumour cell kill whilst minimizing normal tissue damage.

Table 1 Types of external beam radiation

	Energy	Source	Clinical use
X-rays			
Superficial	50–150 kV	X-ray tube	Skin tumour
Orthovoltage	250–500 kV	X-ray tube	Superficial sites e.g. breast, rib, sacrum
Megavoltage	> 1 MV (usually 4–16 MV)	Linear accelerator	Main source of therapeutic beams for sites other than skin (Megavoltage and Gamma rays)
Gamma rays	2.5 MV	Cobalt	
Electrons	4–30 MV	Linear accelerator	Superficial sites e.g. skin, lymph nodes (depth depends upon electron energy)

Aspects of radiation delivery

The most common means of delivering radiotherapy to a patient is by the use of an external beam of radiation directed at the site of interest. The different types of external beam radiation are outlined in Table 1. Ionizing radiation can also be delivered by the application of a radioactive source into or around the tumour site. This is known as brachytherapy. Examples of this are shown in Table 2.

Because radiation is damaging to normal tissues it is important that it is directed as accurately as possible to the area requiring treatment, minimizing the amount of sensitive, normal tissue within the treated area. For superficial lesions which are visible or palpable, the area to be localized can be easily defined on clinical examination but deep-seated tumours require radiographic localization using a treatment simulator. This is an X-ray machine identical to the therapy machine in its geometric specifications and movements but which differs by emitting a diagnostic X-ray beam producing an image of the proposed therapeutic beam. X-ray localization of deep structures and the definition of internal organs can be enhanced by coupling this process with CT scanning; this is of particular value in certain sites such as the bladder, prostate, and pancreas. In addition to accurate localization, it is vital that if an area is to be treated more than once in a course of treatment the beam position relative to the patient can be accurately reproduced from day to day. This is ensured by both careful measurement of the beam position and indelible marking of accurately defined skin entry points on the patient. Immobilization of the patient using sandbags or plastic shells may be necessary, particularly for sites which can easily change position from day to day, such as limbs or regions within the head and neck area.

Table 2 Clinical use of radioisotopes

Intracavity	Caesium Colbalt Iridium	Intrauterine Intravaginal Endo-oesophageal Endobronchial
Interstitial	Caesium needles Iridium wire	Tongue/floor of mouth Buccal mucosa Breast Anus/vulva
Internal	Iodine Phosphorus Strontium	Thyroid cancer Polycythaemia (Bone pain) Bone metastases

Most radiotherapy treatments will last for only a few minutes and have no accompanying symptoms at the time of delivery. It is important, however, to facilitate patient compliance with the procedure which involves some co-operation in positioning and lying still. The judicious administration of analgesia or anxiolytic drugs prior to treatment should be considered for those experiencing specific pain or anxiety.

Palliative compared with radical radiotherapy

The aim of radical radiotherapy is to cure local tumour by the complete eradication of tumour cells with minimum associated normal tissue damage; the aim of palliative radiotherapy is to control local symptoms with minimum associated acute radiation reaction.

Curative radiotherapy requires lengthy treatments of up to 6 or 7 weeks' duration in which the total dose of radiation is built up through small daily doses or fractions. An alternative approach uses hyperfractionation and accelerated fractionation in which two or three treatments per day are given, each smaller and therefore less damaging than the usual daily fraction (hyperfractionation) but by giving multiple treatments per day the overall treatment time is reduced (acceleration). In situations where extensive tumour regression is necessary for symptom control, for instance in the head and neck region, this high dose treatment may be necessary but it is often not appropriate for palliative therapy, particularly for patients with advanced metastatic disease whose survival may be measured in terms of only weeks or a few months. In this group, the aim of therapy is to delay tumour growth, relieve pain, and arrest haemorrhage. This can usually be achieved with relatively low doses of radiation delivered in a single treatment or a short course over 1 to 2 weeks. By reducing total doses, acute reactions are kept to a minimum whilst being compatible with the control of local symptoms.

Side-effects of radiotherapy

Radiotherapy side-effects are manifest as acute toxicity and late radiation damage. These are distinct events.

Acute toxicity represents loss of surface epithelial cells resulting in skin erythema or desquamation, mucositis, oesophagitis, cystitis, or gastrointestinal irritation. Re-epithelialization of the denuded surface occurs once treatment is completed, provided that sufficient underlying stem cells are maintained. Recovery usually occurs within a period of a few days or weeks from treatment. On rare occasions there may be persistent damage, particularly in certain vulnerable sites such as the lower leg or back and after infection or trauma when re-epithelialization fails. In these rare cases radionecrosis may occur.

Late radiation damage is potentially far more serious than the acute reaction. It may develop several months or years after treatment and is mainly due to progressive vascular changes in small blood vessels (endarteritis obliterans). The clinical manifestations of this range from the relatively minor such as the commonly observed appearance of skin atrophy and telangiectasia at a site of entry of a radiation beam, to the potentially fatal as seen with damage to bowel or bladder, resulting in perforation and fistula formation, or necrosis of the central nervous system. Such serious, late radiation damage is related to both high total doses and the delivery of radiation in large fractions over a relatively short period. Common clinical manifestations of acute and late radiation toxicity are shown in Table 3.

Table 3 Clinical manifestations of acute and late radiation toxicity

Site	Acute effects	Late effects[a]
Skin	Erythema Desquamation	Atrophy, fibrosis Telangiectasia Necrosis
Gastrointestinal tract	Nausea, anorexia vomiting, diarrhoea	Bowel stricture, haemorrhage, perforation, fistula
Bladder	Sterile cystitis	Reduced bladder volume Haematuria from bladder telangiectasia Urethral stricture Fistula
Head and neck	Mucositis Dry mouth Taste loss	Mucosal atrophy Telangiectasia Dental caries
Lungs	Pneumonitis	Pulmonary fibrosis
Central nervous system	Lhermitte's sign Local oedema	Myelitis Necrosis

[a] In most patients only minor late effects are seen. These are minimized by limiting the radiation dose to remain within tolerance of the surrounding tissues. Late effects are not usually seen after palliative radiation doses.

Management of the acute effects of radiotherapy is conservative, aiming to provide relief of symptoms whilst allowing the affected area to heal.

Mild skin reactions require no active treatment. Local irritation can be relieved by application of aqueous or 1 per cent hydrocortisone cream. Desquamation is conventionally treated with topical gentian violet. Talcum powder and proprietary creams containing metal salts should be avoided during treatment as these may enhance the reaction but starch powder, as found in proprietary baby powders, is often helpful in keeping the skin dry and comfortable.

Nausea during irradiation to the abdomen or pelvis will usually respond to simple antiemetic therapy such as metoclopramide (10 mg every 6–8 h). More severe symptoms may be helped by ondansetron (8 mg twice daily) or prednisolone (10–30 mg daily). Diarrhoea will respond to codeine phosphate (30 mg 2–3 times daily) or loperamide taken as required.

Radiation cystitis is more difficult to control and there is no satisfactory local treatment. It is important to exclude coexisting infection. Potassium citrate may be prescribed but is often unhelpful; systemic analgesics may be of value.

Local relief from mucositis of the oropharyngeal region may be achieved by the use of soluble aspirin or benzydamine mouthwashes. It is important to maintain a high level of oral hygiene using regular chlorhexidine mouthwashes and to treat the first signs of oropharyngeal candidiasis aggressively with nystatin suspension or clotrimazole gel. Any irradiation of the oral cavity or salivary glands should be preceded by careful dental assessment and correction of any dental problems, and fluoride dental gel is also often recommended during radiotherapy. Irritants, including alcohol and smoking, should be avoided. Rarely, in severe cases of mucositis in the gastrointestinal tract or oral cavity feeding through a nasogastric fine bore tube may be required to maintain nutrition during therapy.

Pneumonitis, presenting with a dry cough and dyspnoea, may be seen up to 4 months after radiotherapy which has included the lungs. It is diagnosed by the classic appearance on chest radiograph (Fig. 1) and should be treated with a 2 to 3 week course of systemic steroids, and antibiotics if there is secondary infection.

Finally it is important to anticipate probable acute side-effects, explain their likelihood to the patient, and encourage the prophylactic use of antiemetics, antidiarrhoeal drugs, and mouthwashes. The patient should also be reassured that they will resolve following completion of radiotherapy.

Combined modality treatment

Radiotherapy may be used alone but also in combination with drugs. Four types of radiation drug interaction have been

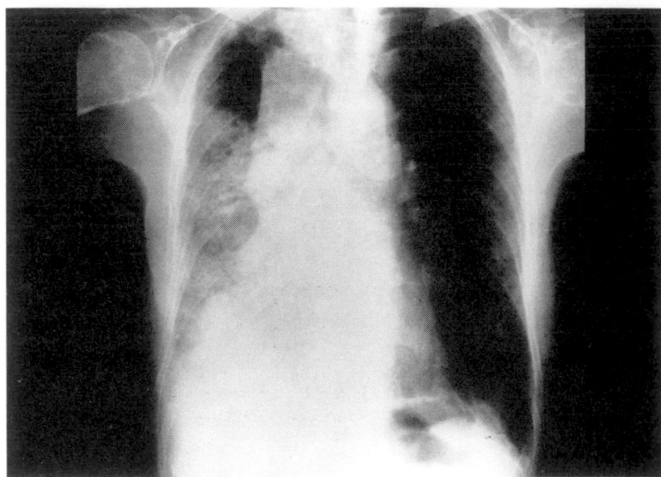

Fig. 1 Interstitial pneumonitis in the right mid and lower zones on chest radiograph after palliative irradiation for carcinoma of the bronchus.

described:[1] additive independent cell kill, spatial co-operation, enhancement of cell kill (e.g. radiosensitization), and protection of normal tissues. Common examples of combined modality therapy usually reflect spatial co-operation with control of micrometastases using systemic treatment and local control of bulky disease ensured with radiotherapy. This is used, for example, in the management of breast cancer, small-cell lung cancer, and lymphomas. True radiosensitization is rare but may occur in the use of combinations of radiotherapy with 5-fluorouracil and mitomycin C in the treatment of anal carcinoma, and cisplatin with radiotherapy in the treatment of non-small-cell lung cancer. Few, if any, of these treatments, however, fall readily within the scope of palliative medicine.

Other agents which may modify the radiation response have been developed and include misonadizole and nimorazole, which reduce tissue hypoxia, and nicotinamide, which influences tumour blood flow. Whilst effective in animal models, these agents have yet to be translated into routine clinical use.

Specific indications for radiotherapy in symptom control

Bone metastasis

Bone pain

Radiotherapy is the most effective treatment of local metastatic bone pain. Some degree of pain relief occurs in around 80 per cent of patients after treatment and complete pain relief is seen in a significant proportion. The majority of patients with bone metastases survive for less than 1 year and a simple, short treatment schedule is therefore most appropriate; in most situations a single treatment delivering a dose of 8 Gy is adequate and, as shown in Fig. 2, this has been found to be equivalent to more prolonged courses of treatment. The alternative is to deliver a fractionated course of 20 to 30 Gy over 1 to 2 weeks which may be given particularly when there is concern over possible fracture or nerve compression.

Superficial bones such as the clavicle, ribs, and sacrum may be treated with a direct field using orthovoltage X-rays (250–300 kV); other sites will usually be treated using a linear accelerator or cobalt beam. Under optimal conditions the site will be localized using a treatment simulator based on clinical examination and radiographic or bone scan evidence of metastatic disease. It is particularly important to document carefully the field margins in the spine where metastases at several levels may necessitate treatment of different areas at different times. Overlap of fields in the spine will result in overdosage to the spinal cord and possible subsequent radiation myelitis with irreversible neurological deterioration.

When accurate prospective assessments of pain have been used to monitor the response to local irradiation of a painful bone metastasis, an increasing incidence of pain relief is seen up to 4 weeks from the time of treatment with around half of responders achieving pain relief within the first 2 weeks (Fig. 2).[2] Immediate pain relief after local irradiation is relatively unusual in contrast with that seen after hemibody irradiation. The timing of the response is important when considering patients for reirradiation or adding alternative pain control methods. If pain returns to a previously irradiated site, retreatment is often feasible particularly after single dose treatments. There is now evidence that retreatment responses occur and are similar to those after primary treatment; these occur in over 80 per cent of retreatments and are even seen on second or third retreatments to a single site.[3] Alternative approaches may be more appropriate, however, for patients who fail to respond to initial radiotherapy.

The majority of patients with bone metastases will have multiple sites of disease and pain is sometimes not well localized but presents as a diffuse symptom affecting several sites. These patients may be better treated with wide field irradiation in which a single dose of 6 Gy is delivered to the upper body or 8 Gy is delivered to the lower body. This is associated with greater toxicity than local field irradiation; around two-thirds of patients have gastrointestinal symptoms of nausea, vomiting, or diarrhoea and the majority have a period of bone marrow suppression following treatment. A more serious consequence of upper hemibody irradiation is the development of radiation pneumonitis. Limiting the dose to 6 Gy, after correction for increased transmission of the X-ray beam through the lungs, will usually avoid this complication but occasional cases still occur and are usually progressive and fatal. Despite this, hemibody irradiation is a valuable tool for the treatment of widespread bone pain with response rates consistently around

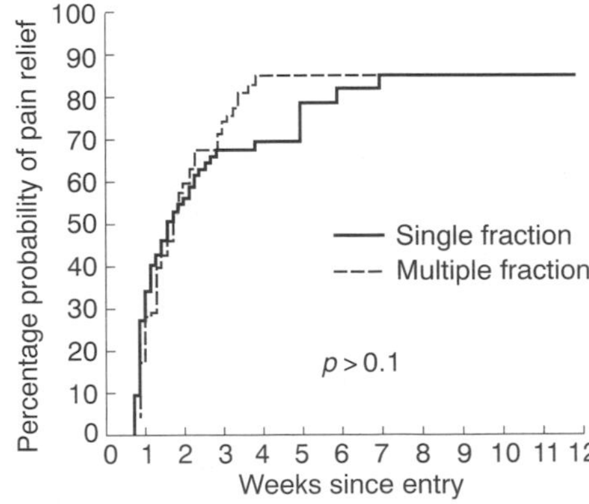

Fig. 2 Onset of pain relief following radiotherapy for local bone pain after either a single dose of 8 Gy or 30 Gy in 10 fractions over 2 weeks. No difference is seen between the two randomly allocated treatment groups. (Reproduced with permission from Price *et al*. 1986.[2])

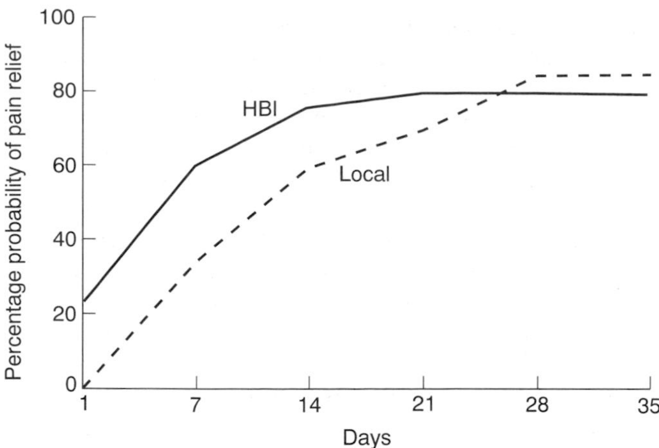

Fig. 3 Comparison of onset of pain relief following hemibody irradiation (HBI) and local irradiation for bone pain. (After Salazar, *et al.* 1986,[4] reproduced with permission.)

80 per cent, which are maintained in the majority of patients until death.

Pain relief after hemibody irradiation is often seen at a much earlier stage than after local field irradiation with many patients achieving pain relief within 24 to 48 h, as shown in Fig. 3.[4] This may suggest an alternative mechanism of action in achieving pain relief when hemibody irradiation is used compared to that seen after local irradiation.

An alternative approach to the treatment of multiple sites of bone pain is the administration of a bone seeking radioactive isotope which will be concentrated in a bone metastasis at sites of osteoblastic activity. The isotopes used deliver their radiation dose by the release of beta particles with a short range of only a few millimetres, thereby concentrating their dose within the immediate area of uptake.

In the specific case of differentiated thyroid cancer, radio-iodine administered orally is taken up by functioning tumour and is concentrated at the sites of bone metastasis. Unfortunately, however, published series report a disappointingly low response in terms of bone pain relief after radio-iodine and external beam therapy is better in this setting.[5]

For other tumours, radioisotopes taken up by actively mineralizing bone have been used. Radioactive phosphorus (^{32}P) is taken up non-selectively and is an effective agent in widespread bone pain but may be associated with considerable bone marrow depression which has limited its use. This has now been largely superseded by the development of radioactive strontium (^{89}Sr) which is selectively taken up at sites of osteoblastic activity in bone corresponding to areas of bone invasion by tumour cells. Transient bone marrow depression may also be seen with ^{89}Sr but is rarely of clinical significance and it is otherwise free from side-effects provided there is adequate renal function to clear the isotope. Effective pain relief is seen in around 80 per cent of patients and strontium treatment, which is given as a single intravenous outpatient injection, can be repeated at three-monthly intervals if appropriate.[6]

Other new radioisotopes under evaluation include samarium complexed in a tetraphosphonate compound to enable its concentration in bone (^{153}Sm-EDTMP) and rhenium (^{186}Re) complexed in a diphosphonate compound (^{186}Re-DP).

The mechanism by which irradiation achieves pain control is not clear. Tumour cells are undoubtedly killed, even after small single doses of radiation which result in pain relief, but other factors may be important. Evidence suggesting that tumour shrinkage itself may not be necessary include: the observation that rapid pain relief may result within 24 h of treatment, particularly after hemibody irradiation (Fig. 3); that no relation has been shown between the response in terms of pain relief and different histological types of tumour correlating with variations in radiosensitivity; and that no clear dose response relationship above very small single doses of 4 Gy[7] have been shown for the onset or duration of pain relief. This implies that local effects upon the host tissue, possibly affecting the release of pain mediating humoral agents, and osteoblast/osteoclast interaction are important cofactors in achieving and maintaining pain relief.

Prophylaxis

There has been considerable interest in the role of radiation in preventing the development and subsequent morbidity from bone metastasis. Inadvertent irradiation of certain sites, such as the thoracic spine when a breast is irradiated, has been shown to reduce the incidence of subsequent metastatic events in bones in this area. More recently, the value of hemibody irradiation at the time of presentation of localized bone pain has been evaluated and a reduction in subsequent episodes of bone pain demonstrated.[8] Similarly, the use of radioactive strontium (^{89}Sr) has been explored when bone metastases first present and this also has been shown to reduce or delay the need for further treatment for bone pain.[9] As yet, however, the evidence has not been sufficiently strong to justify routine use of hemibody irradiation or strontium in patients presenting with localized bone metastases since the gains are relatively modest—hemibody irradiation resulting in a 16 per cent reduction in requirements for additional local radiotherapy and strontium delaying the median time to further radiotherapy for a site of bone pain by 15 weeks.

Pathological fracture

Pathological fracture at a site of bone metastasis may occur spontaneously or as a result of minor trauma, particularly in weight-bearing bones. Internal fixation by surgical means is the preferred management in long bones but there will be situations, including vertebral collapse and fractures of the rib and girdle bones, where surgery is not feasible and other situations, where a patient has advanced disease and poor performance status, when surgery is inappropriate. In these cases, local irradiation remains a valuable palliative tool, both to achieve local pain relief and to enable bone healing.

When the object of treatment is pain relief alone, a single dose of 8 Gy is adequate treatment. Following irradiation, around two-thirds of patients with pathological fracture will achieve pain relief. There are no comparative data defining the optimum dose to achieve bone healing after pathological fracture. Remineralization is reported in one-third of patients after doses of 40 to 50 Gy delivered in 4 to 5 weeks but it is also seen after lower doses of only

20 Gy in 2 weeks. In practice, most patients will receive courses delivering 20 to 30 Gy in 5 to 10 fractions over 1 to 2 weeks.

Radiotherapy may also be indicated postoperatively, following internal fixation, to prevent further progression of the remaining metastatic tumour and enable healing of the bone around the prosthesis. Conventionally, fields covering the entire length of the prosthesis or intramedullary nail are used because of the potential risk of dissemination through the marrow cavity, although this approach has not been subject to critical evaluation. Patients with widespread metastatic disease and limited survival whose pain is controlled postoperatively gain little benefit from postoperative radiotherapy and this should be deferred unless local pain develops.

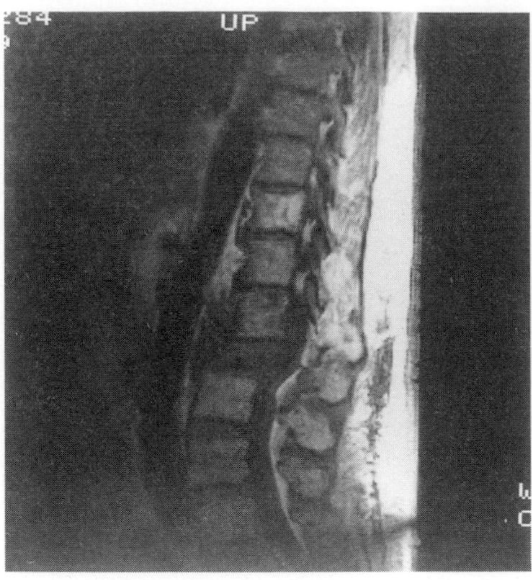

Fig. 4 Magnetic resonance imaging of spinal cord compression demonstrating the superior definition of bone and soft tissue compared to myelography or CT.

Neurological symptoms

Spinal cord and cauda equina compression

The clinical picture of spinal cord or cauda equina compression arises due to tumour growth within the spinal canal. The initial events are predominantly vascular with venous engorgement and oedema followed by mechanical compression of the nervous tissue. Magnetic resonance imaging of spinal cord compression demonstrates around one-quarter of these cases to be due to direct encroachment of the spinal canal by tumour arising in a vertebral body with the remainder attributable to blood-borne extradural or intradural metastasis.[11] Approximately 70 per cent of cases involve thoracic cord, 20 per cent the lumbosacral region, and 10 per cent the cervical cord.

Early diagnosis is essential in this condition and it is a major determinant of outcome. It should be considered and excluded in any patient presenting with sensory or motor changes in the limbs or urinary symptoms, in particular when there is associated backache. Metastases in the vertebrae may be demonstrated on plain radiograph or isotope bone scan but early confirmation of the precise anatomical site of compression should be obtained by urgent imaging of the spinal canal. In recent years, magnetic resonance imaging has superseded the use of myelography, giving superior definition of the anatomical structures and more readily demonstrating the full length of the cord; this is an important feature in view of the incidence of multiple levels of compression in many patients. It also has the advantage of being simpler for the patient, requiring no invasive procedures, in contrast to myelography where spinal lumbar puncture is required to introduce dye into the subarachnoid space. An example of spinal cord compression shown on T_1 weighted magnetic resonance imaging is given in Fig. 4 and is contrasted with the more conventional picture at myelography shown in Fig. 5. In centres where magnetic resonance imaging is not available, myelography remains an adequate tool for the urgent diagnosis of spinal canal compression and is superior to magnetic resonance imaging in demonstrating small epidural lesions, cauda equina lesions, and carcinomatous meningitis.[12]

Pathological diagnosis is essential before embarking upon definitive treatment. In many patients there will already be an underlying diagnosis of metastatic malignancy but in one series 48 per cent of patients presenting with spinal cord compression had no previous history of malignant disease.[13] Using accurate localization with the CT scanner, in most cases the diagnosis can be made by fine needle aspiration cytology or needle biopsy avoiding the morbidity of laminectomy.[14] Where a patient with known metastatic disease presents with spinal cord compression it is usually reasonable to assume that this is a manifestation of the known malignancy unless there are atypical features to suggest a second primary.

Both radiotherapy and decompressive surgery are effective in the initial management of spinal cord compression. No advantage of surgery over radiotherapy has been demonstrated in published series where patients have a previously confirmed diagnosis of malignant disease and no evidence of vertebral collapse.[15] Initial

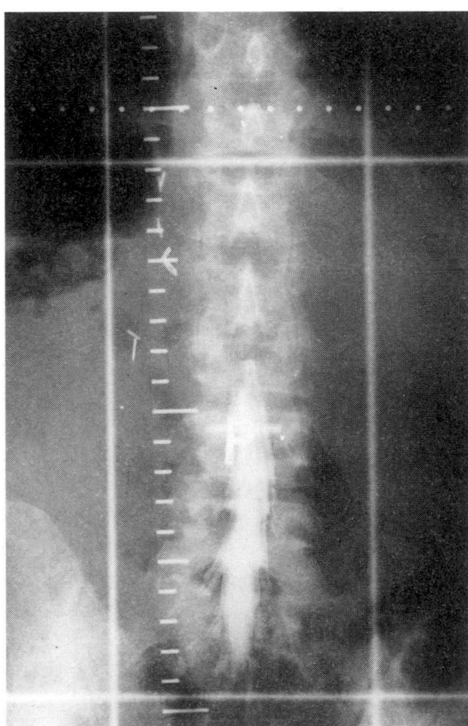

Fig. 5 Spinal cord compression demonstrated by complete block on myelogram with radiation fields to treat the area of compression outlined by the wires of the treatment simulator.

management for most patients, therefore, should be using high dose dexamethasone* and local irradiation to the spinal site. Certain histological types of tumour may be considered for primary treatment with chemotherapy, in particular lymphoma and small cell lung cancer.

Radiotherapy will be given through a single posterior field in most cases, although the cervical spine is better treated with lateral opposed fields. These should be localized using a treatment simulator, together with the information from MR scanning or myelography, to ensure accurate definition of vertebral levels. Where there is a large paravertebral mass, more complex planning may be required using two or three angled fields to cover the tumour volume and taking care to avoid sensitive paravertebral structures, in particular the kidneys in the lower thoracic and upper lumbar regions. Doses delivered in this situation vary. There is some evidence that single doses of 10 to 12 Gy are adequate but more usual practice is to deliver 20 to 30 Gy in 5 to 10 fractions over 1 to 2 weeks. In selected cases, particularly those with a localized potentially curable tumour such as a solitary plasmacytoma or localized non-Hodgkin's lymphoma, higher doses of up to 40 to 50 Gy over 3 to 5 weeks may be delivered.

In a small group of patients who develop spinal cord compression and in these patients a return to mobility is not an appropriate goal, particularly those with widespread advanced disease whose life expectancy is very short and those who present late with established paraplegia. Local irradiation may still be of value in these patients to achieve pain relief where there is local bony back pain or nerve root irritation. Similar doses to those mentioned above will be used.

The outcome of treatment depends primarily upon the speed of diagnosis and neurological status at initiation of treatment. When patients present ambulatory, 79 per cent are still ambulant following radiotherapy treatment; in contrast, of those presenting with paraparesis, only 42 per cent become ambulant and 20 to 25 per cent will suffer significant neurological deterioration during treatment by radiotherapy alone.[15] Where pain relief is the goal of treatment, radiotherapy will achieve this in over three-quarters of patients. Histology may influence outcome—patients with myeloma and lymphoma having a better outcome than those with breast cancer who in turn respond better than those with lung or kidney primary tumours.

In patients who have extensive vertebral collapse with intrusion into the spinal canal, radiotherapy is of little value in re-establishing neurological function. It is in this group of patients that surgery has its main application, with the use of anterior spinal surgery involving resection and spinal stabilization. This represents a more invasive procedure with significant operative morbidity and mortality but results in series of selected patients are superior to either laminectomy or radiotherapy alone, with between 62 and 83 per cent of patients being able to walk following anterior surgery and pain relief being achieved in 71 per cent.[16,17] Many of these patients, however, have poor general condition as shown by a 30 per cent mortality in one series of 26 consecutive patients operated on for pain or neurological deficits,[17] and careful selection of patients for surgical referral is therefore required.

* Readers are reminded that different authors in this textbook recommend widely differing doses of dexamethasone. [Editors].

Since the outcome of treatment for spinal cord compression is best when the diagnosis is made very early, there would be considerable advantages in predicting those patients at risk of spinal cord compression and treating them pre-emptively with prophylactic irradiation. It is possible using magnetic resonance imaging to detect metastases in vertebral bodies at very early stages of development and minor encroachment into the spinal canal which is often clinically asymptomatic and not detectable on plain radiographs. Prophylactic irradiation of such lesions may well be indicated although there is no published analysis of the natural history of such lesions and the incidence of clinical spinal cord compression related to these appearances. Other predictors for spinal cord compression reported in small cell lung cancer are local back pain associated with a positive bone scan in the spine or cerebral metastasis with a positive bone scan. These situations are associated with cord compression in 36 per cent and 25 per cent respectively.[18]

The most important issue in the management of spinal cord compression remains high awareness of the condition and a low threshold for investigating relatively minor symptoms, particularly in patients with known vertebral metastases or disease in the nervous system.

Brain metastasis

Up to 10 per cent of all cancers metastasize to the brain, the most common primary sites being the lung and the breast; approximately one-third will be solitary, the remainder are multiple throughout the substance of the brain. Disability from brain metastases tends to be disproportionate to the bulk of the tumour, for example a very small deposit on the motor cortex may have catastrophic results for the patient whilst a deposit of similar size would have little effect in the lung or liver. In general, therefore, active treatment of brain metastases as soon as they have presented is indicated. Confirmation of the diagnosis should be obtained by CT or magnetic resonance scanning. Initial management usually includes the use of steroids, for example dexamethasone, to reduce and control raised intracranial pressure, and where symptoms are due to oedema rather than tumour infiltration some initial improvement in neurological deficit is often seen.

Radiotherapy is well established as an effective palliative treatment for cerebral metastases, improving symptoms at presentation and preventing progressive neurological deficits. Overall headache, motor and sensory loss, and confusion will respond to treatment by cranial irradiation in around 80 per cent of patients with a complete response rate of between 35 and 55 per cent.[19]

The median survival after irradiation for brain metastases is less than 6 months; this reflects the fact that brain metastases herald advanced disease and systemic spread and the majority of patients die from the combined effect of distant metastases rather than progressive disease in the nervous system. Twenty per cent of patients who embark upon a course of radiotherapy fail to complete the course and this argues for careful selection in determining which patients may benefit from radiotherapy. In particular, those with multiple metastases outside the central nervous system, those with poor performance status, and those with rapidly progressive disease are most likely to succumb within the period of treatment. Factors influencing survival after irradiation are shown in Table 4.

Table 4 Factors influencing survival after irradiation of brain metastases

Increased survival	Decreased survival
Brain first site of relapse	Multiple lobes involved
Long disease-free interval prior to relapse in brain	Meningeal disease
Primary site in breast	
Early response to irradiation	

Because of the very limited survival in these patients, lengthy courses of treatment should be avoided unless there is clear benefit to be gained. There is no evidence that doses greater than 30 Gy in 10 fractions over 2 weeks are of any benefit. Lower doses may be equally effective and recognized schedules include 20 Gy in five daily fractions over 1 week, 12 Gy in two fractions over 2 days and 10 Gy as a single dose. In patients with advanced disease, the shorter schedules are likely to be of most benefit and a recent, large, randomized comparison of 12 Gy in two fractions with 30 Gy in ten fractions has shown no clinically significant difference between the two schedules (T Priestman, personal communication).

Solitary metastases usually reflect a more favourable prognosis and in selected patients with no detectable systemic disease elsewhere surgical removal gives best local and long-term control. This is further improved by postoperative radiotherapy. A prospective randomized study of 48 patients with solitary metastases comparing radiotherapy alone with surgery and postoperative radiotherapy showed that median survival was increased from 15 weeks after radiotherapy alone to 40 weeks following surgery and radiotherapy.[20] Localized high-dose radiotherapy using new stereotactic techniques to enable accurate focusing of an X-ray beam on a small spheroidal volume around the metastasis may give equivalent results to surgery without the need for the morbidity of a surgical procedure.[21] However, it is a time-consuming and technically very demanding treatment with limited availability. Despite the local effectiveness of surgery or stereotactic irradiation (radiosurgery), most patients still ultimately succumb to the effects of distant metastases and careful selection and screening is still required before considering aggressive local therapy of this type.

There is usually little acute toxicity from a short palliative course of cranial irradiation. Mild scalp erythema may occur, particularly around the external pinnae, but it is rarely significant in palliative doses. An unfortunate, but unavoidable, effect of cranial irradiation is complete alopecia. Hair regrowth does occur but requires a period of 2 to 3 months. In the presence of raised intracranial pressure and cerebral oedema high dose steroids (dexamethasone, 12–16 mg daily) are recommended to control the pressure. Transient rises in intracranial pressure are reported during radiotherapy which may be troublesome if pressure is already raised. In these situations, steroid dose should be increased to a maximum of 16 mg dexamethasone daily and, where this is not sufficient, intravenous mannitol may be required to maintain control.

At completion of cranial irradiation it is important to reduce, and if possible, discontinue steroids in order to minimize long-term side-effects provided that there is no neurological deterioration whilst doing so.

The majority of patients with multiple cerebral metastases will die from widespread metastatic disease outside the central nervous system but around a quarter will suffer persistent or recurrent symptomatic cerebral metastases. Steroids may achieve short-term control of symptoms but significant side-effects may occur. Retreatment following a dose of 20 to 30 Gy in 1 to 2 weeks carries a risk of radiation damage and there is often reluctance to consider reirradiation of the brain for recurrent disease. Without treatment, however, progressive morbidity and ultimately death from brain metastases will occur and neurological sequelae from radiation damage may take many months, if not years, to be manifest. On this basis, therefore, low-dose retreatment delivering a further 20 to 30 Gy in 2 to 3 weeks may be beneficial for selected patients who have had a good initial response to treatment.

Primary brain tumours

Primary brain tumours (including low grade (1 or 2) astrocytoma, oligodendroglioma, ependymoma, and meningioma) will, in most cases, be treated by surgery, radiotherapy, or both with curative intent. However, high grade astrocytomas (grade 3 or 4) are extremely malignant, incurable tumours with, untreated, a prognosis of only a few months. Palliative radiotherapy may be of value in this situation for selected patients with good performance status. Conventionally, relatively high doses of 45 to 60 Gy over 4 to 6 weeks are delivered with the aim of prolonging the symptom-free interval and survival. Adjuvant chemotherapy has also been advocated but, despite treatment, only 10 per cent of patients with high grade astrocytoma will be alive 2 years after treatment. Such treatment for those aged over 60 years with major neurological deficits and poor performance status has little benefit and is of doubtful value.[22]

Malignant meningitis

Diffuse meningeal carcinomatosis is generally a preterminal event with a median survival of only a few weeks if untreated. It commonly presents with multiple spinal root symptoms and signs and multiple cranial nerve palsies. Raised intracranial pressure may occur, resulting in headache and other symptoms. Common primary sites to develop this condition include carcinoma of the breast and lung. It may also be seen in cerebral lymphoma which is typically multifocal and spreads throughout the central nervous system—a condition of increasing frequency because of its relation to HIV infection. Central nervous system relapse of leukaemia also typically presents with a malignant meningitis.

Intensive treatment may be indicated where there is a treatable underlying malignancy. In the case of acute leukaemia and lymphoma sustained remissions may be achieved by the use of intrathecal chemotherapy using methotrexate and cytosine arabinoside, often combined with craniospinal irradiation (radiotherapy to the entire brain and spinal cord). Such treatment is no small undertaking and may be associated with morbidity due to bone marrow depression and nausea, vomiting, and alopecia from the radiotherapy. In children there are also the associated issues of impaired spinal growth and intellectual development. It is unfortunately the case that despite initial remission, central nervous system relapse of lymphoma or leukaemia or primary central nervous system lymphoma is generally associated with a poor overall prognosis with subsequent relapse and death, often within a few months.[23]

The outlook for carcinomatous meningitis from other primary sites, however, is even worse and whilst untreated the median survival is only a few weeks even intensive treatment with intrathecal chemotherapy and craniospinal irradiation will extend this to no more than a few months, much of which may be taken up with treatment.[24] On this basis judicious local irradiation to specific sites causing symptoms, such as the skull base if cranial nerves are involved or the segments of spinal cord where there may be spinal root irritation, delivering doses of 20 Gy in five fractions offers a more pragmatic approach, achieving effective palliation whilst minimizing the morbidity and duration of treatment in a universally fatal condition.

Cranial nerve palsies

Cranial nerve symptoms and signs due to metastatic cancer may arise from intrinsic metastases in the brain stem and mid-brain, infiltration of the leptomeninges, compression by extradural deposits, or bone involvement in the skull base. The management of intrinsic metastases and leptomeningeal metastases has been discussed above; results of whole brain irradiation for cranial nerve deficits due to cerebral metastases show an overall response rate of 78 per cent and a complete response rate of 42 per cent.[19] Local irradiation of the skull base is of value where diffuse bone involvement has resulted in cranial nerve compression. Symptomatic improvement is reported in between 50 and 78 per cent of patients and is maintained until death in around 80 per cent of these. In general, patients with skull base metastases will have a better prognosis than those with intrinsic central nervous system metastases; their median survival is between 10 and 20 months.[25,26]

Peripheral nerve symptoms

Involvement of peripheral nerves will typically result in nerve root pain and loss of motor function in the distribution of that nerve. This may be due to compression of the nerve by tumour at any point from the spinal root canal to its peripheral receptors. A common form of spinal root compression is that of cauda equina compression from encroachment into the spinal canal, as discussed in the section above. Outside the spinal canal, symptoms may arise because of direct tumour compression and infiltration, particularly in the brachial plexus from apical lung tumours or metastatic lymph nodes and at the lumbosacral plexus from pelvic tumours of the bowel, bladder, ovary, or uterus. Lumbosacral neuropathic pain will respond to palliative doses of radiotherapy, with complete pain relief within 1 month reported in 85 to 100 per cent of patients.[27] Pelvic irradiation for pain relief from recurrent colorectal cancer is successful in up to 80 per cent of patients[28] with no difference detected between a 3 week course of treatment delivering 45 Gy and a single dose of 10 Gy.[29]

Choroidal and orbital metastasis

Metastases to the eye are unusual but may cause distressing symptoms of proptosis, pain, and visual disturbance. The most common intraocular site is the choroid where over 50 per cent of metastases arise from primary breast cancer, 30 per cent from lung cancer, and around 25 per cent are bilateral. The diagnosis is made on fundoscopy or a slit lamp examination. Untreated, there is progressive deterioration and ultimately loss of vision. Local treatment with radiotherapy, delivering doses of 30 to 40 Gy in 2 to 4 weeks, results in stabilization and improvement of vision in 70 to 85 per cent of patients.[30] Metastases at other intraorbital sites are less common and may arise not only from blood-borne metastasis but also as a result of direct invasion from other head and neck sites, particularly nasopharynx, nasal cavity, and sinuses. Palliative local irradiation is again of value in preventing and relieving local symptoms from pressure and infiltration.

Radiotherapy to the eye and orbit require meticulous attention to technique, avoiding as far as possible direct irradiation of the cornea, which can result in painful keratitis, and shielding the lens, where appropriate. Radiation cataracts may occur after small doses of only 5 to 10 Gy to the lens but these may take many years to evolve and in the context of palliative treatment are unlikely to be seen.

Obstructive symptoms

Mediastinal compression and superior vena cava obstruction

The syndrome of superior vena cava obstruction may arise due to occlusion by extrinsic compression, intraluminal thrombosis, or direct invasion of the vessel wall. The majority of cases are due to malignant tumour within the mediastinum but other rare causes which should be excluded include aortic aneurysm, chronic mediastinitis, trauma, or thrombosis following central venous catheterization. Approximately 3 per cent of patients with carcinoma of the bronchus and 8 per cent of those with lymphoma will develop superior vena cava obstruction, and of the patients who present with this syndrome 75 per cent will have primary bronchial carcinomas (40 per cent of which will be small-cell lung cancer) and 15 per cent will have mediastinal lymphoma.

The clinical effects arise as a result of increased venous pressure above the site of obstruction. The extent to which this produces symptoms will depend on the efficiency of collateral vessels (particularly the internal mammary vessels, pulmonary veins, and the thoracic and vertebral venous plexuses) which may bypass the obstruction. Because of this, obstruction above the azygous vein will have less effect than obstruction below this level. A wide variety of presenting symptoms may result including headache, somnolence, and dizziness together with effects of oedema within the mediastinum causing dysphagia, dyspnoea, cough, or hoarseness; more rarely convulsions may result from cerebral hypertension. Examination may reveal fixed engorgement of arm and neck veins with visible dilatation of superficial skin veins, cyanosis, and facial oedema. Management requires both alleviation of symptoms and shrinkage of the intrathoracic tumour to relieve the obstruction. Conventionally, superior vena cava obstruction has been regarded as an oncological emergency requiring immediate treatment. More recently, however, this approach has been tempered by the need to obtain an accurate histological diagnosis in order to establish the correct, effective therapy. It is particularly important not to compromise potentially curable situations, such as mediastinal lymphoma or germ cell tumour, by inappropriate emergency treatment and also to identify those patients with small cell lung cancer who may be better treated with chemotherapy than radiotherapy. A large review of 1986 patients with superior vena cava obstruction reports only one death directly attributable to venous obstruction which occurred as a result of inhalation from an epistaxis.[31] This was despite a policy of delaying treatment until a definitive tissue diagnosis was achieved.

There are theoretical problems in performing a biopsy within a region of raised venous pressure, because of the risk of increased haemorrhage, but in practice bronchoscopy, mediastinoscopy, or lymph node biopsy are performed without major complications and should be part of the initial management before definitive treatment unless there is life-threatening large airways obstruction. During the acute phase of investigation, steroids may be of value in high doses (dexamethasone 12–16 mg daily) although there is no good, objective data to support this practice.

Radiotherapy will be the definitive treatment of choice for patients in whom malignancy is confirmed, except for those having a primary small-cell lung cancer, germ cell tumour, or lymphoma when chemotherapy is often more appropriate. Radiotherapy is given to the mediastinum covering the tumour mass and adjacent lymph node areas where appropriate. In the patient with impaired respiratory function this may present some technical difficulties if they are unable to lie flat for treatment and on occasions it is necessary to compromise on technique, treating the patient sitting up until symptoms improve. It is usual to treat this situation with doses of 20 to 30 Gy in 1 to 2 weeks and there is little published evidence for the use of alternative radiation schedules.[32] There may also be instances where the primary tumour is localized and radical treatment would otherwise be indicated. Superior vena cava obstruction is not a contraindication to proceeding with radical doses of radiotherapy in such patients.

Symptomatic relief following irradiation is reported variously in 50 to 95 per cent of patients within the first 2 weeks of treatment. The survival of patients presenting with superior vena cava obstruction is determined by their underlying disease rather than the syndrome itself, with the exception of the relatively rare instance of large airway obstruction or cerebral oedema when urgent treatment is required. Postmortem data suggest treatment has little effect upon the obstruction to blood flow in the superior vena cava, which persists in three-quarters of patients, with the implication that the development of collaterals is most important in achieving the observed clinical improvement rather than the physical release of compression from the superior vena cava.[31]

Lung collapse secondary to bronchial obstruction

Collapse of a segment of lung may occur due to intrinsic bronchial obstruction and is a common presentation of carcinoma of the bronchus. Obstruction may also occur as a result of extrinsic compression by mediastinal lymph nodes secondary to bronchial or other epithelial cancers or lymphoma. Dyspnoea will result particularly when collapse is an acute event. Local irradiation to restore the bronchial lumen will enable lung expansion and relieve dyspnoea provided this is initiated within a short time from the occlusion. Tumours presenting with bronchial obstruction are not in themselves excluded from radical treatment, thus chemotherapy (for a lymphoma or small-cell lung cancer) or radical primary radiotherapy (for non-small-cell lung cancer) may be indicated . In most cases of bronchial carcinoma, however, there will be mediastinal lymphadenopathy and often distant metastasis precluding radical treatment. In this setting, palliative external beam irradiation will be the treatment of choice.

Palliative radiotherapy for carcinoma of the bronchus, which is indicated not only for lung collapse but also for haemoptysis (see below), cough, pain, or dysphagia, may be given in short treatment courses. Randomized studies by the Medical Research Council in the United Kingdom have shown that two treatments, 1 week apart, delivering a total dose of 17 Gy are as effective as more prolonged schedules[32] and that in patients with a poor performance status a single dose of 10 Gy is equally effective as 17 Gy.[33] In selected patients, however, with good performance status and limited intrathoracic disease there may be some advantage to delivering higher doses and a course over 2 to 5 weeks delivering between 30 and 40 Gy may be considered.

An alternative method of delivering radiotherapy into the bronchial lumen is using the technique of endobronchial irradiation. This may be particularly appropriate for patients relapsing after previous external beam irradiation and involves the insertion of a fine plastic catheter through the area of tumour involvement under direct vision using a bronchoscope. The area is then irradiated by introducing a radioactive source along the catheter to deliver a dose of radiation to a defined length covering the area of tumour involvement. Where there is complete bronchial obstruction this may be usefully preceded by either laser therapy or cryotherapy to re-establish the bronchial lumen. The results of this approach are comparable to that reported using external beam treatment and one large series reports relief of stridor in 92 per cent of patients, dyspnoea in 60 per cent, and reinflation of pulmonary collapse in 46 per cent at 6 weeks after treatment.[35] The major advantage is that it can be delivered in a single procedure combining the bronchoscopy with radiation treatment, which is often possible without hospital admission.

Dysphagia

Difficulty in swallowing is a common symptom in patients with advanced cancer. This may be related to intrinsic tumour arising from the wall of the oesophagus or extrinsic compression by mediastinal lymph nodes or a tumour arising in an adjacent structure, in particular the bronchus. Post mortem data has shown that in around 80 per cent of cancer patients presenting with dysphagia this will be due to intrinsic tumour within the oesophagus and one study has demonstrated multiple levels of obstruction in almost a quarter of these patients.[36] Whilst pain relief and fine bore nasogastric tube feeding or intravenous feeding may alleviate the immediate crisis, conservative treatment will not re-establish swallowing in these cases. Surgical intervention may be considered in selected patients and has the advantage of rapid symptom relief if successful. There is, however, a significant morbidity and procedure-related mortality associated with surgery. External beam irradiation may be effective in relieving dysphagia, both in the case of intrinsic tumour obstruction and extrinsic compression from a primary bronchial tumour or mediastinal lymph nodes. A typical radiation field for this is shown in Fig. 6, the usual dose delivered to such an area being 20 to 30 Gy in 1 to 2 weeks, which will re-establish swallowing in over 80 per cent of patients and this will be maintained for a mean duration of 6 months.[37] Relief is not immediate and may take several weeks to occur, which is one disadvantage of radiotherapy in this setting as compared to surgery.

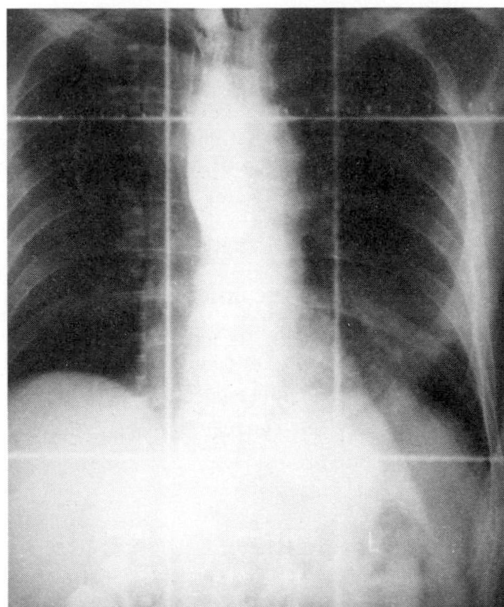

(a)

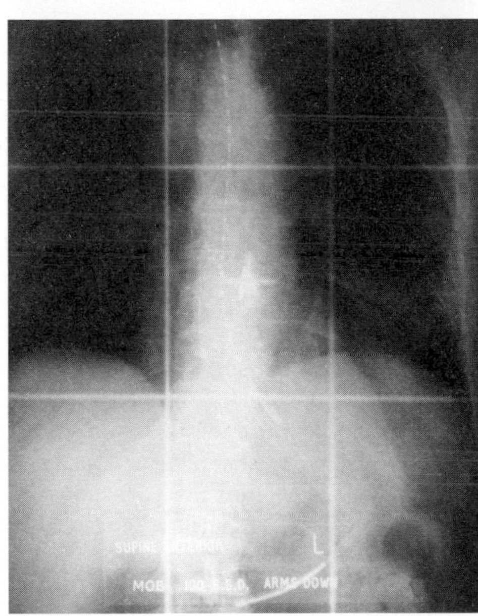

(b)

Fig. 6 Radiation field for external beam treatment of oesophageal cancer causing dysphagia. The area of obstruction has been defined at the time of simulation by barium swallow (a). Retreatment in this patient was possible using the endo-oesophageal technique. The catheter in position containing dummy sources to check its position prior to loading is shown in (b).

There is some evidence that higher doses of 50 Gy in 5 weeks or more may give a higher and more durable response rate[38] and this should be considered for patients who have good performance status and limited disease in whom a longer prognosis might be expected.

Acute toxicity from treatment may result in oesophagitis, and swallowing may become more difficult during the course of treatment. Simple topical medication such as soluble aspirin in a viscous mucilage or a local anaesthetic analgesic such as Mucaine (Wyeth Laboratories, Maidenhead, United Kingdom) is indicated for this. Oesophageal stricture may occur as a late complication of treatment requiring subsequent dilatation, although this is often a sign of persisting or recurrent tumour. After palliative doses of radiotherapy, more severe complications such as perforation and fistula are unusual unless related to recurrent tumour.

An alternative technique to external beam irradiation is endo-oesophageal radiotherapy in which a tube is passed through the area of oesophageal constriction and a radioactive source is passed along the tube (Fig. 6). Modern techniques use remote afterloading with either a medium dose rate caesium source or high dose rate iridium source. The latter has the advantage of a small diameter source of only 2 mm and a short treatment time of 20 to 30 min enabling this procedure to be performed on an outpatient basis. Used alone, relief of dysphagia was reported in 65 per cent of 40 patients with minimal associated treatment morbidity;[39] more recently, intraluminal therapy has been used in conjunction with external beam irradiation to achieve high local doses and one large series of 171 patients reports an improvement in swallowing for 3 or more months in 90 per cent, with 56 per cent achieving complete restoration of normal swallowing and a late stricture incidence of 35 per cent.[40] Clearly such intensive schedules are only indicated in good performance status patients with limited disease.

Urinary tract obstruction

The urinary tract may be obstructed by a primary or a metastatic tumour at any point along its length from renal pelvis to urethral orifice.

In the absence of distant metastases the most satisfactory means of re-establishing renal drainage is a surgical procedure to bypass the obstruction using a nephrostomy, ureteric stents, or transurethral resection of an intrinsic urethral tumour.

The role of radiotherapy in relieving urinary tract obstruction is restricted to those patients in whom surgery is either not technically possible or otherwise inappropriate. This may include those with locally advanced cancer of the cervix, bladder, or prostate or recurrence of a colorectal tumour. Lymphoma and germ cell tumours represent a special case where the underlying cause may be curable. In these patients (following surgical relief of drainage) radiotherapy, or more often chemotherapy, with curative intent should be initiated. Primary tumours of the cervix, prostate, or bladder causing urinary tract obstruction may be treated with varying schedules all of which will attempt to deliver a relatively high radiation dose to achieve tumour shrinkage and re-establish urinary flow. This may mean doses of 50 to 55 Gy in 4 weeks or 60 to 65 Gy in 6 to $6\frac{1}{2}$ weeks.

In some instances, intraluminal or interstitial radiotherapy may also be possible. A specific example is that of a suburethral metastasis from endometrial carcinoma (which has a recognized pattern of spread through submucosal vaginal lymphatics to the urethral meatus) for which an interstitial implant will enable high dose local treatment to be delivered.

Limb oedema

Limb oedema in a patient with advanced cancer may result from venous obstruction, lymphatic obstruction, or both. This may be compounded by general debility, immobility, and poor nutrition with accompanying hypoalbuminaemia. In a proportion of patients, particularly those with upper limb oedema due to carcinoma of the breast, postradiation changes may have caused lymphatic obstruction; ipsilateral arm oedema is seen in over 30 per cent of patients undergoing both axillary surgery and radiotherapy to the axilla for breast cancer.

Local radiotherapy may be of value in the treatment of limb oedema where enlarged malignant axillary, inguinal, or pelvic nodes are the cause of obstruction. Best results are obtained with early treatment when the circulatory obstruction can be reversed. Relatively low doses of 20 to 30 Gy in 1 to 2 weeks are used, taking care to preserve, wherever possible, a channel of unirradiated skin and soft tissue through which lymph drainage can be maintained despite postradiation changes.

Hydrocephalus

Obstructive hydrocephalus is an uncommon manifestation of cancer within the central nervous system and may result from primary or secondary tumours which obstruct the cerebrospinal fluid at any point in the ventricular system. Typically, it occurs when tumours of either the midbrain or the posterior fossa obstruct the aquaduct or fourth ventricle; it may also be secondary to malignant meningitis. Patients present with features of raised intracranial pressure together with focal neurological symptoms, depending upon the site of the tumour. Rapid relief of hydrocephalus may be gained by inserting an intraventricular shunt and patients with advanced disease may need no further treatment to achieve temporary symptom control. Where surgery is not feasible, or where there are multiple intracerebral lesions, palliative radiotherapy should be given in the same way as discussed for the management of brain metastases in the previous section.

Advanced primary central nervous system tumours of the midbrain and posterior fossa are also treated by radiotherapy, usually delivering doses of 50 to 55 Gy given over 6 to 7 weeks.

Haemorrhage

Haemoptysis

Haemoptysis is a common symptom of bronchial carcinoma, occurring in around 50 per cent of patients at presentation. It may also accompany pulmonary metastases and is distressing for the patient, although it is rarely of haemodynamic significance. It is life-threatening only when a major vein or bronchial artery is eroded and it is then usually beyond all treatment. Haemoptysis is otherwise an indication for local radiotherapy and control rates of up to 80 per cent are reported with palliative doses. There is no evidence that, for this indication, a single dose of 10 Gy is any less effective than more prolonged schedules.[34] An alternative approach to delivering radiotherapy for haemoptysis is to use intraluminal treatment, with a bronchial catheter being passed at bronchoscopy which is used to direct an iridium afterloading treatment source to the site of bleeding. A response rate of 88 per cent is reported from one large series, which is similar to the reported control rates after external beam irradiation.[35]

It is important to remember that haemoptysis as a presenting symptom of bronchial carcinoma is not, in itself, a contraindication to radical treatment in patients having localized disease which can be radically resected or encompassed in a high-dose radiation volume. Screening for this possibility should always occur prior to embarking upon palliative irradiation at primary presentation.

The management of haemoptysis due to pulmonary metastases is more difficult. Local irradiation is only of value where a specific site of haemorrhage can be identified or where there is only a solitary metastasis. Bronchoscopic confirmation of the origin of bleeding is, therefore, needed where there are multiple metastases; arbitrary irradiation of a particular area of metastatic disease is not to be recommended although low-dose whole-lung irradiation delivering a dose of 25 Gy in 20 fractions over 4 weeks has been used in the past for widespread metastases from radiosensitive tumours such as Ewing's sarcoma or Wilms' tumour. In general, however, chemotherapy or hormone therapy is the preferred treatment in this setting and only when this has failed should palliative irradiation be explored.

There is no proven advantage in terms of survival for treating the asymptomatic patient with inoperable lung cancer. There is, however, some evidence that tumours greater than 10 cm in diameter, whether primary or metastatic, carry a significant risk of haemorrhage and it has been suggested that such lesions should receive prophylactic irradiation.

Haematuria

Haematuria in patients with advanced cancer is usually caused by bleeding from a local bladder tumour which may be primary or secondary to local infiltration of an advanced rectal or uterine carcinoma. Other causes that may be relevant to the cancer patient are infective cystitis, chemical cystitis associated with certain chemotherapy agents such as cyclophosphamide or ifosphamide, bladder telangiectasis as a late change following high-dose radiotherapy to the bladder, and as a manifestation of thrombocytopenia or other coagulation defect. Haematuria may also be due to bleeding from primary or metastatic disease at any site along the urinary tract from the renal pelvis to the urethra. Thus, before embarking upon palliative treatment, careful localization of the site of bleeding (including intravenous urography, CT scanning, or cystoscopy) is vital.

The main role for radiotherapy in this setting is to achieve haemostasis in patients with inoperable or recurrent tumours. Haematuria may settle with conservative measures such as bladder irrigation, administration of antifibrinolytic drugs such as tranexamic acid, and cystoscopic diathermy. Where this fails, modest doses of irradiation delivered to a small volume encompassing the site of haemorrhage will usually be successful.

In the case of the bladder, careful localization using a cystogram or CT scan is advised and simple field arrangements can be used to deliver a palliative dose of treatment. The optimal dose to be used in this circumstance is uncertain. Single doses of 8 to10 Gy may be effective and a control rate of 59 per cent is reported after 17 Gy in two fractions.[41] Earlier work[42] suggested a higher control rate of around 65 per cent when doses greater than 40 Gy were delivered. On the basis of a large series reporting a 52 per cent control rate after 21 Gy in three fractions,[43] there is currently a multicentre trial in the United Kingdom comparing 21 Gy in three fractions to 35 Gy in ten fractions.

As with other sites, haematuria may be the presentation of a potentially curable primary bladder or prostatic carcinoma and, therefore, screening for this possibility should proceed. Radical treatment to the bladder or prostate will aim to deliver doses of 50 to 55 Gy in 4 weeks or 60 to 65 Gy in 6 to $6\frac{1}{2}$ weeks.

Haematuria due to locally advanced inoperable renal carcinoma may also benefit from local irradiation. The tolerance of the normal kidney to radiation is low and damage may occur even with modest palliative doses. It is, therefore, important to ensure that renal function from the contralateral kidney is normal before treatment.

Doses of 10 Gy single dose or 30 or 40 Gy in 2 to 3 weeks will usually be given.

Treatment to the bladder or prostate may result in diarrhoea because of the inevitable inclusion of some of the rectum in the treatment volume. Similarly, treatment of the kidney may include stomach or small bowel resulting in nausea, vomiting, or diarrhoea. Pre-emptive treatment with antidiarrhoeal agents and antiemetics will usually avoid major toxicity.

Uterine and vaginal bleeding

Tumours of the uterus, including endometrial and cervical cancer and uterine sarcomas, frequently present with abnormal vaginal bleeding. This is rarely excessive and is readily managed conservatively before embarking upon definitive treatment. Occasionally, major haemorrhage may be the presenting feature of a uterine tumour and this requires urgent treatment. Haemorrhage in patients with advanced and metastatic cancer is commonly due to recurrent tumour in the pelvis or mucosal deposits along the vaginal wall. Haemorrhagic mucosal deposits are a particular feature of vulval or vaginal melanoma.

The initial management of acute haemorrhage entails control of bleeding by pressure using a vaginal pack and resuscitation with intravenous fluids, blood, or plasma. Radiotherapy is of value in obtaining definitive control of bleeding and either external beam irradiation or intracavity treatment with a vaginal source is effective.

Where previous radical irradiation has been given to the pelvis only a limited dose may be tolerated but haemostasis will often be obtained using doses of only 8 to 20 Gy in one to five fractions. Where vaginal bleeding is the primary presentation of a tumour it is again important to screen the patient for the possibility of localized disease meriting radical treatment. Where this is not possible, external beam treatment delivering 20 to 30 Gy in 1 to 2 weeks is usually effective.

Where bleeding is from small volume disease, such as nodules at the vaginal vault or along the vaginal mucosa, intracavity treatment may be preferable. Vaginal sources (ovoids or a vaginal tube or dobby) can be introduced at the time of vaginal packing so that haemostasis can be achieved and definitive treatment delivered in a single manoeuvre (see Fig. 7). This technique enables a high dose to be given to the mucosal surface but with a rapid fall off in dose away from the source; critical structures such as bladder and rectum are relatively spared from radiation. This may be of particular value in a patient who has received previous radiotherapy to the pelvis.

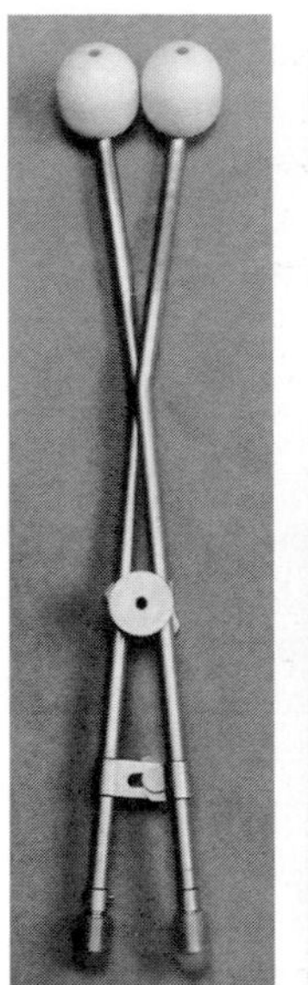
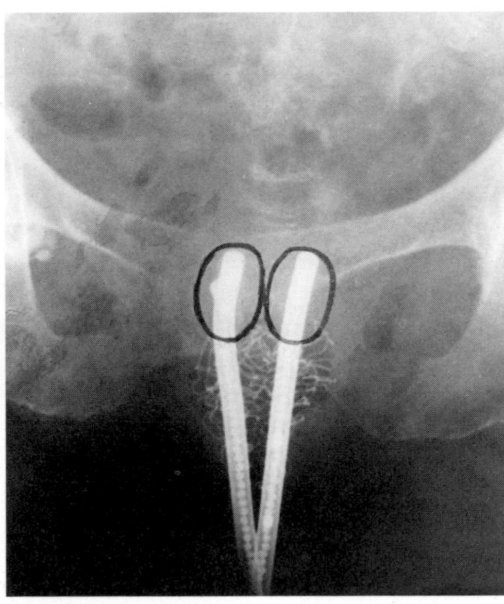

(a) (b)

Fig. 7 Intracavity applicators for vaginal vault irradiation. The two ovoids and their source carriers are shown in (a). Following insertion, a radiograph is taken to define their precise position as shown in (b). Dummy sources have been placed in the source carriers to improve imaging and to enable dosimetry calculations to be made prior to loading with active sources.

Gastrointestinal haemorrhage

Symptomatic gastrointestinal haemorrhage may arise from either the upper or lower gastrointestinal tract resulting in haematemesis, melaena, or rectal bleeding. The underlying tumour may be a primary neoplasm arising within the gastrointestinal tract, most commonly from the stomach, large bowel, or rectum, or a result of direct invasion by a locally advanced tumour in adjacent structures such as the uterus or bladder. Blood borne metastases to the bowel are rare but metastatic malignant melanoma is a recognized cause of haemorrhagic deposits within the small bowel wall.

As in other sites, local radiotherapy in modest doses to a site of haemorrhage within the bowel will often achieve effective and durable haemostasis. In the lower bowel, tumours in the rectum and colon are usually readily identified and localized within a treatment volume. Treatment to the stomach may be more difficult, both because it can be a relatively mobile structure and also because of the sensitivity of surrounding tissues (in particular liver, small bowel, and kidneys). Similarly, localization of tumours within the small bowel for radiotherapy can be difficult and radiation to this organ can have considerable associated morbidity with nausea, vomiting, and diarrhoea.

Results for such treatment are mainly based upon reports from recurrent colorectal cancer when an overall response rate of 85 per cent, with a complete control rate of 63 per cent, has been reported after palliative irradiation for rectal bleeding, delivering 30 to 35 Gy in ten fractions over 2 weeks.[44]

Chest wall and other skin lesions

Locoregional recurrence remains a significant problem in patients with breast cancer, occurring in 7 to 10 per cent of those with early disease and up to 40 per cent of those presenting with advanced local disease. Postoperative irradiation at the time of primary treatment significantly reduces the likelihood of locoregional relapse but despite this a number of patients with recurrent metastatic breast cancer will have progressive tumour recurrence on the chest wall which will fungate and bleed.

Where total mastectomy is possible this may be the best procedure but in many cases the tumour will be fixed and inoperable with multiple nodules across the chest. If no previous radiotherapy has been given and the area of recurrent disease is localized within the chest wall without distant metastasis, high dose local irradiation may be appropriate delivering doses of up to 60 Gy in 6 weeks. In patients with distant metastases and a poor prognosis, shorter schedules of from 10 Gy in one fraction up to 30 Gy in 2 weeks may be more appropriate.

Where there has been recurrence despite previous irradiation, further radiotherapy may be possible to a limited area of symptomatic tumour since the risks of skin necrosis are negligible compared with the effects of progressive fungating tumour within the skin. Superficial X-ray treatment or low energy electrons to fungating or bleeding chest wall nodules is often highly effective and a single dose of 8 to 10 Gy or a course of treatment delivering 20 to 30 Gy over 1 to 2 weeks will be usually be considered.

Skin nodules may also be a manifestation of primary tumours in other sites and, once established, may fungate and bleed. These will, by definition, reflect blood borne metastases, therefore radical treatment will be inappropriate but local treatment to isolated symptomatic nodules is often of value using techniques and doses similar to those mentioned above for recurrent breast cancer. Again, local irradiation of skin nodules or fungating lymph nodes may have palliative value using doses described above. Skin nodules from melanoma may be treated with higher doses delivering total radiation doses of 30 Gy in five to six fractions given twice weekly.

Other local tumour effects

Fungation

Fungation of a superficial tumour mass is a distressing feature of locally advanced cancer. It is seen most commonly in chest wall recurrence after breast carcinoma and with metastatic lymph nodes in the neck or groin. Local irradiation is most valuable in the prevention of fungation at a time when the overlying skin is intact. A palliative course of treatment delivering 20 to 30 Gy in 1 or 2 weeks will usually delay growth in a tumour mass sufficiently to prevent fungation. In certain instances where local tumour is the sole manifestation of malignancy, higher doses may be appropriate. The most common scenario of this type is the presence of a cervical lymph node containing squamous carcinoma but no apparent primary tumour on full examination of the ear, nose, and throat region. Radical doses of radiotherapy to the neck may achieve long-term control in this setting with overall 5 year survival figures of 20 to 30 per cent in selected series.[45]

Once fungation has occurred successful treatment is more difficult but, alongside nursing care and administration of analgesics and antibiotics, local irradiation may be of value in reducing the underlying tumour bulk, arresting surface haemorrhage, and drying the surface as the process of healing is allowed to commence. This will make nursing care simpler and relieve the patient from the distress of local haemorrhage.

Kaposi's sarcoma

Kaposi's sarcoma was until recent years a rare malignancy presenting in the skin of the lower limbs in European men. It has become increasingly important because of its association with HIV infection and is the most common AIDS related malignancy. Typically, it presents with multiple skin lesions but extracutaneous disease is also common, affecting the oral cavity and gastrointestinal tract. The characteristic purplish raised plaques may bleed and ulcerate. In contrast to other soft tissue sarcomas, Kaposi's sarcoma is markedly radiosensitive and small doses of irradiation will result in complete regression of lesions in up to 70 per cent of patients.[46]There is good evidence that single doses are as effective as more prolonged schedules and superficial irradiation delivering 8 Gy to symptomatic sites is recommended (see Chapter 20.1).

Liver metastasis

In most instances, the presence of liver metastases heralds the terminal phases of advanced cancer. Clinical symptoms are mainly systemic including anorexia, malaise, and weight loss, but local pain and discomfort may arise from massive hepatic enlargement, rapid expansion of the liver, or haemorrhage into a metastasis. Local treatment may be of value in this setting, particularly in those patients with good performance status and normal bilirubin where the primary site is other than stomach or pancreas.[47] If the primary tumour is chemosensitive this is usually the first line of approach and where there are solitary metastases resection may occasionally be considered. For the majority of patients, however, palliative low-dose radiotherapy may provide valuable relief of symptoms. Two prospective randomized trials have demonstrated relief of hepatic pain in 80 per cent of patients, with complete relief in 55 per cent, and improvements in nausea, vomiting, fever, and night sweats in 45 per cent.[47,48]

The liver has limited tolerance to radiation and so hepatic radiotherapy may be associated with morbidity. With doses greater than 30 Gy there is a risk of inducing radiation hepatitis. The toxicity from local irradiation is related not only to the dose but also the volume of liver included and, unless there is diffuse infiltration of the entire organ, a portion of uninvolved liver should be shielded. With doses of 30 Gy delivered in 2 to3 weeks relatively mild self-limiting toxicity is reported, mainly in the form of lethargy and nausea.

Splenomegaly

Symptomatic splenomegaly from malignant disease is usually associated with haematological malignancies, in particular lymphoma and chronic leukaemias. Surgical removal of the spleen is the preferred management but in advanced disease or in patients with poor performance status this may not be appropriate and local irradiation to the spleen is an effective means of palliation. Symptoms due to local bulk (causing pain and discomfort) and hypersplenism (causing consumption of red cells and platelets) benefit from treatment. The spleen containing lymphoma or leukaemia is extremely sensitive to radiation and high doses should be avoided as these may precipitate pancytopenia and rapid tumour lysis. Total doses of between 3 and 10 Gy delivered in multiple small fractions are frequently given and even at these low doses precautions should be taken against the effects of rapid tumour lysis with active hydration and the administration of allopurinol to prevent hyperuricaemia.

Hypercalcaemia

Hypercalcaemia complicates the clinical course of around 10 per cent of all patients with malignant disease, particularly those with common epithelial tumours such as breast and lung cancer. Whilst hypercalcaemia frequently occurs in patients with widespread metastatic disease, no clear correlation with the extent of bone metastases is usually demonstrated and it is thought that many cases arise due to the production of chemical agents promoting osteoclastic reabsorbtion of bone; these may include parathyroid hormone related protein (PTHrP), transforming growth factor alpha (TGFα), Interleukin 1 and tumour necrosis factor (TNF).[49] The initial management of a patient with hypercalcaemia secondary to advanced cancer includes rehydration, diuresis, and the introduction of calcium lowering agents. However, whilst initial reduction of serum calcium is usually achieved, rebound hypercalcaemia frequently follows requiring further intensive treatment and often a refractory phase is entered after several episodes. Where a potential source of the chemical agent can be identified, such as a locally advanced inoperable bronchial carcinoma, local irradiation to reduce its production and enable maintenance of blood calcium levels may be of value. Standard palliative doses are usually delivered as described above and, whilst anecdotally a valuable treatment in this setting, no published data are available for accurate estimates of response.

Paraneoplastic phenomena

Certain conditions may be seen in patients with malignancy which are not directly related to the process of tumour growth, invasion, and metastasis but are nonetheless associated with the malignant process. Their severity often mirrors the extent of the associated tumour. The most common association is with primary carcinoma of the bronchus when paraneoplastic symptoms arise in around 2 per cent of patients and include neuropathies, myopathies, myasthenia (the Eaton–Lambert syndrome), and cutaneous manifestations such as acanthosis nigricans, erythema gyratum, or 'hairy man syndrome'. It is probable that these symptoms reflect secretion of a humoral agent, possibly an autoantibody. The paraendocrine syndromes are associated with ectopic production of ACTH, ADH, human chorionic gonadatrophin (HCG), 5-hydroxytryptamine (5HT), or thyroid stimulating hormone (TSH), as well as those mentioned above in the context of hypercalcaemia. Where there is an identifiable local tumour, and where surgical excision is not possible or appropriate, local irradiation may result in improvement and resolution of the paraneoplastic symptoms as the tumour regresses. In advanced disease, only palliative doses may be appropriate but in localized disease the presence of a paraneoplastic syndrome should not exclude consideration of radical treatment. As with hypercalcaemia, there are no good data on precise response rates to treatment in this setting.

Conclusion

Local irradiation is a valuable treatment for palliation of local symptoms with consistently high response rates in the relief and control of bone pain, neurological symptoms, obstructive symptoms, and haemorrhage. Short treatments and simple techniques can minimize disruption and acute morbidity for the patient with advanced cancer whilst enabling control of symptoms.

References

1. Steel GG. The search for therapeutic gain in the combination of radiotherapy chemotherapy. *Radiotherapy and Oncology*, 1988; **11**: 31–53.
2. Price P, Hoskin PJ, Easton D, Austin D, Palmer S, Yarnold JR Prospective randomised trial of single and multifraction radiotherapy schedules in the treatment of painful bone metastases. *Radiotherapy and Oncology*, 1986: **6**; 247–55.
3. Mithal N, Needham PR, Hoskin PJ. Retreatment with radiotherapy for painful bone metastases. *International Journal of Radiation Oncology Biology Physics*, 1994; **29**: 1011–14.
4. Salazar, *et al.* Single dose hemibody irradiation in palliation of multiple bone metastases from solid tumours. *Cancer*, 1986: **58**; 29–36.
5. Brown AP, Greening, WP, McCready VR, Shaw, H, Harmer CL. Radioiodine treatment of metastatic thyroid carcinoma: The Royal Marsden Hospital experience. *British Journal of Radiology*, 1984; **57**: 323–7.
6. Hoskin PJ. Strontium. In: Dollery C, ed. *Therapeutic Drugs*, Suppl 2. Edinburgh: Churchill Livingstone, 1994: 223–7.
7. Hoskin PJ, Price P, Easton D, Austin D, Palmer SG, Yarnold JR. A prospective randomised trial of 4Gy or 8Gy single doses in the treatment of metastatic bone pain. *Radiotherapy and Oncology*, 1992; **23**: 74–8.
8. Poulter C, *et al.* A Phase III study of whether the addition of single dose hemibody irradiation to standard fractionated local field irradiation is more effective than local field irradiation alone in the treatment of symptomatic osseous metastases. *International Journal of Radiation Oncology Biology Physics*, 1992; **23**: 207–14.
9. Porter, *et al.* Results of a randomised Phase III trial to evaluate the efficacy of Strontium-89 adjuvant to local field external beam irradiation in the management of endocrine-resistant metastatic prostate cancer. *International Journal of Radiation Oncology Biology Physics*, 1993; **25**: 805–13.
10. Reider K, Kober B, Mende U, zum Winkel K. Strahlentherapie pathologischer frakturen und frakturge fahrdeter skelettlasionen. *Strahlentherapie Onkology*, 1986; **162**: 742–9.
11. Pigott K, Baddeley H, Maher EJ. Pattern of disease in spinal cord compression on MRI scan and implications for treatment. *Clinical Oncology*, 1994; **6**: 7–10.
12. Williams MP, Cherryman GR, Husband JE. Magnetic resonance imaging in suspected metastatic spinal cord compression. *Clinical Radiology* 1989; **40**: 286–90.
13. Shaw MDM, Rose JE, Paterson A. Metastatic extradural malignancy of the spine. *Acta Neurochirurgica*, 1980; **52**: 113–20.
14. Findlay GFG, Sandeman DR, Buxton P. The role of needle biopsy in the management of cervical metastases. *British Journal of Neurosurgery*, 1988; **2**: 479–84.
15. Findlay GFG. Adverse effects of the management of malignant spinal cord compression. *Journal of Neurology, Neurosurgery and Psychiatry*, 1984; **47**: 761–8.
16. Siegal T, Siegal T. Surgical decompression of anterior and posterior malignant epidural tumours compressing the spinal cord: a prospective study. *Neurosurgery*, 1985; **17**: 424–32.
17. Moore AJ, Uttley D. Anterior decompression and stabilisation of the spine in malignant disease. *Neurosurgery*, 1989; **24**: 713–17.
18. Goldman JM, *et al.* Spinal cord compression in small cell lung cancer: a retrospective study of 610 patients. *British Journal of Cancer*, 1989; **59**: 591–3.
19. Borgelt B, *et al.* The palliation of brain metastases: final results of the first two studies by the Radiation Therapy Oncology Group. *International Journal of Radiation Oncology, Biology, Physics*, 1982; **6**: 1–9.
20. Patchell RA, *et al.* A randomised trial of surgery in the treatment of single metastases to the brain. *New England Journal of Medicine*, 1990; **322**: 494–500.
21. Brada M, Hoskin PJ. New approaches in the management of brain metastases. *Critical Reviews in Neurosurgery*, 1995; **5**: 42–9.
22. Bleehen N, *et al.* A Medical Research Council trial of two radiotherapy doses in the treatment of grades 3 and 4 astrocytoma. *British Journal of Cancer*, 1991; **64**: 769–74.
23. De Angelis LM, Yahalom J, Thaker HT, Kher V. Combined modality therapy for primary CNS lymphoma. *Journal of Clinical Oncology*, 1992; **10**: 635–43.
24. Wasserstrom WR, Glass JP, Posner JB. Diagnosis and treatment of leptomeningeal metastases from solid tumours. *Cancer*, 1982; **49**: 759–72.
25. Vikram B, Chu F. Radiation therapy to metastases to the base of the skull. *Radiology*, 1979; **130**: 465–8.
26. Hall S, Buzdar A, Blumenschein G. Cranial nerve palsies in metastatic breast cancer due to osseous metastases without intracranial involvement. *Cancer*, 1983; **52**: 180–4.
27. Russi EG, Pergolizzi S, Gaeta M, Mesiti M, D'Aquino A, Delia P. Palliative radiotherapy in lumbosacral carcinomatous neuropathy. *Radiotherapy and Oncology*, 1993; **26**: 172–3.

28. James RD, Johnson RJ, Eddleston B, Zheng GL, Jones JM. Prognostic factors in locally recurrent rectal carcinoma treated by radiotherapy. *British Journal of Surgery*, 1983; **70**: 469–72.
29. Allum WH, Mack P, Preistman TJ, Fielding JWL. Radiotherapy for pain relief in locally recurrent colorectal cancer. *Annals of the Royal College of Surgeons of England*, 1987; **69**: 220–1.
30. Dobrowsky W. Treatment of choroidal metastases. *British Journal of Radiology*, 1988; **61**: 140–2.
31. Ahman FR. A reassessment of the clinical implications of the superior vena caval syndrome. *Journal of Clinical Oncology*, 1984; **2**: 961–8.
32. Sculier JP, Feld R. Superior vena cava obstruction syndrome: recommendations for management. *Cancer Treatment Reviews*, 1985; **12**: 209–18.
33. MRC Lung Cancer Working Party. Inoperable non-small cell lung cancer (NSCLC): a Medical Research Council randomised trial of palliative radiotherapy with two fractions or ten fractions. *British Journal of Cancer*, 1991; **63**: 265–70.
34. MRC Lung Cancer Working Party. A Medical Research Council (MRC) randomised trial of palliative radiotherapy with two fractions or a single fraction in patients with inoperable non-small cell lung cancer (NSCLC) and poor performance status. *British Journal of Cancer*, 1992; **65**: 934–41.
35. Gollins SW, Burt PA, Barber PV, Stout R. High dose rate intraluminal radiotherapy for carcinoma of the bronchus: outcome of treatment of 406 patients. *Radiotherapy and Oncology*, 1994; **33**: 31–40.
36. Sykes NP, Baines M, Carter RL. Clinical and pathological study of dysphagia conservatively managed in patients with advanced malignant disease. *Lancet*, 1988; **ii**: 726–8.
37. Wara M, Mauch PM, Thomas AN, Philips TL. Palliation for carcinoma of the oesophagus. *Radiology*, 1976; **121**: 717–20.
38. Leslie MD, *et al.* The role of radiotherapy in carcinoma of the thoracic oesophagus: an audit of the Mount Vernon experience 1980–1989. *Clinical Oncology*, 1992; **4**: 114–18.
39. Rowland CG, Pagliero KM. Intracavity irradiation for palliation of carcinoma of the oesophagus and cardia. *Lancet*, 1985; **ii**: 981–3.
40. Flores AD, *et al.* The impact of new radiotherapy modalities in the surgical management of cancer of the oesophagus and cardia. In: Martinez AA, Orton CG, Mould RF, eds. *Brachytherapy HDR and LDR*. Columbia: Nucletron, 1990: 27–43.
41. Srinivasan V, Brown CH, Turner AG. A comparison of two radiotherapy regimes for the treatment of symptoms from advanced bladder cancer. *Clinical Oncology*, 1994; **6**: 11–13.
42. Green N, George FW. Radiotherapy of advanced localised bladder cancer. *Journal of Urology*, 1974; **111**: 611–12.
43. Wijkstrom H, Naslund J, Ekman P, Kohler C, Nilsson B, Norming U. Short-term radiotherapy as palliative treatment in patients with transitional cell bladder cancer. *British Journal of Urology*, 1991; **67**: 74–8.
44. Taylor RE, Kerr GR, Arnott SJ. External beam radiotherapy for rectal adenocarcinoma. *British Journal of Surgery*, 1987; **74**: 455–9.
45. Fletcher GH. Controversial views in the management of cervical metastases. *International Journal of Radiation Oncology, Biology, Physics*, 1990; **19**: 1101–2.
46. Munro AJ, Stewart JSW. Aids: Incidence and management of malignant disease. *Radiotherapy and Oncology*, 1989; **14**: 121–31.
47. Leibel SA, *et al.* A comparison of misonidazole sensitised radiation therapy to radiation therapy alone for the palliation of hepatic metastases: results of a Radiation Therapy Oncology Group randomised study. *International Journal of Radiation Oncology, Biology, Physics*, 1987; **13**: 1057–64.
48. Borgelt BB, Gelber R, Brady LW, Griffin T, Hendrickson FR. The palliation of hepatic metastases: results of the Radiation Therapy Oncology Group pilot study. *International Journal of Radiation Oncology, Biology, Physics*, 1981; **7**: 587–91.
49. Mundy GR. Pathophysiology of cancer-associated hypercalcaemia. *Seminars in Oncology*, 1990; **17**: 10–15.

9.1.3 Surgical palliation

Adrian B. S. Ball, M. Baum, Nicholas M. Breach, John H. Shepherd, R.J. Shearer, J. Meirion Thomas, T.G. Allen-Mersh, Peter Goldstraw, and Ugo Pastorino

General introduction

In spite of an enormous financial commitment into the research and treatment of cancer there is evidence that the incidence of, and mortality from, the disease in the developed world is increasing, rather than decreasing.[1] Admittedly this might be a paradox resulting from an ageing population, which in itself will increase the incidence of the disease, together with refinement in diagnosis which may artificially enhance the prevalence of the disease. Furthermore, more accurate classification of causes of death within cancer registries might artificially inflate mortality from cancer but, whichever way you look at it, it is very difficult to determine that modern cancer treatment is contributing to a reduction in mortality for cancer. Does this mean therefore that the activity of surgeons, radiotherapists, and other oncologists over the last century have been in vain? Nothing could be further from the truth because crude cancer statistics as generated by the National Cancer Registries take no account of the way cancer therapy improves the quality of life and the dignity of dying.

Nowhere is this seen more clearly than in the role of surgery for the palliation of cancer. The surgical oncologist must always play a leading role in the multidisciplinary approach to the management of advanced cancer. Surgeons more than anyone have a clear idea of the natural history of the disease as they are most often involved in the initial evaluation of patients with the commonest malignancies. Thirty per cent of the work of any general surgeon (even without a specialist interest in cancer) involves cancer. It is the function of this chapter to illustrate how the surgical oncologist plays a major role in the palliation of the disease, in addition to the curative treatment they can offer for a depressingly static minority of such cases.

The surgeon has five essential roles in the palliation of advanced cancer:

(1) initial evaluation of the disease;

(2) local control of the disease;

(3) control of discharge or haemorrhage;

(4) control of pain;

(5) reconstruction and rehabilitation.

Evaluation

The initial diagnosis and staging of a cancer is usually in the hands of a surgeon. This might involve upper or lower gastrointestinal endoscopy, cystoscopy, or laparoscopy, all of which may involve tissue sampling for diagnosis. Minor surgery involving biopsy of lymph nodes or other suspicious lumps may establish a diagnosis of a lymphoma or be of value in staging the extent of one of the common solid tumours. A clinical diagnosis together with a result of tissue diagnosis and staging investigations may determine whether the case is inoperable or potentially curable.

Local control of the disease and the control of pain

Even if not curative, surgery is essential to gain control of the local disease for the relief of obstruction to hollow viscera such as the gut, the biliary tract, and the genitourinary system. Debulking a primary tumour may also enhance the effectiveness of radiotherapy and chemotherapy. In addition, removing a primary tumour, even in the presence of distant metastases, may control discharges, fistulas, and haemorrhage. Once a primary tumour has already infiltrated nerve roots it is extremely difficult for surgery in itself to relieve pain but this complication of advanced cancer should always be anticipated and attempts to control the cancer before it infiltrates nerve roots, especially around the brachial and sacral plexus, may prevent the development of intractable pain in the future. The orthopaedic surgeon also cuts across disciplinary boundaries when involved in the prophylactic or therapeutic pinning of metastases in the long bones or laminectomy for decompression of spinal metastases. Similarly, the neurosurgeon may be called upon for symptom relief by decompressing nerves, removing solitary cerebral metastases, and performing tractotomies.

Reconstruction

Just because the patient is facing a limited expectation of life, does not mean that he or she should carry the added burden of physical or functional morbidity. Reconstructive surgery involving the head and neck region and the breast may be of vital importance in allowing a patient to face an uncertain future with equanimity. Furthermore, preserving an intact gastrointestinal and urogenital tract may spare the dying patient the additional burden of a colostomy, ileostomy, or urostomy bag.

The essential role of the surgeon in the palliation of cancer will be illustrated using the specific examples of the head and neck, lung, breast, gastrointestinal, urological, gynaecological, and soft tissue tumour oncology. It should be noted that figures quoted for survival and operative mortality reflect experience in the United Kingdom and may vary in other parts of the world.

Head and neck cancer

It has been estimated that the probable cure rate for patients suffering from cancer in the head and neck region, excluding the skin and central nervous system, lies between 30 and 40 per cent of those treated with curative intent. These are disappointing figures emphasizing the slow progress made in the last 30 years despite earlier diagnosis, improved management techniques, and a greater interest in aetiological factors. Such figures mean that specialists and general practitioners are required to offer some form of palliative treatment to the majority of patients who have been diagnosed as suffering from head and neck cancer.

To those involved in the management of these patients there is often no clear-cut distinction between 'palliative' or 'curative' treatment. In some cases palliative treatment may be so effective that cure becomes feasible. As in all cancer surgery, though, local control must be the primary object of all treatment modalities.

If we look at the role of surgery in the palliation of head and neck cancer, then rehabilitation is of paramount importance. The head and neck region is more complex than many others as there are many essential and social functions that challenge the surgeon's skills, namely breathing, mastication, swallowing, and speech, quite apart from appearance. An end tracheostomy may alleviate breathing difficulties but will limit communication unless a technique for restoring speech is undertaken. Likewise, a gastrostomy or jejunostomy will relieve the need for the patient to masticate and swallow. Loss of the ability to converse and eat, however, are a high price for a patient to pay if the duration of life is limited. The services of a competent speech therapist are essential for all laryngectomy patients.

Surgery for local control

Advanced local disease in the head and neck is debilitating and invariably affects one or more of the essential functions of the region. Whereas surgery for local involvement of skin and/or mucosa may be undertaken whatever the area of involvement, surgery for a similar tumour mass in the maxillary and ethmoid sinuses or nasal cavity compromising vision may have to be declined. Similar reservations may arise when the internal carotid artery is involved by the tumour mass. A hemiparesis, with or without speech impairment, may be a price that neither the patient nor the surgeon is prepared to pay.

A total glossectomy does not necessarily entail laryngectomy. The replacement of the whole tongue with a platform of tissue, a latissimus dorsi myocutaneous flap, can restore the ability to swallow and maintain intelligible speech, as well as relieve the severe pain and discomfort of a tongue tumour. Similarly, advanced hypopharyngeal and pharyngeal tumours, which cause marked problems with the airway and swallowing, may now be resected (albeit incompletely if there is involvement of the prevertebral tissues) and repaired by interposing a jejunal loop. This can be compared with the morbidity of a pharyngolaryngo-oesophagectomy using stomach or large bowel for replacement.

Despite these examples of complex surgery for advanced tumours, less major procedures remain a keystone of palliative treatment.

Debulking surgery and the relief of obstruction in hollow organs

The advent of the laser and cryoprobe in recent years has extended the scope of palliative surgery in debulking tumour and relief of obstruction. Their use has allowed patients to remain ambulant and to be nursed at home in the course of a terminal illness.[2] To be effective the techniques should be used as early as possible.

Debulking a tumour sometimes permits other treatment modalities to be employed. Thus, the effectiveness of radio-iodine in advanced thyroid cancer is enhanced if the residual bulk of the tumour is reduced to a minimum.[3] In other cases, when macroscopic disease remains after surgical excision, a second course of radiotherapy may be appropriate providing the surrounding and overlying tissues can withstand the effects of the radiation. Radiation can be administered by either external beam or an interstitial implant.

Surgery for the control of discharge and haemorrhage

The most debilitating discharge from the upper aerodigestive tract is from a salivary fistula. Spontaneous healing is rare, particularly when radiotherapy has been a primary method of treatment. Repair requires the introduction of healthy tissue, that is a pedicled or free flap.

Haemorrhage can occur from any ulcerated surface. There are two potentially dangerous situations in the head and neck—a 'carotid blow-out' and bleeding into the upper aerodigestive tract causing acute airway obstruction. 'Carotid blow-outs' usually occur when the carotid vessels are relatively unprotected, for example when a neck dissection is required after radiation to the neck. In spite of well designed skin flaps, wound breakdown is not unknown. In such cases consideration must be given to replacement of the neck skin with a deltopectoral flap. When interstitial irradiation is used following radiotherapy it is mandatory to replace the whole of the skin that will overlie the radiation source.[4]

Haemorrhage into the upper aerodigestive tract is usually unexpected and frequently catastrophic. If time permits, vessels supplying the area are ligated—frequently the external carotid artery. The ease with which this can be accomplished depends upon the previous treatment.

Surgery for the control of pain

Head and neck tumours are commonly associated with pain, often referred. Headaches, earache, and orbital pain are presenting symptoms of advanced disease. Chemical nerve blocks are used when tumour resection is neither indicated nor possible. It is rare for surgical division of a nerve or nerve root to be indicated. The sole exception is when cutaneous nerves, divided during surgery, subsequently produce a neuroma causing an area of hypersensitivity. In these cases a nerve may be transposed into muscle thereby removing it from its immediate position beneath the skin.

In most situations the pain associated with advanced disease is controlled using analgesics which will often need to be given by parenteral routes.

Surgery for reconstruction and/or rehabilitation

Reconstructive techniques with pedicled and free tissue transfer must restore, if possible, the essential functions mentioned above. As in most reconstructive surgery attention must be given to an adequate replacement of the excised tissues. Dead space should be eliminated and normal anatomical relationships maintained. When mucosa has to be replaced, whether this be the tongue, floor of mouth, or pharynx, the tissue chosen for repair will be influenced by the space available for the repair. Many pedicled flaps are too bulky, that is the pectoralis major and latissimus dorsi myocutaneous flaps, and would be less than ideal. On the other hand, while free tissue transfer in the form of radial and lateral forearm, groin, or dorsalis pedis flaps allows more accurate replacement of limited tissue loss at specific sites, it may lack the bulk required to eliminate a significant tissue dead space.[5]

Lung cancer

Bronchogenic carcinoma is a major cause of mortality world-wide and the survival rate has not improved significantly in the last 20 years. Over 150 000 new cases of lung cancer are diagnosed in Europe every year but less than 10 per cent are cured even with the best standards of medical treatment. With the exception of a few patients whose small-cell lung cancers may be eradicated by chemotherapy and radiotherapy, the majority of patients with lung cancer can only be cured by complete surgical resection. Unfortunately, the proportion of primary lung cancers amenable to curative surgery is only 10 per cent in the United Kingdom, compared to 20 to 30 per cent in the United States. In the vast majority of cases surgery is not feasible because of the tumour extent (local spread or distant metastases) or the poor general condition of the patient.

In large retrospective series, there are virtually no long-term survivors after resection of T4 or bulky N2-N3 disease.[6] Induction chemotherapy or chemo-radiotherapy is reported to improve the proportion of patients with advanced NSCLC (stage IIIA-B) suitable for resection, resulting in a higher 5-year survival than historical series (18 per cent versus 9 per cent).[7] However, in those with bulky N2 disease the long-term survival after induction chemotherapy was only 4 per cent.

Due to the poor surgical and medical curability of lung tumours, the role of palliative treatment has increased. Only in very rare instances can surgery be usefully combined with other treatment modalities to prolong the survival of patients who otherwise have no chance of cure. Recent technological progress in developing new surgical instruments and minimally invasive techniques have improved the results of palliative treatment. Video assisted bronchoscopy and thoracoscopy now enable the surgeon to perform complex endobronchial and intrathoracic procedures with greater accuracy and safety, without the need for open thoracotomy, and new synthetic materials provide more flexible and durable bronchial stents and other endoprostheses.

Locally advanced or metastatic lung cancer

In the management of primary lung cancer, major surgery is rarely justified for palliation alone. Incomplete or debulking surgery does not influence the patient's life expectancy or improve quality of life. A few long-term survivors can be identified after incomplete resection followed by postoperative radiotherapy, but similar results can be achieved with radiotherapy alone.

To describe complete resection as 'palliative' is misleading, as typical symptoms such as cough, dyspnoea, or chest pain are likely to be worse after surgery than they were before. Radiotherapy with or without chemotherapy is preferable to incomplete resection in patients with locally advanced lung cancer, and symptoms of bronchial obstruction and haemoptysis are better treated by endoscopic resection and/or brachytherapy. Even in the presence of the paraneoplastic syndromes, durable control of hormone related symptoms is only achieved by complete excision of the disease.

Lung abscess or acute sepsis are rare indications for partial resection, and even experienced thoracic surgeons have only anecdotal cases. Salvage resection is sometimes indicated for acute life-threatening complications such as the massive necrosis of heavily irradiated lung parenchyma.

Lung resection in the presence of cytological positive pleural effusion is associated with a mean survival of 3 to 6 months. A similar survival time can be anticipated after resection of T4 tumours invading mediastinal structures such as the superior vena cava, aorta, myocardium, or oesophagus.

Patients presenting with operable lung cancer and a solitary distant metastasis may benefit from resection of both tumour foci. The probability of long-term survival after resection of a brain metastasis and the lung primary is between 10 and 20 per cent at 5 years, with no significant difference in survival between patients with synchronous and metachronous presentation of the brain lesion.[8] Resection of the brain metastasis plus brain irradiation is better than radiotherapy alone in terms of median survival and quality of life. Long-term survivors have also been reported after resection of isolated adrenal metastases.

It is more difficult to assess the prognosis after resection of synchronous intrapulmonary metastases as they are virtually indistinguishable from multiple primary cancers. Clinically, concurrent lung lesions should be considered as independent primary tumours and treated with curative intent whenever possible.

Airway obstruction (see also Chapter 9.5)

Obstruction of the trachea and main bronchi, with severe dyspnoea and stridor, is an infrequent but serious complication of lung cancer, leading to life-threatening respiratory distress. Occasionally patients with a localized endoluminal tumour may be candidates for curative resection.

In the majority of cases, however, obstruction results from compression of the airway due to metastatic involvement of mediastinal nodes at the carina or in the paratracheal chain. Such metastatic spread is common in lung cancer and other extrathoracic malignancies such as breast cancer and lymphoma. Extraluminal compression may be associated with an intraluminal component in lung cancer cases. Palliative therapy is usually best provided by external irradiation. In an emergency however, or if relapse occurs after external irradiation or prior resection, the surgeon may be involved.

If the chief component of airway obstruction is endoluminal, endoscopic resection provides immediate and safe relief of symptoms. This is achieved by various techniques including simple 'core out', Nd:YAG laser photocoagulation, cryotherapy, or diathermy resection.[9] Whilst laser photocoagulation was originally applied through the fibreoptic bronchoscope under local anaesthesia, the use of a rigid bronchoscope and Sanders Venturi ventilation under general anaesthesia offers a number of definite advantages and has now become the accepted approach. Using the rigid bronchoscope it is now possible to maintain adequate ventilation during the whole procedure even when there is significant bleeding, and haemostasis can be secured at the end of resection. Other modalities can be applied at the same time, such as the insertion of an endobronchial stent. The results of endoscopic disobliteration may be consolidated by giving high dose intraluminal radiotherapy within a few days of endoscopic resection.

Where the major component of obstruction is extrinsic compression (resistant or recurrent disease after external irradiation) the insertion of an endobronchial stent can relieve symptoms, and is especially useful in an emergency.

Initial experience of tracheobronchial stenting was based on the Montgomery T tube or T–Y tube, inserted through a tracheostomy incision under bronchoscopic control. This procedure remains a valid option for high tracheal obstructions, being easily managed and tolerated by the patient, even for long periods. A further advance has been the development of fully endobronchial silicone stents, manufactured from T tubes at the time of endoscopy,[10] or commercially available in various shapes. Silicone stents can be easily removed[11] if obstruction is relieved by further irradiation (external or endobronchial) and reinserted in case of relapse.

Expandable wire stents have been used as a alternative to silicone, to provide a larger internal lumen and to avoid displacement (Fig. 1). However, tumour ingrowth is a problem and covered expanding devices have now been developed.

Thus, a combination of therapies can now be applied to treat the intraluminal as well as extrinsic component of the obstruction (Table 1) at a single endoscopic procedure. In our experience, diathermy resection is an effective and safe way of relieving intraluminal obstruction at less financial cost than laser resection, and can be combined with silicone stent insertion if there is an extraluminal component to the obstruction.[6] Multiple sequential bronchoscopies are often required to reassess the disease, resect endobronchial recurrence, and/or reposition the stent. Although the median survival of these patients is 5 to 6 months, occasional long-term survivors have been reported.

Pleural effusion (see also Chapter 9.5)

The aim of palliation is to achieve as complete an expansion of the lung as possible, preferably with permanent pleurodesis to prevent recurrence. Surgical pleurodesis by talc poudrage at thoracoscopy or thoracotomy is the most effective technique, achieving permanent control in over 90 per cent of cases.[12] Medical pleurodesis with intercostal chest drainage and intrapleural instillation of tetracycline or other chemicals is an acceptable alternative in compromised patients, although the success rate is less (50–60 per cent).

A number of factors may interfere with pleurodesis and ultimately result in clinical failure. They include: incomplete drainage of the effusion; an ineffective agent; insufficient contact between agent and pleural surface due to adhesion or fibrin from previous pleural interventions; and failed apposition of the two pleural surfaces.

Surgical pleurodesis cannot succeed when lung expansion is restricted by a malignant or benign cortex as apposition of the two pleural surfaces is essential. In patients in whom the lung will not expand sufficiently to allow apposition, the insertion of a pleuroperitoneal shunt may be effective. Video assisted thoracoscopy is the best way to assess the results and it is then possible to proceed to talc pleurodesis or insertion of a pleuroperitoneal shunt. Both procedures provide reliable long-term control of effusion, without the need for repeated readmission and pleural aspiration.

In our experience of 180 patients treated with either talc pleurodesis or pleuroperitoneal Denver shunt at the Royal Brompton Hospital, effective palliation was achieved in over 95 per cent of patients.[13] In the whole series there was no intraoperative mortality but a few patients (5 per cent) died within the first month due to

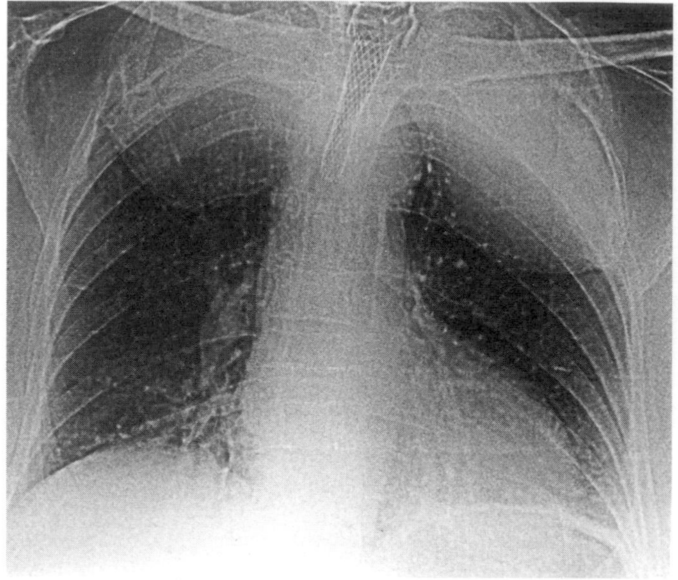

(a)

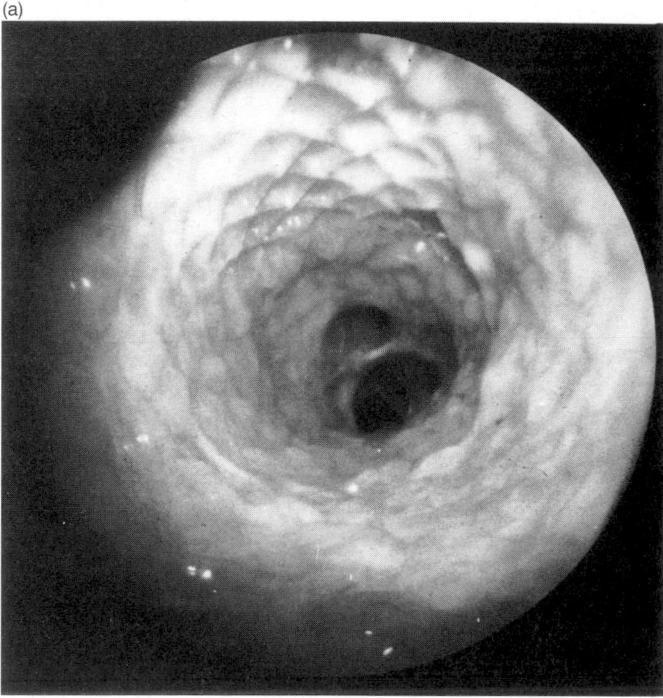

(b)

Fig. 1 Wallstent prosthesis, radiological (a) and endoscopic (b) appearance.

respiratory or multiorgan failure related to their advanced malignant disease. Median survival was 5 months (range 1–53). These results justify the early surgical referral of any patient with good performance status and recurrent malignant effusion.

The cause of dyspnoea in these patients is often complex and multifactorial. It may result from chest wall restriction due to previous surgery or radiotherapy, or infiltration by recurrent breast cancer. There may be bronchial obstruction due to metastatic nodal disease, lymphangitis and pulmonary fibrosis secondary to radiotherapy or airway obstruction. Pleural effusion may be the only correctable component, but it can be difficult to assess its contribution to the dyspnoea prior to treatment.

Tumour recurrence along a the track of a chest drain track or pleuroperitoneal shunt has been occasionally observed in patients with malignant effusions. It seldom causes significant symptoms but radiotherapy may be required to control pain and discourage local progression.

Pericardial effusion

Surgery is often required for patients with malignant pericardial involvement where constriction or effusion causes cardiac tamponade. Pericardiectomy relieves constriction and pericardial fenestration provides effective and continued drainage for effusion. Survival after pericardiectomy for malignant constriction is dismal and surgery is not justified for tumours with a poor prognosis such as lung cancer. Fenestration is possible via thoracotomy or video-assisted thoracoscopy. The subxiphoid approach has been reported to be a safer alternative for pericardial fenestration than the intrathoracic procedure. Other techniques have been used, such as percutaneous balloon pericardiotomy or pericardioperitoneal shunt.

Superior vena cava obstruction

Major surgery has no role in the palliation of superior vena cava syndrome due to advanced lung cancer. Resection and reconstruction of the superior vena cava or innominate vein with polytetrafluoroethylene grafts is only justified for cases of primary germ cell tumours of the mediastinum or invasive thymoma, for whom surgery aims at cure or long-term survival. For other malignancies including lung cancer, chemotherapy and/or radiotherapy offers better palliation than surgery.

The recent development of intravascular stenting techniques provides new possibilities for managing persistent or recurrent superior vena cava obstruction (see Section 8). The percutaneous transvenous insertion of expandable wire stents, with or without prior balloon dilatation, can be a safe and effective alternative to conventional therapy.[14]

Chest wall invasion and Pancoast syndrome

Chest wall resection for locally advanced lung cancer yields excellent results, providing tumour excision is macroscopically and microscopically complete and mediastinal node involvement excluded. The 5-year survival is approximately 50 per cent for T3N0 and 30 per cent for T3N1.[15]

The development of safe techniques for chest wall reconstruction, including polypropylene mesh (Marlex), methyl methacrylate composite prosthesis, and soft tissue reconstruction using myocutaneous flaps, has expanded the role of surgery in this field. Extensive chest wall resections, including total sternectomy, can now be performed with a low operative mortality in selected cases.

Such major surgery is only justified by an intention to cure. There is no symptomatic or survival benefit after incomplete resection and such cases are best treated by radiotherapy alone. Palliative surgery is often advocated in superior sulcus or Pancoast tumours but there is little evidence that incomplete resection in these circumstances affords better control of chest pain than radiotherapy alone. Median survival after incomplete resection of Pancoast tumours is less than 1 year, with 10 to 15 per cent of

Table 1 Endoscopic techniques in the palliation of malignant airways obstruction

Endoscopic techniques		Advantages versus disadvantages
Disobliteration:	Nd:YAG laser	Effective/costly
	Diathermy	Effective/not widely available
	Cryotherapy	Effective/repeated application required
Brachytherapy:	Iridium afterload	Tolerable in previous irradiation, day case treatment/not widely available
Silicone stents:	T or T/Y tubes	Cheap, stable/tracheostomy required
	Endobronchial stents	Cheap/can displace
Metal stents:	Gianturco	Expandable/tumour ingrowth
	Wallstent	Thin wall/tumour ingrowth
	Covered	High internal versus external ratio

patients surviving 3 years and none alive at 5 years. In the unique experience of Memorial Sloan-Kettering, where postoperative brachytherapy has been regularly used as an adjuvant treatment for patients undergoing resection of superior sulcus tumours, 9 per cent of patients survived 5 years after incomplete resection.[16] However, there was no difference in survival between these patients and those who did not undergo resection, and median survival after surgery was only 11 months.

Radiotherapy remains the principal treatment for symptomatic bone metastases. Rib or sternal resection may be sometimes be advised if relapse occurs after radiotherapy and the patient's life expectancy is otherwise reasonable, or if there are no other sites of disease and the primary tumour is controlled.

Dysphagia

In patients with locally advanced lung cancer, oesophageal obstruction may occur as a result of mediastinal lymphadenopathy or direct extension of the primary tumour (at the level of the carina or left main bronchus). Occasionally, tumour spread may be associated with a broncho-oesophageal fistula, which more commonly follows radiotherapy.

Radiation can relieve dysphagia, but local relapse is frequent and recurrent dysphagia may require further management.

The insertion of an endoprosthesis often provides adequate palliation. Various types of prosthesis—Celestin, Wilson-Cook, Atkinson—are available for push-through intubation. Endoscopic insertion is safe and reliable, and complications such as bleeding or perforation are uncommon. Tube displacement is not infrequent, however, and may require removal or repositioning of the tube. New expandable metal stents are now available which are apparently more effective than plastic ones. Early experiences show a lower complication rate and 30-day mortality, and a shorter average hospital stay. The stents may be covered with a membrane, preventing tumour ingrowth. While they are particularly suitable for tracheo-oesophageal fistula, they may be more prone to displacement.

Oesophageal bypass is inadvisable for oesophageal obstruction from primary lung cancer but may be required in patients with tracheo-oesophageal fistula who otherwise have a favourable prognosis and a good performance status.

Conclusion

The thoracic surgeon has a valuable role in the palliation of some manifestations of advanced intrathoracic disease. Survival is usually measured in months but some patients will benefit for years.

Breast cancer

Breast cancer is the commonest female malignancy in the Western world and the commonest cause of death in the age group 35 to 55. In the United Kingdom alone, there are 25 000 cases registered annually, resulting in over 15 000 deaths from the disease each year. Approximately 20 per cent of all cases that present are in the advanced stages, where cure is an unrealistic expectation and of those cases presenting at an early stage (potentially curable) between one-half and two-thirds will relapse with metastatic disease over a 10 to 20 year period of follow-up. Breast cancer is almost unique in its potential for very late relapse for which prolonged vigilance is necessary.

Evaluation

At presentation the surgeon has responsibility for the diagnosis and staging of the disease before determining rational therapy. Outpatient diagnosis is usually easy to achieve using fine needle aspiration cytology or cutting needle histopathology. If the patient is clinically stage I or II (T1,2 NO,1 MO) then no further evaluation is necessary before she undergoes definitive surgery. However, with more locally advanced disease, particularly if supraclavicular or cervical lymph node involvement is suspected, then a staging lymph node biopsy may be indicated. Furthermore, if the patient is judged to be inoperable it may be necessary to take a tumour sample for the measurement of oestrogen receptor before deciding on the relative merits of chemotherapy, tamoxifen, or surgical castration.

Local control and pain relief

It is fashionable these days to dismiss the achievements of William S. Halstead at the turn of the century, having lost sight of the fact that he introduced the radical mastectomy predominantly to achieve local control of locally advanced disease.[17] It also has to be remembered that there is one thing worse than a radical mastectomy and that is an ulcerated, fungating, and malodorous tumour on the chest wall. The radical mastectomy in the days before the availability of radiotherapy or chemotherapy achieved this objective in approximately 70 per cent of cases. These days locally advanced breast cancer is conventionally managed by chemotherapy, endocrine therapy, or radiotherapy. However, radical surgery still has a role. There are occasional rare patients where local control of the disease has not been possible with combinations of systemic therapy and radiotherapy yet the patient is not obviously dying of distant metastases. Under these circumstances a radical operation getting rid of the breast, the affected surrounding skin, and the underlying muscles, together with clearance of involved axillary lymph nodes, may in itself be palliative. Reconstruction of the defect is possible using myocutaneous flaps or an omental graft covered by split skin. This approach may be necessary for the late effects of radio necrosis as well as controlling the ulcerating malignancy.

It should also be remembered that patients, even though they might ultimately relapse with systemic metastases, can avoid the disgusting and painful results of uncontrolled local disease by either a modified radical mastectomy or a quadrantectomy, axillary node dissection, and radiotherapy to the breast. The decision over which approach is to be preferred is determined by the size and position of the original primary in relation to the size of the breast and to some extent the preference of the individual patient. An initial failure to control the disease in the axillary nodes can result in the very worst complications of breast cancer, where the uncontrolled disease grows to obstruct the lymphatics, the axillary vein, and the brachial plexus. This can lead to a painful, useless, and swollen arm.

Patients who present with distant metastases where the primary focus in itself is not a problem should initially be treated with systemic therapy as they are likely to die before the primary becomes a problem. Therefore, local regional therapy with surgery or radiotherapy in combination should be kept in reserve.

Reconstruction

A patient who has had a mastectomy in the past and represents with metastatic disease is not usually a candidate for the consideration of reconstruction. However, any woman who has been submitted to a mastectomy, however poor her long-term prognosis, should be offered reconstruction as part of her psychological rehabilitation. At the same time it must be remembered that there are no good empirical data to support the common-sense notion that breast conservation in itself necessarily improves psychological morbidity of the treatment of the disease.[18]

Techniques for reconstruction have improved enormously over recent years and this has largely depended upon the availability of implantable prostheses. For relatively small-busted women, who have had a simple or modified radical mastectomy in the past, a subpectoral tissue expander can produce pleasing results that will satisfy most patients. However, women who have been submitted to radical mastectomy or mastectomy plus radiotherapy in the past usually fare better with a myocutaneous flap to produce sufficient volume to match up with the contralateral breast (Fig. 2). These flaps can be swung on the latissimus dorsi pedicle or the transverse rectus abdominis (TRAM flap). Occasionally a reduction mammoplasty of the contralateral breast is necessary to achieve a perfect outcome.

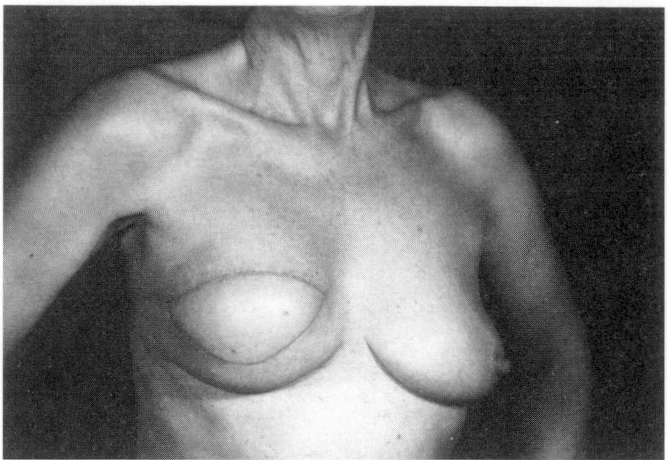

Fig. 2 Latissimus dorsi (LD) flap with underlying prosthesis used to reconstruct breast following mastectomy for breast cancer.

Cancer of the gastrointestinal tract

Malignant tumours of the gastrointestinal tract account for around 40 000 deaths a year in England and Wales—nearly 30 per cent of all deaths from malignancy. Many patients have advanced disease at presentation and the survival figures of those regarded as ostensibly curable suggest many of them already have disseminated disease. While surgery undoubtedly cures patients with minimally invasive tumours, its contribution lies chiefly in symptom relief and local disease control.

The principal symptoms of gastrointestinal malignancy are from obstruction of a hollow conduit, tumour bulk, or blood loss—either acute or chronic. The most effective way to relieve them is to excise the primary tumour completely, even when metastases are unequivocally present. If this is technically feasible, there may be little practical difference between curative and palliative procedures. When complete excision is impossible, or when associated risks are unacceptably high, symptoms from obstruction can still be relieved by surgical bypass or decompression, or by establishing a channel through the tumour by various means. Unless the primary tumour is removed, however, symptoms of obstruction are likely to recur and those caused by other pathological processes, such as bleeding, may become more prominent. Some symptoms, like the pain of malignant infiltration, may not be alleviated by surgery at all; others may be due to metastatic disseminated disease rather than the primary tumour itself. In these circumstances, surgical intervention of any kind may be inappropriate.

Carcinoma of the oesophagus

Oesophageal cancer accounts for 2 per cent of cancer deaths in the United Kingdom a year. Treatment is seldom curative and median survival after diagnosis is 10 months. Most clinicians agree palliation is the most important aspect of management.[19] Surgical excision is possible in over 50 per cent of cases, and there is recent evidence that primary medical therapy may improve resectability, but despite a substantial fall in the operative mortality rate (now 5–10 per cent, largely due to improved anaesthesia and post-operative care), complications are still common. Retrospective studies suggest surgical excision offers better palliation than radical radiotherapy but this may simply reflect the selection of less advanced cases for surgery. The most that can be concluded from uncontrolled studies is that the best results of surgery are achieved by experienced teams in carefully selected cases.

Patients fall broadly into two groups—those without evidence of advanced disease who are fit and those who either have advanced disease or are unfit. Patients in the first group are best served by resection; those in the second group have a variety of options.

Tumours at the gastro-oesophageal junction are approached through a left thoracoabdominal or thoracic incision with incision of the diaphragm. More proximal tumours require the Ivor–Lewis approach via a right thoracotomy after mobilizing the stomach at laparotomy. Some surgeons favour a three-stage procedure to achieve an adequate resection margin with anastomosis in the neck. Cervical anastomoses are more likely to leak, however, and in practice this often occurs in the superior mediastinum, not in the neck, with dire consequences.

In the technique of transhiatal oesophagectomy the oesophagus is removed through cervical and abdominal incisions without opening the chest.[20] Proponents of this approach claim there are less pulmonary complications but there is little evidence to support a reduction in morbidity or mortality and the procedure does not achieve adequate clearance in advanced disease. Endoscopic ultrasonography may assist selection for this procedure and the introduction of minimally invasive techniques now makes it possible to mobilize the thoracic oesophagus under direct vision.[21] The stomach is the most popular organ for oesophageal replacement; the colon and small bowel are alternatives and free jejunal grafts have been used to replace the cervical oesophagus with encouraging results.

Several studies have shown a promising response to radiotherapy and combination chemotherapy with cisplatinum-based regimens in patients with advanced disease. The results have stimulated studies into the use of combined modality treatment preoperatively to improve resectability.[22]

At present oesophageal intubation is the standard way of relieving symptoms in patients with unresectable tumours or malignant tracheo-oesophageal fistulas. Permanent gastrostomy is hardly ever justifiable and palliative radiotherapy, like oesophageal dilatation, provides only temporary symptomatic relief with over 60 per cent of patients experiencing recurrent dysphagia. Bypass procedures are associated with a particularly high operative mortality rate (at least 30 per cent) and should probably be reserved for tumours that prove unresectable at operation contrary to expectation.

Intubation is achieved either by traction at open operation or by pulsion through an endoscope. Endoscopic intubation under fluoroscopic control is safer than surgical intubation and recovery is swifter . The principal tubes employed for open intubation are the Mousseau–Barbin tube, which has a long leading catheter for this purpose, and the Celestin tube. The latter has been modified by the addition of a distal flange, to prevent upward displacement, and adapted for endoscopic insertion using a Nottingham introducer . Intubation carries a 10 per cent risk of perforation but the newer, self-expanding metal stents are less traumatic to insert and easier to maintain.[23]

Patients with oesophageal tubes require a semisolid diet. Steak, unless minced, and fresh bread are particularly liable to stick. Blockage may resolve spontaneously and can be encouraged to do so by administering fizzy drinks. If not, a nasogastric tube should be passed to try to dislodge the bolus before resorting to endoscopy.

Nd: YAG laser therapy is an alternative to intubation and can be undertaken without general anaesthesia. It is only suitable for exophytic tumours. The laser is used to burrow through the tumour on successive occasions or to photocoagulate the entire tumour at one session after preliminary dilatation. Dysphagia is relieved in over 60 per cent of cases, half of whom can take a normal diet, and the complication rate is low. More than half the patients require further courses of treatment, however, sometimes after only a few weeks, and for this reason the technique is unsuitable for patients living a long way from the treatment centre. Additional external beam radiotherapy may reduce the need for frequent treatments.

Similar results to those achieved by laser have been reported using absolute alcohol given by injection endoscopically, and an increasing number of studies report the value of combining tumour destruction with intubation. Another development is the introduction of photodynamic therapy using the argon laser after presensitization with intravenous haematoporphyrin derivative. Haematoporphyrin derivative is retained by malignant tissue and activated by light of wavelength 630 nm, producing cytotoxic free radicals. Accidental oesophageal perforation is less likely with photodynamic therapy and, as healing apparently occurs by tissue regeneration rather than by fibrosis, strictures are supposed to develop less frequently.

Carcinoma of the stomach

Several retrospective studies have shown that patients with incurable gastric cancer have better symptomatic relief and a longer life expectancy after resection than after bypass procedures or no treatment at all. While the results may simply reflect a selection bias, there is little doubt that symptoms due to mechanical obstruction or haemorrhage are relieved more successfully by resection than by procedures which leave the tumour in place.

The operative mortality rate of palliative resection is related to the type of operation performed. Figures vary widely but within the last decade mortality rates have fallen: figures of 5 per cent or less have been consistently reported after subtotal gastrectomy for tumours of the cardia and gastric antrum, and figures of 10 per cent after total gastrectomy for tumours of the body of the stomach. Total gastrectomy can be followed by severe nutritional deficiencies but the majority of patients have a good or satisfactory quality of life after surgery.

There is currently great interest in the use of preoperative combination chemotherapy in patients with advanced gastric cancer. Response rates of 70 per cent (complete remission >10 per cent) have been obtained with epirubicin-cisplatinum-fluoracil in patients with advanced disease enabling some of them (>50 per cent) to proceed to surgery and successful resection.[22]

For patients with unresectable tumours options are limited. Tumours confined to the cardia can be treated by intubation or laser therapy, as described above, but palliation is more difficult if the tumour is extensive. Simple bypass of antral tumours offers temporary relief from vomiting but gastric emptying can be unsatisfactory and the Devine antral exclusion operation may be preferable.

Malignant obstructive jaundice

Surgical resection or bypass for pancreatic cancer is being undertaken more frequently nowadays because of substantially lower operative mortality rates (<10 per cent). Exploratory laparotomy on the other hand is becoming less common because of better preoperative assessment, including laparoscopy. Survival time after resection is improving (mean 17 months) but it is not clear how much this is due to earlier diagnosis and patient selection. Improved survival is limited to patients with tumours of the head of the pancreas; the prospects for those with distal tumours remain dismal.

Most patients with carcinoma of the pancreas present with obstructive jaundice. Relief of biliary obstruction results in a prolonged and more comfortable survival, free of distressing pruritus. Percutaneous transhepatic endoprostheses are associated with a lower mortality rate and fewer early complications than surgical bypass. Later complications of recurrent jaundice and cholangitis are avoided using self-expanding metallic endoprostheses, though these are difficult to remove[23] (see Section 8).

Endoscopic biliary stenting with Teflon, polyethylene, or polyurethane endoprostheses has similar results to percutaneous stenting and surgical bypass. The mortality rate of this procedure is less than that reported for surgical bypass and recovery is quicker, but occlusion of the stent within a few months is not uncommon and may require further admission to hospital for the stent to be changed. Even so, the total period spent in hospital may still be less than after surgery, especially if the survival time is short. A recent study showed no significant survival difference between surgery and stenting but fewer early treatment-related complications after stenting (14 per cent versus 3 per cent) and fewer late complications after surgery (7 per cent versus 17 per cent).[24] Non-operative measures are appropriate for elderly and high-risk patients without evidence of duodenal obstruction whose life expectancy is short. In other cases surgery offers the advantages of providing a definitive diagnosis, confirming irresectability, providing permanent biliary and gastric drainage, and treating intractable pain all at once.

There is some evidence that survival is better after palliative resection than after bypass. Palliative resection is only justifiable, however, if operative mortality and morbidity rates can be kept extremely low. Bypass is customarily accomplished by cholecystojejunostomy except when the cystic duct is occluded by tumour, in which case the jejunum is joined to the hepatic duct by means of a Roux loop (Figs 3 and 4). The procedures are technically straightforward but recurrent jaundice or cholangitis occur more often than after anastomosis of the divided common bile duct with a jejunal loop–choledochojejunostomy (20 per cent versus 8 per cent). The latter procedure is preferred by biliary surgeons in whose hands the mortality rate is low (<10 per cent).

Duodenal obstruction occurs in 5 per cent of patients at presentation and in a further 15 to 30 per cent within 12 months. Most surgeons, therefore, perform a gastroenterostomy at the same time as the biliary bypass, the addition of which is not associated with a greater mortality rate or a longer recovery period.

Injecting the coeliac plexus with 40 ml of 5 per cent phenol (chemical splanchnicectomy) has been found to be an effective way of relieving pain arising from tumour infiltration. Slightly less favourable results have been achieved with 20 to 30 ml of 50 per cent ethanol (60 per cent versus 80 per cent) though a controlled study has not been done. Injection can be performed at the time of surgery and repeated later by percutaneous injection. Because peroperative chemical splanchnicectomy is simple, effective, and safe it can be recommended whenever pain is a prominent feature. Persistent pain may respond to external beam radiotherapy (see Chapters 9.2.6 and 9.2.10).

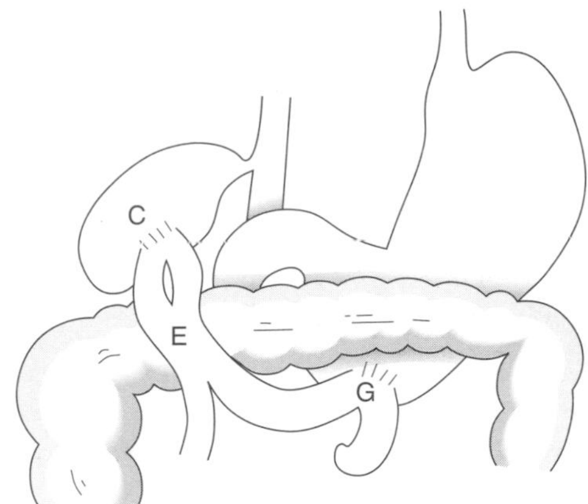

Fig. 3 Triple bypass: C, cholecystojejunostomy; E, enteroenterostomy; G, gastroenterostomy.

Advanced tumours of the distal bile duct and ampulla are treated the same way as pancreatic carcinoma. Those of the gallbladder carry an extremely poor prognosis. Unresectable tumours of the proximal biliary tree can be managed by surgical bypass or by intubation and drainage. Surgery is claimed to provide better symptomatic relief as it avoids the need for a prosthetic implant but this has yet to be established by comparative trials. Bypass is achieved by joining a Roux loop to the intrahepatic biliary tree which is found by following the round ligament into the umbilical fissure or by removing the anterior portion of the quadrate lobe. Interstitial irradiation using iridium wires inserted by either route may provide further useful palliation.

Malignant tumours of the small intestine are uncommon. As a rule they can be resected or bypassed with little difficulty.

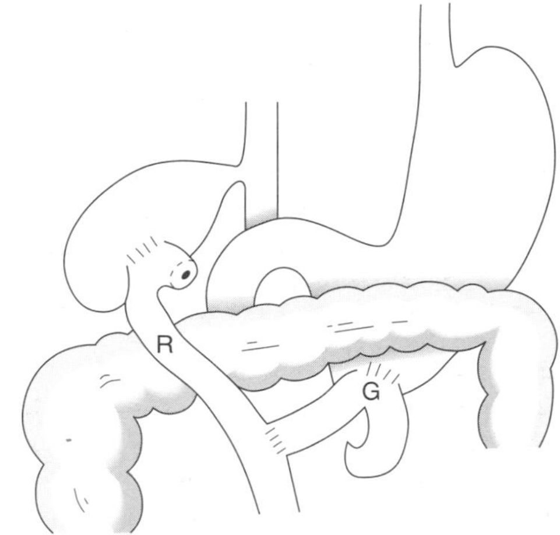

Fig. 4 Cholecystojejunostomy-en-Y: R, Roux loop; G, gastroenterostomy.

Colorectal cancer

Colorectal cancer is the second commonest cause of cancer death in the United Kingdom, where an estimated 27 000 new cases occur each year with a 37 per cent 5-year survival, which has improved little in recent years. Death occurs either from locoregional disease progression (in 10–15 per cent of patients) or from disseminated disease, particularly involving the liver (in 50 per cent of patients). Therefore, palliation of colorectal cancer involves treatment of both local and disseminated disease.

Local disease

The primary tumour is locally advanced with involvement of adjacent viscera at initial presentation in roughly 20 per cent of cases. Complete surgical excision is the only effective treatment for locally advanced colorectal cancer,[25] and offers a chance of cure which is comparable to similar stage disease that has not invaded adjacent tissues. The most useful preoperative test for assessment of extent of local invasion is the computerized tomography (**CT**) scan,[26] although tumour fixity on rectal examination suggests extramural involvement with 60 per cent accuracy in palpable rectal tumours. Preoperative irradiation of locally advanced disease,[27] particularly in the rectum, reduces local recurrence without increasing the risks of surgery.

Recurrent disease after primary tumour resection occurs solely at the site of tumour excision in 30 per cent of cases but is associated with distant metastases in 70 per cent of cases of local recurrence.[28] In addition to abdominal CT, which provides the most comprehensive assessment of the site and extent of local recurrence, sacral magnetic resonance imaging (**MRI**) is particularly useful where there is unexplained pelvic pain which is usually due to sacral nerve involvement with recurrent disease after rectal cancer excision.

Surgical excision of local recurrence helps symptom control in about 10 per cent of cases and should be considered in appropriately fit patients with limited disease. Further resection is not feasible for most cases in whom continued uncontrolled growth produces obstruction, bleeding, and pain. Localized duodenal or small bowel obstruction can be relieved with intestinal bypass, but this is rarely helpful when there are multiple areas of hold-up requiring multiple bypasses. When the diagnosis of multiple areas of obstruction can be made before laparotomy, for example from barium follow through or abdominal CT scan, the patient is probably better managed by non-operative measures.

Distal colonic or rectal obstruction can be relieved by a defunctioning colostomy proximal to the site of obstruction. Rectal or distal colonic obstruction can also be relieved by endoluminal diathermy or laser resection, sometimes with metal stent insertion, but these procedures do not control pelvic pain.[29] Control of pain and bleeding can be achieved by irradiation of areas of local recurrence,[30] but this is better used where obstruction has first been resolved by one of the approaches mentioned above.

Disseminated disease

The commonest site of metastasis in colorectal cancer is the liver, which is involved in about 80 per cent of patients with disseminated disease. It is thought that secondary metastasis from the liver to other sites is the main source of general dissemination.[31]

Uncontrolled liver metastases produce pain, abdominal distension, jaundice, and inferior vena cava obstruction. The only curative treatment for colorectal liver metastases is surgical resection which is technically feasible in about 20 per cent of affected patients.[28] Since only 20 to 25 per cent of patients undergoing liver metastasis resection will survive 5 years, it appears that at most 5 per cent of patients with colorectal cancer can be offered long-term survival by liver resection. Criteria indicating suitable patients for metastasis resection are fewer than four liver metastases, a node-negative primary tumour, and an observation interval of 3 months from diagnosis of metastasis during which time additional disease has not developed. The perioperative mortality from metastasis resection should be less than 5 per cent[32] but increases with patients age, coexisting disease, and extent of resection. Recurrent disease develops within the liver in 25 per cent and elsewhere in 50 per cent of patients who have previously undergone liver metastasis resection.[33]

The majority of liver metastasis patients cannot be helped by resection. Although other metastasis ablation techniques involving freezing and laser are being developed, the only treatment of proven benefit is chemotherapy. The most effective agents are fluorinated pyrimidines. A 23 per cent partial response rate is achieved with 5-fluorouracil and there is probable survival benefit when combined with the thymidylate kinase inhibitor folinic acid.[34] Regional administration of the 5-fluorouracil analogue floxuridine via the hepatic artery produces a 50 per cent partial response rate and significant survival benefit.[35] Seventy per cent of patients treated with regional floxuridine die of disease progression outside the liver. Therefore, palliation of the symptoms of liver metastasis growth can be achieved in most cases with this technique.

Systemic, 5-fluorouracil based chemotherapy can now be administered by continuous infusion as an outpatient, and intrahepatic floxuridine is likewise administered by continuous infusion via a totally implanted pump. Chemotherapy can thus prolong survival and delay the onset of symptoms with little treatment-associated inconvenience. The benefits of treatment are greater in fit patients with a good quality of life and treatment should be considered at this stage, before patients reach a terminal stage when chemotherapy is usually inappropriate. Follow-up, relying on identifying patients with liver pain or palpable liver metastases, identifies liver metastases at a late stage (35–40 per cent liver replacement) which reduces the benefits of intrahepatic floxuridine chemotherapy. More benefit can be achieved, even allowing for lead time bias, if metastases are diagnosed sooner (15 per cent liver replacement) by routine liver ultrasound scan or serum carcinoembryonic antigen estimation. These are recommended in routine follow-up of suitable patients at high risk of developing liver metastases. Corticosteroids can be used in patients with advanced liver metastases to reduce liver capsule pain.

Disseminated disease can also be temporarily controlled with systemic 5-fluorouracil and folinic acid chemotherapy to produce a quality of life benefit.[36] Rarely, resection of an isolated lung metastasis can produce long-term survival, but the development of lung, bone, or brain metastases usually indicates that the disease is incurable. The pain of bone metastases can usually be controlled by irradiation, and prophylactic bone fixation may be required for metastases affecting long bones. Cerebral irradiation plus high dose corticosteroids can reduce intracerebral pressure and delay neurological deterioration.

Since most patients with colorectal carcinoma are not cured, it could be argued that the majority of patients receive palliative treatment. Careful judgement is required in deciding the correct mixture of radical surgery, radiotherapy, and chemotherapy to produce the best chance of prolonged, high-quality survival.[37]

Advanced epidermoid carcinoma of the anal canal may respond sufficiently well to systemic chemotherapy and irradiation to permit local excision of residual tumour with conservation of the anus. Local excision is usually adequate for tumours of the anal margin but extensive tumours may still require abdominoperineal resection. Recurrent tumour in the perineum following surgery and irradiation is an extremely distressing problem and one that is particularly difficult to treat. Although further recurrence is almost inevitable, it is occasionally possible to provide temporary palliation by excising the bulk of malignant tissue and closing the defect with a myocutaneous flap based on an inferior epigastric pedicle.

Palliative urological surgery

In advanced malignancy of the urinary tract massive local recurrence requiring heroic surgery is uncommon, although judicious endoscopic surgery may be of significant palliative value.

Renal adenocarcinoma

The characteristic pattern of disseminated renal adenocarcinoma is of multiple metastases to lung and/or bone, often with lymphadenopathy. Reports of spontaneous remission of metastases after nephrectomy are poorly documented and there is little real evidence that it confers any advantage, although in patients with small numbers of soft tissue metastases confined to one organ survival may be prolonged by nephrectomy. In patients with pulmonary metastases confined to one lobe nephrectomy can be combined with lobectomy either synchronously or, more commonly, nephrectomy can be followed after some 3 months by pulmonary lobectomy if repeat staging investigations show that no new lesions have developed.

Palliative nephrectomy for local symptoms should be considered only after other measures such as renal artery embolization have failed.

Transitional cell carcinoma of the upper urinary tract

Prognosis in carcinoma of the renal pelvis or calices is related to tumour grade and stage rather than therapeutic endeavour and surgery (nephroureterectomy, partial nephrectomy, percutaneous or endoscopic) is therefore presumed to be curative until proved otherwise by the pathologist or subsequent events. Haematuria, if metastases are present, should be controlled, if possible, by renal artery embolization or radiotherapy before resorting to nephrectomy.

Similarly, ureteric tumours are presumed to be curable until proved otherwise. In the elderly, frail patient unfit for nephroureterectomy simple resection with ligation of the proximal ureter is an option. Endoscopic surgery can also be considered.

Carcinoma of the bladder

The first therapeutic choice in patients with locally recurrent muscle invasive bladder cancer is 'salvage' cystectomy. Operable patients will, however, be only a minority and radical local surgery is not often possible. Transurethral resection, which may need to be repeated, can be effective for the relief of haematuria or the frequency, strangury, and outflow obstruction of a large exophytic tumour recurrence.

Severe haematuria in patients with metastatic disease can sometimes be controlled by bilateral internal iliac arterial embolization but cystectomy may be necessary. If the bladder is fixed and inoperable, internal iliac ligation may be possible. Continuous intravesical infusion of alum solution is sometimes effective in controlling haemorrhage. Postirradiation bleeding may be controlled by sublingual administration of sodium pentosan polysulphate.

Transurethral resection as the only therapy in the frail, elderly patient unfit for more aggressive treatment will often result in prolonged relief of symptoms with little operative risk. It can be repeated although rapid recurrence of a poorly differentiated tumour after transurethral resection is an indication for cautious palliative radiotherapy.

Carcinoma of the prostate

Carcinoma of the prostate is predominately a disease of the elderly, and only about 20 per cent of patients are likely to benefit from radical local therapy. Management is, therefore, palliative in the majority of cases.

Obstructive prostatic symptoms or urinary retention are best treated in the first instance by transurethral resection. Symptomatic local recurrence after radiotherapy or androgen deprivation can also be treated by transurethral resection though if, as is often the case, there is invasion of the bladder base, frequency and urgency may prove refractory.

Symptomatic metastatic carcinoma of the prostate is effectively palliated in 80 to 85 per cent of patients by androgen deprivation with a median response duration of 15 months. Since the recognition of the dangers of oestrogens, surgical orchidectomy has been the principal method of androgen deprivation, although luteinizing-hormone-releasing hormone analogues provide an effective alternative.[38]

A small sub-group of patients present with spinal cord compression from a solitary metastasis and respond well to a combined approach of surgical decompression and radiotherapy to the spine followed by orchidectomy. In contrast, patients with pre-existing prostatic carcinoma who develop cord compression usually have metastatic disease too extensive for effective surgical decompression, and prognosis is very poor.

Penile carcinoma

Total amputation of the penis, even in the presence of lymphatic or distant metastatic disease, is the most effective palliative manoeuvre for the extensive, ulcerating infected carcinoma of the penis.

Secondary tumours

Any primary tumour can produce secondary deposits in the urinary tract. The commonest presentation will be ureteric obstruction (see below) or haematuria. Most parts of the urinary tract are now accessible endoscopically or percutaneously and secondary tumours should be treated by minimally invasive surgical techniques. Major open surgery is rarely needed.

Relief of ureteric obstruction

Most malignant tumours are capable of ureteric obstruction from retroperitoneal metastases, lymphadenopathy, or direct invasion. Relief of obstruction seldom confers survival advantage and quality of life is significantly impaired both by the effects of the tumour and the morbidity of the urinary diversion required. Death from renal failure appears (at least to the observer) to be easier and more peaceful than death with uncontrolled pelvic malignancy. Ureteric obstruction in the presence of untreatable malignancy should, in general, not be relieved unless relief of obstruction will permit effective palliative chemotherapy or radiotherapy.

Once a decision to undertake relief of obstruction is made, the method employed should be as minimally invasive as possible. The optimal technique is the endoscopic insertion of a ureteric stent under radiological control. This has the advantage of requiring no external appliance or stoma, but may be technically impossible if the ureteric orifices are obscured or the course of the ureter distorted by tumour masses. Stent insertion usually requires a general anaesthetic and is more difficult the more distal the obstruction. Antegrade placement of a ureteric stent under radiological control via a percutaneous approach can be undertaken. Occasionally, a combined antegrade/retrograde technique is helpful. Less satisfactory, though it can be done under local anaesthetic, is the insertion of a percutaneous nephrostomy tube under radiological or ultrasound control. Nephrostomy drainage can rarely be maintained for longer than 6 weeks; there are frequent problems with infection and blockage or displacement of the nephrostomy tube; the quality of life provided by long-term nephrostomy drainage is low. It is particularly indicated in patients with relatively acute obstruction in whom other treatment offers a reasonable prospect of tumour regression or in those in the early stage of radiotherapy where oedema may have converted partial into complete obstruction. Open nephrostomy or ureterostomy is never indicated.

'Permanent' methods of diversion (e.g. ileal conduit or catheterizable stomata) are rarely indicated.

The management of urinary fistulas

The rule against diversion in the presence of untreatable distal malignancy should be relaxed in patients with malignant or postradiotherapy vesicovaginal or vesicocolic fistulas. Although in the very ill or dying patient bilateral nephrostomy drainage may be adequate, the arguments against nephrostomy advanced above are still valid; long stent insertion is unlikely to be effective and formal open diversion is almost mandatory, with or without an attempt to remove the bulk of the tumour mass. If the fistula involves the rectum, a colostomy will be needed.

Surgery for urinary pathology in non-urological malignancy

Many male patients with cancer are in the age range in which prostatic pathology occurs. Acute urinary retention should be treated either by transurethral resection or the insertion of an endoprostatic stent since the alternative, an indwelling urethral catheter, carries a significant morbidity and impaired quality of life. Transurethral laser ablation of the prostate may be effective with less morbidity than transurethral resection. Prostatism may need no treatment but transurethral resection can be considered. Chronic retention is often unresponsive to transurethral resection; there is little alternative to catheterization. Incidentally-found prostatic carcinoma will need no treatment unless symptomatic.

Asymptomatic stones are unlikely to need treatment unless associated with persistent infection. Symptomatic stones, usually ureteric, should be treated by appropriate, minimally invasive techniques—external shock wave lithotripsy, percutaneous, or endoscopic treatment.

Gynaecological and pelvic cancer

Approximately 15 000 gynaecological malignancies occur every year in the United Kingdom. Of these, more than 8000 will die either from their cancer or with the malignancy implicated in their death. Surgery has an important part to play in the management of these cases.

Women with terminal pelvic cancer of the lower genital tract suffer from various complications depending upon the type of primary lesion. Those with recurrent ovarian cancer develop progressive intestinal obstruction and cachexia leading to death. Those with progressive and recurrent cervical carcinoma develop obstructive uropathy and renal failure. Some suffer from fistulas and haemorrhage. Progressive and recurrent vulval cancer leads to a fungating tumour with subsequent sepsis.

Obstruction (see Chapter 9.3.4)

Over 75 per cent of patients who develop ovarian cancer ultimately die of their disease, despite current advances in management. Intestinal obstruction may be recurrent and is usually subacute. It may result from multiple metastases, postoperative adhesions, postirradiation strictures, or a new primary tumour. Initially, conservative treatment should be instituted with intravenous fluids, nasogastric suction, and aspiration to defunction the gastrointestinal tract. Suitable analgesia, antiemetics, and antispasmodic agents should be administered.

Sometimes, more active treatment is worthwhile. Chemotherapy for primary or recurrent disease can be effective and occasionally high-dose therapy with bone marrow rescue is worth considering. Total parenteral nutrition is needed while the response is assessed, after which the question of surgical exploration with debulking of tumour and relief of the obstruction can be reviewed. Ideally, a radical oophorectomy should be carried out but this is not always practical. A partial debulking procedure with resection of tumour and affected bowel and primary anastomosis may be possible. If not, diversion either by bypass or colostomy may be necessary. The creation of a colostomy or other stoma may be indicated for palliative reasons but it is not usually justified as a prophylactic measure. The natural history of ovarian cancer is such that progressive obstruction occurs with proximal extension along the gastrointestinal tract so that an ileostomy and then jejunostomy may become necessary. Repeated surgical exploration for obstruction will ultimately necessitate gastrostomy but this should only be reserved for special cases after very careful consideration and full discussion with the patient.

There are several reasons for debulking ovarian cancer.

(1) to improve the response to chemotherapy and radiotherapy;

(2) to reverse immunosuppression and to encourage immunological enhancement;

(3) to prevent inevitable complications involving the gastrointestinal and urogenital tracts (reduction in tumour bulk also helps prevent the development of ascites and uncomfortable abdominal distension);

(4) the psychological advantage of removing a huge abdominopelvic mass.

Fistulas

The development of a vesicovaginal or rectovaginal fistula typically complicates cervical carcinoma. On occasions a 'three-way' fistula can develop in the form of a cloaca. This may be due to tumour but more often results from tumour progression following radiotherapy and radionecrosis. The ideal management is excision of the fistula with primary repair but this is seldom practical. Small fistulas without marked radionecrosis may be dealt with in this way, using healthy tissue from the omentum or a labial fat pad as in a Martius rotational graft. More usually, urinary diversion will be needed—either an ileal conduit or a nephrostomy. Rarely, an indwelling catheter can be used to relieve incontinence from a vesicovaginal fistula, and a ureteric stent to bypass a ureteric fistula.

For fistulas involving the large bowel diversion by colostomy is usually the most practical treatment. Although a double-barrelled colostomy allows drainage of the distal limb via a type of mucous fistula, it doubles the size of the stoma and complicates control of the appliance. Under these circumstances, an end colostomy is more practical with or without resection of the distal limb or tumour site. If needed, a separate mucous fistula can be developed at the inferior margin of the abdominal incision.

Local fungation

With recurrent and progressive vulvar cancer it is important to balance the advantages and disadvantages of surgical excision against the possibility of controlling the tumour and the patient's symptoms by palliative radiotherapy. The mainstay of treatment for vulvar cancer is surgery but recent evidence shows these tumours are radiosensitive when modified radiotherapy is given in conjunction with sensitizing chemotherapy. This has been shown to be effective with anal cancer, utilizing the NIGRA regimen of combination chemotherapy with 5-fluorouracil and mitomycin C and planned radiotherapy. This approach can provide considerable symptomatic control and even result in resolution of the tumour. If unsuccessful, surgery needs to be considered. Wide, local excision of fungating groin nodes and tumours involving the vulva and introitus gives symptomatic relief from discharge and pain but it is not always possible to obtain primary skin closure under these circumstances and a musculocutaneous graft may have to be created to fill any defect. This can be taken from the gluteus maximus, tensor fascia lata, or rectus abdominus muscle. The latter gives a considerable amount of healthy tissue outside any previously treated area, either by surgery or radiotherapy.

Discharge

Recurrent pelvic cancer can be associated with profuse discharge, a foul odour, and sometimes bleeding. Symptoms are due to necrotic tumour and may be partly affected by previous radiotherapy and associated with local infection. Treatment is symptomatic and involves reducing any infection present by local toilet measures, using for example povidone iodine. Metronidazole is useful for its effects on anaerobic organisms. The odour should be isolated if it is arising from a localized wound and the use of charcoal dressings or a colostomy bag may help. If the discharge is from a fistula or arising from the colostomy itself, then local treatment and isolation is relatively simple. Discharge from the vagina often heralds recurrence associated with radiation necrosis and is more difficult to deal with. If the discharge comes from the rectum, it is important to exclude faecal impaction which may be precipitated by opioid analgesics.

It is important to protect the skin around the discharge site using barrier creams or a zinc oxide paste. Local corticosteroids may help. Tampons may be useful when the discharge comes from the vagina, particularly if social engagements are contemplated.

Further treatment with radiotherapy may be considered using an intracavity source, but combining this with hyperbaric oxygen has not proved successful. Local diathermy and cryosurgery is of little value and may lead to worse symptoms but, in future, laser surgery may help in the in symptomatic control of inoperable disease.

Haemorrhage

Haemorrhage from recurrent pelvic cancer may be either acute, occurring during a surgical procedure, or chronic, complicating recurrent tumour with or without the effects of radiation and further necrosis.

Severe haemorrhage may occur during pelvic exenteration, particularly if previous radiotherapy has been given. Haemostasis should be attempted in the routine way using clamps, diathermy, and transfixion sutures but if this fails, the pelvis should be packed whilst the patient is resuscitated. To continue to use an excessive number of clamps and sutures may be counterproductive and it may be necessary to leave clamps or packs in the pelvis to create a tamponade. These may be removed 48 to 72 h later. Suitable antibiotic cover will need to be given, but repeat delayed primary haemorrhage or indeed early secondary haemorrhage is rarely a complication providing any clotting disorder is corrected.

Local pressure and packing may help control chronic blood loss and intracavity radiotherapy may often reduce bleeding from a localized site even if it has been used in the past. If it is possible to isolate the bleeding source radiologically, embolization may be considered but this is not without risk. Surgical ligation of the internal iliac vessels may sometimes be of great benefit, especially if persistent haemorrhage is occurring from a pelvic source. This, however, requires a laparotomy or at least a bilateral extraperitoneal approach to the pelvic side-walls.

Ascites

Ascites is now much less of a problem because of more effective chemotherapy. However, it may still lead to troublesome abdominal distension when a tumour is chemoresistant. Paracentesis may then be required for symptomatic relief and the introduction of intraperitoneal chemotherapeutic agents. Peritoneovenous shunts have been used for palliative relief and provide interim relief but lead to further dissemination of tumour. Monoclonal antibodies have been used therapeutically to target therapy. For persistent and recurring ascites, resistant to other modalities, this has been shown to be effective.[39,40] The management of ascites is considered in detail in Chapter 9.3.7.

Soft tissue sarcoma

Soft tissue sarcomas are rare tumours accounting for less than 2 per cent of new adult cancers. There are approximately 5000 new cases annually in the United States and about 1000 in the United Kingdom. The tumours arise in connective tissue, can occur anywhere in the body, and affect males and females equally. The commonest group are collectively referred to as extremity sarcomas (60 per cent) occurring in the limb and limb girdles, while 30 per cent of sarcomas occur in the trunk, and 10 per cent in the head and neck. They are best treated by an experienced multidisciplinary team.

About half the patients with soft tissue sarcoma die of their disease, invariably of pulmonary metastases, although this dissemination is usually undetectable at the time of presentation. Poor prognostic factors at the time of presentation include large tumour size, high histological grade, and sites (such as head/neck, mediastinum, and retroperitoneum) where adequate surgical clearance cannot be achieved.

All patients with a normal CT scan of thorax at the time of presentation are potentially curable providing the primary disease can be permanently eradicated. For extremity sarcomas this means aggressive primary treatment by surgery alone or in combination with radiotherapy with an emphasis on limb conservation and preservation of function. Small, low-grade tumours at sites where adequate clearance can be achieved may be treated by surgery alone. Local failure is due to inadequate margins of clearance and the value of radiotherapy in improving local control after surgery is well proven. Large primary tumours at relatively inaccessible sites, where it can be predicted that adequate surgical margins cannot be achieved, are treated by preoperative radiotherapy, accepting the consequence of delayed or poor wound healing with 10 per cent of patients suffering major wound breakdown. Unfortunately, at the present time, there is probably no effective adjuvant chemotherapy for soft tissue sarcomas, as the results of many randomized clinical trials have shown conflicting results. For many patients with resectable primary tumours at presentation, certain prognostic factors may indicate a poor chance of cure, but these patients must still be offered potentially curative treatment as the only method of identifying those who can be salvaged.

Palliative surgery

Although around 50 per cent of patients with soft tissue sarcoma will die of their disease, few have demonstrable metastatic disease at the time of presentation, making it difficult to determine prospectively when surgery is palliative. In the presence of established metastatic disease, or surgically incurable local disease, surgery still has a role to play in palliation as well as in achieving the occasional cure. Because of the diverse clinical situations the subject will be discussed under four headings.

(1) post-treatment recurrences at the primary site

(2) amputation

(3) metastasectomy

(4) management of retroperitoneal sarcomas.

Post-treatment recurrences at the primary site

Following primary treatment of resectable extremity sarcomas in specialist units, the local recurrence rate is of the order of 15 per cent. The recurrence rate for patients who have received inadequate primary treatment is greater than this, but these patients can often be rendered free of local disease more easily because factors other than biology of the tumour are responsible for the recurrence. Thus, at one end of the spectrum are patients with recurrence who have received minimal surgery and no radiotherapy at initial diagnosis, who can be treated conventionally, while at the other end of the spectrum are patients with recurrence that is surgically inaccessible or in previously irradiated tissues in which case even amputation may not be an option. Further radical treatment should be undertaken whenever possible and the availability and application of a variety of reconstructive techniques, when necessary, is essential. Skin and subcutaneous tissues most often require reconstruction, and the transfer of unirradiated well-vascularized tissues promotes healing and permits wound closure without tension. Major nerve trunks may need to be sacrificed and, rarely, vascular reconstruction is necessary. Bone and joint involvement by recurrent tumour is usually an indication for amputation, if feasible. Because of the natural distribution of extremity sarcomas, most recurrences occur at or close to limb girdles, so that myocutaneous flaps (or transposed muscle with split skin graft) are frequently the reconstructive technique of choice. The inferiorly based rectus abdominis myocutaneous flap is extremely useful to reconstruct and promote healing of wounds in the groin and upper thigh. At more peripheral sites, free tissue transfer with microvascular anastomosis will prevent the need for amputation.

Amputation

Amputation is reserved for locally unresectable disease, and is usually a secondary procedure after failed limb-conserving treatment. Unless absolutely essential for palliation, amputation should be avoided in the presence of metastatic disease. The site of amputation should always be proximal to the involved compartment, because sarcomas spread along tissue planes within compartments and transcompartmental amputations run the risk of stump recurrence. For major ablative procedures, such as fore-quarter and hind-quarter amputations, careful clinical and radiological assessments of operability is necessary because stump recurrence after such procedures is so distressing. In patients with buttock and pelvic tumours, considered for hind-quarter amputation, it is essential to be certain that tumour does not extend significantly through the greater sciatic notch into the pelvis or encroach on the site of the most proximal possible bone section at the sacroiliac joint. When feasible, preamputation radiotherapy may reduce tumour bulk to make amputation technically less difficult and this may also reduce the risk of stump recurrence. Counselling, full informed consent, preamputation assessment at limb fitting centres, and early, energetic rehabilitation are essential aspects of patient care. In the presence of metastatic disease, palliative amputation may be necessary to control local pain, fungation, or the threat of major haemorrhage.

Metastasectomy

Long term survival of patients with isolated or few pulmonary metastases is well documented. For patients whose primary disease is controlled, metastasectomy must always be considered given that the best chemotherapy regimens for soft tissue sarcoma offer a response rate of about 45 per cent and achieve complete remission in only 10 per cent of patients. Both CT scan and tomography detect about half the number of metastases subsequently found at operation and similarly half the patients with apparently unilateral disease are found to have bilateral metastases at the time of surgery. These findings have led to the suggestion that pulmonary metastasectomy should always be performed by median sternotomy rather than by thoracotomy. In a recent series, the median post-thoracotomy survival time was 20 months which was slightly greater for patients with four metastases or less and for those rendered disease free by surgery via medial sternotomy. Postoperative chemotherapy made little difference to survival. Patients with a disease-free interval (time from resection of primary tumour to detection of first pulmonary metastasis) of greater than 1 year fared better than those with a shorter disease free interval. The efficacy of metastasectomy has never been tested by randomized prospective study but historically controlled patients with untreated pulmonary metastases survive a median time of 12 months.

Retroperitoneal sarcoma

The lowest recurrence rates for soft tissue sarcomas are achieved by a combination of surgery with adequate clearance and sufficient radiotherapy. Retroperitoneal sarcomas, which account for about 12 per cent of all sarcomas, carry a particularly ominous prognosis. This is not because the biology of the disease at this site is any different but because wide clearance can only be achieved infrequently and because an adequate dose of radiotherapy is prohibited by tolerance of surrounding normal tissues such as gut, kidney, spinal cord, and liver. Wide excision can be achieved in about 30 per cent of patients and even then the 5 year disease-free survival is only about 30 per cent. Operability and the chances of a wide excision can be predicted from the CT scan by the site of the tumour and its proximity and relationship to surrounding structures. With the exception of the rare low-grade tumour, which is compatible with long-term survival, the prognosis of retroperitoneal sarcoma is so poor that one of the main purposes of surgery is to confirm the diagnosis and to exclude more treatable conditions such as lymphoma, metastatic teratoma, or fibromatosis. The natural history of retroperitoneal sarcoma should affect treatment decisions. For example it may not be in the best interests of an asymptomatic patient with recurrent sarcoma to undergo further surgery if the disease-free interval is, for example, shorter than 1 year and if it can be predicted from the CT scan that the recurrence is either multifocal or unlikely to be amenable to wide excision. Laparotomy may be indicated purely with palliative intent, to temporarily overcome mechanical intestinal obstruction and to debulk for comfort.

In conclusion, surgery, radiotherapy, and chemotherapy are often used in complementary fashion to palliate advanced soft tissue sarcomas and joint consultations between these disciplines is mandatory. Involvement of clinicians with expertise in pain relief and continuing care and of nursing staff with counselling skills completes this team approach.

Conclusion

Palliative cancer surgery carefully considered on an individual basis may usefully relieve symptoms and improve quality of life. It is important to treat the patient first and the cancer second. This involves a team approach covering all aspects of cancer management both in the home environment (with community care) and in hospital.

References

1. Marshall E. Experts clash over cancer data: news and comment. *Science*, 1990; **250**: 900–2.
2. Rhys Evans PH, Frame JW, Brandrick J. A review of carbon dioxide laser surgery in the oral cavity and pharynx. *Journal of Laryngology and Oncology*, 1986; **C (1)**: 69–77.
3. Lennquist S. Surgical strategy in thyroid cancer—a clinical review. *Acta Chirurgica Scandinavica*, 1986; **152**: 321–38.
4. Shaw HJ. Palliation in head and neck cancer: a discussion paper. *Journal of the Royal Society of Medicine*, 1986; **79**: 84–6.
5. Hendrickson FR. Strategy of palliative treatment. *International Journal of Radiation Oncology Biology Physics*, 1982; **8**: 155–6.
6. Van Raemdonck DE, Schneider A, Ginsberg RJ. Surgical treatment for higher-stage non-small-cell lung cancer. *Annals of Thoracic Surgery*, 1992; **54**: 999–1013.
7. Martini N, Kris MG, Flehinger BJ, Gralla RJ, Bains MS, Burt ME, Heelan R, McCormack PM, Pisters KM, Rigas JR, *et al.* Preoperative chemotherapy for stage IIIa (N2) lung cancer: the Sloan-Kettering experience with 136 patients. *Annals of Thoracic Surgery*, 1993; **55**: 1365–73.
8. Burt M, Wronski M, Arbit E, Galichich GH. Resection of brain metastasis from non-small cell lung carcinoma. *Journal of Thoracic and Cardiovascular Surgery*, 1992; **103**: 399–410.
9. Cavaliere S, Foccoli P, Farina PL. Nd-YAG laser bronchoscopy. A five-year experience with 1396 applications in 1000 patients. *Chest*, 1988; **94**: 15–21.
10. Tsang V, Goldstraw P. Endobronchial stenting for anastomotic stenosis after sleeve resection. *Annals of Thoracic Surgery*, 1989; **48**: 568–71.
11. Petrou M, Kaplan D, Goldstraw P. Bronchoscopic diathermy resection and stent insertion: a cost effective treatment for tracheobronchial obstruction. *Thorax*, 1993; **48**: 1156–9.
12. Webb WR, Ozmen V, Moulder PV, Shabahang B, Breaux J. Iodized talc pleurodesis for the treatment of pleural effusions. *Journal of Thoracic and Cardiovascular Surgery*, 1993; **103**: 881–6.
13. Petrou M, Kaplan D, Goldstraw P. The management of recurrent malignant pleural effusion: the complementary role of talc pleurodesis and pleuroperitoneal shunting. *Cancer*, 1995; **75**: 801–5.
14. Watkinson AF, Hansell DM. Expandable Wallstent for the treatment of obstruction of the superior vena cava. *Thorax*, 1993; **48**: 915–20.
15. Shah SS, Goldstraw P. *Thorax*, 1995; **50**: 782–4.
16. Ginsberg RJ, Martini N, Zaman M, Armstrong JG, Bains MS, Burt ME, McCormack PM, Rusch VW, Harrison LB. Influence of surgical resection and brachytherapy in the management of superior sulcus tumor. *Annals of Thoracic Surgery*, 1994; **57**: 1440–5.
17. Halsted WJ. The Results of radical operations for the cure of cancer of the breast. *Annals of Surgery*, 1907; **46**: 1–27.
18. Fallowfield LJ, Baum M, Maguire GP. Effects of breast conservation on

psychological morbidity associated with the diagnosis and treatment of early breast cancer. *British Medical Journal*, 1986; **293**: 1331–4.

19. Cukingnan RA, Carey JS. Carcinoma of the oesophagus. *Annals of Thoracic Surgery*, 1978; **26**: 274–85.
20. Orringer M. Transhiatal oesophagectomy without thoracotomy for carcinoma of the thoacic oesophagus. *Annals of Surgery*, 1984; **200**: 282–8.
21. Thoracic procedures. In: Cushieri A, Buesss G, Perissat J, eds. *Operative Manual of Endoscopic Surgery*. Berlin: Springer-Verlag, 1992.
22. Findlay M, Cunninham D, Norman A, Mansi J, Nicolson M, Hickish T, Nicolson V, Nash A, Sacks N, Ford H, Carter R, Hill A. A phase II study in advanced gastroeoesophageal cancer using epirubicin and cisplatin in combination with continuous infusion 5-fluorouracil (ECF). *Annals of Oncology*, 1994; **5**: 609–16.
23. Alderson D, Blazeby JM. Expanding metal stents in the gastrointestinal tract. *British Journal of Surgery*, 1995; **82**: 1441–3.
24. Smith AC, Dowsett JF, Russell RCG, Hartfield ARW, Cotton PB. Randomized trial of endocopic stenting versus surgical bypass in malignant low bile-duct obstruction. *Lancet*, 1994: **344**: 1655–60.
25. Enker WE, Laffer UT, Block GE. Enhanced survival of patients with colon and rectal cancer is based upon wide anatomic resection. *Annals of Surgery*, 1979; **190**: 350–60.
26. Butch RJ, Stark DD, Wittenberg J, Tepper JE, Saini S, Simeone JF, Mueller PR, Fernicci JT. Staging rectal cancer by MRI and CT. *American Journal of Roentgenology*, 1986; **146**: 1155–60.
27. Pahlman L, Glimelius B. Preoperative radiotherapy is better than post-operative radiotherapy in patients with colorectal cancer. *Annals of Surgery*, 1990; **211**: 187–95.
28. August DA, Ottow RT, Sugarbaker PH. Clinical perspective of human colorectal cancer metastases. *Cancer Metastasis Reviews*, 1984; **3**: 303–24.
29. Berry AR, Souter RG, Campbell WB, Mortensen NJMcC, Kettlewel MGW. Endoscopic transanal resection of rectal tumours—a preliminary report of its use. *British Journal of Surgery*, 1990; **77**: 134–7.
30. Taylor RE, Kerr GR, Arnott SJ. External beam radiotherapy for rectal adenocarcioma. *British Journal of Surgery*, 1987; **74**: 455–9.
31. Allen-Mersh TG. Improving survival after large bowel cancer—surgeons should look for the occult. *British Medical Journal*, 1991; **303**: 595–6.
32. Vetto JT, Hughes KS, Rosenstein R, Sugarbaker PH. Morbidity and mortality of hepatic resection for metastatic colorectal carcinoma. *Diseases of the Colon and Rectum*, 1990; **33**: 408–13.
33. Ekberg H, Tranberg KG, Andersson R, Landstedt C, Hagerstrand I, Ranstam J, Bengmark S. Determinants of survival in liver resection for colorectal secondaries. *British Journal of Surgery*, 1986; **73**: 727–31.
34. Advanced colorectal cancer metaanalysis project. Modulation of fluorouracil in patients with advanced colorectal cancer; evidence in terms of response rate. *Journal of Clinical Oncology*, 1992; **10**: 896–903.
35. Allen-Mersh TG, Earlam S, Fordy S, Abrams K, Houghton J. Quality of life and survival with continuous hepatic artery floxuridine infusion for colorectal liver metastases. *Lancet*, 1994; **344**: 1255–60.
36. Nordic Gastrointestinal Tumour Adjuvant Therapy Group. Expectancy or primary chemotherapy in patients with advanced asymptomatic colorectal cancer—a randomised trial. *Journal of Clinical Oncology*, 1992; **10**: 904–11.
37. Allen-Mersh TG. Improving palliation for patients with gastrointestinal cancer. For debate. *British Journal of Surgery*, 1994; **81**: 86.
38. Peeling WB. Stage 3 studies to compare busrelin with orchidectomy and with methylstilboestrol in the treatment of prostrate cancer. *Urology*, 1989; **33** (Suppl): 45.
39. Crowther ME, Britton KE, Granowska M, Shepherd JH, Monoclonal antibodies and their usefulness in epithelial ovarian cancer. A Review. *British Journal of Obstetrics and Gynaecology*, 1989; **96**: 516–21.
40. Ward BG, Malther S, Shepherd JH, Crowther M, Hawkins LA, Britton K, Slevin M. The treatment of interperitoneal malignant disease with monoclonal antibody guided 131–1-radiotherapy. *British Journal of Cancer*, 1988; **58**: 658–62.

9.2 Management of pain

9.2.1 Pathophysiology of pain in cancer and other terminal diseases

Richard Payne and Gilbert R. Gonzales

Pathophysiology of pain: inferences from clinical syndromes

Recent advances in the understanding of fundamental neurobiological mechanisms of nociception have provided insights into the evaluation and treatment of clinical pain.[1] Pain caused by cancer and other medical illnesses may be caused by direct effects of the disease (e.g. tumour infiltration of pain sensitive structures in cancer, infarction of tissue in sickle cell anaemia) or by the treatment associated with the disease which injures visceral, musculoskeletal, and nervous tissues. For example surgery, chemotherapy, and radiation therapy which are necessary to treat cancer are all associated with potentially painful sequelae.[2]

Acute pain serves the purpose of alerting the organism to the presence of harmful (or potentially harmful) stimuli in the internal or external environment. Acute pain may be repetitive in circumstances in which recurrent and/or progressive tissue injury is experienced. This is typically the case when pain accompanies medical disorders such as cancer, sickle cell disease, haemophilia, multiple sclerosis, etc. Although these conditions cause pain extended over a period of time, and are often referred to as chronically painful conditions, they should be distinguished from the chronic 'pain state'. The latter term is usually used in the context of patients who report pain on a long-term basis, with no apparent tissue injury component or at least no apparent evidence of persistent nociceptor activation. Pain in this setting serves no known useful biological purpose. The psychological counterparts to the chronic pain state include depression, anxiety, and other affective states, and are key to understanding the disability associated with this condition.[3]

It is therefore important to recognize that chronic pain is not merely a temporal extension of acute pain. New data emerging from studies evaluating the central modulation of nociception, indicate that a major distinction between acute and chronic pain may be found in the differences in central neural responses induced by the chronic afferent neural impulses of nociceptor activity.[3] Changes in central neural processing induced by these impulses activate *N*-methyl-D-aspartate (**NMDA**) receptors, and other biochemical and physiological processes, which may allow a persistent pain sensation to occur in the presence of diminishing nociceptive activity, or even in the absence of such activity (see below).

Much recent experimental evidence suggests that acute persistent pain (such as that induced by experimental arthritis production in animals) may promote biochemical, physiological, and pharmacological changes in the peripheral and central nervous systems which may promote the continuation of pain.[4] These data are detailed in the sections below dealing with inflammatory and neuropathic pain models. Although acute pain may be associated with profound psychological reactions such as anxiety and fear, and may also be accompanied by activation of the sympathetic nervous system, many of these physiological and psychological reactions become habituated as pain persists. Adaptation of sympathetic activity and the development of chronic vegetative signs, including a decrease in appetite, malaise, sleep disturbances, and irritability, characterize chronic pain.

Traditionally, the cancer patient has served as a model for acute and chronic pain in man, and several broad 'physiological' types of pain have been distinguished: somatic, visceral, and neuropathic, and perhaps even sympathetically-maintained pain. Somatic or nociceptive pain occurs as a result of activation of nociceptors in cutaneous and deep musculoskeletal tissues. This pain is typically well localized and may be felt in superficial cutaneous or deeper musculoskeletal structures. Examples of somatic pain include bone metastasis, postsurgical incisional pain, and pain accompanying myofascial or musculoskeletal inflammation or spasm (Table 1).

Table 1 'Physiological' pain categories

Type of pain	Examples	Putative mechanisms
Nociceptive	Arthritis; fracture; bone metastasis; cellulitis	Activation of nociceptors
Visceral	Pancreatitis; peptic ulcer; myocardial infarction	Activation of nociceptors
Neuropathic	Herpes zoster; diabetic neuropathy; post-stroke pain; trigeminal neuralgia	Ectopic discharges within nervous system; spontaneous activity in nerves; neuroma formation; others
Complex regional pain syndromes[a]	Persistent focal pain following trauma with or without evidence of sympathetic involvement	Sensitization of spinal neurones; ephaptic transmission; others

[a] See Stanton-Hicks *et al.*, 1995, ref. 12

Visceral pain is also common in the cancer patient and results from infiltration, compression, distension, or stretching of thoracic and abdominal viscera (e.g. liver metastasis and pancreatic cancer). This type of pain is poorly localized, often described as 'deep, squeezing' and 'pressure' and may be associated with nausea, vomiting, and diaphoresis, particularly when acute. Visceral pain is often referred to cutaneous sites which may be remote from the site of the lesion (e.g. shoulder pain with diaphragmatic irritation). Tenderness and pain on touching the referred cutaneous site may occur.[5]

Neuropathic pain results from injury to the peripheral and/or central nervous systems.[6] Pain resulting from lesions to the peripheral nerves (especially those which are traumatic in origin and which partially or completely interrupt afferent sensory transmission between the peripheral and central nervous systems) has sometimes been termed 'deafferentation' pain. Pain resulting from injury to the spinal cord or brain, especially pain complicating strokes, is usually termed 'central pain'. The terms 'deafferentation' and 'central' pain are forms of neuropathic pain and are often used to denote pain following injury or dysfunction to peripheral or central neural structures respectively.

In the cancer patient, neuropathic pain most commonly occurs as a consequence of tumour compression or infiltration of peripheral nerves, nerve roots, or the spinal cord. In addition surgical trauma, chemical, or radiation-induced injury to peripheral nerves or the spinal cord from cancer therapies may also result in this type of pain. Examples of common neuropathic pains include metastatic or radiation-induced brachial or lumbosacral plexopathies, epidural spinal cord and/or cauda equina compression, postherpetic neuralgia, and painful vincristine, cisplatin, or placitaxel neuropathy. Pain resulting from neural injury is often severe and is different in quality as compared to somatic or visceral pain. It is typically described as a constant dull ache, often with a pressure or 'vice-like' quality; superimposed paroxysms of burning and/or electrical shock-like sensations are common. These paroxysms of pain may be associated with spontaneous and ectopic activity in the peripheral[7] and central nervous systems.[8]

Although much is now known about the biochemical and neurophysiological processes associated with activation of nociceptors, a complete understanding of the pathophysiology of pain in specific patients is seldom possible. Although different physiological mechanisms of pain frequently coexist in patients with advanced cancer and other chronic medical illnesses, their recognition often has direct diagnostic and therapeutic implications.[1] This is particularly true for neuropathic pain. For example the presence of paroxysmal or lancinating pain may indicate the appearance of spontaneous action potential propagation, and usually leads the clinician to suspect a neuropathic aetiology, even in the absence of compelling evidence for neural injury. Anticonvulsant medications which inhibit these discharges (such as phenytoin, carbamazepine, valproic acid, gabapentin, or clonazepam) may successfully manage this lancinating pain when traditional analgesics such as opioids or non-steroidal anti-inflammatory analgesics have failed. On the other hand, continuous burning dysaesthetic pains which commonly accompany toxic metabolic polyneuropathies (e.g. diabetic neuropathy) may respond better to tricyclic antidepressants than to either anticonvulsants or opioids. Although the mechanisms by which the dysaesthesias are generated are not well understood, the clinician can make important treatment decisions based on the quality of the pain, which is likely to reflect differences in the pathophysiology of different forms of neuropathic pain.

Injury to nervous tissue may activate nociceptive systems and produce pain without stimulating nociceptors. Pain which occurs as a result of neurological injury is often qualitatively different from somatic or visceral pain, which results from activation of nociceptors in the setting of a normal nervous system. Given the different mechanisms and quality of neuropathic pain, it is not surprising that this pain may respond to drugs such as anticonvulsants, which are not useful in somatic or visceral pain.

The sympathetic nervous system may be involved in these pain states (particularly acute visceral and neuropathic pain), although its role is poorly understood.[9] Evidence for the involvement of the sympathetic nervous system in pain include:

(1) the improvement of some forms of pain with sympathetic nerve blocks or with adrenergic blocking drugs such as propranolol and phenoxybenzamine;

(2) increase in pain with sympathetic stimulation in some patients with causalgia and other reflex sympathetic dystrophies;

(3) animal studies of peripheral nerve injury which show the development of new α-adrenergic receptors and the sensitivity of regenerating nerve sprouts to systemic or locally applied catecholamines and sympathetic nerve blocks.[10]

However, the primary role of the sympathetic nervous system in chronic pain states has been challenged recently.[11] A recent review of this subject suggested that a new term, 'complex regional pain syndrome' be used rather than 'reflex sympathetic dystrophy' or 'sympathetically-maintained pain' to avoid any inferences regarding mechanisms of sympathetic involvement in these pain states that are not conclusively determined.[12]

Nociceptors and peripheral nerve physiology

Sensory receptors that are preferentially sensitive to noxious (tissue damaging) or potentially noxious stimuli are prevalent in skin, bone, muscle, connective tissues, thoracic, abdominal, and pelvic viscera.[13] The free nerve endings which transduce these noxious stimuli conduct electrical discharges to the spinal cord utilizing two types of nerve fibres, Aδ- and C-fibres. Aδ-fibres are thinly myelinated, about 2.5 μm thick, and conduct action potentials at a rate of 5 m/s or less. Activation of these fibres by electrical stimulation is typically associated with sharp, stinging painful sensations. C-fibres are unmyelinated, about 0.3 μm thick, and conduct action potentials at a rate of 2 m/s or less. Patterns of electrical activity in C-fibres evoked by noxious stimuli are often associated with vaguely localized pain of a 'dull' and 'burning' quality. In human cutaneous peripheral nerves 10 per cent of all myelinated fibres carry nociceptive information, and more than 90 per cent of all unmyelinated fibres are nociceptive (Figs 1 and 2).[14]

Cutaneous nociceptors and hyperalgesia

Cutaneous nociceptors are defined morphologically by their appearance in light and electron microscopy, and physiologically by

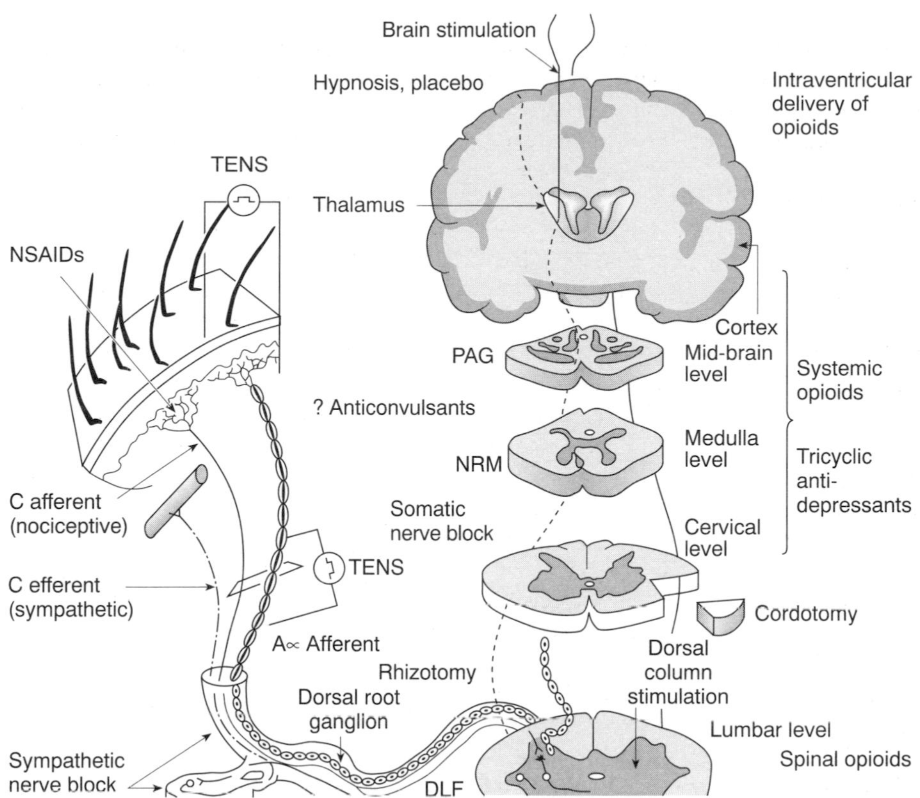

Fig. 1 Diagram of ascending and descending neural pathways involved in nociception.

their patterns of response to mechanical, thermal, and chemical cutaneous stimuli.[15] On this basis, nociceptors have been classified as Aδ mechanical nociceptors, C-polymodal nociceptors, and silent or sleeping nociceptors, the latter being discovered only recently.[16] The silent nociceptor is mechanically insensitive and is only active when tissue is injured. Several research strategies have been used to correlate verbal reports of pain with patterns of electrical activity in these units. For example one can correlate pain responses to laser heat applied to human skin (in which nerve fibre activity cannot be measured easily) with recordings from afferent C-fibres in the primate stimulated by the identical stimulus.[17] Using this paradigm, it has been demonstrated that human judgements of pain following a brief laser burn injury to the skin (i.e. defined as primary hyperalgesia) were most closely matched by increased responses in Aδ rather than C-afferent fibres. This demonstrates that burning pain and hyperpathia are not exclusively mediated by unmyelinated C-fibre units as had been previously thought (Fig. 3).[17]

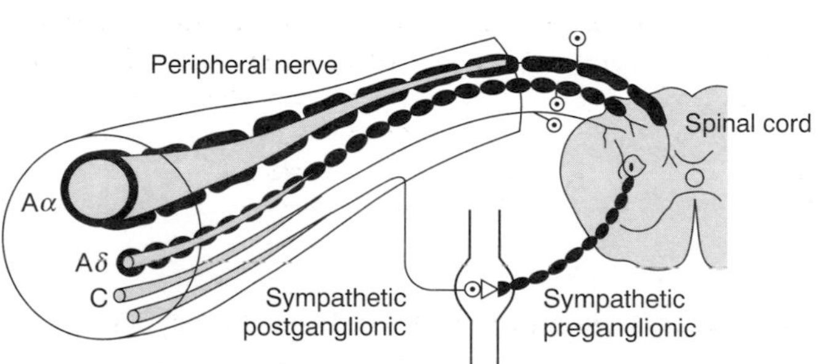

Fig. 2 Diagram of peripheral nerve mosaic 'cables'.

Another strategy used to investigate more directly the relationship between peripheral nerve activity in man and unpleasant or painful sensations involves the use of microneurography.[18] This technique allows the stimulation and recording from single afferent or efferent fibres in peripheral nerves of conscious patients or volunteers, and also allows the correlation of electrical activity in afferent nociceptive fibres with verbal reports of pain. Microneurographic techniques have shown that activation of a single myelinated nociceptor is sufficient to cause pain, and direct electrical stimulation of unmyelinated nociceptors to discharge frequencies greater than 1.5/s is associated with a dull, burning, or aching pain.[14] Microneurographic recordings have confirmed that positive symptoms and signs of peripheral nerve disease such as Tinel's sign, Lhermitte's symptom, or positive straight leg raising in S1 root compression are associated with spontaneous activity in peripheral nerves. Paraesthesias are represented by ectopic paroxysmal activity and high frequency (>220 Hz) discharges in peripheral nerves as observed in microneurographic recordings.[19]

Nociceptors are not spontaneously active but may show sensitization, particularly after thermal injury to the skin.[17] Sensitization is manifested as:

(1) decreased threshold of activation after injury;

(2) increased intensity of a response to a noxious injury;

(3) the emergence of spontaneous activity.

Sensitization of nociceptors may occur within minutes after a thermal injury and may last for hours. Sensitization of nociceptors produces the clinical phenomenon of hyperalgesia, defined as an increased response to a stimulus that is normally painful.

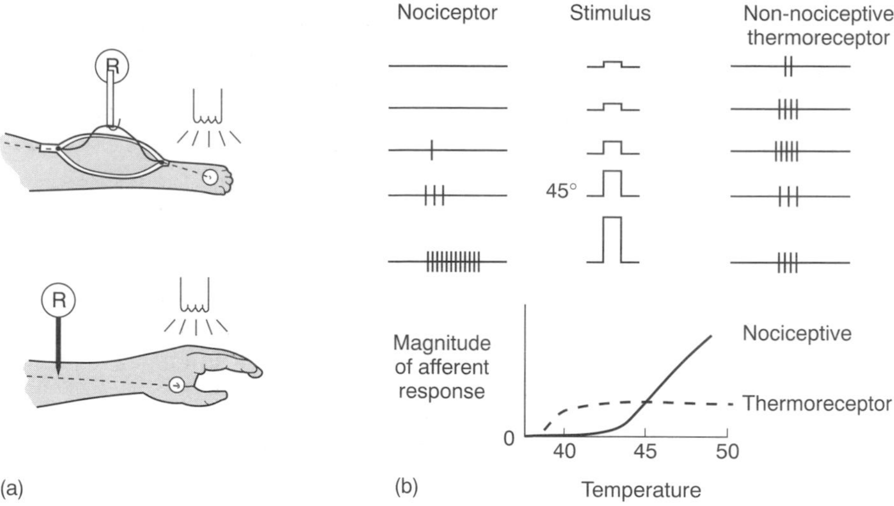

Fig. 3 Graph of a nociceptor versus a simple thermoreceptor.

Sensitization of nociceptors may be mediated by efferent sympathetic activity (see below) as well as by chemical substances which are liberated by tissue injury and inflammation—potassium, adenosine triphosphate, bradykinin and prostaglandins, tachykinins, and other peptides.[20],[21]

Nociceptor sensitization is the physiological correlate of primary hyperalgesia which occurs after tissue injury, and is a mechanism of persistent pain in man. Secondary hyperalgesia results from central nervous system changes induced by tissue injury and nociceptor sensitization. The clinical expression of secondary hyperalgesia includes expansion of the zone of cutaneous hyperalgesia outside of the area of initial injury. This phenomenon is caused by hyperexcitability or 'central sensitization' of the second-order neurones in the spinal cord, upon which the nociceptive afferents terminate. Central sensitization is mediated by a complex set of biochemical and physiological events in which NMDA receptors play an important role.[22]

Central sensitization is dependent on NMDA receptor activation.[22] The amino acid glutamate binds postsynaptically to the NMDA receptor. When coupled with glutamate, the NMDA receptor is activated and functions as a divalent cation channel regulator, admitting Ca^{2+} and Mg^{2+} cations into the cell. Glutamate and NMDA receptors are found in high concentration in the dorsal horn of the spinal cord. Glutamate depolarizes spinal cord neurones when applied iontophoretically and is known to be released from spinal cord preparations following electrical stimulation or noxious chemical stimulation *in vivo*. Blockade of NMDA receptors by drugs such as ketamine, dextrophan, phencyclidine, and MK-801 reduces windup (e.g. progressive increase in the number of spikes evoked by a single stimulus in response to repeated stimulation of peripheral C-fibres) to C-fibre stimulation, and can also prevent or terminate central sensitization once it has begun. Spinal administration of non-steroidal anti-inflammatory drugs block the hyperalgesia produced by formalin injection into the hind paw in animal models of pain, indicating that prostaglandins are important to the central as well as peripheral anti-inflammatory actions of this group of analgesics.[23]

A second type of excitatory amino acid receptor, α-amino-3-hydroxy-5-methyl-4-isoxazoleproprionic acid (**AMPA**), has also been implicated in analgesia. This receptor admits Na^+ and K^+ when activated; blockade of AMPA receptors by selective antagonists such as CNQX (cyano-7-nitroquinoxaline-2,3-dione) appears to be antinociceptive in animals. Thus, pharmacological agents which are very selective antagonists at NMDA and AMPA receptors hold great promise for future development as analgesics.

Synthesis of a great body of recent work on central nervous system modulation of nociception has shown that the NMDA receptor modulation has many clinical implications. It is apparent that several pre- and postsynaptic systems converge to provide a complex network of interactions that may contribute to the persistence of pain, even in the absence of ongoing nociceptive stimulation. Better understanding of these systems has major implications for:

(1) explaining the persistent or chronic pain in the absence of ongoing nociception;

(2) new opportunities for analgesic drug development;

(3) opportunities for pre-emptive analgesia to prevent hyperalgesia and chronic pain.

The synthesis of nitric oxide, a gaseous neurotransmitter, is accomplished by activation of the enzyme nitrous oxide synthetase. This enzyme is activated by Ca^{2+}; the calcium gains access to the cell via activation of A receptors, which is a calcium channel ionophore. Nitric oxide is an excitatory neurotransmitter, and as a gas can diffuse across the synaptic cleft to induce retrograde effects such as release of glutamate and other neurotransmitters. It also appears to interact with adjacent neurones and glia. Thus, the synthesis of nitric oxide has important, widespread ramifications (Fig. 4).[24,25]

Visceral and bone nociceptors and deep pain

Bone pain from metastatic disease is perhaps they most common cause of pain in advanced cancer. Tumour metastasis to bone is associated with bone destruction and new bone formation and prostaglandins are important in this.[26] Myelinated and

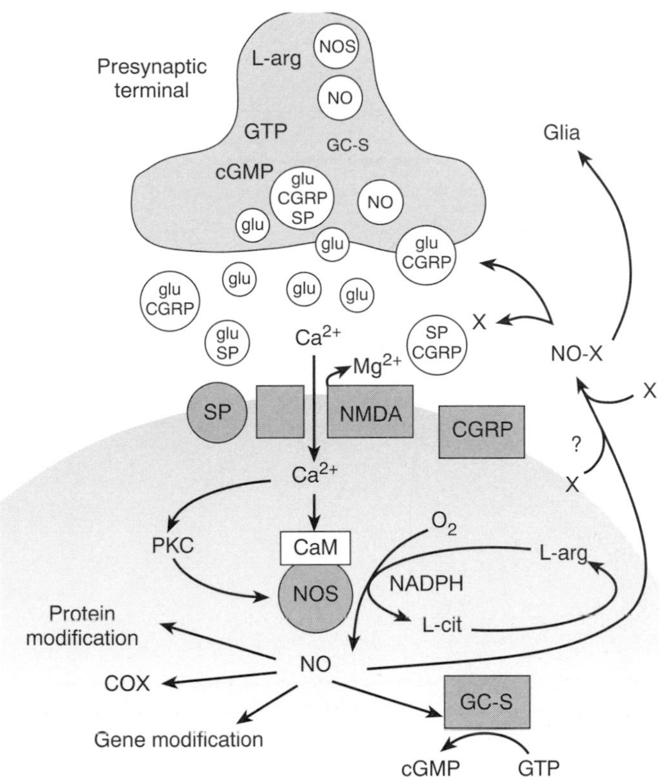

Fig. 4 Pre- and postsynaptic mechanisms of NMDA and nitric oxide systems.

unmyelinated afferent fibres exist in bone and are in highest density in the periosteum; prostaglandins E_1 and E_2 are known to sensitize nociceptors and produce hyperalgesia.[27]

Deep pain originating from bone and visceral structures in the thoracic, abdominal, and pelvic cavities is, in fact, more common than cutaneous pain. Although much less well studied than their cutaneous counterparts, muscle and visceral nociceptors do exist in almost all organs studied thus far and appear to have different physiological properties than do cutaneous nociceptors, including the property of referred pain.[5] When normal human viscera are cut or otherwise manipulated, pain is usually not elicited—thus, unlike their cutaneous counterparts, visceral nociceptors appear to have a different function for the organism than as a simple 'acute warning system' for the presence of harmful tissue damaging stimuli. The types of stimuli which are sufficient to cause visceral pain include such things as chemical or mechanical irritation of the mucosal and serosal surfaces or torsion, traction, and distension of the mesentery or a hollow viscus. It has been emphasized recently that visceral nociceptors have a wide range of responsiveness, and so-called 'silent' nociceptors may be recruited in the presence of inflammation.[5]

Visceral pain has a deep (rather than superficial) and aching quality, is poorly localized, and often referred to a cutaneous point (which may be tender). Common examples of referred pain in cancer patients include back pain and paraspinal muscle tenderness which occurs with pancreatic and endometrial cancer, right shoulder pain which occurs with hepatoma or liver metastasis, and abdominal or leg pain, occurring in prostatic cancer. The mechanism of referred pain is not fully understood, but may be related to convergence of cutaneous and visceral sensory input onto common spinothalamic tract cells in the spinal cord.[28] It is hypothesized that pain is referred to the skin because the brain 'misinterprets' the source of the input, since cutaneous non-nociceptive afferent stimulation is so common. Another explanation for referred pain is that some afferent fibres innervate both somatic and visceral structures, thus activation of visceral nociceptors would cause antidromic activation of cutaneous sensory fibres and could release algesic substances to excite cutaneous nociceptors. Also many spinothalamic tract cells in the thalamus receive convergent input from skin, muscle, viscera, or all three—these cells may also contribute to the phenomenon of referred pain. There is evidence for all of these mechanisms for referred pain.[28]

Inflammatory pain models

Nociceptors exist in periarticular joint surfaces and much recent work has reported on the time course and physiology of the response of these nociceptors to experimentally-induced arthritis. The inflammatory reaction is often induced by direct injection of Freund's adjuvant or another immunogen (i.e. carrageenan, yeast extract, formalin, etc.) into a joint or foot pad, and is associated with pain-related behaviours (e.g. limping, guarding of the limb, circling, etc.) in the animal. As discussed below, inflammation also exposes opioid receptors on peripheral nerves and causes the migration of immune cells which have opioid receptors on their surface.

These inflammatory pain models thus offer an alternative to the more traditional, static and acute models (e.g. tail flick) that are dependent on reflex spinal activity rather than more highly organized animal behaviours, and thus allow one to study pain states which may more closely reproduce human conditions. For example the ability to produce persistent pain states in animals using inflammatory models has demonstrated that peripheral noxious stimulation could induce gene expression in central nervous system neurons.[29] Thus, it has been demonstrated that unilateral inflammatory pain may induce expression of a proto-oncogene resulting in opioid gene expression for dynorphin ipsilateral to the side of the inflammatory lesion.[30] In addition, the proto-oncogene *c-fos* mRNA may act as a messenger molecule in signal transduction systems of preproencephalin and preprodynorphin, which then may regulate the production of the endogenous opioids methionine and leucine encephalin and dynorphin in response to noxious stimuli.[31] Exogenously administered opioids are also known to influence the regulation and expression of opioid peptide gene expression.[32] These experimental techniques allow activated cells to be identified and potentially targeted for pharmacological manipulation to control pain.

Cytokines produced by immune cells are potent activators of nociceptors.[77] Current concepts of the function of the immune system emphasize its importance as a 'diffuse sensory organ', signalling important information to the brain about events, particularly inflammatory events, in the periphery. (Fig. 5). Injury to the skin and inflammatory changes cause the elaboration of many cytokines, particularly tumour necrosis factor and interleukin 1 (**IL-1**) and 6 (**IL-6**), which are released from mast cells, keratinocytes, fibroblasts, and macrophages. IL-1 binds to the peripheral nerve causing release of substance P, which initiates a positive feedback loop because substance P can stimulate the release of these cytokines from immune cells. This process produces hyperalgesia

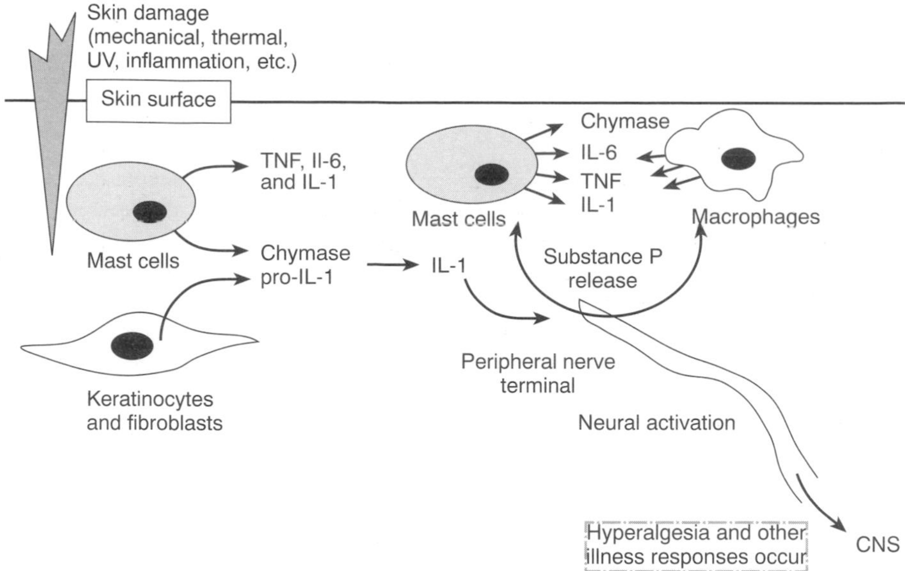

Fig. 5 Cartoon illustrating the interaction of cytokines and nociceptors.

that can be diffuse in its distribution, even though the pathological process may have been initiated from a very focal injury. These phenomena have obvious clinical relevance. For example specific antagonists of IL-1 have been shown to block hyperalgesia in the rat,[77] thereby pointing to the possibilities of new analgesic agents.

Peripheral opioid effects

It is now apparent that opioids have peripheral antinociceptive and anti-inflammatory effects.[33] Peripheral opioid receptors of the μ (morphine-preferring), δ (encephalin-preferring), and κ (dynorphin-preferring) subtypes appear to be located on primary afferents, especially C-fibre afferents. One can demonstrate antinociceptive effects of opioids which are administered topically to peripheral tissues at sites of inflammation and the excitability of the afferent fibre is reduced. The release of substance P is also inhibited.[34]

Peripheral opioid effects can be observed within minutes of an inflammatory response but are not observed in the absence of inflammation.[35] The relatively brief time course needed for expression of peripheral analgesic effects and binding studies suggest that these opioid receptors are pre-existing on peripheral nerves and are not dependent on *de novo* synthesis. It appears that inflammation may disrupt the perineurium and expose the receptors.[36]

Several human studies have demonstrated analgesia to intra-articular injection of morphine for the treatment of postoperative pain.[37] In fact, intra-articular injection is more effective than perineural injection of morphine. The observation that opioid receptors are transported from the cell body in the dorsal root ganglion down the peripheral nerve axon to the terminal during inflammatory injury may explain this observation, since axonal receptors appear to be in transit and probably less functional.[35]

Opioid receptors are also present on immunocompetent cells which migrate to inflamed tissue.[38] Local application of opioids which are polar and which do not cross the blood–brain barrier would be advantageous in order to avoid adverse central nervous system effects such as sedation, nausea, respiratory depression, and mental clouding, and require direct investigation in inflammatory pain states in man.

Animal models of neuropathic pain

Several models of neuropathic pain have been described.[39–42] These models have been helpful in dissection of the physiological and pharmacological mechanisms of neuropathic pain. The chronic constriction model of Bennett and Xie is of particular interest because it produces unilateral spontaneous pain within 4 days of tying a loose ligature around the rat sciatic nerve. In addition to pain behaviours which are inferred by the guarding of the extremity, hyperalgesia, and allodynia to sensory testing, a temperature abnormality in the nerve-injured limb also occurs. Thus, this animal model of neuropathic pain appears to mimic many important clinical findings that are seen in peripheral nerve injury in man. Recent quantitative neuropathological analysis of the nerve injury indicates that, initially, oedema produces a four fold increase in the fasicular area; later, myelinated fibres are decreased to less than 0.5 per cent of their control values by day 14 after injury.[43] Unmyelinated fibres decrease in the first 5 days, but increase thereafter secondary to nerve fibre sprouting. Macrophage invasion occurs over time. It appears that Wallerian degeneration and macrophage activation are important peripheral components of hyperalgesia.

Although peripheral nerve injuries can be produced and quantified in these animal models, it is apparent that there are important changes occurring in the central nervous system as a consequence of the nerve lesions, and the ubiquitous NMDA receptors and the excitatory amino acid glutamate have been implicated in these changes. For example one can demonstrate the presence of 'dark neurones' in the spinal cords ipsilateral to nerve injury, which are thought to be caused by NMDA-mediated excitatoxicity.[44] Blockade of NMDA receptors may reduce this cytotoxicity by decreasing spontaneous discharges in the peripheral nerve following the injury.[45] In addition, the thermal hyperalgesia that occurs after the nerve injury is mediated by nitric oxide.[46]

Dorsal horn circuitry and the spinothalamic tracts

Afferent fibres from nociceptors enter the spinal cord laterally in the dorsal root and ascend or descend one to two segments in Lissauer's tract to synapse in the dorsal horn. The dorsal horn consists of six laminas with lamina I, the marginal zone, being the most dorsal. Lamina II and III together comprise the substantial gelatinosa, which is an important site of integration of nociceptive and non-nociceptive input into the spinal cord (Fig. 6).[47] However, as many as 30 per cent of afferent fibres are also known to enter through the ventral root; this is an explanation for the failure of dorsal rhizotomy to relieve pain permanently.[48]

Dorsal horn neurones receiving input from primary afferent fibres can have two types of responses: (1) nociceptive-specific, and (2) wide dynamic range (Fig. 7).[13] Similar responses can also be observed in thalamic and cortical cells receiving projections from the spinothalamic tract. Both types of neuronal responses appear important in pain perception. The wide dynamic range neurone responds to innocuous and noxious stimuli of many types and increases its firing pattern in proportion to the intensity of the stimulus. These neurones probably provide the central nervous system with information relative to the quality of the perceived painful stimulus. The nociceptive-specific neurone responds only to intense noxious stimulation; they probably signal the central nervous system with respect to the presence or absence of tissue damaging stimuli. The dorsal horn is the site of much of the modulation of the nociceptive stimulus mediated by opioid, NMDA, and nitric oxide mechanisms discussed above.

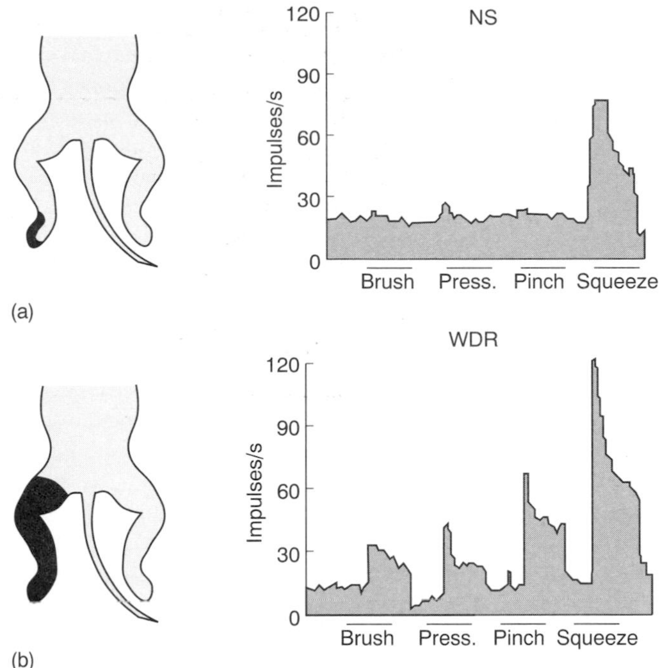

Fig. 7 Wide dynamic range versus nociceptive-specific neurones.

Spinothalamic tracts and other ascending nociceptive systems

Axons from lamina I and V neurones decussate in the central grey of the spinal cord and become the ascending projections of the neo- and paleospinothalamic tracts. The spinothalamic tract is located in the anterolateral segment of the spinal cord, and is a composite of two ascending systems—the neospinothalamic tract and the paleo-spinothalamic tracts. The neospinothalamic tract has a large component of myelinated nociceptive fibres (Aδ) which project monosynaptically to the ventroposterolateral nucleus of the thalamus. These fibres subserve the functions of stimulus localization and pain intensity. C-fibre activity is transmitted in the paleospinothalamic tract with projections branching off to the brainstem reticular formation and to the medial regions of the thalamus before their ultimate termination in ventroposterolateral nucleus. Recently a distinct nucleus in the posterior thalamus in the brains of monkey and humans, has been identified which receives topographic projections from spinothalamic tract neurones in lamina I.[49] This posterior nucleus appears to be a specific thalamic nucleus for pain and temperature sensation. The ventrobasilar complex (ventroposterolateral nucleus, ventroposteromedial thalamic nucleus) axons project to the parietal somatosensory cortex. The medial thalamic nuclear group projects to the striatum and cerebral cortex.

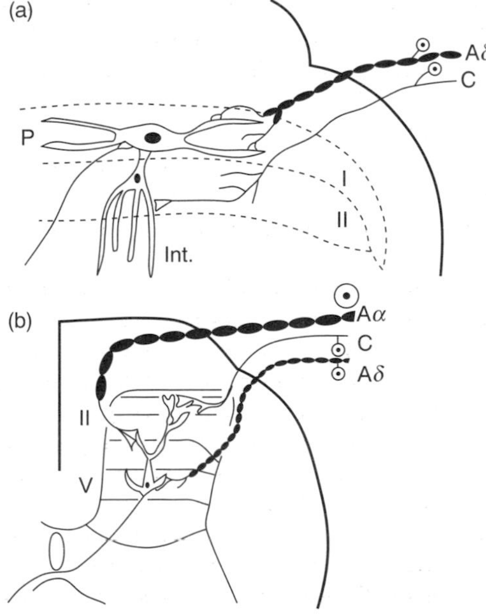

Fig. 6 Dorsal horn circuitry.

Several other ascending spinal tracts have been identified including the spinohypothalamic tract, spinoreticular tract, spinopontoamygdala tract, and the dorsal column tract.[50] The spinoreticular tract, which projects to the brainstem reticular formation, and the spinocervicothalamic tract ascend in the ipsilateral dorsolateral quadrant and travel with the spinothalamic tract in the medial lemniscus. Dorsal column fibres transmit both proprioceptive and nociceptive information and ascend in the ipsilateral medial lemniscus to the thalamus.[51] In fact, recent neurophysiological and neuroanatomical studies also indicate a convergence of somatic and visceral afferent information in this tract.[78] The multiple ascending non-spinothalamic tracts may be responsible for the recurrence of painful symptoms following ablative procedures such as cordotomy.

The composition of the spinothalamic tracts suggests functional diversity.[52] The neospinothalamic tract probably subserves the sensory–discriminatory aspects of pain perception (stimulus localization and intensity). The phylogenetically older paleospinothalamic tract appears to subserve the arousal, emotional, and affective/suffering components of pain. In addition to receiving inputs from the paleospinothalamic tracts, the intralaminar nuclear complex of the thalamus also receives afferents from the cerebellum and projects efferent fibres to the striatum. This suggests that this system is also important in mediating the inevitable reflex withdrawal responses that accompany the reaction to unexpected painful stimuli.[11]

The trigeminal subnucleus caudalis (spinal trigeminal nucleus) and adjacent reticular formation are the equivalent of the spinal dorsal horn, and modulate nociceptive information entering the nervous system from head and neck structures. This nucleus has a similar laminar structure and afferent synaptic connections as the spinal dorsal horn. Descending fibres in the spinal trigeminal tract convey pain, thermal, and tactile information from the ipsilateral face, forehead, and mucous membranes of the nose and mouth. The spinal trigeminal nucleus appears to be the only part of the trigeminal complex uniquely concerned with pain and thermal sensation. It has a laminated structure and neurones within laminas I and V and the adjacent reticular formation encodes nociceptive information in the same manner as do spinal dorsal horn neurones. Second-order neurones cross to the other side of the brainstem and ascend in the contralateral medial leminiscus, eventually terminating in the ventroposteromedial thalamic nucleus.[11]

Cerebral cortex and pain

Lesions of the cerebral cortex which are large and destroy the somatosensory area have been reported to produce minimal or no pain, while small and highly localized cortical lesions outside of this area can be associated with increased pain perception. Clinically, it is clear that cortical lesions can produce central pain and cortical stimulation rarely has been demonstrated to produce pain.[53] The primary somatosensory cortex receives projections from ventroposterolateral and ventroposteromedial thalamic nuclei—areas which receive heavy input from nociceptive systems. A syndrome of 'asymbolia for pain' has been described which is associated with lesions of the insular cortex.[54] These patients have normal thresholds to experimental cutaneous pain stimuli contralateral to the insular lesion, but do not generate emotional responses to the stimuli and appear not to perceive the stimuli as noxious.

A lesion anywhere in the first-, second-, or third-order neurones of the spinothalamic and thalamocortical projections may result in central pain symptoms. Thus, lesions affecting the spinal cord, brainstem, and cortex may impact on critical thalamic functions to induce central pain.[55] For example a recent report of a central pain complicating a toxoplasmosis abscess in the internal capsule and thalamus indicates the range of pathologies that can cause this syndrome.[56] However, mass lesions such as primary or metastatic tumours involving the brainstem, thalamus, and cortex only very rarely produce pain of this type. Brain tumours may be associated with headache when accompanied by increased intracranial pressure, but this is not considered to be central pain. Hypoalgesia (i.e. reduced appreciation of painful stimuli such as pinprick) is a common accompaniment of central pain, and in the case of ischaemic thalamic injury decreased temperature sensation of the affected area is an almost invariable accompaniment.[55]

The loss of inhibitory influences on excitatory pathways has been proposed to be the mechanism for the initiation of central pain. Lhermitte proposed that the thalamus acts as a gating mechanism on sensory fibres along the route to the cortex.[57] Electrophysiological studies in animal models suggest that removal of inhibition exerted by the neospinothalamic system (lateral thalamus) on the paleospinothalamic system (medial thalamus) might be important in the aetiology of some cases of central pain.[55] Although the lateral thalamus is often destroyed in cases of thalamic pain, it is difficult to assign a single thalamic structure as the only centre for initiation of all cases of central pain.

Endogenous pain suppression pathways and the neuropharmacology of nociception

Neuroanatomical pathways which arise in the brainstem and descend to the spinal cord function to modulate activity in the ascending nociceptive pathways (Fig. 1).[58] One such pathway begins in the periaqueductal grey of the midbrain and descends to the nucleus raphe magnus in the medulla. From the nucleus raphe magnus there is a projection to the dorsal horn of the spinal cord via the dorsal longitudinal fasciculus. This pathway terminates in laminas I, II, and IV of the spinal cord to modulate afferent nociceptive impulses. A second, more laterally placed descending pathway, starting in the nucleus reticularis paragigantocellularis in the pons, projects to the dorsal horn via the dorsal longitudinal fasciculus. Electrical stimulation or microinjection of morphine into these brainstem and/or spinal cord sites produces analgesia in the absence of motor, sensory, or autonomic blockade.

Serotonin and noradrenaline are putative neurotransmitters in these brainstem endogenous pain suppression pathways in animals and man, and drugs which affect their pharmacological actions may have analgesic activity. For example tricyclic antidepressant compounds, such as amitriptyline, block the presynaptic uptake of both chemicals, thus augmenting their postsynaptic actions in the descending pain suppression pathways. The actions of both noradrenaline and serotonin appear to be important for analgesia, since antagonists of these amines partially block analgesia.[59] However, noradrenaline appears to be the more important of the two neurotransmitters in the mediation of analgesia because relative 'pure' serotonin reuptake inhibitors, such as zimelidine, appear not to be as effective as amitriptyline,[60] and relatively 'pure' noradrenaline reuptake blocks such as desipramine have demonstrated analgesic actions in randomized controlled clinical trials in postherpetic neuralgia.[61] Drugs such as clonidine, which are α_2-agonists at adrenergic receptors in the spinal cord, produce analgesia when delivered directly into the spinal epidural space.[62]

Amitriptyline has analgesic properties independent of its antidepressant effects and has been used for the management of many painful conditions, including postherpetic neuralgia and painful diabetic neuropathy. Amitriptyline may also augment the effects of morphine analgesia in animals.[63] It is postulated that activation of these descending systems by opioid medications, such as morphine,

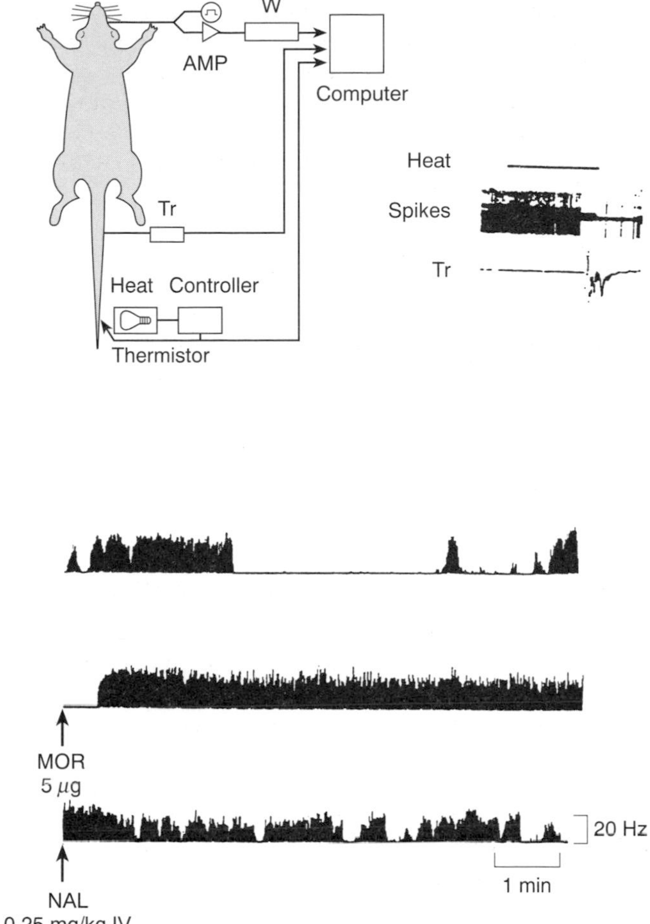

Fig. 8 On–off cells and morphine analgesia.

or by endogenous substances, such as serotonin, methionine and leucine encephalin, or dynorphin, leads to the release of putative neurotransmitter agents such as serotonin which then modulate the activity of ascending spinothalamic pathways. For example it has been reported recently that an important action of morphine is to activate 'off cells' in the brainstem, which then inhibit phasic electrical activity in the descending systems, thereby permitting ascending transmission of nociceptive stimuli (Fig. 8).[58] Also, it has been suggested that activation of this descending control system by the action of endogenous opioids such as β-endorphin and encephalin may account for the phenomenon of placebo and acupuncture analgesia.[58] However, the reversibility of these phenomena by naloxone and the true role of endogenous opioid systems in their production is still in doubt.

Acute and chronic pain in medical disorders

Many chronic, incapacitating, and/or ultimately fatal disease processes may be accompanied by severe pain, especially in their terminal phases. Cancer is the most obvious and widely discussed condition, but AIDS, multiple sclerosis, central pain following stroke, and musculoskeletal pain secondary to joint immobility, and arthritis complicating neurodegenerative dementing illnesses such as Parkinson's disease, amyotrophic lateral sclerosis, and Alzheimer's disease are but a few other examples of this problem. In addition, birth defects attendant to prematurity and birth-related trauma, which produce catastrophic neurological deficits that lead to disability and death, may be associated with pain in the neonate which is particularly problematic to assess and treat. This is so because the physiology of nociception in the developing nervous system has only been investigated recently, and the assessment of pain in preverbal children is difficult.[64] The following section highlights specific examples of pain in these clinical conditions which are likely to be encountered by physicians involved in palliative care of terminally-ill patients.

Painful conditions complicating HIV infection and AIDS

Pain is now recognized as a significant problem in patients with acquired immunodeficiency syndrome (**AIDS**).[65] Statistics on the prevalence of pain in AIDS ranges from 30 to 97 per cent. A recent study estimated that 50 per cent of pain syndromes in AIDS patients are directly related to HIV infection and 30 per cent are related to the therapy for HIV disease.[65] There are many potential mechanisms by which this may occur, but neuropathic symptoms in AIDS patients with peripheral neuropathy is an important and frequent cause.[66] Acute and chronic polyneuropathy, symmetric distal sensory neuropathy, brachial plexopathy, herpetic neuralgia, cranial neuropathy, and headaches from acute and chronic meningitis are common and may be associated with pain.[67] As noted above, AIDS patients with central pain from cerebral abscesses have been treated.[56]

Other complications of AIDS such as infectious gastrointestinal disease causing oesophagitis and abdominal pain, chest pain from pneumocystis pneumonia, and generalized myalgias are not uncommon and can be incapacitating to the patient.

Pain and sickle cell disease

Haemoglobinopathies producing the sickle cell phenotype may produce acute episodic and chronic pain.[68] In fact, episodes of vaso-occlusion which cause ischaemia and infarction resulting in severe acute focal bone, muscle, and visceral pain characterize the homozygous recessive form of the disease, which is particularly prevalent in Africans and African-Americans.[68] A recent, large study undertaken to describe the natural history of sickle cell anaemia, confirmed that frequent episodes of vaso-occlusion and pain is a poor prognostic variable, since less than 50 per cent of adult patients who experienced three or more episodes of vaso-occlusive crises were alive beyond the age 40.[69] Recently, hydroxyurea has been shown to decrease the frequency of vaso-occlusive episodes.[70] Hydroxyurea increases the production of fetal haemoglobin, which decreases the tendency of deoxygenated haemoglobin to sickle when present in at least 20 per cent of the total haemoglobin.

Pain syndromes in multiple sclerosis

It is generally accepted that pain in patients with multiple sclerosis is common. As many as 55 to 82 per cent of multiple sclerosis patients have pain complaints.[71] A possible pathophysiological mechanism of pain in multiple sclerosis includes ectopic spontaneous discharges in central demyelinated axons. This has been proposed to be the cause of paroxysmal pain in conditions such as trigeminal neuralgia complicating multiple sclerosis. The pain associated with optic neuritis and periorbital pain with eye movement has been suggested to be due to traction on the meninges which envelops the swollen optic nerve.[72] Extremity pain, especially with a dysaesthetic component and painful electric shock-like sensations (i.e. Lhermitte's sign associated with neck flexion) is thought to be due to posterior column demyelination and ephaptic conduction of impulses (i.e. cross excitation of nerves by shunting of current between fibres in close apposition). Other causes of extremity pain and low back pain in multiple sclerosis have been attributed to musculoskeletal abnormalities which become secondarily irritated or develop spasm as a result of abnormal gait and posturing because of the neurological abnormalities.

Cerebrovascular disease

As many as 1 to 2 per cent of stroke patients may develop central poststroke pain. Decreased temperature sensation on the affected side may be an absolute accompaniment in these patients.[55] The onset of pain may be delayed for several years after the stroke, and the pain may be superficial or deep. The pain is often severe in intensity and may be accompanied by hyperalgesia and allodynia. Paroxysms of severe pain may occur and may be elicited by emotional episodes and movement. Another common cause of pain in the hemiplegic poststroke patient is mechanical shoulder pain unrelated to the central injury.[55]

Spinal cord injury

Central pain may occur from a traumatic injury at any level of the spinal cord. Central pain usually occurs in the area of spinal cord or root somatosensory deficit.[72] If the nerve root is injured, neuropathic pain in a radicular distribution may add to the central pain of spinal cord origin. The pathophysiology of central pain caused by a spinal cord lesion is not known and not everyone with similar lesions develops pain. The traumatic spinal cord lesions that have been reported to cause central pain include: traumatic hemisection of the cord, traumatic haematomyelia of the cervical cord, post-traumatic vascular lesions, and syringomyelia. High-dose corticosteroids administered within hours of the injury may ameliorate acute pain and aid recovery of neurological function.[73]

Pathophysiology of pain in special circumstances

Pain in the infant or preverbal child

Although this is not a common circumstance in palliative medicine, the assessment and treatment of pain in the very young child poses significant challenges. However, it is now clear that in the human fetus the neuroanatomic pathways necessary for pain perception are developed, and analysis of the behavioural and physiological responses to putatively painful stimuli suggest that the human neonate can, indeed, perceive pain.[74] The available evidence suggests that analgesic and anaesthetic agents should be used in procedures and operations which are known to be painful in older individuals or when the infant is responding in a way which is consistent with discomfort. Unique issues with respect to the pharmacokinetic and pharmacodynamic responses to analgesic and anaesthetic agents in this age group in comparison to older individuals is beyond the scope of this chapter; however, this is also under intense study.

Pain in the elderly and demented patient

Chronic pain in patients over the age of 65 has been reported to occur in 20 per cent of people in this age group.[75] Patients in this age group have been considered to have a greater sensitivity to medications with sedative effects such as opioids, tricyclic antidepressants, anticonvulsants, and benzodiazepines. Body fluid volume decreases with age and this may affect the distribution and concentration of drugs such as morphine in the elderly patient.[76]

Acute confusional states may occur with many medications, especially in the patient with abnormal baseline cortical function, that is the demented individual. Adverse effects of the opioids which may be enhanced in the elderly include constipation, hypotension, and, with certain opioids such as pethidine, the accumulation of toxic metabolites (especially in the setting of renal dysfunction) which may cause convulsions, myoclonic jerks, hallucinations, agitation, and psychotomimetic effects. There is also an increased risk of drug interactions. In general, opioids and other drugs with short plasma half-lives (e.g. morphine, hydromorphone, or oxycodone) should be used in elderly patients, as opposed to those with longer plasma half-lives (e.g. methadone or levorphanol), as there is less likelihood of accumulation with repetitive dosing and therefore less chance to cause confusion.

Summary

There have been major advances in our understanding of fundamental neurobiological processes involved in nociception. The increased understanding offers the opportunity for new therapeutic agents to treat pain in patients in all stages of diseases, including terminal illnesses. Evaluation of the pathophysiological mechanisms of pain in specific patient populations may also improve our ability to target treatment strategies for optimal outcomes.

References

1. Payne R. Cancer pain—anatomy, physiology and pharmacology. *Cancer*, 1989; **63**: 2266–74.
2. Foley KM. Pain syndromes in patients with cancer. In: Portency RK, Kanner RM, eds. *Contemporary Neurology Series: Pain Management: Theory and Practice*, Vol. 48. Philadelphia: F.A. Davis, 1996: 215.
3. Cleeland CS, Syrjala KL. How to assess cancer pain. In: Turk DC, Melzack R, eds. *Handbook of Pain Assessment*. New York: Guilford Press, 1992: 360–87.
4. Woolf CS. Central mechanisms of acute pain. In: *Proceedings of the VIth World Congress on Pain*. Amsterdam: Elsevier, 1990: 25–34.
5. Cervero F, Morrison JFB, eds. *Visceral Sensation*. Amsterdam: Elsevier Science, 1986.
6. Elliott K, Foley KM. Neurologic pain syndromes in patients with cancer. *Neurologic Clinics*, 1989; **7**: 333–60.
7. Wall P, Gutnic M. Ongoing activity in peripheral nerves: the physiology and pharmacology of impulses originating from a neuroma. *Experimental Neurology*, 1974; **43**: 580–93.
8. Albe-Fessard DG, Lombard MC. Use of an animal model to evaluate the origin of and protection against deafferentation pain. In: Bonica JJ, Lindblom ULF, Iggo A, eds. *Advances in Pain Research and Therapy*, Vol. 5. New York: Raven Press, 1983: 691–738.
9. Nathan OW. Pain and the sympathetic nervous system. *Journal of Autonomic Nervous System*, 1983; **7**: 363–70.

10. Bennett GJ. An animal model of neuropathic pain: a review. *Muscle and Nerve*, 1993; **16**: 1040–8.
11. Verdago RJ, Ochoa JL. Sympathetically maintained pain I. Phentolamine block questions the concept. *Neurology*, 1994; **44**: 1003–10.
12. Stanton-Hicks M, Janis W, Hassenbusch S, Haddox JD, Boas R, Wilson P. Reflex sympathetic dystrophy: changing concepts and taxonomy. *Pain*, 1995; **63**: 127–33.
13. Willis WD. *The Pain System: The Neural Basis of Nociceptive Transmission in the Mammalian Nervous System*. Basil: S Karger, 1985.
14. Torebjork HE, Hallin RG. Identification of afferent C units in intact human skin nerves. *Brain Research*, 1974; **67**: 387–403.
15. Burgess PR, Perl ER. Cutaneous mechanoreceptors and nociceptors. In: A Iggo, ed. *Handbook of Sensory Physiology*, Vol. II: *Somatosensory System*. Berlin: Springer-Verlag, 1973: 29–78.
16. Schmidt R, Schmelz M, Forer C, Ringkamp M, Torbejork E. Novel classes of responsive and unresponsive C-nociceptors in human skin. *Journal of Neuroscience*, 1995; **15**: 333–41.
17. Raja S, Meyer RA, Campbell JN. Hyperalgesia and sensitization of primary afferent fibers. In: Fields HD, ed. *Pain Syndromes in Neurology*. London: Butterworth, 1990:19–45.
18. Burke D. Microneurography: impulse conduction and parasthesia. *Muscle and Nerve*, 1993; **16**: 1025–32.
19. Torebjork HE, Ochoa JL. Specific sensations evoked by activity in single identified sensory units in man. *Acta Physiologica Scandinavica*, 1980; **110**: 445–7.
20. Levine JD, Fields HL, Basbaum AI. Peptides and the primary afferent nociceptor. *Journal of Neuroscience*, 1993; **13**: 2273–86.
21. Walker K, Perkins M, Dray A. Kinins and kinin receptors in the nervous system. *Neurochemistry International*, 1995; **26L**: 1–16.
22. Gordh T, Kaarlsten R, Kristensen J. Intervention with spinal NMDA, adenosine, and NO systems for pain modulation. *Annals of Medicine*, 1995; **27**: 229–34.
23. Malmberg AB, Yaksh TL. Hyperalgesia mediated by spinal glutamate or substance P receptor blocked by spinal cyclooxygenase inhibition. *Science*, 1992; **257**: 1276–9.
24. Bredt DS, Snyder SH. Nitric oxide: a physiologic messenger molecule. *Annual Review of Biochemistry*, 1994; **63**: 175–95.
25. Meller ST, Pechman PS, Gebhart GF, Maves TJ. Nitric oxide mediates the thermal hyperalgesia produced in a model of neuropathic pain in the rat. *Neuroscience*, 1992; **50**: 7–10.
26. Galasko CSB. Mechanism of bone destruction in the development of skeletal metastasis. *Nature*, 1976; **263**: 507–10.
27. Ferreira SH, Nakamura M, Castro MSA. The hyperalgesic effects of prostacyclin and protaglandin E_2. *Prostaglandins*, 1978; **16**: 31–7.
28. Milne RJ, Foreman RD, Giesler GJ, *et al.* Convergence of cutaneous and pelvic visceral nociceptive inputs onto primate spinothalamic neurons. *Pain*, 1981; **11**: 163–81.
29. Hunt SP, Pini A, Evan G. Induction of c-fos like protein in spinal cord neurons following sensory stimulation. *Nature*, 1987; **328**: 632–4.
30. Iadorola JJ, Douglass J, Civelli O, Naranjo JR. Differential activation of spinal cord dynorphin and enkephalin neurons during hyperalgesia: evidence using cDNA hybridization. *Brain Research*, 1988; **455**: 205–12.
31. Draisci G, Iadarola M. Temporal analysis of increases in c-fos, preprodynorphin and preproenkephalin in mRNAs in rat spinal cord. *Molecular Brain Research*, 1989; **6**: 31–7.
32. Crosby G, Chaar M, Uhl GR. Subarachnoid morphine alters opiate peptide gene expression. *Pain*, 1990; (suppl. 5): S455.
33. Stein C. The control of pain in peripheral tissues by opioids. *New England Journal of Medicine*, 1995; **332**: 1685–90.
34. Stein C, Millan MJ, Shippenberg TS, Peter K, Herz A. Peripheral opioid receptors mediating antinociception in inflammation. Evidence for involvement of mu, delta and kappa receptors. *Journal of Pharmacology and Experimental Therapy*, 1989; **248**: 1269–75.
35. Stein C, Schafer M, Hassan AHS. Peripheral opioid receptors. *Annals of Medicine*, 1995; **27**: 219–21.
36. Antonijevic I, Mousa SA, Schafer M, Stein C. Perineural defect and peripheral opioid analgesia in inflammation. *Journal of Neuroscience*, 1995; **15**: 165–72.
37. Stein C, Comise K, Haimerl E, *et al.* Analgesic effect of intraarticular morphine after arthroscopic knee surgery. *New England Journal of Medicine*, 1991; **325**: 1123–6.
38. Sibinga NES, Goldstein A. Opioid peptides and opioid receptors in cells of the immune system. *Annual Review of Immunology*, 1988; **6**: 219–49.
39. Wall PD, Devor M, Inbal R, Scadding JW, Schonfeld D, Seltzer Z, Tomkiewicz MM. Autotomy following peripheral nerve lesions: experimental anesthesia dolorosa. *Pain*, 1979; **7**: 103–9.
40. Bennett GJ, Xie Y-K. A peripheral mononeuropathy in the rat that produces disorders of pain sensation like those seen in man. *Pain*, 1988; **33**: 87–107.
41. Kim SH, Chung JM. An experimental model for peripheral neuropathy produced by segmental spinal nerve ligation in the rat. *Pain*, 1992; **50**: 355–63.
42. Seltzer Z, Dubner R, Shir Y. A novel behavioral model of neuropathic pain disorders produced by partial sciatic nerve injury. *Pain*, 1990; **43**: 205–18.
43. Sommer C, Lalonde A, Heckman HM, Rodriguez M, Myers RR. Quantitative neuropathology of a focal nerve injury causing hyperalgesia. *Journal of Neuropathology and Experimental Neurology*, 1995; **54**: 635–43.
44. Sugiomoto T, Bennett GJ, Kajander KC. Transynaptic degeneration in the superficial dorsal horn after sciatic nerve injury: effects of a chronic constriction injury, transection and strychnine. *Pain*, 1990; **42**: 205–13.
45. Tal M, Bennett GJ. Dextrorphan relieves neuropathic heat-evoked hyperalgesia. *Neuroscience Letters*, 1993; **151**: 107–10.
46. Meller ST, Penchman PS, Gebhart GF, Maves TJ. Nitric oxide mediates the thermal hyperalgesia produced in a model of neuropathic pain in the rat. *Neuroscience*, 1992; **50**: 7–10.
47. Cervero F, Iggo A. The substantia gelatinosa of the spinal cord. A critical review. *Brain*, 1980; **103**: 717–22.
48. Coggeshall RE. Afferent fibers in the ventral root. *Neurosurgery*, 1979; **4**: 443–8.
49. Craig DD, Bushnell MC, Zhang E-T, Blomqvist A. A thalamic nucleus specific for pain and temperature sensation. *Nature*, 1994; **372**: 770–3.
50. Giesler GJ, Katter JT, Dado RJ. Direct spinal pathways to the limbic system for nociceptive information. *Trends in Neuroscience*, 1994; **17**: 244–50.
51. Besson JM, Chaouch A. Peripheral and spinal mechanisms of nociception. *Physiological Review*, 1987; **67**: 67–185.
52. Mehler WR, Feferman ME, Nanta WJH. Ascending axon degeneration following anterolateral cordotomy: an experimental study in the monkey. *Brain*, 1960; **83**: 718–750.
53. Penfield W, Boldrey E. Somatic motor and sensory representation in the cerebral cortex of man as studied by electrical stimulation. *Brain*, 1937; **60**: 389–443.
54. Bertheier M, Startstein S, Leiguanrda R. Asymbolia for pain: a sensory-limbic disconnection syndrome. *Annals of Neurology*, 1988; **24**: 41–9
55. Casey KL. *Pain and Central Nervous System Disease: The Central Pain Syndromes*. New York: Raven Press, 1991.
56. Gonzales GR, Herskovitz S, Rosenblum M, Kanner R, Foley KM, Portenoy R, Brown A. Clinicopathologic correlation of Dejerine-Roussy syndrome (DRS) caused by CNS toxoplasmosis in patients with AIDS. *Neurology*, 1990; **40** (suppl. 1): 117: 437.
57. Lhermitte J. Physiologie des ganglions centraux. Les corps stries. La couche optique. Les formations sous-thalamiques. In: Roger, Binet J, eds. *Traite de Physiologie Normale et Pathologique*, Vol. 9. Paris: Masson, 1933: 357–402.
58. Fields HL, Besson JM, eds. Pain modulation. *Progress in Brain Research*, **77**, 1986.
59. Taiwo YO, Fabian H, Pazoles CJ, Fields HL. Potentiation of MS antinociception by monoamine reuptake inhibitors in rat spinal cord. *Pain*, 1985; **21**: 329–37.
60. Watson CPN, Evans RJ. A comparative trial of amitriptyline and zimelidine in post-herpetic neuralgia. *Pain*, 1985; **23**: 387–94.

61. Kishore KR, Max MB, Schafer SC, Ganghan MA, Smoller B, Gracey RH, Dubner R. Desipramine relieves postherpetic neuralgia. *Clinical and Pharmacological Therapy*, 1990; **47**: 305–12.
62. Eisenach JC, DuPen S, Dubois M, Miguel R, Allin D, Payne R, and the Epidural Clonidine Study Group. Epidural clonidine analgesia for intractable cancer pain. *Pain*, 1995; **61**: 391–9.
63. Botney M, Fields HL. Amitriptyline potentiates morphine analgesia by a direct action on the central nervous system. *Annals of Neurology*, 1983; **13**: 160–4.
64. Anand KJS, Hickey PR. Pain and its effects in the human neonate and fetus. *New England Journal of Medicine*, 1987; **317**: 1321–9.
65. Breitbart W, Patt R. Pain management in patients with AIDs. *Annals of Hematology-Oncology*, 1995; **2**: 391–9.
66. Lipton SA. HIV-related neuronal injury. Potential therapeutic intervention with calcium channel antagonists and NMDA antagonists. *Molecular Neurobiology*, 1994; **8**: 181–96.
67. Britton CB, Miller JR. Neurologic complications in acquired immunodeficiency syndrome (AIDS). *Neurolologic Clinics*, 1984; **2**: 315.
68. Patt RB, Payne R. Management of pain. In: Collier BS, Kipps TS, eds. *Williams' Textbook of Hematology*. McGraw-Hill, 1995: 203–8.
69. Platt OS, Branbilla DJ, Rosse WF. Mortality in sickle cell disease. Life expectancy and risk factors for early death. *New England Journal of Medicine*, 1994; **330**:1639–44.
70. Charche S. *et al.* Effect of hydroxyurea on the frequency of painful crises in sickle cell anemia. *New England Journal of Medicine*, 1995; **332**: 1317–22.
71. Moulin DE. Pain in multiple sclerosis. *Neurologic Clinics*, 1989; **7**: 321–31.
72. Tasker RR. Pain resulting from central nervous system pathology (central pain). In: JJ Bonica, ed. *The Management of Pain*, 2nd edn. Philadelphia: Lea and Febiger, 1990: 267–83.
73. Akdemir H, Pasaoglu A. Histopathology of experimental spinal cord trauma. Comparison of treatment with TRH, naloxone and dexamethasone. *Research in Experimental Medicine*, 1992; **192**: 177–83.
74. Owen JA, Sitar DS, Berger L, *et al.* Age related morphine kinetics. *Clinical Pharmacology and Therapy*, 1983; **34**: 364–8.
75. Crook J, Hideout E, Brown G. The prevalence of pain complaints in a general population. *Pain*, 1984; **18**: 299–314.
76. Payne R, Pasternak G. Pain and pain management. In: CK Cassel, DE Riesenberg, LB Sorensen, JR Walsh, eds. *Geriatric Medicine*, 2nd edn. Springer-Verlag: New York, 1990: 585–606.
77. Watkins LR, Maier SF, Goehler LE. Immune activation: the role of pro-inflammatory cytokines in inflammation, illness responses and pathological pain states. *Pain*, 1995; **63**: 289–302.
78. Berkley KJ, Hubscher CH. Are there separate central nervous system pathways for touch and pain? *Nature Medicine*, 1995; **1**: 766–73.

9.2.2 Pain assessment and cancer pain syndromes

Kathleen M. Foley

Introduction

Adequate assessment is the critical first step to define a treatment strategy for the patient with pain. The major goal of an assessment strategy is to use the most appropriate diagnostic and therapeutic approaches to define the cause of the pain and to direct its treatment. Advances in our understanding of the pathophysiology of cancer pain, coupled with the availability of validated pain measurement tools, facilitates such an assessment.[1-9] Identification and categorization of a wide range of distinct, yet characteristic, pain syndromes provide the clinical basis for choosing specific therapeutic strategies.[1,3,8,9] Advances in our knowledge about cancer pain need to be integrated into daily clinical practice. Such an approach has been advocated by the World Health Organization (WHO) in the formulation of its Cancer Pain Relief Programme.[10,11] This programme provides an approach for the management of cancer pain as part of broad national cancer control programmes. Its major thrust is based upon the construct that nothing would have a greater impact on the quality of life of patients with pain and cancer than the dissemination and implementation of existing knowledge on pain assessment and treatment. To this end, the WHO Cancer Pain Relief Programme has expanded its mission to include a broad programme of pain relief and palliative care, recognizing that the goal of palliative care is the achievement of the best possible quality of life for patients and their families. Freedom from pain is seen as a right of every cancer patient, and access to pain therapy is a measure of respect for this right. Cancer pain relief cannot be considered in isolation but should be seen as part of a comprehensive programme of palliative care. Numerous international pain and palliative care organizations have worked closely with the WHO to facilitate wide dissemination of its guidelines for pain assessment and treatment.[11] Before reviewing the specific principles of assessment and cancer pain syndromes, an overview of the epidemiology of cancer pain and the barriers to its effective treatment are summarized.

Epidemiology of pain

Extent of the problem

Prevalence data indicates that there are currently about 17 million people living with cancer world-wide. Numerous studies have demonstrated that the prevalence of pain increases with progression of disease, and that the intensity, type, and location of pain varies according to the primary site of cancer, extent of disease, progression, and the treatments employed.[12-26]. Several country-wide surveys have reported comparable epidemiological data, suggesting consistent prevalence rates of 30 to 40 per cent of patients in active therapy reporting pain and 70 to 90 per cent of patients with advanced disease reporting pain.[18,20,24,26,27] In the United States survey of 1308 oncology outpatients treated by the Eastern Co-operative Oncology Group, 67 per cent reported recent pain, with 36 per cent describing pain severe enough to impair function.[27,28] In a similar survey undertaken in France, 69 per cent of the cancer patients surveyed rated their worse pain to be at a level that impaired their ability to function.[20,29]

Studies that have attempted to look at the global impact of pain in cancer patients have addressed not only the prevalence of cancer pain, but its impact on function.[5,16] Uncontrolled pain precludes a satisfactory quality of life. Persistent pain markedly interferes with activities of daily living and social interaction. The impact of pain on mood and psychological functioning is complex, but numerous studies point to the increased risk of anxiety, depression, and suicidal ideation.[30] In a study of ambulatory patients with recurrent or metastatic lung or colon cancer, as many as 90 per cent experienced pain more than 25 per cent of the time.[22] More than one-half of the patients reported that pain interfered moderately or more with general activity and work. More than one-half of the patients reported moderate or greater pain interference with sleep, mood, and enjoyment of life. In short, pain is prevalent among well functioning, ambulatory patients and substantially compromises function in about one-half of the patients who experience it.[5,21,22,28]

In a study to validate the Memorial Symptom Assessment Scale, Portenoy *et al.* reported pain was present in 63 per cent of 246 randomly selected inpatients and outpatients undergoing active treatment for prostate, colon, breast, or ovarian cancers and was rated moderate-to-severe by 43 per cent of respondents.[5] In surveys of patients admitted to palliative care or hospice services, pain was inadequately relieved in 64 to 80 per cent of patients at the time of intake.[24,25] These numbers vary considerably. For example data from the National Hospice Report, which was based on 1754 terminal cancer patients, revealed that 25 per cent of patients interviewed within 2 days of death had persistent and severe pain.[31] Although the majority of patients admitted to such palliative care or hospice facilities report pain, Shannon *et al.* tested the feasibility of standardized pain instruments in a population of patients with far advanced cancer at the time of admission to a specialty hospital.[32] Only 26 per cent of patients could use the assessment tools. The other patients were cognitively impaired and either reported no pain or were unable to state whether or not they had pain. This study points to the difficulty of pain assessment in the cognitively impaired patient with advanced disease and suggests that there may well be an underestimation of the prevalence of pain in such patient populations because of their inability to report this symptom.[33]

In a survey combining epidemiological with ethnographic data, 2266 cancer patients who were referred to an anaesthesiology-based pain service were prospectively evaluated.[18] On referral, 98 per cent of patients suffered pain, with the average pain intensity on the day prior to admission rated as severe-or-worse by 70 per cent of the patients, despite 92 per cent of patients having been previously treated with analgesics or coanalgesics.

These various studies point out the wide variation in assessing the prevalence of pain in various populations of patients with cancer. They do, however, point to the fact that cancer pain is a major problem and significantly impacts quality of life. To understand better the reasons for inadequate pain management, numerous barriers have been identified that focus on how difficulty in pain assessment impacts on pain treatment.

Barriers to pain assessment and adequate pain management

Lack of knowledge about pain assessment methodology is one of the common barriers associated with inadequate pain treatment. Physicians, patients, and the public, through a series of well-validated surveys, have defined the numerous barriers that interfere with inadequate cancer pain management.[26–29,34–36,41,42] These barriers have been categorized broadly as; patient-related, physician-related, and institution-related. They exist, in part, because of the multidimensional nature of the subjective complaint of pain and a lack of a clearly defined language of pain.

The patient-related barriers include:

(1) patient's reluctance to report pain;

(2) patient's reluctance to follow treatment recommendations;

(3) patient's fear of tolerance and addiction;

(4) patient's concern about side-effects;

(5) patient's belief that pain is an inevitable consequence and must be accepted;

(6) patient's fear of disease progression;

(7) patient's fear of injections.

In a study by Ward *et. al.* evaluating these barriers, 37 to 85 per cent of patients had comparable concerns.[38,39] A higher level of concern was associated with the elderly, the less educated, and those with lower incomes and was correlated with under medication and higher levels of pain. Several cross-cultural studies have demonstrated similar barriers in various cultures.[29,37,39,40]

Closely allied to these patient-related barriers are physician-related issues. Again, numerous surveys have demonstrated the failure of clinicians to evaluate or appreciate the severity of the pain problem.[26,27,29] Grossman *et al.* reported that when patients rate their pain as moderate-to-severe, oncology fellows failed to appreciate the severity of the problem in 73 per cent of cases.[42] In both the Eastern Co-operative Oncology Group survey by Von Roenn *et al.* and in a study of French physicians, the discrepancy between patient and physician evaluation of the severity of the problem was a major predictor of inadequate relief.[27] Other surveys have validated that poor physician and nursing assessment results in inadequate treatment of pain. Knowledge deficits in cancer pain assessment and treatment have been well identified.[26,27,29] In this recent study of French oncologists, not only major knowledge deficits related to assessment and analgesic therapy were identified, but a major discrepancy between their actual and perceived knowledge was revealed.[29] Several studies have revealed very low correlation between self-evaluation of clinical skills in pain therapy and correct responses to clinical vignettes.[29,34] Identification of physicians' lack of perception about their lack of knowledge provides necessary information to develop strategies to improve physician self-evaluation skills that more closely mimic their true knowledge.[34]

Institutional-related barriers include the lack of a language of pain and the failure to use validated pain measurement tools in clinical practice.[43] The lack of time committed to pain as a priority, lack of economic resources committed to its treatment, and the serious legal restrictions to drug prescribing and drug availability add further impediments to adequate pain treatment. These impediments have been widely discussed in the literature.[43–45] There is good evidence that making pain visible and incorporating a pain measurement tool into institutional daily practice can heighten awareness of pain and its treatment. For example making pain one of the integral parts of a vital sign chart in hospitals (Fig. 1) can influence its treatment.[46]

To address these various barriers, specific programmes have been developed that focus on broad educational efforts to change attitudes, behaviours, and knowledge deficits in patients, physicians, and institutions. The use of continuous quality improvement programmes has been demonstrated to be effective in providing the framework for initiatives for change.[46,47]

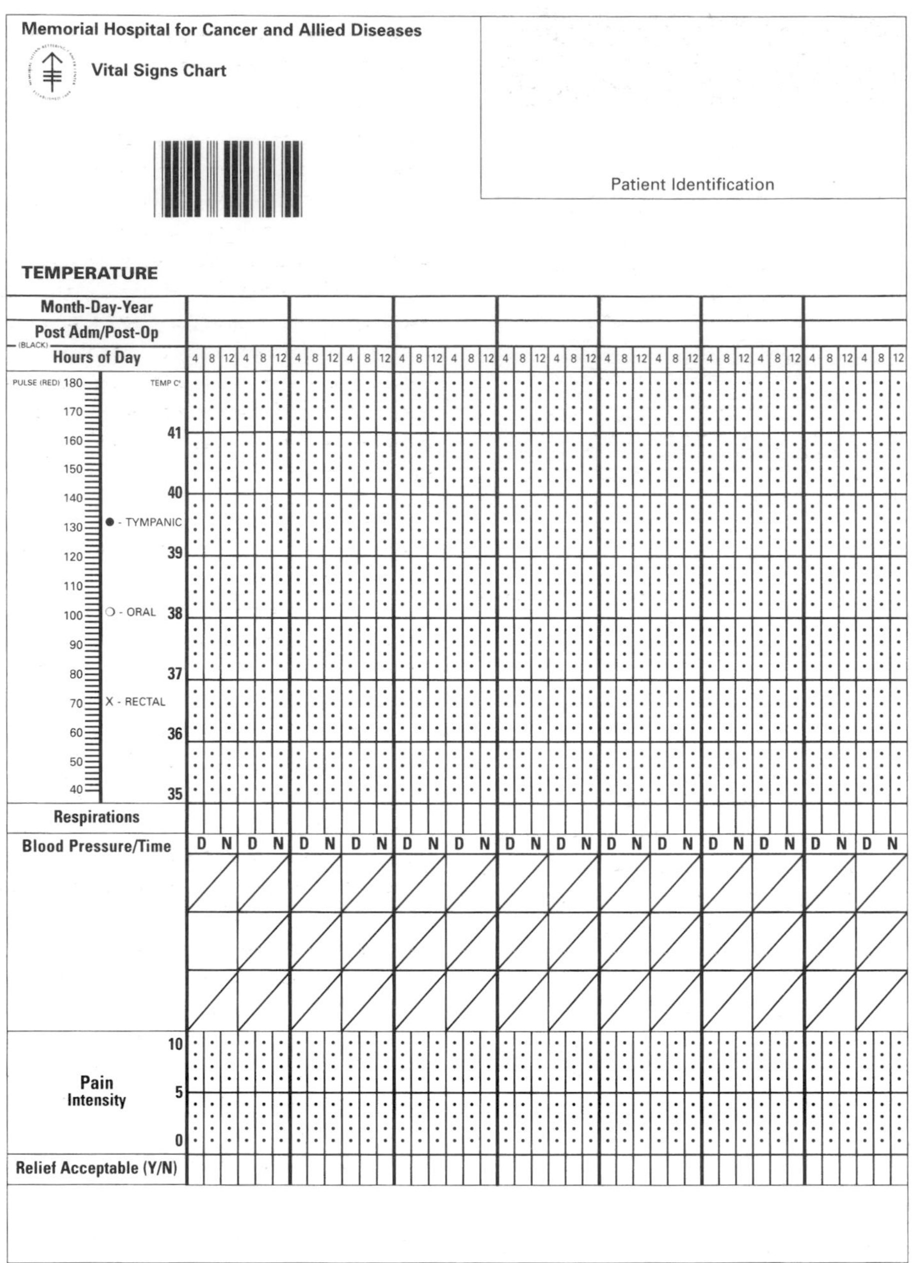

Memorial Hospital for Cancer and Allied Diseases

Vital Signs Chart

Patient Identification

TEMPERATURE

Month-Day-Year

Post Adm/Post-Op

(BLACK)

Hours of Day

4 8 12 4 8 12

PULSE (RED)

TEMP C°

180 170 160 150 140 130 120 110 100 90 80 70 60 50 40

41 40 39 38 37 36 35

● - TYMPANIC

O - ORAL

X - RECTAL

Respirations

Blood Pressure/Time

D N D N

Pain Intensity

10 5 0

Relief Acceptable (Y/N)

Fig. 1 The Memorial Hospital Vital Sign Sheet containing a pain intensity scale.

A recent multicentre study of cancer pain and its treatment in France combined a study of pain prevalence with an evaluation of predictive factors for inadequate management.[20,29] This study, which was similar to the studies published by Von Roenn *et al.* and Cleeland *et al.*, demonstrated that despite the increased attention to the treatment of cancer pain in France and the publication in 1986 by the French government of clinical guidelines on pain and palliative care, little attention had been focused on learning about the prevalence of the cancer pain problem and accumulating data on the adequacy of management from the perspective of patients and their doctors. The results of these surveys are summarized in Tables 1, 2, and 3, and provide a useful example of the epidemiological data, from 273 patients, on types of cancer, severity of pain by site of cancer and disease stage, and treatment of cancer pain. This study is a good model to define the magnitude of the problem.[20] Table 4 lists French physicians' attitudes and knowledge and provides one approach to combine studies of pain prevalence with pain management.[29] The French data are quite similar to data collected from American physicians.[28]

The basic principles of pain assessment

Definition of pain

The International Association for the Study of Pain defines pain as 'an unpleasant sensory and emotional experience associated with actual or potential tissue damage or described in terms of such damage'.[47] Pain is always subjective. There is no definitive way to distinguish pain occurring in the absence of tissue damage and pain

Table 1 Patients with pain due to cancer by type of cancer; values are percentages (proportions) unless stated otherwise[29]

	Total number	Pain during past week[a]	Pain at its worst ≥5[a,b]
Breast	211	56 (117/209)	67 (74/111)
Gastrointestinal	108	56 (59/106)	77 (44/57)
Genitourinary	80	58 (46/80)	63 (29/46)
Lung	77	58 (45/77)	72 (31/43)
Head and neck	57	67 (38/57)	69 (25/36)
Lymphoma	26	35 (9/26)	71 (5/7)
Other	46	57 (26/46)	64 (16/25)
Total	605	57 (340/601)	69 (224/325)

[a] No patient answered every question; patients were excluded if their responses or those of their doctors were incomplete on these variables.
[b] On scale of 0 to 10 where 0=no pain and 10=extreme pain.

resulting from damaged tissue. Pain as a somatic delusion or a masked depression is rare in patients with cancer, and the presence of pain usually implies a pathological process.

Types of pain

There are numerous ways to categorize the types of pain that occur in patients with cancer. These include definitions based on the neurophysiological mechanisms of pain, its temporal aspects, its intensity, the categories of patients with pain, and on the specific pain syndromes that occur in patients with cancer. These categories have practical value because they capture the multidimensional aspects of pain.

Neurophysiological mechanisms of pain

Three types of pain—somatic, visceral, and neuropathic—have been described, based on their neurophysiological mechanisms.[1,2,8] These have been discussed in Chapter 9.2.1.

Temporal pattern of pain

Pain may also be defined on a temporal basis. It is well recognized that cancer patients have both acute and chronic pain. This division is based on our increased understanding of pain mechanisms and on the recognition that the central modulation for these types of pain states may be different and that the clinical management of, and response to, treatment is different.

Acute pain

Acute pain is characterized by a well-defined, temporal pattern of pain onset, generally associated with subjective and objective physical signs with hyperactivity of the autonomic nervous system. These signs provide the health-care professional with objective evidence that substantiates the patient's complaint of pain. Acute pain is usually self limited and responds to treatment with analgesic drug therapy and treatment of its precipitating cause. Acute pain can be further subdivided into subacute and intermittent or episodic types. Subacute pain describes pain that comes on over several days, often with increasing intensity, and represents a pattern of progressive pain symptomatology. Episodic pain refers to pain that occurs during confined periods of time, on a regular or irregular basis. Intermittent pain is an alternative word to describe episodic pain. All of the pains in this category of acute pain usually have associated autonomic hyperactivity.

Chronic pain

In contrast, chronic pain is defined as pain that persists for more than 3 months, often with a less well-defined temporal onset.[47] Adaptation of the autonomic nervous system occurs and patients with chronic pain lack the objective signs common to the patient with acute pain. Chronic pain is associated with significant changes in personality, lifestyle, and functional ability. Such patients require a management approach that encompasses not only the treatment of the cause of the pain, but also treatment of the complications that have ensued in their functional status, social lives, and personalities.[3] Treatment of chronic pain is especially challenging because it requires careful assessment of both the intensity of the pain as well as the degree of psychological distress.

Breakthrough pain

More recently, a language using more specific terms to define and convey pain that occurs in cancer patients with both acute and chronic pain states has been implemented. Baseline pain is defined as that pain reported by patients as the average pain intensity experienced for 12 h or more during a 24-h period.[45] Breakthrough pain is characterized by a transient increase in pain to greater than moderate intensity, occurring on a baseline pain of moderate intensity or less. In a study of 70 adult cancer inpatients, 41 (65 per cent) reported breakthrough pain.[48] The median number of reported pains was four, with a wide range. The majority of pains were characterized by both a rapid onset and a brief duration. Breakthrough pain has a diversity of characteristics. In some patients, it characterizes pain onset or marked worsening of pain at the end of the dosing interval of the regularly scheduled analgesic. In other patients, it is caused by an action of the patient and referred to as incident pain. In some patients, the incident pains have a non-volitional precipitate, such as flatulence. The majority of breakthrough pains are usually thought to be associated with a known malignant cause but, of interest in the Portenoy study, one-fifth were associated with tumour therapy and 4 per cent were unrelated to either the cancer or its treatment.

Intensity of pain

Pain may also be defined on the basis of intensity and there is an extensive literature on the use of words to describe pain intensity.[6,27,33] However, it is well recognized that there are limitations to a unidimensional concept of pain which is described solely in terms of pain intensity. In a study by Cleeland *et al.*, 451 cancer patients were instructed to describe their pain using their own words.[49] A total of 129 distinct words were used by patients to describe their pain, with each patient using an average of 1.8 words. Ten words accounted for 67 per cent of total word usage. Patients with specific pain aetiologies could not be differentiated using word descriptors. In fact, the nature of the word did not define either the pain syndrome nor its affective component.

Specific categorical scales of pain intensity have been used, in which patients are asked to describe their pain as mild, moderate, severe, or excruciating.[50] Visual analogue scales have also been used.[51] These are often a 10-cm line anchored on either end by two points—'no pain' or 'worst possible pain'—and the patient is asked to mark on the line the intensity of their pain. Numerical scales are often commonly used, asking patients to rate their pain as a number

Table 2 Severity of cancer pain[a] in 529 patients with cancer by site of primary disease and stage of disease[29]

Type of cancer	Number of patients	Mean average pain (standard deviation)	Mean worst pain (standard deviation)
Breast			
No metastasis	83	4·08 (2·14)	5·22 (2·31)
Metastasis	126	4·99 (2·52)	5·95 (2·55)
Gastrointestinal			
No metastasis	39	3·80 (2·01)	5·40 (2·53)
Metastasis	67	4·57 (2·03)	6·19 (2·45)
Genitourinary			
No metastasis	18	3·22 (3·15)	5·56 (2·88)
Metastasis	62	4·83 (2·41)	6·00 (2·64)
Lung			
No metastasis	38	4·86 (1·85)	6·29 (2·51)
Metastasis	39	4·78 (2·22)	6·00 (2·58)
Head and neck			
No metastasis	35	4·25 (2·36)	5·25 (2·61)
Metastasis	22	4·88 (2·63)	6·06 (3·00)

[a] index ranges from 0 (no pain) to 10 (extreme pain).

between one ('no pain') and ten ('worst possible pain'). These different scales to capture a patient's experience of pain have their limitations but they are part of a series of validated instruments that include a measure of pain intensity as one of the components of the pain experience to be defined. In a study of understanding by physicians and nurses of the language to describe pain experiences, there was a close correlation among them in the level of intensity that is meant by the terms ache, hurt, or pain.[52] Although health-care professionals may understand a common language of pain, there is enormous discrepancy between health-care professionals' assessment and the patient's report of pain, particularly when patients report pain as moderate or severe. In a study by Peteet *et al.*, in which both cancer patients and physicians were interviewed to obtain complete and direct information about pain treatment and the reasons for inadequate pain relief in individual cases, a comparison of ratings of pain severity by patients with those of physicians indicated that patients tend to rate their pain as more intense than their physician's rating.[53] In a study by Grossman *et al.* the cancer patient's report of pain and physicians' concurrent observations of the patient's pain had a close correlation when patients reported mild pain.[42] However, when patients reported moderate to severe pain, the correlation with the nurse, house officer, and oncology fellow differed significantly from that of the patient, with the concordance dropping from 78 per cent for those patients with mild pain to a correlation of 27 per cent for patients with moderate to severe pain. These problems in communication about pain intensity strongly support the construct that multiple dimensions of the pain experience should be used to assess it adequately. Fig. 2 depicts the cancer patients' rating of average pain in the French study of 605 patients with the rating given by each clinic's doctors.[20] The diagonal in the figure represents a theoretically 'perfect' correlation between a patient's rating and the rating of the institutions where they were treated. Each dot represents a group of at least 10 patients treated at one institution. Across all institutions (cancer centres, university hospitals, state hospitals, private clinics, and one home care setting) patients consistently rated their pain as being more severe than did their doctors, indicating that French physicians underestimate the severity of their patients cancer pain.

Table 3 Drug treatment of cancer pain[a] in 273 patients with cancer by severity of pain[b]; values are numbers (percentages) of patients[29]

Treatment	Mild (*n*=77)	Moderate (*n*=61)	Severe (*n*=135)
None	47 (61)	15 (25)	15 (11)
Aspirin type	11 (14)	12 (20)	11 (8)
Codeine type	12 (16)	23 (38)	54 (40)
Strong opioids	7 (9)	11 (18)	55 (41)

[a] According to doctors' reports of strongest pain relief prescribed.

[b] No patient answered every question; patients were excluded if their responses or those of their doctors were incomplete on treatment variables.

Pain intensity assessment must be made appropriate to the population under study; for example in children the measurement of pain intensity includes various age-specific methods.[54] Symptom measurement including the measurement of pain is discussed in much greater detail in Section 6.

Pain setting

Pain can also be defined by the setting in which it occurs; for example postoperative pain, pain associated with trauma, and labour pain. Both postoperative pain and traumatic pain occur in patients with cancer, and are usually described as acute pain in which there is an identifiable cause and associated therapy.

Special groups of patients with pain

Pain can also be described by the special groups of patients in which it occurs—pain in children, pain in the elderly, pain in the mentally incompetent. It is beyond the scope of this chapter to

Table 4 French physicians' attitudes and knowledge about cancer pain management[20]

	Oncologists *n*=300 (%)	Primary care physicians *n*=600 (%)	*p* value
Personal experience with cancer pain	34.7	32.5	0.80
Estimated cancer pain prevalence in own practice (median %)	21–30	10–20	0.00001
Satisfied with own practice of cancer pain management	93.2	85.3	0.0007
Satisfied with cancer pain management in France	50.5	60.3	0.005
Prescribes morphine frequently or very frequently	42.5	48.3	0.03
Experiences pharmacists as reluctant to fill morphine prescription	30.0	20.0	0.0008
Relies on patient to assess pain (% agree)	89.7	88.2	0.50
Uses the WHO analgesic ladder systematically	25.7	17.8	0.006
Administers analgesics by the clock (% agree)	70.3	61.8	0.01
No upper limit to morphine prescription (% agree)	42.4	27.3	0.00001
Morphine can be prescribed at any stage (% agree)	66.0	55.2	0.002
Received training in cancer pain management	38.7	27.3	0.0006

WHO: World Health Organization.

define these different pains, but each of these groups of individuals are represented in the cancer-patient population and their specific features influence both the assessment and therapeutic perspective.

Types of patients with pain

A series of specific types of patients with pain has been described in the cancer population (Table 5). Group I comprises patients with acute cancer-related pain. A subgroup in this category includes patients in whom pain is the major symptom leading to the diagnosis of cancer. For this group, pain has a special meaning as a harbinger of their illness. The occurrence of pain during the course of the illness or after successful therapy has the immediate implication of recurrent disease. Determination of the cause of the pain may present a diagnostic problem but effective treatment of the cause, for example radiation therapy for bone metastases, is usually possible and associated with dramatic pain relief in the majority of patients. The second subgroup includes patients who have acute pain associated with their cancer therapy; for example pain after surgery or secondary to the acute effects of chemotherapy. The cause of the pain is readily identified and its course is predictable and self limited. Such patients endure pain for the promise of a successful outcome. This is most readily observable in studies of patients undergoing bone marrow transplant who commonly undermedicate themselves for oral mucositis pain.[55]

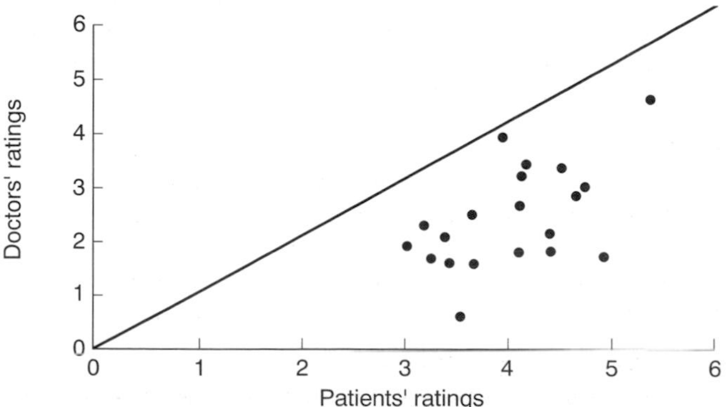

Fig. 2 Comparison of patients' ratings of average pain with those of doctors; each dot represents a group of at least 10 patients at one institution.[29]

Group II consists of patients with chronic cancer-related pain with difficult diagnostic and therapeutic problems. The group can be subdivided into patients with chronic pain associated with tumour progression and those with chronic pain related to cancer treatment. Both subgroups have pain that has persisted for more than 3 months. In patients with chronic pain associated with the progression of disease, such as those with carcinoma of the pancreas,[56] the pain escalates in intensity and combinations of antitumour therapy, analgesic drug therapy, anaesthetic blocks, and behavioural approaches to pain control are all attempted with varying degrees of success.[57] Psychological factors play an important role in this group of patients in whom palliative anticancer therapy may be of little value and is physically debilitating. The sense of hopelessness and fear of impending death may add to and exaggerate the pain, which then contributes to the overall suffering of the patient.[58] Identification of both the pain and the suffering component is essential for the provision of adequate therapy. It is for this group of patients that Cicely Saunders has used the phrase 'total pain' to describe the aetiological components other than the noxious physical stimulus, including emotional, social, bureaucratic, financial, and spiritual pain.[59] Those caring for this group of patients must be concerned with all aspects of distress and discomfort if the experience of physical pain is to be alleviated. The chronicity of the pain is associated with a series of psychological signs—disturbances in sleep, reduction in appetite, impaired concentration, and irritability—and with the clinical signs and symptoms mimicking a depressive disorder. Patients with chronic pain associated with cancer therapy usually require treatment directed at the symptoms not the cause. Treatment of the pain is often limited by the lack of available methods to remove the cause of the pain. This group of patients closely parallels those in the general population with chronic intractable pain. Identification of this group of patients is imperative because recognition of the cause of

Table 5 Types of patients with cancer pain

Group I	Patients with acute cancer-related pain Associated with the diagnosis of cancer Associated with the cancer therapy (surgery, chemotherapy, and radiation therapy)
Group II	Patients with chronic cancer-related pain Associated with cancer progression Associated with cancer therapy (surgery, chemotherapy, and radiation therapy)
Group III	Patients with pre-existing chronic pain and cancer-related pain
Group IV	Patients with a history of drug addiction and cancer-related pain Actively involved in illicit drug use In methadone maintenance programme With a history of drug abuse
Group V	Dying patients with cancer-related pain

the pain as independent of the cancer markedly alters the patient's therapy, prognosis, and psychological state. All approaches intended to maintain the functional status of the patient should be employed. Approaches other than drug therapy provide effective alternatives for pain management. This group is increasing in size and accounts for up to 25 per cent of patients referred to one cancer pain clinic.[8]

Group III includes patients with a history of chronic non-malignant pain who have cancer and associated pain. Psychological factors play an important part in this group of patients whose psychological and functional status is already compromised. They are at risk of further functional incapacity and escalating chronic pain. However, their history should not be used in a punitive way to minimize their complaints. Identification of this group of patients as a high-risk group helps to improve their psychological assessment and intervention.

Group IV includes patients with a history of drug addiction who have a cancer-related pain. Three subgroups can be identified:

(1) patients actively involved in illicit drug use and drug-seeking behaviour;

(2) those receiving methadone in a maintenance programme;

(3) those who have not used drugs for several years.

Under-treatment with analgesic drugs occurs most commonly in this group of patients. Assessment of reported pain by physicians and nurses is coloured by the fact that the pain symptoms are confused with drug-seeking behaviour.[60] Attention to the medical and psychological needs of these patients requires individualized assessment and consultation with experts in drug-related problems. The first subgroup represents a major management problem, straining the most tolerant of medical care systems. Pain in the other two subgroups is readily managed with the recognition that the psychological stresses consequent to the pain and cancer may place the patient at high risk for recidivism.

Group V includes dying patients with pain. In his group, diagnostic and therapeutic considerations should be directed at maintaining the comfort of the patient. The issues of hopelessness and of death and dying become prominent, and the suffering component of the illness must be addressed. Inadequate control of pain exacerbates the suffering and demoralizes both the family and the medical personnel, who feel that they have failed in treating the patient's pain at a time when adequate treatment may matter most. Rapid escalation of analgesic drug therapy and attempts to ameliorate the psychological symptoms should be employed. The risk/benefit ratios associated with analgesic approaches become less of an issue when the goal of pain therapy is the comfort of the patient. A clear understanding of the common associated symptoms that occur in this population of patients, and the use of approaches that actively search out and provide appropriate symptom control, are particularly important in this group of patients.[61]

Clinical assessment of pain

Certain general principles should be adhered to when evaluating all cancer patients who complain of pain (Table 6). Lack of attention to these general principles is the major cause for misdiagnosis of the specific pain syndrome.

Table 6 Clinical assessment of pain

1. Believe the patient's complaint of pain
2. Take a careful history of the pain complaint to place it temporally in the patient's cancer history
3. Assess the characteristics of each pain, including its site, its pattern of referral, its aggravating and relieving factors, and its impact on activities of daily living and quality of life
4. Clarify the temporal aspects of the pain; acute, subacute, chronic, baseline, intermittent, breakthrough, or incident
5. List and prioritize each pain complaint
6. Evaluate the response to previous and current analgesic and antitumour therapies
7. Evaluate the psychological state of the patient
8. Ask if the patient has a past history of alcohol or drug dependence
9. Perform a careful medical and neurological examination
10. Order and personally review the appropriate diagnostic procedures
11. Treat the patient's pain to facilitate the necessary work-up
12. Design the diagnostic and therapeutic approach to suit the individual
13. Provide continuity of care from evaluation to treatment, to ensure patient compliance and to reduce patient anxiety
14. Reassess the patient's response to pain therapy
15. Discuss advance care planning with the patient and the family

Believe the patient's complaint of pain

Critical to the management of the patient with cancer pain is the establishment of a trusting relationship with the physician. The complaint of pain is a symptom, not a diagnosis. Pain perception is not simply a function of the amount of physical injury sustained by the patient but is a complex state determined by multiple factors. It is important to remember that the diagnosis of the specific pain syndrome and a complete understanding of the psychological state of the patient is not always made on the initial evaluation. In fact, it may take several weeks to define its nature because of the lack of radiological or pathological verification. It may take a similar period to fully comprehend the psychological make-up of the individual patient. There are numerous examples in the assessment of patients with pain and cancer that point out the limitation of the diagnostic procedures. It is not uncommon for patients with tumour infiltration of the brachial plexus from either lung or breast cancer to have pain for several weeks or months prior to the onset of objective radiological and neurological findings.[62] A comprehensive evaluation involves taking a careful history, performing a detailed medical, neurological, and psychological evaluation, developing a series of diagnosis-related hypotheses, and ordering the appropriate diagnostic studies.

Take a careful history of the pain complaint

This should include the patient's description of:

(1) the site of the pain;

(2) quality of pain;

(3) exacerbating and relieving factors;

(4) its temporal pattern;

(5) its exact onset;

(6) the associated symptoms and signs;

(7) interference with activities of daily living;

(8) impact on the patient's psychological state;

(9) response to previous and current analgesic therapies.

Multiple pain complaints are common in patients with advanced disease and need to be ordered in terms of priority and classified.[18,25]

Evaluate the psychological state of the patient

It is imperative to clarify the patient's current level of anxiety and depression and to learn whether he/she experienced such feelings before his illness. Knowing whether he has been treated by a psychiatrist or has been an inpatient for psychiatric care helps to clarify the patient's psychological risk. Does the patient have a past history, or family history, of acute or chronic pain? Information on how he/she handled previous painful events may provide insight into whether the patient has demonstrated chronic illness behaviour. A personal or family history of alcohol or drug dependence may explain why the patient may be fearful or refuses to take opioid drugs. Has the patient seen someone die a painful death? From our experience, patients who have had such an experience are particularly fearful of their own death.

Since each patient has their own understanding of the meaning of pain, it is useful to have the patient elaborate this meaning. Do they think it represents recurrent tumour or are they convinced that it is simply arthritis? There is good evidence to suggest that when patients have a clear understanding of the meaning of their pain as representing recurrent tumour, they have increased psychological distress.[63]

The importance of defining the patient with pain is supported by a variety of studies which have focused on the impact of suffering in patients with pain.[64] A taxonomy of suffering has been described and the interface between pain and suffering is discussed in Chapter 9.2.9 and Section 11. Psychological factors play a significant role in accounting for the differences in pain experiences in patients with cancer. A series of psychiatric syndromes have been described for patients with cancer. Depression occurs in as many as 25 per cent.[66] The depression presents either as an acute stress response or as a major depression. Awareness of the common psychiatric syndromes when evaluating the pain complaint may expand the physician's understanding of such a complaint. Although it is critical to know as much as possible about each individual patient with pain, such information may not be readily available on the first interview and, in some instances, may never be available because of the lack of intellectual competence on the part of the patient to define clearly these various components of the pain complaint. It is also necessary to verify the history from a family member who may provide information that the patient is unable or unwilling to provide; the family member may be more objective in assessing the disability of the patient who under reports his symptoms. Similarly, in a patient who is a poor historian, the family member may be able to provide essential information that may alter the diagnostic approach. All attempts should be made to compile a careful history and to define the medical, neurological, and psychological profile of the pain complaint.

As the patient becomes more active in defining advance directives and as he focuses on the issues of quality of life, it is critical to ask him to define what he would do if the pain is intractable or intolerable. Does he have suicidal thoughts or a pact with a family member? Does he have a family history of suicide? Does he have drugs in reserve for such an event, or a gun in the house which he might use if he feels desperate? Such questions may allow the patient to discuss openly enormous fears of death and the need to take matters into his own control rather than trust the health-care professional. Such open discussion can allow the treating physician better to define for the patient his options for care, and reassure the patient of his commitment to care. Patients will rarely offer this information unless requested by physicians. Therefore, it is critical that a repertoire of specific questions be developed that can be integrated readily into the initial history-taking by the physician.[66,67]

Perform a careful medical and neurological examination

The medical and neurological examination helps to provide the necessary data to substantiate the history. Knowledge of the referral patterns of pain in the common cancer pain syndromes can direct the examination. The characteristics of pain in breast cancer patients with brachial plexopathy are so specific that they can help define the diagnosis of tumour infiltration of the brachial plexus from radiation fibrosis of the brachial plexus.[62] Similarly, the commonly described postmastectomy pain syndrome in patients with breast cancer is readily separable from pain due to tumour infiltration of the brachial plexus.[68,69] The physical and neurological examination also allows one to inspect visually and palpate the site of pain, and to look for the associated physical and neurological signs that might help improve the definition of the nature of the pain symptom. Defining the degree of motor or sensory changes can help define the specific site in the nervous system that may be involved. Similarly, in patients with sensory loss, the presence of allodynia and hyperaesthesia can further define the nature of the sensory problem. Moreover, the degree of muscle spasm, gait instability, and impaired co-ordination can only be assessed fully by such an evaluation.

Order and personally review the appropriate diagnostic studies

Diagnostic studies confirm the clinical diagnosis and define the site and extent of tumour infiltration in those patients with metastatic disease. Computed transaxial tomography (**CT**) and magnetic resonance imaging (**MRI**) represent the most useful diagnostic procedures in evaluating patients with pain and cancer. The CT scan provides a detailed visualization of bone and soft tissue in a two-dimensional view, and is most useful in defining early bony changes. MRI is particularly useful in evaluating vertebral body involvement in epidural spinal cord compression, as well as parenchymal brain metastases. CT is also useful in directing the needle placement for biopsies and for anaesthetic procedures such as coeliac plexus block.

Although plain radiographic films are useful screening procedures, they should not be used to overrule a clinical diagnosis if they are negative. They are inadequate for the assessment of areas of the body where bone shadows overlap and where specific pain syndromes may arise, such as the base of the skull, vertebral bodies—specifically C2, C7 to T1, and the sacrum. Similarly, the bone scan, although it provides a more sensitive method for demonstrating abnormalities in bone before changes appear on plain radiographs, does not, if positive, establish a diagnosis of metastatic disease, because patients with osteoporosis and collapsed vertebral bodies may have positive bone scans without any metastatic disease. Infections and disuse atrophy are also associated with positive bone scans. A negative bone scan does not rule out bony metastatic disease; we have evaluated a large number of patients with cancer who had proven bony disease and negative bone scans in both carcinoma of the lung and malignant melanoma.[51] The physician, when ordering the necessary diagnostic procedures, should review them personally with the radiologist to correlate any pathological change with the site of pain.

Evaluation of the extent of metastatic disease may help to discern the relationship of the pain complaint to possible recurrent disease; for example the postmastectomy pain syndrome that occurs secondary to the interruption of the intercostobrachial nerve is never causally associated with recurrent disease. In contrast, in a patient with carcinoma of the lung, the presence of recurrent disease is closely associated with the appearance of a late post-thoracotomy pain syndrome following initial resolution of the postoperative pain.[59] The use of tumour markers (including carcinogenic embryonic antigen (CEA) Ca-125 and Ca-15-3 and prostate specific antigen (PSA)) can be very useful for gastrointestinal, lung, ovarian, breast cancer, and prostate cancer.

Treat the pain to facilitate the appropriate work-up

No patient should be evaluated inadequately because of a significant pain problem. Early management of the pain while investigating the source will markedly improve the patient's ability to participate in the necessary diagnostic procedures.[79] During the initial evaluation of the pain complaint, the use of alternative methods of pain control, including anaesthetic and neurosurgical approaches, should be considered; for example the temporary use of local anaesthetics via an epidural catheter to manage sacral pain, or the use of a percutaneous cordotomy in a patient with unilateral pain below the waist from a lumbosacral plexopathy.[71] These approaches should not be considered for use only when all else fails but should be an integral part of the assessment of the patient with pain.

Reassess the patient's response to therapy

Continual reassessment of the response of the patient's pain complaint to the prescribed therapy provides the best method to validate the initial diagnosis as correct. However, in those patients in whom the effect of therapy is less than predicted or in whom exacerbation of the pain occurs, reassessment of the treatment approach or a search for a new cause of the pain should be considered. An example is the patient with epidural spinal cord compression who develops a second block proximal to the one being irradiated, with neurological signs mimicking those of the original block.

Design the diagnostic and therapeutic approach to suit the individual

The evaluation of the patient must also be closely allied to the patient's level of function, ability to participate in a diagnostic work-up, willingness to undergo the necessary diagnostic approaches, objective evidence that treatment approaches may be beneficial, and life expectancy. Careful judgement should be employed in the use of diagnostic approaches that will have a direct impact on the choice of the therapeutic strategy or answer a specific question. The random use of diagnostic procedures in this group of patients is inappropriate, and may have an adverse effect on the quality of life for such patients. Open discussion with the patient about the need for assessment as well as the therapeutic options is critical, to provide the necessary dialogue that will allow the patient to be part of the decision-making process. In some patients, diagnostic procedures, such as myelography or MRI, are inappropriate because they simply confirm the existence of disease for which there are no treatments available, or in whom the treatments are major surgical procedures (for example vertebral body resection, which would be inappropriate for the dying patient). Patient refusal of evaluation or treatment must be respected when the physician has fully explained the options to the patient and is convinced that the patient has an accurate understanding of the implications of no further work-up and/or treatment.

Discuss advance directives with the patient and family

Lastly, it is critical in developing approaches for treatment that there be an open discussion about advance directives, so that the physician has a clear understanding of the patient's goal for therapy or ambivalence in developing a therapeutic strategy. The physician must have unconditional positive regard for the patient, placing the control of symptoms of pain and treatment of their psychological distress in highest regard. Knowledge of the patient's decisions about resuscitation, living wills, and symptom management, should he or she become incompetent, improves the physician's ability to care for the patient with advanced disease appropriately and humanely.[61] Discussions related to the sedative effects of opioid therapy should help clarify patient's perspective on their cognitive status during the course of their pain management. The discussion should include patient input on whether they would accept being sleepy as a consequence of pain therapy if their pain could not be controlled with them awake and cognitively intact.[64,66]

The impact of a comprehensive evaluation on the management of cancer pain

Although the need for a comprehensive medical and neurological evaluation in the treatment of cancer pain is well described, the full impact of such an approach has only recently been formally studied. In a retrospective review of 226 consultations in a total of 190 patients, and in 50 consultations evaluated prospectively in 46 patients, a pain diagnosis was derived which included the delineation of a somatic, visceral, or neuropathic lesion based on the history, examination, and results of imaging procedures.[72] Sixty per cent of the consultations were requested in patients with known metastatic disease. A new lesion was identified through the pain evaluation performed by the consultant in 64 per cent of retrospectively studied consultations and 64 per cent of consultations evaluated prospectively. More than 50 per cent of diagnoses were neurological with the most common diagnosis being epidural spinal cord compression. The Memorial Sloan-Kettering Cancer Center Pain Service evaluation resulted in changes of treatment and provided an opportunity for primary antineoplastic therapies to be considered. Radiation therapy was offered to 19 per cent of the retrospective group and to 12 per cent of prospective study patients. Two per cent of patients from both studies received chemotherapy and 1 per cent of retrospective study patients were referred to surgery on the basis of pain evaluation. The prospective survey also tabulated specific neurological diagnoses both related and unrelated to the pain complaint. Thirty-four per cent (17 patients) had a neurological diagnosis prior to evaluation by the pain consultant. Nine of the 17 diagnoses were confirmed and the consultation led to a new neurological diagnosis in an additional 18 patients. Thus, neurological evaluation by the pain consultant confirmed neurological diagnoses in 54 per cent of patients, and the most prevalent of these were epidural spinal cord compression in nine patients and lumbosacral plexopathy in another nine patients. Eight new cases of malignant lumbosacral plexopathy were identified by the pain consultant, far more than any other neurological condition in this group of patients. Such neurological pain syndromes are discussed in Chapter 9.12.

This study supports the construct that new pathology is commonly identified through a comprehensive assessment of pain in cancer patients. Equally important, many of these lesions are amenable to primary therapy which may have direct analgesic consequences. Approximately one-fifth of the patients received primary antineoplastic therapy based upon the pain evaluation, and another 6 per cent received antibiotics. Although the high prevalence of neurological diagnosis may represent a bias in the Memorial study, it is essential to recognize that neurological lesions comprise a substantial proportion of painful lesions in the cancer population.

In a prospective study of the neurological symptoms, neurological diagnoses, and primary tumours in all patients with a history of systemic cancer (referred to the Memorial Sloan-Kettering Cancer Center Department of Neurology's consultation service), the three most common symptoms in 851 patients were:

(1) back pain (18.2 per cent);

(2) altered mental status (17.1 per cent);

(3) headache (15.4 per cent).[73]

The most common neurological diagnosis was brain metastasis (15.9 per cent) followed by metabolic encephalopathy (10.2 per cent), pain associated with bone metastases only (9.9 per cent), and epidural extension or metastasis of tumour (8.4 per cent), as had been emphasized previously. Physicians evaluating patients with cancer pain need to have sufficient knowledge of the neurological complications of cancer to evaluate and treat this group of patients appropriately.

In a very extensive, prospective survey of cancer patients referred to an anaesthesiology-based pain service, a total of 4542 anatomically distinct pain syndromes were identified for 2266 patients.[18] This study points out the complexity of pain assessment in a cancer pain population. Thirty per cent of patients presented with one, 39 per cent with two, and 31 per cent with three or more pain conditions. The greatest number of pain syndromes was described in patients with breast cancer. The most frequent pain localizations were lower back, abdominal region, thoracic region, and lower limbs. This study was the first to use the International Association for the Study of Pain Classification. Table 7 summarizes the localization, aetiology, and type of pain syndromes in 2118 patients for whom these data were available. Of interest, pain of a somatic type, originating most commonly from bone or soft tissue, was the aetiology of pain in 35 per cent of patients. Patients had mixed somatic and visceral, somatic and neuropathic, and visceral neuropathic pain syndromes, with neuropathic pain occurring in up to 47 per cent of patients either alone or in combination with other types of pain. In using the International Association for the Study of Pain classification the authors only classified pain syndromes caused by cancer in these surveys (Table 8). The authors importantly note that the International Association for the Study of Pain classification limits the coding of important information regarding pain intensity, aetiology, and pathophysiology and regarding multiple, distinct pain syndromes. However, it did provide important information on the temporal characteristics of pain, the organ systems involved, and pain intensity. These data support the previous observations that tumour infiltration of bone, soft tissue, or nerve is the most common cause of cancer-related pain. The authors also confirmed that the pain most commonly evaluated was somatic, followed by visceral and neuropathic pain.

The authors looked at the impact of the pain consultation on the reported pain intensity of this population of patients. At the time of referral, 77 per cent of patients rated their pain intensity as severe or worse, 17 per cent of patients suffered pain for more than 6 months and 44 per cent for 1 to 6 months despite 64 per cent of patients having already received treatment with non-opioid analgesics, 55 per cent with second step weak opioids, 20 per cent with third step strong opioids, and 18 per cent with coanalgesics. In the majority of these patients, adequate pain relief could be achieved

Table 7 Aetiology and pathophysiological type of pain syndromes—the number of pain syndromes and the percentage of patients (in parentheses) are given[18]

	HNR (*n*=377)	GIT (*n*=663)	RES (*n*=218)	BRS (*n*=227)	GUS (*n*=379)	LHS (*n*=114)	SBC (*n*=121)	OTH (*n*=167)	Total (*n*=2266)
Caused by cancer	514 (81)	946 (85)	340 (87)	398 (88)	617 (88)	178 (82)	166 (76)	279 (84)	3438 (85)
Bone (somatic)	70 (17)	89 (12)	117 (39)	259 (67)	216 (38)	86 (45)	48 (31)	96 (41)	981 (30)
Soft tissues/myofascial (somatic)	283 (62)	214 (28)	68 (28)	54 (20)	135 (31)	32 (25)	60 (39)	57 (28)	903 (34)
Visceral	30 (7)	504 (56)	68 (24)	24 (9)	140 (29)	22 (16)	19 (12)	48 (23)	855 (29)
Neuropathic	124 (31)	123 (15)	71 (27)	56 (22)	112 (25)	33 (22)	36 (24)	74 (34)	629 (23)
Unknown	7 (1)	16 (2)	16 (6)	5 (2)	14 (3)	5 (3)	3 (2)	4 (2)	70 (3)
Related to treatment	162 (31)	140 (17)	44 (16)	40 (14)	53 (11)	11 (8)	42 (24)	24 (11)	516 (17)
Bone (somatic)	8 (2)	6 (1)	6 (3)	1 (0)	3 (1)	1 (1)	3 (2)	3 (2)	31 (1)
Soft tissue/myofascial (somatic)	102 (24)	69 (10)	15 (5)	22 (9)	14 (3)	4 (4)	20 (13)	11 (6)	257 (10)
Visceral	0 (0)	36 (5)	8 (3)	0 (0)	16 (4)	1 (1)	0 (0)	1 (1)	62 (2)
Neuropathic	51 (11)	23 (3)	11 (4)	16 (6)	19 (4)	5 (4)	16 (11)	7 (3)	148 (5)
Unknown	1 (0)	6 (1)	4 (2)	1 (0)	1 (0)	0 (0)	3 (2)	2 (1)	18 (1)
Associated with cancer disease	19 (5)	72 (9)	13 (6)	29 (11)	45 (10)	16 (12)	9 (7)	20 (11)	223 (9)
Bone (somatic)	2 (1)	5 (1)	1 (0)	4 (2)	5 (1)	2 (2)	0 (0)	5 (3)	24 (1)
Soft tissue/myofascial (somatic)	5 (1)	25 (4)	7 (3)	14 (6)	24 (6)	4 (4)	4 (3)	4 (2)	87 (4)
Visceral	0 (0)	34 (4)	3 (1)	1 (0)	12 (3)	1 (1)	1 (1)	4 (2)	56 (2)
Neuropathic	10 (2)	6 (1)	1 (0)	10 (4)	4 (1)	9 (6)	3 (3)	6 (3)	49 (2)
Unknown	2 (1)	2 (0)	1 (0)	0 (0)	0 (0)	0 (0)	1 (1)	1 (1)	7 (0)
Unrelated to cancer or treatment	37 (7)	97 (12)	30 (10)	18 (6)	39 (8)	16 (11)	11 (7)	21 (8)	269 (9)
Bone (somatic)	14 (3)	32 (4)	12 (4)	6 (2)	13 (3)	6 (5)	4 (3)	5 (3)	92 (4)
Soft tissue/myofascial (somatic)	5 (1)	19 (3)	3 (1)	2 (1)	10 (3)	3 (3)	5 (2)	5 (2)	52 (2)
Visceral	1 (0)	7 (1)	3 (1)	1 (0)	1 (0)	0 (0)	0 (0)	0 (0)	13 (1)
Neuropathic	11 (3)	27 (4)	4 (1)	9 (3)	13 (3)	6 (5)	1 (1)	6 (3)	77 (3)
Unknown	6 (1)	12 (2)	8 (3)	0 (0)	2 (1)	1 (1)	1 (1)	5 (2)	35 (1)
Unknown	20 (4)	14 (2)	11 (4)	10 (3)	12 (3)	6 (4)	16 (7)	7 (4)	96 (3)
Bone (somatic)	2 (1)	0 (0)	2 (1)	3 (0)	2 (1)	1 (1)	1 (1)	1 (1)	12 (0)
Soft tissue/myofascial (somatic)	3 (1)	1 (0)	1 (0)	2 (1)	3 (1)	0 (0)	4 (3)	3 (1)	17 (1)
Visceral	1 (0)	2 (0)	1 (0)	0 (0)	2 (1)	2 (2)	1 (1)	0 (0)	9 (0)
Neuropathic	4 (1)	3 (0)	1 (0)	4 (2)	3 (1)	1 (1)	4 (3)	2 (1)	22 (1)
Unknown	10 (2)	8 (1)	6 (2)	1 (0)	2 (1)	2 (2)	6 (2)	1 (1)	36 (1)
Total	752 (100)	1269 (100)	438 (100)	495 (100)	766 (100)	227 (100)	244 (100)	351 (100)	4542 (100)
Bone (somatic)	96 (22)	132 (18)	138 (45)	273 (71)	239 (42)	96 (49)	56 (36)	110 (47)	1140 (35)
Soft tissue/myofascial (somatic)	398 (76)	328 (41)	94 (35)	94 (32)	186 (41)	43 (33)	93 (54)	80 (38)	1316 (45)
Visceral	32 (8)	583 (63)	83 (30)	26 (10)	171 (34)	26 (19)	21 (13)	53 (25)	995 (33)
Neuropathic	200 (47)	182 (23)	88 (32)	95 (35)	151 (33)	54 (38)	60 (40)	95 (41)	925 (34)
Unknown	26 (5)	44 (6)	35 (12)	7 (3)	19 (4)	8 (5)	14 (8)	13 (7)	166 (6)

Up to three pain syndromes could be coded, multiple selections possible.

HNR, head and neck region; GIT, gastrointestinal tract; RES, respiratory system; BRS, breast; GUS, genitourinary system; LHS, lymphatic-haematopoeitic system; SBC, skin, bones, connective tissue; OTH, others or more than 1.

within 1 week using the WHO guidelines for cancer pain relief.[74] This study points out the great variety of pain syndromes encompassed in the term 'cancer pain' and the importance of comprehensive assessment, not only for anticancer therapies but also for symptomatic pain management.

In order to use this extensive information to look at treatment effectiveness, investigators have proposed various methodologies to compare studies. Bruera has stressed the need for a cancer pain classification that would aid clinical trials research. He has developed the Edmonton Staging System for Cancer Pain.[75] Using prognostic factors, he has argued that the outcome of treatment can be better assessed and has advocated for validation of his measurement tool. By using specific, known prognostic factors like neuropathic pain, incidental pain, psychological distress, rapid tolerance and history of drug addiction or alcohol abuse, and the stage of disease, patients can be compared during treatment protocols. Such studies are currently in progress. Cleeland *et al.* have employed the pain management index to assess outcomes of pain treatment.[28] This index compares the analgesic drug used by a patient labelled according to the conventional position in the WHO analgesic ladder with the level of reported pain. The index is computed by subtracting the pain score from the analgesia score. Pain scores were categorized as 0 no pain, 1 mild pain, 2 moderate pain, and 3 severe pain. Analgesic drugs prescribed were scored for 0 no drugs for pain relief, 1 non-opioids, 2 weak opioids, and 3 strong opioids. The range varies from −3 (a patient with severe pain receiving no analgesic drugs) to 3, a patient receiving morphine or similar opioids and reporting no pain. Negative scores are a conservative indicator of undertreatment.

Mercadante *et al.* have used a variety of scales to relate pain assessment to treatment outcome.[76] They use an effective analgesic score which monitors the analgesic consumption to pain relief

Table 8 International Association for the Study of Pain classification of main pain syndrome—the percentage of patients is given[18]

	HNR (*n*=377)	GIT (*n*=663)	RES (*n*=218)	BRS (*n*=227)	GUS (*n*=379)	LHS (*n*=114)	SBC (*n*=121)	OTH (*n*=167)	Total (*n*=2266)
Axis I: Regions									
0 Head, face, mouth	68	1	1	2	1	4	12	11	14
1 Cervical region	17	1	4	1	0	2	4	4	4
2 Upper shoulder, upper limbs	3	2	9	14	3	9	12	8	6
3 Thoracic region	3	11	48	19	7	15	14	13	14
4 Abdominal region	0	45	6	8	19	13	5	14	20
5 Lower back, lumber spine, sacrum, coccyx	2	13	11	21	26	26	17	19	15
6 Lower limbs	1	4	5	6	11	11	17	9	6
7 Pelvic region	1	4	1	8	14	3	10	6	6
8 Anal, perianal, genital region	0	12	0	0	9	1	0	1	5
9 More than three major sites	3	6	14	19	9	14	8	14	9
Missing value	2	1	1	2	1	2	1	1	1
Axis II: Systems									
0 Nervous system (physical)	11	8	12	8	10	17	17	16	11
1 Nervous system (psychological)	1	0	0	1	1	1	1	1	1
2 Respiratory, cardiovascular system	6	1	22	2	1	2	1	4	4
3 Musculoskeletal system, connective tissue	43	17	43	60	39	56	52	45	38
4 Cutaneous, subcutaneous, glands	10	1	1	6	0	4	11	1	4
5 Gastrointestinal system	7	60	3	4	10	4	4	11	22
6 Genitourinary system	0	1	0	0	22	0	0	2	4
7 Other organs, viscera	9	2	3	1	3	12	4	5	4
8 More than one system	11	8	16	16	14	4	9	13	11
Missing value	2	2	0	2	0	0	1	2	1
Axis III: Temporal characteristics: pattern of occurrence									
0 Not recorded/not available	4	5	5	6	3	3	7	8	6
1 Single episode, limited duration	0	0	0	1	0	1	0	1	0
2 Continuous, non-fluctuating	36	35	33	34	33	29	33	32	34
3 Continuous, fluctuating	33	33	43	37	40	39	39	35	36
4 Recurring, irregularly	9	7	6	7	5	5	5	7	7
5 Recurring, regulary	2	5	1	4	4	4	2	1	3
6 Paroxysmal	1	2	0	0	1	2	2	1	1
7 Sustained with paroxysms	14	12	11	11	11	17	12	15	12
8 Other combinations	1	1	1	0	2	0	0	0	1
9 None of the abovel	0	0	0	0	1	0	0	0	0
Axis IV: Intensity: time since onset									
0 Not recorded/not available	2	5	5	4	3	4	4	6	3
1 Mild, < 1 month	0	1	1	1	1	0	1	1	1
2 Mild, 1–6 months	2	2	0	2	1	1	0	2	1
3 Mild, > 6 months	1	0	2	0	0	0	1	1	1
4 Medium, < 1 month	11	11	5	4	10	10	11	7	9
5 Medium, 1–6 months	13	11	11	12	11	7	11	13	12
6 Medium, > 6 months	5	6	2	3	4	5	7	5	5
7 Severe, < 1 month	26	23	27	31	24	32	31	24	26
8 Severe, 1–6 months	30	32	34	30	33	32	25	30	31
9 Severe, > 6 months	10	9	13	13	13	9	9	11	11
Axis V: Aetiology									
0 Genetic, congenital disorders	1	0	0	0	0	0	1	1	0
1 Trauma, operations, burns	9	8	6	5	5	2	14	5	7
2 Infective, parasitic	0	0	0	1	1	4	1	1	1
3 Inflammatory, immune reactions	0	1	1	1	0	0	2	1	1
4 Neoplasm	82	80	80	85	85	80	75	80	81
5 Toxic, metabolic, radiation	4	2	1	3	4	3	2	2	3
6 Degenerative, mechanical	1	2	1	1	1	4	1	2	1
7 Dysfunctional	0	1	1	1	0	0	0	2	1
8 Unknown or other	1	3	6	0	2	6	3	5	3
9 Psychological	1	0	0	0	0	0	0	0	0
Missing value	1	3	4	3	2	1	1	1	2

Abbreviations as given in Table 7.

ratios. He has also developed a formula to track opioid escalation index per cent using methodological formulas. He presents an alternative method to the Bruera and Cleeland approaches to compare patients during clinical trials to improve our understanding of pain management outcome.

Cancer pain syndromes

Cancer pain has also been classified according to a series of common pain syndromes and their pathophysiological mechanisms. The pain syndromes that occur commonly in patients with cancer have been evaluated in both inpatients and outpatient settings, and have been divided into three major categories:[1,2,3,8,9]

1. The first and most common cause of pain in patients with cancer is that associated with direct tumour involvement. This accounted for 78 per cent of pain problems in a survey of the Memorial Sloan-Kettering Cancer Center inpatient population and for 62 per cent of the problems in an outpatient survey. Metastatic bone disease, nerve compression or infiltration, and hollow viscus involvement are the most common causes of pain from direct tumour involvement.

2. The second group of pain syndromes are those associated with cancer therapy. This group accounts for approximately 19 per cent of pain problems in an inpatient population and 25 per cent of problems in an outpatient population. It includes pain that occurs in the course of, or as a result of, surgery, chemotherapy, or radiation therapy.

3. The third category of pain syndromes includes those unrelated to the cancer or the cancer therapy. Approximately 3 per cent of inpatients have pain unrelated to their cancer or their cancer therapy and this figure increases to 10 per cent when an outpatient population is surveyed.

These data reflect information about the prevalence of pain symptoms in adults with pain and cancer. Several other authors have noted comparable figures and have demonstrated that direct cancer involvement is the major cause of pain in cancer patients.[13,16,17] Studies of an inpatient population of children with cancer demonstrated that one-third of children in active therapy and two-thirds with advanced disease have significant pain.[8] Of interest, in children in active therapy, the major cause of pain is procedure-related pain, in contrast to tumour-related pain.

Specific pain syndromes in patients with cancer

In this section a series of acute and chronic pain syndromes that have been described in the cancer patient are briefly summarized. Some of the common or unique syndromes are considered to alert the reader to the wide spectrum of clinically relevant syndromes. They have been classified as acute or chronic, based on the review of Cherny and Portenoy and integrating the original Foley classification.[1,8,9] Tables 9 and 10 are comprehensive lists of these clinical syndromes.[9] The major, common neurological pain syndromes in cancer patients are discussed in Chapter 9.12.

Acute pain syndromes associated with cancer

There is a series of well-described, cancer-related acute pain syndromes that occur most commonly due to diagnostic or therapeutic interventions. Pain from tumour is typically chronic and may be recurrent. However, some tumour-related pains have an acute onset, such as pain from a metastatic bone fracture. Effective treatment for the underlying lesion is the common approach for management of such acute pain problems.

Acute pain associated with diagnostic intervention

Common, acute pain syndromes include pain following bone marrow aspiration and postlumbar puncture headache. Postlumbar puncture headache is an acute pain syndrome which is typically precipitated by assuming an upright posture.[77] The incidence of headache is related to the calibre of the lumbar puncture needle and to the amount of cerebrospinal fluid removed. Persistent lumbar puncture headache is thought to be related to continuous cerebrospinal fluid leak, with reduced cerebrospinal fluid volume and traction on the meninges secondary to the loss of volume. It usually occurs hours to several days following the procedure and is most commonly described as a dull pain, usually with associated neck and shoulder pain. Persistent headache may necessitate application of an epidural blood patch, but assuming a recumbent position will dramatically relieve the pain.[78,79]

Acute pain associated with invasive therapeutic intervention

These include the pain associated with tumour embolization, chemical pleurodesis, and the most common acute pain—postoperative pain. Each of these pain syndromes has a known aetiology and is associated with transient pain which slowly improves; for example with postoperative pain this occurs in a matter of several days to 1 week.[77]

Similarly, there are acute pain syndromes associated with analgesic techniques, ranging from the pain following injection by either the intramuscular or subcutaneous route or the pain induced in certain patients sensitive to histamine release. Opioid-induced headache is a rare complication of opioid drug therapy and appears to occur in a selective population of patients. Switching from morphine to drugs with less histamine release, such as oxymorphone or fentanyl, can often obviate this acute pain syndrome.[1] Spinal opioid hyperalgesia is a rare pain syndrome that occurs in patients following either epidural or intrathecal injections of high doses of opioids. It is typically characterized by hyperaesthesia and diffuse pain in the perineal, buttock, or both legs and may include segmental myoclonus and priapism.[80,81] The use of naloxone or a benzodiazepine has been reported anecdotally to provide relief. Reduction in the drug by its removal from the cerebrospinal fluid is associated with dramatic pain relief.

Acute pain associated with cancer therapy

Acute pain syndromes associated with chemotherapy ***Intravenous infusion pain*** Four intravenous infusion-related pain syndromes have been described; venospasm, chemical phlebitis, vesicant extravasation, and anthracycline-associated flare.[82,83]

Hepatic artery infusion pain Hepatic arterial infusion for patients with hepatic metastasis may be associated with a diffuse abdominal pain syndrome.[84] The pain is usually self-limiting and stops with discontinuation of the infusion. In rare instances, continuous infusions may be associated with a persistent pain syndrome. Some studies report that reduction in the infusion to a lower dose may ameliorate the syndrome.[85]

Intraperitoneal chemotherapy pain Approximately 25 per cent of patients receiving intraperitoneal chemotherapy reported transient, mild abdominal pain associated with a sensation of fullness and

Table 9 Cancer-related acute pain syndromes[9]

Acute pain associated with dignostic and therapeutic interventions

- Acute pain associated with diagnostic intervention
  - Lumbar puncture headache
  - Arterial or venous blood sampling
  - Bone marrow biopsy
  - Lumbar puncture
  - Colonoscopy
  - Myelography
  - Percutaneous biopsy
  - Thoracocentesis
- Acute postoperative pain
- Acute pain caused by other therapeutic interventions
  - Pleurodesis
  - Tumour embolization
  - Suprapubic catheterization
  - Intercostal catheter
  - Nephrostomy insertion
- Acute pain associated with analgesic techniques
  - Injection pain
  - Opioid headache
  - Spinal opioid hyperalgesia syndrome
  - Epidural injection pain

Acute pain associated with anticancer therapies

- Acute pain associated with chemotherapy infusion techniques
  - Intravenous infusion pain
    - Venous spasm
    - Chemical phlebitis
    - Vesicant extravasation
    - Anthracycline associated flare reaction
  - Hepatic artery infusion pain
  - Intraperitoneal chemotherapy abdominal pain
- Acute pain associated with chemotherapy toxicity
  - Mucositis
  - Corticosteroid-induced perineal discomfort
  - Steroid pseudorheumatism
  - Painful peripheral neuropathy
  - Headache
    - Intrathecal methotrexate meningitic syndrome
    - L-Asparaginase associated dural sinuses thrombosis
    - Trans-retinoic acid headache
  - Diffuse bone pain
    - Trans-retinoic acid
    - Colony stimulating factors
  - 5-flurouracil-induced anginal chest pain
  - Postchemotherapy gynaecomastia
- Acute pain associated with hormonal therapy
  - Luteinizing hormone releasing factor tumour flare in prostate cancer
  - Hormone-induced pain flare in breast cancer
- Acute pain associated with immunotherapy
  - Interferon-induced acute pain
- Acute pain associated with radiotherapy
  - Incident pain associated with positioning
  - Oropharyngeal mucositis
  - Acute radiation enteritis and proctocolitis
  - Early onset brachial plexopathy
  - Subacute radiation myelopathy

Acute pain associated with infection

- Acute herpes zoster

bloating. Another 25 per cent report moderate or severe pain necessitating opioid analgesia or discontinuation of the therapy.[86] The differential diagnosis of moderate to severe pain is either chemical peritonitis or infection. Certain drugs such as mitoxantrone and doxorubicin can produce chemical peritonitis. In those patients who develop fever and leucocytosis, an infectious peritonitis must be ruled out.[87,88]

Acute pain associated with chemotherapy toxicity Severe mucositis is the most common consequence of chemotherapy and/or radiotherapy. Grading systems for the severity of mucositis have

Table 10 Cancer-related chronic pain syndromes[9]

Tumour-related pain syndromes

- Bone pain
  - Multifocal or generalized bone pain
    - Multiple bony metastases
    - Marrow expansion
  - Vertebral syndromes
    - Atlantoaxial destruction and odontoid fractures
    - C7-T1 syndrome
    - T12-L1 syndrome
    - Sacral syndrome
  - Back pain and epidural compression
  - Pain syndromes of the bony pelvis and hip
    - Hip joint syndrome
- Headache and facial pain
  - Intracerebral tumour
  - Leptomeningeal metastases
  - Base of skull metastases
    - Orbital syndrome
    - Parasellar syndrome
    - Middle cranial fossa syndrome
    - Jugular foramen syndrome
    - Occipital condyle syndrome
    - Clivus syndrome
    - Sphenoid sinus syndrome
  - Painful cranial neuralgias
    - Glossopharyngeal neuralgia
    - Trigeminal neuralgia
- Tumour involvement of the peripheral nervous system
  - Tumour-related peripheral neuropathy
  - Cervical plexopathy
  - Brachial plexopathy
    - Malignant brachial plexopathy
    - Idiopathic brachial plexopathy associated with Hodgkin's disease
    - Malignant lumbosacral plexopathy
  - Paraneoplastic painful peripheral neuropathy
    - Subacute sensory neuropathy
    - Sensorimotor peripheral neuropathy
- Pain syndromes of the viscera and miscellaneous tumour-related syndromes
  - Hepatic distension syndrome
  - Midline retroperitoneal syndrome
  - Chronic intestinal obstruction
  - Peritoneal carcinomatosis
  - Malignant perineal pain
    - Malignant pelvic floor myalgia
  - Ureteric obstruction

Chronic pain syndromes associated with cancer therapy

- Post-chemotherapy pain syndromes
    - Chronic painful peripheral neuropathy
  - Avascular necrosis of femoral or humeral head
  - Plexopathy associated with intra-arterial infusion
  - Gynaecomastia with hormonal therapy for prostate cancer
- Chronic postsurgical pain syndromes
  - Postmastectomy pain syndrome
  - Postradical neck dissection pain
  - Post-thoracotomy pain
  - Postoperative frozen shoulder
  - Phantom pain syndromes
    - Phantom limb pain
    - Phantom breast pain
    - Phantom anus pain
    - Phantom bladder pain
  - Stump pain
  - Postsurgical pelvic floor myalgia
- Chronic postradiation pain syndromes
    - Radiation-induced peripheral nerve tumour
    - Radiation-induced brachial and lumbosacral plexopathies
  - Chronic radiation myelopathy
  - Chronic radiation enteritis and proctitis
  - Burning perineum syndrome
  - Osteoradionecrosis

been developed and its treatment usually requires the use of both local and systemic analgesic therapies. Superinfection with fungal or viral micro-organisms is common and careful attention to such infections is necessary to prevent systemic sepsis.[89]

Corticosteroid-induced perineal burning This pain syndrome is characterized by a transient burning sensation in the perineum following the rapid intravenous infusion of doses of dexamethasone. This transient pain lasts through the infusion time only and is usually associated with the use of large doses of dexamethasone in the range of 20 to 100 mg per intravenous bolus.[68]

Steroid pseudorheumatism This is another pain syndrome associated with the use of corticosteriods. It manifests as diffuse arthralgia and myalgia with muscle and joint tenderness following withdrawal from steroids. The symptoms occur with rapid or slow withdrawal, and may occur in patients who have been taking corticosteroids for long or short periods of time. The pathogenesis of this syndrome is poorly understood but it has been speculated that steroid withdrawal may sensitize joint and muscle mechanoreceptors and nociceptors. Treatment consists of reinstituting steroids at a higher dose and withdrawing them more slowly.[90]

Painful neuropathy or mononeuropathy A variety of chemotherapeutic agents may produce a toxic peripheral neuropathy. The syndrome is manifest by painful paraesthesia and hyper-reflexia and, less frequently, by motor and sensory loss or autonomic dysfunction. The drugs most commonly associated with peripheral neuropathy are the vinca alkaloids, especially vincristine, cisplatin, and procarbazine, and, more rarely, misonidazole and hexamethylmelamine. Dysaesthesias and paraesthesia occur in up to 100 per cent of patients treated with vinca alkaloids.[91-94] The painful sensations in patients with neuropathy are usually localized to the hands and feet, are burning in quality, and frequently exacerbated by cutaneous stimulation of the distal extremities. Many patients complain of a significant hyperaesthesia and may develop associated autonomic changes.

In patients with severe peripheral neuropathy and significant autonomic changes, sympathetic blocks may be indicated. In patients receiving intra-arterial infusion of a chemotherapeutic agent, such as cisplatin, into the iliac artery, the therapy may result in a lumbosacral plexopathy or mononeuropathy. In this syndrome, patients develop symptoms within 48 h of the procedure, characterized by the acute onset of pain, weakness, and paraesthesia in the distribution of the lumbosacral plexus. This syndrome is thought to be due to small vessel damage and infarction of the plexus or nerve at the site of injection. The prognosis for neurological recovery has not been fully established. Such patients have a pain syndrome of a neuropathic type, characterized by burning dysaesthetic pain in the leg, in an area with both motor and sensory dysfunction.

Chemotherapy-induced headache An acute meningitic syndrome can occur in 5 to 50 per cent of patients treated for leukaemia or leptomeningeal metastases with intrathecal methotrexate. Headache is the prominent symptom and may be associated with vomiting, nuchal rigidity, fever, irritability, and lethargy.[93,94] The symptoms usually begin within hours following the treatment and persist for several days. The cerebrospinal fluid examination reveals a pleocytosis which may mimic a bacterial meningitis. Patients at risk for the development of this syndrome include those who have received multiple intrathecal injections and those patients undergoing treatment for proven leptomeningeal metastases. A second syndrome associated with headache following chemotherapy administration is L-asparaginase-induced thrombosis of the cerebral veins or dural sinuses.[95] This occurs in upwards of 1 to 2 per cent of patients receiving this treatment as a result of the depletion of asparagine which leads to the reduction of plasma proteins involved in coagulation and fibrinolysis. Headache followed by seizures, hemiparesis, delirium, vomiting, or cranial nerve palsies may occur. The diagnosis is established by gradient-echo sequences on MR scan or by angiography. A third chemotherapeutic agent, trans-retinoic acid therapy, which is used in the treatment of acute promyelocytic leukaemia, can cause a transient severe headache.[96] The mechanism may be related to pseudo tumour induced by hypervitaminosis A.

Diffuse bone pain Acute bone pain is another common adverse effect of trans-retinoic acid therapy in patients with acute promyelocytic leukaemia. The pain is generalized, variable in intensity, and closely associated with a transient neutrophilia.[97] A similar pain syndrome occurs following the administration of colony stimulating factors.[98] The aetiology at the present time remains unclear.

5-Fluorouracil-induced anginal chest pain 5-Fluorouracil in continuous infusion may be associated with the development of ischaemic chest pain.[99,100] Coronary vasospasm is the underlying mechanism and studies with continuous ambulatory electrocardiograph monitoring of patients demonstrate a near three-fold increase in ischaemic episodes over pretreatment recordings. These electrocardiography changes were more common among patients with known coronary artery disease.

Postchemotherapy gynaecomastia Painful gynaecomastia can occur as a delayed complication of chemotherapy.[101] It occurs most commonly in testicular cancer and resolves spontaneously. It is thought to be secondary to cytotoxic-induced disturbance of androgen secretion and it needs to be differentiated from tumour-related gynaecomastia, which may herald early recurrence of a testicular tumour.

Acute pain associated with hormonal therapy *Luteinizing hormone releasing factor hormonal therapy* Initiation of luteinizing hormone releasing factor hormonal therapy in patients with prostate cancer can produce a transient flare in pain symptoms in 5 to 25 per cent of patients.[102] Exacerbation of bone pain or urinary retention are the most common associated symptoms. This syndrome occurs typically within the first week of therapy and lasts upwards of 1 to 3 weeks. Co-administration of an androgen antagonist at the start of luteinizing hormone releasing factor agonist therapy can prevent this tumour flare from occurring.

Hormone-induced pain flare in breast cancer Various hormonal therapies for the treatment of metastatic breast cancer can precipitate a sudden onset of diffuse musculoskeletal pain, commencing within hours to weeks of initiation of therapy.[103] Erythema around cutaneous lesions, changes in liver function studies, and hypercalcaemia are other manifestations of this hormone-induced tumour flare. The underlying mechanism is not understood.

Acute pain associated with immunotherapy *Interferon-induced acute pain* Virtually all patients treated with interferon experience an acute syndrome consisting of fever, chills, myalgia, arthralgia, and headache that often begin shortly after initial dosing and improves with continuous administration of the drug.[104] The severity of symptoms is related to the type of interferon, route of administration, schedule, and doses.

Acute pain associated with radiotherapy Oral pharyngeal mucositis, stomatitis, and/or pharyngitis are radiotherapy induced-acute pain syndromes involving the oral mucosa. They occur with doses above 1000 cGy.[105]These occur following radiation therapy to the head and neck region and are associated with inflammation and ulceration of mucus membranes. Acute cystitis, proctitis, and vaginitis can similarly occur with local radiation therapy to the perineal region. These syndromes occur several days to a week after the initiation of radiation therapy and may take several weeks to clear. The prevalence of these syndromes varies. There are data to suggest that following abdominal and pelvic radiotherapy 50 per cent of patients may develop an acute radiation proctocolitis associated with rectal pain, tenesmus diarrhoea, mucus discharge, and bleeding. A subacute radiation myelopathy may also occur and Lhermitte's sign has been reported as an early, acute pain syndrome in patients receiving radiation therapy to an area that includes the cervical or thoracic spinal cord.[106] It is most frequently observed after radiation therapy for head and neck cancers and Hodgkin's disease. It is characterized by a painful shock-like sensation in the neck precipitated by neck flexion. Such pains radiate down the spine and into one or more extremities. This syndrome usually begins weeks to months after the completion of radiotherapy and typically resolves within 3 to 6 months.

Acute pain associated with an infection

Cancer patients have a high incidence of viral infection, most commonly associated with the varicella virus and the clinical syndrome of acute herpetic neuralgia. Acute herpes zoster is characterized by the onset of pain or itch followed by the development of a dermatomal rash occurring in the trigeminal distribution or in the cervical thoracic or lumbar region. Pain is initially dull and aching, progressing to continuous, and is often associated with an acute, lancinating component. Postherpatic neuralgia is the term used to describe pain persisting beyond the clearance of the skin lesions. Progressive therapy with antiviral medications within 72 h of the eruptions has been demonstrated to reduce the prevalence of chronic pain syndromes secondary to this viral infection. In some instances acute herpes zoster may appear in an area overlying a malignancy and it occurs twice as frequently in previously irradiated dermatomes as in non-irradiated areas.[107,108]

Chronic pain syndromes associated with cancer

Chronic pain syndromes associated with direct tumour involvement

This category includes those syndromes associated with the common sites for tumour invasion of bone, hollow viscus, and nerve. Bone tumours, either primary or metastatic, are the most common cause of pain in patients with cancer. Tumour involvement of bone produces pain in one of two ways—by direct involvement of the bone and activation of nociceptors locally or by compression of the adjacent nerves, soft tissues, or vascular structures. (Bone pain is reviewed in detail in Chapters 9.1.2 and 9.2.11. The bone pain syndromes associated with neurological signs and symptoms are reviewed in Chapter 9.12.)

Pain from tumour invasion of a hollow viscus, with or without pleural or peritoneal involvement, is the second most common cause of pain in patients with cancer.[109,110] These syndromes have been described in the discussions of different tumour types (lung, pancreas, gynaecological) and are addressed in several of the chapters related to symptom control and intestinal obstruction.[64–68] A detailed description of these syndromes is beyond the scope of this chapter.

Tumour infiltration of nerve is the third most common cause of pain from direct tumour infiltration. Many of these are described in Chapters 9.2.1 and 9.2.10. Table 10 lists the common chronic pain syndromes evaluated by an inpatient and outpatient pain consultation service and by a supportive care programme in a comprehensive cancer centre.[1,8,9,15]

Hepatic distension syndrome Gross hepatomegaly or expanding intrahepatic metastasis may produce pain in the right subcostal region and occasionally in the right midback or flank.[111] The pain may be referred to the right neck or shoulder or in the region of the right scapula. The pain is typically described as dull and aching and maybe exacerbated by movement, pressure on the abdomen, and deep inspiration. It is commonly associated with anorexia and nausea. The pain originates from stretching of the hepatic capsule or from distension or compression of vessels in the biliary tract. Appropriate imaging of the liver and retroperitoneal space can determine the aetiology of the pain and steroids may be effective in treating tumour-induced hepatic distension.

Midline retroperitoneal syndrome Tumour infiltration of the pancreas or lymph node enlargement in the paravertebral and retroperitoneal spaces are the most common causes of pain referred to the posterior abdominal wall and bilateral flank region. The pain may also be referred anteriorly to the epigastrium. It is commonly dull and boring in character exacerbated by lying down and improved by sitting. CT or MRI scanning of the abdomen are the diagnostic procedures of choice. This syndrome needs to be differentiated from epidural cord compression which shares characteristic pain features with retroperitoneal tumour invasion.

Chronic intestinal obstruction Diffusive abdominal pain is a common complication of chronic gastrointestinal obstruction.[109] These syndromes and their treatment are discussed in Chapter 9.3.4.

Peritoneal carcinomatosis This syndrome occurs most commonly associated with colonic and ovarian cancer and is commonly associated with peritoneal inflammation, malignant adhesions, and ascites.[110] CT scanning may demonstrate evidence of a bowel infiltration and peritoneal nodules.

Malignant perineal pain Tumours of the gastrointestinal, genitourinary, and reproductive tract are commonly associated with perineal pain.[112] The pain is often characterized as constant and aching, aggravated by sitting or standing and maybe associated with tenesmus or bladder spasms. Characteristically, the tumour may spread by perineal invasion or by compression and infiltration of the musculature of the deep pelvis. CT and MRI scanning can provide an appropriate diagnosis, but many patients commonly complain of pain for long periods of time before radiological documentation of recurrent tumour. In this setting tumour markers can sometimes be used to document the progression of disease without radiological documentation.

Ureteric obstruction Tumour infiltration paravertebrally and within the pelvis is commonly associated with ureteric obstruction. Gastrointestinal, genitourinary, and gynaecological cancers are most commonly associated with progressive obstruction of the ureters.[112] The pain is commonly unilateral, radiating from the flank anteriorly to the groin region and exacerbated by standing and partially relieved by sitting. In some instances the pain maybe associated with acute spasms. The use of ultrasound, CT, or MRI can demonstrate the presence of hydronephrosis and define the site of compression. Ureteral stents can often dramatically improved this unilateral pain syndrome.

Chronic pain syndromes associated with cancer therapy

Postsurgical pain syndromes In assessing a patient with a postsurgical pain syndrome, knowledge of the exact time of onset of the syndrome is critical to help differentiate it from recurrent tumour. Postsurgical syndromes are characterized by either persistent pain following a surgical procedure or recurrent pain after the initial surgical pain has cleared. Several postsurgical pain syndromes have been characterized in cancer patients undergoing common surgical procedures.

Postmastectomy pain syndrome Four to 10 per cent of women who undergo any surgical procedure on the breast, from lumpectomy to radical mastectomy, are at risk to develop this syndrome. The pain can occur immediately, several days following the procedure, or as late as 6 months following the surgery.[68,113,114] Pain is characterized by a constricting, burning sensation localized to the posterior arm, axilla, and anterior chest wall in the area of sensory loss. It is aggravated by arm movement and relieved by immobilization. Patients often develop a frozen shoulder because they posture the arm in a flexed position, close to the chest wall, to reduce the pain associated with movement. In the majority of patients, a trigger point in the axilla or anterior chest wall can often be palpated and corresponds to the site of a traumatic neuroma. Following a series of anatomical studies, the aetiology of postmastectomy pain is believed to be a neuroma originating from the intercostobrachial nerve, a cutaneous sensory branch of T1, T2. The nature of the pain and the clinical symptoms should distinguish it readily from tumour infiltration of the brachial plexus. There is marked anatomical variation in the size and distribution of the intercostobrachial nerve, accounting for its variable appearance in patients undergoing mastectomy. The syndrome appears to occur more commonly in patients who have had postoperative complications at the time of their breast surgery, such as local haematoma, infection, or problems in wound closure. Those patients who demonstrated an increased risk for the development of keloids may also be at risk for this syndrome. The neuropathic quality of the pain is often reported by patients as dysaesthetic and hyperaesthetic and, on examination, a significant degree of allodynia may be demonstrated. In those patients complaining of a tight constricting sensation, breast reconstruction does not alter this phenomenon. Management of this pain syndrome includes physical therapy, local trigger point injections, sympathetic blocks, topical application of capsaicin, and, in isolated cases, surgical exploration of the area of traumatic neuroma.

Postradical neck dissection pain This pain results from injury to the cervical nerves and cervical plexus at the time of surgery. A sensation of tightness with burning dysaesthesias in the area of sensory loss are the characteristic symptoms. Patients typically report acute lancinating pain in the area of sensory loss. They may also complain of a second type of pain, resulting from the musculoskeletal imbalance that occurs in the shoulder following surgical removal of neck muscles, similar to the droopy shoulder syndrome. Thoracic outlet symptoms and signs of suprascapular nerve entrapment can occur.[115,116] Selective weakness and wasting of the supraspinatus muscles, with or without aching discomfort in the shoulder, are the characteristic clinical signs and symptoms. Escalating pain in this group of patients may signify recurrent tumour or soft-tissue infection. The latter is often difficult to diagnose in tissue damaged by radiation and surgery. Empirical treatment with antibiotics in patients with head and neck tumours and escalating pain has been reported to be associated with dramatic resolution of symptoms.[117] The diagnostic approach to these patients depends upon repeated CT scans through the area of pain and frequent head and neck examinations to rule out the presence of recurrent tumour. The treatment of patients with post-radical neck dissection pain includes physical therapy, trigger point injections, and appropriate bracing of the shoulder and back, as well as pharmacological approaches.

Post-thoracotomy pain This pain is typically characterized as an aching and burning sensation in the distribution of the thoracotomy incision, often associated with sensory loss and occasionally with autonomic changes. Patients complain of exquisite point tenderness at the most medical and apical points of the scar. The pain results from traction or disruption of the intercostal nerve following surgery on the chest wall. The intercostal neurovascular bundle (vein, artery, and nerve) courses along a groove in the inferior border of the rib. Traction on the ribs and rib resection are the common causes of nerve injury during a surgical procedure of the chest. Studies by Kanner, in a series of 126 patients undergoing thoracotomy at the Memorial Sloan-Kettering Cancer Center, have defined the pattern of pain following thoracotomy.[70] Kanner identified three groups of patients:

1. Group I consisted of patients with immediate postoperative pain that diminished by 2 months after surgery. When pain recurred in this group of patients, in all cases the pain was due to recurrence of tumour.
2. In Group II, in whom pain persisted following the thoracotomy and then increased during the follow-up period; local recurrences of disease and infection were the most common causes of increasing pain.
3. Group III had stable or decreasing pain, which gradually resolved over and 8-month period, although recurrence of the tumour was noted.

Late post-thoracotomy pain, which characterized patients in Group I and Group II, was due to recurrent or persistent tumour or infection. Thus, the persistence of pain for more than 8 months, the recurrence of pain after initial improvement, and the persistent escalating pain during the postoperative recovery all suggest recurrent tumour and, less commonly, infection as aetiological factors in this pain symptomatology. This is in contrast to patients with postmastectomy pain, where both a recurrent tumour and infection are rarely, if ever, associated with escalating pain symptomatology. Chest radiographs are insufficient to evaluate recurrent chest disease, and a CT scan through the chest, with bone and soft-tissue windows, is the diagnostic procedure of choice. The CT scan is also necessary prior to the consideration of an intercostal nerve block in the management of pain in these syndromes. If pain management is inadequate or patients are not actively rehabilitated following surgery, a frozen shoulder and a secondary reflex sympathetic dystrophy involving the arm may develop.

Phantom limb and stump pain Pain following surgical amputation of a limb is of two types—pain in the phantom limb and stump pain. Preamputation limb pain influences the development of phantom pain.

Phantom limb pain The incidence of phantom pain is significantly lower in patients with short-lasting preamputation pain and in patients who do not have pain in the limb the day before the amputation.[118,119] After amputation, phantom limb pain may initially magnify and then slowly fade over time. The pain has a paroxysmal burning or shooting quality and may be associated with bothersome paraesthesias. The phantom limb often assumes painful and unusual postures and, with time, telescopes as it approaches the stump. Preoperative lumbar epidural blockade significantly reduces the incidence of phantom limb pain in the first years after the amputation, and preoperative analgesic control appears to be the treatment of choice as multiple medical therapies, including antidepressants, opioids, anticonvulsants, sympathetic blockade, and transcutaneous electrical nerve stimulation (TENS), have met with limited success once the pain is well established.

Stump pain Stump pain occurs at the site of the surgical scar several months to years following amputation. It results from the development of a traumatic neuroma at the site of the nerve section. The pain is characterized by burning dysaesthesias, which are often exacerbated by movement and blocked by the injection of a local anaesthetic. Careful assessment of the patient with pain will help distinguish stump pain from phantom pain. Stump pain is treated by identifying the triggerpoint site and treating it locally, readjusting the prosthesis, and using drugs to suppress neuronal firing, such as anticonvulsants and antidepressants. Recurrence of pain in a phantom limb is an ominous sign, and should alert the physician to reassess the patient for proximal recurrence of tumour. We have evaluated several patients who began to complain of phantom leg pain several years after leg resection for primary tumours of bone. The pain proved to be the first symptom of recurrent disease in the pelvis following below-the-knee or above-the-knee amputation.[68]

Other phantom pain syndromes Several phantom pain syndromes have been described following surgical procedures.[120,121] These include phantom breast pain following mastectomy, which occurs in 15 to 30 per cent of patients and appears to occur most commonly in those patients who report preoperative pain. The pain tends to start in the region of the nipple and spread to the entire breast. Boas has reported a phantom anus syndrome occurring in 15 per cent of patients who undergo abdominal perineal resection. This pain syndrome may occur in the early postoperative period or after a latency of months to years. Of note, late onset pain is almost always associated with tumour recurrence.[121]

Postradiation pain syndromes Pain occurring as a complication of radiation therapy is less common than postchemotherapy and metastatic pain syndromes.[94] Pain occurs following damage to a peripheral nerve or the spinal cord, either as a result of changes in the microvasculature of the connective tissue surrounding the peripheral nerve, from fibrosis and chronic inflammation in connective tissues, or from demyelination and focal necrosis of white and grey matter in the spinal cord. These syndromes occur late in the course of a patient's illness and the differential diagnosis always includes recurrent tumour. In all instances, pain is a component of the syndrome but usually it is not as prominent a complaint as when the syndrome is associated with recurrent tumour.

Radiation fibrosis of the brachial plexus Pain in the distribution of the brachial plexus following radiation therapy is due to fibrosis of surrounding connective tissue and secondary nerve injury.[114,122,123] Pain occurs in only 18 per cent of patients at the time of presentation. Radiation changes in the skin, lymphoedema, and weakness in the C5, C6 distribution typically occur. This disorder may begin as early as 6 months or as late as 20 years after the radiation therapy. The neurological deficits are relentlessly progressive and ultimately result in a useless, often oedematous limb. In contrast to malignant infiltration, electromyogram studies show myokymic discharges. The CT scan usually demonstrates diffuse infiltration that cannot be distinguished from tumour infiltration. The MRI scan demonstrates diffuse soft-tissue changes that do not enhance with gadolinium. A careful history, knowledge of the radiation ports and total dose of radiation therapy, and a clear assessment of the patient's extent of disease, coupled with radiological and electrodiagnostic studies, can help in making the diagnosis.

Radiation fibrosis of the lumbosacral plexus Radiation fibrosis of the lumbosacral plexus is rare but may present from 1 to 30 years following radiation treatment.[124] The use of intracavity radium implants with pelvis radiation for carcinoma of the cervix may be an additional risk factor. Presenting symptoms include weakness of the legs, associated with sensory symptoms and numbness and paraesthesias. Pain occurs in only 10 per cent of patients. Symptoms and signs are usually bilateral upon presentation, and weakness commences distally in the L5, S1 segments and slowly progresses. Radiation necrosis of the pelvic bone commonly accompanies this disorder and can help in furthering the diagnosis.

Radiation myelopathy Pain may be an early symptom and is localized in the area of spinal cord damage. It is characterized as a typical central pain, burning in quality, associated with pain and temperature loss. This particular pain is often refractory to therapy and associated with significant motor and sensory neurological findings. MRI scan may demonstrate an area of hypointensity in the spinal cord. The aetiology is thought to be changes in both the vascular supply and myelin in the spinal cord.[94]

Radiation-induced peripheral nerve tumours Malignant peripheral nerve tumours and secondary primary tumours in a previously irradiated site may occur and present as a painful, expanding mass in a patient with a history of previously treated cancer. Patients with neurofibromatosis have an increased risk of developing malignant peripheral nerve tumours following radiation therapy.[123] The diagnosis may be difficult in a patient presumed cured of his underlying malignancy who presents with progressive pain, with or without a palpable mass in the plexus. The use of MRI scan can be helpful, particularly if there is evidence of gadolinium enhancement, but often the diagnosis is made by surgical exploration and pathological confirmation.

References

1. Foley KM. Management of cancer pain. In: DeVita VT, Hellman S, Rosenberg SA, eds. *Cancer: Principles and Practice of Oncology.* 5th edn. Philadelphia: J. Lippincott, 1996.
2. Portenoy RK. Cancer pain: pathophysiology and syndromes. *Lancet*, 1992; **339**: 1026–31.
3. Bonica JJ. *Management of Pain*. Philadelphia: Lea and Febiger, 1953.
4. Ingham, J, Portenoy R. Symptom assessment. *Hematology/Oncology Clinics of North America*. Philadelphia: W.B. Saunders, 1996; **10**: 21–39
5. Portenoy RK, *et al.* The Memorial Symptom Assessment Scale: an instrument for the evaluation of symptom prevalence, characteristics and distress. *European Journal of Clinical Oncology*, 1994; **30**: 1326–36.
6. Fishman B, *et al.* The Memorial Pain Assessment Card: a valid instrument for the assessment of cancer pain. *Cancer*, 1986; **60**: 1151–7.
7. Daut RL, Cleeland CS, Flanery RC. The development of the Wisconsin Brief Pain Questionnaire to assess pain in cancer and other diseases. *Pain*, 1983; **17**: 197–210.
8. Foley KM. Pain syndromes in patients with cancer. In: Bonica JJ, Ventafridda V, eds. *Advances in Pain Research and Therapy.* Vol 2. International Symposium on Pain in Advanced Cancer. New York: Raven Press, 1979: 59–76.
9. Cherny N, Portenoy RK. Cancer pain: principles of assessment and syndromes. In: Wall PD, Melzack R, eds. *Textbook of Pain.* 3rd edn. Edinburgh: Churchill Livingstone, 1994: 787–823.
10. World Health Organization. *Cancer Pain Relief.* 2nd edn. Geneva: World Health Organization, 1995.
11. World Health Organization. *Cancer Pain Relief and Palliative Care.* Geneva: World Health Organization, 1990.
12. Ahles TA, Ruckdeschel JC, Blanchard EB. Cancer-related pain –1. Prevalence in an outpatient setting as a function of stage of disease and type of cancer. *Journal of Psychosomatic Research*, 1984; **28**: 115–19.
13. Banning A, Sjogren P, Henriksen H. Pain causes in 200 patients referred to a multidisciplinary cancer pain clinic. *Pain*, 1991; **45**: 45–8.
14. Brescia FJ *et al.* Hospitalized advanced cancer patients: a profile. *Journal of Pain and Symptom Management*, 1990; **5**: 221–7.
15. Coyle N *et al.* Character of terminal illness in the advanced cancer patient: pain and other symptoms during the last four weeks of life. *Journal of Pain and Symptom Management*, 1990; **5**: 83–93.
16. Daut RL, Cleeland CS. The prevalence and severity of pain in cancer. *Cancer*, 1982; **50**: 1913–18.
17. Greenwald HP, Bonica JJ, Bergner M. The prevalence of pain in four cancers. *Cancer*, 1987; **60**: 2563–9.
18. Grond S, Zech D, Diefenbach C, Radbruch L, Lehmann K. Assessment of cancer pain: a prospective evaluation in 2266 cancer patients referred to a pain service. *Pain*, 1996; **64**: 107–14.
19. Kelsen DP, Portenoy RK, Thaler HT, Niedzwiecki D, Passik SD, Tao Y, *et al.* Pain and depression in patients with newly diagnosed pancreas cancer. *Journal of Clinical Oncology*, 1995; **13**: 748–55.
20. Larue F, Colleau SM, Brasseur L, Cleeland CS. Multicentre study of cancer pain and its treatment in France. *British Medical Journal*, 1995; **310**: 1034–7.
21. Portenoy RK, Kornblith AB, Wong G, Vlamis V, Lepore JM, Loseth DB, *et al.* Pain in ovarian cancer patients: prevalence, characteristics, and associated symptoms. *Cancer*, 1994; **74**: 907–15.
22. Portenoy RK, Miransky J, Thaler HT, Hornung J, Bianchi C, Cibas-Kong I, *et al.* Pain in ambulatory patients with lung or colon cancer: prevalence, characteristics and impact. *Cancer*, 1992; **70**: 616–24.
23. Stjernsward J, Teoh N. The scope of the cancer pain problem. In: Foley KM, Bonica JJ, Ventafridda V, eds. *Advances in Pain Research and Therapy.* Vol 16. Second International Congress on Cancer Pain. New York: Raven Press, 1990: 7–12.
24. Tay WK, Shaw RJ, Goh CR. A survey of symptoms in hospice patients in Singapore. *Annals of the Academy of Medicine Singapore*, 1994; **23**: 191–6.
25. Twycross RG, Fairfield S. Pain in far advanced cancer. *Pain*, 1982; **14**: 303–10.
26. Zenz M, Zenz T, Tryba M, Strumpf M. Severe undertreatment of cancer pain: a 3 year survey of the German situation. *Journal of Pain and Symptom Management*, 1995; **10**: 187–91.
27. Von Roenn JH, Cleeland CS, Gonin R, Hatfield A, Pandya KJ. Physicians' attitudes and practice in cancer pain management: A survey from the Eastern Cooperative Oncology Group. *Annals of Internal Medicine*, 1993; **119**: 121–6.
28. Cleeland CS, Gonin R, Hatfield A, Edmonson MD, Blum RH, Stewart JA, *et al.* Pain and its treatment in outpatients with metastatic cancer. *New England Journal of Medicine*, 1994; **330**: 592–6.
29. Larue F, Colleau SM, Fontaine A, Brasseur L. Oncologists and primary care physicians' attitudes towards pain control and morphine prescribing in France. *Cancer*, 1995; **76**: 2181–5.
30. Breitbart W. Psychiatric management of cancer pain. *Cancer*, 1989; **63**: 2336–42.
31. Morris JN *et al.* The effects of treatment settings and patient characteristics on pain in terminal cancer patients: a report from the National Hospice Study. *Journal of Chronic Diseases*, 1986; **39**: 27–35.
32. Shannon M, Ryan M, D'Agostino N, Brescia F. Assessment of pain in advanced cancer patients. *Journal of Pain and Symptom Management*, 1995; **10**: 274–8.
33. DeConno F, Caraceni A, Gamba A, Mariani L, Abbattista A, Brunelli C, La Mura A, Ventafridda V. Pain measurements in cancer patients: a comparison of six methods. *Pain*, 1994; **57**: 151–66.
34. Cherny N, Catane R. Professional negligence in the management of cancer pain. *Cancer*, 1995; **76**: 2181–4.
35. Foley KM. Pain relief into practice: rhetoric without reform. *Journal of Clinical Oncology*, 1995; **13**: 2149–51.
36. Levin DN, Cleeland CS, Dar R. Public attitudes toward cancer pain. *Cancer*, 1985; **56**: 2337–9.
37. Lin CC, Ward SE. Patient-related barriers to cancer pain management in Taiwan. *Cancer Nursing*, 1995; **18**: 16–22.
38. Wallace K, Reed B, Pasero C, Olsson G. Staff nurses' perceptions of barriers to effective pain management. *Journal of Pain and Symptom Management*, 1995; **10**: 204–13.
39. Ward SE, Goldberg N, Miller-McCauley V, Mueller C, Nolan A, Pawlik-Plank D, *et al.* Patient related barriers to management of cancer pain. *Pain*, 1993; **52**: 319–24.
40. Zenz M, Willweber-Strumpf A. Opiophobia and cancer pain in Europe. *Lancet*, 1993; **341**: 1075–6.
41. Elliott T, *et al.* Physician knowledge and attitudes about cancer pain management: a survey from the Minnesota cancer pain project. *Journal of Pain and Symptom Management*, 1995; **10**: 494–504.
42. Grossman SA, Sheidler VR, Swedeen K, Mucenski J, Piantadosi S. Correlation of patient and caregiver ratings of cancer pain. *Journal of Pain and Symptom Management*, 1991; **6**: 53–7.
43. Max M, Donovan M, Miaskowski C, *et al.* American pain society quality improvement guidelines for the treatment of acute and chronic pain. *Journal of the American Medical Association*, 1995; **274**: 1874–80.
44. Joranson DE, Cleeland CS, Weissman DE, *et al.* Opioids in chronic cancer and non- cancer pain: A survey of state medical board members. *Federal Bulletin: Journal of Medical Licensure and Discipline*, 1992; **79**:15–49.
45. Hill CS, Fields S, eds. *Advances in Pain Research and Therapy. Drug Treatment of Cancer Pain in a Drug-Oriented Society.* Vol. 11. New York: Raven Press, 1989.
46. Bookbinder M, Coyle N, Thaler H, *et al.* Implementing national standards for cancer pain management: program model and evaluation. *Oncology Nursing Forum*, 1995.
47. International Association for the Study of Pain. Classification of chronic pain. *Pain*, 1986; Suppl. 3: 51–226.
48. Portenoy RK, Hagen NA. Breakthrough pain: definition, prevalence and characteristics. *Pain*, 1990; **41**: 273–82.
49. Tearnan J, Blake H, Cleeland CS. Unaided use of pain descriptors by patients with cancer pain. *Journal of Pain and Symptom Management*, 1990; **5**: 228–32.

50. Wallenstein SL. Measurement of pain and analgesia in cancer patients. *Cancer*, 1984; **53**: 2217–384.
51. Ahles TA, Ruckdeschel JH, Blanchard EB. Cancer-related pain–II. Assessment with visual analogue scales. *Journal of Psychosomatic Research*, 1984; **28**: 121–4.
52. Norvell C, Turner K, Gaston-Johansson F, Fannie, Zimmerman L. Pain description by nurses and physicians. *Journal of Pain and Symptom Management*, 1990; **5**:11–17.
53. Peteet J, *et al.* Pain characteristics and treatment in an outpatient cancer population. *Cancer*, 1986; **57**: 1259–65.
54. McGrath PJ, Beyer J, Cleeland C, Eland J, McGrath PA, Portenoy RK. Report of the subcommittee on assessment and methodologic issues in the management of pain in childhood cancer. *Pediatrics*, 1990; **86**: 813–34.
55. Chapman CR, Hill HF. Prolonged morphine self-administration and addiction liability. *Cancer*, 1989; **63**: 1636–44.
56. Salzburg D, Foley KM. The management of pancreatic cancer pain. In: Reber H, ed. *Surgical Clinics of North America*. Philadelphia: W.B. Saunders, 1989: 629–50.
57. Portenoy RK, Foley KM, Inturrisi CE. The nature of opioid responsiveness and its implications for neuropathic pain: new hypotheses derived from studies of opioid infusions. *Pain*, 1990; **43**: 273–86.
58. Cassell EJ. The nature of suffering and the goals of medicine. *New England Journal of Medicine*, 1982; **306**: 639–45.
59. Saunders C. *The Management of Terminal Illness*. London: Edward Arnold, 1967.
60. Portenoy RK, Payne R. Acute and chronic pain. In: Lowinson J, Ruiz P, Millman R. *Substance Abuse*. Baltimore: Williams and Wilkins, 1992.
61. Foley KM, Cherny NI. Guidelines for the care of the dying. In: Cherny NI, Foley KM, eds. *Hematology/Oncology Clinics of North America*. Philadelphia: W.B. Saunders, 1996: 261–86.
62. Cherny NI, Foley KM. Bachial plexopathy in patients with breast cancer. In: Harris JR, Hellman S, Henderson IC, Kinne D, eds. *Breast Diseases*. 3rd edn. Philadelphia: JP Lippincott, 1996: 796–808.
63. Spiegel D, Bloom JR. Pain in metastatic breast cancer. *Cancer*, 1983; **52**: 341–5.
64. Cherny NI, Coyle N, Foley KM. Suffering in the advanced cancer patient. Part I: A definition and taxonomy. *Journal of Palliative Care*, 1994; **10**: 57–70.
65. Roth A, Breitbart W. Psychiatric emergencies in terminally ill cancer patients. *Hematology/Oncology Clinics of North America*. Philadelphia: W.B. Saunders, 1996; **10**: 235–59.
66. Cherny NI, Coyle N, Foley KM. The treatment of suffering when patients request elective death. *Journal of Palliative Care*, 1994; **10**: 71–9.
67. Foley KM. The relationship of pain and symptom management to patient requests for physician-assisted suicide. *Journal of Pain and Symptom Management*, 1991; **6**: 289–97.
68. Elliott K, Foley KM. Neurologic pain syndromes in patients with cancer. *Neurologic Clinics*, 1989; **7**: 333–60.
69. Kanner RW, Martini N, Foley KM. Epidural spinal cord compression in Pancoast syndrome (superior pulmonary sulcus tumor): clinical presentation and outcome. *Annals of Neurology*, 1981; **10**: 77.
70. Kanner R, Martini N, Foley KM. Nature and incidence of post-thoracotomy pain. *Proceedings of the American Society of Clinical Oncology*, 1982; **1**: 152.
71. Cherny NI, Arbit E, Jain S. Invasive techniques in the management of cancer pain. In: Cherny NI, Foley KM, eds. *Hematology/Oncology Clinics of North America. Pain and Palliative Care*. Philadelphia: W.B. Saunders, 1996; **10**: 121–37
72. Gonzalez GR, Elliott KJ, Portenoy RK, Foley KM. Impact of a comprehensive evaluation in the management of cancer pain. *Pain*, 1991; **47**: 141–4.
73. Clouston P, DeAngelis L, Posner JB. The spectrum of neurologic disease in patients with systemic cancer. *Annals of Neurology*, 1992; **31**: 268–73.
74. Zech D, Grond S, Lynch J, Hertel D, Lehmann K. Validation of World Health Organization Guidelines for cancer pain relief: a 10-year prospective study. *Pain*, 1995; **63**: 65–76.
75. Bruera E, MacMillan K, Hanson J, MacDonald RN. The Edmonton staging system for cancer pain: a preliminary report. *Pain*, 1989; **37**: 203–9.
76. Mercadante S. Celiac plexus block versus analgesics in pancreatic cancer pain. *Pain*, 1993; **52**: 187–92.
77. Raskin NH. Lumbar puncture headache: a review. *Headache*, 1990; **30**: 197–200.
78. Heide W, Diener HC. Epidural blood patch reduces the incidence of post lumbar puncture headache. *Headache*, 1990; **30**: 280–1.
79. Acute Pain Management Guideline Panel. *Acute Pain Management: Operative or Medical Procedures and Trauma: Clinical Practice Guideline*. AHCPR Pub. No. 92–0032. Rockville, MD: US Public Health Service, Agency for Health Care Policy and Research, 1992.
80. Stillman MJ, Moulin DE, Foley KM. Paradoxical pain following high-dose spinal morphine. *Pain*, 1987; suppl. 4: 389.
81. DeConno F, Caracenti A, Martini C, Spoldi E, Salvetti M, Ventafridda V. Hyperalgesia and myoclonus with intrathecal infusion of high-dose morphine. *Pain*, 1991; **47**: 337–9.
82. Molloy HS, Seipp CA, Duffey P. Administration of cancer treatments: practical guide for physicians and oncology nurses. In: DeVita VT, Hellman S, Rosenberg SA, eds. *Cancer: Principles and Practice of Oncology*, 3rd edn. Philadelphia: Lippincott, 1989: 2369–402.
83. Curran CF, Luce JK, Page JA. Doxorubicin-associated flare reactions. *Oncology Nursing Forum*, 1990; **17**: 387–9.
84. Kemeny N, Cohen A, Bertino J, Sigerson ER, Botet J, Oderman P. Continuous intrahepatic infusion of floxuridine and leucovorin through an implantable pump for the treatment of hepatic metastases from colorectal carcinoma. *Cancer*, 1990; **65**: 2446–50.
85. Botet JF, Watson RC, Kemeny N, Daly JM, Yeh S. Cholangitis complicating intraarterial chemotherapy in liver metastasis. *Radiology*, 1985; **156**: 335–7.
86. Almadrones L, Yerys C. Problems associated with the administration of intraperitoneal therapy using the Port-A-Cath system. *Oncology Nursing Forum*, 1990; **17**: 75–80.
87. Fitsch E, Sevelda P, Schmidl S, Salzer H. First experiences with intraperitoneal chemotherapy in ovarian cancer. *European Journal of Gynaecological Oncology*, 1990; **11**: 19–22.
88. Markman M, Howell SB, Lucas WE, Pfeifle CE, Green MR. Combination intraperitoneal chemotherapy with cisplatin, cytarabine, and doxorubicin for refractory ovarian carcinoma and other malignancies principally confined to the peritoneal cavity. *Journal of Clinical Oncology*, 1984; **2**: 1321–6.
89. Chapko MK, Syrjala KL, Schilter L, Cummings C, Sullivan KM. Chemoradiotherapy toxicity during bone marrow transplantion: time course and variation in pain and nausea. *Bone Marrow Transplantion*, 1990; **4**: 181–6.
90. Rotstein J, Good RA. Steroid pseudorheumatism. *Archives of Internal Medicine*, 1957; **99**: 545–55.
91. Mollman JE *et al.* Cisplatin neuropathy: risk factors, prognosis and protection by WR- 2721. *Cancer*, 1988; **61**: 2192–5.
92. Mollman JE *et al.* Unusual presentation of cis-platinum neuropathy. *Neurology*, 1988; **38**: 488–90.
93. Weiss HD, Walker MD, Wiernik PH, *et al.* Neurotoxicity of commonly used antineoplastic agents. *New England Journal of Medicine*, 1974; **291**: 75–81.
94. Posner J. *Neurologic Complications of Cancer*. Philadelphia: F.A. Davis Company, 1995.
95. Feinberg WM, Swenson MR. Cerebrovascular complications of L-asparaginase therapy. *Neurology*, 1988; **38**: 127–33.
96. Huang ME, Ye YC, Chen SR, *et al.* Use of all-trans retinoic acid in the treatment of acute promyelocytic leukemia. *Blood*, 1988; **72**: 567–72.
97. Castaigne S, Chomienne C, Daniel MT, *et al.* All-trans retinoic acid as a differentiation therapy for acute promyelocytic leukemia. I. Clinical results. *Blood*, 1990; **76**: 1704–9.
98. Balmer CM. Clinical use of biologic response modifiers in cancer treatment: an overview. Part II. Colony-stimulating factors and interleukin-2. *DICP*, 1991; **25**: 490–8.

99. Freeman NJ, Costanza ME. 5-Fluorouracil-associated cardiotoxicity. *Cancer*, 1988; **61**: 36–45.
100. Eskilsson J, Albertsson M. Failure of preventing 5-fluorouracil cardiotoxicity by prophylactic treatment with verapamil. *Acta Oncologica*, 1990; **29**: 1001–3.
101. Trump DL, Anderson SA. Painful gynecomastia following cytotoxic therapy for testis cancer: a potentially favorable prognostic sign? *Journal of Clinical Oncology*, 1983; **1**: 416–20.
102. Thompson IM, Ziedman EJ, Rodriguez FR. Sudden death due to disease flare with luteinizing hormone-releasing hormone agonist. *Journal of Urology*, **144**: 1479–80.
103. Henderson, JC, Harris JR. Principles in the management of metastatic disease. In: Harris JR, Hellman S, Henderson IC, Kinne D, eds. *Breast Diseases*, 2nd edn. Philadelphia: J.B. Lipincott.
104. Quesada JR, Talpaz M, Rios A, Kurzrock R, Gutterman JU. Clinical toxicity of interferons in cancer patients: a review. *Journal of Clinical Oncology*, 1986; **4**: 234–43.
105. Rider CA. Oral mucositis. A complication of radiotherapy. *New York State Dental Journal*, 1990; **56**: 37–9.
106. Earnist DL, Trier JS. Radiation enteritis and colitis. In: Sleisenger MH, Fordtran JS, eds. *Gastrointestinal Disease: Pathophysiology Diagnosis Management* Vol. 2. Philadelphia: Saunders, 1989: 1369–82.
107. Watson CPN, Watt VR, Chipman M, Birkett N, Evans RJ. Prognosis with post-herpetic neuralgia. *Pain*, 1991; **46**:195–9.
108. Portenoy RK, Duma C, Foley KM. Acute herpetic and postherpetic neuralgia: clinical review and current management. *Annals of Neurology*, 1986; **20**: 651–64.
109. Baines M, Oliver DJ, Carter RL. Medical management of intestinal obstruction in patients with advanced malignant disease: a clinical and pathological study. *Lancet*, 1985; **2**: 990–3.
110. Cherny N, Foley KM. Colorectal and anal cancer pain: pathophysiology, assessment, syndromes and management. In: Cohen AM, Winawer SJ, Friedman MA, Gunderson LL, eds. *Cancer of the Colon, Rectum, and Anus*. New York: McGraw-Hill, 1994: 1075–117.
111. Mulholland MW, Debas H, Bonica JJ. Diseases of the liver, biliary system and pancreas. In: Bonica JJ, ed. *The Management of Pain*. Vol. 2. Philadelphia: Lea and Febiger, 1990: 1214–31.
112. Stillman MJ. Perineal pain: diagnosis and management, with particular attention to perineal pain of cancer. In: Foley KM, Bonica JJ, Ventafridda V, eds. *Advances in Pain Research and Therapy*. Vol 16. Second International Congress on Cancer Pain. New York: Raven Press, 1990: 359–78.
113. Granek I, Ashikari R, Foley KM. Postmastectomy pain syndrome: Clinical and anatomic correlates. *Proceedings of the American Society of Clinical Oncology*, 1983; 3:122.
114. Vecht CJ. Arm pain in the patient with breast cancer. *Journal of Pain and Symptom Management*, 1990; **5**: 109–17.
115. Cailliet R. *Shoulder Pain*. Philadelphia: FA Davis, 1966.
116. Swift TR, Nichols FT. The droopy shoulder syndrome. *Neurology*, 1984; **34**: 212–15.
117. Bruera E, Macdonald N. Intractable pain in patients with advanced head and neck tumors: A possible role of local infection. *Cancer Treatment Reports*, 1986; **70**: 691–2.
118. Bressler B, Cohen SJ, Magnussen S. The problem of phantom breast and phantom pain. *Journal of Nervous and Mental Disorders*, 1955; **123**: 181–7.
119. Frederiks JAM. Phantom limb and phantom limb pain. In: Fredericks JAM, ed. *Handbook of Clinical Neurology*. Vol 1, *Clinical Neuropsychology*. New York: Elsevier Science Publishers, 1985: 395–404.
120. Kroner K, Krebs B, Skov J, Jorgensen HS. Immediate and long-term phantom breast syndrome after mastectomy: incidence, clinical characteristic relationship to pre-mastectomy breast pain. *Pain*, 1989; **36**: 327–35.
121. Boas RA. Phantom anus syndrome. In: Bonica JJ, Lindblom U, Iggo A, eds. *Proceedings of the Third World Congress on Pain. Advances in pain research and therapy*. Vol 5. New York: Raven Press, 1983: 947–51.
122. Foley KM. Brachial plexopathy in patients with breast cancer. In: Harris JR, Hellman S, Henderson IC, Kinne D, eds. *Breast Diseases*. Philadelphia: JP Lippincott, 1987: 532–7.
123. Foley KM, Woodruff JM, Ellis FT. Radiation-induced malignant and atypical peripheral nerve sheath tumors. *Archives of Neurology*, 1980; **7**: 311–18.
124. Glass JP, Foley KM. Harmful effects of radiation. In: Asbury AK, McKhann GM, McDonald WI, eds. *Diseases of the Nervous System*. Philadelphia: WB Saunders, 1986: 1188–202.

9.2.3 Opioid analgesic therapy

Geoffrey Hanks and Nathan Cherny

Introduction

Treatment with analgesic drugs is the mainstay of cancer pain management.[1-3] Although concurrent use of other approaches and interventions may be appropriate in many patients, and necessary in some, analgesic drugs are needed in almost every case. Drugs whose primary clinical action is the relief of pain are conventionally classified on the basis of the site of activity at opioid receptors as either opioid or non-opioid analgesics. A third class, the adjuvant analgesics, are drugs with other primary indications that can be effective analgesics in specific circumstances. The major group of drugs used in cancer pain management are the opioid analgesics.

During the last 20 years there has been a dramatic increase in our knowledge of the sites and mechanism of action of the opioids.[4] The development of analytical methods has also been of great importance in facilitating pharmacokinetic studies of the disposition and fate of opioids in patients. These studies have begun to offer us a better understanding of some of the sources of variation between individuals in the response to opioids and to suggest ways of minimizing some of their adverse effects.[5] Although there are gaps in our knowledge of opioid pharmacology, the rational and appropriate use of these drugs is based on the knowledge of their pharmacological properties derived from well-controlled clinical trials.[6-9]

Terminology

In this chapter and throughout this text we have adopted the following conventions in terminology.

Opiate is a specific term which is used to describe drugs (natural and semisynthetic) derived from the juice of the opium poppy.[10] For example, morphine is an opiate but methadone (a completely synthetic drug) is not.

Opioid is a general term which includes naturally occurring, semisynthetic, and synthetic drugs which produce their effects by combining with opioid receptors and are stereospecifically antagonized by naloxone. In this context we refer to opioid agonists, opioid antagonists, opioid peptides, and opioid receptors.

Narcotic is commonly used to describe morphine-like drugs and other drugs of abuse. The term is derived from the Greek

Table 1 Responses mediated by activation of opioid receptors

Receptor	Response on activation
μ	Analgesia, respiratory depression, miosis, euphoria, reduced gastrointestinal motility
κ	Analgesia, dysphoria, psychotomimetic effects, miosis*, respiratory depression*
δ	Analgesia†

* Less intense than with μ activation.
† Not yet defined in humans.

narke, meaning numbness or torpor. Since this is an imprecise and pejorative term that is not useful in a pharmacological context, its use with reference to opioids is discouraged. The term narcotic is not used in this book.

Opioid receptors

Opioids are agonists at highly specific receptor sites, and there is general agreement on the existence of at least three types of opioid receptor: the morphine receptor μ (mu), the receptor κ (kappa) at which the prototype agonist is ketocyclazocine, and the enkephalin receptor δ (delta).[11] A fourth receptor, σ (sigma), was originally identified by Martin *et al.*,[12] but it is not a true opioid receptor because actions mediated through it are not reversed by naloxone. The μ receptors have been further subclassified into two distinct subtypes (μ_1 and μ_2), as have the δ receptors (δ_1 and δ_2). Kappa receptors have been divided into κ_1, κ_2, and κ_3 subtypes. Recently, several of these receptors have been successfully cloned.[13-16]

Table 1 shows the putative effects mediated by the three main opioid receptors;[17] this classification is based on the original description by Martin *et al.*[12] The effects presumed to be mediated at μ receptors have been defined as a result of numerous human and animal studies, while the effects mediated at κ receptors derive predominantly from animal responses. κ receptors mediate analgesia that persists in animals made tolerant to δ agonists; κ agonists produce less respiratory depression and miosis than μ agonists. The effects mediated by δ receptors are extrapolated entirely from animals. It is assumed that opioid receptors mediate the sedative and mental clouding effects of opioids, in addition to their other pharmacological actions.

Opioid receptors are found in several areas of the brain, particularly in the periaqueductal grey matter, and throughout the spinal cord. Supraspinal systems have been described for μ_1, κ_3, and δ_2 receptors, whereas μ_2, κ_1, and δ_1 receptors modulate pain at the spinal level.[11] Although our understanding of the effect profiles of opioid receptors is incomplete, the available information can be used to explain the apparently complex effects of the mixed agonist–antagonist group of opioid analgesics.

Agonists, antagonists, potency, and efficacy

Based on their interactions with the various receptor subtypes, opioid compounds can be divided into agonist, agonist–antagonist, and antagonist classes (Table 2)

Agonists

An agonist is a drug which has affinity for and binds to cell receptors to induce changes in the cell which stimulate physiological activity. The agonist opioid drugs have no clinically relevant ceiling effect to analgesia. As the dose is raised, analgesic effects increase in a log linear function, until either analgesia is achieved or dose-limiting adverse effects supervene. Efficacy is defined by the maximal response induced by administration of the active agent. In practice, this is determined by the degree of analgesia produced following dose escalation through a range limited by the development of adverse effects. Potency, in contrast, reflects the dose–response relationship. Potency is influenced by pharmacokinetic factors (i.e. how much of the drug enters the body systemic circulation and then reaches the receptors) and by affinity to drug receptors.

The concepts of efficacy and potency are illustrated in Fig. 1 which shows the dose–response for two drugs A and B. If the logarithm of dose is plotted against response an agonist will produce an S-shaped or sigmoid curve. The efficacy of the two drugs, defined by maximum response is the same. Drug A produces

Table 2 Classification of opioid analgesics into agonist, agonist–antagonist and antagonist classes

Agonists	Partial agonists
Morphine	Buprenorphine
Codeine	
Oxycodone	
Dihydrocodeine	**Agonist–antagonists**
Oxymorphone	Pentazocine
Pethidine	Butorphanol
Levorphanol	Nalbuphine
Hydromorphone	Dezocine
Methadone	Meptazinol
Fentanyl	
Dextropropoxyphene	
Diamorphine (heroin)	**Antagonists**
Tramadol	Naloxone
Phenazocine	Naltrexone
Dextromoramide	
Dipipanone	

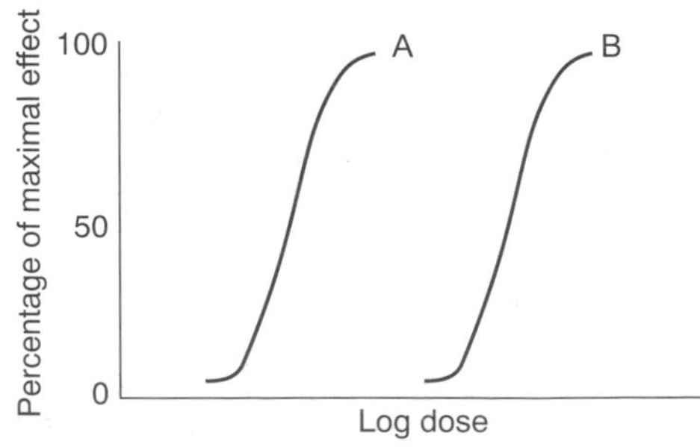

Fig. 1 Dose–response curves for two full opioid agonists (A and B) similar in efficacy but different in potency (A is more potent than B).

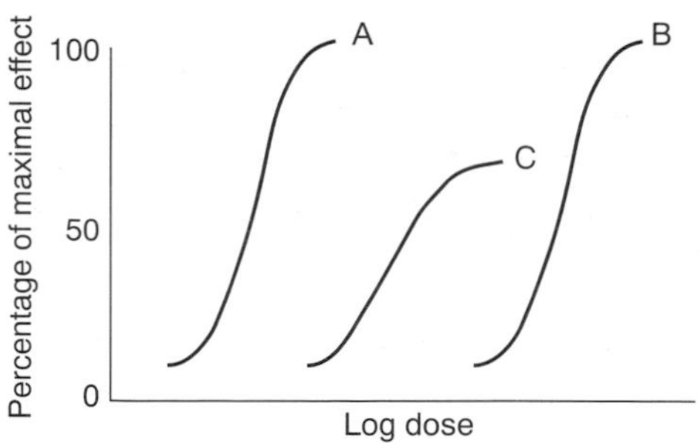

Fig. 2 Dose–response curves for two full opioid agonists (A and B) and a partial opioid agonist C.

the same response as B but at a lower dose, and therefore is described as more potent.

Antagonist

Antagonist drugs have no intrinsic pharmacological action but can interfere with the action of an agonist. Competitive antagonists bind to the same receptor and compete for receptor sites, whereas non-competitive antagonists block the effects of the agonist in some other way.

Agonist–antagonist

The agonist–antagonist analgesics can, in turn, be subdivided into the mixed agonist–antagonists and the partial agonists, a distinction also based on specific patterns of drug-receptor interaction.[4,17] Both the partial agonist and agonist–antagonist drugs have a ceiling effect for analgesia, and although they produce analgesia in the opioid-naïve patient, they can precipitate withdrawal in patients who are physically dependent on morphine-like drugs. For these reasons they have a limited role in the management of patients with cancer pain.

Mixed agonist–antagonists

The mixed agonist–antagonist drugs produce agonist effects at one receptor and antagonist effects at another. Pentazocine is the prototype agonist–antagonist: it has agonist effects at κ receptors and weak μ antagonist actions. Thus in addition to analgesia, pentazocine may produced κ-mediated psychotomimetic effects not seen with full or partial μ agonists. When a mixed agonist–antagonist is administered together with an agonist, the antagonist effect at the μ receptor can generate an acute withdrawal syndrome.

Partial agonists

A partial agonist has low intrinsic activity (efficacy) so that its dose–response curve exhibits a ceiling effect at less than the maximum effect produced by a full agonist. Buprenorphine is the main example of a partial agonist opioid. Increasing the dose of such a drug above its ceiling level does not result in any further increase in response. This phenomenon is illustrated in Fig. 2 in which C is a partial agonist. C is more potent than B (in the lower part of the curve it will produce the same response at a lower dose), but is less effective than both A and B because of its ceiling effect.

When a partial agonist is administered together with an agonist, displacement of the agonist can cause a net reduction in pharmacological action which may be sufficient to generate an acute withdrawal syndrome. When buprenorphine is used, this effect is most likely when it is administered to a patient receiving high doses of a pure agonist. This can occur when buprenorphine is administered to a patient receiving morphine. Buprenorphine, the more potent drug, displaces morphine at the μ receptors (potency is a measure of the affinity of a drug for receptors — the more potent the drug the greater the affinity). At low doses of morphine this merely means that the buprenorphine rather than the morphine is producing the μ-receptor effect, and so nothing changes. However, if a patient is receiving high doses of morphine and buprenorphine is added, the morphine is displaced from the receptors, the net pharmacological action is reduced, and an acute withdrawal syndrome may ensue.

Relative potency and equianalgesic doses

Relative potency is the ratio of the doses of two analgesics required to produce the same analgesic effect. By convention the relative potency of each of the commonly used opioids is based upon a comparison with 10 mg of parenteral morphine.[18] Data from single-dose and repeated-dose studies in patients with acute or chronic pain have been used to develop an equianalgesic dose table (Table 3) that provides guidelines for dose selection when the drug or route of administration is changed. The information contained in the equianalgesic dose table does not represent standard doses, nor is it intended as an absolute guideline for dose selection. Numerous variables may influence the appropriate dose for an individual patient, including intensity of pain, prior opioid exposure (and the degree of cross-tolerance that this confers), age, route of administration, level of consciousness, and metabolic abnormalities (see below).

Dose–response relationship

As noted above, there is no ceiling to the analgesic effects of full agonist opioids. As the dose is raised, analgesic effects increase as a log linear function. In practice, the appearance of adverse effects, including confusion, sedation, nausea, vomiting, or respiratory depression, imposes a limit on the useful dose of an opioid agonist. Thus the efficacy of any particular drug in an individual patient will be determined by the degree of analgesia produced following dose escalation to intolerable and unmanageable side-effects.[19]

The role of opioids in the management of cancer pain

Analgesic therapy with opioids, non-opioids, and adjuvant analgesics is developed for the individual patient through a process of continuous evaluation so that a favourable balance between pain relief and adverse pharmacological effects is maintained.

An expert committee convened by the Cancer and Palliative Care Unit of the World Health Organization (WHO) has proposed a useful approach to drug selection for cancer pain, which has become known as the WHO analgesic ladder.[1,2] Emphasizing that the intensity of pain, rather than its specific aetiology, should be the prime consideration in analgesic selection, the approach advocates three basic steps (Fig. 3):

1. Patients with mild cancer-related pain should be treated with a non-opioid analgesic, which should be combined with adjuvant drugs if a specific indication for these exists.

Table 3 Opioid analgesics: equianalgesic doses, half-life, and duration of action

Drug	Dose (mg) equianalgesic to 10 mg IM/SC morphine		IM/SC:PO ratio	Half-life (h)	Duration of action (h)
	IM/SC	PO			
Morphine	10	20–30 60*	2/3:1 6:1*	2–3.5	3–6
Codeine	130	200	1.5:1	2–3	2–4
Oxycodone	15	30	2:1	3–4	2–4
Propoxyphene	—	100	—		2–4
Hydromorphone	1.5	7.5	5:1*	2–3	2–4
Methadone	10	20	2:1	15–120	4–8
Pethidine	75	300	4:1	2–3	2–4
Oxymorphone	1	10	10:1	2–3	3–4
Diamorphine	5	20–30 60	2/3:1 6:1‡	0.05†	3–4
Levorphanol	2	4	2:1	12–16	4–8
Fentanyl	0.1§	—	—	1–2¶	1–3¶
Tramadol	100	120	1.2:1	?	4–6
Phenazocine	—	6	—	3	4–8
Dextromoramide	—	15	—	?	2–1
Dipipanone	—	60	—	?	3–4
Buprenorphine	0.4	0.8	—	2–3	6–9

Abbreviations: IM, intramuscular; SC, subcutaneous; PO, by mouth.
* Derived from single-dose studies (see text).
† Rapidly biotransformed to morphine and acetyl morphine (see text).
‡ Single doses.
§ Empirically, transdermal fentanyl 100 μg/h = 2–4 mg/h intravenous morphine.
¶ Single-dose data. Continual infusion produces lipid accumulation and prolonged terminal excretion.

2. Patients who are relatively non-tolerant and present with moderate pain, or who fail to achieve adequate relief after a trial of a non-opioid analgesic, should be treated with an opioid conventionally used for mild to moderate pain (a 'weak' opioid). This group includes codeine, hydrocodone, dihydrocodeine, or propoxyphene. These drugs are typically combined with a non-opioid and may be coadministered with an adjuvant analgesic.

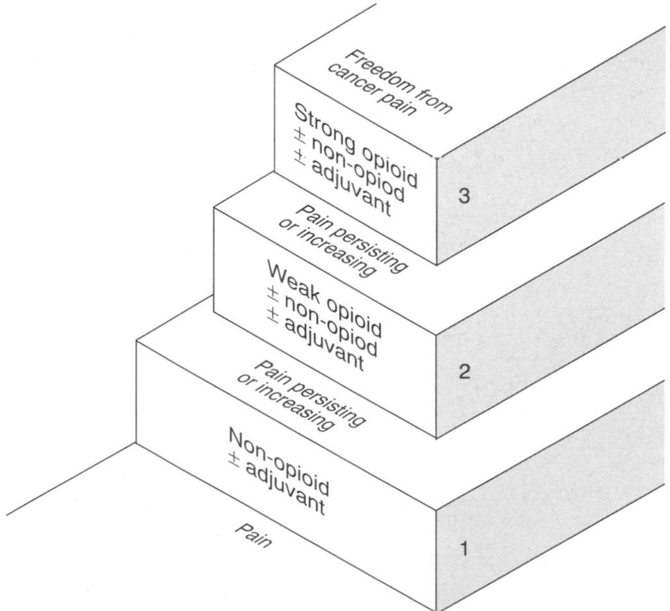

Fig. 3 The WHO three-step analgesic ladder. (Reproduced with permission from ref. 2.)

3. Patients who present with severe pain, or who fail to achieve adequate relief following appropriate administration of drugs on the second step of the analgesic ladder, should receive an opioid conventionally used for moderate to severe pain (a 'strong' opioid). This group includes morphine, diamorphine, fentanyl, oxycodone, phenazocine, hydromorphone, methadone, levorphanol, and oxymorphone. These drugs may also be combined with a non-opioid analgesic or an adjuvant drug.

According to these guidelines, a trial of opioid therapy should be administered to all patients with pain of moderate or greater severity. Patients who present with severe pain are usually treated with an opioid customarily used in step 3 of the analgesic ladder. Patients with moderate pain are commonly treated with a combination product containing paracetamol (acetaminophen) or aspirin plus a conventional step 2 opioid (codeine, dihydrocodeine, hydrocodone, or propoxyphene).[1,2] The doses of these combination products can be increased until the maximum dose of the non-opioid analgesic is attained (e.g. 4000–6000 mg paracetamol); beyond this dose, the opioid contained in the combination product could be increased as a single agent, or the patient could be switched to an opioid conventionally used in step 3.

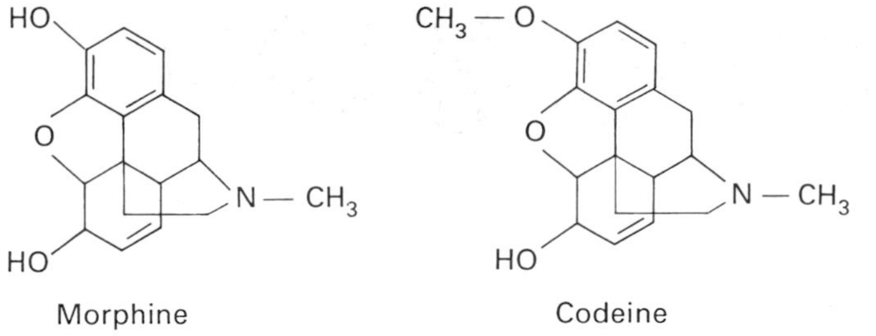

Fig. 4 The chemical structures of morphine and codeine.

The efficacy of the WHO method for cancer pain relief

When combined with appropriate dosing guidelines, this approach is capable of providing adequate relief to roughly 80 per cent of patients.[20-22] This figure has been derived from a number of validation studies involving several thousand patients in different countries and different clinical settings. The validity of this figure has recently been challenged in a systematic review of these same studies.[23] The authors highlighted the lack of detail regarding outcome assessment, the retrospective nature of some of the studies, and other deficiencies such as short and variable follow-up and high withdrawal rates. No data are adduced or reasons provided for concluding that the response rates achieved with the WHO method are likely to be very different from those reported. Indeed, the weight of anecdotal clinical evidence supports the conclusion that most cancer pain can be adequately managed with analgesic drugs. The method was never intended to be used in isolation or to exclude other treatment modalities, and is more a statement of principles than a rigid framework.

Opioid analgesics

The division of opioid agonists into 'weak' or 'strong' opioids, which was incorporated into the original analgesic ladder proposed by the WHO,[1] was not based on fundamental differences in the pharmacology of the agonist opioids, but rather reflected the customary manner in which these drugs were used. It is evident that low-dose morphine produces effects indistinguishable from that of the opioids commonly used in step 2 so that it is inaccurate arbitrarily to classify them differently. In this chapter we shall refer to opioids for mild to moderate pain and opioids for moderate to severe pain rather than 'weak' or 'strong' opioids. This terminology is now incorporated into the current version of the WHO analgesic ladder.[2]

Opioids for mild to moderate pain

Codeine

Codeine (methylmorphine) is a naturally occurring opium alkaloid (Fig. 4) used as an analgesic, antitussive, and antidiarrhoeal agent. Codeine is much less potent than morphine and produces its analgesic effects in part by binding to μ opioid receptors but with low affinity. It is also biotransformed to morphine, and it has been suggested that this contributes the major part of its analgesic effects. However, there are conflicting data. In a study in post-operative (cholecystectomy) patients the morphine-to-codeine ratio (comparing areas under the curve of plasma concentration versus time) was less than 3 per cent.[24] Earlier investigations have indicated similar figures of 2 to 6 per cent, although one study showed a somewhat greater (10 per cent) transformation to morphine.[25] Data from animal models indicate that in the absence of cytochrome P450 2D1, which is necessary for the *o*-demethylation of codeine to morphine, codeine lacks significant analgesic activity.[26] In contrast, a randomized study of patients undergoing third molar tooth extraction showed a significant difference between oral doses of 45 and 90 mg codeine.[27] Four patients were unable to demethylate codeine to produce detectable plasma levels of morphine, but all four showed a better analgesic effect with 90 mg than with 45 mg codeine. Thus in these patients conversion to morphine obviously did not play a role in the enhanced analgesia with the higher dose. Overall the data suggest that biotransformation to morphine may contribute to the analgesic effects of codeine, but to a variable and unpredictable extent, and that the parent compound has analgesic activity in its own right.

Codeine phosphate is absorbed well from the gastrointestinal tract, but oral bioavailability varies considerably between individuals (from 12 to 84 per cent in one study.[24]) The main metabolite is codeine-6-glucuronide, with much smaller amounts of norcodeine, morphine, and morphine 3- and 6-glucuronides also being produced.[28] The usual oral dose of codeine is 30 to 60 mg and its duration of action is 4 to 6 h. Its ratio of oral to parenteral potency is 2:3,[29] which is greater than that of most other opioid analgesics, but parenterally codeine is less than one-twelfth as potent as morphine.[30] There are differing views about the effective dose range of codeine. Early studies showed that the analgesic effect of parenteral codeine levels off above 60 mg and that 120 mg fails to equal the effect of 10 mg morphine, whilst others have shown a progressive increase in analgesia with intramuscular doses up to 360 mg.[31] However, such high parenteral doses are rarely used.

Codeine is not generally given as a single agent when used orally as an analgesic, but is usually combined with a non-opioid (see below). Recently, however, a sustained-release formulation of codeine has been developed. Efficacy in moderate cancer pain has been established in a placebo-controlled randomized double-blind crossover study. In this study patients used a mean daily codeine dose of 277 mg (range 200–400 mg).[32] When changing from regular administration of a codeine–non-opioid combination to morphine, patients receiving a total daily dose of 240 to 360 mg codeine are usually started on 60 mg morphine daily.

Dihydrocodeine

Dihydrocodeine is a semisynthetic analogue of codeine that was first synthesized in 1911. Like codeine, dihydrocodeine is used as an analgesic, antitussive, and antidiarrhoeal agent. Its relative analgesic potency by subcutaneous injection has been variously reported in different studies which have shown doses ranging from 30 to 70 mg as being equivalent to 10 mg of morphine.[33] It appears from these early studies that 60 mg dihydrocodeine produces greater analgesia than 30 mg, but with a corresponding increase in side-effects, whereas there is little difference in analgesia between doses of 60 and 90 mg but a further increase in adverse effects. These data suggest that dihydrocodeine is roughly twice as potent as codeine when given parenterally, although no direct comparison is available. However, when given by mouth the two drugs appear to be equipotent.[34] This may be explained by the consistently poorer bioavailability of dihydrocodeine (20 per cent) which probably results from hepatic presystemic metabolism.[35]

The usual starting dose is 30 mg every 4 to 6 h (by mouth), and this may be increased to 60 mg. However, dihydrocodeine appears to have a narrower therapeutic range than codeine, with a high incidence of adverse effects at the 60-mg dose. A comparison of 30 and 60 mg dihydrocodeine with ibuprofen 400 mg in the treatment of pain following extraction of the third molar tooth showed significantly greater analgesia with the larger dose, but this was accompanied by a significant increase in adverse effects.[36] Overall, ibuprofen was the most effective analgesic in this study and produced far fewer unwanted effects than either dihydrocodeine dose.

A controlled-release formulation of dihydrocodeine is available in several countries, and there are a few published reports of open evaluations in chronic cancer pain but no controlled studies.

There have been a number of reports of severe toxicity associated with dihydrocodeine in patients with impaired renal function.[37] The mechanism is not clear because of the limited data available on the pharmacokinetics of this drug, althought it seems most likely that the cause is accumulation of active glucuronide metabolites, as occurs with morphine.

There is considerable confusion about the relative analgesic potency of dihydrocodeine. One author notes four different recommendations from four different sources,[38] and this is a reflection of the variable data from the early comparative studies. It seems reasonable to assume that oral dihydrocodeine is roughly equipotent to oral codeine, and to use a similar conversion ratio when changing to morphine.

Dextropropoxyphene

Propoxyphene is a synthetic derivative of methadone, and its dextrorotatory stereo-isomer dextropropoxyphene is responsible for its analgesic activity. Dextropropoxyphene is a μ agonist with low receptor affinity similar to that of codeine.[39] Dextropropoxyphene produces typical opioid effects but its main therapeutic use is as an analgesic; it is rarely employed as an antitussive or antidiarrhoeal agent.

Dextropropoxyphene is readily absorbed from the gastrointestinal tract with peak serum levels about 2 h after administration. The mean elimination half-life is about 15 h, with steady state levels being reached after 3 to 4 days of regular administration every 6 to 8 h. The half-life may be very long (over 50 h) in elderly patients.[40]

Dextropropoxyphene undergoes extensive first-pass metabolism. Its principal metabolite is norpropoxyphene, which is active but penetrates the brain to a much lesser extent and has much weaker opioid effects. Norpropoxyphene has a longer half-life (about 23 h) than dextropropoxyphene itself and accumulates in plasma.[41] Both dextropropoxyphene and norpropoxyphene reach plasma concentrations in the steady state which are five to seven times greater than those found after the first dose.

The analgesic efficacy and relative potency of dextropropoxyphene have been questioned. However, the analgesic effect of dextropropoxyphene hydrochloride in doses of 65 mg or more has been established in a number of placebo-controlled studies.[42] Beaver[31] equates lower doses with aspirin and estimates that the relative potency of dextropropoxyphene is half to two-thirds that of codeine. Both salt forms (dextropropoxyphene napsylate and dextropropoxyphene hydrochloride) contain the same amount of active ingredient (i.e. dextropropoxyphene). The larger dose of the napsylate is required solely to accommodate the greater weight of this anion compared with hydrochloride.

Single-dose studies comparing aspirin, paracetamol, and non-steroidal anti-inflammatory drugs, including ibuprofen 400 mg, mefenamic acid 250 mg, and fenoprofen 50 mg, have shown dextropropoxyphene to be a less effective analgesic.[42] However, single-dose studies may be misleading, as is the case with single-dose studies of oral morphine. Dextropropoxyphene undergoes extensive first-pass metabolism, but this is dose dependent: the systemic availability of the drug increases with increasing oral doses.[43] Thus, with regular administration, there is enhanced bioavailability and some degree of accumulation because of the long elimination half-lives of the parent drug and its main metabolite. Dextropropoxyphene is probably more effective when given in repeated dosage. The usual starting dose of morphine for patients receiving dextropropoxyphene–paracetamol combinations every 4 to 6 h (representing 390–260 mg of dextropropoxyphene daily) is 60 mg/day.

Toxicity of dextropropoxyphene

For a long time a combination of dextropropoxyphene and paracetamol was the most commonly prescribed analgesic in the United Kingdom and some Scandinavian countries, but it received much adverse publicity because of its lethal effects in overdose and fears about its addiction potential.[44] Part of this concern was stimulated by its very widespread use. The preparation has remained popular, particularly in the United Kingdom, despite recent evidence that dextropropoxyphene remains the single most common cause of death from analgesic poisoning in some parts of the country.[15] Another recent report also suggests that hepatoxicity due to dextropropoxyphene may be much more common than previously suspected.[46] At present, however, there is insufficient evidence to conclude that dextropropoxyphene is inherently more toxic than codeine or other opioids of similar efficacy, and there are no grounds for recommending one over another.

Oxycodone

Oral oxycodone is an opioid analgesic that is equipotent with morphine. It is commonly formulated in a low dose (5 mg) in combination with aspirin or paracetamol, suitable for use as a step 2 opioid.

Tramadol

Tramadol is a centrally acting analgesic which possesses opioid agonist properties and may also activate monoaminergic spinal inhibition of pain.[47] It has modest affinity with μ opioid receptors, with weak affinity to δ and κ receptors, and its analgesic effect is reversed by naloxone.[47] Unlike other opioids, it also inhibits the uptake of noradrenaline and serotonin, and in an animal model systemically administered yohimbine or ritanserin blocked tramadol-induced analgesia,[47] suggesting that this effect contributes significantly to the drug's analgesic action.

Tramadol can be administered orally, rectally, intravenously, subcutaneously, or intramuscularly. Tramadol given parenterally appears to be as effective as pethidine in postoperative pain and labour pain.[48,49] In a study of patients with pain following dental surgery, 75 mg tramadol administerd orally was less effective than paracetamol and dextropropoxyphene, but 150 mg was more effective.[50].

Although tramadol has been available in some European countries for almost 20 years, there is little published data on its use in chronic cancer pain and only one randomized study.[51] This suggested that oral tramadol was generally not quite as effective as oral morphine, but better tolerated. Data from comparative studies in non-cancer patients with chronic pain[52] and from open evaluations in cancer patients[53] indicate that tramadol is closer to the codeine-like opioids in terms of analgesic efficacy. The majority of cancer patients treated with tramadol for pain need to change to morphine as their disease progresses.[53]

Thus tramadol appears to offer a useful alternative to the standard step 2 opioid analgesics. It has a similar side-effect profile, but may cause less constipation and respiratory depression at equianalgesic doses. The usual oral dose is 50 to 100 mg every 4 to 6 h. Parenteral tramadol has about one-tenth the potency of morphine. There are insufficient data for a reliable assessment of its relative analgesic potency when given orally, but patients whose pain is uncontrolled on 400 mg/day will normally start on 10 to 20 mg morphine every 4 h.

Opioids in combination with non-opioids

The use of an opioid analgesic in combination with a non-opioid can achieve additive analgesia and a consequent reduction in dose-related side-effects associated with increasing doses of the opioid.[54,55] Most of the step 2 opioids are available in formulations where they are combined with aspirin or paracetamol. However, these combinations have frequently proved to be relatively ineffective because the dose of opioid was too low. For example, there are several codeine–paracetamol combinations where the codeine dose is only 8 mg. Thus even two tablets of such a combination would constitute a subtherapeutic dose of codeine.

The most frequently employed step 2 analgesics in cancer pain management are combination preparations containing 300 to 500 mg paracetamol with 30 mg codeine, 32.5 mg dextropropoxyphene, or 5 mg oxycodone. The combination of dextropropoxyphene with paracetamol (coproxamol in the United Kingdom) has theoretical disadvantages of pharmacokinetic incompatibility (dextropropoxyphene has a much longer elimination half-life than paracetamol) and accumulation of dextropropoxyphene and its active metabolite norpropoxyphene. However, neither problem appears to have any clinical consequence in practice and this combination remains the most widely used step 2 opioid in the United Kingdom. Codeine and paracetamol are pharmacokinetically more compatible, and at present either combination would be an appropriate choice.

Recent studies comparing single doses of opioid–non-opioid combinations with various non-steroidal anti-inflammatory drugs in postoperative pain models have shown advantages for the latter in terms of greater efficacy and less adverse effects.[56-58] Chronic use of non-steroidal anti-inflammatory drugs may negate any advantage in terms of unwanted effects, although at present there are no comparative data for chronic cancer pain. It may be that non-steroidal anti-inflammatory drugs could play a greater role as step 2 analgesics in the future.

The second step of the analgesic ladder

Traditionally, patients with moderate pain have been treated with codeine, dihydrocodeine, hydrocodone, oxycodone, and dextropropoxyphene in low-dose formulations combined with either aspirin or paracetamol (acetaminophen). All these drugs have a short half-life and their duration of action is typically 2 to 4 h. Using these formulations, the dose of these combination products can be increased until the maximum dose of the non-opioid coanalgesic is attained (e.g. 4000–6000 mg paracetamol). The major drawback of this approach has been the need for frequent dosing to maintain control of continuous pain.

Experience derived from patients with severe pain indicates that the convenience of administration is a major patient concern. Sustained-release formulations of codeine, dihydrocodeine, oxycodone, and tramadol are currently available or under development, and in some countries controlled-release morphine is available in a low-dose formulation suitable for moderate pain. Although experience with most of these formulations is still very limited, they are likely to provide a more convenient alternative to regular four-hourly dosing with conventional preparations. Since many patients with moderate pain are at a relatively early stage of their illness and some find it more acceptable to be treated with a drug which is not morphine, the traditional step 2 analgesics, codeine, dextropropoxyphene, dihydrocodeine, oxycodone, or tramadol may be preferred.

Opioids for moderate to severe pain

Morphine-like agonists

The morphine-like agonist drugs (Table 2) are widely used to manage cancer pain. Although they may differ from morphine in quantitative characteristics they qualitatively mimic the pharmacological profile of morphine, including both desirable and undesirable effects.[3] Controversy has developed over the choice of an opioid drug, in part because of the dearth of well-controlled studies comparing the efficacy and side-effects of these drugs during chronic administration, and in part because of the large amount of survey data and anecdotal reports supporting one drug over another.

Morphine

Morphine is a potent μ-agonist drug that was first introduced into clinical use almost 200 years ago. It is the main naturally occurring alkaloid of opium derived from the poppy *Papaver somniferum* and is available for therapeutic use as the sulphate, hydrochloride, and tartrate. Recent evidence suggests that biosynthetic pathways for morphine exist in animal and even human tissues such as liver, blood, and brain.[59] Its chemical structure is shown in Fig. 4. Because of its availability and familiarity to clinicians, morphine has been designated as the prototype opioid for step 3 of the 'analgesic ladder'.[1] The World Health Organization has placed oral morphine on the Essential Drug List, and preparations are available for oral, rectal, parenteral, and intraspinal administration.

Bioavailability

Morphine is available in four oral formulations: an elixir, an immediate-release tablet, a controlled-release tablet (of which there are now several preparations using different controlled-release

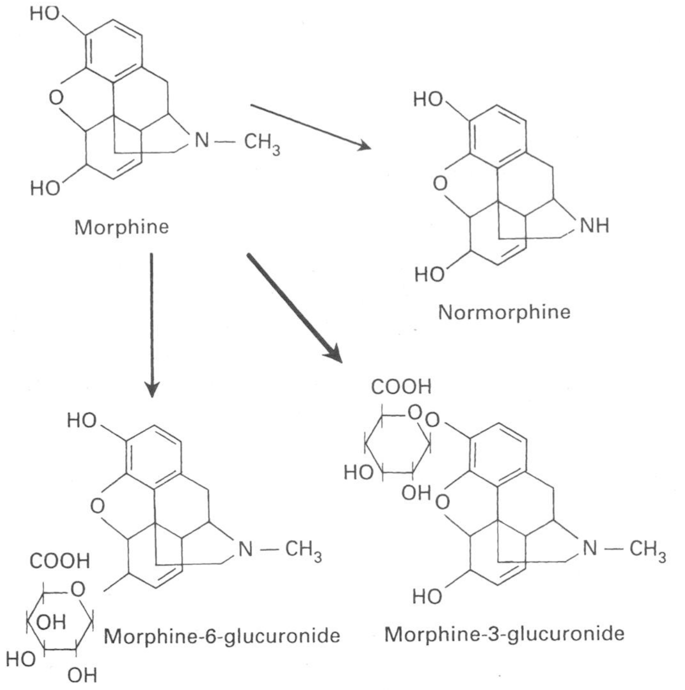

Fig. 5 The metabolites of morphine.

mechanisms), and controlled-release suspensions. Absorption of morphine after oral administration occurs predominantly in the alkaline medium of the upper small bowel (morphine is a weak base) and is almost complete. After oral administration, extensive presystemic elimination of the drug occurs during its passage across the small bowel wall and through the liver. In healthy volunteers and cancer patients the average bioavailability for oral morphine is 20 to 30 per cent.[60–62] The relative contribution of the gut and the liver to this first-pass effect in humans is not known. Like all other pharmacokinetic parameters, bioavailability demonstrates marked interindividual variability. In patients with normal renal function the plasma half-life (2–3 h) is somewhat shorter than the duration of analgesia (4–6 h). The pharmacokinetics remain linear with repetitive administration, and there does not appear to be autoinduction of biotransformation even following large chronic doses.[3,63]

Morphine is relatively hydrophilic and, when administered epidurally or intrathecally, it is not rapidly absorbed into the systemic circulation. This results in a long half-life in cerebrospinal fluid (90–120 min) and extensive rostral redistribution.[64]

Metabolism

About 90 per cent of morphine is converted into metabolites (Fig. 5), principally the glucuronide conjugates morphine-3-glucuronide and morphine-6-glucuronide; minor metabolites include codeine, normorphine, and morphine ethereal sulphate. The liver appears to be the predominant site for metabolism in humans, although in animal models extrahepatic metabolism has been demonstrated in the small bowel and the proximal renal tubule of rodents. These sites may become important where liver function is impaired. Morphine-3-glucuronide is the major metabolite,[63] and in recent years there has been some controversy about its possible role as an opioid antagonist or in mediating some of the adverse effects of morphine. This is discussed elsewhere in this section (Chapter 9.2.10). Viewed overall, the current evidence suggests that morphine-3-glucuronide plays no significant role in the pharmacodynamics of morphine and has no significant opioid antagonist effects in humans.

Morphine-6-glucuronide binds to opioid receptors[65] and produces potent opioid effects in animals[65–67] and humans.[65,68–70] Morphine-6-glucuronide excretion by the kidney is directly related to calculated creatinine clearance;[69] its elimination half-life is 2 to 3 h in patients with normal renal function (similar to that of morphine) but becomes progressively longer with deteriorating function, resulting in significant accumulation.[71] In patients with impaired renal function, morphine-6-glucuronide may accumulate in blood and cerebrospinal fluid,[72] and high concentrations of this metabolite have been associated with toxicity.[68,73] Although further studies are needed to clarify the clinical importance of morphine-6-glucuronide and other metabolites, the data available are sufficient to recommend caution when administering morphine to patients with renal impairment. Patients who are receiving regular morphine and develop acute renal failure in a previously stable situation (e.g. a rapidly developing obstructive uropathy in a patient with pelvic malignancy) may develop a sudden onset of signs and symptoms of opioid toxicity, necessitating temporary withdrawal of the morphine and subsequent dose reduction.

Oral to parenteral relative potency

Single-dose studies of morphine in postoperative cancer patients demonstrated an oral-to-intramuscular potency ratio of 1:6.[7] However, empirical clinical practice using chronically administered oral morphine in cancer patients has generated a different ratio of 1:3 or 1:2.[74,75] The reason for the discrepancy between relative potency estimates derived from single-dose versus chronic dosing studies is probably associated with both methodology[76] and the pharmacokinetics and pharmacodynamics of morphine-6-glucuronide.[74] It is possible that morphine-6-glucuronide accumulation relative to morphine may be greater with oral than with parenteral administration; this would lead to an increase in the relative potency of the orally administered drug when given on a chronic basis.

The important principle for clinical practice is that there is a difference in relative analgesic potency when the route of administration is changed, and that adjustment of dose is necessary in order to achieve an equivalent effect and to avoid either underdosing or toxicity. The usual practice when converting from oral morphine to subcutaneous morphine (or diamorphine) is to divide the oral dose by two or three.

Parenteral morphine

The inorganic salts of morphine (morphine sulphate and morphine hydrochloride) have limited solubility. Standard formulations are available up to 20 mg/ml, and morphine can be constituted from lyophilized power up to 50 mg/ml. Morphine tartrate is substantially more soluble and, in some countries, is formulated in a concentration of 80 mg/ml.

Slow-release morphine preparations

The development of slow-release morphine preparations has had a major impact on clinical practice. These preparations, which are usually administered on a 12-h schedule, provide a much more convenient means of administering oral morphine.[77] They were first introduced in the United Kingdom in 1981, and the original formulation (and others) are now widely available worldwide with a range of tablet strengths (10, 15, 30, 60, 100, and 200 mg depending on the country), allowing considerable flexibility in their use. A controlled-release suspension is available in addition to the tablets.[78]

In contrast with morphine elixir or immediate-release tablets, where peak plasma concentrations are achieved within the first hour followed by a rapid decline with an elimination half-life of 2 to 4 h, controlled-release morphine typically achieves peak plasma concentrations 3 to 6 h after administration, the peak is attenuated, and plasma concentrations are sustained over a 12-h period.[79,80] The pharmacokinetics varies depending on the specific formulation and individual factors, and more recent preparations may allow once-daily dosing.[81] The type and incidence of adverse effects with controlled-release morphine and immediate-release oral morphine appear to be similar with the currently available formulations.

Although some clinicians advocate the use of controlled-release morphine when initiating morphine therapy in cancer patients, an immediate-release preparation is generally recommended in the dose titration period.[82] Initial dose titration using controlled-release morphine is difficult because of the delay in achieving peak plasma concentrations, the attenuation of peak concentrations, and the long duration of action. In this situation, dose finding is performed more efficiently with a short-acting morphine preparation. Once the effective dose is identified using an immediate-release formulation, this may be changed to a controlled-release preparation using a milligram-to-milligram conversion. For the same reasons, controlled-release morphine is not appropriate for the treatment of acute pain or 'breakthrough' pain. An immediate-release morphine preparation should be provided to patients stabilized on controlled-release morphine to be used 'as required' for breakthrough pain.[82]

Diamorphine (heroin)

Diamorphine (diacetylmorphine) is a semisynthetic analogue of morphine and has a long tradition of use for cancer pain in the United Kingdom. It is only available for legal medicinal use in the United Kingdom and Canada. Diamorphine does not bind to the opioid receptor but must be biotransformed to 6-acetylmorphine and morphine to produce its analgesic effect.[83] Therefore it is classified as a prodrug. Following oral administration of diamorphine, only morphine can be measured in the patient's blood. The use of oral diamorphine is an inefficient way of delivering morphine to the systemic circulation. There is no good basis to believe that there is any difference between these two drugs when given by mouth. Sublingual administration of diamorphine has been advocated by some but, as discussed below, this route is not appropriate for either morphine or diamorphine because of poor absorption.

Since diamorphine is more soluble and lipophilic than morphine, it does have some advantages in the setting of parenteral administration. When administered by subcutaneous or intramuscular injection, diamorphine is approximately twice as potent as morphine.[84] There are also differences between diamorphine and morphine administered by intravenous injection: diamorphine has a marginally quicker onset of action, produces greater sedation, and possibly less vomiting.[84] The high solubility of diamorphine (shared also with hydromorphone and morphine tartrate) is of particular advantage for patients who require large doses of subcutaneous opioids.

Methadone

Methadone is a synthetic opioid with an oral-to-parenteral potency ratio of 1:2 and an oral bioavailability greater than 85 per cent. In single-dose studies methadone is only marginally more potent than morphine; however, with repeated administration it is several times more potent.[85,86] The plasma half-life of methadone is long, averaging approximately 24 h (with a range from 13 to over 100 h). However, most patients require dosing at intervals of 4 to 8 h,[87] and this discrepancy between plasma half-life and duration of effect may place patients at increased risk of drug accumulation when treatment is initiated or the dose is increased.[88,89] Sedation, confusion, and even death can occur if patients are not carefully monitored.[90]

Methadone may be a useful alternative to morphine, but its safe administration requires knowledge of its pharmacology and experience. In the opioid-naïve patient, initial doses must be titrated carefully and the patient must be followed closely until there is reasonable certainty that a steady state plasma concentration has been approached (approximately 1 week).[89] Serious adverse effects can be avoided if the initial period of dosing is accomplished with 'as needed' administration and patients are carefully monitored.[91] Patients usually need frequent doses when first starting on methadone because of the short duration of analgesia, but the intervals between dosing will become progressively longer such that maintenance treatment is usually achieved with two to four doses daily. Experimental methods have been developed that allow simple pharmacokinetic measures to predict the appropriate dose, but these have not been used in routine clinical settings. Oral and parenteral preparations of methadone are available. However, the subcutaneous route is not generally recommended because infusion of methadone is often associated with the development of local skin toxicity.[92]

Pethidine (meperidine)

Pethidine is a synthetic opioid with agonist effects similar to those of morphine but a profile of potential adverse effects that limits its utility as an analgesic for chronic cancer pain. Intramuscular pethidine 75 mg is equivalent to 10 mg of intramuscular morphine. Pethidine has an oral bioavailability of 40 to 60 per cent, and its oral-to-parenteral potency ratio is 1:4. It is more lipophilic than morphine, and produces a faster onset and shorter duration of analgesia. Its duration of action after parenteral dosing is 2 to 3 h.

Pethidine is *N*-demethylated to norpethidine, which is an active metabolite that is twice as potent as a convulsant and half as potent as an analgesic compared with its parent compound. Accumulation of norpethidine after repetitive dosing of pethidine can result in central nervous system excitability characterized by subtle mood effects, tremors, multifocal myoclonus, and occasionally seizures.[93-95] Naloxone does not reverse pethidine-induced seizures, and it is possible that its administration to patients receiving pethidine chronically could precipitate seizures by blocking the depressant action of pethidine and allowing the convulsant activity of norpethidine to become manifest.[96] If naloxone is necessary in this situation, it should be diluted and slowly titrated while appropriate seizure precautions are taken.

Although accumulation of norpethidine is most likely to affect patients with overt renal disease, toxicity is sometimes observed in patients with normal renal function.[93,95,97] These potential adverse effects contraindicate pethidine for the management of chronic cancer pain. Given the availability of alternative drugs that lack these toxicities, its use in acute pain management is not recommended.[98]

Hydromorphone

Hydromorphone is another morphine congener. It is five times more potent than morphine and can be administered by the oral, rectal, parenteral, and intraspinal routes. Its oral bioavailability varies from 30 to 40 per cent, and its oral-to-parenteral potency ratio is 1:5.[99] Its half-life is 1.5 to 3 h and it has a short duration of action. Its solubility, the availability of a high-concentration preparation (10 mg/ml), and high bioavailability by continuous subcutaneous infusion (78 per cent)[100] make it particularly suitable for subcutaneous infusion. In the United States it is routinely available in oral, rectal, and injectable formulations, and a sustained-release formulation of oral hydromorphone is now widely available.[101] For patients who require very high opioid doses via the subcutaneous route, hydromorphone can be constituted in concentrations of up to 50 mg/ml from lyophilized powder. It has also been administered via the epidural and intrathecal routes to manage acute and chronic pain.[102] Hydromorphone is hydrophilic and, when administered via the epidural route, its pharmacokinetics, including its long half-life and extensive rostral distribution in cerebrospinal fluid, is similar to those of morphine.[103]

Levorphanol

Levorphanol is a morphine congener with a long half-life (12–16 h).[104] It is five times more potent than morphine and has an oral-to-parenteral potency ratio of 1:2.[105] Like methadone, the discrepancy between plasma half-life (12–16 h) and duration of analgesia (4–6 h) may predispose to drug accumulation following the initiation of therapy or dose escalation. Although dose titration needs to be done carefully in the opioid-naïve patient, problems with drug accumulation appear to be less than those produced by methadone.

In the United States levorphanol is generally used as a second-line agent in patients with chronic pain who cannot tolerate morphine. The possibility that this drug may be particularly useful in morphine-tolerant patients has been proposed on the basis of its affinity for receptors (κ_3 and δ) that are presumably not involved in morphine analgesia.[106] It is no longer available in the United Kingdom or Canada.

Oxycodone

Oxycodone is a synthetic morphine congener which has a high oral bioavailability (60–90 per cent) and an analgesic potency that is comparable with that of morphine.[107–109] It has a short half-life (2–4 h) and is excreted predominantly by the kidney. Oral oxycodone, in combination with aspirin or paracetamol in products that provide 5 mg of oxycodone per tablet, is a useful drug for moderate pain in step 2 of the analgesic ladder. It is also available as a single tablet or syrup, and doses can be escalated for the effective management of severe pain.[110] In currently available oral formulations, this drug usually requires to be administered every 3 to 4 h. Oxycodone pectinate is available in the United Kingdom as a 30-mg rectal suppository which has a delayed absorption and prolonged duration of effect.[111] An oral controlled-release preparation of this drug has recently been introduced in the United States. There are limited data to suggest that oxycodone is associated with a lower likelihood of hallucinations than morphine.[108]

Oxymorphone

Oxymorphone is a lipophilic congener of morphine. It is currently most widely used in suppository form, infrequently used parenterally on a chronic basis, and is not available orally. The injectable formulation is 10 times more potent than morphine.[112] A rectal formulation which is approximately equipotent with parenteral morphine is also available in the United States. The plasma half-life of oxymorphone is 1.2 to 2 h, and its duration of action is 3 to 5 h. It is less likely to produce histamine release than morphine,[113] and may be particularly useful for patients who develop itch in response to other opioids.[114] Oxymorphone is currently unavailable in the United Kingdom.

Fentanyl

Fentanyl is a semisynthetic opioid which interacts predominantly with the μ receptor. It is highly potent; its relative potency compared with parenteral morphine is approximately 80:1 in the non-tolerant acute pain patient.[17] It is also extremely lipophilic and is extensively taken up into fatty tissue. Its elimination half-life ranges from 3 to 12 h and is influenced by the duration of prior administration and the extent of fat sequestration. Fentanyl is used parenterally as a premedication for painful proceedures[98] and in continuous infusions.[115] The development of a transdermal system has broadened its clinical utility for the management of cancer pain.[116–119]

Transdermal fentanyl

A transdermal formulation of fentanyl that delivers 25, 50, 75, or 100 μg/h is now widely available. The transdermal system consists of a drug reservoir that is separated from the skin by a copolymer membrane that controls the rate of drug delivery to the skin surface. The drug is released at a nearly constant amount per unit time along a concentration gradient from the patch to the skin. After application of the transdermal system, serum fentanyl concentration increases gradually, usually levelling off after 12 to 24 h, and then remaining stable for a time before declining slowly. When the patch is removed, serum concentration falls 50 per cent in approximately 17 h (range 13–22 h).[120] The slow onset of effect after application and an equally slow decline in effect after removal are consistent with the development of a subcutaneous depot of drug that maintains the plasma concentration. There is significant interindividual variability in fentanyl bioavailability by this route and dose titration is necessary. The dosing interval for each system is usually 72 h, but interindividual pharmacokinetic variability is large[120] and some patients require a dosing interval of 48 h.

Familiarity with the kinetics of the transdermal system is essential for optimal use. Since peak analgesia is not approached until 8 to 12 h after initial administration, it is essential to provide alternative analgesia for the initial 12 h following administration. It is prudent to apply the patch in the early hours of the day so that the patient can be observed as blood levels rise over the ensuing 12 h to minimize the risk of overdosing during sleep. Significant concentrations of fentanyl can remain in the plasma for up to 24 h after removal of the patch because of delayed release from tissue and subcutaneous depots. Neither age nor patch location appear to affect fentanyl absorption from the transdermal system. There is a potential for temperature-dependent increases in fentanyl release from the system associated with increased skin permeability in patients with fever, who should be monitored for opioid side-effects.[117] Patients should also avoid exposing the patch to direct external heat.

Empirically, the indications for the transdermal route include intolerance of oral medication, poor compliance with oral medication, and occasionally the desire to provide a trial of fentanyl to patients who have reacted unfavourably to other opioids. However, there are a number of limitations. The delay in onset of analgesia and in the establishment of steady state blood levels require the liberal use of an alternative short-acting opioid (usually morphine) for breakthrough pain during the early treatment period. Transdermal fentanyl is generally unsuitable for patients with unstable pain, and if a patient's pain goes out of control management may be complicated because of the delay in re-establishing steady state. If dose reductions are required or discontinuation is indicated, the continuing absorption following patch removal must be taken into account. Poor patch adhesion may be a problem in some patients. Set against these considerations are the putative advantages in terms of convenience and compliance. Transdermal fentanyl may be preferred to oral opioids for patients with stable pain.

Empirical observations suggest that a 100-μg/h fentanyl patch is approximately equianalgesic to 2 to 4 mg/h of intravenous morphine (or equivalent). The relative potency ratio that is applicable when converting patients from oral morphine to transdermal fentanyl has been the subject of some controversy,[121] but the dosing recommendations of the manufacturer seem about right. The patch should be placed in an area where skin movement is limited, such as the upper anterior chest wall or either side of the midline on the back, preferably the lower back. Studies have shown that all areas of skin absorb the drug at roughly the same rate. Since the adhesive strips on these patches are less than optimal, securing the patch with non-irritant tape is often necessary.

Data from open evaluations of transdermal fentanyl in advanced cancer patients suggest that constipation may be less of a problem than with conventional oral opioids. However, at present there are no comparative data from randomized studies to substantiate this potential advantage.

Phenazocine

Phenazocine is a synthetic opioid structurally related to morphine with strong binding to the σ receptor. One 5-mg tablet is equivalent to 25 mg of oral morphine, which means that there is less flexibility in its use. Phenazocine is associated with less sedation and fewer psychotomimetic side-effects than morphine[122] and may be given sublingually, although administration by this route is usually avoided because of its bitter taste and variable absorption. In the United Kingdom it is often used for patients who are unable to tolerate oral morphine.

Other drugs

Dextromoramide

Dextromoramide is a potent agonist and is approximately twice as potent as morphine when taken by mouth. Few data on its pharmacokinetics are available because of difficulties in accurately assaying the drug, but in clinical practice in cancer pain it has a rapid onset of action but a shorter duration than morphine.[123] Tolerance to dextromoramide seems to develop rapidly in humans and, although the duration of analgesia may initially be 2 to 4 h, with repeated administration this may be reduced to only 1 or 2 h. For this reason it is unsuitable for maintenance treatment in chronic cancer pain, although it has been used successfully as a short-acting strong analgesic for breakthrough pain in some patients. It does not have any particular advantages over morphine used in this way, and in general the use of dextromoramide in chronic cancer pain is not recommended.

Papaveretum

Papaveretum contains 50 per cent morphine hydrochloride; the remainder consists of the hydrochlorides of other opium alkaloids (predominantly noscapine with small quantities of codeine and papaverine). Morphine has the strongest analgesic activity of these, and this mixture of alkaloids has no advantages over morphine alone. Recently there has been concern that noscapine may be genotoxic. For this reason papaveretum is now contraindicated in women of childbearing potential.

Dipipanone

Dipipanone is a diphenylpropylamine structurally related to both dextromoramide and methadone. As an analgesic it is approximately half as potent as morphine, and in the United Kingdom it is only available in a combination tablet containing 10 mg dipipanone and 30 mg cyclizine. For many patients this results in excessive sedative and anticholinergic side-effects related to cyclizine when adequate analgesic doses are given, and thus it has only limited application in the management of chronic cancer pain.[124]

Agonist–antagonist opioid analgesics

The agonist–antagonist opioid analgesics are a heterogeneous group of drugs with moderate to strong analgesic activity, comparable with that of the agonist opioids such as codeine and morphine but with a limited effective dose range.[125] The group includes drugs which act as an agonist or partial agonist at one receptor and as an antagonist at another (pentazocine, dezocine, butorphanol, nalbuphine) — 'the mixed agonist–antagonists' — and drugs acting as a partial agonist at a single receptor (buprenorphine). These two groups of drugs can be also classified as nalorphine-like or morphine-like. Meptazinol fits neither classification and occupies a separate category.

Mixed agonist–antagonist analgesics

The agonist–antagonists produce analgesia in the opioid-naïve patient but may precipitate withdrawal in patients who are physically dependent on morphine-like drugs. Therefore, when used for chronic pain, they should be tried before repeated administration of a morphine-like agonist drug.

Pentazocine, butorphanol, and nalbuphine are μ antagonists and κ agonists or partial agonists. All three drugs are strong analgesics when given by injection: pentazocine is one-sixth to one-third as potent as morphine, nalbuphine is roughly equipotent with morphine, and butorphanol is 3.5 to 7 times as potent. The duration of analgesia is similar to that of morphine (3 to 4 h). Oral pentazocine is closer in analgesic efficacy to aspirin and paracetamol (acetaminophen) than the weak opioid analgesics, such as codeine. Neither nalbuphine nor butorphanol is available as an oral formulation, and butorphanol is no longer available in any form in the United Kingdom.

At usual therapeutic doses nalbuphine and butorphanol have respiratory depressant effects equivalent to that of morphine (although the duration of such effects may be longer with butorphanol). Unlike morphine, there appears to be a ceiling to both the respiratory depression and the analgesic action.

All three drugs have a lower abuse potential than the agonist opioid analgesics such as morphine. However, all have been subject to abuse and misuse, and pentazocine (but not the others) is subject to controlled drug restrictions. In North America the oral preparation of pentazocine is marketed in combination with naloxone (but is available without naloxone elsewhere).

Meptazinol is a synthetic hexahydroazepine derivative with opioid agonist and antagonist properties, but is unlike either the nalorphine-type agonist–antagonists or buprenorphine. Meptazinol has central cholinergic properties which may account at least in part for its analgesic effects. Receptor binding studies show it to be a specific μ_1 agonist. Meptazinol is one-tenth as potent as morphine by intramuscular injection and has a duration of action of about 4 h. Some studies have shown adverse effects to be more frequent than with morphine, although respiratory depression and constipation appear to be less.

In therapeutic doses, the mixed agonists–antagonists may produce certain self-limiting psychotomimetic effects in some patients; pentazocine is the most common drug associated with these effects.[125] These drugs play a very limited role in the management of chronic cancer pain[3,125] because the incidence and severity of the psychotomimetic effects increase with dose escalation, and nalbuphine and butorphanol are only available for parenteral use.

A transnasal formulation of butorphanol is now on the market in the United States, but there is no reported experience of its use in the management of chronic cancer pain.

Partial agonist analgesics

Buprenorphine (Table 2) is a potent partial agonist at the μ receptor, and when administered by intramuscular injection is 30 times as potent as morphine. A ceiling to the analgesic effect of buprenorphine has been demonstrated in animals and is also claimed in humans. However, there are no reliable data available to define the maximum dose of buprenorphine in humans. A practical ceiling exists for sublingual use in that the maximum dose formulation is a 400-μg tablet and few patients will accept more than two or three of these in a single dose. The duration of analgesia, at 6 to 9 h, is longer than that of morphine. The sublingual form is not available in the United States.

There have been suggestions that buprenorphine causes less respiratory depression than morphine, but, viewed overall, the evidence suggests that in equianalgesic doses the two drugs have similar respiratory-depressant effects. Naloxone is relatively ineffective in reversing serious respiratory depression caused by buprenorphine.[126] Coadministration of buprenorphine to patients receiving high doses of a morphine-like agonist may precipitate withdrawal symptoms. Buprenorphine does not produce the psychotomimetic effects seen with the mixed agonist–antagonists.

Buprenorphine has a lower abuse potential than morphine, but misuse of this drug has been a growing problem in some areas. It is now a controlled drug in many countries. It has been studied in cancer patients with pain, and is useful for moderate to severe pain requiring an opioid analgesic. We would see sublingual buprenorphine as an alternative to oral morphine in the lower-dose range. Since progression to morphine will invariably be required, the usefulness of buprenorphine in cancer pain is limited.

Principles of opioid administration

The effective clinical use of opioid drugs requires familiarity with drug selection, routes of administration, dosing guidelines, and potential adverse effects.

Indications

A trial of opioid therapy should be administered to all patients with pain of moderate or greater severity, irrespective of the underlying pathophysiological mechanism.[3,19] As discussed in Chapter 9.2.10, the suggestion that some forms of pain, such as neuropathic pain, are intrinsically refractory to opioid analgesia has been refuted by several studies that demonstrate that pain mechanisms do not accurately predict analgesic outcome from opioid therapy.[19] Given the variability of response, all opioid trials in the clinical setting should include dose titration until adequate analgesia occurs or intolerable adverse effects supervene. This approach will identify those responders who can gain substantial clinical benefit from opioid therapy.

Patients whose pain is not easily controlled with an opioid analgesic may benefit from alternative strategies. A different opioid agonist (such as methadone or phenazocine) may achieve good analgesia without disabling side-effects in patients who are poorly controlled on oral morphine. If analgesia is adequate but side-effects are limiting, other drugs are added (e.g. an antiemetic or, in some patients, a central stimulant) to reduce side-effect intensity. If the patient continues to experience adverse effects, spinal administration of morphine or another opioid should be tried. At the same time a variety of adjuvant drugs or non-drug measures should be considered, as described in Chapters 9.2.5 and 9.2.6.

Drug selection

The factors that influence opioid selection include pain intensity, pharmacokinetic considerations and type of formulation, previous adverse effects, and the presence of coexisting disease.

Pain intensity

Patients who present with severe pain are usually treated with an opioid customarily used in step 3 of the analgesic ladder (morphine, hydromorphone, oxycodone, oxymorphone, fentanyl, methadone, or levorphanol). Patients with moderate pain are conventionally treated with a combination product containing paracetamol or aspirin plus a conventional step 2 opioid (codeine, dihydrocodeine, hydrocodone, oxycodone (low dose), and propoxyphene). The doses of these combination products can be increased until the maximum dose of the non-opioid analgesic is attained (e.g. 4000 mg paracetamol); beyond this dose the opioid contained in the combination product could be increased as a single agent, or the patient could be switched to an opioid conventionally used in step 3.

Pharmacokinetic considerations and type of formulation

Any of the available agonist opioids can be selected for the opioid-naïve patient without major organ failure. Short-half-life opioids (morphine, hydromorphone, fentanyl, oxycodone, or oxymorphone) are generally favoured because they are easier to titrate than the long-half-life drugs which require a longer period to approach steady state plasma concentrations. Among the short-half-life opioids, the range of available formulations often influences specific drug selection. For example, although oxycodone is a versatile opioid agonist, the oral formulations currently available cannot be conveniently administered in the high doses frequently required by patients with severe pain, and no parenteral formulation is available. For ambulatory patients who are able to tolerate oral opioids, morphine sulphate is generally preferred since it has a short half-life and is easy to titrate in its immediate-release form; it is also available as controlled-release preparations that allow 12-h and 24-h dosing intervals. The long-half-life opioids methadone and levorphanol are not usually considered for first-line therapy because they can be difficult to titrate and present challenging management problems if delayed toxicity develops as plasma concentrations gradually rise following dose increments. For the reasons previously described, the use of pethidine, dextromoramide, and dipipanone for the management of cancer pain is discouraged.

When the oral route of opioid administration is contraindicated, the available routes of administration may become an important consideration in opioid selection. Fentanyl is the only opioid available for administration by the transdermal route. Although most of the full agonist drugs are well absorbed by subcutaneous infusion, some (like morphine tartrate, hydromorphone, and diamorphine) are more suitable by virtue of their high solubility and low irritability. Methadone and fentanyl may produce significant local irritation when administered by the subcutaneous route. For cultural and aesthetic reasons these routes are often preferred to rectal administration of morphine, oxycodone, oxymorphone, methadone, or hydromorphone. Subcutaneous infusion may be also preferable in patients at the end of life because it is less disruptive than using intermittent analgesic suppositories when nursing a sick patient.

Response to previous trials of opioid therapy

It is always important to review the response to previous trials of opioid therapy. If the current opioid is well tolerated, it is usually continued unless difficulties in dose titration occur or the required dose cannot be administered conventionally. If dose-limiting side-effects develop, a trial of an alternative opioid should be considered. The existence of different degrees of incomplete cross-tolerance to various receptor-mediated opioid effects (analgesia and side-effects) may explain the utility of these sequential trials.[127] It is strongly recommended that clinicians be familiar with at least three opioid drugs used in the management of severe pain and have the ability to calculate appropriate starting doses using equianalgesic dosing data.

Coexisting disease

Pharmacokinetic studies of pethidine, pentazocine, and propoxyphene have revealed that liver disease may decrease the clearance and increase the bioavailability and half-lives of these drugs.[128,129] These changes may result in above-normal plasma concentrations. Mild or moderate hepatic impairment has only a minor impact on morphine clearance;[130] however, advanced disease may be associated with reduced elimination.[131]

Patients with renal impairment may accumulate the active metabolites of propoxyphene (norpropoxyphene), pethidine (norpethidine), and morphine (morphine-6-glucuronide). Particular caution is required in the administration of these drugs to such patients.[68,71,132] Until more data are available it may be wise to assume that other opioids with active metabolites may produce similar problems of toxicity in patients with impaired renal function.

Routes of administration

Opioids should be administered by the least invasive and safest route capable of providing adequate analgesia. In a survey of patients with advanced cancer, more than half required two or more routes of administration prior to death, and almost a quarter required three or more.[133]

Oral administration

The oral route of opioid administration remains the most important and appropriate in routine practice. Orally administered drugs have a slower onset of action, a delayed peak time, and a longer duration of effect compared with parenterally administered drugs. The time to peak effect depends on the drug and the nature of the formulation. For most immediate-release oral formulations, peak effect is typically achieved within 60 min. The oral route of drug administration is inappropriate for patients who have impaired swallowing or gastrointestinal obstruction, and for some patients who require a rapid onset of analgesia. For patients who require very high doses, the inability to prescribe a manageable oral opioid regimen may be an indication for the use of a non-oral route.

When given orally the opioids differ substantially with respect to their relative analgesic potency compared with parenteral administration. To some extent, this reflects differences in presystemic metabolism, i.e. the degree to which they are inactivated as they are absorbed from the gastrointestinal tract and pass through the liver into the systemic circulation. As indicated in Table 3, morphine, diamorphine, pethidine, hydromorphone and oxymorphone, have ratios of oral to parenteral potency ranging from 1:3 to 1:12. Methadone, levorphanol, and oxycodone are subject to less presystemic elimination and also demonstrate a lower oral-to-parenteral potency ratio of at least 1:2. Failure to recognize these differences may result in a substantial reduction in analgesia when a change from parenteral to oral administration is attempted without upward titration of the dose, or toxic effects when changing in the opposite direction.

Rectal administration

The rectal route is a non-invasive alternative to parenteral routes for patients unable to use oral opioids. Rectal suppositories containing morphine, hydromorphone and oxymorphone, and oxycodone are available. The pharmacokinetics and bioavailability of drugs given rectally may differ from that of oral administration because of delayed or limited absorption and partial bypassing of presystemic hepatic metabolism. In practice, however, the potency of opioids administered rectally is approximately equal to that achieved by oral dosing.[134] In contrast with morphine, rectal oxycodone appears to have a delayed absorption and prolonged duration of action.

The rectal route has been the usual first alternative for patients unable to take oral medication who need continuous regular opioid administration. However, for many patients it may be more convenient to convert directly to a subcutaneous infusion of opioid using a portable syringe driver or similar device.

Parenteral administration

Bolus injections

Parenteral routes of administration are considered for patients who have impaired swallowing or gastrointestinal obstruction, those who require a rapid onset of analgesia, and those who require very high doses that cannot be conveniently administered by other methods. Repeated parenteral bolus injections, which can be delivered by the intravenous, intramuscular, or subcutaneous routes, may be complicated by the occurrence of untoward 'bolus' effects (toxicity at peak concentration and/or pain breakthrough at the trough). Intravenous bolus provides the most rapid onset; the time to peak effect correlates with the lipid solubility of the opioid, ranging from 2 to 5 min for methadone and 10 to 15 min for morphine. Although repetitive intramuscular injections are commonplace in some countries, they are painful and offer no pharmacokinetic advantage, and their use is not recommended.[82,135] Repeated bolus doses, if required, can be accomplished without frequent skin punctures by using an indwelling intravenous or subcutaneous infusion device. To deliver repeated subcutaneous injections, a 25–27 gauge 'butterfly' can be left under the skin for up to a week.[136] The discomfort associated with this technique is partially related to the volume to be injected; it can be minimized by the use of concentrated formulations.

Continuous infusions

Continuous infusions avoid the problems associated with the 'bolus effect' and can be administered intravenously or subcutaneously.[136–138] Continuous subcutaneous infusion using a portable battery-operated syringe driver or other similar device was originally devised to administer infusions of desferrioxamine to patients with thalassemia, but was subsequently used to deliver diamorphine to patients with advanced cancer who were unable to take oral drugs.[139] This technique is now well established in palliative care and is used to administer analgesics, antiemetics, anxiolytic sedatives, and dexamethasone.

Ambulatory infusion devices vary in complexity, cost, and ability to provide patient-controlled 'rescue doses' as an adjunct to a continuous basal infusion. A variety of devices have been employed, all designed to be lightweight and portable, and in one case disposable.[136] Opioids suitable for continuous subcutaneous infusion must be soluble, well absorbed and non-irritant. Extensive experience has been reported with morphine, diamorphine, hydromorphone, fentanyl, and oxymorphone.[100,137,140] Methadone[92] and fentanyl appear to be relative irritants and are best avoided by this route.

Studies suggest that dosing with subcutaneous administration can proceed in a manner identical to continuous intravenous infusion: a postoperative study comparing patients who received an identical dose of morphine by either intravenous or subcutaneous infusion found no difference in blood levels,[141] and a controlled study of hydromorphone calculated a bioavailability of 78 per cent for the subcutaneous route and observed that analgesic outcome was identical during intravenous or subcutaneous infusion.[100] To maintain the comfort of an infusion site, the subcutaneous infusion rate should not exceed 5 ml/h. Patients who require high doses may benefit from the use of concentrated solutions which, in selected cases, can be made up specifically for continuous subcutaneous infusion; diamorphine, morphine tartrate, and hydromorphone are particularly useful in this setting. Subcutaneous infusion has become the first choice when parenteral analgesia is required in palliative care patients.

Continuous intravenous infusion may be the most appropriate way of delivering an opioid for patients with a pre-existing implanted central line, when there is a need for infusion of a large volume of solution, or when using methadone. If continuous intravenous infusion must be continued on a long-term basis, a permanent central venous port is recommended.

Continuous infusions of drug combinations may be indicated when pain is accompanied by nausea, anxiety, or agitation. In such cases an antiemetic, neuroleptic, or anxiolytic may be combined with an opioid provided that it is non-irritant, miscible, and stable in combined solution. Experience has been reported with infusions of an opioid combined with metoclopramide, haloperidol, hyoscine (scopolamine), cyclizine, methotrimeprazine, ondansetron, and midazolam (see Sections 7 and 17 and Chapter 9.3.1). In all cases chemical compatibility and stability should be confirmed.

Epidural, intrathecal, and intraventricular administration

The discovery of opioid receptors in the dorsal horn of the spinal cord led to the development of intraspinal opioid delivery techniques.[142] In general, they provide a longer duration of analgesia at doses lower than required by systemic administration. The delivery of low opioid doses near the sites of action in the spinal cord may decrease supraspinally mediated adverse effects. Opioid selection for intraspinal delivery is influenced by several factors. Hydrophilic drugs, such as morphine and hydromorphone, have a prolonged half-life in cerebrospinal fluid and significant rostral redistribution.[64,103,143] Lipophilic opioids, such as fentanyl and sufentanil, have less rostral redistribution and may be preferable for segmental analgesia at the level of spinal infusion. The addition of a low concentration of a local anaesthetic, such as 0.125 to 0.25 per cent bupivacaine, to an epidural[144,145] or intrathecal opioid[146,147] has been demonstrated to increase the analgesic effect without increasing toxicity. There are no trials comparing the intrathecal and epidural routes in cancer pain. The epidural route is generally preferred because the techniques to accomplish long-term administration are simpler. A combined analysis of adverse effects observed in numerous trials of epidural or intrathecal administration suggests that the risks associated with these techniques are similar[148] (see Chapter 9.2.6). The potential morbidity for these procedures indicates the need for a well-trained clinician and long-term monitoring.

Limited experience suggests that the administration of an opioid into the cerebral ventricles can provide long-term analgesia in selected patients.[149] This technique has been used for patients with upper-body or head pain or with severe diffuse pain. Schedules have included both intermittent injection via an Ommaya reservoir and continual infusion using an implanted pump.

The indication for the spinal routes of administration of opioid analgesics in palliative care patients is discussed in more detail in Chapter 9.2.6.

Other routes and modes of administration

As previously described, fentanyl is available in a transdermal formulation and its use is discussed above. At present, no other opioids are available for transdermal administration.

Sublingual absorption could potentially occur with any opioid, but bioavailability is very poor with drugs that are not highly lipophilic.[150] A sublingual preparation of buprenorphine is available in some countries, although not in the United States. Anecdotally, sublingual morphine has also been reported to be effective; given the poor sublingual absorption of this drug,[150] this efficacy may be related in part to swallowing of the dose.[151] Both fentanyl and methadone are well absorbed sublingually, but no preparations are currently available for clinical use. Thus the sublingual approach has limited value owing to the lack of true sublingual formulations, poor absorption of most drugs, and the inability to deliver high doses or to prevent swallowing of the dose.[152] Sublingual administration of an injectable formulation is occasionally used in patients requiring low doses of opioids who temporarily lose the option of oral dosing.

An oral transmucosal formulation of fentanyl citrate (OTFC) has been developed and is licensed in the United States as an anaesthetic premedicant. It is currently being evaluated in a multicentre trial for the treatment of breakthrough pain in cancer patients. The so-called fentanyl 'lollipop' consists of a fentanyl-impregnated raspberry-coloured lozenge on a plastic handle. As the patient consumes the lollipop and it dissolves in the saliva, a proportion of the fentanyl diffuses across the oral mucosa and the remainder is swallowed and partially absorbed in the gastro-intestinal tract. Total bioavailability of this administration system is about 50 per cent.[153] OTFC is currently available in 200-, 300-, and 400-μg dosage units. In this formulation, fentanyl is absorbed rapidly through the oral mucosa with peak plasma concentrations occurring 22 min after the start of administration.[153] In a study of cancer patients being treated for breakthrough pain the average time to pain relief was 9.5 min.[154] Transmucosal fentanyl may provide a non-invasive rapid-onset alternative for patients with poor oral or venous access who would otherwise require parenteral administration to combat breakthrough or incident pain,.

Changing the route of administration

As described above, when changing from the oral to parenteral routes, or vice versa, an adjustment in dose is required to avoid either toxic effects or a reduction in analgesia. The ratios of oral to parenteral relative potency given in Table 3 are estimates and should not be taken as precise figures but used as guidelines. There is considerable variation between patients, and doses will need to be carefully adjusted for individual patients. When patients are switched from one route of administration to another, it is the lack of attention to the route-dependent differences in opioid dose that accounts for the common reports of undermedication of patients. The slower onset of analgesia after oral administration often requires some adaptation on the part of a patient who is accustomed to the more rapid onset seen after parenteral opioid. In some patients the problems associated with switching from the parenteral to the oral route of opioid administration may need to be minimized by slowly reducing the parenteral dose and increasing the oral dose over a 2 to 3 day period.

Usually, no dose adjustment is required when patients are switched from the subcutaneous to the intravenous route or vice versa.

Scheduling opioid administration

'Around-the-clock' dosing

To provide the patient with continuous relief by preventing the pain from recurring, patients with continuous or frequent pain are usually scheduled for 'around-the-clock' dosing. In the hospital setting, this approach may prevent the usual medical and nursing delays that occur when a patient on an 'as-needed' schedule requires medication. However, clinical vigilance is required in patients with no previous opioid exposure and those administered drugs with long half-lives. With long-half-life drugs, such as methadone, delayed toxicity may develop as plasma concentration rises slowly toward steady state levels.[90]

Rescue doses

All patients who receive an around-the-clock opioid regimen should also be offered a 'rescue dose', i.e. a supplemental dose given on an as-needed basis to treat pain that breaks through the regular schedule.[82] The integration of scheduled dosing with rescue doses provides a method for safe and rational stepwise dose escalation and is applicable to all routes of opioid administration. The rescue dose drug is typically identical to that administered on a continuous basis, with the exception of transdermal fentanyl and methadone; the use of an alternative short-half-life opioid is recommended for the rescue dose when these drugs are used. The frequency with which the rescue dose can be administered depends on the time to peak effect for the drug and the route of administration. Oral rescue doses can be offered up to every 60 to 90 min, and parenteral rescue doses can be offered up to every 15 to 30 min. Clinical experience suggests that the size of the rescue dose should be equivalent to one-sixth of the 24-h baseline dose, i.e. the same as the four-hourly dose of opioid.

Scheduling with controlled-release formulations

Controlled-release formulations can reduce the inconvenience associated with around-the-clock administration.[77] These formulations should not be used for rapid titration of the dose in patients with severe pain. Controlled-release oral morphine sulphate and, to a somewhat lesser extent, transdermal fentanyl are now widely used, and new controlled-release formulations of codeine, oxycodone, and hydromorphone have been introduced recently in various countries.

An immediate-release formulation of a short-half-life opioid (usually the same drug) is generally used as the rescue medication. Controlled-release and immediate-release formulations of oral morphine are dose equivalent; switching from one to the other is done on a milligram-for-milligram basis after the daily dose requirement is identified using an immediate-release formulation.

As-needed dosing

In some limited situations an as-needed dosing regimen alone can be recommended. This type of dosing provides additional safety during the initiation of opioid therapy in the opioid-naïve patient, particularly when rapid dose escalation is needed or a long-half-life drug is administered. This technique is strongly recommended when starting methadone therapy[155] and for patients with acute renal failure.

Patient-controlled analgesia

Patient-controlled analgesia is a technique of parenteral drug administration in which the patient controls a pump that delivers bolus doses of an analgesic according to parameters set by the physician. Use of a patient-controlled analgesia device allows the patient to titrate the opioid dose carefully to his or her individual analgesic needs. Long-term patient-controlled analgesia in cancer patients is accomplished via subcutaneous or intravenous routes using an ambulatory infusion device. The more technologically advanced of these devices have programmable variables, including infusion rate, rescue dose, and lock-out interval.[136] The option for bolus dosing is typically used in conjunction with continuous opioid infusion.[156]

Dose selection and adjustment

Initial dose selection

A patient with severe pain that is not controlled with a step 2 opioid–non-opioid combination in full dose should begin one of the opioid agonists at a dose equivalent to 10 to 20 mg oral morphine sulphate every 4 h.

Dose adjustments when switching opioids

When patients are switched from one opioid analgesic to another, lack of attention to the drug-dependent differences in opioid dose may result in undermedication or overdose. In this setting familiarity with the use of the equianalgesic dose table (Table 3) is essential. For patients with good pain control the starting dose of the new drug should be reduced to 50 to 75 per cent of the equianalgesic dose to account for incomplete cross-tolerance. However, if the patient had inadequate pain control on the previous opioid, a smaller dose reduction is used and the starting dose of the new drug can be usually 75 to 100 per cent of the equianalgesic dose. Clinical experience suggests that additional caution is needed when the change is to methadone; a reduction to 25 to 33 per cent of the equianalgesic dose is prudent. After any change from one opioid to another, patients must be monitored to assess the adequacy of analgesia and to detect the development of side-effects. Subsequent dose adjustments are usually necessary.

This information has been gained empirically but is based upon the concept that cross-tolerance is not complete among opioids and conforms to our recognition that the relative potency of some of the opioid analgesics may change with repetitive dosing, particularly those opioids with a long plasma half-life.

Dose titration

Inadequate pain relief should be addressed by gradual escalation of the opioid dose until adequate analgesia is reported or intolerable side-effects (that cannot be managed by simple interventions) supervene. Because analgesic response to opioids increases linearly with the logarithm of the dose, dose escalations of less than 30 to 50 per cent are not likely to improve analgesia significantly. Clinical experience indicates that a dose increment of this order of magnitude is safe and is large enough to observe a meaningful change in effects. In most cases, gradual dose escalation identifies a favourable balance between analgesia and side-effects which remains stable for a prolonged period.[157] While doses can become extremely large during this process, the absolute dose is immaterial as long as the balance between analgesia and side-effects remains favourable. In a retrospective study of 100 patients with advanced cancer, the average daily opioid requirement was equivalent to 400 to 600 mg of intramuscular morphine, but approximately 10 per cent of patients required more than 2000 mg and one patient required over 30 000 mg every 24 h.[133]

A simple method of dose titration using oral morphine is to prescribe a dose of immediate-release morphine every 4 h and the same dose for rescue (for breakthrough pain). The rescue dose can be given as often as required (e.g. every hour) and the total dose of morphine can be reviewed daily. The regular dose can then be adjusted according to how many rescue doses have been given.[82]

Rate of dose titration

The severity of the pain should determine the rate of dose titration. Patients with very severe pain can be managed by repeated parenteral dosing every 15 to 30 min until pain is partially relieved[158] when an oral dosing regimen should be started.

Tolerance

Patients vary greatly in the opioid dose required to manage pain. The need for escalating doses is a complex phenomenon. Most patients reach a dose that remains constant for prolonged periods.[157,159,160] When the need for dose escalation arises, any of a variety of distinct processes may be involved. Clinical experience suggests that true analgesic tolerance is a much less common reason than disease progression or increasing psychological distress. Changes in the pharmacokinetics of an analgesic drug could also be potentially involved.

True pharmacological tolerance probably involves changes at the receptor level,[161,162] and in this situation continued drug administration itself induces an attenuation of effect. Clinically, tolerance to the non-analgesic effects of opioids appears to occur commonly albeit at varying rates for different effects.[161] For example, tolerance to respiratory depression, somnolence, and nausea generally develops rapidly, whereas tolerance to opioid-induced constipation develops very slowly, if at all.[161] Tolerance to these opioid side-effects is not a clinical problem, and indeed is a desirable outcome that allows effective dose titration to proceed.

From the clinical perspective, the concern is that tolerance to the analgesic effect of the drug will develop and that this will necessitate rapid dose escalation which may continue until the drug is no longer useful. Induction of true analgesic tolerance which could compromise the utility of treatment can only be said to occur if a patient manifests a need for increasing opioid doses in the absence of other factors (e.g. progressive disease) that would be capable of explaining the increase in pain. Extensive clinical experience suggests that most patients who require an escalation in dose to manage increasing pain have demonstrable progression of disease.[157,161,163].

This conclusion has two important implications: concern about tolerance should not impede the use of opioids early in the course of the disease, and worsening pain in a patient receiving a stable dose of opioid should not be attributed to tolerance but taken as presumptive evidence of disease progression or, less commonly, increasing psychological distress.

Opioid pharmacokinetic factors that may influence drug dosing

Hepatic and renal impairment

The impact of hepatic and renal impairment on opioid metabolism and excretion has been described previously. Neither hepatic nor renal dysfunction is a contraindication to the use of opioid analgesics in cancer pain. Care is required, particularly in patients with renal impairment, but most situations can be managed without complex or exceptional measures. Opioids may exacerbate the central nervous system signs and symptoms in patients with very severe hepatic or renal dysfunction. A high level of clinical vigilance is required, and clinical signs and symptoms are more important than biochemical data in indicating the need for caution.

Drug interactions

The tricyclic antidepressants clomipramine and amitriptyline may increase plasma morphine levels as measured by an increase in bioavailability and the half-life of morphine in cancer patients.[164] The concurrent administration of drugs that induce the hepatic mixed function oxidase system can alter the disposition of certain opioids. The metabolism of pethidine is increased by phenobarbitone and phenytoin, and that of methadone is increased by phenytoin[165] and rifampicin. Methadone has also been reported to induce its own metabolism.[166]

The potential for additive side-effects and serious toxicity from drug combinations must be recognized. The sedative effect of an opioid may add to that produced by numerous other centrally acting drugs such as anxiolytics, neuroleptics, and antidepressants. Likewise, the constipating effects of opioids are probably worsened by drugs with anticholinergic effects. A severe adverse reaction, including excitation, hyperpyrexia, convulsions, and death, has been reported after the administration of pethidine to patients treated with a monoamine oxidase inhibitor.[5]

Advanced age

It appears that all phases of pharmacokinetics are affected by the ageing process.[167] Absorption may be influenced by decreases in gastric acid, intestinal blood flow, mucosal cell mass, and intestinal motility[168]. The clearance of morphine,[169,170] fentanyl, and nalbuphine are decreased in the elderly, and this age-related difference in pharmacokinetics may partially explain the greater sensitivity of older patients to therapeutic opioid doses compared with younger patients. Pharmacodynamic responses may also be altered in older patients. Increased receptor sensitivity and concurrent alterations in mental status may account in part for the increased response shown by elderly patients to opioid analgesics. In practice, reducing the dose or lengthening the time interval between doses for the elderly patient will minimize the development of serious adverse effects.

Children

The management of pain in children with opioid analgesics follows the same principles as described for the adult patient (see Chapter 19.1). The oral and intravenous routes are commonly used to avoid repetitive needle injections. Continuous subcutaneous infusion has also been used in the terminally ill child. Individualization of doses and titration to the needs of the child are essential.

Adverse effects of opioid analgesics

There are a number of side-effects associated with the use of opioid analgesics. The most common are sedation, constipation, and nausea and vomiting, but there are other adverse effects including confusion, hallucinations, nightmares, urinary retention, multifocal myoclonus, dizziness, and dysphoria. The mechanisms that underlie these various adverse effects, even the most common, are only partly understood and, as discussed above, appear to depend upon a number of factors including age, extent of disease and organ dysfunction, concurrent administration of certain drugs, prior opioid exposure, and the route of drug administration. Studies comparing the adverse effects of one opioid analgesic with another in this population are lacking. Similarly, controlled studies comparing the adverse effects produced by the same opioid given by various routes of administration are also lacking.

As a general rule, caution is required when using opioids in patients in acute pain with impaired ventilation, bronchial asthma, or raised intracranial pressure; the same caveats do not usually limit dose titration in chronic cancer pain management.

Sedation and other central nervous system effects

The opioid analgesics produce dose-related sedation; stupor is a predictable effect of dose escalation. While this effect may be useful in certain clinical situations (e.g. preanaesthesia), it is not usually a desirable concomitant of analgesia, particularly in ambulatory patients.

Daytime drowsiness, dizziness, or mental clouding commonly occur at the start of treatment with morphine, but these symptoms soon resolve (usually within a few days) in the majority of patients once they are stabilized. Hallucinations and confusion are relatively unusual but may occur, particularly in elderly patients.

The central nervous system depressant actions of these drugs can be expected to be at least additive with the sedative and respiratory depressant effects of sedative–hypnotics such as alcohol and the benzodiazepines.

The mixed agonist–antagonist opioids, particularly pentazocine, and pethidine in repeated doses are associated with an elevated risk of adverse central nervous system effects. The likelihood of delirium following the start of therapy or rapid dose escalation may also be greater with drugs that have a long half-life, such as methadone or levorphanol, or a metabolite with a long half-life, such as pethidine[94] and propoxyphene, which may accumulate with repeated dosing and produce plasma concentrations associated with adverse effects. There are insufficient data to draw definitive conclusions regarding the relative likelihood of adverse central nervous system effects with the other full agonists. Some preliminary data suggest that fentanyl and oxycodone[108] may be associated with less drowsiness and a lower likelihood of hallucinations than morphine. Further controlled studies are required to elucidate the relative central nervous system toxicities of these agents.

Persistent confusion attributable to an opioid alone occurs, but is uncommon. More often opioids are a contributing factor in a delirium that is multifactorial (see Chapter 9.2.10).

Morphine and driving

The ability to continue driving is very important to maintaining the quality of life of many patients with advanced cancer. Many assume that they must stop driving whilst taking regular potent opioid analgesics, but this is not necessarily so. The usual advice to patients is that they should not drive or engage in other skilled activities such as operating machinery when they first start on morphine or a similar opioid, or when they increase the dose. However, once the initial sedative effects have resolved and both the patient and physician are confident that cognitive and psychomotor performance are no longer impaired, driving and other similar activities may restart.

This advice is based to a large extent on empirical experience and there have been few objective data to substantiate it. However, recent studies confirm, perhaps surprisingly, that morphine produces little measurable impairment of cognitive and psychomotor function,[171] particularly in patients receiving continuous treatment with stable doses. In one study which used a battery of performance tests designed specifically to assess functions related to driving ability, chronic morphine use was associated with slower reaction times, more mistakes, and a slowing in ability to process visual information and perform motor sequences, but these changes were not statistically significant compared with a control group of cancer patients not taking morphine.[172] These data support the clinical impression that stable doses of morphine are unlikely to cause substantial impairment of the psychomotor skills required for driving, and allow us to continue to advise patients to this effect.

Central stimulants and morphine-induced sedation

Concurrent administration of dextroamphetamine in oral doses of 2.5 to 5.0 mg twice daily has been reported to reduce the sedative effects of opioids. Methylphenidate has also been shown to increase the analgesic effect and decrease sedation in cancer patients receiving opioids,[173] although significant tolerance may develop after periods as short as 1 month.[174] The use of central stimulants as adjuvant analgesics is discussed in more detail in Chapter 9.2.5.

We have noted different practices with these drugs in different parts of the world. In general, their use in conjunction with opioids in a palliative care setting is restricted to a small proportion of patients.

Constipation

The most common adverse effect of the opioid analgesics is constipation (see also Chapter 9.3.3). These drugs act at multiple sites in the gastrointestinal tract and spinal cord to produce a decrease in intestinal secretions and peristalsis, resulting in a dry stool and constipation. Tolerance to the smooth muscle effects of opioids develops very slowly, so that constipation will persist when these drugs are used for chronic pain.

Constipation must be anticipated and treated prophylactically with adequate laxatives. Usually a peristaltic stimulant (e.g. senna, bisacodyl, or phenolphthalein) in combination with a stool softener (such as docusate) will be required for maintenance treatment. The doses of these drugs should be increased as necessary, and an osmotic laxative (e.g. lactulose or a magnesium salt) can be added if necessary.

Oral naloxone has been investigated as a treatment for opioid-induced constipation, on the basis that the constipating effect of opioids is at least partially mediated by receptors in the gastrointestinal tract. Naloxone undergoes extensive presystemic metabolism when administered by mouth, such that its bioavailability is less than 1 per cent, and therefore it is unlikely to antagonize the systemic effects of the opioids. However, it may still be able to block gastrointestinal opioid receptors. Several clinical studies have confirmed that oral naloxone does have a laxative effect in morphine-induced constipation,[175] but also has a significant potential to cause systemic opioid withdrawal effects. Therefore its use in this way is not recommended at present.

Nausea and vomiting

Nausea and vomiting (see also Chapter 9.3.1) occurs in half to two-thirds of patients taking oral morphine, is variable in intensity, and is usually easy to control if it does develop. In many patients it is an initiation side-effect and resolves with continued use. A small proportion of patients experience severe nausea and vomiting which may be difficult to control. Three mechanisms underlie this side-effect: stimulation of the chemoreceptor trigger zone in the medulla, increased vestibular sensitivity, and delayed gastric emptying.

The ability of opioid analgesics to produce nausea and vomiting appears to vary with drug and patient, so that there may be some advantage in switching to another opioid in patients with severe nausea and vomiting which is difficult to control with concurrent antiemetics. For some patients initiating treatment by the parenteral route and then switching to the oral route may reduce the emetic symptoms.

Urinary retention

Because the opioid analgesics increase smooth muscle tone, they can cause bladder spasm and an increase in sphincter tone leading to urinary retention. This is most common in elderly patients, and is also generally more likely to occur after spinal (epidural, intrathecal) administration of opioids.

Multifocal myoclonus

At high doses, all the opioid analgesics can produce multifocal myoclonus. This complication is most prominent with repeated administration of large parenteral doses of pethidine (e.g. 250 mg or more per day). As previously discussed, accumulation of norpethidine is responsible for this toxicity. It is unclear whether active metabolites of other opioids play a similar role (see also Chapter 9.2.10).

If the myoclonus is symptomatic and distressing, it should be treated. If dose reduction is impossible, options include either a switch to an alternative opioid[176] or empirical treatment with a low dose of a benzodiazepine (clonazepam[177]), dantrolene,[178] a barbiturate, or sodium valproate.

Respiratory depression (see also Chapter 9.5)

Respiratory depression is potentially the most serious adverse effect of strong opioids. The morphine-like agonists act on brainstem respiratory centres to produce, as a function of dose, increasing respiratory depression to the point of apnoea. In humans, death due to overdose of a morphine-like agonist is nearly always due to respiratory arrest.

Therapeutic doses of morphine may depress all phases of respiratory activity (rate, minute volume, and tidal exchange). However, as CO_2 accumulates, it stimulates central chemoreceptors, resulting in a compensatory increase in respiratory rate which masks the degree of respiratory depression. For these reasons, individuals with impaired respiratory function or bronchial asthma are at greater risk of experiencing clinically significant respiratory depression in response to usual doses of these drugs. At equianalgesic doses, the morphine-like agonists produce an equivalent degree of respiratory depression.

Respiratory depression and CO_2 retention result in cerebral vasodilation and an increase in cerebrospinal fluid pressure unless $P\text{CO}_2$ is maintained at normal levels by artificial ventilation.

When respiratory depression occurs, it is usually in opioid-naïve patients following acute administration of an opioid and is associated with other signs of central nervous system depression, including sedation and mental clouding. Although tolerance to this effect may develop rapidly,[161] the observation that some patients on stable opioid therapy develop respiratory depression after anaesthetic or neurodestructive procedures[179] suggests that other pain-related factors may also play a role in the ability to tolerate high-dose opioid therapy in the management of chronic cancer pain without significant risk of respiratory depression. Indeed, clinically important respiratory depression is a very rare effect in the cancer patient whose opioid dose has been titrated against pain. When respiratory depression occurs in such patients, alternative explanations (e.g. pneumonia or pulmonary embolism) should be sought. However, opioid-induced respiratory depression can occur if pain is suddenly eliminated (as may occur following neurolytic procedures) and the opioid dose is not reduced.

Clinically significant respiratory depression is always accompanied by other signs of central nervous system depression, including somnolence, mental clouding, and bradypnoea. Respiratory distress associated with tachypnoea and anxiety is never a primary opioid event but may be associated with infection or pulmonary embolism. It is rarely necessary to use the specific opioid antagonist naloxone to reverse respiratory depression in the palliative care setting. Reduction in dose or temporary withdrawal of the opioid is usually all that is required.

If the patient is becoming progressively obtunded, cannot be roused, or has severe respiratory depression, naloxone should be administered using small bolus injections of dilute solution (0.4 mg in 10 ml saline) which are titrated against respiratory rate.[180] Since partial reversal of respiratory depression with naloxone does not prove that the opioid was the primary cause of the event, it does not obviate the need for a careful patient evaluation for a decompensating cardiopulmonary process. Since naloxone has a short half-life, patients receiving controlled-release morphine, transdermal fentanyl, or methadone may require repeated doses or a naloxone infusion to prevent recurrence of respiratory depression.

Naloxone should be used with caution. Injudicious administration may precipitate an acute severe opioid withdrawal reaction which may be extremely distressing.

'Allergy' and intolerance to morphine

Morphine and other opioids cause histamine release, and this is said to contribute to asthma or urticaria in allergic patients. There is no published information on the incidence of this phenomenon and, in our experience, it is very rare.

However, it is not uncommon for patients to claim that they are 'allergic' to morphine. This usually means that they have had a bad experience with the drug but, on investigation, what they describe are its common side-effects. There is no doubt that most patients experience some adverse effects when they first start regular morphine treatment. Invariably this is sedation, and in some it is nausea and less often vomiting. All patients must be warned about this and appropriate measures must be taken, as described above. If patients are not warned and experience unpleasant adverse effects they will be discouraged from continuing with the drug, and if they do not understand what is going on they may assume they that are 'allergic' to it.

Some adverse effects with opioids may be more likely in the absence of pain. Pain may act as an 'antagonist' of the central nervous system depressant effects of opioid analgesics,[181,182] and clinically this can be demonstrated in relation to respiratory depression.[183] Clinical experience suggests that this rule does not apply to respiratory depression only. It appears that a balance is usually achieved between pain and the central nervous system adverse effects of opioid analgesics, so that analgesia is achieved without intolerable unwanted effects. Usually the balance between analgesia and unwanted effects produced by opioids weighs very much towards analgesia. In patients where the balance is in the other direction and adverse effects dominate the clinical picture, re-evaluation of the patient and his or her pain and the specific drug therapy are required.

The opioid-dependent patient: definitions and misconceptions

Confusion about physical dependence and addiction underlies the fear of opioid drugs and contributes to physician reluctance to prescribe opioids and patient reluctance to use them.[184] To understand these phenomena as they relate to opioid treatment of cancer pain, it is useful first to present a concept that might be called 'therapeutic dependence'. Patients who require a specific drug therapy to control a symptom or disease process are clearly dependent on the therapeutic efficacy of the drugs in question. Examples of this 'therapeutic dependence' include the requirements of patients with congestive cardiac failure for cardiotonic and diuretic medication or the reliance of insulin-dependent diabetics on insulin therapy. In these patients undermedication or withdrawal of treatment would result in serious untoward consequences. Patients with chronic cancer pain have an analogous relationship to their analgesic therapy. This relationship may or may not be associated with the development of physical dependence, but is virtually never associated with addiction.

Psychological dependence, physical dependence, and 'addiction'

The properties of the opioid analgesics that are most likely to lead to their being misused, or the patient mistreated, are effects mediated in the central nervous system and seen following chronic administration, including psychological and physical dependence. It must be emphasized that, while the development of physical dependence and tolerance are predictable pharmacological effects seen in humans and laboratory animals in response to repeated administration of an opioid, these effects are distinct from the behavioural pattern seen in some individuals and described as 'addiction'.[185] Physical dependence and tolerance may occur with other therapeutic agents which are not drugs of abuse, for example antihypertensives. 'Addiction' implies something distinct and is characterized by psychological dependence. This latter term is used to mean a pattern of drug use characterized by a continued craving for an opioid which is manifest as compulsive drug-seeking behaviour leading to an overwhelming involvement with the use and procurement of the drug. Within these definitions anyone who is addicted to opioids is likely to be physically dependent. However, the term addiction is not interchangeable with physical dependence; it is possible to be physically dependent on an opioid analgesic without being addicted. Fear of addiction is a major consideration limiting the use of appropriate doses of opioids in hospital inpatients in pain. Some patients are reluctant to take even small doses of opioids for fear of becoming addicted. However, surveys in medical patients[186] and burn patients in hospital,[187] and an analysis of the patterns of drug intake in cancer patients receiving chronic opioids,[157] suggest that medical use of opioids rarely, if ever, leads to drug abuse or iatrogenic opioid addiction.

Physical dependence

Physical dependence is the term used to describe the phenomenon of withdrawal when an opioid is abruptly discontinued or an opioid antagonist is administered. The severity of withdrawal is a function of the dose and duration of administration of the opioid just discontinued (i.e. the patient's prior opioid exposure). The administration of an opioid antagonist to a physically dependent individual produces an immediate precipitation of the withdrawal syndrome. Patients who have received repeated doses of a morphine-like agonist to the point where they are physically dependent may experience an opioid withdrawal reaction when given a mixed agonist–antagonist. It can be shown that prior exposure to a morphine-like drug greatly increases a patient's sensitivity to the antagonist component of a mixed agonist–antagonist. Therefore, when used for chronic pain, the mixed agonist–antagonists should be tried before prolonged administration of a morphine-like agonist is initiated.

The abrupt discontinuation of an opioid analgesic in a patient with significant prior opioid experience will result in signs and symptoms characteristic of the opioid withdrawal or abstinence syndrome. The onset of withdrawal is characterized by the patient's report of feelings of anxiety, nervousness and irritability, and alternating chills and hot flushes. A prominent withdrawal sign is 'wetness' including salivation, lacrimation, rhinorrhoea, sneezing, and sweating, as well as gooseflesh.[185] At the peak intensity of withdrawal patients may experience nausea and vomiting, abdominal cramps, insomnia, and, rarely, multifocal myoclonus. The time course of the withdrawal syndrome is a function of the elimination half-life of the opioid on which the patient has become dependent. Abstinence symptoms will appear within 6 to 12 h and reach a peak at 24 to 72 h following cessation of a short-half-life drug such as morphine, while onset may be delayed for 36 to 48 h with methadone which has a long half-life. Therefore it is important to emphasize that, even in a patient in whom pain has been completely relieved by a procedure (e.g. a cordotomy), it is necessary to decrease the opioid dose slowly to prevent withdrawal.[157]

Experience indicates that the usual daily dose required to prevent withdrawal is equal to 75 per cent of the previous daily dose. Following this rule of thumb, doses can be gradually titrated down until the drug is discontinued.

'Pseudoaddiction'

Some cancer patients who continue to experience unrelieved pain manifest intense concern about opioid availability and drug-seeking behaviour that is reminiscent of addiction but ceases once pain is relieved, often through opioid dose escalation. This behaviour has been termed 'pseudoaddiction'.[188] Pain relief usually produced by dose escalation eliminates this aberrant behaviour and distinguishes the patient from the true addict. Misunderstanding of this phenomenon may lead the clinician inappropriately to stigmatize the patient with the label 'addict' which may compromise care and erode the doctor–patient relationship. In the setting of unrelieved pain the request for increases in drug doses requires careful assessment, renewed efforts to manage pain, and avoidance of stigmatizing labels.

Management of cancer pain in patients with a history of drug abuse

Patients with a history of abuse of opioid analgesics may develop cancer and severe pain. The management of such patients is, in principle, exactly the same as that outlined in this chapter.[189] Our approach is to maintain such patients on oral medication if possible, even though they may require very much larger doses than normal. If parenteral medication is required, continuous subcutaneous infusion remains the mode of administration of choice.

For patients receiving therapy for drug abuse, with or without opioid maintenance therapy (e.g. methadone maintenance), it is essential that the issues relating to the use of opioid analgesics for pain management are discussed not only with the patient but also with his or her family and drug abuse counsellors, so that the patient's support group reaches a consensus on the utility and appropriateness of analgesic therapy.[190] An open and supportive approach, and the use of concomitant psychotropic medication as appropriate, will aid the effective management of these patients.

In managing these patients clinicians should be aware of several common issues that may confound therapy.[190,191] Mental clouding, either as an effect of disease progression or as an iatrogenic adverse effect, commonly raises concerns about the relapse or recurrence of psychological dependence. A request for escalation of their opioid dose may be generated by increased psychological stress rather than pain alone. Aberrant drug-seeking behaviour such as acquisition of opioids from multiple sources, 'loss' of prescribed drugs or prescriptions, unsanctioned dose escalation, and prescription fraud must be recognized as suggestive of true addiction and addressed openly as such. In all cases one clinician should be identified as responsible for pain management, and these patients should be reviewed frequently.

Conclusions

Optimal therapy for the cancer patient with pain depends on a comprehensive assessment of his or her pain, medical condition, and psychosocial status as well as an understanding of the clinical pharmacology of analgesic drugs. It must be emphasized that cancer patients with pain vary greatly in their response to analgesics. Pharmacokinetic and pharmacodynamic factors, as well as psychological factors, will influence the effectiveness of an analgesic in an individual patient. Through a process of repeated evaluation and continuous review, analgesic therapy with opioids, non-opioids, and adjuvant analgesics is individualized so that a favourable balance between pain relief and adverse pharmacological effects is maintained.

References

1. World Health Organization. *Cancer Pain Relief.* Geneva: WHO, 1986.
2. World Health Organization. *Cancer Pain Relief.* 2nd edn. Geneva: WHO, 1996.
3. Foley KM. The treatment of cancer pain. *New England Journal of Medicine*, 1985; **313**:84–95.
4. Dickenson AH. Mechanisms of the analgesic actions of opiates and opioids. *British Medical Journal,* 1991; **47**:690–702.
5. Inturrisi CE. Effects of other drugs and pathologic states on opioid disposition and response. In: Benedetti C, Giron G, Chapman CR, eds. *Advances in Pain Research and Therapy*, Vol. 14. New York: Raven Press, 1990:171–80.
6. Beaver W, Wallenstein S, Houde R, Rogers A. Comparison of the analgesic effects of pentazocine and morphine in patients with cancer. *Clinical Pharmacology and Therapeutics*, 1966; **7**:740–51.
7. Houde RW, Wallenstein S, Beaver WT. Clinical measurement of pain. In: de Stevens G, ed. *Analgetics.* New York: Academic Press, 1965: 75–122.
8. Houde RW. Analgesic effectiveness of narcotic agonist–antagonists. *British Journal of Clinical Pharmacology,* 1979; **7**:297–308.
9. Inturrisi CE, Portenoy RK, Max MB, Colburn WA, Foley KM. Pharmacokinetic–pharmacodynamic relationships of methadone infusions in patients with cancer pain. *Clinical Pharmacology and Therapeutics,* 1990;**47**:565–77.
10. Hughes J, Kosterlitz HW. Introduction (to opioid peptides). *British Medical Bulletin,* 1983; **39**:1–3.
11. Pasternak GW. Pharmacological meachanisms of opioid analgesics. *Clinical Neuropharmacology,* 1993; **16**:1–18.
12. Martin WR, Eades CG, Thompson JA, Huppler RE, Gilbert PE. The effects of morphine and nalorphine-like drugs in the non-dependent and morphine-dependent spinal dog. *Journal of Pharmacology and Experimental Therapeutics,* 1976; **197**:517–32.
13. Knapp RJ, *et al.* Identification of a human delta opioid-receptor: cloning and expression. *Life Sciences*, 1994; **54**:9.
14. Zhu J, Chen C, Xue JC, Kunapulis, DeRiel JK, Liu CL. Cloning of a human kappa opioid receptor from the brain. *Life Sciences,* 1995; **56**:7.
15. Simonin F, *et al.* The human delta-opioid receptor: genomic organization , cDNA cloning, functional expression, and distribution in human brain. *Molecular Pharmacology,* 1994; **46**:1015–21.
16. Wang JB, Imai Y, Eppler CM, Gregor P, Spivak CE, Uhl GR. Mu opiate receptor: cDNA cloning and expression. *Proceedings of the National Academy of Sciences of the United States of America*, 1993; **90**:10 230–4.
17. Reisine T, Pasternak G. Opioid analgesics and antagonists. In: Hardman JG, Limbird LE, Molinoff PB, Ruddon RW, Gilman AG, eds. *Goodman and Gilman's Pharmacological Basis of Therapeutics.* 9th edn. New York: McGraw-Hill, 1996:521–55.
18. Houde RW, Wallenstein SL, Beaver WT. Evaluation of analgesics in patients with cancer pain. In: Lasagna L, ed. *International Encyclopaedia of Pharmacology and Therapeutics*, Vol. 1. New York: Pergamon Press, 1966:59–67.
19. Portenoy RK, Foley KM, Inturrisi CE. The nature of opioid responsiveness and its implications for neuropathic pain: new hypotheses derived from studies of opioid infusions. *Pain,* 1990; **43**:273–86.
20. Ventafridda V, Tamburini M, Caraceni A, DeConno F, Naldi F. A validation study of the WHO method for cancer pain relief. *Cancer,* 1987; **59**:851–6.
21. Takeda F. Japan's WHO cancer pain relief program. In: Foley KM, Bonica JJ, Ventafridda V, Callaway MV, eds. *Advances in Pain Research and Therapy,* Vol. 16. New York: Raven Press, 1990:475–83.
22. Zech DFJ, Grond S, Lynch J, Hertel D, Lehman KA. Validation of World Health Organization guidelines for cancer pain relief. A 10 year prospective study. *Pain,* 1995; **63**:65–76.
23. Jadad AR, Browman GP. The WHO analgesic ladder for cancer pain management. *Journal of the American Medical Association,* 1995; **274**:1870–3.
24. Persson K, Hammarlund-Udenaes M, Mortimer O, Rane A. The post-operative pharmacokinetics of codeine. *European Journal of Clinical Pharmacology,* 1992; **42**:663–6.
25. Findlay JWA, Jones EC, Butz RF, Welch RM. Plasma codeine and morphine concentrations after therapeutic oral doses of codeine-containing analgesics. *Clinical Pharmacology and Therapeutics*, 1978; **24**:60–8.
26. Cleary J, Mikus G, Somogyi A, Bochner F. The influence of pharmacogenetics on opioid analgesia: studies with codeine and oxycodone in the Sprague–Dawley/Dark Agouti rat model. *Journal of Pharmcology and Experimental Therapeutics,* 1994; **271**:1528–34.
27. Quiding H, Lundqvist G, Boreus LO, Bondesson U, Ohrvik J. Analgesic effect and plasma concentrations of codeine and morphine after two dose levels of codeine following oral surgery. *European Journal of Clinical Pharmacology,* 1993; **44**:319–23.
28. Vree TB, Verwey-van Wissen CP. Pharmacokinetics and metabolism of codeine in humans. *Biopharmaceutics and Drug Disposition,* 1992; **13**:445–60.
29. Beaver WT, *et al.* Analgesic studies of codeine and oxycodone in patients with cancer: I. Comparisons of oral with intramuscular codeine and of oral with intramuscular oxycodone. *Journal of Pharmacology and Experimental Therapeutics*, 1978; **207**:92–100.
30. Lasagna L, Beecher KH. The analgesic effectiveness of codeine and meperdine (Demerol). *Journal of Pharmacology and Experimental Therapeutics*, 1954; **112**:306–11.
31. Beaver WT. Mild analgesics: a review of their clinical pharmacology (part II). *American Journal of Medical Science*, 1966; **251**:576–99.
32. Dhaliwal HS, *et al.* Randomized evaluation of controlled-release codeine and placebo in chronic cancer pain. *Journal of Pain and Symptom Management,* 1995; **10**:612–23.
33. Palmer RN, Eade OE, O'Shea PJ, Cuthbert MF. Incidence of unwanted effects of dihydrocodeine bitartrate in healthy volunteers. *Lancet* 1966; **ii**: 620–1.
34. Anonymous. Dihydrocodeine (tartrate). In: Dollery C, ed. *Therapeutic Drugs.* Edinburgh: Churchill Livingstone, 1991:D133–6.
35. Rowell FJ, Seymour RA, Rawlins MD. Pharmacokinetics of intravenous and oral dihydrocodeine and its acid metabolites. *European Journal of Clinical Pharmacology,* 1983; **25**:419–24.
36. McQuay HJ, Carroll D, Guest PG, Robson S, Wiffen PJ, Juniper RP. A multiple dose comparison of ibuprofen and dihydrocodeine after third molar surgery. *British Journal of Oral and Maxillofacial Surgery,* 1993; **31**:95–100.

37. Barnes JN, Williams AJ, Tomson MJF, Toseland PA, Goodwin FJ. Dihydrocodeine in renal failure: further evidence for an important role of the kidney in the handling of opioid drugs. *British Medical Journal*, 1985; **290**:740–2.
38. Martin M. Converting to morphine. *Pharmaceutical Journal*, 1989; **242**:181.
39. Nickander RC, Emmerson JL, Hynes MD, Steinberg MI, Sullivan HR. Pharmacologic and toxic effects in animals of dextropropoxyphene and its major metabolite norpropoxyphene: a review. *Human Toxicology*, 1984; 3:13S–36S.
40. Crome P, Gain R, Ghurye R, Flanagan RJ. Pharmacokinetics of dextropropopoxyphene and nordextropropoxyphene in elderly hospital patients after single and multiple doses of Distalgesic. Preliminary analysis of results. *Human Toxiciology*, 1984;3:41S–8S.
41. Inturrisi CE, Colburn WA, Vereby K, Dayton HE, Woody GE, O'Brien CP. Propoxyphene and norpropoxyphene kinetics after single and repeated doses of propoxyphene. *Clinical Pharmacology and Therapeutics*, 1982; **31**:157–67.
42. Beaver WT. Analgesic efficacy of dextropropoxyphene and dextropropoxyphene-containing combinations: a review. *Human Toxicology*, 1984; 3:191S–220S.
43. Perrier D, Gibaldi M. Influence of first-pass effect on the systemic availability of propoxyphene. *Journal of Clinical Pharmacology*, 1972; **12**:449–52.
44. Anonymous. Dangers of dextropropoxyphene (Editorial). *British Medical Journal*, 1977; **i**:668.
45. Obafunwa JO, Busuttil A. Deaths from substance overdose in the Lothian and Borders region of Scotland (1983–1991). *Human and Experimental Toxicology*, 1994; **13**:401–6.
46. Rosenberg WM, Ryley NG, Trowell JM, McGee JO, Chapman RW. Dextropropoxyphene induced hepatotoxicity: a report of nine cases. *Journal of Hepatology*, 1993; **19**:470–4.
47. Raffa RB, Friderichs E, Reimann W, Shank RP, Codd EE, Vaught JL. Opioid and non-opioid components independently contribute to the mechanism of action of tramadol, an 'atypical' opioid analgesic. *Journal of Pharmacology and Experimental Therapeutics*, 1992; **260**:275–85.
48. Vickers MD, O'Flaherty D, Szekely SM, Read M, Yoshizumi J. Tramadol: pain relief by an opioid without depression of respiration. *Anaesthesia*, 1992; **47**:291–6.
49. Viegas OAC, Khaw B, Ratnam SS. Tramadol in labour pain in primiparous patients. A prospective comparative clinical trial. *European Journal of Obstetrics and Gynaecology and Reproductive Biology*, 1993: **49**:131–5.
50. Brown P, Mehlisch DR, Minn F. Tramadol hydrochloride: efficacy compared to codeine sulfate, acetaminophen with dextropropoxyphene and placebo in dental-extracetion pain. *British Journal of Pharmacology*, 1989; **98**:441.
51. Wilder Smith CH, Schimke J, Osterwalder B, Senn HJ. Oral tramadol, a mu-opioid agonist and monoamine reuptake-blocker, and morphine for strong cancer-related pain. *Annals of Oncology*, 1994; **5**:141–6.
52. Rauck RL, Ruoff GE, McMillen JI. Comparison of tramadol and acetaminophen with codeine for long-term pain management in elderly patients. *Current Therapeutic Research*, 1994; **55**: 1417–31.
53. Grond S, Zech D, Lynch J, Schug S, Lehmann KA. Tramadol—a weak opioid for relief of cancer pain. *Pain Clinic*, 1992; **5**:241–7.
54. Beaver WT. Aspirin and acetaminophen as constituents of analgesic combinations. *Archives of Internal Medicine*, 1981; **141**:293–300.
55. McQuay HJ, Carroll D, Watts PG, Juniper RP, Moore RA. Codeine 20 mg increases pain relief from ibuprofen 400 mg after third molar surgery. A repeat-dosing comparison of ibuprofen and an ibuprofen-codeine combination. *Pain*, 1989; **37**: 7–13.
56. Lysell L, Anzen B. Pain control after third molar surgery—a comparative study of ibuprofen (Ibumetin) and a paracetamol/codeine combination (Citodon). *Swedish Dental Journal*, 1992; **16**:151–60.
57. Dionne RA, Snyder J, Hargreaves KM. Analgesic efficacy of flurbiprofen in comparison with acetaminophen, acetaminophen plus codeine, and placebo after impacted third molar removal. *Journal of Oral and Maxillofacial Surgery*, 1994; **52**:919–24.
58. Naidu MU, *et al.* Evaluation of ketorolac, ibuprofen–paracetamol, and dextropropoxyphene–paracetamol in postoperative pain. *Pharmacotherapy*, 1994; **14**:173–7.
59. Benyhe S. Morphine: new aspects in the study of an ancient compound. *Life Sciences*, 1994: **55**:969–79.
60. Sawe J, Dahlstrom B, Paalzow L, Rane A. Morphine kinetics in cancer patients. *Clinical Pharmacology and Therapeutics*, 1981: **30**:629–35.
61. Hoskin PJ, Hanks GW, Aherne GW, Chapman D, Littleton P, Filshie J. The bioavailability and pharmacokinetics of morphine after intravenous, oral and buccal administration in healthy volunteers. *British Journal of Clinical Pharmacology*, 1989; **27**:499–505.
62. Gourlay GK, Plummer JL, Cherry DA, Purser T. The reproducibility of bioavailability of oral morphine from solution under fed and fasted conditions. *Journal of Pain and Symptom Management*, 1991; **6**:431–6.
63. Sawe J, Svensson JO, Rane A. Morphine metabolism in cancer patients on increasing oral doses —no evidence for autoinduction or dose dependence. *British Journal of Clinical Pharmacology*, 1983; **16**:85–93.
64. Max MB, Inturrisi CE, Kaiko RF, Grabinski PY, Li CH, Foley KM. Epidural and inthrathecal opiates: cerebrospinal fluid and plasma profiles in patients with chronic cancer pain. *Clinical Pharmacology and Therapeutics*, 1985; **38**:631–41.
65. Paul D, Standifer KM, Inturrisi CE, Pasternak GW. Pharmacological characterization of morphine-6-beta-glucuronide, a very potent morphine metabolite. *Journal of Pharmacology and Experimental Therapeutics*, 1989; **251**:477–83.
66. Shimomura K, *et al.* Analgesic effect of morphine glucuronides. *Tohoku Journal of Experimental Medicine*, 1971; **105**:45–52.
67. Pasternak GW, Bodnar RJ, Clark JA, Inturrisi CE. Morphine-6-glucuronide, a potent mu agonist. *Life Sciences*, 1987; **41**:2845–9.
68. Osborne JR, Joel SP, Slevin ML. Morphine intoxication in renal failure: the role of morphine-6-glucuronide. *British Medical Journal*, 1986; **292**:1548–9.
69. Osborne R, Thompson P, Joel S, Trew D, Patel N, Slevin ML. The analgesic activity of morphine-6-glucuronide. *British Journal of Clinical Pharmacology*, 1992; **34**:130–8.
70. Portenoy RK, Thaler HT, Inturrisi CE, Friedlander-Klar H, Foley KM. The metabolite, morphine-6-glucuronide, contributes to the analgesia produced by morphine infusion in pain patients with normal renal function. *Clinical Pharmacolgy and Therapeutics*, 1992; **51**:422–31.
71. Portenoy RK, *et al.* Plasma morphine and morphine-6-glucuronide during chronic morphine therapy for cancer pain: plasma profiles, steady state concentrations and the consequences of renal failure. *Pain*, 1991; **47**:13–19.
72. D'Honneur G, Gilton A, Sandouk P, Scherrmann JM, Duvaldestin P. Plasma and cerebrospinal fluid concentrations of morphine and morphine glucuronides after oral morphine. The influence of renal failure. *Anesthesiology*, 1994; **81**:87–93.
73. Lehmann KA, Zech D. Morphine-6-glucuronide a pharmacologically active morphine metabolite: a review of the literature. *European Journal of Pain*, 1993; **12**:28–35.
74. Hanks GW, Hoskin PJ, Aherne GW, Turner P, Poulain P. Explanation for potency of repeated oral doses of morphine? *Lancet*, 1987; **ii**:723–5.
75. Twycross RG. The therapeutic equivalence of oral and subcutaneous/intramuscular morphine sulphate in cancer patients. *Journal of Palliative Care*, 1988; **2**:67–8.
76. Kaiko RF. Commentary: equianalgesic dose ratio of intramuscular/oral morphine, 1:6 versus 1:3. In: Foley KM, Inturrisi CE, eds. *Advances in Pain Research and Therapy*, Vol. 8. New York: Raven Press, 1986: 87–93.
77. Hanks GW. Controlled-release morphine (MST Contin) in advanced cancer: the European experience. *Cancer*, 1989; **623**:2378–82.
78. Forman WB, Portenoy RK, Yanagihara RH, Hunt C, Kush R, Shepard K. A novel morphine sulphate preparation: clinical trial of a controlled-release morphine suspension in cancer pain. *Palliative Medicine*, 1993; **7**:301–6.
79. Savarese JJ, Goldenheim PD, Thomas GB, Kaiko RF. Steady-state pharmacokinetics of controlled release oral morphine sulphate in healthy subjects. *Clinical Pharmacokinetics*, 1986; **11**:505–10.

80. Poulain P, *et al.* Relative bioavailability of controlled release morphine tablets (MST Continus) in cancer patients. *British Journal of Anaesthesia*, 1988; **61**:569–74.
81. Cherry DA, Gourley G, Plummer JL, Onley MM, Russell A, Beaumont AC. A comparison of Kapanol® (a new sustained release morphine formulation) and MST Continus® and morphine solution in cancer patients: morphine metabolite profiles and renal function. *Abstracts, 7th World Congress on Pain.* Seattle: IASP Publications, 1993:abstract 999.
82. Hanks GW, *et al.* Morphine in cancer pain: modes of administration. *British Medical Journal,* 1996; **312**:823–6.
83. Inturrisi CE, Max MB, Foley KM, Schultz M, Shin S-U, Houde RW. The pharmacokinetics of heroin in patients with chronic pain. *New England Journal of Medicine*, 1984; **210**:1213–17.
84. Kaiko RF, Wallenstein SL, Rogers AG, Grabinski PY, Houde RW. Analgesic and mood effects of heroin and morphine in cancer patients with postoperative pain. *New England Journal of Medicine*, 1981; **304**:1501–5.
85. Ventafridda V, Ripamonti C, Bianchi M, Sbanotto A, DeConno F. A randomized study on oral administration of morphine and methadone in the treatment of cancer pain. *Journal of Pain and Symptom Management,* 1986; **1**:203–8.
86. Twycross RG, Lack SA. *Symptom control in far-advanced cancer: pain relief.* London: Pitman, 1984:244–7.
87. Grochow L, Sheidler V, Grossman S, Green L, Enterline J. Does intravenous methadone provide longer lasting analgesia than intravenous morphine? A randomized double-blind study. *Pain,* 1989; **38**:151–7.
88. Inturrisi CE, Colburn WA, Kaiko RF, Houde RW, Foley KM. Pharmacokinetics and pharmacodynamics of methadone in patients with chronic pain. *Clinical Pharmacology and Therapeutics,* 1987; **41**:392–401.
89. Inturrisi CE, Portenoy RK, Max MB. Colburn WA, Foley KM. Pharmacokinetic–pharmacodynamic (PK–PD) relationships of methadone infusions in patients with cancer pain. *Clinical Pharmacology and Therapeutics,* 1990; **47**:565–70.
90. Fainsinger R, Schoeller T, Bruera E. Methadone in the management of cancer pain: a review. *Pain,* 1993; **52**:137–47.
91. Ettinger DS, Vitale PJ, Trump DL. Important clinical pharmacologic considerations in the use of methadone in cancer patients. *Cancer Treatment Reports*, 1979; **63**:457–9.
92. Bruera E, Fainsinger R, Moore M, Thibault R, Spoldi E, Ventafridda V. Local toxicity with subcutaneous methadone. Experience of two centers. *Pain,* 1991; **45**:141–145.
93. Szeto HH, Inturrisi CE, Houde R, Saal R, Cheigh J, Reidenberg MM. Accumulation of normeperidine an active metabolite of meperidine, in patients with renal failure or cancer. *Annals of Internal Medicine,* 1977; **86**:738–41.
94. Eisendrath SJ, Goldman B, Douglas J, Dimatteo L, Van DC. Meperidine-induced delirium. *American Journal of Psychiatry,* 1987; **144**:1062–5.
95. Hagmeyer KO, Mauro LS, Mauro VF. Meperidine-related seizures associated with patient-controlled analgesia pumps. *Annals of Pharmacotherapy,* 1993; **27**:29–32.
96. Umans JG, Inturrisi CE. Antinociceptive activity and toxicity of meperidine and normeperidine in mice. *Journal of Pharmacology and Experimental Therapeutics*, 1982; **223**:203–6.
97. Kaiko RF, *et al.* Central nervous system excitatory effects of meperidine in cancer patients. *Annals of Neurology,* 1983; **13**:180–5.
98. Agency for Health Care Policy and Research: Acute Pain Management Panel. *Acute Pain Management: Operative or Medical Procedures and Trauma.* Washington, DC: US Department of Health and Human Services, 1992.
99. Houde RW. Clinical analgesic studies of hydromorphone. In: Foley KM, Inturrisi CE, ed. *Advances in Pain Research and Therapy,* Vol. 8. New York: Raven Press, 1986:129–36.
100. Moulin DE, Kreeft JH, Murray PN, Bouquillon AI. Comparison of continuous subcutaneous and intravenous hydromorphone infusions for management of cancer pain. *Lancet,* 1991; **337**:465–8.
101. Hays H, *et al.* Comparative clinical efficacy and safety of immediate release and controlled release hydromorphone for chronic severe pain. *Cancer,* 1994; **74**:1808–16.
102. Coombs DW, Saunders RL, Fratkin JD, Jensen LE, Murphey CA. Continuous intrathecal hydromorphone and clonidine for intractable cancer pain. *Journal of Neurosurgery,* 1986; **64**:890–4.
103. Brose WG, Tanalian DL, Brodsky JB, Mark JBD, Cousins MJ. CSF and blood pharmacokinetics of hydromorphone and morphine following lumbar epidural administration. *Pain,* 1991; **45**:11–17.
104. Dixon R, Crews T, Inturrisi CE, Foley KM. Levorphanol: pharmacokinetics and steady-state plasma concentrations in patients with pain. *Research Communications in Chemistry, Pathology and Pharmacology,* 1983; **41**:3–17.
105. Wallenstein SL, Rogers AG, Kaiko RF, Houde RW. Clinical analgesic studies of levorphanol in acute and chronic cancer pain. In: Foley KM, Inturrisi CE, ed. *Advances in Pain Research and Therapy,* Vol 8. New York: Raven Press, 1986: 211–15.
106. Moulin DE, Ling GS, Pasternak GW. Unidirectional cross tolerance between morphine and levorphanol in the rat. *Pain,* 1988; **33**:233–9.
107. Kalso E, Vainio A. Morphine and oxycodone hydrochloride in the management of cancer pain. *Clinical Pharmacology and Therapeutics,* 1990; **47**:639–46.
108. Poyhia R, Vainio A, Kalso E. A review of oxycodone's clinical pharmacokinetics and pharmacodynamics. *Journal of Pain and Symptom Management,* 1993; **8**:63–7.
109. Leow KP, Smith MT, Williams B, Cramond T. Single-dose and steady-state pharmacokinetics and pharmacodynamics of oxycodone in patients with cancer. *Clinical Pharmacology and Therapeutics,* 1992; **52**:487–95.
110. Glare PA, Walsh TD. Dose-ranging study of oxycodone for chronic pain in advanced cancer. *Journal of Clinical Oncology,* 1993; **11**:973–8.
111. Leow KP, Cramond T, Smith MT. Pharmacokinetics and pharmacodynamics of oxycodone when given intravenously and rectally to adult patients with cancer pain. *Anesthesia and Analgesia,* 1995; **80**:296–302.
112. Eddy NB, Lee LE. The analgesic equivalence and relative side action liability of oxymorphone. *Journal of Pharmacology and Experimental Therapeutics,* 1959; **125**:116–21.
113. Hermens JM, Hanifin JM, Hirshman CA. Comparison of histamine release in human skin mast cells by morphine, fentanyl and oxymorphone. *Anesthesiology,* 1985; **62**:124–9.
114. Rogers A. Considering histamine release in prescribing opioid analgesics. *Journal of Pain and Symptom Management,* 1991; **6**:44–5.
115. Singer M, Noonan KR. Continuous intravenous infusion of fentanyl: case reports of use in patients with advanced cancer and intractable pain. *Journal of Pain and Symptom Management,* 1993; **8**:215–20.
116. Varvel JR, Shafer SL, Hwang SS, Coen PA, Stanski DR. Absorption characteristics of transdermally administered fentanyl. *Anesthesiology,* 1989; **70**:928–34.
117. Southam MA. Transdermal fentanyl therapy: system design, pharmacokinetics and efficacy. *Anti-Cancer Drugs,* 1995; **6**(Supplement 3):26–34.
118. Simmonds MA, Richenbacher J. Transdermal fentanyl: long-term analgesic studies. *Journal of Pain and Symptom Management,* 1992; **7**:S36–9.
119. Zech DFJ, Grond SUA, Lynch J, Dauer HG, Stollenwerk W, Lehmann KA. Transdermal fentanyl and initial dose-finding with patient-controlled analgesia in cancer pain. A pilot study with 20 terminally ill cancer patients. *Pain,* 1992; **50**:293–301.
120. Portenoy RK, *et al.* Transdermal fentanyl for cancer pain: repeated doses pharmacokinetics. *Anesthesiology,* 1993; **78**:36–43.
121. Storey P. More on the conversion of transdermal fentanyl to morphine. *Journal of Pain and Symptom Management*, 1995; **10**:581–2.
122. Anonymous. Phenazocine. *Drug Therapy Bulletin*, 1979; **18**:70.
123. Anonymous. Dextromoramide (tartrate). In: Dollery C, ed. *Therapeutic Drugs.* Edinburgh: Churchill Livingstone, 1991:D66–9.
124. Faull C, McKechnie E, Riley J, Ahmedzai S. Experience with dipipanone elixir in the management of cancer related pain: case study. *Palliative Medicine,* 1994; **8**:63–5.
125. Hoskin PJ, Hanks GW. Opioid agonist antagonist drugs in acute and chronic pain states. *Drugs,* 1991; **41**:326–44.

126. Gal TJ. Naloxone reversal of buprenorphine-induced respiratory depression. *Clinical Pharmacology and Therapeutics*, 1989; **45**:6–71.
127. Galer BS, Coyle N, Pasternak GW, Portenoy RK. Individual variability in the response to different opioids: report of five cases. *Pain*, 1992; **49**:87–91.
128. Neal EA, Meffin PJ, Gregory PB, Blaschke TF. Enhanced bioavailability and decreased clearance of analgesics in patients with cirrhosis. *Gastroenterology*, 1979; **77**:96–102.
129. Giacomini KM, Giacomini JC, Gibson TP, Levy G. Propoxyphene and norpropoxyphene plasma concentrations after oral propoxyphene in cirrhotic patients with and without surgically contructed portacaval shunt. *Clinical Pharmacology and Therapeutics*, 1980; **28**:417–24.
130. Patwardhan RV, *et al.* Normal metabolism of morphine in cirrhosis. *Gastroenterology*, 1981; **81**:1006–11.
131. Hasselstrom J, Eriksson LS, Persson A, Rane A, Svensson J, Sawe J. The metabolism and bioavailability of morphine in patients with severe liver cirrhosis. *British Journal of Clinical Pharmacology*, 1990; **29**:289–97.
132. Chan GL, Matzke GR. Effects of renal insufficiency on the pharmacokinetics and pharmacodynamics of opioid analgesics. *Drug Intelligence in Clinical Pharmacology*, 1987; **21**:773–83.
133. Coyle N, Adelhardt J, Foley KM, Portenoy RK. Character of terminal illness in the advanced cancer patient: pain and other symptoms during last four weeks of life. *Journal of Pain and Symptom Management*, 1990; **5**:83–9.
134. Hanning CD. The rectal absorption of opioids. In: Benedetti C, Chapman CR, Giron G, eds. *Advances in Pain Research and Therapy*, Vol. 14. New York: Raven Press, 1990:259–69.
135. Agency for Health Care Policy and Research: Cancer Pain Management Panel. *Management of Cancer Pain. Clinical Practice Guideline 9*. Washington, DC: US Department of Health and Human Services, 1994.
136. Coyle N, Cherny NI, Portenoy RK. Subcutaneous opioid infusions in the home. *Oncology*, 1994; **8**:21–27.
137. Oliver DJ. The use of the syringe driver in terminal care. *British Journal of Clinical Pharmacology*, 1985; **20**:515–16.
138. Portenoy RK. Continuous intravenous infusions of opioid drugs. *Medical Clinics of North America*, 1987; **71**:233–41.
139. Russell PSB. Analgesia in terminal malignant disease. *British Medical Journal*, 1979; **i**:1561.
140. Bruera E, Brenneis C, Michaud M, MacMillan K, Hanson J, MacDonald RN. Patient-controlled subcutaneous hydromorphone versus continuous subcutaneous infusion for the treatment of cancer pain. *Journal of the National Cancer Institute*, 1988; **80**:1152–4.
141. Waldmann CS, Eason JR, Rambohul E, Hanson GC. Serum morphine levels. A comparison between continuous subcutaneous infusions and intravenous infusions in post-operative patients. *Anaesthesia*, 1984; **39**:768–71.
142. Yaksh TL. Spinal opiate analgesics: characteristics and principal action. *Pain*, 1981; **11**:293–346.
143. Moulin DE, Inturrisi CE, Foley KM. Epidural and intrathecal opioids: cerebrospinal fluid and plasma pharmacokinetics in cancer pain patients. In: Foley KM, Inturrisi CE, eds. *Pain Research and Therapy*, Vol 8. New York: Raven Press, 1986:369–384.
144. Du Pen S, Williams AR. Management of patients receiving combined epidural morphine and bupivacaine for the treatment of cancer pain. *Journal of Pain and Symptom Management*, 1992; **7**:125–7.
145. Hogan Q, Haddox JD, Abram S, Weissman D, Taylor ML, Janjan N. Epidural opiates and local anesthetics for the mangement of cancer pain. *Pain*, 1991; **46**:271–9.
146. Van Dongen RT, Crul BJ, De Bock M. Long-term intrathecal infusion of morphine and morphine/bupivacaine mixtures in the treatment of cancer pain: a retrospective analysis of 51 cases. *Pain*, 1993; **55**:119–23.
147. Goucke R. Continuous intrathecal analgesia with opioid/local anaesthetic mixtures for cancer pain. *Anaesthesia and Intensive Care*, 1993; **21**:222–3.
148. De Castro MD, Meynadier MD, Zenz MD. *Developments in Critical Care Medicine and Anesthesiology*, Vol. 20. Dordrecht: Kluwer Academic, 1991.
149. Cramond T, Stuart G. Intraventricular morphine for intractable pain of advanced cancer. *Journal of Pain and Symptom Management*, 1993; **8**:465–73.
150. Weinberg DS, *et al.* Sublingual absorption of selected opioid analgesics. *Clinical Pharmacology and Therapeutics*, 1988; **44**:335–42.
151. Hirsch JD. Sublingual morphine sulphate in chronic pain management. *Clinical Pharmacy*, 1984; **3**:585.
152. Ripamonti C, Bruera E. Rectal, buccal and sublingual narcotics for the management of cancer pain. *Journal of Palliative Care*, 1991; **7**:30–5.
153. Streisand JB, *et al.* Absorption and bioavailability of oral transmucosal fentanyl citrate. *Anesthesiology*, 1991; **75**:223–9.
154. Fine PG, Marcus M, DeBoer AJ, Van der Oord B. An open label study of oral transmucosal fentanyl citrate (OTFC) for the treatment of breakthrough cancer pain. *Pain*, 1991; **45**:149–55.
155. Sawe J, *et al.* Patient-controlled dose regimen of methadone for chronic cancer pain. *British Medical Journal*, 1981; **282**:771–3.
156. Citron ML, Kalra JM, Seltzer VL, Chen S, Hoffman M, Walczak MB. Patient-controlled analgesia for cancer pain: a long-term study of inpatient and outpatient use. *Cancer Investigation*, 1992; **10**:335–41.
157. Kanner RM, Foley K. Patterns of narcotic drug use in a cancer pain clinic. *Annals of the New York Academy of Science*, 1981; **362**:161–72.
158. Lichter I. Accelerated titration of morphine for rapid relief of cancer pain. *New Zealand Medical Journal*, 1994; **107**:488–90.
159. Twycross RG. Clinical experience with diamorphine in advanced malignant disease. *International Journal of Clinical Pharmacology, Therapeutics and Toxicology*, 1974; **9**:184–98.
160. Brescia FJ, *et al.* Pain, opioid use, and survival in hospitalized patients with advanced cancer. *Journal of Clinical Oncology*, 1992; **10**:149–55.
161. Foley KM. Clinical tolerance to opioids. In: *Towards a New Pharmacotherapy of Pain, Dahlem Konfrenzen*. Chichester: Wiley, 1991:81–204.
162. Lufty K, Yoburn BC. The role of opioid receptor density in morphine tolerance. *Journal of Pharmacology and Experimental Therapeutics*, 1991; **256**:575–80.
163. Foley KM. Changing concepts of tolerance to opioids: what the cancer patient has taught us. In: Chapman CR, Foley KM, eds. *Current and Emerging Issues in Cancer Pain: Research and Practice*. New York: Raven Press, 1993:331–50.
164. Ventafridda V, Ripamonti C, DeConno F, Bianchi M, Pazzuconi F, Panerai AE. Antidepressants increase bioavailability of morphine in cancer patients. *Lancet*, 1987; **i**:1204.
165. Tong TG, Pond SM, Kreek MJ, Jaffery NF, Benowitz NL. Phenytoin-induced methadone withdrawal. *Annals of Internal Medicine*, 1981; **94**:349–51.
166. Nilsson MI, Angaard E, Holstrand J, Gune L-M. Pharmacokinetics of methadone during maintenance treatment: adaptive changes during the induction phase. *European Journal of Clinical Pharmacology*, 1982; **22**:343–9.
167. Morgan J, Furst DE. Implications of drug therapy in the elderly. *Clinics in the Rheumatic Diseases*, 1986; **12**:244.
168. Geokas MC, Haverbek BJ. The aging gastrointestinal tract. *American Journal of Surgery*, 1969; **117**:881.
169. Kaiko RF. Age and morphine analgesia in cancer patients with post-operative pain. *Clinical Pharmacology and Therapeutics*, 1980; **28**:823–6.
170. Sear JW, Hand CW, Moore RA. Studies on morphine disposition: plasma concentrations of morphine and its metabolites in anesthetized middle-aged and elderly surgical patients. *Journal of Clinical Anesthesia*, 1989; **1**:164–9.
171. Zacny JP. A review of the effects of opioids on psychomotor and cognitive functioning in humans. *Experimental and Clinical Psychopharmacology*, 1993; **3**:432–66.
172. Vainio A, Ollila J, Matikainen E, Rosenberg P, Kalso E. Driving ability in cancer patients receiving long-term morphine analgesia. *Lancet*, 1995; **346**:667–70.
173. Bruera E, Chadwick S, Brenneis C, Hanson J, MacDonald N. Methylphenidate associated with narcotics in the treatment of cancer pain. *Cancer Treatment Reports*, 1987; **71**:67–70.

174. Bruera E, Brenneis C, Paterson AH, MacDonald N. Use of methylphenidate as an adjuvant to narcotic analgesics in patients with advanced cancer. *Journal of Pain and Symptom Management,* 1989; **4**:3–6.
175. Sykes NP. An investigation of oral naloxone to correct opioid related constipation in patients with advanced cancer. *Palliative Medicine,* 1996; **10**:135–44.
176. Cherny NI, *et al.* Opioid pharmacotherapy in the management of cancer pain: a survey of strategies used by pain physicians for the selection of analgesic drugs and routes of administration. *Cancer,* 1995; **76**:1283–93.
177. Eisele JH, *et al.* Clonazepam treatment of myoclonic contractions associated with high dose opioids: a case report. *Pain,* 1992; **49**: 231–2.
178. Mercadante S. Dantrolene treatment of opioid-induced myoclonus. *Anesthesia and Analgesia,* 1995; **81**:1307–8.
179. Hanks GW, Twycross RG, Lloyd JW. Unexpected complication of successful nerve block. Morphine induced respiratory depression precipitated by removal of severe pain. *Anaesthesia,* 1981; **36**:37–9.
180. Bradberry JC, Reabel MA. Continuous infusion of naloxone in the treatment of narcotic overdose. *Drug Intelligence and Clinical Pharmacy,* 1981; **15**:85–90.
181. Hanks GW, Twycross RG. Pain, the physiological antagonist of opioid analgesics. *Lancet,* 1984; **i**:1477–8.
182. McQuay HJ. Potential problems of using both opioids and local anaesthetic. *British Journal of Anaesthesia,* 1988; **61**:121.
183. Borgbjerg FM, Nielsen K, Franks J. Experimental pain stimulates respiration and attenuates morphine-induced respiratory depression: a controlled study in human volunteers. *Pain,* 1996; **64**:123–8.
184. Cleeland CS. Pain control: public and physician's attitudes. *Drug Treatment of Cancer Pain in a Drug-Oriented Society.* New York: Raven Press, 1989:81–9.
185. O'Brien CP. Drug addiction and drug abuse. In: Hardman JG, Limbird LE, Molinoff PB, Ruddon RW, Gilman AG, eds. *Goodman and Gilman's Pharmacological Basis of Therapeutics.* 9th edn. New York: McGraw-Hill, 1996:557–80.
186. Porter J, Jick H. Addiction rare in patients reated with narcotics. *New England Journal of Medicine,* 1980; **302**:123.
187. Perry S, Heidrich G. Mangement of pain during debridement: a survey of U.S. burn units. *Pain,* 1982; **13**:267–80.
188. Weissman DE, Haddox JD. Opioid pseudoaddiction—an iatrogenic syndrome. *Pain,* 1989; **36**:363–6.
189. Payne R. Pain in the drug abuser. In: Foley KM, Payne R, eds. *Current Therapy of Pain.* Philadelphia, PA: Decker, 1989:46–54.
190. Gonzales GR, Coyle N. Treatment of cancer pain in a former opioid abuser: fears of the patient and staff and their influence on care. *Journal of Pain and Symptom Management,* 1992; **7**:246–9.
191. Portenoy RK, Payne R. Acute and chronic pain. In: Lowinson JH, Ruiz P, Millman RB, eds. *Comprehensive Textbook of Substance Abuse.* Baltimore, MD: Williams and Wilkins, 1992: 697–721.

9.2.4 Non-opioid analgesics

M. D. Rawlins

Non-opioid analgesics encompass the non-steroidal anti-inflammatory drugs (**NSAIDs**), paracetamol (acetominophen), and nefopam. They are used widely in the management of mild-to-moderate pain, particularly pain of somatic origin, and have an important place in palliative medicine. Drugs such as glucocorticoids, antidepressants, and some anticonvulsants also have a role in the management of pain in palliative medicine but are not, formally, analgesics. They are discussed elsewhere in this book.

Chemistry

NSAIDs are a heterogeneous group of compounds, often chemically unrelated, but which share common pharmacological properties. They are classified, conventionally, in relation to their chemical structure and Table 1 depicts those most widely used in clinical medicine. The proprionic acid NSAIDs are isomers and their pharmacological activity resides in one (*S*) enantiomer with the other (*R*) entantiomer being inactive. Naproxen is marketed as the *S* enantiomer, but the others are formulated as racemic mixtures. To complicate matters further there is considerable interisomeric conversion (*R* to *S*), in man, of some members of the group. Whether there are any significant consequences to the use of racemates, when compared to pure enantiomers, has yet to be established. Excluded from Table 1 are NSAIDs of the pyrazolone class(oxyphenbutazone, aminopyrine, dipyrone), which have largely been abandoned in developed countries but which remain freely available in some developing countries. In the author's opinion the toxicity of these agents (particularly their adverse effects on blood and blood-forming organs), and the availability of other equally effective but safer products, renders them obsolete. They are not discussed further. Paracetamol is the major active metabolite of acetanilide and phenacetin. It has almost entirely replaced these older analgesics because of its relative lack of toxicity. Nefopam is a benzoxazocine with chemical similarities to orphenadrine and diphenhydramine.

Table 1 Classification of non-steroidal anti-inflammatory drugs

Chemical class	Therapeutic agents
Salicylates	Aspirin
	Benorylate
	Diflunisal
Acetates	Diclofenac
	Etodolac
	Indomethacin
	Sulindac
	Tolmetin
Proprionates	Fenbufen
	Fenoprofen
	Flurbiprofen
	Ibuprofen
	Ketoprofen
	Naproxen
	Tiaprofenic acid
	Ketorolac
Fenamates	Flufenamic acid
	Meclofenamate sodium
	Mefenamic acid
Oxicams	Piroxicam
	Tenoxicam
Pyrazolones	Azapropazone
	Phenylbutazone
Butazones	Nabumetone

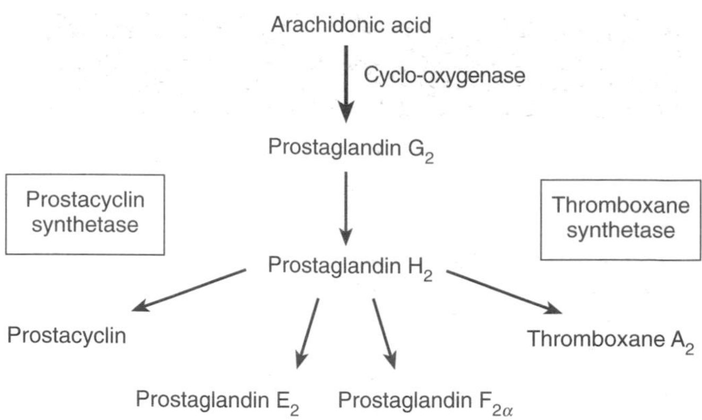

Fig. 1 Metabolism of arachidonic acid by cyclo-oxygenase.

Pharmacology

Non-steroidal anti-inflammatory drugs

The NSAIDs all possess anti-inflammatory, analgesic, and antipyretic actions at therapeutic doses. There is now abundant confirmation of the hypothesis, originally advanced in 1971 by Vane,[1] that NSAIDs exert their pharmacological effects primarily by inhibition of cyclo-oxygenase. This enzyme (Fig. 1) catalyses the conversion of arachidonic acid to an unstable endoperoxide (PGG_2) which is the sole substrate for the formation of prostacyclin, prostaglandins, and thromboxane. Although most tissues can form prostaglandin endoperoxides from arachidonic acid, the subsequent fate of these unstable intermediates in an individual tissue appears to depend on the presence (or otherwise) of other enzymes (Fig. 1). Thus, in platelets, the main end-product of cyclo-oxygenase activity is thromboxane A_2 (via the action of thromboxane synthetase); in vascular endothelium, the end-product is primarily prostacyclin (via the action of prostacyclin synthetase); and some organs, such as lung and spleen, are able to synthesize a wide range of cyclo-oxygenase products.

Individual NSAIDs have differing modes of inhibitory activity on cyclo-oxygenase.[2] Aspirin acetylates serine at the active site of the enzyme, forming a covalent bond, and prostaglandin formation can only be resumed after further synthesis of cyclo-oxygenase. This probably explains the susceptibility of platelets to the action of aspirin, since they possess little or no capacity for protein biosynthesis. Most NSAIDs appear to be so-called competitive, irreversible inhibitors of cyclo-oxygenase and exert their effects by interacting with an allosteric site on the enzyme and impeding its catalytic activity in a time-dependent manner.

The inhibition of cyclo-oxygenase activity by NSAIDs largely explains their pharmacological and toxicological properties. First, the products of the metabolism of arachidonic acid by cyclo-oxygenase are intimately involved in the pathogenesis of inflammation, the production of pain, and the development of fever.[2] Secondly, NSAIDs inhibit prostaglandin production, in man, at therapeutic doses. Thirdly, there is a reasonable rank order correlation between the inhibition of cyclo-oxygenase activity by NSAIDs and their anti-inflammatory activity. Fourthly, NSAIDs have common toxic effects attributable to their actions in other organs, resulting particularly in adverse gastrointestinal and renal effects and bronchospasm. There is emerging evidence that cyclo-oxygenase exists in (at least) two forms (COX-1 and COX-2) and that conventional NSAIDs inhibit both. The therapeutic actions of NSAIDs appear to be mediated as a result of their inhibition of COX-2, whilst their toxic effects occur as a result of their activity on COX-1.[3] There is thus a real possibility that selective NSAIDs, acting on COX-2 rather than COX-1, could offer significant therapeutic advantages.

Although NSAIDs clearly inhibit prostaglandin biosynthesis, they have other pharmacological properties which, it has been suggested, may contribute to their therapeutic efficacy.[4] Some, such as diclofenac and indomethacin, inhibit lipoxygenase enzymes and decrease production of leukotrienes by leucocytes and synovial cells. Others, such as piroxicam, inhibit the production of hydrogen peroxide by activated neurophils. Individual NSAIDs have also been shown to interfere with the synthesis of proteoglycans by chondrocytes, transmembrane ion fluxes, and cell-cell binding. While these non-prostaglandin actions of NSAIDs have rarely been demonstrated in man, they may explain the variability in responses, both between patients and between NSAIDs, that are seen in clinical practice.

Paracetamol

The mechanism of action of paracetamol is poorly understood. It possesses analgesic and antipyretic activity, but its anti-inflammatory actions can only be demonstrated in animals at inappropriately high doses. It is a potent inhibitor of cyclo-oxygenase within the brain and this might explain its antipyretic action.[5] It is, however, only a weak inhibitor of the enzyme elsewhere, and has little or no clinical anti-inflammatory activity. Two hypotheses are currently advanced to explain its analgesic effects. First, studies in animals suggest that it may exert a non-opioid action on pain pathways within the central nervous system.[6] Secondly, paracetamol may have a peripheral effect on the formation, or action, of chemical mediators of pain. Recently, it has been shown that both aspirin and paracetamol, when placed in tooth sockets at doses that have no systemic effect, produce significant analgesia after dental extraction.[7]

Nefopam

Nefopam has neither opioid nor NSAID-like properties, and is devoid of anti-inflammatory or antipyretic actions. Its mechanism of action is unknown but is presumed to be within the brain. It also possesses anticholinergic (antimuscarinic) properties which are unrelated to its analgesic action.

Clinical pharmacodynamics

Non-steroidal anti-inflammatory drugs

In man, NSAIDs show qualitatively similar profiles of anti-inflammatory, analgesic, and antipyretic activities to those in animals. The anti-inflammatory properties of NSAIDs are particularly apparent in patients with inflammatory arthropathies, where their administration is associated not only with a reduction in pain but also evidence of diminished joint swelling. Some NSAIDs also influence systemic markers of inflammation, such as causing a fall in the erythrocyte sedimentation rate or a reduction in acute-phase proteins in patients with rheumatoid arthritis. Despite their anti-inflammatory properties NSAIDs have no influence, in man, on the natural history of inflammatory arthropathies and do not prevent erosive joint destruction.

NSAIDs possess analgesic activity (in mild-to-moderate pain) independent of their anti-inflammatory properties.[8] They are effective, after oral administration, in relieving pain in patients with inflammatory arthropathies, sprains and strains, non-articular musculoskeletal disorders (capsulitis, bursitis, tendonitis, low back pain), dysmenorrhoea, headaches, and dental pain. NSAIDs are also effective in the treatment of postoperative pain resulting from episiotomy, minor orthopaedic surgery, and in postpartum pain.

The antipyretic activity of NSAIDs is shared by all members of the class. It is mediated by an action in the anterior hypothalamus to reduce the 'set-point' which is elevated in all fevers of inflammatory origin. Consequently, NSAIDs have no effect on normal body temperature, nor on hyperpyrexial states induced by other means.[9]

NSAIDs, by inhibiting the formation of thromboxane A_2 in platelets, have significant effects on platelet function in man. This has been studied most fully in relation to aspirin. Administration of low doses of aspirin in man results in *ex vivo* inhibition of platelet aggregation induced by ADP, collagen, or arachidonic acid, and prolonged *in vivo* bleeding time.[10] The effect of aspirin on platelet function is presumed to be the basis for its efficacy in patients with cerebrovascular and coronary artery diseases.

NSAIDs promote renal salt and water retention. By impeding the prostaglandin-induced inhibition of both the renal tubular reabsorption of chloride and the action of antidiuretic hormone, they may cause oedema in some patients.[11] This is especially likely to occur in patients with heart failure or decompensated hepatic cirrhosis. Retention of salt and water by NSAIDs also commonly leads to antagonism of the effects of antihypertensive agents and diuretics.

Paracetamol

Although paracetamol shows, in man, significant analgesic and antipyretic activities, it has virtually no anti-inflammatory properties. Its analgesic activity is generally regarded to be less than that achieved by full doses of NSAIDs. It is, however, effective in the treatment of mild pain, including headache, dental pain, and dysmenorrhoea. Paracetamol is also an effective antipyretic by a mechanism that probably involves the inhibition of cyclo-oxygenase activity in the central nervous system.[12] Paracetamol has no effect on platelet function, bleeding time, or renal salt and water excretion.

Nefopam

Nefopam has been shown to be effective in mild to moderate pain, including dental and musculoskeletal pain. It has no anti-inflammatory or antipyretic activity, but its antimuscarinic effects may give rise to adverse effects after oral or parenteral administration.

Clinical pharmacokinetics

Non-steroidal anti-inflammatory drugs

NSAIDs may be administered orally, parenterally, or topically.

Systemic administration

After oral administration, NSAIDs are well absorbed. Although food may delay absorption and, possibly, by a buffering action, reduce the incidence of dyspepsia, the extent of absorption is not generally impaired. Some NSAIDs are formulated as prodrugs (for example, fenbufen, sulindac, and nabumetone) which require metabolic conversion (by the liver) to yield their respective active metabolites.

Table 2 Pharmacokinetic parameters of non-steroidal anti-inflammatory drugs

Drug	Half-life (h)	Protein binding (%)	Urinary excretion (%)	Active metabolite
Aspirin	0.25	70	<5	+
Azapropazone	13	99	60	–
Diclofenac	1.5	99	<5	?
Diflunisal	5–20[a]	99	5	–
Etodolac	3	99	5	
Fenbufen	10	99	5	+
Fenoprofen	3	99	5	?
Flufenamic acid	9	90	<5	
Flurbiprofen	3.5	99	10	
Ibuprofen	2.5	99	<5	
Indomethacin	5	90	15	
Ketoprofen	1–5	95	25	
Ketorolac	5	99	60	
Mefenamic acid	3.5	high	10	
Nabumetone	26	99	<5	+
Naproxen	14	99	10	
Phenylbutazone	70	99	<5	+
Piroxicam	45	99	10	
Salicylate	2–30[a]	85	10	
Sulindac	7	96	<5	+
Tenoxicam	72	99	<5	
Tiaprofenic acid	2	98		
Tolmetin	1	99	5	

[a] Dose-dependent elimination.

All NSAIDs are highly protein bound (Table 2) and their free fractions may therefore be increased in patients with hypoalbuminaemia.[13] The distribution of NSAIDs in synovial fluid has been studied extensively.[14] Trans-synovial transport occurs through passive diffusion, but NSAID concentrations in the synovial fluid are much higher than their free concentrations in plasma because of binding to protein in synovial fluid. Total NSAID concentrations in synovial fluid are therefore about 60 per cent of those in plasma and fluctuate much less between doses than would be anticipated from changes in plasma concentrations. Consequently, although slow-release preparations of NSAIDs with short half-lives may reduce interdose fluctuations of drug concentrations in plasma they have little effect on fluctuations in synovial fluid concentrations.[4]

NSAIDs tend to divide into two types on the basis of their plasma elimination half-lives (Table 2). Short half-life NSAIDs (less than 6 h) include aspirin, diclofenac, ketorolac, and indomethacin, and long half-life NSAIDs (more than 10 h) are exemplified by naproxen and piroxicam. Acemetacin is mainly metabolized to indomethacin. Caution needs to be taken, however, in interpreting the half-lives of NSAIDs with active metabolites such as fenbufen and sulindac, since these may be substantially longer than their parent compounds. Because steady-state plasma concentrations during regular dosing are only achieved after administration over approximately five half-lives, maximum clinical efficacy may not be seen until a week after starting a drug such as piroxicam. By contrast, short half-life NSAIDs will reach steady-state within a day or so of starting regular treatment.

All NSAIDs undergo extensive metabolism (Table 2). A variety of metabolic pathways are involved, including hydrolysis (aspirin), glucuronidation (salicylate, naproxen, ketoprofen), and oxidation (diclofenac, piroxicam). Some NSAIDs, such as ibuprofen and indomethacin, undergo both oxidation and glucuronidation to a significant extent. Studies of the enterohepatic circulation of NSAIDs are limited but there is evidence for substantial biliary excretion of indomethacin and sulindac.[4] There is also a potential for enterohepatic recycling of glucuronide conjugates of NSAIDs with reabsorption of the parent drug following hydrolysis by gut flora.

Since only azapropazone and ketorolac undergo significant renal clearance, it might erroneously be assumed that impaired renal function had little influence on the elimination of other NSAIDs. There is, however, emerging evidence that the glucuronide conjugates of NSAIDs, such as ketoprofen and naproxen, accumulate in renal impairment; that they undergo enterohepatic recycling with hydrolysis by gut flora; and that the effective half-life of such drugs may be significantly prolonged in the face of reduced renal function. This, at least in part, underpins the empirical use of lower doses of NSAIDs in patients with renal impairment.

Topical administration

In order to achieve significant local NSAID concentrations, without exposing patients to the risks of systemic therapy, several topical formulations are now available (ibuprofen, diclofenac, felbinac). There is now evidence from randomized controlled clinical trials that topical NSAIDs, applied to an affected area, produce modest benefit. Successful studies, generally, have been those where topical application is made adjacent to the damaged area, such as superficial joints (fingers, knees) and musculoligamentous injuries (calves, knees, ankles). There is controversy, however, as to whether this represents a true local effect or whether the NSAID reaches the affected area via the systemic circulation.[15]

Paracetamol

Paracetamol is rapidly and completely absorbed although there is incomplete (70–90 per cent) systemic availability due to dose-dependent, first-pass metabolism.[16] The rate of absorption varies with the formulation but mainly with the rate of gastric emptying. Paracetamol is rapidly and uniformly distributed throughout total body water, with less than 5 per cent bound to plasma protein.

The elimination half-life of paracetamol averages about 4 h, with renal excretion of the unchanged drug contributing little (less than 5 per cent) to its overall clearance. Paracetamol undergoes hepatic metabolism predominantly to glucuronide and sulphate conjugates. After therapeutic doses, a small proportion (<10 per cent) is converted by hepatic microsomal (cytochrome-P450) oxidation to a reactive metabolite, which is rapidly conjugated with reduced glutathione and then excreted. Large overdoses of paracetamol saturate glucuronidation and sulphation, resulting in the formation of an excessive amount of the reactive intermediate, which depletes intrahepatic glutathione and causes liver cell necrosis.

Table 3 Type A reactions to non-steroidal anti-inflammatory drugs

Organ	Clinical reaction
Gastrointestinal tract	Dyspepsia Haemorrhage Peptic ulceration Perforation
Kidney	Salt and water retention Interstitial nephritis
Lung	Bronchospasm

Nefopam

There is little published information about the pharmacokinetics of nefopam. It appears to be rapidly absorbed[17] and then eliminated, with a half-life of about 4 h. It is extensively metabolized by hepatic oxidation and glucuronidation.

Adverse effects

Adverse drug reactions can be categorized[18] into type A (augmented) effects, which are predictable, dose-dependent manifestations of the normal pharmacological or toxicological properties of the compound; and type B (bizarre), unpredictable reactions, independent of dose, which are qualitatively abnormal responses to the drug. Non-opioid analgesics display both type A and B reactions.

Type A reactions

Type A reactions to NSAIDs are believed to occur as a consequence of cyclo-oxygenase inhibition (Table 3).

Gastrointestinal toxicity

This is the most common adverse reaction to NSAIDs. Upper gastrointestinal symptoms (dyspepsia, nausea, vomiting) occur in 10 to 20 per cent of patients. Occult bleeding after oral administration is an almost inevitable consequence of the mucosal changes produced by these drugs, and may give rise to symptomatic anaemia.

More significantly, NSAIDs may precipitate overt gastrointestinal perforation or haemorrhage[19] either as a result of acute mucosal injury, or from a peptic ulcer. A number of formal epidemiological studies have recently been undertaken comparing the relative risks of overt upper gastrointestinal haemorrhage with NSAIDs.[20–25]. Whilst the individual relative risks show significant differences between studies, the overall ranking of gastrointestinal toxicities are similar. On the basis of these investigations, azapropazone appears to be associated with the highest risk and ibuprofen with the lowest. Piroxicam, ketoprofen, indomethacin, naproxen, and diclofenac are in the intermediate category though the risks with piroxicam may be higher.[26]

The balance of evidence[19] strongly suggests that cyclo-oxygenase inhibition, within the gastroduodenal mucosa, is responsible for the upper gastrointestinal toxicity of NSAIDs. Moreover, the prostaglandin E_1 analogue, misoprostol, not only heals peptic ulcers but also protects against aspirin-induced acute mucosal injury and prevents NSAID-induced gastric ulceration in man.[27] There is, however, controversy about whether these adverse effects are mediated by a direct, local effect of NSAIDs in contact with the gastrointestinal mucosa; or whether the gastrointestinal toxicity follows systemic absorption. Although there is some evidence that microscopic blood loss and dyspepsia may be reduced with enteric-coated products, there is also substantial data suggesting that rectal or parenteral NSAIDs may precipitate overt upper gastrointestinal haemorrhage. The incidence of duodenal ulceration, but not gastric ulceration, in patients on NSAIDs can also be reduced significantly with ranitidine.[28] There is no evidence that paracetamol or nefopam share any of the gastrointestinal toxicity of NSAIDs.

In patients for whom NSAID therapy is particularly indicated, but who are at risk for developing gastrointestinal complications (patients with a prior history of peptic ulcer disease, patients over the age of 65, and those with concomitant serious cardiovascular disease), there are two approaches which should be considered:

1. If the patient has dyspepsia, another agent may be better tolerated and, therefore, changing to an alternative NSAID from a different class (Table 1) can be helpful. Antacids and H_2 antagonists may suppress the dyspepsia associated with NSAID therapy, but they do not prevent serious adverse gastrointestinal events; indeed, in one study, their use was associated with high risk of these events.[29]
2. Prophylactic therapy with misoprostol is recommended.[30] Misoprostol, a prostaglandin analogue, has been demonstrated to protect older patients with rheumatoid arthritis from serious NSAID-induced upper gastrointestinal complications.[31]

Nephrotoxicity

Renal syndromes with NSAIDs include[11] fluid retention, interstitial nephritis, and papillary necrosis. Salt and water retention (as above) is particularly relevant in oedematous patients, and those on diuretics or antihypertensive drugs. In patients with reduced renal plasma flow (e.g. volume depletion), where renal prostaglandins play a major role in maintaining renal perfusion, NSAIDs may precipitate impairment of renal function. Interstitial nephritis and papillary necrosis are almost universal in laboratory animals given NSAIDs at high doses for prolonged periods of time. Interstitial nephritis also occurs occasionally in patients receiving NSAIDs, but whether its pathogenesis is the same is unclear. Papillary necrosis, although usually attributed to phenacetin, has been described in association with many NSAIDs. A causal relationship, however, is difficult to confirm and it is unclear whether cyclo-oxygenase inhibition is involved. Paracetamol, at therapeutic doses, is not nephrotoxic.

Bronchospasm

Bronchospasm may be precipitated (Table 3) by aspirin, or other NSAIDs, in up to 20 per cent of asthmatic individuals when given oral challenge tests.[19] There is evidence to indicate that this results from inhibition of cyclo-oxygenase, and several mechanisms have been proposed;[19] all postulate that NSAIDs induce asthma by damaging a controlling mechanism mediated by products of cyclo-oxygenase activity. Irrespective of the mechanism, NSAIDs should be used with considerable care in asthmatic patients, and avoided in those with a history of aspirin intolerance. Paracetamol, which does not cross-react with aspirin in precipitating asthma, can be a useful alternative.

Table 4 Type B reactions to non-steroidal anti-inflammatory drugs

Organ/system	Reaction	NSAIDs
Skin	Morbilliform rash	Fenbufen
	Angioedema	Ibuprofen
		Azapropazone
		Piroxicam
Blood	Thrombocytopenia	Diclofenac
		Ibuprofen
		Piroxicam
	Haemolytic anaemia	Mefenamic acid
		Diclofenac
	Agranulocytosis	Phenylbutazone
	Aplastic anaemia	Phenylbutazone
Central nervous system	Aseptic meningitis	Ibuprofen
Liver	Reye's syndrome	Aspirin
	Hepatitis	Diclofenac
		Piroxicam
Gastrointestinal	Diarrhoea	Mefenamic acid
		Flufenamic acid
Immunological	Anaphylaxis	Most NSAIDs

Inhibition of platelet aggregation

This occurs with all NSAIDs. It is of clinical significance, however, in patients receiving anticoagulants, or those with significant coagulopathies (such as haemophilia). In the latter, NSAIDs should be avoided unless the coagulation defect is under good therapeutic control and there is no prior history of peptic ulcer disease. In patients on anticoagulants, the cautious administration of ibuprofen, starting at doses of no more than 200 mg thrice daily, may provide sufficient analgesia without precipitating gastrointestinal bleeding.

Type B reactions

A variety of atypical, bizarre responses (Table 4) to NSAIDs are occasionally observed as idiosyncratic reactions. It is presumed that many of these (although not all) are mediated by immunological mechanisms, but direct evidence is lacking. The mechanisms underlying the development of blood dyscrasias is unknown.

Paracetamol is virtually devoid of type B reactions. There are a few case reports of thrombocytopenia and anaphylaxis but the incidence of these is extraordinarily low.

Non-opioid analgesics in palliative medicine

Non-opioid analgesics have three main uses in palliative medicine: as occasional treatment for intercurrent pain, as regular treatment in the management of cancer pain, and as specific treatment for painful bony metastases.

Treatment of intercurrent mild-to-moderate pain

Patients with malignant disease are as likely as anyone else to suffer minor aches and pains, which are unrelated to their underlying disease. In such circumstances paracetamol (500–1000 mg) or ibuprofen (220–400 mg) are reasonable choices and rarely cause significant adverse effects in these circumstances.

Regular treatment of cancer pain

Paracetamol or NSAIDs are first-time agents for the management of mild-to-moderate cancer pain.[32,33] While they do not result in tolerance or physical dependence, they have a ceiling effect. Unlike the opioids, therefore, there is no therapeutic gain to increasing dosages beyond those recommended for other conditions. NSAIDs are also useful in combination with opioids, but there is no good evidence that they truly potentiate their effects.

There have been very few well-conducted clinical trials of NSAIDs in cancer pain. The range of available NSAIDs, however, is considerable, and therefore the choice of NSAID has to be determined largely by extrapolation from use in other conditions. Five broad principles apply.

1. It is sensible to restrict the choice of NSAID in cancer pain to drugs with shorter half-lives (Table 2). The time taken to reach steady-state plasma levels with the oxicams is too great to permit flexible dosage adjustment in this indication.
2. The analgesic and toxic (type A) potencies of individual NSAIDs are broadly parallel. Ibuprofen, probably the safest but least effective NSAID, is likely to be of limited value in the treatment of most patients with cancer pain. Aspirin at fully effective doses has an incidence of gastrointestinal adverse effects that are intolerable to many patients. Claims by a manufacturer for a superior risk–benefit profile of one NSAID over others should be examined with exquisite care. Because of its gastrointestinal and other toxicities, azapropazone is unacceptable.[24] The type B reactions of some NSAIDs occur sufficiently often as to place an additional (and unreasonable) burden on patients with cancer pain. The NSAIDs falling into this category include the fenamates (diarrhoea), fenbufen (rashes), and both phenylbutazone and azapropazone (blood dyscrasias).
3. In order to maximize the efficacy and minimize the toxicity of NSAIDs in patients with cancer, treatment should begin at the lowest recommended dose. Dosage increases of short half-life NSAIDs can reasonably be made every 2 to 3 days in the light of the clinical response.
4. Patients vary widely in their response to NSAID therapy[34] and there is an inevitable element of trial and error. In patients intolerant or refractory to one NSAID, it seems reasonable to change to another from a different chemical class. Familiarity by individual prescribers with several members of the class is essential if patients are not to be denied effective and safe treatment.
5. It is wiser to avoid newer NSAIDs until their safety, and especially their profile of type B reactions, has been fully evaluated during wider usage in other indications. Products such as ketorolac, whose indications are confined solely to short-term use (e.g. postoperative pain), should also be avoided.
6. Patients should be reassessed, at regular intervals, to ensure that the therapeutic objectives are being maintained. In the light of these principles, NSAID therapy can reasonably be started with either naproxen or diclofenac and changed to the other if patients are intolerant or refractory. It is wise to restrict indomethacin, probably the most potent but most toxic NSAID, to patients who fail to respond to those of lesser potency.

Special treatment of bone pain

Although formal evidence from randomized, controlled trials is lacking, there is sufficient body of evidence to suggest the use of NSAIDs for their specific effect in the treatment of bone pain.

There is experimental evidence to show that the osteolytic activity of a number of malignant cell lines can be inhibited by aspirin at concentrations comparable to those achieved during treatment. Furthermore, both human breast tumour cells and bone metastases associated with these cells have high concentrations of prostaglandin-like material.[35] Published studies of the effects of NSAIDs in the treatment of painful bony metastases have more frequently used naproxen or indomethacin. Evidence[36] from a short-term (3 day) randomized, parallel group clinical trial suggests that higher doses (550 mg, 8-hourly) of naproxen are more effective than low ones (275 mg, 8-hourly), but at the inevitable cost of a higher incidence (16 per cent versus 7 per cent) of adverse reactions.

Future trends

Continued advances in the relief of pain in palliative medicine with non-opioid analgesics can be expected, achieved both by learning how to use our existing drugs better and by developing new compounds with novel actions.

Improved knowledge about the relative merits of different NSAIDs, and the reasons for individual variation in response, could do much to help optimize their use. There would seem to be little merit, however, in continuing to develop compounds with the broad spectrum of activity of current NSAIDs. Compounds with greater specificity for COX-2, or with activity against other chemical mediators of pain and inflammation, offer a much better hope for the future.

References

1. Vane JR. Inhibition of prostaglandin synthesis as a mechanism of action for aspirin-like drugs. *Nature*, 1971; **231**: 232–5.
2. Flower RJ, Moncada S, Vane JR. Analgesic-antipyretics and anti-inflammatory agents. In: Gilman AG, Goodman LS, Rall TW, Murad F, eds. *The Pharmacological Basis of Therapeutics*, 7th edn. New York: Macmillan, 1985: 674–715.
3. Mitchell JA, Akaarasereenot P, Thierermann C, Flower RJ, Vane JA. Selectivity of non-steroidal anti-inflammatory drugs as inhibitors of constitutive and inducing cyclo-oxygenases. *Proceedings of the National Academy of Sciences, USA*. 1993; **90**: 11693–7.
4. Brooke PM, Day RO. Non-steroidal anti-inflammatory drugs—differences and similarities. *New England Journal of Medicine*, 1991; **324**: 1716–25.

5. Glenn EM, Bowman BJ, Rohloff A. Anti-inflammatory and PG-inhibitory effect of phenacetin and acetaminophen. *Agents and Actions*, 1977; **7**: 513–16.
6. Carlson K, Monzel W, Junra I. Depression by morphine and the non-opioid analgesic agents, metazimol (dipyrone), lysine acetylsalicylate and paracetamol, of activity in rat thalamic neurones evoked by electrical stimulation of nociceptins afferents. *Pain*, 1988; **32**: 313–26.
7. Moore UK, Seymour RA, Rawlins MD. The efficacy of locally applied aspirin and paracetamol in postoperative pain after third molar surgery. *Clinical Pharmacology and Therapeutics*, 1992; **52**: 292–6.
8. Brodgen RN. Non-steroidal anti-inflammatory anagesics other than salicylates. *Drugs*, 1986; **32** (suppl. 4): 27–45.
9. Cranston WI, Hellow RF, Lull RH, Rawlins MD, Rosendorff C. Observations on the mechanism of salicylate-induced antipyresis. *Journal of Physiology*, 1970; **210**: 593–600.
10. Rainsford KD. *Aspirin and the Salicylates*. London: Butterworth, 1984.
11. Clive DM, Staff JS. Renal syndromes associated with non-steroidal anti-inflammatory drugs. *New England Joumal of Medicine*, 1984; **310**: 563–72.
12. Milton AS. Prostagiandins in fever and the mode of action of antipyretic drugs. In: Milton AS, ed. *Pyretics and Antipyretics: Handbook of Experimental Pharmacology*, Vol. 60. Berlin: Springer-Verlag, 1982: 257–303.
13. Lin JH, Cocchetto DM, Duggen DE. Protein binding as a primary determinant of the clinical pharmacokinetic properties of non-steroidal anti-inflammatory drugs. *Clinical Pharmacokinetics*, 1987; **12**: 402–32.
14. Netter P, Bannwarth B, Royer-Morrot M-J. Recent findings on the pharmacokinetics of non-steroid anti-inflammatory drugs in synovial fluid. *Clinical Pharmacokinetics*, 1987; **17**: 145–62.
15. Radermacher J, Hentsch D, Scholl MA, Lustinetz T, Frolich JC. Diclofenac concentrations in synovial fluid and plasma adter cutaneous application in inflammatory and degenerative joint disease. *British Journal of Clinical Pharmacology*, 1991; **31**: 537–41.
16. Rawlins MD, Henderson DB, Hijab AR. Pharmacokinetics of paracetamol (acetaminophen) after intravenous and oral administration. *European Journal of Clinical Pharmacology*, 1977; **11**: 283–6.
17. Heel RC, Brogden RN, Pakes GE, Speight TM, Avery GS. Nefopam: a review of its pharmacological properties and therapeutic efficacy. *Drugs*, 1980; **19**: 249–67.
18. Rawlins MD, Thompson JW. Pathogenesis of adverse drug reactions. In: Davis DM, ed. *Textbook of Adverse Drug Reactions*. Oxford: Oxford University Press, 1977: 11–34.
19. Rawlins MD. Metablic and adverse effects of drugs. In: Cohen RD, Lewis B, Alberta KGMM, Denman AM, eds. *The Metabolic and Molecular Basis of Acquired Disease*. London: Ballière Tindall, 1990: 1149–66.
20. Laporte JR, Carne X, Vidal X, Morena M, Juan J. Upper gastrointestinal bleeding in relation to previous use of analgesics and non-steroidal anti-inflammatory drugs. *Lancet*, 1991; **337**: 85–9.
21. Somerville K, Faulkner G, Langton MJS. Non-steroidal anti-inflammatory drugs and bleeding peptic ulcer. *Lancet*, 1986; **i**: 452–4.
22. Kaufman DW, Kelly JP, Sheeban JE, *et al.* Non-steroidal anti-inflammatory drug use in relation to major upper gastrointestinal bleeding. *Clinical Pharmacology and Therapeutics*, 1993; **53**: 485–94.
23. Garcia Rodriguez LA, Jick H. Risk of upper gastrointestinal bleeding and perforation associated with individual non-steroidal anti-inflammatory drugs. *Lancet*, 1994; **343**: 769–72.
24. Langman MJS, Weil J, Wainwright P, Lawson DH, Rawlins MD, Logan RFA, Murphy M, Vessey MP, Colin-Jones DG. Risks of bleeding peptic ulcer associated with individual non-steroidal anti-inflammatory drugs. *Lancet*, 1994; **343**: 1075–8.
25. Belton KJ, Lewis SC, Matthews JNS, Rawlins MD. Systematic overview of upper gastrointestinal haemorrhage associated with non-steroidal anti-inflammatory drugs. In: *Perspectives in Pharmacotoxicology and Pharmacovigilance*. Amsterdam: 105 Press, 1994: 322–30.
26. Committee on Safety of Medicines and Medicines Control Agency. Relative safety of oral non-aspirin NSAIDS. *Current Problems in Pharmacovigilance*, 1994; **20**: 9–11.
27. Graham DY, Agrawal NM, Roth SH. Prevention of NSAID-induced gastric ulcer with misprostol: a multicentre, double-blind, placebo-controlled trial. *Lancet*, 1988; **ii**: 1277–80.
28. Ehsanullah RSB, Page MC, Tildesley G, Word JR. Prevention of gastroduodenal damage induced by non-steroidal anti-inflammatory drugs: controlled trial of ranitidine. *British Medical Journal*, 1988; **287**: 1017–21.
29. Singh *et al.* Gastrointestinal complications of nonsteroidal anti-inflammatory drug treatment in rheumatoid arthritis—a prospective observational. *Archives of Internal Medicine*, 1996; **156**: 1530–6.
30. American College of Rheumatology Ad Hoc Committee on Clinical Guidelines. Guidelines for Monitoring Drug Therapy in Rheumatoid Arthritis. *Arthritis and Rheumatism*, 1996; **39**: 723–31.
31. Silverstein FE *et al.* Reduction by misoprostol of clinically detected serious gastrointestinal complications associated with NSAID use in older patients with rheumatoid arthritis. *Annals of Internal Medicine*, 1995; **123**: 241–9.
32. Foley KM. The treatment of cancer pain. *New England Journal of Medicine*, 1985; **313**: 84–95.
33. Twycross RG, Lack SA. *Therapeutics in Terminal Cancer*, 2nd edn. Edinburgh: Churchill Livingstone, 1990.
34. Day RO, Brooks PM. Variations in response to non-steroidal drugs. *British Journal of Clinical Pharmacology*, 1987; **23**: 655–8.
35. Bennet A, McDonald AM, Simpson JS, Stanford IF. Breast cancer, prostaglandins and bone metastases. *Lancet*, 1975; **i**: 608–10.
36. Levick S, Jacobs C, Loukas D, Gorden DR, Meyskens FL, Uhm K. Naproxen sodium in the treatment of bone pain due to metastatic cancer. *Pain*, 1988; **35**: 253–8.

9.2.5 Adjuvant analgesics in pain management

Russell K. Portenoy

The term 'adjuvant analgesic' describes any drug that has a primary indication other than pain, but is analgesic in some painful conditions. In the palliative care literature, this term is often used synonymously with 'coanalgesic' to refer to a drug that is administered with a primary analgesic, usually an opioid, to enhance pain relief, treat pain that is refractory to the analgesic, or allow reduction of the analgesic dose for the purpose of limiting side-effects.

This terminology is widely accepted, but can be problematic. In the palliative care setting, adjuvant analgesics are a subset of a much larger group of 'adjuvant drugs,' which are co-administered with analgesics for a variety of reasons. Adjuvant drugs may be administered to treat the side-effects produced by the analgesic or manage other symptoms associated with the pain. In this sense, laxatives and antiemetics are adjuvant drugs.

It may also be confusing to note that the term 'adjuvant' itself can be a misnomer. The adjuvant analgesics are often used alone—not as adjuvant to any other therapy. Indeed, this group includes some drugs that are non-specific, multipurpose analgesics and others that are commonly used in selected disorders as primary analgesics. This is particularly true in populations with chronic pain unrelated to cancer or other progressive medical diseases.

Given this imprecise terminology and the expanding use of adjuvant analgesics as non-traditional primary analgesics, it is important to understand the pharmacology of these drugs and their therapeutic role in varied patient populations. In this way, the use of the adjuvant analgesics can be optimized, both as 'add-on' therapy to an opioid regimen and as distinct, primary therapy in those painful disorders that are likely to demonstrate a good response.

General considerations

Several principles guide the administration of all adjuvant analgesics. These emphasize the importance of a comprehensive patient assessment and a broad foundation in analgesic pharmacotherapy.

Comprehensive assessment

The selection of a drug and optimal dosing regimen depends on a systematic assessment of the patient.[1,2] This assessment requires a careful history and review of records, physical examination, and appropriate laboratory and imaging studies. The information obtained includes the following:

(1) characteristics of the pain, including severity, location, temporal features, quality, and syndrome;

(2) aetiology of the pain and its relationship to the underlying disease;

(3) inferences about the predominating type of pain pathophysiology, for example nociceptive or neuropathic (see Chapter 9.2.10);

(4) impact of pain on function and quality of life;

(5) impact of associated factors on quality of life, including physical and psychological symptoms, functional impairments, psychiatric disorder, family or social disruption, financial problems, and spiritual or religious concerns.

The need for systematic assessment continues during the course of therapy with an adjuvant analgesic. Over time, changes in pain, side-effects, or any of the broader quality of life concerns may impel a shift in therapeutic strategy. The use of adjuvant analgesics in the management of pain is a 'labour intensive' endeavour, which requires frequent contact with the patient to ensure continuous, appropriate administration of the drug.

Positioning of treatment

Extensive experience in the cancer population indicates that the adjuvant analgesics are, as a group, less reliable analgesics than opioids. This characteristic may be determined by a smaller proportion of treated patients who respond adequately, a higher likelihood of troublesome side-effects, or a slower onset of analgesic effect for most drugs (perhaps due to the need to initiate therapy at low doses to avoid side-effects). For example, in contrast to survey data that demonstrate a favourable outcome within days for 70 to 90 per cent of cancer patients who receive opioid therapy,[3-14] studies of the tricyclic antidepressants show that these drugs require treatment for weeks to obtain optimal results and offer 50 per cent, or greater, relief to 50 to 75 per cent of patients with neuropathic pain.[15,16]

This observation suggests that most patients in the palliative care setting who experience moderate or severe pain and have no relative contraindications to opioid therapy should not receive an adjuvant analgesic until opioid therapy has been optimized. Although some clinicians attempt to improve patient response by initiating therapy with an opioid and an adjuvant analgesic concurrently, this approach increases the risk of additive toxicity. With rare exceptions, the safest and most efficient approach involves the addition of an adjuvant analgesic to an opioid regimen that is yielding inadequate analgesia despite dose escalation to limiting side-effects.

Table 1 Therapeutic options when opioid therapy regimen fails due to dose-limiting toxicity

Approach	Therapeutic options
I. Pharmacological techniques to reduce systemic opioid requirement	Use of adjuvant analgesics Use of spinal opioids
II. Identifying an opioid with a more favourable balance between analgesia and side-effects	Sequential opioid trials
III. Improving the tolerability of the opioid regimen to allow further dose escalation	More aggressive side-effect management (e.g. psychostimulants for opioid-induced somnolence)
IV. Non-pharmacological techniques to reduce the systemic opioid requirement	Anaesthetic approaches Surgical approaches Rehabilitative approaches Psychological approaches

This positioning of the adjuvant analgesics must be understood in relation to the other options that exist in this situation (Table 1). In the absence of data from comparative clinical trials, the decision to use an adjuvant analgesic drug instead of an alternative therapy, such as a trial of spinally administered opioids or a nerve block, is usually a matter of clinical judgement.

The selection of a specific adjuvant analgesic is usually suggested by the characteristics of the pain (see below) or, in some instances, by the existence of another symptom concurrent with pain that may be amenable to a non-analgesic effect of the drug. In many situations, multiple options exist and priorities for therapeutic trials must also be developed on the basis of a comprehensive assessment of the patient and best clinical judgement.

Pharmacological characteristics

To select and properly administer an adjuvant analgesic, the clinician must be familiar with the drug's actions, approved indications, unapproved indications accepted in medical practice, likely side-effects and potential serious adverse effects, usual time–action relationship, pharmacokinetics, and specific dosing guidelines for pain. Very few of the adjuvant analgesics have been studied in the palliative care setting and the information used to develop dosing guidelines is usually extrapolated from other patient populations.

Caution is usually appropriate as adjuvant analgesics are used in a medically ill population. Low initial doses and gradual dose escalation may avoid early side-effects, allow acclimatization to the drug, and identify dose-dependent analgesic effects that can be explored to optimize the balance between pain relief and adverse effects. The use of low initial doses and dose titration may delay the onset of analgesia, and patients must be forewarned of this possibility to improve compliance with the therapy.

Interindividual and intraindividual variability

There is great variability in the response to all adjuvant analgesics. Although specific patient characteristics, such as advanced age or coexistent major organ failure, may increase the likelihood of some (usually adverse) responses, it is nonetheless true that neither favourable effects nor specific side-effects can be reliably predicted in the individual patient. Additionally, there is remarkable intra-individual variability in the response to different drugs, including those within the same class. Implicit in both these observations is the potential utility of sequential trials of adjuvant analgesics. The process of sequential drug trials, like the use of low initial doses and dose titration, should be explained to the patient at the start of therapy to enhance compliance and reduce the distress that may occur as treatments fail.

Risks and benefits of polypharmacy

Adjuvant analgesics are typically administered to patients who are receiving several other drugs. Although this is widely regarded as appropriate care in the palliative care population, the potential for additive side-effects and unpredictable adverse effects must be anticipated by the practitioner whenever an adjuvant is added to an existing drug regimen. The decision to add, or continue, a therapy must be based on a careful assessment of outcomes and a clear understanding of the goals of care. If a treatment yields demonstrable benefit without serious risk, and without cumulative side-effects that otherwise impair function or quality of life, there is ample justification for continuing. Additional pain relief at the price of somnolence or mental clouding is not acceptable for patients whose goals include restoration of function, but may be completely appropriate for those who seek comfort as the only goal.

The risks of additive toxicity from polypharmacy derive from both pharmacokinetic and pharmacodynamic changes. For example the addition of a tricyclic antidepressant to a morphine regimen may produce somnolence due to an increase in morphine plasma concentration[17] or a pharmacodynamic interaction independent of changes in drug concentration.

Adjuvant analgesics

The adjuvant analgesics comprise an extraordinarily diverse group of drug classes (Table 2). A generally useful, broad classification distinguishes those that may be considered non-specific, multipurpose analgesics from those used for more specific indications. A review of the evidence supporting the analgesic efficacy of agents in each class provides the foundation for the development of clinical guidelines.

Table 2 Adjuvant analgesics: major classes

Antidepressants
Alpha-2 adrenergic agonists
Corticosteroids
Neuroleptics
Local anaesthetics
Anticonvulsants
Gamma aminobutyric acid agonists
Sympatholytics
N-methyl-D-aspartate receptor blockers
Osteoclast inhibitors
Radiopharmaceuticals
Muscle relaxants
Benzodiazepines

Multipurpose analgesics

The data supporting the analgesic efficacy of some drug classes derive from numerous studies of very diverse syndromes. The range of positive outcomes for these drugs suggests that they can be considered multipurpose analgesics, fundamentally similar to the opioid and non-opioid analgesics (Table 3). This designation is appropriate even if these drugs are used only for selected indications in the palliative care setting.

Antidepressant drugs

As reviewed recently,[18-24] there is compelling evidence that the tricyclic antidepressants are analgesic in a variety of chronic pain syndromes. The efficacy of the tertiary amine compounds has been demonstrated in a large number of controlled and uncontrolled trials. Amitriptyline was effective in migraine and other types of headache,[25-31] arthritis,[32] chronic low back pain,[33] postherpetic neuralgia,[34,35] fibromyalgia,[36,37] painful diabetic polyneuropathy,[15,38,39] central pain,[40] chronic facial pain,[41] cancer pain,[42] and psychogenic pain.[43] Imipramine was useful for arthritis,[44-46] headache,[29] painful diabetic neuropathy,[38,47-49] low back pain,[50] and idiopathic chest pain.[51] Doxepin relieved coexistent pain and depression,[52,53] headache,[31,54] and low back pain.[55] Clomipramine

Table 3 Non-specific multipurpose adjuvant analgesics

Class	Examples
Antidepressants	
Tricyclic antidepressants	Amitriptyline, doxepin, imipramine, clomipramine, desipramine, nortriptyline
Monoamine oxidase inhibitors	Phenelzine
Non-tricyclic antidepressants	Paroxetine, trazodone, maprotiline
Alpha-2-adrenergic agonists	Clonidine
Corticosteroids	Dexamethasone, prednisone, methylprednisolone
Neuroleptics	Methotrimeprazine

was analgesic in various neuropathic pains and idiopathic pain[56-59] and dothiepin was effective in fibromyalgia and psychogenic pain.[60,61]

Analgesic efficacy has also been demonstrated for the secondary amine tricyclic antidepressants. In controlled trials, desipramine was analgesic in postherpetic neuralgia and painful diabetic neuropathy.[16,39,59] Nortriptyline was effective in mixed neuropathic pains[56] and, combined with fluphenazine, in painful diabetic polyneuropathy.[62]

The non-tricyclic antidepressants have also been studied, with somewhat more equivocal results. The analgesic efficacy of maprotiline has been established in controlled comparisons against clomipramine in idiopathic pain[58] against amitriptyline in postherpetic neuralgia.[35] Although a trial of trazodone for dysaesthetic pains in patients with traumatic myelopathy did not demonstrate a favourable effect,[63] benefits were suggested in another controlled trial performed in patients with cancer pain.[42]

Convincing evidence of analgesic effects, albeit rather weak, have also been observed in recent controlled trials of two selective serotonin reuptake inhibitors—paroxetine[64] and citalopram.[65] Both drugs were studied in populations with painful diabetic neuropathy. Zimelidine was found to be analgesic in a controlled trial of patients with mixed organic and psychogenic pain syndromes,[66] but was ineffective for postherpetic neuralgia in an open-label comparison against amitriptyline.[67] Although case reports suggested that fluoxetine has analgesic effects,[68-70] a controlled trial in patients with diabetic neuropathy failed to demonstrate benefit from this drug.[39] Other serotonin reuptake inhibitors have not been systematically studied as analgesics in patient populations.

Few clinical trials have specifically evaluated the efficacy of antidepressants as analgesics for cancer pain. Nonetheless, several partially controlled[17,42,71] and many uncontrolled trials[72-79] generally confirm the analgesic potential of the tricyclic antidepressants in the cancer population. An open-label survey of patients treated with alprazolam, a benzodiazepine with antidepressant effects, suggested that this drug may also be analgesic in patients with neuropathic pain due to cancer.[80]

Monoamine oxidase inhibitors have been evaluated in limited clinical settings. A controlled trial of phenelzine demonstrated analgesic efficacy in patients with atypical facial pain[81] and several favourable uncontrolled trials of either phenelzine or tranylcypromine have also been reported.[82]

In summary, there is very substantial evidence that antidepressant drugs have analgesic effects in diverse types of chronic pain. Given the range of pain syndromes that are potentially responsive, it is appropriate to classify these drugs as non-specific, multipurpose analgesics. The strongest evidence of analgesic efficacy is found in the numerous controlled trials of the tertiary amine drugs, the best studied of which has been amitriptyline. Although less abundant data support the efficacy of the secondary amine tricyclic drugs, desipramine has been carefully studied and has clear analgesic potential. Drugs with more selective actions at specific monoaminergic synapses are also analgesic and there is particularly strong clinical interest in the serotonin reuptake inhibitors because of their relatively good side-effect profile.[83-85] Among the serotonin reuptake inhibitors, current evidence supports the analgesic efficacy of citalopram and paroxetine, but is equivocal or absent for the others. The serotonin reuptake inhibitors appear to be weaker analgesics than the tricyclics, a finding confirmed in one controlled comparison.[64]

Mechanism of action

Although effective treatment of concurrent depression can contribute to a favourable outcome from antidepressant therapy in patients with chronic pain, the analgesic effect of these drugs is not dependent on their antidepressant activity. Controlled studies have demonstrated that the usually effective analgesic dose is often lower than that required to treat depression, and the onset of analgesia typically occurs much sooner, usually within 1 week.[34,40,47,49,56,57,59,64] Moreover, non-depressed patients can experience analgesia and depressed patients can report pain relief without a change in mood.[15,16,39,40,50,64] Finally, single-dose studies of amitriptyline in animal models have demonstrated dose-dependent antinociception,[86-89] further suggesting an independent analgesic effect from these drugs.

Several hypotheses may be proposed to explain the analgesia produced by the antidepressants. The most widely accepted postulates that their ability to block the reuptake of monoamines increases activity in endogenous monoamine-mediated pain modulating pathways, the best characterized of which descend from the brainstem and use serotonin or norepinephrine as transmitters.[90-92] Interestingly, favourable clinical studies with drugs that have selective serotonergic or noradrenergic effects suggest that increased neurotransmitter availability in either pathway can yield analgesic effects.

Animal studies have demonstrated that the acute antinociceptive effects produced by tricyclic antidepressants can be partially blocked by the specific opioid antagonist, naloxone.[87-89] Although this finding suggests that activation of opioid receptors by these drugs could be involved in their mechanism of action, it is more likely that opioid mechanisms are actually enhanced by the increased availability of monoamines in pathways that interact with endogenous opioid systems. The affinity of the tricyclic compounds for the opioid receptor itself is low.[93]

When a tricyclic antidepressant is co-administered with an opioid, some of the benefit may relate to a pharmacokinetic interaction that results in higher opioid concentrations. Such an interaction has been demonstrated when clomipramine or amitriptyline is added to a morphine regimen.[17] Neither the importance of this mechanism in comparison to other effects on pain modulation nor the degree to which this pharmacokinetic interaction occurs with other drugs is known.

The tricyclic antidepressants are not highly selective and they also interact with other types of receptors (e.g. acetylcholine and histamine) that may be important in the development of analgesia.[94-97] Further elucidation of these mechanisms awaits additional investigations using more selective drugs.

Adverse effects

Although serious adverse effects are uncommon at the doses of antidepressant usually administered for pain, such morbidity occurs rarely and less serious side-effects are frequent.[83,84,98] Dose-related side-effects can occur even at low doses, particularly in patients who may be predisposed to adverse effects due to major organ dysfunction or the use of multiple other drugs. Moreover, some patients who receive low doses of the tricyclic antidepressants actually attain relatively high plasma drug concentrations,[99] and this pharmacokinetic variability may also account for some cases of toxicity.

The most serious adverse effect of the tricyclic antidepressants, cardiotoxicity, is very uncommon.[100] Patients who have significant heart disease, including conduction disorders, arrhythmia, or failure, should not be selected for treatment. To minimize the risk for those who are treated, initial doses should be low, dose escalation should be gradual, and the electrocardiogram should be monitored as doses reach relatively high levels. Concern about cardiotoxicity may justify the selection of a drug associated with less risk. If the patient cannot tolerate a tricyclic compound (a preferred choice, given the better evidence of analgesic efficacy), a secondary amine drug, such as desipramine, should be administered. If the risk of cardiotoxicity contraindicates a tricyclic, treatment with one of the newer antidepressants or a monoamine oxidase inhibitor is still possible. In such cases, the selection of an analgesic serotonin reuptake inhibitor, such as paroxetine, may be most sensible.

Orthostatic hypotension is far more common than cardiac toxicity during treatment with a tricyclic antidepressant.[100] Of the tricyclic compounds, nortriptyline is the least likely to cause this, and should be considered for patients who develop orthostatic dizziness following treatment with another tricyclic or are otherwise predisposed to this symptom.[101] Orthostatic hypotension appears to be more likely in the elderly and, combined with the sedative effects of these drugs, probably accounts for an increased risk of hip fracture in this population.[102] Again, patients who are predisposed to orthostasis, such as those with autonomic neuropathy, may be better candidates for one of the newer analgesic antidepressants—specifically a serotonin reuptake inhibitor.

Somnolence and mental clouding are common side-effects of the tricyclic antidepressants. An acute delirium occurs rarely. The likelihood of these effects is increased in the elderly and those with pre-existing encephalopathy due to disease (e.g. dementia, brain metastases, or metabolic encephalopathy), prior treatments (e.g. cranial radiotherapy), or concurrent use of other centrally-acting drugs. Within the class of tricyclic antidepressants, desipramine is perhaps the least likely to cause somnolence or confusion and nortriptyline is less problematic than the tertiary amine drugs, such as amitriptyline.

Although somnolence or confusion can occur during treatment with a serotonin reuptake inhibitor, this side-effect is uncommon. Indeed, patients who receive one of the serotonin reuptake inhibitors are more likely to report a sense of activation,[83,84] which, in some cases, is experienced as distressing anxiety, tremulousness, akathisia, or insomnia. The serotonin reuptake inhibitors are also less likely to cause mental clouding.[86]

Anticholinergic side-effects are also common during treatment with the tricyclic antidepressants. These effects are more likely during treatment with the tertiary amine drugs than the secondary amine drugs; they are not characteristic of the serotonin reuptake inhibitors. When relatively mild, anticholinergic side-effects (such as dry mouth, blurred vision, or constipation) can usually be managed or tolerated. Occasional patients are distressed enough to warrant a trial of a less anticholinergic drug.

Rarely, more serious anticholinergic toxicity can occur, including precipitation of acute angle closure glaucoma, tachycardia, severe constipation, or urinary retention. The likelihood of urinary retention can be reduced in male patients by inquiring about symptoms of prostatism prior to therapy and using a compound with less anticholinergic effects (such as desipramine) in those at risk. Acute angle closure glaucoma is a largely preventable ophthalmological emergency that may occur in a patient who has a shallow anterior chamber of the eye. It is prudent to screen patients prior to treatment for the depth of the anterior chamber;[103] should side illumination of the eye with a penlight held at the limbus fail to light the entire iris, the patient may have a shallow chamber and thus be at risk for acute glaucoma. These patients, and all those already under treatment for either narrow angle or open angle glaucoma, should be evaluated by an ophthalmologist prior to treatment with a tricyclic antidepressant.

Indications

As multipurpose analgesics, antidepressant drugs could potentially be considered for the treatment of any chronic pain syndrome. The available evidence does not support their use as analgesics for acute pain,[104,105] despite the demonstrated efficacy of selected tricyclic antidepressants in animal models of acute nociception[86–89] and human experimental pain.[106]

As discussed previously, treatment with an adjuvant analgesic, such as an antidepressant drug, is usually considered in the palliative care setting when a favourable balance between analgesia and side-effects cannot be attained with an opioid. There are many potential reasons for a poor response to an opioid,[107] among which is a 'neuropathic' pathophysiology (see Chapter 9.2.10).[108,109] Given the established benefit of the antidepressants in patients with diverse types of neuropathic pains,[15,16,34,35,39,40,48,49,56,59,64,65,67] these drugs may be particularly valuable in painful conditions related to such mechanisms. Thus, the strongest indication for the use of an antidepressant as an adjuvant analgesic in palliative care occurs in the patient with neuropathic pain whose response to opioids has been inadequate.

There is great heterogeneity in the range of symptoms presented by patients with neuropathic pains. Conceivably, specific symptoms may indicate the existence of mechanisms that respond differently to drugs with varying modes of action. Although there has been little systematic investigation of this possibility, the clinical literature has guidelines, based on anecdotal observation, that reflect this perspective. For example it is generally accepted that antidepressants are more useful for neuropathic pains characterized by continuous dysaesthesias, regardless of the specific syndrome, than pains described as lancinating (stabbing). This impression continues, notwithstanding controlled trials that have demonstrated the efficacy of amitriptyline and desipramine for continuous and lancinating dysaesthesias in patients who are experiencing both.[15,16] The latter data suggest that antidepressant trials may be considered for patients with predominating lancinating neuropathic pains who have failed other specific adjuvant analgesics (see below).

Early use of an adjuvant analgesics is also considered when pain is accompanied by a comorbid condition that may respond to a non-analgesic effect of the drug. Antidepressants are commonly used when pain is complicated by depression and the sedative tricyclic antidepressants are often added when pain is accompanied by insomnia.

Dosing guidelines

Given the extensive data from controlled clinical trials, amitriptyline should be considered first when an antidepressant trial is selected for a pain indication. If treatment with amitriptyline has failed or is not indicated due to concerns about toxicity, there are numerous options remaining. The tricyclic compounds are generally better analgesics than the non-tricyclics,[35,39,64] and a trial with an alternative tricyclic antidepressant is the most appropriate second-line approach. For example desipramine might be considered in such cases because of its favourable side-effect profile and substantive evidence of analgesic efficacy.[16,39]

Patients who cannot tolerate any tricyclic compound, or have a contraindication to these drugs, may be a candidates for a therapeutic trial with one of the non-tricyclic antidepressants. The serotonin reuptake inhibitors have the most favourable side-effect profiles and might be considered in this circumstance. The evidence suggests that these drugs do vary in analgesic efficacy and it is prudent to select one, such as paroxetine,[64] that has established analgesic effects.

Anecdotal observation and very limited empirical data[35] suggest that there is substantial variability in the analgesic response to the different antidepressants. Failure of a drug due to inefficacy, therefore, might reasonably be followed by a trial of an alternative drug. There are no guidelines for drug selection during these sequential trials and the process usually proceeds by trial and error.

The starting dose of the tricyclic antidepressants should be low, 10 mg in the elderly and 25 mg in younger patients. The initial dosing increments are usually the same size as the starting dose. Doses can be increased every few days. The usual effective dose range for amitriptyline or desipramine is 50 to 150 mg; some patients will benefit from doses below or above this range. Although most patients can be treated with a single night-time dose, some patients have less morning 'hangover' and some report less late afternoon pain if doses are divided.

Given evidence of dose dependent analgesic effects, at least for the tricyclic antidepressants,[15,49] it is reasonable to continue upward dose titration beyond the usual analgesic doses in patients who fail to achieve benefit and have no limiting side-effects. This course is clearly justified in patients with a coexistent depression, but should be considered even in patients without evidence of this disorder. There is currently no justification for increasing doses beyond the levels associated with antidepressant effects.

Although current data are insufficient to define concentration–effect models for antidepressant analgesia, it is useful to monitor plasma drug concentration during therapy, if feasible. In non-responders, low plasma drug concentration suggests either poor compliance or an unusually rapid metabolism; in the latter case, doses can be increased while repeatedly monitoring the plasma drug level. Likewise, non-responders whose plasma concentration is not very low, but is lower than the antidepressant range, should be considered for a trial of higher doses if side-effects are not a problem. For patients who are benefiting from therapy, plasma levels provide a baseline for comparison should pain recur in the future.

Changes in pain, mood, cognitive status, sleep pattern, and other clinical effects must be carefully monitored during dose escalation. There are limited, anecdotal observations that suggest the existence of a therapeutic window for analgesia during dose escalation with some tricyclic drugs. That is, it is possible that analgesic effects could decline as the dose is increased above some threshold and that dose reduction from this level could regain analgesia. This potential for a therapeutic window emphasizes the importance of careful monitoring during dose escalation.

A favourable analgesic effect is usually observed within a week after achieving an effective dosing level and, in some patients, maximal effect appears to evolve over days or weeks thereafter. This delay, combined with the many days required to increasethe dose to a therapeutic level, may result in a prolonged period during which patients experience unsatisfactory effects from the therapy, and sometimes experience uncomfortable side-effects. Unless the patient is well informed about this potential, non-compliance is likely.

Corticosteroids

Corticosteroid drugs have many potential indications in the palliative care setting. Numerous studies have suggested that these drugs may improve appetite, nausea, malaise, and overall quality of life.[110–119] Although concern about toxicity has generally limited chronic use to patients with advanced disease and short life expectancies, there is a substantial anecdotal experience with both short-term and long-term administration for a variety of clinical problems, including pain.

Data from controlled trials and clinical series supports the classification of corticosteroids as multipurpose analgesics. Efficacy has been suggested in reflex sympathetic dystrophy, a type of neuropathic pain,[120] and diverse types of cancer pain, including: bone pain; neuropathic pain from infiltration or compression of neural structures; headache due to increased intracranial pressure; arthralgia; and pain due to obstruction of a hollow viscus (e.g. bowel or ureter).[113,115,117,121–125]

Analgesic effects have been described for a variety of corticosteroids and a broad range of doses. A placebo-controlled trial in patients with far-advanced cancer demonstrated that relatively low doses of methylprednisolone (16 mg twice daily) were analgesic but that these effects waned over a 20 day evaluation period.[115] Low dose prednisone (7.5–10 mg) produced substantial improvement in bone pain and quality of life in an uncontrolled survey of patients with metastatic prostate cancer.[117] A survey of patients administered high doses of dexamethasone (96 mg/day for 2 weeks) for malignant epidural spinal cord compression observed pain relief in 64 per cent within hours of the initial dose.[123] A recent randomized trial confirmed that dexamethasone was profoundly analgesic in spinal cord compression but could not identify any difference between a high (100 mg) and low (10 mg) initial dose.[126] Symptoms related to bowel obstruction have been shown to respond to dexamethasone 8 to 60 mg/day[124,125] and methylprednisolone 30 to 50 mg/day.[113]

This accumulated experience establishes the analgesic potential of corticosteroid drugs in a variety of chronic pain syndromes. Differences among drugs have not been discerned, and there are no data by which to judge dose–response relationships, relative potencies among drugs, and long-term efficacy.

Mechanism of action

The mechanism of analgesia produced by corticosteroids is unknown. Any of several processes may be involved. Compression of pain sensitive structures may be relieved by reduction of peritumoural oedema[127] or, in the case of steroid-responsive neoplasms, by shrinkage of tumour masses themselves.[128] Activation of nociceptors may be lessened by reduced tissue concentrations of some inflammatory mediators—specifically prostaglandins and leukotrienes. Aberrant electrical activity in damaged nerves may also be tempered by these agents.[129]

Adverse effects

Well recognized adverse effects are associated with short-term and long-term administration of corticosteroids, and with the withdrawal of these drugs following chronic use.[130,131] The risk of serious toxicity increases with the dose of the drug, the duration of therapy, and predisposing factors associated with the medical condition of the patient.

Although acute toxicity is possible, transitory corticosteroid therapy is usually well tolerated. The potential toxicities include adverse neuropsychological effects, hyperglycaemia, fluid retention (which can lead to hypertension or volume overload in predisposed patients), and gastrointestinal disturbances ranging from dyspepsia to frank ulceration. A recent study of a high-dose dexamethasone regimen for epidural spinal cord compression (96 mg intravenously, followed by 96 mg orally for 3 days, then a taper for 10 days) noted three cases of serious toxicity among the 27 patients randomized to the steroid therapy (11 per cent); one patient became hypomanic, one developed a confusional state, and one developed a perforated gastric ulcer.[132]

The neuropsychological toxicity associated with corticosteroid therapy ranges from frank delirium to relatively isolated changes in mood, cognitive functioning, or perception. Mood disturbances can themselves vary from euphoria to depression. In another study of patients who received a high-dose dexamethasone regimen for epidural spinal cord compression (100 mg followed by 24 mg every 6 h), the overall rate of psychiatric disorders was no greater than a comparison group, but there was a greater incidence of major depressive disorders and a trend toward a greater incidence of delirium in the steroid-treated group; those who received steroids also had more depressive and anxious symptomatology.[133] Although neuropsychological toxicity is usually observed early during treatment and when relatively high doses are administered, these adverse effects can complicate any steroid regimen at any time. There is no proven association with any specific drug and the occurrence of acute toxicity during one course of therapy does not predict a similar response during subsequent courses.

Chronic administration of a corticosteroid can produce: a cushingoid habitus; changes in integument, subcutaneous tissues, and connective tissues; weight gain; hypertension; severe osteoporosis; myopathy; increased risk of infection; hyperglycaemia; gastrointestinal toxicity; and late neuropsychological effects.[130,131] In the palliative care setting, however, long-term treatment with relatively low doses is generally well tolerated. A study of advanced cancer patients chronically administered prednisolone or dexamethasone at varying doses observed oropharyngeal candidiasis in approximately one-third of patients and oedema or cushingoid habitus in less than one-fifth; dyspepsia, weight gain, neuropsychological changes, and ecchymoses occurred in 5 to 10 per cent and the incidence of other adverse effects, such as hyperglycaemia, myopathy, and osteoporosis, was even lower than this.[119]

Chronic administration of a corticosteroid approximately doubles the risk of peptic ulcer.[134] This risk is increased further by coadministration of a non-steroidal anti-inflammatory drug.[135] This potentiation of gastrointestinal toxicity relatively contraindicates the combined use of a corticosteroid and a non-steroidal anti-inflammatory drug in the palliative care setting. Steroid use also increases the risk of gastrointestinal perforation, even during short-term therapy.[136,137] This complication may be associated with constipation.[136]

Steroid withdrawal following chronic therapy can produce a syndrome of myalgia and arthralgia known as steroid 'pseudorheumatism'.[138] Withdrawal may also produce other symptoms, such as malaise, headache, and mood disturbance, or yield a flare of the symptoms for which steroid therapy had been initiated previously. Following a reduction to low doses, patients also may be at risk for disturbances associated with hypocortisolism, particularly during a period of intercurrent stress such as systemic infection.

The symptoms associated with steroid withdrawal can occur with either dose reduction or discontinuation of therapy. In some cases, symptoms appear after a relatively modest decline in a relatively high baseline dose. Escalation of the steroid dose can provide relief, and a slower, more gradual taper may avoid recurrence.

Indications

Corticosteroids are used acutely in the management of epidural spinal cord compression, raised intracranial pressure, and superior vena cava syndrome. Pain may accompany each of these syndromes and symptomatic relief is one of the goals of therapy.

On the basis of anecdotal experience, corticosteroids are also administered for many other painful syndromes, including metastatic bone pain, neuropathic pain due to compression or infiltration of peripheral nerves or nerve plexus, painful lymphoedema, pain due to obstruction of a hollow viscus, and pain due to organ capsule distension. Like other adjuvant analgesics, corticosteroids are usually added to an opioid regimen following dose escalation to limiting toxicity. Patients who present with these pain syndromes commonly have other symptoms that could potentially be improved by steroid therapy, such as nausea or malaise, and corticosteroid therapy may be considered earlier if primarily indicated by these other symptoms.

Dosing guidelines

The relative risks and benefits of the various corticosteroids are unknown. In the United States, dexamethasone is usually selected, a choice that gains theoretical support from the relatively low mineralocorticoid effects of this drug. Prednisone and methylprednisolone have also been used.

On the basis of clinical experience, corticosteroids are usually administered either in a high-dose regimen or a low-dose regimen. A high-dose regimen (e.g. dexamethasone 100 mg followed initially by 96 mg per day in divided doses) has been used for patients who experience an acute episode of very severe pain that cannot be promptly reduced with opioids, such as that associated with a rapidly worsening malignant plexopathy.[110] This regimen may also be appropriate when treating an oncological emergency that may be steroid-responsive, such as superior vena cava syndrome or epidural spinal cord compression. The dose can be tapered over weeks, concurrent with the initiation of other analgesic approaches such as radiotherapy.

A low-dose corticosteroid regimen (e.g. dexamethasone 1–2 mg once or twice daily) has been used for patients with advanced medical illness who continue to have pain despite optimal dosing of opioid drugs. In most cases, long-term therapy is planned. Although the risks associated with prolonged steroid use in this setting are more than balanced by the need for enhanced comfort, repeated assessments are required to ensure that benefits are sustained.[112] Ineffective regimens should be tapered and discontinued and, in all cases, the lowest dose that yields the desired results should be sought.

Alpha-2 adrenergic agonists

Classification of the alpha-2 adrenergic agonists as non-specific, multipurpose analgesics is supported by both animal and human studies. Strong antinociceptive effects in animals can be produced by clonidine, a partial agonist at the alpha-2 adrenergic receptor,[139-141] and by both medetomidine, a full alpha-2 agonist,[142] and dexmedetomidine, the active d-isomer of medetomidine.[143] These effects can be observed in a variety of experimental models, including models of neuropathic pain.[141,143] In humans, analgesic effects in diverse pain syndromes have been established in controlled studies of systemic dexmedetomidine,[144] and both systemic and intraspinal clonidine.[145-149] These and other reports suggest that clonidine can be beneficial in pain syndromes that may be relatively less opioid-responsive, including chronic headache, nonmalignant neuropathic pains,[145,148-154] and some cancer pain syndromes (including neuropathic cancer-related pain).[146,156-158]

Two recent controlled trials have illuminated the role of clonidine as an analgesic. The first study used an 'enriched enrolment' design, in which an open-label phase was used to identify patients with painful diabetic polyneuropathy who might be potential clonidine responders; these patients were then tested in a controlled trial of transdermal clonidine.[145] This trial confirmed an earlier report[150] in demonstrating that less than one-quarter of patients are potential responders, and that those who do respond can experience analgesia that is both substantial and sustained.

The second study compared a 14 day epidural infusion of clonidine (30 μg/h) with an epidural placebo infusion in patients with cancer pain who were receiving titrated intraspinal opioids via epidural morphine patient-controlled analgesia.[146] Overall, clonidine reduced pain but not opioid consumption. Therapeutic success, defined as either reduced opioid requirement or pain reduction, occurred in 45 per cent of those who received clonidine and 21 per cent of those who received placebo. Remarkably, most of this difference in success rates was due to the response of patients with neuropathic pain; in this subgroup, success was achieved by 56 per cent of those who received clonidine and only 5 per cent of those who received placebo.

These data provide evidence that clonidine is a multipurpose analgesic that may be particularly useful in the management of neuropathic pain. Both systemic administration, by the oral or transdermal route, and epidural administration can yield favourable effects. Although a minority (less than one-quarter during systemic administration) are likely to respond, those that do can experience clinically meaningful effects.

Mechanism of action

The mechanism of clonidine analgesia has not been established and is likely to be complex.[141] Noradrenergic receptors are clearly important in the modulation of nociceptive processing and it is possible that interaction with alpha-2 receptors in the spinal cord[143,159] or brainstem[160] activates endogenous systems that reduce nociceptive input to the central nervous system. Presumably, these systems may be relatively more or less involved in the processing of different types of noxious stimuli[141] or the development of different types of pain syndromes.

It is also possible that clonidine may produce analgesia in some cases through interference with the mechanisms that perpetuate so-called sympathetically-maintained pain, a subtype of neuropathic pain (more specifically, this type of pain is usually observed to be a subtype of reflex sympathetic dystrophy or causalgia).[155] Clonidine may reduce sympathetic tone and, in this way, ameliorate pains that are sustained, at least in part, by circulating catecholamines or efferent activity in the sympathetic nervous system.

Adverse effects

In placebo-controlled trials, the most common adverse effects associated with systemic or epidural clonidine administration have been somnolence, hypotension (usually orthostatic), and dry mouth.[145,146] In patients without severe concurrent medical illness, the major toxicity produced by clonidine is usually somnolence. The medical frailty of palliative care patients may increase the risk of adverse effects, however, and the potential for serious hypotension during therapy must be recognized. The controlled trial of epidural clonidine in cancer pain demonstrated that the drug produced sustained hypotensive effects in almost one-half of the patients;[146] six of the 38 patients (16 per cent) who received clonidine experienced serious blood pressure changes associated with dizziness, hypotension, or rebound hypertension.

Indications

Like other multipurpose analgesics, clonidine can be considered for a therapeutic trial in any chronic pain state. In the palliative care setting, anecdotal experience has generally been limited to patients with opioid-refractory pains, typically neuropathic pains. Due to the potential for adverse effects, treatment trials should be limited to patients who are haemodynamically stable, not predisposed to serious hypotension (e.g. by severe autonomic neuropathy, intravascular volume depletion, or concurrent therapy with potent hypotensive agents), and not markedly somnolent from other causes. Given limited experience with the drug in the palliative care setting, it is generally used after other adjuvant analgesics, such as the antidepressants, oral local anaesthetics, and anticonvulsants, have failed.

Dosing guidelines

Although there is strong evidence that intraspinal clonidine is an effective therapy for some patients with refractory pain, this route of administration is not generally available. Hence, treatment trials generally proceed using the oral or transdermal route. Currently, there is no evidence that one of these routes is better than the other, and the choice is usually based on patient preference.

To limit the risk of adverse effects, starting doses should be low (for example, 0.1 mg/day, orally). If doses lower than those commercially available are desirable, the transdermal system can be cut into pieces without change in its delivery properties.

Monitoring of both pain and adverse effects is necessary during gradual dose escalation. Neither dose-dependent effects nor the potential for a ceiling dose has been evaluated during systemic clonidine therapy. Consequently, gradual dose escalation should continue until significant side-effects occur or blood pressure declines to a degree that is worrisome. Anecdotally, some patients have benefited from relatively high doses (as high as 2 mg/day in rare cases), and it is reasonable to continue upward dose titration until dose-limiting toxicity is encountered.

Neuroleptics

The demonstration of antinociceptive effects in animal models[161] and the favourable results of several controlled clinical trials in diverse pain syndromes[162–166] suggest that the neuroleptics, or some neuroleptics, might be considered non-specific, multipurpose analgesics. None the less, there is relatively little evidence of analgesic activity for most neuroleptic compounds and their role as adjuvant analgesics is limited by this lack of definitive data and the potential for adverse effects.[167]

Controlled trials have yielded mixed results. The strongest evidence of analgesic efficacy has been acquired in studies of the phenothiazine, methotrimeprazine. Favourable studies of this drug have been conducted in patients with cancer pain, other chronic pain states (including some with neuropathic pain), and acute pain following surgery or myocardial infarction.[162–164,168,169] In these studies, the analgesic potency of methotrimeprazine 10 to 20 mg approximated morphine 10 mg in patients with little or no prior opioid exposure.

A controlled comparison of pimozide (4–12 mg/day) and carbamazepine in patients with trigeminal neuralgia demonstrated that pimozide has analgesic efficacy in this lancinating neuropathic pain syndrome.[166] Unfortunately, a very high incidence of disturbing side-effects, including physical and mental slowing, tremor, and parkinsonian symptoms, limited the value of this therapy. The analgesic efficacy of fluphenazine in headache was similarly suggested in a controlled, multiple dose (1 mg/day) study of 50 patients with chronic tension headache.[165]

The analgesic efficacy of neuroleptic drugs was not confirmed in other, single dose controlled studies. These evaluated chlorpromazine,[170] promethazine,[171] and haloperidol [172] in varied pain models.

The possibility of neuroleptic-mediated analgesic effects has also been suggested in numerous anecdotal reports. Trifluoperazine, chlorprothixine, haloperidol, and fluphenazine have been administered for a variety of pain syndromes, including chronic headache and neuropathic pains,[173–183] and various neuroleptics have been reported to be coanalgesic when added to another psychotropic or an opioid.[62,71,183–185] An opioid-sparing effect has been described in several,[71,183] but not all,[186] surveys of patients with cancer pain.

Thus, the available data establish the analgesic potential of one neuroleptic, methotrimeprazine, and suggest that others may be similarly characterized. The evidence is limited, however, and some well controlled studies have failed to confirm this effect.

Mechanism of action

The mechanism of neuroleptic analgesia is unknown, but may involve the effect of dopaminergic blockade on endogenous pain modulating systems. Dopamine receptors, specifically the D_2 subtype, are represented among the numerous pathways that subserve pain modulation.[187] Studies in animals have suggested that selective dopamine antagonists can potentiate morphine analgesia[161,188] and controlled clinical trials have demonstrated that metoclopramide, a relatively selective blocker of the D_2 receptor, is analgesic in humans.[189,190] This evidence, however, does not confirm that a dopaminergic mechanism underlies the analgesic effects of neuroleptic drugs, because all these drugs interact with other receptors that could potentially mediate analgesic effects. Even metoclopramide has effects on another central nervous system receptor, specifically the 5-HT_3 serotonin receptor subtype, that could mediate analgesia.[191]

Adverse effects

Common side-effects of neuroleptic drugs include sedation, orthostatic dizziness, and anticholinergic effects. Some patients experience mental clouding or confusion. Phenothiazines, such as chlorpromazine and fluphenazine, are more likely to produce these effects than other subclasses, such as the butyrophenones (e.g. haloperidol). The sedation produced by the neuroleptics can be additive to other central nervous system depressants. Rare, idiosyncratic reactions include blood dyscrasias, dermatoses (including photosensitivity), and hepatic damage.

The possibility of extrapyramidal side-effects is perhaps the greatest concern in the clinical use of neuroleptic drugs. The incidence of these disorders varies with the drug, duration of therapy, and dose.[98] Compared to other neuroleptics, both fluphenazine and haloperidol are relatively more likely to produce these effects.

The most serious extrapyramidal reaction is the neuroleptic malignant syndrome, which is characterized by rigidity, autonomic instability, and encephalopathy.[192] Successful management requires prompt diagnosis, discontinuation of the neuroleptic, and intensive supportive measures. The use of dantrolene and bromocriptine has been suggested in severe cases.[175]

Some extrapyramidal effects tend to occur early in therapy. These include acute dystonic reactions (e.g. trismus, torticollis, and even opisthotonos), akathisia, and parkinsonism. The management of these complications usually involves discontinuation of the neuroleptic, with or without the administration of an anticholinergic drug, such as benztropine. Akathisia has also been managed anecdotally with a benzodiazepine.

Tardive syndromes, including dyskinesias and the less common dystonias, occur late and may become intractable. Tardive dyskinesia is more common in the elderly and women. Although believed to be related to the quantity of the neuroleptic consumed, it has been observed even in those consuming low doses for a period of months. Treatment of a tardive syndrome usually requires tapering and then discontinuation of the drug. Rarely, tapering of the neuroleptic will be accompanied by the development of worsening dyskinesias (so-called 'withdrawal emergent dyskinesias'), which are usually transient. This phenomenon should not prevent a trial of a drug-free period.

Indications

In the palliative care setting, neuroleptics are used commonly in the management of delirium. Their specific use as analgesics has been limited by concerns about toxicity and the availability of alternative, safer drugs. Nonetheless, some indications have evolved on the basis of anecdotal experience.

Methotrimeprazine may be useful in bedridden patients with advanced cancer, who experience pain associated with anxiety, restlessness, or nausea. Consistent with the view of neuroleptics as possible non-specific, multipurpose analgesics, the type of pain in this setting should have no bearing on the decision to use this drug. For patients with advanced disease, the sedative, anxiolytic, and antiemetic effects of this drug can be highly favourable, and side-effects, such as orthostatic hypotension, are less of an issue.

The efficacy of pimozide in patients with trigeminal neuralgia[166] has suggested a role for this drug in the treatment of patients with refractory neuropathic pains characterized by a predominating lancinating or paroxysmal component. Given its side-effect liability, this drug is used after failed trials of other adjuvant analgesics that may be helpful in this setting (see below). Other neuroleptics, such as haloperidol and fluphenazine, are sometimes considered for patients with various neuropathic pains that have not responded to opioids or preferred adjuvant analgesics (such as antidepressants), local anaesthetics, or anticonvulsants.

Dosing guidelines

With known dose-related toxicity and no confirmation of dose-dependent efficacy, the neuroleptics are prudently dosed to some arbitrary ceiling based on published reports, then discontinued if no analgesia ensues. For example low initial doses of fluphenazine can be escalated to 1 to 2 mg three times daily, and the dose of haloperidol can be slowly increased to 2 to 5 mg two to three times a day.

In the United States, methotrimeprazine is approved only for repetitive intramuscular administration, but extensive experience has affirmed that it may also be given by continuous subcutaneous administration,[193] subcutaneous bolus injection, or brief intravenous infusion (administration over 20–30 min). A useful dosing schedule begins with 5 mg every 6 h, or a comparable dose delivered by infusion, which is gradually increased as needed. Most patients will not require more than 20 mg every 6 h to gain desired effects.

Table 4 Adjuvant analgesics typically selected for neuropathic pain with predominating continous dysaesthesias

Class	Examples
First line	
Tricyclic antidepressants	See Table 3
Non-tricyclic antidepressants	
Oral local anaesthetics	Mexiletine, tocainide, flecainide
For refractory cases	
Alpha-2 adrenergic agonists	Clonidine
Anticonvulsants	Carbamazepine, phenytoin, valproate, clonazepam
Topical agents	Capsaicin, local anaesthetics
Neuroleptics	Prochlorperazine, haloperidol
N-methyl-D-aspartate receptor antagonists	Dextromethorphan, ketamine
Calcitonin	
Baclofen	

Table 5 Adjuvant analgesics typically selected for neuropathic pain with predominating lancinating or paroxysmal dysaesthesias

Class	Examples
First line	
Anticonvulsants	Carbamazepine, phenytoin, valproate, clonazepam
Baclofen	
For refractory cases	
Oral local anaesthetics	Mexiletine, tocainide, flecainide
Tricyclic antidepressants	See Table 3
Non-tricyclic antidepressants	
Neuroleptics	Pimozide
Alpha-2 adrenergic agonists	Clonidine
Topical agents	Capsaicin, local anaesthetics
N-methyl-D-aspartate receptor antagonists	Dextromethorphan, ketamine
Calcitonin	

Other adjuvant analgesics used for neuropathic pain

As noted previously, the focus on neuropathic pain as a target for the adjuvant analgesics in the palliative care setting derives from the relatively poor response of these pain syndromes to opioid drugs.[107-109,194-197] Inadequately relieved neuropathic pain is the usual indication for a trial of a multipurpose adjuvant analgesic. Indeed, the antidepressant analgesics are a first-line approach in this situation, particularly for neuropathic pain syndromes characterized by continuous dysaesthesias. The antidepressants are complemented by many other drugs that may be administered for the same indication (Table 4). On the basis of clinical experience, the strategy used for neuropathic pains characterized by predominating lancinating or paroxysmal pain may emphasize the first-line use of other adjuvant analgesics, specifically the anticonvulsants, for first-line therapy (see below and Table 5).

Oral and parenteral local anaesthetics

Many clinical series and controlled studies have established the analgesic potential of systemically administered local anaesthetic drugs in patients with acute pain and various chronic pain syndromes.[198,199] Although the possibility of benefit in such diverse pains suggests that these drugs are multipurpose analgesics, both the controlled trials and a large clinical experience has focused on the management of neuropathic pains.

Numerous surveys[200-205] and several controlled trials[206-209] have demonstrated that a brief intravenous infusion of lignocaine (lidocaine) or procaine can relieve acute postoperative pain and pain due to burns. Other surveys suggest that this treatment can be effective in a variety of chronic pains, including neuropathic pains, arthritis, musculoskeletal pains, and headache.[210–221] A single-blind, placebo-controlled trial suggested that intravenous lignocaine can relieve migraine but not tension headache[222] and another, similarly designed trial suggested benefit from this therapy in central pain.[223] Other well controlled studies yielded conflicting results: whereas intravenous lignocaine acutely reduced the pain of postherpetic neuralgia[224] and painful diabetic neuropathy,[225] it did not relieve neuropathic cancer pain.[226,227]

Prolonged relief of pain following a brief local anaesthetic infusion may be possible.[215] Long-term subcutaneous administration of lignocaine has also been used anecdotally to yield sustained relief of refractory neuropathic pain in cancer patients.[228]

Long-term systemic local anaesthetic therapy became widely available with the advent of the oral formulations of these drugs. A survey of cancer patients suggested that flecainide can be effective in the treatment of pain due to tumour infiltration of nerves.[229] In controlled trials, tocainide was effective for trigeminal neuralgia[230] and mexiletine lessened the pain of diabetic neuropathy.[231]

These data establish the analgesic potential of systemic local anaesthetic therapy. They suggest that diverse types of pain can potentially respond. Controlled trials have emphasized the value of this therapy in neuropathic pain, and this is the use that has been pursued in clinical practice.

Mechanism of action

It is well known that local anaesthetic drugs block sodium channels and thereby impose a non-depolarizing conduction block of the action potential.[232] A profound conduction block can be produced in peripheral axons following the local instillation of these drugs, a phenomenon exploited in regional anaesthesia. This type of peripheral effect, however, does not explain the analgesia produced by systemic administration of these drugs. Non-toxic systemic doses of local anaesthetics do not block the peripheral action potential, although amplitudes are decreased to a degree.[233]

Studies of experimental models have revealed that systemic administration of local anaesthetic drugs suppresses the activity of dorsal horn neurones that are activated by C fibre input,[234] as well as the spontaneous firing of neuromas and dorsal root ganglion cells.[235,236] Thus, systemic local anaesthetic drugs probably produce analgesic effects in neuropathic pain states through suppression of aberrant electrical activity or hypersensitivity in neural structures involved in the pathogenesis of the pain. These may include sensitized central neurones, neuroma associated with damaged peripheral axons, or both.

Adverse effects

The major dose-dependent toxicities associated with the local anaesthetics affect the central nervous system and the cardiovascular system. The central nervous system effects generally occur at a lower concentration than cardiac changes. Dizziness, perioral numbness and other paraesthesias, and tremor usually occur first; at higher plasma concentrations, progressive encephalopathy develops and seizures may occur.[232] There is a correlation between the local anaesthetic potency and the dose required to produce this central nervous system toxicity.[237]

Toxic concentrations of local anaesthetic drugs can produce cardiac conduction disturbances and myocardial depression.[232] The effect on the conduction system is first observed as prolongation of the PR interval and the QRS duration. At higher concentrations, bradycardia and other arrhythmias occur. If severe enough, the depression of myocardial contractility can result in pump failure. Similar to the central nervous system effects of these drugs, the likelihood of cardiovascular toxicity with relatively low doses is correlated with local anaesthetic potency.

Thus, all local anaesthetics share a spectrum of serious, dose-dependent adverse effects, the existence of which mandates caution in dose selection and titration. Although variability across drugs in the propensity to produce these effects may be clinically relevant, comparative trials of systemically administered local anaesthetic drugs have not been performed and clinical guidelines based on adverse effect data are largely inferential.

Long-term systemic treatment with a local anaesthetic is usually accomplished with one of the oral formulations; mexiletine, tocainide, or flecainide. In the United States, flecainide has not been used commonly due to an association with sudden death during a trial of therapy for patients immediately postmyocardial infarction.[238] Neither the general applicability of this risk of sudden death to other medical settings nor the degree to which it reflects a specific effect of flecainide are known. Nonetheless, flecainide does have relatively potent local anaesthetic effects and greater negative inotropic effects than the other oral local anaesthetics, and these pharmacological actions, combined with the association with sudden death, has tended to place it in a negative light as a therapy for chronic pain. In the absence of comparative safety data, it is reasonable to consider flecainide less preferred as a potential adjuvant analgesic than other oral local anaesthetics.

Troublesome side-effects occur commonly during therapy with mexiletine or tocainide and serious adverse effects also have been described.[239] A survey of patients administered tocainide for arrhythmia noted nausea in 34 per cent, dizziness in 31 per cent, light-headedness in 24 per cent, tremors in 22 per cent, palpitations in 17 per cent, vomiting in 16 per cent, and paraesthesias in 16 per cent.[240] Rare serious reactions include interstitial pneumonitis, severe encephalopathy, blood dyscrasia, hepatitis, and dermatological reactions;[239–242] of these, the pulmonary disorder appears to be most frequent.[239] Mexiletine often produces nausea and vomiting (diminished by ingesting the drug with food), tremor, dizziness, unsteadiness, and paraesthesias, which may induce discontinuation of dosing in up to 40 per cent of patients.[239,243] Serious side-effects, including liver damage and blood dyscrasias are very rare, however.

Indications

Data from controlled trials and clinical experience suggest that any type of neuropathic pain can be considered a potential indication for systemic local anaesthetic therapy. A survey of patients treated with a brief lignocaine infusion found that neuropathic pains related to disorders of the peripheral nervous system are more likely to respond than pains related to a central nervous system lesions, but some patients with central pain do attain at least partial relief.[211] Both continuous and lancinating dysaesthesias can be ameliorated.[230,231]

The oral local anaesthetic drugs are usually considered for the long-term management of opioid-refractory neuropathic pain. There have been no comparative clinical trials to help define the appropriate use of these drugs in relation to the many other adjuvant analgesics that may be used for this indication. Based on the limited data available concerning long-term safety and efficacy, it is appropriate to position the local anaesthetics as second-line drugs for neuropathic pain. Specifically, a trial with an oral local anaesthetic is warranted in patients with continuous dysaesthesias who fail to respond adequately or who cannot tolerate the antidepressant analgesics, and in patients with lancinating pains who have been refractory to trials of anticonvulsant drugs or baclofen (see below).

The role of brief intravenous local anaesthetic infusions is even less well defined. Some patients experience immediate analgesia with this technique and favourable effects have been observed to continue for some period in a minority. Although it is reasonable to conjecture that the analgesic response to an intravenous infusion could predict the response to oral local anaesthetic treatment, this has not been adequately studied for pain and the intravenous approach cannot be advocated for this purpose.

On the basis of clinical experience, a trial of a brief local anaesthetic infusion is sometimes implemented in patients with severe neuropathic pain that has not responded promptly to an opioid and requires immediate relief. This technique, therefore, may be a useful approach to the uncommon circumstance of 'crescendo' neuropathic pain.

Dosing guidelines

On the basis of the limited data available, mexiletine appears to be the oral local anaesthetic least likely to produce serious toxicity. Although intraindividial variability in the response to different drugs in this class has not been systematically assessed, such variability has been observed commonly with other drug classes and is likely to exist with the oral local anaesthetics as well. Thus, if mexiletine does not provide relief to a patient with severe neuropathic pain that has already proved refractory to opioids and other adjuvants, trials with tocainide or flecainide are justified.

There have been no controlled comparisons of the analgesic effects produced by brief intravenous infusions of the various parenteral anaesthetics. The published experience is greatest with procaine and lignocaine, and it is reasonable to consider these drugs first.

All local anaesthetic drugs must be used cautiously in patients with pre-existing heart disease. It is prudent to avoid this therapy in those patients with cardiac rhythm disturbances, those who are receiving antiarrhythmic drugs, and those who have cardiac insufficiency. Patients who have significant heart disease should undergo cardiological evaluation before local anaesthetic therapy is administered.

Low initial doses and dose titration may reduce the likelihood of adverse effects. In the absence of contrary information, overall dosing levels should conform to those employed in the treatment of cardiac arrhythmias. For example, mexiletine should usually be started at 150 mg once or twice per day. This and subsequent doses are better tolerated when taken with food. If intolerable side-effects do not occur, the dose can be increased by a like amount every few days until the usual maximum dose of 300 mg three times per day is reached. Plasma drug concentrations, if available, can provide useful information as described previously for the tricyclic antidepressants.

There has been no systematic evaluation of the safety or efficacy of the combination of an oral local anaesthetic and other adjuvant drugs, such as a tricyclic antidepressant or anticonvulsant. Based on clinical experience, trials of such combinations, undertaken with close clinical monitoring, can be justified in patients with refractory neuropathic pain. If administration of the local anaesthetic has yielded meaningful partial analgesia, it should be continued as a trial with another drug is initiated. If there is a risk of drug interactions, or additive toxicities, dosing must be very cautious and monitoring must be intensified.

Dosing guidelines for local anaesthetic infusion are derived from the large clinical experience with this approach and a limited number of trials in patients with neuropathic pain. Lignocaine infusions have been administered at varying doses, typically within a range of 2 to 5 mg/kg infused over 20 to 30 min.[199] In the medically frail patient, it is prudent to start at the lower end of this range.

Anticonvulsant drugs

There is good evidence that several anticonvulsant drugs are useful in the management of lancinating (stabbing) neuropathic pains.[244] Clinical experience also suggests that these agents may be useful in patients with other types of episodic neuropathic pains (particularly those that have paroxysmal onset) and in occasional patients with continuous dysaesthesias.

The efficacy of carbamazepine in the treatment of neuropathic pain was suggested in numerous uncontrolled trials,[245-261] and confirmed in controlled studies of patients with trigeminal neuralgia,[262-265] postherpetic neuralgia (in which an effect against lancinating but not continuous pains was demonstrated),[264] and painful diabetic neuropathy.[266] Among the other lancinating dysaesthesias that have been reported to respond are glossopharyngeal neuralgia, tabetic lightning pains, paroxysmal pain in multiple sclerosis, postsympathectomy pain, so-called 'flashing' dysaesthesias in spinal cord injured patients, stabbing pains following laminectomy, and lancinating pains due to cancer and post-traumatic mononeuropathy.[253-261] These data suggest that carbamazepine has analgesic efficacy in lancinating neuropathic pain, regardless of the specific pathology that induces it.

In controlled trials, phenytoin was an effective analgesic for painful neuropathy in Fabry's disease[267] and painful diabetic neuropathy.[268] Surveys and case reports also suggested efficacy in trigeminal neuralgia, diabetic neuropathy, glossopharyngeal neuralgia, tabetic lightning pains, paroxysmal pain in postherpetic neuralgia, central pain, postsympathectomy pain and post-traumatic neuralgia.[251,253-255,269-275] These neuropathic pains were all characterized by a prominent lancinating component.

Uncontrolled surveys and a number of case reports have suggested that clonazepam and sodium valproate may also be useful in lancinating neuropathic pain. Clonazepam was reported to be effective in patients with trigeminal neuralgia,[276] paroxysmal post-laminectomy pain,[277] and post-traumatic neuralgia;[255] valproate was beneficial for patients with trigeminal neuralgia[278] and postherpetic neuralgia.[279]

Newer anticonvulsants have also been administered for pain. In a published series, gabapentin therapy appeared to help some patients with reflex sympathetic dystrophy.[280] Lamotrigine was effective in reducing hyperalgesia in an animal model;[281] it has yet to be described as an analgesic in humans. Felbamate has been used anecdotally to treat hemifacial spasm,[282] a painless syndrome characterized by paroxysmal contraction of facial muscles; although this observation and successful anecdotal treatment of a small number of patients with pain initially raised expectations, there have been no follow-up studies of this drug and its recently recognized potential for lethal aplastic anaemia has tempered enthusiasm for its use.

Of these newer anticonvulsants, anecdotal experience has been most favourable with gabapentin. This drug is now widely used by pain specialists in the United States to treat neuropathic pain of various types. The pharmacological profile of gabapentin includes properties that suggest a relatively high degree of safety, including no hepatic metabolism, no known drug–drug interactions, and a pharmacokinetic ceiling dose due to saturation of a transport system. Based on clinical experience, treatment is usually initiated at a dose of 300 mg/day or less, then gradually increased to a usual dose range of 900–3200 mg/day in three divided doses. Analgesic effects appear to be dose dependent, and it is reasonable to continue dose escalation until pain relief occurs, side-effects are reported, or a dose at or above the usual maximum is attained. Several controlled trials are now under way to evaluate the efficacy and safety of gabapentin in a variety of neuropathic pains.

In summary, selected anticonvulsant drugs can relieve some types of dysaesthesias in diverse neuropathic pain syndromes. The evidence of this effect is best for carbamazepine, but published reports and clinical experience suggest that phenytoin, clonazepam, and valproate may have similar effects. Newer anticonvulsants, particularly gabapentin, may also have some analgesic potential in neuropathic pain but experience is as yet too limited to judge their utility.

Mechanism of action

The efficacy of anticonvulsant drugs has been most clearly established for episodic lancinating pains, which are acute in onset, peak very rapidly, and remit after a brief period. The benefits of these drugs for neuropathic pains that are non-lancinating but have a paroxysmal onset is supported by extensive clinical experience. Anecdotally, continuous dysaesthesias appear to respond occasionally, but there is little evidence of benefit comparable to that attained in lancinating dysaesthesia. These observations suggest that pain phenomenology, such as the complaint of paroxysmal pain, associates with specific mechanisms and that these mechanisms, in turn, have relatively selective responses to drugs with differing modes of action. Specifically, it may be hypothesized that mechanisms associated with paroxysmal pains respond relatively well to drugs that stabilize membranes, such as anticonvulsant drugs.

The specific mechanisms of the analgesia produced by the anticonvulsant drugs are not known, but presumably relate to those actions underlying anticonvulsant effects. These include suppression of paroxysmal discharges and their spread from the site of origin, and reduction of neuronal hyperexcitability.[283] It can be postulated that the aberrant electrical activity that has been recorded from different levels of the neuraxis in experimental models of nerve injury[129,235,236,284-286] and in patients with chronic neuropathic pains[287-289] is the pathophysiological substrate for the experience of lancinating pains, and that the suppression of these discharges by anticonvulsant drugs results in analgesia.

Adverse effects

Carbamazepine commonly causes sedation, dizziness, nausea, and unsteadiness. These effects can be minimized by low initial doses and gradual dose titration. The intensity diminishes in most patients maintained on the drug for several weeks. Of much greater concern is that carbamazepine causes leucopenia and/or thrombocytopenia in approximately 2 per cent of patients; aplastic anaemia is a rare complication.[290] A complete blood count should be obtained prior to the start of therapy, again after several weeks, then every 3 to 4 months thereafter. A leucocyte count below 4000 is usually considered to be a contraindication to treatment, and a decline to less than 3000 (or an absolute neutrophil count of less than 1500) during therapy should lead to discontinuation of the drug. Other rare adverse effects of carbamazepine include hepatic damage, hyponatremia due to inappropriate secretion of antidiuretic hormone, and congestive heart failure.[291,292] Baseline liver and renal function tests should also be obtained prior to therapy.

Most of the common side-effects of phenytoin are dose-dependent. These include sedation or mental clouding, dizziness, unsteadiness, and diplopia.[293] These effects usually occur at plasma concentrations above the therapeutic range for seizure control. Occasional patients experience toxicity at lower concentrations. Ataxia, progressive encephalopathy, and even seizures can occur at toxic levels.[294] Of the idiosyncratic effects, the most serious are hepatotoxicity and exfoliative dermatitis. The occurrence of a maculopapular rash, which can be the harbinger of the more severe cutaneous reactions, should lead to discontinuation of the drug. A rare permanent cerebellar degeneration has been reported in patients with chronic phenytoin intoxication.[295]

At usual therapeutic doses, the side-effects of valproate are usually mild, consisting of sedation, nausea, tremor, and sometimes increased appetite.[296] An enteric coated tablet minimizes gastrointestinal disturbances, and dose-dependent side-effects are reduced by the use of low initial doses and gradual upward dose titration. Hepatotoxicity, encephalopathy, dermatitis, alopecia, and a rare hyperammonaemia syndrome are among the reported idiosyncratic reactions.[297] The hyperammonaemia syndrome can occur without abnormalities in other liver function tests. The development of confusion or any symptoms or signs compatible with hepatic dysfunction during valproate therapy should be evaluated with both liver function tests and serum ammonia level.

Drowsiness, the most common and troubling side-effect of clonazepam, is usually additive to that produced by other drugs, including alcohol. Tachyphylaxis to this effect often develops within weeks after dosing has begun. Occasional patients develop ataxia, particularly at higher doses. Idiosyncratic reactions, including dermatitis, hepatotoxicity, and haematological effects, appear to be very rare. Like other benzodiazepine drugs, a withdrawal syndrome may occur with abrupt discontinuation of relatively high doses.

The newer anticonvulsant drugs, including gabapentin, lamotrigine, and felbamate, are generally associated with a favourable side-effect profile.[298-301] Experience with these drugs is limited, however, and the recognized spectrum of toxicities is evolving. In the United States, felbamate has been associated with rare fatal aplastic anaemia and liver failure, which has limited its use to patients with refractory epilepsy. This potential toxicity suggests that felbamate should not be administered for neuropathic pain unless other reasonable therapeutic options have been exhausted.

Indications

Lancinating and other episodic paroxysmal neuropathic pains are generally considered to be the primary indication for trials of anticonvulsant drugs. These drugs are often administered as a first-line approach for pains of this type. The treatment of lancinating or paroxysmal neuropathic pain may also be undertaken with other selected adjuvant analgesics (Table 5). As noted previously, data from controlled studies do suggest that the tricyclic antidepressants can ameliorate pain of this type,[15,16] but conventional practice continues to view these drugs as a second-line approach in patients with predominating lancinating dysaesthesias.

Dosing guidelines

There have been no studies comparing the relative efficacy of the various anticonvulsant drugs in patients with neuropathic pain. The variability in the response to these drugs is great, and sequential trials in patients with refractory pain is amply justified by clinical experience.

Many practitioners begin with carbamazepine because of the extraordinarily good response rate observed in trigeminal neuralgia. The use of carbamazepine is contraindicated, however, in patients with leukopenia, and the drug must be used cautiously in those with thrombocytopenia, those at risk for marrow failure (e.g. following chemotherapy), and those whose blood counts must be monitored to determine disease status. Patients with chronic pain associated with anxiety or insomnia might be considered for an early trial of clonazepam, which may also be effective for these symptoms.

Dosing guidelines employed in the treatment of seizures are typically extrapolated for the management of pain. Low initial doses are appropriate for carbamazepine, valproate, and clonazepam, but the administration of phenytoin often begins with the presumed therapeutic dose (e.g. 300 mg/day) or a prudent oral loading regimen (e.g. 500 mg twice, separated by hours). When low initial doses are used, dose escalation should ensue until favourable effects occur, intolerable side-effects supervene, or plasma drug concentration has reached some arbitrary level (customarily at the upper end of the therapeutic range for seizures).

Baclofen and other drugs for lancinating neuropathic pain

As noted previously, several non-anticonvulsant drugs have been used in the management of lancinating or paroxysmal neuropathic pains, including the neuroleptic pimozide,[166] systemically administered local anaesthetics, and the tricyclic antidepressants.[15,16] Baclofen is another alternative, a trial of which typically precedes these other therapies (Table 5).

Baclofen, an agonist at the gamma aminobutyric acid type B ($GABA_B$) receptor, has been conclusively demonstrated to have efficacy in trigeminal neuralgia[302] and is widely considered to be the second-line pharmacological approach in this condition, following carbamazepine.[303] Other neuropathic pains characterized by an episodic lancinating or paroxysmal phenomenology have also been reported to respond to this drug.[304–306] Although there have been a few observations that suggest a broader analgesic potential,[307] baclofen is generally considered to have a relatively selective efficacy for lancinating or paroxysmal neuropathic pain.

The administration of baclofen for pain is undertaken in a manner similar to the use of the drug for its primary indication, spasticity. A starting dose of 5 mg two to three times per day is gradually escalated to the range 30 to 90 mg/day, and sometimes higher if side-effects do not occur. It is appropriate to continue dose escalation until pain is relieved or limiting side-effects occur. The common side-effects (dizziness, somnolence, and gastrointestinal distress) are minimized by low starting doses and gradual dose escalation. The potential for a serious withdrawal syndrome, including delirium and seizures, exists with abrupt discontinuation following prolonged use;[308] doses should always be tapered before discontinuation of the drug.

N-methyl-D-aspartate receptor blockers

Excitatory amino acids, such as glutamate and aspartate, are released by primary afferent neurones in response to noxious stimuli and are important in the central processing of pain-related information. Interactions at the *N*-methyl-D-aspartate (NMDA) receptor are involved in the development of central nervous system changes that may underlie chronic pain and modulate opioid mechanisms—specifically tolerance.[309] Preclinical studies have established that the *N*-methyl-D-aspartate receptor is involved in the sensitization of central neurones following injury and the development of the 'wind-up' phenomenon, a change in the response of central neurones that has been associated with neuropathic pain.[310,311]

Antagonists at the *N*-methyl-D-aspartate receptor may offer another novel approach to the treatment of pain. Although there is evidence that such drugs may be multipurpose analgesics, which could potentially ameliorate acute pain[312] and diverse types of chronic pain,[313–316] the most intense interest has focused on their role as new therapies for neuropathic pain. The treatment of neuropathic pain may become an indication for the use of these drugs in the palliative care setting.

A variety of *N*-methyl-D-aspartate receptor antagonists are currently undergoing intensive investigation as potential analgesics. At the present time, there are two commercially available drugs, the antitussive dextromethorphan and the general anaesthetic ketamine. Both have been shown to have analgesic effects in controlled studies of experimental pain.[317,318] Although a controlled trial of low dose dextromethorphan in patients with neuropathic pain failed to demonstrate efficacy,[319] both case reports[315,316] and controlled studies of short-term dosing[320,321] with ketamine indicate analgesic efficacy in neuropathic pain. Sustained analgesia during long-term administration of ketamine has been observed anecdotally; some of these reports describe patients with cancer pain (Mercadante *et al.*, in press).[315,316,322]

Although information on the role of *N*-methyl-D-aspartate receptor antagonists in the management of chronic pain is evolving, current data are sufficient to justify a trial of one of the commercially available drugs in patients with neuropathic pain that has been refractory to other measures. Dextromethorphan has an extremely good safety profile and has been administered at doses higher than 1 g/day. At high doses, sedation or confusion can occur. Based on clinical experience, a trial of dextromethorphan may be initiated using a proprietary cough suppressant (ensuring that this product contains no alcohol or other active drugs). A prudent starting dose is 45 to 60 mg daily, which can be gradually escalated until favourable effects occur, side-effects supervene, or a conventional maximal dose of 1 g is achieved.

Clinicians who are experienced in the use of parenteral ketamine may also consider this option in patients with refractory pain. In the palliative care setting, this treatment may be useful, for example in patients who have advanced disease and severe neuropathic pain that has not responded adequately to opioids. The side-effect profile of ketamine, which includes delirium, nightmares, hallucinosis, and dysphoria, can be daunting, particularly in the frail, medically ill. However, the likelihood of serious toxicity is low at the relatively small, subanaesthetic doses used to treat pain and the risks may be justified when pain has been intractable to many routine approaches.

Typically, ketamine therapy for pain has been initiated at low doses given subcutaneously, such as 0.1 to 0.15 mg/kg by brief infusion or 0.1 to 0.15 mg/kg/h by continuous infusion. The dose can be gradually escalated, with close monitoring of pain and side-effects. Long-term therapy has been maintained using continuous subcutaneous infusion or repeated subcutaneous injections.

New *N*-methyl-D-aspartate receptor antagonists are in development and may ultimately prove useful for a variety of medical indications. Advances in this area have occurred rapidly and it is likely that the role of these agents in the management of pain will be much better defined within a few years.

Calcitonin

Calcitonin is an interesting drug that may have several pain-related indications in the palliative care setting. Its potential role in bone pain is discussed below. In recent years, evidence has accumulated that calcitonin may also have efficacy in neuropathic pain states. Favourable controlled trials have been reported in populations with sympathetically-maintained pain (see below)[323] and acute phantom pain.[324] Although the mechanisms that may be responsible for these analgesic effects are unknown, these observations justify an empirical trial of calcitonin in refractory neuropathic pain of diverse types.

The optimal dose and dosing frequency for calcitonin are unknown, and the durability of favourable effects, if they occur, has not been evaluated systematically. Anecdotally, therapy is usually initiated with a low dose, such as 25 IU/day intramuscularly. This may reduce the incidence of nausea, the major side-effect. Skin testing with 1 IU prior to the start of therapy is sometimes recommended due to the small risk of serious hypersensitivity reactions. After therapy begins, gradual dose escalation may identify a minimal effective dose. The usual maximum dose, which is recommended solely on the basis of clinical experience, is in the range of 100 to 200 IU/day. The dosing frequency is usually daily at the start of therapy, then reduced, if possible, to the fewest weekly doses required to sustain effects.

Other drugs for sympathetically-maintained pain

Sympathetically-maintained pain is a form of neuropathic pain in which dysaesthesias are believed to be sustained through efferent activity in the sympathetic nervous system.[325] This type of pain is believed to occur most often in patients with a clinical syndrome consistent with reflex sympathetic dystrophy or causalgia. The latter syndromes are characterized by the occurrence of focal autonomic dysregulation (e.g. swelling, vasomotor disturbances, and sweating abnormalities), focal motor disturbances (e.g. tremor or dystonia), or trophic changes (e.g. focal osteoporosis, atrophy of skin or subcutaneous tissues, and changes in nail or hair growth) in the region of the pain. Sympathetic nerve blocks are an important diagnostic test, and, if positive, a first-line of treatment. Drug therapy is usually considered if nerve blocks fail or are contraindicated.

Drug treatments for pain that is presumed to be sympathetically maintained may involve the non-specific use of any of the aforementioned classes of adjuvant analgesics, either multipurpose drugs or drugs used specifically for neuropathic pain. Alternatively, therapy may focus on trials of drugs that either influence sympathetic function or have been specifically studied in this condition.

As noted previously, calcitonin has been evaluated as a treatment for reflex sympathetic dystrophy in a controlled trial.[323] The findings from this study suggest that this drug may be useful when combined with physical therapy. A trial for neuropathic pains that may be sympathetically maintained is warranted.

Drugs that modulate sympathetic nervous system function have been explored in single cases or small series of patients. The analgesic effects that have been associated with phentolamine infusion, which has been developed as a diagnostic tool for sympathetically-maintained pain,[326] indicate the potential viability of this therapeutic strategy. In separate surveys, phenoxybenzamine, prazosin, and guanethidine were reported to be effective for patients with causalgia.[327–329] Although propranolol has been recommended on the basis of uncontrolled observations,[330,331] another survey yielded disappointing results.[332] The risk of orthostatic hypotension may limit the utility of all these treatments.

Nifedipine, a calcium-channel blocker, has also been reported to have favourable effects in a small survey of patients with reflex sympathetic dystrophy.[333] This finding may be illuminated by both experimental evidence linking calcium channels and nociception[334–337] and clinical data that suggest a role for another calcium-channel blocker, nimodipine, as a potentiator of morphine.[338]

Topical analgesics

Topical therapies for neuropathic pain have been used for those syndromes characterized by both a predominating peripheral mechanism and continuous dysaesthesia. Available topical therapies include capsaicin preparations, formulations containing aspirin or a non-steroidal anti-inflammatory drug, and local anaesthetic preparations.[339] A case report that suggested benefit from topical prostaglandin E_1 ointment has not been replicated.[340]

The potential value of topical capsaicin in both painful mononeuropathies and polyneuropathies has been suggested from surveys of patients with postherpetic neuralgia or postmastectomy pain[341–343,347] and controlled trials in populations with postherpetic neuralgia[344] or painful diabetic neuropathy.[345,346] In an open-label series of 12 patients with trigeminal neuralgia, topical capsaicin provided sustained relief in 10 (six complete and four partial).[348] Other controlled trials, which demonstrate that topical capsaicin may relieve the pain associated with osteoarthritis of the finger joints,[349] also suggest that some painful somatic disorders may be amenable to this therapy. The benefit of topical capsaicin in painful diabetic neuropathy and osteoarthritis, as well as one non-painful condition, psoriasis, was confirmed in a meta-analysis of available controlled trials.[350]

Presumably, topical capsaicin lessens pain by reducing the concentration of small peptides in primary afferent neurones. These peptides, which include substance P, may activate nociceptive systems in the dorsal horn of the spinal cord. Their depletion may reduce the central transmission of information about noxious stimuli or reduce peripheral input to sensitized central neurons.[351]

Numerous anti-inflammatory drugs have been investigated for topical use in populations with neuropathic pain, particularly postherpetic neuralgia, and results have generally been mixed. Although one small controlled trial demonstrated efficacy greater than placebo for topical aspirin, indomethacin, and diclofenac in patients with acute herpetic neuralgia or postherpetic neuralgia,[352] another controlled trial found no efficacy whatsoever for topical treatment with a benzydamine cream in a similar patient population.[353] Survey data are similarly conflicting.[339] These limited data suggest that the efficacy of topical anti-inflammatory drugs for neuropathic pain remains unproved.

A commercially available mixture of local anaesthetics, which contains a 1:1 mixture of prilocaine and lignocaine, is capable of penetrating the skin and producing a dense local cutaneous anaesthesia. This product, known as eutectic mixture of local anaesthetics (EMLA®) is widely used to prevent the pain of needle puncture or incision. A limited study in patients with postherpetic neuralgia suggests its utility in the management of some chronic neuropathic pains.[354] Surveys of relatively high concentrations of topical lignocaine,[339,355] and a controlled trial of 5 per cent lignocaine gel,[356] have also been positive in patients with postherpetic neuralgia. Anecdotal experience with commercially available, relatively low concentration local anaesthetic products has not been favourable, however, unless the painful area involves mucosal surfaces.

On the basis of these data, a trial of a topical drug may be considered for neuropathic pains presumed to be sustained, at least in part, by peripheral input. With the exception of topical capsaicin in the treatment of osteoarthritis, the utility of these treatments for other peripherally-driven pain syndromes, including nociceptive pains due to injury of the skin, subcutaneous tissues, muscle, or joint, has not been clarified. Nonetheless, a trial in one of the latter pain syndromes is often warranted by the potential advantages of topical therapy in medically ill patients, who are often predisposed to side-effects from systemically administered drugs.

The adverse effects associated with topical analgesic therapy have been minimal. Capsaicin can cause local burning, which is sometimes intense. Although this symptom is not related to tissue damage and poses no risk to the patient, it can create significant discomfort and lead to discontinuation of the treatment. For those who are able to tolerate the burning initially, it may disappear with repeated administrations over days to weeks. Some patients are able to tolerate the drug if administration is preceded by application of a local anaesthetic or ingestion of an analgesic.

There is a very remote risk of toxicity from systemic absorption of a topical local anaesthetic.[354,356] When the eutectic mixture of local anaesthetics is used, there is also a small risk of methaemoglobinuria from prilocaine application in predisposed patients. This rare event suggests that the drug should be used cautiously in infants, patients with prior histories of methaemoglobinaemia, and those who are coadministered drugs that may also cause this complication, such as sulphonamides.[357]

There have been no comparative trials of the various topical therapies. Most clinicians begin with a trial of capsaicin, a local anaesthetic, or both applied concurrently. In the United States, capsaicin is available in 0.025 per cent and 0.075 per cent concentrations. The latter concentration has been tested most often in controlled trials[350] and it is reasonable to use this compound in most circumstances. Based on clinical observations, an adequate trial is usually considered to be 3 to 4 applications per day for a minimum of 4 weeks.

Guidelines for a trial of topical local anaesthetic are ill defined. To create an area of dense sensory loss using the eutectic mixture of lignocaine and prilocaine, a relatively thick application must remain in contact with the skin under an occlusive dressing for at least 1 h. This mode of administration may be difficult if the painful area is large or adjacent to the face or a mobile region of the body. There is no evidence in populations with neuropathic pain that cutaneous anaesthesia is necessary to gain benefit from a topical local anaesthetic and, anecdotally, some patients seem to respond favourably to a thin application applied without a dressing. In the absence of any systematic evaluation of dosing techniques, the patient should be encouraged to try various modes of administration in an effort to identify a salutary approach. If possible, one of these trials should include an occlusive dressing of some type (ordinary plastic wrap can be used for large areas) and a duration of application of at least 1 h.

A trial of a topical anti-inflammatory drug is usually implemented by application on the painful area of a solution in which aspirin (or other drugs in published reports) is dissolved in ether or chloroform. The solvent evaporates, leaving the drug in contact with the skin.

Anticholinesterase drugs

Anecdotal reports have described the successful use of a variety of anticholinesterase drugs in patients with diverse types of neuropathic pain.[358,359] Physostigmine has also been reported to have favourable effects when combined with morphine during the treatment of acute pain.[360] The mechanism of the putative benefits produced by these drugs is not established and treatment is associated with the potential for serious adverse effects, such as bradycardia. A trial of one of these drugs should only be considered for medically stable patients with severe refractory pain.

Vinca alkaloids

Iontophoretic delivery of vinca alkaloids has been reported to benefit some patients with postherpetic neuralgia.[361] This technique, the results of which could potentially relate to neuroablation of peripheral nerves or their central connections, has not been systematically evaluated and must be considered experimental at the present time.

Benzodiazepines for neuropathic pain

As noted previously, the benzodiazepines clonazepam[255,276,277] and alprazolam[80] have been used in the management of lancinating and cancer-related neuropathic pains, respectively. These data suggest a broad role for the benzodiazepines as adjuvant analgesics for neuropathic pain. Unfortunately, critical reviews of the current information about these drugs do not support this position.[362,363] In

Table 6 Adjuvant analgesics used for malignant bone pain[a]

Corticosteroids
Calcitonin
Bisphosphonates
Clodronate
Pamidronate
Radionuclides
Strontium-89 (^{89}Sr)
Rhenium-186 (^{186}Re)
Samarium-153(^{153}Sm)
Gallium nitrate

[a] Anecdotal data suggets that non-steroidal anti-inflammatory drugs are also useful in bone pain.

contrast to these anecdotal reports and favourable single dose studies of diazepam and midazolam in postoperative pain,[364,365] negative findings have been reported in a controlled trial of lorazepam for postherpetic neuralgia[366] and a small controlled repeated dose study of oral chlordiazepoxide for chronic pain.[367] In a human experimental pain paradigm, the addition of alprazolam to a morphine infusion did not potentiate analgesia[368] and another study of diazepam in a model of laboratory-induced pain suggested that the analgesic effects produced by diazepam were attributable to a change in response bias—the psychological inclination to describe a nociceptive stimulus as painful—rather than a change in the sensorineural processing of the stimulus.[369]

Thus, the evidence for benzodiazepine analgesia is limited and conflicting. Although a trial of clonazepam or alprazolam can be justified in refractory neuropathic pain on the basis of anecdotal experience, the relative safety of these drugs, and the common coexistence of pain and anxiety, wider use of benzodiazepines as adjuvant analgesics is not warranted. Clinical experience with clonazepam has generally been most favourable in those patients with lancinating or paroxysmal pain.

Adjuvant analgesics used for bone pain

Bone pain is a common problem in the palliative care setting. Radiation therapy is usually considered when bone pain is focal and poorly controlled with an opioid, or is associated with a lesion that appears prone to fracture on radiographic examination. Anecdotally, multifocal bone pain has been observed to benefit from treatment with a non-steroidal anti-inflammatory drug or a corticosteroid.[370] Other adjuvant analgesics that are potentially useful in this setting include calcitonin, bisphosphonate compounds, gallium nitrate, and selected radiopharmaceuticals (Table 6). There have been no comparative trials of these adjuvant analgesics for bone pain and the selection of one over another is usually based on convenience, patient preference, and the clinical setting.

Calcitonin

The use of calcitonin in the treatment of various neuropathic pains has been described previously.[323,324] Bone pain may be another indication for this compound in the palliative care setting.

Calcitonin has ameliorated bone pain in some,[371,372] but not all,[373] controlled trials. Clinical experience with this drug suggests that it is relatively safe and can occasionally produce substantial pain relief. The optimal dose, dosing frequency, and duration of therapy are unknown. Skin testing with 1 IU may be prudent to screen for hypersensitivity reactions. Nausea is the major side-effect, the severity of which may be reduced by gradual escalation from a low starting dose (e.g. 25 IU/day IM). Based on anecdotal experience, a dose of 100 to 200 IU/day IM for approximately 1 week should be sufficient to determine analgesic efficacy. If benefits occur, the dose can be gradually lowered to the minimum required to maintain effects. Periodic monitoring of calcium and phosphorus is prudent during treatment.

Intrathecal calcitonin has also been suggested to produce analgesic effects,[374] presumably independent of its putative mechanism of action in bone pain, but the long-term risks and benefits of this approach are not known and this approach should be considered experimental at the present time.

Bisphosphonates

Bisphosphonates (previously known as diphosphonates) are analogues of inorganic pyrophosphate that inhibit osteoclast activity and, consequently, reduce bone resorption in a variety of illnesses. Many surveys and several controlled trials have established the analgesic efficacy of these compounds, particularly pamidronate and clodronate.[375-389] For example, a recent, controlled, dose-ranging study of pamidronate[388] noted that 60 mg every 2 to 4 weeks and 90 mg every 4 weeks produced at least partial pain relief in 50 per cent of patients; almost one-third of those who received the highest dose became pain-free. Although analgesic effects from sodium etidronate have been suggested,[380] the benefits of this drug were not demonstrated in a controlled trial.[390]

The bisphosphonates may also reduce other skeletal morbidity. For example, a placebo-controlled trial of oral clodronate in patients with metastatic breast cancer recorded a significant reduction in the number of hypercalcaemic episodes, number of terminal hypercalcaemic events, incidence of vertebral fractures, rate of vertebral deformity, and combined rate of all morbid skeletal events. A similar improvement in skeletal morbidity was demonstrated in a recent placebo-controlled evaluation of intravenous pamidronate (90 mg every month).[453] Another recent placebo-controlled trial evaluated the addition of clodronate to antitumour therapy in women with recurrent breast cancer and no known bony metastases. During the follow-up period, treated patients had significantly fewer bone metastases, hypercalcaemic episodes, vertebral deformities, and overall rate of morbid skeletal events.).[454] Although the latter study did not reveal a survival advantage from clodronate therapy, the results suggest that prophylactic bisphosphonate therapy may influence the presentation of metastatic disease and, in turn, reduce the likelihood of adverse disease-related outcomes.

Optimal dosing regimens for the bisphosphonates have only begun to be clarified. The dose-ranging trial of pamidronate demonstrated efficacy and an acceptable safety profile for three different dosing regimens (60 mg every 2 weeks, 60 mg every 4 weeks, and 90 mg every 4 weeks).[388] This study also suggested that analgesia can begin after a period of weeks after treatment is initiated (as early as 2 weeks in some cases) and that several doses may be needed to judge the full efficacy of the drug.[388]

Radiopharmaceuticals

Radionuclides that are absorbed at areas of high bone turnover have been evaluated as potential therapies for metastatic bone disease.[391,392] The first radionuclide introduced into clinical practice was phosphorus-32 orthophosphate. Numerous series suggest that this drug can relieve bone pain in as many as 80 per cent of patients.[393] Bone marrow suppression is the major toxicity, and the desire for a compound with a better therapeutic index has spurred the development of several new radionuclides.

Many newer radionuclides have been advocated as potential therapies for bone pain.[391,392] Strontium chloride-89, rhenium-186 hydroxyethylenediphosphonic acid, and samarium-153 ethylenediaminetetramethylenephosphonic acid have been most promising thus far. Surveys of patients with bone metastases from a variety of tumour types have provided strong evidence that these compounds can reduce bone pain without undue risk to bone marrow or other vital structures.[394–402]

Strontium-89, which is commercially available in the United States, has been most extensively evaluated as a treatment for bone pain. Favourable effects have been reported in numerous surveys[394–396] and confirmed in placebo-controlled trials.[403,404] The larger of these controlled trials evaluated strontium-89 as an adjunct to conventional radiotherapy in 126 patients with advanced prostate cancer; treatment reduced the need for both radiotherapy and analgesic drugs.[403] Strontium-89 has also been shown to compare favourably with hemibody irradiation in a randomized trial.[405]

Reviews of the extensive clinical experience with strontium-89 suggest that pain relief occurs in approximately 80 per cent of patients, 10 per cent of whom attain complete relief.[406,407] Initial clinical response occurs in 7 to 21 days and peak response may be delayed for a month or more. Approximately 5 to 10 per cent of patients experience a transitory pain flare immediately after treatment. The usual duration of benefit is 3 to 6 months, after which retreatment may regain a favourable effect. Following treatment, clinically significant leucopenia or thrombocytopenia occur in approximately 10 per cent and 33 per cent of patients, respectively.[403] The nadir of bone marrow effects occurs 4 to 8 weeks after injection and usually undergoes at least partial return to baseline by 12 weeks.

In the absence of comparative trials, the profile of clinical effects produced by strontium-89 can help clarify its role in relation to the other strategies used for bone pain. Strontium-89 is only potentially effective in the treatment of pain due to osteoblastic bone lesions or lesions with an osteoblastic component. An osteoblastic component should be confirmed by positive bone scintigraphy before treatment with this drug. Given the delayed onset and peak effects, treatment should not be administered unless patients have a life expectancy greater than 3 months. This delay also implies that treatment should not be considered as the sole approach for patients with severe pain.

Due to the potential for bone marrow toxicity, treatment with strontium-89 should not be considered unless adequate bone marrow reserve has been documented. In the case of strontium-89, this is usually considered to be a platelet count above 60 000 and a white blood cell count above 2400.[407] Patients who continue to be candidates for myelosuppressive chemotherapy should not be treated because the effects on bone marrow may worsen the toxicity of later cytotoxic therapy or limit the ability to rebound after therapy.

Other drugs for bone pain

Gallium nitrate is another osteoclast inhibitor that may be analgesic for multifocal malignant bone pain. Experience is currently limited to a series of cases.[408] Future studies are need to clarify the value of this drug.

Anecdotal reports have suggested that L-dopa can ameliorate metastatic bone pain.[409] More recent experience, however, has been disappointing,[410,411] and the approach cannot be recommended for routine trials.

Adjuvant analgesics used for bowel obstruction

The management of symptoms associated with malignant bowel obstruction may be challenging.[412] If surgical decompression is not feasible, the need to control pain and other obstructive symptoms, including distension, nausea, and vomiting, becomes paramount. The use of opioids may be problematic due to dose-limiting toxicity (including gastrointestinal toxicity) or the intensity of breakthrough pains. Anecdotal reports suggest that anticholinergic drugs, the somatostatin analogue octreotide, and corticosteroids may be useful adjuvant analgesics in this setting. The use of these drugs may also ameliorate non-painful symptoms and minimize the number of patients who must be considered for chronic drainage using nasogastric or percutaneous catheters.

Anticholinergic drugs

Anticholinergic drugs could theoretically relieve the symptoms of bowel obstruction by reducing propulsive and non-propulsive gut motility and decreasing intraluminal secretions. There have been no controlled trials of this therapy and anecdotal experience is limited.

Some patients appear to benefit from the administration of hyoscine (scopolamine).[413,414] In some countries, hyoscine is only commercially available as the hydrobromide salt, which readily crosses the blood–brain barrier. Although this formulation can be delivered via a transdermal system, which simplifies treatment in patients with bowel obstruction, it is likely to be associated with a relatively higher incidence of central nervous system side-effects, such as somnolence and confusion, than an anticholinergic drug with less penetration through the blood–brain barrier. A small series demonstrated that hyoscine butylbromide, which is less likely to pass the blood–brain barrier due to low lipid solubility, can be effective for obstructive symptoms, including pain.[415] Glycopyrrolate has a pharmacological profile similar to hyoscine butylbromide, but has not been systematically evaluated in a population with symptomatic bowel obstruction. In medically ill patients who are predisposed to central nervous system toxicity, a trial of one of the latter drugs may be warranted on theoretical grounds.

Octreotide

The somatostatin analogue octreotide inhibits the secretion of gastric, pancreatic, and intestinal secretions and reduces gastrointestinal motility. These effects probably underlie the analgesic effects that have been observed anecdotally in the symptomatic treatment of bowel obstruction.[416] Octreotide has also been used to manage severe diarrhoea due to enterocolic fistula, high output jejunostomies or ileostomies, or secretory tumours of the gastrointestinal tract.[417–419]

Octreotide has a good safety profile but is expensive. In some settings, however, the cost may be balanced by an excellent clinical result or the avoidance of the costs involved in the use of a gastrointestinal drainage procedure.

Corticosteroids

As discussed previously, the symptoms associated with bowel obstruction may improve with corticosteroid therapy. The mode of action is unclear and the most effective drug, dose, and dosing regimen is unknown. A broad range of doses have been described anecdotally. For example dexamethasone has been used for this indication in a dose range of 8 to 60 mg/day[124,125] and methylprednisolone has been administered in a dose range of 30 to 50 mg/day.[113] The potential for complications during long-term therapy, including an increased risk of bowel perforation,[136,137] may limit this approach to patients with short life expectancies.

Adjuvant analgesics used for musculoskeletal pain

Although pains that originate from injury to muscle or connective tissue are prevalent in the medically ill,[420] there has been no systematic evaluation of analgesic therapies for this problem. In the management of acute traumatic sprains or strains in the non-medically ill, non-opioid and opioid analgesics are commonly supplemented by treatment with so-called muscle relaxant drugs or benzodiazepines. The role of the latter drugs for opioid-refractory musculoskeletal pains in populations with advanced medical illness remains ill defined.

Muscle relaxants

The so-called muscle relaxants include drugs in a variety of classes, all of which are marketed for the treatment of acute musculoskeletal pain. In the United States, this group includes drugs that are also administered as antihistamines (e.g. orphenadrine), tricyclic compounds structurally similar to the tricyclic antidepressants (e.g. cyclobenzaprine), and other types of drugs (e.g. carisoprodol, chlorzoxazone, and methocarbamol).

The efficacy of the muscle relaxant drugs in common musculoskeletal pains has been established in placebo-controlled studies.[421–424] Some studies have demonstrated analgesic effects that are superior to either aspirin or acetaminophen, and others have shown that the combination of a muscle relaxant and one of the latter drugs provides better analgesia than does aspirin or acetaminophen alone. There have been no controlled comparative trials or studies that have directly compared the efficacy and side-effect profiles of these drugs with either non-steroidal anti-inflammatory drugs or opioids.

Although muscle relaxant drugs can relieve musculoskeletal pains, these effects may not be specific and do not depend on relaxation of skeletal muscle. The label 'muscle relaxant' notwithstanding, there is actually no evidence that these drugs relax skeletal muscle in the clinical setting. They do inhibit polysynaptic myogenic reflexes in animal models, but the relationship between this action and analgesia is not known.

Thus, the muscle relaxant drugs are best viewed as alternatives to the anti-inflammatory drugs and opioids, which may be indicated in musculoskeletal pains because of the evidence of analgesic efficacy in these conditions. These drugs should not be administered in the mistaken belief that they relieve muscle spasm.

The muscle relaxant drugs are generally well tolerated, but have sedative effects that may be additive to other centrally acting drugs, including the opioids. Anecdotally, some patients report differences among drugs in analgesic efficacy or sedative side-effects, and it is reasonable to switch to an alternative drug if treatment is initially ineffective. Although the dose–response relationships of the muscle relaxant drugs have not been systematically explored, there are probably dose-dependent effects and the use of a low initial dose followed by gradual dose escalation can be recommended as a means to identify the most salutary balance between analgesia and side-effects. Experience with these drugs is too limited to pursue dose escalation beyond the usual recommended range.

Benzodiazepines for musculoskeletal pain

As discussed previously, there are relatively few data that support the existence of analgesic effects for benzodiazepine drugs.[362,363] Based on a favourable anecdotal experience, selected drugs, most often clonazepam, are used in the management of some neuropathic pains. In a similar way, diazepam is sometimes administered for acute musculoskeletal pains, particularly those characterized by spasm. This use is based on a favourable clinical experience and evidence that this drug, unlike the so-called muscle relaxants, actually reduces myotonic activity.[425]

Other adjuvant analgesics

Many other drugs have analgesic effects, but are not usually administered for pain in the palliative care setting. Some, such as the psychostimulants, are given for alternative indications; others have been disappointing in clinical practice or are yet too new to confirm safety and efficacy in the medically ill population.

Psychostimulants

There is substantial evidence that psychostimulant drugs have analgesic effects. Controlled, single dose studies have established the analgesic efficacy of dextroamphetamine in postoperative pain,[426] methylphenidate in pain associated with Parkinson's disease[427] or cancer,[428] and caffeine in headache, sore throat, and oral surgery pain.[429–432] Analgesic effects were not identified in a well-controlled, single dose, postoperative study of cocaine,[433] but intranasal cocaine (the so-called sphenopalantine ganglion block) has produced analgesia in several such trials.[434,435]

Controlled trials of methylphenidate in the cancer population have established that this drug can reduce opioid-induced somnolence and cognitive impairment.[428,436] The management of central nervous system side-effects is an important issue, and, accordingly, the practical use of psychostimulants in the palliative care setting has focused on this indication, rather than the treatment of unrelieved pain.

Both dextroamphetamine and methylphenidate have been widely used to reverse opioid-induced somnolence, and there has been some anecdotal experience with the related compound, pemoline. The latter drug has relatively minor sympathomimetic effects and is available in a chewable tablet, characteristics that may increase its utility in the palliative care setting.

The psychostimulants are usually well tolerated. A survey of 50 patients treated with methylphenidate observed early toxicity in 2 patients (hallucinations and a paranoid reaction, respectively) and no late toxicity.[437] Anecdotal experience suggests that the other psychostimulants have a similarly favourable therapeutic index. Recently, pemoline has been associated with a rare hepatopathy, which has been fatal in 3 cases;[438] this association has not been reported with other psychostimulants drugs and suggests that pemoline should be considered a second-line drug in the medically ill.

Treatment with methylphenidate or dextroamphetamine is typically begun at 2.5 to 5 mg in the morning and again at midday, if necessary, to keep the patient alert during the day and not interfere with sleep at night. The second dose is usually needed. Doses are increased gradually until efficacy is established. Although few patients require more than 40 mg/day in divided doses, occasional patients benefit from higher doses. Some patients require dose escalation later in the course of therapy.[436]

Antihistamines

Controlled, single-dose studies have established that diphenhydramine, hydroxyzine, orphenadrine, phenyltoloxamine, and pyrilamine can have analgesic effects.[421,423,439–444] Favourable effects from antihistamine-containing proprietary pain relievers have also been observed.[445] These data suggest that antihistaminic drugs may be non-specific analgesics.

Clinical experience, however, has been disappointing. The reason for this disparity is not evident, but the failure to observe substantial analgesia from the addition of an antihistamine suggests that treatment should be considered only for patients who have indications other than pain. Hydroxyzine, for example, is sometimes administered to patients with pain complicated by anxiety, nausea, or itch in the hope that analgesia will be augmented while these other symptoms are relieved. The use of these agents must also be tempered by the potential for side-effects (e.g. somnolence) that add to those produced by other centrally acting drugs, including the opioids.

Cannabinoids

Cannabinoids have antinociceptive effects in animal models[446,447] and single dose studies of intramuscular levonantradol in post-operative pain and oral delta-9-tetrahydrocannabinol in cancer pain demonstrated clear analgesic effects.[448,449] In the study of cancer pain, for example, 10 mg of delta-9-tetrahydrocannabinol was well tolerated and produced analgesic effects similar to 60 mg codeine, but a higher dose yielded severe side-effects in many patients.[448] Thus, the therapeutic window for this drug appears narrow and maximal efficacy at tolerable doses is limited. For these reasons, cannabinoids have not become accepted as adjuvant analgesics in palliative care.

Other drugs

The efficacy of sucralfate as a therapy for the acute and late effects of pelvic irradiation has been evaluated in a placebo-controlled trial.[450] Sucralfate, 1 g, was administered 6 times per day for 6 weeks, beginning 2 weeks after the start of radiotherapy. Although cramping was not significantly affected, both acute and long-term (1 year later) problems with diarrhoea were ameliorated by the drug, and the need for treatment with loperamide was reduced. This approach may help prevent an uncomfortable chronic toxicity associated with radiotherapy.

A recent study of adenosine in the postoperative setting suggests that this compound may have analgesic effects.[451] A clinical role for adenosine is yet to be clarified, but the finding exemplifies the ongoing process by which basic studies of the enormously complex neuropharmacology of nociception[452] are translated into the development of clinical tools for the treatment of pain.

Conclusions

Although the use of adjuvant analgesics in palliative care remains largely guided by anecdotal experience, controlled clinical trials have begun to provide a scientific rationale for many therapies. Future investigations of nociceptive processes and pain pathophysiology will undoubtedly lead to the development of novel drugs. For example the adjuvant analgesics may one day include drugs that modulate peripheral nociceptive processes, such as substance P or bradykinin antagonists, or drugs that alter central processing by interacting with gangliosides or second messenger systems activated by excitatory amino acids. Although opioid drugs continue to be the major approach to the treatment of pain in the palliative care setting, adjuvant analgesics offer opportunities for improved outcomes in the substantial group of patients who cannot attain an acceptable balance between pain relief and side-effects.

References

1. Cherny NI, Portenoy RK. Cancer pain: principles of assessment and syndromes. In: Wall PD, Melzack R, eds. *Textbook of Pain*, 3rd edn. Edinburgh: Churchill Livingstone, 1994: 787–823.
2. Gonzales GR, Elliot KJ, Portenoy RK, Foley KM. The impact of a comprehensive evaluation in the management of cancer pain. *Pain*, 1991; **47**: 141–4.
3. Jorgensen L, Mortensen M-J, Jensen N-H, Eriksen J. Treatment of cancer pain patients in a multidisciplinary pain clinic. *The Pain Clinic*, 1990; **3**: 83–9.
4. Moulin DE, Foley KM. Review of a hospital-based pain service. In: Foley KM, Bonica JJ, Ventafridda V, eds. *Advances in Pain Research and Therapy*, vol 16, Second International Congress on Cancer Pain. New York: Raven Press, 1990: 413–27.
5. Portenoy RK. Cancer pain: epidemiology and syndromes. *Cancer*, 1989; **63**: 2298–307.
6. Schug SA, Zech D, Dorr U. Cancer pain mangement according to WHO analgesic guidelines. *Journal of Pain and Symptom Management*, 1990; **5**: 27–32.
7. Schug SA, Zech D, Grond S, Jung H, Meurser T, Stobbe B. A long-term survey of morphine in cancer pain patients. *Journal of Pain and Symptom Management*, 1992; **7**: 259–66.
8. Takeda F. Results of field testing in Japan of the WHO draft interim guidelines on relief of cancer pain. *The Pain Clinic*, 1986; **1**: 83–9.
9. Toscani F, Carini M. The implementation of WHO guidelines for the treatment of advanced cancer pain at a district general hospital in Italy. *The Pain Clinic*, 1989; **3**: 37–48.
10. Ventafridda V, Tamburini M, DeConno F. Comprehensive treatment in cancer pain. In: Fields HL, Dubner R, Cervero F, eds. *Advances in Pain Research and Therapy*, vol 9, Proceedings of the Fouth World Congress on Pain. New York: Raven Press, 1985: 617–28.
11. Ventafridda V, Tamburini M, Caraceni A, *et al.* A validation study of the WHO method for cancer pain relief. *Cancer*, 1990; **59**: 850–6.
12. Vijayaram S, Bhargava K, *et al.* Experience with oral morphine for cancer pain relief. *Journal of Pain and Symptom Management*, 1989; **4**: 130–4.
13. Walker VA, Hoskin PJ, Hanks GW, White ID. Evaluation of WHO analgesic guidelines for cancer pain in a hospital-based palliative care unit. *Journal of Pain and Symptom Management*, 1988; **3**: 145–9.

14. World Health Organization. *Cancer Pain Relief and Palliative Care*, Geneva: World Health Organization, 1990.
15. Max MB, *et al.* Amitriptyline relieves diabetic neuropathy pain in patients with normal or depressed mood. *Neurology*, 1987; **37**: 589–96.
16. Kishore-Kumar R, *et al.* Desipramine relieves postherpetic neuralgia. *Clinical Pharmacology and Therapeutics*, 1990; **47**: 305–12.
17. Ventafridda V, *et al.* Studies on the effects of antidepressant drugs on the antinociceptive action of morphine and on plasma morphine in rat and man. *Pain*, 1990; **43**: 155–62.
18. Atkinson JH, Slater MA. Psychopharmacologic agents. In: Tollison CD, Kriegel ML, eds. *Interdisciplinary Rehabilitation of Low Back Pain*. Baltimore: Williams and Wilkins, 1989: 169–202.
19. Monks R. Psychotropic drugs. In: Wall PD, Melzack R, eds. *Textbook of Pain*. 3rd edn. New York: Churchill Livingstone, 1994: 963–90.
20. France RD, Krishnan KRR. Psychotropic drugs in chronic pain. In: France RD, Krishnan KRR, eds. *Chronic Pain*. Washington, DC: American Psychiatric Press, 1988: 322–74.
21. Onghena P, Van Houdenhove B. Antidepressant-induced analgesia in chronic nonmalignant pain: a meta-analysis of 39 placebo-controlled studies. *Pain*, 1992; **49**: 205–19.
22. Egbunike IG, Chaffee BJ. Antidepressants in the management of chronic pain syndromes. *Pharmacotherapy*, 1990; **10**: 262–70.
23. Getto CJ, Sorkness CA, Howell T. Antidepressants and chronic non-malignant pain: a review. *Journal of Pain and Symptom Management*, 1987; **2**: 9–18.
24. Magni G. The use of antidepressants in the treatment of chronic pain: a review of the current evidence. *Drugs*, 1991; **42**: 730–48.
25. Gobel H, Hamouz V, Hansen C, Heininger K, Hirsche S, Lindner V, Heuss D, Soyka D. Chronic tension-type headache: amitriptyline reduces clinical headache duration and experimental pain sensitivity but does not alter pericranial muscle activity readings. *Pain*, 1994; **59**: 241–50.
26. Couch JR, Ziegler DK, Hassanein R. Amitriptyline in the prophylaxis of migraine: effectiveness and relationship of antimigraine and antidepressant effects. *Neurology*, 1976; **26**: 121–7.
27. Diamond S, Baltes BJ. Chronic tension headache—treatment with amitriptyline—a double-blind study. *Headache*, 1971; **11**: 110–16.
28. Gomersall JD, Stuart A. Amitriptyline in migraine prophylaxis. *Journal of Neurology, Neurosurgery and Psychiatry*, 1973; **3C**: 684–90.
29. Lance JW, Curran DA. Treatment of chronic tension headache. *Lancet*, 1964; **1**: 1236–9.
30. Indaco A, Carrieri PB. Amitriptyline in the treatment of headache in patients with Parkinson's disease: a double-blind placebo-controlled study. *Neurology*, 1988; **38**: 1720–2.
31. Okasha A, Ghaleb AA, Sadek A. A double-blind trial for the clinical management of psychogenic headache. *British Journal of Psychiatry*, 1973; **122**: 181–3.
32. Frank RG, *et al.* Antidepressant analgesia in rheumatoid arthritis. *The Journal of Rheumatology*, 1988; **15**: 1632–8.
33. Ward NG. Tricyclic antidepressants for chronic low back pain: mechanism of action and predictors of response. *Spine*, 1986; **11**: 661–5.
34. Watson CPN, Evans RJ, Reed K, Merskey H, Goldsmith L, Warsh J. Amitriptyline versus placebo in postherpetic neuralgia. *Neurology*, 1982; **32**: 671–3.
35. Watson CPN, Chipman M, Reed K, Evans RJ, Birkett N. Amitriptyline versus maprotiline in postherpetic neuralgia: a randomized double-blind, crossover trial. *Pain*, 1992; **48**: 29–36.
36. Carrette S, *et al.* Evaluation of amitriptyline in primary fibrositis. *Arthritis and Rheumatism*, 1986; **29**: 655–9.
37. Dinerman H, Felsen D, Goldenberg D. A randomized clinical trial of naproxen and amitriptyline in primary fibromyalgia. *Arthritis and Rheumatism*, 1985; **159**(S): 28–33.
38. Turkington RW. Depression masquerading as diabetic neuropathy. *Journal of the American Medical Association*, 1980; **243**: 1147–50.
39. Max MB, Lynch SA, Muir J, Shoaf SE, Smoller B, Dubner R. Effects of desipramine, amitriptyline, and fluoxetine on pain in diabetic neuropathy. *New England Journal of Medicine*, 1992; **326**: 1250–6.
40. Leijon G, Boivie J. Central post-stroke pain: a controlled trial of amitriptyline and carbamazepine. *Pain*, 1989; **36**: 27–36.
41. Sharav Y, Singer E, Schmidt E, Dionne RA, Dubner R. The analgesic effect of amitriptyline on chronic facial pain. *Pain*, 1987; **31**: 199–209.
42. Ventafridda V, Bonezzi C, Caraceni A, *et al.* Antidepressants for cancer pain and other painful syndromes with deafferentation component: comparison of amitriptyline and trazadone. *Italian Journal of Neurological Science*, 1987; **8**: 579–87.
43. Pilowsky I, Hallett EC, Bassett DL, Thomas PG, Penhall RK. A controlled study of amitriptyline in the treatment of chronic pain. *Pain*, 1982; **14**: 169–79.
44. McDonald-Scott WA. The relief of pain with an antidepressant in arthritis. *Practitioner*, 1969; **202**: 802–7.
45. Gringas M. A clinical trial of tofranil in rheumatic pain in general practice. *Journal of International Medical Research*, 1976; **4**: 41–9.
46. Glick EN, Fowler PD. Imipramine in chronic arthritis. *Pharmacology and Medicine*, 1979; **1**: 94–6.
47. Kvinesdal B, Molin J, Froland A, Gram LF. Imipramine treatment of painful diabetic neuropathy. *Journal of the American Medical Association*, 1984; **251**: 1727–30.
48. Sindrup SH, Ejlertsen B, Froland A, Sindrup EH, Brosen K, Gram LF. Imipramine treatment in diabetic neuropathy: relief of subjective symptoms without changes in peripheral and autonomic nerve function. *European Journal of Clinical Pharmacology*, 1989; **37**: 151–3.
49. Sindrup SH, Gram LF, Skjold T, Froland A, Beck-Nielsen H. Concentration-response relationship in imipramine treatment of diabetic neuropathy symptoms. *Clinical Pharmacology and Therapeutics*, 1990; **47**: 509–15.
50. Alcoff J, Jones E, Rust P, Newman R. Controlled trial of imipramine for chronic low back pain. *Journal of Family Practice*, 1982; **14**: 841–6.
51. Cannon RO, Quyyumi AS, Mincemoyer R, *et al.* Imipramine in patients with chest pain despite normal coronary angiograms. *New England Journal of Medicine*, 1994; **330**: 1411–17.
52. Ward NG, Bloom VL, Friedel RP. The effectiveness of tricyclic antidepressants in the treatment of coexisting pain and depression. *Pain*, 1979; **7**: 331–41.
53. Evans W, Gensler F, Blackwell B, Galbrecht C. The effects of antidepressant drugs on pain relief and mood in the chronically ill. *Psychosomatics*, 1973; **14**: 214–9.
54. Morland TJ, Storli OV, Mogstad TE. Doxepin in the treatment of mixed vascular and tension headaches. *Headache*, 1979; **19**: 382–3.
55. Hameroff SR, *et al.* Doxepin effects on chronic pain, depression and plasma opioids. *Journal of Clinical Psychiatry*, 1982; **43**: 22–7.
56. Panerai AE, Monza G, Movillia P, Bianchi M, Francucci BM, Tiengo M. A randomized, within-patient crossover, placebo-controlled trial on the efficacy and tolerability of the tricyclic antidepressants chlorimipramine and nortriptyline in central pain. *Acta Neurologica Scandinavica*, 1990; **82**: 34–8.
57. Langohr HD, Stohr M, Petruch F. An open and double-blind crossover study on the efficacy of clomipramine (Anafranil) in patients with painful mono- and polyneuropathies. *European Neurology*, 1982; **21**: 309–17.
58. Eberhard G, *et al.* A double-blind randomized study of clomipramine versus maprotiline in patients with idiopathic pain syndromes. *Neuropsychobiology*, 1988; **19**: 25–34.
59. Sindrup SH, Gram LF, Skjold T, Grodum E, Brosen K, Beck-Nielsen H. Clomipramine vs. desipramine vs. placebo in the treatment of diabetic neuropathy symptoms. A double-blind cross-over study. *British Journal of Clinical Pharmacology*, 1990; **30**: 683–91.
60. Caruso I, *et al.* Double-blind study of dothiepin versus placebo in the treatment of primary fibromyalgia syndrome. *Journal of International Medical Research*, 1987; **15**: 154–7.
61. Feinman C, Harris M, Cawley R. Psychogenic facial pain: presentation and treatment. *British Medical Journal*, 1984; **288**: 436–8.
62. Gomez-Perez FJ, Riell JA, Dies H, Rodriguez-Rivera JG, Gonzalez-Barranco J, Lozano-Castaneda O. Nortriptyline and fluphenazine in the symptomatic treatment of diabetic neuropathy. A double-blind crossover study. *Pain*, 1985; **23**: 395–400.

63. Davidoff G, Guarracini M, Roth E, Sliwa J, Yarkony G. Trazodone hydrochloride in the treatment of dysesthetic pain in traumatic myelopathy: a randomized, double-blind, placebo-controlled study. *Pain*, 1987; **29**: 151–61.
64. Sindrup SH, Gram LF, Brosen K, Eshoj O, Mogensen EF. The selective serotonin reuptake inhibitor paroxetine is effective in the treatment of diabetic neuropathy symptoms. *Pain*, 1990; **42**: 135–44.
65. Sindrup SH, Bjerre U, Dejgaard A, *et al*. The selective serotonin reuptake inhibitor citalopram relieves the symptoms of diabetic neuropathy. *Clinical Pharmacology and Therapeutics*, 1992; **52**: 547–52.
66. Johansson F, Von Knorring L. A double-blind controlled study of a serotonin uptake inhibitor (zimelidine) versus placebo in chronic pain patients. *Pain*, 1979; **7**: 69–78.
67. Watson CPN, Evans RJ. A comparative trial of amitriptyline and zimelidine in postherpetic neuralgia. *Pain*, 1985; **23**: 387–94.
68. Diamond S, Frietag FG. The use of fluoxetine in the treatment of headache. *Clinical Journal of Pain*, 1989; **5**: 200–1.
69. Geller SA. Treatment of fibrositis with fluoxetine hydrochloride (Prozac). *American Journal of Medicine*, 1989; **87**: 594–5.
70. Walsh TD. Controlled study of imipramine and morphine in chronic pain due to advanced cancer. *Proceedings of the American Society of Clinical Oncology*, 1986; **5**: 237.
71. Breivik H, Rennemo F. Clinical evaluation of combined treatment with methadone and psychotropic drugs in cancer patients. *Acta Anaesthetica Scandinavica*, 1982; **74**: 135–40.
72. Magni G, Arsie D, DeLeo D. Antidepressants in the treatment of cancer pain: a survey in Italy. *Pain*, 1987; **29**: 347–53.
73. Adjan M. Uber therapeutischen Beeinflussung des Schmerzsumptoms bei unheilbaren Tumorkranken. *Therapie der Gergenwart*, 1970; **10**: 1620–7.
74. Barjou B. Etude du Tofranil sules douleurs en chirugie. *Revue Medicine de Tours*, 1971; **6**: 473–82.
75. Deutschmann W. Tofranil in der schmerzbehandlung de krebskranken. *Medizinische Welt*, 1971; **22**: 1346–7.
76. Hugues A, Chauvergne J, Lissilour T, Lagarde C. L'imipramine utilisee comme antalgique majeur en carcinologie: etude de 118 cas. *Presse Medicale*, 1963; **71**: 1073–4.
77. Gebhardt KH, Beller J, Nischik R. Behandlung des Karzinomschmerzes mit Chlorimipramin (Anafranil). *Mediziniche Klinik*, 1969; **64**: 751–6.
78. Bernard A, Scheuer H. Action de la clomipramine (Anafranil) sur la douleur des cancers en pathologie cervico-faciale. *Journal Francais d'Oto-rhino-laryngologie*, 1972; **21**: 723–8.
79. Fiorentino M. Sperimentazione controllata dell'imipramina come analgesico maggiore in oncologia. *Rivista Medica Trentina*, 1967; **5**: 387–96.
80. Fernandez F, Adams F, Holmes VF. Analgesic effect of alprazolam in patients with chronic, organic pain of malignant origin. *Journal of Clinical Psychopharmacology*, 1987; **3**: 167–9.
81. Lascelles RG. Atypical facial pain and depression. *British Journal of Psychiatry*, 1966; **122**: 651–9.
82. Anthony M, Lance JW. Monoamine oxidase inhibitors in the treatment of migraine. *Archives of Neurology*, 1969; **21**: 263–8.
83. Cooper GL. The safety of fluoxetine: an update. *British Journal of Psychiatry*, 1988; **153**(suppl 3): 77–86.
84. Boyer WF, Blumhardt CL. The safety profile of paroxetine. *Journal of Clinical Psychiatry*, 1992; **53**(suppl 2): 61–6.
85. Kerr JS, Fairweather DB, Mahendran R, Hindmarch I. The effects of paroxetine, alone and in combination with alcohol on psychomotor performance and cognitive function in the elderly. *International Clinical Psychopharmacology*, 1992; **7**: 101–8.
86. Spiegel K, Kalb R, Pasternak GW. Analgesic activity of tricyclic antidepressants. *Annals of Neurology*, 1983; **13**: 462–5.
87. Biegon A, Samuel D. Interaction of tricyclic antidepressants with opiate receptors. *Biochemistry and Pharmacology*, 1980; **29**: 460–2.
88. Isenberg KE, Cicero TJ. Possible involvement of opiate receptors in the pharmacological profiles of antidepressant compounds. *European Journal of Pharmacology*, 1984; **103**: 57–63.
89. De Felipe MC, de Ceballow ML, Fuentes JA. Hypoalgesia induced by antidepressants in mice: a case for opioids and serotonin. *European Journal of Pharmacology*, 1986; **125**: 193–9.
90. Besson JM, Chaouch A. Peripheral and spinal mechanisms of nociception. *Physiological Reviews*, 1987; **67**: 67–186.
91. Basbaum AI, Fields HL. Endogenous pain control systems: brainstem spinal pathways and endorphin circuitry. *Annual Review of Neuroscience*, 1984; **7**: 309–38.
92. Yaksh TL. Direct evidence that spinal serotonin and noradrenaline terminals mediate the spinal antinociceptive effects of morphine in the periaqueductal gray. *Brain Research*, 1979; **160**: 180–5.
93. Hall H, Ogren SO. Effects of antidepressant drugs on different receptors in the brain. *European Journal of Pharmacology*, 1981; **70**: 393–407.
94. Richelson E. Tricyclic antidepressants and neurotransmitter receptors. *Psychiatric Annals*, 1979; **9**: 186–94.
95. Charney DS, Menkes DB, Heninger FR. Receptor sensitivity and the mechanism of action of antidepressant treatment. *Archives of General Psychiatry*, 1981; **38**: 1160–80.
96. Potter WZ, *et al*. Selective antidepressants and cerebrospinal fluid: lack of specificity in norepinephrine and serotonin metabolites. *Archives of General Psychiatry*, 1985; **42**: 1171–7.
97. Cross JA, Horton RW. Effects of chronic oral administration of the antidepressants, desmethylimipramine and zimelidine on rat cortical GABA-B binding sites: a comparison with 5HT2 binding site changes. *British Journal of Pharmacology*, 1988; **93**: 331–6.
98. Baldessarini RJ. Drugs and the treatment of psychiatric disorders. In: Gilman AG, Rall TW, Nies AS, Taylor P, eds. *The Pharmacological Basis of Therapeutics*, 8th edn. New York: Pergamon Press, 1990: 383–435.
99. Preskorn SH, Irwin HA. Toxicity of tricyclic antidepressants—kinetics, mechanism, intervention: a review. *Journal of Clinical Psychiatry*, 1982; **43**: 151–6.
100. Glassman AH, Bigger JT. Cardiovascular effects of therapeutic doses of tricyclic antidepressants. *Archives of General Psychiatry*, 1981; **38**: 815–20.
101. Roose SP, *et al*. Nortriptyline in depressed patients with left ventricular impairment. *Journal of the American Medical Association*, 1986; **256**: 3253–7.
102. Ray WA, Griffin MR, Schaffner W, Baugh DK, Melton LJ. Pyschotropic drug use and the risk of hip fracture. *New England Journal of Medicine*, 1987; **316**: 363–9.
103. Lieberman E, Stoudemire A. Use of tricyclic antidepressants in patients with glaucoma. Assessment and appropriate precautions. *Psychosomatics*, 1987; **28**: 145–8.
104. Kerrick JM, Fine PG, Lipman AG, Love G. Low-dose amitriptyline as an adjunct to opioids for postoperative orthopedic pain: a placebo-controlled trial trial. *Pain*, 1993; **52**: 325–30.
105. Gordon NC, Heller PH, Gear RW, Levine JD. Interactions between fluoxetine and opiate analgesia for postoperative dental pain. *Pain*, 1994; **58**: 85–8.
106. Poulsen L, Arendt-Nielsen L, Brosen K, Nielsen KK, Gram LF, Sindrup SH. The hypoalgesic effect of imipramine in different human experimental pain models. *Pain*, 1995; **60**: 287–93.
107. Bruera E, Schoeller T, Wenk R, MacEachern T, Marcelino S, Hanson J, Suarez-Almazor M. A prospective multi-center assessment of the Edmonton staging system for cancer pain. *Journal of Pain and Symptom Management*, 1995; **10**: 348–55.
108. Arner S, Meyerson BA. Lack of analgesic effect of opioids on neuropathic and idiopathic forms of pain. *Pain*, 1988; **33**: 11–23.
109. Portenoy RK, Foley KM, Inturrisi CE. The nature of opioid responsiveness and its implications for neuropathic pain: new hypotheses derived from studies of opioid infusions. *Pain*, 1990; **43**: 273–86.
110. Ettinger AB, Portenoy RK. The use of corticosteroids in the treatment of symptoms associated with cancer. *Journal of Pain and Symptom Management*, 1988; **3**: 99–103.
111. Watanabe S, Bruera E. Corticosteroids as adjuvant analgesics. *Journal of Pain and Symptom Management*, 1994; **9**: 442–5.
112. Needham PR, Daley AG, Lennard RF. Steroids in advanced cancer: survey of current practice. *British Medical Journal*, 1992; **305**: 999.

113. Farr WC. The use of corticosteroids for symptom management in terminally ill patients. *American Journal of Hospice Care*, 1990; **7**: 41–6.
114. Wilcox JC, Corr J, Shaw J, Richardson M, Calman KC. Prednisolone as an appetite stimulant in patients with cancer. *British Medical Journal*, 1984; **288**: 27.
115. Bruera E, Roca E, Cedaro L, Carraro S, Chacon R. Action of oral methylprednisolone in terminal cancer patients: a prospective randomized double-blind study. *Cancer Treatment Report*, 1985; **69**: 751–4.
116. Della Cuna GR, *et al.* Effect of methylprednisolone sodium succinate on quality of life in preterminal cancer patients. A placebo-controlled multicenter study. *European Journal of Clinical Oncology*, 1989; **25**: 1817–21.
117. Tannock I, *et al.* Treatment of metastatic prostatic cancer with low-dose prednisone: evaluation of pain and quality of life as pragmatic indices of response. *Journal of Clinical Oncology*, 1989; **7**: 590–7.
118. Popiela T, Lucchi R, Giongo F. Methylprednisolone as palliative therapy for female terminal cancer patients: the Methylprednisolone Female Preterminal Cancer Study Group. *European Journal of Cancer*, 1989; **25**: 1823–9.
119. Hanks GW, Trueman T, Twycross RG. Corticosteroids in terminal cancer. *Postgraduate Medical Journal*, 1983; **59**: 702–6.
120. Kozin F, Ryan LM, Carerra GF, Soin LS, Wortmann RL. The reflex sympathetic dystrophy syndrome (RSDS). III. Scintigraphic studies, further evidence for the therapeutic efficacy of systemic corticosteroids, and proposed diagnostic criteria. *American Journal of Medicine*, 1981; **70**: 23–9.
121. Schell HW. Adrenal corticosteroid therapy in far advanced cancer. *Geriatrics*, 1972; **27**: 131–41.
122. Moertel CG, *et al.* Corticosteroid therapy of preterminal gastrointestinal cancer. *Cancer*, 1974; **33**: 1607–9.
123. Greenberg HS, Kim J, Posner JB. Epidural spinal cord compression from metastatic tumor: results with a new treatment protocol. *Annals of Neurology*, 1980; **8**: 361–6.
124. Reid DB. Palliative management of bowel obstruction. *Medical Journal of Australia*, 1988; **148**: 54.
125. Fainsinger RL, Spanchynski K, Hanson J, Bruera E. Symptom control in terminally ill patients with malignant bowel obstruction. *Journal of Pain and Symptom Management*, 1994; **9**: 12.
126. Vecht Ch.J, Haaxma-Reiche H, van Putten WLJ, de Visser M, Vries EP, Twijnstra A. Initial bolus of conventional versus high-dose dexamethasone in metastatic spinal cord compression. *Neurology*, 1989; **39**: 1255–7.
127. Yamada K, *et al.* Effects of methylprednisolone on peritumoral brain edema. *Journal of Neurosurgery*, 1983; **59**: 612–19.
128. Posner JB, Howieson J, Cvitkovic E. 'Disappearing' spinal cord compression: oncolytic effects of glucocorticoids (and other chemotherapeutic agents) on epidural metastases. *Annals of Neurology*, 1977; **2**: 409–13.
129. Devor M, Govrin-Lippman R, Raber P. Corticosteroids reduce neuroma hyperexcitability. In: Fields HL, Dubner R, Cervero F, eds. *Advances in Pain Research and Therapy*, vol 9, Proceedings of the Fourth World Congress on Pain. New York: Raven Press, 1985: 451–5.
130. Haynes RC. Adrenocorticotrophic hormone: adrenocortical steroids and their synthetic analogs: inhibitors of the synthesis and actions of adrenocortical hormones. In: Gilman AG, Rall TW, Nies AS, Taylor P, eds. *The Pharmacological Basis of Therapeutics*, 8th edn. New York: Pergamon Press, 1990: 1431–62.
131. Weissman D, *et al.* Corticosteroid toxicity in neuro-oncology patients. *Journal of Neurooncology*, 1987; **5**: 125–8.
132. Sorensen PS, Helweg-Larsen S, Mouridsen H, Hansen HH. Effect of high-dose dexamethasone in carcinomatous metastatic spinal cord compression treated by radiotherapy: a randomized trial. *European Journal of Cancer*, 1994; **30A**: 22–7.
133. Breitbart W, Stiefel F, Kornblith AB, Pannulo S. Neuropsychiatric disturbance in cancer patients with epidural spinal cord compression receiving high dose corticosteroids: a prospective comparison study. *Psycho-oncology*, 1993; **2**: 233–45.
134. Messer J, Reitman D, Sacks HS, Smith H, Chalmers T. Association of adrenocorticosteroid therapy and peptic ulcer disease. *New England Journal of Medicine*, 1983; **309**: 21–4.
135. Piper JM, Ray WA, Daugherty JR, Griffin MR. Corticosteroid use and peptic ulcer disease—role of nonsteroidal anti-inflammatory drugs. *Annals of Internal Medicine*, 1991; **114**: 735–40.
136. Fadul CE, Lemann W, Thaler HT, Posner JB. Perforation of the gastrointestinal tract in patients receiving steroids for neurologic disease. *Neurology*, 1988; **38**: 348–52.
137. ReMine SG, McIlrath D. Bowel performation in steroid-treated patients. *Annals of Surgery*, 1980; **192**: 581–6.
138. Dixon RA, Christy NP. On the various forms of corticosteroid withdrawal syndrome. *American Journal of Medicine*, 1980; **68**: 224–30.
139. Eisenach JC, Dewan DM, Rose JC, Angelo JM. Epidural clonidine produces antinociception, but not hypotension in sheep. *Anesthesiology*, 1987; **66**: 496–501.
140. Yaksh TL, Reddy SVR. Studies in the primate on the analgesic effects associated with intrathecal actions of opiates, alpha adrenergic agonists and baclofen. *Anesthesiology*, 1981; **54**: 451–67.
141. Kayser V, Desmeules J, Guilbaud G. Systemic clonidine differentially modulates the abnormal reactions to mechanical and thermal stimuli in rats with peripheral mononeuropathy. *Pain*, 1995; **60**: 275–85.
142. Pertovaara A, Kauppila T, Tukeva T. The effect of medetomidine, an alpha-2 adrenoceptor agent in various pain tests. *European Journal of Pharmacology*, 1990; **179**: 323–8.
143. Puke MJC, Wiesenfeld-Hallin Z. the differential effects of morphine and the alpha 2 adrenoceptor agonists clonidine and dexmedetomidine on the prevention and treatment of experimental neuropathic pain. *Anesthesia and Analgesia*, 1993; **77**: 104–9.
144. Aho MS, Erkola OA, Scheinin H, Lehtinen AM, Korttila KT. Effect of intravenously administered dexmedetomidine on pain after laparoscopic tubal ligation. *Anesthesia and Analgesia*, 1991; **73**: 112–18.
145. Byas-Smith MG, Max MB, Muir H, Kingman A. Transdermal clonidine compared to placebo in painful diabetic neuropathy using a two-staged 'enriched enrollment' design. *Pain*, 1995; **60**: 267–74.
146. Eisenach JC, Du Pen S, Dubois M, Miguel R, Allin D, and the Epidural Clonidine Study Group. Epidural clonidine analgesia for intractable cancer pain. *Pain*, 1995; **61**: 391–400.
147. Carroll D, Jadad A, King L, Wiffen P, Glynn C, McQuay H. Single-dose, randomized, double-blind, double-dummy, cross-over comparison of extradural and i.v. clonidine in chronic pain. *British Journal of Anaesthesiology*, 1993; **7**: 665–9.
148. Max MB, Schafer SC, Culnane M, Dubner, R, Gracely, RH. Association of pain relief with drug side effects in postherpetic neuralgia: a single dose study of clonidine, codeine, ibuprofen and placebo. *Clinical Pharmacology and Therapeutics*, 1988; **43**: 363–71.
149. Tan Y-M, Croese J. Clonidine and diabetic patients with leg pains. *Annals of Internal Medicine*, 1986; **105**: 633.
150. Shafar J, Tallett ER, Knowlson PA. Evaluation of clonidine in prophylaxis of migraine. *Lancet*, 1972; **i**: 403–7.
151. Boisen E, *et al.* Clonidine in the prophylaxis of migraine. *Acta Neurologica Scandinavica*, 1978; **58**: 288–95.
152. Petros AJ, Wright RMB. Epidural and oral clonidine in domiciliary control of deafferentation pain. **Lancet**, 1987; **1**: 1034.
153. Zeigler D, Lynch SA, Muir J, Benjamin J, Max MB. Transdermal clonidine versus placebo in painful diabetic neuropathy. *Pain*, 1992; **48**: 403–8.
154. Glynn CJ, Teddy PJ, Jamous MA, Moore RA, Lloyd JW. Role of spinal noradrenergic system in transmission of pain in patients with spinal cord injury. *Lancet*, 1986; **2**: 1249–50.
155. Rauck RL, Eisenach JC, Jackson K, Young LD, Southern J. Epidural clonidine treatment for refractory reflex sympathetic dystrophy. *Anesthesiology*, 1993; **79**: 1163–9.
156. Coombs DW, Saunders R, Gaylor M, LaChance B, Jensen L. Clinical trial of intrathecal clonidine for cancer pain. *Regional Anesthesia*, 1984; **9**: 34–5.
157. Coombs DW, Saunders RL, LaChance D, Savage S, Ragnarsson TS, Jensen LE. Intrathecal morphine tolerance: use of intrathecal clonidine,

DADLE and intraventricular morphine. *Anesthesiology*, 1985; **62**: 357–63.

158. Coombs DW, Saunders RL, Fratkin JD, Jensen LE, Murphy CA. Continuous intrathecal hydromorphone and clonidine for intractable cancer pain. *Journal of Neurosurgery*, 1986; **64**: 890–4.
159. Yaksh TL. Pharmacology of spinal adrenergic systems which modulate spinal nociceptive processing. *Pharmacology, Biochemistry and Behavior*, 1985; **22**: 845–58.
160. Sagen J, Proudfit H. Evidence for pain modulation by pre- and post-synaptic noradrenergic receptors in the medulla oblongata. *Brain Research*, 1985; **331**: 285–93.
161. Yjritsy-Roy JA, Standish SM, Terry LC. Dopamine D-1 and D-2 receptor antagonists potentiate analgesic and motor effects of morphine. *Pharmacology, Biochemistry and Behavior*, 1989; **32**: 717–21.
162. Bloomfield S, Simard-Savoie S, Bernier J, Tetreault L. Comparative analgesic activity of levomepromazine and morphine in patients with chronic pain. *Canadian Medical Association Journal*, 1964; **90**: 1156–9.
163. Beaver WT, Wallenstein S, Houde RW, Rogers A. A comparison of the analgesic effects of methotrimeprazine and morphine in patients with cancer. *Clinical Pharmacology and Therapeutics*, 1966; **7**: 436–46.
164. Lasagna L, DeKornfeld TJ. Methotrimeprazine, a new phenothiazine derivative with analgesic properties. *Journal of the American Medical Association*, 1961; **178**: 887–90.
165. Hakkarainen H. Fluphenazine for tension headache: double-blind study. *Headache*, 1977; **17**: 216–8.
166. Lechin F, van der Dijs B, Lechin ME, *et al.* Pimozide therapy for trigeminal neuralgia. *Archives of Neurology*, 1989; **9**: 960–2.
167. Patt RB, Proper G, Reddy S. The neuroleptics as adjuvant analgesics. *Journal of Pain and Symptom Management*, 1994; **9**: 446–53.
168. Davidson O, Lindenberg O, Walsh M. Analgesic treatment with levomepromazine in acute myocardial infarction. *Acta Medica Scandinavica*, 1979; **205**: 191–4.
169. Montilla E, Frederick WS, Cass, LJ. Analgesic effects of methotrimeprazine and morphine. *Archives of Internal Medicine*, 1963; **111**: 725–8.
170. Houde RW and Wallenstein SL. Analgesic power of chlorpromazine alone and in combination with morphine. *Federation Proceedings*, 1966; **14**:353.
171. Keats AS, Telford J, Kurosu, Y. Potentiation of meperidine by promethazine. *Anesthesiology*, 1961; **22**: 31–41.
172. Judkins KC, Harmer M. Haloperidol as an adjuvant analgesic in the management of postoperative pain. *Anaesthesia*, 1982; **37**: 1118–20.
173. Davis JL, Lewis SB, Gerich JE, Kaplan RA, Schultz TA, Wallin JD. Peripheral diabetic neuropathy treated with amitriptyline and fluphenazine. *Journal of the American Medical Association*, 1977; **238**: 2291–2.
174. Margolis LH, Gianascol AJ. Chlorpromazine in thalamic pain syndrome. *Neurology*, 1956; **6**: 302–4.
175. Kocher R. Use of psychotropic drugs for the treatment of chronic severe pain. In: Bonica JJ, Albe-Fessard D, eds. *Advances in Pain Research and Therapy*, vol 1. Raven Press: New York, 1976: 579–82.
176. Farber GA, Burks JW. Chlorprothixene therapy for herpes zoster neuralgia. *Southern Medical Journal*, 1974; **67**: 808–12.
177. Nathan PW. Chlorprothixene (Taractan) in postherpetic neuralgia and other severe pains. *Pain*, 1978; **5**: 367–71.
178. Raft D, Toomey T, Gregg JM. Behavior modification and haloperidol in chronic facial pain. *Southern Medical Journal*, 1979; **72**: 155–9.
179. Schubert DSP, Patterson MB, Long C. Phenothiazine analgesics in a patient with psychotic symptoms. *Psychosomatics*, 1983; **24**: 599–600.
180. Daw JL, Cohen-Cole SA. Haloperidol analgesia. *Southern Medical Journal*, 1981;**74**: 364–5.
181. Polliack J. Chronic recurrent headaches. *South African Medical Journal*, 1979; **56**: 980.
182. Merskey H, Hester RA. The treatment of chronic pain with psychotropic drugs. *Postgraduate Medical Journal*, 1976; **48**: 594–8.
183. Cavenar JO, Maltbie AA. Another indication for haloperidol. *Psychosomatics*, 1976; **17**: 128–30.
184. Weis O, Sriwatanakul K, Weintraub M. Treatment of postherpetic neuralgia and acute herpetic pain with amitriptyline and perphenazine. *South African Medical Journal*, 1982; **62**: 274–5.
185. Taub A. Relief of postherpetic neuralgia with psychotropic drugs. *Journal of Neurosurgery*, 1973; **39**: 235–9.
186. Hanks GW, Thomas PJ, Trueman T, Weeks E. The myth of haloperidol potentiation. *Lancet*, 1983; **2**: 523–4.
187. Yaksh TL, Malmberg AB. Central pharmacology of nociceptive transmission. In: Wall PD, Melzack R, eds. *Textbook of Pain*, 3rd edn. Edinburgh: Churchill Livingstone, 1994: 165–200.
188. Bodnar RJ, Nicotera N. Neuroleptic and analgesic interactions upon pain and activity measures. *Pharmacology, Biochemistry and Behavior*, 1982; **16**: 411–6.
189. Rosenblatt WH, Cioffi AM, Sinatra R, Saberski LR, Silverman DG. Metoclopramide: an analgesic adjunct to patient-controlled analgesia. *Anesthesiology and Analgesia*, 1991; **73**: 553–5.
190. Kandler D, Lisander B. Analgesic action of metoclopramide in prosthetic hip surgery. *Acta Anaesthesiologica Scandinavica*, 1993; **37**: 49–53.
191. Moss HE, Sanger GJ. The effects of granisetron, ICS 205–930 and ondansetron on the visceral pain reflex induced by duodenal distension. *British Journal of Pharmacology*, 1990; **100**: 497–501.
192. Caroff S. The neuroleptic malignant syndrome. *Journal of Clinical Psychiatry*, 1980; **41**: 79–83.
193. Storey P, Hill HH, St. Louis R, Tarver EE. Subcutaneous infusions for control of cancer symptoms. *Journal of Pain and Symptom Management*, 1990; **5**: 33–41.
194. Cherny NI, Thaler HT, Friedlander-Klar H, *et al.* Opioid responsiveness of cancer pain syndromes caused by neuropathic or nociceptive mechanisms. *Neurology*, 1994; **44**: 857–61.
195. Mercadante S, Maddaloni S, Roccella S, Salvaggio L. Predictive factors in advanced cancer pain treated only by analgesics. *Pain*, 1992; **50**: 151–5.
196. McQuay HJ, Jadad AR, Carroll D, *et al.* Opioid sensitivity of chronic pain: a patient-controlled analgesia method. *Anaesthesia*, 1992; **47**: 757–67.
197. Jadad AR, Carroll D, Glynn CJ, Moore RA, McQuay HJ. Morphine responsiveness of chronic pain: double-blind randomised crossover study with patient-controlled analgesia. *Lancet*, 1992; **339**: 1367–71.
198. Glazer S, Portenoy RK. Systemic local anesthetics in pain control. *Journal of Pain and Symptom Management*, 1991; 6: 30–9.
199. Backonja M. Local anesthetics as adjuvant analgesics. *Journal of Pain and Symptom Management*, 1994; **9**: 491–9.
200. Barbour CM, Tovell RM. Experiences with procaine administered intravenously. *Annals of Internal Medicine*, 1948; **10**: 514–23.
201. Graubaud DJ, Peterson MC. The therapeutic uses of intravenous procaine. *Annals of Internal Medicine*, 1949; **10**: 175–87.
202. Gordon RA. Intravenous novocaine for analgesia in burns. *Canadian Medical Association Journal*, 1943; **49**: 478–81.
203. Gordon RA. Intravenous procaine: clinical applications. *Canadian Medical Association Journal*, 1948; **59**: 534–5.
204. McLachlin JA. The intravenous use of novocaine as a substitute for morphine in postoperative care. *Canadian Medical Association Journal*, 1945; **52**: 383–6.
205. Gilbert CRA, Hanson IR, Brown AB, Hingson RA. Intravenous use of xylocaine. *Current Research in Anesthesia and Analgesia*, 1951; **30**: 301–13.
206. Cassuto J, Wallin G, Hogstrom S, Faxen A, Rimback G. Inhibition of postoperative pain by continuous low dose infusion of lidocaine. *Anesthesia and Analgesia*, 1985; **64**: 971–4.
207. Birch K, Jorgensen B, Chraemer-Jorgensen B, Kehlet H. Effect of i.v. lignocaine on pain and the endocrine metabolic responses after surgery. *British Journal of Anaesthesia*, 1987; **59**: 721–4.
208. Bartlett EE, Hutaserani O. Xylocaine for the relief of postoperative pain. *Anesthesia and Analgesia*, 1961; **40**: 296–304.
209. Keats AS, D'Allessandro GL. A controlled study of pain relief by intravenous procaine. *Journal of the American Medical Association*, 1951; **147**: 1761–3.
210. Edwards WT, Habib F, Burney RG, Begin G. Intravenous lidocaine in the management of various chronic pain states. *Regional Anesthesia*, 1985; **10**: 1–6.
211. Galer BS, Miller KV, Rowbotham MC. Response to intravenous lidocaine

infusion differs based on clinical diagnosis and site of nervous system injury. *Neurology*, 1993; **43**: 1233–5.

212. Petersen P, Kastrup J, Zeeburg I, Boysen G. Chronic pain treatment with intravenous lidocaine. *Neurology Research*, 1986; **8**: 189–90.
213. Petersen P, Kastrup J. Dercum's disease (adiposa dolorosa): treatment of severe pain with intravenous lidocaine. *Pain*, 1987; **28**: 77–80.
214. Juhlin L. Long-standing pain relief of adiposa dolorosa (Dercum's disease) after intravenous infusion of lidocaine. *Journal of the American Academy of Dermatology*, 1986; **15**: 383–4.
215. Atkinson RL. Intravenous lidocaine for the treatment of intractable pain of adiposis dolorosa. *International Journal of Obstetrics*, 1982; **6**: 351–7.
216. Iwane T, Masanori M, Matsuki M, Ito Y, Shimoji K. Management of intractable pain in adiposis dolorosa with intravenous administration of lidocaine. *Anesthesia and Analagesia*, 1976; **55**: 257–9.
217. Graubard DJ, Kovacs J, Ritter HH. The management of destructive arthritis of the hip by means of intravenous procaine. *Annals of Internal Medicine*, 1948; **28**: 1106–16.
218. Marton R, Spitzer N, Steinbrocker O. Intravenous procaine as an analgesic and therapeutic procedure in painful, chronic neuromusculoskeletal disorders. *Annals of Internal Medicine*, 1949; **10**: 629–33.
219. Rosner S. A simple method of treatment for acute headache. *Headache*, 1984; **24**: 50.
220. Arner S, Lindblom U, Meyerson BA, Molnar C. Prolonged relief of neuralgia after regional anesthestic blocks: a call for further experimental and systemic clinical studies. *Pain*, 1990; **43**: 287–97.
221. Boas RA, Covino BG, Shahnarian A. Analgesic responses to IV lignocaine. *British Journal Anaesthesia*, 1982; **54**: 501–5.
222. Maciewicz R, Chung RY, Strassman A, Hochberg F, Moskowitz M. Relief of vascular headache with intravenous lidocaine: clinical observations and a proposed mechanism. *Clinical Journal of Pain*, 1988; **4**: 11–16.
223. Backonja M, Gombar K. Response of central pain syndromes to intravenous lidocaine. *Journal of Pain and Symptom Management*, 1992, **7**: 172–8.
224. Rowbotham MC, Reisner-Keller LA, Fields HL. Both intravenous lidocaine and morphine reduce the pain of postherpetic neuralgia. *Neurology*, 1991; **41**: 1024–8.
225. Kastrup J, Petersen P, Dejgard A, Angelo HR, Hilsted J. Intravenous lidocaine infusion—a new treatment for chronic painful diabetic neuropathy. *Pain*, 1987; **28**: 69–75.
226. Bruera E, Ripamonti C, Brenneis C, MacMillan K, Hanson J. A randomized double-blind crossover trial of intravenous lidocaine in the treatment of neuropathic cancer pain. *Journal of Pain and Symptom Management*, 1992; **7**: 138–40.
227. Elleman K, Sjogren P, Banning A, Jensen TS, Smith T, Geertsen P. Trial of intravenous lidocaine on painful neuropathy in cancer patients. *Clinical Journal of Pain*, 1989; **5**: 291–4.
228. Brose WG, Cousins MJ. Subcutaneous lidocaine for treatment of neuropathic cancer pain. *Pain*, 1991; **45**: 145–8.
229. Dunlop R, Davies RJ, Hockley J, Turner P. Letter to the Editor. *Lancet*, 1989; i; 420–1.
230. Lindstrom P, Lindblom U. The analgesic effect of tocainide in trigeminal neuralgia. *Pain*, 1987; **28**: 45–50.
231. Dejgard A, Petersen P, Kastrup J. Mexiletine for treatment of chronic painful diabetic neuropathy. *Lancet*, 1988; **i**: 9–11.
232. Covino BG. Local anesthetics. In: Ferrante FM, VadeBoncouer TR, eds. *Postoperative Pain Management*. New York: Churchill Livingstone, 1993: 211–53.
233. deJong RH, Nace R. Nerve impulse conduction during intravenous lidocaine injection. *Anesthesiology*, 1968; **29**: 22–8.
234. Woolf CJ, Wiesenfeld-Halli Z. The systemic administration of local anesthetic produces a selective depression of C-afferent evoked activity in the spinal cord. *Pain*, 1985; **23**: 361–74.
235. Chabal C, Russell LC, Burchiel KJ. The effect of intravenous lidocaine, tocainide and mexiletine on spontaneously active fibers originating in rat sciatic neuromas. *Pain*, 1989; **38**: 333–8.
236. Devor M, Wall PD, Catalan N. Systemic lidocaine silences ectopic neuroma and DRG discharge without blocking nerve conduction. *Pain*, 1992; **48**: 261–8.
237. Liu PL, Feldman HS, Giasi R, *et al.* Comparative CNS toxicity of lidocaine, etidocaine, bupivacaine, and tetracaine in awake dogs following rapid intravenous administration. *Anesthesia and Analgesia*, 1983; **62**: 375.
238. CAST (Cardiac Arrhythmia Suppression Trial) Investigators: Preliminary report: effect of encainide and flecainide on mortality in a randomized trial of arrhythmia suppression after acute myocardial infarction. *New England Journal of Medicine*, 1989; **321**: 406–12.
239. Kreeger W, Hammill SC. New antiarrhythmic drugs: tocainide, mexiletine, flecainide, encainide and amiodarone. *Mayo Clinic Proceedings*, 1987; **62**: 1033–50.
240. Horn HR, Hadidian Z, Johnson JL, Vasallo HG, Williams JH, Young MD. Safety evaluation of tocainide in an American emergency use program. *American Heart Journal*, 1980; **100**: 1037–40.
241. Vincent FM, Vincent T. Tocainide encephalopathy. *Neurology*, 1985; **35**: 1804–5.
242. Stein MG, Demarco T, Gamsu G, Finkbeiner W, Golden J. Computed tomography: pathologic correlates in lung disease due to tocainide. *American Review of Respiratory Diseases*, 1988; **137**: 458–60.
243. Campbell RWF. Mexiletine. *New England Journal of Medicine*, 1987; **316**: 29–34.
244. Swerdlow M. Anticonvulsant drugs and chronic pain. *Clinical Neuropharmacology*, 1984; **7**: 51–82.
245. Blom S. Tic douloureaux treated with new anticonvulsant. *Archives of Neurology*, 1963; **9**: 285–90.
246. Spillane JD. The treatment of trigeminal neuralgia. *Practitioner*, 1964; **192**: 71–7.
247. Lloyd-Smith DL, Sachdev KK. A long-term, low dosage study of carbamazepine in trigeminal neuralgia. *Headache*, 1969; **9**: 64–72.
248. Taylor JC, Brauer S, Espir MLE. Long-term treatment of trigeminal neuralgia with carbamazepine. *Postgraduate Medical Journal*, 1980; **57**: 16–18.
249. Tomson T, Bertilsson L. Potent therapeutic effects of carbamazepine-10,11-epoxide in trigeminal neuralgia. *Archives of Neurology*, 1984; **41**: 598–601.
250. Chakrabarti AK, Samantaray SK. Diabetic peripheral neuropathy. Nerve conduction studies before, during and after carbamazepine therapy. *Australia/New Zealand Journal of Medicine*, 1976; **6**: 565–8.
251. Hatangdi VS, Boas RA, Richards EG. Postherpetic neuralgia: management with antiepileptic and tricyclic drugs. In: Bonica JJ, Albe-Fessard D, eds. *Advances in Pain Research and Therapy*, vol 1. New York: Raven Press, 1976: 583–7.
252. Gerson GR, Jones RB, Luscombe DK. Studies on the concomitant use of carbamazepine and clomipramine for the relief of postherpetic neuralgia. *Postgraduate Medical Journal*, 1977; **53**: 104–9.
253. Taylor PH, Gray K, Bicknell RG, Rees JR. Glossopharyngeal neuralgia with syncope. *Journal of Laryngology and Otology*, 1977; **91**: 859–68.
254. Raskin NH, Levinson SA, Hoffman PM, Pickett JBE, Fields HL. Postsympathectomy neuralgia: amelioration with diphenylhydantoin and carbamazepine. *American Journal of Surgery*, 1974; **128**: 75–8.
255. Swerdlow M, Cundill JG. Anticonvulsant drugs used in the treatment of lancinating pains. A comparison. *Anesthesia*, 1981; **36**: 1129–32.
256. Ekbom K. Carbamazepine in the treatment of tabetic lightning pains. *Archives of Neurology*, 1972; **26**: 374–8.
257. Elliot F, Little A, Milbrandt W. Carbamazepine for phantom limb phenomena. *New England Journal of Medicine*, 1976; **295**: 678.
258. Espir MLE, Millac P. Treatment of paroxysmal disorders in multiple sclerosis with carbamazepine (Tegretol). *Journal of Neurology, Neurosurgery and Psychiatry*, 1970; **33**: 528–31.
259. Mullan S. Surgical management of pain in cancer of the head and neck. *Surgical Clinics of North America*, 1973; **53**: 203–10.
260. Dunsker SB, Mayfield FH. Carbamazepine in the treatment of flashing pain syndrome. *Journal of Neurosurgery*, 1976; **45**: 49–51.

261. Martin G. Recurrent pain of a pseudotabetic variety after laminectomy for a lumbar disc lesion. *Journal of Neurology, Neurosurgery and Psychiatry*, 1980; **43**: 283–4.
262. Campbell FG, Graham JG, Zilkha KJ. Clinical trial of carbamazepine (Tegretol) in trigeminal neuralgia. *Journal of Neurology, Neurosurgery and Psychiatry*, 1966; **29**: 265–7.
263. Rockliff BW, Davis EH. Controlled sequential trials of carbamazepine in trigeminal neuralgia. *Archives of Neurology*, 1966; **15**: 129–36.
264. Killian JM, Fromm GH. Carbamazepine in the treatment of neuralgia. Use and side effects. *Archives of Neurology*, 1968; **19**: 129–36.
265. Nicol CF. A four year double-blind study of carbamazepine in facial pain. *Headache*, 1969; **9**: 54–7.
266. Rull JA, *et al.* Symptomatic treatment of peripheral diabetic neuropathy with carbamazepine (Tegretol): double-blind cross-over trial. *Diabetologia*, 1969; **5**: 215–8.
267. Lockman LA, Hunninghake DB, Drivit W, Desnick RJ. Relief of pain of Fabry's disease by diphenylhydantoin. *Neurology* (Minneap), 1973; **23**: 871–5.
268. Chadda VS, Mathur MS. Double-blind study of the effects of diphenylhydantoin sodium in diabetic neuropathy. *Journal of the Association of Physicians of India*, 1978; **26**: 403–6.
269. Green JB. Dilantin in the treatment of lightning pains. *Neurology* (Minneap), 1961; **11**: 257–8.
270. Cantor FK. Phenytoin treatment of thalamic pain. *British Medical Journal*, 1972; **2**: 590.
271. Ianmore A, Baker AR, Morrell F. Dilantin in the treatment of trigeminal neuralgia. *Neurology*, 1958; **8**: 126–8.
272. Braham J, Saia A. Phenytoin in the treatment of trigeminal and other neuralgias. *Lancet*, 1960; **ii**: 892–3.
273. Ellenberg M. Treatment of diabetic neuropathy with diphenylhydantoin. *New York State Journal of Medicine*, 1968; **68**: 2633–55.
274. Mladinich EK. Diphenylhydantoin in the Wallenberg Syndrome. *Journal of the American Medical Association*, 1974; **230**: 372–3.
275. Hallag IY, Harris JD. The syndrome of postherpetic neuralgia: complications and an approach to therapy. *Journal of the American Osteopathic Association*, 1968; **681**: 1265–8.
276. Caccia MR. Clonazepam in facial neuralgia and cluster headache: clinical and electrophysiological study. *European Neurology*, 1975; **13**: 560–3.
277. Martin G. The management of pain following laminectomy for lumbar disc lesions. *Annals of the Royal College of Surgeons of England*, 1981; **63**: 244–52.
278. Peiris JB, Perera GLS, Devendra SV, Lionel NDW. Sodium valproate in trigeminal neuralgia. *Medical Journal of Australia*, 1980; **2**: 278.
279. Raftery H. The management of postherpetic pain using sodium valproate and amitriptyline. *Journal of the Irish Medical Association*, 1979; **72**: 399–401.
280. Mellick GA, Mellick LB. Gabapentin in the management of reflex sympathetic dystrophy. *Journal of Pain and Symptom Management*, 1995; **10**: 265–6.
281. Nakamura-Craig M, Follenfant RL. Lamotrigine and analogs: a new treatment for chronic pain? In: Gebhardt GF, Hammond DL, Jensen TS, eds. *Progress in Pain Research and Management*, vol 2. Seattle:IASP Press, 1994: 725–30.
282. Mellick GA. Hemifacial spasm: successful treatment with felbamate. *Journal of Pain and Symptom Management*, 1995; **10**: 392–5.
283. Weinberger J, Nicklas WJ, Berl, S. Mechanism of action of anticonvulsants. *Neurology* (Minneap), 1976; **26**: 162–73.
284. Devor M. The pathophysiology of damaged peripheral nerves. In: Wall PD, Melzack R, eds. *Textbook of Pain*. Edinburgh: Churchill Livingstone, 1994: 79–100.
285. Albe-Fessard D, Lombard MC. Use of an animal model to evaluate the origin of deafferentation pain and protection against it. In: Bonica JJ, Lindblom U, Iggo A, eds. *Advances in Pain Research and Therapy*, vol 5. New York: Raven Press, 1982: 691–700.
286. Guilbaud G, Benoist JM, Levante A, Gautron M, Willer JC. Primary somatosensory cortex in rats with pain-related behaviours due to a peripheral mononeuropathy after moderate ligation of one sciatic nerve: neuronal responsivity to somatic stimulation. *Experimental Brain Research*, 1992; **92**: 227–45.
287. Lenz FA, Kwan HC, Dostrovsky JO, Tasker RR. Caracteristics of the bursting pattern of action potentials that occurs in the thalamus of patients with central pain. *Brain Research*, 1989; **496**: 357–60.
288. Nystrom B, Hagbarth KE. Microelectrode recordings from transected nerves in amputees in phantom limb pain. *Neuroscience Letters*, 1981; **27**: 211–16.
289. Loeser JD, Ward AA, White LE. Chronic deafferentation of human spinal cord neurons. *Journal of Neurosurgery*, 1968; **29**: 48–50.
290. Hart RG, Easton JD. Carbamazepine and hematological monitoring. *Annals of Neurology*, 1982; **11**: 309–16.
291. Flegel KM, Cole CH. Inappropriate antidiuresis during carbamazepine treatment. *Annals of Internal Medicine*, 1977; **87**: 722–3.
292. Terrence CF, Fromm GH. Congestive heart failure during carbamazepine therapy. *Annals of Neurology*, 1980; **8**: 200–1.
293. Ramsey RE, Wilder BJ, Berger JR, Bruni J. A double-blind study comparing carbamazepine and phenytoin as initial seizure therapy in adults. *Neurology*, 1983; **33**: 904–10.
294. Troupin A and Ojemann LM. Paradoxical intoxication: a complication of anticonvulsant administration. *Epilepsia*, 1975; **16**: 753–8.
295. Ghatak NR, Santoso RA, McKinney WM. Cerebellar degeneration following long-term phenytoin therapy. *Neurology*, 1976; **26**: 818–24.
296. Egger J, Brett EM. Effects of sodium valproate in 100 children with special reference to weight. *British Medical Journal*, 1981; **283**: 577–81.
297. Schmidt D. Adverse effects of valproate. *Epilepsia*, 1984; **25**: 44S–9.
298. Goa KL, Sorkin EM. Gabapentin: a review of its pharmacological properties and clinical potential in epilepsy. *Drugs*, 1993; **46**: 409–27.
299. Fraught E. Sacdeo RC, Remler MP, *et al.* Felbamate monotherapy for partial-onset seizures: an active control trial. *Neurology*, 1993; **43**: 688–92.
300. Matsuo F, Bergen D, Faught E, *et al.* Placebo-controlled study of the efficacy and safety of lamotrigine in patients with partial seizures. *Neurology*, 1993; **43**: 2284–91.
301. Messenheimer J, Ramsay RE, Willmore LJ, *et al.* Lamotrigine therapy for partial seizures: a multicenter, placebo-controlled, double-blind, cross-over trial. *Epilepsia*, 1994; **35**: 113–21.
302. Fromm GH, Terrence CF, Chattha AS. Baclofen in the treatment of trigeminal neuralgia: double-blind study and long-term follow-up. *Annals of Neurology*, 1984; **15**: 240–4.
303. Fromm GH. Baclofen as an adjuvant analgesic. *Journal of Pain and Symptom Management*, 1994; **9**: 500–9.
304. Ringel RA, Roy EP. Glossopharyngeal neuralgia: successful treatment with baclofen. *Annals of Neurology*, 1987; **21**: 14–15.
305. Fromm GH, Graff-Radford SB, Terrence CF, Sweet WH. Pretrigeminal neuralgia. *Neurology*, 1990; **40**: 1493–5.
306. Terrence CF, Fromm GH, Tenicela R. Baclofen as an analgesic in chronic peripheral nerve disease. *European Neurology*, 1985; **24**: 380–5.
307. Corli O, Roma G, Bacchini M, *et al.* Double-blind placebo-controlled trial of baclofen, alone and in combination, in patients undergoing voluntary abortion. *Clinical Therapeutics*, 1984; **6**: 800–7.
308. Kofler M and Leis AA. Prolonged seizure activity after baclofen withdrawal. *Neurology*, 1992; **42**: 697.
309. Mao J, Price DD, Mayer DJ. Experimental mononeuropathy reduces the antinociceptive effects of morphine: implications for common intracellular mechanisms involved in morphine tolerance and neuropathic pain. *Pain*, 1995; **61**: 353–4.
310. Woolf CJ, Thompson SWN. The induction and maintenance of central sensitization is dependent on N-methyl-D-aspartic acid receptor activation: implications for the treatment of post-injury pain hypersensitivity states. *Pain*, 1991; **44**: 293–9.
311. Dickenson AH, Sullivan AF. Evidence for a role of the NMDA receptor in the frequency dependent potentiation of deep dorsal horn nociceptive neurons following C fibre stimulation. *Neuropharmacology*, 1987; **26**: 1235–8.
312. Jahangir SM, Islam F, Aziz L. Ketamine infusion for postoperative

analgesia in asthmatics: a comparison with intermittent meperidine. *Anesthesia and Analgesia*, 1993; **76**: 45–9.

313. Mathisen LC, Skjelbred P, Skoglund LA, Oye I. Effect of ketamine, an NMDA receptor inhibitor, in acute and chronic orofacial pain. *Pain*, 1995; **61**: 215–20.
314. Cherry DA, Plummer JL, Gourlay GK, Coates KR, Odgers CL. Ketamine as an adjunct to morphine in the treatment of pain. *Pain*, 1995; **62**: 119–21.
315. Persson J, Axelsson G, Hallin RG, Gustafsson LL. Beneficial effects of ketamine in a chronic pain state with allodynia, possibly due to central sensitization. *Pain*, 1995; **60**: 217–22.
316. Stannard CF, Porter GE. Ketamine hydrochloride in the treatment of phantom limb pain. *Pain*, 1993; **54**: 227–30.
317. Price DD, Mao J, Frenk H, Mayer DJ. The N-methyl-D-aspartate antagonist dextromethorphan selectively reduces temporal summation of second pain in man. *Pain*, 1994; **59**: 165–74.
318. Park KM, Max MB, Robinovitz E, Gracely RH, Bennett GJ. Effects of intravenous ketamine and alfentanil on hyperalgesia induced by intradermal capsaicin. In: Gebhardt GF, Hammond DL, Jensen TS, eds. *Proceedings of the 7th World Congress on Pain*. Seattle: IASP Press, 1994: 647–55.
319. McQuay HJ, Carrol D, Jadad AR, Glynn CJ, Jack T, Moore RA, Wiffen PJ. Dextromethorphan for the treatment of neuropathic pain: a double-blind, randomised controlled crossover trial with integral n-of-1 design. *Pain*, 1994; **59**: 127–34.
320. Backonja M, Arndt G, Gombar KA, Check B, Zimmerman M. Response of chronic neuropathic pain syndromes to ketamine: a preliminary study. *Pain*, 1994; **56**: 51–7.
321. Eide PK, Jorum E, Stubhaug A, Bremnes J, Breivik H. Relief of post-herpetic neuralgia with the N-methyl-D-aspartic receptor antagonist ketamine: a double-blind, cross-over comparison with morphine and placebo. *Pain*, 1994; **58**: 347–54.
322. Oshima E, Tei K, Kayazawa H, Urabe N. Continuous subcutaneous injection of ketamine for cancer pain. *Canadian Journal of Anaesthesia*, 1990; **37**: 385–92.
323. Gobelet C, Waldburger M, and Meier JL. The effect of adding calcitonin to physical treatment on reflex sympathetic dystrophy. *Pain*, 1992; **48**: 171–5.
324. Jaeger H, Maier C. Calcitonin in phantom limb pain: a double blind study. *Pain*, 1992; **48**: 21–7.
325. Backonja M. Reflex sympathetic dystrophy/sympathetically-maintained pain/causalgia: the syndrome of neuropathic pain with dysautonomia. *Seminars in Neurology*, 1994; **14**: 263–71.
326. Raja SN, Treede RD, Davis KD, Campbell JN. Systemic alpha-adrenergic blockade with phentolamine: a diagnostic test for sympathetically-maintained pain. *Anesthesiology*, 1991; **74**: 691–8.
327. Ghostine SY, Comair YG, Turner DM, Kassell NF, Azar CG. Phenoxybenzamine in the treatment of causalgia. *Journal of Neurosurgery*, 1984; **60**: 1263–8.
328. Abram SE, Lightfoot RW. Treatment of longstanding causalgia with prazosin. *Regional Anesthesia*, 1981; **6**: 79–81.
329. Tabira T, Shibasaki H, Kuroiwa Y. Reflex sympathetic dystrophy (causalgia) treatment with guanethidine. *Archives of Neurology*, 1983; **40**: 430–2.
330. Simson G. Propranolol for causalgia and Sudek's atrophy. *Journal of the American Medical Association*, 1974; **227**: 327.
331. Meyers FH and Meyers FJ. Patients with neuropathic pain regularly benefit from treatment with propranolol. *American Journal of Pain Management*, 1992; **2**: 89–92.
332. Scadding JW. Clinical trial of propranolol in post-traumatic neuralgia. *Pain*, 1982; **14**: 283–92.
333. Prough DS, *et al.* Efficacy of oral nifedipine in the treatment of reflex sympathetic dystrophy. *Anesthesiology*, 1985; **62**: 796–9.
334. Contreras E, Tamayo L, Amigo M. Calcium channel antagonists increase morphine-induced analgesia and antagonize morphine tolerance. *European Journal of Pharmacology*, 1988; **148**: 463–6.
335. Lux E, Welch SP, Brase DA, Dewey WL. Interaction of morphine with intrathecally administered calcium and calcium antagonists: evidence for supraspinal endogenous opioid mediation of intrathecal calcium-induced antinociception in mice. *Journal of Pharmacology and Experimental Therapeutics*, 1988; **246**: 500–7.
336. Miranda HF, Bustamante D, Kramer V, *et al.* Antinociceptive effects of Ca2+ channel blockers. *European Journal of Pharmacology*, 1992; **217**: 137–41.
337. Del Pozo, E, Ruiz-Garcia C, Baeyens JM. Analgesic effects of diltiazem and verapamil after central and peripheral administration in the hot-plate test. *General Pharmacology*, 1990; **21**: 681–5.
338. Santillan R, Maestre JM, Hurle MA, Florez J. Enhancement of opiate analgesia by nimodipine in cancer patients chronically treated with morphine: a preliminary report. *Pain*, 1994; **58**: 129–32.
339. Rowbotham MC. Topical analgesic agents. In: Fields HL, Liebeskind JC (eds). *Pharmacological Approaches to the Treatment of Chronic Pain: New Concepts and Critical Issues.* Seattle: IASP Press, 1994: 211–29.
340. Mashimo T, Tomi K, Pak M, Demizu A, Yyoshiya I. Relief of causalgia with prostaglandin E_1 ointment. *Anesthesia and Analgesia*, 1991; **72**: 700–1.
341. Bernstein JE, Bickers RR, Dahl MV, Roshal JY. Treatment of chronic postherpetic neuralgia with topical capsaicin. A prelminary study. *Journal of the American Academy of Dermatology*, 1987; **17**: 93–6.
342. Watson CPN, Evans RJ, Watt VR. Postherpetic neuralgia and topical capsaicin. *Pain*, 1988; **33**: 333–40.
343. Watson CPN, Evans RJ, Watt VR. The post-mastectomy pain syndrome and the effect of topical capsaicin. *Pain*, 1989; **38**: 177–86.
344. Watson CPN, Tyler KL, Bickers DR, Millikan LE, Smith S, Coleman E. A randomized vehicle-controlled trial of topical capsaicin in the treatment of postherpetic neuralgia. *Clinical Therapeutics*, 1993; **15**: 510–26.
345. Tandan R, Lewis GA, Krusinski PB, Badger GB, Fries TJ. Topical capsaicin in painful diabetic neuropathy. Controlled study with long-term follow-up. *Diabetes Care*, 1992; **15**: 8–14.
346. Capsaicin Study Group. Treatment of painful diabetic neuropathy with topical capsaicin. A multicenter, double-blind, vehicle-controlled study. *Archives of Internal Medicine* 1991; **151**: 2225–9.
347. Watson CPN, Evans RJ. The postmastectomy pain syndrome and topical capsaicin: a randomized trial. *Pain*, 1992; **51**: 375–9.
348. Fusco BM, Alessandri M. Analgesic effect of capsaicin in idiopathic trigeminal neuralgia. *Anesthesia and Analgesia*, 1992; **74**: 375–7.
349. McCarthy GM, McCarty DJ. Effect of topical capsaicin in the therapy of painful osteoarthritis of the hands. *Journal of Rheumatology*, 1992;**19**: 604–7.
350. Zhang WY, Li Wan Po A. The effectiveness of topically applied capsaicin: a meta-analysis. *European Journal of Clinical Pharmacology*, 1994; **46**: 517–22.
351. Dubner R. Topical capsaicin therapy for neuropathic pain. *Pain*, 1991; **47**: 247–8.
352. DeBenedittis G, Besana F, Lorenzettit A. A new topical treatment for acute herpetic neuralgia and postherpetic neuralgia: the aspirin/diethyl ether mixture. An open-label study plus a double-blind controlled clinical trial. *Pain*, 1992; **48**: 383–90.
353. McQuay HJ, Carroll D, Moxon A, Glynn CJ, Moore RA. Benzydamine cream for the treatment of postherpetic neuralgia: minimum duration of treatment periods in a cross-over trial. *Pain*, 1990; **40**: 131–5.
354. Stow PJ, Glynn CJ, Minor B. EMLA cream in the treatment of post herpetic neuralgia: efficacy and pharmacokinetic profile. *Pain*, 1989; **39**: 301–5.
355. Rowbotham MC, Fields HL. Topical lidocaine reduces pain in post-herpetic neuralgia. *Pain*, 1989; **38**: 297–302.
356. Rowbotham MC, Davies PS, Fields HL. Topical lidocaine gel relieves postherpetic neuralgia. *Annals of Neurology*, 1995; **37**: 246–53.
357. Frayling IM, Addison GM, Chattergee K, Meakin G. Methaemoglobinaemia in children treated with prilocaine-lignocaine cream. *British Medical Journal*, 1990; **301**: 153–4.
358. Schott GD, Loh L. Anticholinesterase drugs in the treatment of chronic pain. *Pain*, 1984; **20**: 201–6.

359. Hampf G, Bowsher D, Nurmikko T. Distigmine and amitriptyline in the treatment of chronic pain. *Anesthesia Progress*, 1989; **36**: 58–62.
360. Weinstock M, Davidson JT, Rosin AJ, Schnieden H. Effect of physostigmine on morphine-induced postoperative pain and somnolence. *British Journal of Anaesthesia*, 1982; **54**: 429–34.
361. Rossano C, De Lucat LF, Firetto V, *et al.* Vinca alkaloids administered by iontophoresis in postherpetic pain: preliminary report. *The Pain Clinic*, 1989; **3**: 31–6.
362. Dellemijn PLI, Fields HL. Do benzodiazepines have a role in chronic pain management. *Pain*, 1994; **57**: 137–52.
363. Reddy S, Patt RB. The benzodiazepines as adjuvant analgesics. *Journal of Pain and Symptom Management*, 1994; **9**: 510–4.
364. Singh PN, Sharma P, Gupta PK, Pandey K. Clinical evaluation of diazepam for relief of postoperative pain. *British Journal of Anaesthesia*, 1981; **53**: 831–6.
365. Miller R, *et al.* Midazolam as an adjunct to meperidine analgesia for postoperative pain. *Clinical Journal of Pain*, 1986; **2**: 37–43.
366. Max MB, Schafer SC, Culnane M, Scholler B, Dubner R, Gracely RH. Amitriptyline, but not lorazepam, relieves postherpetic neuralgia. *Neurology*, 1988; **38**: 1427–32.
367. Yosselson-Superstine S, Lipman AG, Sanders SH. Adjunctive antianxiety agents in the management of chronic pain. *Israel Journal of Medical Science*, 1985; **21**: 113–17.
368. Coda BA, Mackie A, Hill HF. Influence of alprazolam on opioid analgesia and side effects during steady-state morphine infusions. *Pain*, 1992; **50**: 309–16.
369. Yang JC, *et al.* Analgesic action and pharmacokinetics of morphine and diazepam in man: an evaluation by sensory decision theory. *Anesthesiology*, 1979; **51**: 495–502.
370. Payne R. Pharmacologic management of bone pain in the cancer patient. *Clinical Journal of Pain*, 1989; **5**: S43–50.
371. Hindley AC, Hill AB, Leyland MJ, Wiles AE. A double-blind controlled trial of salmon calcitonin in pain due to malignancy. *Cancer Chemotherapy Pharmacology*, 1982; **9**: 71–4.
372. Roth A, Kolaric K. Analgesic activity of calcitonin in patient with painful osteolytic metastases of breast cancer: results of a controlled randomized study. *Oncology*, 1986; **43**: 283–7.
373. Blomquist C, Elomaa I, Porkka L, Karonen SL, Lamberg-Allardt C. Evaluation of salmon calcitonin treatment in bone metastases from breast cancer—a controlled trial. *Bone*, 1988; **9**: 45–51.
374. Fraioli F, *et al.* Calcitonin and analgesia. In: Benedetti C, Chapman CR, Moricca G, eds. *Advances in Pain Research and Therapy*, vol 7. New York: Raven Press, 1984: 37–50.
375. Paterson AHG, Powles TJ, Kanis JA, McCloskey E, Hanson J, Ashley S. Double-blind controlled trial of oral clodronate in patients with bone metastases from breast cancer. *Journal of Clinical Oncology*, 1993; **11**: 59–65.
376. Elomaa I, *et al.* Long-term controlled trial with diphosphonate in patients with osteolytic bone metastases. *Lancet*, 1983; **1**: 146–9.
377. Siris ES, *et al.* Effects of dichloromethylene diphosphonate on skeletal mobilization of calcium in multiple myeloma. *New England Journal of Medicine*, 1980; **302**: 310–15.
378. Adami S and Mian M. Clodronate therapy of metastatic bone disease in patients with prostatic carcinoma. *Cancer Research*, 1989; **116**: 67–72.
379. Schnur W. Relief of metastatic bone pain with etidronate disodium. *Ohio Medical Journal*, 1987; **83**: 62–5.
380. Carey PO, Lippert MC. Treatment of painful prostatic bone metastases with oral etidronate disodium. *Urology*, 1988; **32**: 403–7.
381. Ernst DS, MacDonald RN, Paterson AHG, Jensen J, Brasher P, Bruera E. A double blind, cross-over trial of IV clodronate in metastatic bone pain. *Journal of Pain and Symptom Management*, 1992; **7**: 4–11.
382. Kanis JA, McCloskey EV, Taube T, *et al.* Rationale for the use of bisphosphonates in bone metastases. *Bone*, 1991; **12**: 8–13.
383. Coleman RE, Woll PJ, Miles M, *et al.* Treatment of bone metastases from breast cancer with (3 amino-1-hydroxypropylidene)-1,1-bisphosphonate (APD). *British Journal of Cancer*, 1988; **58**: 621–5.
384. Thiebaud D, Leyvraz S, von Fliedner V, *et al.* Treatment of bone metastases from breast cancer and myeloma with pamidronate. *European Journal of Cancer*, 1991; **27**: 37–41.
385. van Holten-Verzantvoort AT, Kroon HM, Bijvoet OL, *et al.* Palliative pamidronate treatment in patients with bone metastases from breast cancer. *Journal of Clinical Oncology*, 1993; **11**: 491–8.
386. Clarke NW, Holbrook IB, McClure J, *et al.* Osteoclast inhibition by pamidronate in metastatic prostate cancer: a preliminary report. *British Journal of Cancer*, 1991; **63**: 420–3.
387. Morton AR, Cantrill JA, Pillai GV, *et al.* Sclerosis of lytic bony metastases after aminohydroxypropylidene bisphosphonate (APD) in patients with breast cancer. *British Medical Journal*, 1988; **297**: 772–3.
388. Glover D, Lipton A, Keller A, *et al.* Intravenous pamidronate disodium treatment of bone metastases in patients with breast cancer. *Cancer*, 1994; **74**: 2949–55.
389. Averbuch SD. New bisphosphonates in the treatment of bone metastases. *Cancer*, 1993; **72**: 3443–52.
390. Smith JA. Palliation of painful bone metastases from prostate cancer using sodium etidronate: results of a randomized, prospective, double-blind, placebo-controlled study. *Journal of Urology*, 1989; **141**: 85–7.
391. Holmes RA. Radiopharmaceuticals in clinical trials. *Seminars in Oncology*, 1993; **20**: 22–6.
392. Serafini AN. Current status of systemic intravenous radiopharmaceuticals for the treatment of painful metastatic bone disease. *International Journal of Radiation Oncology and Biological Physics*, 1994; **30**: 1187–94.
393. Silberstein EB. The treatment of painful osseous metastases with phosphorus-32-labeled phosphates. *Seminars in Oncology*, 1993; **20**: 10–21.
394. Laing AH, Achery DM, Bayly RJ, *et al.* Strontium-89 chloride for pain palliation in prostatic skeletal malignancy. *British Journal of Radiology*, 1991; **64**: 816–22.
395. Robinson RG, Spicer JA, Preston DF, *et al.* Treatment of metastatic bone pain with strontium-89. *Nuclear Medicine Biology*, 1987; **14**: 219–22.
396. Silberstein EB and Williams C. Strontium-89 therapy for the pain of osseous metastases. *Journal of Nuclear Medicine*, 1985; **26**: 345–8.
397. Maxon HR, *et al.* Initial experience with 186-Re(Sn)-HEDP in the treatment of painful skeletal metastases. *Journal of Nuclear Medicine*, 1988; **29**: 776.
398. Turner JH, Claringbold PG. A phase II study of treatment of painful multifocal skeletal metastases with single and repeated dose samarium-153 ethylenediaminetetramethylene phsophonate. *European Journal of Cancer*, 1991; **27**: 1084–6.
399. Maxon HR, Thomas SR, Hertzberg VS, *et al.* Rhenium-186 hydroxyethylidene diphosphonate for the treatment of painful osseous metastases. *Seminars in Nuclear Medicine*, 1992; **22**: 33–40.
400. Turner JH, Claringbold PG, Hetherington EL, *et al.* A phase I study of samarium-153 ethylenediamenetramethylene phosphonate therapy for disseminated skeletal metastases. *Journal of Clinical Oncology*, 1989; **7**: 1926–31.
401. Farhanghi M, Holmes RA, Volkert WA, Logan KW, Singh A. Samarium-153-EDTMP: pharmacolkinetic, toxicity and pain response using an escalating dose schedule in treatment of metastatic bone pain. *Journal of Nuclear Medicine*, 1992; **33**: 1451–8.
402. Holmes PA. [153Sm]EDTMP: a potential therapy for bone cancer pain. *Seminars in Nuclear Medicine*, 1992; **22**: 41–5.
403. Porter AT, EcEwan AJ, Powe JE, *et al.* Results of a randomized phase-III trial to evaluate the efficacy of strontium-89 adjuvant to local field external beam irradiation in the management of endocrine resistant metastatic prostate cancer. *Interntional Journal of Radiation, Oncology, and Biologic Physics*, 1993; **25**: 805–13.
404. Lewington VJ, McEwan AJB, Ackery DM, *et al.* A prospective, randomized double-blind cross-over study to examine the efficacy of strontium-89 in pain palliation in patients with advanced prostate cancer metastatic to bone. *European Journal of Cancer*, 1991; **27**: 954–58.
405. Quilty PM, Kirk D, Bolger JJ, *et al.* A comparison of the palliative effects of strontium-89 and external beam radiotherapy in metastatic prostate cancer. *Radiotherapy and Oncology*, 1994; **31**: 33–40.
406. Robinson RG, Preston DF, Baxter KG, Dusing RW, Spicer JA. Clinical

experience with strontium-89 in prostatic and breast cancer patients. *Seminars in Oncology*, 1993; **20**: 44–8.

407. Robinson RG, Preston DF, Schiefelbein M, Baster KG. Strontium-89 therapy for the palliation of pain due to osseous metastases. *Journal of the American Medical Association*, 1995; **274**: 420–4.
408. Warrell RP, Lovett D, Dilmanian FA, *et al.* Low-dose gallium nitrate for prevention of osteolysis in myeloma: results of a pilot randomized study. *Journal of Clinical Oncology*, 1993; **11**: 2443–50.
409. Minton JP. The response of breast cancer patients with bone pain to L-dopa. *Cancer*, 1974; **33**: 358–63.
410. Hanks GW. The pharmacological treatment of bone pain. *Cancer Surveys*, 1988; **7**: 87–101.
411. Sjolin S, Trykker H. Unsuccessful treatment of severe pain from bone metastases with Sinemet 25/100. *New England Journal of Medicine*, 1985; **302**: 650–1.
412. Ripamonti C. Management of bowel obstruction in advanced cancer patients. *Journal of Pain and Symptom Management*, 1994; **9**: 193–200.
413. Baines M, Oliver DJ, Carter RL. Medical management of intestinal obstruction in patients with advanced malignant disease: a clinical and pathological study. *Lancet*, 1985; **ii**: 990–3.
414. Ventafridda V, Ripamonti C, Caraceni A, Spoldi E, Messina L, De Conno F. The management of inoperable gastrointestinal obstruction in terminal cancer patients. *Tumori*, 1990; **76**: 389–93.
415. De Conno F, Caraceni A, Zecca E, Spoldi E, Ventafridda V. Continuous subcutaneous infusion of hyoscine butylbromide reduces secretions in patients with gastrointestinal obstruction. *Journal of Pain and Symptom Management*, 1991; **6**: 484–6.
416. Mercadante S, Maddaloni S. Octreotide in the management of inoperable gastrointestinal obstruction in terminal cancer patients. *Journal of Pain and Symptom Management*, 1992; **7**: 496–8.
417. Mercadante S. Treatment of diarrhea due to enterocolic fistula with octreotide in a terminal cancer patient. *Palliative Medicine*, 1992; **6**: 257–9.
418. Mulvihill S, Pappas TN, Passaro E, Debas HT. The use of somatostatin and its analogues. *Surgery*, 1986; **100**: 467–76.
419. Ladefoged K, Christensen KC, Hegnhoj J, Jarnum S. Effect of a long acting somatostatin analogue SMS 201–995 on jejunostomy effluents in patients with severe short bowel syndrome. *Gut*, 1989; **30**: 943–9.
420. Twycross RG, Fairfield S. Pain in far-advanced cancer. *Pain*, 1982; **14**: 303–10.
421. Batterman RC. Methodology of analgesic evaluation: experience with orphenadrine citrate compound. *Current Therapeutic Research*, 1965; **7**: 639–47.
422. Bercel NA. Cyclobenzaprine in the treatment of skeletal muscle spasm in osteoarthritis of the cervical and lumbar spine. *Current Therapeutic Research*, 1977; **22**: 462–8.
423. Birkeland IW, Clawson DK. Drug combinations with orphenadrine for pain relief associated with muscle spasm. *Clinical Pharmacology and Therapeutics*, 1958; **9**: 639–46.
424. Gold RH. Treatment of low back pain syndrome with oral orphenadrine citrate. *Current Therapeutic Research*, 1978; **23**: 271–6.
425. Tseng TC, Wang SC. Locus of action of centrally-acting muscle relaxants, diazepam and tybamate. *Journal of Pharmacology and Experimental Therapeutics*, 1971; **178**: 350–60.
426. Forrest WH, *et al.* Dextroamphetamine with morphine for the treatment of postoperative pain. *New England Journal of Medicine*, 1977; **296**: 712–15.
427. Cantello R, *et al.* Analgesic action of methylphenidate on parkinsonian sensory symptoms. Mechanisms and pathophysiological implications. *Archives of Neurology*, 1988; **45**: 973–6.
428. Bruera E, Chadwich S, Brenneis C, Hanson J, MacDonald RN. Methylphenidate associated with narcotics for the treatment of cancer pain. *Cancer Treatment Report*, 1987; **71**: 67–70.
429. Sawynok J. Pharmacological rationale for the clinical use of caffeine. *Drugs*, 1995; **49**: 37–50.
430. Schachtel BP, Fillingim JM, Lane AC, Thoden WR, Baybutt RI. Caffeine as an analgesic adjuvant: a double-blind study comparing aspirin with caffeine to aspirin and placebo in patients with severe sore throat. *Archives of Internal Medicine*, 1991; **151**: 733–7.
431. Laska EM, *et al.* Caffeine as an analagesic adjuvant. *Journal of the American Medical Association*, 1984; **251**: 1711–18.
432. Forbes JA, Beaver WT, Jones KF, *et al.* Effect of caffeine on ibuprofen analgesia in postoperative oral surgery pain. *Clinical Pharmacology and Therapeutics*, 1991; **49**: 674–84.
433. Kaiko RF, *et al.* Cocaine and morphine interaction in acute and chronic cancer pain. *Pain*, 1987; **31**: 35–45.
434. Marbach JJ, Wallenstein SL. Analgesia, mood and hemodynamic effects of intranasal cocaine and lidocaine in chronic facial pain of deafferentation and myofascial origin. *Journal of Pain and Symptom Management*, 1988; **3**: 73–9.
435. Yang JC, Clark WC, Dooley JC, Mignogna FV. Effect of intranasal cocaine on experimental pain in man. *Anesthesia and Analgesia*, 1982; **61**: 358–61.
436. Bruera E, Miller MJ, Macmillan K, Kuehn N. Neuropsychological effects of methylphenidate in patients receiving a continuous infusion of narcotics for cancer pain. *Pain*, 1992; **48**: 163–6.
437. Bruera E, Brenneis C, Paterson AH, MacDonald RN. Use of methylphenidate as an adjuvant to narcotic analgesics in patients with advanced cancer. *Journal of Pain and Symptom Management*, 1989; **4**: 3–6.
438. Berkovitch M, Pope E, Phillips J, Koren G. Pemoline-associated fulminant liver failure: testing the evidence for causation. *Clinical Pharmacology and Therapeutics*, 1995; **57**: 696–8.
439. Campos VM, Solis EL. The analgesic and hypothermic effects of nefopam, morphine, aspirin, diphenhydramine and placebo. *Journal of Clinical Pharmacology*, 1980; **20**: 42–9.
440. Hupert C, Yacoub M, Turgeon LR. Effect of hydroxyzine on morphine analgesia for the treatment of postoperative pain. *Anesthesia and Analgesia*, 1980; **59**: 690–6.
441. Stambaugh JE, Lance C. Analgesic efficacy and pharmacokinetic evaluation of meperidine and hydroxyzine, alone and in combination. *Cancer Investigation*, 1983; **1**: 111–17.
442. Beaver WT, Feise G. Comparison of the analgesic effect of morphine, hydroxyzine and their combination in patients with postoperative pain. In: Bonica JJ, ed. *Advances in Pain Research and Therapy*, vol 1. New York: Raven Press, 1976: 553–7.
443. Sunshine A, *et al.* Augmentation of acetaminophen analgesia by the antihistamine phenyltoloxamine. *The Journal of Clinical Pharmacology*, 1989; **29**: 660–4.
444. McColl JD, Durkin W. The effect of pyrilamine on relief of symptoms of the premenstrual syndrome (PMS) and primary dysmenorrhea. *Federation Proceedings*, 1982; **41**: 5572.
445. Gilbert MM. The efficacy of Percogesic in relief of musculoskeletal pain associated with anxiety. *Psychosomatics*, 1976; **17**: 190–3.
446. Wilson RS, May EL, Martin BR, Dewey WL. 9-nor-9-hydroxyhexahydrocannabinols. Synthesis, some behavioral and analgesic properties, and comparison with the tetrahydrocannabinols. *Journal of Medicinal Chemistry*, 1976; **19**: 1165–7.
447. Chesher GB, Dahl CJ, Everingham M, Jackson DM, Marchant-Williams H, Starmer GA. The effect of cannabinoids on intestinal motility and their antinociceptive effect in mice. *British Journal of Pharmacology*, 1973; **49**: 588–94.
448. Noyes R, Brunk SF, Avery DH, Canter A. The analgesic properties of delta-9-tetrahydrocannabinol and codeine. *Clinical Pharmacology and Therapeutics*, 1976; **18**: 84–9.
449. Jain AK, Ryan JR, McMahon FG, Smith G. Evaluation of intramuscular levonantradol and placebo in acute postoperative pain. *Journal of Clinical Pharmacology*, 1981; **21**: 320S–6.
450. Henriksson R, Franzen L, Littbrand B. Effects of sucralfate on acute and late bowel discomfort following radiotherapy of pelvic cancer. *Journal of Clinical Oncology*, 1992; **10**: 969–75.
451. Segerdahl M, Ekblom A, Sandelin K, Wickman M, Sollevi A. Perioperative adenosine infusion reduces the requirements for isoflurane and postoperative analgesics. *Anesthesia and Analgesia*, 1995; **80**: 1145–9.

452. Duggan AW, Weihe E. Central transmission of impulses in nocicieptors: events in the superficial dorsal horn. In: Basbaum AI, Besson J-M, eds. *Towards a New Pharmacotherapy of Pain*. Chichester: John Wiley and Sons, 1989: 35–67.
453. Theriault R, Lipton A, Leff R, *et al*. Reduction of skeletal related complications in breast cancer patients with osteolytic bone metastases receiving hormone therapy by monthly pamidronate sodium. (Aredia) infusion. *Proceedings of ASCO*, 1996; **15**: 122.
454. Paterson AHG, McCloskey EV, Ashley S, Powles TJ, Kanis JA. Reduction of skeletal morbidity and prevention of bone metastases with oral clodronate in women with recurrent breast cancer in the absence of skeletal metastases. *Proceedings of ASCO*, 1996; 15: 104.

9.2.6 Anaesthetic techniques for pain control

Robert A. Swarm and Michael J. Cousins

The role of the anaesthetist and anaesthetic techniques in palliative medicine

Except for the past 100 years, medicinal attempts at pain relief relied upon the oral administration of systemically active agents. Although the drugs used in early civilization varied, these agents (mandragora, opium, alcohol, cocaine, and various hallucinogens) probably provided only partial analgesia, at the price of significant depression of the central nervous system. Appropriately, modern clinical practice has continued to rely on the oral administration of analgesics as the first-line choice of analgesic drug delivery. Analgesic alternatives to the systemic administration of agents acting upon the central nervous system only became possible after the first demonstration of local anaesthetic blockade of nerve conduction in 1884. Subsequently, many techniques have been adapted from the evolving practice of anaesthesia, to provide analgesia without excessive central nervous system depression. Local anaesthetic or neurolytic nerve conduction blockade is generally not associated with any degree of sedation or general central nervous system depression. Other techniques, such as spinal opioid administration, may be associated with some central nervous system depression, but potentially offer more profound analgesia with less depression than systemic analgesic administration.[1]

Local anaesthetic and neurolytic conduction blockade of peripheral nerves and sympathetic ganglia, in the management of pain inadequately controlled by systemic analgesics, were previously the major contribution of anaesthetic techniques to pain management and continue to have a significant role. Through the recent advances in understanding the neurophysiology of pain, it has become evident that current analgesic medications do not block mechanisms of hypersensitization and, as in the case of morphine, may actually contribute to the development of hyperalgesia.[2,3] These potential limits to the effectiveness of current systemic analgesics highlight the ongoing utility of neuronal conduction block in pain management. The demonstration[4] and clinical utilization[5–7] of spinal opioid administration has begun to shift and broaden the focus of anaesthetic pain management techniques from simple neuronal conduction blockade to diverse techniques of regional administration of pharmacological agents that modulate neuronal transmission. The predominant, current example of this regional modulation of neuronal transmission in clinical practice is spinal opioid administration, but intrathecal baclofen for spasticity and the spinal administration of non-opioid analgesics are of increasing clinical importance.

The majority of patients receiving palliative care will not require anaesthetic techniques, just as the majority of cancer patients can obtain adequate pain relief through an appropriate regimen of oral analgesics and adjuvant medications.[8] Fewer than 10 per cent of patients with cancer pain will require spinal opioids or neurolytic blocks. However, if systemic administration of agents acting on the central nervous system has proven ineffective or is associated with unacceptable adverse effects, combined approaches directed at more than one level of the nervous system should be considered. Combinations of various medical and anaesthetic techniques may include:

(1) agents directed at the level of peripheral pain receptors (anti-inflammatory drugs);

(2) techniques to block axonal transmission (local anaesthetic or neurolytic conduction blockade);

(3) blockade of the sympathetic nervous system (local anaesthetic or neurolytic blockade);

(4) agents to decrease central nervous system reception and transmission of pain signals (systemic, spinal, or intraventricular administration of opioids and other agents).

Those patients whose pain is inadequately relieved by systemic agents may benefit from anaesthetic techniques of pain management. Over the last one or two decades, pain management has become a recognized area of subspecialization for anaesthetists. By extension of their basic knowledge and skills in surgical anaesthesia, anaesthetists with pain management training and expertise can make considerable contributions to the palliative care of selected patients. In addition to technical skills, a pain management anaesthetist has knowledge of the indications, contraindications, and patient selection and management factors crucial to the successful application of anaesthetic techniques. Anaesthetists also have wide-ranging experience in the clinical use of opioid and non-opioid analgesics, numerous sedatives, antiemetics, and other drugs useful in some palliative care settings. Not all anaesthetists have the time, interest, and commitment to contribute, and such attributes are as important as the pharmacological knowledge and technical skill required for the successful application of anaesthetic techniques to palliative care.

Descriptions of anaesthetic techniques with clinical utility are grouped below, according to the major anatomical divisions of the nervous system. The medications, potential benefits, and potential complications of anaesthetic techniques are discussed, but in-depth description of technical details of procedures is beyond the scope of this text, though relevant references are provided.

Table 1 Administration sites for spinal analgesia

Spinal	All routes of administration near or within the spinal meninges ('spinal anaesthesia' is generally used to indicate subarachnoid administration of local anaesthetic)
Epidural	Immediately outside the dura mater, within the vertebral spinal canal
Intrathecal	Inside the thecal sac or dura mater. Intrathecal is often used synonymously with subarachnoid, but anatomically intrathecal also includes the subdural space
Subdural	Between the dura mater and arachnoid mater
Subarachnoid	Inside the arachnoid mater. This space contains the cerebrospinal fluid

Techniques for pain control: the central nervous system

Spinal opioid administration

The spinal administration of opioid analgesics is now used extensively and has an established role in the management of severe pain in many settings. In the setting of acute pain,[9] cancer-related pain,[10] and selected but diverse settings of non-cancer chronic pain[11] spinal opioids have been used to provide profound analgesia. 'Spinal' opioid includes both epidural and intrathecal or subarachnoid routes of opioid administration (Table 1). The rationale for spinal administration of opioid is to provide improved analgesia through enhanced delivery of drug to opioid receptors within the spinal cord, as compared with systemic routes of administration.

Although a relatively recent addition to anaesthetic techniques for pain control, the spinal administration of opioid is likely to play an important role in pain therapies for many years to come. In the mid-1970s, electrophysiological evidence for naloxone-reversible interruption of nociceptive signals by iontophoretic application of morphine to the dorsal horn region of the spinal cord[12,13] was followed by the demonstration of intrathecal morphine-induced analgesic behaviour in experimental animals.[4] After the first clinical reports of spinal opioid analgesia in 1979,[5-7] the use of spinal opioid analgesic techniques quickly became widespread and common.

The initial enthusiasm for the use of spinal opioids was soon tempered by the recognition of potential adverse effects,[14-16] the problem of opioid tolerance, and various technical limitations to long-term spinal opioid therapy. Further clinical experience has shown that with careful patient selection, opioid dose adjustment, and anticipation and management, adverse effects from spinal opioids generally can be reasonably controlled. Furthermore, in patients previously receiving systemic opioids and therefore with some degree of opioid tolerance, as is generally the case in palliative pain management, adverse effects from spinal opioid are less common than in opioid-naive patients.[16,17] The technical complexity of spinal opioid administration continues to be clinically challenging, but the problems of opioid tolerance and management of pain resistant to spinal opioids may well be addressed by the application of new spinal analgesic agents (see below). In the future, spinal opioid is likely to play an important role in pain management as a mainstay of diverse spinal analgesic therapies.

Spinal action of opioids

Opioid receptors are present within the spinal cord, predominantly within the dorsal horns of the spinal grey matter.[18,19] The dorsal horns are the location of the important synapses between primary afferent sensory neurones responsible for pain transmission (A_δ- and C-fibres), and the second-order spinal neurones. These spinal opioid receptors are one of a large number of receptor types now thought to modulate pain transmission across the dorsal horn synapses.[20] The binding of spinal opioid agonist agents (opioid analgesics) to opioid receptors within the dorsal horns, inhibits synaptic transmission between the primary afferent nociceptors and the second-order spinal neurones. By their presence on both the presynaptic (peripheral afferent nociceptor) and postsynaptic (second-order spinal neurone) nerve terminals, spinal opioid receptors are strategically positioned to inhibit nociceptive transmission. Spinal routes of administration have been shown to be an effective way to deliver opioid analgesics to the spinal dorsal horns to decrease nociceptive transmission.[7]

Both spinal and brain[21] opioid receptors are likely to contribute to opioid-mediated analgesia regardless of the route of opioid administration. Analgesia from systemically applied opioids relates, in large part, to their effect on spinal opioid receptors.[22,23] Similarly, spinally administered opioids may spread beyond spinal receptors. The vascular uptake following epidural administration of opioids results in plasma levels comparable to those following parenteral administration,[24,25] and is likely to result in a systemic contribution to the analgesia following epidural opioid administration. In addition, the normal cephalad migration of cerebrospinal fluid may deliver spinally-administered opioid to medullary and brain opioid receptors.[26] Separating the contribution of spinal opioid receptors, from the contribution of brain and other receptors to the total analgesia observed, is difficult, and perhaps unimportant in clinical palliative care.

Studies in humans have documented spinal cerebrospinal fluid opioid concentrations far in excess of blood or plasma opioid concentrations, following lumbar spinal opioid administration.[25-28] The time course of the onset and duration of analgesia following epidural opioid administration follows that of the spinal cerebrospinal fluid opioid concentrations rather than that of blood or plasma opioid concentrations.[1] Spinal opioid administration enables the clinician to focus analgesic therapy towards the spinal opioid receptors. In palliative care, when systemically administered opioids fail to provide adequate analgesia and/or are associated with unacceptable adverse effects, optimization of opioid delivery to spinal opioid receptors, through spinal administration routes, may result in enhanced analgesia.

Pharmacokinetic model of spinal opioids

There is considerable variation in the pharmacokinetics of different opioids when administered spinally—variation related largely to differences in lipid solubility.[19,26-28] Following epidural administration (Fig. 1), opioid must be transferred across the dura, spread within the cerebrospinal fluid, and penetrate into the spinal cord to reach opioid receptors within the dorsal horns of the spinal cord.

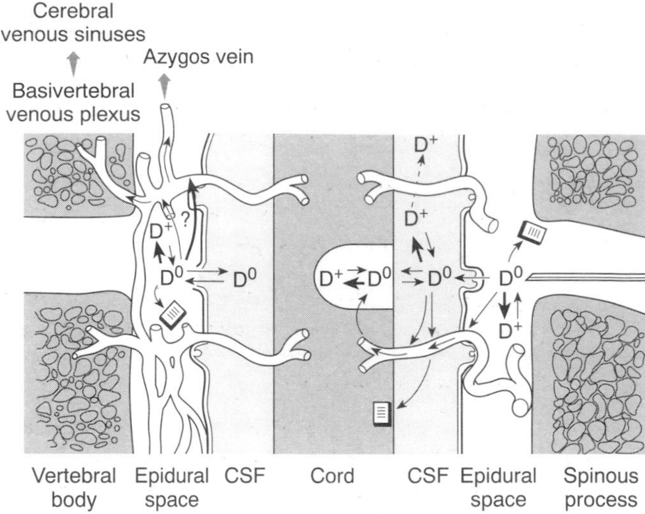

Fig. 1 Pharmacokinetic model of spinal opioid administration. An epidural needle (right) is shown delivering a hydrophilic opioid, such as morphine, to the epidural space. Within the epidural space, cerebrospinal fluid (CSF), and spinal cord equilibria of D^o (non-ionized moiety of drug) and D^+ (ionized, hydrophilic moiety) are shown. Non-specific lipid binding sites are indicated by the shaded squares. The role of spinal arteries, in proximity to arachnoid granulations, in drug delivery is speculative. Epidural veins are the major point of clearance of epidural drugs. (Reproduced with permission from Cousins MJ and Bridenbaugh PO, eds. *Neural Blockade in Clinical Anaesthesia and Management of Pain*. 2nd edn. Philadelphia: J. B. Lippincott, 1988.)

Vascular uptake and absorption into fat and other tissue binding sites reduces the quantity of drug available to reach the spinal cord. Differences in pharmacokinetics form the basis for the use of different spinal opioids under different circumstances. In general, pharmacokinetic considerations indicate that morphine has the most favourable characteristics for chronic spinal administration.

Morphine is a hydrophilic drug and, under physiological conditions, is also highly ionized. Following epidural injection (Fig. 1), only a low concentration of the more lipid-soluble, non-ionized moiety will be present in solution; however, it is through this low concentration of non-ionized moiety that morphine diffuses into lipid-rich structures (such as meninges, spinal cord, and vessel walls). The movement of the non-ionized moiety of morphine across the dura, as well as in and out of the spinal cord, is a slow process effected by small concentration gradients. As a result, epidurally administered morphine does not reach a peak concentration in cerebrospinal fluid until 90 min after injection. From the aqueous cerebrospinal fluid, hydrophilic morphine will move slowly into the lipid-rich spinal cord. Similarly, morphine reaching spinal receptors will tend to have a long duration of effect, as egress from the spinal cord will be inhibited by the prolonged presence of (hydrophilic) morphine in the cerebrospinal fluid. This pharmacokinetic model[1] is in keeping with the delayed peak and prolonged duration of analgesia and cerebrospinal fluid morphine concentration following epidural morphine injection.

After epidural administration of a less-ionized, lipophilic opioid (such as fentanyl or pethidine (meperidine)) a greater proportion of the drug will be present as a more lipid-soluble, non-ionized moiety in solution. This results in a more rapid transfer of the drug across the dura,[27] as well as in and out of the spinal cord. From the cerebrospinal fluid, lipophilic opioid passes readily into the lipid-rich spinal cord, resulting in a rapid onset of analgesia. Egress from spinal receptors will be enhanced by rapid systemic redistribution of opioid due to vascular uptake, as well as by binding to non-specific tissue sites. This model[1] is in keeping with the observed rapid onset and short duration of analgesia, as well as the limited cephalad migration, of lipophilic opioids[28] as compared with hydrophilic opioid (morphine).

The long duration of analgesia with the spinal administration of some very lipophilic opioids, such as sufentanil, may relate to non-specific binding of opioid to spinal cord lipid, as well as a higher drug affinity for opioid receptors.[29,30] By comparison with morphine, sufentanil is a high-efficacy opioid agonist, in that to produce a comparable effect it need occupy a smaller fraction of available receptors. It has been suggested that the use of high-efficacy agonists may reduce the rate of tolerance development, as well as increase the potency of spinal opioid analgesia.[31] Perhaps due to its relatively high cost, sufentanil has not become widely used for chronic spinal administration; however, it has been useful as a second choice agent when tolerance or insufficient effect limits spinal morphine analgesia.[32]

Drug uptake and distribution following subarachnoid opioid administration is similar to that of epidural administration once the opioid is present within the cerebrospinal fluid. Following subarachnoid administration, opioid is not subject to initial uptake by the epidural vasculature and epidural non-specific tissue binding sites, so subarachnoid doses of opioid are generally 10 per cent of doses required for epidural administration. There is a decrease in the time to onset of analgesia and a prolongation of analgesic effect following bolus subarachnoid, as compared with epidural, opioid administration.[1]

The prolonged presence of morphine in the cerebrospinal fluid following epidural or subarachnoid administration, results in migration of morphine from the spinal level of injection, due to the normal circulation of cerebrospinal fluid.[33] This migration of morphine to other spinal segments, and to supraspinal or brain structures, extends the level of analgesia and increases the utility of spinal morphine in the management of chronic pain. Unless cerebrospinal fluid circulation is blocked[34,35] (by, for example, tumour, congenital malformation, or arachnoiditis), spinal morphine need not be administered at the spinal segmental level of the pain. Although somewhat more lipophilic than morphine, following epidural administration, hydromorphone appears to be pharmacokinetically similarly to epidural morphine,[36] especially with regard to the similar degree of cervical migration of hydromorphone in cerebrospinal fluid following lumbar administration.

Clinical studies of epidural morphine administration have reported large interindividual variability in the ratio of morphine concentration in cerebrospinal fluid and plasma or blood.[26] A component of this variability may be related to individual differences in the transdural delivery of opioid from the epidural space to the cerebrospinal fluid. A sheet of fibrous or scar tissue around chronically implanted epidural catheters has been documented in post mortem studies.[37] Such epidural fibrosis appears to be a variable process that may limit delivery of the injected opioid to the epidural space[38–40] and may account for some of the observed variability in cerebrospinal fluid opioid concentrations following lumbar epidural administration. Fibrosis does not seem to occur to a significant degree around subarachnoid spinal catheters.

Appropriate palliative care applications of spinal opioids

Chronic administration of spinal opioid, with or without simultaneous administration of local anaesthetic, has been used most commonly in the management of severe, cancer-related pain. In the appropriate settings, however, spinal analgesia may also be used with considerable benefit in the palliation of otherwise intractable, non-cancer pain. In general, indications for the use of spinal opioids in palliative care are the same as the indications for their use in cancer pain:

(1) in patients treated with systemic opioids with effective pain relief, but with unacceptable adverse effects, such as clouding of consciousness, nausea, and vomiting;

(2) in patients whose pain cannot be controlled adequately with the use of systemic opioids.

In both indications, it is assumed that prior analgesic trials included appropriate adjuvant drugs, in combination with adequate opioid. Ongoing chemotherapy or radiotherapy is not a contraindication to the placement of a spinal catheter and initiation of spinal opioid therapy. Adequate analgesia, perhaps with spinal opioid administration, may allow patients with otherwise intractable pain to undergo appropriate palliative antitumour therapy.

In the management of both cancer and non-cancer pain, the nature of the underlying disease(s), the character of the pain, and the predicted patient survival are important factors when considering spinal opioid therapy. In the management of cancer pain, the best response to spinal opioids is obtained in patients with deep, constant somatic pain. Other types of cancer pain are variably responsive, as are cutaneous pain, intermittent somatic pain (pathological fracture), intermittent visceral pain (intestinal obstruction), and coexistent cancer-related and non-cancer pain.[41] In settings where the potential benefit of spinal opioid administration is uncertain, it may be useful to carry out a trial of epidural opioid through a standard percutaneous catheter, before embarking on the more invasive implantation of a permanent system for long-term spinal opioid therapy.

Patients with severe, intractable pain not responsive to systemic analgesics may have a significant component of neuropathic pain. Previously it was felt that 'central' pain, neuropathic pain, and deafferentation pain were not responsive to opioid therapy, so that such patients may not have been considered candidates to receive spinal opioids. Although neuropathic pain may be less sensitive to opioid therapy than nociceptive pain, it now seems likely that the type of pain is simply an additional factor to be considered in the titration of opioid analgesics for each patient, and is not a reliable predictor of opioid responsiveness.[42] In both acute and chronic trials, spinal opioids (with and without simultaneous administration of other spinal analgesics) have been used to good effect in selected cases of intractable neuropathic and deafferentation pain.[17,43–46]

Spinal opioids have applications in addition to the management of cancer pain. Spinal analgesia has been utilized in the management of intractable non-cancer pain, and other symptoms, in the setting of:

(1) severe, inoperable peripheral vascular disease with ischaemic extremity rest pain;[17,47]

(2) vertebral crush fractures and stress rib fractures in patients with severe osteoporosis, often on chronic steroid therapy for control of chronic lung disease or autoimmune disease;[11,17]

(3) medically intractable and inoperable myocardial ischaemia may be improved and angina successfully treated;[48–50]

(4) painful urinary bladder spasms due to tumour, chronic catheterization, or infection,[51] and hyperactive micturition reflexes in patients with spinal cord lesions;[52]

(5) muscle spasticity due to lesions of the central nervous system (intrathecal baclofen may be more potent—see below);[53]

(6) neuropathic pain following spinal cord injury;[44]

(7) various other conditions including postherpetic neuralgia, nephrolithiasis, thrombophlebitis, multiple sclerosis, phantom limb pain, reflex sympathetic dystrophy (complex regional pain syndrome, Type I), and intractable back pain including inoperable spinal stenosis.[11,17]

The contraindications for spinal opioid therapy are similar to those for any regional anaesthetic technique, with a few additional concerns due to the chronicity of spinal opioid use.

1. Bleeding diathesis would increase the risk of epidural haematoma and possible neurological deficit due to compression of the spinal cord or nerve roots.

2. Septicaemia is practically an absolute contraindication, due to the risk of spreading infection to the spinal opioid delivery system, perhaps resulting in epidural abscess, meningitis, and neurological deficit.

3. Local, cutaneous infection is only a contraindication if a reasonable site for implantation of the spinal catheter system, free of infection, cannot be found.

4. Patients with known immune suppression may be at higher risk of infection of the spinal catheter system, but this is only a relative contraindication as spinal catheter infections are uncommon.

5. Insulin-dependent diabetics seem to have an increased susceptibility to infection of spinal catheters.[54]

6. If appropriate support for the ongoing management of spinal opioid administration is not available, then spinal opioid therapy is inappropriate.

The known presence of epidural or spinal metastasis deserves special consideration. While anaesthetists generally consider spinal metastasis to be a contraindication for neuraxial regional anaesthetic techniques, patients with such lesions may have severe pain and require spinal analgesia. The concern is that, at least theoretically, trauma to a friable tumour mass during spinal catheterization could result in haemorrhage, epidural haematoma, and neural compression. To avoid such trauma, spinal catheters should be inserted away from spinal metastases, perhaps under fluoroscopy. Furthermore, the potential for eventual obstruction of cerebrospinal fluid circulation, by expansion of a tumour mass, should encourage the placement of spinal catheters cephalad to known, or suspected, epidural or spinal metastases.[34]

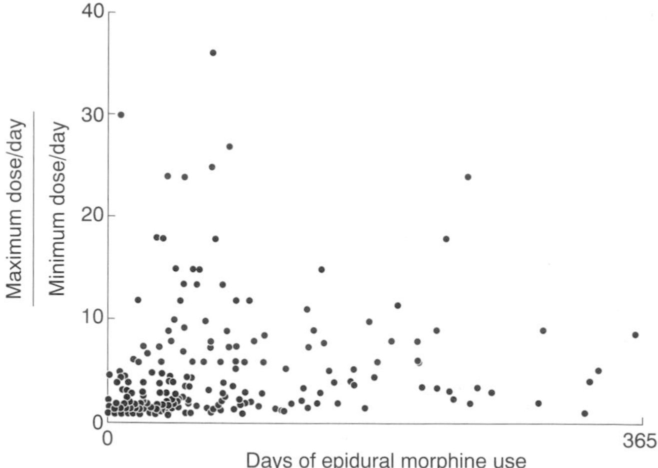

Fig. 2 Epidural opioid via a 'portal': long-term follow-up relationship between dose escalation (ratio of maximum daily morphine dose to minimum daily morphine dose) and duration of epidural morphine treatment in 240 patients with cancer. There is a poor correlation between dose escalation and duration of treatment. (Reproduced, with permission, from Plummer, *et al.*[17].)

An anticipated long duration of analgesic therapy (many months) is not necessarily a contraindication to the use of spinal opioids. Opioid requirement may change and generally increases over time, but chronic spinal analgesia does not inexorably lead to continued dose escalation (Fig. 2).[17] As with systemic opioid therapy, it is generally recognized that an increase in opioid requirement, due to deteriorating analgesia, is likely to indicate an exacerbation or progression of the underlying disease rather than simple opioid tolerance.[55] There are numerous reported clinical series documenting the analgesic efficacy of chronic spinal analgesia in excess of 1 to 2 years.[17,38,56–58] Epidural fibrosis (the formation of scar tissue around an implanted epidural catheter) may limit the efficacy of injected opioid, but may be managed by replacement of the epidural catheter or revision to a subarachnoid delivery system. The low risk of spinal catheter infection, and the risk of opioid tolerance and abuse, should only be practical considerations (not theoretical proscriptions) in the application and long-term use of spinal analgesia.

Adverse effects and complications of spinal opioids

Adverse effects and complications which may be associated with the use of spinal opioids are a result of the physiology and pharmacology of spinal opioids, or a consequence of the devices and techniques employed to deliver the opioids spinally (see technical considerations below). As in the successful application of any invasive therapy, patients for spinal opioids must be selected carefully and followed closely to minimize the incidence and consequence of complications.

The most common adverse effects of the spinal administration of opioids are those of opioid therapy in general. Fortunately, respiratory depression, nausea and vomiting, dysphoria, urinary retention, and pruritus are not commonly reported following the spinal administration of opioids to patients with pain in palliative care, since such patients usually have been previously treated chronically with systemic opioids and will likely have become tolerant to such adverse effects. If present, these adverse effects are usually self-limiting or can be successfully managed by adjustment of the opioid dose.[1] During a period of dose reduction, these adverse effects, if severe, may be managed with small doses of naloxone, often without reversal of spinal opioid analgesia. In this setting, naloxone is best administered initially as an intravenous loading dose, given in 40 μg increments, followed by an intravenous infusion of approximately 1 to 5 μg/kg.h, titrated to effect.

Cephalad migration of morphine within the cerebrospinal fluid appears to explain the delayed respiratory depression (onset 3 to 20 h) that has been rarely reported following spinal morphine administration in opioid-naïve patients with acute pain.[14] Significant, delayed respiratory depression has not been reported when epidural fentanyl was the only opioid administered.[59] Even with spinal morphine, following appropriate patient selection,[1] respiratory depression is uncommon but is particularly rare in patients previously treated chronically with systemic opioids.[16] Thus, with appropriate patient selection, there appears to be a very low risk of respiratory depression with the use of spinal opioids, including morphine, as typically employed in palliative care.

Not all the effects of spinal opioids are antagonized by naloxone. Very high doses of subarachnoid morphine in rats may produce either convulsive seizures of the hind limbs or generalized intense motor rigidity that is not antagonized by naloxone; the mechanism is unknown, but may result from non-analgesic effects of spinal opioids.[19] Hyperaesthesia has been reported with high doses of spinal morphine in patients with cancer pain.[60,61] High doses of subarachnoid opioids have been reported to result in severe myoclonic jerks.[61,62] These motor and sensory effects of spinal opioids indicate the need for caution in the use of exceptionally high doses of spinal opioids.

Upon initiation of spinal opioid therapy, patients previously treated chronically with systemic opioids may experience an opioid withdrawal response, if opioid administration via the systemic route is suddenly ceased when pain relief is obtained from spinal opioids. Opioid withdrawal has been reported following initiation of either epidural morphine[63] or subarachnoid morphine[64,65] following systemic opioid therapy. Withdrawal symptoms may also develop if chronic epidural opioid administration is replaced with subarachnoid administration. Withdrawal symptoms in these settings, which seem to confirm some selective spinal analgesic action of spinally administered opioids, are readily managed with tapering doses of systemic opioids, while continuing to provide analgesia through spinal opioid administration.

Spinal local anaesthetic administration

When spinal opioid administration is associated with inadequate analgesia, either due to opioid tolerance or the extreme characteristics of the pain,[41,66] the addition of spinal local anaesthetic may significantly potentiate spinal opioid analgesia.[67,68] In addition to the obvious, immediate analgesic effect of neuraxial local anaesthetic conduction blockade, decreasing the nociceptive input to the spinal dorsal horns may decrease spinal mechanisms of hypersensitization. With carefully adjusted, low-dose epidural local anaesthetic administration,[32,69,70] it is generally possible to achieve good analgesia without significant impairment of motor or sensory function. This differential blockade of pain, rather than other sensory and motor function, is more readily obtained with epidural than subarachnoid local anaesthetic administration, and is one of the main clinical advantages of the epidural route of administration.

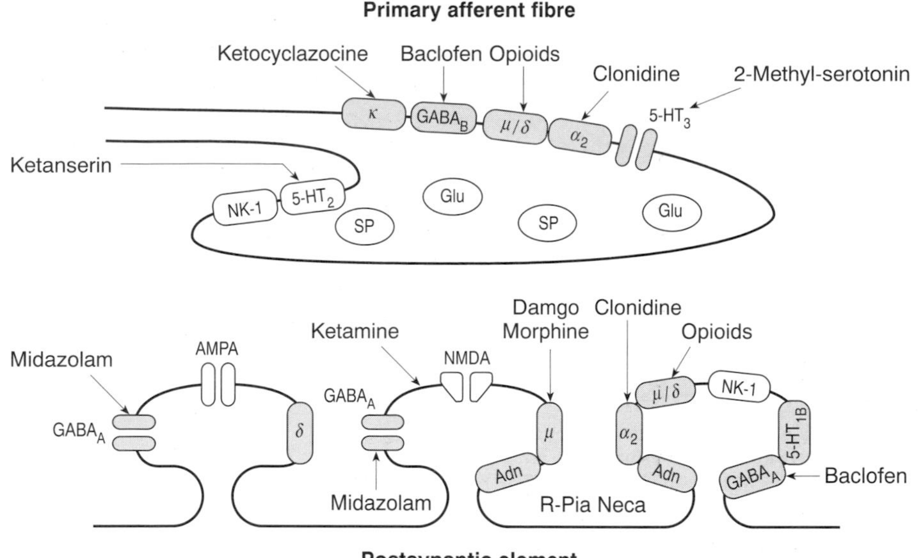

Fig. 3 Summary of neurotransmission from primary afferent sensory fibres to second-order spinal neurones (postsynaptic element) in the spinal dorsal horns. Neurotransmitters (open circles) include the excitatory amino-acid transmitters (i.e. glutamine = Glu) and neurokinins (i.e. substance P = SP). Activation of postsynaptic, excitatory amino-acid receptors (classified by their response to *N*-methyl-D-aspartate (NMDA) and α-amino-3-hydroxy-5-methyl-4-isoxazoleproprionic acid (AMPA)), as well as neurokinin receptors (NK-1), results in depolarization of the postsynaptic membrane. Excitatory receptors (open ovals) are also located presynaptically, where activation results in enhanced transmitter release (5-HT$_2$ = excitatory serotonin receptors). Activation of inhibitory receptors (filled ovals), located both pre- and postsynaptically, decreases the release and effectiveness of transmitters (κ, μ, δ, opioid; GABA, γ-aminobutyric acid; 5-HTβ, inhibitory serotonin receptor; α$_2$, α$_2$-adrenergic; Adn, Adenosine). The drugs shown affect pain transmission, at least experimentally, and are believed to be active at the sites indicated (arrows). (Reproduced with permission from Cousins MJ, Bridenbaugh PO, eds. *Neural Blockade in Clinical Anaesthesia and Management of Pain*. 3rd edn. Philadelphia: J. B. Lippincott, in press.)

However, subarachnoid local anaesthetic administration[56,58] has been used to good analgesic effect, without significant motor block, if doses of local anaesthetic are low (less than 30 mg/day subarachnoid bupivacaine). In extreme cases, continuous spinal anaesthesia, with dense blockade of sensory and motor function from higher doses of subarachnoid local anaesthetic, may be the only available means of providing adequate pain relief.[71,72]

Spinal local anaesthetic blockade has only a limited role in the diagnosis of chronic pain.[73] As with peripheral local anaesthetic blockade,[74] there is a poor correlation between the results of spinal local anaesthetic blockade and neurodestructive procedures. Spinal blockade may provide information regarding the spinal segmental level of pain, and be somewhat helpful in differentiating between peripheral nociceptive and central, deafferentation pain; however, central pain may temporarily respond to alterations in afferent input, and nociceptive and deafferentation pain may respond to systemically absorbed local anaesthetic.[75–77] These factors may confound attempts at interpreting patient response to nerve blocks and thereby limit the 'diagnostic' utility of such procedures in determining the aetiology of pain. Despite these limitations, occasional unfortunate attempts have been made to use patient response to local anaesthetic blocks to differentiate 'real' from 'psychogenic' pain. Spinal local anaesthetic blocks, or other anaesthetic techniques, have no utility in the diagnosis of rare psychiatric illness presenting as chronic pain.

Other spinal analgesics

One outgrowth of recent advances in understanding of the neurophysiology of nociception has been the recognition of the potential analgesic efficacy of the spinal administration of non-opioid drugs, acting at dorsal horn neurone receptors (Fig. 3). Non-opioid analgesics inhibiting different aspects of pain neurotransmission might be used synergistically with other agents, including opioids, to reduce the incidence of adverse effects. Such agents also might prove useful in the management of patients with pain resistant to opioid analgesics.[78] Agents affecting spinal neurotransmission have a potential for neurotoxicity, as described for spinal somatostatin administration.[79] Clearly, the analgesic efficacy, as well as systemic and local toxicity, of potential spinal analgesics must be evaluated carefully before clinical use.

Epidural butamben

Butamben (n-butyl-*p*-aminobenzoate) is a highly lipid soluble congener of the local anaesthetic benzocaine, that may eventually play an important role in palliative pain management. Although butamben is available from various chemical suppliers, suspensions appropriate for epidural administration are not currently commercially available. Due to its limited water solubility, injected butamben persists as a slowly-dissolving reservoir of local anaesthetic. Epidural administration of butamben has been described as an alternative to neurolytic blockade, in the management of intractable cancer pain. In the cases reported, patients with intractable pain despite systemic opioid[80] or epidural opioid with or without local anaesthetic,[81] received fair to complete pain relief. Although two to four epidural injections were generally required to obtain pain relief, analgesia then persisted for many days to weeks, often lasting until the patient's death.

Epidural butamben appears to be well tolerated. Despite a long duration of effect for pain relief, only brief periods of motor weakness, lasting less than 24 h, have been reported. One study in dogs described histopathological evidence of dorsal spinal nerve root degeneration following epidural butamben administration,[82] but another study found no such toxicity.[83] Human histopathological data is limited,[81,83] but suggests that epidural butamben is not neurotoxic, although small, focal areas of necrosis of the outer aspect of the dura have been reported.[82] Subarachnoid injection of butamben should be avoided, as this resulted in adhesive arachnoiditis in dogs.[83] In addition to epidural administration, butamben has been used for peripheral nerve block.[80]

Most published reports of epidural butamben administration describe a 10 per cent suspension, but some authors[84] have used a 5 per cent suspension due to difficulties with the 10 per cent suspensions. Descriptions of preparation techniques for butamben suspensions for epidural administration have been published,[80,85] but a commercial preparation (Abbott Laboratories) is under clinical trials, and may be available soon.

Spinal α-adrenergic agonists

α_2-Adrenergic agonists, including clonidine and dexmedetomidine, have received considerable attention as analgesic agents,[86,87] though clonidine has been used more extensively clinically. Systemic administration of these agents has been shown to have analgesic efficacy[88] and to potentiate the analgesic effects of opioids. Spinal administration of clonidine and dexmedetomidine has also been shown to have analgesic effect that is independent of,[89] and that potentiates,[90] opioid analgesia. The spinal analgesic effect appears to be mediated by the inhibitory effects of pre-and postsynaptic α_2-adrenergic receptor stimulation on the neurotransmission of primary afferent nociceptor projections onto second-order spinal neurones within the spinal dorsal horns.[91,92] Adverse effects, including sedation and hypotension, clearly limit the analgesic utility of systemically administered α_2-adrenergic agonists, and these adverse effects may also limit the effectiveness of these agents given via spinal routes of administration.[93-95] However, α_2 agonists have clear analgesic effect with limited cross tolerance with opioids,[96,97] and clonidine is without known neurotoxicity from spinal administration.[98] Although still in early clinical development, spinal clonidine, and perhaps other α_2 agonists, may come to have an important role in the management of opioid-tolerant[99] or opioid-resistant[44,100,101] pain.

Subarachnoid baclofen

The clinical management of severe spasticity, due to upper motor neurone lesions resulting from central nervous system injury or disease, is a challenging and complex undertaking.[102] Oral administration of baclofen, a γ-aminobutyric acid (GABA) analogue, is widely and successfully used to treat such spasticity. Baclofen binding at presynaptic ($GABA_B$) receptors on afferent neurones results in inhibition of calcium influx into presynaptic terminals, suppressing release of excitatory neurotransmitters. Perhaps through these presynaptic effects[103] or other mechanisms,[104] baclofen results in inhibition of monosynaptic and polysynaptic spinal motor reflexes, clinically observed as a reduction in spasticity. Other medications, including benzodiazepines, dantrolene, and spinal opioids,[53,105] are used in the management of spasticity, but baclofen has generally been found to be more effective with fewer adverse effects. Especially with higher doses of oral baclofen, sedation and other adverse effects may limit patient tolerance.

In patients with severe spasticity unresponsive to oral baclofen, or with intolerable adverse effects from this medication, subarachnoid administration of baclofen has been shown to be a useful management technique.[103] Baclofen is hydrophilic and has low blood–brain barrier permeability. As a result, subarachnoid administration of baclofen results in significantly higher spinal fluid baclofen concentrations than does oral administration, even though clinical subarachnoid baclofen doses are 100 to 1000 times less than oral doses.[106] With each patient, the effectiveness of subarachnoid baclofen is generally evaluated through trial bolus subarachnoid administration before proceeding with chronic administration. Chronic administration is achieved with implanted systems, either a manually-activated pump,[107] or a computer-controlled infusion pump.[103] These implanted systems are the same as may be used for subarachnoid opioid administration. Although highly reliable, the cost and technical complexity of these systems is considerable (see technical considerations below).

Several studies of patients with spinal spasticity resistant to oral baclofen have documented beneficial reduction of spasticity with subarachnoid baclofen,[108,109] but this technique also appears to have utility in the management of spasticity due to brain injury,[110] and perhaps also in the management of post-stroke central pain syndromes.[111] Although there have been no human histopathological evaluations of subarachnoid baclofen, animal studies have not documented neurotoxicity.[112] Human clinical studies, with several years follow-up, indicate that this therapy is reasonably well tolerated.[103,113]

As with other invasive techniques, subarachnoid baclofen must be used with caution and is best reserved for those familiar with its use and the management of potential complications. Finding the appropriate dose of subarachnoid baclofen is critical and may require frequent adjustment: too little drug could lead to the erroneous conclusion of ineffectiveness, while an excessive dose may result in generalized muscle weakness or hypotonia.[114] Accidental overdose may result in respiratory arrest through generalized weakness and/or central nervous system depression. When patients who have received an accidental overdose have been appropriately supported, including temporary mechanical ventilation, no long-term complications have been reported.[115]

Experimental spinal analgesics

Spinal cholinergic agonists

Subarachnoid injection of cholinergic agonists has produced dose-dependent antinociception in experimental animals[116] and healthy human volunteers.[117] Subarachnoid administration of cholinergic agonists, together with α_2-adrenergic or opioid analgesics, also results in potentiation of α_2-adrenergic-mediated and opioid-mediated analgesia,[118] and counteracts α_2-adrenergic-induced hypotension.[119] One experimental technique of enhancing spinal cholinergic effects has been the subarachnoid administration of the acetylcholinesterase-inhibitor neostigmine. Subarachnoid neostigmine has been studied in experimental animals and was shown to produce significant antinociception without evidence of neurotoxicity.[120,121] Following appropriate neurotoxicology studies,[122] preliminary human trials have been conducted, showing significant analgesic effect of subarachnoid neostigmine, although this was associated with significant nausea and vomiting, and lower extremity weakness.[117] Further clinical trials with neostigmine, and animal studies with various cholinergic agonists may elucidate a significant analgesic role for spinal cholinergic agonists either alone or in combination with other analgesic agents.[123]

Dextromethorphan

Dextromethorphan, the dextro-isomer of the codeine analogue of levorphanol, is commonly used as a cough suppressant but had been thought to have little analgesic effect following systemic administration. Recent data indicates that dextromethorphan has an *N*-methyl-D-aspartate (NMDA) receptor antagonist activity.[124,125] In experimental animals, subarachnoid[126] and systemic[127] dextromethorphan has an antinociceptive effect consistent with the proposed NMDA receptor antagonism. In a human experimental model of acute pain, oral dextromethorphan reduced temporal summation of second pain ('wind-up'),[128] but in a clinical trial involving patients with various types of neuropathic pain, equivalent or higher doses of oral dextromethorphan did not provide significant analgesia.[129] Higher doses of systemic dextromethorphan may be associated with systemic adverse effects (drowsiness, nausea)[129] and, although rare, there does appear to be some potential for abuse.[130] Although there have been no clinical trials to date, it may be that spinal administration of dextromethorphan may serve to potentiate the analgesic efficacy, and decrease the tolerance to, traditional spinal or systemic opioid analgesics.[126]

Calcitonin

Calcitonin, the parafollicular thyroid hormone which acts peripherally to control serum calcium concentration by limiting bone resorption, also has analgesic efficacy. While its systemic effect on bone metabolism may contribute to its analgesic action in patients with Paget's disease of bone, and in patients with diffuse bony metastases, calcitonin also exists in the central nervous system and subarachnoid administration of calcitonin has an antinociceptive effect.[131,132] The central nervous system mechanism of calcitonin antinociception is unknown, but does not appear to be directly mediated through opioid receptors.[133,134] Spinal administration of calcitonin has been used in humans for relief of acute[135] and chronic[136] pain, but may be associated with significant adverse effects, including nausea and vomiting. Furthermore, animal data suggests that spinal calcitonin may be associated with significant toxicity.[137] Pending further animal trials regarding toxicity and efficacy, the spinal administration of calcitonin for pain management should be considered experimental (see Chapter 9.2.5).

Calcium-channel blocking agents

Voltage-sensitive calcium channels (VSCC) in the neurone cell membrane play a key role in neuronal function. In response to neuronal membrane depolarization, VSCC open and selectively allow entry of Ca^{2+} into the cell, where the increasing Ca^{2+} concentration triggers a wide variety of intracellular responses. VSCC translate neurone surface-membrane electrical activity into intracellular chemical signals.[138] Different types of VSCC have been characterized, depending on their selective response to medications (i.e. L-type VSCC blocked by nifedipine, nimodipine) or toxins. N-type VSCC are selectively blocked by polypeptide toxins from marine *Conus* snails (ω-conopeptides).

N-type VSCC appear to be important in nociceptive transmission. Release of neurotransmitter from the presynaptic nerve terminal is, in part, triggered by an increase in intracellular calcium, some of which results from influx of calcium via N-type VSCC. Some of the effect of opioid analgesics appears to be due to indirect inhibition of N-type VSCC.[139] This indirect (G-protein mediated) opioid inhibition of N-type VSCC, results in decreased intracellular Ca^{2+} and decreased release of neurotransmitter from the presynaptic nerve terminal.

Agents that directly and selectively block (inhibit) N-type VSCC may have utility as analgesics. Subarachnoid administration of synthetic ω-conopeptides (SNX-111, SNX-239) produces an antinociceptive effect in standard rat models of nociception.[140] No tolerance developed to the antinociceptive effect of chronically infused ω-conopeptide, compared with the virtually complete tolerance observed with chronic subarachnoid morphine infusion.[141] This lack of tolerance suggests that antinociceptive agents acting directly at VSCC regulating neurotransmitter release may offer some benefit over indirect-acting (membrane-bound, G-protein mediated) opioid analgesics.

N-type VSCC inhibitors (ω-conopeptides) promise to be useful in further studies of nociception and may lead to a useful alteration in clinical pain management. VSCC are widespread in the central nervous system and it remains to be determined whether or not a calcium-channel blocker can be found with appropriate selectivity, and other requisite characteristics of a clinically useful analgesic. An initial clinical trial of subarachnoid infusion of SNX-111 in terminal cancer patients with intractable pain suggests that this is a potent analgesic worthy of further investigation.[142]

Technical considerations in long-term spinal analgesia

Various technical considerations may be as important to the successful application of spinal analgesic therapy as the theoretical and clinical factors discussed above. In practice, long-term spinal analgesia requires catheter access to the subarachnoid or epidural space: the catheter may be a simple, percutaneous catheter for intermittent injection via a syringe or part of a totally implanted, computer-controlled infusion pump system. No one spinal administration system is appropriate for all clinical settings, but any spinal system may be associated with complications such as infection, catheter dislodgement, or other technical failure, which must be properly assessed and managed. Before beginning with spinal analgesia for long-term use, it is essential to ensure that appropriate nursing and social support will be available to assist with the management of the patient and spinal analgesia system.

The simplest means of providing long-term spinal analgesia is with a percutaneous epidural catheter, as may be typically used for surgical anaesthesia or acute pain management. Percutaneous epidural catheters can be used for long periods of time (months)[143] and, with careful observation and technique, have a reasonably low risk of infection. For long-term use, totally implanted subcutaneous epidural catheters attached to a subcutaneous injection portal (Fig. 4) may be preferable, as these devices are less likely to become dislodged and may have a lower infection rate than simple percutaneous catheters.[144] Implanted under local anaesthesia,[54] these epidural catheter injection portal systems have been used extensively in various settings[17] and are reliable for use with either intermittent bolus analgesic administration or continuous infusion via an external infusion pump. An alternative to the epidural portal

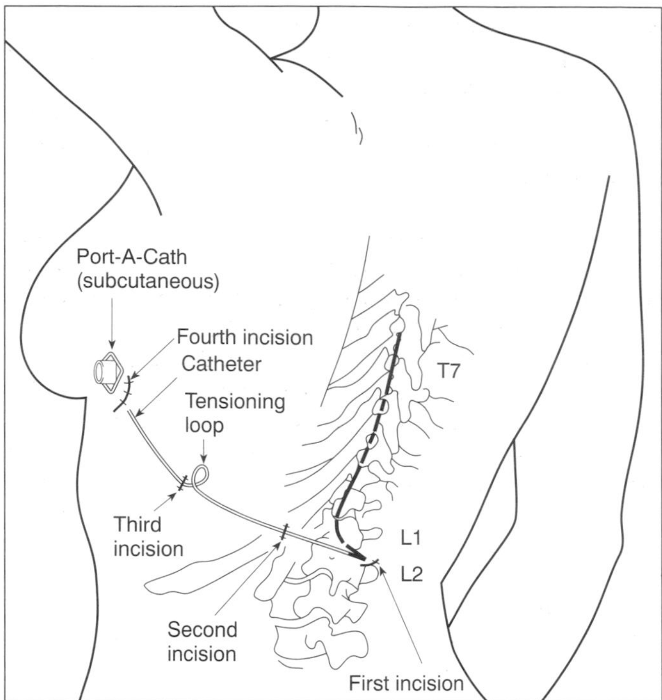

Fig. 4 Epidural catheter tunnelled subcutaneously to an implanted injection portal (Port-A-Cath, Pharamacia) for chronic epidural access. (Reproduced with permission from Cousins MJ and Bridenbaugh PO, eds. *Neural Blockade in Clinical Anesthesia and Management of Pain*. 2nd edn. Philadelphia: J. B. Lippincott, 1988.)

system is a modified percutaneous epidural catheter.[145] Adapted from Hickman and Broviac venous catheter technology, these catheters function well and also have a low infection rate.[146]

Infusion pumps are a significant cost factor in spinal analgesia. Ranging in cost and sophistication from totally implanted, computer-controlled, programmable pumps to simple, externally applied mechanical syringe-drivers, all infusion systems are more expensive than intermittent bolus dosing, with needle and syringe, into a percutaneous catheter or subcutaneous injection portal. Short-acting agents, such as fentanyl or local anaesthetics, may be best used with continuous infusion, but long-acting agents, such as morphine, may be given either as a bolus or infusion. In a prospective, randomized comparison of repeated bolus doses versus continuous infusion of epidural morphine, no difference in adequacy of pain relief was observed.[147] Patients receiving epidural morphine infusion did have a slight, but statistically significantly higher degree of dose escalation than patients receiving bolus doses (Fig. 5). In view of the lower cost and lower dose escalation, bolus morphine administration may be preferable to continuous infusion in some clinical settings.

One factor which may limit the long-term efficacy of epidural analgesia is the potential for formation of a sheath of fibrous scar tissue around the catheter, within the epidural space.[37–39,148] The formation of this sheath of scar tissue, or epidural fibrosis, is a variable process that appears to be clinically significant in a minority of patients, but may develop within 2 weeks of epidural catheter placement. Epidural fibrosis limits the spread of analgesic solution within the epidural space and may result in pain on injection. Lack of good epidural spread of analgesic solution may also result in loss of analgesic efficacy.[40] Management of epidural fibrosis requires repositioning the catheter within the epidural space or replacing the epidural catheter with a subarachnoid catheter.

Some centres routinely use subarachnoid, rather than epidural, delivery systems because subarachnoid administration results in more efficient delivery of analgesics to the cerebral spinal fluid and avoids the problem of epidural fibrosis.[149,150] Histopathological studies in animals[30] and humans,[151] together with extensive clinical experience, point to the apparent lack of neurotoxicity from long-term subarachnoid opioid and/or local anaesthetic infusions. The primary concern with simple percutaneous subarachnoid catheters and implanted portals attached to subarachnoid catheters is the risk of fulminant bacterial meningitis, which may prove fatal.[152,153] By strict attention to techniques limiting opportunities for contamination of subarachnoid percutaneous catheter systems, including limiting the frequency of infusion pump refills and catheter dressing changes, reasonably low rates of infection have been reported recently.[56,58,66]

In order to minimize the risk of meningitis from the spread of cutaneous organisms to the subarachnoid catheter, a totally implanted delivery system, with a subcutaneous infusion pump, may be the best option for long-term subarachnoid analgesia.[57,154] The main drawbacks to the use of these pumps are their high cost (US$10 000 plus costs of implantation and maintenance) together with the technical complexity of programming these computer-controlled devices. Some of the initial high cost of implanted pumps may be balanced by the potentially lower long-term drug costs with subarachnoid administration due to the remarkable efficiency of subarachnoid opioids compared with systemic or epidural routes of administration. The same pumps may be used for subarachnoid baclofen administration for control of spasticity.[103] These implantable pumps have an analgesic solution reservoir which can be refilled percutaneously via a built in

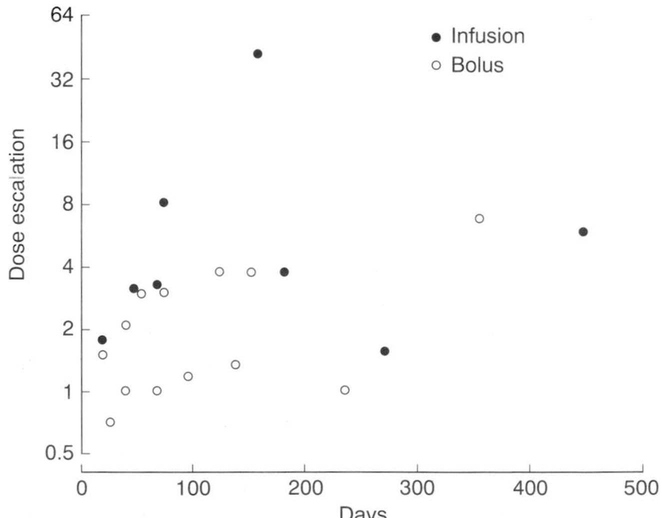

Fig. 5 Epidural infusion ('infusaid') versus repeated doses (via 'portal') of opioid. Dose escalation (measured as the ratio of the maximum morphine dose to the initial, stabilized dose) was slightly, but significantly, greater in patients with cancer pain receiving epidural morphine by infusion (closed circles) compared with those receiving epidural morphine by repeated bolus doses (open circles). (Reproduced with permission from Gourlay, *et al.*[147])

injection portal. When used for opioid or baclofen infusion, typically the pumps require filling approximately once a month.

The small size of the medication reservoir in implanted pumps (18 ml, SynchroMed infusion pump, Medtronic) limits the utility of these devices for subarachnoid local anaesthetic administration, at least using standard, commercially available solutions of local anaesthetic (i.e. bupivacaine 0.5 per cent or 0.75 per cent), due to the need to refill the reservoir too frequently. Clearly, the advantage of a totally implanted system regarding lower risk of infection may be lost if the device is accessed frequently. Suitable alternatives may be the use of highly concentrated lignocaine preparations (10 to 20 per cent, marketed for the preparation of intravenous infusions for cardiac arrhythmias), or powdered tetracaine. Unfortunately, no published clinical trials have documented the utility of these agents for chronic subarachnoid infusion. Some authors have chosen to bypass the limitation of reservoir size and the high cost of implantable pumps by using simple, tunnelled percutaneous subarachnoid catheters (with specific, careful attention to technical details to minimize the risk of infection), especially when it is anticipated that higher-volume, local anaesthetic-containing solutions will be required.[56,58]

Infections of epidural catheters (simple percutaneous catheters, modified percutaneous catheters, and epidural portals) are generally limited to the skin entry site, subcutaneous catheter, or injection portal.[17] Although meningitis is an extremely rare complication following epidural analgesia,[38,155] infections of epidural systems should be treated aggressively (immediate, complete removal of the epidural catheter system, initiation of appropriate bacterial cultures, followed by antibiotic therapy) to avoid epidural abscess. When infections are treated aggressively, epidural abscess is rare, but failure to remove the infected system may result in neurological compromise of the patient.[156] In contrast to the management of epidural catheter infections, meningitis associated with implanted subarachnoid infusion pumps has been successfully treated, after taking appropriate cultures, with subarachnoid infusion of antibiotics via the implanted infusion pump,[157,158] without pump removal. If the meningitis does not resolve promptly and permanently with antibiotic therapy, the pump (foreign body) should be removed.

The spinal segmental level of the catheter tip can be an important factor in the success of spinal analgesia. It is essential that spinal local anaesthetics be administered as close as possible to the spinal segmental level of innervation to the painful area. When spinal administration of hydrophilic opioid (i.e. morphine) is planned, a lumbar level of catheter spinal placement is often used regardless of the segmental level of pain, due to the technical ease of placing spinal catheters at the lumbar level and the potential for hydrophilic opioid to be dispersed to higher spinal segments by the circulation of cerebral spinal fluid.[1] Lumbar spinal administration of hydrophilic compounds does result in subarachnoid dispersion of compound to higher spinal levels, but the highest concentrations are found at the level of drug administration and there is a marked decline in drug concentration at more cephalad spinal segments.[26,33,159] Placement of catheters in close proximity to the spinal segmental level of pain may be advantageous, even for administration of hydrophilic opioid. On the other hand, experimental animals with chronic subarachnoid catheters had, on histopathological examination, mild deformation and local demyelination where the catheter was in contact with the spinal cord.[30] This complication was not seen in a post mortem study of cancer patients with subarachnoid analgesia,[151] but the animal data does suggest the need for caution in selecting long-term subarachnoid catheterization at a spinal level overlying the spinal cord, especially for benign conditions.

To avoid potential complications from the spinal administration of possibly neurotoxic preservatives, only preservative-free drug preparations are recommended for spinal administration. Suitable preparations of morphine, other opioids,[36] and local anaesthetics are widely available for either epidural or subarachnoid use, but the specific solutions to be used should be carefully evaluated to avoid unintentional administration of solutions with neurotoxic additives.[160] Where required formulations are not commercially available, a hospital pharmacy may be able to prepare drug solutions suitable for chronic spinal administration. An alternative, though perhaps less desirable approach, is to use carefully selected, commercially available solutions containing low concentrations of those preservatives or antioxidants felt to have little or no potential for neurotoxicity,[151,160] although this practice is controversial.[161] Spinal administration of solutions containing phenols and alcohols must be avoided except in the controlled setting of intentional neurolytic blockade.[159,162]

Malfunctions in spinal delivery systems can result in the deterioration of previously acceptable analgesia. Loss of analgesia may be gradual in onset (as with the development of epidural fibrosis, described above), or may be abrupt (infusion pump malfunction). Patients may report uncontrolled pain and/or symptoms of opioid withdrawal. Accurate functioning of infusion devices, implanted or external, must be verified. Epidurography, the injection of contrast medium via an in-dwelling epidural catheter, has been used to verify adequate epidural spread of the injected solution.[38,145] Similarly, myelography may be used to verify subarachnoid spread of contrast medium injected through subarachnoid catheters. Plain radiographs may be used to evaluate the structural integrity of spinal analgesic delivery systems.

When spinal analgesia systems malfunction, are removed to manage infectious complications, or must otherwise be discontinued, the patient is likely to require systemic opioid analgesics for pain relief and prevention of withdrawal symptoms. Management of pain, in this setting, with systemic opioids may prove to be unsatisfactory since, generally, inadequate analgesia from systemic medication will have been the primary indication for the initiation of spinal analgesia. If an epidural catheter has malfunctioned due to epidural fibrosis (documented by epidurogram or clinically diagnosed based on decreased analgesic efficacy and pain on injection), it is likely that the patient's pain can be managed equally well with systemic opioid at the same rate of administration (the epidural fibrosis prevents spinal absorption of injected analgesic, and the medication may have been absorbed systemically from the perivertebral tissues). If the epidural system has been functioning well, and delivering analgesics to the epidural space efficiently, simply administering similar doses of opioid systemically is likely to be insufficient; however, systemic administration of prior epidural doses of opioid may at least prevent withdrawal symptoms while other analgesic measures are put into place. As a general rule, subarachnoid morphine doses are approximately 10 per cent of epidural doses, and as low as 2 per cent to 3 per cent of systemic

Table 2 Equivalent morphine dose by administration route

Administration route	Morphine dose approximate	Dosing interval
Oral	300 mg	4 h
Intravenous	100 mg	4 h
Epidural	10 mg	6–8 h
Subarachnoid	1 mg	12–24 h

Doses are approximate and must be applied to individual patients with caution and close observation. In general, these ratios do not apply to other opioids.

The conversion factors, based on systemic pharmacokinetics, commonly used to estimate equipotent doses of various opioids for systemic administration will not predict equipotency of opioid doses for spinal administration due to variations in spinal pharmacokinetics between different opioids.

(parenteral) doses, but these are estimates only and must be used cautiously to prevent significant under or over-dosing of patients (Table 2). When spinal administration of local anaesthetic has been previously added due to lack of efficacy of spinal opioid alone, it is especially unlikely that systemic opioid will provide reasonable analgesia should the spinal delivery system fail: additional anaesthetic or neurosurgical techniques for pain management (see below) are likely to be necessary. An intravenous or subcutaneous infusion of low-dose ketamine, the NMDA-receptor antagonist analgesic/anaesthetic, may be utilized to temporarily control otherwise intractable pain while other measures are initiated. Ketamine administration may be associated with dysphoric hallucinations, which may necessitate coadministration of a benzodiazepine. The incidence of psychotomimetic adverse effects is dose-related, and recent studies describe good analgesic effect from low-dose infusions of ketamine (0.1–0.2 mg/kg per h) without significant dysphoria.[163]

The patient's ability to participate in his own care, whether the patient requires inpatient treatment, and the availability of family and/or nursing support may be overriding factors in decisions regarding spinal opioid therapy. Once implanted and the dose adjusted, systems using implanted subcutaneous infusion pumps have the advantage of only requiring attention for pump refill every few weeks, but refills require physician or skilled nursing personnel. Percutaneous catheters or implanted injection portal systems may be managed readily by the majority of patients and/or family members, but do require bolus dosing two to four times daily.[17] Recently, the successful initiation of spinal analgesia in patients at home has been described.[164] Adequate availability of skilled nursing assistance is essential to the successful application of spinal analgesia,[165] and can be accomplished through intermittent office evaluations, home visits, or inpatient treatment, depending on other aspects of the patient's care requirements.

Management of pain resistant to spinal analgesics

The management of pain resistant to spinal analgesia must begin with a thorough re-evaluation of the aetiology of the pain, with special attention to the possible progression of the underlying disease, malfunction of the spinal analgesia delivery system, and the development of neuropathic rather than purely nociceptive pain. Exacerbation of cancer pain may often be related to tumour progression,[55] and further antitumour therapy, if possible, may be of analgesic benefit. The development of neuropathic pain may arise from disease progression or therapy resulting in nerve injury or involvement. In addition to spinal opioids, tricyclic antidepressants and antiseizure medications, as well as mexiletine[166] or systemic local anaesthetic infusions,[75,77,167] may be useful in neuropathic pain management. Exacerbations of pain in non-malignant disease may also indicate the need for further disease-specific therapy (e.g. ischaemic pain from atherosclerosis and pain of infection in AIDS).

The management of severe pain not controlled by spinal analgesics and adjuvant drugs may well require the application of techniques directed against other aspects of the neural transmission of pain. As described below, intraventricular opioid, spinal neurolytic block, blockade of peripheral nerves or sympathetic ganglia, either separately or in combination with other manoeuvres, may be necessary in the management of selected patients with otherwise intractable pain.

Intraventricular opioid administration

Techniques similar to those used for spinal opioid administration have been used to provide opioid analgesia through the administration of opioid directly into the cerebral ventricles. There are several clinical reports of patients with severe, intractable cancer pain in whom intraventricular opioid therapy provided good to excellent analgesia,[168–170] although few studies have defined the role of this technique.[171] The proportion of patients in palliative care for whom intraventricular opioid therapy is necessary and appropriate is exceedingly small, yet for those few patients with otherwise intractable pain, this is an important and useful analgesic technique.

Spinal and intraventricular opioid administrations are similar, in that these techniques provide analgesia through enhanced delivery of opioid to both spinal and brain receptors,[33,172] yet intraventricular opioid administration results in much higher ventricular cerebrospinal fluid concentrations of opioid than lumbar cerebrospinal fluid concentrations.[173] Indications for intraventricular opioid therapy include intractable pain (usually cancer-related pain) resistant to systemic opioid and adjuvant therapy in terminally ill patients, who also have:

(1) inadequate analgesia through less complicated techniques;[99]

(2) inaccessible spinal epidural and subarachnoid spaces;

(3) known spinal obstruction to the circulation of cerebrospinal fluid; and/or

(4) intractable head and neck pain.[170,174]

Techniques have included intermittent injection of opioid into a subcutaneously implanted portal system, as well as the use of implanted infusion pumps.[175]

Neurolytic blockade of the central nervous system

General consideration for neurolytic blockade

In general, neurolytic blocks are suitable for patients with short life expectancy and well-localized nociceptive pain that has proven difficult to control with other measures.[176] Systemic or spinal analgesics (opioid) may be more efficacious than localized, neurolytic blockade in patients with widespread pain. Deafferentation (neurogenic) pain responds poorly, if at all, to neurolytic procedures. Somatic neurolytic blocks may in fact result in sufficient denervation to result in deafferentation pain, but incomplete neural destruction by neurolytic block may also produce a neuralgic type of pain. Such neuropathic pain may be a sequela in as many as 14 to 30 per cent of patients undergoing peripheral neurolytic block,[177] as compared to only 1 to 3 per cent of patients undergoing subarachnoid neurolysis.[178] Neuropathic pains following attempts at neurolysis are most appropriately treated with transcutaneous electrical nerve stimulation, centrally acting drugs, or, less commonly, spinal cord stimulation,[179,180] rather than further attempts at neurolysis. Appropriate injections of suspensions of the long-acting local anaesthetic butamben (see above) may prove to be a valuable alternative to neurolytic block, as is spinal administration of opioid and/or non-opioid analgesics (see above).

Prior to attempting pain relief through neurolytic blockade, a similar local anaesthetic block may be of prognostic value, regarding both the degree of pain relief and potential complications associated with the proposed neurolytic block.[181] Unfortunately, local anaesthetic blocks are not entirely predictive of the results of neurolytic block; systemically absorbed local anaesthetic, analgesic and sedative medications given during the nerve-block procedure, spread of local anaesthetic to adjacent neural structures, neural plasticity effects, and placebo response may all variably contribute to the temporary success of local anaesthetic blocks. Furthermore, in terminally ill patients with severe pain, the combination of a prognostic local anaesthetic block, followed by neurolysis, may exceed the patient's willingness or ability to undergo medical procedures. In such cases, if at least significant partial pain relief is likely to be achieved through neurolysis, it may be reasonable to omit the prognostic block and proceed directly to the neurolytic procedure.

The neurolytic agents in most frequent clinical use are ethyl alcohol (ethanol) and phenol.[182] Glycerol is also used for trigeminal ganglion block, where it appears to have unique advantages in the management of trigeminal neuralgia. Phenol has local anaesthetic, as well as neurolytic effects, resulting in near painless injection. Large systemic doses of phenol, or accidental intravascular injection, may cause convulsions, followed by central nervous system depression and cardiovascular collapse. Clinical doses of phenol are unlikely to cause systemic toxicity,[180] but should be limited to 1 to 10 ml of 6 to 10 per cent solution for peripheral or sympathetic blocks, or 1 to 3 ml for subarachnoid injection. Similarly, as used for neurolytic alcohol block, there are few significant adverse effects from the systemic absorption of the ethanol injected.[183] There are few comparative data on which to base a choice of neurolytic agent.

Prior to considering neurolytic blockade, it is essential that as thorough an evaluation, as is reasonably possible, be carried out to accurately determine the aetiology of the pain. Especially when considering neuraxial neurolysis for management of cancer pain, radiographic evaluation should be carried out (if possible) to determine the extent of spinal spread of tumour. Needle trauma to spinal or epidural tumour poses a risk of bleeding that may result in spinal cord compression and neurological deficit. In addition, tumour distortion of the spinal spaces may lead to an unpredictable, unacceptable spread of neurolytic solution.

Table 3 Results of subarachnoid block with alcohol

Author	Number of cases	Percentage results: Good	Fair	Poor
Dogliotti[186]	150	50	25	16
Greenhill[187]	> 100	60	10	30
Hay[188]	252	46	32	22
Kuzucu[189]	322	58.2	26.1	15.7
Combined series				
Drechsel[185]	1908	60	21	19

(Data from original articles and ref. 184.)

Subarachnoid neurolytic block

The subarachnoid injection of a neurolytic agent is an effective method of pain control, which ideally should be restricted to patients with advanced malignancy, in whom the pain is limited in extent to a few spinal segments. The aim is to produce a chemical posterior rhizotomy, thereby interrupting the pain pathways from the affected area.[184] Subarachnoid neurolytic blocks are best used for bilateral saddle (perineal) pain in patients with colostomy and permanent bladder catheter, or in relatively localized (unilateral) somatic pain of the chest wall or trunk.[185] It should be used with great caution when the pain is widespread, or when the pain is of undiagnosed aetiology, even when the patient is known to have malignant disease. Particular care must be taken to avoid increasing the patient's disability through motor weakness, sphincteric incompetence, and loss of position sense. In limb pain, use of subarachnoid neurolytic block is seldom justified, in view of the risk of producing an insensate, immobile extremity.[180]

An assessment of the reported results of neurolytic blockade is limited by the subjective nature of the patient's response, the generally progressive nature of the underlying pain problem, and the variability of inclusion criteria and duration of follow up, in the reported series. In the hands of skilled experts, the results of phenol and alcohol subarachnoid block are probably similar, with good results in approximately 60 per cent of patients. In Table 3, 'good' means complete relief of pain for more than 1 month; 'fair' means complete relief of pain for less than 1 month, or reduction of pain for more than 1 month; 'poor' means relief for several days or no relief. Some patients may obtain pain relief for up to 12 months.[180] Provided that the selection of patients is appropriate and the technique is meticulous, complication rates are reported to be in the range of 1 to 14 per cent. These complications may be an acceptable 'price' for some patients. For example, if a bladder catheter is in use, bladder incontinence may be of no consequence;

however, ambulatory patients will almost never accept incontinence as a complication even if pain relief by alternative methods is inferior.

In rare, extreme cases of lower body and/or lower extremity pain, generally in bed-bound, terminally ill patients with advanced cancer, usually with significant nerve root or spinal cord tumour involvement, the typically described techniques of neuraxial neurolysis may be insufficient. The management of such situations is always complex and must be designed for each individual, but chemical transection of the spinal cord at the upper lumbar or lower thoracic dermatomal level may be a reasonable alternative to terminal sedation (see below) or continuous local anaesthetic spinal anaesthesia (see above). As the intent of chemical cord transection is fundamentally different than the more selective techniques of spinal neurolysis, much larger volumes (3–5 ml) of neurolytic solution are utilized. Depending on the baricity of the neurolytic solution compared with cerebrospinal fluid, appropriate patient position must be used to prevent unwanted spread of the large volume of neurolytic solution. In general, with hypobaric solutions (ethanol), the patient must be kept in a head-down recumbent position with elevation of the (painful) lower body ('Trendelenburg's position'). With hyperbaric solutions (phenol), a head-up, recumbent position should be used with the (painful) lower body in a dependent position ('reverse Trendelenburg's position'). It is essential that all those involved understand the implications of chemical cord transection: the goal of this intervention is the destruction of spinal cord function below the mid-thoracic level. Despite the extreme degree of this neurolytic procedure, its use in the appropriate setting may offer high quality relief of otherwise intractable pain.

Epidural and subdural neurolytic blockade

Pain within the cervical segments may be difficult to relieve with subarachnoid neurolytic block, due to the rapid dilution of neurolytic solution by the faster rate of cerebrospinal fluid circulation in the neck.[180] Similarly, cerebrospinal fluid circulation may cause neurolytic solution to spread in an undesirable manner to adjacent neural structures. Epidural and subdural injections may have an advantage in cervical and upper thoracic neurolytic block as solutions are placed outside the cerebrospinal-fluid-containing subarachnoid space and are therefore not so affected by cerebrospinal fluid circulation, as with subarachnoid block.

In addition to using epidural neurolytic block for cervical and upper thoracic blockade, epidural neurolysis has also been used at the lower thoracic level (for upper abdominal pain)[190] and at the lumbar level. Although the duration and intensity of pain relief may be less with epidural phenol than with subarachnoid neurolysis, these problems have been reported to be overcome by carrying out a short (daily) series of epidural phenol injections via a chemically-resistant percutaneous epidural catheter.[191] The potential advantage of epidural phenol neurolysis may be a lower incidence of complications, such as motor weakness, than with subarachnoid neurolysis, though comparative trials are not available. Epidural butamben may become an attractive alternative to epidural neurolysis.

The subdural space is a potential space between the dura and the arachnoid: injection of fluid into the space converts this potential space into an actual space that may extend cranially to the foramen magnum and caudally to the level of termination of the dura at S2. The subdural space is wider in the cervical region and thus easier to enter there than at other spinal levels.[180] Cervical neurolytic subdural block has been reported to be useful for pain due to neoplastic disease of the ear, nose, and throat, as well as by other tumours encroaching on the cervical region, such as in Pancoast's syndrome and cervical vertebral metastases. The safety, efficacy, and utility of epidural and subdural neurolytic blockade has not been studied in comparative trials.

Although most problems of spasticity due to central nervous system disease may be managed medically, or with spinal baclofen (see below), there appears to be a role for subarachnoid[192–194] and epidural[191] neurolytic block in the palliative management of intractable spasticity.[195] In some patients, spasticity may be of a severity that even routine nursing and hygiene manoeuvres become nearly impossible, and flaccid paralysis through neurolytic block may be desirable. Relief of severe spasticity may be necessary to provide an opportunity for closure or healing of decubitus ulcers.[196]

Neurolytic trigeminal nerve block

Neurolytic block of the trigeminal nerve and its branches has been used effectively in the management of chronic pain. Maxillary and mandibular nerve blocks are particularly useful in controlling pain of malignant origin arising from structures that these nerves supply. In the past, injection of the trigeminal (Gasserian) ganglion with alcohol was widely used in the treatment of trigeminal neuralgia, but medical treatment with carbamazepine and other methods, such as glycerol injection,[197] surgical rhizotomy, and thermogangliolysis, have largely superseded this technique. Trigeminal ganglion blockade is usually achieved via the foramen ovale, using fluoroscopic control.[198] The utility of glycerol trigeminal neurolysis in the management of cancer-related pain is unclear. Studies comparing trigeminal neurolysis with spinal opioid administration or other therapies for management of intractable facial pain of malignant origin have not been published.

Spinal cord stimulation

In spinal cord stimulation, stimulating electrodes are implanted in the epidural space, overlying the posterior aspect of the spinal cord, at a dermatomal level corresponding to the site of pain. Adjustable electrical stimulation is provided by either a totally implanted battery and pulse generator or an external battery and pulse generator electromagnetically linked to the implanted stimulating electrodes.[179] Spinal cord stimulation is perceived by the patient as a mild, tingling paraesthesia in the area of pain. This paraesthesia, in the appropriate clinical setting, may be associated with significant pain relief. As with the related electrical neurostimulation techniques of transcutaneous electrical nerve stimulation (**TENS**) and deep brain stimulation, the analgesic mechanism of action of spinal cord stimulation has not been fully elucidated. Spinal cord stimulation analgesia is thought to result from interruption of nociceptive afferents through activation of non-nociceptive afferents, as predicted in the gate control theory.[199]

The main drawbacks to spinal cord stimulation include high cost and difficulty in predicting which patients, with appropriate pain problems, will gain lasting benefits. Spinal cord stimulation systems cost US$ 6000 to 18 000, not including the costs and fees associated with implantation. Implantation of a permanent spinal cord stimulation system is preceded by a temporary trial of spinal cord stimulation. This temporary trial adds to the cost of spinal cord stimulation, but is helpful in determining the potential analgesic benefit of spinal cord stimulation for a given patient. Even when a permanent spinal cord stimulation implantation is predicated on satisfactory results of a trial period, good, long-term analgesic efficacy may be experienced in only 20 to 80 per cent of patients.[179] Such analgesic failures may be due to various technical difficulties, placebo response during initial trial, development of tolerance to spinal cord stimulation, or progression of underlying pathology. If programmable arrays of multiple electrodes are used,[200] the loss of appropriate distribution of stimulation paraesthesia due to electrode migration may be overcome by using alternate combinations of electrodes. Spinal cord stimulation has been used in many clinical settings, including chronic back and/or leg pain following lumbar surgery ('failed back syndrome'),[201] various neuropathic conditions (reflex sympathetic dystrophy),[202] postherpetic neuralgia,[203] intractable angina,[204] and (with limited success) spasticity.[102] Unfortunately, there are no controlled trials comparing spinal cord stimulation with other therapies in any of these conditions.

An example of one controversial use of spinal cord stimulation is in the management of patients with severe, inoperable peripheral vascular disease. This clearly is a matter of palliative care, as these patients are generally elderly, have systemic atherosclerosis and/or other advanced disease, severe ischaemic pain with chronic ulceration, and perhaps face impending lower extremity amputation. The use of spinal cord stimulation in this setting has been reported to result in decreased pain and improved functioning[205-207] with a possible limb-saving effect.[205] The benefits of spinal cord stimulation in severe ischaemia are probably due to improved microvascular blood flow.[208] In animals, spinal cord stimulation has produced changes in microvascular blood flow comparable to those of complete surgical sympathectomy.[209] Although these reports are promising, there has been no comparison of spinal cord stimulation with the less expensive, simpler technique of chemical lumbar sympathectomy, the effectiveness of which, in relieving pain and enhancing peripheral blood flow in severe peripheral vascular disease, has been well documented (see below).

The controversies and uncertainties of its use notwithstanding, spinal cord stimulation has been used successfully in a number of settings (above). The spinal cord stimulation electrodes can be inserted percutaneously through an epidural needle, and the entire implantation procedure can be carried out under local anaesthesia. Spinal cord stimulation is an anaesthetic technique worthy of consideration when the palliation of appropriate symptoms has been resistant to other measures.

Techniques for pain control: the peripheral nervous system

Somatic local anaesthetic blockade

Local anaesthetic blockade of the peripheral nervous system is probably most important in the management of severe somatic pain, such as pathological fracture. Individual block techniques, perhaps with modification to include placement of a catheter to allow continuous infusion of local anaesthetic, can be of considerable analgesic benefit.[210] Such techniques may be used temporarily to facilitate patient preparation for other therapy (surgery for fracture stabilization, radiation therapy, or neurolytic block), or may be used as the primary analgesic therapy. Because long-term use of continuous peripheral nerve block catheters may be complicated by catheter-associated infection, displacement of the catheter, or other technical difficulties, these local anaesthetic techniques are typically used on a temporary basis or for terminally ill patients. Suspensions of the local anaesthetic butamben have been reported to provide long-lasting pain relief following peripheral nerve block,[80] but the role of this interesting agent in peripheral neural blockade is unclear.

Somatic neurolytic blockade

The use of neurolytic somatic neural blockade is often tempered by the significant incidence (up to 30 per cent)[177] of resultant neuralgia that may be worse than the original pain. Despite this concern, there are occasions in palliative care in which the use of these techniques is indicated.[211] Examples of analgesic use of neurolytic peripheral block include trigeminal, intercostal, and sacral nerve, brachial plexus block, and intralesional neurolytic injection for bony metastases.[212] The incidence of inadequate analgesia, as well as that of neuralgia, may be lessened by careful technique, perhaps assisted by the use of a nerve stimulator.[180]

Patients with spasticity resulting from central nervous system damage may experience a considerable reduction in spasticity when treated with neurolytic blockade of appropriate peripheral nerves[213-215] or motor points.[216] Neurolysis of specific peripheral nerves may allow more selective neurodestruction than neuraxial neurolysis; this may be of clear importance in continent, ambulatory patients. Unfortunately, the risk of neuralgia following peripheral neurolysis for control of spasticity is similar to that following peripheral neurolysis for pain relief.

Cryoanalgesia

Cryoanalgesia is the destruction of neural tissue, by the application of extreme cold, to produce pain relief. Modern techniques are based on the use of a cryo needle, which is chilled by the rapid expansion of nitrous oxide gas within the needle tip.[217] Cryoanalgesia must be used with caution. Cryolesions produce complete loss of function in peripheral nerves, and result in wallerian axonal degeneration and breakup of the myelin sheath. There is minimal disruption of the endoneurium and less fibrous tissue reaction after cryoanalgesia than with other forms of neurolysis; this may be related to the decreased, but existent,[218] incidence of neuralgia following cryoanalgesia. Although there is functional recovery following a cryolesion,[217] nerve recovery is not completely normal.[219] Cryoanalgesia is best used when motor function is not of great importance. One palliative care role for cryoanalgesia may be for intercostal nerve blockade, in the management of pain from stress rib fractures in patients with advanced osteoporosis resulting from chronic steroid therapy for chronic lung disease or autoimmune disorders. Cryolesioning should be carried out with caution in the paraspinal area, since it may cause vascular spasm or irreversible damage to spinal nutrient vessels, perhaps resulting in paraplegia.

Peripheral opioid analgesia

In the future, the peripheral nervous system may come to be utilized as a target of opioid analgesic techniques. Opioid receptors are present on the peripheral terminals of primary afferent neurones, where they are likely to play a role in the modulation of nociceptive neural transmission.[220] Peripheral opioid receptors appear to be up-regulated, by a number of mechanisms, in the setting of tissue inflammation, and are likely to be activated by endogenous opioids produced by peripheral immune cells. In selected settings (especially intra-articular administration of morphine following knee surgery), exogenous opioids provide significant peripherally-mediated analgesia.[221] Development of peripherally acting opioid analgesics, that would not cross the blood–brain barrier, is currently the focus of considerable pharmaceutical research. Theoretically, such analgesics might provide significant analgesia, especially in the management of pain associated with significant tissue inflammation, without the central nervous system adverse effects of opioid analgesics.

Techniques for pain control: the sympathetic nervous system

Interruption of the sympathetic nervous system, either coincident with peripheral nerve blocks or spinal blockade or through block techniques specifically directed towards the sympathetic nervous system, may have a significant analgesic effect, depending on the aetiology of the pain. The sympathetic chain and ganglia receive the efferent sympathetic fibres from the central nervous system, but are traversed (without synapse) by the visceral afferent nociceptive fibres. In various clinical settings, sympathetic block techniques may be used to block either the sympathetic efferent and/or the visceral nociceptive afferent fibres:

(1) blockade of the afferent visceral nociceptive fibres may reduce or eliminate visceral pain;

(2) blockade of the sympathetic (efferent) fibres may interrupt the interaction between nociception and the sympathetic nervous system that is especially important in sympathetically maintained pain;

(3) sympathetic blockade may provide relief of ischaemic pain, produce vasodilatation, and facilitate the healing of chronic ulceration in the palliation of inoperable peripheral vascular disease.

In the clinical management of neuropathic pain, interruption of the sympathetic nervous system innervation to the area of pain may be of diagnostic, prognostic, and therapeutic utility.[222] Neuropathic pain relieved by a trial of sympatholysis may be termed sympathetically maintained pain, whereas neuropathic pain which persists despite sympathetic blockade may be termed sympathetically independent pain. Sympatholysis may be induced through either regional local anaesthetic blockade of the sympathetic nervous system or infusion of sympathetic antagonist medications (intravenous regional guanethidine,[223] systemic intravenous phentolamine infusion[224]). In sympathetically maintained pain, nociceptors apparently develop adrenergic sensitivity following soft tissue and/or nervous tissue injury. Subsequently, pain-mediated reflex activation of efferent sympathetic stimulation may result in further nociceptor activation, perhaps contributing to other mechanisms of nociceptor sensitization and hyperalgesia. Sympathetic blockade is an accepted technique in the management of sympathetically maintained pain, though aspects of the interactions between the sympathetic nervous system and nociception remain speculative.[225]

Both local anaesthetic and neurolytic techniques are used for blockade of the cervicothoracic ganglia, which are usually blocked at the stellate ganglion (for pain in the head, neck, upper extremity, and upper thorax), the coeliac plexus (upper abdominal visceral pain), the lumbar sympathetic chain (lower extremity pain), and the superior hypogastric plexus (pelvic visceral pain); however, neurolytic stellate ganglion block is infrequently carried out due to the proximity of, and potential for damage to, somatic nerves, vascular structures, and the brain stem.[223]

Local anaesthetic sympathetic blockade

Local anaesthetic sympathetic blockade may have both diagnostic and therapeutic utility. Demonstration that a given patient's neuropathic pain can be relieved by sympathetic blockade is an important diagnostic step, since there may be therapeutic benefit from the use of further sympathetic blockade in such cases of sympathetically maintained pain. Local anaesthetic sympathetic blockade may have prognostic value in indicating the potential for benefit from neurolytic sympathetic blockade. However, such prognostic blocks must be assessed carefully.[73] Differentiation of the systemic versus sympatholytic effects of injected local anaesthetic may be aided by the comparison of the effectiveness and duration of pain relief following systemically (intravenously) administered local anaesthetic and regional sympathetic blockade. In addition to the management of sympathetically maintained pain, local anaesthetic sympathetic blockade is of therapeutic benefit in the management of acute exacerbations of chronic problems such as renal colic or ischaemic crises in Raynaud's disease and other obliterative arteriopathies.[223]

Local anaesthetic sympathetic blockade is an effective technique for management of the acute pain of herpes zoster.[226] The potential utility of sympathetic blockade in the prevention of postherpetic neuralgia is less clear. Although some clinical trials have suggested a reduction in the incidence of postherpetic neuralgia in patients treated early with local anaesthetic sympathetic blockade,[227,228] a beneficial effect has not been found in all studies[229] and remains contested.[230,231] Until adequate prospective controlled trials are published, it seems reasonable to use local anaesthetic sympathetic blockade in the management of acute herpes zoster and in new onset postherpetic neuralgia (less than 2 months duration), particularly when pain can not be reasonably controlled with systemic analgesics. Sympathetic blockade has not been shown to have a significant role in the management of established postherpetic neuralgia.

Neurolytic sympathetic blockade

In the management of abdominal and pelvic visceral pain, usually in the setting of advanced malignancy, neurolytic coeliac plexus and superior hypogastric plexus blocks offer the greatest potential for pain relief in patients with primarily visceral pain. Patients with mixed somatic and visceral pain, perhaps due to local tumour

Table 4 Results of 'classic' coeliac plexus block with alcohol

Author	Indication	Number of cases	Percentage results		
			Good	Fair	Poor
Brown *et al.*[234]	Pancreatic cancer	136	85[a]	—	15.0
Black and Dwyer[235]	Pancreatic cancer	20	70	30.0	0.0
	Other abdominal malignancy	37	70	17.0	13.0
Bridenbaugh *et al.*[236]	Upper abdominal cancer	41	73	24.5	2.5

[a] In 75 per cent of patients, good pain relief lasted through their remaining life. The success of repeat blocks was also 85 per cent.

invasion of somatic structures or distant metastases, are likely to have incomplete pain relief following sympathetic blockade. Such combined somatic and visceral pain is perhaps better managed by other analgesic techniques, but in some patients, even partial pain relief through sympathetic blockade may improve the overall quality of pain relief, allow reduction of opioid dose, and reduction in opioid-related adverse effects. Especially in such complicated cases, a local anaesthetic sympathetic blockade may be helpful in determining the potential benefit of neurolytic sympathectomy.

Neurolytic coeliac plexus block

Currently the only significant use in palliative care for neurolytic coeliac plexus block is for the management of severe, upper abdominal visceral pain, usually of malignant origin, especially that resulting from carcinoma of the pancreas. Severe pain is a common problem in patients with pancreatic cancer,[232] but the pain is often well controlled by neurolytic coeliac plexus block[233] (Table 4). In a prospective randomized trial, neurolytic coeliac plexus block was shown to provide equivalent pain relief, with significantly fewer adverse effects, than systemic analgesics in the management of pancreatic cancer pain.[237] The appropriate use of neurolytic coeliac plexus block, therefore, appears to be for the management of cancer-related upper abdominal visceral pain that has not been reasonably controlled with analgesic medications. In general, the long-term management of pain from chronic (non-cancer) pancreatitis is not improved by neurolytic coeliac plexus block[238] due to the limited duration of analgesia and the risk of complications, but there may be some role for its use in the palliative care of patients with intractable visceral abdominal pain of various aetiologies.

Following neurolytic coeliac plexus block, the most common adverse effects are orthostatic hypotension and increased gastrointestinal motility. These adverse effects are usually self-limiting and temporary, and are expected consequences of interruption of the sympathetic efferent innervation to the abdominal viscera. Rarely patients may require oral ephedrine (30 mg, three times daily) to control orthostatic hypotension or oral opioid to decrease gastrointestinal motility. Fortunately, the incidence of other complications of neurolytic coeliac plexus block is low (Table 5), but there is a small risk of major neurological complication. Even using radiographic imaging of needle placement, there have been reports of paraplegia following neurolytic coeliac plexus block.[240,241] It has been postulated that paraplegia has resulted from vascular injury,[242] perhaps vasospasm of the artery of Adamkiewicz,[243] resulting in ischaemic injury to the spinal cord. The true incidence and aetiology of such catastrophic complications are unknown, but in view of the several hundred patients reported to have undergone local anaesthetic and/or neurolytic coeliac plexus block safely,[233] the incidence appears to be quite low. Epidural butamben (see above) has been compared with coeliac plexus neurolysis for the management of pancreatic cancer pain[244] and may prove to be an alternative therapy.

Careful patient selection and meticulous technique[239] are the most important factors in the successful application of neurolytic coeliac plexus block. Radiographic imaging, to verify needle placement, is recommended. Fluoroscopy is sufficient for most cases and has the potential advantage of allowing continual observation of the spread of neurolytic agent during injection (if mixed with radiographic contrast medium). However, imaging by computerized tomography may be of assistance if there are significant anatomical abnormalities due to tumour spread, hepatomegaly, prior surgery, if prior neurolytic coeliac plexus block has been ineffective,[245,246] or if it is required in a young child.[245,247]

Chemical lumbar sympathectomy

In patients with inoperable peripheral vascular disease, ischaemia and cellulitis often produce severe pain. This pain may lead to increased sympathetic discharge, resulting in sensitization of nociceptors, as well as peripheral vasospasm; both of these, in turn, may lead to further pain and sympathetic discharge. Neurolytic lumbar sympathetic block, or chemical lumbar sympathectomy, may result in vasodilatation due to blockade of sympathetic efferent fibres modulating lower-extremity vascular tone, but may also interrupt

Table 5 Complications of coeliac plexus blockage

Weakness or numbness T10–L2	8%
Lower chest pain	3%
Failure of ejaculation	2%
Urinary retention	1%
Postural hypotension	1%[a]
Diarrhoea, pneumothorax, paraplegia	?%

Data from ref. 235.
[a] Temporary postural hypotension occurs in 30 to 60 per cent of patients (ref. 239).

the cycle of pain and reflex increase in sympathetic discharge. Chemical lumbar sympathectomy has been shown to reduce ischaemic rest pain, increase blood flow, and enhance healing of chronic ulceration in inoperable vascular disease.[248–250] The results of chemical lumbar sympathectomy are comparable to those following surgical lumbar sympathectomy, including a mean duration of effect of approximately 6 months. Chemical lumbar sympathectomy is less invasive, is associated with lower morbidity, mortality, and cost,[249] and is more easily repeated than surgical sympathectomy.[223] While the risk of significant complications following chemical lumbar sympathectomy appears to be reasonably low, radiographic imaging is recommended to verify needle positioning and document appropriate spread of radiographic-contrast-containing neurolytic solution.[248] When carefully applied in appropriate patients, chemical lumbar sympathectomy is of real potential utility in the palliative management of inoperative peripheral vascular disease.

Neurolytic hypogastric plexus block

Neurolytic blockade of the superior hypogastric plexus for control of cancer-related pelvic visceral pain[251,252] appears to be an appropriate extension of previously existing techniques of sympathetic plexus neurolysis. A majority of patients with inadequate control of pelvic pain due to malignancy, despite systemic analgesics, received an improved quality of pain relief with fewer adverse effects following superior hypogastric plexus neurolysis.[252] Due to a significant somatic component of pain as a result of tumour invasion of the pelvic wall, many patients with severe cancer-related pelvic pain may have incomplete pain relief following superior hypogastric plexus block; however, in patients with predominantly visceral pain, this appears to be a useful analgesic technique worthy of careful consideration and further investigation.

Neurolytic blockade of the ganglion impar

Neurolytic blockade of the terminal sympathetic ganglion (ganglion impar) has been described for management of intractable perineal pain.[242,253] Pending further investigation, this may prove to be a useful analgesic technique, but currently should be considered investigational.

Miscellaneous techniques of pain management

Trigger point injections

Myofascial pain syndromes (**MPS**) are a common cause of muscular pain and tenderness that potentially involve any skeletal muscle in any region of the body. Myofascial pain syndromes may be the primary cause of severe pain or may be secondary to other significant pathology (i.e. vertebral compression fracture). As a common cause of chronic pain, myofascial pain syndromes may be a prevalent cause of the described problem of chronic non-cancer pain that may coexist with cancer-related pain.[254] Appropriate diagnosis of myofascial pain syndromes requires careful physical examination for muscular 'trigger points'; a hyperirritable spot, usually within a taut band of skeletal muscle, that is tender to palpation and gives rise to characteristic referred pain and autonomic phenomena.[255,256] The aetiology of myofascial pain syndromes is not fully known, but myofascial trigger points apparently arise from cycles of sustained muscle contraction, impaired metabolic activity, and ischaemia, together with local sensitization of nociceptors. Nociceptor sensitization and receptive field changes are also felt to account for the characteristic but often complex patterns of referred pain that may complicate accurate diagnosis of myofascial pain syndromes.[257] Management of myofascial pain syndromes is best directed at relief of pain (i.e. trigger point injections, acupuncture, spray and stretch, analgesics) and removal of underlying or perpetuating factors (i.e. physical therapy for postural or muscular abnormalities, appropriate orthotic devices to compensate for structural abnormalities).[258] Trigger point injections, with local anaesthetic, are most effective if carried out at the specific trigger point, rather than at the area of maximum tenderness. Appropriate recognition and management of myofascial pain syndromes is an important component of comprehensive pain management; myofascial pain may be quite severe but management techniques are largely non-invasive and are often successful.

Interpleural analgesics

The use of an interpleural catheter for injection or infusion of local anaesthetic was initially described for management of acute post-thoracotomy pain,[259] but subsequently has been also used for upper abdominal,[260] upper extremity, and neck pain.[261] The mechanism of action of interpleural local anaesthetic is unclear; analgesia may result from blockade of intercostal nerves, systemic local anaesthetic absorption, sympathetic blockade, and/or effects at the spinal level. Interpleural analgesia may be used temporarily to allow patients with severe upper abdominal or thoracic pain to undergo necessary procedures (such as radiographic imaging, radiation therapy, or coeliac plexus block). With techniques similar to those used for chronic epidural access, including simple percutaneous catheters,[262] as well as subcutaneously implanted injection portals,[263] interpleural local anaesthetic has been reported to provide successful outpatient analgesia for several weeks to months. The interpleural injection of phenol has been described, in a single case report,[264] as successfully controlling previously intractable thoracic and upper abdominal cancer pain; however, until further investigated, interpleural neurolysis should be considered experimental. Although complications, including infections, fibrosis, and intrapulmonary catheter migration, do occur rarely,[263] local anaesthetic interpleural analgesia is a useful analgesic technique in appropriate settings.

The management of intractable pain: when all else fails

The management of resistant, unrelieved pain must always begin with a thorough re-evaluation of the patient, with special attention to new possible aetiologies of pain.[55] Pain uncontrolled due to opioid tolerance often can be managed with an increased dose of opioid or switching to an alternate opioid analgesic.[265] In general, exacerbations of pain probably reflect progression of the underlying pathology. When possible, the most effective pain-relieving therapy may be therapeutic management of the underlying disease. Severe, resistant pain problems are generally multifactorial and reappraisal may lead to new insights regarding possible alternative therapies to address previously untreated or inadequately treated components of the total pain problem.[266,267]

There are clearly pain problems of an intensity such that

adequate relief can not be provided by standard analgesic techniques, and instead, truly anaesthetic techniques are required. For example, with pathological fracture, it may be the case that no amount or adjustment of opioid analgesic, by any route of administration, will result in sufficient pain relief to allow movement necessary for patient care. In such cases, local anaesthetic or neurodestructive techniques may be required. In patients with diffuse pain, however, there may be no suitable or feasible combination of regional anaesthetic or neurodestructive techniques to adequately control pain. In addition to pain, other symptoms, such as dyspnoea, delirium, or intractable vomiting from bowel obstruction, may fail to be reasonably controlled with management techniques typically employed in palliative care.[268]

Just as sedation techniques, ranging from conscious sedation to general anaesthesia, are widely used to aid patients through various medical diagnostic and therapeutic procedures, when intolerable symptoms in palliative care are refractory to therapy, there is a role for symptom control through sedation. Such techniques are generally based on benzodiazepine or barbiturate infusions, but may also include opioids or various tranquillizers.[269-271] Before proceeding with palliative terminal sedation of patients with uncontrolled symptoms, it is imperative that careful consideration be given to establishing whether the patient's symptoms are merely difficult to control or truly refractory to reasonable palliative intervention. Appropriate distinction between 'difficult' and 'refractory' symptoms will spare patients with refractory symptoms unnecessary, futile interventions, as well as avoid unnecessary sedation in patients with controllable symptoms.[271]

Palliative terminal sedation may be provided, using various techniques, depending on the clinical setting.[271] Benzodiazepines, neuroleptic sedatives, and barbiturates are the most commonly used agents for palliative sedation, either singly or in combination, and can be given by various routes of administration. The new anaesthetic agent propofol appears to have utility in this setting; it is generally very well tolerated, has significant antiemetic properties, and has a short duration of effect (which can facilitate rapid titration of continuous infusion).[272,273] Unfortunately, propofol is significantly more expensive than other sedatives, causes painful irritation unless infused into a large vein, and (due to a very short elimination half-life) must be given by (costly) continuous infusion. The use of barbiturates and other sedatives in palliative terminal sedation may incorrectly raise the spectre of euthanasia (the intentional termination of life).[269] The goal of palliative terminal sedation is to provide the dying patient relief of otherwise refractory, intolerable symptoms, and it is therefore firmly within the realm of good, supportive palliative care and is not euthanasia.

Recent advances and future direction in pain management techniques

Recent advances in the understanding of the neurophysiology and consequences of nociception hold the potential for profound and fundamental changes in the management of patients with pain. Because of spinal cord plasticity (alteration of function in response to previous neural activity), nociception modifies spinal cord function and may facilitate further pain transmission.[274] Such changes may result in the temporal[274] and/or spatial[275] summation nociceptive input, as well as alteration of gene regulation in the dorsal horn neurone. Similar mechanisms of facilitation may also play a role in the development of neuropathic pain and opioid tolerance.[2] Analgesic techniques to prevent or decrease such spinal hyperalgesia are currently under development. The need for improved techniques of pain management is increasingly clear; uncontrolled pain is a maleficent force that has significant, broad, adverse effects on patients and, in some cases, it appears that 'pain can kill'.[276,277]

'Wind-up' is the progressive increase in dorsal horn neuronal response to rapidly repeated, noxious stimuli. Timing of the stimuli, so that the dorsal horn neuronal response to one stimulus does not decay prior to subsequent stimuli, results in temporal summation of stimuli, producing a cumulative depolarization of the dorsal horn neurone. This relative depolarization results in increased responsiveness, or even spontaneous firing of the neurone, and may persist for many minutes. 'Wind-up' appears to be mediated by the *N*-methyl-D-aspartate (**NMDA**) and neurokinin receptors,[278] and can be reduced by NMDA receptor antagonists (such as ketamine, MK-801, and possibly dextromethorphan).[128,279]

Long-term potentiation is another mechanism of facilitation of dorsal horn neuronal responsiveness that generally is associated with NMDA-receptor activation-induced transient increases in intracellular calcium. As a result of intracellular calcium increase, an apparent cascade of events is initiated to bring about long-lasting (hours to months) increases in neuronal activity.[274] NMDA-receptor antagonists may prevent long-term potentiation but are ineffective in reversing established long-term potentiation, suggesting a potential limitation to the clinical effectiveness of NMDA antagonists in the management of chronic pain. Induction of long-term depression may be one way to manage established long-term potentiation associated pain. Stimulation-induced long-term depression, also apparently produced by a rise in intracellular calcium, results in persistent decrease in neuronal excitability. One suggested mechanism for the analgesic effect of low-frequency TENs is the induction of long-term depression.[274] The relationship of spinal cord stimulation analgesia to long-term depression is unknown.

Alteration of gene expression in dorsal horn neurones, such as the induction of the proto-oncogene *c-fos* appears to result from noxious stimuli lasting seconds to minutes.[280,281] Activation of the *c-fos* gene results in the production of the nuclear phosphoprotein Fos, an intranuclear messenger molecule, which appears to be involved in regulation of adjacent genes encoding neuropeptides.[282] Activation of the *c-fos* gene is, therefore, a potential mechanism coupling short-term receptor activation to long-term alteration in dorsal horn neuronal function.[283] *C-fos* induction appears to be reduced by NMDA antagonists[284] and opioids.[281]

Recent reports have highlighted and summarized the similarities between the neuronal mechanisms of neuropathic hyperalgesia and morphine tolerance,[2] including activation of NMDA receptors with subsequent activation of intracellular protein kinase C and nitric oxide production. Opioid tolerant animals demonstrate thermal hyperalgesia[285] and, conversely, animals with partial nerve injuries demonstrate morphine tolerance,[286] but both effects are blocked by NMDA receptor antagonists. Given apparent similarities between mechanisms of neuropathic hyperalgesia and morphine tolerance, the frequently noted opioid resistance of clinical neuropathic pain should be anticipated.[42] These suggested similarities are consistent with the observed limits of opioid therapy seen when markedly opioid-tolerant individuals develop diffuse hyperalgesia to exceedingly high doses of systemic[3] or spinal[63] opioid. The neuropathic hyperalgesia associated with opioid tolerance underscores the potential utility of non-opioid based techniques for pain management (non-opioid analgesia, conduction block, neurostimulation, etc.).

Severe physiological stress, including pain, can result in impaired immune function.[287] Immunocompetence is an important factor in host defence against tumour progression. In experimental animals, repeated painful footshock decreases cytotoxic activity of natural killer cells,[288] and similar stress has been shown to result in accelerated growth of transplanted tumours.[289] In a related rat experiment, an analgesic dose of morphine decreased laparotomy-induced enhancement of tumour progression.[277] It is apparent that prompt, consistent, adequate pain relief is not simply a humane endeavour; there is now a growing body of evidence detailing the potential medical consequences of unrelieved pain.[290]

Over the last few years, the clinical application of analgesic therapies has evolved greatly, and the recent developments in the understanding of the neurophysiology of pain suggest numerous future developments in pain management techniques. There are experimental[291] and clinical[292] data suggesting the possibility of preventing severe pain through early or prophylactic analgesic therapy, and the importance of improved pain management has been clarified. Fortunately, the vast majority of people now with, or soon to develop, severe pain need not wait for the clinical application of recent discoveries for pain relief. Consistent and timely application of available therapies, including analgesic anaesthetic techniques, has the potential for significantly reducing the incidence, severity, and consequences of acute and chronic pain.

References

1. Cousins MJ, Cherry DA, Gourlay GK. Acute and chronic pain: use of spinal opioids. In: Cousins MJ, Bridenbaugh PO, eds. *Neural Blockade in Clinical Anesthesia and Management of Pain*. 2nd edn. Philadelphia: J. B. Lippincott, 1988: 955–1029.
2. Mao J, Price DD, Mayer DJ. Mechanisms of hyperalgesia and morphine tolerance: a current view of their possible interactions. *Pain*, 1995; **62**: 259–74.
3. Sjogren P, Jonsson T, Jensen NH, Drenck NE, Jensen TS. Hyperalgesia and myoclonus in terminal cancer patients treated with continuous intravenous morphine. *Pain*, 1993; **55**: 93–7.
4. Yaksh TL, Rudy TA. Analgesia mediated by a direct spinal action of narcotics. *Science*, 1976; **192**: 1357–8.
5. Wang JK, Nauss LA, Thomas JE. Pain relief by intrathecally applied morphine in man. *Anesthesiology*, 1979; **50**: 149–51.
6. Behar M, Magora F, Oshwang D, Davidson JT. Epidural morphine in treatment of pain. *Lancet*, 1979; **i**: 527–8.
7. Cousins MJ, Mather LE, Glynn CJ, Wilson PR, Graham JR. Selective spinal analgesia. *Lancet*, 1979; **1**: 1141–2.
8. Ventafridda V, Tamburini M, DeConno F. Comprehensive treatment in cancer pain. In: Fields H, *et al.*, eds. *Advances in Pain Research and Therapy*. Vol 9. New York: Raven Press, 1985: 617–28.
9. VadeBoncouer TR, Ferrante FM. Epidural and subarachnoid opioids. In: Ferrante FM, VadeBoncouer TR, eds. *Postoperative Pain Management*. New York: Churchill Livingstone, 1993: 279–303.
10. Waldman SD, Leak DW, Kennedy LD, Patt RB. Intraspinal opioid therapy. In: Patt RB, ed. *Cancer Pain*. Philadelphia: J. B. Lippincott, 1993: 285–328.
11. Murphy TM, Hinds S, Cherry D. Intraspinal narcotics: non-malignant pain. *Acta Anaesthesiologica Scandinavica*, 1987; **31**(suppl. 85): 75–6.
12. Calvillo O, Henry JL, Neuman RS. Effects of morphine and naloxone on dorsal horn neurones in the cat. *Canadian Journal of Physiology and Pharmacology*, 1974; **52**: 1207.
13. Duggan AW, Hall JG, Headley PM. Morphine, enkephalin, and the substantia gelatinosa. *Nature*, 1976; **264**: 456.
14. Glynn CJ, Mather LE, Cousins MJ, Wilson PR, Graham JR. Spinal narcotics and respiratory depression. *Lancet*, 1979; **ii**: 356.
15. Boas RA. Hazards of epidural morphine. *Anaesthesia and Intensive Care*, 1980; **8**: 377.
16. Coombs DW, Maurer LH, Saunders RL, Gaylor M. Outcomes and complications of continuous intraspinal narcotic analgesia for cancer pain control. *Journal of Clinical Oncology*, 1984; **2**: 1414.
17. Plummer JL, Cherry DA, Cousins MJ, Gourlay GK, Onley MM, Evans KHA. Long-term spinal administration of morphine in cancer and non-cancer pain: a retrospective study. *Pain*, 1991; **44**: 215–20.
18. Atweh SF, Kuhar MJ. Autoradiographic localization of opiate receptors in rat brain. I. Spinal cord and lower medulla. *Brain Research*, 1977; **124**: 53.
19. Yaksh TL, Noueihed R. The physiology and pharmacology of spinal opiates. *Annual Review of Pharmacology and Toxicology*, 1985; **25**: 443.
20. Yaksh TL. New horizons in our understanding of the spinal physiology and pharmacology of pain processing. *Seminars in Oncology*, 1993; **20**(2 Suppl. 1): 6–18.
21. Heinricher MM, Morgan MM, Tortorici V, Fields HL. Disinhibition of off-cells and antinociception produced by an opioid action within the rostral ventromedial medulla. *Neuroscience*, 1994; **63**: 279–88.
22. Johnson SM, Duggan AW. Evidence that opiate receptors at the substantia gelatinosa contribute to the depression by intravenous morphine of the spinal transmission of impulses in the unmyelinated primary afferents. *Brain Research*, 1981; **207**: 223.
23. Kitahata LM, Collins JG. Spinal action of narcotic analgesics. *Anesthesiology*, 1981; **54**: 153.
24. Gustafsson LL, Johannisson J, Garle M. Extradural and parenteral pethidine as analgesia after total hip replacement: Effects and kinetics. A controlled clinical study. *European Journal of Clinical Pharmacology*, 1986; **29**: 529.
25. Max MB, Inturrisi CE, Kaiko RF, Grubinski PY, Li CH, Foley KM. Epidural and intrathecal opiates: cerebrospinal fluid and plasma profiles in patients with chronic cancer pain. *Clinical Pharmacology and Therapeutics*, 1985; **38**: 631–41.
26. Gourlay GK, Cherry DA, Cousins MJ. Cephalad migration of morphine in CSF following lumbar epidural administration in patients with cancer pain. *Pain*, 1985; **23**: 312.
27. Gourlay GK, Cherry DA, Plummer JL, Armstrong PJ, Cousins MJ. The influence of drug polarity on the absorption of opioid drugs into CSF and subsequent cephalad migration following lumbar epidural administration: application to morphine and pethidine. *Pain*, 1987; **31**: 297–305.
28. Gourlay GK, Murphy TM, Plummer JL, Kowalski SR, Cherry DA, Cousins MJ. Pharmacokinetics of fentanyl in lumbar and cervical CSF following lumbar epidural and intravenous administration. *Pain*, 1989; **38**: 253–9.
29. Mather LE. Clinical pharmacokinetics of fentanyl and its newer derivatives. *Clinical Pharmacokinetics*, 1983; **8**: 422.
30. Yaksh TL, Noueihed RY, Duran AC. Studies of the pharmacology and pathology of intrathecally administered 4-aminopiperidine analogues and morphine in the rat and cat. *Anesthesiology*, 1986; **64**: 54.
31. Yaksh TL. Mechanisms of analgesic action of spinal opioids. In: Stanley TH, Asburn MA, Fine PG, eds. *Anaesthesiology and Pain Management*. Dordrecht: Kluwer Academic, 1991: 93–102.
32. Hassenbusch SJ, Stanton-Hicks MD, Soukup J, Covington EC, Boland MB. Sufentanil citrate and morphine/bupivacaine as alternative agents in chronic epidural infusions for intractable non-cancer pain. *Neurosurgery*, 1991; **29**: 76–81.
33. Payne R, Inturrisi CE. CSF distribution of morphine, methadone and sucrose after intrathecal injection. *Life Science*, 1985; **37**: 1137–44.

34. Cherry DA, Gourlay GK, Cousins MJ. Extradural mass associated with lack of efficacy of epidural morphine and undetectable CSF morphine concentrations. *Pain*, 1986; **25**: 69.
35. Rodan BA, Cohen FL, Bean WJ, Martyar SN. Fibrous mass complicating epidural morphine infusion. *Neurosurgery*, 1985; **16**: 68.
36. Brose WG, Tanelian DL, Brodsky JB, Mark JBD, Cousins MJ. CSF and blood pharmacokinetics of hydromorphone and morphine following lumbar epidural administration. *Pain*, 1991; **45**: 11–15.
37. Coombs DW, Fratkin JD, Frederick AM, Nierenberg DW, Saunders RL. Neuropathologic lesions and CSF morphine concentrations during chronic continuous intraspinal morphine infusion. A clinical and postmortem study. *Pain*, 1985; **22**: 337–51.
38. Arner S, Rawal N, Gustafsson LL. Clinical experience of long-term treatment with epidural and intrathecal opioids—a nationwide survey. *Acta Anaesthesiologica Scandinavica*, 1988; **32**: 253–9.
39. Cherry DA, Gourlay GK. CT contrast evidence of injectate encapsulation after long-term epidural administration. *Pain*, 1992; **49**: 369–71.
40. Plummer JL, *et al.* Leakage of fluid administered epidurally to rats into subcutaneous tissue. *Pain*, 1990; **42**: 121–4.
41. Arner S, Arner B. Differential effects of epidural morphine in the treatment of cancer-related pain. *Acta Anaesthesiologica Scandinavica*, 1985; **29**: 32.
42. Portenoy RK, Foley KM, Inturrisi CE. The nature of opioid responsiveness and its implications for neuropathic pain: new hypothesis derived from studies of opioid infusions. *Pain*, 1990; **43**: 273–86.
43. Jacobson L., Chabal C, Brody MC, Mariano AJ, Chaney EF. A comparison of the effects of intrathecal fentanyl and lidocaine on established postamputation stump pain. *Pain*, 1990; **40**: 137–41.
44. Siddall PJ, Gray M, Rutkowski S, Cousins MJ. Intrathecal morphine and clonidine in the management of spinal cord injury pain: a case report. *Pain*, 1994; **59**: 147–8.
45. Aguilar JL, Espachs P, Roca G, Samper D, Cubells C, Vidal F. Difficult management of pain following sacrococcygeal chordoma; 13 months of subarachnoid infusion. *Pain*, 1994; **59**: 317–20.
46. Leiphart JW, Dills CV, Zikel OM, Kim DL, Levy RM. A comparison of intrathecally administered narcotic and nonnarcotic analgesics for experimental chronic neuropathic pain. *Journal of Neurosurgery*, 1995; **82**: 595–9.
47. Layfield DJ, Lemberger RJ, Hopkinson BR, Makin GS. Epidural morphine for ischemic rest pain. *British Medical Journal*, 1981: **282**: 697.
48. Skoeld M, Gillberg L, Ohlsson O. Pain relief in myocardial infarction after continuous epidural morphine analgesia. *New England Journal of Medicine*, 1985; **312**: 650.
49. Kock M, Blomberg S, Emanuelsson H, Lomsky M, Stromblad SO, Ricksten SE. Thoracic epidural anesthesia improves global and regional left ventricular function during stress-induced myocardial ischemia in patients with coronary artery disease. *Anesthesia and Analgesia*, 1990; **71**: 625–30.
50. Blomberg SG. Long-term home self-treatment with high thoracic epidural anesthesia in patients with severe coronary artery disease (see comments). *Anesthesia and Analgesia*, 1994; **79**: 413–21.
51. Olshwang D, Shapino A, Perlberg S, Magora F. The effect of epidural morphine on ureteral colic and spasm of the bladder. *Pain*, 1984; **18**: 97.
52. Herman RM, Wainberg MC, DelGiudice PF, Willscher MK. The effect of a low dose of intrathecal morphine on impaired micturition reflexes in human subjects with spinal cord lesions. *Anesthesiology*, 1988; **69**: 313–8.
53. Erickson DL, Blacklock J, Michaelson M, Sperling KB, Lo JN. Control of spasticity by implantable continuous flow morphine pump. *Neurosurgery*, 1985; **16**: 215–7.
54. Cherry DA, Gourlay GK, Cousins MJ, Gannon BJ. A technique for the insertion of an implantable portal system for the long term epidural administration of opioids in the treatment of cancer pain. *Anaesthesia and Intensive Care*, 1985; **13**: 145.
55. Gonzales GR, Elliott KJ, Portenoy RK, Foley KM. The impact of a comprehensive evaluation in the management of cancer pain. *Pain*, 1991; **2**: 141–4.
56. Van Dongen RT, Crul BJ, De Bock M. Long-term intrathecal infusion of morphine and morphine/bupivacaine mixtures in the treatment of cancer pain: a retrospective analysis of 51 cases. *Pain*, 1993; **55**: 199–23.
57. Krames ES. Intrathecal infusional therapies for intractable pain: patient management guidelines. *Journal of Pain and Symptom Management*, 1993; **8**: 36–46.
58. Sjoberg M, Nitescu P, Appelgren L, Curelaru I. Long-term intrathecal morphine and bupivacaine in patients with refractory cancer pain. Results from a morphine:bupivacaine dose regimen of 0.5:4.75 mg/ml. *Anesthesiology*, 1994; **80**: 284–97.
59. Ahuja BR, Strunin L. Respiratory effects of epidural fentanyl. *Anaesthesia*, 1985; **40**: 949.
60. Yaksh TL, Harty GJ, Onofrio BM. High dose of spinal morphine produces a non-opiate receptor-mediated hyperesthesia: clinical and theoretic implications. *Anesthesiology*, 1986; **64**: 590–7.
61. DeConno F, Caraceni A, Martini C, Spoldi E, Salvetti M, Ventafridda V. Hyperalgesia and myoclonus with intrathecal infusion of high-dose morphine. *Pain*, 1991; **47**: 337–9.
62. Parkinson SK, Bailey SL, Little WL, Mueller JB. Myoclonic seizure activity with chronic high-dose spinal opioid administration. *Anesthesiology*, 1990; **72**: 743–5.
63. Tanelian DL, Cousins MJ. Failure of epidural opioid to control cancer pain in a patient previously treated with massive doses of intravenous opioid. *Pain*, 1989; **36**: 359–62.
64. Messahel FM, Tomlin PJ. Narcotic withdrawal syndrome after intrathecal administration of morphine. *British Medical Journal of Clinical Research*, 1981; **283**: 471.
65. Tung AS, Tenicela R, Winter PM. Opiate withdrawal syndrome following intrathecal administration of morphine. *Anesthesiology*, 1980; **53**: 340.
66. Sjoberg M, *et al.* Long-term intrathecal morphine and bupivacaine in 'refractory' cancer pain. I. Results from the first series of 52 patients. *Acta Anaesthesiologica Scandinavica*, 1991; **35**: 30–43.
67. Penning JP, Yaksh TL. Interaction of intrathecal morphine with bupivacaine and lidocaine in the rat. *Anesthesiology*, 1992; **77**: 1186–2000.
68. Krames ES. The chronic intraspinal use of opioid and local anesthetic mixtures for the relief of intractable pain: when all else fails. *Pain*, 1993; **55**: 1–4.
69. Hogan Q, Haddox JD, Abram S, Weissman D, Taylor ML, Janjan N. Epidural opiates and local anesthetics for the management of cancer pain. *Pain*, 1991; **46**: 271–9.
70. Du Pen SL, *et al.* Chronic epidural bupivacaine-opioid infusion in intractable cancer pain. *Pain*, 1992; **49**: 293–300.
71. Berde CB, Sethna NF, Conrad LS, Hershenson MB, Shillito J Jr. Subarachnoid bupivacaine analgesia for seven months for a patient with a spinal cord tumour. *Anesthesiology*, 1990; **72**: 1094–6.
72. Hunt M, Massolino J. Spinal bupivacaine for the pain of cancer. *Medical Journal of Australia*, 1989; **150**: 350.
73. Boas RA, Cousins MJ. Diagnostic neural blockade. In: Cousins MJ, Bridenbaugh PO, eds. *Neural Blockade in Clinical Anaesthesia and Management of Pain*, 2nd edn. Philadelphia: J. B. Lippincott, 1988: 885–98.
74. Loeser JD. Dorsal rhizotomy for the relief of chronic pain. *Journal of Neurosurgery*, 1972; **36**: 745.
75. Brose WG, Cousins MJ. Subcutaneous lidocaine for treatment of neuropathic cancer pain. *Pain*, 1991; **45**: 145–8.
76. Glazer S, Portenoy RK. Systemic local anesthetics in pain control. *Journal of Pain and Symptom Management*, 1991; **6**: 30–9.
77. Abram SE, Yaksh TL. Systemic lidocaine blocks nerve injury-induced hyperalgesia and nociceptor-driven spinal sensitization in the rat. *Anesthesiology*, 1994; **80**: 383–91.
78. Sosnowski M, Yaksh TL. Spinal administration of receptor-selective drugs as analgesics: new horizons. *Journal of Pain and Symptom Management*, 1990; **5**: 204–13.
79. Yaksh TL. Spinal somatostatin for patients with cancer: risk-benefit assessment of an analgesic. *Anesthesiology*, 1994; **81**: 531–3.
80. Shulman M. Treatment of cancer pain with epidural butyl-amino-benzoate suspension. *Regional Anesthesia*, 1987; **12**: 1–4.

81. Korsten HH, *et al.* Long-lasting epidural sensory blockade by n-butyl-p-aminobenzoate in the terminally ill intractable cancer pain patient. *Anesthesiology*, 1991; **75**: 950–60.
82. Korsten HH, *et al.* Long-lasting epidural sensory blockade by n-butyl-p-aminobenzoate in the dog: neurotoxic or local anesthetic effect? *Anesthesiology*, 1990; **73**: 491–8.
83. Shulman M, Joseph NJ, Haller CA. Effect of epidural and subarachnoid injections of a 10 per cent butamben suspension. *Regional Anesthesia*, 1990; **15**: 142–6.
84. Shulman M, Greenlee W, Kim T, Lubenow T, Ivankovich A. Magnetic resonance imaging of epidural butamben injections. *Regional Anesthesia*, 1995; **20** (suppl.2): 134.
85. Grouls RJE, Ackerman EW, Machielsen EJA, Korsten HHM. Butyl-p-aminobenzoate: preparation, characterization and quality control of a suspension injection for epidural analgesia. *Pharmaceutisch Weekblad* (scientific edition), 1991; **13**: 13–7.
86. Quan DB, Wandres DL, Schroeder DJ. Clonidine in pain management. *Annals of Pharmacotherapy*, 1993; **27**: 313–5.
87. Sabbe MB, Penning JP, Ozaki GT, Yaksh TL. Spinal and systemic action of the α_2 receptor agonist dexmedetomidine in dogs. Antinociception and carbon dioxide response. *Anesthesiology*, 1994; **80**: 1057–72.
88. Jaakola ML, Salonen M, Lehtinen R, Scheinin H. The analgesic action of dexmedetomidine—a novel α_2-adrenoceptor agonist—in healthy volunteers. *Pain*, 1991; **46**: 281–5.
89. Glynn C, Dawson D, Sanders R. A double-blind comparison between epidural morphine and epidural clonidine in patients with chronic non-cancer pain. *Pain*, 1988; **34**: 123–8.
90. Drasner K, Fields HL. Synergy between the antinociceptive effects of intrathecal clonidine and systemic morphine in the rat. *Pain*, 1988; **32**: 309–12.
91. Holz GG, Kream RM, Spiegel A, Dunlap K. G proteins couple alpha-adrenergic and $GABA_B$ receptors to inhibition of peptide secretion from peripheral sensory neurons. *Journal of Neuroscience*, 1989; **9**: 657–66.
92. Murata K, Nakagawa I, Kumeta Y, Kitahata L, Collins J. Intrathecal clonidine suppresses noxiously evoked activity of wide dynamic range neurons in cats. *Anesthesia and Analgesia*, 1989; **69**: 185–91.
93. Penon C, Ecoffey C, Cohen SE. Ventilatory response to carbon dioxide after epidural clonidine injection. *Anesthesia and Analgesia*, 1991; **72**: 761–4.
94. Bonnett F, Boico O, Rostaing S, Loriferne JF, Saada M. Clonidine-induced analgesia in postoperative patients: epidural versus intramuscular administration. *Anesthesiology*, 1990; **72**: 423–7.
95. Coombs DW, Saunders RL, Fratker JD, Jensen LE, Murphy CA. Continuous intrathecal hydromorphone and clonidine for intractable cancer pain. *Journal of Neurosurgery*, 1986; **64**: 890–4.
96. Solomon RE, Gebhart GF. Intrathecal morphine and clonidine: anti-nociceptive tolerance and cross tolerance and effects on blood pressure. *Journal of Pharmacology and Experimental Therapeutics*, 1988; **245**: 444–54.
97. Stevens CW, Monasky MS, Yaksh TL. Spinal infusion of opiate and α_2 agonists in rats: tolerance and cross-tolerance studies. *Journal of Pharmacology and Experimental Therapeutics*, 1988; **244**: 63–70.
98. Gordh T, Post C, Olsson Y. Evaluation of the toxicity of subarachnoid clonidine, guanfacine, and a substance P-antagonist on rat spinal cord and nerve roots: light and electron microscopic observations after chronic intrathecal administration. *Anaesthesia and Analgesia*, 1986; **65**: 1301–11.
99. Coombs DW, Saunders AL, LaChance D, Savage S, Ragnarson TS, Jansen L. Intrathecal morphine tolerance: use of intrathecal clonidine, DADLE, and intraventricular morphine. *Anesthesiology*, 1985: **62**: 358.
100. Rauck RL, Eisenach JC, Jackson K, Young LD, Southern J. Epidural clonidine treatment for refractory reflex sympathetic dystrophy. *Anesthesiology*, 1993; **79**: 1163–9.
101. Glynn CJ, Jamous MA, Teddy PJ. Cerebrospinal fluid kinetics of epidural clonidine in man. *Pain*, 1992; **49**: 361–7.
102. Katz RT. Management of spasticity. *American Journal of Physical Medicine and Rehabilitation*, 1988; **67**: 108–16.
103. Coffey RJ, *et al.* Intrathecal baclofen for intractable spasticity of spinal origin: results of a long-term multicenter study. *Journal of Neurosurgery*, 1993; **78**: 226–32.
104. Azouvi P, Roby-Brami A, Biraben A, Thiebaut JB, Thurel C, Bussel B. Effect of intrathecal baclofen on the monosynaptic reflex in humans; evidence for a postsynaptic action. *Journal of Neurology, Neurosurgery, and Psychiatry*, 1993; **56**: 515–9.
105. Chabal C, Jacobson L, Terman G. Intrathecal fentanyl alleviates spasticity in the presence of tolerance to intrathecal baclofen. *Anesthesiology*, 1992; **76**: 312–4.
106. Penn RD, *et al.* Intrathecal baclofen for severe spinal spasticity. *The New England Journal of Medicine*, 1989; **320**: 1517–21.
107. Patterson V, Watt M, Byrnes D, Crowe D, Lee A. Management of severe spasticity with intrathecal baclofen delivered by a manually operated pump. *Journal of Neurology, Neurosurgery, and Psychiatry*, 1994; **57**: 582–85.
108. Lewis KS, Meuller WM. Intrathecal baclofen for severe spasticity secondary to spinal cord injury. *The Annals of Pharmacotherapy*, 1993; **27**: 767–74.
109. Latash ML, Penn RD, Corcos DM, Gottlieb SL. Effects of intrathecal baclofen on voluntary motor control in spastic paresis. *Journal of Neurosurgery*, 1990; **72**: 388–92.
110. Rifici C, Kofler M, Kronenberg M, Kofler A, Bramanti P, Saltuari L. Intrathecal baclofen application in patients with supraspinal spasticity secondary to severe traumatic brain injury. *Functional Neurology*, 1994; **9**: 29–34.
111. Taira T, Tanikawa T, Kawamura H, Iseki H, Takakura K. Spinal intrathecal baclofen suppresses central pain after a stroke. *Journal of Neurology, Neurosurgery, and Psychiatry*, 1994; **57**:381–2.
112. Sabbe MB, Grafe MR, Pfeifer BL, Mirzai THM, Yaksh TL. Toxicity of baclofen continuously infused into the spinal intrathecal space of the dog. *Neurotoxicology*, 1993; **14**: 397–410.
113. Ochs G, *et al.* Intrathecal baclofen for long-term treatment of spasticity: a multi-centre study. *Journal of Neurology, Neurosurgery, and Psychiatry*, 1989; **52**: 933–9.
114. Lazorthes Y, Sallerin-Caute B, Verdie JC, Bastide R, Carillo JP. Chronic intrathecal baclofen administration for control of severe spasticity. *Journal of Neurosurgery*, 1990; **72**: 393–402.
115. Dralle D, Neuhauser G, Tonn JC. Intrathecal baclofen for cerebral spasticity. *Lancet*, 1989; **2**: 916.
116. Gordh T, Jansson I, Hartvig P, Gillberg PG, Post C. Interactions between nonadrenergic and cholinergic mechanisms involved in spinal nociceptive processing. *Acta Anaesthesiologica Scandinavica*, 1989; **33**: 39–47.
117. Hood DD, Eisenach JC, Tuttle R. Phase I safety assessment of intrathecal neostigmine methylsulfate in humans. *Anesthesiology*, 1995; **82**: 331–43.
118. Naguib M, Yaksh TL. Antinociceptive effects of spinal cholinesterase inhibition and isobolographic analysis of the interaction with mu and α_2 receptor systems. *Anesthesiology*, 1994; **80**: 1338–48.
119. Williams JS, Tong C, Eisenach JC. Neostigmine counteracts spinal clonidine-induced hypotension in sheep. *Anesthesiology*, 1993; **78**: 301–7.
120. Hood DD, Eisenach JC, Tong C, Tommasi E, Yaksh TL. Cardiorespiratory and spinal cord blood flow effects of intrathecal neostigmine methylsulfate, clonidine, and their combination in sheep. *Anesthesiology*, 1995; **82**: 428–35.
121. Yaksh TL, Grafe MR, Malkmus S, Rathbun ML, Eisenach JC. Studies on the safety of chronically administered intrathecal neostigmine methylsulfate in rats and dogs. *Anesthesiology*, 1995; **82**: 412–27.
122. Foley KM, Yaksh TL. Another call for patience instead of patients: developing novel therapies for chronic pain. *Anesthesiology*, 1993; **79**: 637–40.
123. Abram SE, Winne RP. Intrathecal acetyl cholinesterase inhibitors produce analgesia that is synergistic with morphine and clonidine in rats. *Anesthesia and Analgesia*, 1995; **81**: 501–7.
124. Choi DW. Dextrorphan and dextromethorphan attenuate glutamate neurotoxicity. *Brain Research*, 1987; **403**: 333–6.
125. Church J, Lodge D, Berry SC. Differential effects of dextrorphan and

levorphanol on the excitation of rat neurons by amino acids. *European Journal of Pharmacology*, 1985; **111**: 185–90.

126. Dickenson AH, Sullivan AF, Stanfa LC, McQuay HJ. Dextromethorphan and levorphanol on dorsal horn nociceptive neurones in the rat. *Neuropharmacology*, 1991; **30**: 1303–8.
127. Elliott KJ, Brodsky M, Hynansky AD, Foley KM, Inturrisi CE. Dextromethorphan suppresses both formalin-induced nociceptive behavior and the formalin-induced increase in spinal cord *c-fos* mRNA. *Pain*, 1995; **61**: 401–409.
128. Price DD, Mao JR, Frenk H, Mayer DJ. The N-methyl-D-aspartate receptor antagonist dextromethorphan selectively reduces temporal summation of second pain in man. *Pain*, 1994; **59**: 165–74.
129. McQuay HJ, *et al.* Dextromethorphan for the treatment of neuropathic pain: a double-blind randomized controlled crossover trial with integral n-of-1 design. *Pain*, 1994; **59**: 127–33.
130. Wolfe TR, Caravati EM. Massive dextromethorphan ingestion and abuse. *American Journal of Emergency Medicine*, 1995; **13**: 174–6.
131. Spampinato S, Romualdi P, Candeletti S, Cavicchini E, Ferri S. Distinguishable effects of intrathecal dynorphins, somatostatin, neurotensin and s-calcitonin on nociception and motor function in the rat. *Pain*, 1988; **35**: 95–104.
132. Maeda Y, Yamada K, Hasegawa T, Iyo M, Fukui S, Nabeshima T. Inhibitory effects of salmon calcitonin on the tail-biting and scratching behavior induced by substance P and three excitatory amino acids. *Journal of Neural Transmission*, General Section, 1994; **96**: 125–33.
133. Spampinato S, Candeletti S, Cavicchini E, Romualdi P, Speroni E, Ferri S. Antinociceptive activity of salmon calcitonin injected intrathecally in the rat. *Neuroscience Letters*, 1984; **45**: 135–9.
134. Collin E, Bourgoin S, Gorce P, Hamon M, Cesselin F. Intrathecal porcine calcitonin enhances the release of (Met5)enkephalin-like material from the rat spinal cord. *European Journal of Pharmacology*, 1989; **168**: 201–8.
135. Miralles FS, Lopez-Soriano F, Puig MM, Perez D, Lopez-Rodriguez F. Postoperative analgesia induced by subarachnoid lidocaine plus calcitonin. *Anesthesia and Analgesia*, 1987; **66**: 615–18.
136. Blanchard J, Menk E, Ramamurthy S, Hoffman J. Subarachnoid and epidural calcitonin in patients with pain due to metastatic cancer. *Journal of Pain and Symptom Management*, 1990; **5**: 42–5.
137. Eisenach JC. Demonstrating safety of subarachnoid calcitonin: patients or animals? *Anesthesia and Analgesia*, 1988; **67**: 298.
138. McCleskey EW. Calcium channels: cellular roles and molecular mechanisms. *Current Opinion in Neurobiology*, 1994; **4**: 304–12.
139. Taddese A, Nah SY, McCleskey EW. Selective opioid inhibition of small nociceptive neurons. *Science*, 1995; **270**: 1366–9.
140. Malmberg AB, Yaksh TL. Voltage-sensitive calcium channels in spinal nociceptive processing: blockade of N- and P-type channels inhibits formalin-induced nociception. *Journal of Neuroscience*, 1994; **14**: 4882–90.
141. Malmberg AB, Yaksh TL. Effect of continuous intrathecal infusion of ω-conopeptides, N-type calcium-channel blockers, on behavior and antinociception in the formalin and hot-plate tests in rats. *Pain*, 1995; **60**: 83–90.
142. Brose WG, Cherukuri S, Longton WC, Gaeta RR, Presley R. Safety and efficacy of intrathecal SNX-111, a novel analgesic, in the management of intractable neuropathic and nociceptive pain in humans: preliminary results. In: American Pain Society. *14th Annual Scientific Meeting* (Program Book), November 1995; abstract number 95821.
143. Zenz M, Schappler-Scheel B, Neuhans R, Piepenrock S, Hilfrich J. Long term peridural morphine analgesia in cancer pain. *Lancet*, 1981; **1**: 91.
144. de Jong PC, Kansen PJ. A comparison of epidural catheters with or without subcutaneous injection ports for treatment of cancer pain. *Anesthesia and Analgesia*, 1994; **78**: 94–100.
145. Du Pen SL, Peterson DG, Bogosian AC, Ramsey DH, Larson C, Omoto M. A new permanent exteriorized epidural catheter for narcotic self-administration to control cancer pain. *Cancer*, 1987; **59**: 986–93.
146. Du Pen SL, Peterson DG, Williams A, Bogosian AJ. Infection during chronic epidural catheterization: diagnosis and treatment. *Anesthesiology*, 1990; **73**: 905–9.
147. Gourlay GK, *et al.* Comparison of intermittent bolus with continuous infusion of epidural morphine in the treatment of severe cancer pain. *Pain*, 1991; **47**: 135–40.
148. Hogan QH. Loculated? Encapsulated? Indented? *Pain*, 1993; **53**: 241–2.
149. Madrid JL, Fatela LV, Lobato RD, Gozalo A. Intrathecal therapy: rationale, technique, clinical results. *Acta Anaesthesiologica Scandinavica*, 1987; **31**(suppl. 85): 60–7.
150. Penn RD, Paice JA. Chronic intrathecal morphine for intractable pain. *Journal of Neurosurgery*, 1987; **67**: 182–6.
151. Sjoberg M, *et al.* Neuropathologic findings after long-term intrathecal infusion of morphine and bupivacaine for pain treatment in cancer patients. *Anesthesiology*, 1992; **76**: 173–86.
152. Devulder J, Ghys L, Dhondt W, Rolly G. Spinal analgesia in terminal care: risk versus benefit. *Journal of Pain and Symptom Management*, 1994; **9**: 75–81.
153. Silbert PL, Stewart-Wynne EG. Surgical procedures for the relief of acute and chronic pain: caution about intermittent intrathecal injection. *Medical Journal of Australia*, 1992; **156**: 439.
154. Andersen PE, Cohen JL, Everts EC, Bedder MD, Burchiel KJ. Intrathecal narcotics for relief of pain from head and neck cancer. *Archives of Otolaryngology—Head and Neck Surgery*, 1991; **117**: 1277–80.
155. Ready LB, Helfer D. Bacterial meningitis in parturients after epidural anesthesia. *Anesthesiology*, 1989; **71**: 988–90.
156. van Diejen D, Driessen JJ, Kaanders JHAM. Spinal cord compression during chronic epidural morphine administration in a cancer patient. *Anaesthesia*, 1987; **42**: 1201–3.
157. Bennett MI, Tai YM, Symonds JM. Staphylococcal meningitis following Synchromed intrathecal pump implant: a case report. *Pain*, 1994; **56**: 243–4.
158. Samuel M, Finnerty GT, Rudge P. Intrathecal baclofen pump infection treated by adjunct intrareservoir antibiotic instillation (letter). *Journal of Neurology, Neurosurgery, and Psychiatry*, 1994; **57**: 1146–7.
159. Kroin JS, Ali A, York M, Penn RD. The distribution of medication along the spinal canal after chronic intrathecal administration. *Neurosurgery*, 1993; **33**: 226–30.
160. Du Pen SL, Ramsey D, Chin S. Chronic epidural morphine and preservative-induced injury. *Anesthesiology*, 1987; **67**: 987–8.
161. Wang BC, *et al.* Are the preservatives sodium bisulfite and ethylene diaminetetraacetate free from neurotoxic involvement? *Anesthesiology*, 1992; **77**: 602–4.
162. Hahn AF, Feasby TE, Gilbert JJ. Paraparesis following intrathecal chemotherapy. *Neurology*, 1983; **33**: 1032–8.
163. Eide PK, Jorum E, Stubhang A, Bremnes J, Breivik H. Relief of post-herpetic neuralgia with the *N*-methyl-D-aspartic acid receptor antagonist ketamine: a double-blind, cross-over comparison with morphine and placebo. *Pain*, 1995: 347–54.
164. Mercadante S. Intrathecal morphine and bupivacaine in advanced cancer pain patients implanted at home. *Journal of Pain and Symptom Management*, 1994; **9**: 201–7.
165. Blue CL, Purath G. Continuing education. Home care of the epidural analgesia patient: the nurse's role. *Home Health Nurse*, 1989; **7**: 23–32.
166. Dejgard A, Petersen P, Kastrup J. Mexiletine for treatment of chronic painful diabetic neuropathy, *Lancet*, 1988; **i**: 9–11.
167. Devulder JE, Ghys L, Dhondt W, Rolly G. Neuropathic pain in a cancer patient responding to subcutaneously administered lignocaine. *Clinical Journal of Pain*, 1993; **9**: 220–3.
168. Lobato RD, Madrid JL, Fatela LV, Sarabia R, Rivas JJ, Gozalo A. Intraventricular morphine for intractable cancer pain: rationale, methods, clinical results. *Acta Anaesthesiologica Scandinavica*, 1987; **31**(suppl. 85): 68–74.
169. Obbens EA, Hill CS, Leavens ME, Ruthenbeck SS, Otis F. Intraventricular morphine administration for control of chronic cancer pain. *Pain*, 1987; **28**: 61–8.
170. Cramond T, Stuart G. Intraventricular morphine for intractable pain of advanced cancer. *Journal of Pain and Symptom Management*, 1993; **8**: 465–73.

171. Lazorthes Y, Verdie JC, Bastide R, Lavados A, Descouens D. Spinal versus intraventricular chronic opiate administration with implantable drug delivery devices for cancer pain. *Applied Neurophysiology*, 1985; **48**: 234–41.
172. Tafani JA, *et al.* Human brain and spinal cord scan after intracerebroventricular administration of iodine-123 morphine. *International Journal of Radiation Applications and Instrumentation Part B, Nuclear Medicine and Biology*, 1989; **16**: 505–9.
173. Sandouk P, Serrie A, Urtizberea M, Debray M, Got P, Scherrmann JM. Morphine pharmacokinetics and pain assessment after intraventricular administration in patients with terminal cancer. *Clinical Pharmacology and Therapeutics*, 1991; **49**: 442–8.
174. Lenzi A, Gali G, Ganddfini M, Marini G. Intraventricular morphine in paraneoplastic painful syndrome of the cervicofacial region. Experience in thirty-eight cases. *Neurosurgery*, 1985; **17**: 6–11.
175. Dennis GC, DeWitty RL. Long-term intraventricular infusion of morphine for intractable pain in cancer of the head and neck. *Neurosurgery*, 1990; **26**: 404–7.
176. Cousins MJ. Introduction to acute and chronic pain: implications for neural blockade. In: Cousins MJ, Bridenbaugh PO, eds. *Neural Blockade in Clinical Anesthesia and Management of Pain*. 2nd edn. Philadelphia: J. B. Lippincott, 1988: 739–90.
177. Swerdlow M. Complications of neurolytic neural blockade. In: Cousins MJ, Bridenbaugh PO, eds. *Neural Blockade in Clinical Anesthesia and Management of Pain*. 2nd edn. Philadelphia: J. B. Lippincott, 1988: 719–35.
178. Wood KM. The use of phenol as a neurolytic agent: a review. *Pain*, 1978; **5**: 205–29.
179. Tasker R. Neurostimulation and percutaneous neural destructive techniques. In: Cousins MJ, Bridenbaugh PO, eds. *Neural Blockade in Clinical Anesthesia and Management of Pain*. 2nd edn. Philadelphia: J. B. Lippincott, 1988: 1085–118.
180. Cousins MJ. Chronic pain and neurolytic neural blockade. In: Cousins MJ, Bridenbaugh PO, eds. *Neural Blockade in Clinical Anesthesia and Management of Pain*. 2nd edn. Philadelphia: J. B. Lippincott, 1988: 1053–84.
181. Bonica JJ, Buckley FP. Regional analgesia with local anesthetics. In: Bonica JJ, ed. *The Management of Pain*. 2nd edn. Philadelphia: Lea and Febiger, 1990: 1886.
182. Myers RR, Katz J. Neuropathy of neurolytic and semi-destructive agents. In: Cousins MJ, Bridenbaugh PO, eds. *Neural Blockade in Clinical Anesthesia and Management of Pain*. 2nd edn. Philadelphia: J. B. Lippincott, 1988: 1031–52.
183. Noda J, Umeda S, Mori K, Fukunaga T, Mizoi Y. Acetaldehyde syndrome after celiac plexus alcohol block. *Anesthesia and Analgesia*, 1986; **65**: 1300–2.
184. Swerdlow M. Intrathecal and extradural block in pain relief. In: Swerdlow M, Charlton JE, eds. *Relief of Intractable Pain*. 4th edn. Amsterdam: Elsevier, 1989: 223–57.
185. Drechsel U. Treatment of cancer pain with neurolytic agents. *Recent Results of Cancer Research*, 1984; **89**: 137–47.
186. Dogliotti AM. Traitement des syndrome douloureux de la peripheric par l'alcoolisation subarachnoidienne des racines posterieurs a leur émergencede las moelle épinière. *Presse Médicale*, 1931; **39**: 1249.
187. Greenhill JP. Sympathectomy and intra-spinal alcohol injections for relief of pelvic pain. *British Medical Journal*, 1947; **2**: 859.
188. Hay RC. Subarachnoid alcohol block in control of intractable pain. Report of 252 patients. *Anesthesia and Analgesia*, 1962; **41**: 12.
189. Kuzucu EY, Derrick WS, Wilber SA. Control of intractable pain with subarachnoid alcohol block. *Journal of the American Medical Association*, 1966; **195**: 541.
190. Korevaar WC. Transcatheter thoracic epidural neurolysis using ethyl alcohol. *Anesthesiology*, 1988; **69**: 989–93.
191. Arter OE, Racz GB. Pain management of the oncologic patient. *Seminars in Surgical Oncology*, 1990; **6**: 162–72.
192. Kelly RE, Gautier-Smith PC. Intrathecal phenol in the treatment of reflex spasms and spasticity. *Lancet*, 1959; **2**: 1102–5.
193. Chabal C, Jacobson L, White J. Electrical localization of spinal roots for the treatment of spasticity by intrathecal alcohol injection. *Anesthesia and Analgesia*, 1989; **68**: 527–9.
194. Loubser PG. Intrathecal alcohol injection guided by electrical localization of spinal roots. *Anesthesia and Analgesia*, 1990; **70**: 119–21.
195. Bonica JJ. Neurolytic blockade and hypophysectomy. In: Bonica JJ, ed. *The Management of Pain*. 2nd edn. Philadelphia: Lea and Febiger, 1990: 2035.
196. Scott BA, Weinstein Z, Chiteman R, Pulliam MW. Intrathecal phenol and glycerin in metrizamide for treatment of intractable spasms in paraplegia: case report. *Journal of Neurosurgery*, 1985; **63**: 125–7.
197. DeLaPorte C, Verlooy J, Veeckmans G, Parizel P, deMoor J, Selosse P. Consequences and complications of glycerol injection in the cavum of Meckel: a series of 120 consecutive injections. *Stereotactic and Functional Neurosurgery*, 1990; **54–5**: 73–5.
198. Gomoro JM, Rappaport ZH. Transovale trigeminal cistern puncture: modified fluoroscopically guided technique. *American Journal of Neuroradiology*, 1985; **6**: 93.
199. Melzack R, Wall PD. Pain mechanisms: a new theory. *Science*, 1965; **150**: 971–9.
200. North RB, Ewend MG, Lawon MT, Piantadosi S. Spinal cord stimulation for chronic, intractable pain: superiority of 'multichannel' devices. *Pain*, 1991; **44**: 119–30.
201. North RB, *et al.* Failed back surgery syndrome: five year follow-up after spinal cord stimulator implantation. *Neurosurgery*, 1991; **28**: 692–9.
202. Barolat G, Schwartzman R, Woo R. Epidural spinal cord stimulation in the management of reflex sympathetic dystrophy. *Stereotactic and Functional Neurosurgery*, 1989; **53**: 29–39.
203. Meglio M, Cioni B, Rossi GF. Spinal cord stimulation in management of chronic pain. *Journal of Neurosurgery*, 1989; **70**: 519–24.
204. de Jongste MJ, *et al.* Effects of spinal cord stimulation on myocardial ischaemia during daily life in patients with severe coronary artery disease. A prospective ambulatory electrocardiographic study. *British Heart Journal*, 1994; **71**: 413–8.
205. Augustinsson LE, Carlsson CA, Holm J, Jivegard L. Epidural electrical stimulation in severe limb ischemia. Pain relief, increased blood flow, and a possible limb-saving effect. *Annals of Surgery*, 1985; **202**: 104–10.
206. Augustinsson LE. Epidural spinal electrical stimulation in peripheral vascular disease. *Pace*, 1987; **10**: 205–6.
207. Franzetti I, *et al.* Epidural spinal electrostimulatory system (ESES) in the management of diabetic foot and peripheral arteriopathies. *Pace*, 1989; **12**: 705–8.
208. Jacobs MJ, Jorning PJ, Joshi SR, Kitslaar PJ, Slaaf DW, Reneman RS. Epidural spinal cord electrical stimulation improves microvascular blood flow in severe limb ischemia. *Annals of Surgery*, 1988; **207**: 179–83.
209. Linderoth B, Gunasekera L, Meyerson BA. Effects of sympathectomy on skin and muscle microcirculation during dorsal column stimulation: animal studies. *Neurosurgery*, 1991; **29**: 874–9.
210. Sato S, Yamashita S, Iwai M, Mizuyama K, Satsumae T. Continuous interscalene block for cancer pain. *Regional Anesthesia*. 1994; **19**: 73–5.
211. Patt RB. Peripheral neurolysis and the management of cancer pain. In: Patt RB, ed. *Cancer Pain*. Philadelphia: J. B. Lippincott, 1993: 359–76.
212. Doyle D. Nerve blocks in advanced cancer. *Practitioner*, 1982; **226**: 539–44.
213. Barnes MP. Local treatment of spasticity. *Baillieres Clinical Neurology*, 1993; **2**: 55–71.
214. Koyama H, Murakami K, Suzuki T, Suzaki K. Phenol block for hip flexor muscle spasticity under ultrasonic monitoring. *Archives of Physical Medicine and Rehabilitation*, 1992; **73**: 1040–3.
215. Petrillo CR, Knoplock S. Phenol block of the tibial nerve for spasticity: a long-term follow-up study. *International Disability Studies*, 1988; **10**: 97–100.
216. Garland DE, Lilling M, Keenan MA. Percutaneous phenol blocks to motor points of spastic forearm muscles in head-injured adults. *Archives of Physical and Medical Rehabilitation*, 1984; **65**: 243–5.
217. Lloyd JW, Barnard JDW, Glynn CJ. Cryoanalgesia: a new approach to pain relief *Lancet*, 1976; **ii**: 932.

218. Conacher ID, Locke T, Hilton C. Neuralgia after cryoanalgesia for thoracotomy. *Lancet*, 1986; **1**: 277.
219. Fasano VA, *et al.* Cryoanalgesia. Ultrastructural study on cryolytic lesion of sciatic nerve in rat and rabbit. *Acta Neurochirurgica, Supplementum (Wien)*, 1987; **39**: 177–80.
220. Stein C. The control of pain in peripheral tissue by opioids. *New England Journal of Medicine*, 1995; **332**: 1685–90.
221. Stein C, *et al.* Analgesic effect of intraarticular morphine after arthroscopic knee surgery. *New England Journal of Medicine*, 1991; **325**: 1123–6.
222. Fields HL. Peripheral neuropathic pain: an approach to management. In: Wall PD, Melzack R, eds. *Textbook of Pain*. 3rd edn. Edinburgh: Churchill Livingstone, 1994: 991–6.
223. Lofstrom JB, Cousins MJ. Sympathetic neural blockade of upper and lower extremity. In: Cousins MJ, Bridenbaugh PO, eds. *Neural Blockade in Clinical Anesthesia and Management of Pain*. 2nd edn. Philadelphia: Lippincott, 1988: 461–502.
224. Raja SN, Treede RD, Davis KD, Campbell JN. Systemic alpha-adrenergic blockade with phentolamine: a diagnostic test for sympathetically maintained pain. *Anesthesiology*, 1991; **74**: 691–8.
225. Campbell JN, Raja SN, Belzberg AJ, Meyer RA. Hyperalgesia and the sympathetic nervous system. In: Boivie J, Hansson P, Lindblom U, eds. *Touch, Temperature, and Pain in Health and Disease: Mechanisms and Assessments*. Seattle: IASP Press, 1994: 249–65.
226. Colding A. The effect of regional sympathetic blocks in the treatment of herpes zoster: a survey of 300 cases. *Acta Anaesthesiologica Scandinavica*, 1969; **13**: 133–41.
227. Winnie AP, Hartwell P. Relationship between time of treatment of acute herpes zoster with sympathetic blockade and prevention of post-herpetic neuralgia: clinical support for anew theory of the mechanism by which sympathetic blockade provides therapeutic benefit. *Regional Anesthesia*, 1993; **18**: 277–82.
228. Milligan NS, Nash TP. Treatment of post herpetic neuralgia: a review of 77 consecutive cases. *Pain*, 1985; **23**: 381–6.
229. Yanagida H, Suwa K, Corssen G. No prophylactic effect of early sympathetic blockade on postherpetic neuralgia. *Anesthesiology*, 1987; **66**: 73–6.
230. Bauman J. Prevention of postherpetic neuralgia. *Anesthesiology*, 1987; **67**: 441–2.
231. Hogan QH. The sympathetic nervous system in post-herpetic neuralgia. *Regional Anesthesia*, 1993; **18**: 271–3.
232. Saltzburg D, Foley KM. Management of pain in pancreatic cancer. *Surgical Clinics of North America*, 1989; **69**:629–49.
233. Eisenberg E, Carr DB, Chalmers TC. Neurolytic celiac plexus block for treatment of cancer pain: a meta-analysis. *Anesthesia and Analgesia*, 1995; **80**: 290–5.
234. Brown DL, Bulley CK, Quiel EL. Neurolytic celiac plexus block for pancreatic cancer pain. *Anesthesia and Analgesia*, 1987; **66**: 869–73.
235. Black A, Dwyer B. Coeliac plexus block. *Anaesthesia and Intensive Care*, 1973; **1**: 315.
236. Bridenbaugh LD, Moore DC, Campbell DD. Management of upper abdominal cancer pain. Treatment with celiac plexus block with alcohol. *Journal of the American Medical Association*, 1964; **190**: 877.
237. Mercadante S. Celiac plexus block versus analgesics in pancreatic cancer pain. *Pain*, 1993; **52**: 187–92.
238. Leung JWC, Bowen-Wright M, Aveling W, Shorvon PJ, Cotton PB. Coeliac plexus block for pain in pancreatic cancer and chronic pancreatitis. *British Journal of Surgery*, 1983; **70**: 730–2.
239. Thompson GE, Moore DC. Celiac plexus, intercostal and minor peripheral blockade. In: Cousins MJ, Bridenbaugh PO, eds. *Neural Blockade in Clinical Anesthesia and Management of Pain*. 2nd edn. Philadelphia: J. B. Lippincott, 1988: 503–32.
240. DeConno F, *et al.* Paraplegia following coeliac plexus block. *Pain*, 1993; **55**: 383–5.
241. Davies DD. Incidence of major complications of neurolytic coeliac plexus block. *Journal of the Royal Society of Medicine*, 1993; **86**: 264–6.
242. Plancarte R, Velazquez R, Patt RB. Neurolytic blocks of the sympathetic axis. In: Patt RB, ed. *Cancer Pain*. Philadelphia: J. B. Lippincott, 1993: 377–425.
243. Brown DL, Rorie DK. Altered reactivity of isolated segmental lumbar arteries of dogs following exposure to ethanol and phenol. *Pain*, 1994; **56**: 139–43.
244. Shulman M, Lubenow T, Rozanski L, Ivankovich A. Comparison of coeliac plexus neurolytic block and epidural butamben injection for the control of pain from metastatic cancer of the pancreas. *Regional Anesthesia*, 1995; **20**(Suppl. 2): 52.
245. Tanelian D, Cousins MJ. Celiac plexus block following high-dose opiates for chronic non-cancer pain in a four year old child. *Journal of Pain and Symptom Management*, 1989; **4**: 82–5.
246. Pateman J, Williams MP, Filshie J. Retroperitoneal fibrosis after multiple coeliac plexus blocks. *Anaesthesia*, 1990; **45**: 309–10.
247. Berde CB, Sethna NF, Fisher DE, Kahn CH, Chandler P, Grier HE. Celiac plexus blockade for a 3 year old boy with hepatoblastoma and refractory pain. *Pediatrics*, 1990; **86**: 779–81.
248. Cousins MJ, Reeve TS, Glynn CJ, Walsh JA, Cherry DA. Neurolytic lumbar sympathetic blockade: duration of denervation and relief of rest pain. *Anesthesia and Intensive Care*, 1979; **7**: 121–35.
249. Walsh JA, Glynn CJ, Cousins MJ, Basedow RW. Bloodflow, sympathetic activity and pain relief following lumbar sympathetic blockade or surgical sympathectomy. *Anaesthesia and Intensive Care*, 1984; **13**: 18–24.
250. Reid W, Watt JK, Gray TG. Phenol injection of the sympathetic chain. *British Journal of Surgery*, 1970; **57**: 45–55.
251. Plancarte R, Amescua C, Patt RB, Aldrete JA. Superior hypogastric plexus block for pelvic cancer pain. *Anesthesiology*, 1990; **73**: 236–9.
252. deLeon-Casasola OA, Kent E, Lema MJ. Neurolytic superior hypogastric plexus block for chronic pelvic pain associated with cancer. *Pain*, 1993; **54**: 145–51.
253. Plancarte R, Amescua C, Patt RB, Allende S. Presacral blockade of the ganglion of Walther (ganglion impar). *Anesthesiology*, 1990; **73**: A751.
254. Foley KM. The treatment of cancer pain. *The New England Journal of Medicine*, 1985; **313**: 84–95.
255. Travell JG, Simons DG. *Myofascial Pain and Dysfunction: The Trigger Point Manual*. Vol 1: The Upper Extremities. Baltimore: Williams and Wilkins, 1983.
256. Travell JG, Simons DG. *Myofascial Pain and Dysfunction: The Trigger Point Manual*. Vol 2: The Lower Extremities. Baltimore: Williams and Wilkins, 1992.
257. Mense S. Nociception from skeletal muscle in relation to clinical muscle pain. *Pain*, 1993; **54**: 241–89.
258. McCain GA. Fibromyalgia and myofascial pain syndromes. In: Wall PD, Melzack R, eds. *Textbook of Pain*. 3rd edn. Edinburgh: Churchill Livingstone, 1994: 475–93.
259. Reiestad F, Stromskag KE. Interpleural catheter in the management of postoperative pain: a preliminary report. *Regional Anesthesia*, 1986; **11**: 89–91.
260. Waldman SD, Allen ML, Cronen MC. Subcutaneous tunneled intrapleural catheters in the long-term relief of right upper quadrant pain of malignant origin. *Journal of Pain and Symptom Management*, 1989; **4**: 86–9.
261. Myers DP, Lema MJ, deLeon-Casasola OA, Bacon DR. Interpleural analgesia for the treatment of severe cancer pain in terminally ill patients. *Journal of Pain and Symptom Management*, 1993; **8**: 505–10.
262. Fineman SP. Long-term post-thoracotomy cancer pain management with interpleural bupivacaine. *Anesthesia and Analgesia*. 1989; **68**: 694–7.
263. Harrison P, Kent EA, Lema MJ. Interpleural analgesia: its use, and a complication, in a quadriplegic patient with chronic benign pain. *Journal of Pain and Symptom Management*, 1993; **8**: 238–41.
264. Lema MJ, Myers DP, deLeon-Casasola O, Penetrante R. Pleural phenol therapy for the treatment of chronic esophageal cancer pain. *Regional Anesthesia*, 1992; **17**: 166–170.
265. Bruera E, Watanabe S, Fainsinger RL, Spachynski K, Suarez-Almazor M, Inturrisi C. Custom-made capsules and suppositories of methadone for patients on high-dose opioids for cancer pain. *Pain*, 1995; **62**: 141–6.

266. Twycross R. *Pain Relief in Advanced Cancer.* Edinburgh: Churchill Livingstone, 1994: 25–9.
267. Cherny NI, Coyle N, Foley KM. The treatment of suffering when patients request elective death. *Journal of Palliative Care*, 1994; **10**: 71–9.
268. Ventafridda V, Ripamonti C, DeConno F, Tamburini M. Symptom prevalence and control during cancer patients' last days of life. *Journal of Palliative Care*, 1990; **6**: 7–11.
269. Truog RD, Berde CB, Mitchell C, Grier HE. Barbiturates in the care of the terminally ill. *The New England Journal of Medicine*, 1992; **327**: 1678–82.
270. Greene WR, Davis WH. Titrated intravenous barbiturates in the control of symptoms in patients with terminal cancer. *Southern Medical Journal*, 1991; **84**: 332–7.
271. Cherny NI, Portenoy RK. Sedation in the management of refractory symptoms: guidelines for evaluation and treatment. *Journal of Palliative Care*, 1994; **10**: 31–8.
272. Mercadante S, DeConno F, Ripamonti C. Propofol in terminal care. *Journal of Pain and Symptom Management*, 1995; **10**: 639–42.
273. Moyle J. The use of propofol in palliative medicine. *Journal of Pain and Symptom Mangement*, 1995; **10**: 643–6.
274. Pockett S. Spinal cord synaptic plasticity and chronic pain. *Anesthesia and Analgesia*, 1994; **80**: 173–9.
275. Woolf CJ. Recent advances in the pathophysiology of acute pain. *British Journal of Anaesthesia*, 1989; **63**: 139–46.
276. Liebeskind JC. Pain *can* kill. *Pain*, 1991; **44**: 1–2.
277. Page GG, Ben-Eliyahu S, Yirmiya R, Liebeskind JC. Morphine attenuates surgery-induced enhancement of metastatic colonization in rats. *Pain*, 1993; **54**: 21–8.
278. Wilcox GL. Excitatory neurotransmitters and pain. In: Bond MR, Charlton JE, Woolfe CJ, eds. *Proceedings of the VIth World Congress on Pain.* Amsterdam: Elsevier, 1991: 97–117.
279. Ren K. Wind-up and the NMDA receptor: from animal studies to humans. *Pain*, 1994; **59**: 157–8.
280. Presley RW, Menetray D, Levine JD, Basbaum AI. Systemic morphine suppresses noxious stimulus-evoked Fos protein-like immunoreactivity in the rat spinal cord. *Journal of Neuroscience*, 1990; **10**: 323–35.
281. Tolle TR, Castro-Lopes JM, Evans G, Zieglgansberger W. *C-fos* induction in the spinal cord following noxious stimulation: prevention by opiates but not by NMDA antagonists. In: Bond MR, Charlton JE, Woolfe CJ, eds. *Proceedings of the VIth World Congress on Pain.* Amsterdam: Elsevier, 1991: 249–305.
282. Sonnenberg JL, Ranscher FR III, Morgan JI, Curran T. Regulation of proenkephalin by Fos and Jun. *Science*, 1989; **246**: 1622–5.
283. Herdegen T, Tolle TR, Bravo R, Zieglgansberger W, Zimmermann M. Sequential expression of JUN B, JUN D, and FOS B proteins in rat spinal neurons cascade of transcriptional operations during nociception. *Neuroscience Letters*, 1991; **129**: 221–4.
284. Kehl LJ, Basbaum AI, Pollock CM, Mayes M, Wilcox GL. The NMDA antagonist MK 801 reduces noxious stimulus-evoked Fos expression in the mammalian spinal dorsal horn. *Pain*, 1990; **5**: S165.
285. Mao J, Price DD, Mayer DJ. Thermal hyperalgesia in association with the development of morphine tolerance in rats: roles of excitatory amino acid receptors and protein kinase C. *Journal of Neuroscience*, 1994; **14**: 2301–12.
286. Mao JR, Price DD, Mayer DJ. Experimental mononeuropathy reduces the antinociceptive effects of morphine—implications for common intracellular mechanisms involved in morphine tolerance and neuropathic pain. *Pain*, 1995; **61**: 353–64.
287. Laudenslager MI, Ryan SM, Drugan RC, Hyson RL, Maier SF. Coping and immunosuppression: inescapable but not escapable shock suppresses lymphocyte proliferation. *Science*, 1983; **221**: 568–70.
288. Shavit Y, Lewis JW, Terman GW, Gale RP, Liebeskind JC. Opioid peptides mediate the suppressive effect of stress on natural killer cell cytotoxicity. *Science*, 1984; **223**: 188–90.
289. Ben-Eliyahu S, Yirmiya R, Shavit Y, Liebeskind JC. Stress-induced suppression of natural killer cell cytotoxicity in the rat: a naltrexone insensitive paradigm. *Behavioural Neuroscience*, 1990; **104**: 235–8.
290. Cousins M. Acute and postoperative pain. In: Wall PD, Melzack R, eds. *Textbook of Pain.* 3rd ed. Edinburgh: Churchill Livingstone, 1994: 357–85.
291. Davar D, Maciewitz R. MK-801 blocks thermal hyperalgesia in a rat model of neuropathic pain. *Neuroscience Abstracts*, 1989; **15**: 472.
292. Bach S, Noreng MF, Tjellden NU. Phantom limb pain in amputees during the first 12 months following limb amputation, after preoperative lumbar epidural blockade. *Pain*, 1988; **33**: 297–301.

9.2.7 Neurosurgical approaches in palliative care

Ehud Arbit and Mark H. Bilsky

Introduction

Due to the availability and effectiveness of pharmacotherapy and the recognized limitations of neurosurgical treatments—specifically, transience of effect and potential neurological sequelae—only a small number of patients with cancer pain are referred for consideration of a neurosurgical procedure.[1], Of approximately 1000 new patients seen annually in consultation by the pain service at Memorial Sloan-Kettering Cancer Center, only 100 (10 per cent) will be referred for interventional therapy. The majority of these, that is 70 patients (7 per cent), will be referred to an anaesthesiologist for a nerve block or epidural block, while roughly 30 patients (3 per cent) will be referred for a neurosurgical procedure.

Neurosurgical procedures are categorized as ablative modalities (e.g. cordotomy, thalamotomy, rhizotomy) and augmentative modalities (e.g. central nervous system or spinal stimulation, spinal or ventricular opioid infusion). In choosing the most appropriate of these, several basic premises should be considered.[2]

1. Ablative procedures should be deferred as long as pain relief is attainable by other means. For example patients with axial or pelvic pain, which can be alleviated by opioids, should receive that treatment in preference to bilateral cordotomy or myelotomy which are also viable approaches for pain in these regions.

2. The procedure most likely to be effective should be performed but, if there is a choice, the one with fewer and less serious potential complications is preferred. For example cordotomy, myelotomy, and spinal opioid infusion are all potentially excellent ways to relieve pain caused by a pelvic malignancy. As spinal opioid infusion is least likely to have permanent sequelae, it is the preferred first choice.

3. If interruption of pain pathways is indicated, the lowest or most peripheral point relative to the location of the pain is the appropriate site for the procedure. For example if a patient has a tumour at the skull base and intractable facial pain in the distribution subserved by the trigeminal nerve, an ablative procedure of the trigeminal nerve, via selective radiofrequency rhizotomy, is preferred to trigeminal tractotomy or thalamotomy.

4. Since many patients referred for pain procedures today have advanced illness, the neurosurgeon usually has a single opportunity to relieve the pain. Thus, the procedure of choice is the one most likely to alleviate pain successfully in one session. Procedures that may require tailoring or adjustments (e.g., deep brain stimulation) are less suitable.

5. In later stages of cancer, pain is likely to be multifocal, as multiple organs and sites become affected by the disease. A procedure aimed at one locus of pain, even if performed flawlessly, is unlikely to provide freedom from pain for the duration of the patient's life. A realistic expectation to have of a neurosurgical procedure is an enduring decrease in pain to a level that is manageable by pharmacotherapy, with minimal side-effects.[3]

Choosing the most appropriate procedure for an individual patient involves two considerations apart from the pain character: the pathophysiological mechanism underlying the pain and the patient's functional and disease status (and expected longevity).

Pathophysiology

Pain may be categorized as either nociceptive or neuropathic; each requires a different approach. The vast majority of pain in the cancer patient population is nociceptive. 'Nociceptive' implies chronic pain commensurate with tissue damage associated with an identifiable somatic or visceral lesion. Its persistence is presumed to be related to ongoing activation of primary afferent neurones responsive to noxious stimuli (nociceptors). Activation of nociceptors in skin or deep tissue results in somatic pains which, characteristically, are well localized, constant, and described as aching, stabbing, throbbing, or pressure-like.

Nociceptive pains often respond to opioid drugs,[4] and they are also the most amenable to ablative treatment, as interventions that either ameliorate or denervate the nerve(s) subserving the lesion will result in pain control. While most cancer-related pain is predominantly nociceptive, at least initially, many patients develop an underlying component of deafferentation pain as well. As the tumour mass increases in size and compresses or encases a nerve or a nerve plexus, irreversible neural damage and denervation ensues, resulting in a dysaesthetic, causalgic pain superimposed on the primary, original nociceptive pain. This parameter of deafferentation pain is often overlooked, which leads to the less than optimal results achieved by procedures aimed at nociceptive pain. By the same token, a component of deafferentation should not dissuade the surgeon from an ablative procedure. Only when the pain is predominantly of the deafferentation type should treatment procedures be focused on deafferentation-related problems as such.

Visceral pain occurs when visceral nociceptors are activated by stretch or distension of intrathoracic or intra-abdominal viscera. Visceral pain is typically poorly localized and experienced as gnawing or cramping, due to the obstruction of a hollow viscus, and aching, sharp, or throbbing, due to the involvement of organ capsules or mesentery. Visceral pain is often associated with nausea, vomiting, and diaphoresis, and may be referred to cutaneous sites distant from the nociceptive lesion. Visceral pain is conducted afferently by visceronociceptive fibres which ascend bilaterally in crossed and uncrossed tracts. As a result of this anatomical pattern, intervention procedures must be carried out either at the peripheral, ganglionic level or bilaterally and more rostral in the spinal cord.

Neuropathic pain is a consequence of damage to the peripheral and/or central nervous system. Such damage is often caused by the tumour or by surgical, radiotherapeutic, or chemotherapeutic treatments. Neuropathic pain is an unfamiliar experience to most people and has been described as a sensation similar to pins and needles, numbness, dysaesthesia, and electric shock. These paroxysms may be related to spontaneous and ectopic impulse conduction at axonal sites of damaged peripheral nerve structures. Ongoing nociception is not a requisite for the occurrence of neuropathic pain, as it is for nociceptive pain; neuropathic pain occurs presumably as the result of a central pain generator or mechanism, and the removal of the nociceptive lesion may not produce relief. Neuropathic pain is regarded as less opioid responsive than organic pain and may be effectively treated with adjuvant analgesics such as antidepressants and anticonvulsants. From the surgical perspective, neuropathic pain is not well served by ablation of a peripheral nerve or pain tract but rather by procedures aimed at deafferentation, such as stimulation of peripheral nerves, the dorsal column, or the medial lemniscal system.

The impact of functional and disease status

Cancer patients may be placed in one of two groups:

(1) terminally ill individuals with widespread, untreatable systemic disease which is likely to be fatal within weeks or a few months;

(2) individuals with potential protracted longevity, whose focal or systemic cancer may be eradicable or controllable for months to years by antineoplastic therapy.

The majority of patients for whom surgical interventions are considered belong to the first group. They are terminally ill with a short prospective survival time. Frequently, they are partially or completely functionally impaired because of neurological deficits, long bone fractures, spinal metastases, or other causes. These patients are unique in that the benefit of pain relief may well outweigh the risks and consequences of further loss of function caused by increased neurological deficit. Faced with one of these patients, the neurosurgeon has a choice between a neurodestructive procedure or the use of spinal opioids assuming that systemic opioids have not been effective. Nevertheless, some neurological complications are unacceptable at any stage of disease, given the short time the patient is expected to survive and the fact that the procedure is performed only in order to improve quality of life. It is the authors' belief that the risk of potential serious complications, however rare (e.g. blindness or oculomotor dysfunction resulting from chemical hypophysectomy), should sway the surgeon to an alternative with less onerous potential risks. An important advantage of destructive procedures is that they are 'once only' events and, unlike cerebrospinal spinal fluid opioids, do not require ongoing attendance and servicing.[5] This fact becomes an advantage if the patient is discharged and subsequently is not followed by a programme with expertise in the management of infusion pumps or ports.

The second group of patients, those with prospective long-term survival, may be further divided into highly functional or functionally impaired individuals. In the highly functional patient with a long prospective survival, it is advisable to choose non-destructive procedures (such as spinal or ventricular opioids) first and to defer destructive procedures for as long as possible. In patients with long prospective survival but with functional impairment, there is a choice between destructive or non-destructive procedures, based on the rationales described above.

Neurosurgical procedures

When judiciously applied, neurosurgical procedures can produce comfort and palliation. The usefulness and indications for ablative and augmentative procedures will be discussed.

Ablative neurosurgery

Peripheral neurectomy

Currently, techniques such as neuraxial opioid infusion or lytic nerve block have slowly replaced peripheral neurectomy for controlling cancer pain. Before considering a patient for neurectomy, several issues should be addressed. Primarily, both motor and sensory fibres overlap in a single nerve, thus adequate sectioning of a single nerve to denervate even a small area is often hindered. Multiple nerves may have to be sectioned and this, in turn, may result in substantial sensory disturbances and motor deficits. Even if pure sensory nerves are sectioned and motor function is left intact, the extremity may still have a severe disability as the sensory nerves that influence movement might be lost.

Chest wall pain is a preferable indication for peripheral neurectomy, since the resulting motor loss is frequently insignificant, especially when a discrete pain-producing lesion can be demonstrated to involve several intercoastal nerves.[6] Pain originating from a paraspinal tumour, involving a nerve or nerves at, or distal to, the neural foramen, may be effectively alleviated by neurectomy which is often performed at the time of a spine operation.

Neuralgias resulting from cancer have selected indications for cranial neurectomies. The trigeminal and glossopharyngeal nerves can be ablated by radiofrequency lesions created by electrodes placed in either the foreamen ovale or the jugular foreamen or by chemical neurolysis at the gasserian ganglion.[7–10]

Dorsal rhizotomy

Dorsal rhizotomy involves sectioning and eliminating all forms of sensory input entering the dorsal spinal cord. Pain resulting from Pancoast tumours of the lung and head and neck tumours[11] appear to be suitable indications for dorsal rhizotomies. The major advantages of this technique include reducing nociceptive perception in the affected area and sparing motor function. Extensive dorsal rhizotomy of all nerve roots supplying the extremity can lead to a useless limb. Preserving one dorsal root may circumvent such an impairment. As a result, this procedure is considered only for localized pain in the trunk or abdomen or, rarely, for an extremity that is preoperatively functionless.[6,12]

Dorsal rhizotomy can be accomplished by chemical neurolysis with radiographic guidance by placing the tip of an infusion catheter at the precise segment within the epidural space.[10] Potential complications from rhizotomy include sexual and bowel and bladder dysfunction.

Commissural myelotomy

Relief from intractable bilateral and midline pelvic or perineal pain can be achieved with commissural myelotomy.[13–15] Commissural myelotomy disrupts pain and thermal fibres in the process of crossing, before reaching the opposite spinothalamic tract. Open myelotomy involves performing an extensive laminectomy using radiographic localization to expose adequate segments of the spinal cord. Longitudinal division of the spinal cord is performed over several segments (preferably two or three segments above the highest level of pain) along the dorsal midline through the anterior white commissure.[16] The procedure may cause bowel and/or bladder and motor disturbances.

Myelotomy can also be performed stereotactically with computerized tomography (**CT**) guidance where a midline incision is made at the cervicomedullary junction.[17] Potential complications arising from stereotactic myelotomy include dysaesthesia and limb apraxia.[18]

Dorsal root entry zone lesions

Dorsal root entry zone lesions are used primarily to treat neuropathic pain including brachial plexus avulsion or carcinomatous invasion, post-herpetic neuralgia, and post-traumatic paraplegia. The anatomic ablative lesion that is created involves the posterior part of the dorsal horn, including the substantia gelatinosa and probably the medial part of the tract of Lissauer. Candidates are patients who have failed transcutaneous stimulation and drug treatments. A standard laminectomy or hemilaminectomy is performed over the affected spinal segments. Several techniques have been described for creating the lesion including thermocoagulation, scalpel dissection, or CO_2 laser.

Pain relief is complete in approximately one-third of patients. Significant pain may be experienced postoperatively from the laminectomy. Pain relief in the immediate postoperative period that persists for 3 to 6 months generally results in permanent relief. Temporary neurological deficits have been reported in up to 50 per cent of patients and permanent deficits in 5 to 10 per cent of patients. These deficits include weakness, ataxia, and sensory loss. Cerebrospinal fluid leaks occurred in 16 per cent of patients who underwent dorsal root entry zone lesions. All of these patients had undergone previous operations at the involved level for attempted control of pain.

Hypophysectomy

Hypophysectomy involves ablation or chemical destruction (stereotactic transsphenoidal) of the pituitary gland. Both procedures can provide equally successful pain relief from bone metastases. The mechanism by which pain relief is achieved is not completely understood, but evidence shows that it is unrelated to suppression of pituitary function, since hormone insensitive and sensitive tumours can also achieve pain relief.[19–23] Instead, stimulation of a hypothalamic pain-suppressing capability prompted by hypophysectomy seems to be a more suitable explanation.[24]

Bilateral or diffuse bone pain from metastatic disease that did not respond well to all other hormonal, radiation, or medical therapies are common settings for hypophysectomy. Potential complications include endocrine deficits, damage to the optic nerves or oculomotor apparatus from the injected chemical agent, and cerebrospinal spinal fluid leakage.[25–27]

Lesions of the brain

Thalamotomy

Although a relatively uncommon procedure, thalamotomy can alleviate midline or bilateral pain from widespread metastatic disease. Like cordotomy or myelotomy, spinothalamic fibres are interrupted but thalamotomy occurs at a higher, central level in the dorsolateral midbrain contralateral to the pain. Stereotactic thalamotomies are recommended[28] since it provides localization with stimulation and the use of local anaesthesia.

Initial pain relief in medial or basal thalamotomies can be achieved in over 80 per cent of patients; unfortunately pain recurs in 30 per cent of patients after 1 year of treatment. Patients with cancer benefit more than those with non-malignant disease.[29] Potential complications, aside from bleeding and infection, include impaired function of the compromised adjacent sensory nuclei. Motor tracts near the outer portions of the thalamus can be affected as a result of ill-placed lesions. Confusion, memory impairment, and disorientation can also occur and, although usually transient, can be permanent.[15]

Cingulotomy

Cingulotomy involves the interruption of the fibre tracts of the cingulate gyri, which interrupts fibres of the cortex, thalamic nuclei, and other components of the thalamic system. In 1962, Foltz and White[30] postulated that creating a lesion in the bilateral frontal lobe or cingulum might modify the patient's emotional response as well as relieve intractable pain. Patients with unresectable, disseminated disease and who have exhausted all other treatment options to relieve severe cancer-related pain are most likely to benefit from this procedure. Cingulotomy done stereotactically can be effectively performed under local anaesthesia with minimal risk to the patient.[31] Due to insufficient reported experience, meaningful success rates for cingulotomy are unavailable but some studies[30,32] have shown this procedure to be well tolerated with no significant side-effects.

Augmentative neurosurgery (non-ablative)

Intracerebral stimulation

Heath and Mickle[33] initially reported pain relief from specific intracerebral stimulation of the septal nucleus in 1960. While intracerebral stimulation has not been used extensively, improved anatomic definition and localization of targets, as well as improved hardware, have made these techniques more attractive in the pain treatment armamentarium. Brain stimulation procedures do not require a permanent destructive lesion that may cause permanent adverse neurological sequelae, as neuroablative procedures do, and are generally reversible once the electrical stimulus is removed.

The major targets for intracerebral stimulation are the ventral posterior medial and ventral posterior lateral somatosensory nuclei of the thalamus, for control of deafferentiation or neuropathic pain, and stimulation of the periaqueductal gray for control of somatic pain. The mechanism of action is different for these stimulation targets. Stimulations of the thalamic nuclei produces localized tingling in a somatotopic distribution that may also inhibit pain in that somatic region. This effect is thought to be mediated by a gait control mechanism at that segmental level which results in a modification of the pain signal. The stimulation does not result in elevated endorphin levels and is not blocked by naloxone. Conversely, periaqueductal gray stimulation does result in an elevation in intraventricular endorphin levels and is inhibited by naloxone. The result of periaqueductal gray stimulation is a reduction in pain and a general sense of well-being, but this does not occur in a somatotopic distribution.

Due to this difference in mechanisms of action, the choice of targets may be made on the basis of the response to a graduated morphine test. Patients who obtain dose-dependent relief from morphine that is reversible with naloxone may benefit from periaqueductal gray stimulation. Those who do not respond to this test are better candidates for thalamic stimulation procedures. Mixed neuropathic and somatic pain syndromes (i.e. arachnoiditis) may require stimulation at both sites for adequate pain relief.

In the series reported by Hosobuchi,[34] 122 patients underwent implantation for chronic pain syndromes. The mean duration of time between the onset of pain and implantation was 6.5 years. All patients had been previously tried on multiple analgesic regimens and/or other pain procedures without success. The leading reasons for implantation in the thalamic nuclei of patients with deafferentiation pain were lumbosacral radiculopathy, thalamic pain, anaesthesia delorosa, and postcordotomy dysaesthesias. Long-term success was achieved in 44 out of 50 patients who underwent internalization of the electrodes. Implantation in the periaqueductal gray for somatic pain was performed in 62 patients. The most common reason was chronic low back pain. Other causes of pain include cancer, cauda equina syndrome, and non-malignant abdominal pain. Fifty patients had good long-term control of their pain. Complications were seen in 11 per cent of patients. These complications included intraventricular haemorrhage (three patients) and intracerebral haemorrhage (two patients). One patient in each of these groups died as a result of their complication. Other rare complications included ventriculitis, subgaleal infection, and subdural empyema. Three patients also developed permanent eye-movement dysfunction.

Choosing the most appropriate neurological procedure

For the most part, destructive surgical procedures have been superseded by minimally invasive stereotactic approaches, that are less taxing on the already debilitated and terminally ill patients, or alternative augmentative modalities which carry a much reduced risk. Neuroablative procedures are now viable options for patients in advanced stages of illness who were not candidates for such therapy before. It should be emphasized that there are situations in which the use of an ablative procedure, especially a one-time procedure, can be less invasive and taxing to the patient than continued aggressive medical management. Cordotomy, which will be described in detail, is considered one of the most commonly used representatives of the ablative modalities.

Cordotomy

Prior to the development of intrathecal delivery of opioids, anterior cordotomy was the most common palliative surgical pain procedure. The anterior spinothalamic tract mediates pain and temperature from the contralateral half of the body. The original procedure was performed by Martin and Spiller in 1912 via an open surgical approach in the thoracic region.[35] Since that time the procedure has undergone a number of modifications. In 1965, Mullan described the high cervical percutaneous approach which was subsequently improved by a number of technical innovations.[36] This approach is most commonly used in cancer patients. Two other approaches which are also warranted on occasion are the open[37] and percutaneous[38] low cervical cordotomy performed via the C5–6 disc space.

Anatomy

Understanding the anatomy of the spinothalamic tract is essential to successful cordotomy. A-delta and C fibres enter the spinal cord through the lateral dorsal root and ascend or descend one to three levels via the tract of Lissauer. The first order neurones synapse on the spinal grey laminae I (marginal zone), II (substantia gelatinosa), and V. The second order neurones generally decussate through the anterior white commissure and ascend via spinothalamic tract in the anterolateral funiculus. The neurones then synapse in the thalamus on the ventroposterior nucleus (ventral posterior lateral), posteromedial portion of the nucleus parafascularis, intralaminar nucleus, and nucleus submedius of the thalamus.

The spinothalamic tract has both a topographic and modality-specific orientation. The lumbar and sacral fibres are predominately posterior and superficial in the spinal cord, and those fibres mediating thoracic and cervical areas are more anterior and deep, in close proximity to the ventral horn. The spinothalamic tract also has modality-specific orientation with superficial pain located in the superficial part of the spinothalamic tract, while temperature and deep visceral pain are located more deeply.

Anatomic variations in the spinothalamic tract may effect the outcome of cordotomy. While fibres generally ascend one to three spinal segments in the tract of Lissauer, they may ascend as many as six to eight segments before synapsing in the spinal grey matter. For this reason, the level of analgesia that was obtained may be considerably lower than that expected from the level in which the cordotomy lesion was made. In Ischia's series of percutaneous high cervical cordotomy performed for thoracic primary and metastatic tumours, including superior sulcal and Pancoast tumours, the level of analgesia that was consistently obtained was below C5, but 12.5 per cent patients obtained a level of analgesia as high as C3. [48] Following low cervical or high thoracic cordotomy, the highest level of analgesia consistently obtained is at approximately T4.

While uncommon, there are a number of reports in the literature of the spinothalamic tract conducting pain and temperature fibres from the ipsilateral side of the body.[7,39,40] Lesioning the spinothalamic tract results in ipsilateral analgesia as opposed to the expected contralateral analgesia. This may be prevented by awake spinal cord stimulation which is routinely used during percutaneous cordotomy.

Indications

Cordotomy is currently indicated primarily for unilateral nociceptive pain below C5. Bilateral cordotomy should be considered for midline or bilateral pain. Cordotomy is not an effective treatment for dysaesthetic pain, postherpetic pain, or causalgia. It has been performed more successfully for pain of malignant origin than for non-malignant disease, because of the often short duration of analgesia achieved and the possibility of developing delayed postcordotomy dysaesthetic pain.

Procedure

The patient is placed in a supine position with his head secured in a strict anteroposterior orientation. Intravenous analgesics are administered throughout the procedure and frequent increased dosages may be required to maintain enough patient comfort to perform the procedure. With fluoroscope guidance, a C1–C2 spinal puncture is performed with the spinal needle aimed horizontally toward the anterior third of the spinal canal. A contrast mixture of metrizamide and cerebrospinal spinal fluid is injected into the subarachnoid space in order to clearly delineate the dentate ligament.

After the dentate ligament has been identified, the cordotomy electrode is introduced through the spinal needle. The needle hub is clamped to a vertical assembly bar and the electrode is advanced toward the cord parenchyma, anterior to the dentate ligament. The procedure is carried out under impedance guidance with the audiotone monitor turned on.

An anteroposterior fluoroscopic view at this stage shows the tip of the electrode at or just beyond the middle of the odontoid process. Paraesthesia or other sensations usually described as heat or cold in the contralateral lower body segments, in response to stimulation at 100 Hz, indicate that the desired location has been reached. Stimulation at 2 Hz and voltage of approximately 2.6 V provokes ipsilateral contractions of cervical myotomes. If these responses do not occur, the electrode must be repositioned.

The lesion is produced in successive steps, between which the depth of analgesia and strength in the patient's legs are checked. A radiofrequency lesion is produced with a thermocouple–monitor electrode, at a temperature of 80°C and a duration of 30 s. The extent of the lesion may be adjusted by using a higher temperature (up to 90°C) and a longer duration (up to 60 s).[41]

Outcomes

Complete analgesia is obtained in 85 to 93 per cent of patients immediately following the unilateral percutaneous cordotomy.[18,42–45] However, over time, analgesic levels may decline. Rosomoff *et al.*[46] reported a series of 1279 unilateral cordotomies in which 90 per cent of patients achieved complete pain relief immediately following the procedure, but at 1 year only 61 per cent had complete relief, 43 per cent at 5 years, and 37 per cent at 10 years. Despite the loss of complete pain relief, 50 per cent of patients continued to have significant long-term relief that improved their daily living. Tasker *et al.*[45] in a series of 244 patients reported a similar trend with 94 per cent showing significant relief in the immediate perioperative period. This figure declined to 78 per cent at the time of discharge. Twenty-four patients in this series were operated on for benign pain. All patients experienced recurrent pain, but this ranged from 1 to 21 years after the initial procedure.[45] Repeat cordotomy is frequently successful in returning a patient's level of analgesia.[44,45,47]

The immediate success seen with bilateral cordotomy approximates that seen with the unilateral procedure, producing pain relief in greater than 90 per cent of patients. However, the long-term relief is less gratifying. Tasker reports that less than 5 per cent of survivors continue to have pain relief at 1 year.[45] Ischia reports a 47 per cent incidence of long-term pain relief in patients, with the majority of the treatment failures occurring contralateral to the second procedure.[48]

Patterns of failure

Several patterns of recurrent pain have been identified following unilateral cordotomy. New pain above the level of previously acquired analgesia results either from a falling level of analgesia, which is commonly seen in the weeks following the procedure, or new disease producing pain above a constant level of analgesia.

Additionally, in the immediate post cordotomy period mirror pain, ipsilateral to the lesion, may be unmasked. This ipsilateral pain may not be appreciated by the patient prior to the cordotomy, because of the overwhelming nature of the contralateral pain. In Ischia's series, 72 per cent of the 58 patients undergoing the procedure for unilateral thoracopulmonary tumour involvement experienced mirror pain that was successfully controlled with analgesics.[45]

As with mirror pain, deafferentation pain may not be appreciated as contributing to the patient's pain picture prior to cordotomy, either because it is masked by the nociceptive pain component or because the quality of the pain is not recognized prior to the procedure. Even if nociceptive pain is successfully alleviated with an appropriate level of anaesthesia below the level of the cordotomy, dysaesthetic pain may persist in 15 to 33 per cent of patients. Frequently, the deafferentation pain will be alleviated for a short time making the cordotomy seem successful, only to be followed by its emergence a few weeks later. Repeat cordotomy is generally not effective in alleviating this pain.

Deafferentation pain may also be produced by the cordotomy itself. This occurs in approximately 1 per cent of patients, generally greater than 1 year after the procedure. This is one of the major contraindications to performing the procedure in patients with benign disease and an extended life expectancy.

Complications

The major complications from cordotomy include respiratory dysfunction, sleep apnoea, hemiparesis, bladder dysfunction, Horner's syndrome, and arterial hypotension.

Respiratory dysfunction is the most significant complication from high percutaneous cervical cordotomy. Respiratory function is mediated through two pathways. Voluntary respiration is controlled by the corticospinal tract which is rarely damaged during cordotomy, if care is taken to remain anterior to the dentate ligament. Autonomic respiration is controlled via the reticulospinal tract, which subserves ipsilateral lung function. These fibres are adjacent to the anteromedial portion of the spinothalamic tract (cervical region) and the anterior horn of the grey matter. High cervical cordotomy may result in disruption of the reticulospinal tract and lead to significant pulmonary compromise. This fibre tract is at highest risk for sectioning when attempting to achieve a cervical or high thoracic level of analgesia. This spinal cord lesion is directly adjacent to the reticulospinal tract.

Patients undergoing high unilateral percutaneous cordotomy are at risk for respiratory decompensation with concomitant pulmonary disease contralateral to the side of the cordotomy. Preoperative pulmonary function tests are useful in predicting which of these patients may be affected. Tencela *et al.*[49] reported a series of patients undergoing unilateral cordotomy in whom forced vital capacity and maximum expiratory flow rate were measured both pre- and postoperatively. While these values were not significantly altered by the unilateral procedure, seven out of 41 patients developed postoperative dyspnoea. These seven patients had pulmonary involvement with cancer and decreased preoperative pulmonary function tests. Of the 12 patients in this study with preoperative forced vital capacity and maximum expiratory flow rate values less than 50 per cent of predicted for normals, six developed postoperative dyspnoea with two succumbing to pneumonia and two others requiring artificial ventilatory assistance.

Bilateral high cervical cordotomy has a higher risk of causing respiratory decompensation than the unilateral procedure and is associated with an additional risk of sleep apnoea. While forced vital capacity and maximum expiratory flow rate were not adversely affected following unilateral high percutaneous cordotomy, both values were significantly reduced following the bilateral procedure.[49] Rosomoff *et al.*[43] likewise demonstrated a significant reduction in other respiratory parameters including tidal volume, minimum volume, and ventilatory response to 5 per cent CO_2.

Sleep apnoea has been reported in 0 to 18 per cent of cases following bilateral cordotomy.[48] Patients appear to have normal respirations while awake because they maintain voluntary control which is mediated by the intact corticospinal tracts. Bilateral reticulospinal tract lesions cause a loss of autonomic respiratory drive when the patient falls asleep. Additionally, these lesions may result in a decreased response to hypercarbia as a stimulus to breathe. This scenario leads to sleep apnoea, or 'Ondine's curse'. Sleep apnoea generally develops within 5 days of the procedure but may occur at any time, often without warning. This condition is often self-limiting but patients may require interim ventilatory support. There is a high mortality from unrecognized sleep apnoea.

A number of technical safeguards have been employed to prevent the development of sleep apnoea. It is recommended to wait at least 1 week between cordotomies to assess for intervening respiratory distress that may be caused by a unilateral reticulospinal tract lesion. Additionally, attempts to produce bilateral anteromedial lesions in order to obtain a high level of analgesia are contraindicated with this approach. Ishchia *et al.*[48] reported a large series of bilateral cordotomy procedures without a single patient developing sleep apnoea. All lesions were produced in the posterolateral quadrant of the spinothalamic tract. The average level of analgesia was T4. Alternatively, a high thoracic or low cervical approach may be used to avoid the risk to the reticulospinal tract.

Hemiparesis or ataxia following percutaneous cordotomy results from involvement of the corticospinal tracts. This is usually a transient finding occurring in 5 to 31 per cent of cases, but decreasing to less than 3 per cent long-term following both unilateral and bilateral cordotomy.

Bladder dysfunction results from interruption of the voluntary and autonomic ascending and descending pathways that are concentrated in a narrow band at the periphery of the anterior horn of the spinal cord. These fibres are crossed, so that unilateral interruption of the fibre tracts does not usually lead to problems. Pre-existing bladder dysfunction may worsen following unilateral cordotomy. Involvement of these fibres following bilateral cordotomy is frequent, occurring in 12 to 40 per cent of patients and may require permanent catheterization.

Arterial orthostatic hypotension may occur following bilateral cordotomy in up to 40 per cent of patients as a result of the bilateral interruption of the reticulospinal fibres. It is frequently transient, but is a major contributing factor to the mortality following bilateral procedures. The bilateral procedure is contraindicated in patients with significant pre-existing heart disease or in patients with a low ejection fraction.

References

1. Gildenberg PL. Functional neurosurgery. In: Schmidek HH, Sweet WH, eds. *Operative Neurosurgical Techniques*, Vol. 2. New York: Grune and Stratton, 1982: 993–1043.
2. Gildenberg PL. Considerations in the selection of patients for surgical treatment of pain caused by malignancy. In: Arbit E, ed. *Management of Cancer-Related Pain*. Mount Kisco NY: Futura, 1993: 221–30.
3. Arbit E. Neurosurgical management of cancer pain. In: Foley KM, Bonica JJ, Ventafridda V, eds. *Proceedings of the Second International Congress on Cancer Pain. Advances in Pain Research and Therapy*, 1990; **16**: 289–301.
4. Arner S, Arner B. Differential effects of epidural morphine in the treatment of cancer-related pain. *Acta Anaesthesiologica Scandinavica*, 1985; **29**: 32–6.
5. Tasker RR. Stereotaxic surgery. In: Wall PD, Melzack R, eds. *Textbook of Pain*, 1st edn. Edinburgh: Churchill Livingstone, 1984: 639–55.
6. Arbit E, Galicich JH, Burt M, *et al.* Modified open thoracic rhizotomy for treatment of intractable chest wall pain of malignant etiology. *Annals of Thoracic Surgery*, 1989; **48**: 820–3.
7. Sweet WH. Treatment of facial pain by percutaneous differential thermal trigeminal rhizotomy. *Progress in Neurological Surgery*, 1976; **7**: 153–79.
8. Giorgi C, Broggi G. Surgical treatment of glossopharyngeal neuralgia and pain from cancer of the nasopharynx. A 20-year experience. *Journal of Neurosurgery*, 1984; **61**: 952–5.
9. Ischia S, Luzzani A, Polati E. Retrogasserian glycerol injection: a retrospective study of 112 patients. *Clinical Journal of Pain*, 1990; **6**: 291–6.
10. Jacox A, Carr DB, Payne R, *et al.* Management of cancer pain. *Clinical Practice Guidelines, No. 9.* AHCPR Publication No. 94–0592. Rockville, MD: Agency for Health Care Policy and Research, U.S. Department of Health and Human Services, Public Health Service, March 1994.
11. Mracek Z. Surgical treatment in intractable pain in advanced malignant tumors of the face, oral cavity, pharynx and larynx. *Ceskoslovenska Otolaryngologie*, 1980; **29**: 104–9.
12. Sindou M, Fischer G, Goutelle A, *et al.* Micro surgical selective posterior rhizotomy. 69 cases. Third World Congress on Pain, Edinburgh Scotland, Sept 4–11, 1981. *Pain*, 1981; (suppl. 1): S289
13. Adams JE, Lippert R, Hosobuchi Y. Commissural myelotomy. In: Schmidek HH, Sweet WH, eds. *Operative Neurosurgical Techniques: Indications, Methods, and Results*, 2nd edn, Vol. 2. Philadelphia PA: WB Saunders, 1988: 1185–9.
14. van Roost D, Gybels J. Myelotomies for chronic pain. *Acta Neurochirurgica*, 1989; **46** suppl.: 69–72.
15. Carson BS. Neurologic and neurosurgical approaches to cancer pain. In: McGuire DB, Yarbro CH, eds. *Cancer Pain Management*. Orlando FL: Grune and Stratton, 1987: 223–43.
16. Jones MW. Commissural myelotomy for relief of intractable pain. In: Arbit E, ed. *Management of Cancer-Related Pain*. Mount Kisco, NY: Futura, 1993: 313–19.
17. Schvarcz JR. Spinal cord stereotactic techniques re: trigeminal nucleotomy and extralemniscal myelotomy. *Applied Neurophysiology*, 1978; **41**: 99–112.
18. Gildenberg PL. Myelotomy and percutaneous cervical cordotomy for the treatment of cancer pain. *Applied Neurophysiology*, 1984; **47**: 208–15.
19. Katz S, Levin AB. Treatment of diffuse metastatic pain by instillation of alcohol into the sella turcica. *Anesthesiology*, 1977; **46**: 115–21.
20. Levin AB, Katz S, Benson RC, *et al.* Treatment of pain of diffuse metastatic cancer by stereotactic chemical hypophysectomy: long term results and observations on mechanism of action. *Neurosurgery*, 1980; **6**: 258–62.
21. Madrid JL. Chemical hypophysectomy. *Advances in Pain Research and Therapy*, 1979; **2**: 381–91.
22. Silverberg GD. Hypophysectomy in the treatment of disseminated prostate carcinoma. *Cancer*, 1977; **39**: 1727–31.
23. Tindall GT, Ambrose SS, Christy JH, *et al.* Hypophysectomy in the treatment of disseminated carcinoma of the breast and prostate gland. *Southern Medical Journal*, 1976; **69**: 579–83.
24. Levin AB. Hypophysectomy in the treatment of cancer pain. In: Arbit E, ed. *Management of Cancer-Related Pain*. Mount Kisco, NY: Futura, 1993: 281–95.
25. Cook PR, Campbell FN, Puddy BR. Pituitary alcohol injection for cancer pain. *Anesthesia*, 1984; **39**: 540–5.
26. Lahuerta J, Lipton S, Miles J, *et al.* Update on percutaneous cervical cordotomy and pituitary alcohol neuroadenolysis: an audit of our recent results and complications. In: Lipton S, Miles J, eds. *Persistant Pain: Modern Methods of Treatment*, Vol. 5. Orlando, FL: Grune and Stratton, 1985: 197–223.
27. Lipton S, Miles J, Williams N, *et al.* Pituitary injection of alcohol for widespread cancer pain. *Pain*, 1978; **5**: 73–82.
28. Hitchcock E, Leece B. Somatotropic representation of respiratory pathways in the cervical cord of man. *Journal of Neurosurgery*, 1967; **27**: 320–9.
29. Nashold BS Jr, Nashold JRB, Foltz RM. Neurosurgical management of pelvic and perineal pain of cancer. In: Arbit E, ed. *Management of Cancer-Related Pain*. Mount Kisco, NY: Futura, 1993: 491–504.
30. Foltz EL, White LE Jr. Pain relief by frontal cingulotomy. *Journal of Neurosurgery*, 1962; **19**: 89–93.
31. Hassenbusch SJ, Pillay PK. Cingulotomy for treatment of cancer-related pain. In: Arbit E, ed. *Management of Cancer-Related Pain*. Mount Kisco, NY, Futura, 1993: 297–312.
32. Hurt RW, Ballantine HT Jr. Stereotactic anterior cingulate lesions for persistent pain: a report of 68 cases. *Clinical Neurosurgery*, 1974; **21**: 334–51.
33. Heath RG, Mickle WA. Evaluation of 7 years' experience with depth electrode studies in human patients. In: Ramey ER, O'Doherty DS, eds. *Electrical Studies in the Anesthetized Brain*. New York: Harper and Row, 1960: 214–47.
34. Hosobuchi Y. Subcortical electrical stimulation for control of intractable pain in humans. Report of 122 cases. *Journal of Neurosurgery*, 1986; **64**: 543–53.
35. Spiller WG, Martin E. The treatment of persistent pain of organic origin in the lower part of the body by division of the anterolateral column of the spinal cord. *Journal of the American Medical Association*, 1912; **58**: 1489–90.
36. Mullan S, Hekmatpanah J, Dobben G, *et al.* Percutaneous, intramedullary cordotomy utilizing the unipolar anodal electrolytic system. *Journal of Neurosurgery*, 1965; **22**: 548–53.

37. Cloward RB. Cervical chordotomy by the anterior approach: technique and advantages. *Journal of Neurosurgery*, 1964; **21**: 19–25.
38. Lin PM, Gildenberg PL, Polakoff PP. An anterior approach to percutaneous lower cervical cordotomy. *Journal of Neurosurgery*, 1960; **25**: 553–60.
39. Voris HC. Ipsilateral sensory loss following cordotomy. Report of a case. *Archives of Neurology and Psychiatry*, 1951; **65**: 95–6.
40. White JC. Cordotomy: assessment of its effectiveness and suggestions for its improvement. *Clinical Neurosurgery*, 1966; **13**: 1–19.
41. Arbit E. Anterolateral cordotomy-percutaneous cordotomy. In: Arbit E, ed. *Management of Cancer-Related Pain*. Mount Kisco, NY: Futura, 1993: 321–32.
42. Ventafridda V, Tamburini M, De Conno F. Comprehensive treatment in cancer pain. In: Fields HL, Dubner R, Cervero F, eds. *Advances in Pain Research and Therapy*. New York, Raven Press, 1985: 617–28.
43. Rosomoff HL, Krieger AJ, Kuperman AS. Effects of percutaneous cervical cordotomy on pulmonary function. *Journal of Neurosurgery*, 1969; **31**: 620–7.
44. Lipton S. Percutaneous cervical cordotomy. *Acta Anaesthesiology Belgica*, 1981; **32**: 81–5.
45. Tasker RR. Percutaneous cordotomy: the lateral high cervical technique. In: Schmidek HH, Sweet WH, eds. *Operative Neurosurgical Techniques: Indications, Methods, and Results*, 2nd edn, Vol. 2. Philadelphia, PA: WB Saunders, 1988: 1191–205.
46. Rosomoff HL, Papo I, Loeser JD, *et al.* Neurosurgical operations on the spinal cord. In: Bonica JJ, ed. *Management of Pain*. Malvern, PA: Lea and Febiger, 1990: 2067–81.
47. Nathan PW. Results of antero-lateral cordotomy for pain in cancer. *Journal of Neurology, Neurosurgery and Psychiatry*, 1963; **26**: 353–62.
48. Ischia S, Luzzani A, Ischia A, *et al.* Bilateral percutaneous cervical cordotomy: immediate and long-term results in 36 patients with neoplastic disease. *Journal of Neurology, Neurosurgery and Psychiatry*, 1984; **47**: 141–7.
49. Tenicela R, Rosomoff HL, Feist J, *et al.* Pulmonary function following percutaneous cervical cordotomy. *Anesthesiology*, 1968; **29**: 7–16.

9.2.8 Transcutaneous electrical nerve stimulation (TENS) and acupuncture

John W. Thompson and Jacqueline Filshie

Introduction

Medical historians and anthropologists have described numerous ways in which painful conditions have been managed by sensory modulation.[1] One common feature in all these folklore techniques, such as cupping, scarification, cauterization, and acupuncture, is that a painful stimulus is applied to abolish the pain. Similarly, electrical stimulation of the human body for therapeutic purposes, particularly for the relief of pain, has been employed since early times. Evidence from cave drawings suggest that the Egyptians of the Fifth Dynasty (2500 BC) used the electric fish *Malapterurus electricus* to relieve pain. Hippocrates, in 400 BC, referred to the use of the electric torpedo for the treatment of headache and arthritis and the Roman physician, Scribonius Largus, almost certainly utilized the electrical ray fish *Torpedo marmorata* for the treatment of gout.

Table 1 Clinical pain conditions that have been treated successfully with TENS

Peripheral nerve disorders
peripheral nerve injury
causalgia
amputation pain
phantom limb pain
postherpetic neuralgia
Spinal cord and spinal root disorders
dorsal root compression and spinal nerve compression
Pain associated with neoplastic lesions
metastatic bone pain
neoplastic pain
Muscle pain
secondary muscle spasm
musculoskeletal disorders
Joint pain
rheumatoid arthritis
osteoarthritis
Acute pain
acute orofacial pain
postoperative pain

Reproduced in an abbreviated form from Woolf, ref. 6.

Transcutaneous electrical nerve stimulations (TENS)

A critical turning point in the history of electrotherapy was the advent of the gate control theory of pain proposed by Melzack and Wall in 1965.[2] This hypothesis was immediately verifiable and was quickly put to the test by Wall and Sweet, who, in 1967, showed that high-frequency (50–100 Hz) percutaneous electrical nerve stimulation relieved chronic neurogenic pain.[3] Further corroboration came in 1967 when Shealy and his colleagues[4] showed that electrical stimulation of the dorsal column was also effective for the relief of chronic pain. In 1973, Long reported the results of transcutaneous electrical nerve stimulation which, up to then, had been used to select patients for dorsal column implantation.[5] It was soon realized that TENS alone was effective, thus largely obviating the need for dorsal column implantation. This situation was facilitated by the advent of solid-state electronics which made it possible to manufacture small battery-operated stimulators and from then on the use of TENS developed rapidly.

More recent developments of TENS have involved the use of different patterns of electrical stimulation, which include pulsed (burst), modulation (ramped), random, and complex waveforms, all designed with the aim of improving the efficacy of TENS. Clinical pain conditions that are now commonly treated with TENS are listed in Table 1.

Techniques

Several forms of TENS are now in common use. These may be classified as in Table 2. The way in which these different types of

Table 2 Forms of TENS in common use

Form	Pulse	Effects		
	Pattern	Frequency	Amplitude	
1. Continuous = 'conventional'	Continuous	High 40–150 Hz	Low 10–30 mA	Non-painful paraesthesia as directed into area supplied by stimulated nerve(s)
2. Pulsed = 'burst'	Bursts	Low Bursts of 100 Hz at 1–2 Hz	Low 10–30 mA	As for 1 but felt in bursts
3. Acupuncture-like = high-intensity pulsed	Bursts	Low Bursts of 100 Hz at 1–2 Hz	High 15–50 mA	As for 1 but accompanied by non-painful phasic twitching of muscles in those myotomes stimulated

Note
(1) On some stimulators pulsed forms of TENS (2 and 3) are available in a modulated or ramped form so that the amplitudes of each set of shocks making up the pulses or burst are not equal but form a rising staircase of increasing intensity. This pattern of pulsing produces a stroking sensation which is more comfortable for the patient.
(2) On some stimulators a randomized continuous output is available, the purpose of which is to reduce the development of tolerance to TENS which may occur more readily with a regular pattern of stimulation due to habituation of the nervous system.
(3) Stimulators are now available that produce complex wave forms designed to operate with a single pair of electrodes (LIKON) or multiple electrodes activated randomly (CODETRON), and it is hoped that their role in TENS therapy, especially for palliative care, will soon become clear.

TENS are used is described below (see below, Practical use and indications for TENS therapy).

Equipment

TENS equipment consists essentially of the stimulator (including connecting leads) and the electrodes.

During the past 15 years or so the number of stimulators designed specifically for TENS therapy has steadily increased on a worldwide basis. Stamp and Wood[8],[9] have published two comparative evaluations of transcutaneous stimulators which survey the type of equipment available (summarized in Table 3). Since this is a profitable market, new models appear frequently but before making a purchase the potential buyer should check that any stimulator under consideration has as a minimum the following features:

(1) compact, lightweight, conveniently shaped, sturdily built, and easily attachable to belt or pocket;

(2) on–off/amplitude (strength) and frequency controls of convenient size and shape, easily adjustable yet sufficiently protected from accidental knocking or disturbance;

(3) availability of pulse patterns—continuous (conventional) and pulsed (burst) patterns essential; modulation (ramped) and random patterns desirable;

Table 3 Main characteristics of stimulators for transcutaneous electrical nerve stimulation (TENS) currently available[7,8]

Country of origin:	Finland, Israel, Japan, UK, USA
Dimensions:	6 x 4.9 x 1.78 cm (smallest)–12 x 8.5 x 3.6 cm (largest)
Weight, including battery:	55–220 g
Pulse width:	200 μs fixed or 100–500 μs adjustable
Pulse frequency:	1.5–100 Hz adjustable; rarely fixed In some instruments 'packets' or 'bursts' of pulses available at 2 Hz
Channels:	1 or 2
Battery type (with or without optional rechargeable kit):	PP3, 2 x AA, or special
Battery life:	40–120 h (occasionally 4–16 h)
Guarantee:	0.5–2 years
Costs:	£70–£250 + VAT (UK) (NB Stimulators used for the relief of chronic pain conditions are usually eligible for relief from Value Added Tax under Group 14 of Schedule 5 to the Value Added Tax Act 1983).

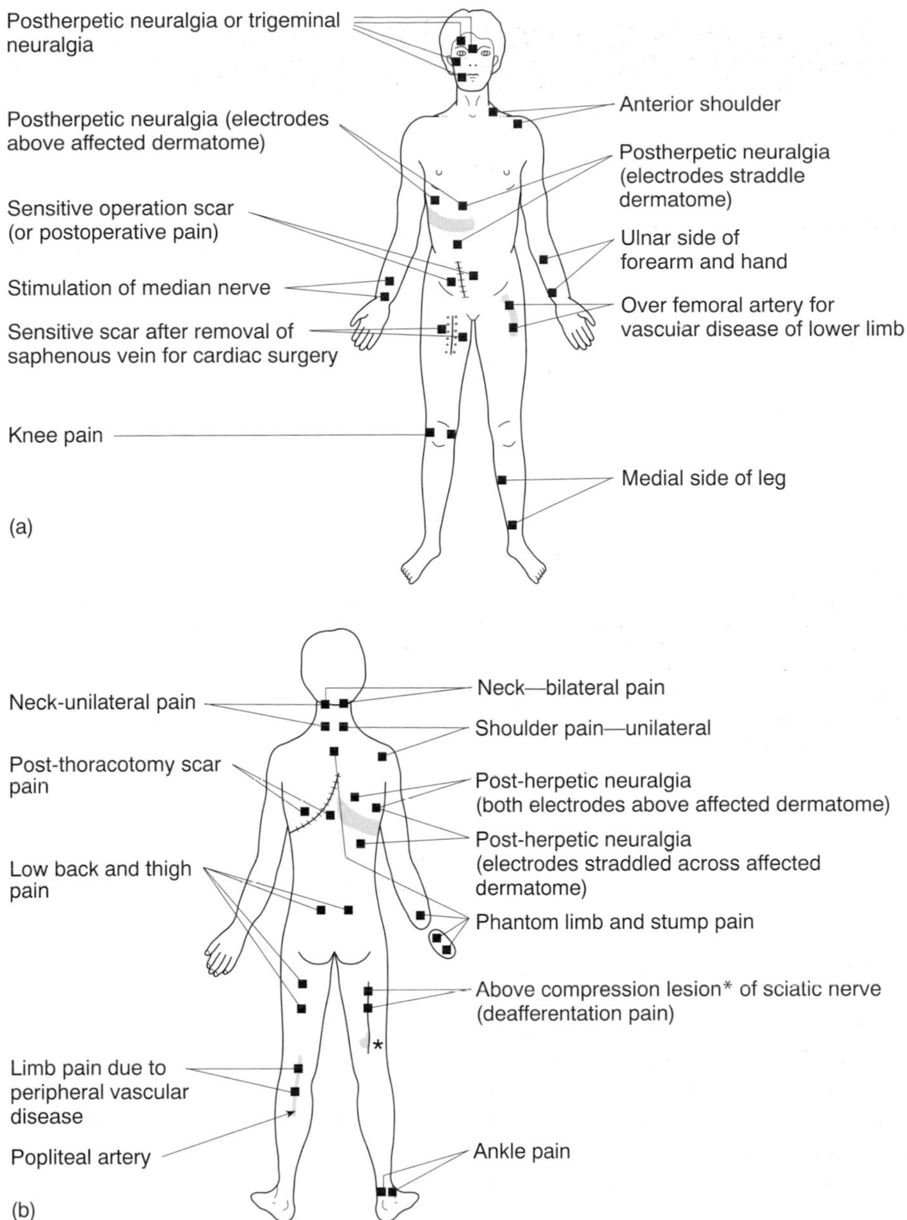

Fig. 1 Drawing of electrode positions commonly used for TENS. (a) Anterior aspect. (b) Posterior aspect.

(4) connecting lead(s)—lightweight, flexible, and will connect to all standard types of electrodes;

(5) low battery drain; where necessary can be used with rechargeable batteries and is supplied with a simple, compact mains battery charger;

(6) simple, lucid instruction manual;

(7) minimum 2 year guarantee;

(8) reliable and rapid maintenance service.

A policy recommended for any pain clinic is to standardize on two or three models of stimulator which have been found by patients, nurses, and medical staff to be effective, reliable, and economical. This can be a much more satisfactory arrangement than the alternative of purchasing a mixture of stimulators of different design and manufacture, each with its own idiosyncrasies and electrical incompatibilities with respect to the others. In many pain clinics it is the normal practice for stimulators to be loaned out to a patient for an initial trial period of, say, 1 month. If the trial of TENS proves successful then the stimulator can be either rented or purchased by the patient with the aid of public or private support.

Practical use

For many pain conditions, standard electrode positions have been worked out on a dermatomal basis, combined with trial and error. When starting a patient on a trial of TENS therapy it is important to check that the electrode positions used initially are appropriate to the pain condition being treated (see Fig. 1). Nevertheless, it is also important to establish that the electrode positions employed are optimum; and this can only be achieved by encouraging the patient to alter the sites of application within reasonable limits.

For pain conditions where there are no standard electrode positions the following procedure should be adopted:

1. Initially, place electrodes over the painful site and stimulate.

2. If initial placement brings inadequate relief, relocate electrodes over next largest nerve which innervates the affected area. Restimulate.

For all positions continue as follows:

3. The stimulus sensation should be directed into the painful area.

4. The sensation produced by TENS should be 'strong but comfortable' and not just tolerable.

5. Neither continuous (conventional) TENS nor pulsed (burst) TENS should be permitted to produce muscle twitching or spasm. By contrast, acupuncture-like TENS (Acu-TENS) is deliberately adjusted to a strength that evokes muscle twitching (see Table 2).

6. To treat large areas of pain, multiple electrodes may be needed.

Use of electrodes

TENS electrodes are either reusable or disposable and can be classified as follows:

Reusable

1. Conducting rubber pads used with electrode jelly and tape. Common sizes (mm): 40×40 (small), 93×42 (large), 210×40 (postoperative), 28 or 50 circular (for face).

2. Self-adhesive conductive polymer pads (i.e. do not require jelly or tape). Available in same range of sizes as for 1, conducting rubber pads. The anticipated life of these electrodes varies with manufacturers but is usually about 10 to14 days. However, in practice and with care the useful life can be substantially longer.

Disposable

These are self-adhesive conductive polymer pads available in the same range of sizes as for conducting rubber pads but each electrode has an anticipated life of about 2 to 4 days. It should be noted that:

1. Conducting rubber pads can be converted into self-adhesive electrodes by the use of Karaya pads (double sided sticky) and thereby eliminate the need for jelly and tape.

2. Some disposable electrodes are now available using pregelled silver/silver chloride construction in order to avoid polarization. However, with stimulators of modern design the latter is not usually a problem.

3. Other uncommon types of electrodes are available such as cotton pads and stainless steel but these are rarely used.

Treatment plan

As with any other form of therapy, it is important to have a treatment plan as follows.

Diagnosis before treatment

As with all other forms of therapy, it is essential to diagnose the cause of the pain before deciding to treat it. However, it is not always possible to make a precise diagnosis, particularly with chronic pain. What must be done then, especially when using TENS for pain caused by a neoplasm, is to ensure that the condition does not require some form of urgent and/or more radical therapy.

It cannot be emphasized too strongly that for some pain conditions, including those of neoplastic origin, it may take a considerable amount of time and patience on the part of both patient and therapist to establish effective electrode positions. During this session it is also important to check that TENS does not aggravate the pain condition, which occasionally occurs, and usually indicates that this form of treatment is unsuitable for the patient.

Extended trial period

Experience has shown that the best way to find out whether or not TENS will produce effective pain relief is to loan the patient a clinic stimulator for a trial period of 1 month, for example, so that it can be given an exhaustive test under normal everyday conditions of the patient's life. The following are typical directions given to the patient:

(1) 'use all day initially or for a minimum of 1 hour's treatment three times a day'

(2) 'adjust according to need'

(3) 'use as much as you like'

(4) 'try comparing the pain relieving effect of continuous, burst, and modulated TENS, if available, and then use the form which is best for you, or all forms if necessary'

(5) 'you may get a bonus of pain relief after the stimulator has been switched off' (post-TENS analgesia)

(6) 'if you have any problems with the treatment, for example with the stimulator or the electrodes, contact the clinic immediately'.

During the month's trial period, the patient is encouraged to contact the clinic to report progress.

Review

Initially each patient on TENS therapy should be reviewed at monthly intervals and thereafter according to need.

Indications for TENS therapy

Many different acute and chronic pains, including those associated with cancer, have been treated successfully with TENS (Table 1 contains a representative list). Any pain that occurs in a patient suffering from cancer may well respond to TENS. The pain may be:

(1) directly due to the cancer;

(2) indirectly due to the cancer;

(3) related to the treatment of the cancer;

(4) unrelated to the cancer or treatment.

As with all other pains, it is important to try to discover the cause of the pain but treatment should not be withheld pending the completion of investigations.

TENS can be used to treat pain in any or all of the above four categories. Contrary to some earlier impressions, it has become abundantly clear that it is not possible to predict whether a particular pain problem in a particular patient will respond to TENS.[10] This situation also applies to the use of TENS for cancer-related pain.[11] When embarking on a course of TENS for a patient it is important not to raise excessive expectations but to indicate firmly that 'a trial of TENS is well worthwhile and may result in useful and possibly very effective pain relief'.

As discussed in other sections of this book, there are two main types of pain for which the current preferred terms are 'nociceptive' and 'neurogenic or neuropathic'. Nociceptive pain is the consequence of tissue damage and is due to excitation of nociceptive nerve endings (subserved by Aδ and C neurones). It is characteristically described as pricking or aching pain. Neurogenic or neuropathic pain is the consequence of malfunction of the peripheral nerve trunks and/or nerve pathways in the central nervous system. These effects may be due to physical damage (e.g. trauma, surgery, infection, or cerebrovascular accident) or to functional damage (e.g. trigeminal neuralgia or causalgia).[12] It is characteristically described as 'burning' or 'scalding' in nature and is sometimes accompanied by shooting or stabbing pains. It is frequently accompanied by hyperaesthesia, dysaesthesia, and allodynia, singly or in combination, and there is usually an associated sensory deficit. Nociceptive and neurogenic pain are not mutually exclusive but often coexist, even though one type may dominate the clinical picture.

In addition to separating pains into predominantly nociceptive and neurogenic categories, it is also important to determine whether a particular pain is influenced by the sympathetic nervous system. Thus, some pains are sympathetically maintained pains whereas others are sympathetically independent pains. The contrasting diagnostic features of these pains have been described elsewhere in this book. Fortunately TENS is often effective in the treatment of both types of pain, irrespective of whether or not the pain is sympathetically maintained or sympathetically independent.

There are several pain conditions associated with cancer that, in our experience, respond particularly well to TENS and these are as follows.

Predominantly nociceptive pains

1. Pain from metastatic bone disease. The electrodes should be sited near the painful metastatic deposit or on healthy skin within the affected dermatome.
2. Pain caused by initial compression of nerve roots following vertebral collapse. The electrodes should be placed in the affected dermatome or on an adjacent dermatome.
3. Pain in the abdomen including that due to an enlarged liver caused by secondary deposits. The electrodes should be placed over or near the painful area.

Predominantly neurogenic pains

1. Pain due to compression of a nerve by a neoplasm, for example a lumbar nerve by a retroperitoneal tumour. The electrodes should be placed on skin innervated by the affected nerve but proximal to the site of compression and at a level where sensory function has been preserved.
2. Pain due to postherpetic neuralgia. Apply electrodes to skin of the same or an adjacent dermatome in vicinity of (but not on) the affected area.
3. Pain due to infiltration of nerves, for example brachial plexus. Electrodes should be placed on skin of the dermatome(s) that are adjacent (cephalad) to those affected.
4. Postchemotherapy neuropathy. Electrodes placed paravertebrally at or above the level of affected nerve roots and on affected limbs using modulated mode can produce effective analgesia. (Muscle power can also increase in hypotonic muscles with these peripheral placements.)

Choosing the form of TENS

Without doubt, trial and error is the best method by which to discover the optimum form of TENS (see Table 2) for treating a particular pain. As a rough guide, continuous (conventional) TENS may be found better for those pains which are predominantly nociceptive, namely skeletal, paravertebral, and joint pains and also visceral referred pain. On the other hand, pulsed and acupuncture-like TENS may be better for neurogenic or neuropathic pain, especially where hyperaesthesia or dysaesthesia are prominent features.[13]

Efficacy

There is now an extensive world literature on TENS and most of it supports the view that this is a useful form of analgesia, particularly for chronic pain.[7,14,15] A small but slowly increasing number of controlled clinical trials have been carried out to test this therapy. There are those sceptics who hold the view that any useful effect of TENS is the result of a placebo response. It is true that there is a placebo component to every form of therapy and TENS is no exception.[16] Nevertheless, there is strong evidence that TENS acts upon pain mechanisms to produce an analgesic action. Furthermore, a recent study by Marchand *et al*[17] clearly differentiated the effect of TENS on pain intensity and pain unpleasantness.

When a patient is started on TENS and pain is relieved, it is not possible at this stage to distinguish whether this response is likely to be maintained or is likely to wane. If the latter occurs it may be due to a change in the level of pain or a change in the response of the patient.

Changes in the level of pain

This may be due to an actual increase in the intensity of the pain for which TENS is being used or it may be due to a change in the emotional response of the patient to his or her pain. Alternatively, the increase may be due to a change in the quality of pain, for example the addition of a neurogenic component to an existing nociceptive pain. Finally, the increase may be due to the addition of one or more new pains to the original pain. This situation highlights the importance of continuously monitoring the site(s) and cause(s) of pain, especially in patients suffering from advanced cancer.

Changes in the response of the patient to TENS

There are three main causes that need to be considered.

1. The initially favourable response to TENS may have been due to a placebo response as discussed earlier. The hallmark of a placebo response is that it is likely to fade rapidly, even abruptly, commonly within a week of starting treatment, although sometimes taking a little longer.[7]

2. The waning response may be due to the development of tolerance, a term that conceals a considerable amount of ignorance as to its mechanism. Tolerance develops more slowly and insidiously than a placebo response and indeed may not occur for weeks or months after starting treatment. It appears to be akin to drug tolerance which, of course, may develop slowly over the course of weeks (e.g. opioid tolerance) or over the course of months or years (e.g. insulin tolerance). Tolerance to TENS may involve several possible mechanisms which could include some or all of the following: dysfunction of pain-inhibitory neuronal pathways (e.g. waning neurotransmitter release or down-regulation of receptors concerned with opioid peptides, 5-hydroxytryptamine, or noradrenaline); interference by the production of increasing amounts of endogenous opioid antagonists (e.g. the octapeptide form of cholecystokinin, CCK-8).[18]

The effectiveness of these possible mechanisms whereby tolerance to TENS develops may depend upon the establishment of regular patterns of neuronal activity in the nerve pathways involved. This, in turn, may be linked to the well-known phenomenon of habituation, which the regular pulse patterns of TENS may help to establish. For this reason some stimulators are now constructed with the option of a random pulse output. This development has been carried to the furthest degree by the development of the Codetron stimulator, which applies randomly distributed pulses to a set of six electrodes (instead of the usual pair) and is claimed to be more effective than ordinary TENS.[11] It is possible that random stimulation may help to delay or reverse tolerance, and that when it does so it achieves it through delaying or reversing the regular patterns of neuronal activity which perhaps form an integral part of the tolerance mechanism, as suggested above.

3. The response to TENS may be antagonized by concurrent medication. There is some equivocal clinical evidence to suggest that the concurrent use of opioids (more especially when opioid dependence is well developed), corticosteroids, or benzodiazepines may interfere with the efficacy of TENS.[14,19] However, these drugs are commonly prescribed to patients who obtain an excellent therapeutic response with TENS and it therefore seems unlikely that medication is a common cause of TENS failure. Nevertheless, it is possible that when the onset of failure with TENS therapy coincides with some change in medication with one of these (or other) drugs, that such a mechanism be considered and appropriate action taken.

In a recent survey of 179 patients,[10] the average length of use of TENS was 4 years (range 3 months to 9 years) during which time 47 per cent of them found it reduced their pain by more than half. Furthermore, TENS analgesia was rapid both in onset (less than 30 min in 75 per cent) and offset (less than 30 min in 75 per cent), with one-third utilizing this therapy for over 61 h/week. It is also well known that in patients who suffer from more than one type of pain condition, TENS may be very effective for one and yet totally ineffective for another. All the foregoing evidence mitigates strongly against the view that TENS analgesia is a placebo response.

Unfortunately, tolerance to TENS occurs and may develop slowly or suddenly so terminating what has previously been effective analgesia. The reasons for this are not fully understood but sometimes it is possible to overcome this problem by changing the type of stimulation (see above). It is also important to note that some patients are non-responders to TENS. The results of recent research suggests that the response to TENS may depend upon the level of cortical responsivity, which is significantly lower in non-responders.[20]

Table 4 summarizes the results of TENS for the treatment of malignant disease and is an updated version of the table published by Ostrowski.[21] It indicates the apparent wide range of efficacy for good (15–99 per cent) or partial (2–44 per cent) pain relief, which may be due to many variables including the severity of disease, the mode of application of TENS, and differences in methods of assessing pain relief. These results indicate the urgent need for further controlled trials of TENS in palliative medicine.

Complications and contraindications

Complications of TENS therapy may be related to the response of the patient or the performance of the equipment.

1. Serious complications due to TENS therapy are rare. The majority of complications related to TENS therapy are due to skin irritation, skin burn, or allergy to the electrode (or associated conducting jelly, tape, or gum). Skin irritation can be minimized by ensuring that the skin area to which electrodes are applied is kept dry, clean, and free from grease (e.g. cosmetics). By this means electrical resistance between the electrode and skin is kept low and evenly distributed, thus avoiding 'hot spots' (caused by uneven current flow). This is important both for electrodes requiring electrode jelly and also for those that are self-adhesive. In a recent survey of nearly 200 patients using TENS regularly,[10] the only common problem was skin irritation. This occurred in a third, probably due in part to drying out of electrode jelly.[30,31]

2. Equipment failure due to faulty leads, stimulator, battery, or charger is uncommon. When modern, well-designed, and properly constructed equipment is used in accordance with the manufacturers instructions these problems are unusual and are most likely to be due to failure of the leads, the weakest link in the chain. It should also be remembered that disposable batteries have a finite life and that rechargeable batteries cannot be recharged indefinitely.

Contraindications to TENS therapy are few and may be listed as follows:

1. DO NOT place electrodes on inflamed, infected, or otherwise unhealthy skin.
2. DO NOT stimulate over the anterior part of the neck. This is to avoid the possibility of stimulating the nerves of the carotid sinus or the larynx which could produce hypotension or laryngeal spasm, respectively.
3. DO NOT stimulate over a pregnant uterus (except when TENS is being used for obstetric analgesia).
4. DO NOT use the stimulator in the presence of a cardiac

Table 4 TENS for the treatment of malignant disease

Author	Good or complete pain relief	Partial pain relief or reduction of analgesics	No relief	Total (comments)
Long (1974)[22]	3 (60%)	–	2 (40%)	5 malignancies out of total series of 197 cases
Hardy (1975)[23]	2 (50%)	–	2 (50%)	4 out of 53
Loeser *et al* (1975)[24]	–	3 (42%)	4 (57%)	7 out of 198
Campbell and Long (1976)[25]	1 (25%)	–	3 (75%)	4
Ostrowski (1979)[21]	4 (44%)	4 (44%)	1 (11%)	9
Ventafridda (1979)[26]	36 (97%) 1–10 days	–	1 (3%)	37
	4 (11%) at 30 days		33 (89%) at 30 days	37
Bates and Nathan (1980)[16]	4 (80%) (all longer than 1 week)	–	1 (20%)	5
Avellanosa and West 1982[27]				
2 weeks	17 (28%)	22 (37%)	21 (35%)	60
3 months	9 (15%)	11 (18%)	40 (67%)	60
Dil-din *et al* (1985)[28]	11 (100%)	–	–	11 (abstract only available)
Rafter (1986)[29] quoted by Librach and Rapson (1988)[11]	34 (70%)	1 (2%)	4 (8%)	49
Range	15–99%	2–44%	3–75%	

pacemaker. This restriction applies especially to an on-demand pacemaker but in order to err on the side of safety the manufacturers of TENS equipment apply this as a general restriction. It is not uncommon to operate fixed rate pacemakers in the presence of a TENS machine, but this should only be done after consulting the cardiologist responsible for the patient and also, if necessary, the manufacturers of the pacemaker and the TENS equipment.

5. DO NOT try to force the use of TENS on a non-compliant patient, for example one who is senile or has a low IQ. In addition, some patients will be found to have a congenital fear of, rooted objection to, or inability to use electricity in any form for medical treatment, including TENS.

Acupuncture

Introduction

Acupuncture was apparently first recorded in the stone age, when flint needles were used.[32] This ancient Chinese system of healing was first described in *The Yellow Emperor's Classic of Internal Medicine*. This text was translated into English by Dr Ilsa Veith.[33] The Yellow Emperor or Huang Ti was a much worshipped figure and reigned approximately 2600 BC. He wanted the secrets of medicine to be passed to his sons and his grandsons and the records to be made known to posterity. Eastern style acupuncture involves a sophisticated and elaborate system of diagnosis and subsequent selection of acupuncture points for stimulation by the insertion of fine needles in order to effect a 'cure'. Western practitioners, in general, rely on conventional means of diagnosis by history, examination, and special investigations and use a simplified form of point selection.

Techniques of acupuncture

The techniques employed by an individual acupuncturist vary enormously, not only on the selection of acupuncture points but also on the mode and length of stimulation (Table 5).

Traditional Chinese acupuncture

The Chinese describe a circulation of vital energy Qi or Chi. Qi is partly fuelled by food and respiration and partly represents innate energy. Qi circulates in the body in deep channels and along meridians. Meridians are invisible lines joining a series of acupuncture points on the surface of the body. There are twelve paired, two unpaired, and several extra meridians. After taking a history, each radial artery is palpated carefully in three superficial and three deep sites and, from this, disease can be subtly diagnosed in 12 distant organs. The meridians and their associated organs bear little or no relationship to organs of the same name known to western medicine (for example pericardium and spleen meridians).

The Yellow Emperor believed that forces of opposite polarities were present in nature—Yin and Yang, negative and positive, dark and light, feminine and masculine. These were the basic principles of the entire universe and these forces, Yin and Yang, should be present in appropriate quantities and balanced in each organ for healthy function. The Qi circulates round the body along the meridians to nourish both Yin and Yang components of organs in the following sequence; the lungs, large intestine, stomach, spleen, heart, small intestine, bladder, kidneys, pericardium (circulation),

Table 5 Techniques of acupuncture

Traditional Chinese medicine	Qi vital energy Yin and Yang in balance Pulse and tongue diagnosis ± Moxibustion
Western acupuncture	Manual acupuncture minimal stiumulation up to 20 min maximal stimulation up to 5 min Electroacupuncture 2–4 Hz low frequency 50–200 Hz high frequency
Acupuncture analgesia	Vigorous manual stimulation or electroacupuncture (used for <10% of operations in China)
Laser acupuncture	No needles, advantageous in paediatrics
Acupressure	No needles, less effective than needling
Auricular acupuncture	Needles inserted in tender regions or 'recipe' points
Ryodoraku	Reduced skin impedance treated electrically
Veterinary	± Electroacupuncture Unlikely to be a placebo

triple energizer (metabolism), gallbladder, and liver (Fig. 2). Clinical examination of the tongue assumes great importance in traditional Chinese medicine, possibly partly on account of its accessibility. Even now entire textbooks are available on diagnosis based on the colour and consistency of the tongue.

Several laws of acupuncture also help to guide the traditional acupuncturist to the correct diagnosis, including the law of the five vital elements of nature, wood, fire, earth, metal, and water. This and many other laws are invoked to select which points to 'tonify' or 'sedate' if a deficiency or excess were found in any meridian. Chosen acupuncture points are manually stimulated with a needle until the patient feels a sensation of De Qi or Teh Chi, a feeling of aching, numbness, tingling, heaviness, and fullness. Less than 1 per cent of patients experience a propagated sensation from the needle point along the pathway of a meridian.[34] Needles are often thermally stimulated in addition, usually by the combustion of the pith of *Artemesia japonica* (moxa) applied to the end of the needle. This is termed moxibustion. Some acupuncture points are slightly tender in health and many more become tender in disease states. These points appear commonly in 'recipes' for treatment of various conditions.

It is not surprising that such a seemingly bizarre system of diagnosis and treatment arose when one realizes that the study of formal anatomy only became possible in China early this century. Further history and philosophical background is available elsewhere.[35,36] However, one account of the history of acupuncture challenges the date of emergence of acupuncture as being approximately AD 100, based on archaeological and literary evidence.[37]

Western acupuncture

Western trained doctors rely on conventional history taking, examination, and special investigations as necessary before making a diagnosis. Such abstract concepts as Qi and Yin and Yang are unacceptable to many Western trained doctors and have contributed to the scepticism with which many still view acupuncture. Recent neuropharmacological and neurophysiological advances have given acupuncture a sound scientific basis and clinical credibility. In many western pain clinics, acupuncture has become a standard complementary form of treatment in addition to more orthodox methods. A mixture of Eastern established acupuncture points and locally selected segmental, tender, or trigger points are used for many conditions. Some use minimal stimulation for up to 20 minutes and do not attempt to elicit De Qi. Some use more vigorous manual stimulation of the needles for up to 5 minutes. It has been noticed that some patients are more sensitive to acupuncture than others, so called 'strong reactors' and require shorter, gentle treatments.[38]

Patients, in the main, are treated somewhat empirically and treatment intensified or reduced on a trial and error basis, depending on individual progress. A wide variety of techniques are both available and effective. These range from a traditional Chinese approach on the one hand, in which point selection is a fine art utilizing many laws and principles,[39,40] to the other extreme, in which some respected Western practitioners frankly do not believe in the special properties associated with all the formal Eastern acupuncture points and who teach a simplified yet effective system of needling.[38,41,42]

Electroacupuncture

Electroacupuncture was first established as a substitute for the manual, vigorous stimulation required for intraoperative acupuncture or acupuncture analgesia. An electric current is applied to the needles to stimulate chosen points. This is a stronger stimulus than TENS, as the stimulus is transmitted through the skin; this is in contrast to TENS, when electrodes are only stimulated on the skin surface. Low frequency electroacupuncture (2–4 Hz) is more

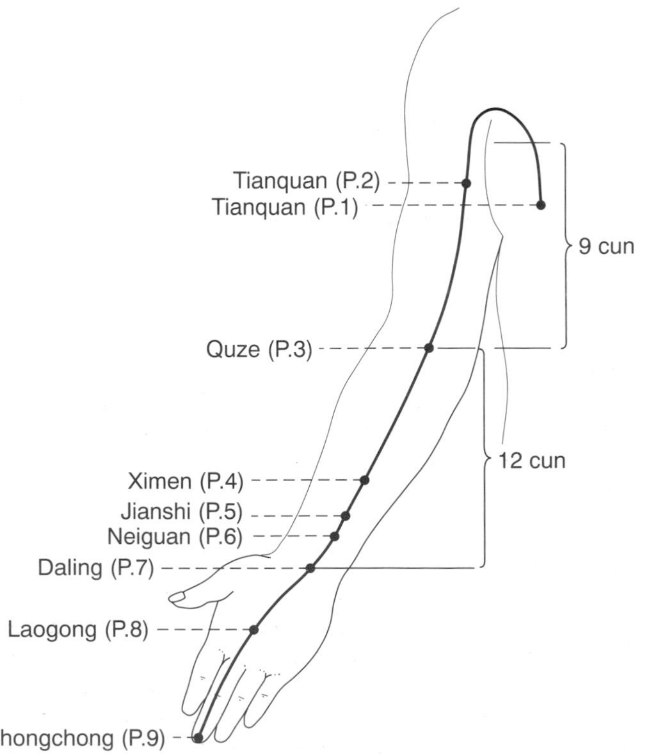

Fig. 2 The 'pericardium' meridian in traditional Chinese medicine.

likely to stimulate the release of enkephalins and cortisol, whereas high frequency (50–200 Hz) releases serotonin (5-HT) and dynorphin.[43] Electroacupuncture is mainly used for the treatment of acute pain and difficult pain problems such as fibromyalgia.[44]

Acupuncture analgesia

Acupuncture performed in a vigorous manner with or without electrical stimulation can raise pain tolerance to both experimental and surgically induced pain.[45] Acupuncture analgesia was introduced in 1958 and became popular in China for perioperative analgesia for many years.[46,47] The lengthy induction time, coupled with inadequate analgesia in many cases which required opioid supplementation, diminished its popularity. It is currently used for less than 6 per cent of operations in China. Nevertheless, it has had proven benefit as an adjunct to modern anaesthesia in diminishing postoperative analgesic requirements[48] and can help to reduce morbidity.[49]

Laser therapy

The use of external laser probes to deliver stimulation is gaining acceptance. It is not strictly acupuncture as no needles are involved and is more acceptable to paediatric patients and veterinary subjects.[50] However, the mechanisms of action are uncertain and it may be misleading to include it with acupuncture. Nevertheless, statistically significant reduction of pain intensity was found in patients with trigeminal neuralgia in one controlled trial[51] and in rheumatoid arthritis.[52,53] Further work is to be encouraged in this area.

Acupressure

Acupressure involves the massage of traditional acupuncture points. It is believed to be less effective than acupuncture with needles.

Auricular acupuncture

In traditional Chinese acupuncture the ear is very closely connected with channels to internal organs. Nogier developed auricular acupuncture further in the 1950s.[54] In his system, different parts of the external helix are supposed to represent different parts of the body. In one study, tender areas on palpation of the ear with a probe were found to correspond to distant pain sites and could be relieved of pain when those auricular sites were needled.[55]

Ryodoraku

This is a Japanese form of electroacupuncture. The skin impedance is measured and if abnormal can be altered electrically.[56]

Veterinary acupuncture

This is being used increasingly for domestic and farm animals.[57] Electroacupuncture and laser probes are often used. The effectiveness of treatment in animals further supports the view that acupuncture is more than merely an elaborate placebo.

Equipment

Numerous wall charts and models are available which depict traditional acupuncture points for accurate localization purposes. Acupuncture needles are usually made of surgical stainless steel and are disposable or reusable. As the quality control of sterilization techniques is variable, it should be standard practice to use disposable needles. The size, length, and gauges of needles vary according to practitioner preferences. Many use a plastic introducing guide tube to facilitate a quick and relatively painless insertion.

There is an enormous selection of electrical and laser equipment available. It is beyond the scope of this book to include this topic in any depth so the reader is advised to consult standard textbooks and suppliers for further details.

Indications

In China, acupuncture is first-line treatment for hundreds of minor and major complaints.[39,41]. In 1979, The World Health Organization published a list of conditions which are recognized to be helped by acupuncture.[58] It is steadily gaining popularity in the West because of its success in treating a host of common ailments, in many cases obviating the need for medication and its risk of side-effects. Selected topics have been chosen for their relevance to palliative medicine. The quality of referenced articles is rather variable but this is not surprising as it is only comparatively recently that the subject has been subjected to scientific scrutiny.

Pain

Acupuncture has been found to help a wide variety of pain conditions with 40 to 86 per cent symptomatic improvement.[59] The shorter the duration of the problem, the better the response. Old age and multiple illnesses reduce the benefit.[60] Treatment of acute and chronic musculoskeletal complaints and many cases of headache, such as tension and migraine, are particularly successful.[61] Some chronic pain, such as that caused by rheumatoid arthritis, is treated with partial success only.[62]

Cancer pain

Many advances have been made over recent years in the treatment of cancer pain. However, despite an adequate trial of analgesics and coanalgesics, a significant minority have pain inadequately controlled in late stage disease.[63] The failure of pharmacological means alone to control pain has led to the use of many non-drug treatments, including TENS and acupuncture.[64] They may improve pain control sufficiently to permit a reduction of dosage and side-effects of analgesics and coanalgesics. A patient who exhibits excessive side-effects with low doses of exogenous opioids will frequently respond favourably to acupuncture and/or TENS, in our experience. There is some experimental evidence to suggest that diffuse noxious inhibitory control mechanisms, by which acupuncture partly works, are extremely sensitive to the administration of low doses of morphine.[65] Some patients on morphine respond well to acupuncture and others do not. There are also anecdotes about patients obtaining a reduced response to acupuncture after starting a course of steroids, but many will respond. As with TENS, concurrent medication should not prevent a doctor from using a course of acupuncture when pain has been inadequately controlled by conventional means.

Two retrospective studies on patients attending a pain clinic in a cancer hospital showed that 339 were given acupuncture.[66,67] This was as a result of failure of conventional medication or relative intolerance to drugs such as opioids. This heterogeneous group of patients were referred by oncologists, radiotherapists, and surgeons. They had well documented disease, had been appropriately investigated, and continued to attend referring clinics in addition to the pain clinic. Drug treatment was not stopped initially but patients could be weaned off original medication if treatment was successful. Minimal stimulation manual acupuncture was used in all cases and three initial weekly acupuncture treatments were considered an adequate therapeutic trial. Out of the two studies, over 50 per cent of patients had worthwhile improvement of their pain for at least 7 days.[66,67] Multiple treatments were necessary either two, three, or four weekly in general. Up to 30 per cent had short lived pain relief of 2 days or less or an increase in mobility alone. This was of insufficient duration for outpatient based patients but could be useful with more frequent treatments in inpatients. Patients with cancer treatment related pain, such as postsurgery pain and postirradiation fibrosis, derived longer analgesia than patients who had metastatic tumour related pain. However, the diagnostic distinction between malignant and non-malignant pain is not always clear cut as can be demonstrated by patients with brachial plexus lesions.[68] In the two retrospective studies, neurogenic pain was helped in one-third of patients with tumour related pain and two-thirds of patients with cancer treatment related pain. Bone pain, persisting despite radiotherapy or chemotherapy, was sometimes helped with improvement in mobility and exercise tolerance. Such empirical use of acupuncture with consistent beneficial results in over 50 per cent of patients with problematic cancer pain seems worthy of more careful scrutiny.

Mobility

A dramatic increase in mobility often occurred with or without pain relief.[66,67]

Muscle spasm

Painful muscle spasm and visceral bladder spasm were especially helped by acupuncture.

Vascular problems

Vascular problems were helped by acupuncture. The most dramatic example of this was two radionecrotic ulcers (which classically never heal) but which healed completely using acupuncture.[64] Chronic ulcers have been healed by acupuncture, for example those due to venous stasis.[34]

Tolerance

It is interesting to note that practically all the patients required multiple treatments—two, three, or four weekly in general. This is in marked contrast to patients with non-malignant disease who cope well with increasing intervals between treatments. Some patients, in addition, exhibited a reduced response to acupuncture with time. In fact, almost an inverse relationship was noted between tumour size and longevity of acupuncture response.[66,67] The larger the tumour burden, or the more active the disease, the shorter the beneficial effect of acupuncture. Advanced disease may have accounted for the 30 per cent of patients who only exhibited short-lived pain relief of 2 days or less in the two studies. Sudden tolerance occurring in a patient who had previously been acupuncture responsive was considered to be a sinister sign. Tolerance in such a patient was the reason for the patient to be immediately referred back to the oncologists for further investigation, as 17 out of 27 such patients had developed further metastases. Not only that, if metastatic disease was found and treated successfully by chemotherapy or radiotherapy, the patient could revert back to being acupuncture responsive again. Tolerance has been described in animal models when the opioid antagonists angiotensin 2[69] and cholecystokinin[70] were released with prolonged electroacupuncture. It is possible that patients with malignant disease and pain already had an increased or maximal output of endogenous opioids, which would prevent them from gaining an optimal response when treated.

A general acupuncturist who fails to get long lived analgesia in a patient should perhaps refer the patient for investigation of possible malignancy.

The study on 29 patients by Wen[71] emphasizes the need for frequent treatments in a variety of cancer pain syndromes in the terminal stages. These patients were given several electroacupuncture treatments on the first day and then three treatments a day gradually reducing to one treatment per day, pain relief permitting. Pain medication could also be reduced with this regimen. It could be postulated that patients in the two studies [66,67] who only exhibited short-lived pain relief of 2 days or less with acupuncture might have been adequately treated with daily treatment. In 1973, Felix Mann also described short lived relief in eight patients with intractable cancer pain.[72]

Acupuncture and TENS

TENS can often be used as a back-up for acupuncture, if the acupuncture effect wears off between outpatient visits. The responses are not necessarily interchangeable, some patients responding to acupuncture alone and others to TENS.

The use of acupuncture for other symptoms

Phantom limb pain

Acupuncture can both elicit phantom limb sensations in absent limbs[73] as well as alleviate pain, abnormal sensations, and stump pain.[73,74] Neurophysiological studies of the phantom sensation propagated along channels show the parietal cortex to be the most likely 'meridian' centre in the brain.[73] Pain relief can be instant and dramatic in selected patients but again tolerance to acupuncture may occur with time.

Dyspnoea

In a randomized, controlled trial of patients with chronic obstructive pulmonary disease, the traditional Chinese acupuncture-treated group showed significant benefit in subjective breathlessness and 6-min walking distance.[75] Objective measures of lung function were unchanged in both the treated and placebo acupuncture groups. A prospective single blind trial of acupuncture, real and sham, showed that both attenuated exercise-induced asthma in children.[76] Its benefit in patients with endstage lung disease is encouraging, when current therapeutic options are limited.[77] The observation that acupuncture gave subjective improvement in shortness of breath in several cases with advanced cancer in a pain clinic lead to a pilot study.[78]

The short-term effects of acupuncture were studied in 20 patients with breathlessness at rest where the symptom was directly related to primary or secondary malignancy. Two simple sternal needles (Fig. 3) and two traditional acupuncture points (large intestine 4) were used. Outcome measures showed significant improvement in VAS scores of breathlessness, relaxation, and anxiety at 90 min. There was also a significant reduction in the respiratory rate which was sustained for the objective treatment period. Seventy per cent (14/20) of the patients reported marked symptomatic benefit from treatment. Eight of these patients elected to have two indwelling studs inserted on to the sternal points in an attempt to prolong the response (Fig. 4). This gave patients control by enabling them to massage the studs during breathless 'panic attacks' or prior to any, even trivial, exercise. All eight reported varying degrees of benefit lasting up to 2 weeks. It was successful in patients who had failed to respond to multiple treatments for shortness of breath including steroids, opioids, various nebulizers, and oxygen. Further prospective studies should be performed.

The mechanisms of action of acupuncture for dyspnoea remain speculative, but the sedative action of endogenous opioid peptide release may be contributory. Acupuncture also has widespread effects on autonomic function[79] which has, in turn, major influence on the respiratory system.

Nausea and vomiting

The late Professor John Dundee looked closely at claims made for acupuncture using modern methods of evaluation and analysis. He has shown that single point acupuncture to the P6 point on the pericardium meridian (Fig. 2) is a clinically useful antiemetic in postoperative nausea and vomiting, morning sickness, and as an additional antiemetic for patients having cytotoxic drugs.[80,81,82] Transcutaneous electrical methods of stimulation have also been used to increase the scope of treatment beyond needling techniques.[83,84] As to the possible mechanisms of action of acupuncture for nausea and vomiting, there is no clear cut explanation so far.

Acupuncture is infrequently a cause of nausea and vomiting which may be due simply to release of opioid peptides. When the provocative agent is a cytotoxic drug for example, it may have excited vomiting through some indirect mechanism involving activation of nerve pathways depending upon such transmitters as 5-hydroxytryptamine, dopamine, or opioid peptides (or possibly all three). Under these circumstances the release of opioid peptides by acupuncture may switch on various inhibitory pathways which block the emetic pathway to the chemoreceptor trigger zone and/or the vomiting centre. An alternative explanation is that there may be significant antagonistic interaction between opioid peptides released by acupuncture such that when one group is present in high concentration (thus causing the emetic effect) that the release of other opioid peptides (by acupuncture treatment) may release peptides which act as antagonists to the emetic-producing peptides. Yet another possibility is that under conditions in which opioid peptide concentration is high (causing the emetic effect) the antiemetic effect of acupuncture is due to the release of other antagonistic substances such as, for example, cholecystokinin.[18]

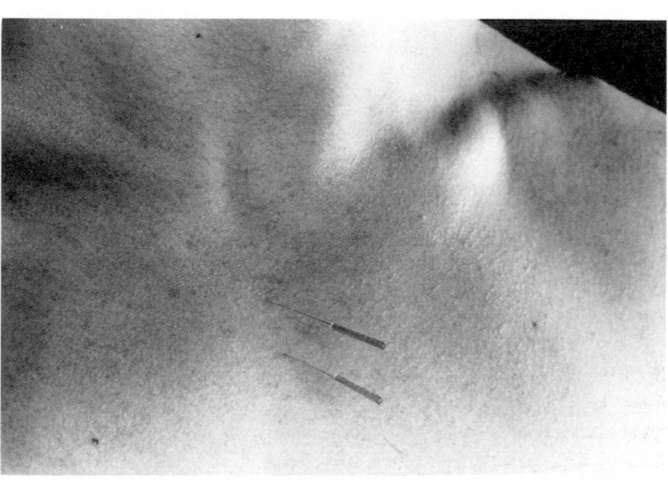

Fig. 3 Two needles inserted at the top of the sternum.

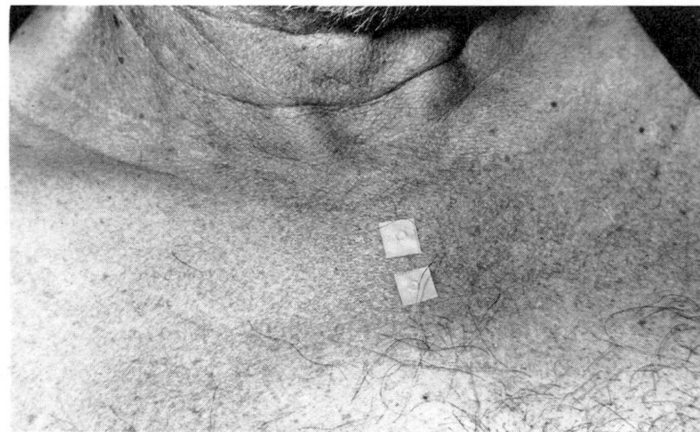

Fig. 4 Two semipermanent indwelling acupuncture needles which can be massaged to give relief in panic attacks or prior to activity.

Stroke

In a randomized, controlled trial of 78 patients treated within 10 days of a severe stroke, the group receiving acupuncture (sensory stimulation) twice a week for 10 weeks recovered faster and spent less time in hospital.[85] Motor function, balance, activities of daily living, and quality of life were measured up to 12 months after stroke onset. In addition, rehabilitation costs were $US26 000 less for hospital and nursing care per patient in the treatment group. The Swedish government is currently sponsoring further work in this area. Barbro Johansson's group has also studied the same survivors, at 2.7 years mean time after the stroke, for postural control.[86] The sensory stimulation group had enhanced recovery of postural function 2 years after the lesion and treatment. The patients who had acupuncture and who could perform all the tests showed no difference between themselves and age matched healthy subjects in contrast to the control group. Two further related papers describe functional recovery and rehabilitation in this type of patient.[87,88]

Miscellaneous

Inability to swallow is common with oesophageal obstruction and acupuncture has given some immediate relief and can be a useful temporary source of palliation.[89] Treatment of intractable hiccup is referenced in most acupuncture textbooks and it may be effective for this disabling and distressing symptom.[90,91] Acupuncture reduced radiation proctitis following radiotherapy for carcinoma of the cervix.[92] Acupuncture was found to be equally as helpful as tricyclic drugs in depression in two studies.[93,94] Acupuncture has been used for drug addicts to wean them off opioid medication.[95] Experimentally induced itch has been helped by acupuncture[96] as has uraemic pruritus.[97]

AIDS

People with AIDS are turning to alternative medicine for a perceived 'cure' or symptomatic relief. Spurious claims of symptomatic relief have been made[98,99] and should be treated with caution, as practitioner qualifications and details of needle sterilization techniques are incomplete or inadequate. This is an obvious reason for the use of disposable needles, as patients may not know their diagnosis or fail to reveal it when seeking advice.

Efficacy

Although acupuncture has been used therapeutically for thousands of years, it is only in the past two decades that it has been subjected to Western scientific scrutiny. The results of clinical trials on acupuncture have been conflicting and this is probably due, in part, to the difficulties involved in constructing controlled trials on treatments such as acupuncture. The generally accepted method of establishing the efficacy of a new treatment is to subject it to a randomized double blind placebo controlled trial. It is difficult to see how a trial of acupuncture could be truly double blind as this would require an unskilled acupuncturist with little or no knowledge of the treatment he was attempting to give, which would be ethically unacceptable. However, it can mean blinding of both patient and independent observer.

The nature of the placebo used may also affect results of any trial since placebo response rates have been shown to vary from study to study and the placebo effect can be deliberately improved if attention is paid to the psychological impact.[100] Indeed, it has been suggested by cynics that acupuncture is no more than a 'supreme placebo'.

Four basic types of study can be identified in the literature—uncontrolled, no treatment control, alternative treatment control, and placebo control.

Uncontrolled trials

Unfortunately these represent a considerable part of the acupuncture literature and show that acupuncture gives a 50 to 70 per cent successful response.

There are no no-treatment control trials or alternative treatment control trials relevant to palliative medicine at present.

Placebo-controlled studies

In these studies, the choice of an effective placebo treatment remains problematic. This varies from rubbing a needle against the skin or tapping an introducer tube on to the skin, to 'sham' acupuncture using needles in non-acupuncture points, to minimal acupuncture or 'dummy' dead TENS battery as a control.[46] From a neurophysiological point of view both minimal acupuncture and sham acupuncture might be expected to have effects in their own right. This helps to explain why some controlled studies have shown rather equivocal results, with both placebo and treatment giving higher success rates than expected with conventional placebo results. Jobst has attempted to address this subject in a recent article on acupuncture for pulmonary disease.[101] In 1986, Richardson and Vincent comprehensively reviewed all controlled trials of acupuncture in chronic pain[102] and concluded that the overall quality was poor; many were seriously flawed by methodological problems, poor design, inadequate outcome measures, poor (or absent) statistical data, and a lack of follow-up data. In a series of articles,[103,104,105] Dutch epidemiologists reported a meta-analysis of 86 controlled trials of acupuncture for pain, asthma, and addiction conditions. They concluded that the better the study technique, the less likely acupuncture was to surpass a placebo. Another meta-analysis looking only at randomized trials of acupuncture in chronic pain concluded that whilst the potential sources of bias, including problems with blindness, precluded a conclusive finding, most results favoured acupuncture.[106]

Clearly, more clinical trials are required, but these need to be of high quality—well designed with adequate numbers and credible control groups.

Complications and contraindications

Complications

Acupuncture is said to be a safe method of treatment with no side-effects, when general precautions are taken.[40] Rampes has recently completed a review on the side-effects of acupuncture.[107] The incidence of side-effects is generally considered to be much lower than side-effects of medication.

Non-serious side-effects include postneedling pain, bleeding, bruising, sleepiness or euphoria (possibly due to endorphin release), occasional syncope, and local skin reactions. Exacerbation of migraine, vertigo, or dizziness can also occur as can needle breakage. Although rare, anatomical damage to most organs and structures have been reported, such as lungs (unilateral and bilateral pneumothorax), heart, liver, spleen, kidney, vessels and nerves, etc. Some traditional Chinese textbooks include diagrams with alarmingly deep needling techniques, which are more likely to cause damage. Some complications are life-threatening and arrhythmias and cardiac arrests have been reported. Burns from moxibustion and faulty electrical apparatus have also been described.

Infectious complications via inadequately sterilized needles are also a major hazard. Disposable needles are the best way of reducing the risks and should be compulsory. Bacterial infection, including bacterial endocarditis, has been described.[108] Prophylactic antibiotics may reduce the risks in a patient with pre-existing valvular disease but acupuncture could be contraindicated in these patients. The most serious viral infections include hepatitis B[109,110] and HIV infection.[111,112] There are still clinics in both East and West who do not use adequate sterilization techniques and this practice has obvious implications.

An unusual complication of indwelling gold needles in one patient with rheumatoid arthritis and thyroid cancer caused artifacts to bone and I-131 scans similar to metastases.[113]

Masking of symptoms due to a serious underlying cancer by giving symptomatic relief is a potential danger. This is more likely to happen with non-medically qualified practitioners. Any patient who gets persistent short-lived relief from acupuncture merits further investigation.

Finally, many patients describe the coincidental improvement of a wide variety of other conditions after treatment of pain; for example hay fever, migraine, dumping syndrome, psoriasis, and prostatism, and many more—a contrast of welcome side-effects!

Contraindications

Acupuncture needling is contraindicated in the area of an unstable spine in a patient with good neurological function below that level. There is a serious, theoretical danger of removal of the protective muscle spasm around the unstable area, with ensuing danger of further compression or transection.[67] TENS is a useful alternative for local pain relief in these cases. However, acupuncture given to the legs of a patient has relieved excruciating hyperpathia associated with vertebral metastasis and cord compression, and helped the pain disappear for up to 2 weeks per treatment. The mechanism may be similar to the use of regional sympathetic blockade in a limb to relieve central pain states.[64] It is inadvisable to needle superficial sites of tumour growth and the affected limbs of a patient with moderate to severe lymphoedema. In practice, very gentle treatment does not seem to be problematic in an area of mild lymphoedema for pain conditions. Grossly abnormal clotting function is a contraindication and particularly if a patient bruises spontaneously. Superficial needling in patients with a platelet count above 20 000 may be permissible, as with patients with a prolonged prothrombin time, within reason. It is contraindicated to use electroacupuncture in patients with a pacemaker, and many practitioners beware of treating patients during pregnancy in case of inducing a miscarriage.

Neuroanatomy and neuropharmacology of TENS and acupuncture

During the past two decades considerable progress has been made with the study of the neuroanatomy and neuropharmacology of nociceptive systems including the possible mechanisms of both TENS and acupuncture. Several reviews are available on both aspects of this subject.[114-120]

Figure 5 shows a diagram of the neuroanatomical and neuropharmacological basis of pain and the way in which this is modified by TENS and acupuncture. The diagram is based on the writings of Duggan and Foong,[115] Bowsher,[116,118] Han and Terenius,[114] Le Bars *et al*, [121]Fields and Basbaum,[122] and Jones *et al.*[123] So-called 'first', 'rapid', or 'aversive' pain is due to the activation of small myelinated Aδ fibres whereas 'second', 'slow', or 'tissue damage' pain is due to activation of mostly unmyelinated C fibres with activation of some Aδ fibres.[116]

There are four conditions to be considered:

1. Pathways for tissue damage pain. Peripheral polymodal nociceptor afferents (C) are activated as the result of, for example, a painful scar (as depicted in Fig. 3). The C-fibre afferents terminate in the substantia gelatinosa (lamina II) where their axon terminals secrete substance P or vasoactive intestinal peptide, according to whether these arise from skin or viscera, respectively. The substantia gelatinosa indirectly excites transmission cells deep in the spinal grey matter whose axons form the spinoreticular tract and which forms one component of the crossed anterolateral funiculus which ascends to the brain. The spinoreticular tract sends collaterals to the hypothalamus (triggering autonomic responses to pain) and then synapses in the thalamus. In the latter, it excites other neurones which are distributed widely over the cerebral cortex including the frontal cortex and also the limbic system, which give rise to the conscious sensation and emotional experience of tissue-damage (second) pain.

2. TENS. Electrical stimulation excites Aβ afferents connected to tactile receptors. After entering the spinal cord these afferents ultimately ascend in the dorsal columns. However, at spinal cord level these Aβ afferent fibres give collaterals which synapse with short interneurons, the endings of which are in proximity to the terminations of the C fibres as the latter synapse with substantia gelatinosa cells. These interneurons probably release gamma amino butyric acid which causes presynaptic blockade of the C afferents, thereby preventing them from exciting the substantia gelatinosa cells and so blocking the onward transmission of nociceptive information. The elegant demonstration by Garrison and Foreman[117] that TENS decreases the activity of spontaneous and noxiously evoked dorsal horn cells is in accord with this explanation.

3. Segmental acupuncture. High-threshold mechanoreceptors connected to small myelinated primary afferents (Aδ) are activated by acupuncture. One central branch of the Aδ afferent excites the inhibitory enkephalinergic interneuron (on the borders of laminae I and II), releasing enkephalin (Enk) which produces post-synaptic block of the substantia gelatinosa cell. This prevents the onward transmission of noxiously-generated information. This mechanism would explain segmental acupuncture.

4. Extra-segmental acupuncture. Waldeyer cells in lamina I of the spinal grey matter are excited by acupuncture via another central branch of Aδ primary afferents. The axons of the Waldeyer cells constitute another component (spinothalamic tract) of the crossed anterolateral funiculus and convey pin-prick information to consciousness through the ventral posterolateral nucleus of the thalamus and thence to the somatosensory cortex (where there is somatotopic representation). Collaterals excite the periaqueductal grey which in its turn projects to the nucleus raphe magnus, situated in the midline of the lower brainstem reticular formation.

Serotoninergic (5-hydroxytryptamine) and adrenergic (noradrenaline) axons of nucleus raphe magnus cells descend through the dorsolateral funiculus of the spinal cord to synapse eventually with the cells described above and so block the onward transmission of noxiously generated information in the same way as does segmental acupuncture. However, this descending inhibitory pathway gives off these connections at all levels of the spinal cord thereby explaining the extra segmental effect of acupuncture.

A striking and puzzling difference between analgesia produced by TENS and acupuncture is the duration of pain relief. Whereas TENS usually produces analgesia for minutes or hours, acupuncture can, and often does, produce analgesia for weeks. The mechanisms discussed previously cannot account for the prolonged analgesia commonly seen after acupuncture and so some additional mechanisms must be involved. One recently suggested by Professor Jisheng Han of Beijing Medical University postulates that acupuncture sets up a so-called mesolimbic loop of analgesia[124] formed by the periaqueductal grey, the nucleus accumbens, and the habenula. Han and his colleagues have suggested that acupuncture may set in motion this particular loop of neuronal activity which, whilst it is in motion, blocks the upward transmission of nociceptive impulses from the spinal cord to the thalamus and cortex. In support of this hypothesis, Han and his colleagues[125] have shown that acupuncture analgesia can be blocked by injecting naloxone into any one of the main neuronal stations on the loop. It seems unlikely that naloxone would have this effect unless these areas operate as a loop and are thus interdependent in this way. Presumably, once the loop has been set in motion it takes some time to slow down and it is during this time that analgesia occurs, and so

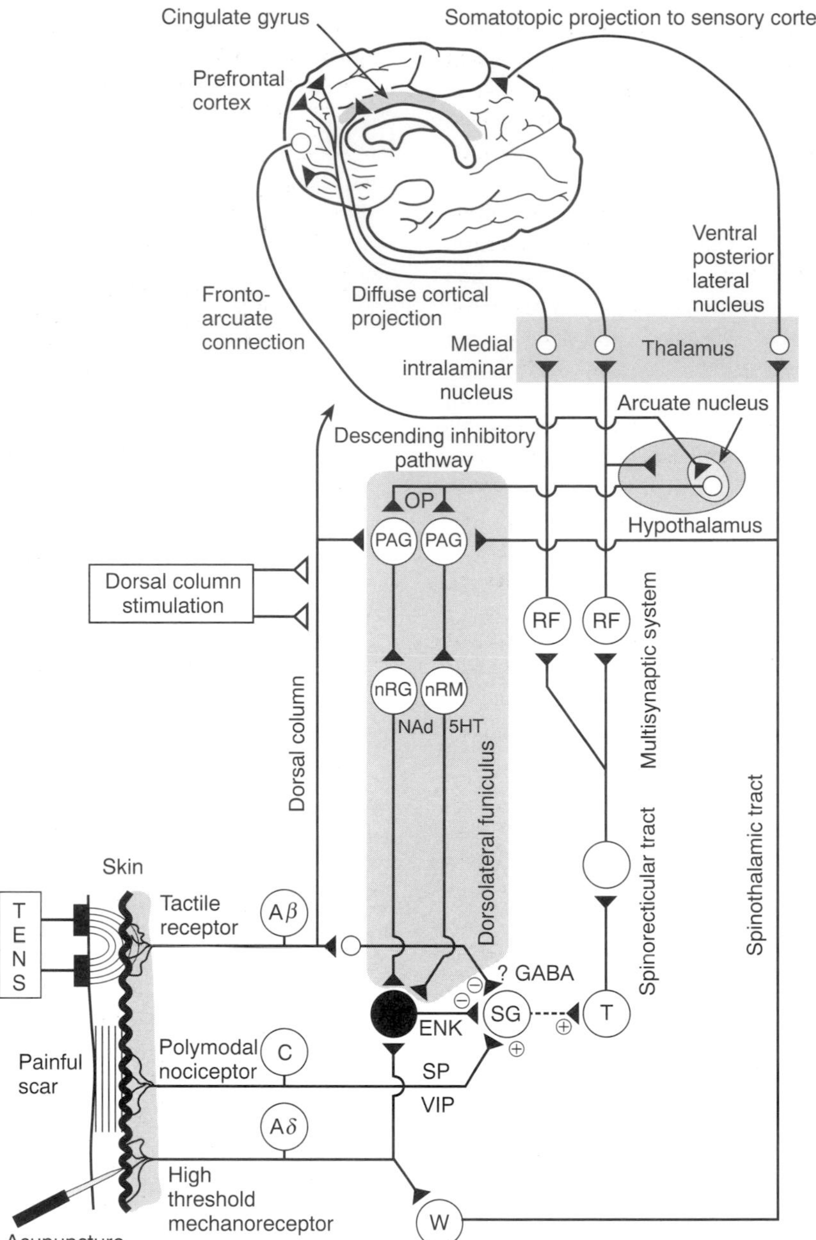

Fig. 5 Diagram to show neuronal circuits involved in TENS and acupuncture analgesia. The afferent pathways involved in transmitting nociceptive information from a painful scar to the higher centres via the dorsal horn, the ascending tracts, and the thalamus are shown. The connections to the descending inhibitory pathways which descend in the dorsolateral funiculus are also shown. The connections to the hypothalamus are indicated. Abbreviations Aβ, C, and Aδ represent the posterior root ganglion cells of Aβ, C, and Aδ fibres, respectively; SP = substance P; VIP = vasoactive intestinal polypeptide; GABA = γ-amino-butyric acid; OP = opioid peptides; SG = cell in the substantia gelatinosa (lamina II); Enk = enkephalinergic neurone; T = transmission cell; W = Waldeyer cell; PAG = periaqueductal grey; mRG = cell in the nucleus raphe gigantocellularis; nRM = cell in the nucleus raphe magnus; NAd = noradrenaline; 5-HT = 5-hydroxytryptamine. For full details see text.

giving its prolonged effect. It is an exciting and novel concept but it remains to be substantiated by further experiments.

Factors that limit the pace of advances: research and future trends

As has been described earlier, acupuncture and TENS can provide useful and effective analgesia in the field of palliative care. However, there is a need to improve the efficacy of both for a number of reasons. Every attempt should be made to find ways of increasing the depth and the duration of analgesia, especially that following a single treatment. The latter problem is more pertinent to acupuncture because with TENS the stimulator can be kept switched on for as long as need be (provided rules of electrode care are observed).

The development of a form of effective non-invasive or needleless acupuncture would be a great step forward not only for the patient but also because it would make it available for use by doctors and other health professionals untrained as acupuncturists. TENS can often prolong analgesia following acupuncture but the optimum conditions for this synergism have yet to be determined. It would also be extremely useful if some method could be discovered to predict positive responses to acupuncture and TENS, although it may always need to depend upon trial and error, as with analgesic drugs.

The potential for development of TENS is great in view of the large number of variables (pulse amplitude, width, frequency, pattern, etc.) that can be controlled precisely with TENS. The appearance of stimulators with outputs incorporating biphasic waves (H-wave) or complex waveforms, such as the Codetron and the Likon, are evidence of advances taking place in this area, although their exact role in TENS therapy has yet to be determined. The latest development is transcutaneous spinal electroanalgesia (TSE) which utilizes very brief pulses (duration not more than 4 microseconds at 600 Hz) that permit the application of a high voltage (400 volts) to the skin, via electrodes overlying the spinal cord, without causing any sensation.[126] For all these therapies, controlled trials, difficult though these may be to design, would seem to be mandatory.

However, it should be noted that it has recently been suggested that the treatment of back pain with TENS is so impressive that it may well be irrelevant to subject TENS to further clinical trials.[127] The need to find individuals who are able and motivated to carry out research in these areas is obvious. In the meantime, information about acupuncture and TENS is scattered widely in the literature, and it would make for economy of time and effort if a databank were to be set up to collect the world literature on these subjects so that palliative care (as well as other branches of medicine) could derive the maximum benefit.

Acupuncture and TENS are not only of importance in their own right but also because both have acted as important catalysts in the study of the neuropharmacology of pain. They may thus help to lead the way not only to a better understanding of the mechanism of pain and analgesia but also to the development of better analgesic agents.

References

1. Melzack R. Folk medicine and the sensory modulation of pain. In: Melzack R, Wall PD, eds. *Textbook of Pain*. 3rd edn. Edinburgh: Churchill Livingstone, 1994: 1209–17.
2. Melzack R, Wall PD. Pain mechanisms. *Science*, 1965; **150**: 971–9.
3. Wall PD, Sweet W. Temporary abolition of pain in man. *Science*, 1967; **155**: 108–9.
4. Shealy CN, Mortimer JT, Reswick JB. Electrical inhibition of pain by stimulation of the dorsal column: preliminary clinical reports. *Anaesthesia and Analgesia*, 1967; **46**: 488–91.
5. Long DM. Electrical stimulation for relief of pain from chronic nerve injury. *Journal of Neurosurgery*, 1973; **39**: 718–22.
6. Woolf CJ. Segmental afferent fibre-induced analgesia: transcutaneous electrical nerve stimulation (TENS) and vibration. In: Wall PD, Melzack R, eds. *Textbook of Pain*. 2nd edn. Edinburgh: Churchill Livingstone, 1989: 884–6.
7. Woolf CJ, Thompson JW. Stimulation-induced analgesia: transcutaneous electrical nerve stimulation (TENS) and vibration. In: Wall PD, Melzack R, eds. *Textbook of Pain*. 3rd edn. Edinburgh: Churchill Livingstone, 1994: 1191–208.
8. Stamp JM, Wood D. A *Comparative Evaluation of Transcutaneous Electrical Nerve Stimulators*. Sheffield: Sheffield University and Area Health Authority (T), 1981.
9. Stamp JM, Rose BA. *A Comparative Evaluation of Transcutaneous Electrical Nerve Stimulators (TENS) Part II*. Sheffield: Sheffield University and Area Health Authority, 1984.
10. Johnson, MI, Ashton CH, Thompson JW. An in-depth study of long term users of transcutaneous electrical nerve stimulation (TENS). Implications for clinical use of TENS. *Pain*, 1981: **44**: 221–9.
11. Librach SI, Rapson LM. The use of transcutaneous electrical nerve stimulation (TENS) for the relief of pain in palliative care. *Palliative Medicine*, 1988; **2**: 15–20.
12. Bowsher D. Neurogenic pain syndromes and their management. *British Medical Bulletin*, 1991; **47**: 644–6.
13. Sjolund BH, Eriksson M, Loeser JD. Transcutaneous and implanted electrical stimulation of peripheral nerves. In: Bonica JJ, ed. *The Management of Pain* Vol II. 2nd edn. Philadelphia and London: Lea and Febiger, 1990: 1852–61.
14. Mannheimer JS, Lampe GN. *Clinical Transcutaneous Electrical Nerve Stimulation*. Philadelphia: FA Davis, 1984.
15. Sjolund B, Eriksson M. *Relief of Pain by TENS* (English translation). Chichester and New York: John Wiley and Sons, 1985.
16. Bates JAV, Nathan PW. Transcutaneous electrical nerve stimulation for chronic pain. *Anaesthesia*, 1980; **35**: 817–22.
17. Marchand S, Charest J, Li J, Chenard J-R, Lavignolle B, Laurencelle L. Is TENS purely a placebo effect? A controlled study on chronic low back pain. *Pain*, 1993; **54**: 99–106.
18. Wang X-J, Wang X-H, Han J. Cholecystokinin octapeptide antagonise opioid analgesia mediated by mu- and kappa but not delta-receptors in the spinal cord of the rat. *Brain Research*, 1990; **523**: 5–10.
19. Thompson JW. Pharmacology of transcutaneous electrical stimulation (TENS). *Journal of the Intractable Pain Society*, 1989; **7**: 33–40.
20. Johnson MI, Ashton CH, Thompson JW. A prospective investigation into factors related to patient response to transcutaneous electrical nerve stimulation (TENS)—the importance of cortical responsivity. *European Journal of* Pain, 1993; **14**: 1–9.
21. Ostrowski MJ. Pain control in advanced malignant disease using transcutaneous nerve stimulation. *British Journal of Clinical Practice*, 1979; **33**: 157–62.
22. Long DM. External electrical stimulation as a treatment of chronic pain. *Minnesota Medicine*, 1974; **57**: 195–8.
23. Hardy RW. Current techniques in the management of pain. *Cleveland Clinical Quarterly*, 1975; **41**: 177–83.
24. Loeser JD, Black RG, Christman A. Relief of pain by transcutaneous stimulation. *Journal of Neurosurgery*, 1975; **42**: 308–14.
25. Campbell JN, Long DM. Peripheral nerve stimulation in the treatment of intractable pain. *Journal of Neurosurgery*, 1976; **45**: 692–9.
26. Ventafridda V. Transcutaneous nerve stimulation in cancer pain. In: Bonica JJ, Ventafridda V, eds. *Advances in Pain Research and Therapy*. New York: Raven Press, 1979: 509–15.
27. Avellanosa AM, West CR. Experience with transcutaneous nerve stimulation for relief of intractable pain in cancer patients. *Journal of Medicine*, 1982; **13**: 203–13.
28. Dil-din AS, Tikhonova GP, Kozvov SV. Transcutaneous electro-stimulation method leading to a permeation system of electroanalgesia in oncological practice. *Vopr-Onkologica*, 1985; **31**: 33–6.
29. Rafter J. *TENS and Cancer Pain*. Paper read to the Acupuncture Foundation of Canada Congress on Acupuncture and Related Techniques. Toronto, Canada, November 19–36. (Quoted by Librach and Rapson[11]).
30. Mason JL, Mackay NAM. Pain sensations associated with electrocutaneous stimulation. *IEEE Transactions on Biomedical Engineering*, 1976; **23**: 405–9.
31. Yamamoto T, Yamamoto Y, Akiharu Y. Formative mechanisms of current concentration and breakdown phenomena dependent on direct current flow through skin by a dry electrode. *IEEE Transactions on Biomedical Engineering*, 1986; **33**: 396–404.
32. Mann F. Acupuncture. In: Lipton S, ed. *Persistent Pain*. Vol 1. London: Academic Press, 1977.
33. Veith I. *The Yellow Emperor's Classic of Internal Medicine*. Berkeley: University of California Press, 1972.

34. MacDonald AJ. Acupuncture analgesia and therapy. In: Melzack R, Wall PD. *Textbook of Pain*. 2nd edn. Churchill Livingstone, 1989: 906–19.
35. Lu GD, Needham J. *Celestial Lancets. A History and Rationale of Acupuncture and Moxa*. Cambridge University Press, 1980.
36. Mann F. *Acupuncture: The Ancient Chinese Art of Healing*. 2nd edn. London: Heinemann, 1972.
37. Lim J. Understanding Acupuncture. Cambridge University, 1989. Ph.D.Thesis.
38. Mann F. *Reinventing Acupuncture*. Oxford: Butterworth and Heinemann, 1992.
39. *Essentials of Chinese Acupuncture*. Beijing College: Foreign Languages Press, 1980.
40. Stux G, Pomeranz B. *Acupuncture Textbook and Atlas*. Springer-Verlag, 1987.
41. Mann F. *Textbook of Acupuncture*. London: Heinemann, 1987.
42. Baldry PE. *Acupuncture, Trigger Points and Musculoskeletal Pain*. 2nd edn. Churchill Livingstone, 1993.
43. Stux G, Pomeranz B. *Basics of Acupuncture*. Springer-Verlag, 1988.
44. Deluze C, Bosia L, Zirbs A, Chantraine A, Vischer TL. Electro-acupuncture in fibromyalgia; results of a controlled trial. *British Medical Journal*, 1992; **305**: 1249–52.
45. Price DD, Rafii A, Watkins LT, Buckingham B. A psychophysical analysis of acupuncture analgesia. *Pain*, 1984; **19**: 27–42.
46. Murphy TM, Bonica JJ. Acupuncture analgesia and anaesthesia. *Archives of Surgery*, 1977; 896–902.
47. Kho HG, Edmond J, Van Zhuang CF, Liu GF, Zhang GL. Acupuncture anaesthesia. Observations on its use for removal of thyroid ademona and influence on recovery and morbidity in a chinese hospital. *Anaesthesia*, 1990; **45**: 480–6.
48. Christensen PA, Noreng M, Anderson PE, Nielsen JW. Electro-acupuncture and post-operative pain. *British Journal of Anaesthesia*, 1989; **62**: 258–62.
49. Li Qi-song, Cao Su-ha, Xie Guomin, Gan Yu-hong, Ma Hong-jian, Lu Ji-zheng, Zhang Zhao-huan. Relieving effects of chinese herbs, ear acupuncture and epidural morphine on postoperative pain in liver cancer. *Chinese Medical Journal*, 1994; **107**: 289–95.
50. Woolley-Hart A. *Handbook for Low Power Lasers and their Medical Application*. London: East Asia Company, 1988.
51. Walker JB, Akhanjee LK, Cooney MM, *et al*. Laser therapy for pain of trigeminal neuralgia. *Clinical Journal of Pain*, 1987; **3**: 183–7.
52. Goldman JA, Chiapella J, Casey H, Bass N, *et al*. Laser therapy of rheumatoid arthritis. *Lasers in Surgery and Medicine*, 1980; **1**: 93–101.
53. Walker JB, Akhanjee LK, Cooney MM, Goldstine J, *et al*. Laser therapy for pain of rheumatoid arthritis. *Clinical Journal of Pain*, 1987; **3**: 54–9.
54. Nogier PFM. *Treatise of Auriculotherapy*. Maisonneuve, France, 1972.
55. Oleson TD, Kroening RJ, Bresler DE. An experimental evaluation of auricular diagnosis; the somatotopic mapping of musculoskeletal pain at ear acupuncture points. *Pain*, 1980; **8**: 217–29.
56. Yoshino N, Kumio Y. *Ryodoraku Acupuncture*. Ryodoraku Research Institute Limited, 1977.
57. Klide AM, Shin HK. *Veterinary Acupuncture*. 3rd reprint. University of Pennsylvania Press, 1986.
58. Bannerman R. *Acupuncture: The World Health Organisation View*. World Health, 27th/28th December, 1979: 24–9.
59. Filshie J, Morrison PJ. Acupuncture for chronic pain: a review. *Palliative Medicine*, 1988; **2**: 1–14.
60. Sodipo JOA. Therapeutic acupuncture for chronic pain. *Pain*, 1979; **7**: 359–65.
61. Loh L, Nathan PW, Schott GD, Zilka KJ. Acupuncture versus medical treatment for migraine and muscle tension headaches. *Journal of Neurology, Neurosurgery and Psychiatry*, 1984; **47**: 333–7.
62. Bhatt-Sanders D. Acupuncture for rheumatoid arthritis: an analysis of the literature. *Seminars in Arthritis and Rheumatism*, 1985; **14**: 225–31.
63. Hanks GW. Pain and Cancer. *Cancer Surveys*, 1988; **7**: 1–224.
64. Filshie J. The non-drug treatment of neuralgic and neuropathic pain of malignancy. *Cancer Surveys*, 1988; **7**: 161–93.
65. Le Bars D, Villanueva L, Willer JC, Bouhassira D. Diffuse noxious inhibitory controls (DNIC) in animals and in man. *Acupuncture in Medicine*, 1991; **9**: 47–58.
66. Filshie J, Redman D. Acupuncture and malignant pain problems. *European Society of Surgical Oncology*, 1985; **2**: 389–94.
67. Filshie J. Acupuncture and malignant pain problems. *Acupuncture in Medicine*, 1990; **8**: 38–9.
68. Kori SH, Foley K, Posner JB. Brachial plexus lesions in patients with cancer: 100 cases. *Neurology*, 1981; **31**: 45–50.
69. Wang K, Han J. Accelerated synthesis and release of angiotensin in the rat brain during electroacupuncture tolerance. *Science in China* (Series B), 1990; **33**: 686–93.
70. Zhou Y, Sun YH, Shen JM, Han JS. Increased release of immunoreactive CCK-8 by electroacupuncture and enhancement of electroacupuncture analgesia by CCK-B antagonist in rat spinal cord. *Neuropeptides*, 1993; **24**:139–44.
71. Wen HL. Cancer pain treated with acupuncture and electrical stimulation. *Modern Medicine of Asia*, 1977; **13**: 12–16.
72. Mann F, Bowsher D, Mumford J, Lipton S, Miles J. Treatment of intractable pain by acupuncture. *Lancet*, 1973; **ii**: 57–60.
73. Xue CC. Acupuncture induced phantom limb and meridian phenomenon in acquired and congenital amputees. A suggestion of the use of acupuncture as a method for investigation of phantom limb. *Chinese Medical Journal*, 1986; **3**: 247–52.
74. Monga TN, Jaksic T. Acupuncture in phantom limb pain. *Archives of Physical Medicine and Rehabilitation*, 1981; **62**: 229–31.
75. Jobst K, Chen JH, McPherson J, *et al*. Controlled trial of acupuncture for disabling breathlessness. *Lancet*, 1986; **ii**: 1417–19.
76. Fung KP, Chow OKW, So SY. Attenuation of exercise-induced asthma by acupuncture. *Lancet*, 1986; **ii**: 1419–21.
77. Editorial. Acupuncture, asthma and breathlessness. *Lancet*, 1986; **ii**: 1427–8.
78. Filshie J, Penn K, Ashley S, Davis CL. Acupuncture for the relief of cancer related breathlessness. *Palliative Medicine*, 1996; **10**:145–50.
79. Han JS, ed. *The Neurochemical Basis of Pain Relief by Acupuncture*. Beijing: Medical Science Press of China, 1987.
80. Dundee JW. Belfast experience with P6 acupuncture antiemesis. *Ulster Medical Journal*, 1990; **59**: 63–70.
81. Dundee JW, Chaly RG, Yang J. Scientific observations on the antiemetic action of stimulation of the P6 acupuncture point. *Acupuncture in Medicine*, 1990; **7**: 2–5.
82. Dundee DW. Prolongation of the antiemetic action of P6 acupuncture by acupressure in patients having cancer chemotherapy. *Journal of the Royal Society of Medicine*, 1990; **83**: 360–2.
83. McMillan CM, Dundee JW. The role of transcutaneous electrical stimulation of neiguan antiemetic acupuncture point in controlling sickness after cancer chemotherapy. *Physiotherapy*, 1991; **77**: 499–502.
84. McMillan CM, Dundee JW, Abram WP. Enhancement of the antiemetic action of Ondansetron by transcutaneous electrical stimulation of P6 antiemetic points in patients having emetic cytotoxic drugs. *British Journal of Cancer*, 1991; **64**: 971–2.
85. Johansson K, Lindgren I, Widner H, Wiklund I, Johansson BB. Can sensory stimulation improve the functional outcome in stroke patients? *Neurology*, 1993; **43**: 2189–92.
86. Magnusson M, Johansson R, Johansson BB. Sensory stimulation promotes normalization of postural control after stroke. *Stroke*, 1994; **25**: 1176–80.
87. Johansson BB, Grabowski M. Functional recovery after brain infarction: Plasticity and neural transplantation. *Brain Pathology*, 1994; **4**: 85–95.
88. Johansson BB. Has sensory stimulation a role in stroke rehabilitation? *Scandinavian Journal of Rehabilitation Medicine*, 1993; **29**: 87–96.
89. Ruzhen F. Relief of oesophageal carcinomatous obstruction by acupuncture. *Journal of Traditional Chinese Medicine*, 1984; **4**: 3–4.
90. Liansheng Y. Treatment of persistent hiccupping with electro-acupuncture at 'hiccup- relieving' point. *Journal of Traditional Chinese Medicine*, 1988; **8**: 29–30.
91. Wong SSA. Treatment of hiccough by acupuncture—a report of two cases. *Medical Journal of Malaysia*, 1983; **38**: 80–1.

92. Zaohua Z. Effect of acupuncture on 44 cases of radiation rectitis following radiation therapy for carcinoma of the cervix uteri. *Journal of Traditional Chinese Medicine*, 1987; **7**: 139–40.
93. Hechun L, Yunkui J, Li Z. Electro-acupuncture vs. amitriptyline in the treatment of depressive states. *Journal of Traditional Chinese Medicine*, 1985; **5**: 3–8.
94. Han JS. Electroacupuncture; an alternative to antidepressants for treating affective diseases. *International Journal of Neuroscience*, 1986; **29**: 79–92.
95. Kroening RJ, Oleson TD. Rapid narcotic detoxification in chronic pain patients. *International Journal of the Addictions*, 1985; **20**: 1347–60.
96. Lundeberg T, Bondesson L, Thomas M. Effect of acupuncture on experimentally induced itch. *British Journal of Dermatology*, 1987; **117**: 771–7.
97. Duo LJ. Electrical needle therapy of uraemic pruritus. *Nephron*, 1987; **47**: 179–83.
98. Yi L. A report of 2 cases of type B Aids treated with acupuncture. *Journal of Traditional Chinese Medicine*, 1989; **9**: 95–6.
99. Boping W. Recent development of studies on traditional chinese medicine in prophylaxis and treatment of Aids. *Journal of Traditional Chinese Medicine*, 1992; **12**: 10–20.
100. Richardson PH. Pain and the placebo effect. *Frontier of Pain*, 1990; **2**: 1–2.
101. Jobst KA. A critical analysis of acupuncture in pulmonary disease: efficacy and safety of the acupuncture needle. *Journal of Alternative and Complementary Medicine*, 1995; **1**: 57–85.
102. Richardson PH, Vincent CA. Acupuncture for the treatment of pain; a review of evaluative research. *Pain*, 1986; **24**: 15–40.
103. Ter Riet G, Kleinjen J, Knipschild P. Acupuncture and chronic pain: a criteria-based meta-analysis. *Journal of Clinical Epidemiology*, 1990; **43**: 1191–9.
104. Ter Riet G, Kleijnen J, Knipschild P. Acupuncture and asthma: a review of controlled trials. *Thorax*, 1991; **46**: 799–802.
105. Ter Riet G, Kleijnen J, Knipschild P. A meta analysis of studies into the effect of acupuncture on addiction. *British Journal of General Practice*, 1990; **40**: 379–82.
106. Patel M, Gutzwiller D, Paccaud F, Marazzi A. A meta-analysis of acupuncture for chronic pain. *International Journal of Epidemiology*, 1989; **18**: 900–6.
107. Rampes H, James R. Complications of acupuncture. *Acupuncture in Medicine*, 1995; **13**: 26–33
108. Spelman DW, Weinmann A, Spicer WJ. Endocarditis following skin procedures. *Journal of Infection*, 1993; **26**: 185–9.
109. Keng GP, Brondum B, Keenlyside RA, LaFazia LM, Scott HD. A large outbreak of acupuncture-associated hepatitis B. *American Journal of Epidemiology*, 1988; **127**: 591–8.
110. Slater PE, *et al.*. An acupuncture associated outbreak of hepatitis B in Jerusalem. *European Journal of Epidemiology*, 1988; **4**: 322–5.
111. Vittecoq D, Mettetat JF, Rouzioux C, Bach JF. Acute HIV infection after acupuncture treatments. *New England Journal of Medicine*, 1989; **320**: 250–1.
112. Cheng TO. Acupuncture and acquired immunodeficiency syndrome. *American Journal of Medicine*, 1989; **87**: 489.
113. Otusaka N, Fukunaga M, Morita K, Ono S, Nagai K, Katagiri M, Harada T, Morita R. Iodine-131 uptake in a patient with thyroid cancer and rheumatoid arthritis during acupuncture treatment. *Clinical Nuclear Medicine*, 1990; **15**: 29–31.
114. Han JS, Terenius L. Neurochemical basis of acupuncture analgesia. *Annual Review of Pharmacology and Toxicology*, 1982; **22**: 193–220.
115. Duggan AW, Foong FW. Bicuculline and spinal inhibition produced by dorsal column stimulation in the cat. *Pain*, 1985; **22**: 249–59.
116. Bowsher D. Sensory mechanisms. *Clinical Neuropsychology*, 1985; **45**: 227–44.
117. Garrison DW, Foreman RD. Decreased activity of spontaneous and noxiously evoked dorsal horn cells during transcutaneous electrical nerve stimulation (TENS). *Pain*, 1994; **58**: 309–15.
118. Bowsher D. The physiology of acupuncture. *Journal of the Intractable Pain Society of Great Britain and Ireland*, 1987; **5**: 15–18.
119. Thompson JW. The role of transcutaneous electrical nerve stimulation (TENS) for the control of pain. In: Doyle D, ed. *International Symposium on Pain Control*. Royal Society of Medicine Services International Congress and Symposium series, 1987.
120. Pomeranz B, Stux G, eds. *Scientific Bases of Acupuncture*. Berlin, Heidelberg, New York: SpringerVerlag, 1989.
121. Le Bars D, Dickenson AH, Besson JM. Diffuse noxious inhibitory controls (DNIC). II Lack of effect on non-convergent neurons, supraspinal involvement and theoretical implications. *Pain*, 1979; **6**: 283–304.
122. Fields HL, Basbaum AL. Central nervous system mechanisms of pain modulation. In: Wall PD, Melzack R, eds. *Textbook of Pain*, 3rd edn. Edinburgh: Churchill Livingstone, 1994.
123. Jones AKP, Brown WD, Friston KT, Qi L, Frackowiak RSJ. Cortical and subcortical localisation of response to pain in man using positron emission tomography. *Proceedings of the Royal Society of London*, Series B, 1991; **244**: 29–44.
124. Han JS, Yu LC, Shi Y. A Mesolimbic loop of analgesia. III A neuronal pathway from nucleus accumbens to periaquaductal grey. *Asian Pacific Journal of Pharmacology*, 1986: **1**: 17–22.
125. Zhou ZF, Xuan YT, Han JS. Analgesic effect of morphine injected into habenula, nucleus accumbens or amygdala of rabbits. *Acta Pharmacologica Sinica*, 1984; **5**: 1150–3.
126. Macdonald AJR, Coates TW. The discovery of transcutaneous spinal electroanalgesia and its relief of chronic pain. *Physiotherapy*, 1995; **81**: 653–61.
127. Leading article. TENS for chronic low-back pain. *Lancet*, 1991; **337**: 462–3.

9.2.9 Psychological and psychiatric interventions in pain control

William Breitbart, Steven Passik, and David Payne

Introduction

Effective management of pain in patients with advanced cancer or AIDS requires a multidisciplinary approach, enlisting expertise from a wide variety of clinical groups.[1-3] The utilization of psychiatric interventions in the treatment of cancer and AIDS patients with pain and psychological distress has now also become an integral part of such a comprehensive approach.[4-6]

The scope of the problem:

Prevalence of pain in cancer and AIDS

Pain is a common problem for cancer patients, with approximately 70 per cent of patients experiencing severe pain at some time in the course of their illness.[2] It has been suggested that nearly 75 per cent of patients with advanced cancer have pain[7] and that 25 per cent of cancer patients die in severe pain.[8] There is considerable variability in the prevalence of pain amongst different types of cancer. For example approximately 5 per cent of leukaemia patients experience pain during the course of their illness as compared to 50 to 75 per cent of patients with tumours of the lung, gastrointestinal tract, or genitourinary system. Patients with cancers of the bone or cervix have been found to have the highest prevalence of pain, with as many as 85 per cent of patients experiencing significant pain during the course of their illness.[1] Yet, despite its prevalence, studies have shown that pain is frequently underdiagnosed and inadequately treated.[9,2] It is important to remember that pain is frequently only one of several symptoms present in cancer patients. In addition to pain, patients were found, in a survey of symptoms, to suffer from an average of three additional troubling physical symptoms.[10] A global evaluation of the symptom burden allows for a more complete understanding of the impact of pain for the cancer patient.

Pain is a significant and often neglected problem in patients with AIDS. Estimates of the prevalence of pain in AIDS generally range from 40 to 60 per cent, with prevalence of pain increasing as the disease progresses.[11] A recent retrospective chart review of hospitalized patients with AIDS revealed that over 50 per cent of patients required treatment for pain, with pain being the presenting complaint in 30 per cent (second only to fever).[12] In this study, chest pain occurred in 22 per cent, headache in 13 per cent, oral cavity pain in 11 per cent, abdominal pain in 9 per cent, and peripheral neuropathy in 6 per cent. A second retrospective review of pain in an AIDS population reported abdominal pain, peripheral neuropathy, and Kaposi's sarcoma as the three most frequent pain problems, which affected 15 per cent of patients.[13] Other reviews report that between 5 and 30 per cent of AIDS patients have painful peripheral neuropathy.[14–16] In a hospice setting, Schofferman and Brody[17] described pain in patients with far advanced AIDS. Fifty-three per cent of patients surveyed had pain, most commonly peripheral neuropathy, abdominal pain, headache, and Kaposi's sarcoma (skin pain). In an ambulatory AIDS population, 43 per cent of patients reported pain of at least 2 weeks duration.[18] Painful neuropathy accounted for 50 per cent of pain diagnoses and lower extremity pain related to Kaposi's sarcoma was found in 45 per cent. While pains of a neuropathic nature are an important clinical problem that has attracted a great deal of attention, the evolving literature on AIDS pain syndromes suggests that pains of somatic and visceral aetiologies make up the bulk of the cases of pain in AIDS. Recent work suggests that of the pains experienced by ambulatory patients with AIDS, approximately 33 per cent are somatic, 35 per cent are visceral, and 33 per cent are neuropathic. In addition, somatic, visceral, and neuropathic pains often occur concurrently, and neuropathic pain is not often the predominant pain.[19]

Multidimensional concept of pain in terminal illness

Pain, and especially pain in advanced cancer and AIDS, is not a purely nociceptive or physical experience, but involves complex aspects of human functioning including: personality, affect, cognition, behaviour, and social relations.[20] A more enlightened description of the pain resulting from a terminal illness coined by Cecily Saunders[21] is 'total pain,' a label that attempts to describe the all encompassing nature of this type of pain. It is important to note that the use of analgesic drugs alone does not always lead to pain relief.[22] In a recent study[23] it has been demonstrated that psychological factors play a modest but important role in pain intensity. The interaction of cognitive, emotional, socioenvironmental, and nociceptive aspects of pain shown in Fig. 1 illustrates the multidimensional nature of pain in terminal illness and suggests a model for multimodal intervention.[3] The challenge of untangling and addressing both the physical and psychological issues involved in pain is essential to developing rational and effective management strategies. Psychosocial therapies directed primarily at psychological variables have profound impact on nociception, while somatic therapies directed at nociception have beneficial effects on the psychological aspects of pain. Ideally, such somatic and psychosocial therapies are used simultaneously in the multidisciplinary approach to pain management in the terminally ill.[4]

Psychological factors in pain experience

The patient with cancer or AIDS faces many stressors during the course of their illness including dependency, disability, and fear of painful death. Such fears are universal; however, the level of psychological distress is variable and depends on medical factors, social supports, coping capacities, and personality. Pain has profound effects on psychological distress in cancer patients, and psychological factors such as anxiety, depression, and the meaning of pain can intensify cancer pain experience. Daut and Cleeland[24] showed that cancer patients who attribute a new pain to an unrelated benign cause report less interference with their activity and pleasure than cancer patients who believe their pain represents progression of disease. Spiegel and Bloom[25] found that women with metastatic breast cancer experience more intense pain if they believe their pain represents spread of their cancer, and if they are depressed. Beliefs about the meaning of pain and the presence of a mood disturbance are better predictors of level of pain than is the site of metastasis.

In an attempt to define the potential relationships between pain and psychosocial variables, Padilla *et al.*[26] found that there were pain-related quality of life variables in three domains:

(1) physical well-being;

(2) psychological well being consisting of affective factors, cognitive factors, spiritual factors, communication, coping, and meaning of pain or cancer;

(3) interpersonal well-being focusing on social support or role functioning.

The perception of marked impairment in activities of daily living has been shown to be associated with increased pain intensity.[27,28] Measures of emotional disturbance have been reported to be

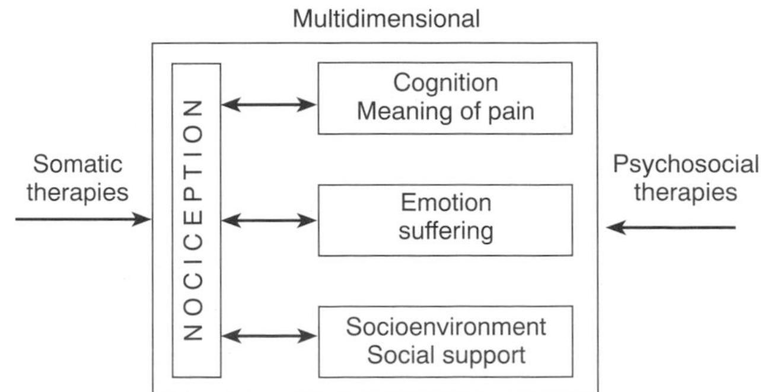

Fig. 1 The multidimensional nature of pain in terminal illness.

Table 1 Rates of DSM-III psychiatric disorders and prevalence of pain observed in 215 cancer patients from three cancer centres*

Diagnostic category	Number in diagnostic class	Percentage of psychiatric diagnoses	Number with significant pain[a]
Adjustment disorders	69	(32%)	68
Major affective disorders	13	(6%)	13
Organic mental disorders	8	(4%)	8
Personality disorders	7	(3%)	7
Anxiety disorders	4	(2%)	4
Total with psychiatric diagnosis	101	(47%)	39 (39%)
Total with no psychiatric diagnosis	114	(53%)	21 (19%)
Total patient population	215	(100%)	60 (28%)

[a] Score greater than 50 mm on a 100 mm VAS for pain severity.

predictors of pain in late stages of cancer, and cancer patients with less anxiety and depression are less likely to report pain.[29,30] Both cancer and AIDS patients who report negative thoughts about their personal or social competence report increased pain intensity and emotional distress.[27,28] In a prospective study of cancer patients it was found that maladaptive coping strategies, lower levels of self-efficacy, and distress specific to the treatment or disease progression were modest but significant predictors of reports of pain intensity.[23]

Psychological variables—such as the amount of control people believe they have over pain, emotional associations and memories of pain, fear of death, depression, anxiety, and hopelessness—contribute to the experience of pain in people with AIDS and can increase suffering.[31] We recently reported[27] that negative thoughts related to pain are associated with greater pain intensity, psychological distress, and disability in ambulatory patients with AIDS. Pain appears to have a profound impact on levels of emotional distress and disability. In a pilot study of the impact of pain on ambulatory HIV-infected patients,[32] depression was significantly correlated with the presence of pain. In addition to being significantly more distressed and depressed, those with pain were twice as likely to have suicidal ideation (40 per cent) as those without pain (20 per cent). HIV-infected patients with pain were more functionally impaired. Such functional interference was highly correlated to levels of pain intensity and depression. Those who felt that pain represented a threat to their health reported more intense pain than those who did not see pain as a threat. Patients with pain were more likely to be unemployed or disabled, and they reported less social support. Singer and colleagues[11] also reported an association among the frequency of multiple pains, increased disability, and higher levels of depression.

All too frequently, however, psychological variables are proposed to explain continued pain or lack of response to therapy when in fact medical factors have not been adequately appreciated. Often, the psychiatrist is the last physician to consult on a cancer or AIDS patient with pain. In that role one must be vigilant that an accurate pain diagnosis is made and be able to assess the adequacy of the medical analgesic management provided. Psychological distress in terminally ill patients with pain must initially be assumed to be the consequence of uncontrolled pain. Personality factors may be quite distorted by the presence of pain, and relief of pain often results in the disappearance of a perceived psychiatric disorder.[33,9]

Psychiatric disorders and pain in the terminally ill

There is an increased frequency of psychiatric disorders found in cancer patients with pain. In the Psychosocial Collaborative Oncology Group Study[34] on the prevalence of psychiatric disorders in cancer patients, of the patients who received a psychiatric diagnosis (see Table 1), 39 per cent reported significant pain, while only 19 per cent of patients without a psychiatric diagnosis had significant pain. The psychiatric disorders seen in cancer patients with pain include primarily adjustment disorder with depressed or anxious mood (69 per cent) and major depression (15 per cent). This finding of increased frequency of psychiatric disturbance in patients with cancer pain has been reported elsewhere.[35,36]

Epidural spinal cord compression is a common neurological complication of systemic cancer that occurs in 5 to 10 per cent of patients with cancer and can often present with severe pain. These patients are often treated with a combination of high-dose dexamethasone and radiotherapy. Patients who receive this high-dose regimen are exposed to as much as 96 mg/day of dexamethasone for up to a week, and continue on a tapering course for up to 3 or 4 weeks. Stiefel *et al.*[37] recently described the psychiatric complications seen in cancer patients undergoing such treatment for epidural spinal cord compression. Twenty-two per cent of patients with epidural spinal cord compression had a major depressive syndrome diagnosed as compared to 4 per cent in the comparison group. Also, delirium was much more common in the dexamethasone treated patients with epidural spinal cord compression, with 24 per cent diagnosed with delirium during the course of treatment as compared to only 10 per cent in the comparison group.

Cancer patients with advanced disease are a particularly vulnerable group. The incidence of pain, depression, and delirium increases with greater debilitation and advanced stages of illness.[38] Approximately 25 per cent of all cancer patients experience severe depressive symptoms, with the prevalence increasing to 77 per cent in those with advanced illness. The prevalence of organic mental disorders (delirium) among cancer patients requiring psychiatric consultation has been found to range from 25 to 40 per cent, and to be as high as 85 per cent during the terminal stages of illness.[39] Opioids can cause confusional states, particularly in the elderly and terminally ill.[40]

Breitbart and Passik[18] described the psychological impact of pain in an ambulatory AIDS population. AIDS patients with pain reported significantly greater depression and functional impairment than those without pain. Psychiatric disorders, in particular the organic mental disorders such as AIDS dementia complex, can occasionally interfere with adequate pain management in AIDS patients. Opioid analgesics, the mainstay of treatment for moderate to severe pain, may worsen dementia or cause treatment-limiting sedation, confusion, or hallucinations in patients with neurological complications of AIDS. The judicious use of psychostimulants to diminish sedation and neuroleptics to clear confusional states can be quite helpful. Other psychiatric disorders that have an impact on pain management in the AIDS population include substance abuse and personality disorders.

Pain and suicide

Uncontrolled pain is a major factor in suicide and suicidal ideation in cancer and AIDS patients.[41–43] Cancer is perceived by the public as an extremely painful disease compared with other medical conditions. In Wisconsin, a study revealed that 69 per cent of the public agreed that cancer pain could cause a person to consider suicide.[44] The majority of suicides observed among patients with cancer had severe pain, which was often inadequately controlled or tolerated poorly.[45] Although relatively few cancer patients commit suicide, they are at increased risk.[46,44] Patients with advanced illness are at highest risk and are the most likely to have the complications of pain, depression, delirium, and deficit symptoms. Psychiatric disorders are frequently present in hospitalized cancer patients who attempt suicide. A review of the psychiatric consultation data at Memorial Sloan-Kettering Cancer Center showed that one-third of cancer patients who were seen for evaluation of suicide risk received a diagnosis of major depression; approximately 20 per cent met criteria for delirium; and more than 50 per cent were diagnosed with an adjustment disorder.[41]

Thoughts of suicide probably occur quite frequently in the clinical context, particularly in the setting of advanced illness,[47] and seem to act as a steam valve for feelings often expressed by patients as 'If it gets too bad, I always have a way out.' It has been our experience working with terminally ill pain patients that once a trusting and safe relationship develops, patients almost universally reveal that they have had occasionally persistent thoughts of suicide as a means of escaping the threat of being overwhelmed by pain. Recent published research reports, however, suggest that persistent suicidal ideation is relatively infrequent in cancer and is limited to those who are significantly depressed. Silberfarb *et al.*[48] found that only 3 of 146 breast cancer patients had suicidal thoughts, whereas none of the 100 cancer patients interviewed in a Finnish study expressed suicidal thoughts.[49] A study conducted at St. Boniface Hospice in Winnipeg, Canada, demonstrated that only 10 of 44 terminally ill cancer patients were suicidal or desired an early death, and all 10 were suffering from clinical depression.[50] At Memorial Sloan-Kettering Cancer Center, suicide risk evaluation accounted for 8.6 per cent of psychiatric consultations, usually requested by staff in response to patients verbalizing suicidal wishes.[41] In the 71 cancer patients who had suicidal ideation with serious intent, significant pain was a factor in only 30 per cent of cases. In striking contrast virtually all 71 suicidal cancer patients had a psychiatric disorder (mood disturbance or organic mental disorder) at the time of evaluation.[41]

We recently examined the role of cancer pain in suicidal ideation by assessing 185 cancer patients with pain involved in ongoing research protocols of the Memorial Sloan-Kettering Cancer Center Pain and Psychiatry Services.[51] Suicidal ideation occurred in 17 per cent of the study population with the majority reporting suicidal ideation without intent to act. Interestingly, in this population of cancer patients who all had significant pain, suicidal ideation was not directly related to pain intensity but was strongly related to degree of depression and mood disturbance. Pain was related to suicidal ideation indirectly in that patients' perception of poor pain relief was associated with suicidal ideation. Perceptions of pain relief may have more to do with aspects of hopelessness than pain itself. Pain plays an important role in vulnerability to suicide; however, associated psychological distress and mood disturbance seem to be essential cofactors in raising the risk of suicide in cancer patients. Pain has adverse effects on patients' quality of life and sense of control and impairs the family's ability to provide support. Factors other than pain, such as mood disturbance, delirium, loss of control, and hopelessness, contribute to cancer suicide risk.[45]

A study of men with AIDS in New York City[52] demonstrated a relative risk of suicide 36 times greater than that of males in the general population. Many of these patients had advanced AIDS with Kaposi's sarcoma and other potentially painful conditions. However, the role of pain in contributing to increased risk of suicide was not specifically examined. Our group at Memorial Sloan-Kettering Cancer Center has also examined the prevalence of suicidal ideation in an ambulatory AIDS population, and examined the relationship between suicidal ideation, depression, and pain.[43] Suicidal ideation in ambulatory AIDS patients was found to be highly correlated with the presence of pain, depressed mood (as measured by the Beck Depression Inventory), and low T4 (CD4) lymphocyte counts. While 20 per cent of ambulatory AIDS patients without pain reported suicidal thoughts, over 40 per cent of those with pain reported suicidal ideation. Only 2 subjects in the sample (n=110) reported suicidal intent. One of these two men was in the pain group; however, both scored quite highly on measures of depression. No correlations were observed between suicidal ideation and pain intensity or pain relief. The mean visual analogue scale measure of pain intensity for the group overall was 49 mm (range 5–100 mm), thus falling predominantly in the moderate range. As with cancer patients with pain, suicidal ideation in AIDS patients with pain is more likely to be related to a concomitant mood disturbance than to the intensity of pain experienced. Although AIDS patients are frequently found to have suicidal ideation, these thoughts are more often context-specific, occurring almost exclusively during exacerbations of the illness, often accompanied by severe pain, or at times of bereavement.[53]

Inadequate pain management: assessment issues in the treatment of pain

While recent studies suggest that pain in cancer is still being undertreated,[54] pain in AIDS is markedly undertreated. Although still preliminary in nature, reports of marked undertreatment of pain in AIDS are appearing in the literature.[55,56] These studies suggest that opioid analgesics are underused in the treatment of pain in AIDS. Our group has reported that in our cohort of AIDS patients, only 6 per cent of individuals reporting pain in the severe range (8–10 on a numerical rating scale) received a strong opioid, such as morphine,[57] as recommended in the WHO Analgesic Ladder. This degree of undermedication far exceeds published reports of undermedication of pain in cancer patient populations.[54] As with cancer, we have found that factors influencing the undertreatment of pain in AIDS include gender (women are more undertreated), education, substance abuse history, and a variety of patient-related barriers.[57] While opioid analgesics are underused, it is also clear from our work and the work of others that adjuvant agents, such as the antidepressants, are also dramatically underused.[55,56,58] Only 6 per cent of subjects in a sample of AIDS patients reporting pain received an adjuvant analgesic drug (i.e. an antidepressant). This class of analgesic agents is a critical part of the WHO Analgesic Ladder and is vastly underused.

Inadequate management of pain is often due to the inability to assess pain properly in all its dimensions.[4,2,8] All too frequently, psychological variables are proposed to explain continued pain or lack of response to therapy, when in fact medical factors have not been adequately appreciated. Other causes of inadequate pain management include:

(1) lack of knowledge of current pharmaco- or psychotherapeutic approaches;

(2) focus on prolonging life rather than alleviating suffering;

(3) lack of communication between doctor and patient;

(4) limited expectations of patients to achieve pain relief;

(5) limited capacity of patients impaired by organic mental disorders to communicate;

(6) unavailability of opioid analgesics;

(7) doctors' fear of causing respiratory depression;

(8) and, most importantly, doctors' fear of amplifying addiction and substance abuse.

In advanced cancer, several factors have been noted to predict the undermanagement of pain including: a discrepancy between physician and patient in judging the severity of pain; the presence of pain that physicians did not attribute to cancer; better performance status; age of 70 or over; and female sex.[54]

Fear of addiction affects both patient compliance and physician management of opioid analgesics, leading to undermedication of pain in cancer and AIDS patients.[8,59,60,3] Studies of the patterns of chronic opioid analgesic use in patients with cancer have demonstrated that, although tolerance and physical dependence commonly occur, addiction (psychological dependence) is rare and almost never occurs in an individual without a history of drug abuse prior to cancer illness.[61] Escalation of opioid analgesic use by cancer patients is usually due to progression of cancer or the development of tolerance. Tolerance means that a larger dose of opioid analgesic is required to maintain an original analgesic effect. Physical dependence is characterized by the onset of signs and symptoms of withdrawal if the opioid is suddenly stopped or an opioid antagonist is administered. Tolerance usually occurs in association with physical dependence but does not imply psychological dependence. Psychological dependence, or addiction, is not equivalent to physical dependence or tolerance and is a behavioural pattern of compulsive drug abuse characterized by a craving for the drug and overwhelming involvement in obtaining and using it for effects other than pain relief. The cancer pain patient with a history of intravenous opioid abuse presents an often unnecessarily difficult management problem. Macaluso *et al.*[60] reported on their experience in managing cancer pain in such a population. Of 468 inpatient cancer pain consultations, only eight (1.7 per cent) had a history of intravenous drug abuse, but none had been actively abusing drugs in the previous year. All eight of these patients had inadequate pain control and more than half were intentionally undermedicated because of concern by staff that drug abuse was active or would recur. Adequate pain control was ultimately achieved in these patients by using appropriate analgesic dosages and intensive staff education.

More problematic, however, is the management of pain in the growing segment of the AIDS population that is actively abusing intravenous drugs.[62] Such active drug use, in particular intravenous opioid abuse, poses several pain treatment difficulties including:

(1) high tolerance to opioid analgesics;

(2) drug-seeking and manipulative behaviour;

(3) lack of compliance or reliability of patient history;

(4) the risk of spreading HIV while high and disinhibited.

Unfortunately, the patient's subjective report is often the best or only indication of the presence and intensity of pain as well as the degree of pain relief achieved by an intervention. Physicians who believe they are being manipulated by drug-seeking individuals are hesitant to use opioids in appropriate dosages for adequate control of pain, often leading to undermedication. Most clinicians experienced in working with this population of AIDS patients recommend clear and direct limit setting. While that is an important aspect of the care of AIDS patients who are abusing drugs, it is by no means the whole answer. As much as possible, clinicians should attempt to eliminate the issue of drug abuse as an obstacle to pain management by dealing directly with the problems of opioid withdrawal and drug abuse treatment. Often specialized substance abuse consultation services are available to help manage such patients and initiate drug rehabilitation. One should avoid making the analgesic drugs the focus of a battle for control between the patient and physician, especially in terminal stages of illness. Err on the side of believing patients when they complain of pain, and utilize your knowledge of the specific pain syndrome seen in AIDS patients to corroborate the patient's report if you feel it is unreliable.

The risk of inducing respiratory depression is too often overestimated and can limit appropriate use of opioid analgesics for pain and symptom control. Bruera *et al.*[63] demonstrated that, in a population of terminally ill cancer patients with respiratory failure

Table 2 Psychotherapy in patients with advanced disease and pain

Goals	Form
Support — provide continuity **Knowledge** — provide information **Skills** — relaxation cognitive coping use of analgesics communication	**Individuals** — supportive/ crisis intervention **Family** — patient and family are the unit of concern **Group** — share experiences identify successful coping strategies

and dyspnoea, administration of subcutaneous morphine actually improved dyspnoea without causing a significant deterioration in respiratory function.

The adequacy of cancer pain management can be influenced by the lack of concordance between patient ratings or complaints of their pain and those made by caregivers. Persistent cancer pain is often ascribed to a psychological cause when it does not respond to treatment attempts. In our clinical experience we have noted that patients who report their pain as 'severe' are quite likely to be viewed as having a psychological contribution to their complaints. Staff members' ability to empathize with a patient's pain complaint may be limited by the intensity of the pain complaint. Grossman *et al.*[64] found that while there is a high degree of concordance between patient and caregiver ratings of patient pain intensity at the low and moderate levels, this concordance breaks down at high levels. Thus, a clinician's ability to assess a patient's level of pain becomes unreliable once a patient's report of pain intensity rises above 7 on a visual analogue rating scale of 0 to 10. Physicians must be educated as to the limitations of their ability to objectively assess the severity of a subjective pain experience. Additionally, patient education is often a useful intervention in such cases. Patients are more likely to be believed and adequately treated if they are taught to request pain relief in a non-hysterical, business-like fashion.

Psychiatric management of pain in advanced disease

Optimal treatment of pain associated with advanced disease is multimodal and includes pharmacological, psychotherapeutic, cognitive-behavioural, anaesthetic, neurostimulatory, and rehabilitative approaches. Psychiatric participation in pain management involves the use of psychotherapeutic, cognitive-behavioural, and psychopharmacological interventions, usually in combination, that are described below.

Psychotherapy and pain

The goals of psychotherapy with medically ill patients with pain are to provide support, knowledge, and skills (Table 2). Utilizing short-term supportive psychotherapy focused on the crisis created by the medical illness, the therapist provides emotional support, continuity, information, and assists in adaptation. The therapist has a role in emphasizing past strengths, supporting previously successful coping strategies, and teaching new coping skills such as: relaxation, cognitive coping, use of analgesics, self-observation, documentation, assertiveness, and communication skills. Communication skills are of paramount importance for both patient and family, particularly around pain and analgesic issues. The patient and family are the unit of concern, and need a more general, long-term, supportive relationship within the health-care system in addition to specific psychological approaches dealing with pain and dying, that a psychiatrist, psychologist, social worker, chaplain, or nurse can provide.

Psychotherapy with the dying patient in pain consists of active listening with supportive verbal interventions and the occasional interpretation.[65] Despite the seriousness of the patient's plight, it is not necessary for the psychiatrist or psychologist to appear overly solemn or emotionally restrained. Often, it is only the psychotherapist, of all the patient's caregivers, who is comfortable enough to converse light-heartedly and allow the patient to talk about his life and experiences, rather than focus solely on impending death. The dying patient who wishes to talk or ask questions about death and pain and suffering should be allowed to do so freely, with the therapist maintaining an interested, interactive stance. It is common for the dying patient to benefit from pastoral counselling. If a chaplaincy service is available, it should be offered to the patient and family. As the dying process progresses, psychotherapy with the individual patient may become limited by cognitive and speech deficits. It is at this point that the focus of supportive psychotherapeutic interventions shifts primarily to the family. In our experience, a very common issue for family members at this point is the level of alertness of the patient. Attempts to control pain are often accompanied by sedation that can limit communication between patient and family. This can sometimes become a source of conflict, with some family members disagreeing amongst themselves or with the patient about what constitutes an appropriate balance between comfort and alertness. It can be helpful for the physician to clarify the patient's preferences as they relate to these issues early, so that conflict can be avoided and work related to bereavement can begin.

Group interventions with individual patients (even in advanced stages of disease), spouses, couples, and families are a powerful means of sharing experiences and identifying successful coping strategies. The limitations of using group interventions for patients with advanced disease are primarily pragmatic. The patient must be physically comfortable enough to participate and have the cognitive capacity to be aware of group discussion. It is often helpful for family members to attend support groups during the terminal phases of the patient's illness. Passik *et al.*[66] have worked with spouses of brain tumour patients in a psychoeducational group that has included spouses at all phases of the patient's illness. They have demonstrated how bereavement issues are often a focus of such interventions from the time of diagnosis onwards. The group members benefit from one another's support into widowhood. The leaders have been impressed by the increased quality of patient care that can be given at home by the spouse (including pain management and all forms of nursing care) when the spouses engage in such support.

Psychotherapeutic interventions that have multiple foci may be most useful. Based upon a prospective study of cancer pain, cognitive behavioural and psychoeducational techniques based upon increasing support, self-efficacy, and providing education may prove to be helpful in assisting patients in dealing with increased pain.[67] Results of an evaluation of patients with cancer pain indicate psychological and social variables are significant predictors of pain. More specifically, distress specific to the illness, self-efficacy, and coping styles were predictors of increased pain.

Utilizing psychotherapy to diminish symptoms of anxiety and depression, factors that can intensify pain, has beneficial effects on the experience of cancer pain. Spiegel and Bloom[68] demonstrated, in a controlled randomized prospective study, the effect of both supportive group therapy for metatastatic breast cancer patients in general and, in particular, the effect of hypnotic pain control exercises. Their support group focused not on interpersonal processes or self-exploration, but rather on a series of themes related to the practical and existential problems of living with cancer. Patients were divided into two treatment groups and a control group. The treatment group patients experienced significantly less pain than the control patients, and the control group showed a large increase in pain.

While psychotherapy in the cancer pain setting is primarily non-analytical and focuses on current issues, exploration of reactions to cancer often involve insights into earlier more pervasive life issues. Some patients choose to continue a more exploratory psychotherapy during extended illness-free periods or survivorship.

Cognitive-behavioural techniques

Cognitive-behavioural techniques can be useful as adjuncts to the management of pain in cancer and AIDS patients (Table 3). Such techniques include passive relaxation with mental imagery, cognitive distraction or focusing, progressive muscle relaxation, biofeedback, hypnosis, and music therapy.[69–71,33] The goal of treatment is to guide the patient toward a sense of control over pain. Some techniques are primarily cognitive in nature, focusing on perceptual and thought processes, and others are directed at modifying patterns of behaviour that help cancer patients cope with pain. Behavioural techniques for pain control seek to modify physiological pain reactions, respondent pain behaviours, and operant pain behaviours (see Table 4 for definitions).

Primarily, cognitive techniques for coping with pain are aimed at reducing the intensity and distress that are part of the pain experience. This may be accomplished by the utilization of a number of techniques including the modification of thoughts the patient has about their pain or psychological distress, introduction of more adaptive coping strategies, and instruction in relaxation techniques. Cognitive modification (cognitive restructuring) is an approach derived from cognitive therapy for depression or anxiety and is based on how one interprets events and bodily sensation. It is assumed that patients have dysfunctional automatic thoughts that are consistent with underlying assumptions and beliefs. In populations of both cancer and AIDS patients with pain, negative thoughts about pain have been shown to be significantly related to pain intensity, degree of psychological distress, and level of interference in functional activities.[27,28] By identifying and challenging dysfunctional automatic thoughts and underlying beliefs by restructuring or modifying thought processes, a more rational response to pain can occur.[69] Examples of such automatic thoughts that have been shown to worsen pain experience are: 'The intensity of my pain will never diminish' or 'Because my pain limits my activities, I am completely helpless'. Patients can be taught to recognize and interrupt such thoughts and proceed to develop a view of the pain experience as time-limited and themselves as functional despite periods in which they are limited.

Table 3 Cognitive-behavioural techniques used by pain patients with advanced disease

Psychoeducation
- preparatory information
- self-monitoring

Relaxation
- passive breathing
- progressive muscle relaxation

Distraction
- focusing
- controlled mental imagery
- cognitive distraction
- behavioural distraction

Combined techniques (relaxation and distraction)
- passive/progressive relaxation with mental imagery
- systematic desensitization
- meditation
- hypnosis
- biofeedback
- music therapy

Cognitive therapies
- cognitive distortion
- cognitive restructuring

Behavioural therapies
- modelling
- graded task management
- contingency management
- behavioural rehearsal

Although cognitive restructuring may be a useful technique in the earlier stages of cancer and AIDS, the goals change in the palliative care context. In this setting the goal is not necessarily to change the patient's maladaptive thoughts but to utilize techniques designed to diminish the patient's frustration, anxiety, and anger. Helping patients to employ more adaptive coping strategies, that is the avoidance of anticipating a catastrophe and encouraging an increase in problem solving skills, may be helpful at this stage.[72–74]

Aside from modifying dysfunctional thoughts and attitudes, the most fundamental behavioural technique is self-monitoring. The development of the ability to monitor one's behaviour allows a person to notice their dysfunctional reactions to the pain experience and learn to control them. Systematic desensitization (see Table 4) is useful in extinguishing anticipatory anxiety, which leads to avoidant behaviour, and in remobilizing inactive patients. Graded task assignment is essentially systematic desensitization as it is applied to patients who are encouraged to take small steps gradually so as to perform activities more readily. Contingency management is a method of reinforcing 'well' behaviour only, thus modifying dysfunctional operant pain behaviours associated with secondary gain.[70,71]

Table 4 Cognitive-behavioural techniques: definitions and descriptions*

Technique	Definition and description
Behavioural therapy	The clinical use of techniques derived from the experimental analysis of behaviour i.e. learning and conditioning for the evaluation, prevention, and treatment of physical disease or physiological dysfunction.
Cognitive therapy	A focused intervention targeted at changing maladaptive beliefs and dysfunctional attitudes. The therapist engages the client in a process of collaborative empiricism, where these underlying beliefs are challenged and corrected.
Operant pain	Pain behaviours resulting from operant learning or conditioning. Pain behaviour is reinforced and continues because of secondary gain, i.e. increased attention and caring.
Respondent pain	Pain behaviours resulting from respondent learning or conditioning. Stimuli associated with prior painful experiences can elicit increased pain and avoidance behaviour.
Cognitive restructuring	Redefinition of some or all aspects of the patient's interpretation of the noxious or threatening experience, resulting in decreased distress, anxiety, and hopelessness.
Self-monitoring (pain diary)	Written or audiotaped chronicle that the patient maintains to describe specific agreed-upon characteristics associated with pain.
Contingency management	Focusing of patient and family member responses that either reinforce or inhibit specific behaviours exhibited by the patient. Method involves reinforcing desired 'well' behaviours.
Grade task assignments	A hierarchy of tasks, i.e. physical, cognitive, and behavioural, are compartmentalized and performed sequentially in manageable steps ultimately achieving an identified goal.
Systematic desensitization	Relaxation and distraction exercises paired with a hierarchy of anxiety-arousing stimuli presented through mental imagery, or presented *in vivo*, resulting in control of fear.

Cognitive-behavioural interventions that are useful in the setting of advanced illness include a variety of techniques ranging from preparatory information and self-monitoring to systematic desensitization and methods of distraction and relaxation.[75] Most often, techniques such as hypnosis, biofeedback, or systematic desensitization utilize both cognitive and behavioural elements such as muscular relaxation and cognitive distraction.

Patient selection for cognitive-behavioural interventions for pain

Many cancer and AIDS patients fear that focus on their pain will distract their physicians from treating the underlying causes of their disease and consequently are highly motivated to learn and practice cognitive-behavioural techniques. These techniques are often effective not only in pain control, but in restoring a sense of self control, personal efficacy, and active participation in their care. It is important to note that these techniques must not be used as a substitute for appropriate analgesic management of pain, but rather as part of a comprehensive multimodal approach. The lack of side-effects of these techniques makes them attractive in the palliative care setting as a supplement to medication regimens that are already complicated. The successful use of these techniques should never lead to the erroneous conclusion that the pain was of psychogenic origin and as such not 'real.' The mechanisms by which these cognitive and behavioural techniques relieve pain are not known; however, they all seem to share the elements of relaxation and distraction. Distraction or redirection of attention helps reduce awareness of pain, and relaxation reduces muscle tension and sympathetic arousal.[70]

Most patients with advanced illness and pain are appropriate candidates for the useful application of these techniques; the clinician, however, should take into account the intensity of pain and the mental clarity of the patient. Ideal candidates have mild to moderate pain and can expect benefit, whereas patients with severe pain can expect limited benefit from psychological interventions unless somatic therapies can lower the level of pain to some degree. Confusional states interfere dramatically with a patient's ability to focus attention and thus limit the usefulness of these techniques.[71] Occasionally, these techniques can be modified so as to include even mildly cognitive-impaired patients. This often involves the therapist taking a more active role by orienting the patient, creating a safe and secure environment, and evoking a conditioned response to the therapist's voice or presence.

Barriers to engaging patients in cognitive-behavioural therapies can be divided into physician/nurse-based barriers and patient-based barriers. The health-care provider who works with patients with advanced illness may have particular difficulty in becoming comfortable with the use of behavioural therapies. Pharmacotherapy is highly effective in the management of pain and seems simpler and easier to use by physicians than labour intensive and time consuming non-pharmacological interventions. Physicians and nurses have typical concerns about the practice of behavioural interventions such as: 'What if the patient laughs, doesn't buy it?', or 'It seems too theatrical, unscientific, non-medical; too New Age!' Overcoming such obstacles will be greatly rewarded. It is imperative that physicians working with patients with advanced illness are aware of the effective non-pharmacological interventions for pain available, and that they are able to make appropriate referrals to practitioners who can provide such interventions.

Patients themselves may be uncertain about the utility of behavioural therapies. Some may ask, 'How can breathing take away my pain?'. They may be frightened by the word 'hypnosis' and it's connotations. Hypnosis, as patients conceptualize it, is often associated with powerful and magical properties; some patients become frightened at the prospect of losing control or being under the influence of someone else. We generally attempt to introduce behavioural interventions only after we've been able to establish some rapport with a patient and engage them in an alliance with us. Occasionally, some patients may benefit from a discussion of the theoretical basis of these interventions, however we stress that it is not important to understand why a technique works, but rather to use the technique that works. Apprehensions must be affirmed and dealt with. Patients must also feel in control of the process at all times and be reassured that they can stop at any time.

General instructions

A general approach to using cognitive-behavioural interventions with patients with advanced illness and pain involves the following:

(1) assessment of the symptom;

(2) choosing a cognitive-behavioural strategy;

(3) preparing the patient and the setting.

The main purpose of conducting a cognitive-behavioural assessment of pain is to determine what, if any, behavioural interventions are indicated.[71] One must initially engage the patient and establish a therapeutic alliance. A history of the pain symptom must be taken. One should review previous efforts to treat the patient's pain, and collect data regarding the nature of the pain and its impact on the patient and their family.

The assessment process will lead to a variety of potential behavioural interventions. Choosing the appropriate behavioural strategy involves taking into consideration the patient's medical condition and physical and cognitive limitations, as well as issues such as time constraints and practical matters. For instance, patients with cognitive impairment or delirium will probably be unable to keep a pain diary or employ techniques that involve cognitive manipulation.

Relaxation techniques

Several techniques can be used to achieve a mental and physical state of relaxation. Muscular tension, autonomic arousal, and mental distress exacerbate pain.[70,71] Some specific relaxation techniques include:

(1) passive relaxation focusing attention on sensations of warmth and decreased tension in various parts of the body;

(2) progressive muscle relaxation involving active tensing and relaxing of muscles;

(3) meditation.

Other techniques that employ both relaxation and cognitive techniques include hypnosis, biofeedback, and music therapy and are discussed later in this chapter.

Passive relaxation, focused breathing, and passive muscle relaxation exercises involve the focusing of attention systematically on one's breathing, on sensations of warmth and relaxation, or on release of muscular tension in various body parts. Verbal suggestions and imagery are used to help promote relaxation. Muscle relaxation is an important component of the relaxation response and can augment the benefits of simple focused breathing exercises, leading to a deeper experience of relaxation and self-control.

Progressive or active muscle relaxation involves the active tensing and relaxing of various muscle groups in the body, focusing attention on the sensations of tension and relaxation. Clinically, in the hospital setting, relaxation is most commonly achieved through the use of a combination of focused breathing and progressive muscle relaxation exercises. Once patients are in a relaxed state, imagery techniques can then be used to induce deeper relaxation and facilitate distraction from or manipulation of a variety of cancer-related symptoms.

The following script is a generic relaxation exercise, utilizing passive relaxation or focused breathing, that is based on and integrates the work of Erickson,[76] Benson,[77] and others.[71]

Script for passive relaxation (focused breathing)

'Why don't you begin by finding a comfortable position. It could be in a bed or in a chair. Slowly allow your body to unwind and just let it go. That's it . . . I wonder if you can allow your body to become as calm as possible . . . just let it go, just let your body sink into that bed (or chair) . . . feel free to move or shift around in any way that your body needs to, to find that comfortable position. You need not try very hard, simply and easily allow yourself to follow the sound of my voice as you allow your body to find itself a safe, comfortable position to relax in.'

'If you like, (patient's name here), you can gently allow your eyes to close, just let the lids cover your eyes . . . allow your eyes to sink back deeply into their sockets . . . that's it, just let them go, falling back gently and deeply into their sockets as your lids begin to feel heavier and heavier. As you allow your head to fall back deeply into the pillow, feeling the weight of your head sinking into the pillow as you breath out, just breath out, one big breath. Slowly, if you can begin to turn your attention to your breathing. Notice your breath for a few moments, how much air you take in, how much air you let out, and just breath evenly and naturally, and with the sound of my voice I wonder if you can begin to take in more air, breathing in and out, in and out, that's it, gradually breathing in and out . . . in and out . . . Breathing in calmness and quietness, breathing out tiredness and frustration, that's it . . . let it go, its not important to you now . . . breathing in quietness and control, breathing out fear and tension . . . breathing in and out . . . in and out . . . you can enjoy breathing in this relaxed way for as long as you need to. You are peaceful now as you continue to observe your even and steady breathing that is allowing you to feel gentle and calm, breathing that is allowing you to feel a gentle calm, that's it, breathing relaxation in and tension out . . . in and out . . . breathing in quietness and control, breathing out tiredness and tension . . . that's it (patient's name here) as you continue to notice the quietness and stillness of your body, Why don't you take a few quiet moments to experience this process more fully.'

It may be helpful for the clinician to mark the end of an exercise by increasing the pace, raising the volume of voice, and shifting position. Additionally it is helpful for the clinician to both pace and model for the patient. This includes positioning yourself as similarly to the patient as possible (e.g. closing eyes, assuming a position of relaxation, and breathing at the same rate). If the patient exhibits any visible anxiety or agitation, this can be briefly explored verbally, and then, if appropriate, the exercise can be continued.

Script for active or progressive muscle relaxation

This exercise involves the patient actively tensing and then relaxing specific body parts. Once again, it may be helpful if the clinician paces and models for the patient.

'Now, I wonder if you can tense up every muscle in your body . . . that's it, squeeze in the muscles . . . hold it, and then just let it go . . . once more, tense up your muscles . . . make them very tight and tense, hold it, hold it . . . and then breath out, and let your muscles relax, just let them go . . . Now, as your body begins to feel more and more relaxed, clench your jaw, squeeze it tight, clench it and then let it go . . . now open your mouth wide, as wide as it will go, stick out your tongue, stick it way out, hold it and then let it go. Feel your head becoming more and more relaxed, as it sinks down into the pillow, allowing all the tension and tightness to drift out of it . . . Now, I wonder if you can lift up your shoulders, lift them up, up to your ears, hold them there, squeezing them tightly, squeeze, and then let them drop down, just let them go . . . and then once more lift them up . . . hold it . . . then let them go . . . as you feel all the tightness and tension in your shoulders begin to drain away . . . Now, I wonder if you can clench your hands into a fist, make a tight fist as your whole arm tightens, tense your arms as you squeeze in your fingers tighter and tighter . . . and now just let them go, once more now make a fist, a tight fist, hold it, and then let it go.'

As with passive muscle relaxation, the clinician guides the patient through the exercise, requesting the patient to tense and release specific muscles in a progressive order.

Imagery/distraction techniques

Clinically, relaxation techniques are most helpful in managing pain when combined with some distracting or pleasant imagery. The use of distraction or focusing involves control over the focus of attention and can be used to make the patient less aware of the noxious stimuli.[78] One can employ imaginative inattention by picturing oneself on a beach. Mental distraction can be used and is similar to the practice of counting sheep to aid sleep. Keeping oneself busy is a form of behavioural distraction. Imagery, that is using one's imagination while in a relaxed state, can be used to transform pain into a warm or cold sensation. One can also imaginatively transform the context of pain, that is imagining oneself in battle on the football field instead of the hospital bed. Disassociated somatization can be employed by some patients whereby they imagine that a painful body part is no longer part of their body.[3,4,69,71] It is important to note that not every patient finds these techniques acceptable, and the therapist must try out a number of approaches to determine which are consistent with the patient's style.

Imagery (often referred to as guided imagery) is most effective when the specific image is obtained from the patient. The clinician may ask the patient to close his or her eyes and think of a place, an activity, or an experience where the patient felt most safe and secure. The clinician may provide suggestions for the patient such as a favourite beach scene, or a room in a house, or riding a bicycle in a park. Once the patient identifies the scene, the clinician may ask the patient to elaborate upon the scene, asking for specific details such as the temperature, season, time of day, type of ocean (calm, or with big waves), etc. The clinician then utilizes this information and describes an image for the patient in detail. The skill is for the clinician to be as flexible and as creative as possible, and to elaborate upon the scene, utilizing all aspects of the senses and bodily sensations such as 'feel the suns rays touch your skin, allow your skin to feel warm and tingly all over . . .'or, ' breath in the fresh, clear air, allow it to fill your lungs with its freshness . . .' or, ' feel the fresh dew of the grass under your feet'. The clinician can focus on 'aromas in the garden' or the 'sounds of birds singing' always reminding the patient to breath evenly and steadily as he or she feels more and more relaxed and more and more in control. If possible, the clinician should avoid volunteering an image or scene for the patient because the clinician is unaware of the association or meaning the image may have for the patient. For example a patient may have a fear of the water, and therefore a beach scene may invoke feelings of fear and loss of control.

Script for pleasant distracting imagery

'Once you are in a comfortable position, I wonder if you can continue lying there with your eyes closed, continuing to breath in and out . . . in and out to the sound of my voice. Let your mind wander . . . just let it go . . . and if any unwanted thoughts come into your mind, you can allow then to pass out as easily as they came in . . . You don't need them now . . . they are not important to you now. You have the ability to control your thoughts. You have the ability to be in control.'

The clinician now begins to describe a specific image in detail as originally suggested by the patient.

'Slowly, I wonder if you can allow your mind to travel . . . to travel far away to your favourite beach. The beach that you have many fond memories of. I wonder if you can imagine that it's almost the end of the day and the beach is deserted . . . and the sun, while setting, is still warm, as it beats down . . . and makes your skin feel tingly and warm all over. As you begin to walk on the sand, you can feel the granules underneath your feet. Step evenly and steadily along the sand. As you look around, you can see the different colours in the sky. You can see for miles off into the distance and you feel exhilarated and free because no one is around you. You are alone and in control. As you walk closer to the edge of the ocean the sand is becoming a little damp and you can feel the dampness underneath your feet—it feels refreshing. As you continue walking, you may notice a few odds and ends on the sand—maybe something that the ocean brought in . . . some shells perhaps. They may be broken from being knocked against the rocks . . . or there may be a few bits of seaweed or some jellyfish. You stop to notice them as you walk past . . . marvelling at the wonders of nature. As you get to the edge of the ocean, you can feel the tiny little ripples of water washing over your feet . . . bouncing over your feet making you feel light and fresh. The water is warm—it soothes your feet. Washing back and forth . . . back and forth. As you keep walking you see your rubber raft. This is your old dependable rubber raft. You get to the raft and you secure it in your hands and lie down on it letting your whole body sink into the raft—just let it go . . . that's it. Slowly you kick off as the raft begins to take you away. The ocean is very calm and very gentle. Your whole body begins to unwind and sink deeper and deeper into the raft as you feel more and more relaxed. This raft allows you to drift off . . . and underneath you can feel the ripples of the ocean . . . rocking back and forth . . . back and forth as you continue to float away evenly and gently. You can become aware of the sun beating down in your skin. You are aware of the sounds around you—you can hear the ocean washing against the rocks as the waves rock back and forth . . . back and forth. You can hear the gulls crying in the distance. There is a very tiny protected bay that you are floating away in. It is a very calm and peaceful day, and you are feeling more and more relaxed. You are in control now . . . and as you continue to sail away, all your troubles and problems wash right out of you. They're not important to you now. You don't need them now. What's important is that your whole body, from the tip of your toes all the way up to the top of your head, is relaxed and calm in this very safe and private place that is your own. You can continue to lie here as you rock back and forth . . . back and forth for as long as you need to.'

'When you are ready, you can slowly readjust yourself to the sound of my voice and I am going to count slowly backwards from ten and with each count backwards, you can become more and more familiar with where you are. Perhaps when I get to number five you may want to open your eyes or you can keep then closed for as long as you need to. Ten, nine . . . become aware of the sounds around you . . . eight, seven . . . become aware of the temperature of the room—how does it feel, how does your body feel? . . . six, five . . . you can open your eyes now if you want to or you can keep them closed . . . four, three, two, one. You can stay in this relaxed position for as long as you need to. When you feel ready you may slowly prepare to sit up.'

Hypnosis

Hypnosis can be a useful adjunct in the management of cancer pain.[68,79–82] In a controlled trial comparing hypnosis with cognitive-behavioural therapy in relieving mucositis following a bone marrow transplant, patients utilizing hypnosis reported a significant reduction in pain compared to patients who used cognitive behavioural techniques.[67] The hypnotic trance is essentially a state of heightened and focused concentration, and thus it can be used to manipulate the perception of pain. The depth of hypnotizability may determine the effectiveness as well as the strategies employed during hypnosis. One-third of cancer patients are not hypnotizable, and it is recommended that other techniques be employed for them. Of the two-thirds of patients who are identified as being less, moderately, and highly hypnotizable, three principles underlie the use of hypnosis in controlling pain:[78] (1) use self-hypnosis; (2) relax, do not fight the pain; and (3) use a mental filter to ease the hurt in pain. Patients who are moderately and highly hypnotizable can often alter sensations in a painful area by changing temperature sensation or experiencing tingling. Less hypnotizable patients can often utilize an alternative focus by concentrating on a sensation in a non-affected body part or on a mental image of a pleasant scene. The main disadvantage of hypnosis for cancer patients is that the technique frequently requires more attention capacity than these patients generally have.

Biofeedback

Fotopoulos *et al.*[83] noted significant pain relief in a group of cancer patients who were taught electromyographic and electroencephalographic biofeedback-assisted relaxation. Only two out of 17 were able to maintain analgesia after the treatment ended. A lack of generalization of effect can be a problem with biofeedback techniques. Although physical condition may make a prolonged training period impossible, especially for the terminally ill, most cancer patients can often utilize electromyographic and temperature biofeedback techniques for learning relaxation-assisted pain control.[70]

Music, aroma, and art therapies

Munro and Mount[84] have written extensively on the use of music therapy with cancer patients, documenting clinical examples and suggesting mechanisms of action. Music can often capture the focus of attention like no other stimulus, it offers patients a new form of expression, and helps patients distract themselves from their perception of pain, while expressing themselves in meaningful ways[85] (see Chapter 2.6).

Aromas have been shown to have innate relaxing and stimulating qualities. Our colleagues at Memorial Hospital have recently begun to explore the use of aromatherapy for the treatment of procedure-related anxiety (that is anxiety related to magnetic resonance imaging scans). Utilizing the scent heliotropin, Manne *et al.*[86] reported that two-thirds of the patients found the scent especially pleasant and reported much less anxiety than those who were not exposed to the scent during magnetic resonance imaging scans. As a general relaxation technique, aromatherapy may have an application for pain management but this is as yet unstudied.

Art therapy allows the less verbally skilled adults or children to express the fears and concerns that they have in a more comfortable fashion. The creative experience can be used as both an important means of providing support and also as an avenue for providing patients with psychological insights into their experience.[87]

Psychotropic adjuvant analgesics for pain in the patient with advanced illness

The patient with advanced disease and pain has much to gain from the appropriate and maximal utilization of psychotropic drugs. (An extensive review of the subject of adjuvant analgesic drugs can be found in Chapter 2.5.) Psychotropic drugs, particularly the tricyclic antidepressants, are useful as adjuvant analgesics in the pharmacological management of cancer pain and neuropathic pain. Table 5 lists the various psychotropic medications with analgesic properties, their routes of administration, and their approximate daily doses. These medications are not only effective in managing symptoms of anxiety, depression, insomnia, or delirium that commonly complicate the course of advanced disease in patients with cancer or AIDS who are in pain, they also potentiate the analgesic effects of the opioid drugs and have innate analgesic properties of their own.[88]

Antidepressants

The current literature supports the use of antidepressants as adjuvant analgesic agents in the management of a wide variety of chronic pain syndromes, including cancer pain.[89–96] While clinically useful as adjuvant analgesics in managing AIDS-related pain (e.g. HIV neuropathies), there are no published, controlled clinical trials of antidepressants as analgesics.[62,97] Amitriptyline is the tricyclic antidepressant most studied, and has proven to be effective as an analgesic in a large number of clinical trials, addressing a wide variety of chronic pains.[98-102] Other tricyclic antidepressants that

Table 5 Psychotropic adjuvant analgesic drugs for pain in patients with advanced disease

Generic name	Approximate daily dosage range (mg)	Route
Tricyclic antidepressants		
amitriptyline	10–150	PO, IM, PR
nortriptyline	10–50	PO
imipramine	12.5–150	PO, IM
desipramine	12.5–150	PO
clomipramine	10–150	PO
doxepin	12.5–150	PO, IM
Non-cyclic antidepressants		
trazodone	25–300	PO
fluoxetine	20–60	PO
paroxetine	20–60	PO
Monamine oxidase inhibitors		
phenelzine	45–75	PO
Amine precursors		
L-tryptophan	500–3000	PO
Psychostimulants		
methylphenidate	2.5–20 b.i.d.	PO
dextroamphetamine	2.5–20 b.i.d.	PO
pemoline	18.75–75 b.i.d.	PO
Phenothiazines		
fluphenazine	1–3	PO, IM
methotrimeprazine	10–20 q6h	PO, IM, IV SC
Butyrophenones		
haloperidol	1–3	PO, IM, IV SC
pimozide	2–6 b.i.d.	PO
Antihistamines		
hydroxyzine	50 q4–6h	PO, IM, IV
Benzodiazepines		
alprazolam	0.25–2.0 t.i.d.	PO
clonazepam	0.5–4 b.i.d.	PO

PO, per oral; IM, intramuscular; PR, parenteral; IV, intravenous; q6h, every 6h–; q4–6h, every 4 to 6h–; t.i.d., three times a day; b.i.d., two times a day.

have been shown to have efficacy as analgesics include imipramine,[103-105] desipramine,[106,107] nortriptyline,[108] clomipramine,[109,110] and doxepin.[111] Table 6 is a compilation of the studies, both controlled and uncontrolled, that demonstrate adjuvant analgesic efficacy of antidepressants for cancer pain. In a placebo controlled, double-blind study of imipramine in chronic cancer pain, Walsh[112] demonstrated that imipramine had analgesic effects independent of its mood effects, and was a potent coanalgesic when used along with morphine. In general, the tricyclic antidepressants are utilized in cancer pain as adjuvant analgesics, potentiating the effects of opioid analgesics, and are rarely used as the primary analgesic.[112,94,113] Ventafridda *et al.*[94] reviewed a multicentre clinical experience with antidepressant agents (trazodone and amitriptyline) in the treatment of chronic cancer pain that included a deafferentation or neuropathic component. Almost all of these patients were already receiving weak or strong opioids and experienced improved pain control. A subsequent randomized, double-blind study showed both amitriptyline and trazodone to have similar therapeutic analgesic efficacy.[94] Magni, *et al.*[95] reviewed the use of antidepressants in Italian cancer centres and found that a wide range of antidepressants were used for a variety of cancer pain syndromes, with amitriptyline being the most commonly prescribed. In nearly all cases, antidepressants were used in association with opioids. There is some evidence that there may be subgroups of patients who respond differentially to tricyclics and, therefore, if amitriptyline fails to alleviate pain, another tricyclic should be tried.[114] The tricyclic antidepressants are effective as adjuvants in cancer pain through a number of mechanisms (see Table 6) that include: (1)

Table 6 Studies of antidepressants for cancer pain

Study	Drug	Efficacy of pain relief (%)
134	Clomipramine	67
135	Clomipramine	90
136	Clomipramine + Neuroleptic	87
135	Imipramine	80
137	Imipramine	75
138	Imipramine	70–80
139	Imipramine	80
140	Imipramine	
141	Imipramine[a]	p
112	Imipramine[a]	p
94	Amitriptyline[a] versus	p
	Trazodone[a]	p
95	Amitriptyline	
	Imipramine	51–98
	Clomipramine	
	Trazodone	
	Doxepin	
142	Amitriptyline	67
143	Amitriptyline	0
	Trimipramine	0
144	Amitriptyline	70–80
145	Alprazolam	75

[a] Controlled study
p = Drug more effective than placebo

antidepressant activity,[89] (2) potentiation or enhancement of opioid analgesia,[113,115,116] and (3) direct analgesic effects.[117].

The heterocyclic and non-cyclic antidepressant drugs (such as trazodone, mianserin, maprotiline, and the newer serotonin specific reuptake inhibitors fluoxetine and paroxetine) may also be useful as adjuvant analgesics for cancer patients with pain; however, clinical trials of their efficacy as analgesics have been equivocal.[118-122] There are several case reports suggesting that fluoxetine may be a useful adjuvant analgesic in the management of headache,[123] fibrositis,[124] and diabetic neuropathy.[125] In a recent clinical trial, fluoxetine was shown to be no better than placebo as an analgesic in painful diabetic neuropathy.[126] Paroxetine is the first serotonin specific re-uptake inhibitor shown to be a highly effective analgesic in the treatment of neuropathic pain,[127] and may be a useful addition to our armamentarium of adjuvant analgesics for cancer pain. Newer antidepressants such as sertraline, velafaxine, and nefazodone may also eventually prove to be clinically useful as adjuvant analgesics. Nefazodone, for instance, has been demonstrated to potentiate opioid analgesics in an animal model.[128] (See Section 15 for more detailed information on the use of antidepressant drugs in patients with advanced disease.)

At this point, it is clear that many antidepressants have analgesic properties. There is no definite indication that any one drug is more effective than the others, although the most experience has been accrued with amitriptyline and this remains the drug of first choice. In terms of appropriate dosage, there is evidence that the therapeutic analgesic effects of amitriptyline are correlated with serum levels just as the antidepressant effects are, and analgesic treatment failure is due to low serum levels.[98,99,129] A high dose regimen of up to 150 mg, or higher, of amitriptyline is suggested.[130,101] As to the time course of onset of analgesia with antidepressants, there appears to be a biphasic process, with immediate or early analgesic effects that occur within hours or days[110,117,113] and later, longer analgesic effects that peak over a 4 to 6 week period.[98-100]

Treatment should be initiated with a small dose of amitriptyline; for instance 10 to 25 mg at bedtime, especially in debilitated patients, and increased slowly by 10 to 25 mg every 2 to 4 days towards 150 mg with frequent assessment of pain and side-effects until a beneficial effect is achieved. Maximal effect as an adjuvant analgesic may require continuation of the drug for 2 to 6 weeks. Serum levels of the antidepressant drug, when available, may also help in management to assure that therapeutic serum levels of the drug are being achieved. Both pain and depression in cancer patients often respond to lower doses (25–100 mg) of antidepressant than are usually required in the physically healthy (100–300 mg); most likely because of impaired metabolism of these drugs. The choice of drug often depends on the side-effect profile, existing medical problems, the nature of depressive symptoms if present, and past response to specific antidepressants. Sedating drugs like amitriptyline are helpful when insomnia complicates the presence of pain and depression in a cancer patient. Anticholinergic properties of some of these drugs should also be kept in mind. Occasionally, in patients who have limited analgesic response to a tricyclic, potentiation of analgesia can be accomplished by lithium augmentation.[131]

Monoamine oxidase inhibitors are less useful in the cancer setting because of dietary restriction and potentially dangerous interactions between monoamine oxidase inhibitors and opioids such as pethidine (meperidine). Amongst the monoamine oxidase inhibitor drugs available, phenelzine has been shown to have adjuvant analgesic properties in patients with atypical facial pain and migraine.[132,133]

Psychostimulants

The psychostimulants, dextroamphetamine and methylphenidate, are useful antidepressant agents prescribed selectively for medically ill cancer patients with depression.[146,147] Psychostimulants are also useful in diminishing excessive sedation secondary to opioid analgesics, and are potent adjuvant analgesics. Bruera *et al.*[148-150] demonstrated that a regimen of 10 mg methylphenidate with breakfast and 5 mg with lunch significantly decreased sedation and potentiated the analgesic effect of opioids in patients with cancer pain. Dextroamphetamine has also been reported to have additive analgesic effects when used with morphine in postoperative pain.[151] In relatively low dose, psychostimulants stimulate appetite, promote a sense of well being, and improve feelings of weakness and fatigue in cancer patients.

Treatment with dextroamphetamine or methylphenidate usually begins with a dose of 2.5 mg at 8:00 a.m. and at noon. The dosage is slowly increased over several days until a desired effect is achieved or side-effects (overstimulation, anxiety, insomnia, paranoia, confusion) intervene. Typically a dose greater than 30 mg/day is not necessary although occasionally patients require up to 60 mg/day. Patients, usually, are maintained on methylphenidate for 1 to 2 months, and approximately two-thirds will be able to be withdrawn from methylphenidate without a recurrence of depressive symptoms. Those in whom symptoms do recur can be maintained on a psychostimulant for up to 1 year without significant abuse problems. Tolerance will develop and adjustment of dose may be necessary.

A strategy that we have found useful in treating cancer pain associated with depression is to start a psychostimulant (starting dose of 2.5 mg of methylphenidate at 8 a.m. and noon) and then to add a tricyclic antidepressant after several days to help prolong and potentiate the short effect of the stimulant. Pemoline is a unique, alternative psychostimulant that is chemically unrelated to amphetamine, but may have similar usefulness as an antidepressant and adjuvant analgesic in cancer patients (Breitbart and Mermelstein, in press). Advantages of pemoline as a psychostimulant in cancer pain patients include:

(1) the lack of abuse potential;

(2) the lack of federal regulation through special triplicate prescriptions (in the United States);

(3) the mild sympathomimetic effects;

(4) the fact that it comes in a chewable tablet form that can be absorbed through the buccal mucosa and thus used by cancer patients who have difficulty swallowing or have intestinal obstruction.

In our clinical experience, pemoline is as effective as methylphenidate or dextroamphetamine in the treatment of depressive symptoms and in countering the sedating effects of opioid analgesics. There are no studies of pemoline's capacity to potentiate the analgesic properties of opioids. Pemoline can be started at a dose of 18.75 mg in the morning and at noon, and increased gradually over days. Typically, patients require 75 mg/day or less. Pemoline should be used with caution in patients with liver impairment, and liver function tests should be monitored periodically with longer-term treatment.[152]

Neuroleptics

Methotrimeprazine is a phenothiazine that is said to be equianalgesic to morphine, has none of the opioid effects on gut motility, and probably produces analgesia through alpha-adrenergic blockade.[153] In patients who are opioid tolerant, it provides an alternative approach in giving analgesia by a non-opioid mechanism. It is a dopamine blocker and so has antiemetic as well as anxiolytic effects. Methotrimeprazine can produce sedation and hypotension and should be given cautiously by slow intravenous infusion, though in the United Kingdom and Europe it is usually given orally or subcutaneously. Other phenothiazines such as chlorpromazine and prochlorperazine are useful as antiemetics in cancer patients, but probably have limited use as analgesics.[154] Fluphenazine in combination with tricyclic antidepressants has been shown to be helpful in neuropathic pains.[109] Haloperidol is the drug of choice in the management of delirium or psychoses in cancer patients, and has clinical usefulness as a coanalgesic for cancer pain.[154] Pimozide, a butyrophenone, has been shown to be effective as an analgesic in the management of trigeminal neuralgia, at doses of 4 to 12 mg/day.[155]

Anxiolytics

Hydroxyzine is a mild anxiolytic with sedating and analgesic properties that are useful in the anxious cancer patient with pain.[156,157] This antihistamine has antiemetic activity as well. A dose of 100 mg of parenteral hydroxyzine has analgesic activity approaching 8 mg of morphine, and has additive analgesic effects when combined with morphine. Benzodiazepines have not been felt to have direct analgesic properties, although they are potent anxiolytics and anticonvulsants.[158] Some authors have suggested that their anticonvulsant properties make certain benzodiazepine drugs useful in the management of neuropathic pain. Recently, Fernandez *et al.*[145] showed that alprazolam, a unique benzodiazepine with mild antidepressant properties, was a helpful adjuvant analgesic in cancer patients with phantom limb pain or deafferentation (neuropathic) pain. Clonazepam may also be useful in the management of lancinating neuropathic pains in the cancer setting, and has been reported to be an effective analgesic for patients with trigeminal neuralgia, headache, and post-traumatic neuralgia.[159,160] With the use of midazolam by intravenous injection with a patient controlled dosage, there was no reduction in the use of post-operative morphine requirements or in the patient's perception of pain.[161] Intrathecal midazolam in animal models, however, has been shown to potentiate morphine analgesia.[162]

Placebo

A mention of the placebo response is important in order to highlight the misunderstandings and relative harm of this phenomenon. The placebo response is common, and analgesia is mediated through endogenous opioids. The deceptive use of placebo response to distinguish psychogenic pain from 'real' pain should be avoided. Placebos are effective in a portion of patients for a short period of time only and are not indicated in the management of cancer pain.[2]

References

1. Foley KM. Pain syndromes in patients with cancer. In: Bonica JJ, Ventafriddi V, Fink RB, Jones LE, Loeser JD, eds. *Advances in Pain Research and Therapy*, vol 2. New York: Raven Press, 1975: 59–75.
2. Foley KM. The treatment of cancer pain. *New England Journal of Medicine*, 1985; **313**: 845.
3. Breitbart W, Holland J. Psychiatric aspects of cancer pain. In: K.M. Foley, *et al.* eds. *Advances in Pain Research and Therapy*, vol. 16. New York: Raven Press Ltd, 1990: 73–87.
4. Breitbart W. Psychiatric management of cancer pain. *Cancer*, 1989; **63**: 2336–42.
5. Breitbart W. Psychiatric aspects of pain and HIV disease. *Focus: A Guide to AIDS Research and Counseling*, 1990; **5**: 1–2.
6. Massie MJ, Holland JC. The cancer patient with pain: psychiatric complications and their mangement. *Medical Clinics of North America*, 1987; **71**: 243–58.
7. Bonica JJ. Cancer Pain. In: Bonica JJ, ed. *The Management of Pain*, 2nd edn, Vol 1. Philadelphia: Lea and Febiger, 1990: 400–60.
8. Twycross RG, Lack SA. *Symptom Control in Far Advanced Cancer: Pain Relief.* London: Pitman Brooks, 1983.
9. Marks RM, Sachar EJ. Undertreatment of medical inpatients with narcotic analgesics. *Annals of Internal Medicine*, 1973; **78**: 173–81.
10. Grond S, Zech D, Diefenbach C, Bischoff A. Prevalence and pattern of symptoms in patients with cancer pain: A prospective evaluation of 1635 cancer patients referred to a pain clinic. *Journal of Pain and Symptom Management*, 1994; **9**: 372–82.

11. Singer EJ, Zorilla C, Fahy-Chandon B, Chi S, Syndulko K, Teunteliotte W. Painful symptoms reported for ambulatory HIV-infected men in a longitudinal study. *Pain*, 1993; **54**: 15–19.
12. Lebovits AH, Lefkowitz M, McCarthy D, Simon R, Wilpon H, Jung R, Fried E. The prevalence and management of pain in patients with AIDS. A review of 134 cases. *The Clinical Journal of Pain*, 1989; **5**: 245–8.
13. Newshan G, Wainapel S, Schmitz D. Pain related syndromes and their treatment in persons with AIDS. (Abstract) *Eighth Annual Scientific Meeting of the American Pain Society, Phoenix, AZ, 1989.*
14. Levy RM, Bredesen DE, Rosenblum ML. Neurological manifestations of the AIDS experience at UCSF and review of the literature. *Journal of Neurosurgery*, 1985; **62**: 475–95.
15. Snider WD, Simpson DM, Nielsen S, *et al.* Neurological complications of AIDS; analysis of 50 patients. *Annals of Neurology*, 1983; **14**: 403–18.
16. Cornblath DR, McArthur IC. Predominantly sensory neuropathy in patients with AIDS and AIDS-related complex. *Neurology*, 1988; **38**: 794–6.
17. Schofferman J, Brody R. Pain in far advanced AIDS. In: KM Foley, *et al.* eds. *Advances in Pain Research and Therapy*, Vol. 16. New York: Raven Press, Ltd. 1990: 379–86.
18. Breitbart W, Passik S. Pain in AIDS: Prevalence and psychosocial impact. (Abstract) *Biopsychosocial Aspects of HIV Infection: 1st International Conference. Amsterdam, The Netherlands, September 22–25, 1991.*
19. Hewitt D, Breitbart W, Rosenfeld B, McDonald M, Portenoy R. Pain syndromes in the ambulatory AIDS patient. 13th Annual Scientific Meeting, Miami, FL, November 1994 (Abstract) *American Pain Society*, 1994.
20. Stiefel F. Psychosocial aspects of cancer pain. *Supportive Care in Cancer*, 1993; **1**: 130–4.
21. Saunders C M. *The Management of Terminal Illness.* Hospital Medicine Publications, 1967.
22. Hanks G W. Opioid responsive and opioid non-responsive pain in cancer. *British Medical Bulletin*, 1991; **47**: 718–31.
23. Syrjala K, Chapko M. Evidence for a biopsychosocial model of cancer treatment-related pain. *Pain*, 1995; **61**: 69–79.
24. Daut RL, Cleeland CS. The prevalence and severity of pain in cancer. *Cancer*, 1982; **50**: 1913–18.
25. Spiegel D, Bloom JR. Pain in metastatic breast cancer. *Cancer*, 1983; **52**: 341–5.
26. Padilla G, Ferrell B, Grant M, Rhiner M. Defining the content domain of quality of life for cancer patients with pain. *Cancer Nursing*, 1990; **13**: 108–115.
27. Payne D, Jacobsen P, Breitbart W, Passik S, Rosenfeld B, McDonald M. Negative Thoughts related to pain are associated with greater pain, distress, and disability in AIDS pain. 1994 *Presentation American Pain Society*, Miami, Florida, 1994.
28. Payne D. *Cognition in Cancer Pain*, 1995. Unpublished dissertation.
29. McKegney FP, Bailey CR, Yates JW. Prediction and management of pain in patients with advanced cancer. *General Hospital Psychiatry*, 1981; **3**: 95–101.
30. Bond MR, Pearson IB. Psychological aspects of pain in women with advanced cancer of the cervix. *Journal of Psychosomatic Research*, 1969; **13**: 13–19.
31. Breitbart W, Passik S, Rosenfeld B, Portenoy RK, McDonald M, Thaler H. Pain intensity and its relationship to functional interference in patients with AIDS. 13th Annual Scientific Meeting, Miami, FL, November 1994. (Poster) *American Pain Society,* 1994.
32. Breitbart W, Passik S, Bronaugh T, Zale C, Bluestine S, Gomez M. Pain in the ambulatory AIDS patient: Prevalence and psychosocial correlates (Abstract) *38th Annual Meeting, Academy of Psychosomatic Medicine, 1991.*
33. Cleeland CS, Tearnan BH. Behavioral control of cancer pain. In: Holzman D, Turk D, eds. *Pain Mangement.* New York: Pergamon Press, 1986: 193–212.
34. Derogatis LR, Morrow GR, Fetting J, *et al.* The prevalence of psychiatric disorders among cancer patients. *Journal of the American Medical Association*, 1983; **249**: 751–7.
35. Ahles TA, Blanchard EB, Ruckdeschel JC. The multidemensional nature of cancer related pain. *Pain*, 1983; **17**: 277–88.
36. Woodforde JM, Fielding JR. Pain and cancer. *Journal of Psychosomatic Research*, 1970; **14**: 365–70.
37. Stiefel FC, Breitbart W, Holland JC. Corticosteroids in cancer: Neuropsychiatric complications. *Cancer Investigation*, 1989; **7**: 479–91.
38. Bukberg J, Penman D, Holland J. Depression in hospitalized cancer patients. *Psychosomatic Medicine*, 1984; **43**: 119–122.
39. Massie JM, Holland JC, Glass E. Delirium in terminally ill cancer patients. *American Journal of Psychiatry,* 1983; **140**: 1048–50.
40. Bruera E, MacMillan K, Kachin N, *et al.* The cognitive effects of the administration of narcotics. *Pain*, 1989; **39**: 13–16.
41. Breitbart W. Suicide in cancer patients. *Oncology*, 1987; **1**: 49–53.
42. Breitbart W. Cancer pain and suicide. In: KM Foley, *et al.* eds. *Advances in Pain Research and Therapy*, Vol. 16. New York: Raven Press, Ltd, 1990: 399–412.
43. Sison A, Eller K, Segal J, Passik S, Breitbart W. Suicidal ideation in ambulatory HIV-infected patients: The roles of pain, mood, and disease status. (Abstract) *Current Concepts in Psycho-oncology IV, New York, October 10–12, 1991.*
44. Levin DN, Cleeland CS, Dan R. Public attitudes toward cancer pain. *Cancer*, 1985; **56**: 2337–9.
45. Bolund C. Suicide and cancer: II. Medical and care factors in suicide by cancer patients in Sweden. 1973–1976. *Journal of Psychosocial Oncology*, 1985; **3**: 17–30.
46. Farberow NL, Schneidman ES, Leonard CV. *Suicide Among General Medical and Surgical Hospital Patients with Malignant Neoplasms.* Medical Bulletin 9, Washington D.C., U.S. Veterans Administration, 1963.
47. Massie M, Gagnon P, Holland J. Depression and Suicide in Patients with Cancer. *Joural of Pain and Symptom Management*, 1994; **9**: 325–31.
48. Silberfarb PM, Manrer LH, Cronthamel CS. Psychological aspects of neoplastic disease, I: Functional status of breast cancer patients during different treatment regimens. *American Journal of Psychiatry*, 1980; **137**: 450–5.
49. Achte KA, Vanhkonen ML. Cancer and the psych. *Omega*, 1971; **2**: 46–56.
50. Brown JH, Henteleff P, Barakat S, Rowe JR. Is it normal for terminally ill patients to desire death. *American Journal of Psychiatry*, 1986; **143**: 208–11.
51. Saltzburg D, Breitbart W, Fishman B, *et al.* The relationship of pain and depression to suicidal ideation in cancer patients (abstract). *ASCO Annual Meeting. May 21–23, San Francisco, 1989.*
52. Marzuk P, Tierney H, Tardiff K, Gross G, Morgan E, Hsu M, Mann J. Increased risk of suicide in persons with AIDS. *Journal of the American Medical Association*, 1988; **259**: 1333–7.
53. Rabkin J, Remien R, Katoff L, Williams J. Suicidality in AIDS long-term survivors: what is the evidence? *AIDS-Care*, 1993; **5**: 401–11.
54. Cleeland C, Gonin R, Hatfield A, Edmonson J, Blum R, Stewart J, Pandya K. Pain and its treatment in outpatients with metastatic cancer. *New England Journal of Medicine*, 1994. **330**: 592–6.
55. Lebovits AK, Lefkowitz M, McCarthy D. The prevalence and management of pain in patients with AIDS. A review of 134 cases. *The Clinical Journal of Pain*, 1989; **5**: 245–8.
56. McCormack JP, Li R, Zarowny D, Singer J. Inadequate treatment of pain in ambulatory HIV patients. *The Clinical Journal of Pain*, 1993; **9**: 279–83.
57. Breitbart W, Passik R, Rosenfeld B, Portenoy R, McDonald M, Thaler H. AIDS specific patient-related barriers to pain management. 13th Annual Scientific Meeting, Miami, FL, November 1994 (Poster) *American Pain Society, 1994.*
58. Breitbart W, Passik S, Rosenfeld B, Portenoy R, McDonald M, Thaler H. Undertreatment of pain in AIDS. 13th Annual Scientific Meeting, Miami, FL, November 1994. (Poster) *American Pain Society, 1994.*
59. Charap AD. The knowledge, attitudes, and experience of medical personnel treating pain in the terminally ill. *Mount Sinai Journal of Medicine*, 1978; **45**: 561–80.

60. Macaluso C, Weinberg D, Foley KM. Opioid abuse and misuse in a cancer pain population. (Abstract) *Second International Congress on Cancer Pain, July 14–17, Rye, New York, 1988.*
61. Kanner RM, Foley KM. Patterns of narcotic use in a cancer pain clinic. *Annals of the New York Academy of Science*, 1981; **362**: 161–72.
62. Breitbart W, Patt R. Pain management in the patient with AIDS. *Hematology/Oncology Annals*, 1994; **2**: 391–9.
63. Bruera E, MacMillan K, Pither J, MacDonald RN. Effects of morphine on the dyspnea of terminal cancer patients. *Journal of Pain and Symptom Management*, 1990; **5**: 341–4.
64. Grossman SA, Sheidler VR, Sweden K, Mucenski J, Piantadosi S. Correlations of patient and caregiver ratings of cancer pain. *Journal of Pain and Symptom Management*, 1991; **6**: 53–7.
65. Cassem NH. They dying patient. In: Hackett TP, Cassem NH, eds. *Massachusetts General Hospital Handbook of General Hospital Psychiatry*, 2nd edn. Littleton, Mass: PSG Publishing Co. Inc., 1987: 332–52.
66. Passik S, Horowitz S, Malkin M, Gargan R. A psychoeducational support program for spouses of brain tumor patients. (Abstract) *Symposium on New Trends in the Psychological Support of the Cancer Patient. American Psychiatric Association Annual Meeting, New Orleans, La., May 7–12, 1991.*
67. Syrajala K, Cummings C, Donaldson G. Hypnosis or cognitive behavioral training for the reduction of pain and nausea during cancer treatment: a controlled trial. *Pain*, 1992; **48**: 137–46.
68. Spiegel D, Bloom JR. Group therapy and hypnosis reduce metastatic breast carcinoma pain. *Psychosomatic Medicine*, 1983; **4**: 333–9.
69. Fishman B, Loscalzo M. Cognitive-behavioral interventions in the management of cancer pain: principles and applications. *Medical Clinics of North America*, 1987; **71**: 271–87.
70. Cleeland CS. Nonpharmacologic management of cancer pain. *Journal of Pain and Symptom Management*, 1987; **2**: 523–8.
71. Loscalzo M, Jacobsen PB. Practical behavioral approaches to the effective management of pain and distress. *Journal of Psychosocial Oncology*, 1990; **8**: 139–69.
72. Turk D, Fernendez E. On the Putative Uniqueness of cancer pain: Do psychological principles apply? *Behaviour Research and Therapy*, 1990; **28**: 1–13.
73. Fishman B. The treatment of suffering in patients with cancer pain. In: Foley K, Bonica J. Ventafridda V. eds. *Advances in Pain Research and Therapy*, vol 16. New York: Raven Press, 1990: 301–16.
74. Jensen M, Turner J, Romano J, Karoly C. Coping with chronic pain: a critical review of the literature. *Pain*, 1991; **47**: 249–83.
75. Breitbart W, Holland JC. Psychiatric complications of cancer. In: Brain MC, Carbone PP, eds. *Current Therapy in Hematology Oncology-3*. Toronto and Philadelphia: B.C. Decker Inc., 1988: 268–74.
76. Erickson MH. Hypnosis in painful terminal illness. *American Journal of Clinical Hypnosis*, 1959; **1**: 1117–21.
77. Benson H. *The Relaxation Response*. New York: William Morrow, 1975.
78. Broome M, Lillis P, McGahhe T, Bates T. The use of distraction and imagery with children during painful procedures. *Oncology Nursing Forum*, 1992; **19**: 499–502.
79. Spiegel D. The use of hypnosis in controlling cancer pain. *Ca-A Cancer Journal for Clinicians*, 1985; **4**: 221–31.
80. Redd WB, Reeves JL, Storm FK, Minagawa RY. Hypnosis in the control of pain during hyperthermia treatment of cancer. In: Bonica JJ, *et al.*, eds. *Advances in Pain Research and Therapy*, Vol. 5. New York: Raven Press, 1982: 857–61.
81. Barber J, Gitelson J. Cancer Pain: Psychological management using hypnosis. *Ca-A Cancer Journal for Clinicians*, 1980; **3**: 130–6.
82. Levitan A. The use of hypnosis with cancer patients. *Psychiatry and Medicine*, 1992; **10**: 119–31.
83. Fotopoulos SS, Graham C, Cook MR. Psychophysiologic control of cancer pain. In: Bonica JJ, Ventafridda V, eds. *Advances in Pain Research and Therapy*. Vol 2. New York: Raven Press, 1979: 231–44.
84. Munro SM, Mount B. Music therapy in palliative care. *Canadian Medical Association Journal*, 1978; **119**: 1029–34.
85. Schroeder-Sheker T. Music for the dying: a personal accountof the new field of music thanatology—history, theories, and clinical narratives. *Advances*, 1993; **9**: 36–48.
86. Manne S, Redd W, Jacobsen P, Georgiades I. Aroma for treatment of anxiety during MRI scans. (Abstract). *Symposium on New Trends in the Psychological Support of the Cancer Patient. American Psychiatric Association Annual Meeting, New Orleans, La., May 7–12, 1991.*
87. Connell C. Art therapy as part of a palliative cancer program. *Palliative Medicine*, 1992; **6**: 18–25.
88. Breitbart W. Psychotropic adjuvant analgesics for cancer pain. *Psycho-Oncology*, 1992; **5**: 133–45.
89. France RD. The future for antidepressants: treatment of pain. *Psychopathology*, 1987; **20**: 99–113.
90. Getto CJ, Sorkness CA, Howell T. Antidepressants and chronic non-malignant pain: a review. *Journal of Pain and Symptom Management*, 1987; **2**: 9–18.
91. Walsh TD. Antidepressants and chronic pain. *Clinical Neuropharmacology*, 1983; **6**: 271–95.
92. Walsh TD. Adjuvant analgesic therapy in cancer pain. In: K M Foley, *et al.* eds. *Advances in Pain Research and Therapy*, Vol. 16. Second International Congress on Cancer Pain. New York: Raven Press Ltd., 1990: 155–65.
93. Butler S. Present status of tricyclic antidepressants in chronic pain therapy. In: Benedetti C, *et al.*, eds. *Advances in Pain Research and Therapy*. Vol 7. New York: Raven Press, 1986: 173–96.
94. Ventafridda V, Bonezzi C, Caraceni A, DeConno F, Guarise G, Ramella G, Saita L, Silvani V, Tamburini M, Toscani F. Antidepressants for cancer pain and other painful syndromes with deafferentation component: Comparison of Amitriptyline and Trazodone. *Italian Journal of Neurological Science*, 1987; **8**: 579–87.
95. Magni G, Arsie D, DeLeo D. Antidepressants in the treatment of cancer pain. A survey in Italy; *Pain*, 1987; **29**: 347–53.
96. Onghena P, Van Houdenhove B. Antidepressant-induced analgesia in chronic non-malignant pain: a meta-analysis of 39 placebo-controlled studies. *Pain*, 1992; **49**: 205–19.
97. Lefkowitz M, Breitbart W. Chronic pain and AIDS. In Weiner RS, ed. *Innovations in Pain Medicine*. Orlando FL: Paul M. Deutsch Press, 1992: ch. 36: 1–18.
98. Max MB, Culnane M, Schafer SC, Gracely RH, Walther DJ, Smoller B, Dubner R. Amitriptyline relieves diabetic-neuropathy pain in patients with normal and depressed mood. *Neurology*, 1987; **37**: 589–96.
99. Max MB, Schafer SC, Culnane M, Smollen B, Dubner R, Gracel RH. Amitriptyline, but not lorazepam, relieves postherpetic neuralgia. *Neurology*, 1988; **38**: 427–32.
100. Pilowsky I, Hallett EC, Bassett DL, Thomas PG, Penhall RK. A controlled study of amitriptyline in the treatment of chronic pain. *Pain*, 1982; **14**: 169–79.
101. Sharav Y, Singer E, Schmidt E, Dione RA, Dubner R. The analgesic effect of amitriptyline on chronic facial pain. *Pain*, 1987; **31**: 199–209.
102. Watson CP, Evans RJ, Reed K, Merskey H, Goldsmith L, Warsh J. Amitriptyline versus placebo in post herpetic neuralgia. *Neurology*, 1982; **32**: 671–73.
103. Kvindesal B, Molin J, Froland A, Gram LF. Imipramine treatment of painful diabetic neuropathy. *Journal of the American Medical Association*, 1984; **251**: 1727–30.
104. Young RJ, Clarke BF. Pain relief in diabetic neuropathy: The effectiveness of imipramine and related drugs. *Diabetic Medicine*, 1985; **2**: 363–6.
105. Sindrup SH, Ejlertsen B, Froland A, *et al.* Imipramine treatment in diabetic neuropathy: relief of subjective symptoms without changes in peripheral and autonomic nerve function. *European Journal of Clinical Pharmacology*, 1989; **37**: 151–3.
106. Max MB, Kishore-Kumar R, Schafer SC, *et al.* Efficacy of desipramine in painful diabetic neuropathy: a placebo-controlled trial. *Pain*, 1991; **45**: 3–10.
107. Gordon N, Heller P, Gear R, Levine J. Temporal factors in the enhancement of morphine analgesic by desipramine. *Pain*, 1993; **53**: 273–6.
108. Gomez-Perez FJ, Rull JA, Dies H, *et al.* Nortriptyline and fluphenazine

in the symptomatic treatment of diabetic neuropathy. A double-blind cross-over study. *Pain*, 1985; **23**: 395–400.

109. Langohr HD, Stohr M, Petruch F. An open and double-blind crosover study on the efficacy of clomipramine (anafranil) in patients with painful mono- and polyneuropathies. *European Neurology*, 1982; **21**: 309–15.
110. Tiegno M, Pagnoni B, Calmi A, Rigoli M, Braga PC, Panerai AE. Chlorimipramine compared to pentazocine as a unique treatment in post-operative pain. *International Journal of Clinical and Pharmacological Research*, 1987; **7**: 141–3.
111. Hammeroff SR, Cork RC, Scherer K, *et al.* Doxepin effects on chronic pain, depression and plasma opioids. *Journal of Clinical Psychiatry*, 1982; **2**: 22–6.
112. Walsh TD. Controlled study of imipramine and morphine in chronic pain due to advanced cancer. (Abstract) *ASCO May 4–6, Los Angeles*, 1986.
113. Botney M, Fields HC. Amitriptyline potentiates morphine analgesia by direct action on the central nervous system. *Annals of Neurology*, 1983; **13**: 160–4.
114. Watson C, Chipan M, Reed K, Evans R, Birket N. Amitriptyline versus maprotiline in postherpetic neuralgia: a randomized double-blind crossover trial. *Pain*, 1992; **48**: 29–36.
115. Malseed RT, Goldstein FJ. Enhancement of morphine analgesics by tricyclic antidepressnts. *Neuropharmacology*, 1979; **18**: 827–9.
116. Ventafridda V, Bianchi M, Ripamonti C, *et al.* Studies on the effects of antidepressant drugs on the antinociceptive action of morphine and on plasma morphine in rat and man. *Pain*, 1990; **43**: 155–62.
117. Spiegel K, Kalb R, Pasternak GW. Analgesic activity of tricyclic antidepressants. *Annals of Neurology*, 1983; **13**: 462–5.
118. Davidoff, G, Guarracini M, Roth E, *et al.* Trazodone hydrochloride in the treatment of dysesthetic pain in traumatic myelopathy: a randomized, double-blind, placebo-controlled study. *Pain*, 1987; **29**: 151 61.
119. Costa D, Mogos I, Toma T. Efficacy and safety of mianserin in the treatment of depression of woman with cancer. *Acta Psychiatrica Scandinavica*, 1985; **72**: 85–92.
120. Eberhard G, *et al.* A double-blind randomized study of clomipramine versus maprotiline in patients with idiopathic pain syndromes. *Neuropsychobiology*, 1988; **19**: 25–32.
121. Feighner JP. A comparative trial of fluoxetine and amitriptyline in patients with major depressive disorder. *Journal of Clinical Psychiatry*, 1985; **46**: 369–72.
122. Hynes MD, Lochner MA, Bemis K, *et al.* Fluoxetine, a selective inhibitor of serotonin uptake, potentiates morphine analgesia without altering its descriminative stimulus properties or affinity for opioid receptors. *Life Sciences*, 1985; **36**: 2317–23.
123. Diamond S, Frietag FG. The use of fluoxetine in the treatment of headache. *Clinical Journal of Pain*, 1989; **5**: 200–1.
124. Geller SA. Treatment of fibrositis with fluoxetine hydrochloride (Prozac). *American Journal of Medicine*, 1989; **87**: 594–5.
125. Theesen KA, Marsh WR. Relief of diabetic neuropathy with fluoxetine. *DICP, The Annals of Pharmacotherapy*, 1989; **23**: 572–4.
126. Max MB, Lynch SA, Muir J, Shoaf SE, Smoller B, Dubner R. Effects of desipramine, amitriptyline, and fluoxetine on pain in diabetic neuropathy. *New England Journal of Medicine*, 1992; **326**: 1250–6.
127. Sindrup SH, Gram LF, Brosen K, Eshoj O, Mogenson EF. The selective serotonin reuptake inhibitor paroxetine is effective in the treatment of diabetic neuropathy symptoms. *Pain*, 1990; **42**: 135–44.
128. Pick CG, Paul D, Eison MS, Pasternak G. Potentiation of opioid analgesia by the antidepressant nefazodone. *European Journal of Pharmacology*, 1992 :375–81.
129. McQuay H, Carroll D, Glynn C. Dose-respose for analgesic effect of amitriptyline in chronic pain. *Anesthesia*, 1993; **48**: 281–5.
130. Watson CP, Evans RJ. A comparative trial of amitriptyline and zimelidine in post-herpetic neuralgia. *Pain*, 1985; **23**: 387–94.
131. Tyler MA. Treatment of the painful shoulder syndrome with amitriptyline and lithium carbonate. *Canadian Medical Association Journal*, 1974; **111**: 137–40.
132. Lascelles RG. Atypical facial pain and depression. *British Journal of Psychology*, 1966; **122**: 651.
133. Anthony M, Lance JW. MAO inhibition in the treatment of migraine. *Archives of Neurology*, 1969; **21**: 263.
134. Gebhardt KH, Beller J, Nischk R. Behandlung des karzinomschmerzes mit chlorimipramin (Anafranil). *Medizíniche Klinik*, 1969; **64**: 751–6.
135. Adjan M. Uber therapeutischen beeinflussung des schmerzsmptoms bei unheilboren tumorkranken. *Therapie der Gergenwart*, 1970; **10**: 1620–7.
136. Bernard A, Scheuer H. Action de la clomipramine (Anafranil) sur la douleur des cancers en pathologie cervico-faciale. *Journal Francais d'Oto-rhino-laryngologie*, 1972; **21**: 723–8.
137. Monkemeir D, Steffen U. Zur schmerzbehandlung mit Imipramin bei krebserkrankungen. *Medíziniche Klinik*, 1970; **65**: 213–15.
138. Barjou B. Etude du Tofranil sules douleurs en chirugie. *Revue de Medicine de Tours*, 1971; **6**: 473–82.
139. Deutschmann W. Tofranil ider schmerzbehandlung de krebskranken. *Medizinsche Welt*, 1971; **22**: 1346–7.
140. Hughes, A. Chauverghe J, Lissilour T, Lagarde C. L'imipramine utilisee comme antalgique majeur en carcinologie: Etude de 118 cas. *Presse Medicale*, 1963; **71**: 1073–4.
141. Fiorentino M. Sperimentazione controllata dell' Imipramina come analgesico maggiore in oncologia. *Rivista Medica Trentina*, 1969; **5**: 387–96.
142. Breivik H, Rennemo F. Clinical evaluation of combined treatment with methadone and psychotropic drugs in cancer patients. *Acta Anaesthesiologica Scandinavica Supplementum*, 1982; **74**: 135–40.
143. Bourhis A, Boudouresue G, Pellet W, Fondarai J, Ponzio J, Spitalier JM. Pain, infirmity and psychotropic drugs in oncology. *Pain*, 1978; **5**: 263–74.
144. Carton M, Cabarrot E, Lafforque C. Interest de l'amitriptyline utilisee commee antalgique en cancerologie. *Gazette Medicale de France*, 1976; **83**: 2375–8.
145. Fernandez F, Adams F, Holmes VF. Analgesic effect of alprazolam in patients with chronic, organic pain of malignant origin. *Journal of Clinical Psychopharmacology*, 1987; **3**: 167–9.
146. Fernandez F, Adams F, Holmes VF, *et al.* Methylphenidate for depressive disorders in cancer patients. *Psychosomatics*, 1987; **28**: 455–61.
147. Kaufmann MW, Murray GB, Cassem NH. Use of psychostimulants in medically ill depressive patients. *Psychosomatics*, 1982; **23**: 817–9.
148. Bruera E, Chadwick S, Brennels C, Hanson J, MacDonald RN. Methylphenidate associated with narcotics for the treatment of cancer pain. *Cancer Treatment Reports*, 1987; **71**: 67–70.
149. Bruera E, Brenneis C, Paterson AH, MacDonald RN. Use of Methylphenidate as an adjuvant to narcotic analgesics in patients with advanced cancer. *Journal of Pain and Symptom Management*, 1989; **4**: 3–6.
150. Bruera E, Fainsinger R, MacEachern T, Hanson J. The use of methylphenidate in patients with incident cancer pain receiving regular opiates: a preliminary report. *Pain*, 1992; **50**: 75–7.
151. Forrest WH, *et al.* Dextroamphetamine with morphine for the treatment of post-operative pain. *New England Journal of Medicine*, 1977; **296**: 712–15.
152. Nehra A, *et al.* Pemoline associated hepatic injury. *Gastroenterology*, 1990; **99**: 1517–19.
153. Beaver WT, Wallenstein SL, Houde RW, *et al.* A comparison of the analgesic effect of methotrimeprazine and morphine in patients with cancer. *Clinical Pharmacology and Therapeutics*, 1966; **7**: 436–46.
154. Maltbie AA, Cavenar JO, Sullivan JL, *et al.* Analgesia and haloperidol: A hypothesis. *Journal of Clinical Psychiatry*, 1979; **40**: 323–6.
155. Lechin F, *et al.* Pimozide therapy for trigeminal neuralgia. *Archives of Neurology*, 1989; **9**: 960–4.
156. Beaver WT, Feise G. Comparison of the analgesic effects of morphine, hydroxyzine and their combination in patients with post-operative pain. In: Bonica JJ, Albe-Fessard D, eds. *Advances in Pain Research and Therapy*. New York: Raven Press, 1976: 533–57.
157. Rumore M, Schlichting D. Clinical efficacy of antihistamines as analgesics. *Pain*, 1986; **25**: 7–22.
158. Coda B, Mackie A, Hill H. Influence of alprazolam on opioid analgesia and side effects during steady-stage morphine infusions. *Pain*, 1992; **50**: 309–16.

159. Caccia MR. Clonazepam in facial neuralgia and cluster headache: clinical and electrophysiological study. *European Journal of Neurology*, 1975; **13**: 560–3.

160. Swerdlow M, Cundill JG. Anticonvulsant drugs used in the treatment of lancinating pains: a comparison. *Anesthesia*, 1981; **36**: 1129–34.

161. Egan K, Ready L, Nessly M, Greer B. Self administration of midazolam for post-operative anxiety: a double blinded study. *Pain*, 1992; **49**: 3–8.

162. Liao J, Takemori A. Quantitative assessmentof antinociceptive effects of midazolam, amitriptyline, and carbamazepine alone and in combination with morphine in mice. *Anesthesiology*, 1990; **73**: 753.

9.2.10 Difficult pain problems

Geoffrey Hanks, Russell K. Portenoy, Neil MacDonald, and Karen Forbes

Introduction

Cancer pain in general responds in a predictable way to analgesic drugs and studies from specialist units have demonstrated that roughly 80 per cent of patients with cancer pain respond to pharmacological management.[1,2] Pain relief may be sustained for the duration of the illness, which may be weeks, months, or even years. Such good results are not always obtained. The main reasons for failure are lack of knowledge of the simple principles of effective analgesic use, which are described in earlier chapters in this section, and inexperience. That this is still the case is evident from a recent United Kingdom study which indicated that nearly half (of 1678) patients treated for pain by their general practitioners and one-third (of 1220) patients treated by hospital doctors were reported to have received treatment that only partially controlled their pain, if at all.[3] These figures could be considerably improved merely by applying existing knowledge.

Not all pain in cancer is so easily relieved, however. Certain types of pain are invariably difficult to manage even for specialist practitioners. This chapter focuses on these difficult pain problems.

Opioid-responsive and opioid poorly-responsive pain

A proportion of cancer patients have pain that does not respond well to conventional analgesic management. Because opioid analgesics are the most important part of this pharmacological approach a terminology has developed which centres around whether or not pain will respond to opioid analgesics.

The terms 'opioid non-responsive' or 'opioid resistant' pain have been used to describe the phenomenon of a poor response to opioid analgesics. In a study which had considerable influence on this debate, patients with neuropathic pain or other types of pain for which there was no identifiable painful stimulus (that is patients with so called non-nociceptive pain) appeared not to respond to opioid analgesics whereas patients with nociceptive pain did.[4] This stimulated a controversy, which has now largely resolved, over whether this lack of response is absolute or relative, so that if a sufficient dose of opioid is used at least a partial response will be obtained. The controversy has centred particularly around neuropathic pain and is discussed in more detail later in this chapter. Some have suggested unequivocally that neuropathic pain does not respond to opioid analgesics[5,6] but others have noted the fact that, clinically, the situation is rarely clear cut, as far as the so called non-responders are concerned.[7] This is because the end point when titrating dose against pain with opioid analgesics is not simply pain relief or lack of relief; adverse effects may limit dose titration.

The wide interindividual variation in dose requirements has also to be taken into account. It is not possible to define any particular dose of opioids above which a patient can be said to have non-responsive pain because the dose of morphine, for example, needed by one patient may vary a thousand-fold from that required by another. Similarly, patients have an unpredictable predilection to develop adverse effects with morphine. Some patients may be able to tolerate very large doses of morphine without developing the common adverse effects such as sedation or nausea and vomiting, whereas others may do so at very small doses.

Morphine appears to have no clinically relevant ceiling effect to analgesia. As the dose is raised analgesic effects increase as a log linear function. A point may be reached at which higher doses could theoretically produce greater analgesia but dose escalation is not possible because adverse effects supervene, thus effectively defining the responsiveness of the pain syndrome in that particular patient.[7]

It follows, therefore, that opioid responsiveness is a continuum that might be influenced by any of a large number of patient and drug related, as well as pain related, factors. The terms opioid non-responsive or opioid-resistant pain are misleading, implying that a pain either does respond to opioid analgesics or does not. If the terminology is to be used at all it is preferable to talk in terms of opioid poorly-responsive pain and a pragmatic definition is that opioid poorly-responsive pain is pain that is inadequately relieved by opioid analgesics given in a dose that causes intolerable side-effects despite optimal measures to control them.

Paradoxical pain

'Paradoxical pain' is a recently introduced term which has caused some confusion. The confusion results, to some extent, from the different definitions given by the originators of the concept. Paradoxical pain was first described as 'pain which ceases to be relieved or is worsened by further administration' of morphine of diamorphine.[8] The idea that some patients pain could be made worse by continued administration of morphine runs counter to the prevailing clinical wisdom that there is no arbitrary ceiling to the dose of morphine that may be required by an individual patient and that it is safe to titrate up the dose until pain relief is achieved or side-effects supervene. The suggestion thus raises anxiety about the potential harm which may be done if the morphine dose is titrated too far.

There are some animal data which show that high-dose intrathecal morphine may cause hyperalgesia and allodynia,[9,10] supported by some human case reports of similar signs and symptoms associated with continuous intravenous infusion of morphine.[11] There are no reports associating these effects with oral or subcutaneous administration of morphine, whatever the dose. The syndrome is ill-defined and, if it is a real entity, seems rare, given the paucity of reports in humans in the light of the very large numbers of patients treated with morphine.

It is significant that paradoxical pain was defined somewhat differently in a subsequent paper as 'nociceptive pain which is not receptive to opioid analgesics'[12] and the idea that pain could be made worse by high doses of morphine was not repeated. The proposed explanation for this lack of response was abnormal metabolism of morphine occurring in some patients whereby one of the metabolites (morphine-3-glucuronide, **M3G**) was produced in excessive amounts resulting in high cerebrospinal fluid levels and antagonism of the analgesic effects of the parent compound and adverse effects due to excessive central nervous system excitation.

Morphine-3-glucuronide

Two of the major metabolites of morphine are M3G and morphine-6-glucuronide (**M6G**) and conjugation takes place largely in the liver but probably also to a significant extent in the gastrointestinal tract (see Chapter 9.2.3). For many years, it has been assumed that M3G is inert as is the case with most glucuronide metabolites.[13] Recent behavioural studies in rodents, however, suggested that M3G produces a functional antagonism of the analgesic effects of morphine and its active metabolite M6G.[14,15] There is also some evidence in animal models that M3G may be responsible for the central nervous system excitatory adverse effects seen with morphine, such as myoclonus.[10,16] The proponents of the concept of paradoxical pain suggested that M3G is produced in huge quantities in some patients and is thus responsible for the lack of response to morphine and excessive adverse effects. Though the mechanism was not clear, they suggested that M3G binds to opioid receptors and potentially antagonizes the parent compound and M6G in this way.

There is evidence which tends to contradict these assertions.[17] It is now agreed that M3G almost certainly does not bind to opioid receptors.[18] Data from electrophysiological animal models indicate no evidence of an antagonistic effect of M3G.[19] In patients with poor renal function the glucuronide metabolites, which are normally excreted in the urine, accumulate and it is well established that patients with impaired renal function are much more sensitive to the analgesic effects of morphine and at risk of developing sedation and respiratory depression.[20] This is attributed to the accumulation of the active metabolite M6G. In renal impairment there is also massive accumulation of M3G, in substantially greater amounts than M6G.[20] If M3G truly had an effect in antagonizing the analgesic and other pharmacodynamic effects of morphine and M6G, patients with renal failure should behave in exactly the opposite way to that which is observed, that is they should exhibit reduced analgesia and no central nervous system depressant effects. Thus, there is animal and human evidence to indicate no significant antagonistic effect of M3G.

Viewed overall, the currently available evidence suggests that M3G plays no significant role in the pharmacodynamics of morphine and is not responsible for the phenomenon of opioid poorly-responsive pain. It seems likely that both the concept of paradoxical pain as a distinct entity and the purported explanation are spurious. There is no persuasive evidence that high-dose administration of morphine or diamorphine by conventional routes (oral or subcutaneous) makes pain worse. What has been described as paradoxical pain is what we would call opioid poorly-responsive pain according to the definition given above. In some patients this uncontrolled pain may be complicated by delirium and hyperexcitability, characterized by multifocal myoclonus and other signs of central nervous system excitation (tremulousness and occasionally seizures) which may be associated with other opioids not just morphine (as discussed later in this chapter).

Alternative opioid agonists

The proponents of the concept of paradoxical pain suggested that methadone was a useful alternative opioid to use for patients with pain of this type because it has no active metabolites. As will be discussed in this chapter, the use of alternative opioids may well be a beneficial strategy in patients who show a poor response to one particular opioid agonist. However, the strategy seems to work because there is incomplete cross-tolerance between opioid agonists rather than because of differences in metabolism. This is discussed in more detail below.

Opioid-irrelevant pain

In some patients the complaint of pain is more a reflection of social, psychological, or spiritual turmoil than a result of physical injury or damage. Such pain is not best treated with morphine and has been characterized as 'opioid-irrelevant pain' by Hinton (quoted by Kearney[21]). Such pain may appear to be an opioid non-responsive pain. It may dominate a particular individual or, more commonly, may form a component of many patients' complaints of pain. This emphasizes the need to keep in mind the 'total pain' concept, which encompasses physical, social, psychological, and spiritual factors, when managing cancer patients in pain. Patients whose pain remains a problem despite careful dose titration with an opioid analgesic, or who appear unduly sensitive to adverse effects, need careful reassessment of the mechanisms underlying their pain with particular attention to possible psychological factors.

Difficult pain problems

In this chapter we have selected examples of cancer pain which usually present the most difficult management problems. Each is illustrated by a case history which is based on a real patient. The reader will note some differences in clinical practice because these case histories come from Europe and North America. For example hydromorphone is widely prescribed in the United States and Canada but has only recently become available in the United Kingdom, and is still little used. These differences in detail should not obscure the overall approach to each problem and the principles of management.

Neuropathic pain

Patients with chronic neuropathic pain are over-represented amongst those who are refractory to routine analgesic measures, including opioid therapy.[22,23,24] The clinical challenge presented by such patients may be daunting as illustrated by the following case.

Case history: A 66-year-old man presented with progressive scapula pain. A computerized tomography (**CT**) scan demonstrated a mass that arose from the lung apex and abutted the chest wall; enlarged lymph nodes were identified in the mediastinum. A needle biopsy revealed squamous cell carcinoma. Radiotherapy was scheduled and pain was effectively treated with an oxycodone/aspirin combination preparation. The pain was completely relieved by the radiotherapy.

Two months later, an intermittent stabbing pain began in the medial forearm. Within weeks severe aching in the elbow and burning sensations in the hand began. CT revealed that the apical mass had extended superiorly into the region of the brachial plexus. The mediastinal tumour had increased and there were new metastatic deposits in both lungs. Further antitumour therapy was offered but the patient declined.

Little pain relief was provided by the oxycodone/aspirin regimen, and the patient was switched to oral morphine in a dose of 30 mg 4 hourly. Pain continued to be severe and the morphine dose was gradually increased to 150 mg 4 hourly. The pain improved but sedation and confusion became intolerable. Morphine was discontinued and a trial of oral hydromorphone was begun in a dose equianalgesic to two-thirds of the dose of morphine. Pain relief was much improved although still inadequate and daytime sedation lessened. Higher doses, however, produced hallucinations without improving analgesia.

Oral hydromorphone was continued at the initial dose and amitriptyline was added in a dose of 10 mg nightly. There was no effect on pain but sedation and confusion worsened. The amitriptyline was discontinued and desipramine was substituted at the same dose. This drug was better tolerated and the dose was gradually increased to 100 mg nightly. Pain improved slightly but further dose increases were precluded by worsening sedation. The desipramine was discontinued and the antiarrythmic mexiletine (an oral local anaesthetic) was administered in a starting dose of 150 mg/day. During the ensuing week the dose was increased in a step-wise manner to 900 mg/day in divided doses. Improvement was noted with each dose increase and no side-effects occurred. At the highest dose pain was still constant but its usual intensity was mild and severe episodes were both less intense and less frequent. The patient perceived these residual symptoms to be tolerable and therapy was continued.

Six weeks later, pain in the shoulder, elbow, and hand escalated rapidly. Nutritional status had been poor and the patient was troubled by progressive asthenia, dyspnoea on exertion, and cough. A small increase in the hydromorphone dose produced confusion and the patient was admitted to hospital. As the patient's medical status was stabilized, consecutive trials of carbamazepine, sodium valproate, and clonidine were administered but each was limited to a relatively low dose due to the onset of worsening cognitive impairment.

A stellate ganglion block was performed ipsilateral to the painful limb but produced no change in the pain. A percutaneous epidural catheter was then placed with the tip of the catheter situated just caudal to the cervical enlargement. A trial of morphine and then a morphine/local anaesthetic mixture was initiated. The dose of morphine was increased until confusion worsened without impact on the pain. The addition of the local anaesthetic initially yielded substantial improvement but this persisted for only 3 days. The patient developed a fever and the catheter was removed.

The risks and potential benefits of neurolytic procedures, including rhizotomy, cordotomy, and cingulotomy, were discussed with the patient, who refused invasive approaches. Following discussion with the patient and family, it was decided that the opioid dose would be increased and that other neuroleptic or sedative drugs would be used to manage the delirium that would ensue. This was done and the patient was transferred to a hospice 2 weeks later, where he remained deeply sedated until his death a few days later.

The problem

The term 'neuropathic pain' is applied to a diverse group of syndromes in which the sustaining mechanisms for the pain are presumed to be related to aberrant somatosensory processes in the peripheral nervous system, central nervous system, or both. These pains are usually precipitated by overt injury to neural structures but, once established, are often far in excess of any overt peripheral pathology.

This category of pain syndromes is part of a broader taxonomy based on inferred pain mechanisms[25] which also includes the so-called nociceptive pains and psychogenic pains. Nociceptive pain refers to pain that is perceived to be due to ongoing activation of primary afferent nerves that respond to noxious stimuli (nociceptors). These nerves innervate both somatic and visceral structures; somatic pain and visceral pain are considered subtypes. Psychogenic pain, for which an alternative psychiatric classification can be used,[26] refers to pain that is at least partially sustained by primary psychological processes.

Although this approach to classification by inferred pain mechanisms is undoubtedly a gross simplification of the complex pathophysiologies that result in chronic pain, it is clinically relevant and widely accepted by practitioners. As discussed below, such inferences can help guide patient assessment and therapeutic decision-making.

The patient in the case report described aching shoulder pain and dysaesthesias (abnormal pain sensations) in the arm. The nature of these pains and the position and extent of the tumour mass suggest that the pain syndrome resulted from both nociceptive processes (activation of somatic nociceptors by direct infiltration of the chest wall) and neuropathic processes (caused by brachial plexus injury). The experience of multiple types of pain in the same patient is very common in the palliative care setting. A psychological contribution is probably quite common in such settings but was not prominent in this case. As time passed, the predominating and most challenging aspect of the pain was its neuropathic component.

The clinical challenge associated with the management of neuropathic pain derives from the observation that these pains respond less well to opioid drugs than nociceptive pains. The patient described in the case report, for example, failed to respond satisfactorily to two opioids (morphine and hydromorphone) and the same opioid (morphine) by two routes of administration.

The observation that at least some types of neuropathic pain are relatively less responsive to opioid drugs has strong empirical support from both clinical studies[4,7,23,25,27-30] and experimental data.[31] As discussed in the introduction current evidence does not indicate that neuropathic pains are generically 'opioid-resistant,' but it is likely that a neuropathic mechanism (or some types of neuropathic mechanisms) increases the likelihood of an unfavourable opioid response.[23,24]

Given the discouragement that many clinicians experience when encountering patients with neuropathic pain, it is important to emphasize that favourable responses to opioid drugs do occur in

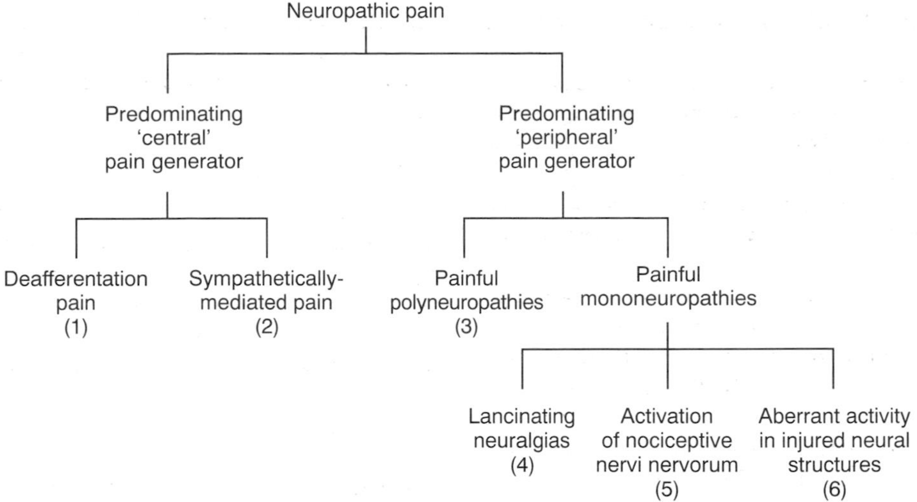

Fig. 1 Classification of neuropathic pains by inferred pathophysiology. (1) Can be precipitated by either peripheral or central nervous system injury. (2) Is most strongly associated with reflex sympathetic dystrophy/causalgia and may be considered a subclass of these syndromes; the possibility of this pathophysiology is suggested by the development of focal autonomic dysregulation (e.g. oedema, vasomotor disturbances), motor impairment, and trophic changes in the region of the pain, but is confirmed by improvement with sympathetic nerve block. (3) Multiple mechanisms probably involved. (4) The patterns of peripheral activity, or peripheral and central interaction, that yield the lancinating quality of these pains are unknown. (5) Nociceptive nervi nervorum (small afferents that innervate larger nerves) may account for neuropathic pain accompanying nerve compression or inflammation. (6) Injury to axons may be followed by neuroma formation, a source of aberrant activity likely to be involved in pain. (Adapted from Portenoy 1991.[25])

such cases. Indeed, clinical experience suggests that properly administered opioid therapy often yields a satisfactory outcome. This potential for a favourable opioid response has been affirmed through surveys of patients with malignant and non-malignant pain,[22,32,33,34] a controlled trial of morphine in patients with postherpetic neuralgia,[30] systematic studies of morphine self-administration in patients with different types of pain,[27] and pharmacokinetic–pharmacodynamic studies of opioid infusions in patients with diverse neuropathic pain syndromes.[7] Together, these observations strongly support the value of a trial of opioids in patients with neuropathic pain, notwithstanding the relatively greater likelihood of an unfavourable outcome.

Clinical spectrum and pathophysiology

Neuropathic pains comprise numerous distinctive clinical entities which vary in presentation, specific pathophysiological factors, and, to a lesser extent, treatment.[35] Although taxonomies based on syndrome identification or lesion localization are often used, classification by putative mechanism[25] (Fig. 1) may be particularly useful in fashioning treatment strategies (see below). Such a classification begins with the division of neuropathic pains into those predominantly sustained by mechanisms in the peripheral nervous system and those sustained by mechanisms in the central nervous system. The evidence for this conceptualization, like that for the broader construct of neuropathic pain itself, is largely conjectural (Table 1) but clinically relevant.

Neuropathic pains sustained by a peripheral mechanism

A diverse group of neuropathic pains results from pathological processes that develop at the site of peripheral nerve injury. These pains may be divided into painful mononeuropathies and painful polyneuropathies. Syndromes characterized by intermittent stabbing pains, which can be termed 'lancinating neuralgias', may also be distinguished, since the unique characteristics shared by these pains probably relates to a unique pathophysiology. Both painful polyneuropathies (such as that caused by neurotoxic chemotherapy) and painful mononeuropathies (such as the brachial plexopathy described in the case report) are common in the palliative care setting.

A variety of pathophysiological processes presumably underlie different peripheral neuropathic pain syndromes. The best studied are those associated with painful mononeuropathies. These may include activation of nociceptive nervi nervorum (small primary afferent nerves that invest the trunks of larger nerves) by compression or inflammation of the nerve, sensitization of the primary afferent neurone, and neuroma formation following axonal transection.[36,37] Studies of neuromas have demonstrated spontaneous electrical activity associated with pain reports in humans, as well as exaggerated responses to both mechanical deformation and some chemical stimuli, such as noradrenaline.

Injury to peripheral nerve can cause persistent changes in the central nervous system, which may contribute further to the pain. Indeed, it may be hypothesized that a process of 'central sensitization' is pivotal in many cases of refractory neuropathic pain.[38] Sensitization of central neurones appears to be a complex process that results from interactions between multiple receptors and both neurotransmitters and neuromodulators. Recent studies have suggested that a fundamental mechanism may involve activation of the *N*-methyl-D-aspartate receptor by excitatory amino acids released by primary afferent neurones.[39]

The identification of a predominating peripheral pathogenesis for a neuropathic pain may have important therapeutic implications. Some of these pains may be relieved by a peripheral intervention, such as decompression of a nerve, resection of a neuroma, or proximal denervation via a neurolytic procedure.

Neuropathic pains sustained by a central mechanism

Neuropathic pains primarily sustained by central nervous system mechanisms can be divided into two broad categories: the so-called deafferentation pains and reflex sympathetic dystrophy/causalgia

Table 1 Types of evidence supporting the division of neuropathic pains into those with sustaining mechanisms for the pain located in the central nervous system and those with sustaining mechanisms for the pain located in the peripheral nervous system

	Evidence	Caveat
1.	Surveys of patients undergoing neurolysis suggest that some pains have a central mechanism that causes pain even after the painful part is denervated.	Data are limited and published cases have selection bias; evidence that peripheral pains do reliably respond to neurolysis is meagre.
2.	Correlations in specific syndromes, e.g. abnormal activity in central nervous system structures of patients with deafferentation pain and similar activity on microneuronography of nerves proximal to neuroma.	Correlations between findings and pain do not prove causality; there have been no simultaneous recordings from peripheral and central structures in man.
3.	Animal models suggest that there are changes following nerve injury that may be either central or peripheral, e.g. the neuroma model demonstrates characteristics, such as mechanosensitivity, that correspond to findings in humans with similar pathology.	Relationship between animal models and chronic neuropathic pain in man is highly inferential; studies show that peripheral injury produces substantial changes in the central nervous system and that central nervous system injury may cause changes in the periphery.

This division is inferred and its tentative nature is emphasized by noting the weaknesses in the supporting data. This model remains hypothetical.

syndromes.[35] The latter syndromes include an important subgroup—the sympathetically-maintained pains (Fig. 1). Clinical recognition of these types of neuropathic pain may suggest useful adjunctive strategies to conventional analgesic therapy.

Deafferentation pains

The deafferentation pains include a number of alternatively named syndromes, such as phantom pain, postherpetic neuralgia, root avulsion pain, anaesthesia dolorosa, and central pain.[35] Although these pains vary in the site of nerve injury, presentation, and response to some specific therapies, all are presumably sustained by abnormal processes in the spinal cord or brain. The specific pathophysiological processes are likely to be diverse[40] and may include denervation hypersensitivity of central neurones, ectopic electrogenesis at sites of injured central neurones, changes in the receptive fields of central somatosensory neurones, and loss of central inhibitions.

The remarkable observation that injury to a peripheral nerve can produce either a peripheral painful mononeuropathy (e.g. from neuroma formation) or a deafferentation syndrome (e.g. anaesthesia dolorosa or phantom pain) has important implications for the use of neurolytic procedures in the treatment of refractory pains. It is possible that neurolytic procedures that denervate the painful part could have markedly different results depending upon the underlying mechanism; a peripheral neuropathic pain may be more likely to be relieved by such a procedure and a deafferentation pain might be worsened. In the clinical setting, temporary local anaesthetic nerve blocks are often used to guide treatment when this consideration exists. Patients with neuropathic pain associated with a peripheral nerve lesion who fail to obtain a favourable response following blockade of the nerves between the painful site and the central nervous system are suspected of having pain sustained by central mechanisms and are not subjected to neurolysis.

Although the validity of this observation has not been tested empirically, it is a sensible stance that is widely accepted in practice. Unfortunately, a favourable response to local anaesthetic nerve block neither proves a peripheral mechanism nor predicts successful neurolysis.

Reflex sympathetic dystrophy/causalgia syndrome

The nomenclature of pain syndromes that have traditionally been labelled reflex sympathetic dystrophy or causalgia has continued to evolve and remains confusing. The International Association for the Study of Pain has recently advocated more descriptive language, renaming these syndromes as complex regional pain syndrome type I and type II, respectively.[41] Although the term sympathetically-maintained pain has also been used, this appellation is now preferred only when pain can be reliably relieved with sympathetic nerve block. Only some patients with reflex sympathetic dystrophy or causalgia have sympathetically-maintained pain.

The diagnosis of reflex sympathetic dystrophy (or complex regional pain syndrome type I) may be offered when focal pain accompanied by autonomic dysregulation, motor impairment, and trophic signs occur after injury to bone, joint, or soft tissue. The diagnosis of causalgia (or complex regional pain syndrome type II) is appropriate for the identical syndrome when it is precipitated by injury to a nerve trunk. In both cases the inciting injury may be minor and, in rare cases, the pain and associated features appear without recollection of a prior event.

The pain of reflex sympathetic dystrophy or causalgia is typically dysaesthetic, often constant burning with intermittent paroxysms. The focal autonomic dysregulation may include swelling, vasomotor instability (pallor, erythema or cyanosis, or livedo reticularis), sweating abnormalities, or temperature changes.[35,41,42] Motor phenomena, including stiffness, weakness, and abnormal involuntary movements (tremor, chorea, or dystonias), are common when the lesion involves an extremity. So-called trophic changes, such as thinning of the skin, change in hair or nail growth, atrophy of subcutaneous tissues or muscle, or focal osteoporosis, may also occur.

In some cases reflex sympathetic dystrophy or causalgia is suspected but the routine evaluation does not reveal the autonomic or trophic changes needed to clarify the diagnosis. Autonomic dysfunction may be demonstrated using more sophisticated measures, such as thermography or quantitative sweat testing, and trophic changes may be assessed with bone scintigraphy, radiography, or magnetic resonance imaging.

Although a major analgesic response to sympathetic nerve block suggests that the pain is sympathetically maintained, the interpretation of a test that is performed in varying ways, often without confirmation of physiological change and almost never with a placebo control, is problematical.[43] There have been no studies that clarify the degree or duration of response necessary to attribute the pain to activity in the sympathetic nervous system. The use of a pharmacological approach to sympathetic block, specifically intravenous phentolamine infusion, has recently been introduced as a more specific way of assessing sympathetic efferent function,[43,44] but this may also be difficult to interpret.[45,46]

The controversy surrounding the role of sympathetic efferent function in reflex sympathetic dystrophy or causalgia reflects the broader uncertainty about the pathogenesis of these disorders. Indeed, one recent analysis of the available literature finds little support for the role of sympathetic nerves and suggests that visceral afferent neurones, which travel with the sympathetic nerves, may actually be more important.[47] A peripheral injury almost always precedes the appearance of reflex sympathetic dystrophy or causalgia and peripheral mechanisms, such as those that result in the peripheral painful mononeuropathies discussed previously, may be involved in the pathogenesis of at least some cases. Nonetheless, a central pathogenesis is probably a critical element in the development and persistence of most cases. For example it has been hypothesized that sensitization of central neurones in the dorsal horn of the spinal cord represents the fundamental pathology, and that in many cases the clinical syndrome can be explained by the maintenance of aberrant activity in these neurones by sympathetically-driven activation of non-nociceptive primary afferent neurones.[48]

Regardless of the underlying pathophysiology, the clinical recognition of a reflex sympathetic dystrophy or causalgia has important implications, suggesting the potential therapeutic value of sympathetic interruption. The appearance of local autonomic dysregulation in a region of neuropathic pain is usually sufficient to suggest the diagnosis and justify diagnostic sympathetic blockade. Interruption of sympathetic efferent function is usually performed by sympathetic nerve block. In some cases the response is favourable enough to consider repeated sympathetic nerve blocks as a primary treatment approach. If nerve blocks cannot be performed, phentolamine infusion can be considered as a diagnostic approach, or other sympatholytic agents might be considered for therapeutic trials (see Chapter 9.2.6).

Management of neuropathic pain

Management of neuropathic pain, like other chronic pains encountered in the palliative care setting, begins with a comprehensive assessment.[49,50] This assessment characterizes the phenomenology of the pain, attempts to elucidate the underlying aetiology for the pain and infer contributing pathophysiologies, and determines relevant medical and psychosocial disturbances that either help explain the nature of the pain or demand independent therapy. This assessment usually yields a complex understanding of a range of problems that together undermine quality of life.

The variable constellation of symptoms, medical problems, functional impairments, and psychosocial concerns often encountered in practice suggests the need for a multimodal strategy that targets a group of specific therapies to discrete problems identified by the comprehensive assessment. The use of one or more specific analgesic treatments is typically part of this strategy.

Similar to the management of other types of chronic pain, opioid therapy is considered to be the first-line approach for the treatment of moderate or severe neuropathic pain in the palliative care setting. Guidelines for optimal opioid therapy (discussed in Chapter 9.2.3) stress the need for dose titration to identify a dose associated with a favourable balance between analgesia and side-effects, that is a dose that is squarely in the therapeutic window for the individual patient. This is particularly salient in the treatment of neuropathic pains, which may be less opioid responsive than other pains and thereby demonstrate a narrower therapeutic window. Hence, all patients with moderate or severe neuropathic pain should undergo a trial with an opioid drug, during which doses should be gradually escalated until either favourable effects occur or intolerable and unmanageable side-effects develop.

Failure with one opioid does not necessarily predict an inadequate response to another and trials of other opioids should be considered in the management of refractory cases (Cherny, in press).[34,51]

Patients who fail to obtain adequate analgesia with opioids alone may be candidates for any of a large number of adjunctive approaches. These range from alternative drug therapies to a variety of invasive approaches.

Adjuvant pharmacological approaches

The use of the so-called adjuvant analgesics to treat neuropathic pain is now widely accepted. Numerous drugs in diverse drug classes have been recommended for this indication (Table 2). The pharmacology, indications, and dosing guidelines for these drugs are described in Chapter 9.2.5. Although the potential for favourable effects justifies sequential trials, the clinician must recognize the possibility of adverse effects in a population predisposed to complications by advanced age, concurrent organ dysfunction, and coadministration of drugs with additive side-effects. Trials must be implemented cautiously and monitoring should be intensified.

Anaesthetic approaches (see Chapter 9.2.6)

As noted, a trial of sympathetic blockade should be considered whenever the clinical findings suggest a reflex sympathetic dystrophy or causalgia in a patient with refractory pain. The patient with intractable pain due to malignant brachial plexopathy who develops swelling and erythema of the hand should not be assumed simply to have venous outflow or lymphatic obstruction but, rather, should be considered a potential case of causalgia that may respond to sympathetic nerve block. An experienced anaesthetist on the palliative care team can help optimize decisions about these invasive procedures.

Other anaesthetic techniques are also useful in patients with neuropathic pain. The simplest of these, trigger point injections, may ameliorate the myofascial pains that can be associated with the primary pain complaint. Trigger point injections are within the purview of all clinicians and are probably under used in the palliative care setting.

Occasional patients with neuropathic pain obtain relatively long-lasting benefit from transient somatic nerve blocks using local anaesthetic. In these cases blocks can be repeated at intervals. More often, however, local anaesthetic blocks produce short-lived relief. This type of response may suggest the potential value of subsequent neurolysis, particularly in patients with severe refractory pain and short life expectancies. Neurolysis may be reasonable in these situations despite the concern, described previously, that

Table 2 Adjuvant analgesics used in the management of neuropathic pain (Chapter 9.2.5)

Drug class	Examples
Tricyclic antidepressants	Amitriptyline Doxepin Imipramine Nortriptyline Desipramine
'Newer' antidepressants	Paroxetine Maprotiline Trazodone
Oral local anaesthetics	Mexiletine Tocainide Flecainide
Anticonvulsants	Carbamazepine Phenytoin Valproate Clonazepam Gabapentin
α-2-adrenergic agonists	Clonidine
γ-aminobutyric acid agonists	Baclofen
Neuroleptics	Pimozide
Corticosteroids	Prednisolone Dexamethasone
N-methyl-D-aspartate receptor antagonists	Dextromethorphan Ketamine
Topical agents	Local anaesthetics Capsaicin
Miscellaneous	Calcitonin
Drugs for sympathetically-maintained pain	Phenoxybenzamine Prazosin Propranolol Nifedipine

worsening denervation could exacerbate the pain of an underlying deafferentation syndrome.

Patients with suspected neuroma (e.g. in a surgical scar) may benefit from direct injection of local anaesthetic into the site of the neuroma. Some of these patients gain long-term relief from neurolytic blockade at these sites.[52]

Intraspinal infusion techniques may be useful in some patients with neuropathic pain, particularly those whose pain is situated below mid-thorax. The usual indication for a trial of epidural or intrathecal opioids is similar to pains of other types, namely the development of intolerable central nervous system side-effects (somnolence or confusion) during escalation of systemic opioid doses (see Chapter 9.2.6).

Not surprisingly, there is evidence that intraspinal opioids may be relatively less efficacious in patients with neuropathic pain than nociceptive pain.[53] The use of intraspinal local anaesthetic infusions, usually combined with an opioid, has been observed anecdotally to benefit some patients with refractory neuropathic pain.[54] Recently, a placebo-controlled trial confirmed the value of epidural clonidine in the treatment of cancer-related neuropathic pain.[55] The use of intraspinal drug combinations in the treatment of refractory neuropathic pain should be considered only by experienced practitioners who are able to implement and monitor these interventions.

Neurostimulatory approaches

Non-invasive stimulatory approaches comprise counter-irritation (systematic rubbing of the painful part) and transcutaneous electrical nerve stimulation. Invasive approaches include acupuncture, percutaneous electrical nerve stimulation, dorsal column stimulation, and deep brain stimulation. All of these approaches have been used in the palliative care setting for patients with refractory neuropathic pain but only the non-invasive approaches are used commonly. Like the invasive anaesthetic approaches, invasive stimulatory approaches should be considered only by experienced practitioners, or team of practitioners, who can evaluate the patient comprehensively, optimise non-invasive therapies, and integrate invasive procedures with other treatments.

Transcutaneous electrical nerve stimulation will initially benefit many patients but only a small minority continue to obtain relief from this approach beyond a period of weeks. Nonetheless, the morbidity is extremely low and the existence of an occasional patient who achieves remarkable benefit for prolonged periods impels consideration of a trial in all patients with refractory neuropathic pain (see Chapter 9.2.8). A trial of transcutaneous electrical nerve stimulation that recognizes individual differences in the response to this approach usually requires a period of weeks. The patient should attempt stimulation using various electrode placements, timing of treatment (minutes, hours, or continuously throughout the day), and stimulation parameters (frequency and amplitude of the waveform and stimulus intensity). In this way, the most effective stimulation regimen can be identified.

Rehabilitation therapies

Although the functional benefits possible through rehabilitative techniques are well recognized, the potential analgesic consequences from these treatments are not often appreciated. Physiotherapy may be able to forestall or reduce the myofascial complications that commonly exacerbate neuropathic pain. Occupational therapy may be able to identify methods that allow a patient to regain function without provoking painful episodes. Patients who experience relief only when a limb or torso is partially immobilized may achieve some measure of analgesia through the skilful use of an orthosis.

Surgical approaches

Surgical procedures that are sometimes considered for neuropathic pains include those designed to address nerve injury directly, such as resection of a neuroma or decompression of a peripheral nerve, and those designed to denervate the painful part, such as rhizotomy or cordotomy.[56,57] Clinical observations suggest that the latter procedures, the most useful of which is cordotomy, may be generally less efficacious for neuropathic pains than for nociceptive pains.[40] Nonetheless, some patients with short life expectancies and severe refractory neuropathic pains clearly benefit from surgical neurolysis of nerve pathways proximal to the painful site. Experienced clinicians weigh the risks and benefits in each case and use these approaches for carefully selected patients.

In some cases the decision to try denervation opens the possibility of either an anaesthetic approach (neurolytic nerve block) or a surgical approach. For example rhizotomy can be performed by epidural or subarachnoid instillation of a neurolytic solution or by surgical sectioning of the nerve root. There have been no comparative trials of any of these techniques and the selection of one or another is usually based on the medical status of the patient, technical considerations, or the availability of resources.

Psychological approaches

Specific cognitive approaches, such as hypnosis and distraction techniques, have been used to manage pain in the palliative care setting.[58] There have been no studies of these approaches in patients with neuropathic pain. Given the potential benefits and lack of risk, however, they should certainly be considered in cognitively intact patients, if the expertise exists to apply them.

Conclusion

The management of neuropathic pain syndromes is a compelling clinical challenge, the outcome of which is too often unsatisfactory. Given the variability of the medically ill patients who experience these syndromes, the lack of data about mechanisms and natural history, and the empirical methods used in management, it is remarkable that the outcome achieved with many patients is as favourable as it is. Further improvements depend on basic and clinical investigations that clarify the mechanisms and phenomenology of these syndromes, and provide data that allow a targeting of treatments according to underlying pathophysiology.

Breakthrough pain

Breakthrough pain refers to a transitory exacerbation of pain experienced by the patient who has relatively stable and adequately controlled baseline pain. In the palliative care population, the baseline pain is typically managed with opioid drugs, and breakthrough pain denotes brief periods during which the usual opioid regimen fails to provide adequate analgesia.

Case history: A 72-year-old man with metastatic prostate cancer was receiving hormonal agents when he noted the insidious onset of progressive sacral pain. Metastases to the sacrum and pelvis had been previously documented and a pelvic CT scan revealed some progression of these lesions. Radiotherapy was administered to the painful site, which abolished the pain. He continued hormonal therapy and was asymptomatic for 6 months, at which time he again experienced the onset of pain in the sacrum and left ileum. CT revealed progression of the bony disease and extension of a tumour mass into the presacral soft tissues. The pain was initially controlled with a combination product containing paracetamol and codeine 30 mg. At two tablets every 4 h, the patient noted minimal residual pain except during periods of physical exertion.

Two months later, continuous aching pain increased and episodes of severe pain on sitting and walking began again. Intermittent perineal stabbing pains started soon after. The latter pains, which were paroxysmal and very brief, increased in frequency and intensity and soon became highly distressing. The paracetamol/codeine preparation did not lessen this pain.

Treatment with oral morphine initially yielded an excellent response. At a dose of 30 mg 4 hourly the patient once again became pain free except during periods of exertion. Within a week, however, stabbing perineal pains began again. During the ensuing 2 weeks, the morphine dose was increased to 80 mg 4 hourly. At this dose the perineal stabbing pains became less frequent and severe but function was compromised during pain-free periods by sedation. Reduction in the morphine dose allowed the patient to think more clearly, but immediately resulted in an exacerbation of the stabbing pain.

Carbamazepine was added to the morphine regimen and eliminated the stabbing perineal pain. Within a month, however, the patient reported that the aching sacral pain began to flare intolerably upon sitting or standing for more than a few minutes. Pelvic CT revealed further bony destruction and a large presacral soft tissue mass. Chemotherapy was offered but refused and a surgical consultant could offer no solution.

Higher doses of morphine produced confusion and had no effect on the pain. Use of a supplemental morphine dose, which was to be taken only during exacerbations of pain, failed because pain onset was too abrupt and the patient would promptly recline when the pain occurred severely, thereby eliminating the need for the supplemental dose. The morphine was discontinued and a trial of an alternative opioid, hydromorphone, was initiated. There was no clinical improvement despite adjustment of the dose.

An epidural catheter was inserted. The hydromorphone and carbamazepine were continued at doses below those associated with cognitive impairment. Epidural administration of first morphine and then hydromorphone failed to identify a dose that eliminated the breakthrough pain without producing exacerbation of side-effects. A low concentration of a local anaesthetic, bupivacaine, was added to the epidural opioid but provided no additional relief. Higher concentrations of local anaesthetic ultimately provided enough relief for the patient to sit, but this treatment impaired the patient's ability to walk and produced an unacceptable numbness in the legs and perineum. The catheter was removed.

The options available to manage the refractory breakthrough pain were discussed with the patient. The use of epidural or subarachnoid neurolysis was rejected because of the likelihood of morbidity, specifically the loss of normal micturition and the possibility that the sensory changes and weakness that had been experienced during local anaesthetic instillation might be reproduced. The patient was appraised of the potential risks and benefits of other neurolytic procedures, including bilateral cordotomy and myelotomy, and these options were compared with an alternative outcome in which the patient would accept a bed-bound existence.

The patient requested bilateral cordotomy and this was performed percutaneously in two steps during the following week. The response was initially excellent. The patient could sit and stand comfortably and walk short distances without pain. The opioid dose was reduced by half and cognition cleared fully.

The patient was discharged home and required no additional interventions until 2 months later, at which time the pain flared again. The patient was readmitted to hospital where re-evaluation showed a pathological fracture of the sacrum and newly apparent metastatic deposits in the liver. The dose of hydromorphone was adjusted until the patient was comfortable at rest. The patient accepted the recommendation that he be confined to bed and he was discharged home, where he died 2 weeks later.

The problem

Although there is widespread clinical recognition that episodic or breakthrough pain can be a major impediment to function,[22,59,60] there is no generally accepted nomenclature to describe the phenomenon, and neither its characteristics nor its management have been well defined. Although the term is often used to refer to transient pains in patients whose baseline pain is controlled by opioid drugs, this definition is unnecessarily narrow. Likewise, breakthrough pain is often equated with incident pain, which is typically understood to be induced by some voluntary action of the patient, but this definition is also too limited. Since adherence to the broadest definition is most likely to clarify the problem of transitory pains in the palliative care setting, breakthrough pains are best defined as any acute transient pain that is severe and has an intensity that flares over baseline.

From this perspective, the patient described in the case report experienced two distinct types of breakthrough pain. The first, aching sacral pain on sitting or standing, could also be labelled as incident pain. It was attributable to the destructive lesion of the sacrum and its inferred pathophysiology was nociceptive. The second, intermittent perineal stabbing, was most likely to be a neuropathic pain caused by tumour extension into the sacral plexus. It was not precipitated by a voluntary action and therefore would not be termed an incident pain. Although the two types of breakthrough pains experienced by the patient described in the case report were clearly distinguished by both phenomenology and the response to an anticonvulsant, carbamazepine, there were similarities between them as well. Most importantly, both were partially responsive to opioid drugs and flared at the end of a dosing interval, but neither could be adequately managed with a supplemental opioid dose.

This patient highlights the great variability in the presentation and aetiology of breakthrough pains. This variability, combined with a poor response to many of the routine pharmacological interventions used to manage more continuous baseline pain, complicates the treatment of breakthrough pains.

Clinical spectrum and pathophysiology

The prevalence and characteristics of breakthrough pain have been evaluated in a prospective survey of patients with cancer pain.[59] In this survey, 41 of 63 patients (63 per cent) who were receiving stable doses of an analgesic and had controlled baseline pain described one or more breakthrough pains during the preceding 24 h. Nine patients reported more than one distinct type of breakthrough pain, yielding a total of 51 pains.

The remarkable variability of the breakthrough pains experienced by these patients was evident in every characteristic evaluated. The median number of pains during a 24-h period was four, but the range varied from one to 3600. Twelve of the 41 patients reported seven or more discrete breakthrough pains per day, and one extraordinary patient experienced a brief chest wall pain every minute, which occurred with a paroxysmal cough. The duration of each breakthrough pain ranged from 1 to 240 min (median 30 min). Seventeen (33 per cent) of the breakthrough pains were somatic, 10 (20 per cent) were visceral, 14 (27 per cent) were neuropathic, and 10 (20 per cent) were mixed. Three-quarters of the pains were specifically related to a known neoplastic lesion, but 20 per cent could be attributed to an effect of antineoplastic therapy and 4 per cent were unrelated to the cancer or its treatment.

Similar variability was demonstrated in precipitating events for breakthrough pain. Specifically, precipitants were identified prior to 28 of the 51 (55 per cent) breakthrough pains. Fourteen patients (34 per cent) noted that breakthrough pains occurred or markedly worsened at the end of an analgesic dosing interval. Other precipitants included movement in bed, walking, sitting, standing, touching the painful site, or cough. Some pains were precipitated by non-volitional events, including bowel distension (four pains), ureteral distension (one pain), and regurgitation of analgesic medication (one pain).

In this survey,[59] treatment of breakthrough pains was accomplished through a combination of approaches administered by the staff and those fortuitously discovered by the patients themselves. Sixteen of the 41 patients (39 per cent) reported that the use of a supplemental dose of an opioid drug ('rescue' dose) was an effective treatment approach. Thirteen patients (32 per cent) stated that breakthrough pains were managed through a change in position or some other movement. Other palliative factors included use of a regularly scheduled dose of analgesic drug, defecation, cough suppression, sleep, or the use of an antacid.

Management of breakthrough pain

Many published guidelines for the therapy of cancer pain allude to the problem of transient exacerbation of pain, but none describe the management of this problem beyond the use of supplemental doses of an opioid. The experience detailed in the aforementioned survey[59] suggests that a more comprehensive approach is needed. The following four principles of management are derived from the meagre published data and clinical experience; controlled clinical trials of therapeutic interventions for breakthrough pain are necessary to confirm the utility of this approach.

Comprehensive assessment

Similar in scope to that recommended for other types of cancer pain,[49,50] the evaluation of breakthrough pains should endeavour to characterize fully the pain itself and the clinical status of the patient. Combined with an understanding of the extent of disease and the physical, psychological, and social condition of the patient, this information clarifies the overall approach to treatment.

Treatment of the underlying cause

Primary therapy directed against the cause of the breakthrough pain can eliminate the need for analgesic therapies. For example breakthrough pain on walking due to a spinal metastasis may be resolved by local radiotherapy. The utility of primary therapy is strong justification for an assessment of the disease-related factors underlying the pain.[50]

Primary therapy for the cause of breakthrough pain may be associated with considerable burden or risks for the patient. The appropriate use of primary therapy depends on many factors, including the extent of the disease, the general medical status of the patient, previous treatments, and the overriding goals of care. Treatment for the specific lesion associated with the breakthrough pain should be provided if it is feasible, does not subject the patient to excessive risk, and has a reasonable likelihood of reducing the frequency or intensity of the pain.

Optimizing the analgesic regimen

The observation that some breakthrough pains only occur, or flare dramatically, at the end of the dosing interval suggests that these pains are related to the plasma concentration of the analgesic drug. For such pains, the maintenance of a higher plasma concentration throughout the dosing interval may resolve the problem.

It is likely that some breakthrough pains without a demonstrable relationship to the end of the dosing interval, such as those occurring in patients receiving opioid infusions, would also be responsive to an increase in dose. This speculation suggests that an adjustment in the regularly scheduled analgesic regimen is a reasonable intervention in all patients with breakthrough pain. If the regularly scheduled analgesic is an opioid, the dose should be increased until either favourable effects occur or intolerable and unmanageable side-effects supervene, which usually occurs during the intervals between the severe pains.[60] Breakthrough pains are often improved, but seldom eradicated, by this approach.

Primary analgesic approaches

Although many patients appear to benefit from the administration of primary treatments and adjustment of the scheduled analgesic regimen, most will require specific analgesic interventions directed at the breakthrough pain itself. At the present time, the selection and use of these approaches is also empirical.

'Rescue' dose

The use of a pharmacological 'rescue' dose is widely accepted in the management of breakthrough pain.[61,62] In this technique, a supplemental 'as required' dose of an analgesic drug is offered concurrently with the regularly scheduled analgesic drug. Although neither the pharmacokinetics nor the pharmacodynamics of the rescue dose have been studied, a drug with a short half-life and rapid onset of action can be recommended empirically. This drug can be a non-steroidal anti-inflammatory drug (**NSAID**), but is more often an opioid. If the regularly scheduled opioid has a short half-life, the same drug should be selected for the rescue; if the regularly scheduled opioid has a long half-life or duration of effect (e.g. methadone or controlled release oral morphine), it is preferable to use an alternative short half-life drug as the rescue.

If possible, the same route of administration should be used for both the rescue and the fixed dose. However, occasional patients receiving oral dosing find that the onset of action of an oral rescue dose is too slow to treat the breakthrough pain effectively. Parenteral administration of an opioid can be considered in this situation. The recent advent of patient-controlled analgesia systems in ambulatory infusion devices capable of delivering continuous subcutaneous or intravenous infusion can, if available, expedite the administration of supplemental doses in those receiving opioid infusions. Patients have been provided with an ambulatory infusion device solely to have access to rescue doses that could be administered quickly and parenterally.

The advent of transmucosal formulations may be another method for the quick administration of a supplemental opioid dose. Any highly lipophilic drug may cross nasal or oral mucosal surfaces rapidly enough to meet the needs of patients who require a 'rescue' dose with a prompt onset of action. An intranasal product is commercially available in the United States, but the drug in this formulation, butorphanol, is an agonist–antagonist compound that has little utility in the palliative care setting. Similarly, buprenorphine is available in many countries as a sublingual formulation, but it is a partial agonist with a limited effective dose range. In the United Kingdom, sublingual dextromoramide is often employed as a rescue medication because it is potent and short-acting. An oral transmucosal fentanyl citrate formulation may be useful for breakthrough pain[63] and is undergoing investigation for this indication; this drug has pharmacokinetics consistent with a rapid onset.[64]

The dose of an opioid rescue must reflect the level of the baseline dose. Some clinicians begin with a dose roughly equivalent to 5 to 10 per cent of the total daily opioid intake, which is offered at short intervals, usually between 1 and 3 h, as needed. Another approach in patients receiving 4-hourly oral morphine is to use the same 4-hourly dose for breakthrough pain, administered as frequently as required (or in patients receiving twice daily controlled release morphine, the equivalent 4-hourly dose). Thus, titration of the rescue dose should be viewed as a key principle in the management of breakthrough pain by this approach. In practice, patients with breakthrough pain often are given inadequate doses of rescue medication because the prescribed rescue dose does not keep pace as the regular opioid dose is increased.

Guidelines for the timing of the supplemental dose are similarly empirical. Patients with predictable pain appear to benefit most from a rescue dose taken 30 to 60 min before the precipitating event. Treatment of unpredictable pains with a supplemental dose is most likely to be effective if the medication is administered as soon after the onset of the pain as possible.

Other pharmacological approaches

The importance of the rescue dose in the management of breakthrough pain should not obscure the potential benefits of other pharmacological approaches. For example there is substantial evidence that patients with lancinating neuropathic breakthrough pains may respond well to the administration of an anticonvulsant drug or other specific agent (see Chapter 9.2.5). Similarly, some patients whose breakthrough pain is related to neoplastic invasion of bone or nerve trunk appear to benefit, at least temporarily, from the co-administration of a corticosteroid. Finally, the use of specific drugs to reduce the frequency of precipitating events, such as antitussives, laxatives, antiperistaltic drugs, or agents that reduce muscle spasm, must be considered.

Non-pharmacological approaches

Non-pharmacological approaches may also be useful in patients with breakthrough pain. Physiotherapy, for example, may lessen the musculoskeletal complications that predispose to breakthrough pains, including foreshortening of immobilized muscles, joint ankyloses, and myofascial trigger points. Those patients with severe movement-related pain may be able to benefit from an orthosis that limits the movements that precipitate the pain. Psychological approaches may be used by some patients to reduce the impact of breakthrough pain. Patients with predictable pains may be particularly good candidates for cognitive approaches that assist in preparation for the pain.

It may be necessary to consider invasive approaches in patients with refractory breakthrough pain. Although temporary neural blockade with local anaesthetic seldom provides long-lasting relief from breakthrough pains, successful blocks may suggest benefit from chemical neurolysis. Anaesthetic techniques that provide continuous neural blockade without neurolysis, such as continuous epidural or intrapleural local anaesthetic infusion, may be also useful in the management of some breakthrough pains. Studies are needed to evaluate the safety and efficacy of these invasive approaches to this problem.

Like chemical neurolysis, surgical denervation of the painful part can also be considered in selected patients with refractory breakthrough pain, as illustrated in the case report. Occasional patients may be candidates for primary surgical treatment targeted at the underlying cause. For example, patients with incident pain due to a proximal femoral lesion may obtain excellent analgesia from femoral pinning or hip replacement, and those with intermittent pain from partial bowel obstruction may respond well to surgical decompression. Although the desire for pain relief alone is seldom a strong enough indication to proceed with primary surgical management, the potential analgesic benefits should be considered in clinical decision-making.

Percutaneous injection of methacrylate into bone lesions has recently been under study in a few centres.[65] More experience with this technique is required to establish its place in the management of difficult bone pain.

Conclusion

Given the frequency of breakthrough pain in the palliative care setting, the clinician must be prepared to address the problem with specific interventions. Assessment is a critical first step in this process. Although the use of a rescue dose of analgesic is sufficient in many patients, some will not respond to this intervention and the use of other approaches must be considered. Surveys are needed to clarify the characteristics, causes, and impact of these pains and clinical trials are required to identify the most useful management approaches.

Rectal and bladder pain

Rectal and bladder pain are considered together here. Though there may be obvious differences in presentation and pathophysiology, there are a number of similarities. Tenesmus is 'ineffectual and painful straining at stool or in urinating' and may be difficult to treat, whether it arises from rectum or bladder. Occasional patients experience excruciating spasms of pain in the rectum, or spasms of pain in the bladder or urethra. Less dramatic but more common is the poorly localized perineal pain which may be associated with any intrapelvic malignancy.

Case history: A 63-year-old retired chef presented with a 2-month history of lower abdominal pain and a change in bowel habit. Investigations demonstrated a mass in the rectum and he subsequently had an anterior resection of a 5-cm long rectal tumour. There was no macroscopic evidence of spread at laparotomy, but histological examination showed it to be an adenocarcinoma with local lymph node involvement (Duke's C). His postoperative course was uncomplicated. Adjuvant chemotherapy was advised but he declined.

He remained well for the next 15 months but then developed pain in the perineum extending across the left buttock and down the left posterior thigh. He was unable to sit in comfort for more than 10 to 15 min. The pain in the perineum, buttock, and posterior thigh was described as burning in character. He was constipated and said that he was fearful of opening his bowels as this caused a severe searing perineal and anal pain but at the same time he had a constant feeling of needing to open his bowels.

The distribution of his pain was thought to indicate involvement of S2 to S5 nerve roots, and a CT scan showed a local recurrence of the rectal carcinoma with associated bony erosion of the sacrum. A defuntioning colostomy was considered because of the severe pain on defecation but the patient declined any further surgery.

Coproxamol (paracetamol 325 mg and dextropropoxyphene 32.5 mg) tablets, two 6 hourly, had not controlled his pain. He was started on morphine 10 mg 4 hourly together with dexamethasone 4 mg twice a day, with codanthramer (a combination of danthron and poloxamer) for his constipation. His morphine was titrated to 40 mg 4 hourly. This was well tolerated, apart from some temporary drowsiness, and improved his pain, but he was still unable to sit for long periods. A course of radiotherapy, 30 Gy in 10 fractions over 14 days, was recommended and his morphine was gradually increased.

Following radiotherapy and on a dose of morphine of 100 mg 4 hourly, he was sleeping well and able to sit for up to 1 h with comfort. His steroids were reduced over the next 3 weeks. With the reduction in dexamethasone, a non-steroidal anti-inflammatory drug, naproxen, was added as he began to complain of pain when walking, consistent with the bony erosion of his sacrum. His pain responded well to the naproxen.

Throughout this period the patient and his wife worked through considerable psychological problems. This required frequent exploration, explanation, and reassurance provided mainly by his general practitioner and the community palliative care nurses who visited him at home. His general practitioner who had known him for many years provided valuable insight into the psychodynamics of his family life. The patient had been very dependent all through his adult life. Both he and his wife had consulted their general practitioner frequently over many years for a large variety of somatic symptoms. They had one daughter, who was now married and living away from home, whom they telephoned on average five or six times each day. This dependent behaviour was never challenged by their daughter. They had emigrated from Spain 30 years previously and despite this lapse of time their command of English was very poor, further increasing their dependence on their daughter.

Three months later his pain returned, as did the constant feeling that he needed to open his bowels. A further course of dexamethasone and escalating doses of morphine failed to produce acceptable relief. He had a diagnostic intrathecal block using bupivacaine. This resulted in good relief of the pain and tenesmus and was followed by intrathecal neurolysis with phenol. His pain was successfully relieved and there were no significant side-effects from this procedure.

Over the next 6 weeks his general condition deteriorated (by now he was known to have extensive liver metastases) and he died 2 years after his original presentation.

The problem

In a series of 350 patients admitted to a hospice in the United Kingdom, 11 per cent had intrapelvic pain and in about half of these the pain was associated with cancer of the large bowel.[66] Colorectal cancer is now the second most common cause of cancer-related death in the Western world (after lung cancer). Surgical resection remains the main mode of treatment but, despite improvements in surgical and anaesthetic techniques, 5-year survival rates have changed little over the past 40 years. However, in recent years adjuvant chemotherapy (colon) and radiotherapy (rectum) have been shown to confer survival advantage and decrease the incidence of local recurrence, and are now part of the standard approach to management. Local recurrence is common in patients classified as Duke's C or D at operation and carries a poor prognosis. A small minority of patients with local recurrence may be amenable to further surgery but in the majority (70 per cent) the local recurrence is associated with distant metastases.[67]

Pain is a frequent problem in those with recurrent disease and the most common site of pain is in the rectum (even when it has been removed surgically — so-called 'phantom' rectal pain). The descriptions of the pain in the series described above tended to fall into two categories: either a constant feeling of fullness (a 'tenesmoid' pain) or a severe spasmodic or searing pain.[66]

The incidence of bladder tenesmoid pain and painful bladder spasms in a palliative care patient population has not been accurately documented. They may be associated with bladder or other pelvic tumours, stones or blood clots, infection or retention, or with an indwelling urinary catheter (see Chapter 9.8).

Pathophysiology

Rectal pain rarely occurs in isolation but is usually a component of a complex clinical picture as illustrated by the case history. The patient described here had symptomatic problems which were similar in a number of respects to those of the previous patient, but the underlying pathology was quite different. This emphasizes the need for careful assessment of each patient in order to devise an appropriate and individualized treatment strategy. This man's pain also had both nociceptive and neuropathic components and, in addition, was complicated by the searing anorectal and perineal pain associated with defecation. Added to this was his anxious mental state.

Intermittent anorectal pain of this nature resembles proctalgia fugax and, as in that condition, the precise mechanism underlying the pain is unclear. Spasm of the levator ani and coccygeal musculature or of the anal sphincter itself are probable contributors and may result from direct tumour invasion of the muscles or may be a manifestation of involvement of the sacral plexus. The spasms of pain may occur spontaneously or may be precipitated by a full rectum or defecation.

Rectal tenesmoid pain is usually less severe but is still sufficient to cause considerable distress, and is more likely to be continuous in nature rather than intermittent. It is usually associated with progressively enlarging pelvic tumour and tends to be made worse by anything which increases pressure within the pelvis, such as constipation or sitting.

Since the precise cause of anorectal spasmodic pain or tenesmoid pain is not understood, it is only possible to speculate on their anatomical and physiological basis. Both somatic and autonomic neuronal pathways are implicated. Excessive contraction of smooth muscle or distension of a hollow viscus will give rise to pain transmission in afferent fibres accompanying autonomic nerves, whereas surrounding inflammation may result in pain impulses transmitted in somatic afferents. The anal sphincter has both smooth muscle and skeletal muscle components, and both may be subject to spasm.

Perineal pain which follows abdominoperineal resection of the rectum for the treatment of carcinoma (other than that arising immediately after surgery) is an early sign of recurrence. In a prospective study of 177 patients, Boas and his colleagues describe two underlying causes for perineal pain after rectal amputation.[68] These were either local recurrence of tumour or neuronal deafferentation following surgical excision of the pudendal nerve supply to the lower rectum and anus. Their data indicate that late development of perineal pain is a highly significant indicator of tumour recurrence (but is more likely to respond to analgesic drugs than early onset pain which is more often neuropathic in nature).

Bladder tenesmoid pain is similar to rectal tenesmus and may also be caused by enlarging pelvic tumour arising from within the bladder or from some other pelvic organ. Urinary retention and urinary tract infection may cause similar discomfort but are generally dealt with more easily.

Management: rectal pain

Careful assessment is the basis of effective management. Because rectal pain is difficult to treat pharmacologically, it is particularly important that the temporal characteristics of the pain and aggravating and relieving factors are clearly identified. This will enable simple manoeuvres or changes in behaviour or lifestyle to be instituted to attempt to ameliorate the symptoms before resorting to pharmacological or other treatments for the pain.

The patient described was fearful of opening his bowels because this precipitated excruciating pain. In this situation it is particularly important to pay close attention to keeping the stool soft and maintaining a regular bowel motion.

This patient had considerable psychological problems complicating his pain symptoms. It would be misleading to make generalizations about psychological components of anorectal pain, but this association of symptoms is not unusual and needs always to be kept in mind and dealt with appropriately.

Antitumour therapy

Pelvic radiotherapy should be considered in patients with symptomatic recurrent colorectal cancer, and in other patients with intrapelvic malignancies where tumour mass or infiltration is causing pain or other symptoms. Chemotherapy is also occasionally helpful in this situation.

Analgesics

Conventional analgesics used in a conventional manner are the basis of analgesic management of rectal pain. This patient illustrates a recurring theme of this chapter which is that patients with advanced cancer invariably present complicated clinical problems involving both nociceptive and non-nociceptive pain. In this case the nociceptive (bone and tumour) pain and the neuropathic pain in the perineum, buttock, and thigh were initially well controlled with opioid analgesics. Other strategies were subsequently required for the movement-related bone pain, the dysaesthetic perineal pain, and the spasmodic anorectal pain.

Adjuvant drugs

The burning dysaesthetic pain involving the perineum, left buttock, and left posterior thigh in this patient was presumed to result from compression of the sacral nerve roots by tumour or from malignant infiltration of the nerves and nerve roots of the sacral plexus. The management of such neuropathic pain is outlined in the early part of this chapter. In this patient corticosteroids were used to good effect.

The mode of action of corticosteroids when used in this way is presumed to be essentially mechanical—nerve compression is relieved by a reduction in inflammatory oedema and hyperaemia surrounding a tumour or within an infiltrated nerve bundle (though other systemic effects of corticosteroids may contribute[69]). This means that if a trial of steroids is successful, treatment with pelvic radiotherapy should be considered as a next step.

In the patient described, the combination of opioid analgesics, corticosteroids, and then radiotherapy controlled his pain. After some 3 months his pain returned and at this stage his complaints were dominated by a continuous midline perineal pain (which was no longer burning in nature) and severe anorectal spasms. Two approaches to management were considered: further pharmacological manipulation using adjuvants, as described earlier, or invasive anaesthetic techniques.

Analysis of these pains suggested that the perineal pain was partly nociceptive (caused by enlarging tumour within the tight tissue planes of the pelvis) and partly neuropathic (resulting from damage to the sacral plexus or nerve roots). The muscle spasm pains were presumed to be mainly smooth muscle generated, but with a possible skeletal muscle cramp-like component. This constellation of different pains with different underlying mechanisms made the choice of the next treatment strategy particularly difficult. It was felt that time was short and that a good response to 'conventional' adjuvants was unlikely (particularly as far as the spasmodic pain was concerned). Other possible drug treatments were considered.

Psychotropic drugs, and in particular the phenothiazines, have been advocated for rectal tenesmus and spasm. However, the evidence of efficacy is entirely anecdotal and there is no rationale to support such use.[70] In our experience these drugs offer no specific benefits in this indication. Phenothiazines may have a non-specific role as anxiolytic sedatives in patients with troublesome anorectal pain. However, benzodiazepines are generally preferable for such use in patients with advanced cancer because they are much better tolerated. Benzodiazepines have an additional benefit in that they relax skeletal muscles by inhibiting spinal polysynaptic reflexes (though this effect is probably unlikely to make a major contribution to the management of anorectal pain).

The belladonna alkaloids atropine and hyoscine and related synthetic and semisynthetic antimuscarinic drugs, such as dicyclomine and flavoxate, have a direct smooth muscle relaxant effect. The problem with this group of drugs is that when used in doses which have a significant spasmolytic effect they invariably produce troublesome anticholinergic adverse effects, and this limits their usefulness. There is little documented information about the use of these drugs to treat rectal tenesmus or spasm but they are invariably given a trial as treatment options become progressively limited.

Calcium channel blocking agents have been used as antispasmodic agents[71] and diltiazem has specifically been reported to relieve the pain of proctalgia fugax.[72] As yet no controlled studies have been published, but these reports open up another potential therapeutic option for a symptom which may be unresponsive to any currently available remedy.

When considering the use of adjuvant drugs, and in particular the psychotropics and anticonvulsants, an important point to make is that polypharmacy and iatrogenic problems are major deterrents to their use in this patient population. In patients with neuropathic and other non-nociceptive pains the balance between unwanted drug effects and analgesia from conventional analgesics tends towards unwanted effects. The addition of adjuvant analgesics with potent side-effect-producing potential may make a barely manageable situation quite impossible. These factors must be carefully weighed and the application of antidepressants, anticonvulsants, and other psychotropics should perhaps be a little more cautious than is usual at present. Dosage should start low and, as with morphine, there may be wide interindividual variation in the therapeutic level that may be required. Thus, the dose may need to be titrated through a considerable range for some patients.

For the patient described here it was felt that an anaesthetic procedure should be considered as the next step.

Anaesthetic procedures

Sympathetic dependent pain is a frequent component of neuropathic pain and, as discussed above, the sympathetic nervous system may be specifically involved in mediating rectal pain. In a recently reported series of patients with rectal tenesmoid pain, bilateral chemical lumbar sympathetic block produced complete relief in 10 out of 12 patients.[73] This procedure is discussed in more detail in Chapter 9.2.6, but it is a safe technique associated with low morbidity and should be considered at an early stage in the management of rectal tenesmus or any other pelvic visceral pain. A similar but more selective technique of superior hypogastric plexus block may also be effective in the management of pelvic pain[74] (see Chapter 9.2.6).

Midline perineal pain resulting from pelvic malignancy may be effectively relieved by a neurolytic saddle block. Traditionally, this has been carried out with a hyperbaric agent such as phenol[75] and it is claimed that in experienced hands this can be accomplished without affecting the bladder. However, a recently reported series of nine patients treated with intrathecal phenol for perianal and perineal pain highlights the limitations of this technique.[76] The duration of pain relief was short (17.8 days) and there was a significant incidence of serious adverse effects, including permanent urinary retention in two patients.

Cryoanalgesia also may be effective in the relief of perineal pain.[77] In this technique a needle cryoprobe is inserted through the sacrococcygeal ligament and into the sacral canal. Repeated freeze cycles produce anaesthesia of the lower sacral nerve roots. Though less likely to cause adverse effects than a phenol subarachnoid block, this technique is less predictable and the duration of analgesia (on average 1 month) is generally shorter than that obtained with a phenol block (though this is very variable as indicated in the study cited above). The choice of procedure will depend to a large extent on the available local expertise and facilities.

The patient described underwent a diagnostic block with local anaesthetic, followed by a phenol injection. His pains —both the perineal pain and the anorectal spasm —were considerably improved.

Management: bladder pain

The emphasis of this section is on the management of bladder tenesmoid pain and bladder spasm.

The first step is to identify potentially remediable causes of bladder pain. Infection or direct irritation by catheter, tumour, debris, or blood clot should all be dealt with appropriately. Where nothing can be done about the underlying cause, or where symptoms persist despite appropriate action, symptomatic remedies are applied.

Analgesics

Once again a conventional approach should be adopted as the baseline, progressing from simple analgesics to opioids.

Adjuvants

Corticosteroids may have a place where symptoms are related to tumour mass, but generally have a limited application in bladder pain management.

NSAIDs may be effective in the management of detrusor instability caused by increased bladder activity.[78] This use was prompted by the observation that the prostaglandins PGE_2 and F2α stimulate strips of human bladder muscle *in vitro*.[79] Thus, there is a theoretical basis for using NSAIDs in the management of bladder pain, particularly spasm, because of their prostaglandin-synthetase-inhibitory action. NSAIDs also have intrinsic analgesic actions. A trial of an NSAID (in conjunction with opioid analgesics) is the first option in the management of bladder tenesmus or spasm.

Other pharmacological treatments are generally unsatisfactory. The smooth-muscle relaxant drugs dicyclomine and flavoxate have been mentioned above and are frequently employed, usually with little success, as are the postganglionic anticholinergic agents propantheline and emepronium bromide (now withdrawn in the United Kingdom). The last two are more likely to cause anticholinergic adverse effects such as dry mouth, blurred vision, and urinary retention. The theoretical basis for the use of all these atropine-like drugs is that they block the parasympathetic control of the bladder. Thus, they can lower intravesicular pressure, increase capacity, and reduce the frequency of urinary bladder contractions.[80]

Oxybutynin hydrochloride is a tertiary amine similar to dicyclomine and flavoxate which has been shown to be effective in a variety of unstable bladder conditions.[81] Topical administration by instillation into the bladder may enhance its beneficial effects whilst reducing systemic anticholinergic effects[82] (and this route may also be preferable for administration of other drugs with similar actions such as atropine and phentolamine[83]). A more recent quaternary ammonium compound, trospium, is also claimed to have a more favourable therapeutic ratio after systemic administration with less anticholinergic effects because it does not easily cross the blood–brain barrier.[84] Unfortunately, with all of these drugs it is easier to demonstrate significant effects on objective urodynamic parameters than symptomatic relief in patients with painful bladder spasm.

Pyridium (phenazopyridine) and methylene blue are azo dyes which are said to have analgesic effects on bladder and urinary tract mucosa. These drugs have been used in a non-specific way to treat dysuria and bladder and urethral pain, but there is little information about their efficacy. Neither is now available in the United Kingdom.

In recent years there have been reports of the analgesic effects of intravesical local anaesthetics[85] and capsaicin[86] in various painful bladder conditions, and the former is certainly worth trying in patients with painful bladder or urethral spasm associated with an indwelling catheter. Bupivacaine, 20 ml of 0.25 per cent instilled for 20 min, is recommended[87] but has not been subjected to investigation in controlled trials.

Anaesthetic procedures

No anaesthetic procedure has proved itself to be particularly useful in the management of bladder tenesmus or bladder spasm, though spinal administration of opioids may be preferable to systemic analgesics.[88]

Conclusion

Unlike the situation in most cancer pain, drugs play a relatively minor role in the management of rectal and bladder tenesmus and spasm. A variety of disparate drug groups are employed but most are ineffective and their limitations should be recognized. A multimodal approach using conventional analgesics and adjuvants and non-drug treatments will usually produce some amelioration of these symptoms but the results are often unsatisfactory. Whilst these types of pain represent a very small proportion of those encountered in cancer patients, this is an area ripe for future improvements in practice.

Abdominal pain

Pancreatic pain is considered here as an example of visceral abdominal pain which may be difficult to manage with conventional analgesics.

Case history: A 49-year-old businessman had been an insulin-dependent diabetic since the age of 18. He presented with malaise, loss of appetite, weight loss of 10 lb (4.5 kg) over 3 months, and vague abdominal discomfort, which was worse after eating and was later associated with a gnawing ache in the lower thoracic region in the midline. The patient tried resting after meals but he noted that the pain was sometimes intensified when he was recumbent, with relief on sitting up. He became jaundiced and a CT scan revealed a mass in the head of the pancreas. Laparotomy confirmed the diagnosis of pancreatic cancer and multiple small hepatic metastases were noted. A choledochojejunostomy was carried out.

Postoperative abdominal pain was controlled with parenteral morphine. Coeliac plexus block was performed on the sixth day with total relief of back pain but he continued to experience epigastric pain. The patient was converted to oral morphine plus ibuprofen and was subsequently discharged home.

Over the next 3 weeks his morphine requirements increased. He was treated with palliative radiotherapy together with 5-fluorouracil. Ibuprofen was discontinued and prednisolone, megestrol, and methylphenidate were added to the regimen. The patient enjoyed satisfactory pain control for 6 weeks and felt sufficiently well to take a sea voyage. However, during the last week of his holiday, pain increased. Upon return he was readmitted with severe epigastric pain. He alternated between periods of confusion and agitation and excessive sedation secondary to increments in morphine therapy. He was converted to a continuous subcutaneous infusion of hydromorphone. Methylphenidate was discontinued and the steroid dose was reduced. He was still confused 2 days later but did not appear to be in pain. He gradually recovered his mental faculties and was switched back to oral morphine but his general condition deteriorated and he died 5 weeks later.

The problem

The incidence of adenocarcinoma of the exocrine pancreas has increased in the last 40 years. For unknown reasons, this upward trend has stabilized in the past 5 years,[89] whilst survival rates have improved primarily as a result of better surgical management of the small group of patients with resectable disease.[90] Nevertheless, 80 to 90 per cent of patients with pancreatic cancer will die within a year of diagnosis, and only 3 to 5 per cent will be alive 5 years after diagnosis.[91]

Pain is common but not inevitable, occurring in 75 to 90 per cent of patients at some stage, often at presentation.[92] Pain from carcinoma of the pancreas usually responds to conventional analgesic drugs. Control may be achieved but the scenario often rapidly changes, requiring consideration of other modalities of therapy in addition to analgesics.

Pathophysiology: abdominal pain

Abdominal pain often puzzles the clinician because the pathophysiology of visceral nociception is poorly defined. Thus, perplexing presentations and responses to therapy are common. Abdominal pain is by nature more difficult to assess than cutaneous pain. The patient readily identifies cutaneous sensation, localizes it with precision, and describes it in terms which separate pain from other cutaneous sensations. We do tend not to confuse itch or cutaneous pressure with pain.

In contrast, abdominal pain, particularly in its early chronic stages, is almost always vaguely located and difficult to describe. This is not surprising as the main task of visceral neurones relates to digestion. Except for satiety and rectal sensations, visceral neurones normally mediate digestive events which do not require conscious perception.[93] Visceral pain is often associated with other unpleasant sensations which, while not painful, cause great distress. The patient may say, 'I think I have pain, but what bothers me is the feeling of fullness in my stomach and nausea. It makes me feel very weak'. The patient's confusion and uncertainty is mirrored by that of neurophysiologists. Arguments continue about whether specific bowel nociceptors exist and the mechanisms of referred pain.

Stimuli that elicit pain in other parts of the body may not be nociceptive when applied to the viscera. For example intestinal cutting, burning, or point pressures will not produce acute pain. Electrical stimulation (an unnatural process which is probably not clinically relevant), bowel or duct distension (a very relevant stimulus), and application of various chemicals will cause pain in normal subjects. However, if a viscus is inflamed, stimuli which are normally non-painful, such as pressure, will cause pain which is accentuated if the stimulus is applied for a period of time over a large tissue area.

Thus, we have a model where summation occurs and pain sensations which are poorly appreciated at the onset become agonizing if pain remains unrelieved. As visceral pain intensifies, it tends to localize.

Localization often occurs because of disease extension to a somatically innervated tissue such as the parietal peritoneum. However, distension studies in normal subjects show that localization will occur even in the absence of somatic nerve involvement. The classic sites of localization are well identified for many organs and disorders. Gallbladder pain localizing in the right upper quadrant is one example. Bladder pain presenting in both the hypogastric (suprapubic) area and sacrum, ulcer pain in the epigastrium, renal colic, and testicular torsion provide other commonly recognized patterns.

Involvement of somatic nerves (defined as those serving the parietal peritoneum, muscles surrounding the abdomen, associated bone and connective tissue, and skin) will help localize the site of disease. An example is the classic localization of pain in the right lower quadrant following inflammation of the parietal peritoneum in association with an inflamed appendix.

Pain will also be referred to somatic structures without direct involvement of somatic nerves. Perhaps the best recognized example of this mechanism is the occurrence of ipsilateral shoulder and scapula pain due to phrenic nerve stimulation by diaphragmatic irritation. Other common patterns include right flank pain following renal colic and pain in the T10–L2 back area with pancreatic disease.

The nature of referred pain is not clearly established. Pertinent factors include the possible presence of 'dichotomizing' sensory nerves with endings in both visceral and somatic tissues and, at the spinal cord level, wide ramifications of visceral nerves whose axons also interact with neurones receiving somatic nerve input. As a result, the higher brain centres assign pain to the region from which sensory inputs are normally received.

Based on the excellent review of visceral pain by Ness and Gebhart,[94] several other features of visceral pain which have clinical relevance can be listed.

1. Visceral pain is very commonly associated with activation of autonomic reflexes which in turn can evoke highly unpleasant but confusing symptoms (such as nausea and weakness).
2. The quality or intensity of pain does not differentiate visceral pain arising from different anatomical sites.
3. Resonant 'vicious circles' probably exist whereby pain arising from a distended, inflamed viscus promotes abnormal gut function which in turn accentuates pain. For example a partially obstructed bowel may induce smooth muscle contractions which in turn increase distension and pain. Clinically, dull, abdominal pain interspersed with crampy, severe, episodic pain may be described.
4. The onset of visceral pain may lag behind the stimulus as sensitization of sensory nerves plus persistence of the disease process must be present before pain is recognized.
5. Hyperalgesia may be present over body surfaces to which visceral pain is referred.

For the clinician the message is clear—keep in mind that abdominal pain places you in a region where surprises are common.

Cancer-induced abdominal pain

Intra-abdominal neoplasm can cause pain through a variety of mechanisms. Growth within a closed space (such as the liver) can stretch a capsule. A tumour partially obstructing the bowel can distend an adjacent loop of bowel with consequent local inflammation, release of pain-producing products of inflammation, and secondary occurrence of smooth muscle spasm or inco-ordinate action, which adds a crampy pain component. Tumours directly invading parietal surfaces can be painful. If tumours invade ducts such as the common bile duct or the large pancreatic duct, inflammation, distension, and consequent pain will occur. Within the pancreas the problem is sometimes compounded by the release outside the ducts of pancreatic enzymes, further inflammation, and increased pain.

Regardless of the anatomical site, a combination of distortion, inflammation, smooth muscle abnormality, and ultimately neuronal hypersensitivity is commonly associated with cancer.

Abdominal pain—AIDS

Abdominal pain which is often non-specific in nature and not clearly related to intra-abdominal pathology is also encountered in AIDS patients.[95] Here the aetiology of pain is even less clear than pain associated with cancer. Abdominal cramps are seen in association with enteritis and ileitis.[96] On occasion retroperitoneal adenopathy or tumour involvement of the bowel wall, in particular Kaposi's sarcoma, may be found. However, Kaposi tumours are usually asymptomatic.[97] Sclerosing cholangitis may cause upper abdominal pain, while pancreatitis may occur in patients receiving pentamidine, didanosine, or dideocytidine.[96] Often a specific cause cannot be determined; neuropathies are common in AIDS patients, but a syndrome of painful visceral neuropathy has not been clearly delineated.

Management

Dull aching pain will occur in most patients with carcinoma of the pancreas, with a higher incidence in those with involvement of the pancreatic body or tail. The pain is usually in the epigastrium but diffuse non-localizing abdominal pain or radiation to the back is common. Our patient showed a feature sometimes indicative of pancreatic pain—an increase of pain on recumbency with improvement on changing positions.

Anorexia, general malaise, and 'indigestion' are common accompanying symptoms. Depression is frequently associated with pancreatic cancer with a disproportionate incidence compared with an abdominal tumour with similar presentation, for example stomach cancer.[98] While the patient's awareness of the presence of an undiagnosed serious illness no doubt contributes to the inordinate rate of depression in pancreatic cancer, it also probably represents a true paraneoplastic syndrome of unknown aetiology. All these factors need to be taken into account alongside specific attention to the pain.

Antitumour therapy

There is no evidence that the lives of pancreatic cancer patients are prolonged by chemotherapy or radiotherapy. Potential curative surgery is now an option for 20 to 25 per cent of patients in some series,[91] but cure remains an uncommon event.

Does therapy influence pain? Choledochojejunostomy is commonly performed to relieve bile duct pressure and obstruction, while gastrojejunostomy is sometimes carried out to prevent or alleviate duodenal obstruction. Both palliative procedures can obviously improve patient comfort and delay or obviate catastrophe. Their specific effect on pain is not defined, although many surgeons feel that relief of duct obstruction will also improve pancreatic pain.

Chemotherapy by itself is not analgesic in this condition, but 5-fluorouracil, which was the most commonly employed agent for gastrointestinal cancers, has radiosensitizing actions in the laboratory. It was often used in combination with radiation therapy. The evidence at hand suggests that 5-fluorouracil combined with radiotherapy is superior to radiotherapy alone, relieving pain in 30 to 40 per cent of patients for an uncertain period.[99] The patient may pay a price for pain relief with increased nausea and anorexia. Recently, gemcytabine in a single controlled trial proved superior to 5-fluorouracil (which by itself was ineffective) in relieving pain in a subset of patients (see Chapter 9.1.1).

In the case of the patient described, therapy was reasonably well tolerated and he enjoyed good pain control following radiation treatment. However, during this time he was also treated with steroids and followed closely in the clinic and at home with frequent titration of analgesics.

Analgesics

Oral opioids are the long-term anchor of pancreatic pain management. They can be used at the same time as interventional techniques such as coeliac plexus block or radiotherapy. If these last procedures are effective, opioids can readily be tapered.

The patient received conventional oral opioid therapy with good effect throughout his illness. Morphine contributed to his sedation and confusion but it is likely that this episode was exacerbated by adjuvant drugs. When the patient presented in a confusional state, he was switched from oral morphine to subcutaneous hydromorphone because subcutaneous opioids can be readily titrated and provide constant opioid levels without the 'peaks and valleys' of oral therapy, while opioid rotation may improve confusional states (see below). Hydromorphone was used in place of morphine and it was anticipated that good pain control would be achieved at lower equivalent doses of hydromorphone with a consequent reduction in opioid side-effects.

It is uncertain whether this manoeuvre actually helped the patient. His pain did improve, his mind cleared, and he was able to take oral morphine once again. Probably the simplification of his adjuvant medication plus, possibly, resolution of a superimposed acute pain event were primarily responsible for the improvement.

The ideal sequence for using opioids *vis-à-vis* coeliac plexus block or antitumour therapy has not been determined in clinical trials. Our practice follows the sequence outlined in Table 3. We prefer to carry out a coeliac plexus block at the onset of severe pancreatic cancer pain as the results of the blocks are reasonable, we believe that associated opioid therapy may be more easily maintained at low doses, and the length of pain relief spans the trajectory of illness in this disorder with a very short survival time after diagnosis. We are more selective in patients with other types of upper abdominal cancer where results are less consistent and where life expectancy may be longer.

This patient's confusion in the latter weeks of his life raises the question of treatment with spinal opioids. Theoretically, the use of epidural opioids would reduce the risk of opioid associated sedation and confusion.[100] Whether their use is associated with reduced end stage delirium is not known, although the hypothesis is eminently reasonable. Randomized trials comparing spinal and subcutaneous opioids in the management of abdominal pain are needed.

Adjuvant drugs

NSAIDs have a proven benefit in pancreatic cancer pain.[101] Patients should receive a trial of an NSAID, if not contraindicated.

Table 3 Guidelines for the management of upper abdominal cancer pain

1. Consider a coeliac plexus block
   - At laparotomy
   - Percutaneous
2. Use concomitant analgesic therapy
   - Opioids
   - NSAIDs
   - Corticosteroids
3. Consider trial of chemoradiotherapy (careful framing of objectives and assessments)
4. Adjuvant drugs
   - Methylphenidate—if oversedation
   - Antidepressants—use not proven
     —help both pain and depression?
5. Adjuvant non-pharmacological techniques
   - Behavioural therapy
   - Imagery
   - Hypnosis
   - Distraction
6. Epidural opioids in centres with established programmes

Alternatively, corticosteroids may be used for short-term pain control (but the possibility of steroid-induced diabetes needs to be kept in mind).

The dose of morphine required for pain control in this patient caused distressing sedation which responded to methylphenidate. The methylphenidate, along with the corticosteroids, may have contributed to subsequent dysphoria and confusion.

Pancreatic cancer patients have an increased incidence of depression, and one might think that antidepressants may relieve both the depression and associated pain. This is an intriguing concept which has not been tested. In view of the high incidence of often-missed depression,[98] the concomitant use of antidepressants with analgesic properties should be considered in patients with pancreatic pain. Kelsen and colleagues suggest that the use of a simple visual analogue scale for mood state correlates highly with more complex instruments for measuring depression. The use of this scale in concert with visual analogue pain scales should be considered in routine practice.[92]

The patient also received a progestational agent, megestrol, not for pain but for anorexia. He benefited from this drug with an increase in appetite and stabilization of weight for a 6 to 8-week period.

Anaesthetic procedures: coeliac plexus block

The pain fibres from the pancreas travel primarily with the sympathetic afferents. Therefore, they will gather in the coeliac plexus before dispersing as part of the superior and middle thoracic splanchnic nerves entering the spinal cord. A neurolytic block of the coeliac plexus is a standard technique in the management of pancreatic pain and other upper abdominal pain associated with malignancy.[102] In expert hands, destruction of the coeliac plexus causes few major acute or long-term harmful sequelae. Postural hypotension may occur transiently because of sympathetic nerve damage; a postblock deafferentation syndrome has occasionally been recognized, probably due to the spread of the injected alcohol to somatic nerves. Rarely, serious neurological sequelae (paraplegia, leg weakness) occur, again due to inadvertent diffusion of alcohol or phenol beyond the plexus. Sympathetic pancreatic nerve stimulation increases enzyme release. Theoretically, patients may actually benefit from reduced stimulus to pancreatic enzyme production and associated pancreatitis.

Randomized controlled trials studying percutaneous coeliac plexus block are uncommon. A recent attempt at meta-analysis[103] summarized 24 studies but only one randomized controlled trial (with an enrolment of only 20 patients) which compared coeliac plexus block with analgesic drugs.[104] The meta-analysis of all 24 studies reported 'good to excellent pain relief' in 89 per cent of patients immediately postprocedure, with partial to complete maintenance of pain control for 90 per cent of patients at 3 months postprocedure. While postprocedure transient hypotension or diarrhoea were common, major adverse effects occurred in only 2 per cent of patients.

If percutaneous blocks are usually successful, should the surgeon block the coeliac plexus at laparotomy? Lillemoe describes a randomized trial comparing operative block using 50 per cent alcohol and placebo.[105] This study reports not only on the effects of a block on established pain but also on the role of coeliac block in preventing pain. The patients who had an alcohol block had a significant reduction in pain scores and a delay in the subsequent return of pain. If free of pain at the time of the alcohol block patients remained free of pain for a significant period compared with the saline (placebo) group. They required lower doses of opioids if pain eventually developed. Lillemoe estimated that the necessary operative exposure added 5 min to the time of surgery; an increase in postoperative morbidity did not occur.

Our patient had only partial relief of pain following coeliac plexus block; the posterior component disappeared but an anterior abdominal pain was untouched. Incomplete relief may relate to an incomplete block. Alternatively, as some vagal afferents also transmit pain impulses,[106] perhaps vagal transmission was responsible for our patient's residual pain. The block may have successfully facilitated pain control achieved with opioids and adjuvant drugs.

As is the case with all surgical interventions, results are 'operator dependent'. The excellent results for coeliac block reported in the literature arise presumably from experienced groups. In the author's opinion, patients requiring laparotomy for pancreatic cancer will benefit from contact with surgeons skilled and interested in carrying out intraoperative palliative procedures. For the increasing numbers of patients who have a diagnosis of inoperable cancer established without laparotomy, if they have moderate to severe pain, early consideration of a percutaneous block is desirable.

New approaches

A trial of oral pancreatic enzymes relieved pain in 50 per cent of patients in an open non-randomized trial.[107] Giving trypsin may reduce hyperstimulation of the pancreas by cholecystokinin, thus reducing local inflammation. These results need confirmation.

The results of cytotoxic chemotherapy are disappointing and have stimulated an interest in hormonal therapy for pancreatic cancer. Treatment with octreotide (a synthetic somatostatin analogue) may confer a survival advantage without producing objective tumour shrinkage, to patients with a variety of advanced gastrointestinal cancers.[108] Somatostatin may inhibit sensory neurones. A trial of epidural somatostatin in postoperative pain demonstrated analgesic effects,[109] although another study of subcutaneous octreotide failed to demonstrate a general analgesic effect.[110] In this series one patient with postprandial pancreatic pain did respond.

Conclusion

Pancreatic pain represents one of the few situations in cancer pain management where an invasive procedure, coeliac plexus block, should be considered at an early stage. Upper abdominal pain of other aetiology may also benefit from this block. However, as always, this procedure represents only one part of a comprehensive strategy including anticancer therapy, analgesics, adjuvant drugs, and non-drug treatments.

Pain in the delirious patient

'When sorrows come they come not single spies, but in battalions'.[111] So it seems to family and staff alike when faced with the vexing problem of a delirious patient, often on high doses of medication for management of severe pain, who is restless, moaning, and yet unable to pin-point the root of his distress. Nerves become frayed, families are angry, and each therapeutic approach appears to move one into checkmate.

Case history: A 32-year-old woman presented with recurrent carcinoma of the ovary with widespread metastases throughout the abdomen. Since diagnosis 18 months prior to admission, she had received repeated courses of chemotherapy and two surgical interventions for relief of small bowel obstruction. Six months prior to admission she developed an inoperable small bowel obstruction. Subsequently, she was maintained at home on parenteral nutrition together with a venting percutaneous gastrostomy.

Prior to her final admission to hospital, in addition to chronic intermittent abdominal pain, the patient had developed increasing pain in the left back and hip secondary to lumbar nerve root involvement. At home the patient was receiving subcutaneous hydromorphone delivered via an Edmonton injector.[112] She was admitted to hospital for pain control.

In hospital, the dose of hydromorphone required to control pain increased until she was receiving 65 mg/h. Nevertheless, the patient remained in poor pain control and she became agitated, confused, developed paranoid ideation, and myoclonus. Her cries and moans were thought to be caused by pain, which stimulated further increases in the dose of hydromorphone. The patient had modest alteration in liver function tests but her renal function was normal and there was no obvious metabolic reason for her agitation.

The patient was switched to morphine by continuous intravenous infusion at a rate of 75 mg/h (23 per cent of the equivalent dose of hydromorphone). Within 24 h the myoclonus and agitation cleared and the patient was lucid and her pain was well controlled. Three days after switching to morphine, it was decided that the patient was over-sedated and the rate of morphine infusion was decreased to 60 mg/h and subsequently, on the same day, to 50 mg/h. At this dose her pain was controlled and she was alert but sleepy. Three days later, a secondary infection was thought to be present. The patient remained comfortable but the morphine infusion was increased to 65 and then 90 mg/h. The patient died within the following 24 h.

The problem

What are the components of this patient's problems? First, she is clearly delirious but there are no apparent metabolic causes for her delirium. There are no clinical signs of infection. Her delirium appeared to worsen as the doses of drugs, which usually have a sedative effect, reached high levels—a paradoxical effect which is well known, if not well understood.

The syndrome usually occurs in palliative care patients with multiple comorbid conditions, often receiving many other drugs which may have psychotropic effects. Usually there is not a single identifiable cause for confusional states; more likely, patients will exhibit multiple contributory factors. These include the following.

Opioid hyperexcitability

Possibly all commonly used opioids can induce a state of central hyperexcitability, sometimes associated with delirium. Pethidine (meperidine) is the most likely opioid to induce this syndrome. It certainly can also occur in association with morphine or hydromorphone therapy.[51,113] Pentazocine, a mixed agonist–antagonist opioid with κ-stimulatory properties, may produce psychotomimetic effects. The relative risks associated with other less commonly employed opioids is not clearly established.

Theories on opioid hyperexcitability, some of which have clinical relevance, include:

1. Multiple receptor stimulation. κ-Receptor stimulation can cause dysphoria.[114] This may account for psychotomimetic effects induced by pentazocine which is a κ-partial agonist. Some opioids may interact with σ and phencyclidine receptors. The σ-receptor is not a classical opioid receptor, having different pharmacological properties and anatomical distribution.[115] For example naloxone does not antagonise σ effects. While σ- and phencyclidine receptors mediate different properties, including dysphoria, most drugs binding to one site also bind to the other.[115] Even within a receptor class, such as the μ-receptors, different subclasses mediating analgesia and adverse effects may exist and may be variably activated.[116]

2. Under certain laboratory conditions, opioids may have direct excitatory actions but the clinical relevance of this observation remains to be determined.[117]

3. Opioids generally act as inhibitors of neurotransmission.[118] Therefore, they could inhibit other inhibitory neurotransmitters, thus setting the stage for seizure enhancement and delirium.

4. Opioids or their metabolites (see below) may have variable effects mediating the activity of glutamate, a neuroexcitatory neurotransmitter, through *N*-methyl-D-aspartate receptors.[119]

5. Opioid metabolites are associated with hyperexcitability states. At doses readily reached in clinical practice, norpethidine (a pethidine metabolite) causes central nervous system excitation.[120] Similar metabolites with excitatory effects could exist for other opioids but, if present, probably only show an effect

at high concentrations. A point of considerable clinical relevance is that as there is not complete cross tolerance between opioids, central nervous system side-effects may diminish or clear when opioids are switched.

In summary, the cause of opioid hyperexcitability is not known. A single common pathway probably does not exist; rather, opioids and their metabolites affect multiple receptors with ultimate effects varying from patient to patient.

Metabolic alterations

Many types of chemical imbalance are associated with the onset of a confusional state. These are discussed in other chapters of this textbook. One cause of metabolic abnormalities, renal insufficiency, is of particular importance as it commonly influences levels of a drug and its metabolites, putting the patient at increased risk for the development of a confusional state. For example patients with renal failure who are receiving morphine or hydromorphone will experience a sharp increase in glucuronide metabolites which are normally excreted by the kidney.[20] As a number of these metabolites are active, and as the primary compounds and metabolites of other drugs used in palliative care are also dependent upon excretion by the kidney, impairment of renal function is a common aetiological factor in delirious patients.

Drug–drug interactions

Most palliative care patients are receiving multiple classes of drugs. Many of them will have effects on the central nervous system. Presumably, observed patient cognitive function and behaviours depend upon a complex dynamic interplay of numerous endogenous neurotransmitters. Not surprisingly, perturbation of these systems following addition of multiple pharmaceuticals with unpredictable effects on finely adjusted neurotransmitter balance may have unpredictable adverse outcomes. Some examples are:

1. Anticholinergic drugs interfere with normal mentation. Patients with a long-standing loss of cortical function will be at risk for delirium when agents in this category are used. Thus, combinations of antidepressants and opioids must be carefully monitored in patients with an increased risk of delirium.

2. Delirium is a well known effect of corticosteroids.

3. Methylphenidate is used to reduce the sedative effects of opioids in patients where this side-effect is troublesome. It, together with other amphetamine-like drugs, will induce a psychotic state in a small number of cancer patients. Occasionally a paranoid reaction occurs or a pre-existing unrecognized delirium will be intensified.[121]

4. Benzodiazepines may have a paradoxical effect in some patients. In delirious patients this may occur, in part, because the sedative action of a benzodiazepine interferes with a delirious patient's already thin link with reality. In neurotransmitter terms, the phenomenon is not clearly understood.

5. Mexiletine and other systemic local anaesthetics are increasingly used for the management of neuropathic pain, often in combination with other drugs with central nervous system effects. These agents have variable effects on the central nervous system; the author has encountered otherwise unaccountable acute paranoid reactions and confusional states in patients receiving both antidepressants and mexiletine.

Table 4 A check list for potentially correctable confusion

Does the patient have:

1. Increased intracranial pressure
    - Tumour
    - Trauma
    - Hydrocephalus
2. Hypoxia
3. Infection
4. Drugs—particularly note
    - Anticholinergic drugs
    - Benzodiazepines
    - Chemotherapy
    - Central nervous system stimulants
    - H_2 blockers
    - Opioids
    - Phenothiazines
    - Steroid agents
5. Chemical imbalance, e.g.
    - Hypercalcaemia
    - Hyponatraemia
    - Uraemia
    - Hepatic failure
    - Hypoglycaemia or ketoacidosis
    - Endocrine disorders (e.g. hypothyroidism)
6. Psychotic reaction to illness
7. Avitaminosis
8. Haematological disorders
    - Severe anaemia (note possibility of vitamin B_{12} deficiency)
    - Coagulopathy
    - Very high white blood cell (WBC) count
9. Elimination disorders
    - Constipation
    - Urinary retention
10. Depression
11. History of alcohol or other drug use suggesting possibility of drug withdrawal

A final reminder—probably any centrally acting drug may contribute to delirium in susceptible patients.

Table 4 provides a check list for potentially correctable confusion.

Even after review, however, the cause of confusion in many patients is not apparent—delirium not related to an obvious cause is common in the last days of life.[122] Is this disorder influenced by iatrogenic factors not yet appreciated? While direct comparisons are not possible, Osler's report of end of life events in 500 Johns Hopkins patients contained few examples of agitated delirium.[123]

Management

In the patient described, it was concluded that the principal cause of delirium was hydromorphone in view of its rapid onset in a young woman who had previously been lucid, had no detectable septic or metabolic abnormalities, and who did not have a space occupying lesion in her brain.

A crucial difficulty in the assessment of a delirious patient receiving high doses of analgesics is determining whether or not the patient is in pain. The physicians caring for the patient thought that pain was not well controlled, as the patient moaned and cried out in distress. Hence the decision to escalate drug doses.

In retrospect, these manifestations were probably symptoms of delirium, but how can one separate the agitation caused by uncontrolled pain from delirium? A gold standard test does not exist and the patient cannot tell us the nature of her distress. We are dependent upon a careful physical examination to rule out an acute new cause of pain and discomfort. The history is also critical. Is the onset of agitation acute and correlated with escalation in drug doses? Was there a clear history of escalating pain prior to the onset of delirium? Does the patient have a history of brain metastases? Did the patient have a recent fall? Sepsis is often subtle and difficult to detect in patients with advanced cancer, particularly if they are on steroids. Could sepsis contribute to the problem?

General principles

A systematic approach to the management of the problem of mixed pain and delirium is proposed in this section.

1. Review correctable factors contributing to delirium. Use an aetiology check list (Table 4) to ensure that the review is comprehensive. In particular, if the event is acute, look for infectious causes, hidden trauma, hypoxia, or a recent metabolic alteration. While not causative, faecal impactation or bladder distension will increase agitation.

2. Simplify drug therapy as much as possible and, in particular, remove those with anticholinergic properties. Also, if possible, lower the doses of corticosteroids and discontinue NSAIDs (because of possible interactions affecting the metabolism of other drugs).

3. Take time to discuss the problem with family members and nursing colleagues. Family members will be reassured to learn that you believe that the patient is probably not appreciating severe pain because of mental clouding, a view beginning to have literature support.[124] They will also gain confidence from your calm manner and plan for systematic analysis and management of the problem. Nursing members of the team will need to be fully aware of your approach in order to reinforce your discussions with the family and to follow your plan for drug titration explicitly.

4. Institute the general principles of delirium management as outlined in Section 15. These measures will involve the family members and friends as part of the treatment team. The delirious patient is separated from his environment which is regarded as hostile and alien. The level of contact with reality fluctuates but can be enhanced by constant attention from family members or friends. In some circumstances, clinicians have noted the calming effect of music associated with important past events in the patient's life. Those with religious faith may respond to the presence of their pastor. Volunteers, if available, can share the bedside visiting with family members and nursing attendants.

5. Review the patient's hydration status. While the advantages and disadvantages of hydration are the subject of intense debate at the present time,[125,126] probably all would agree that dehydration with its consequent effects on renal clearance can increase the risk of a confusional state in a patient receiving psychoactive agents, particularly if they have active metabolites. Bruera and his colleagues have recently observed a sharp decrease in the incidence of confusional states in patients on a palliative care unit when a policy of adequate hydration is associated with assessments leading to an early diagnosis of a confusional state and the use of a rotational opioid policy.[127]

6. If the patient is on an opioid, change the type and dose. This manoeuvre was rapidly and dramatically successful in the patient described. Degrees of relative opioid cross tolerance have not been established but animal work suggests that opioid-induced adverse events clearly vary among opioid classes and even within the same opioid receptor class.[128,129] A switch in opioids with consequent amelioration of adverse effects and reduction in required opioid dose has been reported in a number of case studies.[51,130,131]

In patients who develop the need for rapid opioid dose increases, the wisdom of the statement that opioids do not have a ceiling requires further thought. At very high opioid doses, a myriad of poorly understood pharmacological events take place. We recommend switching opioids when rapidly escalating doses of an opioid associated with changes in mentation or myoclonus occur.

The total opioid dose which the patient received after hydromorphone was discontinued was only equivalent to 20 to 25 per cent of the previous day's opioid consumption. Nevertheless, the patient was sedated (no doubt in part as a reaction to prior excitability), in good pain control, and free of myoclonus. Indications for dose adjustments following opioid switch vary from authority to authority; an equivalent dose somewhere between 50 and 75 per cent of the previous morphine equivalent dose is commonly recommended. This figure is based on evidence gathered from patients or volunteers receiving short courses of low-dose opioids. These equivalencies may not hold in delirious patients receiving high doses of opioids. Careful clinical assessment of the selected new opioid dose is required. In a patient on opioids with an agitated delirium the opioid should be switched to an alternate at approximately 25 per cent of the equivalent dose.

7. Delirium is not a classic result of μ agonist activity. Use naloxone with caution. Naxolone will probably not reverse delirium and could accentuate the problem by blocking the μ agonist function of an opioid, resulting in increased pain, reducing sedative μ effects, and allowing full sway for the unfettered excitatory actions of an opioid if non-naloxone sensitive receptors (such as the σ-receptor) are involved. The authors prefer not to use naloxone in delirious patients, reserving its use for patients who are overly sedated with life-threatening respiratory depression.

8. Consider changing the route of administration. If the patient is intermittently confused on bolus doses of an opioid administered periodically, improvement may be noted when the same dose is administered by continuous infusion. The subcutaneous route is preferred as the site is unobtrusive and less likely to be wrenched out by a delirious patient (if it is lost, the site can be readily replaced). A continuous infusion levels out the 'peak and trough' effect characteristic of intermittent drug therapy.

9. Units experienced in the use of spinal opioids believe that delirium is less likely to occur following epidural administration. This technique is difficult to apply in many delirious patients and may be less effective if the patient is already on high systemic doses. A change to a spinal route can be considered in selected patients. The employment of spinal opioids should follow a formal protocol in units with expertise and provision for follow-up.

10. Monitor patients at risk. A number of instruments currently exist for evaluating delirium; a recent review by Smith *et al.*

provides a critique for selection of instruments.[132] Bruera's group use the Folstein Mini Mental Status questionnaire to assess, on a regular basis, the cognitive status of patients on their unit. Identification of cognitive impairment leads to a review of drugs, hydration, and, if the patient is on an opioid, consideration of a switch to an alternate opioid.

Drug treatments

Neuroleptics are considered in detail in Section 15. They are the mainstay of therapy for delirium, helping to control its manifestations while diagnostic considerations are entertained and potentially causative drugs are removed. Haloperidol has fewer anticholinergic effects than the phenothiazines. Methotrimeprazine is a reasonable choice for a bed-bound patient where sedation is welcome. Its use in ambulant patients can be a problem because it causes postural hypotension and may contribute to falls. It is a neuroleptic with demonstrated analgesic properties. Chlorpromazine is similar but less sedative.

Benzodiazepines can be employed to supplement the effects of opioids on pain and neuroleptics on delirium. They may further diminish the patient's link with his environment and increase delirium,[133] but their sedative properties are often needed to provide the patient, family, and staff with needed rest. They are not analgesic agents, but they may blunt the frightening memory of distress.

In states of severe delirium and pain, in the patient near death, use sedation to control symptoms. One regimen employs midazolam (2–5 mg subcutaneously followed by titrated doses 1–4 mg/h by continuous subcutaneous infusion). This agent can be mixed in the same syringe with an opioid.[134,135]

The additive effects of opioids in combination with benzodiazepines may slow respiration. This potential side-effect must be balanced against patient/family distress; observation and titration will protect the patient.

Conclusion

In contrast with the first edition of this textbook, the current account suggests the institution of preventative protocols for identifying and combating confusional states at the earliest possible moment, thus negating the development of the full-blown delirious state. Diagnostic and therapeutic procedures may abort the full manifestation of a devastating endstage event—agitated delirium. When a confusional state is present, the employment of a careful, systematic approach to identifying and correcting the correctable, simplification of drug management, the involvement of family, nursing, and other professional staff, and the recognition of the value of non-pharmacological techniques is recommended. Anxiety levels will be high; families and colleagues benefit from a calm assured manner and reasoned application of investigation and therapy.

References

1. Ventafridda V, Tamburini M, Caraceni A, De Conno F, Naldi F. A validation study of the WHO method for cancer pain relief. *Cancer,* 1987; **59**: 851–6.
2. Zech DFJ, Grond S, Lynch J, Hertel D, Lehmann KA. Validation of World Health Organisation guidelines for cancer pain relief. A 10-year prospective study. *Pain,* 1995; **63**: 65–7.
3. Addington-Hall J, McCarthy M. Dying from cancer: results of a national population-based investigation. *Palliative Medicine,* 1995; **9**: 295–305.
4. Arner S, Meyerson BA. Lack of analgesic effect of opioids on neuropathic and idiopathic forms of pain. *Pain,* 1988; **33**: 11–23.
5. Twycross RG. Opioid analgesics in cancer pain: current practice and controversies. *Cancer Surveys,* 1988; **7**: 29–53.
6. Bowsher D. Neurogenic pain syndromes and their management. *British Medical Bulletin,* 1991; **47**: 644–66.
7. Portenoy RK, Foley KM, Inturrisi CE. The nature of opioid responsiveness and its implications for neuropathic pain: new hypotheses derived from studies of opioid infusions. *Pain,* 1990; **43**: 273–86.
8. Morley JS, Miles JB, Wells JC, Bowsher D. Paradoxical pain. *Lancet,* 1992; **340**: 1045.
9. Woolf CJ. Intrathecal high dose morphine produces hyperalgesia in the rat. *Brain Research,* 1981; **209**: 491–5.
10. Yaksh TL, Harty GJ. Pharmacology of the allodynia in rats evoked by high dose intrathecal morphine. *Journal of Pharmacology and Experimental Therapeutics,* 1987; **244**: 501–7.
11. Sjogren P, Jonsson T, Jensen N-H, Drenck N-E, Jensen TS. Hyperalgesia and myoclonus in terminal cancer patients treated with continuous intravenous morphine. *Pain,* 1993; **55**: 93–7.
12. Bowsher D. Paradoxical pain. *British Medical Journal,* 1993; **306**: 473.
13. Hanks GW. Morphine pharmacokinetics and analgesia after oral administration. *Postgraduate Medical Journal,* 1991; **67** (Suppl 2): S60–3.
14. Smith MT, Watt JA, Cramond T. Morphine-3-glucuronide—a potent antagonist of morphine analgesia. *Life Sciences,* 1990; **47**: 579–85.
15. Gong Q-L, Hedner J, Bjorkman R, Hedner T. Morphine-3-glucuronide may functionally antagonise morphine-6-glucuronide induced antinociception and ventilatory depression in the rat. *Pain,* 1992; **48**: 249–55.
16. Labella FS, Pinsky C, Havlicek V. Morphine derivatives with diminished opiate receptor potency show enhanced central excitatory activity. *Brain Research,* 1979; **174**: 263–71.
17. Dickenson AH. Neurophysiology of opioid-poorly-responsive pain. In: Hanks GW, ed. Palliative medicine: problem areas in pain and symptom management. *Cancer, Surveys,* 1994; **21**: 5–16.
18. Morley JS, Watt J. The significance of M3G in the use of morphine. *Annual Scientific Meeting of the Pain Society of Great Britain and Ireland, Eastbourne April 1995.* Abstracts 47.
19. Hewett K, Dickenson AH, McQuay HJ. Lack of effect of morphine-3-glucuronide on the spinal antinociceptive action of morphine in the rat: an electrophysicological study. *Pain,* 1993; **53**: 59–63.
20. Osborne RJ, Joel SP, Grebenik K, Trew D, Slevin M. The pharmacokinetics of morphine and morphine glucuronides in kidney failure. *Clinical Pharmacology and Therapeutics,* 1993; **54**: 158–67.
21. Kearney MK. Experience in a hospice with patients suffering cancer pain. In: Doyle D, ed. *Opioids in the Treatment of Cancer Pain.* Royal Society of Medicine Services International Congress and Symposium Series. No 146. London: RSM Services Ltd, 1990; 69–74.
22. Moulin DE, Foley KM. A review of a hospital-based pain service. In: Foley KM, Bonica JJ, Ventafridda V, eds. *Advances in Pain Research and Therapy,* Second International Congress on Cancer Pain. New York: Raven Press, 1990; **16**: 413–28.
23. Bruera E, MacMillan D, Hanson J, MacDonald RN. The Edmonton staging system for cancer pain: preliminary report. *Pain,* 1989; **37**: 203–10.
24. Mercandante S, Maddaloni S, Roccella S, Salvaggio L. Predictive factors in advanced cancer pain treated only by analgesics. *Pain,* 1992; **50**: 151–5.
25. Portenoy RK. Issues in the management of neuropathic pain. In: Basbaum A, Besson J-M, eds. *Towards a New Parmacotherapy of Pain.* New York: John Wiley and Sons, 1991: 393–416.
26. American Psychiatric Association. *Diagnostic and Statistical Manual of Mental Disorder,* 4th edn. Washington, D.C.: American Psychiatric Association, 1994.
27. McQuay HJ, Jadad AR, Carroll D, *et al.* Opioid sensitivity of chronic pain: a patient-controlled analgesia method. *Anaesthesia,* 1992; **47**: 757–67.
28. Jadad AR, Carroll D, Glynn CJ, Moore RA, McQuay HJ. Morphine

responsiveness of chronic pain: double-blind randomised crossover study with patient-controlled analgesia. *Lancet*, 1992; **339**: 1367–71.

29. Cherny NI, Thaler HT, Friedlander-Klar H, *et al.* Opioid responsiveness of cancer pain syndromes caused by neuropathic or nociceptive mechanisms: a combined analysis of controlled single dose studies. *Neurology*, 1994; **44**: 857–61.
30. Rowbotham MC, Reisner L, Fields HL. Both intravenous lidocaine and morphine reduce the pain of postherpetic neuralgia. *Neurology*, 1991; **41**: 1024–8.
31. Mao JJ, Price DD, Mayer DJ. Experimental mononeuropathy reduces the antinociceptive effects of morphine: implications for common intracellular mechanisms involved in morphine tolerance and neuropathic pain. *Pain*, 1995; **61**: 353–64.
32. Urban BJ, France RD, Steinberger DL, Scott DL, Maltbie AA. Long-term use of narcotic/antidepressant medication in the management of phantom limb pain. *Pain*, 1986; **24**: 191–7.
33. Zenz M, Strumpf M, Tryba M. Long-term opioid therapy in patients with chronic nonmalignant pain. *Journal of Pain and Symptom Management*, 1992; **7**: 66–77.
34. Galer BS, Coyle N, Pasternak GW, Portenoy RK. Individual variability in the response to different opioids: report of five cases. *Pain*, 1992; **49**: 87–91.
35. Portenoy RK. Neuropathic pain. In: Portenoy RK, Kanner RM, eds. *Pain: Theory and Practice.* Philadelphia: FA Davis, 1996.
36. Devor M. The pathophysiology of damaged nerve. In: Wall PD, Melzack R, eds. *Textbook of Pain*, 3rd edn. New York: Churchill Livingstone, 1994: 79–100.
37. Bennett GJ. Neuropathic pain. In: Wall PD, Melzack R, eds. *Textbook of Pain*, 3rd edn. New York: Churchill Livingstone, 1994: 201–24.
38. Devor M. Mechanisms of neuropathic pain following peripheral injury. In: Basbaum A, Besson J-M, eds. *Towards a New Pharmacotherapy of Pain.* New York: John Wiley and Sons, 1991: 417–40.
39. Woolf CJ, Ghompson SWN. The induction and maintenance of central sensitization is dependent on *N*-methyl-D-aspartic acid receptor activation: implications for the treatment of post-injury pain hypersensitivity states. *Pain*, 1991; **44**: 293–9.
40. Willis WD. Central plastic responses to pain. In: Gebhart GF, Hammond DL, Jensen TS, eds. *Proceedings of the 7th World Congress on Pain.* Seattle: IASP Press, 1994: 301–24.
41. Mersky H, Bogduk N, eds. *Classification of Chronic Pain*, 2nd edn. Seattle: IASP Press, 1994.
42. Schwartzman RJ, McLellan TL. Reflex sympathetic dystrophy: a review. *Archives of Neurology*, 1987; **44**: 555–61.
43. Dellemijn PLI, Fields HL, Allen RR, McKay WR, Rowbotham MC. The interpretation of pain relief and sensory changes following sympathetic blockade. *Brain*, 1994; **117**: 1475–87.
44. Raja SN, Treede RD, Davis KD, Campbell JN. Systemic alpha-adrenergic blockade with phentolamine: a diagnostic test for sympathetically-maintained pain. *Anesthesiology*, 1991; **74**: 691–8.
45. Verdugo RJ, Ochoa JL. Sympathetically-maintained pain. I. Phentolamine block questions the concept. *Neurology*, 1994; **44**: 1003–10.
46. Fine PG, Roberts WJ, Gillette RG, Child TR. Slowly developing placebo responses confound tests of intravenous phentolamine to determine mechanisms underlying idiopathic chronic low back pain. *Pain*, 1994; **56**: 235–42.
47. Schott GD. Visceral afferents: their contribution to 'sympathetic dependent' pain. *Brain*, 1994; **117**: 397–413.
48. Roberts WJ. A hypothesis on the physiological basis for causalgia and related pains. *Pain*, 1986; **24**: 297–311.
49. Cleeland CS. Assessment of pain in cancer: measurement issues. In: Foley KM, Bonica JJ, Ventafridda V, eds. *Advances in Pain Research and Therapy.* Second International Congress on Cancer Pain. New York: Raven Press, 1990; **16**: 47–55.
50. Gonzales GR, Elliot KJ, Portenoy RK, Foley KM. The impact of a comprehensive evaluation in the management of cancer pain. *Pain*, 1991; **47**: 141–4.
51. MacDonald N, Der L, Allan S, Champion P. Opioid hyper-excitability: the application of alternate opioid therapy. *Pain*, 1993; **53**: 353–5.
52. Kirvela O, Nieminen S. Treatment of painful neuromas with neurolytic blockade. *Pain*, 1990; **41**: 161–5.
53. Arner S, Arner B. Differential effects of epidural morphine in the treatment of cancer-related pain. *Acta Anesthesiologica Scandinavica*, 1983; **29**: 32–6.
54. Sjoberg M, Appelgren L, Einarsson S, *et al.* Long-term intrathecal morphine and bupivacaine in 'refractory' cancer pain. *Acta Anesthesiologica Scandinavica*, 1991; **35**: 30–43.
55. Eisenach JC, DuPen S, Dubois M, Miguel R, Allin D, The Epidural Clonidine Study Group (USA). Epidural clonidine analgesia for intractable cancer pain. *Pain*, 1995; **61**: 391–400.
56. Gybels JM, Sweet WH. *Neurosurgical Treatment of Persistent Pain.* Basel: Karger, 1989.
57. Arbit E. *Management of Cancer-Related Pain.* Mount Kisco, N.Y.: Futura, 1993.
58. Fishman B, Loscalzo M. Congnitive-behavioral interventions in the management of cancer pain: principles and applications. *Medical Clinics of North America*, 1987; **71**: 271–88.
59. Portenoy RK, Hagen NA. Breakthrough pain: definition, prevalence and characteristics. *Pain*, 1990; **41**: 273–82.
60. Hanks GW. The pharmacological treatment of bone pain. *Cancer Surveys*, 1988; **7**: 87–101.
61. Jacox A, Carr DB, Payne R, *et al. Management of Cancer Pain. Clinical Practice Guideline No. 9.* ANCPR Publication No. 94–0592. Rockville, MD: Agency for Health Care Policy and Research, U.S. Department of Health and Human Services, Public Health Service, 1994.
62. American Pain Society. *Principles of Analgesic Use in the Treatment of Acute Pain and Cancer Pain*, 3rd edn. Skokie, Ill.: American Pain Society, 1992.
63. Fine PG, Marcus M, DeBoer AJ, *et al.* An open label study of oral transmucosal fentanyl citrate (OFTC) for the treatment of breakthrough cancer pain. *Pain*, 1991; **45**: 149–55.
64. Streisand J, Varvel JR, Stanski DR, *et al.* Absorption and bioavailability of oral transmucosal fentanyl citrate. *Anesthesiology*, 1991; **75**: 223–31.
65. Kaemmerlen P, Thiesse P, Bouvard H, Biron P, Mornex F, Jonas P. Vertebroplastic percutanée dans le traitement des métastases. Technique et résultats. *Journal of Radiology*, 1989; **70**: 557–62.
66. Baines M, Kirkham SR. Cancer pain. In: Wall PD, Melzack R, eds. *Textbook of Pain*, 2nd edn. Edinburgh: Churchill Livingstone, 1989: 590–7.
67. Willett CG, Tepper GE, Cohen AM, Orlow E, Welch CE. Failure patterns following curative resection of colonic carcinoma. *Annals of Surgery*, 1984; **200**: 685–90.
68. Boas RA, Schug SA, Acland RH. Perineal pain after rectal amputation: a 5-year follow-up. *Pain*, 1993; **52**: 67–70.
69. McQuay H. Pharmacological treatment of neuralgic and neuropathic pain. *Cancer Surveys*, 1988; **7**: 141–59.
70. Hanks GW. Psychotropic drugs. *Clinics in Oncology*, 1984; **3**: 135–51.
71. Castell DO. Calcium channel blocking agents for gastrointestinal disorders. *American Journal of Cardiology*, 1985; **55**: 210B–13B.
72. Boquet J, Moore N, Lhuintre JP, Boismare F. Diltiazem for proctalgia fugax. *Lancet*, 1986; **i**: 1493.
73. Bristow A, Foster JMG. Lumbar sympathectomy in the management of rectal tenesmoid pain. *Annals of the Royal College of Surgeons of England*, 1988; **70**: 38–9.
74. Plancarte R, Amescua C, Patt RB, Aldrete JA. Superior hypogastric plexus block for pelvic cancer pain. *Anesthesiology*, 1990; **73**: 236–9.
75. Gibb D, *et al.* Modern concepts in the treatment of chronic pain. *Current Therapeutics*, 1976; **17**: 33–43.
76. Lynch J, Zech D, Grond S. The role of intrathecal neurolysis in the treatment of cancer-related perianal and perineal pain. *Palliative Medicine*, 1992; **6**: 140–5.
77. Evans PJD, Lloyd JW, Jack TM. Cryoanalgesia for intractable perineal pain. *Journal of the Royal Society of Medicine*, 1981; **74**: 804–9.

78. Cardozo LD, Stanton SL. A comparison between bromocriptine and indomethacin in the treatment of detrusor instability. *Journal of Urology*, 1980; **123**: 399–401.
79. Abrams P, Feneley R. The action of prostaglandins on the smooth muscle of the human urinary tract in vitro. *British Journal of Urology*, 1976; **47**: 909–15.
80. Brown JH. Atropine, scopolamine and related antimuscarinic drugs. In: Gilman AG, Rall TW, Nies AS, Taylor P, eds. *The Pharmacological Basis of Therapeutics*, 8th edn. New York: Pergamon, 1990: 150–65.
81. Kirkali Z, Whitaker RH. The use of oxybutynin in urological practice. *International Urology and Nephrology*, 1987; **19**: 385–91.
82. Brendler CB, Radebaugh LC, Mohler JL. Topical oxybutynin chloride for relaxation of dysfunctional bladders. *Journal of Urology*, 1989; **141**: 1350–2.
83. Ekstrom B, Andersson K-E, Mattiasson A. Urodynamic effects of intravesical instillation of atropine and phentolamine in patients with detrusor hyperactivity. *Journal of Urology*, 1993; **149**: 135–8.
84. Madersbacher H, Stohrer M, Richter R, Burgdorfer H, Hachen HJ, Murtz G. Trospium chloride versus oxybutynin: a randomised double-blind, multicentre trial in the treatment of detrusor hyperreflexia. *British Journal of Urology*, 1995; **75**: 452–6.
85. Holmang S, Aldenborg F, Hedelin H. Extirpation and fulguration of multiple superficial bladder tumour recurrences under intravesical lignocaine anaesthesia. *British Journal of Urology*, 1994; **73**: 177–80.
86. Barbanti G, Maggi CA, Beneforti P, Baroldi P, Turini D. Relief of pain following intravesical capsaicin in patients with hypersensitive disorders of the lower urinary tract. *British Journal of Urology*, 1993; **71**: 686–91.
87. Kaye P. *A to Z of Hospice and Palliative Medicine*. Northampton: EPL Publications, 1992: 184.
88. Olshwang D, Shapiro A, Perlberg S, Magora F. The effect of epidural morphine on ureteral colic and spasm of the bladder. *Pain*, 1984; **18**: 97–101.
89. Devesa SS, Blot WJ, Stone BJ, *et al*. Recent cancer trends in the United States. *Journal of the National Cancer Institute*, 1995; **87**: 75–83.
90. Warshaw AL. Pancreatic surgery: a paradigm for progress in the age of the bottom line. *Archives of Surgery*, 1995; **130**: 240–6.
91. Lillemoe KD. Current management of pancreatic cancer. *Annals of Surgery*, 1995; **221**: 133–48.
92. Kelsen DP, Portenoy RK, Thaler HT, *et al*. Pain and depression in patients with newly diagnosed pancreas cancer. *Journal of Clinical Oncology*, 1995; **13**: 748–55.
93. Mayer EA. Gut feelings: what turns them on? *Gastroenterology*, 1995; **108**: 927–40.
94. Ness TJ, Gebhart CF. Visceral pain: a review of experimental studies. *Pain*, 1990; **41**: 167–234.
95. Schofferman J. Pain: diagnosis and management in the palliative care of AIDS. *Journal of Palliative Care*, 1988; **4**: 46–50.
96. O'Neill WM, Sherrard JS. Pain in human immunodeficiency virus disease: a review. *Pain*, 1993; **54**: 3–14.
97. Friedman SL, Wright TL, Altman DF. Gastrointestinal Kaposi's sarcoma in patients with acquired immunodeficiency syndrome. Endoscopic and autopsy findings. *Gastroenterology*, 1985; **89**: 102–8.
98. McDaniel JS, Musselman DL, Porter MR, *et al*. Depression in patients with cancer. Diagnosis, biology and treatment. *Archives of General Psychiatry*, 1995; **52**: 89–99.
99. Moertel CE, *et al*. Therapy of unresectable pancreatic carcinoma: a randomised comparison of high dose radiation alone, moderate dose radiation and high dose radiation plus 5-FU. *Cancer*, 1981; **48**: 1705–10.
100. Cousins MJ, Plummer JL. Spinal opioids in acute and chronic pain. In: Max M, Portenoy R, Laska E, eds. *Advances in Pain Research and Therapy*. New York: Raven Press, 1991; **18**: 472.
101. Moertel CG, *et al*. Aspirin and pancreatic cancer pain. *Gastroenterology*, 1971; **60**: 552–3.
102. Hanna M, Peat SJ, Woodham MJ, Latham J, Gouliaris A, Di Vadi P. The use of coeliac plexus blockade in patients with chronic pain. *Palliative Medicine*, 1989; **4**: 11–16.
103. Eisenberg E, Carr DB, Chalmers TC. Neurolytic coeliac plexus block for treatment of cancer pain: a meta-analysis. *Anesthesia and Analgesia*, 1995; **80**: 290–5.
104. Mercadante S. Celiac plexus block versus analgesics in pancreatic cancer pain. *Pain*, 1993; **52**: 187–92.
105. Lillemoe MD, Cameron JL, Kaufman HS, *et al*. Chemical splanchnicectomy in patients with unresectable pancreatic cancer. A prospective randomized trial. *Annals of Surgery*, 1993; **217**: 447–57.
106. Mayer EA, Gebhart GF. Basic clinical aspects of visceral hyperalgesia. *Gastroenterology*, 1994; **107**: 271–93.
107. Ihse I, Permerth J. Enzyme therapy and pancreatic pain. *Acta Chirurgica Scandinavica*, 1990; **156**: 281–3.
108. Cascinu S, Del Ferro E, Catalano G. A randomized trial of octreotide vs best supportive care only in advanced gastrointestinal cancer patients refractory to chemotherapy. *British Journal of Cancer*, 1995; **71**: 97–101.
109. Taura P, Planella V, Balust J, *et al*. Epidural somatostatin as an analgesic in upper abdominal surgery: a double-blind study. *Pain*, 1994; **59**: 135–40.
110. De Conno F, Saita L, Ripamonti C, *et al*. Subcutaneous octreotide in the treatment of pain in advanced cancer patients. *Journal of Pain and Symptom Management*, 1994; **9**: 34–8.
111. Shakespeare W. *Tragedy of Hamlet, Prince of Denmark*, Act IV, Scene V.
112. Bruera E, MacMillan K, Hanson J, MacDonald N. The Edmonton injector: a simple device for patient-controlled subcutaneous analgesia. *Pain*, 1991; **44**: 167–9.
113. Tiseo PJ, Thaler HT, Lapin J, *et al*. Morphine-6-glucuronide concentrations and opioid-related side-effects: a survey in cancer patients. *Pain*, 1995; **61**: 47–54.
114. Pfeiffer A, Brantl V, Herz A, Emrich HM. Psychotomimesis mediated by kappa opiate receptors. *Science*, 1986; **233**: 774–6.
115. Sonders MS, Keana JFW, Weber E. Phencyclidine and psychotomimetic sigma opiates: recent insights into their biochemical and physiologic sites of action. *Trends in Neuro-Sciences*, 1988; **11**: 37–40.
116. Jang Y, Yoburn BC. Evaluation of receptor mechanisms mediating fentanyl analgesia and toxicity. *European Journal of Pharmacology*, 1991; **197**: 135–41.
117. Crain SM, Shen K F.Opioids can evoke direct receptor-mediated excitatory effects in sensory neurons. *Trends in Pharmacological Sciences*, 1990; **11**: 77–81.
118. Dickinson AM. Mechanisms of the analgesic actions of opiates and opioids. *British Medical Bulletin*, 1991; **47**: 690–702.
119. Chen L, Huang LM. Sustained potentiation of NMDA receptor-mediated glutamate responses through activation of protein kinase C by a μ opioid. *Neuron*, 1991; **7**: 319–26.
120. Kaiko RF, Foley KM, Grabinski PY, *et al*. Central nervous system excitatory effects of meperidine in cancer patients. *Annals of Neurology*, 1983; **13**: 180–5.
121. Bruera E, Brenneis C, Paterson AH, MacDonald N. Use of methylphenidate as an adjuvant to narcotic analgesics in patients with advanced cancer. *Journal of Pain and Symptom Management*, 1989; **4**: 3–6.
122. Bruera E, Miller L, McCallion J, Macmillan K, Krefting L, Hanson J. Cognitive failure in patients with terminal cancer: a prospective study. *Journal of Pain and Symptom Management*, 1992; **7**: 192–5.
123. Osler W. *Science and Immortality*. The Ingersoll Lecture, 1904. Boston: Houghton Millen, 1905.
124. Bruera E, Fainsinger RL, Miller MJ, Kuehn N. The assessment of pain intensity in patients with cognitive failure: a preliminary report. *Journal of Pain and Symptom Management*, 1992; **7**: 267–70.
125. Fainsinger RL, MacEachern T, Miller MJ, Bruera E, *et al*.. The use of hypodermoclysis for rehydration in terminally ill cancer patients. *Journal of Pain and Symptom Management*, 1994; **9**: 298–302.
126. Dunphy K, Finlay N, Rathbone G, Gilbert J, Hicks F. Rehydration in palliative and terminal care: if not—why not? *Palliative Medicine*, 1995; **9**: 221–8.
127. Bruera E, Franco JJ, Maltoni M, Watanabe S, *et al*. Changing pattern of agitated impaired mental status in patients with advanced cancer: association with cognitive monitoring, hydration, and opiate rotation. *Journal of Pain and Symptom Management*, 1995; **10**: 287–91.

128. Russell RD, Chang K-J. Alternated delta and mu receptor activation: a strategem for limiting opioid tolerance. *Pain*, 1989; **36**: 381–4.
129. Moulin DE, Ling GSF, Pasternak GW. Unidirectional analgesic cross-tolerance between morphine and levorphanol in the rat. *Pain*, 1988; **33**: 233–9.
130. Sjogren P, Jensen NH, Jensen TS. Disappearance of morphine-induced hyperalgesia after discontinuing or susbstituting morphine with other opioid agonists. *Pain*, 1994; **59**: 313–16.
131. de Stoutz ND, Bruera E, Suarez-Almazor M. Opioid rotation for toxicity reduction in terminal cancer patients. *Journal of Pain and Symptom Management*, 1995; **10**: 378–84.
132. Smith MJ, Breitbart WS, Platt MM. A critique of instruments and methods to detect, diagnose and rate delirium. *Journal of Pain and Symptom Management*, 1995; **10**: 35–77.
133. Marcantonio ER, Juarez G, Goldman L, Mangione CM, *et al.* The relationship of postoperative delirium with psychoactive medications. *Journal of the American Medical Association*, 1994; **272**: 1518–22.
134. McNamara P, Minton M, Twycross RG. Use of midazolam in palliative care. *Palliative Medicine*, 1991; **5**: 244–9.
135. Bottomley DM, Hanks GW. Subcutaneous midazolam infusion in palliative care. *Journal of Pain and Symptom Management*, 1990; **5**: 259–61.

9.2.11 Orthopaedic principles and management

Charles S.B. Galasko

Palliate is defined in *The Concise Oxford Dictionary* as 'alleviate (disease) without curing'. This applies to much of orthopaedic surgery, but a detailed description of all types of orthopaedic palliative care is beyond the scope of this book.

Rheumatoid arthritis is an incurable, systemic disease which is best treated by a multidisciplinary team. The role of the rheumatologist is to make the diagnosis and supervise the medical management, which may be complex and is aimed at reducing the systemic and inflammatory components. The occupational therapist tries to improve the quality of life of the affected patient by providing suitable aids. The physiotherapist tries to maintain joint movement and prevent contractures. The role of the orthopaedic surgeon is to reduce pain, improve mobility, and improve the quality of life by a variety of surgical techniques. These include: flexor synovectomy to relieve symptoms of a carpal tunnel syndrome if exuberant synovium is compressing the median nerve within the carpal tunnel; dorsal synovectomy in an attempt to prevent attrition ruptures of the extensor tendons and 'dropped' fingers; forefoot arthroplasty with excision of the metatarsal heads to relieve forefoot pain, which often severely limits the walking ability of rheumatoid patients with severe involvement of the metatarsophalangeal joints; and joint replacement. Total hip and knee replacements are very successful operations in patients with rheumatoid arthritis. The operation relieves pain in the vast majority of patients but it is not without its complications and the artificial joints will not last for ever. Shoulder and elbow replacement have been introduced more recently. They also relieve pain in the vast majority of patients. Following a successful joint replacement, the patient regains a reasonable range of movement, although this is less than normal. Metacarpophalangeal joint replacement is another common operation carried out in rheumatoid arthritis, and arthrodesis may be required in other areas. One of the complications of rheumatoid arthritis is cervical instability and, where this is symptomatic, arthrodesis of the affected levels of the cervical spine may be required.

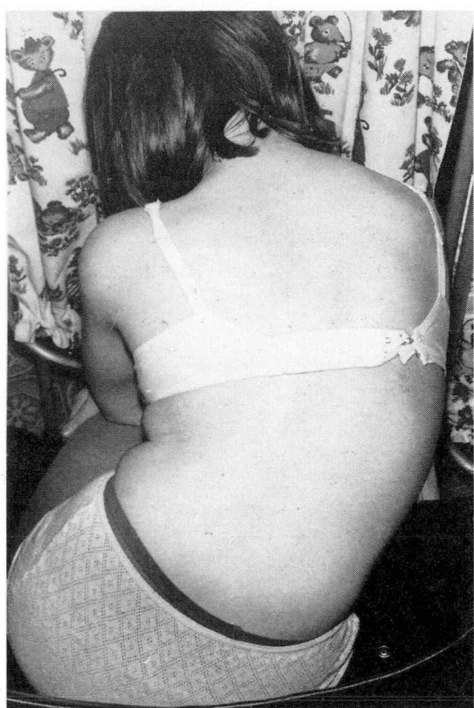

Fig. 1 Patient with Friedreich's ataxia who had developed a collapsing scoliosis and secondary pelvic obliquity. She was unable to sit for more than 30 min because of pain under her right buttock. Following stabilization of her spine, the scoliosis and pelvic obliquity were corrected and sitting became comfortable.

Another large group of patients with incurable illnesses are those with neuromuscular disorders including cerebral palsy, spina bifida, Duchenne's muscular dystrophy, spinal muscle atrophy, etc. Many of these patients develop secondary deformities as a result of: muscle imbalance; unequal growth of abnormal muscle and normal underlying bone resulting in progressive shortening of the muscle during growth; and the effect of gravity where the underlying musculature is extremely weak—for example in the trunk, resulting in scoliosis (Fig. 1); and in the foot resulting in a variety of deformities. These secondary deformities affect the quality of life of the patient. An equinovarus deformity may affect the gait of a patient who otherwise would be independently mobile; a pes cavus deformity may make walking painful; dislocation of the hip secondary to muscle imbalance may be painful and may affect sitting balance; and progressive neuromuscular scoliosis may result in progressive pelvic inequality which may initially make sitting uncomfortable (Fig. 1) and subsequently impossible, and which may predispose to dislocation of the hip and affect lung function in some patients. Kurz *et al.*[1] estimated that in Duchenne's muscular dystrophy there was a 4 per cent reduction in vital capacity for every 10° in scoliosis. The present author has estimated that in spinal muscle atrophy there was a 4.7 per cent reduction in vital capacity for every 10° increase in the scoliosis. [67]The orthopaedic surgeon can do much to improve the quality of life of patients with neuromuscular disease, by trying to prevent the secondary development of deformities and surgical correction of the deformities should they occur.[2,3]

Metabolic bone disease (including Paget's disease of bone, osteoporosis, and osteomalacia) is extremely common. Paget's disease of bone may be associated with secondary arthritis, particularly of the hip, and stress fractures. Osteoporosis predisposes to fractures, most commonly in the proximal femur, distal radius, and spine. In many instances the underlying metabolic disease can be treated medically, for example by the use of bisphosphonates in Paget's disease of bone. The orthopaedic surgeon can do much to improve the quality of life of these patients by treating the complications of these disorders, for example by: joint replacement in patients with Paget's disease and secondary osteoarthritis of the hip; prophylactic stabilisation of a pagetoid bone with impending fracture, internal fixation of pagetoid stress fractures, and osteoporotic proximal femoral fractures; and replacement arthroplasty of some osteoporotic subcapital fractures.

Although less common than the above, the orthopaedic surgeon is also involved in the palliative care of patients with malignant disease. It is this aspect of palliative orthopaedics that will be discussed in greater detail in this chapter.

Primary bone tumours

The treatment depends on the extent of the neoplasm. If it is localized, the emphasis is on radical resection and chemotherapy (the type of resection depending on the type, site, and local dissemination of the tumour) in an attempt to obtain a cure. If the tumour has disseminated, or is inoperable, the treatment is palliative.

Skeletal metastases

The main role of the orthopaedic surgeon in the treatment of neoplastic bone disease is in the treatment of the complications of skeletal metastases.

Pain is the commonest form of presentation of skeletal metastases and occurs in two-thirds of patients with radiographically detectable lesions[4] but pain may develop before the lesion becomes detectable on radiographs. Unless a further complication arises, the orthopaedic surgeon is not usually involved in the treatment of painful skeletal metastases but he may be involved in their early diagnosis as patients with bone pain are frequently referred initially to an orthopaedic surgeon. Magnetic resonance imaging is the most sensitive method of detecting early metastases in the spine but skeletal scintigraphy is probably still the investigation of choice in detecting skeletal metastases elsewhere and in assessing the degree of dissemination.

Radiotherapy is usually indicated for painful skeletal metastases and must be considered.[64] The extent and dose will depend on the age and general condition of the patient, the extent of skeletal involvement, and chemotherapy. Radiotherapy is used in conjunction with optimal analgesic therapy. These techniques are discussed elsewhere in this book. Retreatment with radiotherapy for painful skeletal metastases can be recommended in patients who have relapsed but who initially responded to irradiation of painful bone metastases.[5] Systemic radionuclide therapy (for example using phosphorus-32, strontium-89, samarium-153, and rhenium-186) has also been used successfully (see Chapter 9.12).

Bone pain may be the presenting feature of hypercalcaemia and an increase in bone pain was the commonest symptom of this condition in at least one series.[6]

The orthopaedic surgeon is involved when one of the following complications arise:

(1) impending fracture;

(2) pathological fracture;

(3) spinal instability;

(4) spinal cord or cauda equina compression.

Impending fracture

Large, lytic metastases are evident on plain radiographs and usually present with pain. By the time a large, lytic metastasis has developed there is considerable disruption and the cortex has been involved. The mechanism of pain in these lesions is not fully understood, but may be associated with infractions of the surrounding bone. The risk of fracture is high. Fidler[7] reported a fracture incidence of 3.7 per cent when 25 to 50 per cent of the cortex was involved, 61 per cent when the degree of involvement ranged between 50 and 75 per cent, and 79 per cent if more than 75 per cent of the cortex was involved.

Mirels[8] proposed a scoring system for diagnosing impending fractures. His scoring system was based on the site of the metastasis, the severity of pain, the radiographic appearance of the lesion, and the size of the lesion. The most serious prognostic signs were: lesions in the peritrochanteric region; pain sufficiently severe to interfere with function; lytic lesions; and lesions that involved more than two-thirds of the bone. Hipp *et al.*[9] thought that routine radiographs and CT scans were unreliable in predicting pathological fracture but that new methods, which applied engineering principles to the analysis of quantitative computed tomography, may provide a more objective guideline for determining the treatment strategy for each patient.

Although most fractures are associated with large, lytic metastases, they can also occur in other types of metastases. There are basically three types of bone destruction consequent upon skeletal metastases.[10,11]

Geographic

These are large, solitary, well-defined lytic areas, more than 1 cm. in diameter and usually with a sharply demarcated edge (Fig. 2).

'Moth-eaten'

There are multiple, smaller lytic metastases (2–5 mm) which may coalesce to form larger, confluent areas. The margins are usually ill-defined.

Permeative

There are multiple, tiny lytic areas (usually 1 mm or less) seen principally in cortical bone (Fig. 3). The bone is weakened and such lesions predispose to pathological fracture, even though a large lytic metastasis cannot be seen on the radiographs.

Geographic destruction is usually found in the slowest developing metastases, whereas permeative destruction occurs in the most aggressive lesions. A patient with multiple metastases usually shows one of the three principal patterns.

Management of impending fractures

Radiotherapy relieves pain but could temporarily weaken the bone, probably due to the associated transient resorption. Should this occur, irradiation of a large lytic metastasis could increase the risk of pathological fracture. Biopsy of the metastasis may also predispose to fracture.

Primary internal stabilization of a large lytic deposit, followed by irradiation, has certain advantages. It is easier to fix the bone while it is still intact and the rehabilitation and convalescence are much shorter and easier. Prior to internal stabilization, however, the general fitness of the patient must be assessed, the presence of malignant hypercalcaemia excluded, and the extent of the dissemination of the tumour evaluated. Resection and prosthetic replacement of an isolated skeletal metastasis, with no other evidence of dissemination, must be considered, particularly if the patient has renal carcinoma.

Large, lytic metastases, particularly if secondary to renal carcinoma, may be very vascular and surgery may be associated with torrential haemorrhage. Such lesions may require preoperative arteriography (Fig. 4) and, if necessary, embolization prior to surgery.[12,13]

Where feasible, closed intramedullary nailing is preferred, with interlocking nailing as required for additional stability (Fig. 2). If indicated, a biopsy specimen can be taken using bronchial biopsy forceps or through a separate incision. At the end of the long bones intramedullary nailing provides inadequate stabilization and, in some sites, replacement arthroplasty may be indicated. Care must be taken to avoid producing a fracture when positioning the patient or whilst stabilizing the lesion.

It is essential that the internal stabilization of the lesion provides sufficient strength to allow unsupported use of the limb, including

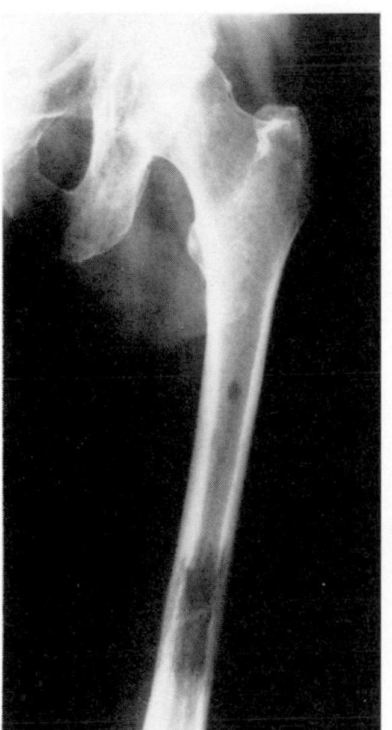

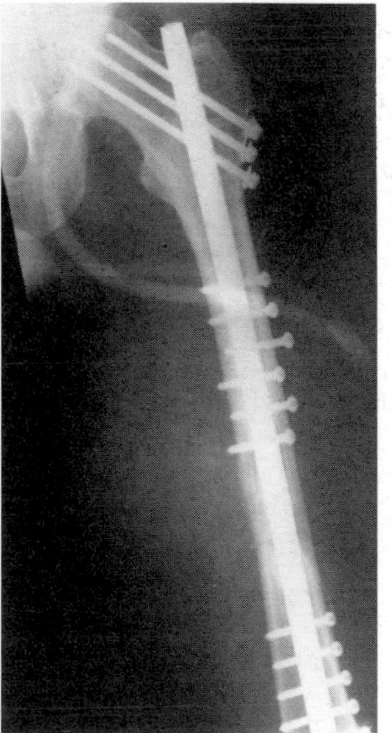

(a) (b)

Fig. 2 (a) Patient with a large 'geographic' metastasis in the mid-shaft of the femur. There is a further metastasis in the proximal femur. Prophylactic stabilization of the femur is indicated, but it is essential that all the lesions in the affected bone should be stabilized. (b) Stabilization of the femur using an interlocking nail, and stabilizing the entire bone. The lesion in the midfemoral shaft has been curetted out and the defect filled with methyl methacrylate.

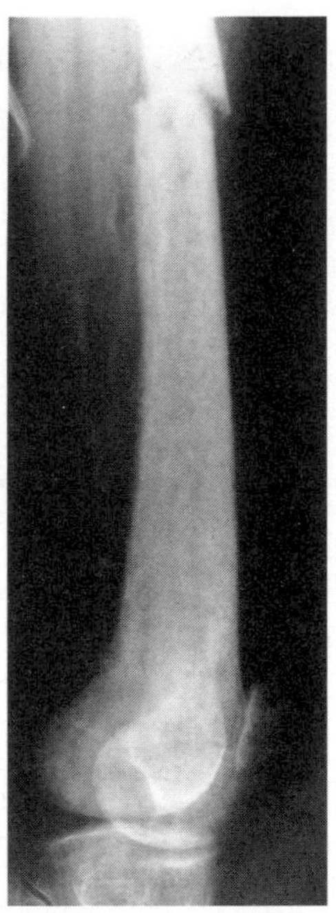

Fig. 3 Patient with multiple 'permeative' metastases. The entire femur was riddled with these tiny lesions. He has developed a pathological fracture through the shaft of the femur.

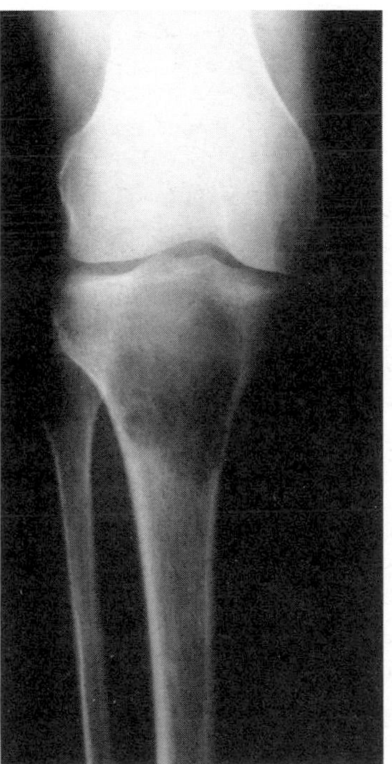

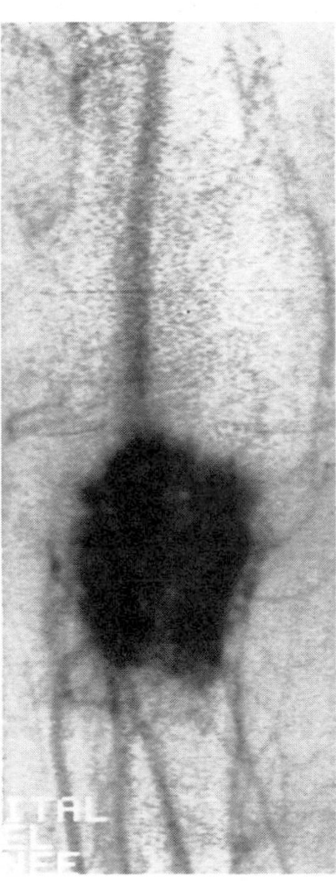

(a) (b)

Fig. 4 Patient with isolated metastasis from renal carcinoma; (a) metastasis in proximal tibia; (b) arteriogram, the lesion is extremely vascular.

weight bearing in the lower limb. If the implant is not likely to provide this, the stabilization should be supplemented with methyl methacrylate. In this case, the tumour is removed, the cavity filled with methyl methacrylate, and the implant fixed across the methyl methacrylate whilst it is still soft, as well as bridging normal bone above and below the lesion.

Irradiation is an essential part of treatment to inhibit further tumour growth, since the latter will result in progressive bone destruction and resultant loosening of the stabilization with increased risk of fracture. There is some evidence to suggest that the incorporation of chemotherapeutic agents in the methyl methacrylate may inhibit local tumour growth.[66] Depending on the primary lesion, the patient may also require endocrine therapy or chemotherapy.

Internal fixation carries the theoretical risk of disseminating tumour cells but there is no evidence that internal fixation causes increased tumour spread, either in the same bone or beyond. Furthermore, there is no evidence that the combined effect of surgical intervention and general anaesthesia has affected the overall prognosis in these patients. On the contrary, there is some evidence to suggest that internal stabilization of these lesions is associated with a lower incidence of pulmonary metastases.[14]

It is important that, prior to treatment, scintigrams and radiographs are obtained of the entire length of the affected bone so that any other metastases, which may subsequently develop into a pathological fracture, are stabilized and are included in the radiotherapy field (Fig. 2). A pathological fracture at the edge of a plate or intramedullary nail, particularly if the implant has been fixed with methyl methacrylate, is more difficult to treat than if there was no implant in the bone. Furthermore, it is extremely difficult to irradiate a metastasis if part of the lesion has been included in the previous field.

Pathological fractures

Although virtually every malignant tumour can metastasize to bone and may be associated with a pathological fracture, mammary carcinoma is responsible for approximately 50 per cent (Table 1), probably because skeletal metastases occur more commonly from mammary carcinoma than from other tumours. Myeloma is the second commonest cause of a malignant pathological fracture.

The commonest site of pathological fracture is in the femur (Table 2), but virtually any long bone is at risk. Although most pathological fractures occur through large lytic metastases, bone that has been significantly weakened by multiple, small, permeative metastases is also liable to fracture (Fig. 3).

The development of a pathological fracture is not necessarily a terminal event. With improvements in chemotherapy and endocrine therapy the average survival has increased during the past two decades. The survival is related to the primary tumour. Virtually no patient with bronchial carcinoma has survived, following a pathological fracture, for more than 6 months[15,16,17] whereas the mean survival for patients with prostatic carcinoma was in excess of two years and many patients with mammary carcinoma live for several years after a pathological fracture has been treated.

There are three aspects to the treatment of pathological fractures:

(1) the orthopaedic management;

(2) localized irradiation;

(3) the treatment of the causative tumour.

The orthopaedic management will be discussed in this chapter. Localized irradiation is an essential part of treatment in an attempt to control the underlying tumour and prevent further osteolysis with loosening of the implant. It can be delayed until the wound has healed but this is not essential. The implant does not appear to affect the irradiation, providing megavoltage is used. Orthovoltage should not be used if there is a metal implant in the bone, because of dose enhancement in the immediate vicinity of the metal and the shielding of tumour cells in the shadow of the implant.

As with impending fractures, the evaluation of a patient with a pathological fracture includes an assessment of the general fitness of the patient, the degree of dissemination of the tumour, the primary tumour, and the presence of other complications. In addition to a careful clinical examination, the evaluation includes appropriate blood tests, radiographs, and a skeletal scintigram. If the primary lesion is not known, or if there is any uncertainty about the origin of a pathological fracture, a biopsy of the lesion is essential. This can be carried out at the time of surgical stabilization.

Orthopaedic management of pathological fractures

The orthopaedic management depends on the site and the type of the fracture. Pathological transcervical femoral fractures do not unite, irrespective of the method of orthopaedic treatment[15] probably due to the effect of irradiation on an area where fractures are associated with impaired vascularity. The failure to unite is irrespective of the degree of displacement. Replacement arthroplasty gives the best results. The type of arthroplasty depends on the degree of tumour involvement. If there are no metastases in the acetabulum a proximal femoral endoprothesis is probably all that is required, although some authors prefer total hip replacement. The endoprothesis should be fixed with methyl methacrylate cement. If

Table 1 Pathological fractures

Primary tumour	Number of patients	Number of fractures
Breast	105	120
Bronchus	25	26
Prostate	22	23
Kidney	8	8
Rectum	6	6
Stomach	4	4
Bladder	3	3
Melanoma	2	2
Uterus	2	2
Thyroid	1	1
Colon	1	1
Oesophagus	1	1
Bile duct	1	1
Cervix	1	1
Penis	1	1
Squamous cell	1	1
Lymphoma	4	5
Leukaemia	6	6
Myeloma	25	35
Not known	5	5
Total	224	252

Personal series

Table 2 Pathological fractures

	Site	Number
Pelvis		3
Femur	Transcervical	60
	Intertrochanteric	26
	Subtrochanteric	29
	Shaft	41
	Distal	10
Humerus	Proximal	20
	Shaft	50
	Distal	3
Tibia	Proximal	2
	Shaft	1
Radius	Shaft	2
Ulna	Shaft	1
Clavicle		3
Mandible		1
Total		252

the acetabulum is involved, a total replacement arthroplasty is indicated. The type of pelvic reconstruction depends on the amount of bone destruction. When it is limited, the tumour is curetted from the acetabulum and a conventional total hip replacement arthroplasty is carried out. If there is more extensive involvement of the acetabulum, reconstruction may be required at the time of arthroplasty[18] Radiographs and scintigrams or MRI should be obtained of the rest of the femur prior to surgery. If there are more distant metastases, these should be stabilized at the time of replacement arthroplasty, a long stemmed femoral component being used. If there are lesions distal to the stem of the prosthesis, additional stabilization of the distal femur may be required. At the time of surgery, the tumour is curetted from the neck of the femur and the defect is filled with methyl methacrylate.

Unstable pathological fractures of the pelvis requiring surgical intervention are uncommon and usually occur in the periacetabular area. Harrington[18] has classified these fractures according to the location and extent of the tumour or radiation lysis.

1. Class I— the lateral cortices and superior and medial acetabular walls are structurally intact. Conventional fixation of a total hip acetabular component is usually successful.

2. Class II —the medial wall is deficient. This requires a reconstructive technique that transfers the stress of weight bearing away from the deficient wall and onto the intact acetabular rim. Some form of protrusion shell is required.

3. Class III —the lateral cortices and the medial and superior acetabular walls are deficient. These require constructive techniques that transmit load-bearing stresses into structurally intact bone in the upper ilium and adjacent to the sacro–iliac joint. Harrington[19] uses Steinman pins, a protrusion shell, and an acetabular component of a total hip replacement with methyl methacrylate to reconstruct such fractures, whereas others use specially constructed modular prostheses with a pelvic saddle prosthesis. Rarely, an allograft can be combined with a prosthesis to form an allograft-prosthetic composite but this carries a higher risk of infection, in addition to non-union, and most authors avoid this in the management of metastatic fractures.

It is sometimes impossible to stabilize a pathological fracture of the proximal humerus because of the lack of bony support proximal to the fracture. Under these circumstances, prosthetic replacement should also be considered.

The indications for endoprosthetic replacement in the management of skeletal metastases are:

(1) resection of a solitary metastasis, usually secondary to a hypernephroma, with the aim of achieving a wide margin of healthy tissue around the tumour;

(2) transcervical femoral fractures;

(3) some proximal humeral fractures;

(4) some metastases or pathological fractures involving the distal femur or proximal tibia;

(5) some failures of previous fixation.

Most intertrochantric fractures are probably best treated by internal-fixation, prosthetic replacement being reserved for those patients where extensive destruction of the proximal femur precludes effective internal stabilization.

Unlike transcervical femoral fractures, the majority of pathological fractures involving the rest of the femur or tibia should be treated with internal fixation, usually supplemented with methyl methacrylate,[20,21] even though this may interfere with callus formation. Internal fixation provides definite advantages over external support. It gives the patient greater and much more rapid relief of pain; it is associated with easier nursing, more comfortable turning of the patient, and prevention of pressure sores; it allows much earlier mobilization of the patient and discharge from hospital. It is also thought to increase the prospects of union. As with impending fractures, it is essential to stabilize the bone adequately, sufficient for weight bearing, at the time of surgery. Methyl methacrylate will not compensate for inadequate mechanical instability due to a poorly positioned implant nor the use of an inadequate implant. The method of internal fixation depends on the site of the pathological fracture. The method of fixation must also stabilize other metastases in the affected bone to avoid the risk of subsequent fracture adjacent to the implant.

Fractures of the femoral shaft are probably best treated with interlocking nails whereas fractures of the intertrochanteric region and supracondylar region may be best treated by implants specifically designed for these sites.

Internal fixation of humeral pathological fractures has also been shown to be of benefit, in that it provides the patient with much greater mobility and earlier use of the limb, and more rapid and greater pain relief. The advantages over conservative treatment, however, are not as marked as with pathological fractures of the lower limb.[22] McCormack *et al.*[23] suggested that a functional brace was indicated if the patient had a limited life expectancy, but for those patients expected to survive for more than three months, internal fixation was the method of choice to ensure pain relief, restoration of function, and avoid later re-fracture. Fractures of the distal humerus might be best treated in a cast brace because of the complexity of internal stabilization. The type of stabilization depends on the site of fracture and includes the Russell-Taylor humeral nail [24] or Ender nails.[25] Harrington [19] advised two Rush rods supplemented by intramedullary methyl methacrylate for supracondylar humeral fractures. In most cases intramedullary fixation is preferable to plating.

Multiple fractures

Some patients present with several pathological fractures and each must be treated on its merits.

Fracture through an isolated metastasis

Occasionally patients present with an isolated skeletal metastasis. They usually present with pain, may present with an impending fracture, and occasionally with a pathological fracture. The commonest primary is renal carcinoma and, provided there is no other evidence of dissemination of the tumour, resection of the lesion should be considered, usually in the form of local resection and prosthetic replacement, including intercalary replacement of the diaphysis. It is easier to excise and replace a metastasis with impending fracture than one that has already fractured. The haematoma consequent upon the latter may cause widespread dissemination of tumour, which may make it impossible to carry out a local resection with adequate margins.

Postoperative irradiation

Local irradiation does not interfere with fracture healing, provided the fracture is adequately immobilized.[16],[26] The optimum time for irradiation is after surgery has been carried out. Preoperative irradiation makes the tissues more friable. Ideally, postoperative irradiation should wait until the wound has settled down. It is not necessary to wait until the sutures have been removed, but the sutures should be retained for 3 to 4 weeks in patients who have undergone surgery for metastatic cancer. Under these circumstances, the radiotherapy can be given at about 12 to 14 days postoperatively.

Townsend *et al.*[27] estimated the probability of achieving normal use of the extremity following internal stabilization was 53 per cent for patients who had had postoperative radiation versus 11.5 per cent for patients who underwent surgery alone ($p<0.01$).

Spinal instability

Back pain is a frequent symptom of disseminated carcinoma and in 10 per cent is due to spinal instability.[28] Carcinoma of the breast is the commonest primary tumour associated with spinal instability, followed by myeloma (Table 3). However, any tumour can metastasize to the spine and can cause sufficient destruction to render the spine unstable. Spinal instability can cause excruciating pain, which is mechanical in nature. In its severe form the patient is only comfortable when lying absolutely still. Any movement, including log-rolling by two or three trained nurses is associated with agonizing pain and the patient may not be able to sit, stand, or walk because of pain, even with the use of a spinal orthosis. In the milder form, the patient may be relatively free from pain when wearing a rigid spinal orthosis but movement of the back, for example turning in bed, sitting, or standing, may be impossible without the support. Plain radiographs show destruction of bone with vertebral collapse of a greater or lesser degree. No discrete fracture can be seen. Nevertheless, spinal instability should be considered the equivalent of a pathological fracture in an appendicular bone, because the pain is due to the instability and not the metastasis. Radiotherapy or chemotherapy will not alleviate the pain. Like pathological fractures of the long bones, stabilization is required for pain relief.

The spine can be stabilized by either a posterior or anterior approach.[29–40] Vascular metastatic lesions require preoperative embolization, particularly if an anterior stabilization is being considered.[13,41]

To date the author has treated 72 patients with spinal instability secondary to metastatic disease (Table 4). Sixty-five patients have

Table 3 Spinal instability

Primary tumour	Number of patients
Breast	35[a] + 1[b]
Myeloma	10
Kidney	5
Bronchus	4
Prostate	2
Melanoma	2
Cervix	2
Colon	1
Bladder	1
Uterus	1
Ovary	1
Vagina	1
Stomach	1
Parotid	1
Lymphoma	1
Chondrosarcoma	1
Histiocytoma	1
Chordoma	1
Unknown	1
Total	72 + 1[b]

[a] One patient's metastatic destruction was too extensive for surgical stabilization.

[b] Lumbar stabilization 22 months after successful dorsal stabilization.

Table 4 Spinal instability results

Destruction too extensive for surgical reconstruction		1
Infection resulting in removal of implant		1
Loosening of implant		2
Relief of pain	complete	65
	partial	3
Complications in the 68 patients with relief of pain		
Paraplegia due to extradural bleed		1
Infection, successfully treated		1
Infection, fatal septicaemia		1
Wound breakdown, successful secondary suture		1
Fracture, L-rod requiring additional anterior stabilization		1
Fracture, Hartshill rectangle at 5 years		1

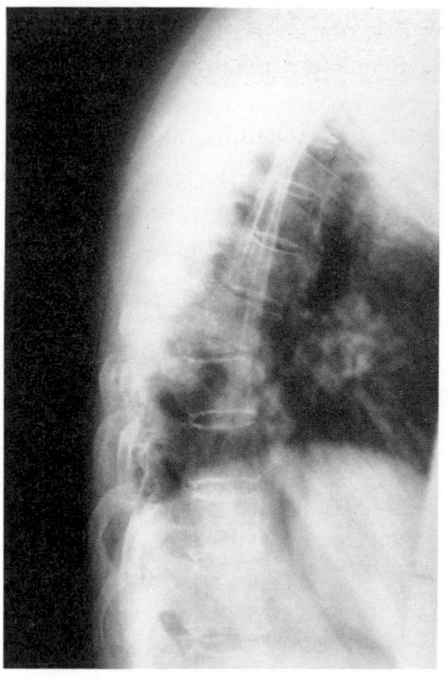
(a)

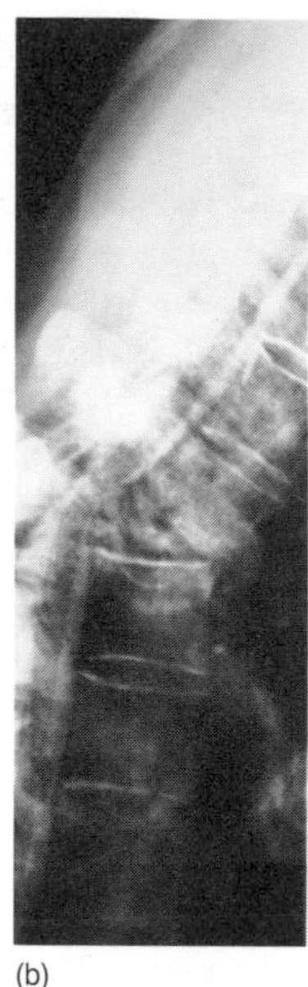
(b)

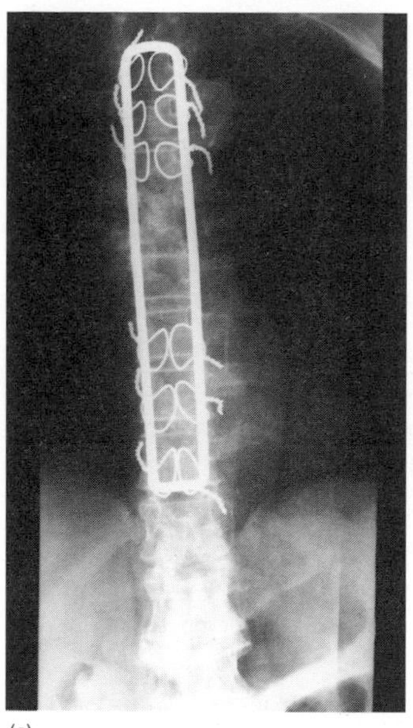
(c)

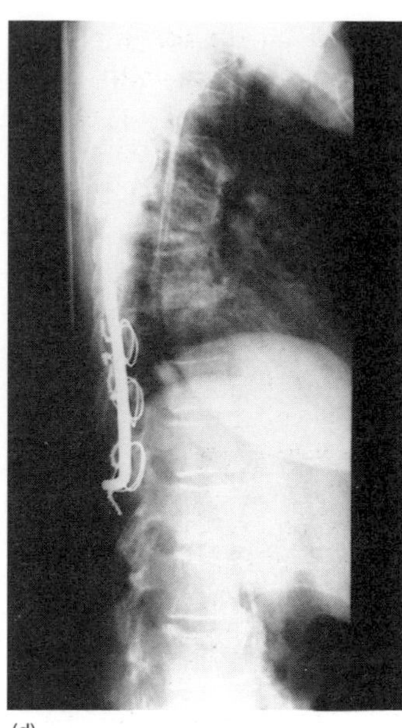
(d)

Fig. 5 Patient with mammary carcinoma. (a) Lateral radiograph of the spine, showing complete collapse of a dorsal vertebra with spinal instability. (b) Myelogram. There is compression of the spinal cord at the level of the lesion. In addition to the agonizing back pain, the patient also had weakness. (c), (d) Anterior-posterior and lateral radiographs following posterior decompression of the spine, stabilization with a Hartshill rectangle, and correction of the kyphus. The patient obtained complete relief of pain and regained full neurological function.

achieved complete relief of pain and three patients achieved partial relief of pain. There were three failures: one patient developed an infection resulting in removal of the implant and in two patients the implant loosened. In one patient the spinal destruction was too extensive for surgical reconstruction.

There were several complications in the patients whose pain was relieved. One patient, who obtained complete relief of pain, developed paraplegia as a result of an extradural bleed despite removal of the clot. Another patient, who also obtained complete relief of pain and who had had preoperative irradiation, developed a wound infection that could not be controlled and died from septicaemia. Five patients required anterior and posterior stabilization because the level of instability was at L5 or L4 and neither anterior stabilization nor posterior stabilization alone was considered to be adequate. These patients underwent two stage combined anterior and posterior stabilization. In the first stage the dura was decompressed anteriorly and the spine stabilized. In the second stage the spine was stabilized posteriorly. In the other patients the spine was stabilized posteriorly. It is essential that the implant adequately stabilizes the spine. Posterior stabilization requires a segmental form of fixation. In these patients the spine should be stabilized for at least two vertebrae above and two vertebrae below the level of instability (Figs 5, 6). Pedicle screw fixation can only be used if the pedicles into which the screws are placed are not involved with metastatic disease. Preoperative magnetic resonance imaging is required and if there is extensive metastatic involvement in adjacent vertebrae these should be stabilized at the same time.

All patients require a preoperative assessment as described above, as well as preoperative skeletal scintigraphy to assess the extent of their skeletal dissemination. Magnetic resonance imaging is indicated to determine whether there is any extradural tumour. If this facility is not available, CT myelography is indicated. If there is any evidence of spinal cord or cauda equina compression, the neural tissues should be decompressed at the time of surgical stabilization, irrespective of whether the patient has developed any signs or symptoms of neurological involvement.

In 34 of the 72 patients, there was some clinical evidence of compression of the spinal cord or cauda equina, usually weakness of the lower limbs severe enough to affect walking or standing (Figs 5, 6). These patients were treated by decompression at the time of stabilization. Twenty three of the 34 (68 per cent) obtained major recovery of neurological function, sufficient to allow them to walk without orthoses and restoration of bladder function where it had

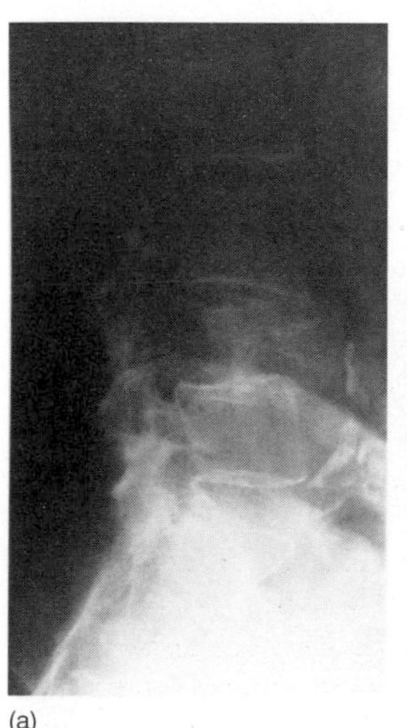
(a)

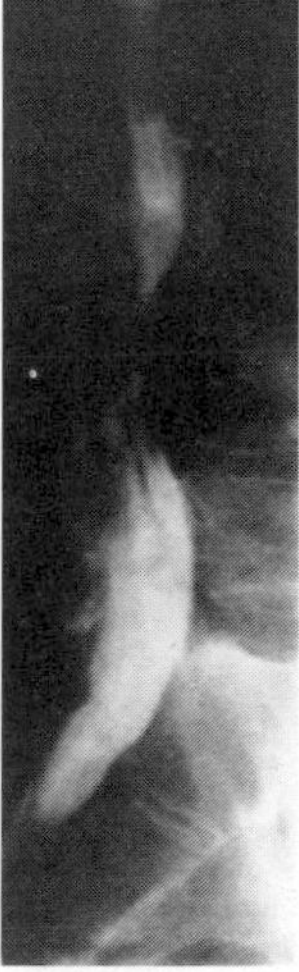
(b)

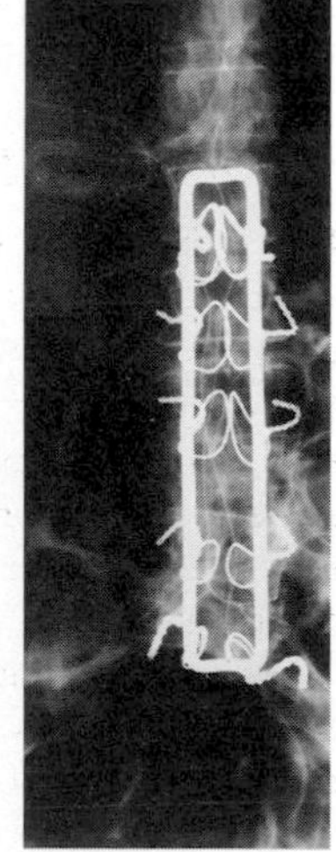
(c)

Fig. 6 Patient with mammary carcinoma who presented with excruciating pain due to spinal instability. Clinical examination revealed significant weakness affecting both lower limbs. (a) Lateral radiograph showing destruction of L4 with spinal instability. (b) Myelogram. Extradural tumour is compressing the cauda equina. (c) The patient was treated with posterior decompression and stabilization using a Hartshill rectangle. She obtained complete relief of pain and made a full neurological recovery.

been compromised. It must be emphasized that these patients presented primarily with pain due to spinal instability. In two patients cord compression recurred 10 and 14 months respectively after decompression.

The first 29 patients have been followed up until death. Their mean survival was 36 weeks, but one patient lived for 3.5 years and one for 4 years. Many of the later patients are alive, some at 5 to 10 years after surgery.

As with pathological fractures, patients should receive postoperative irradiation. There are occasions, however, when the patient has received the maximum tolerable dose preoperatively and any further radiotherapy would put the cord at risk of developing transverse myelitis. The underlying tumour may also be treated by endocrine therapy or chemotherapy.

Instability of the cervical spine is uncommon compared with the involvement of the dorsal or lumbar spine but does occur (Fig. 7). The principles of treatment are the same—namely, spinal stabilization (and decompression if there is any evidence of cord compression), followed by localized irradiation (if feasible) and endocrine therapy or chemotherapy. Minor degrees of cervical instability can be controlled by a collar. However, if this does not control the pain, surgical stabilization is indicated. Several methods of stabilization have been used, including bone grafting, posterior stabilization,[32-34] anterior resection and stabilization,[42,43] and anterior replacement.[44,45]

Compression of the spinal cord or cauda equina

Schaberg and Gainor[46] reported that cord compression occurred in 20 per cent of patients with vertebral metastases. Constans *et al.*[47] thought it likely that 5 to 10 per cent of patients developed symptomatic neurological manifestations of their metastases. Compression of the spinal cord or cauda equina may occur in association with spinal instability (where the treatment of choice is spinal stabilization, decompression, and postoperative radiotherapy) or in isolation. In the latter circumstance the choice of treatment (surgical decompression, radiotherapy, and steroids) depends on the duration, severity, and rapidity of onset of the symptoms. Pain is almost invariable, and persisting and increasing back pain may herald spinal cord compression. Pain is frequently localized to the site of disease and is probably caused by stimulation of pain receptors in the longitudinal ligaments, dura, or periosteum as the tumour expands. Radicular pain is less common. It is important to be aware of the possible significance of localized spinal or radicular pain. Nevertheless, by the time treatment is started up to 50 per cent of patients will no longer be able to walk and 10 to 30 per cent will be paraplegic.[48,49] Other symptoms include weakness, disturbance of gait, paraesthesia, urinary hesitancy or precipitancy, and constipation or spurious diarrhoea. The sequence of events is often pain, motor dysfunction, paraesthesia, and sensory loss. Pinprick and deep pain sensation may be retained until late. Results depend heavily on the neurological status of the patient at the time of starting treatment and it is important, therefore, to make a diagnosis urgently. The assessment of the patient is as described for patients with spinal instability, except that they may have to be carried out as an emergency, outside normal working hours. Ideally, the investigations should only be carried out in a centre where immediate surgical decompression is available. Occasionally, a patient with spinal cord compression will deteriorate abruptly during or following myelography owing to impaction of the compromised cord onto surrounding structures. However, most spinal centres today have available magnetic resonance imaging and so myelography or CT myelography is not required.

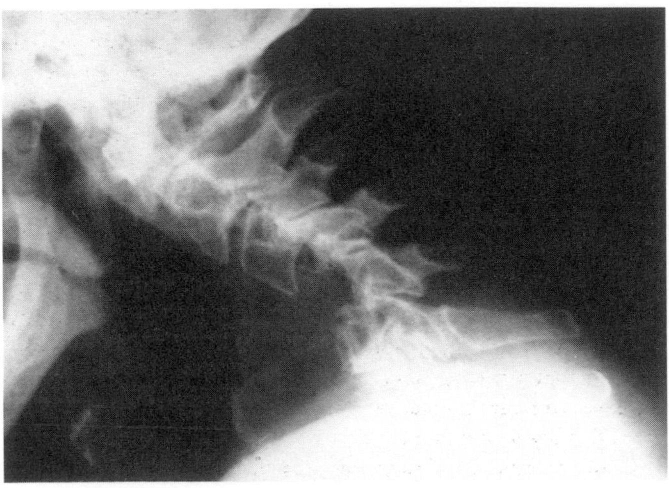
Fig. 7 Instability of the cervical spine following metastatic destruction of C4.

When indicated, surgical decompression is urgent. It is indicated in patients with recent onset of symptoms, particularly a developing paraplegia or urinary retention of less than 24 h duration; a block, shown on the preoperative magnetic resonance image or CT myelogram, localized to no more than two or three segments; and in a patient with a life expectancy of at least two to three months. Once the paraplegia has been established for some days, or urinary retention has been present for more than 30 h, surgical decompression is often associated with some return of sensation and pain relief but not with useful recovery of bladder or motor function. Under these circumstances, irradiation is indicated, as is the case with more extensive blocks. However, occasionally anterior decompression and stabilization may be associated with major neurological recovery in patients with long-standing neurological disturbances, provided the onset of the symptoms has been gradual. In general terms, patients with a gradual onset of neurological disturbances do better than patients who have developed paraplegia and urinary retention extremely rapidly.

Because of the risk of subsequent instability the spine must be stabilized at the time of decompression.[32,50-52] The decompression can be carried out anteriorly[17,29,52-55] or posteriorly[30-32] but it is essential that posterior decompression is associated with stabilization to avoid the development of progressive kyphosis which may produce further compression of the spinal cord and neurological impairment. Laminectomy alone is contraindicated. Laminar removal and replacement has been described.[62]

Treatment (either surgical decompression or radiotherapy) should be combined with a short course of high-dose steroids in order to minimize the oedema, and if surgical decompression is undertaken, postoperative radiotherapy is required. Dexamethasone is usually used. The patient is often given a starting dose in adults of 12 to 20 mg intravenously followed by 4 mg, at 4 to 6 hour intervals. The dosage is reduced within 48 to 72 h after surgery.

Findlay[56] reported that radiotherapy combined with steroids was at least as effective as laminectomy, but as indicated above, laminectomy alone is contraindicated and should not be carried out. Cobb *et al.*[57] found no significant difference in outcome between patients treated initially by laminectomy and those treated by radiotherapy. Gilbert[58] reported that there was no therapeutic advantage of radiotherapy and laminectomy over radiotherapy alone. McBroom[59] recommended that the choice of treatment of spinal cord compression, without deformity or instability, depended on the severity and speed of progression of the neurological symptoms and the radiosensitivity of the tumour. Patients with minor neurological symptoms that had been slow in onset responded favourably to irradiation, irrespective of tumour type. Dense paraparesis or rapid neurological deterioration were poor prognostic indicators, irrespective of the treatment. Under these circumstances the only chance of achieving a functional recovery lay in rapid decompression of the spinal cord. If the tumour was radiosensitive, irradiation could affect cord compression as quickly as surgery. Radioresistant tumours are slow to respond and require urgent surgical decompression. Radiotherapy will not be effective in symptomatic patients with progressive kyphotic spinal deformity, or spinal instability. These patients require decompression and stabilization.

Laminectomy without stabilization will often cause further instability with increasing kyphosis, increasing pain, and increased neurological deficit.

Prevention of bone lysis

The main role of the orthopaedic surgeon, in the palliation of patients with skeletal metastases, is in the treatment of the complications of these lesions. These are usually caused by marked bone lysis resulting in impending fracture, pathological fracture, and spinal instability. The aim of treatment, in the future, must be to prevent this progressive bone destruction. Endocrine therapy and chemotherapy may be effective in some patients. The tumour-induced osteolysis is usually mediated by osteoclasts, the osteoclasts being stimulated by humoral factors secreted by the tumour.[60] A variety of cytokines and growth factors are likely to be involved. Some of these factors may also affect the cell adhesion molecules. For example Evans *et al.*[61] have shown that myeloma inhibits the normal osteoblastic response to bone destruction, this action being mediated by the tumour secreting factors which affect the ability of the osteoblast to adhere to the bone surface. Adhesion molecules may explain why certain tumours metastasize to specific sites—this may be because the tumour cells have the capacity to bind selectively to those organs.

If it is not possible to destroy the cancer cells, the treatment of choice for skeletal metastases may be to inhibit the secondary bone resorption which subsequently occurs and is responsible for much of the morbidity associated with skeletal metastases. The bisphosphonates inhibit osteoclast bone resorption by mechanisms that are still not clearly understood. It may be that with the development of such agents tumour-induced bone lysis will be minimized and the complications that require orthopaedic intervention avoided.

Non-metastatic orthopaedic conditions in patients with malignant disease

Patients with malignant disease may develop benign disorders of the skeleton which mimic metastases. These must be differentiated from metastatic disease, and should be treated on their merits. Like any individual, such a patient may sustain a traumatic fracture. If the patient has a past history of malignancy and there is no evidence of dissemination, a biopsy should be taken from the fracture. In some instances this may be the first manifestation of recurrence of the disease, even though there has been a long disease-free interval. The development of a non-pathological traumatic fracture in such a patient may subsequently be associated with dissemination of the cancer.

Galasko and Sylvester[28] found that a benign lesion was responsible for the back pain that developed in 11 of 31 consecutive patients with an underlying malignant disease. The benign conditions included spondylolisthesis, prolapsed disc, degenerative spondylosis, pyogenic infection, and chronic back strain. The author has treated four patients with a history of malignant disease and who had a prolapsed intervertebral disc, confirmed by radiculography. In one patient the symptoms settled with conservative management; three patients required surgical excision of the disc. In three patients (including the patient who responded to conservative treatment), there was no other evidence of metastatic disease, and two years after treatment the patients were still free from metastases, whereas the fourth patient had disseminated carcinoma. Nevertheless, it was felt that surgical excision of the disc was warranted in view of her severe symptoms, to improve the quality of her remaining life. This patient was alive and asymptomatic one year later.

Painful osteoarthritis and other orthopaedic conditions may occur in patients with malignancy, and in some patients may be secondary to avascular necrosis of the femoral or humeral head as a result of irradiation or steroid treatment. If symptoms warrant it, joint replacement arthroplasty is indicated, even in the presence of disseminated carcinoma.[32]

Conclusions

The development of an impending fracture, pathological fracture, spinal instability, or spinal cord/cauda equina compression in patients with metastatic cancer is not necessarily a terminal event. These lesions are associated with severe pain. The aims of treatment are to alleviate pain and restore mobility and use of the affected limb or spine.

In the vast majority of impending and pathological fractures, this is best achieved by internal stabilization or replacement arthroplasty. The type of stabilization depends on the site of the lesion. If the stabilization is not adequate to provide unsupported use of the limb, which includes weight bearing in a lower limb long bone, it should be supplemented by methyl methacrylate. Postoperative radiotherapy is an essential part of the treatment. The causative tumour should be treated by endocrine therapy or chemotherapy as indicated.

Before treating the lesion, the patient must be carefully evaluated to determine the degree of dissemination of the cancer, and particularly any other areas of involvement in the affected bone, as this may influence the type of surgery and the radiotherapy field. Optimum treatment of these lesions may require major surgery, which should not be carried out if a patient is terminal. The aim of treatment is to palliate the symptoms and improve the patients quality of life. Orthopaedic treatment does not affect the life expectancy. Irrespective of whether surgical reconstruction is possible, the patient should always be made comfortable, kept comfortable, and allowed to die with dignity.

It is hoped that improved understanding of the underlying pathophysiological changes that occur when tumour invades bone may lead to effective osteoclast inhibiting drugs, which may obviate the development of large lytic metastases in the future. The treatment of primary malignant tumours depends on the extent of the tumour, but frequently the emphasis of treatment is on radical resection and chemotherapy.

References

1. Kurz LT, Mubarak SJ, Schultz P, Park SM, Leach J. Correlation of scoliosis and pulmonary function in Duchenne muscular dystrophy. *Journal of Pediatric Orthopedics*, 1983; **3**: 347–53.
2. Galasko CSB. *Neuromuscular Problems in Orthopaedics*. Oxford: Blackwell Scientific Publications, 1987.
3. Galasko CSB. The orthopaedic management of neuromuscular disease. In: Walton J, Karpati G, Hilton-Jones D, eds, *Disorders of Voluntary Muscle*, Edinburgh: Churchill-Livingstone, 1994: 851–77.
4. Galasko CSB. Skeletal metastases and mammary cancer. *Annals of the Royal College of Surgeons of England*, 1972; **50**, 3–28.
5. Mithal NP, Needham PR, Hoskin PJ. Retreatment with radiotherapy for painful bone metastases. *International Journal of Radiation Oncology Biology Physics*, 1994; **29**: 1011–14.
6. Galasko CSB, Burn JI. Hypercalcaemia in patients with advanced mammary cancer. *British Medical Journal*, 1971; **3**: 573–7.
7. Fidler M. Incidence of fracture through metastases in long bones. *Acta Orthopaedica Scandinavica*, 1981; **52**: 623–7.
8. Mirels H. Metastatic disease in long bones: proposed scoring system for diagnosing impending pathologic fractures. *Clinical Orthopaedics and Related Research*, 1989; **249**: 256–64.
9. Hipp JA, Springfield DS, Hayes WC. Predicting pathologic fracture risk in the management of metastatic bone defects. *Clinical Orthopaedics and Related Research*, 1995; **312**: 120–35.
10. Lodwick GS. Reactive response to local injury in bone. *Radiological Clinics of North America*, 1964; **2**: 209–19.
11. Lodwick GS. A systematic approach to the roentgen diagnosis of bone tumours. In: *Tumours of Bone and Soft Tissue*. Chicago: Year Book Publishers, 1965: 49–68.
12. Roscoe MW, McBroom RJ, Louis ESt, Grossman H, Perrin R. Preoperative embolization in the treatment of osseous metastases from renal cell carcinoma. *Clinical Orthopaedics and Related Research*, 1989; **238**: 302–7.
13. Olerud C, Jónsson HJ Jr, Löfberg A-M, Lörelius L-E, Sjöström L. Embolization of spinal metastases reduces peroperative blood loss. Twenty-one patients operated on for renal cell carcinoma. *Acta Orthopaedica Scandinavica*, 1993; **64**: 9–12.
14. Bouma WH, Mulder JH, Hop WCJ. The influence of intramedullary nailing upon the development of metastases in the treatment of an impending pathological fracture: an experimental study. *Clinical and Experimental Metastasis*, 1983; **1**: 205–12.
15. Galasko CSB. Pathological fractures secondary to metastatic cancer. *Journal of the Royal College of Surgeons of Edinburgh*, 1974; **19**: 351–62.
16. Gainor BJ, Buchert P. Fracture healing in metastatic bone disease. *Clinical Orthopaedics and Related Research*, 1983; **178**: 297–302.
17. Harrington KD. Anterior decompression and stabilisation of the spine as a treatment for vertebral collapse and spinal cord compression from metastatic malignancy. *Clinical Orthopaedics and Related Research*, 1988; **233**: 177–97.
18. Harrington KD. The management of acetabular insufficiency secondary to metastatic malignant disease. *Journal of Bone and Joint Surgery*, 1981; **63A**: 653–664.
19. Harrington KD. Orthopaedic management of extremity and pelvic lesions. *Clinical Orthopaedics and Related Research*, 1995; **312**: 136–47.
20. Harrington KD, Johnston JO, Turner RH, Green DL. The use of methylmethacrylate as an adjunct in the internal fixation of malignant neoplastic fractures. *Journal of Bone and Joint Surgery*, 1972; **54A**: 1665–76.
21. Yablon IG, Paul GR. The augmentive use of methylmethacrylate in the management of pathologic fractures. *Surgery, Gynecology and Obstetrics*, 1976; **143**: 177–83.
22. Galasko CSB. The management of skeletal metastases. *Journal of the Royal College of Surgeons of Edinburgh*, 1980; **25**: 143–61.
23. McCormack RR Jr, Glass DB, Lane JM. Functional cast bracing of metastatic humeral shaft lesion. *Orthopedic Transactions*, 1985; **9**: 50–1.
24. Ikpeme JO. Intramedullary interlocking nailing for humeral fractures: experiences with the Russell-Taylor humeral nail. *Injury*, 1994; **25**: 447–55.
25. Hyder N, Wray CC. Treatment of pathological fractures of the humerus with Ender nails. *Journal of the Royal College of Surgeons of Edinburgh*, 1993; **38**: 370–2.
26. Bonarigo BC., Rubin P. Non-union of pathologic fracture after radiation therapy. *Radiology*, 1967; **88**: 889–98.
27. Townsend PW, Rosenthal HG, Smalley SR, Cozad SC, Hassanein RES. Impact of post-operative radiation therapy and other perioperative factors on outcome after orthopaedic stabilization of impending or pathologic fractures due to metastatic disease. *Journal of Clinical Oncology*, 1994; **12**, 2345–50.
28. Galasko CSB, Sylvester BS. Back pain in patients treated for malignant tumours. *Clinical Oncology*, 1978; **4**: 273–83.
29. Harrington KD. The use of methylmethacrylate for vertebral-body replacement and anterior stabilisation of pathological fracture-dislocations of the spine due to metastatic malignant disease. *Journal of Bone and Joint Surgery*, 1981; **63A**: 36–46.
30. Flatley TJ, Anderson MH, Anast GT. Spinal instability due to malignant disease: treatment by segmental spinal stabilisation. *Journal of Bone and Joint Surgery*, 1984; **66A**: 47–52.
31. DeWald RL, Bridwell KH, Prodromas C, Rodts MF. Reconstructive spinal surgery as palliation for metastatic malignancies of the spine. *Spine*, 1985; **10**: 21–6.
32. Galasko CSB. *Skeletal Metastases*. London: Butterworths, 1986.
33. Fidler MW. Pathological fractures of the spine including those causing anterior spinal cord compression: surgical management. In: Galasko CSB, Noble J, eds. *Recent Developments in Orthopaedic Surgery: Festschrift to Sir Harry Platt*. Manchester: Manchester University Press, 1987: 94–103.
34. Heywood AWB, Learmonth ID, Thomas M. Internal fixation for occipito-cervical fusion. *Journal of Bone and Joint Surgery*, 1988; **70B**: 708–11.
35. Sherk HH, Nolan JP, Mooar PA. Treatment of tumours of the cervical spine. *Clinical Orthopaedics and Related Research* , 1988; **233**: 163–7.
36. Bridwell KH, Jenny AB, Saul T, Rich KM, Grubb RL. Posterior segmental spinal instrumentation (PSSI) with posterolateral decompression and debulking for metastatic thoracic and lumbar spine disease: limitations of the technique. *Spine*, 1988; **13**: 1383–94.
37. Cybulski GR. Methods of surgical stabilization for metastatic disease of the spine. *Neurosurgery*, 1989; **25**: 240–52.
38. Galasko CSB. Spinal instability secondary to metastatic cancer. *Journal of Bone and Joint Surgery*, 1991; **73B**: 104–8.
39. Rompe JD, Eysel P, Hopf C, Heine J. Decompression/stabilization of the metastatic spine. Cotrel-Dubousset instrumentation in 50 patients. *Acta Orthopaedica Scandinavica*, 1993; **64**: 3–8.
40. Hosono N, Yonenobu K, Fuji T, Ebara S, Yamashita K, Ono K. Orthopaedic management of spinal metastases. *Clinical Orthopaedics and Related Research*, 1995; **312**: 148–59.

41. Gellad FE, Sadato N, Numaguchi Y, Levine AM. Vascular metastatic lesions of the spine: pre-operative embolization. *Radiology,* 1990; **176**: 683–6.
42. Chadduck WM, Boop WC Jr. Acrylic stabilisation of the cervical spine for neoplastic disease: evolution of a technique for vertebral body replacement. *Neurosurgery,* 1983; **13**: 23–9.
43. Asnis S.E, Lesniewski P, Dowling TJr. Anterior decompression and stabilisation with methylmethacrylate and a bone bolt for treatment of pathologic fractures of the cervical spine. A report of two cases. *Clinical Orthopaedics and Related Research,* 1984; **187**, 139–43.
44. Ono K, Yonenobu K, Ebara S, Fujiwara K, Yamashita K, Fuji T, Dunn EJ. Prosthetic replacement surgery for cervical spine metastasis. *Spine,* 1988; **13**: 817–22.
45. Fidler MW. Radical resection of vertebral body tumours. A surgical technique used in ten cases. *Journal of Bone and Joint Surgery,* 1994; **76B**: 765–72.
46. Schaberg J, Gainor BJ. A profile of metastatic carcinoma of the spine. *Spine,* 1985; **10**: 19–20.
47. Constans JP, de Divitiis E, Donzelli R, Spaziante R, Meder JF, Haye C. Spinal metastases with neurological manifestations. Review of 600 cases. *Journal of Neurosurgery,* 1983; **59**: 111–8.
48. Shaw MDM, Rose JE, Paterson A. Metastatic extradural malignancy of the spine. *Acta Neurochirurgica,* 1980; **52**: 113–20.
49. Shapiro WR, Posner JB. Medical versus surgical treatment of metastatic spinal cord tumours. In: Thompson RA, Green JR, eds. *Controversies in Neurology.* New York: Raven Press, 1983: 57–65.
50. Johnson JR, Leatherman KD, Holt RT. Anterior decompression of the spinal cord for neurological deficit. *Spine,* 1983; **8**: 396–405.
51. Kostuik JP. Anterior spinal cord decompression for lesions of the thoracic and lumbar spine, techniques, new methods of internal fixation, results. *Spine,* 1983; **8**: 512–31.
52. Siegal T, Siegal T. Vertebral body resection for epidural compression by malignant tumours. *Journal of Bone and Joint Surgery,* 1985; **67A**: 375–82.
53. Boland P J, Lane JM, Sundaresan N. Metastatic disease of the spine. *Clinical Orthopaedics and Related Research,* 1982; **169**: 95–102.
54. Turner PL, Prince HG, Webb JK, Sokal MPJW. Surgery for malignant extradural tumours of the spine. *Journal of Bone and Joint Surgery,* 1988; **70B**: 451–6.
55. Moore AJ, Uttley D. Anterior decompression and stabilisation of the spine in malignant disease. *Neurosurgery,* 1989; **24**: 713–17.
56. Findlay GFG. Adverse effects of the management of malignant spinal cord compression. *Journal of Neurology, Neurosurgery and Psychiatry,* 1984; **47**: 761–8.
57. Cobb CAIII, Leavens ME, Eckles N. Indications for non-operative treatment of spinal cord compression due to breast cancer. *Journal of Neurosurgery,* 1977; **47**: 653–8.
58. Gilbert RW, Kim JH, Posner JB. Epidural spinal cord compression from metastatic tumour: diagnosis and treatment. *Annals of Neurology,* 1978; **3**: 40–51.
59. McBroom R. Radiation or surgery for metastatic disease of the spine? *Royal Society of Medicine Current Medical Literature—Orthopaedics,* 1988; **1**: 97–101.
60. Galasko CSB. Mechanisms of bone destruction in the development of skeletal metastasis. *Nature,* 1976; **263**: 507–8.
61. Evans CE, Ward C, Rathour L, Galasko CSB. Myeloma affects both the growth and function of human osteoblast-like cells. *Clinical and Experimental Metastasis,* 1992; **10**: 33–8.
62. Fidler MW, Bongartz EB. Laminar removal and replacement: a technique for the removal of epidural tumour. *Spine,* 1988; **13**: 218–20.
63. Galasko CSB. Diagnosis of skeletal metastases and assessment of response to treatment. *Clinical Orthopaedics and Related Research,* 1995; **312**: 64–75.
64. Hoskin PJ. Radiotherapy in the management of bone pain. *Clinical Orthopaedics and Related Research,* 1995; **312**: 105–119.
65. Traill Z, Richards MA, Moore NR. Magnetic resonance imaging of metastatic bone disease. *Clinical Orthopaedics and Related Research,* 1995; **312**: 76–88.
66. Wang HM, Crank S, Oliver G, Galasko CSB. The effect of methotrexate loaded bone cement on local destruction by the VX_2 tumour. *Journal of Bone and Joint Surgery,* 1996; **78B**: 14–47.
67. Robinson D, Galasko CSB, Delaney C, Williamson JB, Barrie JL. Scoliosis and lung function in spinal muscular atrophy. *European Spine Journal,* 1995; **4**: 268–73.

9.3 Gastrointestinal symptoms

9.3.1 Palliation of nausea and vomiting

Kathryn A. Mannix

Introduction

Nausea and vomiting are unpleasant symptoms which undermine quality of life for people with diseases including cancer, AIDS, and hepatic or renal failure.[1,2] The incidence of these symptoms in patients with advanced cancer is estimated to be between 40 and 70 per cent [3-7] and, unlike pain, this symptom complex has not been reduced in incidence or severity over the last decade. Symptoms may be induced by the disease or by its treatment [8,9] and are ranked as highly distressing by cancer patients.[6]

The neurophysiology of the vomiting reflex is well established in experimental animals[10-12] and is becoming better understood in man.[13-16] Intervention aimed at reducing nausea and vomiting must take into account the cause of the symptom and the central emetogenic pathways involved. Thus, treatment requires knowledge of these pathways, careful assessment of the patient, and prescribing tailored to the cause of the symptoms and to the patient's individual needs.

Pathways involved in emesis

Central pathways involved in emesis

Emesis is mediated centrally by two separate 'centres'. Whilst these are anatomically distinct in experimental animals, in man the neural pathways are more diffuse.

The chemoreceptor trigger zone (CTZ) is located in the area postrema, in the floor of the 4th ventricle, where there is effectively no blood–brain barrier.[10,11] Cerebrospinal fluid which is in chemical equilibrium with blood in locally fenestrated capillaries bathes chemosensitive nerve cell projections. The nature of these chemoreceptors remains obscure.[13,16] Neural pathways project from the CTZ to the nucleus of the tractus solitarius and the reticular formation in the medulla oblongata: these structures are the location of the 'vomiting centre'.

There may be medullary neurones which sustain an antiemetic tone,[16-18] inhibition of which potentiates the CTZ. These neurones may be enkephalinergic, and displacement of enkephalins from their receptors by naloxone[17] or opioids[18] may reduce antiemetic tone, as may inhibition of enkephalin synthesis by chemotherapy,[18] thus potentiating emesis. This interesting hypothesis helps to explain, for example, the different emetogenic potentials of chemotherapeutic agents according to the point at which they interrupt cellular protein synthesis. The importance of medullary antiemetic tone and its influence on the CTZ remains speculative.

The vomiting centre (VC) is a diffuse, interconnecting neural network which integrates emetogenic stimuli with parasympathetic and motor efferent activity to produce the vomiting reflex. This is a complex reflex with respiratory, salivary, vasomotor, and somatic motor components: the VC acts as a central pattern generator.[13,19] It has been proposed that sequential activation of various components of the VC, with amplification at each step, is required to trigger vomiting.[19] Nausea in the absence of vomiting may arise from stimuli which excite the VC without sufficient amplification to trigger the vomiting cascade.[10,21] Thus, nausea usually accompanies the prodromal autonomic effects which precede vomiting. However, the degree of nausea cannot be predicted by the accompanying autonomic changes, for example the relative reduction in gastric contraction.[10] Also, nausea is not always relieved by vomiting: this usually indicates continuing excitation of the central emetogenic pathway.

The VC receives afferents from the cerebral cortex and higher brainstem, thalamus, and hypothalamus, the vestibular system and, via the vagus and splanchnic nerves, the pharynx, gastrointestinal tract, and serosae.[22,23] There is also input from the CTZ, which can only initiate vomiting via the VC[10] (Fig. 1).

At least 17 potential neurotransmitters or receptors have been identified in the CTZ and nucleus of the tractus solitarius.[24] These include dopamine, serotonin, and histamine, and both opioid and cannabinoid receptors.[24,25] The principal receptors at the CTZ are dopamine type 2 (D_2); at the VC the principal receptors are muscarinic cholinergic (Ach_m) and histamine type 1 (H_1). Both sites exhibit serotonin type 3 ($5\text{-}HT_3$) receptors.

Afferent pathways involved in emesis

The interrelationship between CTZ, VC, and their various afferent inputs is summarized in Fig. 1. The major afferent neural pathway from the body to the central structures is the vagus, with additional input via the sympathetic ganglia and the glossopharyngeal nerve.[23,28] The vagus itself is stimulated via mechanoreceptors and chemoreceptors in the gastrointestinal tract, serosae, and viscera.[23]

The VC receives descending fibres from higher centres which may stimulate or inhibit activation of the emetic cascade.[10,13,19] Most vagal afferents terminate at the VC, but there is some vagal input to the CTZ.[29]

Projections from the vestibular nuclei which mediate emesis are incompletely understood; the CTZ may be involved, although D_2

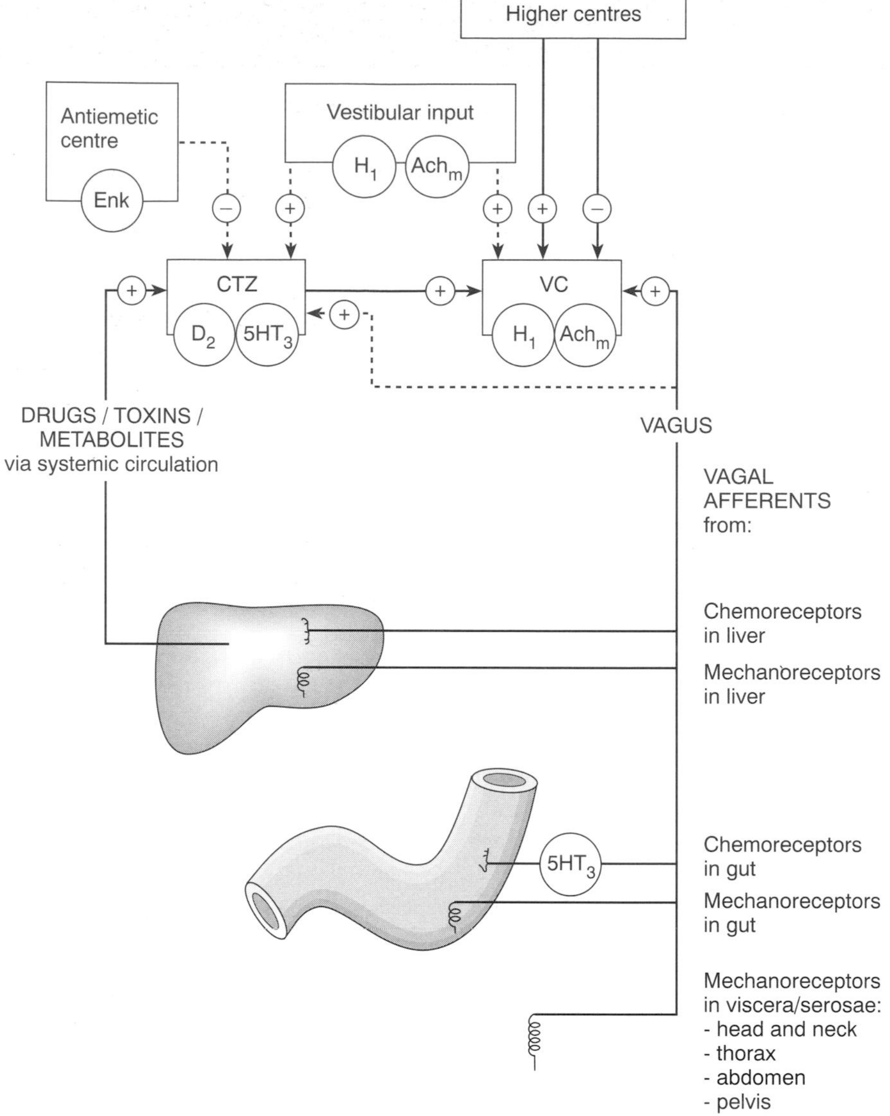

Fig. 1 The interrelationship between CTZ, VC, and their afferent inputs. – , established connections; CTZ, chemoreceptor trigger zone; ... , postulated connections; VC, vomiting centre; D_2, dopamine type 2 receptor; 5-HT_3, serotonin type 3 receptor; Enk, enkephalinergic pathways; H_1, histamine type 1 receptor; Ach_m, muscarinic cholinergic receptor.

antagonists are not potent antiemetics in motion sickness.[30] H_1 and Ach_m antagonists are more potent: they are thought to act on first-order vestibular neurones.[30] Opioids can potentiate sensitivity of the labyrinth.[31]

Choosing an antiemetic

Before prescribing drugs, care should be taken to reduce the stimulus to nausea from the patient's environment. This includes avoidance of cooking smells, attention to unpleasant odours (e.g. from an infected, necrotic tumour), and presentation of small, attractive meals. Cool, fizzy drinks are more palatable than still or hot drinks. Many patients experience a taste change so that previously innocuous foods taste nauseating (see Chapter 9.3.5).

Selection of an appropriate antiemetic strategy involves seven steps, namely:

(1) identify the likely cause(s) of nausea and/or vomiting;

(2) identify the pathway by which each cause triggers the vomiting reflex (Fig. 1);

(3) identify the neurotransmitter receptor involved in the identified pathway;

(4) choose the most potent antagonist to the receptor identified—the binding affinity of a particular antagonist predicts its antiemetic efficacy[26,27] (Table 1);

(5) choose a route of administration which will ensure that the drug reaches its site of action—this often excludes the oral route;

(6) titrate the dose carefully, review the patient frequently, give the antiemetic regularly;

(7) if symptoms persist, review the likely cause(s): additional treatment may be required for an overlooked cause, or alter-

Table 1 Receptor-specific antiemetics of use in palliative care

Drug	Receptor and site (see text)	Indications	Dosage and routes	Side-effects	Notes
Butyrephenones: • haloperidol • droperidol	D_2 -CTZ	opioid induced N; chemical/ metabolic N	haloperidol: 1.5–5.0 mg/day/po; sc (occ up to 20 mg/day)	dystonias dyskinesia akathisia	side-effects unusual at low doses
Prokinetic agents: • metoclopramide	D_2 -CTZ D_2 -GIT 5-HT_4 -GIT	gastric stasis; ileus	10–30 mg 2–4 hourly po, sc, iv	dystonias akathisia oesophageal spasm; colic in GI obstruction	prolonged half-life in renal failure (95)
	5-HT_3 -CTZ 5-HT_3 -GIT (at high doses)	chemotherapy	N/A	frequent at high doses	superseded by 5HT_3 agonists
• domperidone	D_2 -CTZ D_2 -GIT 5-HT_4 -GIT (potentiation)	gastric stasis; ileus	10–30 mg po 4–8 hourly 30–90 mg pr 4–8 hourly	colic if GI obstructed; oesophageal pain	extrapyramidal side-effects are rare
• cisapride	Ach -GIT	gastric stasis; ileus	10 mg po 6–8 hourly 30 mg pr 6–8 hourly	abdominal cramps; diarrhoea; cardiac arrhythmias with systemic azole antifungals (34)	prokinetic throughout GIT
Phenothiazines (including prochlorperazine chlorpromazine, thiethylperazine, Levomepromazine	D_2 -CTZ D_2 -GIT H_1, Ach, α_1Ad { VC, GIT, CVS, CNS with varying potency		prochlorperazine: 5–20 mg po 12.5–25 mg im 25 mg pr 6–8 hourly chlorpromazine: 25–50 mg im 4–6 hourly levomepromazine: 5–12.5 mg/24h po, sc infusion	vary according to spectrum of receptor blockade: see text.	not recommended for routine use, but see text
Antihistamines: • cyclizine • cinnarizine • diphenylhydramine • promethazine	H_1 -VC -vestibular afferents -brain substance Ach_m -VC	intestinal obstruction; peritoneal irritation; vestibular causes; raised ICP	cyclizine: 25–50 mg 8 hourly po/sc/pr only cyclizine is tolerated by sc injection	dry mouth. blurred vision (rare); sedation. cyclizine: skin irritation at sc injection sites in some patients	cyclizine is least sedative therefore the drug of choice
• diphenylhydramine • promethazine					
Anticholinergics: • hyoscine (scopolamine) hydrobromide	Ach_m -VC -GIT	intestinal obstruction; peritoneal irritation; raised ICP; excess secretions	200–400 μg 4–8 hourly subling/sc 500–1500 μg/72 h transdermal patches	dry mouth; ileus; urinary retention; blurred vision; occasionally agitation	useful if N and V coexist with colic
5-HT_3 antagonists: • granisetron • ondansetron • tropisetron	5-HT_3 -GIT -CTZ -(VC)	chemotherapy; abdominal radiotherapy; postoperative nausea and vomiting	granisetron: 3 mg slowly iv up to 8 hourly; ondansetron: 8 mg po or slowly iv 8 hourly; tropisetron 5 mg po or slowly iv daily	headache in 30% constipation diarrhoea	effectiveness increased by combination with dexamethasone

Abbreviations: CTZ = chemoreceptor trigger zone; VC = vomiting centre; GIT = gastrointestinal tract; ICP = intracranial pressure; N = nausea; V = vomiting; po = by mouth; pr = by rectum; sc = by subcutaneous injection; iv = by intravenous injection; im = by intramuscular injection; occ = occasionally.

native treatment may be suggested by a different cause becoming apparent.[20,21]

If several different receptors are involved, use of a potent antagonist for each receptor is preferable to use of one drug which weakly antagonizes several receptors.[22,28]

Antiemetic drugs available

A wide variety of antiemetic drugs is available. Those which have potent, receptor-specific action are summarized in Table 1. The antiemetic efficacy and side-effects of a drug can be predicted by its binding affinity for particular receptors.[26,27]

Drugs with receptor-specific action

Dopamine (D_2) antagonists

Of the dopamine (D_2) antagonists, haloperidol is the most potent at the CTZ.[26] Metoclopramide and domperidone, whilst having some CTZ antidopaminergic activity, act potently in the gut to antagonize D_2 and stimulate 5-HT_4 receptors. Local acetylcholine release, mediated by the 5-HT_4 receptor, appears to play an important role in reversing gastroparesis and bringing about normal peristalsis in the upper gastrointestinal tract.[22, 32] At high doses, metoclopramide blocks 5-HT_3 receptors in the CTZ and gut; extrapyramidal side-effects are common and this mode of use has been superseded by development of specific 5-HT_3 antagonists for cancer chemotherapy-induced emesis.[22,25,33]

The prokinetic agent cisapride acts by potentiating cholinergic activity in the gastrointestinal tract, and thus increases peristalsis from oesophagus to rectum. It has no antidopaminergic activity. Metabolism of cisapride is inhibited by ketoconazole, and potentially cardiotoxic blood levels may occur.[34] The two should not be prescribed together.

Any agent which is prokinetic may induce colic in an obstructed intestine.

Phenothiazines

The phenothiazines are less potent D_2 antagonists. They have varying antagonist activity at other receptors which predicts their side-effects (e.g. chlorpromazine—α_1 adrenergic receptor—may cause hypotension and sedation; diphenhydramine, a phenothiazine antihistamine—Ach_m receptor—may cause sedation and dry mouth).[20,27,35,36] Extrapyramidal reactions occur with all of the D_2 antagonists, although the incidence with domperidone is extremely low.[20] Levomepromazine blocks a wide spectrum of receptors at higher doses; it is highly sedative and causes hypotension but it is a useful antiemetic at lower doses (5–12.5 mg/24h by mouth or subcutaneous infusion). Circumstantial evidence suggests that 5-HT_2 blockage may mediate levomepromazine antiemetic activity (R. Twycross, personal communication).

Antihistamines and anticholinergics

The antihistamines act on H_1 receptors in the VC and on vestibular afferents.[20,26,30] Only cyclizine is suitable for subcutaneous injection. Cyclizine is less sedative than the anticholinergic hyoscine (scopolamine) hydrobromide, which blocks Ach_m receptors in the VC and peripherally.[20,26,28] Hyoscine hydrobromide can be given sublingually, subcutaneously, and transdermally. Its side-effects are those of parasympathetic blockade, which may be beneficial (drying of secretions, reduction of colic) or troublesome (dry mouth, ileus, urinary retention, blurred vision). Drowsiness is not uncommon. Transdermal hyoscine was developed with a view to reducing systemic side-effects, but in the author's experience with cancer and AIDS patients several patches used simultaneously may be required for relief of nausea, with the full complement of anticholinergic side-effects.

Hyoscine butylbromide does not have central antiemetic action. In the gut, however, its anticholinergic properties reduce peristalsis and inhibit exocrine secretions, thus contributing to the palliation of colic and nausea in intestinal obstruction.[37] Glycopyrrolate, a powerful peripheral anticholinergic drug with similar potency to atropine but little penetration into the central nervous system,[38] may be used as an alternative to hyoscine butylbromide.

5-HT_3 receptor antagonists

Receptor-theory based research has reached its zenith in the development of the 5-HT_3 receptor antagonists. Since 1986, when selective blockade of 5-HT 'm' receptors was demonstrated to block cisplatin-related vomiting,[39] there has been a rapid development of new drugs and an increasing understanding of the sites and roles of 5-HT receptors.[13-15,24,25,33,40-42]

5-HT_3 receptors have been demonstrated in the CTZ and VC centrally, and on terminals of vagal afferents in the gut peripherally.[23-27] The bulk of human serotonin is located within enterochromaffin cells in the gut wall; this serotonin is released and metabolized locally in response to various insults including direct abdominal irradiation and highly-emetogenic chemotherapy.[14,43,44] Release appears to be by active secretion,[43] although it is not blocked by octreotide.[14] The emetogenic action of serotonin derived from enterochromaffin cells appears to be by direct stimulation of local vagal 5-HT_3 receptors: high abdominal vagotomy abolishes emesis induced by abdominal irradiation,[28] and blood serotonin levels are rarely raised during emesis, although raised urinary levels of the serotonin metabolite 5-hydroxyindole acetic acid reflect the timing and severity of emesis after chemotherapy.[43] 5-HT_3 antagonists block vagal afferent activity. A reflex increase in vagal efferent activity may be caused, and this has been shown to give rise to temporary (and inconsequential) bradyarrhythmias in patients receiving repeated doses of these drugs, although not in healthy volunteers.[45,46]

Several 5-HT_3 antagonists are currently available (see Table 1). Of these, granistetron is the most specific 5-HT_3 receptor antagonist, ondansetron and tropisetron both showing some affinity for other receptors including α-adrenergic, other 5-HT, and opioid μ receptors.[41,47] Granisetron has the highest potency of these three, with a smoother dose–effect curve and a longer duration of action.[41] In clinical trials which have compared the three drugs, however, there appears to be little to choose between them, although patients who expressed a preference consistently preferred granisetron.[47] All are licensed for use in children, and adverse effects are few.

Although extremely effective for cancer chemotherapy-induced emesis and becoming established for radiotherapy-induced emesis,[48] 5-HT_3 antagonists have yet to find their place in the management of nausea and vomiting from other causes. They do not reverse nausea mediated by dopamine pathways (e.g. opioid-induced) and they remain largely untested in the nausea and vomiting syndromes associated with advanced cancer and AIDS. Some role in postoperative emesis is claimed for them[44,45,49] and ondansetron is licensed in the United Kingdom for this indication. Evidence from controlled trials comparing 5-HT_3 antagonists with less expensive antiemetics is lacking.

Other antiemetic drugs

Corticosteroids

Corticosteroids are known to possess intrinsic antiemetic properties[50–52] and to enhance the effect of other antiemetics.[25,52–55] Their mechanism of action is unclear and may be multiple. Corticosteroids may enhance antiemetic tone in the medulla by:

(1) reducing the permeability of the blood–brain barrier to chemicals which antagonize medullary antiemetic tone, such as chemotherapy agents;

(2) depleting the inhibitory amine γ-aminobutyric acid (GABA) in medullary antiemetic neurones;

(3) reducing leu-enkephalin release in the brainstem.[18]

In addition, capillary permeability changes brought about by corticosteroids may reduce chemical stimulation of the CTZ.

Cannabinoids

Recently, a brainstem cannabinoid receptor[56] and its ligand[57] have been identified. The ligand is an arachidonic acid congener, and its levels may therefore be influenced by the action of corticosteroids on prostaglandin metabolism. In addition, the anti-inflammatory effects of corticosteroids can reduce tumour mass, thereby reducing the stimulus to emesis from autonomic stretch receptors or intracranial tumours.

Anecdotal reports of a lower incidence of chemotherapy-induced emesis amongst marijuana smokers led to trials of cannabinoids. Synthetic cannabinoids with and without psychotropic effects are antiemetic, although marijuana may be more effective than its synthetic analogues.[58] The recent identification of brainstem cannabinoid receptors suggests a site of action for these compounds;[55] however, some of their effects are antagonized by naloxone, leading Harris and Cantwell to suggest that cannabinoids may contribute to medullary antiemetic tone via opioid μ receptors.[18]

The use of the currently licensed cannabinoids is limited by psychotomimetic side-effects, particularly dysphoria in the elderly. This effect can be reduced by low-dose phenothiazines[59] but the resulting drowsiness may undermine any therapeutic advantage of the cannabinoids. Euphoria is more common than dysphoria in younger patients, and there are reports of the successful use of nabilone for intractable nausea in AIDS patients,[60,61] who tend to be younger than adults with cancer, and in children receiving chemotherapy.[62] Larger studies are needed to assess the value of cannabinoids for emesis in advanced disease.

Benzodiazepines

Benzodiazepines have been used in chemotherapy antiemetic combinations. Although they have little antiemetic potency *per se*, in drug combinations they reduce anxiety and akathisia, and reduce the likelihood of anticipatory nausea. These drugs are sedative and sometimes amnesic when used in effective doses, which limits their usefulness for patients with chronic nausea.[25,54,63,64]

Octreotide

Octreotide is a long-acting somatostatin analogue which exerts wide-ranging potent inhibition of endocrine and exocrine secretions and promotes reabsorption of electrolytes in the gut;[65,66] there is clinical evidence of both inhibition and resumption of normal gastrointestinal transit.[67,68] Its combination of effects can be useful in palliating emesis caused by intestinal obstruction: inhibition of exocrine secretion in the gut reduces distension, thus diminishing the stimulus to nausea and to colic.[69–71]

Propofol

Propofol, an intravenous anaesthetic agent, has been noted to protect against postoperative emesis.[72,73] Recent work shows that subhypnotic doses of propofol have antiemetic action in post-anaesthetic and chemotherapy-induced emesis.[74,75,76] The duration of antiemetic action of an intravenous low-dose bolus outlasts the very short duration of hypnosis that would be induced by a far larger dose, suggesting that hypnosis or anxiolysis are not the mechanisms of antiemetic action. Propofol has a widespread central nervous system depressant effect and it is possible that its antiemetic action is at a subcortical level, in either the CTZ or within the VC complex. The observation that propofol is less successful as an antiemetic following vagal-stimulating abdominal surgery[75] suggests that its site of action may be the CTZ.

Opioids

Opioids can induce or block emesis in experimental models; both actions can be antagonized by naloxone.[13] It has been proposed that δ and/or κ opioid receptors are emetogenic, whilst μ receptors are antiemetic.[8] Experimentally, intravenous fentanyl in subanaesthetic doses abolishes emesis due to morphine, cisplatin, and copper sulphate, an effect which is reversed by naloxone.[77] In clinical practice, the nauseating properties of the opioids are well known: it remains to be seen whether more μ-specific drugs can be developed, and whether these may have any role as antiemetics.

Non-drug measures for palliation of nausea and vomiting.

Psychological techniques

Most of the authoritative research on psychological techniques for palliation of emesis has been conducted amongst chemotherapy patients, which is not analogous to the situation of nauseated patients with disease which is not amenable to chemotherapy. However, these studies have shown that patients can learn techniques such as progressive muscle relaxation and guided mental imagery, and use these during the stress of chemotherapy with good effect.[78–80] Cognitive therapy has been used to help relieve the psychological morbidity arising from physical symptoms in advanced cancer.[81] The possibility of adapting such techniques for the needs of nauseated patients with advanced diseases warrants further exploration (see also Chapters 9.2.9 and 15).

Transcutaneous electrical nerve stimulation

Transcutaneous electrical nerve stimulation (TENS) has been shown to enhance the effect of antiemetic drugs: the TENS effect is blocked by naloxone, suggesting that it is mediated by endogenous opioid peptides.[82] (see Chapter 9.2.8)

Acupuncture and acupressure

Acupuncture has also been shown to augment the effect of antiemetics during chemotherapy,[83] although it appears ineffective for postoperative nausea and vomiting.[84] Acupressure prolongs the effect of acupuncture,[85] and the use of TENS in place of traditional acupuncture needles at the P6 acupuncture point is a practical technique for self-use by patients, being only slightly less effective than the use of traditional needles.[86] The P6 (Neiguan) acupuncture point is located in the midline of the palmar aspect of each wrist, approximately 3 cm from the palmar crease.

Clinical syndromes associated with nausea and vomiting

Table 2 summarizes some common or important causes of nausea and vomiting in palliative care patients. They are grouped according to the pathway which mediates emesis, and are similarly grouped in the following discussion.

It must be emphasized, however, that in advanced cancer nausea and vomiting may have more than one cause, stimulating symptoms via more than one pathway. Sometimes apparently appropriate treatment fails to relieve symptoms, necessitating a search for additional and less obvious causes. Sometimes a cause cannot be identified: into this category are likely to fall those with cancer-associated autonomic failure. Growth factors and other tumour products may be emetogenic; their actions are still only partly understood, but it is likely that such factors would act via the CTZ. Tumours arising outside the areas described in the table may generate emesis via the same pathways, for example head and neck tumours cause pressure effects which trigger autonomic relays to the VC. The key to good management of nausea and vomiting is a high index of suspicion, an understanding of the pathways involved, and the setting of realistic goals.

Chemical causes of emesis

Drug induced nausea may arise by chemical action at the CTZ, by serotonin release in the gut, through gastrointestinal irritation or gastric stasis, or a combination of these (Table 3).

Transient nausea mediated by the CTZ accompanies the introduction or increase of opioids in 28 per cent of patients;[87] these patients will benefit from haloperidol, a central D_2 antagonist, during this period. In the United Kingdom and New Zealand, haloperidol is used with good effect; 28 in Northern America metoclopramide is oftern used as an alternative although it has weaker central anti-D_2 activity. 27 The appearance of nausea with other opioid toxicity manifestations (small pupils, drowsiness, myoclonic jerks) in a patient previously tolerant of the same dose of opioid may herald the onset of renal insufficiency: the opioid should be reduced in dose and/or frequency. An alternative opioid may be prescribed, at equianalgesic dose, provided it does not rely on renally excreted metabolites.[88] A proportion of patients experience opioid-induced gastric stasis. Tolerance to this does not develop; a prokinetic agent is required, [88] sometimes in high doses, if change to a different opioid is ineffective or not possible.

Cytotoxic-induced nausea is mediated by the CTZ and by 5-HT_3 receptors on vagal gut afferents. Selective blockade of 5-HT_3 receptors in the gut is highly effective;[33,41] these drugs may also act at the CTZ.[29] Adding antiemetics which work at other sites enhances the effectiveness of treatment,[25,47,54,55] particularly for delayed-onset emesis. Combinations of 5-HT_3 antagonist with a corticosteroid and/or benzodiazepine have been particularly effective, with 65 to 89 per cent complete control of symptoms in patients receiving cisplatin.[47,54,89]

Metabolic causes of nausea include organ failure and hypercalcaemia, which may progress insidiously. Nausea can be controlled using a central D_2 blocker: higher doses of haloperidol may be required (5–20 mg daily)[90] with a consequently higher incidence of extrapyramidal side-effects. These respond to antimuscarinic drugs such as procyclidine and benzatropine, which may be given by slow intravenous injection for relief of acute dystonias. (For the management of hypercalcaemia, see Chapter 9.11.)

Gastrointestinal causes of emesis

Pharyngeal irritation may cause retching, nausea, or cough-induced vomiting. The oropharynx is richly innervated by the glossopharyngeal nerve and vagus, and is highly sensitive to touch. Tenacious sputum or candida overlying the pharyngeal mucosa can stimulate the VC via these afferents; AIDS patients may also have mucosal lesions of cytomegalovirus or herpes simplex. Appropriate antimicrobial therapy is indicated for infections of mouth, pharynx, oesophagus, or respiratory tract. Sticky sputum may be loosened by inhalations, and irritating nocturnal cough causing retching and disturbed sleep may be palliated by application of local anaesthetic spray to the pharynx (with appropriate caution about eating and drinking for the next few hours).

Delayed gastric emptying may arise from physiological abnormalities or mechanical resistance to emptying. Mechanical resistance includes ascites, hepatomegaly, prepyloric inflammation, duodenal ulceration or tumour, and pancreatic cancer. Resistance may be partial or may be complete obstruction. Physiological abnormalities include anticholinergic effects of drugs (Table 3), including opioids, and autonomic failure.[91] The symptoms are listed in Table 2; they may not all occur and the diagnosis can be easily missed.

Complete gastric outlet obstruction is managed as high intestinal obstruction (see Chapter 9.2.4). Other causes of delayed emptying are managed by attention to:

(1) anxiety: explanation of cause and plan of treatment;

(2) optimizing gastric emptying: the prokinetic agents metoclopramide, domperidone; and cisapride increase the rate of gastric and upper intestinal peristalsis (cisapride also stimulates colonic peristalsis), increase lower oesophageal tone (thus reducing reflux), and relax the pylorus; gastric and upper intestinal transit time is shortened;

(3) reducing stimulus to gastric stretch: reduction in volume of meals and drinks and inhibition of gastric secretion using H_2 blockers or omeprazole or octreotide will reduce gastric stretch, thus reducing both the phrenic nerve irritation which gives rise to hiccup and the vagal stimulation which gives rise to nausea and pain.

Two adverse effects of the prokinetic agents are noteworthy. In

Table 2 Common syndromes involving nausea and vomiting in patients requiring palliative care (supplementary information in te

Syndrome	Causes	Key features	Pathway and receptors	Treatment possibiliti
Chemically-induced nausea	• Drugs: opioids digoxin anticonvulsants antibiotics cytotoxics • Toxins: food poisoning ischaemic bowel eg. gut obstruction ? tumour products • Metabolic: organ failure hypercalcaemia ketoacidosis	of drug toxicity or of underlying disease, plus constant nausea, variable vomiting	chemical action stimulates D_2 (±$5HT_3$) in CTZ; chemotherapy→ serotonin release in GI tract → 5-HT_3 receptors on vagus	• stop or reduce the offending drug • treat the underlying cause • haloperidol
Gastric stasis	• anticholinergic drugs, opioids • ascites • hepatomegaly • peptic ulcer • gastritis — stress — drugs — radiotherapy • autonomic failure	epigastric pain, fullness, nausea, early satiety, flatulence acid reflux, hiccup, large volume vomits, (possibly projectile) gastric regurgitation, other features of autonomic failure	gastric mechano-receptors ↓ vagal afferents ↓ VC H_1; Ach_m	• treat the underlying causes • prokinetic agents • reduce gastric secretions: H_2 blocker, omeprazole, octreotide • aid eructation: dimethicone
Stretch/ distortion of GI tract	• constipation • intestinal obstruction • mesenteric metastases	altered bowel habit, nausea, vomiting, may be faeculent, colic	gut/serosal mechanoreceptors ↓ vagal afferents ↓ VC	• treat underlying cause • active bowel management • corticosteroids may reduce the size of tumour mass
serosal stretch/ irritation	• liver metastases • ureteric obstruction • retroperitoneal cancer	of underlying condition, nausea, occasional vomiting	H_1: Ach_m	• cyclizine • hyoscine hydro-bromide if bowel paralysis is acceptable
irritation of GI tract	• e.g. cryptosporidiosis	profuse diarrhoea, nausea, occasional vomiting		
Raised intra-cranial pressure/ meningism	• cerebral oedema • intracranial tumour • intracranial bleeding • meningeal infiltration by tumour • skull metastases • cerebral infection (AIDS)	headache, (diurnal); papilloedema, photophobia may be absent. Nausea may be diurnal; neurological signs may be absent	may be direct stimulation of cerebral H_1 meningeal mechano-receptors ↓ VC H_1; Ach_m	• treat underlying cause • high dose corticosteroids may reduce cerebral oedema/ mass size • cyclizine • levomepromazine
Movement-associated emesis	• opioids (more common in ambulant patients) • gut distortion • gastroparesis → passive regurgitation	nausea and/or sudden vomits on movement/ turning in bed	opioid-induced sensitivity of vestibular afferents H_1; Ach_m gut mechanoreceptors ↓ vagal afferents ↓ VC H_1; Ach_m	• treat the underlying cause • nasogastric aspiration in terminal gastroparesis • cyclizine • cinnarizine • hyoscine hydrobromide
Anxiety - induced emesis	• anxiety —about self —about others —about disease —about symptoms • anticipatory emesis with cytotoxics	nausea of anxiety, may be relieved by distraction, 'waves' of nausea, ± vomiting, reminders trigger nausea	cortex ↓ VC H_1, Ach_m	• address the anxiety • psychological techniques • relaxation • benzodiazepines may be useful

Abbreviations: D_2 = dopamine type 2 receptor; 5-HT_3 = serotonin type 3 receptor; H_1 = histamine type 1 receptor; ACH_m = muscarinic cholinergic receptor; CTZ = chemoreceptor trigger zone; VC = vomiting centre; GI = gastrointestinal.

Table 3 Causes of drug-induced nausea

Mechanism	Drugs	
Activation of chemoreceptor trigger zone	Opioids Digoxin Anticoagulants	Cytotoxics Imidazoles Antibiotics
Gastrointestinal irritation	Non-steroidal anti-inflammatory drugs Iron supplements	Antibiotics Cytotoxics
Gastric stasis	Tricyclics Phenothiazines	Opioids Anticholinergics

a partially obstructed intestine, prokinetic agents may induce colic. Gastric colic may have a long periodicity mimicking ulcer- or tumour-related pain. Action of prokinetic agents in the lower oesophagus may provoke oesophageal spasm; typically this is retrosternal and may mimic angina pectoris. Oesophageal spasm may be relieved by sublingual glyceryl trinitrate.

Stretch and distortion of the gastrointestinal tract activates mechanoreceptors in the bowel wall; similar receptors are present in visceral capsules and in parietal serosal surfaces. Their afferent input is to the VC via the vagus and splanchnic nerves. Mechanoreceptors may be triggered by tumour distorting an organ, stretching or directly invading serosa or mesentery, or by increased transmural pressure in a hollow viscus proximal to a site of obstruction, for example ureter or colon. This is, therefore, a common complication of advanced intra-abdominal, retroperitoneal, or pelvic malignancy. Constipation and resultant colonic stretch is another frequent cause of nausea and anorexia. Local inflammation may potentiate afferent nerve receptors in the gastrointestinal tract, mediating emesis in bowel infections such as cryptosporidiosis in AIDS patients.

If reversal of the cause of emesis is not possible, nausea may be palliated by using antiemetics active at the VC. Control of vomiting may be more difficult to achieve with obstruction in the gastrointestinal tract: this is discussed more fully in Chapter 9.3.4.

Cranial causes of emesis

Raised intracranial pressure may present with nausea and vomiting before headache is apparent. Meningeal irritation can also trigger emesis. Clinical associations are with intracerebral tumours (primary and secondary), bone metastases to skull (base of skull metastases may give rise to cranial nerve symptoms and signs), intracranial bleeding, and cerebral oedema. High dose corticosteroids are the treatment of choice; an antiemetic acting at the VC may be necessary in addition.

Other causes of emesis

Movement-associated emesis may be triggered by distorted or distended viscera exerting increased traction upon their mesentery during movement. Movement-associated nausea may also occur as an unusual side-effect of opioids, related to increased vestibular sensitivity. This centrally-mediated emesis must be distinguished from passive regurgitation of gastric contents during movement of a terminally ill patient, which is usually related to gastroparesis; temporary passage of a nasogastric tube to aspirate the stomach dry of fluid and gas may be necessary to relieve this symptom.

Anxiety-induced emesis is a common experience in health. The patient with advanced disease may be able to identify anxiety as the trigger to nausea, or carers may notice an association between symptoms and stressful situations or conversations. Other causes of emesis must be excluded as far as possible before attributing nausea and vomiting to anxiety. Treatment is by identifying anxiety as a trigger and then working collaboratively with the patient to increase relaxation, identify and challenge anxiety-provoking thoughts and establishing workable coping strategies.[79,81] Benzodiazepines may be useful as short-term adjuvants: it is preferable to select a benzodiazepine with a longer half-life given as a single, evening dose (e.g. diazepam) to prevent as required use of anxiolytics, which is unlikely to be helpful. Some patients benefit from tricyclic antidepressants with secondary anxiolytic properties, for example amitriptyline. Drugs which reduce a patient's ability to concentrate can impair effectiveness or learning of psychotherapeutic techniques.[78]

Anticipatory emesis is a conditioned response in some patients who have suffered nausea and/or vomiting provoked by cytotoxic drugs. Any reminder of their previous experience may trigger emesis, including television pictures of hospitals, hospital smells, or visits by hospital personnel. It can be refractory to treatment and is best avoided by control of emesis from the first cycle of chemotherapy.[78,79] Management is as for anxiety-induced emesis. Systematic desensitization has also been used successfully in these patients.[92]

Intractable nausea

As with pain, the pathways of emesis are probably incompletely documented. Identification of triggers and implementation of receptor-specific antiemetics was successful in 93 per cent of patients in a well-conducted study,[28] but a minority remain for whom nausea continues unabated. There are no published data about these patients, but in the author's experience many of these are younger patients, often with pelvic malignancies and often with complicated psychological overlay to their symptoms. Amongst cachexic patients with chronic nausea, Bruera's group have identified a high incidence of autonomic failure.[91]

Appropriate goal-setting is important. It is unwise to expect or promise total relief of nausea and vomiting. Most patients will be content with major relief of nausea, even if intermittent vomiting continues, provided they have been led to expect this as a possible outcome. It may be helpful to grade emesis or use a tool to measure change in order to assess response to treatment. Patients' perceptions are different from those of nurses observing them,[93] and there is a need for an agreed tool for measurement of nausea and vomiting.[94]

When apparently appropriate measures have failed to relieve symptoms, and combinations of antiemetics directed at different receptors have proved ineffective, empirical use of levomepromazine may offer relief to some patients. Good clinical trials of therapy for such patients are necessary.

Future developments

In order to assess the effects of antiemetic therapies, tools for self-completion by the patient and biological markers of emesis need to be developed and evaluated. Good, controlled clinical trials of therapy are necessary, including further outcome studies of receptor-based prescribing to expand Lichter's welcome work.[28]

Increased understanding of the role of serotonin in emesis suggests that investigation of the use of 5-HT_3 antagonists in patients with vagally-mediated nausea and vomiting may be profitable.

References

1. Coates A, *et al.* On the receiving end—patient perception of the side-effects of cancer chemotherapy. *European Journal of Cancer*, 1983; **19**: 203–8.
2. Bliss JM, Robertson B, Selby PJ. The impact of nausea and vomiting upon quality of life measures. *British Journal of Cancer*, 1992; **66**: S14–23.
3. Grond S, Zech D, Diefenbach C, Bischoff A. Prevalence and pattern of symptoms in patients with cancer pain: a prospective evaluation of 1635 cancer patients referred to a pain clinic. *Journal of Pain and Symptom Management*, 1994; **9**: 372–82.
4. Regnard CFB, Tempest S. *A Guide to Symptom Relief in Advanced Cancer*, (3rd edn). Manchester: Haigh and Hochland, 1992.
5. Fainsinger R, Miller M, Bruera E, Hanson J, Maceachern T. Symptom control during the last week of life on a palliative care unit. *Journal of Palliative Care*, 1991; **7**: 5–11.
6. Dunlop GM. A study of the relative frequency and importance of gastrointestinal symptoms, and weakness in patients with far advanced cancer. *Palliative Medicine*, 1989; **4**: 37–43.
7. Doyle D. Symptom relief in terminal illness. *Medicine in Practice*, 1983; **1**: 694–8.
8. Cooper S, Georgiou V. The impact of cytotoxic chemotherapy—perspectives from patients, specialists and nurses. *European Journal of Cancer*, 1992; **28A**: S36–8.
9. Sims R, Moss V. *Terminal care for people with AIDS*. London: Edward Arnold, 1991.
10. Borison HL and Wang SC. Physiology and pharmacology of vomiting. *Pharmacological Reviews*, 1953; **5**: 192–230.
11. Wang SC. Emetic and antiemetic drugs. In: Root WS, Hofman FG, eds. *Physiological Pharmacology : a Comprehensive Treatise*. Vol II. New York: Academic Press, 1965: 255–328.
12. Esser MJ, Cowles VE, Robinson MD, Schulte WJ, Gleysteen JJ, Condon RE. Effects of vagal cryo-interruption on colon contraction in monkeys. *Surgery*, 1989; **106**: 139–46.
13. Grundberg SM, Hesketh PJ. Control of chemotherapy-induced emesis. *New England Journal of Medicine*, 1993; **329**: 1790–6.
14. Cubeddu LX, Hoffmann IS, Fuenmayor NT, Malave JJ. Changes in serotonin metabolism in cancer patients: its relationship to nausea and vomiting induced by chemotherapeutic drugs. *British Journal of Cancer*, 1992; **66**: 198–203.
15. Oxford AW, Bell JA, Kilpatrick GJ, Ireland SJ, Tyers MB. Ondansetron and related 5-HT_3 antagonists: recent advances. In: Ellis GP, Luscombe DK, eds. *Progress in Medicinal Chemistry* Vol 29. Elsevier Science Publishers, 1992.
16. Harris AL. Cytotoxic-therapy-induced vomiting is mediated via enkephalin pathways. *Lancet*, 1982; **i**: 714–16.
17. Costello DJ, Borison HL. Naloxone antagonises narcotic self-blockade of emesis in the cat. *Journal of Pharmacology and Experimental Therapeutics*, 1972; **203**: 222–30.
18. Harris AL, Cantwell BMJ. Mechanisms and treatment of cytotoxic-induced nausea and vomiting. In: Davis CJ, Lake-Bakaar GV, Grahame-Smith DG, eds. *Nausea and Vomiting: Mechanisms and Treatment*. Berlin: Springer-Verlag, 1986: 78–93.
19. Davis CJ, Harding RK, Leslie RA, Andrews PLR. The organisation of vomiting as a protective reflex. In: Davis CJ, Lake-Bakaar GV, Grahame-Smith DG, eds. *Nausea and Vomiting: Mechanisms and Treatment*. Berlin: Springer-Verlag, 1986: 65–75.
20. Allan SG. Antiemetics. *Gastroenterology Clinics of North America*, 1992; **21**: 597–611.
21. Edwards CM. Chemotherapy induced emesis—mechanisms and treatment. A review. *Journal of the Royal Society of Medicine*, 1988; **81**: 658–62.
22. Lichter I. Which antiemetic? *Journal of Palliative Care*, 1993; **9**: 42–50.
23. Willems JL, Lefebvre RA. Peripheral nervous pathways involved in nausea and vomiting. In: Davis CJ, Lake-Bakaar GV, Grahame-Smith DG, eds. *Nausea and Vomiting: Mechanisms and Treatment*. Berlin: Springer-Verlag, 1986: 56–64.
24. Soukop M, Cunningham D. The treatment of nausea and vomiting induced by cytotoxic drugs. *Ballières Clinical Oncology*, 1987; **1**: 307–26.
25. Kris MG, Baltzer L, Pisters KMW, Tyson LB. Enhancing the effectiveness of the specific serotonin antagonists. *Cancer*, 1993; **72**: 3436–42.
26. Peroutka SJ, Snyder SH. Antiemetics: neurotransmitter binding predicts therapeutic actions. *Lancet*, 1982; **ii**: 658–9.
27. Ison PJ, Peroutka SJ. Neurotransmitter receptor binding studies predict antiemetic efficacy and side effects. *Cancer Treatment Reports*, 1986; **70**: 637–41.
28. Lichter I. Results of antiemetic management in terminal illness. *Journal of Palliative Care*, 1993; **9**: 19–21.
29. Andrews PLR, Davis CJ, Bingham S, Davidson HIM, Hawthorn J, Maskell L. The abdominal visceral innervation and the emetic reflex: pathways, pharmacology and plasticity. *Canadian Journal of Physiology and Pharmacology*, 1990; **68**: 325.
30. Stott JRR. Mechanisms and treatment of motion illness. In: CJ Davis, CV Lake-Bakaar, DG Grahame-Smith, eds. *Nausea and Vomiting: Mechanisms and Treatment*. Berlin: Springer-Verlag, 1986.
31. Gutner LB, Gould WJ, Batterman RC. The effects of potent analgesics upon vestibular function. *Journal of Clinical Investigation*, 1952; **31**: 259–66.
32. Linnik MD, Butler BT, Gaddis RR, Ahmed NK. Analysis of serotonergic mechanisms underlying benzamide-induced gastroprokinesis. *The Journal of Pharmacology and Experimental Therapeutics*, 1991; **259**: 501–7.
33. Jantunen IT, Muhonen TT, Kataja VV, Flander MK, Teerenhovi L. $5HT_3$ receptor antagonists in the prophylaxis of acute vomiting induced by moderately emetogenic chemotherapy—a randomised study. *European Journal of Cancer*, 1993; **29A**: 1669–72.
34. Committee on Safety of Medicines and Medicines Cotrol Agency. Cisapride—interaction with ketoconazole and cardiotoxicity. *Current Problems in Pharmacovigilance*, 1995; **21**: 1.
35. Chlorpromazine (hydrochloride). In: Dollery C, ed. *Therapeutic Drugs*, Vol. 1, Edinburgh: Churchill Livingstone, 1991: C201–6.
36. Diphenhyaramine. In: Dollery C, ed. *Therapeutic Drugs* Vol. 1, Edinburgh: Churchill Livingstone, 1991: D164–8.
37. DeConno F, Caraceni A, Zecca E, Spondi E, Ventafridda V. Continuous subcutaneous infusion of hyoscine butylbromide reduces secretions in patients with gastrointestinal obstruction. *Journal of Pain and Symptom Management*, 1991; **6**: 484–6.
38. Mirakhur RK, Dundee JW. Glycopyrrolate: pharmacology and clinical use. *Anaesthesia*, 1983; **38**: 1195–204.
39. Miner WD, Sanger GJ. Inhibition of cisplatin-induced vomiting by selective 5-hydroxytryptamine m-receptor antagonism. *British Journal of Pharmacology*, 1986; **88**: 497–9.
40. Clarke DE, Craig DA, Fozard JR. The 5-HT_4 receptor: naughty but nice. *Trends in Pharmacological Science*, 1989; **10**: 385–6.
41. Andrews PLR, Bhandari P, Davey P, Bingham S, Marr H, Blower P. Are all 5-HT_3 receptor antagonists the same? *European Journal of Cancer*, 1992; **28A**: S2–6.
42. Van Wijngaarden I, Tulp MTM, Soudijn W. The concept of selectivity in 5-HT_3 receptor research. *European Journal of Pharmacology and Molecular Pharmacology*, 1990; **88**: 301–12.
43. Cubeddu LX, O'Connor DT, Parmer RJ. Plasma chromogranin A: a marker of serotonin release and of emesis associated with cisplatin chemotherapy. *Journal of Clinical Oncology*, 1995; **13**: 681–7.

44. Scarantino CW, Ornitz RD, Hoffman LG, Anderson RF. On the mechanisms of radiation-induced emesis: the role of serotonin. *International Journal of Radiation Oncology, Biology and Physics*, 1994; **30**: 825–30.
45. Watanabe H, Hasegawa A, Shinozaki T, Arita S, Chigira M. Possible cardiac side effects of granisetron, as antiemetic agent, in patients with bone and soft-tissue sarcomas receiving cytotoxic chemotherapy. *Cancer Chemotherapy Pharmacology*, 1995; **35**: 278–82.
46. Upward JW, Archbold BDC, Link C, Pierce DM, Allan A, Tasker TCG. The clinical pharmacology of granisetron (BRL 43694), a novel specific 5-HT_3 antagonist. *European Journal of Cancer*, 1990, **26**: S12–5.
47. Yarker YE, McTavish D. Granistetron: an update of its therapeutic use in nausea and vomiting induced by antineoplastic therapy. *Drugs*, 1994; **48**: 761–93.
48. Roberts JJ, Priestman TH. A review of ondansetron in the management of radiotherapy-induced emesis. *Oncology*, 1993; **50**: 173–9.
49. Kenny G, Rowbotham D, eds. *Postoperative Nausea and Vomiting*. London: Synergy Medical Education, 1992.
50. Cassileth PA, Lusk GJ, Torn S, Dinubile N, Gerson SL. Antiemetic efficacy of dexamethasone therapy in patients receiving cancer chemotherapy. *Archives of Internal Medicine*, 1983; **143**: 1347–9.
51. Jones AL, Hill AS, Soukop M, *et al.* Comparison of dexamethasone and ondansetron in the prophylaxis of emesis induced by moderately emetogenic chemotherapy. *Lancet*, 1991; **338**: 483–7.
52. Aapro MS. Present role of corticosteroids as antiemetics. In*: Recent Results in Cancer Research* Vol. 121. Berlin: Springer-Verlag, 1991: 91–100.
53. Diehl V, Marty M. Efficacy and safety of antiemetics. *Cancer Treatment Reviews*, 1994; **20**: 379–92.
54. Kris MG. Rationale for combination antiemetic therapy and strategies for the use of ondansetron in combinations. *Seminars in Oncology*, 1992; **19**: 61–6.
55. Smith DB, Newlands ES, Rustin GJS, Begent RHJ, Howells N, McQuade B, Bagshawe KD. Comparison of ondansetron and ondansetron plus dexamethasone as antiemetic prophylaxis during cisplatin-containing chemotherapy. *Lancet*, 1991; **338**: 487–90.
56. Gerard CM, Mollereau G, Vassant M, Parmentier M. Molecular cloning of a human cannabinoid receptor which is also expressed in testis. *Biochemical Journal*, 1991; **279**: 129–34.
57. Devane WA, Hanus L, Breuer A, *et al.* Isolation and structure of a brain constituent that binds to the cannabinoid receptor. *Science*, 1992; **258**: 1946–9.
58. Doblin RE and Kleiman MAR. Marijuana as antiemetic medicine: a survey of oncologists' experiences and attitudes. *Journal of Clinical Oncology*, 1991; **9**: 1314–19.
59. Cunningham D, Forrest GJ, Soukop M, *et al.* Nabilone and prochlorperazine: a useful combination for emesis induced by cytotoxic drugs. *British Medical Journal*, 1985; **291**: 864–5.
60. Flynn J, Hanif N. Nabilone for the management of intractable nausea and vomiting in terminally staged AIDS. *Journal of Palliative Care*, 1992; **8**: 46–7.
61. Green ST, Nathwani D, Goldberg DJ, Kennedy DH. Nabilone as effective therapy for intractable nausea and vomiting in AIDS. *British Journal of Clinical Pharmacology*, 1989; **28**: 494–5.
62. Dalzell AM, Bartle HM, Lylleyman JS. Nabilone: an alternative antiemetic for cancer chemotherapy. *Archives of Disease in Childhood*, 1986; **61**: 502–5.
63. Potanovich LM, Pisters KMW, Kris MG, *et al.* Midazolam in patients receiving anticancer chemotherapy and antiemetics. *Journal of Pain and Symptom Management*, 1993; **8**: 519–24.
64. Gordon CJ, Pazdur R, Ziccarelli A, *et al.* Metoclopramide vs metoclopramide and lorazepam: superiority of combined therapy in the control of cisplatin-induced emesis. *Cancer*, 1989; **63**: 578–82.
65. Gordon P, Comi RJ, Maton PN, Go VLW. Somatostatin and somatostatin analogue (SMS 201–995) in treatment of hormone-secreting tumours of the pituitary and gastro-intestinal tract and non-neoplastic diseases of the gut. *Annals of Internal Medicine*, 1989; **110**: 35–50.
66. Fallon MT. The physiology of somatostatin and its synthetic analogue, octreotide. *European Journal of Palliative Care*, 1994; **1**: 20–22.
67. Soudah HC, Hasler WL, Chung O. Effect of octreotide on intestinal motility and bacterial overgrowth in scleroderma. *New England Journal of Medicine*, 1991; **325**: 1461–7.
68. Peeters TL, Janssens J, Vantrappen GR. Somatostatin and the interdigestive migrating motor complex in man. *Regulatory Peptides*, 1983; **5**: 209–217.
69. Riley J, Fallon M. Octreotide in terminal malignant obstruction of the gastrointestinal tract. *European Journal of Palliative Care*, 1994; **1**: 23–5.
70. Mercadante S, Spoldi S, Caraceni A, *et al.* Octreotide in relieving gastrointestinal symptoms due to bowel obstruction. *Palliative Medicine*, 1993; **7**: 295–9.
71. Khoo D, Riley J, Waxman J. Control of emesis in bowel obstruction in terminally ill patients. *Lancet*, 1992; **339**: 375–6.
72. Barst S, McDowall R, Scher C, *et al.* Anesthesia for pediatric cancer patients: ketamine, etomidate, or propofol? *Anaesthesiology*, 1990; **73**: A1114.
73. Raftery S, Sherry E. Total intravenous anaesthesia with propofol and alfentanyl protects against postoperative nausea and vomiting. *Canadian Anaesthetists' Society Journal*, 1992; **39**: 37–40.
74. Scher CS, McDowall RH. Use of propofol for the prevention of chemotherapy-induced nausea and emesis in oncology patients. *Canadian Anaesthetists' Society Journal*, 1992; **39**: 170–2.
75. Borgeat A, Wilder-Smith OHG, Saiah M, Rifat K. Subhypnotic doses of propafol possess direct antiemetic properties. *Anesthesia and Analgesia*, 1992; **74**: 539–41.
76. Borgeat A, Wilder-Smith O, Forni M, Suter PM. Adjuvant propofol enables better control of nausea and emesis secondary to chemotherapy for breast cancer. *Canadian Journal of Anaesthetists*, 1994; **41**: 117–19.
77. Baines NM, Bunce KT, Naylor RJ, Rudd JA. The actions of fentanyl to inhibit drug-induced emesis. *Neuropharmacology*, 1991; **30**: 1073–83.
78. Burish TG, Tope DM. Psychological techniques for controlling the adverse side effects of cancer chemotherapy: findings from a decade of research. *Journal of Pain and Symptom Management*, 1992; **7**: 287–301.
79. Fallowfield LJ. Behavioural interventions and psychological aspects of care during chemotherapy. *European Journal of Cancer*, 1992; **28A**: S39–41.
80. Contach PH. Use of nonpharmacological techniques to prevent chemotherapy-related nausea and vomiting. *Recent Results in Cancer Research*, 1991; **121**: 101–7.
81. Adjuvant psychological therapy in advanced cancer. In: Moorey S, Greer S,. *Psychological Therapy for Patients with Cancer: a New Approach.* Oxford: Heinemann, 1989.
82. Saller R, Hellenbrecht D, Bühring M, Hess H. Enhancement of the antiemetic action of metoclopramide against cisplatin-induced emesis by transdermal electrical nerve stimulation. *Journal of Clinical Pharmacology*, 1986; **26**: 115–19.
83. Dundee JW, *et al.* Acupuncture to prevent cisplatin-associated vomiting. *Lancet*, 1987; **i**: 1083.
84. Weightman WM, Zacharias M, Herbison P. Traditional chinese acupuncture as an antiemetic. *British Medical Journal*, 1987; **295**: 1379.
85. Dundee JW, Yang J. Prolongation of the antiemetic action of P6 acupuncture by acupressure in patients having cancer chemotherapy. *Journal of the Royal Society of Medicine*, 1991; **83**: 360–2.
86. Dundee JW, Yang J, McMillan C. Noninvasive stimulation of the P6 (Neiguan) antiemetic acupuncture point in cancer chemotherapy. *Journal of the Royal Society of Medicine*, 1991; **84**: 210–12.
87. Compora E, Merlini L, Pance M, *et al.* The incidence of narcotic-induced emesis. *Journal of Pain and Symptom Management*, 1991; **6**: 428–30.
88. Twycross R. *Pain Relief in Advanced Cancer.* Edinburgh: Churchill Livingstone, 1994.
89. Sorbe BG. Tropisetron (Novoban) alone and in combination with dexamethasone in the prevention of chemotherapy-induced emesis: the Nordic experience. *Seminars in Oncology*, 1994; **21**: 20–6.
90. Twycross RG, Lack SA. Nausea and vomiting. In: *Therapeutics in Terminal Cancer.* Edinburgh: Churchill Livingstone, 1990: 57–62.
91. Bruera E, Catz Z, Hooper R, Lentle B, MacDonald N. Chronic nausea

and anorexia in advanced cancer patients: a possible role for autonomic dysfunction. *Journal of Pain and Symptom Management*, 1987; **2**: 19–21.

92. Morrow GR, Morrell BS. Behavioural treatment for the anticipatory nausea and vomiting induced by cancer chemotherapy. *New England Journal of Medicine*, 1982; **307**: 1476–80.
93. Olver IN, Matthews JP, Bishop JF, Smith RA. The roles of patient and observer assessments in antiemetic trials. *European Journal of Cancer*, 1994; **30A**: 1223–7.
94. Herrstedt J. We still need common criteria for the assessment of nausea and vomiting. *European Journal of Cancer*, 1994; **30A**: 1217.
95. Bateman DN, Gokal R, Dodd TPR, *et al*. The pharmacokinetics of single doses of metoclopramide in renal failure. *European Journal of Clinical Pharmacology*, 1981; **19**: 437–41.

9.3.2 Dysphagia, dyspepsia, and hiccup

Robert Twycross and Claud Regnard

Dysphagia

Definition

Dysphagia is difficulty in transferring liquids or solids from the mouth to the stomach.

Incidence

At St. Christopher's Hospice, London, where almost all patients have cancer, the incidence in nearly 7000 patients over a 10-year period was 23 per cent,[1] although in a more recent series of 800 patients, the incidence was only 12 per cent.[2] The frequency of dysphagia in patients with head and neck cancer is about 40 per cent on presentation (Table 1), rising to over 80 per cent as the disease progresses.[3,4] In motor neurone disease (amyotrophic lateral sclerosis), the incidence of dysphagia is about 60 per cent,[5] but, despite its progressive nature, it is a fallacy that aspiration is a common cause of death in this condition.[6]

Table 1 Dysphagia on presentation of head and neck cancer

Primary site	Percentage with dysphagia
Glottis	3
Alveoli	4
Floor of mouth	6
Tongue	11
Soft palate	18
Nasopharynx	20
Tonsils	26
Posterior tongue and vallecula	47
Supraglottis	48
Pyriform fossa	66
Posterior wall of pharynx	86
Postcricoid	100

(Reproduced from reference 3, with permission.)

Anatomy and physiology

Although the path taken by fluids and food to the stomach is direct, the mechanism to achieve a smooth and easy passage is complex. It requires intact anatomy, normal mucosa, normal functioning of five cranial nerves and the brainstem, the co-ordination of the cortex, limbic system, basal ganglia, cerebellum, and brainstem centres involved in respiration, salivation, and motor function. Thirty-four skeletal muscles are involved. This complexity reflects the biological necessity for respiration and nutrition, with respiration taking priority. Swallowing comprises four distinct phases.[7] The first two are voluntary; the latter two reflexive:

(1) oral preparatory phase: food is mixed with saliva and chewed to break down larger particles;

(2) oral swallowing phase: the lips are closed to prevent leakage and the anterior tongue retracts and elevates in a wave which pushes the bolus into the oropharynx;

(3) pharyngeal phase: this is triggered by the bolus reaching the posterior tongue. The larynx closes, breathing stops, and a peristaltic wave moves the bolus into the oesophagus in under 1 second. These complex actions are necessary to protect the airway because the pharynx is a shared passage for air and food.

(4) oesophageal phase: reflex peristalsis carries the bolus into the stomach.

Pathophysiology

Any disruption of normal anatomy and physiology may result in dysphagia and consequently there are many causes, sometimes with several concurrent (Table 2). Mechanical obstruction is generally caused by cancer. Tumours of the mouth and upper pharynx cause early symptoms, while those of the lower pharynx and oesophagus are often silent at first. Food will collect proximally and may spill over into an unprotected airway (Fig. 1). Stricture formation may occur following surgery[8] or radiotherapy.

In the absence of mechanical obstruction, severe dysphagia due to functional disturbance can occur. For example inability to raise the posterior tongue because of tumour infiltration may allow food to trickle into the pharynx and into an unprotected airway. Fibrosis following surgery or radiotherapy can also seriously disrupt the swallowing phases. Excessive drowsiness, disinterest, and weakness will result in a poor oral preparatory phase with leakage of food from the mouth, drooling, and possibly aspiration because of poor triggering of the swallowing reflex. Nerve damage is another factor; perineural spread of head and neck cancers can be demonstrated at autopsy in nearly 90 per cent of patients at postmortem.[10] In life, this is often associated with dysaesthesia and pain, particularly in the territories of cranial nerves V and IX. Occasionally, perineural vagal and sympathetic invasion combined with local fibrosis and tumour infiltration causes severe functional dysphagia which is indistinguishable from gross mechanical obstruction.[10] Pharyngeal and laryngeal sensory loss caused by cancer-related damage of the

Table 2 Causes of dysphagia related to advanced disease

Caused by disease process	*Associated with advanced disease*
Obstruction by mass lesion in mouth, pharynx, or oesophagus Infiltration of fibrosis of walls of mouth, pharynx, or oesophagus causing reduced motility ± damage to nerve plexus External compression (e.g. mediastinal tumour) Perineural tumour spread. Upper motor neurone damage (cerebral tumour or infarction) Lower motor neurone damage (motor neurone disease, multiple sclerosis, cranial nerve palsy) Motor or sensory cranial nerve palsy (tumour at base of skull, leptomeningeal infiltration, brainstem metastases or infarction) Cerebellar damage (infarction, surgery, tumour, paraneoplastic) Neuropathy (paraneoplastic) Neuromuscular dysfunction (myasthenic-myopathic syndrome, polymyositis, parkinsonism)	Dry mouth Mucosal infection of mouth, pharynx, or oesophagus (candidiasis, apthous ulceration, herpes simplex, herpes zoster, cytomegalovirus) Dental caries Drowsiness Withdrawal (depression, fear) Dry mouth (anxiety) Extreme weakness (patient moribund) Hypercalcaemia (rare)
Caused by treatment	*Concurrent disease*
Surgery (loss of structure, motor loss, sensory loss, fibrosis, fistula) Radiotheraphy (fibrosis, reduced saliva, mucosal inflammation) Chemotherapy (mucosal inflammation) Drugs (neuroleptics, metoclopramide, anticholinergic drugs)	Benign stricture Reflux oesophagitis (hiatus hernia, gastric stasis) Pain (mucosal, soft tissue, dental, bone)

superior laryngeal nerve will cause silent aspiration. Other neurological and neuromuscular disorders listed in Table 2 can cause severe dysphagia, including motor neurone disease (amyotrophic lateral sclerosis), Parkinson's disease,[11] and multiple sclerosis.

Loss of structures through surgery has varying effects. For example hemilaryngectomy will rarely cause swallowing problems if the epiglottis is preserved, and yet a unilateral supraglottic laryngectomy is likely to result in a chronic swallowing disability.[12]

Oesophageal spasm causes functional obstruction and, if intense, can cause severe central chest pain indistinguishable from ischaemic cardiac pain.[13] Spasm of the lower oesophageal sphincter or the cricopharyngeal muscle can be caused by anxiety.[14] Drugs are another cause of spasm,[15] as demonstrated in the following case report.

A woman aged 87 years presented with a history of progressive high dysphagia and weight loss. A barium swallow showed a smooth narrowing in the upper oesophagus with aspiration, but no abnormality was seen on endoscopy. She was taking prochlorperazine 15 mg daily for dizziness, but once this was stopped the swallowing returned to normal within 2 weeks.[16]

Severe functional dysphagia also occurs as a rare complication of hypercalcaemia.[17] Mucosal inflammation due to infection, radiotherapy or chemotherapy may cause painful dysphagia (odynophagia). Candida may affect the mouth, pharynx, and oesophagus and may present as a reddened mucosa, angular stomatitis, pale patches of chronically infected epithelium, or the classical white patches which leave an erythematous area when rubbed away. Oral candida is found in only 50 per cent of patients with oesophageal candidiasis.[18] The 'moth-eaten' appearances of oesophageal ulceration on barium swallow are characteristic of candida, herpes simplex, or cytomegalovirus infection. Infection in advanced cancer is usually mild, but can be severe and extensive in patients with AIDS. Painful swallowing for any reason can disrupt one or more swallowing phases sufficiently to reduce oral intake.

Evaluation

A basic evaluation can be carried out by the doctor but, if possible, help should be sought from the speech therapist with a special interest in swallowing disorders. In one series of 1000 patients, however, localization by the patient corresponded to the anatomical site of the problem in 99 per cent of patients.[7] The patient's description may also provide additional information (Table 3). Difficulty with certain food consistencies provide some information but is far less specific than is sometimes believed.[19] Even so, obstructing lesions generally produce dysphagia for solids initially with progression to liquids later, whereas neuromuscular disorders may well cause dysphagia for both solids and liquids more or less simultaneously.

Examination includes evaluation of the relevant cranial nerves,

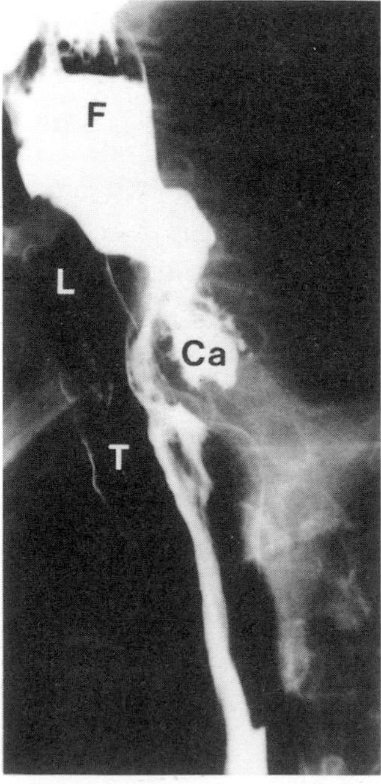

Fig. 1 Lateral view of barium swallow showing an ulcerating squamous cell carcinoma of the upper oesophagus (Ca) with poor pharyngeal emptying demonstrated by the presence of a fluid level in the pharynx (F). Laryngeal (L) and tracheal (T) aspiration of barium can be seen.

looking for evidence of muscle weakness (e.g. drooling or leakage of food, food collecting on palate or lateral sulci), checking for stridor, observing any jaw misalignment during chewing, assessing lip closure by rapidly repeating a syllable such as 'pa', and checking the condition of the teeth and mucosa. Anterior tongue movement is observed easily and posterior tongue movement can be checked by rapidly repeating the syllable 'ka'. Tongue strength can be assessed by asking the patient to push against the examiner's gloved finger. It is generally possible to differentiate between lower motor neurone (bulbar) lesions and upper motor neurone (pseudobulbar) ones (Table 4). A laryngeal mirror can be used when cold to check for mucosal sensation and then used to look for food debris or a pathological condition. The mirror can also be used to check the gag reflex, but the presence or absence of the gag reflex does not reflect of the patient's ability to swallow.[7]

Table 4 Bulbar and pseudobulbar symptoms

	Lower motor neurone (bulbar)	Upper motor neurone (pseudo-bulbar)
Emotions	Normal	Labile
Speech	Nasal escape speech	'Donald Duck' speech
Swallowing	Difficult to initiate, nasal regurgitation, dribbling	Dysphagia
Tongue	Flaccid, fasciculating	Spastic, small
Jaw jerk	Normal or absent	Increased

Reproduced from reference 20, with permission.

A further useful examination is a test swallow using consistencies which the patient finds easiest to swallow. The oropharyngeal transit time is measured from the first tongue movement to the last laryngeal movement. Times of more than 1 second are abnormal. It is also important to know which head positions a patient prefers (Table 3). Coughing, choking, or a 'gargle' quality to the voice after swallowing suggests aspiration.

Table 3 Evaluation of dysphagia

Information provided	Possible interpretation
Leakage from mouth, drooling	Poor lip closure, reduced lip sensation, abnormal tongue movement, or reduced/absent swallowing reflex
Bites cheeks or tongue	Reduced lip or tongue sensation
Frequent nasal regurgitation	Palatal dysfunction
Food collecting:	
in mouth	Poor lip, buccal, or tongue control
in vallecula/pyriform fossae	Reduced/absent swallowing reflex
Patient washes food down with a drink or pushes food in with finger.	Reduced tongue control
Patient tilts head down during swallowing	Delayed swallowing reflex or poor laryngeal closure
Difficulty with solids:	
in triggering swallowing	Poor tongue control
food sticks	Obstruction
Lack of awareness where food is during swallowing	Sensory loss
Difficulty with liquids	Poor tongue control, reduced/absent swallowing reflex, severe obstruction, muscular incooordination, soft palate paralysis or fixation
Coughing, choking:	Aspiration due to:
before swallowing	poor tongue control or delayed or absent swallowing reflex
during swallowing	reduced airway protection
after swallowing	reduced pharyngeal emptying, reduced laryngeal elevation, cricopharyngeus dysfunction, pharyngeal or oesophageal obstruction or tracheo-oesophageal fistula
Voice changes:	
inability to say 'pa'	Poor lip closure
inability to say 'ka'	Poor movement or posterior tongue
'gargle' type voice	Aspiration
'hot potato' voice	Vallecular tumours
'breathy voice/hoarseness	Recurrent laryngeal nerve palsy

Modified from reference 9, with permission.

Although examination may uncover the cause of dysphagia in the oral preparatory phase, accurate evaluation of the remaining phases is best done radiologically. For example aspiration will be missed on clinical evaluation in 40 per cent of patients.[7] Very low volume barium swallows are used initially, if necessary followed with larger volumes.[19] Abnormal pharyngeal phase or disordered oesophageal motility are best assessed by cine- or videofluoroscopy.[21,22]

Management

Clinical decisions

Is hydration and/or feeding appropriate?

Those patients with a very short prognosis (day to day deterioration) are unlikely to need or want feeding and hydration by any route (see Section 17). With slower deterioration, medically assisted hydration is appropriate in many patients with severe dysphagia. In one group of patients with motor neurone disease (amyotrophic lateral sclerosis), however, those with medically assisted feeding were compared with those who had elected to continue with oral feeding. Medically assisted feeding did not improve survival or distressing symptoms and sometimes caused new problems.[23]

The appropriateness of medically assisted feeding and hydration depends on:

(1) speed of deterioration;

(2) patient's opinion;

(3) opinion of family or partner;

(4) opinion of caring staff;

(5) potential advantages of feeding and/or hydration;

(6) feasibility of an alternative route;

(7) potential disadvantages of the route chosen.

Table 5 Indications for choosing an alternative feeding route

	Parenteral route (peripheral long line, central venous line)	Enteral route (nasogastric tube, pharyngostomy, oesophagostomy, gastrostomy, jejunostomy)
Indications		
Oral + pharyngeal transit time > 10 s Failure to modify swallowing technique during treatment to improve muscle control Nutritional support for surgery or chemotherapy	Complete pharyngeal or oesophageal obstruction. Short-term use (< 1 week) Anatomical or functional bowel loss	Long-term use (> 1 week)
Contraindications		
Rapid deterioration Dysphagia due to exhaustion, debility, or weakness caused by malignancy Psychological need of staff or family to provide 'active treatment'	Presence of sepsis Limited or no access to biochemical monitoring Limited or no access to a parenteral nutrition team Poor home cicumstances Long-term use (> 1 week) Superior vena caval obstruction	Nasogastric tube: nasal, pharyngeal, or oesophageal obstruction; cosmetic appearance Pharyngostromy: recently irradiated neck or local tumour Gastrostomy: gastric tumour

Based on reference 9, with permission.

In cases of doubt it is often possible to delay for several days or even weeks. It is easier not to start a treatment than to stop it a short time later.

Is a complete obstruction present?

If hydration is appropriate but there is complete obstruction, parenteral hydration will be required. Parenteral nutrition is rarely appropriate in endstage cancer. Endoscopic dilatation of the obstruction relieves dysphagia in over half of patients but, in malignant obstructions, improvement generally lasts less than 2 weeks.[24] Endoscopic dilatation is therefore used mostly as a short-term measure before radiation, intubation, laser resection, or alcohol injection. Single dose intraluminal radiation (brachytherapy) of oesophageal cancer has a similar initial response rate to endoscopic dilatation, and improvement is maintained for a median of about 4 months.[25] Endoscopic intubation provides another option using either a prosthesis[26] or a stent.[27,28] A prosthesis is better if palliating an oesophagobronchial fistula, whereas a stent is safer when there is a high risk of perforation.

Endoscopic laser therapy produces better relief of dysphagia than intubation[29,30] and, if a retrograde approach is used, improvement may be maintained for a similar length of time to brachytherapy.[31] Several treatments are generally required—more so with prograde resections. In about a quarter of the patients restoration of the lumen does not result in an adequate oral intake.[31] Alcohol injection of malignant obstructions produces similar results to laser therapy and is a useful alternative when laser therapy is not available.[32,33]

Is nutritional support required for surgery or chemotherapy?

Parenteral nutrition may be indicated before surgery or chemotherapy but these are generally not appropriate in patients with advanced disease (Table 5).

Is mucosal infection or a dry mouth present?

The commonest mucosal infection is candidiasis. Effective treatments are ketoconazole 200 mg once daily for 5 days, or a single dose of 150 mg fluconazole, the latter being useful when compliance is difficult.[34] Persistent or recurrent candidiasis will require longer courses (that is, 14 days), and immunosuppressed patients may require long-term prophylaxis with fluconazole 50 to 100 mg daily.[35] Extensive herpes simplex or zoster infections should be treated promptly with systemic acyclovir 200 mg every 4 h for 5 days. Extensive apthous ulceration is helped by tetracycline 250 mg as a 2 min mouthwash three times a day. Persistent apthous ulceration in AIDS patients has been reported to respond to thalidomide (see Chapter 9.10).[36]

If the cause of a dry mouth cannot be reversed, local measures are helpful, for example petroleum jelly to the lips, iced drinks or semifrozen fruit juices, and regular mouth care. Artificial salivas (methylcellulose or porcine mucin) are useful if used frequently by the patient, that is several times every hour. Glycerin or lemon should be avoided as the former dehydrates the mucosa and the latter soon exhausts the salivary glands.

Could drugs be a cause?

Drugs can cause a dry mouth (anticholinergic drugs, opioids), and occasionally oesophageal spasm (neuroleptic drugs, metoclopramide). In these circumstances the dose should be reduced if possible or an alternative drug prescribed.

Is pain affecting swallowing?

Mucosal pain in the mouth can be eased by topical analgesics such as choline salicylate gel or benzydamine mouthwash which are topical non-steroidal anti-inflammatory drugs with a mild local anaesthetic action. Increased local anaesthesia can be obtained with oxethazaine 10 ml 15 min before eating or drinking. This is also

Table 6 Tomato bavarois with yellow pepper coulis

Ingredients

Beef tomatoes	5	Sheets of leaf gelatine	4
Caradom	1	Maxijul powder	60 g
Whipped cream	140 ml	Yellow peppers	2
Beaten egg whites	2	Butter	30 g
Chopped fresh basil leaves	5	Pinch of salt and pepper	

Nutritional content: 169 kcal, 3 g protein, 11 g fat

Instructions

1. Remove the inside of the tomato.
2. Purée the inside of the tomato with caradom, Maxijul, and chopped basil.
3. Warm the puréed tomato and basil in a pan; then add gelatine.
4, When the mixture is nearly set, add whipped cream and beaten egg whites.
5. Gently mix without beating, and then pipe into the tomato skin.
6. To make the yellow pepper coulis:
   - chop the yellow pepper
   - place in a pan with the butter
   - place the lid on the pan
   - cook gently for 1–2 min until tender.
7. Place the tomato on the yellow pepper coulis, and then garnish with fresh basil leaves.

helpful if there is oesophageal pain on swallowing. Pain caused by widespread ulceration secondary to infection, chemotherapy, or radiotherapy is eased with a mucosal protective agent such as sucralfate suspension.[37] Having excluded or treated mucosal infection, the soft tissues need to be considered, particularly in patients with head and neck cancer. The rapid onset of pain over a few hours in such patients may well be caused by infection, but there may be little or no outward signs. Treatment with oral flucloxacillin and metronidazole resolves the infection and the pain within 24 h. Other causes of pain affecting bone, soft tissues, or nerve are treated as described elsewhere (see Section 9.2).

Is anticancer treatment indicated?

This is most commonly intraluminal radiation.[5] Chemotherapy is sometimes helpful in patients with advanced head and neck cancers (see Chapter 9.9).

Is peritumour oedema present?

In the absence of infection, corticosteroids may offer the possibility of easing dysphagia by reducing luminal obstruction, extramural compression, or nerve compression. Patients with dysphagia related to head and neck tumours may respond in the short-term to dexamethasone.[10] This will occur only if oedema is present, but since there is no simple way of assessing this, treatment is often empirical. Dexamethasone 16 mg daily is the typical starting dose and can be given as a single oral or intravenous dose or as a continuous subcutaneous infusion. Any beneficial effect may be present only for a few days or weeks but this is helpful, for example, in a patient awaiting radiotherapy.

Is aspiration occurring?

Since much aspiration is silent, radiological evaluation (generally videofluoroscopy) is necessary to quantify the amount of material aspirated. If this is less than 10 per cent, a swallowing therapist can advise on modifying the swallowing technique. For example, patients with poor anterior tongue movement will need help to position food on the posterior tongue, while those with poor control in the oral phase will need to check if food is collecting in the mouth. Patients with reduced laryngeal closure will aspirate less if they swallow with their head tilted forward because in this position the opened vallecula direct fluids around the glottis. If aspiration is still a problem they can be helped by coughing after each swallow. Aspiration is less likely if a patient remains upright for 15 min after meals to allow residual food to be swallowed. In unilateral pharyngeal paralysis, tilting the head to the same side is helpful.

Once there is a clear understanding of the swallowing problem, several simple measures can be considered. Imaginative food preparation and presentation are vital if unappetizing homogeneous brown sludge is to be avoided each mealtime. Even soft diets can be transformed with care (Table 6). Chilled foods are pleasant and patients with neurological dysfunction find them easier to swallow.

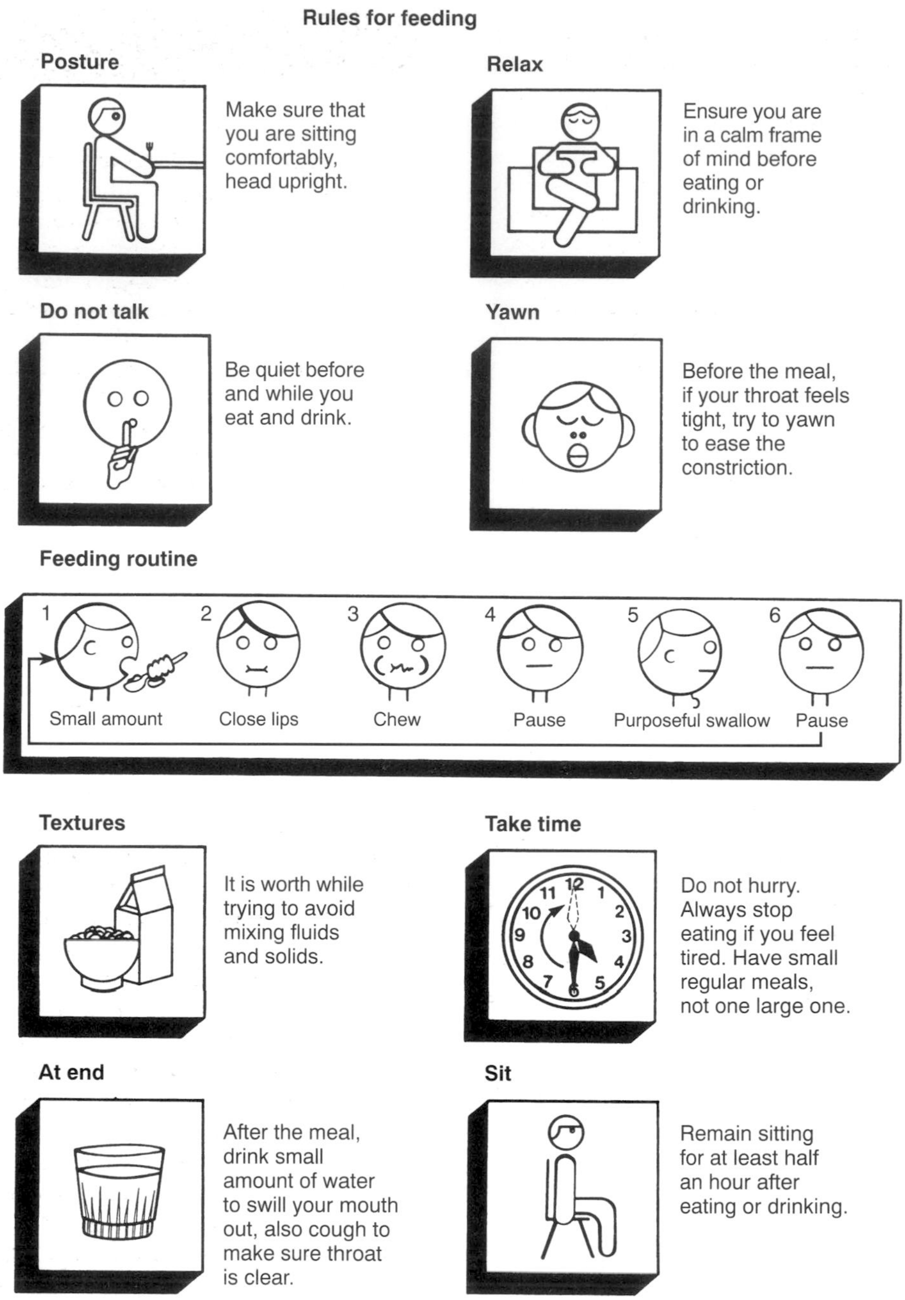

Fig. 2 Helpful hints to aid feeding in patients with dysphagia. (Reproduced with permission of Speech and Language Therapy, Frenchay Hospital, Bristol, United Kingdom.)

Someone with poor muscular control of the head can be helped by stabilizing the head with pillows or a lightweight chin support.[38] Patients may need help with feeding, allowing them to concentrate on swallowing, while the helper concentrates on positioning and transferring the food from plate to mouth.[39,40,41] The patient needs to be helped into a comfortable position and allowed to pause for a few minutes before eating (Fig. 2). Spectacles and hearing aids should be in place and in good working order. Dentures should also be in place, even if chewing is not required. The helper should face the patient so that they can see each other. Small amounts of food or drink should be given slowly. The technique advised by the swallowing therapist is then followed and its effect observed. Patients who are not helped by this or who aspirate more than 10 per cent of swallowed material may require medically assisted feeding.

Is medically assisted feeding needed for more than one month?

If the oral–pharyngeal transit time is longer than 10 s, or if more than 10 per cent of swallowed material is aspirated, medically assisted feeding is often the best option. Standard nasogastric tubes are uncomfortable for more than a few days, whereas fine bore tubes are well tolerated for weeks. Both types, however, may be cosmetically unacceptable. Fine bore tubes are more difficult to replace if displaced and nasogastric tubes may markedly increase oropharyngeal secretions.[23] Parenteral feeding has few indications and several contraindications which invariably preclude its use in endstage disease (Table 5). Because of these problems there has been a search for a better alternative. A pharyngostomy is probably the simplest to insert and maintain,[42] but cannot be used in luminal obstructions of the pharynx or oesophagus, and is unsatisfactory for patients with motor neurone disease.[20] Consequently a percutaneous gastrostomy is now used increasingly. A tube can be inserted either endoscopically under sedation and with local anaesthetic[43,44] or percutaneously under fluoroscopic control after distending the stomach with air or carbon dioxide.[45] Complications are limited to skin infection, tube blockage, or tube displacement. Generally patients with a gastrostomy can be managed at home.[46]

Other considerations

The psychological impact of dysphagia can be profound. This is not surprising because from childhood we are taught that we must eat if we are to keep well and strong, making dysphagia a tangible threat. Anxiety, anger, fear, and depression may result or be exacerbated and will need support and management. Medically assisted hydration and feeding can cause additional problems for the patient and family—both resistance to starting or distress at stopping.

If the patient cannot swallow saliva adequately, drooling is likely to be an embarrassing and troublesome problem. Anticholinergic drugs are helpful and transdermal hyoscine (scopolamine) hydrobromide is convenient, delivering 500 μg over 3 days. Radiation of the salivary glands also helps; 4 to 5 Gy are given initially, repeated if necessary 3 weeks later. In practice, however, this is rarely indicated.

It is inevitable that nutritional deficiencies are a risk in these patients. There is little information on the effect of nutritional deficiencies in patients with terminal illness. Consequently we do not know which specific deficiencies need to be corrected. Until more data are available, it is necessary to rely on advice from a dietician or nutritionist. It is important, however, to avoid a rigid scientific approach which places major burdens on the patient in terms of nutritional demands and/or financial cost.

Dyspepsia

Definition

Dyspepsia is postprandial discomfort or pain centred in the upper abdomen (synonym: indigestion). Dyspepsia encompasses a range of symptoms (Table 7). These vary in intensity and are not present in every patient or in every episode.[47]

Table 7 Symptoms of dyspepsia[47]

Symptom	Comment
Epigastric pain	Mainly postprandial.
Epigastric discomfort	A negative feeling which does not reach the level of pain and which can include any of the symptoms below.
Early satiety	A feeling that the stomach is overfull soon after starting to eat so that the meal cannot be finished.
Postprandial fullness	An unpleasant sensation of persistence of food in the stomach.
Epigastric bloating	Sensation of visceral distension in the upper abdomen; this is not the same as visible abdominal distension.
Belching	
Heartburn	
Hiccup	
Nausea	
Retching	
Vomiting	

Incidence

Dyspepsia is common.[48] In one community survey, a prevalence of nearly 40 per cent was reported over 6 months.[49] In the general population, of those fully investigated about one-third have a peptic ulcer, one-third have no obvious abnormality, and one-third have a variety of other diagnoses including gallstones and irritable bowel syndrome.[50]

Pathogenesis

There are many causes of dyspepsia in advanced cancer (Table 8). Oesophagitis caused by bile acid reflux may occur after total gastrectomy. Functional dyspepsia (i.e. dyspepsia without apparent organic cause) is generally caused by dysmotility. It is seen in about 25 per cent of the normal population and is therefore common in patients with cancer.

Most cases of squashed stomach syndrome[1] and cancer associated dyspepsia syndrome[51] are probably examples of dysmotility exacerbated by opioid-induced delayed gastric emptying, and/or gross hepatomegaly, and/or gross ascites.

A few cancer patients complain of marked early satiety and/or other dyspeptic symptoms without any obvious predisposing cause.[52] This probably relates to paraneoplastic visceral autonomic neuropathy.[53] There is often associated evidence of impaired autonomic control of the cardiovascular system manifesting, for example, as postural hypotension.[54]

Many drugs have an adverse effect on lower oesophageal sphincter tone (Table 9). The onset of heartburn within a day or so of commencing a new drug should alert the doctor to this possibility. The use of morphine and other opioids may lead to reflux secondary to delayed gastric emptying.

An additional cause of gastric distension is swallowed air. Licking one's lips initiates a swallowing reflex which causes air to be sucked into the stomach. A similar association is seen with sniffing, a common concomitant of acute coryza or nasal catarrh. Anxiety and smoking both tend to increase gastric gas because of the associated dry lips which are licked to keep them moist. Up to 15 per cent of laryngectomees give up any attempt at oesophageal speech because of the large volumes of air that are swallowed, preferring silence to abdominal distension and pain.[55]

Evaluation

From a therapeutic perspective, dyspepsia can be divided into four categories:

(1) small stomach capacity;

(2) gassy;

Table 8 Causes of dyspepsia in advanced cancer

Caused by cancer	Related to cancer and/or debility
Small stomach capacity	Oesophageal candidiasis
Large unresected stomach cancer	Minimal food and fluid intake
Massive ascites	Anxiety → aerophagia
Gastroparesis (paraneoplastic visceral neuropathy)	
Caused by treatment	**Concurrent causes**
Postsurgical	Organic dyspepsia
Postgastrectomy	Peptic ulcer
Reflux oesophagitis	Reflux oesophagitis
Radiotherapy	Colelithiasis
Lumbar spine	Renal failure
Epigastrium	Non-ulcer dyspepsia
Drugs	Dysmotility-like
Physical irritant (→ gastritis), e.g.	aerophagia
Iron	
Metronidazole	
Tranexamic acid	
Acid stimulant (→ gastritis), e.g.	
Non-steroidal anti-inflammatory drugs	
Corticosteroids	
Delayed gastric emptying	
Anticholinergics	
Opioids	
Cisplatin	

Table 9 Drugs and the lower oesophageal sphincter

Decrease tone	Increase tone
Alcohol	Antacids
Nicotine	Prokinetic drugs
Carminatives:	Metoclopramide
Mint	Domperidone
Anise	Cisapride
Dill	Parasympathomimetrics
Anticholinergics	Bethanechol
Pethidine/meperidine	
Benzodiazepines	
Oestrogens	
Theophylline	
Nitrates and nitrites:	
Glyceryl trinitrate	
Isosorbide dinitrate	
Calcium channel blockers:	
Verapamil	
Nifedipine	
Diltiazem	
Hydralazine	
Isoproterenol	

Table 10 Characteristics of different types of dyspepsia[56]

Type	Characteristics
Small stomach	Hungry with premature satiety Postprandial epigastric heaviness, fullness, or diffuse pain
Gassy	Bloating, particulary postprandial Repetitive belching Frequent dry swallows and gulping Often related to stress and/or anxiety
Gastro-oesophageal reflux (acid)	Burning retrosternal discomfort particularly: On bending over After large meals On lying flat Recent weight gain Temporary relief from antacids
Ulcer (acid)	Woken by pain at night Pain relief with: Antacids Snacks Meals Localized epigastric discomfort, can identify with 1–2 fingers
Dysmotility	Abdominal distension Hungry with premature satiety Epigastric heaviness or fullness Multiple food intolerances Pain: Diffuse Often more than one site Not at night Nausea prominent Associated features or irritable bowel syndrome

(3) acid (ulcer-like or gastro-oesophageal reflux-like);

(4) dysmotility.

It is important to differentiate between the four types because the treatment differs. Careful history taking and clinical examination generally indicate which type is predominant (Table 10). Patients with dysmotility dyspepsia often have symptoms or a history of irritable bowel syndrome. Barium studies and endoscopy are necessary only in a few patients.

Management

General

As always, treatment begins with explanation. There may be need for advice on diet, smoking, and alcohol. The causal role, if any, of medication should be discussed. Some patients keep over-the-counter proprietary 'indigestion' tablets or mixture in the home. The use of these for occasional dyspepsia can be supported provided the discomfort is relieved. One remedy in the United Kingdom, however, contains aspirin (Alka-Seltzer) and should be discouraged.

The patient's drug regimen should be reviewed. Many patients take several drugs concurrently. These may include ones that delay gastric emptying, stimulate gastric acid secretion, and physically irritate the gastric mucosa (Table 7). Occasional dyspepsia usually does not warrant a change in the drug regimen.

For patients with acid reflux, it may be possible to change to a drug with less anticholinergic properties, for example:

(1) amitriptyline → dothiepin or desipramine;

(2) chlorpromazine or prochlorperazine → haloperidol.

If the prescription of morphine is the precipitating factor, a prokinetic agent should be prescribed (i.e. metoclopramide, domperidone, cisapride).

In non-steroidal anti-inflammatory drug (**NSAID**)-induced dyspepsia, misoprostol (a prostaglandin analogue) is the treatment of choice.[57] If used prophylactically to prevent NSAID gastroduodenal injury in patients with a history of peptic ulceration, 200 μg twice daily is generally adequate. A higher dose, 200 mg thrice daily or 400 mg twice daily, is used to promote healing. The latter regimen sometimes causes diarrhoea; this means misoprostal may act as a 'colaxative' in constipated patients.

H_2-receptor antagonists prevent NSAID-related duodenal ulceration; they do not prevent NSAID-related gastric ulceration.[58] In contrast, they promote the healing of NSAID-related ulceration at both sites. A mucosal protective agent such as sucralfate is effective at both preventing and healing peptic ulceration,[59] including NSAID-induced dyspepsia and ulceration.[60] A proton pump inhibitor (e.g. omeprazole, lansoprazole) may be needed in some patients to treat established ulceration.[61] Other options include:

(1) finding an alternative NSAID which is less irritant—patients who experience dyspepsia with flurbiprofen, for example, may not with diflunisal or naproxen, or vice versa;

(2) reducing the dose;

(3) changing to a shorter-acting drug such as ibuprofen;

(4) administering an antacid regularly;[62]

(5) prescribing a physical mucosal protective agent such as sucralfate or colloidal bismuth subcitrate;

(6) substituting regular paracetamol.

Treatment

Small stomach capacity

If dyspepsia is associated with a small stomach capacity, patients should be advised to separate their main fluid from their main solid intake, and to eat 'small and often', that is take five or six small meals or snacks during the day rather than two or three big meals. Patients with a small stomach capacity may benefit from an antiflatulant after meals—to help clear space in a relatively overfull stomach.

Gassy dyspepsia

Gastric gas is reduced by a defoaming antiflatulent, for example silica activated dimethicone/simethicone.[63] Depending on a patient's individual needs, this can be given as needed, or four times a day, or both. Simethicone is also available alone as a tablet. If anxiety (and air swallowing) is thought to be a significant factor, this should be treated specifically.

Acid dyspepsia

Prescribe an antacid, H_2-receptor antagonist, or a proton pump inhibitor. Of the two commonly available H_2-receptor antagonists, ranitidine is preferable to cimetidine because the likelihood of drug interactions is much less.[64,65] An initial dose of 300 mg at bedtime for 2 weeks followed by 150 mg at bedtime is generally sufficient. A prokinetic to improve gastric emptying should also be considered.

Cimetidine (but not ranitidine) slows the metabolism of pethidine/meperidine.[66,67] Cimetidine also inhibits methadone metabolism; on occasion this has resulted in respiratory depression and coma.[68]

Proton pump inhibitors cause irreversible inhibition of the enzyme adenosine triphosphatase in gastric parietal cells.[69] The induced disturbance of the hydrogen–potassium ion exchange mechanism has a profound inhibitory effect on gastric acid secretion, greater than that achieved by H_2-receptor antagonists. The inhibition is of prolonged duration, and the maximum antisecretory effect occurs several days after starting treatment.

Acid reflux oesophatitis

Objective tests (endoscopy and oesophageal biopsy) demonstrate that an antacid containing simethicone is superior to a plain antacid in the management of reflux oesophagitis,[70] and as least as effective as an antacid containing alginic acid.[71] These findings suggest that simethicone-containing antacids can be regarded as broad-spectrum antacids for all patients troubled by acid-related dyspepsia, whether gastric or oesophageal.

An alginic acid-containing antacid is still commonly prescribed for patients with reflux. Such preparations, however, are more expensive, often have a high sodium content, and are generally weak antacids. Much of the antacid content adheres to the alginate matrix which floats on the surface of the gastric contents. Any neutralization of gastric juice which takes place is localized to the proximal stomach contents, although this is the portion refluxed. A simethicone-containing antacid would seem to be generally preferable.

Bile reflux oesophagitis

This is an unusual but important type of reflux oesophagitis. In a patient with a good prognosis, the best treatment is surgical.[72] A Roux-en-Y procedure results in the amelioration of the symptoms and signs in most patients. The aim of the operation is to divert duodenal secretions and bile into the jejunum about 40 cm distal to the gastrojejunostomy/oesophagojejunostomy.

In palliative care, however, symptomatic measures will be the norm. These include sleeping propped up with three to four pillows and the prescription of bile acid binding agents. Hydrotalcite (magnesium aluminium carbonate hydrate) is a naturally occurring antacid which reversibly binds bile acids, particularly in an acid medium.[73] Thus, although of limited value for bile-reflux oesophagitis after total gastrectomy, it is not valueless and should certainly be tried (e.g. 1 g four times a day). Alginic acid-containing antacids and antiflatulent antacids are ineffectual.[74]

At higher bile acid concentrations, cholestyramine is more efficacious than hydrotalcite.[74] No dose regimen for this condition has been established but it is suggested that 2 g (half a sachet) four times a day (after meals and at bedtime) might be tried.[75] There is a likelihood of steatorrhoea and, if treatment is long-continued,

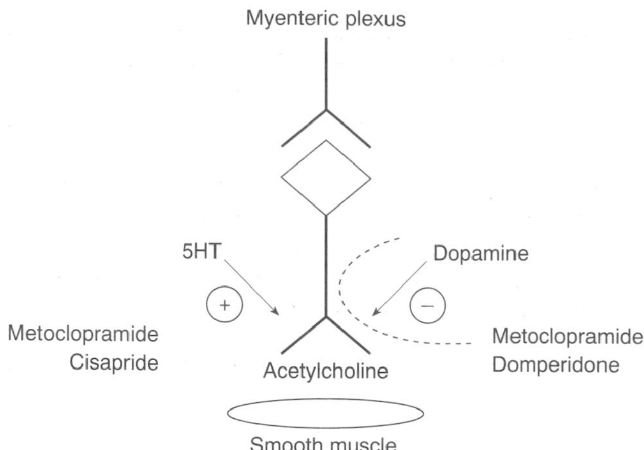

Fig. 3 Schematic representation of drug effects on antroduodenal co-ordination via a postganglionic effect on the cholinergic nerves from the myenteric plexus. + stimulatory effect of 5-HT triggered by metoclopramide and cisapride; – inhibitory effect of dopamine; – – – blockade of dopamine inhibition by metoclopramide and domperidone. (Reproduced from Twycross,[91] with permission.)

supplements of fat-soluble vitamins A, D, E, and K should be considered.

Dysmotility dyspepsia

Dysmotility dyspepsia is not helped by gastric acid reduction,[50] nor by dicyclomine, an anticholinergic drug.[76] It is treated with a prokinetic drug.[77] Tumour-related gastroparesis also benefits from a prokinetic.[78,79] The choice lies between metoclopramide (dopamine antagonist and 5-HT_4 agonist), domperidone (dopamine antagonist) and cisapride (5-HT_4 agonist).[80,81] All trigger a cholinergic system in the myenteric plexus (Fig. 3). Unlike metoclopramide and domperidone, cisapride has no central antiemetic effect.

Despite its dual mechanism of action, metoclopramide is not more potent than domperidone when used in standard doses; that is, 10 mg three or four times per day.[82,83] In functional dyspepsia, cisapride is twice as potent as metoclopramide.[84,85] In diabetic gastroparesis, however, the effect of cisapride 2.5 mg on gastric emptying is greater than that of metoclopramide 10 mg, giving a potency ratio of at least 4.[86] These figures suggest that cisapride is relatively more potent in pathological states than in functional dysmotility. Cisapride has also been shown to be effective in functional dyspepsia resistant to domperidone or metoclopramide, with good or excellent ratings in 65 per cent and 32 per cent of patients respectively.[87,88] The effect of cisapride is maintained long-term better than metoclopramide.[89,85] Cisapride and domperidone have an additive effect on gastric emptying and on symptoms such as epigastric fullness, belching, and nausea.[90]

Morphine and other opioids impede the release of neuronal acetylcholine, and slow gastric emptying. Metoclopramide 10 mg (partly) and cisapride 10 mg (completely) corrects this.[92] Data are not available for domperidone. The maximum plasma concentration of morphine after slow-release 20 mg is significantly greater if given with cisapride 20 mg[93] but not with metoclopramide 10 mg[94]—a smaller prokinetic dose. Paradoxically, greater sedation was noted after metoclopramide[94] but not with cisapride.[93] This suggests that metoclopramide may have its own central sedative effect.

Hiccup

Definition

Hiccup is a pathological respiratory reflex characterized by spasm of one or both sides of the diaphragm, resulting in sudden inspiration and closure of the glottis. Accessory muscles of respiration (anterior scalene, intercostal, abdominal) are occasionally involved.[95]

Incidence

Occasional hiccup is an ubiquitous human experience which rarely warrants designation as a symptom.[96] The incidence of troublesome hiccup in terminal cancer is not known. Rarely, hiccup is a major cause of distress,[97] interrupting talking, eating, and sleeping, and resulting in weight loss, exhaustion, anxiety, and depression. Hiccup is occasionally the presenting symptom of neoplasms of the brainstem and oesophagus.[98,99]

Causes

Over a 28-year period at the Mayo Clinic, 220 patients reported hiccup lasting for more than 2 days; 82 per cent were men.[100] A diagnosis of psychogenic hiccup was made in 36 out of 39 women, compared with 12 out of 181 men. Of the other men, 40 were postoperative and 129 medical. Of the medical patients, 44 had either cerebrovascular or coronary heart disease, 33 had a hiatus hernia, 11 had a duodenal ulcer, and 11 had metabolic disturbances (including four with diabetes mellitus and four with uraemia). Many had two concurrent disorders. Persistent hiccup occurs, therefore, in association with one or more of many diseases (Table 11).

In terminal cancer, clinical experience suggests that gastric distension is the commonest cause. Other relatively common causes

Table 11 Selected causes of hiccups[100-102]

Irritation of the vagus nerve	Irritation of the phrenic nerve
Abdominal branches	Diaphragmatic
Gastric distension	Subphrenic abscess
Gastritis	Tumour
Hepatomegaly	Mediastinal tumour
Gallbladder distension	Cervical tumour
Pancreatitis	
Bowel obstruction	Central nervous system
Peritonitis	
Intra-abdominal haemorrhage	Intracranial tumours
	Brainstem lesions
Tumour	Basilar arterial insufficiency
Thoracic branches	Head injury
Oesophageal reflux	Encephalitis
Oesophageal obstruction	Meningitis
Pneumonia	Toxic
Coronary occlusion	Alcohol
Laryngeal branches	Renal failure
Pharyngeal branches	Psychogenic
Auricular branches	
Meningeal branches	

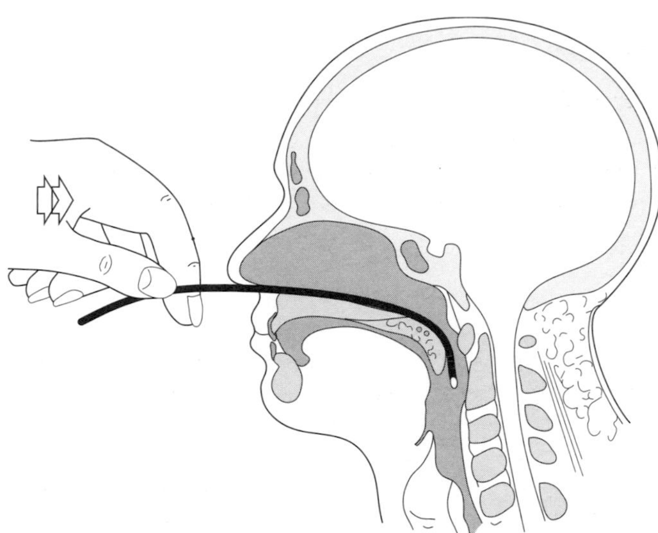

Fig. 4 Pharyngeal stimulation to stop hiccup. A nasal catheter is inserted 8–12 cm so that it is opposite the second cervical vertebra. Jerky to-and-fro movements lead to the immediate cessation of hiccups. Afferent innervation = vagus and glossopharyngeal nerves. (Reproduced from Salem *et al*,[106] with permission.)

include diaphragmatic irritation, and toxicity (uraemic or infection). Less common causes include phrenic nerve irritation and central nervous system tumour.

Pathogenesis

Hiccup is generally considered to be pathological because it appears to serve no useful function.[103] Because of an association with eating, it has been suggested that hiccup may serve to shift food lodged in the oesophagus.[101] The relationship of hiccup to gastric distension, however, probably explains this association. Adults are less prone to hiccup than children.

The reflex arc for hiccup comprises:[104]

(1) the afferent limb: vagus nerve, phrenic nerve or thoracic sympathetic fibres;

(2) the central connections: a non-specific anatomical location in the spinal cord between segments C3 and C5. In addition, there may be complex supraspinal connections between the respiratory centre, phrenic nerve nuclei, reticular formation, and hypothalamus;

(3) the efferent limb: primarily the phrenic nerve.

Occasional patients continue to hiccup after bilateral phrenicectomy.[100] In these, the efferent pathway will involve the accessory muscles of respiration.

Pharyngeal stimulation

Central to an understanding of the treatment of hiccup is the well-established fact that stimulation of the pharynx will normally terminate an episode.[105] As a result, a pharyngeal 'gate-control' mechanism has been proposed.[106]

Stimulation of the pharynx with a plastic or rubber suction catheter was successful in the treatment of hiccup in 84 out of 85 patients, 65 of whom were anaesthetized (Fig. 4). Of the 20 conscious patients, hiccup recurred once in eight patients, and more than once in five. Stimulation of the pharynx by an oral catheter is equally effective. The nasal route is better tolerated in conscious patients.[106] Nebulized saline every 4 hours has been used successfully in one patient whose hiccup failed to respond to various drugs.[107]

Palatal massage is also successful in stopping hiccup.[108] A cotton-wool 'bob' is inserted into the mouth and used to massage the anterior soft palate in the midline for about 1 min.

Most of 'granny's remedies' for hiccup involve pharyngeal stimulation either directly or indirectly:[109]

(1) the rapid ingestion of two heaped teaspoons of granulated sugar;

(2) the rapid ingestion of two glasses of liquid;

(3) swallowing dry bread;

(4) swallowing crushed ice;

(5) drinking from the wrong side of a cup;

(6) a cold key dropped down the collar of one's shirt or blouse;

(7) having someone shout 'Boo!' loudly in order to produce a startle response;

(8) forceful tongue traction sufficient to induce a gag reflex.

Other 'granny's remedies' such as breath holding and rebreathing into a bag are also physiological; the resultant hypercapnia has a central depressant effect and blocks the central component of the reflex.[110]

Management

Most cases of occasional hiccup are probably not reported to a doctor. They either remit spontaneously or respond to one of 'granny's remedies'. Deep breathing and chest physiotherapy also may disrupt the repetitive diaphragmatic spasms.

If reported, explanation should be the initial response and is likely to be focused on the causes and management of gastric distension. If more than occasional, a 2-day trial of a defoaming antiflatulent (e.g. silica activated dimethicone/simethicone in Asilone, Maolox-Plus) before or after meals and at bedtime should be considered. With more troublesome hiccup, a combination of simethicone and a prokinetic drug (metoclopramide, cisapride, domperidone) should be used. In one case cisapride succeeded where metoclopramide failed.[111]

At some centres, peppermint water is used as first line treatment. Although this facilitates belching by relaxing the lower oesophageal sphincter, it does not have a defoaming action on the gastric contents. It is therefore probably less effective than a defoaming antiflatulent, although no controlled trials have been reported. The concurrent use of metoclopramide and peppermint should be discouraged; there is little sense in deliberately combining two drugs with opposing actions on the lower oesophageal sphincter. A defoaming antiflatulent and enhanced belching is preferable to a permanently relaxed oesophageal sphincter.

Various other drugs have been recommended.[112] Baclofen is effective in doses as small as 5 to 10 mg twice a day, although occasionally 20 mg three times a day have been necessary.[112] Alternatively, nifedipine 10 to 20 mg orally or sublingually three times a day may be used.[97,113] One patient with pancreatic cancer required 160 mg a day to stop the hiccup; it was necessary also to give fludrocortisone to maintain normotension.[114] Haloperidol has also been used successfully in resistant cases. It probably acts by depressing activity in the reticular formation in the brainstem. Recommended regimens vary. [115,116]A convenient approach would be to start with 5 mg by mouth or intravenously, followed by maintenance treatment with 5 to 10 mg at bedtime.

Anticonvulsants have been used with occasional success, for example phenytoin 300 mg/day, carbamazepine 800 mg/day, sodium valproate 800 mg/day or more.[96,104] Their use is possibly more appropriate with hiccup of central origin. Intravenous lignocaine 1 mg/kg body weight as a bolus followed by an intravenous infusion of 2 to 4 mg/min has also been used.[117]

In the past, chlorpormazine was widely used for persistent hiccup.[102] Although it almost always works (probably by a diffuse depressant effect on the reticular formation), it does not correct gastric distension. Adverse drug reactions are common (e.g. sedation, dry mouth, postural hypotension) particularly in elderly debilitated patients. If used, chlorpromazine should be given in a test dose of 10 to 25 mg by mouth, and repeated two to three times a day either as needed or prophylactically, according to circumstances. If still intractable, intravenous chlorpromazine 25 mg can be given slowly over 2 or 3 min.[118] This is not without danger, and the patient should lie down for 30 to 60 min, and be warned about drowsiness, light-headedness, and palpitations. The authors have used this approach only two or three times over a period of more than 25 years.

The United Kingdom Datasheet for chlorpromazine (Largactil) suggests a higher oral dose (25 to 50 mg three to four times a day) or 25 to 50 mg intramuscularly and, if this fails, 25 to 50 mg in 500 to 1000 ml of normal saline by slow intravenous infusion.

A recent report details the use of intravenous midazolam 5 to 10 mg to control hiccup in two distressed dying cancer patients in whom various drugs alone or combination had failed, including intramuscular or intravenous chlorpromazine 50 mg.[119] Maintenance treatment was subcutaneous infusion of midazolam 30 to 120 mg per 24 h. Sedation was a concomitant effect but both patients died without hiccups about 2 days later. Surprisingly, both diazepam and midazolam have been reported as causing or exacerbating hiccups.[120,121] Despite this, we recommend a trial of intravenous midazolam in patients with persistent distressing hiccup. On the other hand, because midazolam in the doses used inevitably caused sedation, other possibilities should be considered in patients not close to death.

Other possibilities include glucagon. This is said to help if hiccup is caused by distension of the gallbladder secondary to opioid-induced constriction of the sphincter of Oddi and minimal food.[122] Glucagon has a relaxant effect on the sphincter, strong enough to reverse the opioid effect.

Although destroying the efferent arc of the hiccup reflex by crushing one or both phrenic nerves might seem an attractive option for resistant cases, this has never been necessary in the author's experience. Phrenic nerve stimulation is another possible option.[123] Finally, it is perhaps worth noting that osteopaths sometimes treat hiccup with traction of a leg. This relaxes the ipsilateral psoas muscle and may also terminate spasm of the diaphragm.[115] This may also explain why physical activity sometimes brings about a cessation of hiccups.

References

1. Twycross RG, Lack SA. *Control of Alimentary Symptoms in Far Advanced Cancer.* Edinburgh: Churchill Livingstone, 1986.
2. Sykes NP, Baines M, Carter RL. Clinical and pathological study of dysphagia conservatively managed in patients with advanced malignant disease. *Lancet*, 1988; **2**: 726–8.
3. Robertson MS, Hornibrook J. The presenting symptoms of head and neck cancer. *New Zealand Medical Journal*, 1982; **95**: 337–41.
4. Aird DW, Bihari J, Smith C. Clinical problems in the continuing care of head and neck cancer patients. *Ear Nose and Throat Journal*, 1983; **62**: 10–30.
5. Saunders C, Walsh TD, Smith M. A review of 100 cases of motor neurone disease in a hospice. In: Saunders C, Summers DH, Teller N, eds. *Hospice: the Living Idea.* London: Edward Arnold, 1981: 126–47.
6. O'Brian T, Kelly M, Saunders C. Motor neurone disease: a hospice perspective. *British Medical Journal*, 1992; **304**: 471–3.
7. Logemann JA. *Evaluation and Treatment of Swallowing Disorders.* San Diego: College Hill Press, 1983.
8. Duranceau A, Jamieson G, Hurwitz AL. Alteration in esophageal motility after laryngectomy. *American Journal of Surgery*, 1976; **131**: 30–5.
9. Regnard CFB. Dysphagia. In: Bates T, ed. *Clinical Oncology: Contemporary Palliation of Difficult Symptoms.* Ballière Tindall: London, 1988: 327–55.
10. Carter R, Pittam M, Tanner N. Pain and dysphagia in patients with squamous carcinomas of the head and neck: the role of perineural spread. *Journal of the Royal Society of Medicine*, 1982; **75**: 598–606.
11. Logemann J, Blonsky RE, Boshes B. Dysphagia in Parkinsonism. *Journal of the American Medical Association*, 1975; **231**: 69–70.
12. Weaver AW, Fleming SM. Partial laryngectomy: analysis of associated swallowing disorders. *American Journal of Surgery*, 1978; **136**: 486–9.
13. Vantrappen G, Janssens J, Ghillebert G. The irritable oesophagus—a frequent cause of angina-like pain. *Lancet*, 1987; **1**: 1232–4.
14. Rogers AI, Abrams KS, Presley D. Can emotional stress induce esophageal spasm in man? *Gastroenterology*, 1980; **78**: 1246.
15. Lobo AJ, Dickinson RJ. Oropharyngeal dyskinesia induced by prochlorperazine. *British Medical Journal*, 1987; **295**: 333.
16. Stones M, Kennie DC, Fulton JD. Dystonic dysphagia associated with fluspirilene. *British Medical Journal*, 1990; **301**: 668–9.
17. Grieve R, Dixon P. Dysphagia: a further symptom of hypercalcaemia. *British Medical Journal*, 1983; **286**: 1935–6.
18. Trier JS, Bjorkman DJ. Esophageal, gastric and intestinal candidiasis. *American Journal of Medicine*, 1984; **77**: 39–43.
19. Logemann JA. Aspiration in head and neck surgical patients. *Annals of Otology, Rhinology and Laryngology*, 1985; **94**: 373–6.
20. Leighton SEJ, Burton MJ, Lund WS, Cochrane GM. Swallowing in motor neurone disease. *Journal of the Royal Society of Medicine*, 1994; **87**: 801–5.
21. Ott DJ, Gelfand DW, Wu WC, Chen YM. Radiological evaluation of dysphagia. *Journal of the American Medical Association*, 1986; **256**: 2718–21.
22. Logemann JA, Bytell DE. Swallowing disorders in three types of head and neck surgical patients. *Cancer*, 1979; **44**: 1095–105.
23. Scott AG, Austin HE. Nasogastric feeding in the management of severe dysphagia in motor neurone disease. *Palliative Medicine*, 1994; **8**: 45–9.
24. Aste H, Munizzi F, Martines H, Pugliese V. Esophageal dilation in malignant dysphagia. *Cancer*, 1985; **11**: 2713–5.
25. Brewster AE, Davidson SE, Makin WP, Stout R, Burt PA. Intraluminal brachytherapy using the high dose rate microselectron in the palliation of carcinoma of the oesophagus. *Clinical Oncology*, 1995; **7**: 102–5.

26. Pfleiderer AG, Goodall P, Holmes GKT. The consequences and effectiveness of intubation in the palliation of dysphagia due to benign and malignant strictures affecting the oesophagus. *British Journal of Surgery*, 1982; **69**: 356–8.
27. Ell C, Hochberger J, May A, Fleig WE, Hahn EGH. Coated and uncoated self-expanding metal stents for malignant stenosis in the upper GI tract: preliminary clinical experiences with wallstents. *American Journal of Gastroenterology*, 1994; **89**: 1496–500.
28. Tytgat GNJ, Tytgat S. Esophageal endoprosthesis in malignant stricture. *Journal of Gastroenterology*, 1994; **29** (suppl 7): 80–4.
29. Carter R, Smith JS, Anderson JR. Laser recanalization versus endoscopic intubation in the palliation of malignant dysphagia: a randomized prospective study. *British Journal of Surgery*, 1992; **79**: 1167–70.
30. Lewis-Jones CM, Sturgess R, Ellershaw JE. Laser therapy in the palliation of dysphagia in oesophageal malignancy. *Palliative Medicine*, 1995; **9**: 327–30.
31. Murray FE, Bowers GJ, Birkett DH, Cave DR. Palliative laser therapy of advanced esophageal carcinoma: an alternative perspective. *American Journal of Gastroenterology*, 1988; **83**: 816–20.
32. Nwokolo CU, Payne-James JJ, Silk DBA. Palliation of malignant dysphagia by ethanol induced tumour necrosis. *Gut*, 1994; **35**: 299–303.
33. Chung SCS, Leong HT, Choi CYC, Leung JWC, Li AKC. Palliation of malignant oesophageal obstruction by endoscopic alcohol injection. *Endoscopy*, 1994; **26**: 275–7.
34. Regnard C. Single dose fluconazole versus five day ketoconazole in oral candidiasis. *Palliative Medicine*, 1994; **8**: 72–3.
35. Rabeneck L, Laine L. Esophageal candidiasis in patients infected with the human immunodeficiency virus. *Archives of Internal Medicine*, 1994; **154**: 2705–10.
36. Youle M, Clarbour J, Farthing C. Treatment of resistant apthous ulceration with thalidomide in patients positive for HIV antibody. *British Medical Journal*, 1989; **298**: 432.
37. Solomon MA. Oral sucralfate suspension for mucositis. *New England Journal of Medicine*, 1986; **314**:29–32.
38. Unsworth J. Coping with the disability of established disease. In: Williams AC, ed. *Motor Neuron Disease*. London: Chapman and Hall Medical, 1994: 213–38.
39. Hargrove R. Feeding the severely dysphagic patient. *Journal of Neurosurgical Nursing*, 1980; **12**: 102–7.
40. Kadas N. The dysphagic patient: everyday care really counts. *Registered Nurse*, 1983; **November**: 38–41.
41. Silverman E, Elfant I. Dysphagia. *American Journal of Occupational Therapy*, 1979; **33**: 382–92.
42. Meehan SE, Wood RAB, Cuschieri A. Percutaneous cervical pharyngostomy: a comfortable and convenient alternative to protracted nasogastric intubation. *American Journal of Surgery*, 1984; **148**: 325–30.
43. Ashby M, Game P, Devitt P, Britten-Jones R, Brooksbank M, Davy M, Keam E. Percutaneous gastrostomy as a venting procedure in palliative care. *Palliative Medicine*, 1991; **5**: 147–50.
44. Boyd KJ, Beeken L. Tube feeding in palliative care: benefits and problems. *Palliative Medicine*, 1994; **8**: 156–8.
45. Laing B, Smithers M, Harper J. Percutaneous fluoroscopic gastrostomy: a safe option? *Medical Journal of Australia*, 1994; **161**: 308–10.
46. Campos ACL, Butters M, Meguid MM. Home enteral nutrition via gastrostomy in advanced head and neck cancer patients. *Head and Neck*, 1990; **12**: 137–42.
47. Talley N, Colin-Jones D, Koch K, Nyrea O, Stanghellini V. Functional dyspepsia. A classification with guidelines for diagnosis and management. *Gastroenterology International*, 1991; **4**: 145–60.
48. Grainger SL, Klass HJ, Rake MO, Williams JG. Prevalence of dyspepsia: the epidemiology of overlapping symptoms. *Postgraduate Medical Journal*, 1994; **70**: 154–61.
49. Jones R, Lydeard S. Prevalence of symptoms of dyspepsia in the community. *British Medical Journal*, 1989; **298**: 30–2.
50. Editorial. Non-ulcer dyspepsia. *Lancet*, 1986; **1**: 1306–7.
51. Nelson K, Walsh T, O'Donovan P, Sheehan F, Falk G. Assessment of upper gastrointestinal motility in the cancer-associated dyspepsia syndrome (CADS). *Journal of Palliative Care*, 1993; **9**: 27–31.
52. Armes PJ, Plant HJ, Allbright A, Silverstone T, Slevin ML. A study to investigate the incidence of early satiety in patients with advanced cancer. *British Journal of Cancer*, 1992; **65**: 481–4.
53. Bruera E, Catz Z, Hooper R, Lentle B, MacDonald RN. Chronic nausea and anorexia in advanced cancer patients: A possible role for autonomic dysfunction. *Journal of Pain and Symptom Management*, 1987; **2**: 19–21.
54. Bruera E, Chadwick S, MacDonald N, Fox R, Hanson J. Study of cardiovascular autonomic insufficiency in advanced cancer patients. *Cancer Treatment Reports*, 1986; **70**: 1383–7.
55. Levitt M. Gastrointestinal gas and abdominal symptoms. *Practical Gastroenterology*, 1983; **7**: 6–12.
56. Colin-Jones DG. Management of dyspepsia: report of a working party. *Lancet*, 1988; **1**: 576–9.
57. Fenn GC. An overview of the key role of misoprostol in the prophylaxis of NSAID-associated ulcers and their complications. *Inflammopharmacology*, 1996; **4**: 91–100.
58. Ehsanullah RSB, Page MC, Tildesley G, Wood JR. Prevention of gastroduodenal damage induced by nonsteroidal anti-inflammatory drugs: controlled trial of ranitidine. *British Medical Journal*, 1988; **297**: 1017–21.
59. Lam SK. Why do ulcers heal with sucralfate? *Scandinavian Journal of Gastroenterology*, 1990; **25** (Suppl 173): 6–16.
60. Caldwell JR, Roth SH, Wu WG, Semble EL, Castell DD, Heller MD, March WH. Sucralfate treatment of nonsteroidal anti-inflammatory drug-induced gastrointestinal symptoms and mucosal damage. *American Journal of Medicine*, 1987; **83** (Suppl. 3B): 74–82.
61. Editorial. Misoprostol: ulcer prophylaxis at what cost? *Lancet*, 1988; **2**: 1293–4.
62. Gerber LH, Rooney PJ, McCarthy DM. Healing of peptic ulcers during continuing anti- inflammatory therapy in rheumatoid arthritis. *Journal of Clinical Gastroenterology*, 1981; **3**: 7–11.
63. Bernstein J, Kasich M. A double-blind trial of simethicone in functional disease of the upper gastrointestinal tract. *Journal of Clinical Pharmacology*, 1974; **14**: 614–23.
64. Somogyi A, Gugler R. Drug interaction with cimetidine. *Clinical Pharmacokinetics*, 1982; **7**: 23–41.
65. Mitchard M, Harris A, Mullinger B. Ranitidine drug interactions: a literature review. *Pharmacology and Therapeutics*, 1987; **32**: 293–325.
66. Guay D, Meatherall R, Chalmers J, Grahame G. Cimetidine alter pethidine disposition in man. *British Journal of Clinical Pharmacology*, 1984; **18**: 907–14.
67. Guay D, Meatherall R, Chalmers J. Ranitidine does not alter pethidine disposition in man. *British Journal of Clinical Pharmacology*, 1985; **20**: 55–9.
68. Sorkin E, Ogawa C. Cimetidine potentiation of narcotic action. *Drug Intelligence and Clinical Pharmacy*, 1983; **17**: 60–1.
69. Anonymous. Omeprazole: blocks gastric acid secretion completely. *Drug and Therapeutics Bulletin*, 1990; **28**: 49–52.
70. Ogilvie AL, Atkinson M. Does dimethicone increase the efficacy of antacids in the treatment of reflux oesophagitis? *Journal of the Royal Society of Medicine*, 1986; **79**: 584–7.
71. Smart HL, Atkinson M. Comparison of a dimethicone/antacid (Asilone gel) with an alginate/antacid (Gaviscon liquid) in the management of reflux oesophagitis. *Journal of the Royal Society of Medicine*, 1990; **83**: 554–6.
72. Himal HS. Alkaline gastritis and alkaline oesophagitis: a review. *Canadian Journal of Surgery*, 1977; **20**: 403–12.
73. Watters KJ, Murphy GM, Tomkin GH, Ashford JJ. An evaluation of the bile acid binding and antacid properties of hydrotalcite in hiatus hernia and peptic ulceration. *Current Medical Research Opinion*, 1979; **6**: 85–7.

74. Llewellyn AF, Tomkin GH, Murphy GM. The binding of bile acids by hydrotalcite and other antacid preparations. *Pharmaceutica Acta Helvetiae*, 1977; **52**: 1–5.
75. Keeckner FS, Stahler EJ, Hartzell G, Eicher WP. Esophagitis and gastritis secondary to bile reflux. *Gastroenterology*, 1972; **62**: 890.
76. Stephens CJM, Lever L, Hoare AM. Dicyclomine for idiopathic dyspepsia. *Lancet*, 1988; **1**: 1004.
77. Twycross RG. The use of prokinetic drugs in palliative care. *European Journal of Palliative Care*, 1995; **4**: 141–5.
78. Shivshanker K, Bennett RW, Haynie TP. Tumor-associated gastroparesis: correction with metoclopramide. *American Journal of Surgery*, 1983; **145**: 221–5.
79. Kris M, Yeh SDJ, Gralla RJ, Young CW. Symptomatic gastroparesis in cancer patients. A possible cause of cancer-associated anorexia that can be improved with oral metoclopramide. *Proceedings of the American Society of Clinical Oncology*, 1985; **4**: 267.
80. Sanger GJ, King FD. From metochpramide to selective gut motility stimulants and 5HT3 receptor antagonists. *Drug Design and Delivery*, 1988; **3**: 273–95.
81. Wiseman LR, Faulds D. Cisapride: an updated review of its pharmacology and therapeutic efficacy as a prokinetic agent in gastrointestinal motility disorders. *Drugs*, 1994; **47**: 116–52.
82. Loose FD. Domperidone in chronic dyspepsia: a pilot open study and a multicentre general practice crossover comparison with metoclopramide and placebo. *Pharmatherapeutica*, 1979; **2**: 140–6.
83. Moriga M, A multicentre double blind study of domperidone and metoclopramide in the symptomatic control of dyspepsia. In: Touse G, ed. *Progress with Domperidone. A Gastrokinetic and Anti-emetic Agent*. London: Royal Society of Medicine, 1981: 77–9.
84. Archimandritis A, Tzivras M, Fertakis A, Emmanuel A, Laoudi F. Cisapride, metoclopramide and ranitidine in the treatment of severe nonulcer dyspepsia. *Clinical Therapeutics*, 1992; **14**: 553–61.
85. Fumagalli I, Hammer B. Cisapride versus metoclopramide in the treatment of functional dyspepsia: a double-blind comparative trial. *Scandinavian Journal of Gastroenterology*, 1994; **29**: 33–7.
86. McHugh S, Lico S, Diamant NE. Cisapride vs metoclopramide: an acute study in diabetic gastroparesis. *Digestive Diseases and Science*, 1992; **37**: 997–1001.
87. Van-Outryve M, De-Nutte N, Van-Eeghem P, Gooris JP. Efficacy of cisapride in functional dyspepsia resistant to domperidone or metoclopramide: a double-blind, placebo-controlled study. *Scandinavian Journal of Gastroenterology*, 1993; **28** (suppl 195): 47–53.
88. Dworkin BM, Rosenthal WS, Casellas AR, Girolomo R, Lebovics E, Freeman S, Bennett Clark S. Open label study of long term effectiveness of cisapride in patients with idiopathic gastroparesis. *Digestive Diseases and Sciences*, 1994; **39**: 1395–8.
89. Rothstein RD, Alavi A, Reynolds JC. Electrogastrography in patients with gastroparesis and effect of long term cisapride. *Digestive Diseases and Sciences*, 1993; **38**: 1518–24.
90. Tatsuta M, Iishi H, Nakaizumi A, Okuda S. Effect of treatment with cisapride alone or in combination with domperidone on gastric emptying and gastrointestinal symptoms in dyspeptic patients. *Alimentary Pharmacology and Therapeutics*, 1992; **6**: 221–8.
91. Twycross RG. *Sympton Management in Advanced Cancer*, 1st edn. Oxford: Radcliffe Medical Press, 1995: 338.
92. Rowbotham D, Bamber P, Nimmo W. Comparison of the effect of cisapride and metoclopramide on morphine-induced delay in gastric emptying. *British Journal of Clinical Pharmacology*, 1988; **26**: 741–6.
93. Rowbotham DJ, Milligan K, McHugh P. Effects of cisapride on morphine absorption after oral administration of sustained-release morphine. *British Journal of Anaesthesia*, 1991; **67**: 421–5.
94. Manara AR, Shelly MP, Quinn K, Park GR. The effect of metoclopramide on the absorption of oral controlled release morphine. *British Journal of Clinical Pharmacology*, 1988; **25**: 518–21.
95. Nathan MD, Leshner RT, Keller AP. Intractable hiccups. *Laryngoscope*, 1980; **90**: 1612–18.
96. Launois S, Bizec J, Whitelaw W, Cabane J, Derenne J. Hiccup in adults: an overview. *European Respiratory Journal*, 1993; **6**: 563–75.
97. Mukhopadhyay P, Osman MR, Wajima T, Wallace TI. Nifedipine for intractable hiccups. *New England Journal of Medicine*, 1986; **314**: 1256.
98. Stotka VL, Barclay SJ, Bell HS, Clare FB. Intractable hiccough as the primary manifestation of brain stem tumor. *American Journal of Medicine*, 1962; **32**: 313–15.
99. Kaufman HJ. Hiccups: an occasional sign of esophageal obstruction. *Gastroenterology*, 1982; **82**: 1443–5.
100. Souadjian JV, Cain JC. Intractable hiccup: etiologic factors in 220 cases. *Postgraduate Medicine*, 1968; **43**: 72–7.
101. Wagner HS, Stapczynski JS. Persistent hiccups. *Annals of Emergency Medicine*, 1982; **11**: 24–6.
102. Lewis J. Hiccups: causes and cures. *Journal of Clinical Gastroenterology*, 1985; **7**: 539–52.
103. Fodstad H, Nilsson S. Intractable singultus: a diagnostic and therapeutic challenge. *British Journal of Neurosurgery*, 1993; **7**: 255–62.
104. Rousseau P. Hiccups in terminal disease. *American Journal of Hospice and Palliative Care*, 1994; **11**: 7–10.
105. Howard RS. Persistent hiccups. *British Medical Journal*, 1992; **305**: 1237–8.
106. Salem MR, Baraka A, Rattenborg CC, Holaday DA. Treatment of hiccups by pharyngeal stimulation in anesthetized and conscious subjects. *Journal of the American Medical Association*, 1967; **202**: 126–30.
107. De Ruysscher D, Spaas P, Specenier P. Treatment of intractable hiccup in a terminal cancer patient with nebulized saline. *Palliative Medicine*, 1996; **10**: 166–7.
108. Goldsmith A. A treatment for hiccups. *Journal of the American Medical Association*, 1983; **249**: 1566.
109. Lamphier TA. Methods of management of persistent hiccup (singultus). *Maryland State Medical Journal*, 1977; **November**: 80–1.
110. Saitto C, Gristina G, Cosmi EV. Treatment of hiccups by continuous positive airway pressure (CPAP) in anesthetized subjects. *Anesthesiology*, 1982; **57**: 345.
111. Duffy MC, Edmond H, Campbell K, Fulton JD. Hiccough relief with cisapride. *Lancet*, 1992; **340**: 1223.
112. Ramirez FC, Graham DY. Treatment of intractable hiccup with baclofen: results of a double-blind randomized, controlled, crossover study. *American Journal of Gastroenterology*, 1992; **87**: 1789–91.
113. Lipps DC, Jabbari B, Mitchell MH, Daigh JD. Nifedipine for intractable hiccups. *Neurology*, 1990; **40**: 531–2.
114. Brigham B, Bolin T. High dose nifedipine and fludrocortisone for intractable hiccups. *Medical Journal of Australia*, 1992; **157**: 70.
115. Scarnati RA. Intractable hiccup (singultus): report of case. *Journal of the American Osteopathic Association*, 1979; **79**: 127–9.
116. Ives TJ, Fleming MF, Weart CW, Block D. Treatment of intractable hiccups with intramuscular haloperidol. *American Journal of Psychiatry*, 1985; **142**: 1368–9.
117. Dunst MN, Margolin K, Morak D. Lidocaine for severe hiccups. *New England Journal of Medicine*, 1993; **329**: 890–1.
118. Williamson BWA, MacIntyre IMC. Management of intractable hiccup. *British Medical Journal*, 1977; **2**: 501–3.
119. Wilcock A, Twycross RG. Case report: midazolam for intractable hiccup *Journal of Pain and Symptom Management*, 1996; **12**: 59–61.
120. Fariello RG, Mutani R. Treatment of hiccup. *Lancet*, 1974; **ii**:1201.
121. Mendonica MJTD. Midazolam-induced hiccoughs. *British Dental Journal*, 1984; **157**: 149.
122. Gardner AMN. Glucagon stops hiccups. *British Medical Journal*, 1985; **290**: 822.
123. Aravot DJ, Wright G, Rees A, Maiwand OM, Garland MH. Non-invasive phrenic nerve stimulation for intractable hiccups. *Lancet*, 1989; **ii**: 1047.

9.3.3 Constipation and diarrhoea

Nigel P. Sykes

Constipation

Definition

Constipation is the passage of small hard faeces infrequently and with difficulty. Individuals vary in the weight that they give to the different components of this definition when assessing their own constipation and may introduce other factors, such as flatulence, bloating, or a sensation of incomplete evacuation.

Less than 1 per cent of a healthy British population[1] or 5 per cent of a North American one[2] fail to defaecate at least three times a week, and hence this frequency is often taken as an objective indicator of constipation. Other objective indicators include straining at stool during more than 25 per cent of defaecations and defaecation regularly lasting for more than10 min.

Prevalence of constipation

The first National Health and Nutrition Examination Survey in the United States found that 8 per cent of men and 21 per cent of women reported themselves to be constipated.[3] In a British survey 10 per cent overall said that they were constipated,[1] but again the gender difference was consistent. Both self-reported constipation and laxative consumption increase with ageing.

Physical illness is a risk factor for constipation: 63 per cent of elderly people in hospital have been found to be constipated compared with 22 per cent of the same age group living at home.[4] Constipation is more common in people who are terminally ill with cancer than in those dying of other causes,[5] and about 50 per cent of patients admitted to British hospices complain of it. This is an underestimate of the problem, as some patients will already be receiving effective laxative therapy. Depression is a risk factor for constipation in population surveys,[3] but results of a depression rating scale used on British hospice patients do not correlate with indices of constipation. Confused terminally ill patients appear to be at higher risk of both faecal incontinence and the use of rectal measures.

Pathophysiology

Intestinal motility

The small and large intestines each have their own characteristic motility patterns, but throughout the gut most muscle movements do not propel the contents but mix them. This facilitates enzymatic and bacterial breakdown of food and absorption of the resulting nutrients and of water.

Bursts of propagated motor activity occur in the small gut every 90 to 120 min. This activity is associated with increased gastric, pancreatic, and biliary secretion and is suggested to represent a cleansing mechanism for the small intestine. Feeding abolishes the regularity of this pattern, resulting in an increased variability of the rate of transit of luminal contents. Motor activity in the fed state is apparently random and presumably performs the function of mixing the gut contents in order to allow digestion and absorption of nutrients. Resumption of regular propagated activity correlates closely with the end of gastric emptying; both are delayed by larger or more fatty meals,[6] again suggesting that adequate facilities for digestion are being provided.

The colon shows much less frequent episodes of forward peristalsis which result in mass movements of gut contents. Manometry suggests that this activity occurs about six times per day, but is grouped into two peaks, a larger one associated with wakening and breakfast and a smaller one associated with the midday meal.[7] The frequency is reduced by inactivity.[8]

Food residues normally spend 1 to 2 h in the small intestine, but 2 to 3 days in the colon. In constipation, colonic transit may be greatly prolonged; nearly half of a hospice population had transit times of between 4 and 12 days.[9]

Gut muscle layers form a syncytium through which depolarization spreads from pacemaker areas. The myenteric nerve plexus co-ordinates motility, which is also under external neuronal influence, particularly via the parasympathetic system. High spinal cord transection mainly abolishes the motility response to food, but low cord or pelvic outflow lesions produce colonic dilation and slowing of transit in the descending and distal transverse colon.

Table 1 Opioid effects on the gut

1. Increased tone in ileocaecal and anal sphincters
2. Reduced peristaltic component of motility in small intestine and colon
3. Increased electrolyte and water absorption in small intestine and colon during induced diarrhoea
4. Restoration of colonic capacitance after intracaecal fat infusion
5. Impaired defaecation reflex
    - Reduced sensitivity to distension
    - Increased internal anal sphincter tone

Effects of opioids on intestinal motility

Exogenous opioids are well known to constipate, not by relaxing intestinal muscle but by suppressing forward peristalsis and raising sphincter tone (Table 1). These effects are apparent in both the small and the large intestine. If sufficiently severe, the clinical results on the gut of opioid analgesia produce functional colonic obstruction, a situation whose symptoms have been called the 'narcotic bowel syndrome'[10] but which appears simply to represent severe constipation.

Immunocytochemical work in animals has revealed multiple putative transmitter peptides and amines in myenteric neurones. The two principal neurotransmitters involved in the control of peristalsis appear to be acetylcholine and vasoactive intestinal peptide (VIP). Peristalsis movements have two components, ascending contraction and descending relaxation; acetylcholine mediates the first of these and VIP mediates the second. Anticholinergic drugs tend to constipate because they control part of the peristaltic complex. Both acetylcholine and VIP neurones are modulated by other agents, of which endogenous opioids are one group.

Opioid receptors are present on gut smooth muscle and at all levels of nervous input to the intestine; μ- and δ-receptors are apparently the most important in motility, with the former predominating in the myenteric plexus and the latter in the submucous plexus. Gut opioid effects involve both central and peripheral receptors in animals, but only peripheral opioid activity has been confirmed in humans. This does not imply that parenterally administered opioids are not constipating; it has been found in humans that subcutaneous morphine slows transit and reduces stool frequency.[11] No doubt opioid receptors in the gut wall can be reached by opioids not just in the lumen but also in the circulation. Our data obtained from hospice patients show that when diamorphine is administered by subcutaneous infusion the use of both oral and rectal laxatives is reduced significantly compared with patients receiving oral strong opioids. However, as infusions are used predominantly for patients who are either nauseated or very ill, conclusions regarding the relative constipating effect of opioids delivered by the two routes are hard to draw. Human studies using naloxone suggest that endogenous opioids may exert a basal control of gut motility[11] and, clinically, oral naloxone has been reported to improve idiopathic constipation.[12] Although these results are in line with some animal data they require confirmation and further work with more specific antagonists to clarify the contribution of different opioid receptor populations.

Fluid and electrolyte handling

About 7 litres of fluid enter the jejunum daily from gastric, salivary, pancreatic, and biliary secretions, to which is added a further 1.5 litres of dietary fluid. Approximately 75 per cent of the total volume is absorbed in the small intestine, and all but about 150 ml of the remainder in the colon. The difference between constipation and diarrhoea in terms of fluid excretion is around 100 ml per day, implying a remarkably precise control of water absorption in the colon. The maximum colonic absorptive capacity is 4.5 to 5 litres per day; hence there is a wide tolerance of fluctuations in ileal output, but small variations in colonic absorption can produce diarrhoea. There is no evidence that constipation is accompanied by increased water absorption except by virtue of the extended time that contents remain in the gut.

Gut fluid absorption is an active process, which is chiefly dependent on electrogenic Na^+ transport by the Na^+,K^+-ATPase system at the basolateral surface of the enterocytes. Fluid also follows neutral absorption of Cl^- , in exchange for HCO_3, and of NaCl. Na^+ is also cotransported with glucose and amino acid molecules. At the mucosal surface a cyclic-AMP-dependent system mediates Cl^-, and consequently fluid, secretion.

Non-absorbed solutes retain water in the lumen by osmosis, but luminal factors can also influence active transport. Short-chain fatty acids increase absorption, and bile acids, prostaglandins, bacterial toxins, and some laxatives stimulate secretion. Accordingly, diarrhoea can sometimes be relieved by a bile-acid-binding resin or a prostaglandin inhibitor.

Electrolyte, and hence water, transport is under neuronal control. The basic secretory condition of intestinal epithelium is cholinergic, mediated through changes in intracellular calcium concentrations. Anticholinergic agents and hypercalcaemia tend to constipate, and hypocalcaemia tends to cause diarrhoea.

Lipophilic agents, such as bile salts, could stimulate villous nerve endings directly, but it has been proposed that epithelial 'receptor' cells mediate a defence response of increased secretion and peristalsis to water-soluble toxins.[13] Endogenous opioids inhibit this defence response experimentally and although the physiological significance of such modulation is unclear, it may be a component of the action of exogenous opioids in infective and perhaps other forms of diarrhoea (Table 1).

Defaecation

During defaecation, abdominal pressure is raised by contraction of the abdominal muscles against a closed glottis, a process facilitated by assuming a squatting position. This pressure is transmitted to the rectum and tends to expel a stool positioned in the rectal ampulla. However, once defaecation has been initiated, stools the length of the descending colon can be expelled without abdominal contraction. Such effortless expulsion is probably due to an anocolonic reflex which produces distal colonic contraction in response to anal contact with passing stool. The effort required to pass a stool is inversely proportional to its size, accounting for the straining involved in passing a small constipated stool.[14]

Normal defaecation depends on the ability of receptors in the upper anal canal to detect the presence of stool, and on the relaxation of the involuntary internal anal sphincter and the puborectalis, which also exerts a sphincter function. These actions are abolished by lower motor neurone lesions to produce loss of rectal sensation, decreased rectal tone, and inability to defecate. Upper motor neurone lesions also destroy rectal sensation, but leave intact both reflex relaxation of the internal sphincter and the anocolonic reflex. Hence many patients with high spinal lesions learn to initiate defaecation by digital stimulation of the anal canal.

A physiological role for endogenous opioids in defaecation has yet to emerge, but exogenous opioids inhibit anorectal sphincteric relaxation and diminish anorectal sensitivity (Table 1). Both actions exacerbate constipation. As anorectal sensitivity decreases with age, the constipating effects of opioid therapy are likely to be more pronounced in the elderly.

Causes of constipation in palliative medicine

Constipation in patients with progressive disease is usually multifactorial; for instance an ill person with poor food intake, impaired mobility, and a requirement for opioid analgesia has three reasons to be constipated. A list of the constipating factors most relevant to palliative medicine is given in Table 2. The most important of these are the secondary effects of disease and the use of opioids.

Clinical manifestations and diagnostic considerations in constipation

History

It is important to clarify a complaint of constipation by a careful history. The degree to which constipation predated the present illness should be established, as this may justify wider investigations. Whether it was construed by the patient as constipation or not, the prior stool pattern should be elicited as a basis for comparison. Some necessary questions for taking a constipation history are suggested in Table 3.

Occasionally the patient reports a trick which aids defaecation: a finger inserted in the vagina implies the presence of a rectocoele,

Table 2 Causes of constipation in palliative medicine

Malignancy

Directly due to tumour

- Intestinal obstruction due to i) tumour in the bowel wall
  - ii) external compression by abdominal or pelvic tumour
- Damage to lumbosacral spinal cord, cauda equina or pelvic plexus
- Hypercalcaemia

Due to secondary effects of disease

- Inadequate food intake
- Low-fibre diet
- Dehydration
- Weakness
- Inactivity
- Confusion
- Depression
- Unfamiliar toilet arrangements

Drugs

Opioids

Drugs with anticholinergic effects

- Hyoscine
- Phenothiazines
- Tricyclic antidepressants
- Antiparkinsonian agents

Antacids (calcium and aluminium compounds)

Diuretics

Anticonvulsants

Iron

Antihypertensive agents

Vincristine

Concurrent disease

Diabetes

Hypothyroidism

Hypokalaemia

Hernia

Diverticular disease

Rectocele

Anal fissure or stenosis

Anterior mucosal prolapse

Haemorrhoids

Colitis

Table 3 History-taking in constipation

When were the bowels last opened?

What were the characteristics of the last stool (e.g. loose or formed; thin and ribbon-like or small hard pellets)

Was straining necessary for defaecation?

Was defaecation painful?

How characteristic of recent bowel actions was the last stool?

What is the usual stool frequency now?

Does the patient feel a need to defaecate but is unable to do so (suggests hard stool or rectal obstruction)?

Is the urge to defaecate largely absent (suggests colonic inertia)?

Does the stool emerge part way through a bulging anal outlet after significant straining (suggests haemorrhoids)?

Is there blood or mucus in the stool (suggests tumour obstruction or haemorrhoids or both)?

a finger in the rectum to push away a flap suggests a solitary rectal ulcer, and pressure exerted behind the anus assists defaecation if the levator muscles are weak. All these are distinct from the digital rectal evacuation to which many constipated patients are forced to resort.

Such symptoms as abdominal pain, bloating, flatulence, nausea, malaise, headache, and halitosis are associated with constipation by some patients, but they are non-specific and most can also occur with diarrhoea. It is the frequency and difficulty of defaecation that are the basis for the diagnosis of constipation.

Examination

Abdominal examination and rectal examination, unless there has been a recent full evacuation, are vital, and will help to avoid the major pitfalls in the diagnosis of constipation in palliative medicine. These are discussed below.

Impaction

Impaction, which presents as diarrhoea, often with incontinence, characteristically occurs in elderly patients in whom inattention to the need to defecate, confusion, or rectal insensitivity leads to the formation of a large faecal mass which is impossible to pass spontaneously. Faecal material higher in the colon is broken down into semiliquid form by bacterial action and seeps past the mass, appearing as diarrhoea and, if the closing pressure of the anal sphincters has been exceeded by the mass, faecal leakage or incontinence. Ninety-eight per cent of faecal impactions are said to occur in the rectum and, although it is probable that opioid analgesia alters this distribution, rectal examination will diagnose the great majority.

Intestinal obstruction by tumour or adhesions

Known intra-abdominal malignant deposits, previous intestinal surgery, alternating constipation and diarrhoea, gut colic, and nausea and vomiting combine to suggest the presence of intestinal obstruction. However, a similar picture can occur in severe constipation, of which the 'narcotic bowel syndrome' following use of opioid analgesia is probably one manifestation. The distinction is important, as attempts to clear 'constipation' which is actually obstruction by use of stimulant laxatives can cause severe pain.

Nausea

Some patients rapidly experience nausea, with or without vomiting, in the presence of intestinal hold-up.[15] Unexplained nausea or vomiting should prompt enquiry and examination for constipation.

Abdominal pain

The effort of colonic muscle to propel hard faeces commonly leads to abdominal pain, which is frequently colicky in nature. History and examination usually suggest the cause of the pain, but constipation is still sometimes 'treated' with morphine. Such pain may be particularly marked, and difficult to diagnose, where abdominal or pelvic tumour exists, presumably as a result either of pressure on the tumour from distended gut or because of partial intestinal obstruction.

Palpation of the abdomen may reveal faecal masses in the line of the descending colon and even that of the more proximal colon and caecum. The distinction between tumour and faecal masses can be hard to make. Faeces will usually indent, if the patient will tolerate sufficiently firm pressure, and may give a crepitus-like sensation

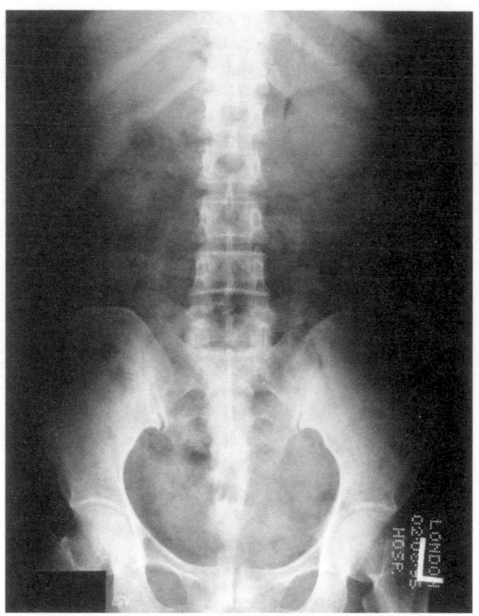

Fig. 1 Constipation in a young woman. There is faecal loading throughout the colon, best seen in the ascending and transverse colon.

because of entrained gas. They also move, given time. Sometimes an abdominal radiograph is needed to distinguish tumour from stool, but this is uncommon.

Digital examination of the rectum may reveal a hard mass of impacted faeces. However, the clinical picture may be of faecal leakage. Alternatively, the complete absence of stool implies colonic inertia. Rectal examination may also uncover rectal tumour, a rectocoele, solitary rectal ulcer, or anal stenosis. A lax anal sphincter may indicate spinal cord damage associated with colonic hypotonia. If a rectocoele or compression from pelvic tumour masses are suspected, vaginal examination may be justifiable.

Examination of the stool can be useful. Small hard pellets suggest slow colonic transit, ribbon-like stools suggest stenosis or haemorrhoids, and blood or mucus suggests tumour, haemorrhoids, or coexisting colitis.

Urinary incontinence

Faecal impaction is well recognized as a precipitant of urinary incontinence in the elderly, and the recent onset of incontinence should indicate abdominal and rectal examination as the first investigative steps.

Investigations

Investigations are rarely needed in the assessment of constipation in palliative medicine. Abdominal radiography may distinguish between constipation and obstruction if there is persisting doubt (Figs. 1, 2), but is rarely necessary and should certainly not be a standard procedure.

Blood tests are confirmatory rather than a screening procedure, but if the clinical picture is suggestive, corrected calcium levels and thyroid function tests should be performed.

Most constipation in palliative medicine is caused by slowing of colonic transit. This can be definitively assessed only by radio-opaque marker studies, which are arduous in ill patients or a hospice unit without its own radiography facilities. Comparison of the stool appearance with a graded chart of descriptions or photographs correlates well with whole-gut transit time[9] and, together with stool frequency, is a simple, non-invasive, and objective measure of gut function.

Management approaches

Prophylaxis

The aetiologies of constipation in patients with progressive disease (Table 1) suggest several prophylactic measures (Table 4). First, there should be good general symptom control, without which no other measures are possible. A key stimulus to colonic peristalsis and defaecation is activity[8] and hence patients should be encouraged and enabled to be as mobile as their physical limitations allow.

Table 4 Prophylaxis of constipation

- Maintain good general symptom control
- Encourage activity
- Maintain adequate oral fluid intake
- Maximize the fibre content of the diet
- Anticipate constipating effects of drugs, altering treatment or starting a laxative prohylactically
- Create a favourable environment

Constipated stools have a relatively low water content, rendering them hard and difficult to pass. This tendency will be exacerbated if the individual is dehydrated, and therefore an adequate fluid intake is helpful. However, the overall comfort of the patient must be kept in view, and constipation does not justify the use of parenteral infusions. Rather, the policy must be to enhance oral intake by encouragement and the provision of drinks that the patient likes—men frequently identify beer as a laxative in its own right.

Ill people have small appetites and what food they do eat tends to be low in fibre. Dietary fibre deficiency has been linked with constipation in Western society, but individuals with severe constipation are not fibre deficient and their gut function responds poorly to added fibre.[16] Work with radiotherapy patients in Oxford suggested that an increase in stool frequency of 50 per cent would require a mean increase in dietary fibre of approximately 450 per cent, well beyond the tolerance of most subjects.[17] Hence, although opportunities should be taken to raise the fibre content of patients' diets, this alone will not correct severe constipation, and the priority remains that food should be as attractive as possible to the person who is expected to eat it.

Doctors should know which drugs are likely to cause constipation (Table 2) and either avoid them or make a laxative available at the time of first prescription, without waiting until constipation is established.

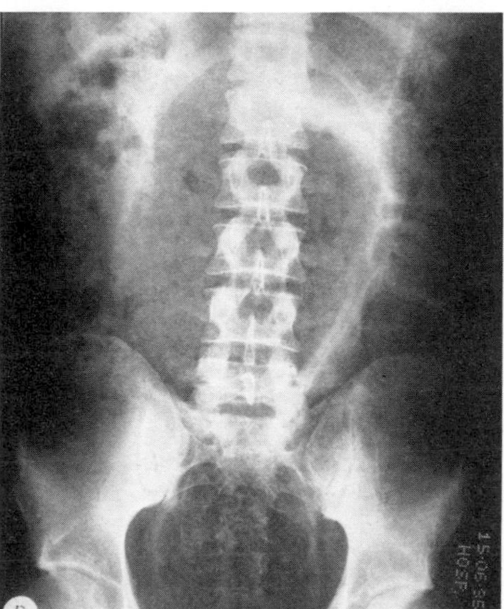

Fig. 2 Extreme constipation, with gross faecal loading throughout the colon, secondary to a chronic sigmoid volvulus.

Institutional lack of privacy for defaecation and the use of bedpans, which impose an inappropriate posture and greatly increase the pressure required to expel a stool, create an environment conducive to constipation. There is evidence that practised patients adapt to such indignities, but it should be a priority to allow patients privacy and the use of a lavatory, or at least a commode, for defaecation.

Use of oral laxative agents

Despite prophylaxis, the majority of patients with advanced disease require laxatives. Nearly 80 per cent of hospice cancer patients need laxatives; this applies to 63 per cent of our patients who do not receive strong opioid analgesia and 87 per cent of those who do, with the former figure being similar to the reported prevalence of constipation in an elderly population of hospital inpatients with non-malignant disease.[4]

There is surprisingly little experimental evidence available to guide choice of laxative type or dosage. If concurrent usage of rectal laxative measures is an indication of the efficacy of an oral laxative regimen, the results seem poor, at least in cancer patients. Forty per cent of Oxford hospice patients receive rectal measures on a continuing basis;[15] in our hospice patients the overall figure is similar, but rises to 57 per cent for those on strong opioid analgesia. In a series of 100 such patients, 67 complained of constipation on admission to the hospice and, despite considerable attention to the problem, 41 remained constipated at the end of their admission, although the subjective severity of constipation had been reduced for almost all of them.

Pending the reports of appropriate trials, the selection of laxatives is most logically made by considering the modes of action of the available agents and the characteristics of the patient's constipation, in particular the consistency of the stool. Hard stool requires an agent that is predominantly softening; excessive stimulation of peristalsis is likely to cause painful colic. Soft stool, which the patient is nevertheless unable to pass, is an indication for a peristaltic stimulant; additional softening produces faecal leakage and incontinence. There is evidence that the combination is effective more often than a predominantly softening agent alone and causes fewer adverse effects than a predominantly peristalsis-stimulating agent given singly.[18]

No drug acts purely to soften the stool or stimulate gut peristalsis. Any drug which softens stool also increases its bulk and thus reflexly stimulates colonic peristalsis. Agents which directly stimulate gut muscle contraction are known to enhance intestinal fluid secretion also and so improve stool consistency. However, the

Table 5 Classification of oral laxatives

Predominantly softening
Liquid paraffin
Bulk-forming laxatives (e.g. methyl cellulose, ispaghula)
Docusate sodium
Lactulose
Saline laxatives (e.g. magnesium hydroxide)
Predominantly peristalsis stimulating
Anthracenes (e.g. senna, danthron)
Polyphenolics (e.g. bisacodyl, sodium picosulphate)

predominance of stool-softening or peristaltic-stimulating actions differs from drug to drug, and so there is scope for logical choice based on clinical findings (Table 5).

The acceptability of laxative therapy will be maximized if previously satisfactory drugs are not changed unnecessarily, even if they are not the unit's standard prescription, and if the patient's preference regarding the choice of a solid or liquid laxative, sweet or less sweet, is heeded. Clinical criteria guide the selection of the class of laxative, but within most classes there are options that can reflect the patient's wishes.

The aim of laxative therapy is comfortable defaecation, not any particular frequency of evacuation. No single laxative dose is adequate for everyone, and many patients are subjected to both rectal interventions and an inadequate oral dose of laxative. The dose needs to be titrated against the response and the advent of adverse effects, remembering the latent period of action of the drug concerned, and should be increased prophylactically if, say, opioids are introduced or their dose is being substantially increased.

As in chronic pain, so in chronic constipation, therapy should be regular, not intermittent. Low doses of laxative are best given at night, but higher doses will need to be divided, usually morning and evening, but sometimes more often. Diarrhoea usually settles promptly by suspending therapy for 24 h and resuming one dose level down.

Lubricant laxatives

- Preparation: liquid paraffin.
- Starting dose:10 ml daily
- Latency of action: 1 to 3 days

Mechanism Liquid paraffin lubricates the stool surface and softens the stool by penetration, allowing easier passage.

Use Liquid paraffin has been blamed for many adverse effects. Those most relevant to palliative medicine are the lipoid pneumonia which may follow paraffin inhalation, and the propensity to cause leakage of oily faecal material with consequent embarrassment and perianal irritation.

There seems to be no justification for reliance on liquid paraffin as the sole laxative. However, its emulsion with magnesium hydroxide, which contains only 25 per cent paraffin, has not been associated with the above adverse effects and has been recommended as an effective and cheap laxative preparation.[19]

Surfactant laxatives

- Preparations: docusate sodium, poloxamer
- Starting dose: docusate sodium 300 mg daily
- Latency of action: 1 to 3 days

Mechanism These agents act as detergents to increase water penetration, and hence softening, of the stool. Docusate also promotes secretion of water, sodium, and chloride in the jejunum and colon;[20] there is a clinical impression that at higher doses it may stimulate peristalsis.

Use Docusate is available alone or in combination with danthron (Codanthrusate) or bisacodyl. Poloxamer is marketed only in combination with danthron (Codanthramer). Docusate's ability as a laxative has been questioned, as it failed to increase colonic output of solids or water in healthy volunteers.[21] However, docusate has been found to be more effective than placebo in clinical trials in elderly or chronically ill patients.[22] Poloxamer has been claimed to be an effective laxative, but in clinical practice there is no opportunity to separate its benefits from those of the danthron with which it is combined. Docusate alone has failed to win popularity in British hospice practice.

Bulk-forming agents

- Preparations: bran, methyl cellulose, ispaghula
- Starting dose: bran 8 g daily; others 3 to 4 g daily
- Latency of action: 2 to 4 days

Mechanism These agents increase stool bulk partly by providing material that resists bacterial breakdown and hence remains in the gut, and partly by providing a substrate for bacterial growth and gas production. The balance between these mechanisms varies from agent to agent. Non-digestible polythene particles will enhance stool bulk and shorten transit time, presumably by a reflex response to stretch or direct mechanical irritation. However, it appears that transit is speeded particularly as a result of fermentation, and is to some degree independent of stool bulking action.[23]

Use Bulking agents are 'normalizers' rather than true laxatives: they will soften a hard stool, but make a loose one firmer. Although they are effective in mild constipation, they are less helpful in palliative medicine for three main reasons. Firstly, they need to be taken with ample water (at least 200–300 ml); this and their consistency are unacceptable to many ill patients. Secondly, if taken with inadequate water, a viscous mass may result which can complete an incipient malignant obstruction. Thirdly, their effectiveness in severe constipation is doubtful.

Osmotic laxatives

- Preparations: lactulose, mannitol, sorbitol
- Starting dose: 15 ml twice daily
- Latency of action: 1 to 2 days

Mechanism These agents are not broken down or absorbed in the small gut, and as a result they exert an osmotic influence to retain water in the lumen. Bacterial degradation in the colon produces short-chain organic acids which lower the intestinal pH, possibly stimulating peristalsis and increasing stool bulk by enlargement of the microbial mass. These acids are absorbed and so the osmotic effect does not extend throughout the colon.

Use Lactulose is the most popular single laxative in British hospices, and probably in British general hospitals also, where its expense has caused concern. It significantly increases faecal weight, volume, water, and frequency, but if used alone in opioid-induced constipation often requires to be given in doses which result in bloating and colic. Flatulence is a problem for about 20 per cent of patients. Its sweet taste is sickly to some. There are suggestions that tolerance to its laxative effects may occur, presumably through changes in bacterial flora. Mannitol and sorbitol are little used as oral preparations, but sorbitol has been reported to be as effective as lactulose, and to be cheaper and less nauseating.[24]

Saline laxatives

- Preparations: magnesium hydroxide or sulphate, sodium sulphate
- Starting dose: 2 to 4 g daily
- Latency of action: 1 to 6 h (dose dependent)

Mechanism These agents are poorly absorbed and, unlike lactulose, exert an osmotic influence throughout the gut. They also increase intestinal water secretion and appear to stimulate peristalsis directly. Magnesium and sulphate ions are the most potent. It has been suggested that the actions of saline laxatives are mediated by cholecystokinin,[25] but other releasers of this substance, such as calcium, lack a purgative effect.

Use Saline laxatives, particularly magnesium sulphate, can produce an undesirably strong purgative action. Therefore they are not regularly used in ill patients, except as a last resort. Magnesium hydroxide is less potent than the sulphate and deserves re-evaluation, either alone or as an emulsion with liquid paraffin, as a cheaper alternative to lactulose and other more popular preparations.[19]

Anthracene and polyphenolic laxatives

- Preparations: senna, danthron (anthracenes); bisacodyl, sodium picosulphate (polyphenolics)
- Starting dose: senna 15 mg daily, danthron 50 mg daily, bisacodyl 10 mg daily, sodium picosulphate 5 mg daily
- Latency of action: 6 to 12 h (bisacodyl suppository 15–60 min)

Mechanism These drugs directly stimulate the myenteric plexus to induce peristalsis; their action can be abolished by local anaesthetic infiltration of the mucosa. Colonic electromyography in humans following oral senna shows an increase in myoelectrical activity of the type seen in diarrhoea. Net absorption of water and electrolytes in the colon is reduced, partly through inhibition of Na^{+},K^{+}-ATPase and probably also by stimulation of cyclic AMP, prostaglandin E_2, and perhaps serotonin synthesis. The effects on water and electrolyte transport may be relatively more important for polyphenolic agents than for the anthraquinones.[26]

Senna contains anthraquinone glycosides, which are almost inactive as laxatives but are converted to the active aglycone forms by colonic bacteria. In consequence, activity is concentrated almost entirely in the colon. The aglycones are absorbed to a limited degree and secreted in the bile, but this circulation is more important for danthron and the polyphenolic agents, which undergo glucuronidation and can then be reconverted in the gut to active drug, prolonging the agent's action.

Use Senna is the second most popular laxative in British hospices after lactulose, and the two drugs are often used in combination. This is a logical practice, as lactulose provides a relatively greater stool-softening effect and senna a relatively greater peristalsis-stimulating effect. Danthron is available in combination with a surfactant agent, either docusate (Codanthrusate) or poloxamer (Codanthramer). Codanthramer is available in two strengths with differing proportions of the constituents; the higher strength contains three times as much danthron as the lower, but five times as much poloxamer. Both Codanthrusate and Codanthramer are available as a capsule or a suspension. It should be noted that in the standard strength of Codanthramer one capsule is equivalent to 5 ml of the suspension, but in the higher strength one capsule is the equivalent of only 2.5 ml of the suspension. Equal proportions of senna liquid and lactulose are significantly more potent than standard Codanthramer, but are probably less potent than higher-strength Codanthramer.[27] Sodium picosulphate is formulated as a single-strength elixir.

Any of the anthraquinones or polyphenolics can cause severe purgation, with colicky abdominal pains. This can generally be avoided by dose titration and combined use of a more specifically stool-softening agent. They are valuable where there is evidence of colonic inertia.

Morphine is known to antagonize the water and electrolyte effects of senna,[28] and it has been suggested that there is a relatively fixed relationship between a dose of codeine and the senna dose that will counteract the resulting constipation.[29] This may be true for a given individual taking relatively low doses of opioid analgesia, but increase of opioid dosage does not proportionately increase constipation. Also, effective doses of polyphenolic laxatives show four-to eightfold variation between individuals[30] and the same seems true of the anthraquinones.

Both classes of agent have been implicated in causing myenteric plexus damage, but neither this nor the unconvincing association of danthron with carcinogenicity in rats is sufficient to influence their use in palliative medicine. However, patients should be warned of the pink discoloration of the urine that can be caused by danthron and watch kept for the perianal rash that it may precipitate, particularly in incontinent patients.

Rectal laxatives

The use of rectal laxatives is undignified for the patient and may be unpleasant for staff, but their short latency of action is satisfying for both parties, who may in consequence come to rely heavily on them. Rectal laxatives may be given as either suppositories or enemas, with the latter usually being used as second-line therapy or for rectal impaction. Any rectal intervention may precipitate defaecation by stimulation of the anocolonic reflex, but more specific mechanisms of action parallel those of oral agents.

Lubricant rectal laxatives

- Enemas: arachis oil, olive oil.

Use These agents are normally used as retention enemas overnight to allow evacuation or manual removal of hard faeces impacted in the rectum. Naturally, their efficacy depends on the patient's ability to retain the oil.

Osmotic rectal laxatives

- Suppositories: glycerine
- Enema: sorbitol

Use Glycerine softens stools by osmosis and is also a lubricant. Presumably, any stimulation of colonic contraction is mechanical. Sorbitol is a constituent of several proprietary microenemas.

Surfactant rectal laxatives

- Enemas: sodium docusate, sodium lauryl sulphoacetate, sodium alkyl sulphacetate

Use Docusate elixir can be used as an enema, but all the above agents are included in different proprietary mini-enemas to aid stool softening by aiding water penetration of the faecal mass.

Saline rectal laxatives

- Suppositories: sodium phosphate
- Enemas: sodium phosphate, sodium citrate

Use In rectal use these agents are claimed to release bound water from faeces, but, as with oral saline laxatives, they may stimulate rectal or distal colonic peristalsis, an action which is presumably aided when an extended enema tube is used to place the liquid as high as possible in the rectum. Repeated use of phosphate enemas can cause hypocalcaemia and hyperphosphataemia. Phosphate enemas can also produce rectal gangrene in ill patients with a history of haemorrhoids.[31] Hence care should be taken in their use.

Sodium phosphate is available in an effervescent base as a suppository (Carbalax). The resultant production of gas is intended to assist defaecation, although as rectal distension by gas is readily distinguishable from that by stool the rationale is unclear.

Polyphenolic rectal laxative

- Suppositories: bisacodyl suppositories 5 mg (paediatric) or 10 mg (adult)

Use Alone among rectal laxative preparations, bisacodyl suppositories act principally by promoting colonic peristalsis. Their latency of action is claimed to be 15 to 60 min, compared with 6 to 12 h when they are administered orally. The difference is probably due to the immediate conversion of bisacodyl to its active desacetyl form by colonic flora in the rectum. As activity depends on bisacodyl's reaching the rectal mucosa, care should be taken that stool does not separate the suppository from the rectal wall.

Bisacodyl suppositories are sometimes inserted in an empty rectum to 'bring the stool down.' A plausible rationale exists for this practice but its efficacy relative to use of oral laxatives, or even a high-phosphate enema, is untested.

Selection of rectal laxatives

As with oral laxatives, there are few data on the comparative efficacy of rectal laxatives. One study showed that the following percentages of patients achieved defaecation within an hour of the rectal intervention: phosphate enema, 100 per cent; mini-enema (Micralax), 95 per cent; bisacodyl suppository, 66 per cent; glycerine suppository, 38 per cent.[32] The approximately equal effectiveness of phosphate and mini-enemas,[33] the speed of action of mini-enemas,[34] and the superiority of bisacodyl suppositories over glycerine suppositories[35] have been confirmed elsewhere. The volume (about 130 ml) and potential adverse effects of phosphate enemas mean that, if an enema is required, the much smaller (5 ml), rather cheaper, and almost as effective mini-enema, of which various proprietary varieties are available, is preferable. If a constipated patient simply requires assistance with an initial evacuation, suppositories may be adequate if only moderate softening is required. A combination of a bisacodyl and a glycerine suppository is often used, as is that of an enema followed by suppositories. Both practices are logical, but no data yet exist to show what advantages they may hold or which categories of patient may benefit.

If none of the rectal laxatives described above proves adequate to remove impacted faeces, rectal lavage with normal saline can be performed. This is cumbersome and messy, requiring about 8 litres of (preferably) warmed saline. Tap-water should not be used because of the risk of circulatory overload, and neither should soap and water which is irritant to the rectal mucosa and can cause hyperkalaemia if a potassium-based soap is employed. In practice, in these circumstances most units will prefer to follow the softening action of an oil retention enema with manual removal of faeces, under cover of diazepam sedation if necessary.

Whenever rectal laxatives have been needed, the doses and types of oral laxatives being taken by the patient should be reappraised and if possible modified to obviate further rectal measures.

An approach to laxative therapy

There is no single correct way of selecting and employing laxatives, but one rational approach is summarized below. Naturally, these situations may succeed one another.

1. Exclude intestinal obstruction: if in doubt use only laxatives with a predominantly softening action (e.g. lactulose, sodium docusate) in order to avoid causing colic. Do not use bulking agents.

2. If the rectum is impacted with hard faeces, spontaneous evacuation is unlikely to be possible without local measures to soften the faecal mass (e.g. glycerine suppositories, olive or arachis oil enema). It may still be necessary to perform a manual rectal evacuation, for which sedation or additional analgesia is often required. Alternatively saline rectal lavage can be given.

3. If the rectum is loaded with soft faeces, a predominantly peristalsis-stimulating laxative (e.g. senna) may be effective alone. If there is rectal discomfort, a mini-enema may assist the initial defaecation. Frequent review is essential, as there is a likelihood that a stool-softening laxative will be required later, given either separately (e.g. lactulose) or as a combination preparation (e.g. Codanthrusate, Codanthramer).

4. If there is little or no stool in the rectum, a peristalsis-stimulating laxative (e.g. senna) is the drug of choice. However, the stools are likely to be hard, and it is a reasonable policy to use a stool-softening laxative (e.g. lactulose) or a combination preparation (e.g. Codanthrusate, Codanthramer) in addition.

New developments and alternative approaches

There is much scope for further work on the comparative efficacy and palatability of conventional laxatives. However, several new developments or alternative approaches are worth mentioning.

There is interest in the use of prokinetic agents to accelerate intestinal transit. Cisapride, which acts by enhancing acetylcholine release from myenteric neurones through 5-HT_4 receptor agonism, is better than placebo in improving stool consistency and frequency in idiopathic constipation.[36] Comparisons with other laxatives or its use in opioid-related constipation have not been reported. It may have value as an adjunct to laxative therapy, and this possibility deserves investigation. Metoclopramide, which also increases gastrointestinal motility by interaction with gut 5-HT_4 receptors, has been shown to be effective in the 'narcotic bowel syndrome' when given by continuous subcutaneous infusion.[37] Oral metoclopramide has not found a place in routine laxative treatment and is less potently prokinetic than cisapride.

Oral erythromycin causes diarrhoea on about 50 per cent of occasions when it is used as an antibiotic.[38] Apart from altering the balance of the gut flora, erythromycin acts as an agonist at motilin receptors, which are responsible for initiating the migrating motor complex in the small bowel. Motilin receptors are also present elsewhere in the gut, and erythromycin reduces the transit time in the right colon in healthy humans.[39] Among the macrolide family of drugs, this prokinetic property is associated with the possession of a 14-carbon lactone ring,[40] and related compounds which are prokinetic without being antibacterial are being developed. Whether these will be effective laxatives or predominantly anti-reflux agents remains to be seen.

Morphine-induced constipation can be counteracted by an opioid antagonist given orally because a major part of the opioid effect on the human gut is mediated peripherally rather than centrally. Naloxone has shown success experimentally in patients receiving strong opioid analgesia.[41,42,43] Oral naloxone has a systemic availability of under 1 per cent, due to first-pass hepatic metabolism, allowing a laxative effect without reversal of analgesia or generalized withdrawal. However, opioid withdrawal can occur occasionally and, although it appears that laxative doses of naloxone are generally 20 per cent or more of the prevailing morphine dose, it seems wise to titrate the naloxone from a starting dose that does not exceed 5 mg. Quaternary derivatives of opioid antagonists, which do not cross the blood–brain barrier, may be an alternative to the use of naloxone itself. Early results with naloxone are encouraging, but further work is needed to clarify the role of opioid antagonists as laxatives.

The specific cholecystokinin antagonist loxiglumide, given orally, significantly accelerated colonic transit in healthy volunteers.[44] This seems an unexpected finding as cholecystokinin itself increases colonic motor activity and can cause purgation. Clarification is needed.

Another possible therapeutic avenue for the management of opioid-induced constipation is suggested by the finding in mice that L-arginine reduces intestinal slowing produced by morphine. This may occur by the release of nitric oxide, which has been identified as a neuromodulator in the gut.[45]

Many plants with laxative properties are known in herbal medicine. Some, such as mulberry and the rheinoside constituents of rhubarb, which are similar to the constituents of senna, are currently under investigation. Patients may prefer such treatments to pharmaceutical laxatives.

Diarrhoea

Definition

Diarrhoea is the passage of frequent loose stools. Objectively, it has been defined as the passage of more than three unformed stools within a 24-h period. However, patients may describe a single loose stool, frequent small stools of normal or even hard consistency, or faecal incontinence as 'diarrhoea'. Therefore, as with constipation, a complaint of diarrhoea requires careful clarification.

Prevalence

Diarrhoea is a complaint of 7 to 10 per cent of cancer patients on admission to a hospice and 6 per cent of similar patients in hospital. Therefore it is a far less common problem in palliative medicine than constipation when cancer patients are being considered. However, 27 per cent of symptomatic HIV-infected patients have been reported to suffer diarrhoea[46] (for management of HIV-related diarrhoea, see Chapter 20.1).

Clinical manifestations and diagnostic considerations

Diarrhoea persisting for more than 3 weeks is said to be chronic and is often linked to serious organic disease. Most diarrhoea is acute, lasting for only a few days, and is generally the result of gastrointestinal infection (Table 6), including overgrowth by Candida.

However, the most common cause of diarrhoea in palliative medicine is an imbalance of laxative therapy.[47] This is particularly likely when laxative doses have been increased to clear a backlog of constipated stool. The diarrhoea normally settles within 24 to 48 h if laxatives are temporarily stopped, after which they should be reinstated at a lower dose. Meanwhile the diarrhoea may be distressing, particularly if it leads to faecal incontinence.

A variety of other common drugs can also precipitate diarrhoea, either commonly, as in the case of antacids and antibiotics, or idiosyncratically, as in the case of non-steroidal anti-inflammatory agents or iron preparations. Sorbitol, which is used as a sweetener in some 'sugar-free' elixirs, is easily overlooked as a cause of diarrhoea in sensitive patients. Those receiving enteral feeding appear particularly prone, with sorbitol being more than twice as likely to be the cause of diarrhoea as the feed itself.[48]

Malignant intestinal obstruction and faecal impaction are the next most common causes of diarrhoea in this patient group. Complete intestinal obstruction produces intractable constipation, but partial obstruction may present with either diarrhoea or alternating diarrhoea and constipation. This clinical picture can also result from severe constipation caused by opioid analgesia, where it has been dubbed the 'narcotic bowel syndrome'.[10] Faecal impaction results in leakage of fluid stool past the mass, often with anal leakage or incontinence. Faecal impaction can account for 55 per cent of instances of diarrhoea in elderly hospital patients with non-malignant disease,[49] emphasizing the need for careful

Table 6 Causes of diarrhoea in palliative medicine

Drugs
Laxatives
Antacids
Antibiotics
Chemotherapy agents, particularly 5-fluorouracil
NSAIDs particularly mefenamic acid, diclofenac, indomethacin
Mitomycin
Iron prepartions
Disaccharide-containing elixirs
Radiation
Obstruction
Malignant
Faecal impaction
Narcotic bowel syndrome
Malabsorption
Pancreatic carcinoma
Gastrectomy
Ileal resection
Colectomy
Tumour
Colonic or rectal carcinoma
Pancreatic islet cell tumours
Carcinoid tumours
Concurrent disease
Diabetes mellitus
Hyperthyroidism
Inflammatory bowel disease
Irritable bowel syndrome
Gastrointestinal infection
Diet
Bran
Fruit
Hot spices
Alcohol

NSAIDs, non-steroidal anti-inflammatory drugs.

attention to regular laxative therapy in any ill and relatively immobile population.

Radiotherapy involving the abdomen or pelvis is liable to cause diarrhoea, with a peak incidence in the second or third week of therapy and continuing for some time after cessation of the course. Damage to intestinal mucosa by radiation results in the release of prostaglandins and the malabsorption of bile salts, both of which increase peristaltic activity. Chronic radiation enteritis rarely presents as diarrhoea.

Malabsorption sufficient to cause diarrhoea may occur in carcinoma of the head of the pancreas or after gastrectomy or ileal resection. Failure of pancreatic secretion leads to reduced fat absorption and consequent steatorrhoea. Gastrectomy can also produce steatorrhoea, presumably as a result of poor mixing of food with pancreatic and biliary secretions. However, the accompanying vagotomy causes increased faecal secretion of bile acids in some patients, resulting in increased water and electrolyte secretion in the colon and hence a chologenic diarrhoea, compounding the problem.

Ileal resection reduces the gut's ability to reabsorb bile acids, of which up to 97 per cent are normally recirculated, again producing chologenic diarrhoea which is characteristically watery and explosive. If less than 100 cm of terminal ileum is removed, fat malabsorption does not generally occur as the liver can compensate for the increased biliary loss. A resection of more than about 100 cm results in relative bile acid deficiency and hence fat malabsorption, exacerbating the diarrhoea. Ileal resection produces a disaccharidase deficiency proportional to the length removed and thus an osmotic diarrhoea due to carbohydrate malabsorption.

Partial colectomy produces little if any persistent diarrhoea. However, total or almost total colectomy results in a high volume of liquid effluent which rapidly diminishes over 7 to 10 days but still remains at 400 to 800 ml/day because the small intestine is unable to compensate fully for the loss of the colon's water-absorbing capacity. Therefore an ileostomy is normally fashioned. Such patients require an average of an extra litre of water and about 7 g of extra salt per day to compensate, with special care needed in hot weather. Iron and vitamin supplementation is also indicated. Similar symptoms can also result from an enterocolic fistula caused either by cancer or as a result of operation.[50]

A colonic or rectal tumour can precipitate diarrhoea by causing partial intestinal obstruction, or loosen stools through increased mucus secretion. Rarely, endocrine tumours cause a secretory diarrhoea. The WDHA syndrome (watery diarrhoea hypokalaemia achlorhydria) is associated with tumours of the pancreatic islet cells and of the sympathetic nervous system, including the adrenal glands. VIP is believed to be the causative hormone both here and in the diarrhoea of the Verner–Morrison syndrome encountered in childhood ganglioneuroblastoma. Diarrhoea also occurs in the Zollinger–Ellison syndrome, in which pancreatic islet cell tumours secrete gastrin, and in carcinoid tumours, where serotonin, prostaglandins, bradykinin, and VIP secretions have all been implicated.[51]

In addition to concurrent gastrointestinal disease (Table 6), the ability of dietary factors to cause diarrhoea should be remembered. Excessive dietary fibre may produce diarrhoea, and fruits may do so both by this means and by their content of specific laxative factors.

Assessment

A complaint of diarrhoea demands a careful history, detailing first of all the frequency of defaecation, the nature of the stools, and the time course of the problem. Together, these often indicate the diagnosis. Defaecation described as 'diarrhoea' which occurs only once or twice a day suggests anal incontinence. Profuse watery stools are characteristic of colonic diarrhoea, whereas the pale fatty offensive stools of steatorrhoea indicate malabsorption due to a pancreatic or small intestinal cause. The sudden advent of diarrhoea following a period of constipation, perhaps with little warning of impending defaecation, should raise the suspicion of faecal impaction.

Both current and recent medication should be investigated. If laxatives are to blame, the error may be insufficiently regular therapy, resulting in alternating constipation and diarrhoea, or an excessive dose. Too much of a predominantly peristalsis-stimulating laxative tends to produce colic and urgency, and too much of a predominantly stool-softening agent may cause faecal leakage, although high doses of lactulose and docusate can produce colic and watery diarrhoea in some patients.

Table 7 Specific treatments for diarrhoea in palliative medicine

Cause	Treatment
Fat malabsorption	Pancreatin (may be more effective if H_2 antagonist given before meals)
Chologenic diarrhoea	Cholestyramine 4–12 g three times daily
Radiation diarrhoea	Cholestyramine 4–12 g three times daily or aspirin
Zollinger–Ellison syndrome	H_2-antagonist (e.g. ranitidine), initially 150 mg three times daily
Carcinoid syndrome	Cyproheptadine, initially 12 mg daily; methysergide 12–20 mg/day
Pseudomembranous colitis	Vancomycin 125 mg four times daily; metronidazole 400 mg three times daily
Ulcerative colitis	Mesalazine 1.2–2.4 g/day; steroids

Examination and investigations

Examination should exclude the possibilities of faecal impaction and intestinal obstruction, and therefore should include rectal examination and abdominal palpation for faecal masses. If there is doubt, an abdominal radiograph will make the distinction, but this is rarely necessary.

Steatorrhoea is generally clearly suggested in the history and readily confirmed on examination of the stool. Persistent watery diarrhoea, without systemic upset which would suggest an infective cause, may be more difficult to diagnose. If in doubt, the stool osmolality and sodium and potassium concentrations should be measured. The anion gap (i.e. the difference between the stool osmolality and twice the sum of the cation concentrations) is over 50 mmol/l in osmotic diarrhoea because of the presence of an additional non-absorbed solute, for example a disaccharide from a medicinal elixir. An anion gap of less than 50 mmol/l shows secretory diarrhoea, resulting from active secretion of fluid and electrolytes, as in the WDHA syndrome. Ileal resection gives rise to a mixed picture, which will become purely secretory if the patient can be fasted.

In any persistent diarrhoea, haematology and blood chemistry should be checked. Other investigations are valuable only in concurrent gastrointestinal disease.

Management approaches

Supportive treatment

Other than in HIV infection, diarrhoea in palliative medicine is rarely of sufficient degree or duration to cause significant risk through dehydration. If rehydration is needed the oral route is superior to the intravenous. Proprietary rehydration solutions, which contain appropriate electrolyte concentrations and a source of glucose to facilitate active electrolyte transport across the gut wall, are adequate for all but the most severe diarrhoea. Any diarrhoea will benefit from a diet of clear liquids, such as flat lemonade or ginger ale, and simple carbohydrates, as in toast or crackers. Some infective causes of diarrhoea cause transient lactase deficiency and so milk should be avoided in these circumstances. Protein and, later, fats are reintroduced gradually to the diet as the diarrhoea resolves.

Specific treatment

Specific treatments exist for several causes of diarrhoea (Table 7). Pancreatin is a combination of amylase, lipase, and protease which is available in several forms for pancreatic enzyme replacement. The effective dose varies widely between individuals and it may be more effective if gastric acidity is reduced with an H_2-receptor antagonist, in which case enteric-coated preparations should not be used.

Cholestyramine is a bile-acid-binding resin which is effective in controlling chologenic diarrhoea provided that ileal resection has not been too extensive. It is often found unpalatable. Both cholestyramine[52] and aspirin[53] have been claimed to be effective in radiation-induced diarrhoea.

Carcinoid syndrome diarrhoea often responds to general anti diarrhoeal agents, but peripheral serotonin antagonists, such as methysergide or the less toxic cyproheptadine, have been claimed to be effective against more severe diarrhoea and, sometimes, the accompanying malabsorption.[51]

General treatment

Non-specific antidiarrhoeal agents, which are absorbent, adsorbent, mucosal prostaglandin inhibitors, or opioids, are numerous. These agents may make illness due to Shigella and *Clostridium difficile* worse, and so they should be used with caution if these organisms are known to be present or if there is blood in the stool or fever.

Absorbent agents

- Preparations: bulk-forming agents (e.g. methyl cellulose; pectin)

Mechanism These agents absorb water to form a gelatinous or colloidal mass which gives a thicker consistency to loose stools. Water is held between the fibres in the case of bulk-forming agents, which are better regarded as 'stool normalizers' than as either laxative or antidiarrhoeal preparations. Pectin produces a viscous colloidal solution with both absorbent and adsorbent properties.

Use Bulk-forming agents may have a delay of up to 48 h before the onset of antidiarrhoeal action and are poorly tolerated in ill patients. They have proved useful in the management of colostomies but exacerbate electrolyte loss from ileostomies.

Pectin can be prepared simply from grated raw apple, but is sometimes combined with the adsorbent kaolin in proprietary antidiarrhoeal mixtures. The use of pectin against diarrhoea is time honoured but there is no evidence for its efficacy.

Adsorbent agents

- Preparations: kaolin, chalk, attapulgite
- Dose: kaolin 2 to 6 g every 4 h, chalk 0.5 to 5 g every 4 h, attapulgite 1.2 g at once followed by 1.2 g after each loose stool up to 8.4 g/day

Mechanism Adsorbents non-specifically take up dissolved or suspended substances, such as bacteria, toxins, and water, onto their surfaces. All are naturally occurring minerals; kaolin is hydrated aluminium silicate and attapulgite is a hydrated magnesium aluminium silicate. The adsorptive capacity of a molecule depends on its surface area, and hence attapulgite, which has a three-layered crystalline structure, is claimed to have 33 times the adsorbent capacity of kaolin. How this translates into relative therapeutic efficacy is unknown.

Use Attapulgite is used alone, but both kaolin and chalk are available in mixtures with morphine; the *British Pharmacopoeia* formulation of chalk with opium mixture contains considerably more morphine (5 mg/10 ml) than that of kaolin with morphine (0.7 mg/10 ml). Any difference in antidiarrhoeal effectiveness between the mixtures must be due to this factor. Indeed, there is no evidence, despite their popularity, of any significant antidiarrhoeal effectiveness of either kaolin or chalk except that of the opiate with which they may be combined. Kaolin is also available in combination with pectin; there is the same dearth of evidence for efficacy. However, attapulgite has been shown to be better than placebo in acute diarrhoea although significantly less effective than loperamide.[54]

Adsorbents may be appropriate for mild non-specific acute diarrhoea in a healthy population. Their modest effectiveness, at best, and the quite large volumes of a rather unattractive liquid which may have to be taken make them unsuitable for general use in palliative medicine.

Mucosal prostaglandin inhibitors

- Preparations: aspirin, mesalazine, bismuth subsalicylate
- Dose: aspirin 300 mg every 4 h up to 4 g/day, mesalazine 1.2 to 2.4 g/day, bismuth subsalicylate 525 mg every 30 min up to 5 mg/day

Mechanism Prostaglandins increase intestinal water and electrolyte secretion, and prostaglandin inhibitors (with exceptions such as mefenamic acid and indomethacin) reduce secretion. Bismuth subsalicylate is said to have a direct antimicrobial effect on enterotoxigenic *Escherichia coli*.[55] The active constituent of mesalazine is 5-amino salicylic acid.

Use Apart from bismuth subsalicylate, which is used for treatment of non-specific acute diarrhoea, these agents are used as specific antidiarrhoeal treatments—aspirin for radiation-induced diarrhoea and mesalazine in ulcerative colitis. All these agents are contraindicated in patients sensitive to salicylate, and the upper dose range of the bismuth compound can produce toxic blood salicylate levels.

Opioid agents

- Preparations: codeine, diphenoxylate, loperamide
- Dose: codeine, 10 to 60 mg every 4 h, diphenoxylate 10 mg at once followed by 5 mg every 6 h, loperamide, 4 mg at once followed by 2 mg after each loose stool up to 16 mg/day
- Duration of action: codeine 4 to 6 h, diphenoxylate 6 to 8 h, loperamide 8 to 16 h

Mechanism The opioids act via specific gut opioid receptors to reduce peristalsis in the colon. They also preserve the fasting pattern of motility in the small intestine after food intake. Their effects on water and electrolyte secretion in man at therapeutic doses are unconvincing. Loperamide is capable of reducing ileal calcium fluxes by a mechanism that is not inhibited by naloxone, but the contribution of this effect to its clinical activity is undetermined. Opioids increase anal sphincter pressure, and loperamide and codeine have been shown to improve continence in patients with diarrhoea suffering from faecal incontinence;[56] diphenoxylate is less effective, even at the same stool frequency.

Alone of the three, loperamide given orally does not reach or cross the blood–brain barrier significantly. In animal studies the relative specificities for antidiarrhoeal as opposed to analgesic effects for codeine, diphenoxylate, and loperamide were 5.24, 23.7 and more than 552 respectively. The relative specificity for morphine was 6.45.[57] Although the recommended maximum daily dose of loperamide is 16 mg, volunteers have received 54 mg/day without ill effects. Diphenoxylate rarely gives significant systemic opioid effects below its recommended maximum of 20 mg/day, but does so at doses of 40 mg/day or more. Therefore it is available only in combination with atropine in order to limit its abuse potential.

Approximate equivalent antidiarrhoeal doses in humans are 200 mg/day for codeine, 10 mg/day for diphenoxylate and 4 mg/day for loperamide.[47]

Use The opioids are the mainstay of general antidiarrhoeal treatment in palliative medicine. A requirement for morphine analgesia may obviate the need for any additional antidiarrhoeal medication. Loperamide is the opioid antidiarrhoeal of choice, as it is significantly more effective than diphenoxylate or codeine and has few adverse effects in adults. It has been reported to cause ileus-like conditions, irritability, drowsiness, and signs of opioid toxicity in children, and therefore more caution is required in its use. Regular therapy can be given for persistent diarrhoea, with the dose being titrated against the clinical response. The drug's duration of action means that it can often be administered twice daily. Loperamide 8 to 12 mg/day significantly reduces ileostomy output,[58] but in some severe chronic diarrhoeas the required dose may need to be higher than usually recommended.

Codeine is prone to cause systemic opioid effects but has the merit of cheapness, which encourages some units to use it for mild diarrhoea. In addition, despite the research evidence, clinical experience suggests that the individual response to opioids for diarrhoea can be as idiosyncratic as that for pain, and in some patients codeine has superior antidiarrhoeal properties to the other opioids without causing excessive nausea or drowsiness.

Diphenoxylate is at least as expensive as loperamide in equally effective doses and appears to hold no advantages.

New developments

Profuse diarrhoea after extensive intestinal resections, or particularly in HIV infection, is still a therapeutic problem. Certain peptides are produced by the gut which reduce intestinal fluid secretion in pathological states. Of these, peptide YY has been used experimentally in humans,[59] and somatostatin has given rise to derivatives which are now in clinical use.

Somatostatin is produced in intestinal D cells and appears to act directly to inhibit secretion and peristalsis. It has been shown to be effective in cryptosporidial diarrhoea and diarrhoea due to the carcinoid, Zollinger–Ellison, and Verner–Morrison syndromes, as well as to ileostomy[60] or enterocolic fistula.[50] The native form has a short half-life, but analogues such as octreotide are available which require only two subcutaneous injections daily.

Subcutaneous injection of octreotide may be painful, but continuous subcutaneous infusion is generally well tolerated and the drug can be combined with morphine, diamorphine, haloperidol, midazolam, or hyoscine without apparent loss of efficacy.[61] Mixing with cyclizine may cause precipitation. Octreotide is now established as an effective therapy for severe secretory diarrhoea, particularly that related to HIV infection. It also improves symptoms of malignant intestinal obstruction in up to 85 per cent of cases at doses which are usually within the range of 300 to 600 mcg/24 h. Although this principally relates to the incidence of vomiting, partial obstruction may produce diarrhoea and a trial of octreotide for this symptom is appropriate in these circumstances.

Bibliography

Ewe K. Diarrhoea and constipation. *Baillière's Clinical Gastroenterology*, 1988; 2:353–84.

Kromer W. Endogenous and exogenous opioids in the control of gastrointestinal motility and secretion. *Pharmacological Reviews*, 1988; **40**:121–62.

Portenoy R. Constipation in the cancer patient: causes and management. *Medical Clinics of North America*, 1987; **71**:303–11.

Twycross RG, Lack SA.. *Control of Alimentary Symptoms in Far Advanced Cancer.* Edinburgh: Churchill Livingstone, 1986.

Walsh TD, O'Shaughnessy C. Diarrhoea. In: Walsh TD, ed. *Symptom Control.* Oxford: Blackwell, 1989:99–116.

References

1. Connell AM, Hilton C, Irvine G, Lennard-Jones JE, Misiewicz JJ. Variation in bowel habit in two population samples. *British Medical Journal*, 1965; **ii**:1095–9.
2. Drossman DA, Sandler RS, McKee DC, Lovitz AJ. Bowel patterns among subjects not seeking health care. *Gastroenterology*, 1982; **83**:529–34.
3. Everhart JE, Go VL, Johannes RS, Fitzsimmons SC, Roth HP, White LR. A longitudinal survey of self-reported bowel habits in the United States. *Digestive Diseases and Sciences*, 1989; **34**:1153–62.
4. Wigzell FW. The health of nonagenarians. *Gerontologia Clinica*, 1969; **11**:137–44.
5. Cartwright A, Hockey L, Anderson JL *Life before Death*. London: Routledge and Kegan Paul, 1973:23.
6. Madsen JL, Dahl K. Human migrating myoelectric complex in relation to gastrointestinal transit of a meal. *Gut*, 1990; **31**:1003–5.
7. Baddotti G, Gaburri M. Manometric investigation of high-amplitude propagated contractile activity of the human colon. *American Journal of Physiology*, 1988; **255**:G660–4.
8. Holdstock DJ, Misiewicz JJ, Smith T, Rowlands EN. Propulsion (mass movements) in the human colon and its relationship to meals and somatic activity. *Gut*, 1970; **11**:91–9.
9. Sykes NP. Methods of assessment of bowel function in patients with advanced cancer. *Palliative Medicine*, 1990; **4**: 287–92.
10. Sandgren JE, McPhee MS, Greenberger NJ. Narcotic bowel syndrome treated with clonidine. *Annals of Internal Medicine*, 1984; **101**:331–4.
11. Kaufman PN *et al.* Role of opiate receptors in the regulation of colonic transit. *Gastroenterology*, 1988; **94**:1351–6.
12. Kreek MJ, Schaefer RA, Hahn EF, Fishman J. Naloxone, a specific opioid antagonist, reverses chronic idiopathic constipation. *Lancet*, 1983; **i**:261–2.
13. Lundgren O. Nervous control of intestinal transport. *Baillière's Clinical Gastroenterology*, 1988; **2**:85–106.
14. Read NW, Timms JM. Defaecation and the pathophysiology of constipation. *Clinics in Gastroenterology*, 1986; **15**:937–65.
15. Twycross RG, Lack SA. Constipation. In: *Control of Alimentary Symptoms in Far Advanced Cancer.* London: Churchill Livingstone, 1986:166–207.
16. Muller-Lissner SA. Effect of wheat bran on weight of stool and gastrointestinal transit time: a meta-analysis. *British Medical Journal*, 1988; **296**:615–17.
17. Mumford SP. Can high fibre diets improve the bowel function in patients on a radiotherapy ward? Cited in: Twycross RG, Lack SA, eds. *Control of Alimentary Symptoms in Far Advanced Cancer.* Edinburgh: Churchill Livingstone, 1986:183.
18. Sykes NP. A volunteer model for the comparison of laxatives in opioid-related constipation. *Journal of Pain and Symptom Management*, 1996; **11**:263–369.
19. Bateman DN, Smith JM. A policy for laxatives. *British Medical Journal*, 1988; **297**:1420–1.
20. Moriarty KJ, Fairclough PD, Clark ML, Dawson AM. Inhibition of glucose and water absorption in the human jejunum by dioctyl sodium sulphosuccinate: a prostaglandin-mediated phenomenon? *Gut*, 1982; **23**:A443.
21. Chapman RW, Sillery J, Saunders DR. Dioctyl sodium sulphosuccinate, 300 mg daily, does not increase human ileal or colonic output. *Gut*, 1984; **25**:A1156.
22. Hyland CM, Foran JD. Dioctyl sodium sulphosuccinate as a laxative in the elderly. *Practitioner*, 1968; **200**:698–9.
23. Read NW. Motility: functional diseases. *Current Opinion in Gastroenterology*, 1990; **6**:9–13.
24. Lederle FA, Busch DL, Mattox KM, West MJ, Aske DM. Cost-effective treatment of constipation in the elderly: a randomised double-blind comparison of sorbitol and lactulose. *American Journal of Medicine*, 1990; **89**: 597–601.
25. Harvey RF, Read NW. Mode of action of the saline purgatives. *American Heart Journal*, 1975; **89**: 810–13.
26. Leng-Peschlow E. Effects of sennosides A+B and bisacodyl on rat large intestine. *Pharmacology*, 1989; **38**:310–18.
27. Sykes NP. A clinical comparison of laxatives in a hospice. *Palliative Medicine*, 1991; **5**:307–14.
28. Verhaeren EH, Geeraerts VC, Lemli J. The antagonistic effect of morphine on rhein-stimulated fluid, electrolyte and glucose movements in guinea-pig perfused colon. *Journal of Pharmacy and Pharmacology*, 1987; **39**:39–44.
29. Maguire LC, Yon JL, Miller E. Prevention of narcotic-induced constipation. *New England Journal of Medicine*, 1981; **305**:1651.
30. Brunton LL. Laxatives. In: Gilman AG, Goodman LS, Rall TW, Murad F, eds. *The Pharmacological Basis of Therapeutics.* 7th edn. New York: Macmillan, 1985:994–1003.
31. Sweeney JL, Hewett P, Riddell P, Hoffmann DC. Rectal gangrene: a complication of phosphate enema. *Medical Journal of Australia*, 1986; **144**:374–5.
32. Sweeney WJ. The use of disposable microenema in obstetrical patients. *Proceedings of a Symposium on the Clinical Evaluation of a New Disposable Microenema, New Brunswick, NJ, June 1963.* Johnson & Johnson, 1963: 7–8.
33. Postlethwait RW. Microenema as evacuant before proctoscopy. *Current Therapeutic Research*, 1965; **7**:7–9.
34. Lieberman W. Rapid patient preparation for sigmoidoscopy by microenema. *American Journal of Proctology*, 1964; **15**:138–41.
35. Mandel L, Silinsky J. Bisacodyl (Dulcolax): an evacuant suppository. A controlled therapeutic trial in chronically ill and geriatric patients. *Canadian Medical Association Journal*, 1960; **83**:384–7.
36. Muller-Lissner SA. Treatment of chronic constipation with cisapride and placebo. *Gut*, 1987; **28**: 1033–8.
37. Bruera E, Brenneis C, Michand M, MacDonald N. Continuous subcutaneous infusion of metoclopramide for treatment of narcotic bowel syndrome. *Cancer Treatment Reports*, 1987; **71**:1121–2.
38. Shanson DC, Akash S, Harris M, Tadayon M. Erythromycin stearate 1.5 g, for the oral prophylaxis of streptococcal bacteraemia in patients

undergoing dental extraction: efficacy and tolerance. *Journal of Antimicrobial Chemotherapy*, 1985; **15**:83–90.
39. Hasler W, Heldsinger A, Soudah H, Owyang C. Erythromycin promotes colonic transit in humans; mediation via motilin receptor. *Gastroenterology*, 1990; **98**:A358.
40. Catnach SM, Fairclough PD. Erythromycin and the gut. *Gut*, 1992; **33**:397–401.
41. Sykes NP. Oral naloxone in opioid-associated constipation. *Lancet*, 1991; **337**:1475.
42. Culpepper-Morgan JA, Inturrisi C, Portenoy RK *et al.* Treatment of opioid-induced constipation with oral naloxone: a pilot study. *ClinicalPharmacology and Therapeutics*, 1992; **52**:90–5.
43. Sykes NP. An investigation of the ability of oral naloxone to correct opioid-related constipation in patients with advanced cancer. *Palliative Medicine*, 1996; **10**:135–44.
44. Meyer BM, Werth BA, Beglinger C *et al.* Role of cystokinin in regulation of gastrointestinal motor functions. *Lancet*, 1989; **ii**:12–15.
45. Calignano A, Moncada S, Di Rosa M. Endogenous nitric oxide modulates morphine-induced constipation. *Biochemical and Biophysical Research Communications*, 1991: **181**:889–93.
46. Rolston KV, Rodriguez S, Hernandez M, Bodey GP. Diarrhoea in patients infected with HIV. *American Journal of Medicine*, 1989; **86**:137–8.
47. Twycross RG, Lack SA. Diarrhoea. In: *Control of Alimentary Symptoms in Far Advanced Cancer.* London: Churchill Livingstone, 1986:208–29.
48. Edes TD, Walk BE, Austin JL. Diarrhoea in tube-fed patients: feeding formula not necessarily the cause. *American Journal of Medicine*, 1990; **88**:91–3.
49. Kinnunen O, Janhonen P, Salokannel J, Kivela SL. Diarrhoea and faecal impaction in elderly long-stay patients. *Zeitschrift Gerontologie*, 1989; **22**:321–3.
50. Mercadante S. Treatment of diarrhoea due to enterocolic fistula with octreotide in a terminal cancer patient. *Palliative Medicine*, 1992; **6**:257–9.
51. Norton JA, Doppman JL, Jensen RT. Cancer of the endocrine system. In: DeVita VT, Hellman S, Rosenberg SA, eds. *Cancer: Principles and Practice of Oncology.* 3rd edn. Philadelphia: Lippincott, 1989:1269–1344.
52. Condon JR, South M, Wolveson RL, Brinkley D. Radiation diarrhoea and cholestyramine. *Postgraduate Medical Journal*, 1978; **54**:838–9.
53. Mennie AT, Dalley VM, Dinneen LC, Collier HO. Treatment of radiation-induced gastrointestinal distress with acetylsalicylate. *Lancet*, 1975; **ii**:942–3.
54. DuPont HL, Ericsson CD, DuPont MW, Luna AC, Mathewson JJ. A randomized, open-label comparison of nonprescription loperamide and attapulgite in the symptomatic treatment of acute diarrhoea. *American Journal of Medicine*, 1990; **88**(Supplement 6A):205–35.
55. Graham DY, Evans MK, Gentry LO. Double-blind comparison of bismuth subsalicylate and placebo in prevention and treatment of ETEC-induced diarrhoea in volunteers. *Gastroenterology*, 1983; **85**:1017–22.
56. Palmer KR, Corbett CL, Holdsworth CD. Double-blind cross-over study comparing loperamide, codeine and diphenoxylate in the treatment of chronic diarrhoea. *Gastroenterology*, 1980; **79**:1272–5.
57. Awouters F, Niemeegers CJE, Janssen PAJ. Pharmacology of antidiarrhoeal drugs. *Annual Reviews of Toxicology and Pharmacology*, 1983; **23**:279–301.
58. Ruppin H. Review: loperamide—a potent antidiarrhoeal drug with actions along the alimentary tract. *Alimentary Pharmacology and Therapeutics*, 1987; **1**:179–90.
59. Playford RJ, Domin J, Beacham J, Parmar KB, Tatemoto K, Bloom SR, Calam J. Preliminary report: role of peptide YY in defence against diarrhoea. *Lancet*, 1990; **335**:1555–7.
60. Fuessl HS *et al.* Treatment of secretory diarrhoea in AIDS with the somatostatin analogue SMS 201–995. *Klinische Wochenschrift*, 1989; **67**:452–5.
61. Riley J, Fallon MT. Octreotide in terminal malignant obstruction of the gastrointestinal tract. *European Journal of Palliative Care*, 1994; **1**:23–5.

9.3.4 The pathophysiology and management of malignant intestinal obstruction

Mary J. Baines

Introduction

Intestinal obstruction is caused by an occlusion to the lumen or a lack of normal propulsion which prevents or delays intestinal contents from passing along the gastrointestinal tract. Obstruction may cause the presenting symptoms of cancer, or may develop during the course of the disease. Any site in the bowel may be involved, from the gastroduodenal junction to the rectum and anus.

While surgery must remain the primary treatment for malignant obstruction, it is now recognized that there is a group of patients with advanced disease or poor general condition who are unfit for surgery and require alternative management to relieve distressing symptoms.

The scope of the problem

The incidence of malignant intestinal obstruction in the general population is not known, nor is its frequency in patients with most common primary tumours. However, epidemiological studies have been undertaken in patients with ovarian cancer, in those presenting with colorectal cancer, and in patients with advanced cancer receiving palliative care (Table 1).

The original series from St Christopher's Hospice was based on 40 consecutive patients (16 men, 24 women) referred to the hospice for terminal care by their general practitioners or hospital consultants. They were aged 26 to 94 years (mean 59 years). The sites of primary tumours are shown in Table 2. Other series show a similar distribution of primary tumours with the majority originating in the large bowel or ovary.

Pathophysiology

As primary tumours of the large intestine enlarge in size they may cause occlusion of the lumen. The likelihood of development of an obstruction depends on the site; 49 per cent of tumours at the splenic flexure obstruct but only 6 per cent of those in the rectum or rectosigmoid junction.[1] Obstruction caused by other primary tumours involving the bowel, or by recurrent colorectal cancer, is probably far more complex, and one or more of the factors given below will be involved.

Intraluminal obstruction

Primary tumours of the right colon may form polypoid lesions large enough to occlude the lumen, or may act as a lead point for a colocolic intussusception. Tumours in both right and left colon can occlude the lumen in an annular fashion so that it is acutely obstructed by faeces. Metastases occasionally form polypoid masses extending into the bowel lumen.

Intramural obstruction

Lateral spread of tumour within the muscular coats of the bowel wall is sometimes present. This is often noted histologically,[4] but sometimes macroscopically; when seen, the bowel appears to be thickened, indurated, and contracted—an 'intestinal linitus plastica'.

Extramural obstruction

Mesenteric and omental masses and malignant abdominal or pelvic adhesions are often present. These cause extrinsic compression of the bowel which produces deformity or kinking on radiological examination.[7]

Certain primary tumours spread directly to the bowel; for example the duodenum from pancreas or stomach, the jejunum and ileum from colon, the rectum from prostate or bladder. These may also cause extramural compression.

Motility disorders

Impaired or absent motility of a segment of bowel (pseudo-obstruction) leads to a similar clinical picture to that of mechanical obstruction, but there is no occlusion of the lumen. This is common in patients with advanced cancer, especially of the ovaries, and is caused by tumour infiltration of the mesentery or bowel muscle or, rarely, involvement of the coeliac plexus. Pseudo-obstruction may also occur as a paraneoplastic neuropathy in patients with lung cancer.[8]

Multiple sites

The majority of patients with advanced ovarian cancer have multiple sites of obstruction; these may involve the small bowel at several levels, or the small and large bowel.[2,9-11] Obstruction at multiple sites is less common in patients with other primary tumours.

Other factors

Inflammatory oedema, faecal impaction, fibrosis, inelasticity and fatigue of intestinal muscle, a change of faecal flora, and the constipating effect of drugs may also contribute to the development of intestinal obstruction.

Thus, the pathophysiology of malignant intestinal obstruction is often multifactorial. There may be a mechanical block from intraluminal tumour or extrinsic compression; a motility disorder may arise from malignant involvement of intestinal muscle or autonomic nerves; obstruction may develop at several sites; and obstruction may be precipitated by inflammatory oedema or by drugs that cause constipation. Strangulation, or ischaemia of the bowel, is common in patients with obstruction due to hernia or adhesions, but it is very rarely found in malignant intestinal obstruction; three series reported an incidence of 4 per cent or less.[12-14]

Clinical features

The symptoms and signs of intestinal obstruction will depend on the level at which it occurs (Table 3). Malignant obstruction may present acutely with the sudden onset of colicky abdominal pain, vomiting, and constipation. More often, however, the onset of obstruction is insidious, over weeks or months. Symptoms may gradually worsen and become continuous but, even without treatment, symptoms may be intermittent and the obstructive episodes resolve spontaneously, if temporarily.

The distinction is often made between complete and partial (subacute) obstruction, but this is far from easy in practice and, clinically, the obstruction may appear to alter from one type to the other on several occasions as the illness progresses.

Investigations

Patients with advanced malignant disease and suspected intestinal obstruction should only be referred for investigations if these will influence the treatment offered. For example it is inappropriate to arrange erect and supine abdominal radiography in an obstructed patient who is too ill to undergo surgery. In practice, there are two clinical situations where radiological investigations are of value. The first is to differentiate between severe constipation and malignant obstruction. The second is to confirm the obstruction and determine its site and nature in the patient who is being considered for surgery.

Constipation and obstruction

Constipation should be suspected if there is a history of increasingly hard faeces, infrequent defecation, and the use of constipating drugs, such as morphine, without a laxative.

Physical examination usually shows a loaded rectum and faecal masses are palpable abdominally. However, the rectum will be

Table 1 Incidence of malignant intestinal obstruction

Author	Primary tumour	Number of patients	Incidence of obstruction (%)	Stage of disease
Phillips *et al.*[1]	Colorectal	713	16	At presentation
Tunca *et al.*[2]	Ovary	518	25	Throughout
Beattie *et al.*[3]	Ovary	105	42	Throughout
Baines *et al.*[4]	Various	1350	3	Terminal illness
Fainsinger *et al.*[5]	Various	100	15	Terminal illness
Reid[6]	Various	461	3	Terminal illness

Table 2 Primary tumours causing obstruction—hospice series[4]

Primary tumour	Number of patients	Male	Female
Ovary	14	0	14
Rectum	8	5	3
Colon	8	7	1
Caecum	2	1	1
Stomach	2	1	1
Endometrium	1	0	1
Prostate	1	1	0
Bladder	1	0	1
Mesothelium (peritoneum)	1	0	1
Unknown	3	1	2

One patient had two primary carcinomas—rectum and colon

empty and ballooned if impaction is high and it may be difficult to distinguish between faecal and malignant masses.

In the patient with severe constipation, abdominal radiographs show gross faecal retention throughout the colon and there may be associated gaseous distension and fluid levels.

Radiological and endoscopic diagnosis of obstruction

The details of these are to be found in specialist textbooks[15,16] and only a brief summary of relevant investigations will be given here.

Barium contrast studies and endoscopy will show the cause in the great majority of patients with duodenal obstruction. Erect and supine abdominal radiographs should be the first investigative procedures in patients with suspected small bowel obstruction. These show the size of bowel loops and the relative amounts of air and fluid within them. Dilation and fluid levels occur proximal to the site of obstruction. Anterograde and retrograde contrast studies using barium are occasionally needed to obtain information regarding the cause of obstruction.

If large bowel obstruction is suspected, abdominal radiographs should be taken with the patient in different positions, to outline different parts of the large bowel. These may be followed by a barium enema and sigmoidoscopy or colonoscopy.

Management

A number of treatment options are now available for the patient with advanced cancer who develops intestinal obstruction. In the following sections, the indications for surgery will be examined, the use of intubation evaluated, and the place of drugs for symptom control described.

Surgery

Surgical treatment, aimed at restoring the continuity of the bowel lumen, should be considered for every patient with cancer who develops intestinal obstruction. A proportion will have a non-malignant cause: in three series, 26 per cent, 32 per cent, and 38 per cent of obstructions were due to a benign cause or an unrelated second primary tumour.[14,17,18]

The knowledge that pharmacological treatment is an effective option must not prevent a patient from receiving palliative surgery which can offer some individuals a long and symptom-free period.

Factors influencing surgical treatment

The decision to operate on a patient with advanced cancer is not easy and each case must be carefully and individually assessed bearing in mind the following poor prognostic factors:

(1) advanced age, poor general medical condition or nutritional status;[10,19]

(2) previous surgical findings showing diffuse peritoneal carcinomatosis;[9,20]

(3) ascites, palpable abdominal masses, or distant metastases;[2,20]

(4) previous radiotherapy to abdomen or pelvis, or combination chemotherapy;[10,21]

(5) multiple small bowel obstructions as shown by prolonged passage time on abdominal radiography or by lack of abdominal distension;[2,22]

(6) small bowel obstruction. This carries a higher mortality and morbidity rate than large bowel obstruction.[9,21,23]

The patient's wishes must be considered carefully and treatment options fully discussed. Many patients will want every chance of prolongation of life, especially if effective chemotherapy is available following surgery. However, others, especially the old or very ill, will chose symptomatic treatment. No patient should be referred for surgery simply to prevent a distressing death from obstruction because the correct use of drugs can prevent this.

Types of surgery

Details of surgical techniques appropriate to each type and site of obstruction are covered in the surgical literature.[24] In summary, they are:

(1) resection and reanastomosis, such as ileal resection and reanastomosis;

(2) decompression, either colostomy or ileostomy;

(3) bypass, such as gastroenterostomy or ileotransverse colostomy;

(4) lysis of adhesions.

If obstructions are present at more than one site, a combination of these methods may be used, such as ileoascending colostomy, partial transverse colectomy, transverse colostomy, and mucous fistula.

Results of palliative surgery

The results of palliative surgery for obstruction due to metastatic carcinoma are shown in Table 4. Not surprisingly, this group of patients has a high mortality. Major complications are common and some patients remain obstructed after surgery or reobstruct at a later date.[10,18-20,23] Between 5 and 18 per cent develop enterocutaneous fistulae, usually in the laparotomy scar, making it difficult to fit the usual appliances. Median survival is measured in months but some individuals will live for 2 years or more.[3] The considerable mortality and morbidity rates associated with surgery

Table 3 Symptoms and signs of intestinal obstruction

Site	Pain	Vomiting	Distension	Bowel sounds
Duodenum	None	Severe; large amounts with undigested food	None	Succussion splash may be present
Small bowel	Upper to central abdominal colic	Moderate to severe	Moderate	Usually hyperactive with borborygmi
Large bowel	Central to lower abdominal colic	Develops late	Great	Borborygmi

Table 4 Results of palliative surgery for obstruction due to metastatic carcinoma

Author	Number of patients	Primary tumours	Operative mortality (%)	Entercutaneous fistulae (%)	Median survival (months)
Aabo *et al.*[9]	41	Various	33	*	4.5
Aranha *et al.*[25]	73	Various	31	10	6 (mean)
Clark-Pearson *et al.*[23]	49	Ovary	14	18	4.5
Krebs and Goplerud[10]	98	Ovary	12	*	4.3
Piver *et al.*[26]	60	Ovary	17	7	2.5
Rubin *et al.*[11]	54	Ovary	16	11	6 (mean)
Soo *et al.*[27]	42	Gynaecological	17	5	2.5
Turnbull *et al.*[19]	89	Various	13	7	4.5 (mean)
Tunca *et al.*[2]	127	Ovary	14	*	7 (mean)
Walsh and Schofield[17]	36	Various	19	*	11

* Not reported

are partly due to poor healing or infection. Since these are likely to be related to the patient's poor nutritional status, some centres administer total parenteral nutrition preoperatively. Results vary; some centres report no benefit, while others indicate some advantage.[10,11,23]

Most patients with ovarian cancer who develop intestinal obstruction will have already received potent chemotherapy so that the likelihood of a further response is small. However, a few patients who obstruct early in the course of their illness will have had minimal or no chemotherapy and so have a good chance of remission with the treatment now available.

Gastrointestinal intubation

The purpose of nasogastric or nasointestinal tube suction is to decompress the stomach and/or intestine in patients with a mechanical or functional obstruction. Suction removes swallowed air and protects against the vomiting of regurgitated fluid in the stomach. After intubation the patient may be observed for a short period for any signs of improvement and be given nothing but intravenous fluids to maintain hydration and correct any electrolyte imbalance. During this time investigations can be carried out and a decision made as to whether to proceed to palliative surgery.

A review of the surgical literature (Table 5) shows that only up to 14 per cent of patients with malignant obstruction respond to conservative treatment. Most authors now recommend early surgery following adequate rehydration.

The place of prolonged conservative treatment in the patient with an unresolved obstruction who is unfit for surgery is controversial. Such treatment involves hospitalization, immobility, and discomfort. It is a barrier between patient and family when they most need each other's closeness and support. It is undoubtedly true that 'Prolonged conservative treatment using nasogastric suction and intravenous fluids only adds to the discomfort of an already terminally ill patient.'[25] With the range of pharmacological treatments now available, intubation should only be needed for patients with a high obstruction and, in these, a venting gastrostomy should be considered as a better tolerated alternative.

Venting gastrostomy

The use of a venting gastrostomy or jejunostomy has been described as a method of relieving nausea and vomiting in patients with inoperable obstruction, and as more effective and acceptable than nasogastric drainage. A gastrostomy tube is sometimes inserted at laparotomy but a percutaneous endoscopic gastrostomy is a simple alternative. It can be undertaken in an endoscopy suite or even at the bedside, under sedation and local anaesthesia. In most series patients treated in this way were placed on a liquid diet, the gastrostomy tube being clamped at meals and for as long

Table 5 Response of obstructed patients to gastrointestinal intubation

Author	Number of patients	Primary tumours	Sustained response (%)	Comment
Aranha *et al.*[25]	51	Various	1	Tube decompression rarely effective
Bizer *et al.*[13]	35	Various	14	Consider early surgery in malignant disease
Krebs and Goplerud[28]	146	Ovary	10[(a)] 2[(b)]	Non-operative therapy is uniformly unsuccessful
Piver *et al.*[26]	60	Ovary	0	No relief by tube decompression
Solomon *et al.*[29]	21	Ovary	0	Surgery after 4 days' conservative treatment

[a] Early response, [b] Sustained response.

afterwards as could be tolerated. Nausea and vomiting were relieved in the majority of patients and, in some, the gastrostomy output was reduced, presumably due to a remission of the obstruction.[30–33]

Although this is theoretically a sound approach to the management of patients with complete obstruction, it would appear from communication with centres in the United Kingdom that it is used surprisingly rarely. This is no longer due to a lack of knowledge of the procedure but from an understandable reluctance on the part of many patients to undergo any further intervention. Most seem to prefer the occasional, or even frequent, vomit to the surgical insertion of a tube. Further studies are required to define 'this small sub-group of patients who do not respond adequately to pharmacological measures and require some form of decompression or venting procedure'.[31] It would be helpful to identify these patients early in their obstructive history so that the required procedure could be carried out without delay.

Symptomatic treatment

The opening of hospices and the development of the specialty of palliative medicine led to the search for pharmacological measures to relieve symptoms in patients with inoperable intestinal obstruction; these patients would previously have been cared for, only in small numbers, in different surgical, gynaecological, and medical wards. The drug regimens to be described have gradually evolved as new treatments have become available, and they can offer good relief to the majority of obstructed patients with advanced disease.

Continuous subcutaneous infusion using a portable syringe driver or other infusion device is the preferred route of drug administration. A combination of drugs can be given and the syringe driver is ideal for use in the home, as it can be loaded every 24 hours by the visiting nurse.[34–36] Other routes are less effective and are now, in developed countries, rarely used. However, if a syringe driver is not available, it is still possible to offer good symptom control. Some analgesics and antiemetics are made in suppository form, these include morphine, oxycodone, prochlorperazine, and chlorpromazine. In addition, tablets can be inserted rectally and be well absorbed. An alternative to the rectal route is sublingual or transdermal administration. Repeated injections are effective, but painful, and should be avoided if possible, as should intravenous infusions.

The incidence of the three main symptoms of obstruction as reported in two series[4,37] is as follows:

intestinal colic	76 per cent	72 per cent
continuous abdominal pain	92 per cent	91 per cent
vomiting	100 per cent	68 per cent

The drugs used to control these symptoms are discussed below.

Analgesic drugs

Diamorphine and morphine are equally effective in the management of continuous abdominal pain. They may relieve intestinal colic but often an antispasmodic is also needed. If diamorphine is available (as in the United Kingdom), it is preferred because of its greater solubility; this is important when drugs are given in the syringe driver. The dose of opioid should be titrated against the response, increasing until pain relief is obtained.

Antispasmodic drugs

Intestinal colic is caused by waves of increased peristalsis against the resistance of a mechanical or functional obstruction. In some patients, colic can be relieved with analgesic drugs alone. However, most patients also require an antispasmodic. Hyoscine hydrobromide 1.2 to 2.4 mg/day was originally used.[4] This is a sedative but it can occasionally cause agitation or hallucinations. Most centres now use hyoscine butylbromide starting at 60 mg/day and increasing up to 380 mg/day if necessary.[37] This drug does not cross the blood–brain barrier and therefore does not cause central side-effects.

Although hyoscine butylbromide has been used for some years to control colicky pain, it has more recently been shown to reduce the frequency and volume of vomits. Patients with inoperable intestinal obstruction, receiving nasogastric drainage, were referred to a palliative care service; they were then given hyoscine butylbromide to relieve colic and it was found that the volume of aspirate from a nasogastric tube was significantly reduced. It was possible to remove the tubes after the first week of treatment in all patients and they were maintained in this way until their death.[38]

Antiemetic drugs

The choice of an antiemetic to control obstructive vomiting and nausea is determined, to a considerable extent, by the possibility of giving it by subcutaneous infusion in the syringe driver. If prochlorperazine or chlorpromazine are given by this method, painful swellings result that may take weeks to subside. Biopsy of these injection sites shows fat necrosis in the subcutaneous tissues.

Both haloperidol 5 to 15 mg/day and cyclizine 150 mg/day are used as first line treatment at different centres and they are sometimes used in combination. Haloperidol is a dopamine antagonist with its main effect at the chemoreceptor trigger zone. Cyclizine acts on histamine and muscarinic cholinergic receptors, its main site of action being the vomiting centre. Despite their different sites of action there is probably little difference in their efficacy, though patients receiving cyclizine often complain of a dry mouth and there is a tendency for this drug to precipitate in the syringe driver.

Methotrimeprazine 12.5 to 150 mg/day is a phenothiazine with antiemetic and analgesic effects. It is of value in obstructive vomiting but high doses cause considerable sedation and should be reserved for very ill patients. Subcutaneous irritation may occur, necessitating changes of site every few days.[39]

Metoclopramide has traditionally been avoided in patients with intestinal obstruction because it is a prokinetic agent that increases peristalsis in the stomach and upper small bowel. This has been shown sometimes to increase colic and could lead to perforation or fistula formation if the obstruction is complete. However, a recent study recommends the use of metoclopramide, given subcutaneously with morphine, in a dose of 60 to 240 mg/day.[40] Metoclopramide has the advantage of being non-sedating but the authors do not give details of the level of symptom control obtained and, in particular, whether colic was an increased problem. Certainly, the doses of morphine used were significantly higher than in a comparable study using haloperidol and hyoscine butylbromide.[37] If metoclopramide is chosen, it is recommended that a 24-h trial is given, stopping treatment if colic occurs.

Ondansetron, and the more recently developed drug granisetron, are 5-HT_3 receptor antagonists that have greatly improved the control of chemotherapy induced vomiting. They have also proved effective in preventing radiotherapy induced emesis. A recent study has shown that patients with advanced ovarian cancer had higher concentrations of serotonin (5-HT) in urine if they were obstructed.[41] This finding, together with some case reports, indicate that ondansetron may be useful in patients with intractable, obstructive vomiting. It can be given by subcutaneous infusion 8 to 16 mg/day, but it is very expensive.

Unfortunately, there have been no controlled clinical trials comparing the efficacy of these antiemetics. Such trials will not be easy as patients are often very ill and the numbers in any centre are small. In addition, obstructive symptoms can be intermittent, even without treatment. But until such trials are conducted there will be little progress to help in the choice of an antiemetic for obstructive vomiting.

Somatostatin analogues

Somatostatin is a naturally occurring hormone, widely distributed in the body and having many physiological functions.[42] Its role in the symptomatic management of intestinal obstruction is due to its effect on gastrointestinal secretions and motility. Somatostatin causes a reduction in the volume of gastrointestinal secretions by increasing the absorption of water and electrolytes and inhibiting their secretion. It also decreases gut peristalsis from the stomach to the large bowel.

Somatostatin itself has a very short half-life and is not used therapeutically. However, the synthetic stable analogue, octreotide, has a half-life of about 1.5 h with a duration of action of 12 h. It can be administered by a 12-hourly injection (though this is sometimes painful) or by continuous subcutaneous infusion using a syringe driver. It has proved possible to mix octreotide with most other drugs with no apparent loss of efficacy. Compatible drugs include diamorphine, haloperidol, metoclopramide, hyoscine hydrobromide, hyoscine butylbromide, and midazolam. Mixing octreotide with cyclizine or corticosteroids is not recommended. However, stability studies on most of these drugs, used in combination in the syringe driver, have not yet been done.

The first reports of the use of somatostatin analogues appeared in 1992.[43-45] Since then, they have been widely used in palliative care and some large series have been reported.[46,47] These suggest that over 70 per cent of patients have complete or good control of vomiting. Abdominal pain and distension are also improved. Significant side-effects have not been noticed in this patient group. The recommended starting dose is 0.3 mg/day; this can be increased to 0.6 mg/day. Much higher doses have been given but they do not seem to improve symptom control.

Unfortunately, octreotide is an expensive drug and, at this stage, probably it should be reserved for patients who have a high obstruction or whose vomiting is not controlled with antiemetics. Hyoscine butylbromide has similar effects in reducing gastrointestinal secretions and motility. A controlled clinical trial is planned to compare these two drugs.

Corticosteroids

Since the anti-inflammatory effect of corticosteroids causes reduction of peritumour inflammatory oedema, steroids have been used for some years in the management of obstructed patients with the expectation that they will cause an opening up of the obstruction and result in relief of symptoms. Small groups of patients have been reported to have benefited[5,6,48] but no clinical trials have been conducted. The intermittent nature of early obstructive symptoms makes it difficult to determine whether any improvement is due to the steroid treatment. The suggested dose of dexamethasone is 8 mg/day or of prednisolone it is 50 mg/day given by injection or subcutaneous infusion, but some centres start with a much higher dose.

Laxatives

Stimulant laxatives are contraindicated in patients with intestinal obstruction. The may cause or worsen colic and may even lead to perforation. Faecal softening laxatives, such as docusate or moderate doses of magnesium hydroxide and liquid paraffin emulsion can be given to patients in whom a single colonic or rectal obstruction is suspected. With the more usual small bowel obstruction there is no role for laxatives.

Antidiarrhoeal drugs

Patients with subacute obstruction or faecal fistulae often complain of diarrhoea. Conventional antidiarrhoeal drugs, such as codeine phosphate or loperamide, may be effective, as also may be medication given for pain and colic.

Summary of symptomatic treatment

In practice, the symptoms of colic, continuous abdominal pain and vomiting usually occur together and a typical prescription, when treatment is started, would be:

diamorphine	30 mg
hyoscine butylbromide	60 mg
haloperidol	5 mg

Given over 24 h in the syringe driver.

If continuous pain or colic are not controlled, the dose of diamorphine or hyoscine butylbromide should be increased. If vomiting is a problem, the dose of haloperidol can be increased, a trial of hyoscine butylbromide at a higher dose can be employed, or a change made to another antiemetic or to octreotide.

Gastroduodenal obstruction

This is much less common than intestinal obstruction and is usually caused by a primary tumour in the stomach or pancreas. The patient has no pain but vomiting is severe, with large volumes containing undigested food.

Pharmacological treatment is less useful than with intestinal obstruction but sometimes, if the obstruction is partial, a prokinetic antiemetic such as metoclopramide 60 to 240 mg/day is effective. If there is no response, a trial of corticosteroids is suggested using dexamethasone 8 mg/day by injection. Octreotide 0.3 to 0.6 mg/day has sometimes proved very effective in controlling this type of vomiting.[47]

If these methods do not give relief, a nasogastric tube should be inserted and a venting gastrostomy considered. Fluids should be given by hypodermoclysis or intravenous infusion unless the patient is in the terminal phase.

Nutrition and hydration

Patients with intestinal obstruction are encouraged to eat and drink as they choose. With good, or even partial, control of nausea and vomiting, most patients will take small, low residue, and mainly fluid meals. These are mostly absorbed in the proximal part of the gastrointestinal tract. With adequate oral fluids, thirst is rarely a problem. A dry mouth is treated with local measures such a providing crushed ice to suck.

A small group of patients, mainly those with high obstruction, continue to vomit profusely in spite of medication. These may benefit from the insertion of a nasogastric tube or venting gastrostomy. Fluids have traditionally been given intravenously but, in this situation, hypodermoclysis (subcutaneous infusion) is recommended.[5,49,50] This route avoids the problem of maintaining venous access, it can be given by any member of staff including a community nurse, and it can be used intermittently. Some patients receive hypodermoclysis overnight and it is removed during the day to allow normal mobility.

Results of symptomatic treatment

Control of continuous abdominal pain and colic is good, with 70 to 90 per cent of patients becoming painfree.[4,37] The management of nausea and vomiting is more difficult, as a proportion of patients continue to vomit about once a day but experience little nausea.

Monitoring of the number of vomits before treatment, 2 days afterwards and 2 days before death (Fig. 1) showed good symptom control except for three patients who had a high obstruction and who required nasogastric tubes.[37]

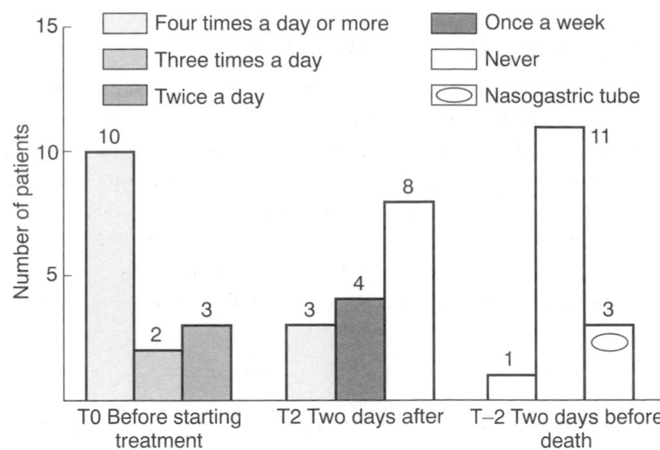

Fig. 1 Number of daily episodes of vomiting before and during treatment. (Reproduced from Ventafridda *et al.*[29] with permission.)

These results were obtained before the widespread use of octreotide and it is to be expected that, with the availability of this drug, the control of intractable vomiting will improve greatly.

Prognosis

The prognosis of patients with malignant obstruction who have undergone palliative surgery, has already been discussed. Many of the studies referred to also give the prognosis for patients unfit for surgery, or who received only laparotomy and biopsy. However, the time spans quoted in these studies date from hospital admission or surgery, not from the onset of the obstruction. In the series from St. Christopher's Hospice, a careful attempt was made to date the first obstructive symptoms so that the natural history of intestinal obstruction, in the absence of relieving surgery, could be determined (Fig. 2). The mean survival was 3.7 months. Seven patients lived with subacute intestinal obstruction for 7 months or more. Factors thought to contribute to survival were chemotherapy in ovarian cancer, faecal fistula formation, and slowly growing colonic cancer in three young patients.[4]

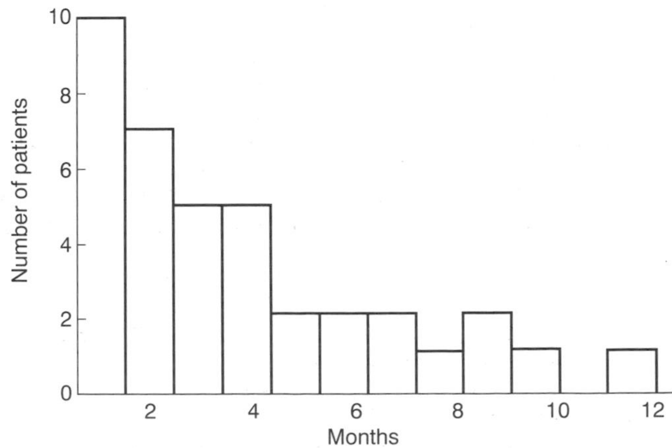

Fig. 2 Survival time (months) of patients with intestinal obstruction.

Summary of management

Some patients develop an obstruction unexpectedly; however, in those with advanced or multifocal abdominal disease this complication can be anticipated and treatment planned in advance. If there is any possibility that surgery will be of benefit, the patient should be treated with nasogastric suction and intravenous fluids while appropriate radiological investigations are performed. The decision to perform surgery should be made bearing in mind the indications and the patient's wishes; if appropriate, it should be undertaken as soon as possible.

Intravenous fluids and nasogastric suction should not be started if it is clear at the outset that palliative surgery is not indicated. Instead, appropriate medication for symptom control should be given by syringe driver. The same symptomatic treatment should be given to the patient who is in hospital receiving conservative treatment when a decision against surgery has been made. In most case, as pain and vomiting are reduced, it will be possible to withdraw the nasogastric tube and intravenous infusion.

Other measures, such as a venting gastrostomy, nasogastric tube, or hypodermoclysis, may need to be considered for the small number of patients, principally with high obstruction, who have refractory symptoms.

References

1. Phillips RKS, Hittinger R, Fry JS, Fielding LP. Malignant large bowel obstruction. *British Journal of Surgery*, 1985; **72**: 296–302.
2. Tunca JC, Buchler DA, Mack EA. The management of ovarian-cancer-caused bowel obstruction. *Gynecologic Oncology*, 1981; **12**: 186–92.
3. Beattie GJ, Leonard RCF, Smyth JF. Bowel obstruction in ovarian cancer: a retrospective study and review of the literature. *Palliative Medicine*, 1989; **3**: 275–80.
4. Baines MJ, Oliver DJ, Carter RL. Medical management of intestinal obstruction in patients with advanced malignant disease: a clinical and pathological study. *Lancet*, 1985; **ii**: 990–3.
5. Fainsinger RL, Spachynski K,Hanson J, Bruera E. Symptom control in terminally ill patients with malignant bowel obstruction. *Journal of Pain and Symptom Management*, 1994; 9:12–18
6. Reid DB. Palliative management of bowel obstruction. *Medical Journal of Australia*, 1988; **1**: 48–54.
7. Yuhasz M, Laufer I, Sutton G, Herlinger H, Caroline D. Radiology of the small bowel in patients with gynecologic malignancies. *American Journal of Radiology*, 1985; **144**: 303–7.
8. Schuffler MD, Baird HW, Flemming CR. Intestinal pseudo-obstruction as the presenting manifestation of small-cell carcinoma of the lung. *Annals of Internal Medicine*, 1983; **98**: 129–34.
9. Aabo K, Pedersen H, Bach F, Knudsen J. Surgical management of intestinal obstruction in the late course of malignant disease. *Acta Chirurgica Scandinavica*, 1984; **150**: 173–6.
10. Krebs H, Goplerud DR. Surgical management of bowel obstruction in advanced ovarian cancer. *Obstetrics and Gynecology*, 1983; **61**: 327–30.
11. Rubin SC, Hoskins WJ, Benjamin I, Lewis JL. Palliative surgery for intestinal obstruction in advanced ovarian cancer. *Gynecologic Oncology*, 1989; **34**: 16–19.
12. Zadeh BJ, Davis JM, Canizaro PC. Small bowel obstruction in the elderly. *American Surgeon*, 1985; **51**: 470–3.
13. Bizer LS, Liebling RW, Delany HM, Gliedman ML. Small bowel obstruction. *Surgery*, 1981; **89**: 407–13
14. Osteen RJ, Guyton S, Steele G, Wilson RE. Malignant intestinal obstruction. *Surgery*, 1980; **67**: 611–15.
15. Ziter FMH. Radiologic diagnosis: small bowel. In: Welch JP, ed. *Bowel Obstruction*. Philadelphia: WB Saunders, 1990: 96–108.
16. Markowitz SK. Radiologic diagnosis: colon. In: Welch JP, ed. *Bowel Obstruction*. Philadelphia: WB Saunders, 1990: 108–121.
17. Walsh HPJ, Schofield PF. Is laparotomy for small bowel obstruction justified in patients with previously treated malignancy? *British Journal of Surgery*, 1984; **71**: 933–5.
18. Ketcham AS, Hoye RC, Pilch YH, Morton DL. Delayed intestinal obstruction following treatment for cancer. *Cancer*, 1970; **25**: 406–10.
19. Turnbull ADM, Guerra J, Starners HF. Results of surgery for obstructing carcinomatosis of gastrointestinal, pancreatic or biliary origin. *Journal of Clinical Oncology*, 1989; **7**: 381–6.
20. Gallick HL, Weaver DW, Sachs RJ, Bouwman DL. Intestinal obstruction in cancer patients. An assessment of risk factors and outcome. *American Surgeon*, 1986; **52**: 434–7.
21. Castaldo TW, Petrilli ES, Ballon SC, Lagasse LD. Intestinal operations in patients with ovarian carcinoma. *American Journal of Obstetrics and Gynecology*, 1981; **139**: 80–4.
22. Taylor RH. Laparotomy for obstruction with recurrent tumour (letter). *British Journal of Surgery*, 1985; **72**: 327.
23. Clarke-Pearson DL, Chin NO, DeLong ER, Rice R, Creasman WT. Surgical management of intestinal obstruction in ovarian cancer. *Gynecologic Oncology*, 1987; **26**: 11–18.
24. Welch JP. *Bowel Obstruction*. Philadelphia: WB Saunders, 1990.
25. Aranha GV, Folk FA, Greenlee HB. Surgical palliation of small bowel obstruction due to metastatic carcinoma. *American Surgeon*, 1981; **47**: 99–102.
26. Piver MS, Barlow JJ, Lele SB, Frank A. Survival after ovarian cancer induced intestinal obstruction. *Gynecologic Oncology*, 1982; **13**: 44–9.
27. Soo KC, Davidson T, Parker M, Paterson I, Paterson A. Intestinal obstruction in patients with gynaecological malignancies. *Annals Academy of Medicine*, 1988; **17**: 72–5.
28. Krebs H, Goplerud DR. The role of intestinal intubation in obstruction of the small intestine due to carcinoma of the ovary. *Surgery, Gynecology and Obstetrics*, 1984; **158**: 467–71.
29. Solomon HJ, *et al.* Bowel complications in the management of ovarian cancer. *Australian and New Zealand Journal of Obstetrics and Gynaecology*, 1983; **23**: 65–8.
30. Malone JM, Koonce T, Larson DM, Freedman RS, Carrasco CHO, Saul PB. Palliation of small bowel obstruction by percutaneous gastrostomy in patients with progressive ovarian carcinoma. *Obstetrics and Gynecology*, 1986; **68**: 431–3.
31. Ashby MA, Game PA, Devitt P, Britten-Jones R, Brooksbank MA, Davy MLJ, Keam E. Percutaneous gastrostomy as a venting procedure in palliative care. *Palliative Medicine*, 1991; **5**: 147–50.
32. McCarthy D. Strategy for intestinal obstruction in peritoneal carcinomatosis. *Archives of Surgery*, 1986; **121**: 1081–2.
33. Gemio B, *et al.* Home support of patients with end-stage malignant bowel obstruction using hydration and venting gastrostomy. *American Journal of Surgery*, 1986; **152**: 100–4.
34. Oliver DJ. The use of the syringe driver in terminal care. *British Journal of Clinical Pharmacology*, 1985; **20**: 515–6.
35. Dover S. Syringe drivers in terminal care. *British Medical Journal*, 1987; **294**: 553–5.
36. Johnson I, Patterson S. Drugs used in combination in the syringe driver—a survey of hospice practice. *Palliative Medicine*, 1992; **6**: 125–30.
37. Ventafridda V, Ripamonti C, Caraceni A, Spoldi E, Messina L, De Como F. The management of inoperable gastrointestinal obstruction in terminal cancer patients. *Tumori*, 1990; **76**: 389–93.
38. De Conno F, Caraceni A, Zecca E, Spoldi E, Ventafridda V. The continuous subcutaneous infusion of hyoscine butylbromide reduces secretions in patients with gastrointestinal obstruction. *Journal of Pain and Symptom Management*, 1991; **6**: 484–6.
39. Oliver DJ. The use of methotrimeprazine in terminal care. *British Journal of Clinical Practice*, 1985; **39**: 339–40.
40. Isbister WH, Elder P, Symonds L. Non-operative management of malignant intestinal obstruction. *Journal of the Royal College of Surgeons of Edinburgh*, 1990; **35**: 369–72.

41. Hutchison SMW, Beattie G, Shearing CH. Increased serotonin excretion in patients with ovarian carcinoma and intestinal obstruction. *Palliative Medicine*, 1995; **9**: 67–8.
42. Fallon MT. The physiology of somatostatin and its synthetic analogue, octreotide. *European Journal of Palliative Care*, 1994; **1**: 20–2.
43. Mercadante S, Maddaloni S. Octreotide in the management of inoperable gastrointestinal obstruction in terminal cancer patients. *Journal of Pain and Symptom Management*, 1992; **7**: 496–8.
44. Koo D, Riley J, Waxman J. Control of emesis in bowel obstruction in terminally ill patients. *Lancet*, 1992; **339**: 375–6.
45. Stiefel F, Morant R. Vapreotide, a new somatostatin analogue in palliative management of obstructive ileus in advanced cancer. *Support Care Cancer*, 1993; **1**: 57–8.
46. Mercadante S, Spoldi E, Caraceni A, Maddaloni S, Simonetti MT. Octreotide in relieving gastrointestinal symptoms due to bowel obstruction. *Palliative Medicine*, 1993; **7**: 295–9.
47. Riley J, Fallon MT. Octreotide in terminal malignant obstruction of the gastrointestinal tract. *European Journal of Palliative Care*, 1994; **1**: 23–5.
48. Farr WC. The use of corticosteroids for symptom management in terminally ill patients. *American Journal of Hospice Care*, 1990; **7**: 41–6.
49. Fainsinger RL, MacEachern T, Miller MJ, Bruera E, Spachynski K, Kuehn N, Hanson J. The use of hypodermoclysis for rehydration in terminally ill cancer patients. *Journal of Pain and Symptom Management*, 1994; **9**: 298–302.
50. Constans T, Dutertre J-P, Froge E. Hypodermoclysis in dehydrated elderly patients: local effects with and without hyaluronidase. *Journal of Palliative Care*, 1991; **7**: 10–2.

9.3.5 The pathophysiology of cancer cachexia

Nora T. Jaskowiak and H. Richard Alexander, Jr

Introduction

The clinical signs that form the hallmark of cancer-associated cachexia are anorexia and weight loss. Cancer cachexia also includes many other clinical features associated with the progressive growth of a cancer, including abnormalities in carbohydrate, fat, protein, and energy metabolism, which are manifest as weakness, fatigue, malaise, and loss of skeletal muscle and adipose tissue. This abnormal metabolism may also be detected by measurements of serum chemistry and haematology profiles, where it appears as anaemia, hypertriglyceridaemia, hypoalbuminaemia, hypoproteinaemia, glucose intolerance, and hyperlacticacidaemia.

Cancer cachexia develops in a majority of patients with advanced malignancy and has been reported to be a major contributing cause of death in up to 50 per cent of these patients (Table 1).[1] The development of effective anticancer therapy, including surgery, chemotherapy, radiation therapy, and immunotherapy, alone or in combination, has produced meaningful improvement in survival for many patients afflicted with cancer. However, patients who are malnourished on the basis of cachexia often cannot tolerate effective therapy and may be more prone to the adverse effects of anticancer treatment. Replenishment of the cachectic patient with enteral or parenteral nutrition has been attempted, and in some circumstances has been effective in interrupting or reversing some of the metabolic sequelae of advancing malignancy.[3–6] However, although total parenteral nutrition appeared to decrease operative morbidity and mortality in patients with gastrointestinal carcinoma[7] and to benefit patients undergoing high-dose chemotherapy and bone marrow transplant,[8] it has not been demonstrated to improve survival in other groups of patients with cancer.[9–12] Other strategies, for example treatment with anabolic hormones, progestins, insulin, growth hormone, and hydrazine sulphate, which is an inhibitor of hepatic gluconeogenesis, are being studied in experimental settings and in humans.[13–17] Although some of these new approaches appear promising, their clinical efficacy and impact on survival have not been established conclusively.

The cachectic changes associated with progressive tumour growth can be carefully observed and quantified in laboratory models, but in studies of cachexia in humans it is much more difficult to measure such parameters under uniform or controlled conditions. A normal rat eats 10 to 12 g of food daily, and after subcutaneous inoculation with a transplantable sarcoma initially consumes a similar amount. However, at approximately 18 to 20 days, the rat begins to eat less food and to lose body weight as the tumour grows progressively (Fig. 1). The tumour has the

Table 1 Frequency of weight loss, relationship to performance status, and impact on survival in patients undergoing chemotherapy for advanced commonly diagnosed cancers

Diagnosis	*n*	Percentage with weight loss in prior 6 months	Percentage with weight loss and normal performance status	Survival of patients with and without weight loss (weeks)		Percentage decrease in survival with weight loss
				With	Without	
Lung, non-small-cell	590	61	56	14	20	30*
Lung, small-cell	436	57	47	27	34	21*
Colon	307	54	45	21	43	51*
Breast	289	36	25	45	70	36*
Prostate	78	56	35	24	46	48*
Gastric, non-measurable	179	83	80	27	41	34*
Gastric, measurable	138	87	86	16	18	11

* $p < 0.05$
Reproduced from ref. 2 with permission.

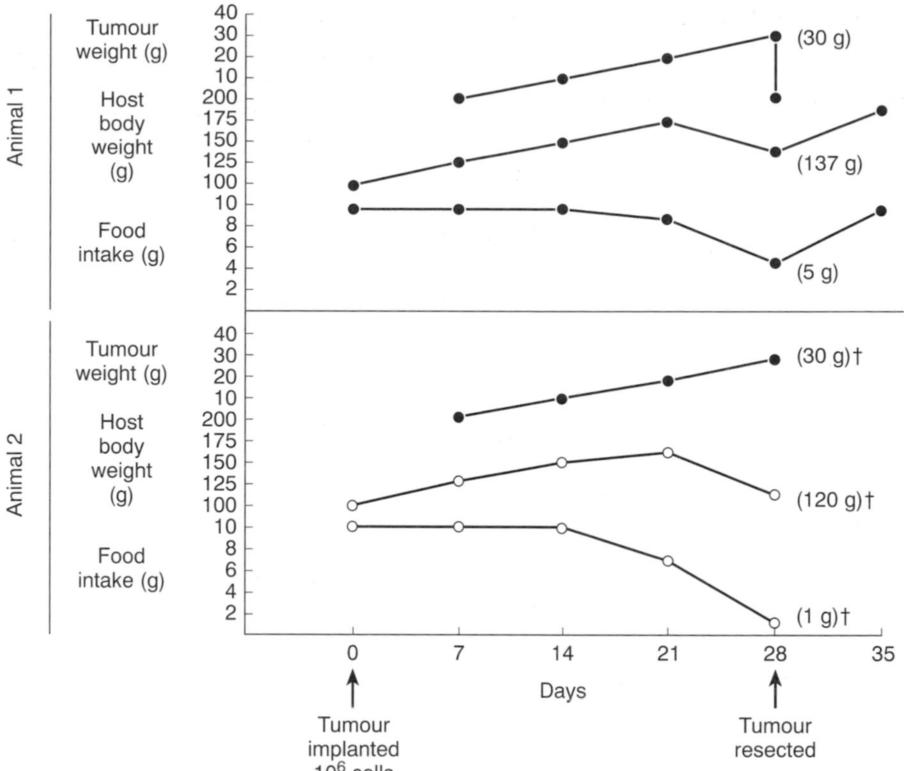

Fig. 1 Tumour weight, host body weight, and food intake in two tumour-bearing rats. Both rats had similar progressive tumour growth, and food intake and body weights in both began to decline approximately 18 days after tumour implantation. The tumour was resected on day 28. Animal 1 showed less weight loss and more food intake, despite the presence of an identical tumour, and survived tumour resection surgery, returning to normal food intake and weight. Animal 2 had a lower food intake and greater weight loss, and died shortly after surgery. The figure illustrates two major points: that cachexia depends on the presence of tumour, and that the magnitude of cachexia adversely affects the outcome of antitumour therapy.

ability to grow progressively at the expense of the host because, despite the fact that the host eats less and less, the tumour gains mass (Fig. 1). Although the sarcoma does not invade or metastasize to vital structures, the rat typically dies 30 to 35 days following tumour transplantation, suggesting that cancer cachexia evolves and progresses until the demise of the tumour-bearing host. Following tumour resection in rats, the anorexia and weight loss is quickly recovered (Fig. 1, animal 1).[18] Cachexia may affect the ability of the animal to tolerate treatment. In the experiment cited, it is clear that a lower food intake and greater weight loss during the perioperative period were correlated with an increased operative death rate (Table 2 and Fig. 1).[18] This is the common pathway to death during progressive malignancy in many other experimental models. Some experimental tumours produce profound cachexia at very small tumour volumes, illustrating that tumours have varying abilities to cause cachexia. This phenomenon is also seen in cancer patients with different tumour histologies.

The complex metabolic changes that occur in tumour-bearing laboratory animals and in patients with cancer have been described meticulously in extensive studies over the past 60 years. Recently, the role of endogenously produced protein cytokines, including tumour necrosis factor, interleukin 1 (IL-1), interleukin 6 (IL-6), leukaemia inhibitory factor, and interferon-γ, in the development of cancer cachexia has been elucidated.[19–23] Plasma and body fluid levels of some of these cytokines have been detected in some patients with malignancy[24,25] but not in others.[26,27] Extensive work with laboratory animal models has detected increased tissue and monocyte gene expression of IL-1, IL-6, and leukaemia inhibitory

Table 2 Factors associated with survival and non-survival following tumour resection in cachectic tumour-bearing rats

	n	**Ratio of host weight to tumour weight**	**Percentage host weight loss**	**Food intake day before resection** (g)	**Tumour weight** (g)
Survivors	19	2.7±0.5	17.6±7.5	2.63±3.35	72.5±9.1
Non-survivors	12	2.3±0.4*	24.4±8.9*	0.7±1.5*	71.6±5.4

Data are mean ± standard deviation.
Host weight is total body weight minus tumour weight.
* < 0.05 compared with survivors.
Reproduced with permission from ref. 18.

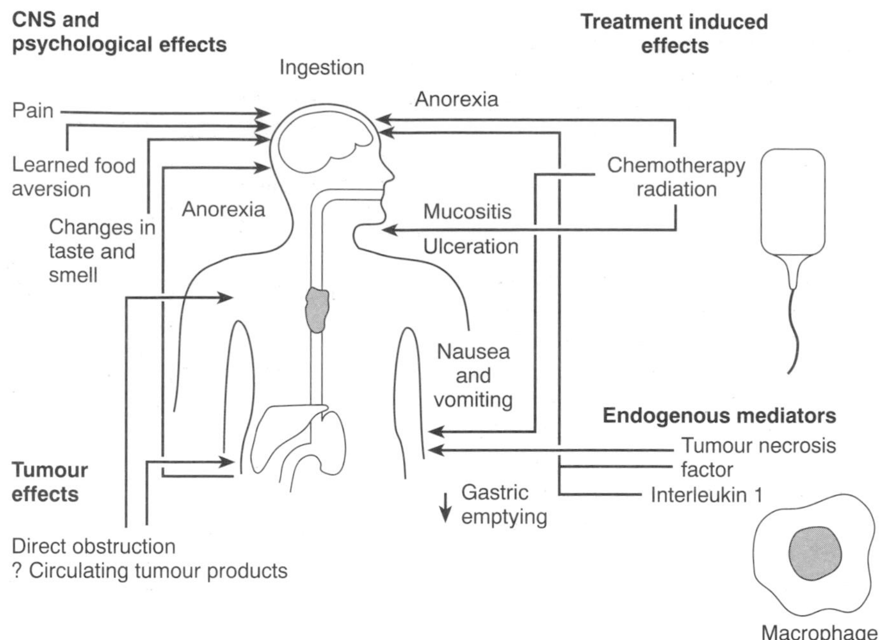

Fig. 2 Multifactorial aetiology of cancer anorexia. The figure demonstrates four different factors that influence the food intake of cancer patients.

factor.[23,28] Furthermore, many of the metabolic effects of cytokines resemble the metabolic changes seen in patients with cancer cachexia, and the administration of recombinant cytokines to laboratory animals produces many of the physiological changes observed in tumour-bearing animals with cancer cachexia.[19,29–31] The administration of antibodies against a variety of cytokines can partially reverse the anorexia, body weight loss, and host protein and fat depletion associated with cachexia in some tumour-bearing laboratory animals.[22,32–34] The current availability of recombinant antibodies or receptor antagonists against endogenous mediators such as tumour necrosis factor, IL-1, interferon-γ, IL-6, and leukaemia inhibitory factor offer exciting potential approaches towards the treatment of cancer cachexia.

Description of cachexia associated with cancer

Anorexia and weight loss

The anorexia of cachexia is relative hypophagia, i.e. a relative decline in food intake such that energy intake falls short of energy expenditure. If the energy and substrate requirements of the organism are not met, the negative energy balance results in wasting of lipid and protein stores. The precise aetiology of anorexia or relative hypophagia is not completely understood, but it is probably multifactorial (Fig. 2).[35] The cancer patient has altered gustatory and olfactory sensations that may decrease appetite because the taste of food is changed or is less appealing.[36] Chemotherapy and radiation therapy may augment hypophagia by causing anticipatory nausea and vomiting or painful mucositis along the upper digestive tract that is exacerbated by food intake. Learned food aversions can develop if certain types of food are given just prior to anticancer treatment, and these will also contribute to the anorexia. Tumors of different histological types may produce more marked degrees of anorexia and/or cachexia.[2] Patients with lung carcinoma may have marked anorexia and weight loss at a relatively early stage of the disease, while patients with breast carcinoma do not reduce their food intake (except as a result of therapy) until a very advanced stage. This suggests that different circulating factors produced either by the tumour or by the host in response to the tumour may cause the anorexia commonly observed with some types of malignancy. In addition, the presence of a large malignant tumour in the aerodigestive tract (such as a squamous cell carcinoma of the oesophagus) may make the ingestion of adequate nutrients impossible, and simple surgical resection or bypass of the tumour may greatly improve the hypophagia.

Abnormal metabolism

Alterations in carbohydrate, protein, lipid, and energy metabolism may be present in the cancer-bearing host prior to the onset of clinically apparent cachexia, indicating that these abnormalities are responsible for the subsequent developtment of cachexia (Table 3). In the 1920s, Cori and Cori[37] observed that the venous effluent from a chick wing bearing a sarcoma had decreased concentrations of glucose and elevated levels of lactate compared with the contralateral non-tumour-bearing wing. This suggested that the sarcoma was using glucose and producing large amounts of lactic acid. Since that initial observation, the metabolic abnormalities present in tumour-bearing laboratory animals and humans have been studied extensively and described carefully. In general, despite anorexia and declining food and energy intake, the cancer-bearing host usually has evidence of accelerated catabolism, with either normal[38] or increased energy expenditure[39–42] and mobilization of peripheral protein and lipid stores with augmented liver gluconeogenesis.[43–48] This may provide substrate and nutrients for the host to combat the tumour or it may provide nutrients for a metabolically active tumour. A number of specific metabolic alterations can be detected in the host at sites remote from the tumour and occur in the presence of a very small tumour burden,[43] suggesting that in the early stages of a growing malignancy either the host response or the tumour itself produces circulating substances that induce the metabolic alterations described. The remarkable similarity of these findings in patients with different types of cancer suggests that the metabolic sequelae of cancer cachexia may be mediated via the host production of specific cytokines.

Carbohydrate metabolism

Specific abnormalities in carbohydrate metabolism have been observed in tumour-bearing laboratory animals and in cancer patients prior to the onset of anorexia and weight loss.[44,49,50] Studies in laboratory animal models have the clear advantage of allowing glucose metabolism to be measured in an untreated animal and at regular intervals in a tumour-bearing host of comparable body weight, sex, and age with a progressively growing tumour. The effects of simple starvation and decreased food intake can be examined by the inclusion of pair-fed controls. However, these findings in laboratory animals may not be applicable to cancer patients, in particular because tumour-bearing animals with cancer cachexia often have a tumour whose mass accounts for 20 to 30 per cent of the total body weight,[51] a proportion that is seldom seen in patients.

Hepatic gluconeogenesis via *de novo* production from amino acids and recycling from lactate has been measured in rats by radiolabelled tracer studies.[44,51-53] The rates of gluconeogenesis and glucose turnover are significantly increased in tumour-bearing animals compared with controls (Fig. 3). In addition, increased rates of futile glucose cycling have been demonstrated in rats with large tumour burdens compared with non-tumour-bearing controls and rats with small tumour burdens.[54] Decreased levels of serum glucose have been detected even in animals with small tumours and levels declined as the tumour burden increased.[51,55] Exactly the opposite finding was observed for lactic acid levels: these may have been slightly elevated in animals with small tumour burdens and

Table 3 Abnormal metabolism in cancer cachexia

Carbohydrate metabolism	
Endogenous glucose production	Increases
Serum glucose	Variable
Lactate recycling	Increases
Hepatic gluconeogenesis	Increases
Glycogen stores	Decrease
Insulin sensitivity	Decreases
Protein metabolism	
Skeletal muscle catabolism	Increases
Skeletal muscle synthesis	Decreases
Hepatic protein synthesis	Increases
Nitrogen balance	Negative
Lipid metabolism	
Lipoprotein lipase activity	Decreases
Lipolysis	Increases
Serum triglyceride level	Increases
Lipid stores	Decrease
Hepatic lipogenesis	Increases
Energy expenditure	Variable

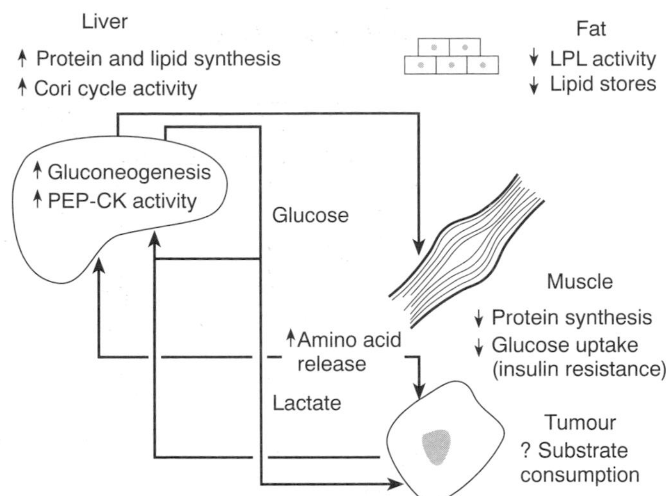

Fig. 3 Abnormal metabolism in cancer cachexia. The metabolic changes of cancer cachexia are shown, with alterations in glucose, fat, and amino acid metabolism in liver, adipose tissues, muscle, and tumour. PEP-CK, phosphoenolpyruvate carboxykinase.

progressively increased as the tumour burden increased.[51,55] Serum levels of glucose were decreased even in the presence of increased gluconeogenesis and increased Cori cycle activity.[44,51] The hepatic activity of gluconeogenic enzymes, including glucose 6-phosphatase and phosphoenolpyruvate carboxykinase, was elevated in tumour-bearing animals. The effect was not secondary to elevated insulin levels, which increase only minimally in cachectic tumour-bearing animals.[44] Increasing phosphoenolpyruvate carboxykinase activity in liver tissue was correlated with increasing tumour burden until the tumour was very advanced.[56] Inhibition of gluconeogenesis from amino acid precursors causes serum levels of glucose to decrease more dramatically in animals with small tumours than in non-tumour-bearing controls. Decreasing serum glucose concentrations associated with an accelerated rate of hepatic gluconeogenesis from amino acid precursors indicate that host tissues may be catabolized to produce glucose for use by the tumour. Some authors have even suggested that inhibition of accelerated gluconeogenesis may provide an effective anticancer therapy by depriving the tumour of glucose.[57] Others have suggested that the possible reduction in Cori cycle activity seen in cancer patients may both inhibit tumour growth and prevent some of the cachectic effects.[58]

The findings in patients with cancer are less clear than those from animal studies since patients comprise a heterogeneous group with respect to age, caloric intake, coexisting medical conditions, and treatment with a variety of anticancer therapies.[59-61] Each of these variables may affect the measured parameters. In addition, control patients without cancer but who are losing weight may have other illnesses that may also alter carbohydrate metabolism. Despite these limitations, consistent abnormalities of glucose metabolism in cancer patients, including accelerated rates of hepatic gluconeogenesis, recycling, and alterations in peripheral glucose utilization, have been found in a number of studies.[46,60] As in animal studies, these changes appear to occur prior to the onset of weight loss or marked anorexia.[49,50] Patients with localized oesophageal cancer and no weight loss have altered forearm glucose metabolism, including increased glucose extraction and lactate release.[44,49]

Similarly, in humans bearing soft-tissue sarcomas of the extremities, glucose uptake is higher in the tumour-bearing limb than in the contralateral non-tumour-bearing limb, and the rate of uptake correlates with the size of the tumour.[60] Although these studies sound similar, each of these findings implies a potentially different mechanism by which glucose utilization may be increased in patients with cancer. The study of patients with oesophageal cancer implies abnormal glucose utilization by host muscle, and the study of extremity sarcoma implies abnormal glucose utilization by the tumour itself. Each of these mechanisms may contribute to the abnormalities of glucose metabolism described.

Cancer patients may also develop glucose intolerance, primarily mediated via insulin resistance. Several different studies using glucose tolerance tests in patients with progressive cancer of various histologies have demonstrated abnormal glucose disposal.[49,50] In patients with metastatic cancer but without weight loss, serum glucose concentrations may be similar to those in non-cancer controls. Following an intravenous glucose infusion, there is an impaired glucose disposal rate despite an appropriate increase in serum levels of insulin, which is comparable to that seen in non-cancer-bearing controls. The presence of metastases appears to make this insulin resistance more pronounced.[50] Sarcoma patients without apparent weight loss or abnormal food intake have also been found to have a similar abnormal glucose tolerance that appears to correlate with tumour burden.[49]

Protein metabolism

Alterations in protein metabolism can be determined from anthropomorphic measurements, nitrogen balance, measurement of serum proteins and/or free amino acid concentrations, urinary excretion of 3-methylhistidine (an amino acid that is released during skeletal muscle catabolism and is not metabolized), and studies of regional or whole-body amino acid kinetics.[62,63] Physical examination and history yield relatively imprecise estimates of protein metabolism, and the determination of nitrogen balance does not provide reliable information about rates of protein synthesis and catabolism. Plasma amino acid levels represent only a minute fraction of the whole-body amino acid pool, and may be altered by factors such as antecedent diet, age, and sex, as well as by renal or hepatic impairment. Measurement of 3-methylhistidine excretion is a relatively simple way of assessing muscle protein catabolism in patients on a meat-free diet.[62] However, it does not measure protein synthesis, nor can it determine the contribution of 3-methylhistidine from visceral protein. Regional and whole-body kinetic studies using labelled amino acids provide the best quantitative information about protein metabolism. However, the metabolism of the tumour itself will need to be measured and considered if the findings are to be interpreted accurately.

Although these methods provide the best information about protein alterations in patients with cancer cachexia, they need to be carefully controlled to be certain that any measured changes are not secondary to starvation or other concomitant illnesses. Protein metabolism in patients with cancer cachexia is quite similar to that seen in patients with acute early starvation.[64] During the early phase of acute starvation, following the depletion of hepatic glycogen stores, the primary source of energy is breakdown of host protein (primarily skeletal muscle) and the conversion of amino acids to glucose in the liver. After several days of starvation, the host adapts to the lack of nutrients by decreasing protein turnover (synthesis and catabolism rates combined), using lipid stores preferentially, and decreasing whole-body energy expenditure. In the catabolic tumour-bearing host, however, the adaptive transfer to lipids as the primary energy source, with relative preservation of protein stores, may not occur, or may occur to a much lesser extent than expected.

Experimental studies of protein metabolism in animals with cachexia offer the same advantages and disadvantages as studies of carbohydrate metabolism.[65] Some investigators have found comparable total plasma amino acid levels in tumour-bearing and control animals,[66] while others have found decreased levels in tumour-bearing animals.[67] Mice bearing a subcutaneously implanted MAC16 colon adenocarcinoma show a progressive decrease in carcass muscle and fat mass that correlates with the size of the tumour.[68] This decrease in carcass mass has been associated with the presence of lipolytic and proteolytic activity in the serum of MAC16 tumour-bearing rats and mice, suggesting that either the tumour produces the factors that cause these changes or the host produces them in response to the tumour.[69,70] These factors have not yet been specifically identified, but further studies with the MAC16 tumour in mice suggests a role for prostaglandin E_2 in the skeletal muscle degradation of cachexia.[71] Increased levels of prostaglandin E_2 were detected in the gastrocnemius muscle of MAC16-bearing mice compared with MAC13-bearing controls (which did not develop cachexia). Further, treatment with the prostaglandin inhibitor indomethacin or with polyunsaturated fatty acid eicosapentanoic acid inhibited the increase in levels of prostaglandin E_2 and blocked muscle protein degradation.[71]

Skeletal muscle contains multiple proteolytic systems. However, which is involved in the upregulated proteolysis of cancer cachexia is unclear. The lysosomal pathway involves four major proteases in muscle, cathepsins B, H, L, and D. Increased cathepsin activities have been described in the muscle of some cancer patients.[72] However, lysosomes are not involved in breakdown of myofibrillar proteins and therefore account for only a minor part of skeletal muscle proteolysis. Two cytosolic proteolytic pathways exist in skeletal muscle: one is calcium dependent and the other is ATP–ubiquitin dependent.[73] Recent experiments suggest that the ATP–ubiquitin-dependent proteolytic pathway is responsible for the proteolysis of most skeletal muscle proteins. Further, mRNA levels for ubiquitin and its carrier protein and proteasome subunits are all increased in the atrophying muscle in cachectic rats bearing Yoshida sarcoma.[73] *In vitro* results demonstrated that depletion of ATP almost completely suppressed the increased proteolysis seen in muscles in this rat model.[73] Therefore, although the mechanism of increased muscle breakdown in cancer cachexia is not yet completely elucidated, understanding of it is increasing.

When hepatic gluconeogenesis is interrupted by administration of phosphoenolpyruvate carboxykinase inhibitors (such as hydrazine sulphate), plasma amino acid levels increase more dramatically in tumour-bearing animals than in controls, suggesting that they are being released more quickly in the former.[67] The rate of conversion of alanine to glucose and the amount of glucose derived from alanine are also higher in tumour-bearing animals.[44,66]

Plasma levels of amino acids in cancer patients without weight loss appear to be preserved and comparable to those of patients without cancer.[74,75] The changes in amino acid concentrations that have been reported in most studies of cancer cachexia include a variety of tumour types and patients with varying amounts of weight loss. Patients with oesophageal cancer and a 20 per cent weight loss have a marked reduction in concentrations of total and individual plasma amino acids, except for branched-chain amino acids.[74] It does not appear that plasma levels of either total or individual amino acids will be of any clinical importance in the assessment and management of cancer cachexia.

Most laboratory and clinical studies have documented an increase in hepatic protein synthesis in cancer patients. Hepatocytes isolated from such patients show a marked increase in protein synthesis compared with patients with benign disease, and this increase is less marked when weight loss is present.[76] The rate of protein synthesis in skeletal muscle is decreased in cancer patients while protein degradation rates are increased, as noted above.[73,74] Together, these findings suggest that the protein metabolism of cancer-bearing animals and patients is markedly abnormal. The mobilization of host protein from skeletal muscle is greater than the increased synthesis of some new proteins in the liver, resulting in overall protein catabolism.

Kinetic studies of whole-body protein metabolism in cancer patients have confirmed that an overall increase in protein turnover can be observed before any other manifestations of cachexia, such as weight loss, decreased food intake, or changes in blood levels of amino acid and protein, are clinically apparent.[77,78] These changes do not appear to be dependent on the presence of metastases.[79] With the onset of anorexia and weight loss, protein turnover remains accelerated and is higher than in non-cancer patients with comparable degrees of weight loss.[80] The increased rate of protein turnover appears to be secondary to both accelerated rates of whole-body protein synthesis and catabolism independent of weight loss. While the physiological importance of accelerated protein turnover in the development of cancer cachexia has not been conclusively demonstrated, it is clear that abnormal protein metabolism plays a significant role in the severe and rapid onset of cachexia seen in conditions such as hepatocellular carcinoma.[81] In addition, these abnormalities in protein metabolism result in loss of functional lean body mass, which is a hallmark of cancer cachexia.

Lipid metabolism

The loss of body fat in patients with progressive cancer is a well-characterized physical finding and may be an indication of poor prognosis. While knowledge of the precise alterations in lipid metabolism in patients with cancer is growing, these alterations have not been as well described as the changes in carbohydrate and protein metabolism. Tumour-bearing rats may have elevated plasma levels of triglycerides and cholesterol before alterations in food intake or weight loss become apparent. Alterations in lipid metabolism that have been characterized in animal models of cancer cachexia include increased rates of free fatty acid and triacylglycerol synthesis, increased rates of lipolysis, and decreased rates of triglyceride clearance from serum.[82,83] These changes in lipid metabolism are dependent on tumour type and are completely reversed after excision of the tumour.[82,84]

Plasma levels of triglycerides and cholesterol may be abnormally high in cancer-bearing rats with weight loss, and circulating and tissue levels of lipoprotein lipase activity are usually decreased.[55,83] Tissue lipoprotein lipase acts to remove triglycerides from the circulation. Elevated plasma levels of triglycerides associated with marked cachexia in rabbits with tularaemia were shown to be secondary to decreased activity of the enzyme lipoprotein lipase. This led to identification of a circulating lipoprotein-lipase-suppressing factor which was called cachectin (later identified as tumour necrosis factor). This factor appears to be a key mediator of the toxicity and cachexia associated with acute and chronic infectious diseases, but whether it is involved in the development of cancer-associated cachexia[85,86] remains a controversial point.

Other factors with lipoprotein-lipase-inhibiting activity have since been identified. IL-1, IL-6, and interferon-γ have all been shown to suppress lipoprotein lipase activity *in vitro* and *in vivo*.[87-90] In addition, a factor with the ability to inhibit lipoprotein lipase was isolated from the conditioned media of a human melanoma cell line known to induce severe cachexia in nude mice.[91] This factor, initially termed melanoma-derived lipoprotein lipase inhibitor, was subsequently identified as leukaemia inhibitory factor, which has been shown to lead to weight loss when injected into experimental animals.[23]

Whole-body rates of lipolysis appear to be elevated in patients with cancer cachexia, as reflected by elevated rates of plasma glycerol turnover.[48] It has long been hypothesized that tumours may produce a factor (or factors) that promotes lipolysis in normal adipocytes. Work in recent years has provided some clues in this area. Studies of specific cytokines have revealed that tumour necrosis factor, interferon-γ, IL-1, and leukaemia inhibitory factor all increase lipolysis rates in cultured murine adipocytes, while IL-6 has minimal effect.[92,93] However, tumour necrosis factor has no effect on cultured human adipocytes, so that its role as a mediator of altered lipid metabolism in cancer patients is less clear.[94] Other lipolysis-promoting factors have also been identified, but have yet to be fully characterized.[95,96] A mechanism of lipolysis promotion has been elucidated by workers who describe increased intracellular accumulation of cAMP. This increase in cAMP was shown to be the result of stimulation of adipose cell adenylate cyclase.[97] The accumulated cAMP stimulates a cAMP-dependent protein kinase, which then activates a cellular triglyceride lipase.[97] This accumulation of cAMP could be blocked by ω-3 polyunsaturated fatty acids via inhibition of adenylate cyclase. *In vivo* studies of mice bearing MAC16 adenocarcinomas showed reduced body weight loss with increased body fat and muscle weight in animals fed ω-3 polyunsaturated fatty acids.[97]

Energy expenditure

Resting energy expenditure, determined by measuring oxygen consumption and carbon dioxide production, can be normal, decreased, or increased in cancer patients, and appears to be influenced by the existence of antecedent weight loss, sex, presence of metastases, and histological tumour type.[38-40,98] Some investigators have found that levels of resting energy expenditure in malnourished cancer patients are higher than those in malnourished controls,[39] but others have shown that measured differences in resting energy expenditure are abolished when the results are corrected for lean body mass.[38] In a study of a homogeneous group of sarcoma patients who had large primary tumours without evidence of metastases or weight loss, the resting energy expenditure was significantly higher than that of controls, even when corrected for lean body mass.[40] Furthermore, the increase in resting energy expenditure was related directly to a decrease in lean body mass, suggesting that, in patients with large primary sarcomas, abnormal increases in resting energy expenditure may cause changes in body composition even before the development of clinically apparent cachexia. In another recent study, patients with pancreatic cancer and weight loss were found to have significantly elevated rates of resting energy expenditure compared with age-matched weight-stable controls.[42] Further, resting energy expenditure was found to be more elevated in cancer patients with evidence of an acute phase response, represented by an elevated serum C-protein level, than in patients with no such response. Clearly, patients with progressive cancer represent a heterogeneous population in whom cachexia may be accompanied by an abnormal increase in resting energy expenditure.

Summary

Host metabolic changes appear to occur early in the course of cancer and at the onset of clinical cachexia. These abnormalities in metabolism usually precede clinically overt manifestations of cachexia and probably contribute to its development. The cachectic tumour-bearing host has increased levels of gluconeogenesis and abnormal serum levels of glucose and insulin. These abnormalities appear to be manifested primarily as insulin resistance, with either stress or infusion-associated hyperglycaemia. Protein turnover is accelerated, with abnormal increases in whole-body protein synthesis and catabolism. This appears to be associated with elevated hepatic protein synthesis and increased skeletal muscle breakdown. Lipogenesis and lipolysis are increased, while there is impaired clearance of plasma triglycerides. Energy expenditure is increased when compared with the normal levels in patients with a clear reduction of food intake. These abnormalities result in abnormal loss of body protein and fat mass and gain in total body water.

Mechanism of cancer cachexia

The mechanisms by which a growing tumour induces cachexia have been the subject of an enormous amount of research over the past two decades. The original hypothesis, that cancer cachexia is secondary to simple starvation, appears unlikely since many of the metabolic derangements that occur in the cachectic state exist prior to the onset of weight loss or anorexia. In addition, simple forced refeeding by enteral or parenteral routes does not reverse all the parameters of cachexia. Furthermore, a large number of laboratory and clinical studies, using weight-stable tumour-bearing hosts or including pair-fed or malnourished non-cancer controls, have uniformly identified cancer-specific alterations in carbohydrate, protein, and lipid metabolism independent of starvation.[43–45,51–53,55]

The consumption of excessive amounts of substrate by the tumour has been suggested to be a major factor contributing to the development of cancer cachexia. Many tumour types have an obligatory requirement for large amounts of glucose and amino acids, and the rate of glucose uptake by some tumours may correlate with the increasing tumour size in sarcoma-bearing humans.[60] Massive substrate consumption by the tumour may play an important role in some animal models of cachexia, in which tumour burden can exceed 10 per cent of body weight prior to development of weight loss or anorexia. Furthermore, it has been demonstrated in rats that the metabolic impact of a large inert mass similar in size to a cachexia-producing tumour may not be inconsequential. However, many animal models of cachexia, particularly those in mice, have relatively small tumour burdens in the setting of significant cachexia. Also, most tumours in humans do not exceed 0.5 or 1 per cent of body weight prior to death, and the basic metabolic rate of neoplastic tissue has been shown to be comparable to that of the tissue from which it originated.[65] In other conditions of excessive energy expenditure or consumption (such as pregnancy or exposure to cold) the host simply consumes more food to meet the metabolic demand.[99,100] However, tumour-bearing hosts consume less rather than more food. Therefore it appears unlikely that the metabolic changes of cachexia in humans are secondary solely to the substrate requirements of the tumour.

Circulating mediators of cancer cachexia

Studies have demonstrated that the anorexia and weight loss of cancer cachexia may be secondary to circulating humoral factors that are produced either by the tumour itself or by the host in response to the presence of tumour. In laboratory animals sharing a surgically created parabiotic circulation (1.5 per cent of cardiac output), the anorexia, weight loss, and other metabolic alterations seen in cancer cachexia were found to be present in both partners of the parabiotic pair despite the fact that only one animal hosted a non-metastasizing tumour.[101] The development of cachexia in parabiotes was altered: the non-tumour-bearing animal lessened the cachexia seen in the tumour-bearing animal, and the parabiotic pair lived significantly longer than a single animal with a tumour. Because the animals shared a small amount of cross-circulation, this experiment suggested that a small stable circulating factor, such as a peptide, was responsible for the cachexia associated with the tumour. However, it was not clear whether this circulating factor was of host or tumour origin. Some human tumours, including small-cell lung cancer, produce blood-borne factors, such as serotonin or bombesin, that can suppress host appetite. Extracts from certain laboratory tumours such as the SEKI melanoma[91] or the MAC16 adenocarcinoma,[69] when injected into laboratory animals, produce anorexia, weight loss, proteolysis, and lipolysis, implying that these tumours produce substances that may cause cancer cachexia. However, it appears that only a minority of laboratory and clinical tumours produce these factors, while evidence of cachexia is present in the vast majority of cancer patients. The reason why some tumours can result in marked anorexia and cachexia is not well understood.

Other research suggests that endogenously produced cytokines are secreted by the host in response to a growing tumour, and these may be important mediators of cancer cachexia; however, some tumour cells may also secrete cytokines. Cytokines, most notably tumour necrosis factor and IL-1, are produced primarily by macrophages and lymphocytes in response to a large variety of invasive stimuli.[19–21,30,31,102–104] These highly conserved protein molecules are pluripotent. They possess a wide range of activities and their effects overlap.[105] Tumor necrosis factor and IL-1 usually work locally through paracrine and autocrine pathways. However, under certain pathophysiological conditions, they may be produced quickly by host cells, enter the circulation, and exert profound endocrine activity. While these molecules certainly have many

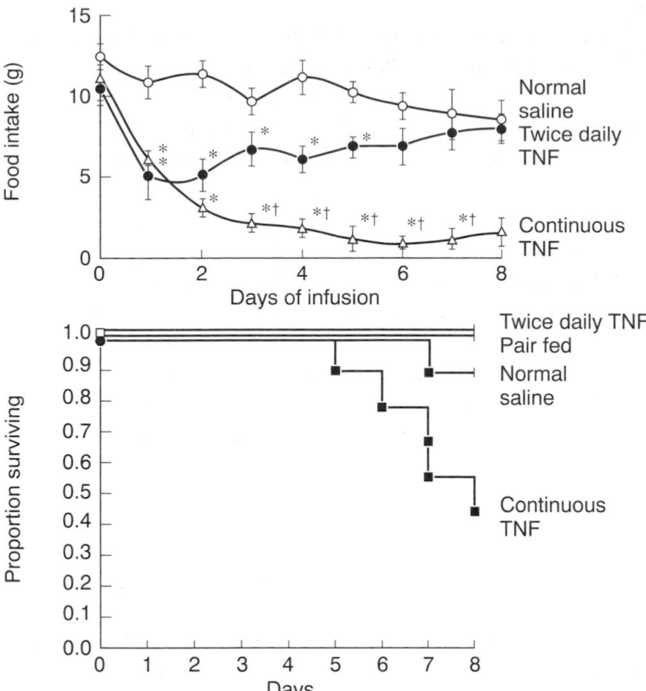

Fig. 4 Development of tolerance to tumour necrosis factor (TNF) is related to the method of administration. Rats were treated with either a continuous intravenous infusion of tumour necrosis factor ((a) △; (b) ■) or the same dose by twice-daily bolus injections (●). The rats given the continuous infusion of tumour necrosis factor had a sustained decreased food intake (a) and 50 per cent mortality during the 8-day infusion (b). However, in rats given the same dose by intermittent bolus injection the food intake recovered to levels similar to those of control animals (a) and there were no deaths from tumour necrosis factor among these rats (b). Therefore tolerance to the anorexia and lethality of tumour necrosis factor develops with bolus intravenous injections but not with continuous intravenous infusion. (Data taken with permission from ref. 109.)

essential functions, they also have potentially detrimental effects, depending on the amount produced and the route through which they act. Recombinant DNA techniques have made tumour necrosis factor and IL-1 available in large quantities and have facilitated the characterization of their wide-ranging biological properties. The possible role in cancer cachexia of other cytokines, such as IL-6, interferon-γ, and leukaemia inhibitory factor, has also been studied.

Tumor necrosis factor

The observation that rabbits infected with a low parasitic burden of *Trypanosoma cruzi* developed anorexia, wasting of host tissues, and lipaemia led to the discovery of a circulating serum lipoprotein-lipase-suppressing factor.[102] This factor, identified as a monocyte/macrophage product and called cachectin, was subsequently found to be the same as a protein previously isolated from the serum of endotoxin-treated BCG-primed mice. This factor induced haemorrhagic necrosis of tumours and was called tumour necrosis factor.[106] Chronic administration of recombinant human tumour necrosis factor to laboratory animals results in marked anorexia and weight loss suggestive of cancer cachexia.[29,107] Interestingly, animals become tolerant to the anorectic effects of this treatment, returning to normal food intake and gaining weight (Fig. 4).[107] Animals receiving continuous doses of tumour necrosis factor through a subcutaneously implanted pump develop a progressive dose-dependent anorexia, weight loss, lean body wasting, and death.[108] Continuous intravenous administration of tumour necrosis factor induces more anorexia and weight loss than an identical dose given as intermittent bolus injections (Fig. 4).[109] Similarly, recombinant human tumour necrosis factor given to rats by continuous infusion will result in death, but intermittent bolus administration of the same dose will not (Fig. 4), indicating that the cachexigenic and toxic effects of tumour necrosis factor are dependent on the dose and route of administration. The anorectic and catabolic effects of tumour necrosis factor are also dependent on its site of production. A subcutaneously implanted tumour transfected with the tumour necrosis factor gene that will continually secrete tumour necrosis factor will cause progressive anorexia, weight loss, lipid depletion, and earlier death than an identical tumour without the gene.[110] If the same tumour is implanted intracerebrally, the anorectic effects are even more marked, but there is relative preservation of host protein stores, more compatible with chronic starvation.[111] Although the degree of anorexia and weight loss seen in advancing malignancy can be reproduced experimentally by administration of tumour necrosis factor, the magnitude of these changes appears to be dependent on the method, dose, route, and frequency of administration.

The chronic administration of increasing sublethal doses of tumour necrosis factor to laboratory animals produces not only anorexia and weight loss, but also inflammatory changes in tissue, hypoproteinaemia, and anaemia, characteristic of changes seen during progressive cachexia (Table 3). Interestingly, the degree of protein depletion is less in laboratory animals pair-fed amounts comparable to the amounts eaten by animals rendered anorectic from chronic tumour necrosis factor administration.[29] This indicates that protein depletion caused by tumour necrosis factor is not simply secondary to decreased food intake, and suggests a direct effect on protein metabolism.

In clinical phase I trials in cancer patients, systemically administered tumour necrosis factor caused significant fever, chills, and malaise.[112-114] The circulating half-life after intravenous injection was just 20 minutes; such a rapid clearance and the infrequent administration may have prevented the development of any significant weight loss. Patients receiving repeated 5-day infusions develop anorexia without weight loss and have elevated serum levels of triglycerides, suggesting that tumour necrosis factor, if administered in sufficiently high doses, could simulate the spectrum of hypophagia and weight loss associated with cachexia in humans.[115]

Receptors for tumour necrosis factor exist on virtually all tissues, except erythrocytes, and some of the physiological actions of tumour necrosis factor simulate those observed in cancer cachexia. *In vitro*, tumour necrosis factor induces a catabolic condition in adipocytes manifested by the decreased production of several lipogenic enzymes, including lipoprotein lipase.[116] Under these conditions, adipocytes will release glycerol and become lipid depleted. In diabetic rats in which lipoprotein lipase activity is suppressed, the administration of tumour necrosis factor produces a progressive increase in serum triglycerides secondary to *de novo* lipogenesis in the liver.[117] Myocytes exposed to tumour necrosis factor increase glucose uptake and become depleted of glycogen stores as glycogenolysis is stimulated.[118] Some of the physiological effects seen with tumour necrosis factor may be caused by the

Table 4 Role of neutralizing antibodies against specific cytokines in cancer cachexia

Treatment	Rationale for use	Effects on food intake	Body weight	Ability to preserve Lipid	Protein
Anti-TNF Ab	TNF detectable in serum of some tumour-bearing hosts, causes cachexia when administered	+	+	+	+
Anti-IL-1 receptor Ab	IL-1 RNA induced in cachexia, *in vivo* effects resemble those observed in cachexia	+	+	+	+
Anti-IFN-γ Ab	IFN-γ has synergy with TNF, causes anorexia in rats	+	+	NA	NA
Anti-IL-6 Ab	IL-6 detectable in serum of some tumour-bearing hosts, causes cachexia when administered	+	+	+	+
Anti-LIF Ab	Human tumours producing LIF cause cachexia in experimental models	NA	NA	NA	NA

Abbreviations: TNF, tumour necrosis factor; Ab, antibodies; IFN, interferon; LIF, leukaemia inhibitory factor; NA, not available

release of other mediators. Although tumour necrosis factor does not directly influence muscle catabolism *in vitro*, it increases whole-body muscle catabolism in laboratory animals.[19,29,119] Hepatocytes treated with tumour necrosis factor *in vitro* develop increased rates of amino acid uptake, acute phase protein synthesis, and gluconeogenesis; these changes are also observed in hepatocytes from patients with cancer cachexia[76,120] and in laboratory animals.[19] Hypoproteinaemia, as manifested by decreased serum levels of albumin, has been observed in cancer patients. Mice implanted with cells transfected with the functional gene for tumour necrosis factor develop decreased serum levels of albumin secondary to decreased albumin synthesis rates.[121] Even prior to the development of cachexia, levels of albumin-specific RNA are significantly reduced in these mice, indicating the selective inhibition of albumin gene expression by tumour necrosis factor. In humans, tumour necrosis factor produces hyperlipidaemia and increased rates of fatty acid turnover and lipolysis,[115] effects which are similar to those described in cancer patients.

The detection of circulating levels of tumour necrosis factor activity in cancer patients has been controversial and inconsistent. Detectable levels have been found in one series of patients with cancer,[24] but not in others.[26,27] RNA specific for tumour necrosis factor is expressed by blood monocytes in a greater proportion of cancer patients than in controls. In laboratory rats with large subcutaneous, methylchlorane-induced sarcomas and marked cachexia, serum levels of tumour necrosis factor correlate with the degree of tumour burden.[122] Animals which are made tolerant to the effects of tumour necrosis factor by chronic administration and are subsequently implanted with the methylchlorane-induced sarcoma survive longer and become less cachectic than non-tolerant tumour-bearing controls, despite similar rates of tumour growth in both groups.[123] Tumour-bearing rats can also be made tolerant to the effects of tumour necrosis factor by repeated intraperitoneal administration of sublethal doses, and this treatment also results in prolonged survival (Fig. 4).[124] This treatment has no antitumour effects but does exhibit marked anticachexia effects.

In one study, but not in another, the administration of antibodies directed against tumour necrosis factor reversed the progressive endstage cachexia seen in tumour-bearing animals (Table 4).[22,32] Reversal of cachexia on administration of antitumour necrosis factor antibodies was also seen in a nude mouse model of cachexia (Table 4). In this model, a human maxilla squamous cell tumour was established in culture and, when implanted in nude mice, led to severe cachexia, hypercalcaemia, and leucocytosis.[125] Plasma levels of tumour necrosis factor were four times higher in tumour-bearing mice than in controls, and administration of antitumour necrosis factor antibody led to increase in body weight. Interestingly, splenectomy in these mice led to decreased tumour growth and decreased cachexia development.[125] Tumour necrosis factor was not detectable in cell culture supernatants of this tumour line, suggesting that normal spleen-derived host cells may interact with the tumour to lead to development of cachexia. Other studies have shown that the chronic administration of antibodies to tumour necrosis factor to mice bearing methylchlorane-induced sarcoma or the Lewis lung adenocarcinoma will attenuate the anorexia, weight loss, and depletion of carcass lipid and protein stores which develop with progressive tumour growth.[32] Other conditions associated with progressive cancer cachexia, such as anaemia, hypoalbuminaemia, and altered serum levels of amyloid P, were not affected by the antibodies, suggesting that either the concentration of antibody in some tissues was insufficient to reverse these changes or that other mediators contribute to the development of cachexia. It is important to appreciate that antibody-treated tumour-bearing mice had smaller tumours than controls, suggesting that amelioration of cachexia may have been partly due to smaller tumour burdens.[32]

Interleukin-1

IL-1 is a protein molecule, originally thought to be a family of proteins named for their physiological activities (leucocyte endogenous mediator and endogenous pyrogen, so named for the ability to activate leucocytes and induce fever) but now known to be the same cytokine.[103,104] The role of IL-1 in the development of cancer cachexia has not been conclusively established, but it shares many of the biological activities of tumour necrosis factor, with which it acts synergistically,[105,126,127] and has been shown to stimulate the release of IL-6 from tumour cells, a pathway through which it may be responsible for cachexia.[128] It is produced in large quantities by macrophages in response to a variety of stimuli that also induce these cells to secrete tumour necrosis factor.[103] Low doses of IL-1 produce fever, inflammation, and anorexia in laboratory animals.[20,30] Anorexia may be primarily induced through the action of IL-1 on the hypothalamus and stimulation of corticotropin-releasing factor.[129]

IL-1 was identified in the plasma of only one of 23 cancer patients compared with five of six patients with bacterial infections,[27] and monocytes from cancer patients release less IL-1 than monocytes from control patients in response to endotoxin. However, plasma tumour necrosis factor was also undetectable in the same series of cancer patients, suggesting that plasma levels may not necessarily reflect the degree of physiologically active IL-1 or tumour necrosis factor in different tissues. Serum levels of IL-1 may not be detected in cachectic tumour-bearing rats, although expression of the gene for IL-1 is markedly augmented in the liver.[28]

IL-1 induces hypoglycaemia in mice and rats, associated with an attendant rise in serum insulin.[130,131] However, in rabbits, the combination of tumour necrosis factor and IL-1 produces hyperglycaemia and increased glucose turnover similar to that seen in cachexia.[132] IL-1 does not appear to have any direct effect on muscle catabolism *in vivo* but does have a synergistic effect with tumour necrosis factor.[132,133] A single dose of IL-1 stimulates hepatic uptake of gluconeogenic amino acids, increases acute phase protein synthesis, and decreases plasma concentrations of many amino acids.[131,134] This effect is comparable to that of tumour necrosis factor and implicates IL-1 as a potential mediator of cancer cachexia.[20,134] IL-1 has been shown to suppress lipoprotein lipase activity *in vitro* and *in vivo*,[87,88] and it increases plasma levels of triglycerides. The effect of IL-1 on glucose, lipid, and protein metabolism is complex, and its lack of effects in some *in vitro* studies indicates that its actions *in vivo* may be enhanced by or expressed through other mediators.

When antibodies to the receptor for IL-1 are chronically administered to mice bearing growing MCA101 sarcoma, less weight loss and protein depletion is seen than in tumour-bearing controls (Table 4).[135] However, tumour growth is also decreased, suggesting that the amelioration of cachectic effects in these mice is partially a result of the smaller tumour burden. Although it is not likely that tumour necrosis factor and IL-1 directly promote tumour growth, it is possible that the endogenously produced factors render local tissue conditions suitable for progressive tumour growth. If these effects are blocked by antibodies to the IL-1 receptor or to tumour necrosis factor, then tumour growth may be impaired.

Interleukin-6

IL-6 is a cytokine with a variety of physiological effects, both alone and in combination with tumour necrosis factor and IL-1.[19,105] Also known as hepatocyte-stimulating factor, IL-6 is secreted by a number of cell types in response to tumour necrosis factor, IL-1, and endotoxin. It has been characterized as an acute phase protein, since it is detectable in plasma during conditions of stress including sepsis and surgery. Recent work supports the role of IL-6 in cancer cachexia, although the mechanism has not yet been fully elucidated.

Circulating IL-6 has been found in tumour-bearing mice.[136] The plasma level appears to correlate with tumour burden and is detectable in animals with a variety of tumour types. Exogenously administered IL-6 demonstrated *in vivo* antitumour activity in a number of tumour types,[137] but has also been shown to be a potent growth factor for malignant B lymphocytes, as in multiple myeloma.[138] IL-6 has been shown to reduce lipoprotein lipase activity in vivo and *in vitro*[90] and to have minimal influence on rates of adipocyte lipolysis.[92,139]

A direct role for IL-6 in cancer cachexia has been a subject of great interest in recent years. Implantation of Chinese hamster ovarian cells transfected with the murine IL-6 gene and constitutively expressing murine IL-6 in nude mice was followed by weight loss.[140] Mice bearing CHO tumours lost approximately 33 per cent of body weight and had measurable circulating levels of IL-6. Strassmann *et al.*[33] demonstrated that a murine colon-26 adenocarcinoma cell line caused cachexia when implanted in Balb C mice. Serum from these mice had measurable levels of IL-6 and increasing levels correlated with increasing cachexia. Further, monoclonal antibodies to murine IL-6 significantly suppressed the development of cachexia in the mouse model (Table 4).[33]

Supportive evidence for the role of human IL-6 came from studies in which Lewis lung carcinoma cells were transfected with hIL-6 cDNA and implanted subcutaneously in mice.[141] Mice with hIL-6 transfected tumours had high serum levels of hIL-6 (but not of tumour necrosis factor or IL-1), marked weight loss, decreased serum albumin levels, and markedly decreased survival. Notably, there was no difference between the growth rates of IL-6-producing tumours and control tumours not producing IL-6.

A relationship between IL-6, hypercalcaemia, and cachexia has been cited in several studies. A human squamous cell tumour of the maxilla from a patient with hypercalcaemia, leucocytosis, and cachexia led to the same triad when implanted in nude mice.[34] High levels of IL-6 were measured in the plasma of the tumour-bearing nude mice and in the culture supernatants of tumour cells. Anti-IL-6 antibodies reversed the hypercalcaemia and prevented further progress of cachexia, while having no effect on tumour growth. The colon-26 tumour line mentioned previously led to hypercalcaemia as well as cachexia in tumour-bearing mice.[142] Treatment of mice bearing colon-26 tumours with 5′-deoxyfluorouridine reduced tumour size and inhibited hypercalcaemia and cachexia, and monoclonal antibodies to IL-6 prevented cachexia and hypercalcaemia in tumour-bearing mice.[142]

Involvement of IL-6 in non-cancer cachexia has also been reported. Monoclonal antibodies against IL-6 attenuated weight loss and reduced hepatic acute phase response in mice with sterile turpentine abscesses.[143]

Administration of anti-IL-6 monoclonal antibodies to humans with lymphoma has recently been reported.[138] While having a mixed effect on tumour growth, the treatment demonstrated a clear effect on cachexia and lymphoma-associated fever. Eleven patients with HIV infection and non-Hodgkin's lymphoma received daily intravenous administration of monoclonal antibodies against hIL-6 for a 21-day period and showed a mean weight gain of 1.4 kg, suggesting a role for IL-6 in human cancer cachexia.

Interferon-γ

Interferon-γ is a product of activated T cells and macrophages[144] which has antiviral and cell-activating capacities. It can act either independently or in concert with tumour necrosis factor and IL-1.[22] Interferon-γ has been shown to inhibit lipoprotein lipase and decrease the rate of fatty acid synthesis in adipocytes,[89] effects comparable to those previously described in cancer cachexia.

The endogenous administration of interferon-γ has clear anorectic effects and causes reduction of weight in non-tumour-bearing rats.[21, 145] Nude mice injected with CHO cells transfected within interferon-γ cDNA develop measurable interferon-γ in serum and significant cachexia.[146] In this model, monoclonal antibodies against interferon-γ, given prior to injection of tumour cells, prevent development of cachexia.[147] Passive immunization of methylchlorane sarcoma-bearing rats with anti-interferon-γ antibodies at the time of established tumour growth and weight loss leads to partial reversal of cachectic changes and prolongs survival without affecting the rate of tumour growth. Interestingly, antibodies to tumour necrosis factor did not reverse anorexia or affect survival in this tumour model (Table 4).[145] These studies implicate interferon-γ as an important mediator of cancer cachexia and suggest a potential therapeutic role for antibodies against it.

Leukaemia-inhibitory factor (D factor)

Leukaaemia inhibiting factor, also called D factor (differentiation factor), is a glycoprotein with a wide range of physiological activities. One of these involves altered lipid metabolism. *In vitro*, leukaemia inhibitory factor produces a dose- and time-dependent inhibition of lipoprotein lipase activity in 3T3-L1 adipocytes and is synergistic with tumour necrosis factor in this inhibition.[139] Mice injected repeatedly with leukaemia inhibitory factor have marked weight loss, based on loss of subcutaneous and abdominal fat.[148] Mice engrafted with CHO cells genetically engineered to produce leukaemia inhibitory factor develop a syndrome involving anorexia, alterations in calcium metabolism, and weight loss.[149] A lipoprotein-lipase-suppressing factor was isolated from the conditioned media of a human melanoma cell line which caused severe cachexia in tumour-bearing mice.[91] This factor was found to be identical to leukaemia inhibitory factor, suggesting that it may be a major factor responsible for cancer cachexia.[23] Further, leukaemia inhibitory factor levels were mildly elevated in malignant effusions and cyst fluids of patients with malignancies.[25] These data suggest that leukaemia inhibitory factor may have a role in the pathophysiology of cancer cachexia.

Host–tumour interactions in cytokine production

The interaction between host immune cells and tumour cells *in vivo* is of intense interest, both for the potential surveillance advantages (i.e. tumour-directed cytotoxicity) and for possible deleterious effects on the host. It has been proposed that host immune cells interacting with tumour cells may lead to augmented tumour cytokine production (Fig. 5). In a model of experimental cancer cachexia using a colon-26 adenocarcinoma, it has been shown that host macrophages interacting with tumour produce IL-1, which then binds to IL-1 receptors on tumour cells and potentiates tumour production of IL-6.[128] It is hypothesized that this augmented cytokine production contributes to cachectic events in this model, which are known to be related to IL-6.[33]

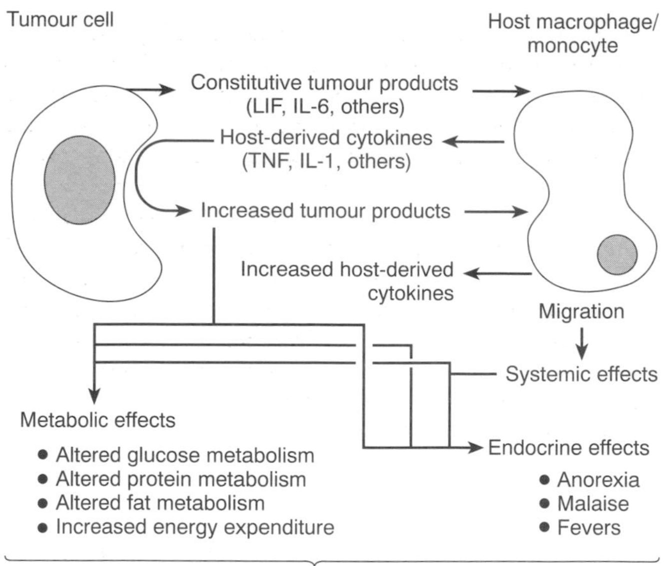

Fig. 5 Proposed pathways of tumour–host interaction in cancer cachexia.

The importance of macrophage–tumour interaction is also supported in work examining the role of tumour location on host metabolism.[150] In this model, tumour was implanted subcutaneously and in the liver, which is rich in macrophages in the form of Kupffer cells. A small liver tumour burden (approximately 1 per cent of body weight) produced the same degree of clinical cachexia and circulating cytokine response as a much greater subcutaneous tumour burden (10 per cent of body weight), suggesting that the macrophage-rich microenvironment of the liver led to potentiated cytokine response in the setting of small tumour burden.

The evidence supporting the role of tumour necrosis factor, IL-1, IL 6, interferon-γ, and leukaemia inhibitory factor as potential mediators in the development of cancer cachexia and the possibility that host–tumour interactions may augment cytokine production is very compelling. Undoubtedly, the combined activities of some or all of these cytokines in a host with a growing malignancy are complex and depend on a number of factors which may ultimately influence their net effect. Research into these cytokines and their role in the pathogenesis of cachexia is proceeding at a remarkable pace, and the increasing availability of recombinant proteins that act as ligands or receptor antagonists against these mediators will provide a potentially powerful approach towards the treatment of cancer cachexia.

Summary

Cancer cachexia is a complex syndrome that afflicts the majority of patients with cancer. It is characterized by anorexia, weight loss, and specific alterations in carbohydrate, protein, and lipid metabolism. Current information implicates endogenously produced cytokines as the principal mediators of cancer cachexia. The presence of progressive cachexia may render a patient unable to respond effectively to aggressive anticancer therapy, and different strategies have been attempted to reverse cancer cachexia and to replete the cancer-bearing host. While some therapies may have measurable and favourable influences on the metabolic parameters in individual patients, no treatment directed towards the amelioration of cachexia has been dramatically successful. Cancer cachexia remains a very difficult therapeutic dilemma, and innovative treatment approaches with antagonists towards endogenous mediators of cachexia and towards abnormal metabolic pathways may provide valuable improvements in response to treatment and survival of patients with cancer.

References

1. Lawson DH, Richmond A, Nixon DW, Rudman D. Metabolic approaches to cancer cachexia. *Annual Review of Nutrition*, 1982; **2**:277–301.
2. DeWys WD, Begg D, Lavin PT. Prognostic effect of weight loss prior to chemotherapy in cancer patients. *American Journal of Medicine*, 1980; **69**:491–9.
3. Daly JM, Copeland EM, Dudrick SJ. Effects of intravenous nutrition on tumor growth and host immunocompetence in malnourished animals. *Surgery*, 1978; **84**:655–8.
4. Bozzetti F, *et al.* Total parenteral nutrition prevents further nutritional deterioration in patients with cancer cachexia. *Annals of Surgery*, 1987; **205**:138–43.
5. Burt ME, Stein TP, Schwade JG, Brennan MF. Whole-body protein metabolism in cancer-bearing patients. *Cancer*, 1984; **53**:1246–52.
6. Tayek, JA, Bistrian BR, Hehir DJ, Martin R, Moldawer LL, Blackburn GL. Improved protein kinetics and albumin synthesis by branched chain amino acid-enriched total parenteral nutrition in cancer cachexia. *Cancer*, 1986; **58**:147–57.
7. Muller JM, Brenner U, Dienst C, Picklmaier H. Preoperative parenteral feeding in patients with gastrointestinal carcinoma. *Lancet*, 1982; **i**:68–71.
8. Ignoffo RJ. Parenteral nutrition support in patients with cancer. *Pharmacotherapy*, 1992; **12**:353–7.
9. Williams RL, *et al.* Myeloid leukaemia inhibitory factor maintains the developmental potential of embryonic stem cells. *Nature, London*, 1988; **336**:684–7.
10. Preshaw RM, Attisha RP, Hollingworth WJ. Randomized sequential trial of parenteral nutrition in healing of colonic anastomoses in man. *Canadian Journal of Surgery*, 1979; **22**:437–9.
11. Lim STK, Choa RG, Lam KH, Wong J, Ong GB. Total parenteral nutrition versus gastrostomy in the preoperative preparation of patients with carcinoma of the oesophagus. *British Journal of Surgery*, 1981; **68**:69–72.
12. Thompson BR, Julian TB, Stremple JF. Perioperative total parenteral nutrition in patients with gastrointestinal cancer. *Journal of Surgical Research*, 1981; **30**:497–500.
13. Loprinzi CL, *et al.* Controlled trials of megestrol acetate for the treatment of cancer anorexia and cachexia. *Journal of the National Cancer Institute*, 1990; **82**:1127–32.
14. Moley JF, Morrison SE, Norton JA. Insulin reversal of cancer cachexia in rats. *Cancer Research*, 1985; **45**:4925–31.
15. Chlebowski RT, Heber D, Richardson B, Block, JB. Influence of hydrazine sulfate on abnormal carbohydrate metabolism in cancer patients with weight loss. *Cancer Research*, 1984; **44**:857–61.
16. Tayek JA, Heber D, Chlebowski RT. Effect of hydrazine sulphate on whole-body protein breakdown measured by ^{14}C-lysine metabolism in lung cancer patients. *Lancet*, 1987; 241–4.
17. Ng B, Wolf RF, Weksler B, Brennan MF, Burt M. Growth hormone adininistration preserves lean body mass in sarcoma-bearing rats treated with doxorubicin. *Cancer Research*, 1993; **53**:5483–6.
18. Moley JF, Morrison SE, Norton JA. Preoperative insulin reverses cachexia and decreases mortality in tumor-bearing rats. *Journal of Surgical Research*, 1987; **43**:21–8.
19. Moldawer LL, Georgieff M, Lundholm K. Interleukin 1, tumour necrosis factor-alpha (cachectin) and the pathogenesis of cancer cachexia. *Clinical Physiology*, 1987; **7**:263–74.
20. Bendtzen K. Interleukin 1, interleukin 6 and tumor necrosis factor in infection, inflammation and immunity. *Immunology Letters*, 1988; **19**:183–92.
21. Evans RD, Argiles JM, Williamson DH. Metabolic effects of tumor necrosis factor-a (cachectin) and interleukin-1. *Clinical Science*, 1991.
22. Langstein HN, Fraker DL, Norton J A. Reversal of cancer cachexia by antibodies to interferon-gamma but not cachectin/tumor necrosis factor. *Surgical Forum*, 1989; **15**:408–10.
23. Mori M, *et al.* Cancer cachexia syndrome developed in nude mice bearing melanoma cells producing leukemia-inhibitory factor. *Cancer Research*, 1991; **51**:6656–9.
24. Balkwill F, *et al.*, Evidence for tumor necrosis factor/cachectin production in cancer. *Lancet*, 1987; **ii**:1229–32.
25. Waring P, Wycherley K, Cary D, Nicola N, Metcalf D. Leukemia inhibitory factor levels are elevated in septic shock and various inflammatory body fluids. *Journal of Clinical Investigation*, 1992; **90**:2031–7.
26. Socher SH, Martinez D, Craig JB., Kuhn J-G, Oliff A. Tumor necrosis factor not detectable in patients with clinical cancer cachexia. *Journal of the National Cancer Institute*, 1988; **80**:595–8.
27. Moldawer LL, Lundholm CD, Lundholm K. Monocytic production and plasma bioactivities of interleukin-1 and tumour necrosis factor. *European Journal of Cell Biology*, 1988; **18**:486–92.
28. Jensen JC, *et al.* Enhanced hepatic cytokine gene expression in cachectic tumor bearing rats. *Surgical Forum*, 1990; **41**:469–72.
29. Tracey KJ, *et al.*Cachectin/tumor necrosis factor induces cachexia, anemia, and inflammation. *Journal of Experimental Medicine*, 1988; **167**:1211–27.
30. Butler LD, *et al.* Interleukin 1-induced pathophysiology: Induction of cytokines, development of histopathologic changes, and immunopharmacologic intervention. *Clinical Immunology and Immunopathology*, 1989; **53**:400–21.
31. Fong Y, *et al.* Cachectin/TNF or IL-1a induces cachexia with redistribution of body proteins. *American Journal of Physiology*, 1989; **256**:R659–65.
32. Sherry BA, *et al.* Anti cachectin/tumor necrosis factor-α antibodies attenuate development of cachexia in tumor models. *FASEB Journal*, 1989; **3**:1956–62.
33. Strassmann G, Fong M, Kenney JS, Jacob CO. Evidence for the involvement of interleukin 6 in experimental cancer cachexia. *Journal of Clinical Investigation*, 1992; **89**:1681–4.
34. Yoneda T, *et al.* Neutralizing antibodies to human interleukin 6 reverse hypercalcemia associated with a human squamous carcinoma. *Cancer Research*, 1993; **53**:737–40.
35. Theologides A. Pathogenesis of anorexia and cachexia in cancer. *Cancer Bulletin*, 1982; **34**:140–9.
36. Bernstein IL, Sigmundi RA. Tumor anorexia: a learned food aversion. *Science*, 1980; **209**:416–18.
37. Cori CF, Cori GT. The carbohydrate metabolism of tumors. II. Changes in the sugar, lactic acid, and CO_2-combining power of blood passing through a tumor. *Journal of Biological Chemistry*, 1925; **66**:397.
38. Hansell DT, Davies JW, Shenkin A, Burns HJ. The oxidation of body fuel stores in cancer patients. *Annals of Surgery*, 1986; **204**:637–42.
39. Lindmark L, Eden E, Ternell M, Bennegard K, Svaninger G, Lundholm K. Thermic effect and substrate oxidation in response to intravenous nutrition in cancer patients who lose weight. *Annals of Surgery*, 1986; **204**:628–36.

40. Peacock JL, *et al.* Resting energy expenditure and body cell mass alterations in noncachectic patients with sarcomas. *Surgery*, 1987; **102**:465–72.
41. Thomson SR, Hirshberg A, Haffejee A. Resting metabolic rate of esophageal carcinoma patients: a model for energy expenditure measurement in a homogeneous cancer patient. *Journal of Parenteral and Enteral Nutrition*, 1990; **14**:119.
42. Falconer JS, Fearon KCH, Plester CE, Ross JA, Carter DC. Cytokines, the acute-phase response, and resting energy expenditure in cachectic patients with pancreatic cancer. *Annals of Surgery*, 1994; **219**:325–31.
43. Alexander HR, Chang TS, Lee JI, Stein TP, Burt ME. Amino acid and protein metabolism in the tumor bearing rat. *Proceedings of the American Association of Cancer Research*, 1989; **30**:22.
44. Burt ME, Lowry SF, Gorschboth C, Brennan MF. Metabolic alterations in a noncachectic animal tumor system. *Cancer*, 1981; **47**:2138.
45. Norton JA, Stamberger R, Stein TP, Milne GWA, Brennan MF. The influence of tumor-bearing on protein metabolism in the rat. *Journal of Surgical Research*, 1981; **30**:456–62.
46. Burt ME, Aoki TT, Gorschboth CM, Brennan MF. Peripheral tissue metabolism in cancer-bearing man. *Annals of Surgery*, 1983; **198**:685–91.
47. Legaspi A, Malayappa J, Starnes HF, Jr, Brennan MF. Whole body lipid and energy metabolism in the cancer patient. *Metabolism*, 1987; **36**:958–63.
48. Eden E, Edstrom S, Bennegard K, Lindmark L, Lundholm K. Glycerol dynamics in weight-losing cancer patients. *Surgery*, 1985; **97**:176–84.
49. Norton JA, Maher M, Wesley R, White D, Brennan, MF. Glucose intolerance in sarcoma patients. *Cancer*, 1984; **54**:3022–7.
50. Copeland GP, Al-Sumidaie AM, Leinster SJ, Davis JC, Hipkin LH. Glucose metabolism in patients with gastrointestinal malignancy but without excessive weight loss. *Euopean Journal of Surgical Oncology*, 1987; **13**:11–16.
51. Inculet RI, Peacock JL, Gorschboth CM, Norton JA. Gluconeogenesis in the tumor-influenced rat hepatocyte: importance of tumor burden, lactate, insulin, and glucagon. *Journal of the National Cancer Institute*, 1987; **79**:1039–46.
52. Lowry SF, Foster DM, Norton JA., Berman M, Brennan MR. Glucose disposal and gluconeogenesis from alanine in tumor-bearing Fischer 344 rats. *Journal of the National Cancer Institute*, 1981; **66**:653–8.
53. Arbeit JM, Burt ME, Rubinstein LV, Gorschboth CM, Brennan MF. Glucose metabolism and the percentage of glucose derived from alanine: response to exogenous glucose infusion in tumor-bearing and non-tumor-bearing rats. *Cancer Research*, 1982; **42**:4936–42.
54. Torosian, MH, Bartlett DL, Chatzidakis C, Stein TP. Effect of tumor burden on futile glucose and lipid cycling in tumor-bearing animals. *Journal of Surgical Research*, 1993; **55**:68–73.
55. Alexander HR, DePippo P, Rao S, Burt ME. Substrate alterations in a sarcoma-bearing rat model : effect of tumor growth and resection. *Journal of Surgical Research*, 1990; **48**:471–5.
56. Gutman A, Thilo E, Biran S. Enzymes of gluconeogenesis in tumor-bearing rats. *Israel Journal of Medical Science*, 1969; **5**:998–1001.
57. Gold J. Proposed treatment of cancer by inhibition of gluconeogenesis. *Oncology*, 1968; **22**:185.
58. Dills WL, Jr. Nutritional and physiological consequences of tumour glycolysis. *Parasitology*, 1993; **107**:S177–86.
59. Waterhouse C, Jeanpretre N, Keilson J. Gluconeogenesis from alanine in patients with progressive malignant disease. *Cancer Research*, 1979; **39**:1968–72.
60. Norton JA, Burt ME, Brennan MF. *In vivo* utilization of substrate by human sarcoma-bearing limbs. *Cancer*, 1980; **45**:2934–9.
61. Holroyde CP, Skutches CL, Boden G, Reichard GA. Glucose metabolism in cachectic patients with colorectal cancer. *Cancer Research*, 1984; **44**:5910–13.
62. Pisters PWT, Brennan MR. Amino acid metabolism in human cancer cachexia. *Annual Review of Nutrition*, 1990; **10**:107–12.
63. Pisters PWT, Pearlstone DB. Protein and amino acid metabolism in cancer cachexia: investigative techniques and therapeutic interventions. *CRC Critical Reviews in Clinical Laboratory Sciences*,1993; **30**:223–72.
64. Brennan MF. Total parenteral nutrition in the cancer patient. *New England Journal of Medicine*, 1981; **305**:375–82.
65. Morrison SD, Moley JF, Norton JA. Contribution of inert mass to experimental cancer cachexia in rats. *Journal of the National Cancer Institute*, 1984; **73**:991.
66. Arbeit JM, Gorschboth CM, Brennan MF. Basal amino acid concentrations and the response to incremental glucose infusion in tumor bearing rats. *Cancer Research*, 1985; **45**:6296.
67. Alexander HR, Lee J-I, Chang T-H, Burt ME. Amino acid and protein metabolism in tumor bearing rats. *Journal of Surgical Research*, 1991.
68. Beck SA, Tisdale MJ. Nitrogen excretion in cancer cachexia and its modification by a high fat diet in mice. *Cancer Research*, 1989; **49**:3800–904.
69. Beck SA, Tisdale MJ. Production of lipolytic and proteolytic factors by a murine tumor-producing cachexia in the host. *Cancer Research*, 1987; **47**:5919–23.
70. Smith KL, Tisdale MS. Increased protein degradation and decreased protein synthesis in skeletal muscle during cancer cachexia. *British Journal of Cancer*, 1993; **67**:680–5.
71. Smith KL, Tisdale MJ. Mechanism of muscle protein degradation in cancer cachexia. *British Journal of Cancer*, 1993; **58**:314–18.
72. Lundholm K, Bylund AC, Holm J. Skeletal muscle metabolism in patients with malignant tumor. *European Journal of Cancer*, 1976; **12**:465–73.
73. Temparis S, *et al.* Increased ATP-Ubiquitin-dependent proteolysis in skeletal muscles of tumor-bearing rats. *Cancer Research*, 1994; **54**:5568–73.
74. Norton JA, Gorschboth CM, Wesley RA, Burt ME, Brennan MF. Fasting plasma amino acid levels in cancer patients. *Cancer*, 1985; **56**:1181–6.
75. Clarke EF, Levies AM, Waterhouse C. Peripheral amino acid levels in patients with cancer. *Cancer*, 1978; **42**:2909–13.
76. Starnes HF, Jr, Warren RS, Brennan MF. Protein synthesis in hepatocytes isolated from patients with gastrointestinal malignancy. *Journal of Clinical Investigation*, 1937; **80**:1384–90.
77. Inculet RI, *et al.* Altered leucine metabolism in noncachectic sarcoma patients. *Cancer Research*, 1987; **47**:4746–9.
78. Kien CL, Camitta BM. Increased whole-body protein turnover in sick children with newly diagnosed leukemia or lymphoma. *Cancer Research*, 1983; **43**:5586–92.
79. Melville S, McNurlan MA, Calder AG, Garlick PJ. Increased protein turnover despite normal energy metabolism and responses to feeding in patients with lung cancer. *Cancer Research*, 1990; **50**:1125–31.
80. Jeevanandam M, Horowitz GD, Lowry SF, Brennan MF. Cancer cachexia and protein metabolism. *Lancet*, 1984; **i**:1423–6.
81. O'Keefe SJD, Ogden J, Ramjee G, Rund J. Contribution of elevated protein turnover and anorexia to cachexia in patients with hepatocellular carcinoma. *Cancer Research*, 1990; **50**:1226–30.
82. Younes RN, Vydelingum NA, Noguchi Y, Brennan MF. Lipid kinetic alterations in tumor-bearing rats: reversal by tumor excision. *Journal of Surgical Research*, 1990; **48**:324–8.
83. Lanza-Jacoby S, Lansey SC, Miller EE, Cleary MP. Sequential changes in the activities of lipoprotein lipase and lipogenic enzymes during tumor growth in rats. *Cancer Research*, 1984; **44**:5062–7.
84. Hollander DM, Ebert EC, Roberts AI, Devereux DF. Effects of tumor type and burden on carcass lipid depletion in mice. *Surgery*, 1986; **100**: 292–7.
85. Beutler B, Cerami A. Tumor necrosis factor in cachexia, shock, and inflammation: a common mediator. *Annual Review of Biochemistry*, 1988; **57**:505–18.
86. Moldawer LL, Sherry B, Lowry SF, Cerami A. Endogenous cachectin/tumor necrosis factor-alpha production contributes to experimental cancer-associated cachexia. *Cancer Survey*, 1989; **8**: 854–9.
87. Price SR, Mizel SB, Pekala PH. Regulation of lipoprotein lipase synthesis and 3T3-L1 adipocyte metabolism by recombinant interleukin 1. *Biochimica et Biophysica Acta*, 1986; **889**:374–81.
88. Argiles JM, Lopez-Soriano FJ, Evans RD, Williamson DH. Interleukin-1 and lipid metabolism in the rat. *Biochemical Journal*, 1989; **259**:673–8.

89. Patton JS, Shepard HM, Wilking H. Interferons and tumor necrosis factor have similar catabolic effects on 3T3LI cells. *Proceedings of the National Academy of Sciences of the United States of America*, 1986; **83**:8313–17.
90. Greenberg AS, Nordan RP, McIntosh J, Calvo JC, Scow RO, Jablons D. Interleukin 6 reduces lipoprotein lipase activity in adipose tissue of mice *in vivo* and in 3T3-LI adipocytes: a possible role for interleukin 6 in cancer cachexia. *Cancer Research*, 1992; **52**:4113–16.
91. Mori M, Yamaguchi K, Abe K. Purification of a lipoprotein lipase-inhibiting protein produced by a melanoma cell line associated with cancer cachexia. *Biochemistry and Biophysics Research Communications*, 1989; **160**:1085–92.
92. Feingold KR, Doerrler W, Dinarello CA, Fiers W, Grunfeld C. Stimulation of lipolysis in cultured fat cells by tumor necrosis factor, interleukin-1, and the interferons is blocked by inhibition of prostaglandin synthesis. *Endocrin*, 1992; **130**:10–16.
93. Marshall MK, Doerrler W, Feingold KR, Grunfeld C. Leukemia inhibitory factor induces changes in lipid metabolism in cultured adipocytes. *Endocrin*, **135**: 1994; 141–7.
94. Kern PA. Recombinant human tumor necrosis factor does not inhibit lipoprotein lipase in primary cultures of isolated human adipocytes. *Journal of Lipid Research*, 1988; **29**:909–14.
95. Taylor DD, Gercel-Taylor C, Jenis LG, Devereux DF. Identification of a human tumor-derived lipolysis-promoting factor. *Cancer Research*, 1992; **52**:829–34.
96. Beck SA, Mulligan HD, Tisdale MJ. Lipolytic factors associated with murine and human cancer cachexia. *Journal of the National Cancer Institute*, 1990; **82**:1922–6.
97. Tisdale MJ. Mechanism of lipid mobilization associated with cancer cachexia: Interaction between the polyunsaturated fatty acid, eicosapentaenoic acid, and inhibitory guanine nucleotide-regulatory protein. *Prostaglandins, Leukotrienes and Essential Fatty Acids*, 1993; **48**:105–9.
98. Dempsey DT, Knox LS, Mullen JL, Miller C, Fdeurer ID, Buzby GP. Energy expenditure in malnourished patients with colorectal cancer. *Arcives of Surgery*, 1986; **121**:789–95.
99. Brobeck JR. Food and temperature. *Recent Progress in Hormone Research*, 1960; **15**:439.
100. Morrison SE. Feeding response to change in absorbable food fraction during growth of Walker 256 carcinosarcoma. *Cancer Research*, 1972; **32**:968.
101. Norton JA, Moley JF, Green MV, Carson RE, Morrison SO. Parabiotic transfer of cancer anorexia/cachexia in male rats. *Cancer Research*, 1985; **45**: 5547–52.
102. Beutler B, Cerami A. Cachectin and tumour necrosis factor as two sides of the biological coin. *Nature, London*, 1986; **320**:584–8.
103. Dinarello CA. Biology of interleukin 1. *FASEB Journal*, 1988; **2**:108–15.
104. Fibbe WE, Schaafsma MR, Falkenburg JHF, Willemze R. The biological activities of interleukin-1. *Blut*, 1989; **59**:147–56.
105. Le J, Vilcek J. Tumor necrosis factor and interleukin 1: cytokines with multiple overlapping biological activities. *Laboratory Investigation*, 1987; **56**:234–48.
106. Carswell EA, Old LJ, Kassel RL, Green S, Fiore N, Williamson B. An endotoxin-induced serum factor that causes necrosis of tumors. *Proceedings of the National Academy of Sciences of the United States of America*, 1975; **72**:3666–70.
107. Fraker DL, Stovroff MC, Merino MJ, Norton JA. Tolerance to tumor necrosis factor in rats and the relationship to endotoxin tolerance and toxicity. *Journal of Experimental Medicine*, 1988; **168**:95–105.
108. Socher SM, Friedman A, Martinez D. Recombinant human tumor necrosis factor induces acute reductions in food intake and body-weight in mice. *Journal of Experimental Medicine*, 1988; **167**:1957–62.
109. Darling G, Fraker DL, Jensen JC, Gorschboth CM, Norton JA. Cachectic effects of recombinant human tumor necrosis factor in rats. *Cancer Research*, 1990; **50**:4008–13.
110. Oliff A, *et al.* Tumors secreting human TNF/cachectin induce cachexia in mice. *Cell*, 1987; **50**:555–63.
111. Tracey KJ, *et al.* Metabolic effects of cachectin/tumor necrosis factor are modified by site of production. *Journal of Clinical Investigation*, 1990; **86**:2014–24.
112. Blick M, Sherwin SA, Rosenblum M. Phase I study of recombinant tumor necrosis factor in cancer patients. *Cancer Research*, 1987; **47**:2986–9.
113. Abbruzzese J-L, Levin B, Ajani JA. Phase I. Trial of recombinant human gamma interferon and recombinant human tumor necrosis factor in patients with advanced gastrointestinal cancer. *Cancer Research*, 1989; **49**:4057–61.
114. Fraker DL, Alexander HR, Pass HI. Biologic therapy with TNF: systemic administration and isolation-perfusion. In: DeVita VT, Jr, Hellman S, Rosenberg SA (ed.). *Biologic Therapy of Cancer*, p.329. Philadelphia, PA: Lippincott, 1995.
115. Sherman ML, Spriggs DR, Arthur KA, Imamura K, Frei E, III, Kufe DW. Recombinant human tumor necrosis factor administered as a five-day continuous infusion in cancer patients: phase I toxicity and effects of lipid metabolism. *Journal of Clinical Oncology*, 1988; **5**:344–50.
116. Torti FM, Dieckmann B, Beutler B, Cerami A, Ringold GM. A macrophage factor inhibits adipocyte gene expression: an in vitro model of cachexia. *Science*, 1985; **229**:867–9.
117. Feingold KR, Grunfeld C. Tumor necrosis factor-alpha stimulates lipogenesis in the rat in vivo. *Journal of Clinical Investigation*, 1987; **80**:184–90.
118. Lee, M.D., Zentella, A., Pekala, P.H., and Cerami, A. Effect of endotoxin-induced monokines on glucose metabolism in the muscle cell line L6. *Proceedings of the National Academy of Sciences of the United States of America*, 1987; **34**: 2590–4.
119. Flores EA, Bistrian BR, Pomposelli JJ, Dinarello CA., Blackburn GL, Istfan NW. Infusion of tumor necrosis factor/cachectin promotes muscle catabolism in the rat. A synergistic effect with interleukin 1. *Journal of Clinical Investigation*, 1989; **83**:1614–22.
120. Warren RS, Donner DB, Starnes HF, Jr, Brennan MF. Modulation of endogenous hormone action by recombinant human tumor necrosis factor. *Proceedings of the National Academy of Sciences of the United States of America*, 1987; **84**:8619–22.
121. Brenner DA, Buck M, Feitelberg SP, Chojkier M. Tumor necrosis factor-α inhibits albumin gene expression in a murine model of cachexia.. *Journal of Clinical Investigation*, 1990; **85**:248–55.
122. Stovroff MC, Fraker DL, Norton JA. Cachectin activity in the serum of cachectic, tumor-bearing rats. *Archives of Surgery*, 1989; **124**:94–9.
123. Stovroff MC, Fraker DL, Swedenborg JA, Norton JA. Cachectin/tumor necrosis factor: a possible mediator of cancer anorexia in the rat. *Cancer Research*, 1988; **48**:4567–72.
124. Sheppard BC, Venzon D, Fraker DL, Langstein HN, Jensen JC, Norton JA. Prolonged survival of tumor-bearing rats with repetitive low-dose recombinant tumor necrosis factor. *Cancer Research*, 1990; **50**:3928–33.
125. Yoneda DM, Alsina MA, Chavez JB, Bonewald L, Nishimura R, Mundy GR. Evidence that tumor necrosis factor plays a pathogenetic role in the paraneoplastic syndromes of cachexia, hypercalcemia, and leukocytosis in a human tumor in nude mice. *Journal of Clinical Investigation*, 1991; **87**:977–85.
126. Waage A, Espevik T. Interleukin-1 potentiates the lethal effect of tumor necrosis factor alpha/cachectin in mice. *Journal of Experimental Medicine*, 1988; **167**:1987–92.
127. Okusawa S, Gelfand JA, Ikejima T, Connolly RJ, Dinarello CA. Interleukin-1 induces a shock like state in rabbits. *Journal of Clinical Investigation*, 1988; **81**:1162–72.
128. Strassmann G, Jacob C, Evans R, Beell D, Fong M. Mechanisms of experimental cancer cachexia interaction between mononuclear phagocytes and colon 26 carcinoma and its relevance to IL-6 mediated cancer cachexia. *Journal of Immunology*, 1992; **148**:3674–8.
129. Uehara A, Sekiya C, Takasugi Y, Namiki M, Arimura A. Anorexia induced by interleukin 1: involvement of corticotropin-releasing factor. *American Journal of Physiology*, 1989; **257**:R613–17.

130. Del Rey A, Besedovsky H. Interleukin-1 affects glucose homeostasis. *American Journal of Physiology*, 1987; **253**:R794–8.
131. Argiles JM, Lopez-Soriano FJ, Wiggins D, Williamson DH. Comparative effects of tumor necrosis factor a (cachectin), interletikin-1-β and tumor growth on amino acid metabolism in the rat in vivo. Absorption and tissue uptake of a-amino [^{14}C]isobutyrate. *Biochemical Journal*, 1989; **261**:357–62.
132. Tredget EE, *et al.* Role of interleukin-1 and tumor necrosis factor in energy metabolism in rabbits. *American Journal of Physiology*, 1988; **255**:E760–8.
133. Pomposelli JJ, Flores EA, Bistrian BR. Role of biochemical mediators in clinical nutrition and surgical metabolism. *Journal of Parenteral and Enteral Nutrition*, 1988; **12**:212–18.
134. Warren RS, Starnes HF, Alcock N, Calvano S, Brennan MF. Hormonal and metabolic response to recombinant human tumor necrosis factor in rat: in vitro and in vivo. *American Journal of Physiology*, 1988; **255**:E206–12.
135. Gelin J, Moldawer LL, Lonnroth C, Sherry B, Chizzonite R, Lundholm K. Role of endogenous tumor necrosis factor of and interleukin 1 for experimental tumor growth and the development of cancer cachexia. *Cancer Research*, 1991; **51**:415–21.
136. Jablons DM, McIntosh JK, Mulé JJ. Induction of interferon-2/interleukin-6 by cytokine administration and detection of circulating interleukin-6 in the tumor bearing state. *Annals of the New York Academy of Sciences*, 1989; **557**:157–60.
137. Mulé JJ, McIntosh JK, Jablons DM. Antitumor activity of recombinant interleukin-6 in mice. *Journal of Experimental Medicine*, 1990; **171**:629–36.
138. Emilie D, *et al.* Administration of an anti-interleukin-6 monoclonal antibody to patients with acquired immunodeficiency syndrome and lymphoma: effect on lymphoma growth and on B clinical symptoms. *Blood*, 1994; **84**:2472–9.
139. Berg M, Fraker DL, Alexander HR. Characterization of differentiation factor/leukaemia inhibitory factor effect on lipoprotein lipase activity and mRNA in 3T3-LI adipocytes. *Cytokine*, 1994; **6**:425–32.
140. Black K, Garrett IR, Mundy GR. Chinese hamster ovarian cells transfected with the murine interleukin-6 gene cause hypercalcemia as well as cachexia, leukocytosis and thrombocytosis in tumor-bearing nude mice. *Endocrin*, 1991; **128**:2657–9.
141. Ohe Y, *et al.* Interleukin-6 cDNA transfected Lewis lung carcinoma cells show unaltered net tumour growth rate but cause weight loss and shorten survival in syngenic mice. *British Journal of Cancer*, 1993; **67**:939–44.
142. Strassmann C, Masui Y, Chizzonite R, Fong M. Mechanisms of experimental cancer cachexia. *Journal of Immunology*, 1993; **150**: 2341–5.
143. Oldenburg HSA, *et al.* Cachexia and the acute-phase protein response in inflammation are regulated by interleukin-6. *European Journal of Immunology*, 1993; **23**:1889–94.
144. Nathan CF. Secretory products of macrophages. *Journal of Clinical Investigation*, 1987; **79**:319–26.
145. Langstein H-N, Doherty GM, Fraker DL, Buresh CM, Norton JA. The roles of interferon-gamma and tumor necrosis factor in an experimental rat model of cancer cachexia. *Cancer Research*, 1991; **51**:2302–6.
146. Matthys P, *et al.* Severe cachexia in mice inoculated with interferon-gamma-producing tumor cells. *International Journal of Cancer*, 1991; **49**:77–82.
147. Matthys P, Heremans H, Opdenakker G, Billiau A. Anti-interferon-gamma antibody treatment, growth of Lewis lung tumors in mice and tumor-associated cachexia. *European Journal of Cancer*, 1991; **27**:182–7.
148. Metcalf D. The leukemia inhibitory factor (LIF). *International Journal of Cell Cloning*, 1991; **9**:95–108.
149. Metcalf D, Gearing DP. Fatal syndrome in mice engrafted with cells producing high levels of the leukemia inhibitory factor. *Proceedings of the National Academy of Sciences of the United States of America*, 1989; **86**:5948–52.
150. Fong Y, *et al.* Tumour location influences local cytokine production and host metabolism. *Surgical Oncology*, 1992; **1**:65–71.

9.3.6 Clinical management of cachexia and anorexia

Eduardo Bruera and R. L. Fainsinger

Introduction

Cachexia–anorexia is a frequent and devastating complication of terminal diseases, particularly cancer[1] and AIDS.[2] The pathophysiology of this extremely complex syndrome has been discussed in Chapter 9.3.5. Although the ideal clinical management of cachexia would be to be able to completely reverse this syndrome, this goal can only be achieved by properly treating the underlying cause. Unfortunately, this cannot be achieved in the overwhelming majority of patients in a palliative medicine practice. Since the main goal of any intervention in palliative medicine is to provide patients with increased comfort, it will be crucial to establish properly the main purpose of any pharmacological or nutritional intervention.

A discussion on the different treatment objectives will be followed by a discussion of the different drugs available that have suggested or demonstrated effects on cancer cachexia. The use of oral, enteral, and parenteral nutrition will be discussed. Finally, areas where future research should focus, both in establishing the symptomatic cost of cachexia and the symptomatic benefit of different treatments, will be discussed.

Treatment objectives

The main objective of any treatment in palliative medicine is to improve the patient's comfort. The two main clinical manifestations of cachexia are anorexia, with resulting decreased food intake, and chronic nausea. In addition, severe asthenia related to the malnutrition and changes in the patients body image are major problems caused by cachexia. In the following paragraphs we will discuss these different clinical findings.

Anorexia

Anorexia is a highly prevalent symptom in patients with advanced and terminal cancer.[3,4] Table 1 summarizes the prevalence of symptoms in 275 consecutive patients admitted to our service.

Table 1 Prevalence of symptoms in 275 consecutive patients

Symptom	Prevalence (percentage)	95 per cent confidence interval
Asthenia	90	81–100
Anorexia	85	78–92
Pain	76	62–85
Nausea	68	61–75
Constipation	65	40–80
Sedation–confusion	60	40–75
Dyspnoea	12	8 –16

Table 2 Causes of anorexia

Tumour factors (toxohormone-L)
Macrophage factors (cachextin–interleukin)
Endogenous peptides (glucagon, calcitonin–cholecystokinins)
Satietins

Anorexia was present in 85 per cent of our patients. It was the second most frequent symptom after asthenia and it was more prevalent than pain in our population. Anorexia is very likely to be a multicausal syndrome, being both partially the cause and also partially the consequence of the metabolic changes and the malnutrition that occurs in advanced cancer.[5-8] A variety of endogenous substances, mainly peptides with a well known physiological spectrum like glucagon, insulin, cholecystokinin, and calcitonin, are capable of inhibiting food intake. A family of α_1-glycoproteins called satietins have recently been described in human and animal serum as having potent and selective anorexic activity. Some of these substances have been identified in tumour-bearing hosts.[7-14] In addition, cytokines frequently produced by macrophages of cancer-bearing hosts, such as tumour necrosis factor/cachectin and interleukin 1, have powerful anorectic effects.[15-17] Finally, chemicals produced directly by the tumour, such as toxohormone-L, appear to cause severe lipolysis by suppressing food and water intake, while the tumour lipolytic factor appears to cause cachexia by direct lipolysis without any significant effects on food intake.[18,19]

In summary, tumour factors, cytokines released by the immune system in response to the presence of the tumour, or a number of endogenous peptides are all capable of causing profound anorexia.

In addition to anorexia, a number of other factors are able to cause a significant decrease in food intake. These factors are summarized in Table 2. Emesis and dysphagia are well recognized causes of starvation. Although decreased taste has been well defined in patients with advanced cancer, the association between decreased taste and cachexia has not been clearly established and it is likely that decreased taste occurs as frequently in patients with cachexia as in those patients with advanced cancer who did not have significant weight loss.[3,20-22] Profound anorexia is one of the frequent manifestations of psychological depression.[23] The contribution that major depressive disorders, adjustment disorders with depressed mood, or simple depressive symptoms could make to decreased food intake is unclear at this time. Cognitive failure, on the other hand, is highly prevalent in advanced cancer and may result in patients being unable to prepare and eat their meals.[24] Finally, severe pain in the mouth and neck can make food intake extremely difficult for patients.

Chronic nausea

Chronic nausea occurs in 68 per cent of patients with advanced cancer admitted to our palliative care programme (Table 1). Reports on chronic nausea and vomiting are somewhat conflicting. Reuben, *et al.*,[25] using data from the National Hospice Study, reported nausea and vomiting in 62 per cent of cancer patients, with the prevalence rate of 40 per cent in the last 6 weeks of life.

Table 3 Frequent causes of chronic nausea in cancer

Bowel obstruction
Delayed chemotherapy-induced emesis
Intracranial pressure
Autonomic failure
Narcotic bowel syndrome
Metabolic abnormalities
Gastric–peptic ulcer
Radiation therapy

Doyle[26] reported a 55 per cent prevalence of nausea and vomiting in terminal cancer patients. Coyle, *et al.*[27] reported 12 per cent of patients with nausea 4 weeks before death with 13 per cent reporting nausea 1 week before death. Lichter[28] reports nausea and vomiting in 14 per cent of patients in the last 48 h of life. Ventafridda, *et al.*[29] did not comment on overall prevalence of nausea and vomiting but did report 4 per cent of patients requiring treatment to the point of sedation because of uncontrollable nausea and vomiting. Fainsinger[30] found that although 71 out of 100 consecutive patients treated in a palliative care unit had chronic nausea, no patients required sedation because of intractable emesis. The difference in prevalence and severity of nausea found by different groups are probably due to different patient characteristics, different treatment, and different methods for the assessment of the presence and intensity of nausea.

Chronic nausea in patients with advanced cancer is also likely to be multicausal, as described in Table 3. Chronic nausea is one of the most frequent manifestations of mechanical bowel obstruction. This subject will be discussed elsewhere in this book. Both radiation therapy, particularly when applied to the abdominal region, and delayed chemotherapy-induced emesis, particularly after cisplatin, are capable of causing chronic nausea.[31]

Although the initiation, or a recent increase in dose, of opioid analgesics can be accompanied by reversible, short-lasting nausea, in some patients, particularly those receiving high doses of narcotics, nausea can become chronic, severe, and be accompanied by abdominal pain, constipation, and gas distension of the large and, occasionally, small bowel.[32,33] In many of these patients, severe constipation aggravates the nausea.

In addition to the previously described causes of chronic nausea, cancer cachexia is associated with chronic nausea in many patients even in the absence of all the previously described factors. In these cases, the most likely cause for chronic nausea is autonomic failure.[34] Autonomic failure is a clinical syndrome including cardiovascular manifestations (postural hypotension, syncope, and fixed heart rate) and gastrointestinal symptoms (nausea, anorexia, constipation, or occasionally diarrhoea).[35-37] This syndrome was originally described in neurological disorders, chronic renal disease, and diabetes mellitus.[34] However, isolated reports had described the presence of autonomic insufficiency in advanced cancer patients.[38-40] Our group studied the incidence of cardiovascular autonomic insufficiency in 43 patients with advanced breast cancer and 20 normal, sex and age-matched controls. Tests for autonomic failure were abnormal in 52 per cent of the cases in the patient group, versus 7 per cent in the control group ($p<0.001$). Among the cancer patients, the tests for autonomic failure were more frequently abnormal in patients with low performance status and malnutrition ($p<0.01$).[41] In a group of five patients with advanced cancer who complained of unexplained chronic nausea and anorexia (>4 weeks), 16 out of 23 tests were abnormal versus 0 out of 25 in five healthy adult controls ($p<0.001$). All patients and controls underwent a gastric emptying scan by giving the patient an egg sandwich with a radioactive labelling. The gastric emptying time was 190 ± 83 min in the patients versus 65 ± 6 min in the control group ($p<0.001$). None of the patients had a history of diabetes or peptic disease, and they were receiving no medication that might affect the autonomic function. Four of the five patients had barium meals and endoscopies that were found to be normal except for mild inflammation of the lower oesophagus in one of the cases. None of the five patients had clinical or laboratory evidence of disseminated disease to the abdomen, including the liver. Therefore, we concluded that gastroparesis was the cause of chronic nausea and anorexia in our patients.[42] Another report found gastric emptying in 10 patients who complained of chronic nausea and anorexia.[43] Some reviews have suggested malnutrition as one of the possible causes of autonomic failure.[34] Elegant studies on animals have suggested that fasting suppresses the activity of the sympathetic nervous system.[44] Studies carried out by Jewish physicians in the Warsaw ghetto during the Second World War showed that victims of starvation demonstrated bradycardia, low arterial blood pressure, and absence of increase in pulse rate or arterial blood pressure after a work stimulus.[45]

The presence of opioid treatment could significantly aggravate autonomic failure.

Asthenia and malnutrition

Asthenia is probably the most prevalent symptom of patients with advanced cancer, as summarized in Table 1. Two different symptoms are usually summarized under the term 'asthenia':

(1) fatigue or lassitude, defined as easy tiring and decreased capacity to maintain adequate performance;

(2) generalized weakness, defined as the anticipatory subjective sensation of difficulty initiating a certain activity.[46]

Although asthenia is recognized as a cause of significant distress to many patients and families, its real incidence, aetiology, and therapy have not been clearly established. The association between asthenia and malnutrition has been clearly established both for malignant and non-malignant populations. Since both malnutrition and asthenia coexist in the great majority of terminally ill cancer and AIDS patients, it is likely that malnutrition significantly contributes to cancer cachexia. Malnutrition has been shown to be able to cause abnormal muscle function.[47,48] Some of the mediators of cachexia, such as cachectin/tumour necrosis factor, interleukin, or interferon, cause significant asthenia when administered to animals and humans.[46] In addition, specific substances have been proposed that might cause asthenia as their main effect.[49]

However, asthenia has also been associated with a number of psychological disorders and it occurs frequently in patients with no evidence of malnutrition.[50]

Table 4 Possible effects of nutritional support

Improved survival (found in only 1 of 14 controlled trials)
Improved tumour response (found in only 1 of 17 controlled trials)
Decreased toxicity (found in none of 15 controlled trials)
Decreased surgical complications (debated)
Tumour growth (demonstrated in animal studies only)
Better quality of life (supporting data lacking)

Body image

Cancer and AIDS-induced cachexia has considerable impact on the patient's body image. It is the most recognizable, external sign of serious illness and it is a major source of concern for both patients and families.

Nutritional approach

Malnourished cancer patients have a reduced response to antineoplastics, diminished tolerance to radiation and chemotherapy, and decreased survival.[51,52] They have also been found to have a higher incidence of infection and added complications after surgical procedures.[53] Finally, there are a variety of symptoms that are related to the presence of cachexia, as described in the previous paragraphs. The successful management of malnutrition might therefore be expected to yield improvements in both life expectancy and the quality of life.

The effects of nourishment are summarized in Table 4. Initial non-controlled studies suggested that aggressive nutritional therapy could improve response to the antineoplastic treatment or decreased complications.[54] However, later randomized controlled studies have suggested that aggressive nutritional therapy has no impact on tumour response, toxicity, or survival. Koretz[55] has reviewed a large number of randomized controlled studies in patients with advanced cancer and has found that parenteral nutrition has not improved general survival (only 1 of 14 controlled trials), tumour response (1 of 17 controlled studies), or toxicity (none of 15 controlled trials). A recent study by a co-operative group also found that aggressive oral nutrition had no influence on survival or tumour response.[56] The effects of aggressive nutritional therapy on the incidence of surgical complications is still debated. Although some controlled trials have suggested that preoperative nutrition could reduce postoperative complications and mortality,[57] a recent review of a large number of controlled clinical trials failed to show significant differences in the incidence of complications and mortality between patients who received aggressive preoperative nutrition and those who had routine oral nutrition.[58]

Animal research has demonstrated that aggressive nutritional therapy can significantly increase tumour growth.[59] Although never demonstrated in human subjects, most of the study patients who received parenteral nutrition were also receiving antineoplastic therapy. This consequence of nutritional therapy, therefore, remains a theoretical concern.

Thus, aggressive nutritional therapy does not significantly influence the outcome of patients with advanced cancer. Nonetheless, its use would still be warranted if the patient's quality of life were significantly improved. Unfortunately, all studies that have assessed the effect of either parenteral or oral aggressive nutrition have not measured the impact of malnutrition or renourishment on patients' symptoms and performance status. Therefore, there is currently no evidence that aggressive nutritional therapy can improve the quality of life of patients with advanced cancer.

The potential advantages of nutritional treatment could be an improvement in the asthenia that frequently occurs in these patients and also an improvement in the patients body image. One randomized double blind trial of megestrol acetate has found improved appetite, caloric intake, and nutritional status after 1 week of megestrol acetate; the authors also found significant improvement in the level of energy reported by patients as compared to placebo.[60] However, it is not possible to establish if the improvement in energy could just be the result of a non-specific steroid effect of megestrol or the effect on muscle function rather than the result of the nutritional improvement. Although it is obvious that the deterioration in body image is very concerning to the patients and their families, there are no effective treatments capable of reversing severe cachexia. Therefore, an improvement in the body image is not a realistic goal of nutritional management of terminally ill patients.

Oral nutrition

Oral nutrition is the ideal management for palliative medicine patients. Although nutritional counselling alone is capable of improving the daily caloric intake by an average of 450 calories/day, the advantages are lost within 3 weeks in most patients.[4] This is due to the fact that terminally ill, malnourished patients have a very high incidence of anorexia and chronic nausea. In some cases, forcing prepared meals or high calorie liquid preparations would only increase the severity of these symptoms without resulting in any improvement in the level of energy or body image of the patients. Adequate counselling of the patients and the families will help decrease the anxiety of the family members about their relative starving to death. Meal times are usually associated by families with social gathering and communication. Poor understanding of the absence of a real need for food can make meal times an extremely unpleasant experience for both the patient and the family. By taking very small servings of enjoyable meals, patients can still participate in family gatherings. As the disease progresses, oral intake will decrease to almost nil. At this stage, adequate mouth care and small sips of ice chips or cold beverages may be adequate for some patients. For patients with symptoms related to dehydration, the use of hypodermoclysis can be very useful in maintaining adequate hydration.[61]

Enteral and parenteral nutrition

Parenteral nutrition has not demonstrated any benefit over enteral nutrition in patients with a functional bowel.[62,63] Enteral nutrition is significantly less expensive than parenteral nutrition and can be easily performed at home by most patients. However, it has been associated with significant morbidity in some cases—mainly due to aspiration, pneumonia, and diarrhoea. The risk of aspiration increases in patients with delayed gastric emptying and can be reduced by frequent aspiration of the gastric contents in the first days of infusion in order to detect gastric stasis. The establishment of a gastrostomy, by either endoscopic or ultrasonographic methods, will make a nasogastric tube unnecessary and will significantly improve the level of comfort and body image of patients. As disease progresses, the tube can also be used for the drainage of the gastrointestinal tract in case of total bowel obstruction. Enteral nutrition can be useful in some cases of patients with advanced head and neck tumours or oesophageal carcinoma who are not able to swallow properly and still have an appetite. Parenteral nutrition has a morbidity of 15 per cent, a high cost estimated at $10 000 per patient,[55] significant difficulties for the maintenance of this treatment in the patient's home, and a significant symptomatic cost given the need to maintain intravenous access, sterility, and comply with the administration of the solutions every day. With the exception of highly selected cases, the use of parenteral nutrition does not have any major role in palliative medicine.

Pharmacological approach

The main purpose of the pharmacological treatment of cachexia will be to antagonize its two main symptoms—anorexia and chronic nausea. Ideally, the improvement in muscle metabolism and asthenia could also be goals of the treatment but it remains to be determined whether new approaches can realize this goal.

The management of chronic nausea has been discussed in Chapter 9.3.1. When chronic nausea occurs in association with cachexia, because of the high incidence of autonomic failure with resulting gastroparesis,[34,35] metoclopramide and other gastric-emptying agents are the drugs of choice.[64,65] New antiemetic agents, such as 5-hydroxytryptamine (5-HT_3) antagonists, have not been found useful in the control of chronic nausea of cancer. As other therapeutic measures for the management of nausea have been discussed in Chapter 9.3.1, the remainder of this section will deal with the pharmacological approach to anorexia.

Corticosteroids

A number of uncontrolled studies have suggested that some symptoms of cancer patients, such as anorexia and asthenia, can be alleviated by corticosteroid treatment, giving patients an increased sensation of well being.[66–69] In 1974, Moertel *et al.*[70] published results comparing dexamethasone at 0.75 and 1.5 mg four times daily to placebo in 116 patients with advanced gastrointestinal cancer. The main purpose of the study was to assess the potential antineoplastic effects of dexamethasone. Although these effects were not found, the authors found a significant symptomatic improvement (appetite and strength) for patients receiving dexamethasone after 2 weeks of treatment, but such improvement disappeared after 4 weeks of treatment. In their trial, toxicity was low with only one case of gastrointestinal haemorrhage.

Willox[71] has reported significant improvement in appetite and well being in a double-blind, crossover trial. The majority of patients in this study were receiving chemotherapy.

Our group designed a 14-day, randomized, double-blind crossover trial comparing oral methylprednisolone 16 mg twice a day versus placebo.[66] The main end points of the study were pain, psychiatric status, appetite, nutritional status, daily activity, and performance. Patients were randomized to receive methylprednisolone or placebo for 5 days. After a 2-day wash-out period, patients were crossed over to the alternative treatment for 5 more days. On day 13, the double-blind phase of the study was completed and all patients received 32 mg of methylprednisolone daily for 20 days.

At the end of the double-blind, crossover phase of the study, the intensity of pain and analgesic consumption had significantly decreased. Appetite, food intake, and a performance status score had also significantly improved. Unfortunately, after the completion of the 20 day open phase trial, all the nutritional parameters had returned to their baseline level. The mechanism of action of methylprednisolone in patients with terminal cancer is not clear; it might be due to its euphoriant activity or to the inhibition of prostaglandin metabolism. Although the number of patients was small, treatment with methylprednisolone was not associated with severe toxicity in any patient. However, prolonged corticosteroid treatment has been associated with weakness, delirium, osteoporosis, and immunosuppression, and all these features are commonly present in advanced cancer patients.[72,73]

Two recent multicentre studies in Europe using intravenous methylprednisolone produced similar results. The first study looked at the quality of life in preterminal cancer patients in a placebo-controlled, multicentre study. The effectiveness of an 8-week, 125 mg/day intravenous course of methylprednisolone sodium succinate (**MPSS**) for improving quality of life in patients with preterminal cancer was investigated. A total of 403 patients were enrolled, with 207 treated with MPSS and 196 with placebo. MPSS was significantly more effective than placebo in improving quality of life with mortality rate being similar for MPSS-treated men, placebo-treated men, and MPSS-treated women; the investigators reporting that women placebo-treated patients had significantly lower mortality rates than their MPSS-treated counterparts. The reason for this lower mortality is unknown and further investigation was suggested.[74] In the second report[75] a total of 173 women terminal cancer patients were randomized to treatment with daily 125 mg infusions of MPSS or placebo for a period of 8 weeks. Significant improvement in quality of life was reported across the 8-week follow-up period in the steroid group. There were no significant differences between treatment groups with regard to overall mortality rates or time to death. The total number of reported adverse effects did not differ significantly between treatment groups. The results of the study confirmed previous reports of steroid efficacy in improving quality of life in terminal cancer patients with absence of any significant effect on mortality and a favourable safety profile, with the authors supporting the use of methylprednisolone as palliative therapy in terminal cancer patients.

Although more trials are needed to establish the optimal dose and modality of administration of corticosteroids, a short course can be given to severely symptomatic, advanced cancer patients who have no major contraindications.

Progestational drugs

Clinical trials on the use of progesterone derivatives for the treatment of hormone-responsive cancers found significant weight gain, both in patients who showed tumour shrinkage and patients who did not show any change in tumour size.[76–78] This finding has, in the last few years, stimulated much research into the use of megestrol acetate for the cachexia/anorexia syndrome in terminally ill patients. Cruz *et al.*[79] reported on 172 patients with advanced breast cancer randomized to receive 160 or 800 mg/day of megestrol acetate. The use of megestrol acetate was associated with weight gain that correlated directly with the dose used, length of treatment, and age of the patient. Von Roenn[80] reported on the use of megestrol acetate in HIV-positive patients. Twenty-two patients were treated with oral megestrol acetate at a dose of 80 mg four times daily. The number of patients gaining weight was 21 out of 22, with 3 patients failing to gain weight on 320 mg/day of megestrol acetate. Appetite stimulation and weight gain was achieved at 460 mg/day in one patient and 640 mg/day in another patient, with the last patient continuing to lose weight despite 480 mg/day of megestrol acetate. The median time to peak weight gain during treatment was 14 weeks. In three out of 22 patients treated, megestrol acetate and zidovudine were started simultaneously and for this group weight gain was potentially associated with the zidovudine treatment. All patients tolerated the drug well. The true effectiveness of megestrol acetate for HIV-related cachexia and the effects of treatment on quality of life still needs to be assessed in a prospective, randomized, double-blind, placebo-controlled trial.

Three trials to evaluate megestrol acetate in patients with cancer anorexia and/or cachexia, all of which were randomized, double-blind, placebo-controlled trials, have recently been reported.[60,81,82] Loprinzi *et al.*[81] report a total of 136 patients with documented cancer anorexia/cachexia randomized to receive megestrol acetate 800 mg/day or placebo. This trial provided convincing evidence that megestrol acetate stimulated both appetite and food intake. In addition, substantial weight gain was observed in a number of the protocol participants, with 11 out of 67 treated with megestrol acetate (16 per cent) gaining 6.75 kg or more compared with only 1 out of 66 placebo treated patients. The observed weight gain did not appear to be caused by fluid accumulation. In 10 out of 11 patients, weight gain did not appear to be related to favourable tumour response. Megestrol acetate was well tolerated in this study which convincingly demonstrated that 800 mg/day can substantially improve patient appetite and food intake in advanced cancer patients and may result in substantial weight gain in a percentage of such subjects.

Tchekmedyian *et al.*[82] report 89 patients with hormone insensitive malignancy treated with megestrol acetate 1600 mg/day or placebo. Monthly evaluations included weight, anthropometrics, prealbumim, questionnaires on quality of life, appetite, and factors affecting food intake. At 1 month, appetite increased significantly more on megestrol acetate, with patient-rated food intake showing a larger increase. Only 53 per cent of patients were evaluable at 2 months, thus limiting analysis beyond 1 month. Prealbumin increased significantly more in megestrol acetate patients. Appetite changes correlated significantly with weight changes, patient-rated food intake, and quality-of-life score. These data suggested that megestrol acetate could be helpful in cancer anorexia and could improve weight as well as nutritional and quality of life parameters.

In the study by Bruera *et al.*,[60] 40 consecutive patients with advanced non-hormone-responsive tumours receiving no antineoplastic treatment were randomized to receive megestrol acetate 480 mg/day versus placebo for 7 days. During day 8 a crossover was made until day 15. Appetite, pain, nausea, depression, energy, and well being was assessed with a visual analogue scale. Measurements were taken on nutritional status, caloric intake, and side-effects. If the patients chose megestrol acetate over placebo or had no choice, they were continued on megestrol acetate until death or they were unable to swallow. Megestrol acetate was chosen over placebo by 66 per cent of patients and 90 per cent of investigators; it was found to improve appetite, caloric intake, and nutritional status to a statistically significant degree. There was good tolerance of megestrol acetate, with mild oedema and nausea in 3 and 2 cases respectively. A likely explanation for the effect of megestrol acetate is a significant increase in appetite. The authors speculate that a potential explanation is the inhibition of some of the macrophage factors recently associated with the production of cachexia, for example cachectin and tumour necrosis factor. It might be beneficial for use in patients likely to develop cachexia due to for example, pancreatic, gastric, and non-small-cell lung cancer. The authors conclude that megestrol acetate is a powerful appetite stimulant with subjective and objective effects on the nutritional status of patients with advanced cancer. The high cost of megestrol acetate (approximately $Can.400.00 for one month's supply at 480 mg/day) is a concern.

Further research is ongoing to establish the ideal dose of megestrol acetate. The Cancer and Leukaemia Group B is now performing a dose–response trial comparing megestrol acetate 160, 800, and 1600 mg/day in patients with advanced lung or colorectal carcinoma who have lost 5 per cent or more of their usual body weight.[83]

The Mayo Clinic and North Central Cancer Treatment Group are currently evaluating the dose–response relationship between megestrol acetate and appetite stimulation, weight gain, nausea, and vomiting.[84] This group is also conducting a clinical trial to evaluate the influence of megestrol acetate on survival duration and quality of life among patients with advanced lung cancer.

The side-effects of progestational drugs are usually mild and consist mostly of oedema and hypercalcaemia and cushingoid fat distribution in patients on high doses. However, preliminary reports have suggested that megestrol might be associated with decreased survival.[85,86] These findings need to be confirmed in prospective studies and might limit the usefulness of megestrol in malnourished cancer patients at an earlier stage of the disease.

Cyproheptadine

Cyproheptadine is an antihistamine with antiserotoninergic properties usually used for allergies.[87] Initial clinical data suggested that it had appetite and weight enhancing effects in both non-cancer patients and in patients with cancer related anorexia and cachexia.[88-90] As a result of these findings, Kardinal *et al.*[91] performed a randomized, placebo-controlled, double-blind clinical trial in 295 patients with advanced malignant disease. Patients were randomly assigned to receive oral cyprophetadine 8 mg three times per day or placebo. The median patient time in this trial was slightly over 1 month, with only 25 per cent of the subjects remaining in the study for 3 months or more. Data suggested that cyproheptadine stimulated patient appetite and food intake mildly. Unfortunately, the drug did not significantly prevent progressive weight loss in this group of patients with advanced malignant disease.

Hydrazine sulphate

Hydrazine sulphate has been found, in human and animal trials, to have a variety of effects. This drug is widely promoted by 'alternative' practitioners, who claim that it has effects on nutrition, energy, and even survival of cancer and AIDS patients.

Hydrazine sulphate has been found to inhibit gluconeogenesis in rats.[92,93] In addition, mice treated with hydrazine sulphate prior to challenge with endotoxin from *Salmonella enteritis*, showed significantly improved survival as compared to a control group.[94] Hughes *et al.*[95] found that hydrazine sulphate inhibits tumour necrosis factor activities and their role in the wasting process.

Tayek *et al.*[96] performed a prospective, double-blind trial of 12 malnourished patients with lung cancer randomized to receive either placebo or hydrazine sulphate 60 mg three time per day for 30 days. Plasma lysine flux did not change significantly in the placebo group but it did show a significant fall in the hydrazine sulphate group, with serum albumin decreasing in the placebo group and unchanged in the hydrazine sulphate group. They conclude that the administration of hydrazine sulphate to reduce amino acid flux may favourably influence the metabolic abnormalities in cancer cachexia.

Two uncontrolled trials,[97,98] in 1975 and in 1981, suggested that hydrazine sulphate could be useful for advanced cancer patients. However, three clinical trials in the 1970s failed to confirm any beneficial effect from hydrazine sulphate.[99-101]

Two recent trials have again tested hydrazine sulphate versus placebo in patients with advanced cancer cachexia. Chlebowski *et al.*[102] evaluated hydrazine sulphate, using 24-h dietary recall and body weight determinations, before and after 30 days of either placebo or hydrazine sulphate, 60 mg three times per day oral administration, in 101 cancer patients with weight loss. After 1 month, 83 per cent of hydrazine sulphate patients, who completed repeat evaluations, maintained or increased their weight, as compared to only 53 per cent of placebo patients. In addition, appetite improvement was more frequent in the hydrazine sulphate group. Hydrazine sulphate toxicity was mild, with 71 per cent of patients reporting no toxic effects. The data from this trial suggested an association between 1 month of hydrazine sulphate administration and body weight maintenance in patients with cancer. The second trial by Chlebowski *et al.*[103] in patients with non-small-cell lung cancer randomly assigned to receive combination chemotherapy plus either placebo or hydrazine sulphate, demonstrated a median survival among the hydrazine sulphate treated patients of 292 days compared to 187 days for those in the placebo group. Although this difference was not statistically significant, patients receiving hydrazine sulphate did have a significant increase in calorie intake and serum albumin levels.

After these initial results, the North Central Cancer Treatment Group designed two prospective, controlled trials on the role of hydrazine sulphate in patients with advanced cancer. In the first study, 127 patients with metastatic colorectal cancer were randomized to receive hydrazine sulphate or placebo in a double-blinded manner. Protocol patients did not concurrently receive any other systemic antineoplastic treatment. Data from the study showed trends to both poorer survival and poorer quality of life in the hydrazine sulphate group. There were no significant differences in the two study arms with regards to anorexia or weight loss. The authors concluded that this trial failed to demonstrate any benefit for hydrazine sulphate.[104]

In the second study, 243 patients with newly diagnosed non-small-cell lung cancer were randomized to receive hydrazine sulphate or placebo in addition to chemotherapy with cisplatin and etoposide. Response rates were similar in the two treatment arms. However, there were trends for worse time to progression and survival in the hydrazine sulphate arm. No significant differences were noted in the two study arms with regards to toxicity or quality of life. The authors concluded that this trial also failed to demonstrated any benefit for patients who received hydrazine sulphate.[105]

The Cancer and Leukaemia Group B also designed a prospective, multicentre study on hydrazine sulphate. In this study, 266 patients with advanced non-small-cell lung cancer were randomized to receive hydrazine sulphate or placebo in addition to chemotherapy including cisplatin and vinblastine. Both survival and objective response rates were similar for the two groups. The toxicity of chemotherapy was similar for both groups. In addition, there were no differences noted between the two groups in degree of anorexia, weight gain or loss, or overall nutritional status. Sensory and motor neuropathy occurred significantly more often in patients treated with hydrazine sulphate. Quality of life was significantly worse in patients who received hydrazine sulphate. The authors concluded that hydrazine sulphate provided no benefit to an effective chemotherapy regimen.[106]

All three aforementioned studies used hydrazine sulphate in the same dose and regimen previously reported by Chlebowski (60 mg three times per day, orally). The results of the last three excellent, multicentre studies suggest very strongly that hydrazine sulphate has no significant effects on nutritional or symptomatic parameters in patients with advanced cancer. At this time, this drug should not be recommended for clinical use and further clinical trials are probably unjustified.

Cannabinoids

Weight gain has been a recognized feature of the use of marijuana and its derivatives. Recent studies including dronabinol have attempted to find whether some of the appetite enhancement could be disassociated from mood effects. Wadleigh *et al.*[107] conducted an open, dose-ranging study in patients with unresectable cancer. After a baseline observation, patients were treated with dronabinol for up to 6 weeks at doses of 2.5 mg daily (n=8), 2.5 mg twice a day (n=9), or 5 mg daily (n=13). Five patients discontinued dronabinol because of adverse effects, with three discontinuing because of progressive disease. Patients in all groups continued to lose weight, although the rate of weight loss decreased with therapy in all doses. Symptomatic improvement was noted in both mood and appetite, although treatment with 2.5 mg daily had no effect. In this open, dose-ranging study, dronabinol appeared to stimulate both mood and appetite at well tolerated doses. Further studies with dronabinol to evaluate dose escalation are still continuing.

Pentoxifylline

Pentoxifylline is a methylxanthine derivative which has been approved by the Food and Drug Administration for treatment of intermittent claudication at a dose of 400 mg three times daily. This drug is able to decrease the tumour necrosis factor mRNA levels in cancer patients and decreases replication of the AIDS virus when administered at a dose of 400 mg every 8 h. These findings could suggest a beneficial role for pentoxifylline on cancer cachexia.

The North Central Cancer Treatment Group randomized 70 patients with a variety of advanced solid tumours and cancer cachexia to receive pentoxifylline or placebo in a double-blind fashion. Patients' weight was monitored and patient questionnaires were used to assess appetite, toxicity, and perception of benefit. Pentoxifylline did not appear to cause any toxicity. However, it failed to improve appetite or weight gain.[108] The results of this multicentre, prospective trial failed to confirm previous anecdotal reports.[109] At the present time, there is no justification for the use of this drug in cancer cachexia.

Clinical guidelines

In the previous paragraphs we have discussed the potential role of different nutritional and pharmacological treatments for cachexia. In the following paragraphs we will attempt to summarize some guidelines based on current knowledge about this subject.

Oral nutrition should be attempted whenever possible. Particular attention should be paid to adequate timing of meals in relation to different medical and nursing procedures as well as in reference to the administration of drugs. In cases in which oral nutrition or hydration is not possible, selected patients may benefit from enteral nutrition or hypodermoclysis. Since parenteral nutrition has not shown any significant survival or comfort improvement, we find no role for its routine use in palliative medicine.

In patients in whom the main symptom associated with cachexia is chronic nausea, adequate management of nausea with the use of different combinations of gastric stimulant agents, with or without corticosteroids and centrally acting antiemetics, will be the primary treatment. In patients in whom profound anorexia is the main manifestation of cachexia, megestrol acetate will be useful if the expected survival of the patient can be measured in weeks to months because of its effects not only on appetite, but also on overall nutritional status. In patients with a shorter survival or those who have problems tolerating progestational drugs, a brief course of corticosteroids may be useful symptomatically. Corticosteroids can be administered both orally and subcutaneously and, in addition to appetite stimulation, they have effects on nausea, pain, and asthenia. However, while progestational agents are able to increase caloric intake and also improve nutritional status, the effects of corticosteroids are short lasting and of merely symptomatic nature.

Future research

An improved knowledge of the pathophysiology of cancer and AIDS-induced cachexia will assist in the development of more effective treatments. The interaction between symptoms of cachexia, such as chronic nausea, anorexia, asthenia, and different psychological syndromes, should also be better established.

Future studies should also aim for a better characterization of the symptomatic effect of different nutritional and pharmacological intervention rather than a simple assessment of the effect of these interventions on calorie intake and nutritional status. These studies should be designed with symptomatic benefit considered to be the main outcome of the study. Newer drugs and 'designer' diets containing different proportions of branch-chain amino acids or fatty acids could prove to have effects on the metabolic changes associated with cachexia.

Finally, the interaction between some of the major syndromes of terminal disease such as pain, cachexia, and cognitive failure should be better established. It is likely that the severity of some of these syndromes will have an impact on the others and that therapeutic interventions aimed to improve pain or neurological syndromes will also have an impact on cachexia and asthenia.

References

1. DeWys WD, Begg C, Lavin PT, Band PR, Bennett JM, Bertino JR, *et al.* Prognostic effect of weight loss prior to chemotherapy in cancer patients. *American Journal of Medicine*, 1980; **69**: 491–7.
2. Kotler D, Wang J, Pierson R. Body composition studies in patients with AIDS. *American Journal of Clinical Nutrition*, 1985; **42**: 1255–65.
3. Bruera E, Roca E, Carraro S. Association between malnutrition and caloric intake, emesis, psychological depression, glucose taste, and tumor mass. *Cancer Treatment Reports*, 1984; **6**: 873–6.
4. Bruera E, MacDonald RN. Nutrition in cancer patients: an update and review of our experience. *Journal of Pain and Symptom Management*, 1988; 3:133–40.
5. Knoll J. Endogenous anorectic agents—satietins. *Annual Review of Pharmacology and Toxicology*, 1988; **28**: 247–68.
6. Williams J, Ali Siddiqui R. Biochemistry of cancer cachexia: Review of results, a new hypothesis and a proposal for treatment. *Medical Science Research*, 1990; **18**: 3–10.
7. Beutler B, Cerami A. Cachectin, cachexia and shock. *Annual Review of Medicine*, 1988; **39**: 75–85.
8. Fearon K, Borland W, Preston T, Tisdale MJ, Shenkin A, Calman KC. Cancer cachexia: Influence of systemic ketosis on substrate levels and nitrogen metabolism. *American Journal of Clinical Nutrition*, 1988; **47**: 42–8.
9. Gibbs J, Young RC, Smith GP. Cholecystokinin decreases food intake in rats. *Journal of Comparative Physiology and Psychology*, 1973; **84**: 488–95.
10. Freed WJ, Perlow MJ, Wyatt RJ. Calcitonin: inhibitory effect on eating in rats. *Science*, 1979; **206**: 850–2.
11. Rizzo AJ, Goltzman D. Calcitonin receptors in the central nervous system of the rat. *Endocrinology*, 1981; **108**: 1672–7.
12. Vijayan E, McCann SM. Suppression of feeding and drinking activity in rats following intraventricular injection of thyrotropin releasing hormone. *Endocrinology*, 1977; **100**: 1727–30.
13. Lotter EC, Krinsky R, McKay JM, Trenner CM, Porte D Jr., Woods CS. Somatostatin decreases food intake of rats and baboons. *Journal of Comparative Physiology and Psychology*, 1981; **95**: 278–87.
14. Schulman JL, Carleton JL, Whitney G, Whitehorn JC. Effect of glucagon on food intake and body weight in man. *Journal of Applied Physiology*, 1957; **11**: 419–21.
15. Bodnar R, Pasternak G, Mann P, *et al.* Mediation of anorexia by human recombinent tumor nercosis factor through a peripheral action in the rat. *Cancer Research*, 1989; **49**: 6280–4.
16. Bachwich P, Chensue S, Larrick J, Kunkel SL. Tumor nercosis factor stimulates interleukin-1 and prostoglandin E, production in resting macrophages. *Biochemical and Biophysical Research Communications*, 1986; **136**: 94–101.
17. Flores EA, Bistrian BR, Pomposelli JJ, Dinarello CA, Blackburn GL, Istfan NW. Infusion of tumor nercosis factor/cachectin promotes muscle catabolism in the rat. A synergistic effect with interleukin-1. *Journal of Clinical Investigations*, 1989; **83**: 1614–22.
18. Masuno H, Yoshimura H, Ogana N, Okuda H. Isolation of lyolytic factor (toxohormonel) from ascites fluid of patients with hepatoma and its effect on feeding behaviour. *European Journal of Cancer and Clinical Oncology*, 1984; **20**:1177–85.
19. Beck S, Mulligan H, Tisdale M. Lipolytic factors associated with murine and human cancer cahcexia. *Journal of the National Cancer Institute*, 1990; **82**: 1922–6.
20. DeWys WD. Taste and feeding behavior in patients with cancer In: Winick M, ed. *Nutrition in Cancer.* Vol 5. *Current Concepts in Nutrition*. New York: Wiley, 1977.
21. DeWys WD, Walters K. Abnormalities of taste sensation in cancer patients. *Cancer,* 1975; **36**: 1888–96.
22. DeWys WD, Costa G, Henkin R. Clinical parameters related to anorexia. *Cancer Treatment Reports,* 1981; **65** (suppl 5): 49–52.
23. Derogatis L, Morrow G, Fetting J, Penman D, Piasetsky S, Schmale AM, *et al.* The prevalence of psychotic disorders among cancer patients. *Journal of the American Medical Association*, 1983; **249**: 751–7.
24. Bruera E, Miller L, McCallion J, Macmillan K, Krefting L. Cognitive failure (CF) in patients with terminal cancer: a prospective study. *Proceedings of the American Society of Clinical Oncology*, 1990; **9**: 308.
25. Reuben DB, Mor V. Nausea and vomiting in terminal cancer patients. *Archives of Internal Medicine*, 1983; **146**: 2021–3.
26. Doyle D. Symptom relief in terminal illness. *Medicine in Practice*, 1983; **1**: 694–8.
27. Coyle N, Adelhardt J, Foley KM, Portenoy RK. Character of terminal illness in the advanced cancer patient: pain and other symptoms during the last 4 weeks of life. *Journal of Pain Symptom Management*, 1990; **5**: 83–93.
28. Lichter I, Hunt E. The last 48 h of life. *Journal of Palliative Care,* 1990; **6**: 7–15.
29. Ventafridda V, Ripamonti C, DeConno F, Tamburini M, Cassileth BR. Symptom prevalence and control during cancer patient's last days of life. *Journal of Palliative Care*, 1990; **6**: 7–11.
30. Fainsinger R, MacEachern T, Hanson J, Miller MJ, Bruera E. Symptom control during the last week of life on a Palliative Care Unit. *Journal of Palliative Care*, 1991; **7**: 5–11.
31. Kris M, Gralla R. Management of vomiting caused by anticancer drugs. *Advances in Pain Research and Therapy*, 1990; **16**: 337–44.
32. Manara L, Bianchetti A. The central and peripheral influence of opioids on gastrointestinal propulsion. *Annual Review of Pharmacology and Toxicology*, 1985; **75**: 249–73.
33. Bruera E, Brenneis C, Chadwick S, Michaud M, MacDonald RN. Continuous subcutaneous infusion of narcotics using a portable disposable device in patients with advanced cancer. *Cancer Treatment Reports*, 1987; **71**: 635–7.
34. Henrich W. Autonomic insufficiency. *Archives of Internal Medicine*, 1982; **142**: 339–44.
35. Ewing D, Campbell I, Clarke B. Assessment of cardiovascular effects of diabetic autonomic neuropathy and prognostic implications. *Annals of Internal Medicine*, 1980; **92**: 308–11.
36. Watkins P, MacKay J. Cardiac denervation in diabetic neuropathy. *Annals of Internal Medicine*, 1980; **92**: 304–7.
37. Hoskins DJ, Bennett T, Hampton JR. Diabetic autonomic neuropathy. *Diabetes*, 1978; **27**: 1043–54.
38. Thomas J, Shields R. Associated autonomic dysfunction and carcinoma of the pancreas. *British Medical Journal*, 1970; **4**: 32.
39. Schuffler M, Baird W, Fleming R, Bell DE, Bouldin TW, Malagelada JR, *et al.* Intestinal pseudo-obstruction or the presenting manifestation of small-cell carcinoma of the lung. *Annals of Internal Medicine*, 1983; **98**: 129–34.
40. Park D, Johnson RH, Crean G, Robinson JF. Orthostatic hypotension in bronchial carcinoma. *British Medical Journal*, 1972; **3**: 510–11.,
41. Bruera E, Chadwick S, MacDonadl N, Fox R, Hanson J. Study of cardiovascular autonomic insufficiency in advanced cancer patients. *Cancer Treatment Reports*, 1986; **70**: 1383–7.
42. Bruera E, Catz Z, Hopper R, Lentle B, MacDonald RN. Chronic nausea and anorexia in advanced cancer patients: A possible role for autonomic dysfunction. *Journal of Pain and Symptom Management,* 1987; **2**: 19–21.

43. Kris M, Yeh S, Gralla R, Young CW. Symptomatic gastroparesis in cancer patients. A possible cause of cancer associated with anorexia. *Proceedings of the American Society of Clinical Oncology*, 1985; **4**: C–1038.
44. Bleich H, Boro E. Fasting, feeding and regulation of the sympathetic nervous system. *New England Journal of Medicine*, 1978; **298**: 1295–300.
45. Apfelbaum-Kowalski E. Pathophysiology of the circulatory system in hunger disease. In: Winnick M, ed. *Hunger Disease*. New York: John Wiley and Sons, 1979: 127–60.
46. Bruera E, MacDonald RN. Asthenia in patients with advanced cancer. *Journal of Pain and Symptom Management,* 1988; **3**: 9–14.
47. Lopes J, Russell D, Whitwell J, Jeejeebhoy KN. Skeletal muscle function in malnutrition. *American Journal of Clinical Nutrition*, 1983; **36**: 602–10.
48. Russell D, Prendergast P, Darby P, Garfinkel PE, Whitwell J, Jeejeebhoy KN. A comparison between muscle function and body composition in anorexia nervosa: the effect of refeeding. *American Journal of Clinical Nutrition*,1983; **38**: 229–37.
49. Theologides A. Anorexins, asthenins and cachectins in cancer. *American Journal of Medicine*, 1985; **81**: 296–8.
50. Bruera E, Brenneis C, Michaud M, Rafter J, Magnan A, Tennant A, *et al.* Association between asthenia and nutritional status, lean body mass, anemia, psychological status, and tumor mass in patients with advanced breast cancer. *Journal of Pain and Symptom Management,*1989; **4**: 59–63.
51. DeWys WD, Begg C, Lavin PT, Bennett JM, Bertino JR, Cohen MH, *et al.* Prognostic effect of weight loss prior to chemotherapy in cancer patients. *American Journal of Medicine*, 1980; **69**: 491–7.
52. Blackburn G, Miller M, Bothe A. Nutritional factors in cancer in medical oncology. In: Calabresi P, Schein P, eds. *Oncology*. New York: MacMillan, 1985: 1406–32.
53. Smale B, Mullen J, Buzby G, Rosato E. The efficacy of nutritional assessment and support in cancer surgery. *Cancer*, 1981; **47**: 2375–81.
54. Issell B, Valdivieso M, Zaren HA, Dudrick SJ, Freireich EJ, Copeland EW, *et al.* Protection against chemotherapy toxicity in IV hyperalimentation. *Cancer Treatment Report*, 1978; **62**: 1139–43.
55. Koretz R. Parenteral nutrition: is it oncologically logical? *Journal of Clinical Oncology*, 1984; **2**: 534–8.
56. Evans W, Nixon D, Daly J. A randomized study of standard or augumented oral nutritional support versus ad lib nutrition intake in patients with advanced cancer. *Clinical and Investigative Medicine* (Abstract), 1986; **9**: A-127.
57. Muller JM, Brenner U, Dienst C, Pickmaier H. Preoperative parenteral feeding in patients with gastrointestinal carcinoma. *Lancet*, 1982; **1**: 68–71.
58. Detsky AS, Baker JP, O'Rourke K, Goel V. Preoperative parenteral nutrition: A meta-analysis. *Annals of Internal Medicine*, 1987; **107**: 195–203.
59. Torosian M, Daly J. Nutritional support in the cancer-bearing host. *Cancer*, 1986; **58**: 1915–29.
60. Bruera E, Macmillan K, Hanson J, Kuehn N, MacDonald RN. A controlled trial of megestrol acetate on appetite, caloric intake, nutritional status, and other symptoms in patients with advanced cancer. *Cancer*, 1990; **66**: 1279–82.
61. Bruera E, Legris MA, Kuehn N, Miller MJ. Hypodermoclysis for the administration of fluids and narcotic analgesics in patients with advanced cancer. *Journal of Pain and Symptom Management*, 1990; **5**: 218–20.
62. Randall H. Enteral nutrition: tube feeding in acute and chronic illness. *Journal of Enteral and Parenteral Nutrition*, 1984; **8**: 113–34.
63. Burt M, Gorschboth C, Brennan M. A controlled prospective, randomized trial evaluating the metabolic effects of enteral and parenteral nutrition in the cancer patient. *Cancer*, 1982; **49**: 1092–105.
64. Schulze-Delriev K. Metoclopramide. *New England Journal of Medicine,* 1981; **305**: 28–32.
65. Montastruc JL, Chamontin B, Senard JL, Rascol A. Domperidone in the management of oathostatic hypotension. *Clinical Neuropharmacology*, 1985; **8**: 191–2.
66. Bruera E, Roca E, Cedaro L, Carraro S, Chacon R. Action of oral methylpredisolone in terminal cancer patients: a prospective randomized double-blind study. *Cancer Treatment Reports*, 1985; **69**: 751–4.
67. Schell H. Adrenal corticosteroid therapy in far-advanced cancer. *Geriatrics,* 1972; **27**: 131–41.
68. Twycross RG. Continuing in terminal care: an overview in advances in pain research and therapy. In: Bonica J, Ventafridda V, eds. *Proceedings of the International Symposium of Pain of Advanced Cancer.* New York: Raven Press, 1979; **2**: 617–34.
69. Pommatau E, Revillard J, Gignous M. Interet de methyl-6-prednisolone hemisuccinate de sodium (Solumedrol) dans les traiments des tumeurs malignes. *Lyon Medicale*, 1962; **49**: 1179–98.
70. Moertel C, Shutt AJ, Reitemeier RJ, Hahn RG. Corticosteroid therapy of preterminal gastrointestinal cancer. *Cancer*, 1974; **33**: 1607–9.
71. Willox J, Corr J, Shaw J, Richardson M, Calman KC, Drennan M. Prednisolone as an appetite stimulant in patients with cancer. *British Medical Journal*, 1984; **200**: 37.
72. Derogatis L, MacDonald R. Psychopharmacologic applications to cancer. *Cancer* 1982; **50**: 1968–73.
73. Haynes R, Murad F. Adrenocorticotropic hormone, adrenocortical steroids and their synthetic analogs. In: Goodman L, Gilman A, eds. *Pharmacological Basis of Therapeutics*. New York: Macmillan, 1980.
74. Robustelli Della Cuna G, Pellegrini A, Piazzi M. Effect of methylprednisolone sodium succinate on quality of life in pre-terminal cancer patients: a placebo controlled, multi-center study. *European Journal of Cancer and Clinical Oncology*, 1989; **25**: 1817–21.
75. Popiela T, Lucchi R, Giongo F. Methylprednisolone as palliative therapy for female terminal cancer patients. *European Journal of Cancer and Clinical Oncology*, 1989; **25**: 1823–9.
76. Cavalli F, Goldhirsch A, Jungi F. Randomized trial of low versus high dose medroxyprogesterone acetate in the treatment of post-menopausal patients with advanced breast cancer. In: Pellegrini A, Robustelli G, eds. *Role of Medroxyprogesterone in Endocrine-Related Tumors.* New York: Raven Press, 1984: 79–90.
77. Tchekmedyian S, Tait N, Moody M, Aisner J. High dose megestrol acetate: A possible treatment for cachexia. *Journal of the American Medical Association*, 1987; **257**: 1195–9.
78. Tchekmedyian S, Tait N, Moody M, Greco FA, Aisner J. Appetite stimulation with megestrol acetate in cachectic cancer patients. *Seminars in Oncology*, 1986; **13**: 37–43.
79. Cruz JM, Mus HB, Brockschmidt JK, Evans GW. Weight changes in women with metastatic breast cancer treated with megestrol acetate: a comparison of standard versus high dose therapy. *Seminars in Oncology*, 1990; **17** (Suppl 9): 63–7.
80. Von Roenn JH, Murphy RL, Wegener N. Megestrol acetate for treatment of anorexia and cachexia associated with human immunodeficiency virus infection. *Seminars in Oncology*, 1990; **17** (Suppl 9): 13–16.
81. Loprinzi CL, Ellison NM, Schaid J, Krook JE, Athmann LM, Dose AM, *et al.* A controlled trial of megestrol acetate treatment of cancer anorexia and cachexia. *Journal of the National Cancer Institute*, 1990; **82**: 1127–32.
82. Tchekmedyian NS, Hariri L, Siau, J, Tait N, Greco FA, Aisner J, *et al.* Megestrol acetate in cancer anorexia and weight loss (Abstract). *Proceedings of the American Society of Clinical Oncology*, 1990; **9**: 336.
83. Aisner J, Parnes H, Tait N, Hickman M, Forrest A, Greco FA, Tchekmedyian S. Appetite stimulation and weight gain with megestrol acetate. *Seminars in Oncology*, 1990; **17** (Suppl 9) 2–7.
84. Loprinzi C, Ellison, NM, Goldberg RN. Alleviation of cancer anorexia and cachexia. Studies of the Mayo Clinic and the North Central Cancer Treatment Group. *Seminars in Oncology*, 1990; **17** (Suppl 9): 8–12.
85. McBeth F, Gregor A, Coltier B. A randomized study of megestrol acetate and prednisolone for anorexia and weight loss in patients with lung cancer. Abstract, *World Conference on Lung Cancer*, 1994.
86. MacDonald RN. Research frontiers in controlling confusin, cachexia and dyspnea. *Western Journal of Medicine*, 1995; **163**: 278–86.
87. Editorial. Cyproheptadine. *Lancet*, 1978; **1**: 368.
88. Shah N. A double blind study on appetite stimulation and weight gain

with cyproheptadine as adjunct to specific therapy in pulmonary tuberculosis. *Current Medical Practice*, 1968; **12**: 861–4.
89. Nobel R. Effect of cyproheptadine on appetite and weight gain in adults. *Journal of the American Medical Association*, 1989; **209**: 2054–5.
90. Pawlowski G. Cyproheptadine: weight gain and appetite stimulation. *Current Therapeutic Research*, 1975; **18**: 673–8.
91. Kardinal C. Loprinzi C, Shaid DJ, Hass AC, Dose AM, Athmann LM, *et al.* A controlled trial of cyproheptadine in cancer patients with anorexia. *Cancer*, 1990; **65**: 2657–62.
92. Ray PD, Hanson RL, Lardy, HA. Inhibition by hydrazine of gluconeogenesis in the rat. *Journal of Biological Chemistry*, 1970; **5**: 690–6.
93. Silverstein R, Bhatia P, Svoboda DS. Effect of hydrazine sulfate on glucose- regulating enzymes in the normal and cancerous rat. *Immunopharmacology*, 1989; **17**: 37–43.
94. Silverstein R, Christofferson CA, Morrison DC. Modulation of endotoxinlethality in mice by hydrazine sulfate. *Infection and Immunity*, 1989; **57**: 2072–8.
95. Hughes TK, Cadet P, Larned CS. Modulation of tumor necrosis factor activities by potential anticachexia compound hydrazine sulfate. *International Journal of Immuopharmacology*, 1989; **11**: 501–7.
96. Tayek JA, Heber D, Chlebowski RT. Effective hydrazine sulfate on whole body protein breakdown measured by 14C-lysine metabolism in lung cancer patients. *Lancet*, 1987; **2**: 241–4.
97. Gold J. Use of hydrazine sulfate in terminal and pre-terminal cancer patients: results of investigation of new drug (IND) study in 84 evaluable patients. *Oncology*, 1975; **32**: 1–10.
98. Gershanovich ML, Danova LA, Ivan BA, Filov VA. Results of clinical study of antitumor action of hydrazine sulfate. *Nutrition and Cancer*, 1981; **3**: 7–12.
99. Spremulli E, Wampler GL, Regelson W. Clinical study of hydrazine sulfate in advanced cancer patients. *Cancer Chemotherapy and Pharmacology*, 1979; **3**: 121- 4.
100. Lener HJ, Regelson W. Clinical trial of hydrazine sulfate in solid tumors. *Cancer Treatment Reports*, 1976; **60**: 959–60.
101. Ocho AM, Wittes RE, Krakoff RH. Trial of hydrazine sulfate (NSC-150014) in patients with cancer. *Cancer Chemotherapy Reports*, 1975; **59**: 1151–4.
102. Chlebowski RT, Bulcavage L, Grosvenor M, *et al.* Hydrazine sulfate in cancer patients with weight loss: a placebo controlled clinical experience. *Cancer*, 1987; **59**: 406–10.
103. Chlebowski RT, Bulcavage L, Grosvenor M, Oktay E, Block JB, Chlebowski JS, *et al.* Hydrazine sulfate influence on nutritional status and survival in non-small-cell lung cancer. *Journal of Clinical Oncology*, 1990: **8**: 9–15.
104. Loprinzi CL, Kuross SA, O'Fallon JR, Gesme Jr DH, Gerstner JB, Rospond RM, *et al.* Randomized placebo-controlled evaluation of hydrazine sulfate in patients with advanced colorectal cancer. *Journal of Clinical Oncology*, 1994; **12**: 1121–5.
105. Loprinzi CL, Goldberg RM, Su JQ, Mailliard JA, Juross SA, Maksymiuk AW, *et al.* Placeob-controlled trial of hydrazine sulfate in patients with newly diagnosed non-small-cell lung cancer. *Journal of Clinical Oncology*, 1994; **12**: 1126–9.
106. Kosty MP, Fleishman SB, Herndon II JE, Coughlin K, Kornblith AB, Scalzo A, *et al.* Cicplatin, vinblastine and hydrazine sulfate in advanced non-small-cell lung cancer: a randomized placebo-controlled, double-blind phase III study of the Cancer and Leukemia Group B. *Journal of Clinical Oncology*, 1994; **12**: 1113–20.
107. Wadleigh R, Spaulding GM, Lumbersky B, Zimmer M, Shepard K, Plasse T. Dronabinol enhancement of appetite and cancer patients (abstract). *Proceedings of the American Society of Clinical Oncology*, 1990; **9**: 1280–331.
108. Goldberg RM, Loprinzi CL, Mailliard JA, O'Fallon JR, Krook JE, Ghosh C, *et al.* Pentoxifylline for treatment of cancer anorexia and cachexia? A randomized, double-blind placebo-controlled trial. *Journal of Clinical Oncology*, 1995; **13**: 2856–9.
109. Dezube BJ, Fridovich-Keil JL, Bouvard I, Lange RF, Pardee AB. Pentoxiphylline and well-being in patients with cancer (letter). *Lancet*, 1990; **335**: 662.

9.3.7 Jaundice, ascites, and hepatic encephalopathy

Vincent G. Bain

Jaundice

The presence of jaundice in the terminally ill patient usually portends a rapid demise; nevertheless, it is important to understand the different underlying mechanisms and causes so that a rational approach can be planned. In some cases, symptomatic treatment of associated symptoms such as pruritus is the only therapeutic goal, whereas in others a more aggressive approach, such as placement of a biliary stent through a malignant stricture, may facilitate a markedly improved quality, and perhaps even duration, of life. The appearance of jaundice in a terminally ill patient serves as an obvious marker of a severe underlying illness; family, friends, and acquaintances may become alarmed and naturally suspect the gravity of the illness. The successful resolution of jaundice can, therefore, have positive psychological and palliative effects which cannot be overestimated. It is important to take a general approach to the patient with jaundice to avoid making the error of equating jaundice with endstage, untreatable disease. We must endeavour to identify those patients whose jaundice can be reversed by relatively simple measures, such as stopping a hepatotoxic medication, and those who might benefit from relief of obstructive jaundice. Clearly, jaundice is not always a direct result of massive infiltration of the liver with malignancy.

Pathophysiology of jaundice

Jaundice can be classified as shown in Table 1 into prehepatic, hepatic, and post-hepatic disorders. Although not completely comprehensive, it includes conditions most likely to be encountered in cancer patients and thereby provides a useful framework for an orderly approach to the patient with jaundice. A prehepatic derangement is defined by an imbalance between the liver's capacity to take up unconjugated bilirubin and the amount being presented from the blood. As the term implies, it is not a hepatic problem at all; common examples include haemolysis, ineffective haematopoiesis, and Gilbert's disease, all of which are characterized by unconjugated hyperbilirubinaemia.

Hepatic causes of jaundice form the largest and most heterogeneous group (see Table 1). Any interference with the liver's capacity to excrete conjugated bilirubin into the biliary system will result in jaundice. In general, this may be secondary to widespread necrosis of hepatocytes (hepatocellular injury) or 'functional' (non-obstructive) impairment of biliary excretion (cholestasis). Extensive hepatic infiltration with malignant cells causes jaundice and is associated with a median survival of only 1 month.[1] In the Western

Table 1 Classification of jaundice

Prehepatic	Hepatic	Posthepatic
Gilbert's disease	Massive tumour infiltration	Malignant
Haemolysis	Viral hepatitis	Pancreas
Ineffective erythropoiesis	Hepatotoxic drugs including alcohol	Ampullary
Haematoma	Cholestasis	Cholangiocarcinoma
	Total parenteral nutrition	Metastatic lymph nodes
	Sepsis	Benign
	Drugs	Gallstones
	Ischaemia	Chronic pancreatitis
	Hepatic artery thrombosis	Biliary stricture
	Left ventricular failure	
	Venous outflow block	
	Severe right heart failure	
	Veno-occlusive disease	
	Budd–Chiari syndrome	

world, this is usually due to metastatic disease from primaries in the gastrointestinal tract (colon, pancreas, stomach), breast, lung, or haematological malignancies.[1] In rare instances, metastatic liver disease may even present as fulminant hepatic failure.[2] Viral hepatitis must always be considered, particularly in patients receiving blood products who are at risk of infection with hepatitis C virus.[3] The risk of acquiring hepatitis C (previously termed non-A, non-B hepatitis) from unscreened blood products was 10 per cent but the routine screening of donors with the hepatitis C virus immunoassay has substantially reduced this risk. Chronic hepatitis B is widely prevalent, especially in Asians; withdrawal of immunosuppressive chemotherapeutic agents may precipitate liver failure in chronic hepatitis B virus carriers.[4] Patients with widespread cancer, like other immunosuppressed individuals, are also at risk of viral hepatitis caused by cytomegalovirus and herpes simplex virus.

Numerous medications can lead to hepatic injury.[5] This usually leads to elevated serum liver enzymes in the absence of jaundice; however, several medications can cause severe hepatocellular injury or cholestasis with jaundice. Examples include commonly used agents such as halothane, erythromycin, amoxycillin/potassium clavulanate, α-methyldopa, isoniazid, prochlorperazine, and chlorpromazine as well as numerous cancer chemotherapeutic agents such as the C-17 alkylated steroids, methotrexate, and, rarely, chlorambucil. Jaundice induced by any of the commonly used sedatives or analgesics (including paracetamol (acetaminophen) at recommended dosage) would be extremely rare.

Intrahepatic cholestasis may be defined as a reduction of bile excretion in the absence of extrahepatic biliary obstruction. Many causes have been identified and cholestasis is often multifactorial; drugs, total parenteral nutrition, sepsis, and the postoperative state may all contribute. Cholestatic jaundice is generally less serious than jaundice secondary to extensive hepatocellular necrosis; however, if it persists, fat malabsorption and fat soluble vitamin deficiency may ensue.

The liver is a highly vascular organ receiving approximately 20 to 25 per cent of the cardiac output from its dual vascular supply of the portal vein (70 per cent) and hepatic artery (30 per cent). Reduced cardiac output secondary to severe impairment of left ventricular function or prolonged hypotension from any cause may lead to hepatic injury;[6] however, in most instances, clinically significant hepatic injury is absent. Similarly, thrombosis of the hepatic artery secondary to catheterization, damage at surgery, or tumour invasion is usually a clinically silent event. In some instances, however, patients develop severe right upper quadrant pain, a marked rise of serum transaminases (often greater than 10 000 IU/l), and, later, jaundice. Portal vein thrombosis may also occur secondary to tumour invasion or hypercoagulable states but usually does not lead to jaundice providing hepatic function is not otherwise compromised.

Blood coming into the liver from the hepatic artery or portal vein percolates through the hepatic sinusoids then passes through the central hepatic veins and exits the liver through the hepatic veins into the inferior vena cava. Obliteration of the small intrahepatic veins (termed veno-occlusive disease) has been associated with radiation, 6-thioguanine, azathioprine, herbal medication, and graft–versus–host disease following bone marrow or renal transplantation. Patients rapidly develop ascites, tender hepatomegaly, and, with progression, jaundice. A similar clinical picture results from the Budd–Chiari syndrome which follows thrombosis of the main hepatic veins as they enter the inferior vena cava. Budd–Chiari syndrome may complicate hypercoagulable states associated with malignancy or it may result from direct tumour invasion, particularly by hepatocellular carcinoma or renal, adrenal, and atrial tumours. The clinical syndrome may develop insidiously or rapidly. Thrombosis may also involve the inferior vena cava which is heralded by massive dependent oedema.

Post-hepatic jaundice results from high grade obstruction to biliary flow at the level of the extrahepatic bile ducts. Malignant causes include cancer of the pancreas, ampullary carcinoma, cholangiocarcinoma, and enlarged lymph nodes at the porta hepatis, but benign causes must also be considered. Gallstones in the common bile duct, acute or chronic pancreatitis, and biliary strictures secondary to previous surgery or hepatic intra-arterial chemotherapy with 5-fluorouracil[7] may also cause obstructive jaundice.

Diagnostic approach

History and physical examination are of paramount importance in narrowing the lengthy differential diagnosis of jaundice and in directing its investigation. It is particularly important to inquire about prior liver disease, alcohol intake, medications, and risk factors for hepatitis. In most patients, jaundice will be painless; however, the presence of associated abdominal pain is compatible with rapid hepatic capsular distension (for example Budd–Chiari syndrome), biliary colic, or pancreatic carcinoma where posterior radiation and exacerbation by recumbency is typical.

Dark or tea-coloured urine results from conjugated hyperbilirubinaemia and is therefore absent in prehepatic causes of jaundice. Acholic stools suggest an hepatic or post-hepatic problem; intermittently acholic stools may be caused by gallstones whereas acholic stools which persist suggests malignant obstruction or a primarily hepatic process such as viral hepatitis. Chills and fever suggest cholangitis but may occasionally accompany acute viral hepatitis. Pruritus is more common with extrahepatic obstruction or cholestasis but, like fatigue, it is not of great diagnostic value.

Deep jaundice is easily detected but more subtle degrees of jaundice will only be appreciated by careful inspection of the sclera and oral mucus membranes under natural light; this assumes even greater importance in dark-skinned individuals. Lymphadenopathy, stigmata of chronic liver disease (e.g. vascular spider naevi and palmar erythema), and oedema are important associated findings. Abdominal examination may reveal hepatomegaly which, if massive, is highly suggestive of direct tumour involvement. Viral hepatitis is associated with a smooth surfaced, tender liver, whereas irregularity of the edge suggests neoplasia or cirrhosis. A palpable gallbladder is compatible with extrahepatic obstruction. Other abdominal masses should be carefully sought. The presence of an arterial bruit over the liver points to hepatoma. Ascites is consistent with hepatic venous outflow obstruction, cirrhosis of any cause, or peritoneal carcinomatosis.

Blood tests

Liver function tests are frequently helpful in assessing the cause and severity of hepatic dysfunction. Although a mixed or intermediate pattern is often seen, derangements of liver function tests can be broadly divided into two patterns suggesting either hepatocellular injury or cholestasis/obstruction. Hepatocellular injury is characterized by a markedly increased aspartate transaminase or alanine transaminase and a variably increased bilirubin level; typical examples include viral hepatitis or injury induced by drugs such as halothane or isoniazid. Intrahepatic cholestasis and biliary obstruction are both associated with normal or only minimally elevated aspartate transaminase and a raised bilirubin. An increased serum alkaline phosphatase is a rather constant finding in obstructive jaundice but varies greatly in different types of cholestasis. Many variations exist, particularly before a given disease process is completely manifest; for example with early incomplete biliary obstruction, the bilirubin will still be normal whereas the alkaline phosphatase will be elevated.

Numerous other blood tests add supplementary information to the above basic liver function tests. Bilirubin fractionation is useful in patients with hyperbilirubinaemia but a normal aspartate transaminase and alkaline phosphatase. A predominant increase in the unconjugated bilirubin fraction is compatible with a prehepatic disorder such as Gilbert's disease or haemolysis, both of which are associated with only low grade hyperbilirubinaemia (less than 120 mmol/l). Since both fractions are increased in hepatic and post-hepatic jaundice, bilirubin fractionation is of little diagnostic aid in most patients with jaundice. Although a rising serum lactic dehydrogenase is often considered a particularly poor prognostic sign, a multivariate analysis of prognostic variables in 175 patients with hepatic metastasis secondary to colorectal carcinoma did not show independent predictive value; other liver function tests, including serum alkaline phosphatase, bilirubin, and albumin, were highly significant predictors of survival.[8] Either a 5′ nucleotidase or a γ-glutamyl transpeptidase determination are useful to confirm the hepatic source of an elevated serum alkaline phosphatase especially in patients with the potential for bony metastasis. Patients with evidence of hepatocellular injury should undergo serological testing for viral hepatitis, particularly types B and C.

Imaging

Non-invasive imaging techniques are of paramount importance in the assessment of jaundice.[9] Abdominal ultrasound, computerized tomography (CT) scanning, and scintiscanning have been studied extensively, are widely available, and are inherently safe. The role of magnetic resonance imaging in the assessment of jaundice remains under active investigation.[10]

Ultrasound and CT scanning

Abdominal ultrasound is an exceedingly useful first investigation in cases of suspected biliary obstruction. Distal common bile duct obstruction, for example secondary to ampullary carcinoma or pancreatic carcinoma, will result in dilatation of the extrahepatic biliary tree, including the gallbladder, and usually the intrahepatic ducts as well. More proximal lesions, for example cholangiocarcinoma at the hilum, will result in intrahepatic bile duct dilatation only. Although the site and nature of the obstruction are usually visualized, this technique may be limited in the following circumstances: obscured visualization of a distal obstructing lesion secondary to duodenal gas; suboptimal examination in the obese; and detection of ductal gallstones where 50 per cent may be overlooked even by experienced radiologists. In addition to detecting obstruction, ultrasound is valuable for the identification of primary and secondary hepatic tumours, occlusion of the hepatic veins in Budd–Chiari syndrome, and in ensuring patency of the hepatic artery and portal vein. This versatility makes the abdominal ultrasound the imaging procedure of first choice in the investigation of jaundice. Abdominal CT provides similar information to ultrasound; biliary obstruction and hepatic tumours are readily diagnosed and, in particular, CT scanning with intravenous contrast enhancement is of special value in the evaluation of hepatic masses. Considering the greater cost of a CT scan, it is best used as a supplement when ultrasound is inconclusive.

Iminodiacetic acid scintograms

Scintiscans employing technetium-labelled iminodiacetic acid (IDA) derivatives (e.g. HIDA scan) can usually make a reliable distinction between hepatocellular dysfunction, in which there is poor hepatic uptake of the isotope, and extrahepatic obstruction, which is characterized by hepatic isotope uptake but lack of secretion into the small bowel.[11] IDA scintograms have not been utilized widely as initial imaging techniques, however, because of poor anatomical resolution compared to ultrasound and CT scanning and due to occasional failure of obstructed livers to concentrate the isotope leading to an erroneous impression of hepatocellular injury. Nevertheless, IDA scintograms are useful in special circumstances, such as to demonstrate a bile leak or to prove biliary obstruction has been relieved (e.g. by stent placement) when the ducts are still dilated.[11]

Cholangiography

In patients with suspected or demonstrated obstruction, a cholangiogram will provide further diagnostic and anatomical details so that corrective or palliative treatment can be planned. A percutaneous transhepatic cholangiogram will successfully opacify the biliary system in over 95 per cent of obstructed patients; serious adverse effects, including bleeding, biliary leakage, and sepsis occur in less than 5 per cent.[12] In patients with severe ascites or coagulopathy, endoscopic retrograde cholangiopancreatography (**ERCP**) is preferred. ERCP is particularly valuable in individuals with suspected pancreatic disease since a pancreatogram can also be obtained. If initial ultrasound and/or CT scanning have failed to exclude a biliary stone or if endoscopic biliary drainage is being entertained, ERCP is clearly the next investigation of choice. In experienced hands, a satisfactory cholangiogram will be obtained in 80 to 90 per cent of cases; periampullary diverticulae, previous Bilroth II gastrectomy, papillary stenosis, or tumour make the procedure more technically difficult. Side-effects occur in 3 per cent of cases and include pancreatitis and cholangitis.[13] Local expertise is also a factor when choosing the most appropriate type of cholangiogram.

Liver biopsy

Liver biopsy is reserved for highly selected patients with unexplained jaundice or liver function test abnormalities in whom obstruction has been excluded or is unlikely. In each case, the possible benefits of accurate diagnosis must be weighed against the risk of biopsy. The most important and potentially lethal complication of liver biopsy is haemorrhage. Recent publication of an experience with almost 10 000 liver biopsies described non-fatal haemorrhage in 0.24 per cent and fatal haemorrhage in 0.11 per cent.[14] Risk factors for haemorrhage included advancing age, number of passes with the biopsy needle, female sex, and, notably, the presence of malignancy. Aspirin and other non-steroidal anti-inflammatory drugs induce platelet dysfunction which may predispose to bleeding; aspirin should be stopped 10 days prior to biopsy. Where liver biopsy is being used as an aid in the diagnosis of infection with hepatic involvement, tissue must also be sent for special stains and cultures for fungal, viral, mycobacterial, and bacterial pathogens. In the diagnosis of metastatic liver disease, diagnostic yield is increased using ultrasound-guided or laparoscopic-directed biopsy.[15]

Management

In view of the vast array of causes of jaundice in the palliative care patient, it is important first to consider remediable, yet potentially rapidly fatal, conditions such as ascending cholangitis. This condition is usually amenable to antibiotic therapy following endoscopic or surgical relief of obstruction. The majority of patients under consideration, however, have jaundice secondary to massive hepatic infiltration with tumours. Nevertheless, the occasional patient has an enlarged lymph node at the porta hepatis which may be responsive to radiotherapy or biliary stenting. Chemotherapy will be a consideration in some patients with potentially responsive tumours including breast cancer, small cell carcinoma of the lung, testicular and ovarian carcinomas, and lymphomas; however, most patients have relatively resistant tumours including gastrointestinal adenocarcinomas, malignant melanoma, and non-small-cell lung carcinomas. The combined use of radiation and chemotherapy has also been generally disappointing.[16]

The use of general measures can greatly add to patient comfort. Patients feel better with the correction of severe anaemia with blood transfusion. Management of pruritus is also an important consideration in patients with malignant biliary obstruction.

Pruritus

The mechanism of pruritus in cholestasis is unknown. Although bile acids have been widely implicated, other possible mediators include histamine, kallikreins, prostaglandins, substance P and, more recently suggested, endogenous opioids[17] and serotonin.[18] Whatever the stimulus, peripheral neurofilaments are activated with transmission of an impulse via unmyelinated C fibres and the spinothalamic tract to the thalamus and cerebral cortex. Although pruritus is most frequently encountered in patients with malignant biliary obstruction, it is also seen in other neoplastic conditions including polycythaemia rubra vera, Hodgkin's lymphoma, systemic mastocytosis, Waldenström's macroglobulinaemia, multiple myeloma, mycosis fungoides, carcinoid syndrome, and various forms of carcinoma.

Pruritus is occasionally refractory to treatment but can usually be at least diminished by the use of general, local, and systemic therapies. As a general measure, an air-conditioned environment may be useful since cool temperatures reduce cutaneous perspiration and lower the itch threshold. Local measures include the use of moistening agents (e.g. oatmeal and oil bath), astringents such as calamine, and the use of steroid creams. Topically applied tricyclic antidepressants, such as doxepin, have been used because of their histamine-inhibiting action with some evidence of benefit in dermatitis but their effect in obstructive jaundice with pruritus is unknown.[19]

Numerous systemic therapies have been tried, although few have been subjected to critical analysis. Most of the drugs used are suggested on the basis of uncontrolled clinical experience or extrapolation from other non-malignant conditions associated with pruritus.

Antihistamines are not uniformly effective, but may be beneficial in some patients; hydroxyzine and cyproheptadine are felt to be the most useful in this class. Similarly, phenothiazines, such as trimeprazine and prochlorperazine, have been widely recommended. Both the antihistamines and phenothiazines are likely to act by depressing the central nervous system rather than a specific peripheral effect. H_2-receptor blockers (particularly cimetidine) have been recommended, but are likely to be ineffective as single agent therapies. Cholestyramine, an ammonium ion exchange resin, at a dose of 4 g one to six times daily is particularly effective in providing relief from pruritus, perhaps by its capacity to bind bile acids and thereby prevent their absorption. At high dose, cholestyramine may impair absorption of fat soluble vitamins by reducing intestinal luminal concentrations of bile acids below a critical micellar level; patients requiring prolonged treatment may require fat soluble vitamin supplementation. There is considerable clinical experience with androgenic steroids such as methyl testosterone which will usually relieve pruritus within 1 week.[17] Norethandrolone and stanozolol may be helpful in some patients, but are not widely available. Paradoxically, these sex steroids may themselves cause cholestasis and worsening jaundice and should be used only in extreme cases. Rifampicin has been useful in alleviating pruritus in chronic cholestasis secondary to primary biliary cirrhosis[20] and other cholestatic disorders.[21] Its mechanism of action is unknown but may relate to its ability to inhibit bile acid uptake into hepatocytes, thereby preventing release of other putative 'pruritogens'.

When pruritus is severe, general and local measures should be combined with systemic drug treatment. Cholestyramine should be tried first since it is most likely to be effective. Histamine (H_1-receptor) blockers and phenothiazines should generally be tried next because they are relatively free of serious side-effects. An H_2-receptor blocker, such as cimetidine, can be added if required. Androgenic steroids or rifampicin can be tried if these first line therapies fail. Since pruritus can be particularly bothersome at night, adequate sedation is a useful added measure. It should be emphasized, however, that pruritus is most effectively palliated by relief of biliary obstruction where possible.

Other agents with reported success but from limited experience include ursodeoxycholic acid,[17] low dose propofol,[22] and ondansetron.[23] Opioid antagonists hold great promise for the relief of pruritus but beware of precipitating a withdrawal-like syndrome in patients receiving opioid analgesia.[17] Both parenteral naloxone and oral nalmefene appear to be effective.[24,25] Phototherapy has been employed in primary biliary cirrhosis with some success. Plasmapheresis has been used effectively in desperate cases of pruritus but is obviously labour intensive, expensive, and inconvenient for the patient.[17]

Relief of biliary obstruction

Patients with biliary obstruction secondary to pancreatic carcinoma, cholangiocarcinoma, and, less frequently, metastatic disease develop jaundice and pruritus and are at risk of ascending cholangitis. Surgical bypass or non-operative stenting (percutaneous or endoscopic) of the malignant stricture provides effective palliation (Fig. 1). These procedures should be performed early for best results and may prolong life, but this is unproven. Surgical bypass is usually achieved by performing either a cholecystojejunostomy or a choledochojejunostomy; the latter may provide superior relief of obstruction.[26] Surgical treatment is associated with a low incidence of recurrent jaundice and, furthermore, in patients with pancreatic carcinoma, it provides the opportunity to perform a gastroenterostomy for prophylaxis against future duodenal obstruction which will otherwise develop in 20 to 40 per cent of patients. However, biliary enteric anastomosis is associated with an operative mortality as high as 33 per cent[27] and a significant hospital stay. This invasive approach is not well suited to older and less well patients who will suffer a particularly high operative morbidity and mortality. Percutaneous transhepatic stent placement is associated with a high risk of sepsis, biliary leakage, and haemorrhage and superior results have been reported using endoscopically placed stents.[28,29] Furthermore, external drainage for preoperative decompression prior to surgical biliary bypass is associated with a higher mortality than immediate surgery.[30] Nevertheless, difficult strictures, including those involving the hepatic hilum, sometimes require transhepatic drainage or a combined approach with a guidewire passed by the percutaneous, transhepatic route through the obstruction into the duodenum followed by endoscopic stent placement over the wire.

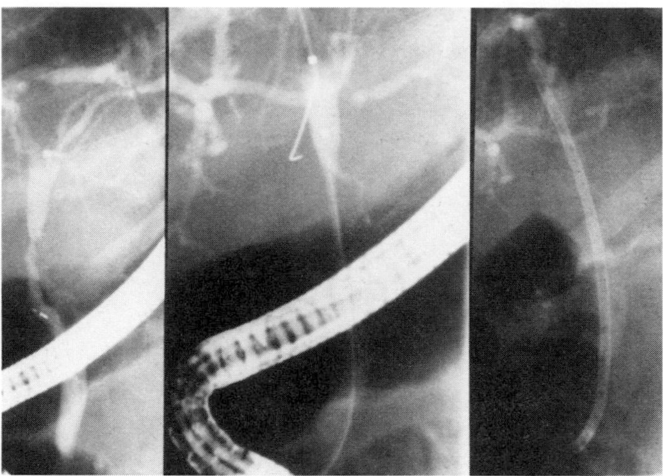

Fig. 1 These cholangiograms are from a 61-year-old male with obstructive jaundice and pruritus. A high grade stricture is shown in the common hepatic duct in the left panel. In the middle panel, the stricture is being dilated with a balloon catheter passed over a guidewire. In the right panel, a large (11.5 French) stent has been placed across the stricture from the duodenum up to the proximal intrahepatic ducts to maintain biliary drainage. His pruritus resolved within 24 h and his jaundice cleared by 10 days.

Results using stents placed endoscopically continue to improve as experience accumulates and as stent clogging is reduced by the use of superior materials (percuflex or polyurethane) and by placement of larger stents (10–12 French).[31,32] Early reports mostly included patients considered non-operable with the most advanced disease and therefore shortest life expectancy. Randomized controlled trials have compared bypass surgery to endoscopic stent placement for the relief of unresectable malignancy involving the bile ducts (principally, pancreatic carcinoma and cholangiocarcinoma).[33–35] The results suggest that endoscopic stent placement is associated with less procedure-related mortality and lower short-term morbidity and mortality than surgery. Readmission rates, however, were higher secondary to stent clogging, requiring replacement, and duodenal obstruction, requiring surgery. Both provided excellent palliation of obstruction but long-term survivals were similar in endoscopically and surgically treated patients. A retrospective cost analysis has compared endoscopical/radiological stent placement to surgical bypass.[36] Total costs including all medical costs from diagnosis to death were 50 per cent higher in the surgical group despite similar survivals in the two groups.

An important advance to reduce stent clogging utilizes expandable metal stents of several available types which can be inserted via the endoscopic or percutaneous transhepatic route (see Section 8).[37] These expand to 10 mm or 30 French! These new types of stents are expensive, but this is blunted by a reduced need for reintervention due to stent clogging. The problem of tumour ingrowth between the struts of the stent is being addressed by new

Table 2 Classification of AIDS hepatopathy

Viral hepatitis
- Hepatitis B virus, hepatitis C virus, hepatitis D virus, cytomegalovirus, Epstein–Barr virus, herpes simplex virus

Malignancy
- Kaposi's sarcoma, lymphoma

Amyloidosis

Opportunistic infection
- Mycobacteria, *Pneumocystis carinii*, cryptococcus

Drug reactions
- Trimethoprim/sulphamethoxazole, isoniazid, zidovudine (AZT), ketoconazole, pentamidine, 2',3'-dideoxyinosine

Biliary tract disease
- Sclerosing cholangitis, biliary stricture, papillary stenosis, acalculous cholecystitis

coatings such as silicone and metal stents without an open framework.

The following general guidelines have been proposed by Cotton for palliation of obstructive jaundice;[38] however, local expertise must also be considered.

1. Fit patients with small tumours should undergo laparotomy to establish unresectability and for biliary enteric bypass; many with pancreatic carcinoma will also be candidates for gastroenteric anastomosis for prophylaxis against future duodenal obstruction.

2. Patients with large tumours and poor general health should undergo endoscopic stenting. These procedures provide effective palliation by reducing jaundice, pruritus, and risk of cholangitis.

3. Moribund patients and those with a very limited life-span should simply be kept comfortable with analgesia and sedation.

4. Optimal treatment for patients lying between these spectrums is controversial and can only be addressed by future randomized controlled studies.

Hepatic abnormalities in AIDS

Despite a lack of hepatic trophism for HIV, hepatic abnormalities are very common in AIDS and have been the subject of several reviews.[39,40,41] Liver disease in AIDS seldom progresses to liver failure; however, clinicians caring for AIDS patients must be familiar with the associated spectrum of liver disease so that treatable conditions can be recognized.

The more frequently encountered afflictions of the liver in AIDS are summarized in Table 2. Due to shared risk factors, AIDS patients are at increased risk for chronic hepatitis secondary to hepatitis B virus and hepatitis C virus; however, because of marked impairment of cellular immune function, hepatic damage is usually limited, particularly for hepatitis B.[42] The liver may be involved secondarily by Kaposi's sarcoma or lymphoma, the two commonest malignancies seen in AIDS. Hepatic amyloidosis has been reported in intravenous drug users with AIDS possibly secondary to chronic suppurative skin infections resulting from dirty needles.[43] A wide variety of fungal and protozoal organisms may infect the liver; however, *Mycobacterium avium-intracellulare* is the commonest opportunistic pathogen detected histologically.[40] As in any patient with hepatic abnormalities, the possibility of a hepatotoxic reaction to self-prescribed or prescription drugs must be considered; such reactions are more common in those with underlying liver disease such as viral hepatitis. AIDS patients are frequently on investigational drugs which may have unknown hepatotoxic potential. For example fulminant hepatic failure was recently attributed to 2′,3′-dideoxyinosine (ddI) in a patient with AIDS.[44] Finally, a wide array of intrahepatic and extrahepatic biliary changes have been described recently in AIDS patients, often in association with cytomegalovirus or cryptosporidial infection.[45] These patients present with symptoms of biliary obstruction and biochemical evidence of biliary stasis.

The temptation aggressively to investigate hepatic abnormalities in AIDS must be tempered by the fact that no effective treatment exists for many of the conditions listed in Table 2. Viral hepatitis is best diagnosed serologically and can often be managed without resort to liver biopsy. The presence of hepatic malignancy can often be surmised from the existence of malignancy elsewhere. Abdominal ultrasound supplemented with CT scanning, if necessary, is useful for the detection of focal masses and to determine the presence of biliary dilatation secondary to obstruction. Biliary dilatation is best investigated by ERCP, where, if required, a therapeutic procedure can be performed concomitantly, such as endoscopic sphincterotomy for papillary stenosis.[45]

In selected patients, use of special stains and cultures on liver biopsy specimens in addition to histological examination provides a unique opportunity for the diagnosis of a wide variety of infectious and other conditions. Liver biopsy will reveal diagnostic findings in about 50 per cent of AIDS patients with abnormal liver function tests;[46,47] however, in some instances, this will only confirm infections involving more readily accessible extrahepatic sites. Liver biopsy will have greatest diagnostic yield when reserved for those patients with unexplained fever, persistently elevated serum alkaline phosphatase, or hepatomegaly.[39] Risk of bleeding should be minimized by checking coagulation status, platelet count, and bleeding time where indicated. Specific and effective therapy is seldom available; however, establishing a diagnosis will prevent further potentially invasive investigation and allows the patient's symptoms to be specifically addressed.

Ascites

The appearance of ascites in a patient with malignancy has always been considered an unfortunate event both in terms of patient comfort and its prognostic implications—1 year survival 40 per cent, 3 year survival less than 10 per cent. It has also been the source of considerable distress for the physician because it places he or she in the unenviable position of having to chose between a variety of therapeutic options that carry appreciable morbidity and mortality rates yet, for the most part, they have not been documented to be efficacious on the basis of data derived from prospective, randomized, controlled trials. Fortunately, the longstanding reluctance of investigators to design and enrol patients with terminal malignancies in such trials has given way to the realization that these data are essential for providing the most appropriate and compassionate care for these unfortunate individuals. As a result, in recent years there have been significant advances in the understanding, diagnosis, and treatment of patients with malignant ascites. These advances have resulted in a more rational approach to diagnostic interventions and an expanding list of safer, more effective therapeutic options.

Incidence of malignant ascites

Malignancy is the underlying cause of ascites in approximately 10 per cent of all cases of ascites and 15 to 50 per cent of patients with malignancy will develop ascites.[48,49] Certain tumours are especially likely to result in malignant ascites. For example the association with ovarian cancer is particularly strong, with 30 per cent of ovarian cancer patients having ascites at presentation and over 60 per cent at the time of death.[50] Other cancers that not uncommonly result in malignant ascites include cancers of the endometrium, breast, large bowel, stomach, and pancreas, which account for approximately 80 per cent of all cases of malignant ascites.[50] Less common causes include mesothelioma, non-Hodgkin's lymphoma, prostatic carcinoma, multiple myeloma, and melanoma.[51]

Classification and pathogenesis of malignant ascites

For diagnostic and therapeutic reasons, malignant ascites can be classified into four relatively distinct subtypes. In the 'central' form of malignant ascites, which constitutes approximately 15 per cent of all cases, the tumour invades the hepatic parenchyma resulting in compression of the portal venous and/or lymphatic systems. The ascites that ensues resembles that formed as a result of primary liver disease; that is, elevated hydrostatic pressure combined with decreased oncotic pressure. In central malignant ascites, however, the decreased oncotic pressure is more the result of limited protein intake and the catabolic state associated with cancer rather than defective hepatic protein synthesis.

In the 'peripheral' form of malignant ascites, which constitutes 50 per cent of cases, deposits of tumour cells are found on the surface of the parietal or visceral peritoneum. As with central ascites the formation of peripheral ascites is largely the result of mechanical interference with venous and/or lymphatic drainage but in this instance the blockage is at the level of the peritoneal space rather than the liver parenchyma. Experimentally, reduced efflux of peritoneal fluid precedes increased fluid influx.[52] There are data to suggest that vasoactive substances released from peritoneal tumour implants and non-malignant monocytes or macrophages increase capillary permeability and thereby contribute to ascites formation.[51,53]

A third form of malignant ascites could be considered a 'mixed' form in which tumour is present both in the liver and on the peritoneal surface. In this form of ascites, which constitutes 15 per cent of all cases, fluid accumulation is the result of combined central and peripheral pathophysiological processes.

The fourth type of malignant ascites is chylous malignant ascites where tumour infiltration of the retroperitoneal space causes obstruction of lymphatic flow through the lymph nodes and/or pancreas. Leakage from the lymphatic channels as a result of direct tumour invasion may also be operative in this form of malignant ascites.

Differential diagnoses

Not all ascites that develops in patients with malignancy is the result of malignancy. Pre-existing advanced liver disease with portal hypertension, portal venous thrombosis, congestive heart failure, nephrotic syndrome, pancreatitis, tuberculosis, hepatic venous obstruction, and bowel perforations should all be considered and are easily ruled out by appropriate clinical investigations.

Clinical features

History

The most frequent complaints of patients with ascites, whether it be malignant or non-malignant in nature, is abdominal bloating and pain.[54] Patients will often describe an unexplained increase in belt size or weight. Nausea and reduced appetite are common. The ascites may also result in increased reflux symptoms of heartburn or water brash. When pronounced, ascites can cause dyspnoea and orthopnoea due to elevation of the diaphragm or leakage of ascitic fluid across diaphragmatic fenestrae into the pleural space.

Physical findings

Two litres of ascitic fluid must be present for bulging of the flanks to be appreciated on physical examination.[54] When the ascites is more extensive, abdominal or inguinal hernia, scrotal oedema, and abdominal venous engorgement may appear.[55] A bruit in the abdomen of a patient with malignant ascites indicates a hypervascular tumour such as hepatocellular carcinoma, carcinoid, islet cell, leiomyosarcoma, or metastases from a renal cell carcinoma.

Extra-abdominal findings may include decreased sweating due to third-space fluid losses, pleural effusions in approximately 5 per cent of individuals with the majority of these being right sided, peripheral oedema which develops as a result of low protein concentrations in the circulation and mechanical impairment of flow in the inferior vena cava, displacement of the cardiac apex in a superiolateral direction, and distension of the neck veins due to increased right atrial and thoracic pressure.[55]

Radiological findings

Plain films of the abdomen characteristically demonstrate hazy or ground glass features, distended and separated loops of bowel, poor definition of the abdominal organs, and loss of the psoas muscle shadows.[54,56]

In general, ultrasound and CT scans of the liver are equally adept at identifying free peritoneal fluid.[57] A collection of fluid around the edge of the liver or in Morrison's pouch are the typical findings with both techniques. It has been reported that gallbladder wall thickness on ultrasound examination may be useful in distinguishing malignant (non-thickened wall) from non-malignant (thickened or double wall) ascites.[58] This is because the gallbladder wall becomes thickened in response to the hypoproteinaemia associated with chronic liver disease or nephrotic syndrome.

Ultrasound may demonstrate a number of abnormalities which serve to heighten the suspicion of malignancy in a patient with ascites. These include visualization of peritoneal metastasis, matted bowel loops, echogenic ascitic fluid, omental matting, lymphadenopathy, or other masses including hepatic metastasis.[59] A negative ultrasound, CT scan, and fluid cytology does not exclude malignant ascites. Laparoscopy will document malignancy in up to 50 per cent of such cases.[60] A modified magnetic resonance imaging technique showed high sensitivity in the diagnosis of malignant ascites in a retrospective series.[61] Specifically, peritoneal tumour was demonstrated in all 21 cases with documented malignancy.

Paracentesis

A diagnostic paracentesis of 50 to 100 ml of fluid should be performed in every case of newly diagnosed ascites. Before proceeding, potential complications should be considered and explained to the patient or next of kin. The most common complication following paracentesis is continued leakage from the puncture site but more serious complications include perforated visci with or without associated haemorrhage and peritonitis.[62] In the absence of midline scars, a site midway between the umbilicus and symphysis pubis should be chosen to minimize the risk of perforation and haemorrhage. The right or left flank in the midanterior axillary line can serve as alternate sites. The paracentesis site should be cleansed carefully and the procedure abandoned for another site if ascitic fluid is not obtained with the initial freezing needle. Ultrasound is helpful to guide paracentesis in difficult cases.

The appearance of the ascitic fluid obtained at paracentesis may provide some indication of the underlying nature of the problem. For example bile stained fluid suggests malignancy or a recent traumatic tap or biopsy.[63] A milky appearance that stains Sudan black positive indicates chylous ascites.[64] Turbid or purulent ascites is consistent with pyogenic or malignant causes.[54,55] Mucinous ascites may be found in patients with pseudomyxoma peritonei, or peritoneal metastasis from colloid carcinoma of the stomach or colon.[54] Bloody ascites is frequent with malignancy but also occurs with tuberculosis.

A number of laboratory tests have been advocated to establish the cause(s) of ascites. Of these, cytology, cell count, Gram stain with culture, and protein (albumin) concentrations have emerged as the most useful.

Cytology

It is stated that cytological examination of ascitic fluid is positive in only 50 per cent of cases where malignancy is the cause.[63] However, this disappointing figure almost certainly reflects the contribution of patients with non-peripheral forms of malignant ascites to most study populations. Indeed, by excluding patients with central or chylous ascites and submitting larger volumes (1 litre) for analysis, the results of ascitic fluid cytological examinations in patients with peripheral or mixed malignant ascites is between 80 and 100 per cent.[48] False positive results are uncommon in experienced laboratories, but when they do occur are often due to exfoliated mesothelial cells resembling malignant cells.[65]

Peritoneal biopsy is less sensitive for diagnosing malignancy (50 per cent) than tuberculosis (100 per cent) which once again may reflect the heterogeneity of malignant ascites study populations.[66]

Cell counts

Cell counts are employed to rule out bacterial peritonitis. A leukocyte count greater than 500 to 750 cells/mm^3 and a neutrophil count greater than 250 to 500 cells/mm^3 are consistent with infection.[67] Monocytosis in the ascitic fluid is often seen in patients with tuberculosis infection of the peritoneal space.

Gram stain and culture

A combination of gram stain and direct inoculation of 10 ml of ascitic fluid into aerobic and anaerobic blood culture tubes at the patient's bedside result in positive identification of the causative organism in approximately 90 per cent of cases compared to only 40 per cent when conventional ascitic fluid culture methods are employed.[68]

Protein (albumin) concentrations

In a patient with malignancy and no underlying hepatic, cardiac, or renal disease, an ascitic fluid protein concentration of less than 25 g/l or 50 per cent that of serum protein (transudative ascites) is suggestive of central or mixed malignant ascites. If on the other hand, the ascitic fluid protein concentration is greater than 25 g/l or 50 per cent that of serum protein (exudative ascites) peripheral malignant ascites is more likely.[48] One must keep in mind, however, that ascitic fluid protein concentrations should not be interpreted in isolation. For example the use of diuretics or albumin infusions prior to paracentesis will increase ascitic fluid protein concentrations and thereby transform transudative ascites to an exudative pattern.[69,70] Similarly, large intravenous infusions of crystalloid will decrease ascitic fluid protein concentrations and in the process transform an exudative ascites to a transudative pattern.[71] A more useful test for determining the type of malignant ascites is the difference between serum and ascitic albumin concentrations where a difference of less than 11 g/l is consistent with peripheral malignant ascites whereas values greater than 11 g/l suggest either central or mixed malignant ascites.[72] In essence, an ascitic–serum difference greater than 11 g/l denotes portal hypertension secondary to hepatic metastasis.

Tests that have been reported to be useful in distinguishing malignant from non-malignant ascites include raised levels of ascitic fluid fibronectin,[73] isoamylase,[74] lactic dehydrogenase,[75] α-fetoprotein,[48] carcinoembryonic antigen,[76] β-human chorionic gonadotrophin,[76] ovarian cancer-associated antigen 125,[77] ferritin,[78] cholesterol, and triglyceride concentrations.[79,80] Unfortunately, in each case the overlap between malignant and non-malignant groups as well as between the different types of malignant ascites, particularly those with central and mixed forms, is such that these tests are often unhelpful individually. Elevated serum alkaline phosphatase levels may be of value in distinguishing patients with central malignant ascites from those with non-malignant ascites secondary to advanced liver disease. The same test may also help to distinguish patients with mixed malignant ascites from those with a peripheral form in whom serum alkaline phosphatase levels are generally normal.[48]

Treatment

Treatment for malignant ascites consists of instituting palliative measures without the expectation that survival might be altered. Exceptions include patients with ovarian cancer in whom survival can be prolonged with surgical intervention and adjuvant therapy,[54] and patients with malignant ascites secondary to lymphoma who respond to radiation and/or chemotherapy.[54] Hormonally sensitive malignancies such as some breast cancers also deserve separate consideration.

Medical therapy

As for ascitic patients with advanced liver disease, patients with the central form (hepatic metastasis with portal hypertension) of malignant ascites often have increased renal sodium and water retention. Therefore, restriction of their sodium intake to 100 mmol/day or less is indicated. Fluid restriction is reserved for patients with moderate to severe hyponatraemia, that is less than 125 mmol/l. Spironolactone (100–400 mg/day) is the diuretic of choice but frusemide (40–80 mg/day) may be required to initiate a diuresis. Care must be taken to avoid overdiuresis which can precipitate electrolyte imbalances, hepatic encephalopathy, and prerenal failure. There is no theoretical reason to expect sodium and fluid restriction or diuretics to be of use in patients with peripheral (peritoneal tumour spread) or chylous forms of malignant ascites and a recent clinical series has borne this out. Furthermore, diuretic complications were frequent in this patient subgroup.[81] However, a trial of sodium restriction and diuretics may prove worthwhile in patients with the mixed form of malignant ascites A low fat diet and an increase in medium chain triglyceride intake may be useful in patients with chylous ascites.[64,82]

Therapeutic paracentesis

Large volume paracentesis significantly shortens the hospital stay for patients with tense ascites (from a mean of 30 days to 10 days) without increasing morbidity or mortality when compared to medical therapy.[83] The removal of 5 l/day until the abdomen is 'dry' is generally well tolerated by patients, particularly those with peripheral oedema who call upon their peripheral reserve of fluid for rapid restoration of effective circulating volume.[84] Intravenous albumin (6 g/l of ascitic fluid removed) should be provided[85,86] and will effectively reduce the complications of hypovolaemia, prerenal failure, and hyponatraemia. Total paracentesis, which consists of complete drainage of all ascitic fluid at one session, affords the ascitic patient the most prompt relief from their discomfort and the earliest possible discharge from hospital,[87,88] but it is important to stress that the data generated to date on large or total volume paracentesis has been derived from patients with non-malignant ascites. Whether the same promising results can be extrapolated to patients with malignant ascites remains to be determined. A reasonable approach is to remove 5 to 10 l of ascitic fluid to provide symptomatic relief. This can usually be accomplished on an outpatient basis.

Peritoneovenous shunts

Peritoneovenous shunts drain ascitic fluid from the peritoneal space into the internal jugular vein. A properly functioning shunt limits the need for dietary or fluid restrictions, diuretics, and hospital admission for paracentesis. The shunt can be inserted during a 30 to 60 min procedure under local anaesthesia. The original studies in cirrhotics with the Denver or LeVeen shunts (the former having a pressure sensitive valve-chamber that can be manipulated manually by the patient) resulted in palliation for 75 to 85 per cent of patients who survived the shunt procedure.[89,90] Unfortunately, the results in patients with malignant ascites have been less impressive, presumably due to the high protein concentrations and decreased flow obtained with the peripheral form of malignant ascites.[91,92] Shunt related operative mortality figures in patients with advanced liver disease are significantly higher (30 per cent) than for patients with malignant ascites (15 per cent) suggesting that operative mortality is primarily due to advanced liver disease rather than the shunt *per se*.[90] Morbidity rates are high (40–60 per cent) in all patients who require this form of therapy.[90,92] Some of the more serious complications include disseminated intravascular coagulation (50 per cent), upper gastrointestinal bleeds (45 per cent), sepsis (20 per cent), pulmonary oedema (14 per cent), thromboembolism (10 per cent), as well as superior vena caval thrombosis, pneumonia, hepatic coma, and neoplastic seeding of subcutaneous tissue but not systemic spread.[89,90] In patients with malignant ascites, disseminated intravascular coagulation may be less frequent.[93] Less serious, but common, complications include shunt malfunction and ascitic fluid leakage around the insertion site. Removal of at least 50 to 70 per cent of ascitic fluid and/or replacement with normal saline at the time of shunt insertion will significantly decrease shunt related morbidity and mortality.[90] Prophylactic antibiotics should be used perioperatively in all patients. Specific contraindications to shunt therapy include haemorrhagic or proteinaceous (more than 45 g/l) ascitic fluid, patients with recent or recurrent bacterial peritonitis or encephalopathy, bilirubin values above 100 μmol/l, advanced coagulopathy, large oesophageal varices, and kidney failure. In brief, severely ill patients are poor candidates for this procedure.

Recently, a non-randomized, controlled experience was reported in 85 patients with malignant ascites. Peritoneovenous shunts (of both LeVeen and Denver type) were compared to non-operative management which utilized primarily diuretics and paracentesis.[93] The authors acknowledged significant selection bias since patients with faster ascites accumulation postparacentesis were most likely to be shunted. In this series, paracentesis and shunting were of equivalent efficacy in improving the patients' quality of life. Shunting preserved serum albumin while paracentesis diminished it. No particular type of shunt was superior with a 50 per cent occlusion rate at 7 months. Tumour type and positive cytology did not affect shunt patency in contrast to previous studies, however, avoidance in blood-stained or pseudomyxomatous ascites was advocated.[93]

Surgical intervention

Surgical intervention for malignant ascites has met with only limited success. The formation of a pedical flap from intestinal mucosa in an attempt to increase absorptive capacity has not been accepted as a worthwhile procedure.[94] Neither has the creation of a peritoneovesicular drain despite promising results and a lack of complications in a small group of patients.[95] A review of 20 patients with pancreatic malignancy and peritoneal carcinomatosis treated surgically found that none of 12 patients with malignancy and ascites survived beyond 30 postoperative days.[96]

Pharmacological therapy

Radioactive isotopes were the first agents to be employed in an attempt to decrease ascitic fluid formation.[97] Although favourable responses were reported (30–70 per cent of cases) with ^{63}Zn, followed by ^{198}Au and then ^{32}P, the high incidence of side-effects (50 per cent) including nausea, pain, fever, and, in the case of ^{198}Au, bone marrow suppression, as well as the risk of radiation exposure to hospital staff, eventually limited their use.[97-100] Moreover, these agents are expensive, have a short half-life and due to radiation safety requirements are confined to use by large treatment centres.

As a result, radioisotopes eventually gave way to trials of sclerosing agents (nitrogen mustard, quinacrine, doxorubicin), mild irritants (bleomycin, tetracycline, cisplatin), and non-sclerosant agents (methotrexate, thiotepa, 5-fluorouracil). The results achieved with these agents are difficult to interpret due to the differences in the parameters of response, small number of patients involved, retrospective nature of the studies and lack of comparative data.[101-106] Due to the potential toxicity of these agents when given intraperitoneally, it seems prudent to avoid their use until the results of prospective controlled clinical trials are available.

Most recently, intraperitoneal α- or β-interferon have been used for malignant ascites in uncontrolled trials. Response rates approximating 40 per cent at 1 month have been reported with recurrence in the majority by 3 months.[100] Side-effects include influenza-like symptoms, local pain, and fever but generally these agents were well tolerated. A preliminary positive experience with intraperitoneal recombinant tumour necrosis factor-α in malignant ascites has been reported as well.[107] A review of intracavity treatments for malignant effusions has been published recently.[100]

A logical approach to the management of malignant ascites, therefore, starts with sodium restriction and diuretics particularly in those with the central form of ascites (liver metastasis) or a serum-ascitic albumin concentration difference greater than 11 g/l. Non-responding patients will benefit from either repeated paracentesis or insertion of a peritoneovenous shunt in highly selected populations where expertise is available. Intraperitoneal agents remain unproven, but some of the biological agents (α- or β-interferon, tumour necrosis factor-α) hold promise and controlled trials are awaited.

Hepatic encephalopathy

Hepatic encephalopathy is a complex neuropsychiatric syndrome characterized by disturbance of consciousness, personality, and intellect together with altered neuromuscular activity and electroencephalographic (**EEG**) abnormalities. It arises most frequently in patients with endstage cirrhosis from any cause but may also occur in patients with extensive hepatic metastasis. Many cirrhotics are not liver transplant candidates and will benefit from the measures described below for cancer patients. In fact, most of the research underlying our current treatments for hepatic encephalopathy was conducted in cirrhotic patients.

Unlike malignant ascites, hepatic encephalopathy is often considered an almost welcome event in the course of the terminally ill patient. Its onset often marks the beginning of a process wherein anxiety and discomfort are attenuated and give way to a peaceful state of repose. The major task facing the physician caring for terminally ill patients with hepatic encephalopathy is to determine whether treatment of the encephalopathy will result in a meaningful survival period or a lightening of the mental state that only serves to allow the patient to become more aware of their suffering.

Pathogenesis

The pathogenesis of hepatic encephalopathy remains unclear. Early hypotheses suggesting that hypoxaemia, hypoglycaemia, or a deficiency of essential nutrients produced by the liver have since been discounted. Similarly, more recent hypotheses regarding ammonia, false neurotransmitters, and GABAergic neurotransmission abnormalities all leave a number of important questions and observations unanswered.[108] The most recent hypothesis implicates endogenous benzodiazepine-like compounds which have been found in increased concentrations in the central nervous system of patients with liver failure.[109] These compounds may increase GABAergic neurotransmission which is inhibitory to many neural processes. Perhaps there is no one encephalopathogenic factor but rather a combination of many if not all the hitherto proposed compounds. A recent review cites mounting evidence for 'neurotransmission failure' possibly as a result of chronic central nervous system exposure to ammonia.[110]

Diagnosis

Clinical features

The most common presenting features of hepatic encephalopathy are drowsiness, reversal of day/night sleep patterns, and difficulty with concentration. As the encephalopathy becomes more advanced, confusion may develop. By this time, abnormalities in spatial diagnosis, as reflected by inability of the patient to draw concentric circles or five-pointed stars, become evident. Other physical signs may include fetor hepaticus (an odd, sweetish smell of breath thought to be secondary to increased mercaptan concentrations), hyperactive tendon reflexes, and, ultimately, decerebrate posturing. The speech of the encephalopathic patient is slow, slurred, and monotonous. Asterixis, an often sought and important clinical feature of hepatic encephalopathy, is tested by fixed extension of the forearms, dorsiflexion of the wrists, and fanning of the digits with eyes opened and then closed. A rapid, forward flexion of the hands at the metacarpophalangeal joints with further fanning of the fingers reflects decreased afferent (proprioceptive) input to the reticular activating system. Once the encephalopathy has advanced to the stage of coma, asterixis, like many of the other motor abnormalities, is no longer present. Prior to overt hepatic encephalopathy more sensitive tests, such as psychometric testing, standard electroencephalograms, or visual evoked potential responses, may detect subclinical abnormalities.

Laboratory tests

Biochemical tests

The laboratory findings that are most useful in establishing the diagnosis of hepatic encephalopathy and at the same time correlate well with the clinical course of the patient are an increase in glutamine and α-ketoglutarate levels in the cerebrospinal fluid.[111] However, these tests are rarely carried out due in part to concerns regarding the performance of a lumbar puncture in patients with severe bleeding diatheses as well as a desire to limit the number of uncomfortable and invasive procedures in terminally ill patients. More readily available, but at the same time less specific, are a series of biochemical abnormalities that include elevated plasma ammonia, aromatic amino acids, short-chain fatty acids, and mercaptan levels and decreased plasma branched chain amino acid concentrations.[112] Of these, the plasma ammonia levels (venous or arterial) are most useful since they are markedly elevated in 90 per cent of encephalopathic patients while only rarely elevated beyond two to three times normal in other conditions which alter cerebral function. Despite helping to distinguish hepatic encephalopathy

Table 3 Differential diagnosis of hepatic encephalopathy

Metabolic	Organ failure	Toxic	Intracerebral
Hypoglycaemia	Cardiac	Drugs	Haemorrhage
Hyponatraemia	Respiratory	Sedatives	Metastasis
Anoxia	Renal	Tranquillizers	Meningitis
Hyperosmolar coma		Diuretics	Abscess
Prerenal azotaemia		Hypnotics	
		Alcohol withdrawal	
		Wernicke–Korsakoff's syndrome	

from other causes of confusion, ammonia levels do not correlate well with the course of the illness or with severity.

Non-biochemical tests

Psychometric tests have been used in diagnosing early (preclinical) hepatic encephalopathy.[113,114] These tests have also been found to be helpful in following the course of the disease, a feature that is becoming increasingly important as new therapeutic modalities are being considered. Of the many psychometric tests that can be applied, the Reitan trail-making or number connection test has achieved the most popularity.[115] This test involves having the patient connect a series of scattered numbers from 1 to 50 while being timed with a stop watch. Their time is compared to standards established for normal, mild, moderate, and severe encephalopathy. It is more sensitive than most other psychometric tests including the five-pointed star construction test, signature test, or subtraction of serial sevens test, and is easier to quantify.

Proton magnetic resonance spectroscopy is very sensitive in the diagnosis of both subclinical and overt hepatic encephalopathy using clinical and neuropsychiatric testing as the gold standard.[116] The specificity of this technique, using encephalopathic patients due to a variety of other disturbances, has not been established.

The EEG abnormalities observed in patients with hepatic encephalopathy are non-specific. Similar if not identical changes are seen in patients with encephalopathy secondary to advanced renal disease or other severe metabolic disturbances which are common with advanced malignancy. Nonetheless, the presence of low-frequency, high-amplitude waveforms in a patient with advanced liver disease, a decreased level of consciousness, and no alternative explanation for the latter finding is strong supportive evidence for the diagnosis of hepatic encephalopathy.[117] Moreover, the extent of the abnormality on EEG correlates well with the patient's clinical status. Although problems with specificity are common, the sensitivity of EEGs are excellent. Indeed, abnormalities compatible with hepatic encephalopathy may be present well prior to the appearance of clinical features and may remain abnormal once clinical features have resolved. In clinical practice, however, the diagnosis is usually made without an EEG on the basis of typical clinical findings in a patient with liver disease or extensive hepatic metastasis.

Differential diagnosis

Table 3 lists disorders which may be difficult to distinguish from hepatic encephalopathy. Fortunately, clinical examination and simple laboratory and/or radiological investigations will often identify their presence. A high index of suspicion is required to consider and exclude these possibilities.

Table 4 Stepwise approach to hepatic encephalopathy

Exclude other causes of encephalopathy (Table 3)
Stop all sedatives, tranquillizers, hypnotics, and diuretics
Correct any precipitating factors: Azotaemia
- Gastrointestinal bleeding
- Hypokalaemia/alkalosis
- Excessive dietary protein
- Infection
- Constipation

Reduce dietary protein to 40 g/day (0.5 g/kg)
Add lactulose or lactitol (oral, nasogastric, or by enema)
If response inadequate, add a non-absorbable antibiotic e.g. neomycin, metronidazole, rifaximine
Other measures:
- Flumazenil
- Sodium benzoate
- Vegetable protein diet

Treatment

In general, if hepatic encephalopathy has clearly been precipitated by an established cause, rather than the result of progressive tumour infiltration of the liver, and the patient was not in distress prior to its onset, treatment should be instituted and a complete return to the pre-encephalopathic state expected. On the other hand, if the onset of encephalopathy is the result of relentless destruction of the liver or the patient was in poor medical condition prior to encephalopathy then instituting specific therapy may not be appropriate. The three most common precipitating factors are: prerenal azotaemia secondary to aggressive use of diuretics and/or persistent vomiting/diarrhoea; over use of tranquillizers, sedatives, or analgesics; and overt or covert gastrointestinal haemorrhage from varices, peptic ulceration, or gastritis.[118] Other precipitating factors include an increased dietary protein intake, hypokalaemic alkalosis (often secondary to diuretics), bacterial infection, and constipation. While searching for and treating these precipitating factors a number of non-specific therapeutic interventions can be employed. A stepwise approach to hepatic encephalopathy is provided in Table 4.

The removal of protein breakdown products from the gut is helpful since gut-derived toxins (e.g. ammonia) play an important role in the pathogenesis. This can be achieved by reducing protein in the diet to approximately 40 g/day, by administering non-absorbable antibiotics active against gram negative and anaerobic intestinal bacteria, and by the use of purgatives. Following protein restriction, the usual approach is to add a non-absorbable disaccharide such as lactulose or lactitol in a dose sufficient to induce one to two loose stools per day. A meta-analysis examining the published randomized controlled trials comparing these two cathartics concluded that they are equally efficacious in the treatment of hepatic encephalopathy and that they have similar side-effect profiles.[119] Nevertheless, patients generally prefer lactitol over lactulose because of better palatability and less flatulence.

In patients not responding to the above measures, a non-absorbable antibiotic can be added, such as neomycin,[120] metronidazole, or rifaximine.[121] This will reduce intraluminal generation of ammonia and possibly other neurotoxins.

The results of early uncontrolled studies suggest that enteral or parenteral administration of branched chain amino acids is effective in patients with hepatic encephalopathy.[122] Subsequently, prospective, randomized, controlled trials, with the possible exception of studies using ketoanalogues, were unable to confirm these early findings.[123] Although perhaps not effective for hepatic encephalopathy, the use of branched chain amino acids appears to be a safe and beneficial, albeit expensive, mode of providing protein calories to the encephalopathic patient with a terminal illness.

A small, randomized crossover study tested the effect of dietary vegetable protein versus animal protein in cirrhotics with chronic encephalopathy despite optimal lactulose therapy. The diet consisting of mainly vegetable protein was associated with improved encephalopathy (clinical grading and psychometric testing) but the effect was not marked.[124]

A randomized controlled trial has shown sodium benzoate, a food preservative and ammonia-lowering agent, to be as effective as lactulose in hepatic encephalopathy at a lower cost;[125] however, clinical experience with sodium benzoate is still limited.

The most recent development in the treatment of hepatic encephalopathy is the use of benzodiazepine antagonists, such as flumazenil, which interfere with the binding of endogenous, benzodiazepine-like ligands to their receptor sites on the GABA receptor complex. These agents have been shown to reverse hepatic encephalopathy in animal models, and to induce marked and rapid, but transient, improvements in humans with chronic liver disease and encephalopathy. Recently, the first randomized trial of flumazenil in cirrhotics has shown improvement in about 45 per cent of cirrhotics with severe hepatic encephalopathy versus no improvement in any of the controls.[126] Unfortunately, the improvement was incomplete and transient, consistent with a multifactorial pathogenesis of hepatic encephalopathy. The role of flumazenil and related investigational compounds in patients with malignancy has not been studied. Possible applications include patients in whom the cause of encephalopathy is unclear, patients having received benzodiazepines, and, possibly, to provide prognostic information.

References

1. Jaffe BM, Donegan WL, Watson F, Spratt JS. Factors influencing survival in patients with untreated liver metastases. *Surgery Gynecology and Obstetrics*, 1968; **127**: 1–11.
2. Myszor MF, Record CD. Primary and secondary malignant disease of the liver and fulminant hepatic failure. *Journal of Clinical Gastroenterology*, 1990; **12**: 441–6.
3. Choo QL, Kuo G, Weiner AJ, Overby LR, Bradley DW, Houghton M. Isolation of a cDNA clone derived from a blood-borne non-A, non-B viral hepatitis genome. *Science*, 1989; **244**: 359–62.
4. Pinto PC, Hu E, Bernstein-Singer M, Pinter-Brown L, Govindarajan S. Acute hepatic injury after the withdrawal of immunosuppressive chemotherapy in patients with hepatitis B. *Cancer*, 1990; **65**: 878–84.
5. Bass NM, Ockner RK. Drug induced liver disease. In: Zakim D, Boyer TD, eds. *Hepatology. A Textbook of Liver Disease*. Philadelphia: WB Saunders Co, 1990: 754–91.
6. Cohen JA, Kaplan MM. Left sided heart failure presenting as hepatitis. *Gastroenterology*, 1978; **74**: 583–7.
7. Shea WJ, Demas BE, Goldberg HI, Hohn DC, Ferrell LD, Kerlan RK. Sclerosing cholangitis associated with hepatic arterial FUDR: Radiographic-histologic correlation. *American Journal of Roentgenology*, 1986; **146**: 717–21.
8. Lahr CJ, *et al*. A multifactorial analysis of prognostic factors in patients with liver metastases from colorectal carcinoma. *Journal of Clinical Oncology*, 1983; **1**: 720–6.
9. Dick R, Dooley J. Jaundice in adults. In: Dooley J, Dick R, Viamonte Jr M, Sherlock S, eds. *Imaging in Hepatobiliary Disease*. Oxford: Blackwell, 1987: 3–36.
10. Kanzer GK, Weinreb JC. Magnetic resonance imaging of diseases of the liver and biliary system. In: The Radiologic Clinics of North America. *Imaging of the Liver and Biliary Tree*. Philadelphia: WB Saunders, 1991; **29**: 1259–84.
11. Drane WE. Nuclear medicine techniques for the liver and biliary system. Update for the 1990's. In: The Radiologic Clinics of North America. *Imaging of the Liver and Biliary Tree*. Philadelphia: WB Saunders, 1991; **29**: 1129–50.
12. Mueller PR, VanSonnenberg E, Simeone JF. Fine needle transhepatic cholangiography. Indication and usefulness. *Annals of Internal Medicine*, 1982; **97**: 567–72.
13. Bilbao MK, Dotter CT, Lee TG, Katon RM. Complications of ERCP. A study of 10 000 cases. *Gastroenterology*, 1976; **70**: 314–20.
14. McGill DB, Rakela J, Zinsmeister AR, Ott BJ. A 21 year experience with major hemorrhage after percutaneous liver biopsy. *Gastroenterology*, 1990; **99**: 1396–1400.
15. Jori GP, Peschle C. Combined peritoneoscopy and liver biopsy in the diagnosis of hepatic neoplasm. *Gastroenterology*, 1972; **63**: 1016–19.
16. Ajlouni MI, Merrick HW, Skeel RT, Dobelbower Jr RR. Concomitant radiation therapy and constant infusion FUDR for unresectable hepatic metastases. *American Journal of Clinical Oncology*, 1990; **13**: 532–5.
17. Khandelwal M, Malet PF. Pruritus associated with cholestasis. A review of pathogenesis and management. *Digestive Diseases and Sciences*, 1994; **39**: 1–8.
18. Richardson BP. Serotonin and nociception. *Annals of the New York Academy of Sciences*, 1990; **600**: 511–20.
19. Anonymous. Doxepin cream for pruritus. *Medical Letter on Drugs and Therapeutics*, 1994; **36**: 99–100.
20. Ghent CN, Carruthers SG. Treatment of pruritus in primary biliary cirrhosis with rifampin. Results of a double-blind crossover randomized trial. *Gastroenterology*, 1988; **94**: 488–93.
21. Gregorio GV, Ball CS, Mowat AP, Mieli-Vergani G. Effect of rifampicin in the treatment of pruritus in hepatic cholestasis. *Archives of Disease in Childhood*, 1993; **69**: 141–3.
22. Borgeat A, Wilder-Smith OH, Mentha G. Subhypnotic doses of propofol relieve pruritus associated with liver disease. *Gastroenterology*, 1993; **104**: 244–7.
23. Radereer M, Muller C, Scheithauer W. Ondansetron for pruritus due to cholestasis (letter). *New England Journal of Medicine*, 1994; **330**: 1540.
24. Bergasa NV, *et al*. A controlled trial of naloxone infusions for the pruritus of chronic cholestasis. *Gastroenterology*, 1992; **102**: 544–9.
25. Jones EA, Bergasa NV. The pruritus of cholestasis and the opioid system. *Journal of the American Medical Association*, 1992; **268**: 3359–62.

26. Rosemurgy AS, Burnett CM, Wasselle JA. A comparison of choledochoenteric bypass and cholcystoenteric bypass in patients with biliary obstruction due to pancreatic cancer. *American Surgeon*, 1989; **55**: 55–60.
27. Schouten JT. Operative therapy for pancreatic carcinoma. *American Journal of Surgery*, 1986; **151**: 626–30.
28. Joseph PK, Bizer LF, Sprayregen SS, Gliedman ML. Percutaneous transhepatic biliary drainage. Results and complications in 81 patients. *Journal of the American Medical Association*, 1986; **255**: 2763–7.
29. Speer AG, *et al.* Randomized trial of endoscopic versus percutaneous stent insertion in malignant obstructive jaundice. *Lancet*, 1987; **2**: 57–62.
30. McPherson GAD, Benjamin IS, Hodgson HJF, Bowley NB, Allison DJ, Blumgart LH. Preoperative percutaneous transhepatic biliary drainage: The results of a controlled trial. *British Journal of Surgery*, 1984; **71**: 371–5.
31. Lammer J, Neumayer K. Biliary drainage endoprosthesis: experience with 201 placements. *Radiology*, 1986; **159**: 625–9.
32. Siegel JH, Pullano W, Kodsi B, Cooperman A, Ramsey W. Optimal palliation of malignant bile duct obstruction: experience with endoscopic 12 French prosthesis. *Endoscopy*, 1988; **20**: 137–41.
33. Andersen JR, Sorensen SM, Kruse A, Rokkjaer M, Matzen P. Randomized trial of endoscopic endoprosthesis versus operative bypass in malignant obstructive jaundice. *Gut*, 1989; **30**: 1132–5.
34. Shepherd HA, Royle G, Ross AP, Diba A, Arthur M, Colin-Jones D. Endoscopic biliary endoprosthesis in the palliation of malignant obstruction of the distal common bile duct: a randomized trial. *British Journal of Surgery*, 1988; **75**: 1166–8.
35. Dowsett JF, *et al.* Malignant obstructive jaundice: a prospective randomized trial of bypass surgery versus endoscopic stenting. *Gastroenterology*, 1989; **96**: A128.
36. Brandabur JJ, *et al.* Nonoperative versus operative treatment of obstructive jaundice in pancreatic cancer: cost and survival analysis. *American Journal of Gastroenterology*, 1988; **83**: 1132–9.
37. Lameris JS, Stoker J. Metal stents for malignant biliary obstruction. *Digestive Diseases*, 1994; **12**: 161–9.
38. Cotton PB. Nonsurgical palliation of jaundice in pancreatic cancer. *Surgical Clinics of North America*, 1989; **69**: 613–27.
39. Lebovics E, Thung SN, Schaffner F, Radensky PW. The liver in the acquired immunodeficiency syndrome: A clinical and histologic study. *Hepatology*, 1985; **5**: 293–8.
40. Schneiderman DJ, Arenson DM, Cello JP, Margaretten W, Weber TE. Hepatic disease in patients with the acquired immune deficiency syndrome. *Hepatology*, 1987; **7**: 925–30.
41. Cappell MS. Hepatobiliary manifestations of the acquired immune deficiency syndrome. *American Journal of Gastroenterology*, 1991; **86**: 1–15.
42. Dworkin BM, *et al.* The liver in acquired immune deficiency syndrome: emphasis on patients with intravenous drug use. *American Journal of Gastroenterology*, 1987; **82**: 231–6.
43. Osick LA, *et al.* Hepatic amyloidosis in intravenous drug abusers and AIDS patients. *Journal of Hepatology*, 1993; **19**: 79–84.
44. Lai KK, Gang DL, Zawacki JK, Cooley TP. Fulminant hepatic failure associated with ddI. *Annals of Internal Medicine*, 1991; **115**: 283–4.
45. Cello JP. Acquired immunodeficiency syndrome cholangiopathy: Spectrum of disease. *American Journal of Medicine*, 1989; **86**: 539–46.
46. Gordon SC, *et al.* The spectrum of liver disease in the acquired immunodeficiency syndrome. *Journal of Hepatology*, 1986; **2**: 475–84.
47. Cappell MS, Schwartz MS, Biempica L. Clinical utility of liver biopsy in patients with serum antibodies to the human immunodeficiency virus. *American Journal of Medicine*, 1990; **88**: 123–30.
48. Runyon BA, Hoefs JC, Morgan TR. Ascitic fluid analysis in malignancy-related ascites. *Hepatolology*, 1988; **8**: 1104–9.
49. Runyon BA. Ascites. In: Schiff L, Schiff ER, eds. *Diseases of the Liver*, 7th edn. Philadelphia, PA: Lippincott Company, 1993: 990–1015.
50. Lifshitz S. Ascites, pathophysiology and control measures. *International Journal of Radiation Oncology Biology and Physiology*, 1982; **8**: 1423–6.
51. Garrison RN, Kaelin LD, Heuser LS, Galloway RH. Malignant ascites: clinical and experimental observations. *Annals of Surgery*, 1986; **203**: 644–51.
52. Nagy JA, Herzberg KT, Dvorak JM, Dvorak HF. Pathogenesis of malignant ascites formation: initiating events that lead to fluid accumulation. *Cancer Research*, 1993; **53**: 2631–43.
53. Yeo KT, *et al.* Vascular permeability factor in guinea pig and human tumour and inflammatory effusions. *Cancer Research*, 1993; **53**: 2912–18.
54. Tabbarah HJ, Casciato DA. Malignant effusions. In: Haskell CM, ed. *Cancer Treatment*. Philadelphia, PA: W.B. Saunders Company, 1990: 815–25.
55. Sherlock S. Ascites. In: Sherlock S, Dooley J, eds. *Diseases of the Liver and Biliary System*, 9th edn. Oxford: Blackwell Scientific Publications, 1993: 114–31.
56. Keeffe EJ, Gagliardi RA, Pfister RC. The roentgenographic evaluation of ascites. *American Journal of Roentgenology*, 1967; **101**: 388–96.
57. Callen PW, Marks WM, Filly RA. Computed tomography and ultrasonography in the evaluation of the retroperitoneum in patients with malignant ascites. *Journal of Computer Assisted Tomography*, 1979; **3**: 581–4.
58. Huan YS, Lee SD, Wu JC, Wang SS, Lin HC, Tsai YT. Utility of sonographic gallbladder wall patterns in differentiating malignant from cirrhotic ascites. *Journal of Clinical Ultrasound*, 1989; **17**: 187–92.
59. Goerg C, Schwerk WB. Malignant ascites: sonographic signs of peritoneal carcinomatosis. *European Journal of Cancer*, 1991; **27**: 720–3.
60. Brady PG, Peebles M, Goldschmid S. Role of laparoscopy in the evaluation of patients with suspected hepatic or peritoneal malignancy. *Gastrointestinal Endoscopy*, 1991; **37**: 27–30.
61. Low RN, Sigeti JS. MR imaging of peritoneal disease: comparison of contrast-enhanced fast multiplanar spoiled gradient recalled and spin—echo imaging. *American Journal of Roentgenology*, 1994; **163**: 1131–40.
62. Runyon BA. Paracentesis of ascitic fluid: a safe procedure. *Archives of Internal Medicine*, 1986; **146**: 2259–61.
63. Malden LT, Tattersall MHN. Malignant effusions. *Quarterly Journal of Medicine*, 1986; **227**: 221–39.
64. Press, OW, Press NO, Kaufman SD. Evaluation and management of chylous ascites. *Annals of Internal Medicine*, 1982; **96**: 358–64.
65. Anonymous. Diagnosis of ascites. *British Medical Journal*, 1981; **282**: 1499.
66. Levine H. Needle biopsy of peritoneum in exudative ascites. *Archives of Internal Medicine*, 1967; **120**: 542–5.
67. Yang CY, *et al.* White count, pH and lactate in ascites in the diagnosis of spontaneous bacterial peritonitis. *Hepatology*, 1985; **5**: 85–90.
68. Runyon BA. Spontaneous bacterial peritonitis: an explosion of information. *Hepatology*, 1988; **8**: 171–5.
69. Hoefs JC. Increase in ascites white blood cell and protein concentrations during diuresis in patients with chronic liver disease. *Hepatology*, 1981; **1**: 249–54.
70. Dykes PW. A study of the effects of albumin infusions in patients with cirrhosis of the liver. *Quarterly Journal of Medicine*, 1961; **30**: 297.
71. Mankin H, Lowell A. Osmotic factors influencing the formation of ascites in patients with cirrhosis of the liver. *Journal of Clinical Investigation*, 1948; **27**: 145.
72. Mauer K, Manzione NC. Usefulness of serum-ascites albumin difference in separating transudative from exudative ascites. Another look. *Digestive Diseases and Sciences*, 1988; **33**: 1208–12.
73. Adamsen S, Jonsson P, Brodin B, Lindberg B, Jorpes P. Measurement of fibronectin concentration in benign and malignant ascites. *European Journal of Surgery*, 1991; **157**: 325–8.
74. Kosches DS, Sosnowik D, Lendvai S, Bank S. Unusual anodic migrating isoamylase differentiates selected malignant from nonmalignant ascites. *Journal of Clinical Gastroenterology*, 1989; **11**: 43–6.
75. Boyer TD, Kahn AN, Reynolds TB. Diagnostic value of ascitic fluid lactic dehydrogenase, protein and WBC levels. *Archives of Internal Medicine*, 1978; **138**: 1103–5.

76. Couch WD. Combined effusion fluid tumour marker assay, carcinoembroyonic antigen (CEA) and human chorionic gonadotropin (hCG), in the detection of malignant tumours. *Cancer*, 1981; **48**: 2475–9.
77. Bergmann JF, Bidart JM, George M, Beaugrand M, Levy VG, Bohuon C. Elevation of CA 125 in patients with benign and malignant ascites. *Cancer*, 1987; **59**: 213–37.
78. Kourouras J, Boura P, Tsapas G, Charsis K, Magoula I, Tsakiri I. Value of ascitic fluid ferritin in the differential diagnosis of malignant ascites. *Anticancer Research*, 1993; **13**: 2441–5.
79. Jungst D, Gerbes AL, Martin R, Paumgartner G. Value of ascitic lipids in the differentiation between cirrhotic and malignant ascites. *Hepatology*, 1986; **6**: 239–43.
80. Colloredo-Mels G, *et al.* Fibronectin, cholesterol and triglyceride ascitic fluid concentrations in the prediction of malignancy. *Italian Journal of Gastroenterology*, 1991; **23**: 179–86.
81. Pockros PJ, Esrason KT, Nguyen C, Dugue J, Woods S. Mobilization of malignant ascites with diuretics is dependent on ascitic fluid characteristics. *Gastroenterology*, 1992; **103**: 1302–6.
82. Lewis JW Jr, Storer EH. The management of iatrogenic chylous ascites. *Henry Ford Hospital Medical Journal*, 1979; **27**: 140–2.
83. Gines P, *et al.* Comparison of paracentesis and diuretics in the treatment of cirrhotics with tense ascites: results of a randomized study. *Gastroenterology*, 1987; **93**: 234–41.
84. Kao HW, Rakov NE, Savage E, Reynolds TB. The effect of large volume paracentesis on plasma volume a cause of hypovolemia? *Hepatology*, 1985; **5**: 403–7.
85. Liebowitz HR. Hazards of abdominal paracentesis in the cirrhotic patient (Part III). *New York State Journal of Medicine*, 1962; **62**: 2223–9.
86. Pinto PC, Amerian J, Reynolds TB. Large-volume paracentesis in nonedematous patients with tense ascites: its effect on intravascular volume. *Hepatology*, 1988; **8**: 207–10.
87. Panos MZ, *et al.* Single, total paracentesis for tense ascites: sequential hemodynamic changes and right atrial size. *Hepatology*, 1990; **11**: 662–7.
88. Tito L, *et al.* Total paracentesis associated with intravenous albumin management of patients with cirrhosis and ascites. *Gastroenterology*, 1990; **98**: 146–51.
89. Gines P, Arroyo V, Rodes J. Treatment of ascites and renal failure in cirrhosis. *Bailliere's Clinical Gastroenterology*, 1989; **3**: 165–86.
90. Epstein M. The LeVeen shunt for ascites and hepatorenal syndrome. *New England Journal of Medicine*, 1980; **302**: 628–30.
91. Holm A, Halpern NB, Aldrete JS. Peritoneovenous shunt for intractable ascites of hepatic, nephrogenic, and malignant causes. *American Journal of Surgery*, 1989; **158**: 162–6.
92. Soderlund C. Denver peritoneovenous shunting for malignant or cirrhotic ascites. A prospective consecutive series. *Scandinavian Journal of Gastroenterology*, 1986; **21**: 1167–72.
93. Gough IR, Balderson GA. Malignant ascites. A comparison of peritoneovenous shunting and non-operative management. *Cancer*, 1993; **71**: 2377–82.
94. McCann WJ, Cappelletti RR, Neumann CG. Ileo-entectropy for ascites associated with ovarian tumours. *Obstetrics and Gynecology*, 1968; **32**: 482–5.
95. Mulvany D. Vesico-coelomic drainage for the relief of ascites. *Lancet*, 1955, Oct 8: 748–9.
96. Chu DZ, Lang NP, Thompson C, Osteen PK, Westbrook KC. Peritoneal carcinomatosis in nongynecologic malignancy. A prospective study of prognostic factors. *Cancer*, 1989; **63**: 364–7.
97. Myers CE, Collins JM. Pharmacology of intraperitoneal chemotherapy. *Cancer Investigation*, 1983; **1**: 395–407.
98. Dybicki J, Balchum OJ, Meneelly, GR. Treatment of pleural and peritoneal effusion with intracavitary colloidal radiogold (^{198}Au). *Archives of Internal Medicine*, 1959; **104**: 802–15.
99. Jacobs ML, Duarte MD. Radioactive colloidal chromic phosphate to control pleural effusion and ascites. *Journal of the American Medical Association*, 1958; **166**: 597–9.
100. Gebbia N, *et al.* Intracavity treatment of malignant pleural and peritoneal effusions in cancer patients. *Anticancer Research*, 1994; **14**: 739–46.
101. Andersen AP, Brincker H. Intracavitary thiotepa in malignant pleural and peritoneal effusions. *Acta Radiological Therapy Physics Biology*, 1968; **7**: 369–77.
102. Bayly TC, *et al.* Tetracycline and quinacrine in the control of malignant pleural effusions. *Cancer*, 1978; **41**: 1188.
103. Fracchia AA, Knapper WH, Carey JT, Farrow JH. Intrapleural chemotherapy for effusion from metastatic breast cancer. *Cancer*, 1970; **26**: 626.
104. Tattersall MHN, Fox RM, Newlands ES, Woods RL. Intracavitary doxorubicin in malignant effusions. *Lancet*, 1979; **1**: 390.
105. Keffort RF, Woods RL, Fox RM, Tattersall MHN. Intracavitary adriamycin, nitrogen mustard and tetracycline in the control of malignant effusions. A randomized study. *Medical Journal of Australia*, 1980; **2**: 447–8.
106. Suhrland LG, Weisberger AS. Intracavitary 5-fluorouracil in malignant effusions. *Archives of Internal Medicine*, 1965; **116**: 431–3.
107. Rath U, *et al.* Effect of intraperitoneal recombinant human tumour necrosis factor alpha on malignant ascites. *European Journal of Cancer*, 1991; **27**: 121–5.
108. Weissenborn K. Recent developments in the pathophysiology and treatment of hepatic encephalopathy. *Bailliere's Clinical Gastroenterology*, 1992; **6**: 609–30.
109. Jones EA, Basile AS, Yurdaydin C, Skolnich P. Do benzodiazepine ligands contribute to hepatic encephalopathy? *Advances in Experimental Biology and Medicine*, 1993, **341**. 57–69.
110. Mousseau DD, Butterworth RF. Current theories on the pathogenesis of hepatic encephalopathy. *Proceedings of the Society for Experimental Biology and Medicine*, 1994; **206**: 329–44.
111. Giguers JF, Butterworth RF. Amino acid changes in regions of the CNS in relation to function in experimental portal-systemic encephalopathy. *Neurochemistry Research*, 1984; **9**: 1307–19.
112. Hoyumpa AM, Jr, Schenker S. Perspectives in hepatic encephalopathy. *Journal of Laboratory and Clinical Medicine*, 1982; **100**: 477–87.
113. Elsass P, Lund Y, Ranek L. Encephalopathy in patients with cirrhosis of the liver: a neuropsychological study. *Scandinavian Journal of Gastroenterology*, 1978; **13**: 241–7.
114. Rikkers L, Jenko P, Rudman D, Freides D. Subclinical hepatic encephalopathy: Detection, prevalence and relationship to nitrogen metabolism. *Gastroenterology*, 1978; **75**: 462–9.
115. Conn HO. Trailmaking and number-connection test in the assessment of mental state in portal systemic encephalopathy. *Digestive Diseases and Sciences*, 1977; **22**: 541–50.
116. Ross BD, *et al.* Subclinical hepatic encephalopathy: proton MR spectroscopic abnormalities. *Radiology*, 1994; **193**: 457–63.
117. Parsons-Smith BG, Summerskill WHJ, Dawson AM, Sherlock S. The electroencephalograph in liver disease. *Lancet*, 1957; **2**: 867–71.
118. Conn HO. Hepatic encephalopathy. In: Schiff L, Schiff ER, eds. *Diseases of the Liver*, 7th edn. Philadelphia: J.B. Lippincott, 1993: 1036–60.
119. Camma C, Fiorello F, Tine F, Marchesini G, Fabbri A, Pagliaro L. Lactitol in treatment of chronic hepatic encephalopathy. A meta-analysis. *Digestive Diseases and Sciences*, 1993; **38**: 916–22.
120. Dawson AM, McLaren J, Serlock S. Neomycin in the treatment of hepatic coma. *Lancet*, 1957; **2**: 1263–8.
121. Bucci L, Palmieri GC. Double-blind, double-dummy comparison between treatment with rifaximin and lactulose in patients with medium to severe degree hepatic encephalopathy. *Current Medical Research and Opinion*, 1993; **13**: 109–18.
122. McGhee A, Henderson JM, Milliken WJ, Bleir J. Comparison of the effect of hepaticaid and casein modular diets on encephalopathy, plasma amino acids and nitrogen balance in cirrhotic patients. *Annals of Surgery*, 1983; **197**: 288–93.
123. Crossley IR, Williams R. Progress in the treatment of chronic portasystemic encephalopathy. *Gut*, 1984; **25**: 85–98.
124. Bianchi GP, *et al.* Vegetable vs animal protein diet in cirrhotic patients with chronic encephalopathy. A randomized cross-over comparison. *Journal of Internal Medicine*, 1993; **233**: 385–92.

125. Sushma S, Dasarathy S, Tandon RK, Jain S, Gupta S, Bhist MS. Sodium benzoate in the treatment of acute hepatic encephalopathy: a double blind randomized trial. *Hepatology*, 1992; **16**: 138–44.

126. Pomier-Layrargues G, *et al*. Flumazenil in cirrhotic patients in hepatic coma: a randomized double-blind placebo-controlled cross-over trial. *Hepatology*, 1994; **19**: 32–7.

9.4 Asthenia

Hans Neuenschwander and Eduardo Bruera

Summary

Asthenia is the most frequent symptom associated with advanced cancer. It is strongly associated with malnutrition and other tumour-related symptom complexes. However, recent research and clinical observations suggest that this symptom has its own pathophysiological mechanisms. As in the case of other symptom complexes, an adequate assessment is crucial before appropriate management can take place. This chapter addresses the importance of multidimensional assessment in attempting to identify reversible causes, in order to evaluate properly the cause–benefit ratio of different treatments. The management of asthenia includes general measures, both pharmacological and non-pharmacological, as well as specific measures addressing reversible underlying causes.

Asthenia, until now, has received limited attention from both clinicians and investigators. More research is badly needed in order to better define epidemiology for this syndrome with the aim to identify adequate techniques for the assessment of asthenia, to better establish pathophysiology of this complex symptom, and for the development of better therapeutic techniques.

Introduction

A variety of symptoms and signs are associated with advanced cancer and/or its treatment such as pain, anorexia, nausea, vomiting, dyspnoea, mucositis, alopecia, and others. In the palliative care setting they are usually addressed independently according to the degree of importance for a given patient. Cancer fatigue or asthenia is commonly recognized as the most frequent symptom. Its onset sometimes precedes the diagnosis of malignancy or may be one of the first manifestations. It may be present during the whole course of the illness, increasing following treatments such as chemotherapy, radiation therapy, or surgery. Asthenia may influence judgement and lead patients to refuse potentially curative treatments. However, in the palliative care setting, it is usually not the target of aggressive assessment and management efforts.

Asthenos (Greek) means absence or loss of strength. Asthenia includes three different major symptoms:

(1) fatigue or lassitude defined as easy tiring and decreased capacity to maintain performance;

(2) generalized weakness defined as the anticipatory sensation of difficulty in initiating a certain activity;

(3) mental fatigue defined as the presence of impaired mental concentration, loss of memory, and emotional lability.[1,2]

The latter condition is commonly similar to the mental status after prolonged mental effort, causing reluctance to retry further efforts. Generalized weakness should be distinguished from localized or regional weakness created by neurological or muscular disorders.

Although there is a great need for more knowledge in this area, over the period between 1980 and 1991 MEDLINE reports just nine references on fatigue and cancer, among which eight were derived from nursing research.[3] Even the first edition of the present textbook did not dedicate a specific chapter to this issue. As in other publications, asthenia was treated within the chapter on cachexia since it is widely believed to be almost exclusively associated with progressive malnutrition. Only in the last few years has the palliative care community developed increased awareness of the importance of asthenia in cancer as a self-standing problem. This delay in perception is a major reason for our limited knowledge about incidence, pathophysiologic mechanisms, and useful therapeutic approaches in the management of asthenia. The purpose of this chapter is to increase awareness of the importance of this symptom, to demonstrate the complex causality and multidimensional aspects of asthenia, to establish the need for continuous assessment, to discuss pharmacological and non-pharmacological approaches to management, and to stimulate an increase in research efforts on this topic.

Significance

It is important to distinguish fatigue as a physiological phenomenon accompanying physical effort or a strong intellectual performance from fatigue as a pathological finding. The first can be considered as beneficial and protective against over-exertion. If it is of reasonable duration and induced by pleasurable activity, it might also be considered a pleasant feeling. Fatigue associated with an infection may be a beneficial mechanism which enforces rest, although it is usually perceived as an unpleasant sensation. Some authors regard infection-induced fatigue as a society-protective device as a contagious subject may remove him/herself from the community and thereby decrease the spread of the disease.[4]

Fatigue as a pathological finding is always a distressing sensation. As in the case of pain, asthenia in chronic diseases such as protracted infection and malignancy serves no beneficial function. No other symptom is perceived as being so closely associated with cancer as asthenia. Therefore, this symptom is often accepted as unavoidable by patients, relatives, and health-care professionals. Some palliative care textbooks have suggested that the best approach is to encourage the patient to accept the symptom and learn to live with it.[5] While, unfortunately, the state of the art may make it necessary for most patients to accept this symptom at the present time, it is important for both caregivers and researchers to consider carefully what can be done today to improve the knowledge on the mechanisms, assessment, and management of this devastating symptom.

In palliative care it is useful to make a priority list of the patients complaints according to their importance. During this exercise, it is common that the patients list will not match with the caregivers relevance list. This is frequently due to different expectations between patients and caregivers with regards to quality of life. In addition, in a given patient, once satisfactory control of more acutely distressing symptoms such as dyspnoea and pain has been achieved, asthenia usually emerges as a main complaint. Institutions that develop adequate guidelines for the assessment of management of symptoms, with well validated therapeutic options for symptoms such as pain or dyspnoea, might find that these will progressively lose relevance over time while, in the meantime, symptoms for which there are more limited diagnostic or therapeutic resources such as psychosocial problems or asthenia will become the most distressing.

Prevalence

Asthenia is universally associated with advanced malignancy. However, there are only a limited number of studies available on prevalence. Most of these studies focus on patients receiving antineoplastic therapy. The prevalence of asthenia in patients receiving chemotherapy has been estimated to be more than 80 per cent (80–96 per cent).[6] Under radiation therapy, asthenia increases over the course of therapy and can outlast the treatment for months.[6]

A retrospective review of 805 cancer patients found generalized weakness in 40 per cent.[7] Almost half of the patients admitted to St Christopher's complained of weakness.[8] Our group found a prevalence of 75 per cent in patients with terminal cancer.[9] In a prospective study we found asthenia present in 72 per cent of patients with advanced breast cancer.[10]

The frequency of asthenia varies widely in the literature. This variation is partially due to the difference in patient groups (type of tumour, stage, tumour mass, institution, etc). However, another major reason for this difference is the lack of a 'gold standard' for the definition and assessment of asthenia, as discussed below.

Pathophysiology

In most patients the aetiology of asthenia is unknown as the basic mechanisms relative to this symptom are poorly understood. Usually, in a given cancer patient, however, there are several potential causes of asthenia coexisting (Table 1). Asthenia may result from one clearly predominant abnormality. Figure 1 summarizes the mechanisms by which the tumour, interacting with the host, results in the production of asthenia.

Abnormalities associated with asthenia

A number of changes in different body systems are consistently associated with asthenia. The three main mechanisms that bring about these changes are:

(1) direct tumour effect;

Table 1 Causes of asthenia in advanced cancer

Causes
Cachexia/malnutrition
Dehydration
Infection (recurrent acute infection, chronic infection such as hepatitis, tuberculosis, brucellosis, mononucleosis, herpes, etc.)
Anaemia
Chronic hypoxia
Neurological disorders (autonomic dysfunction, myasthenia syndrome, parkinsonism, demyelinization)
Psychogenic causes
Metabolic and electrolyte disorders
Endocrine disorders (thyropathy, Addison's disease, diabetes mellitus, etc.)
Insomnia
Over-exertion (chronic/acute)
Pharmacological toxic (narcotics, sedatives, alcohol, chemotherapy, etc.)

(2) tumour-induced products;

(3) other accompanying factors including anaemia, paraneoplastic syndromes, chronic infections, etc.

One or more of these three mechanisms may cause some of the observed abnormalities in a given patient.

There is a strong trend in the literature to associate asthenia with cachexia and anorexia. Although there is no doubt that cachexia is a major cause of asthenia, asthenia may be present without cachexia. However, many of the postulated mechanisms for cachexia are applicable to asthenia. It is now accepted that many cancers release a number of substances capable of significantly altering the intermediary metabolism of the host. It is also accepted that cancers may induce host macrophages to produce and release cachectin and a number of other cytokines (IFN, IL, etc.) which induce the cachexia–anorexia syndrome. Similarly, there might be a

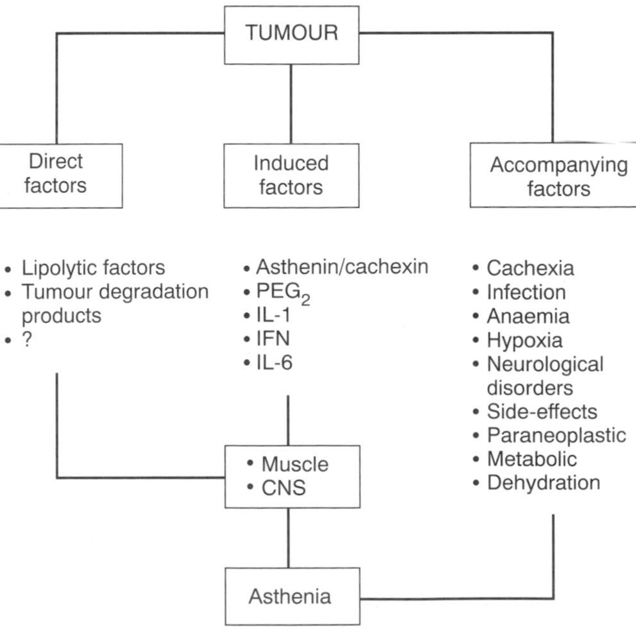

Fig. 1 Mechanisms resulting in asthenia.

release and/or induction of substances by the tumour[11,12] which lead to asthenia. For example if blood from a fatigued subject is injected into a rested subject, manifestations of fatigue are produced. Tumour-free muscle tissue from tumour bearing animals show alterations in the activity of various enzymes, distribution of isoenzymes, and synthesis and breakdown of myofibrillar and sarcoplasmic proteins.[11]

The muscle and the central nervous system can be considered the main target tissues associated with the perception and expression of asthenia. Muscle alterations in tumour bearing patients are well known. Cachexia leads to a loss of muscle and fat. This, at least, may partially explain the cachexia-related asthenia. However, even in the presence of normal caloric intake and a constant body weight and lean body mass, tumour bearing patients present muscle abnormalities. Our group found no correlation between asthenia and nutritional status or weight in a population of breast cancer patients.[13] Tumour free muscle tissue of cancer patients shows excessive lactate production.[14] It is unclear whether lactate is part of the pathogenetic mechanism of weakness or just an epiphenomenon of it. Atrophy of Type-II muscle fibres has been suggested to be a systemic effect of cancer even in early and non-metastatic stages. Type-II muscle fibres are responsible for high anaerobic glycolytic metabolism.[15] Our group found impaired maximal strength, decreased relaxation velocity, and increased fatigue after electrical stimulation of the abductor pollicis muscle via the ulnar nerve in patients with breast cancer as compared to normal controls.[16] These results suggest that at least in some cases, impaired muscle function may be one of the main underlying mechanisms in asthenia. The cause of these abnormalities may relate in part to known abnormalities in cytokine production, but the production of other inducing substances termed 'asthenins' have been postulated.

The asthenia-inducing mechanisms at the central nervous system level are even more hypothetical! It has been suggested that the reticular activating system is responsible for the control of the experience of fatigue. The reticular activating system receives descending stimuli from the cortex on a feedback system base and ascending information from a number of sensory organs.[17,18] Chronic stimuli such as chronic pain may generate fatigue through unremitting reticular stimulation. It has been suggested that 'physiological fatigue' might have an important protective function against over exertion. Cancer asthenia might thus be due to a breakdown of this reticular mediated mechanism by environmental and cortical stimuli as well as humoral factors. This hypothesis is supported by the observation that more than 70 per cent of patients receiving cranial radiotherapy for acute lymphoblastic leukaemia experience fatigue, depression, and somnolence.[19]

Underlying causes of asthenia

Cachexia

As previously discussed, the association between cachexia and asthenia is frequent in cancer patients. Both symptoms coexist in the great majority of terminally ill cancer patients. Therefore, it is likely that malnutrition is one of the major contributors to asthenia (Table 2).[20] However, clinical situations illustrate that the relationship may not be as close as assumed. Asthenia does occur in non-malignant conditions where malnutrition is absent, such as the chronic fatigue syndrome or psychological depression, and also in malignancies that have a low prevalence of malnutrition such as breast cancer or lymphomas. On the other hand, severe malnutrition without asthenia can be observed in patients with anorexia nervosa and in some patient populations with solid tumours (Fig. 2).

Table 2 Prevalence of symptoms in 275 consecutive cancer patients[20]

Symptom	Prevalence (%)	95% Confidence interval
Asthenia	90	81–100
Anorexia	85	78–92
Pain	76	62–85
Nausea	68	61–75
Constipation	65	40–80
Sedation-confusion	60	40–75
Dyspnoea	12	8–16

It is proposed that anorexia and asthenia might be an expression of the major metabolic abnormalities that occur in cancer patients rather than simply an expression of the malnutrition *per se*.[21] This situation would be similar to that experienced when a catabolic state occurs, such as a viral infection or the early postoperative period. In these conditions, patients experience anorexia and asthenia that is secondary to the metabolic abnormalities and not a cause of those abnormalities. Current pharmacological interventions in the area of cachexia are discussed elsewhere in this book. It is currently unknown whether such interventions are able to modify the level of asthenia in cancer patients.

The loss of muscle mass may partially explain the weakness and fatigue. As previously discussed, even in the presence of normal protein and caloric intake and normal body weight, structural and biochemical muscle abnormalities are found in cancer patients.[14,22,23] Similar abnormalities could explain asthenia associated with chronic cardiac and respiratory disease. Some metabolic abnormalities related to cachexia are specifically responsible for muscle breakdown. These include an increased concentration of cathepsin-D (a lysosomal enzyme involved in the intracellular degradation of macromolecules).[24] The administration of factors such as eicosapentaenolic acid (EPA), that are capable of inhibiting protein degradation, might be a promising alternative therapeutic intervention in these patients.[25]

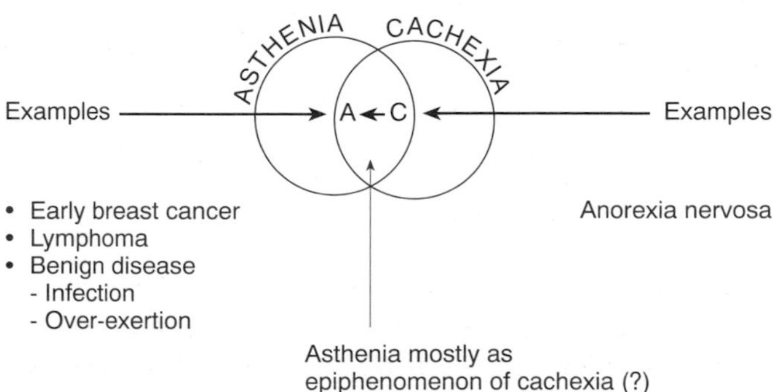

Fig. 2 Cachexia–asthenia. A cause and effect relationship?

Infection

Asthenia often occurs as part of infections, particularly when the course is recurrent or protracted. While it frequently occurs as a prodromic symptom, it may outlast by weeks or months the acute phase of the infection.[26,27] The presence of immunosuppression increases the risk of infectious complications in cancer patients. Chronic infection and cancer induce the same mediators for cachexia, including cachectin/TNFα.[12] It can be hypothesized that they might share similar mediators for asthenia as well.

Anaemia

The role of anaemia is controversial. For many years it was thought to be a main cause. On the other hand, transfusion in anaemic cancer patients doesn't usually result in an improvement of asthenia. Patients with chronic anaemia in the absence of cancer, such as thalassaemia minor, are frequently not asthenic despite a haemoglobin value of approximately 10 g/dl. However, if the haemoglobin value is extremely low or if the drop has been fast, the correction of anaemia might improve the asthenic symptoms.[28]

Neurological changes

As mentioned previously, there are a number of functional alterations in the mid-brain that might be involved in the generation of asthenia. In addition, other neurological syndromes associated with malignancy could contribute. One of these is autonomic dysfunction. This syndrome includes postural hypotension, occasional syncope, fixed heart rate, and gastrointestinal symptoms such as nausea, anorexia, and constipation.[29,30] The association between autonomic failure and asthenia has not been adequately investigated.

Psychological distress

In patients without cancer who present with asthenia, the final diagnosis is psychologic in almost 75 per cent of cases (depression, anxiety, and other psychological disorders).[31] While some depressive symptoms are quite frequent in cancer patients, only a minority of patients develop adjustment disorders and a very small group presents with major depressive or anxiety disorders.[32,34] The diagnosis of a major depressive episode in the terminally ill patient is a major challenge because of the frequent presentation with neuro-vegetative and somatic symptoms that are part of the disease itself. The diagnosis should rely more on the presence of psychological and cognitive signs and symptoms.[33] These have been discussed elsewhere in this book. Patients presenting with an adjustment disorder or a major depressive disorder can have asthenia as one of the prevalent symptoms. Some authors have found an association between asthenia and mood changes in patients with breast cancer that they had attributed to a combination of the disease and therapy.[35]

Metabolic and endocrine disorders

Disorders such as diabetes mellitus, Addison's syndrome, electrolyte disorders such as low sodium, potassium, or magnesium, and hypercalcaemia have to be excluded especially as some of these have simple and effective treatment.

Over-exertion

This is a frequent cause of asthenia in non-cancer patients.[28] It should also be considered in younger cancer patients who are under aggressive antineoplastic treatment, such as radiotherapy and chemotherapy, and who are nevertheless trying to maintain their social and professional activities. Research in sports medicine has shown that for prolonged endurance it is important to provide adequate substrate to the muscles (carbohydrate-loading). Unfortunately, cancer patients frequently present with abnormalities in muscle metabolism that may not allow an adequate utilization of this substrate.[36] In addition, recently sports medicine researchers have been addressing the role of neurotransmitters such as serotonin or choline as mediators of fatigue and depression in athletes suffering from over-exertion.[36] Anecdotal evidence suggest that some of these patient's fatigue may disappear after 48 h of treatment with antidepressants of the serotonin-specific re-uptake inhibitor group.[36] These findings could provide a key to future therapeutic approaches of asthenia.

Side-effects of antineoplastic treatment

Antineoplastic treatments such as surgery, radiation therapy, chemotherapy, and therapy with biological response modifiers are well known causes of asthenia. The mechanism for asthenia related to all these approaches is not well understood.Specifically, biological response modifiers are capable of producing a flu-like syndrome. Fatigue becomes the most important dose-limiting side-effect in these patients.

In addition to antineoplastic drugs, other drugs administered to patients with advanced cancer can aggravate the level of asthenia. For example, opioid agonists such as morphine have significant effects on the reticular system and are capable of inducing sedation, cognitive changes, and asthenia in some patients. In addition, hypnotics are able to cause sedation and asthenia.

Paraneoplastic neurological syndromes

Although they are rare events, they have to be recognized since many of these syndromes precede the clinical appearance of a malignancy and they may be partially reversible with a primary treatment of the tumour. Table 3 summarizes some of the paraneoplastic neurological syndromes associated with asthenia.[37]

Assessment

'What is bothering you the most?'

'As I have told you in the last several days, I have no energy.'

'Yes, I hear you, but what do you exactly mean by that?'

The patient is frustrated because he/she feels the doctor is not getting the point. The doctor is also frustrated since there is no objective, quantifiable evidence that would allow him to justify a diagnostic or therapeutic approach.

Since asthenia is purely a subjective sensation, it is by nature harder to assess than, for example, blood pressure in the case of patients with arterial hypertension. While efforts are being made to try to identify a tool for the assessment of asthenia, there is currently no 'gold standard'. An assessment tool is necessary to determine the characteristics and intensity of asthenia, to monitor

Table 3 Paraneoplastic neurological syndromes associated with asthenia

Syndrome	Comment
Progressive multifocal leucoencephalopathy	Leukaemia, lymphoma
Paraneoplastic encephalomyelitis	70% lung, 30% others
Amyotrophic lateral sclerosis	
Subacute motor neuropathy	Proximal or distal, often asymmetric (e.g. following irradiated lymphoma)
Subacute necrotic myelopathy	Mostly lung cancer
Peripheral paraneoplastic neurological syndrome	Often precedes the primary, similar to Guillain–Barré
Ascending acute polyneuropathy (Guillain–Barré)	Lymphoma
Neuromuscular paraneoplastic syndromes such as:	
dermatomyositis, polymyositis	Associated with malignancy in about 50% Onset within 1 year
Eaton–Lambert syndrome	Strongly associated with small cell lung cancer (6%) Can precede tumour by months Improves under successful treatment
Myasthenia gravis	Thymoma (30%), lymphoma

the progress of the symptom and the response to different therapeutic interventions, and for research purposes. Such an instrument should meet the following criteria:

(1) simple and not time consuming in order to ensure good compliance over time, and use self-assessment as much as possible;

(2) valid;

(3) reliable;

(4) multidimensional.

Some of the characteristics of these tools have been discussed in other chapters of this textbook. Table 4 summarizes some tools that have been proposed for the assessment of asthenia.

It is reasonable to become familiar with the assessment tool that is most suited to the characteristics of the patients and institution where each group operates. Our group has been using the Edmonton Functional Assessment Tool (EFAT)[44] since 1990. This validated instrument assesses asthenia in the context of the functional status of terminally ill patients. It considers the following ten items:

(1) communication

(2) pain

(3) alertness

(4) shortness of breath

(5) balance in a sitting or standing position

(6) mobility

(7) motility

(8) activities of daily living

(9) tiredness

(10) motivation.

In our experience, it is simple for patient and investigator, not very time consuming, and easy to learn. It has been found to have good values for validity and reliability and it seems to adapt appropriately according to the changes in the patients clinical status. The use of a numerical scale, such as EFAT, has the extra advantage of allowing for adequate measurement of the outcome of rehabilitative treatment.

Table 4 Examples for assessment-tools for asthenia

Unidimensional	Rhoten fatigue scale[38] Pearson and Byars fatigue feeling checklist[39] Performance status (Karnofsky, ECOG)[40,41]
Multidimensional	Fatigue symptom checklist of Kogi, adapted by Kobashi[42] Fatigue self-report scale (PFS) of Piper[43] Edmonton functional assessment tool (EFAT)[44]

Management

Since asthenia is a complex, multidimensional symptom, it is crucial for an adequate therapeutic approach to identify and prioritize the different underlying factors. It is clear that in this process prior experience and personal bias will play a significant role. The change in asthenia over time may demonstrate an association with a particular finding (for example does asthenia increase following growth in tumour size, an increase in the serum-

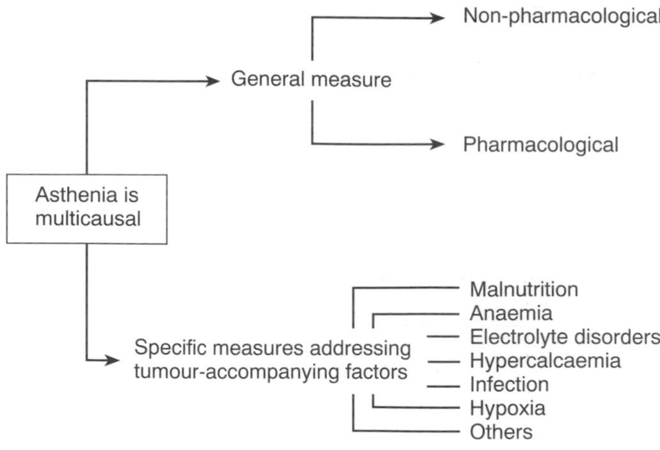

Fig. 3 Therapeutic approach.

calcium, or a change in drug treatment?). This temporal pattern underlines the importance of continuous assessment and monitoring of symptoms and signs in palliative medicine.

In planning the therapeutic approach it is also important to answer the following questions:

1. Is, for this given patient, asthenia a symptom of primary importance?
2. What are the major, probable causes?
3. Are there therapeutic measures available with a reasonable cost/benefit ratio?

The intervention may have a purpose of either decreasing the intensity of asthenia or allowing the patient to express the maximal possible level of function with a stable level of asthenia, or both. Figure 3 summarizes some of the general and specific measures that can be pursued.

General measures

Non-pharmacological measures

It is crucial to keep the patient informed about his/her status, the causes of the loss of energy, and the type of therapeutic options available. This will allow the patient the opportunity to develop realistic expectations. Patients frequently underestimate the side-effect burden at the beginning of chemotherapy. In one study, 8 per cent of patients expected tiredness although 86 per cent experienced it.[45] This suggests a significant information gap that may reduce the ability to develop realistic expectations.

If patients are empowered by correct information and counselling they may combat asthenia by:

(1) adapting activities of daily living (for example decreased housework, allow others to help with physical duties);

(2) rearranging time schedules during the day;

(3) spending more time in bed;

(4) requesting changes in medications perceived as causing loss of energy;

(5) avoiding parasitic energy expending activities.[45]

The caregiver must try to find a balance between more rest, that may decrease the intensity of asthenia, and more dependency that may increase weakness. Unfortunately, all these suggestions are empirical and need to be assessed in clinical research.

Pharmacological measures

In patients with asthenia of unknown origin or in those in whom a specific treatment is not available a number of non-specific pharmacological interventions have been proposed.

Corticosteroids

These drugs have been suggested, by a number of studies, to be able to decrease asthenia in cancer patients. In addition to anecdotal reports,[46] controlled, randomized trials have confirmed the presence of decreased asthenia. The level of activity recorded and the blind preference of patients and investigators identified methylprednisolone 32 mg/day as more effective than a placebo. In this report, however, the duration of the effect was limited to 2 to 3 weeks.[47] Two multicentre European trials have confirmed the effect of corticosteroid therapy in asthenia.[48,49]

The mechanism of action of steroids on asthenia is unknown. Both the inhibition of tumour and tumour-induced substances, as well as a central euphoriant effect, are potential mechanisms.[47] The effects of these drugs are probably not due to their demonstrated appetite stimulation since corticosteroids do not result in significant improvement of the nutritional status.

Amphetamines

In 1977, Forrest reported improved cognition and decreased sedation in postoperative patients receiving dextroamphetamine.[50] In a late open study, 16 advanced cancer patients were treated with dextroamphetamine, of whom 12 appeared to experience improvement in activity.[51] Our group studied mazindol in a double-blind, placebo-controlled study in patients with advanced cancer.[52] This drug was found to have some positive effect on pain, but no significant effect on asthenia. In addition, significant neurotoxicity occurred. In a follow-up study, methylphenidate (a mild short-acting amphetamine derivative) was given to patients receiving higher doses of opioids. In this 3-day, double-blind crossover study, methylphenidate appeared to improve asthenia as compared to placebo. Our experience with methylphenidate and mazindol suggests that these drugs would be useful primarily in those patients in whom asthenia results from increasing doses of opioids and not in order to improve general well being. The use of amphetamine derivatives has been proposed for patients presenting with hypoactive, hypoalert delirium.[53] The role of these drugs in organic brain syndromes has been discussed elsewhere in this book.

In summary, since asthenia was not the main outcome measurement of any of the trials on amphetamines, it is not possible to establish if these drugs have a true effect on asthenia or if it is a question of improvement of other symptoms that coexist in the patient populations.

Specific measures

As previously discussed, asthenia is often multicausal. It may appear as a epiphenomenon of other symptom complexes, such as

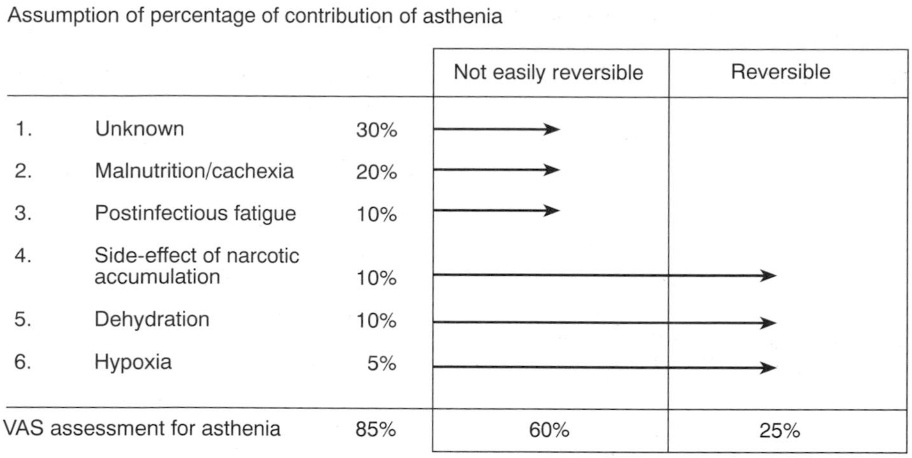

Assumption of percentage of contribution of asthenia

			Not easily reversible	Reversible
1.	Unknown	30%	→	
2.	Malnutrition/cachexia	20%	→	
3.	Postinfectious fatigue	10%	→	
4.	Side-effect of narcotic accumulation	10%	→	→
5.	Dehydration	10%	→	→
6.	Hypoxia	5%	→	→
VAS assessment for asthenia		85%	60%	25%

Fig. 4 Causes of asthenia in an example case.

those related to cachexia, infection, anaemia, etc., rather than as a self-standing, single issue. Any measure able to reverse the underlying abnormality would result in an improvement in asthenia. It is useful to graphically represent the contribution of the different factors, with the aim of identifying reversible causes. Reversible causes such as dehydration, metabolic disorders, or severe anaemia may coexist with non-reversible causes. The list of prescribed drugs must be continuously checked to avoid asthenia as a iatrogenic effect (for example, accumulation of opioids in the presence of renal failure). Psychosocial reasons such as depression, anxiety, or over-exertion can be therapeutically addressed. The treatment of malnutrition as a cause of asthenia in the specific situation of cancer patients remains controversial. Malnourished patients are known to have a significant level of asthenia. However, it has not been clearly demonstrated that attempts to reverse the level of malnutrition are able to result in any significant improvement in the level of asthenia.[54,55] In patients considered to have cachexia as the leading cause of asthenia, a pharmacological trial of megestrol acetate might be useful. Even in cases where megestrol acetate is unable to reverse the catabolic situation, a positive effect on asthenia has been reported. A direct effect of megestrol acetate on asthenia, perhaps independent from its nutritional effects, has also been suggested.[56]

In palliative care, the satisfactory treatment of a symptom such as asthenia does not mean that it is mandatory to eliminate it completely. Even minor improvements would be enough to shift asthenia into a less relevant level in the patient's priority symptom list. Figure 4 summarizes the case of a 60-year-old man with metastatic non-small-cell lung cancer. The patient had lost 6 kg in 4 months and had developed two pneumonias in the last 3 months. His oxygen saturation was 84 per cent, his haemoglobin was 11.5 g/dl and he was clinically dehydrated. He was currently receiving therapy with 180 mg morphine parenterally every 24 h. He was also receiving lorazepam at night because of insomnia. The approach in this patient included the elimination of the toxic effect of opioids, by switching from morphine to another opioid, and rehydration. These changes were able to decrease the intensity of asthenia in the visual analogue scale from 85 to 60. At that time, other symptoms such as shortness of breath became more important than asthenia.

Future research

Asthenia is beginning to be addressed as a symptom that should be studied separately from the cachexia–anorexia complex. In the past, both patients and health care professionals accepted asthenia as an inevitable consequence of cancer. This acceptance reduced interest in the development of asthenia-focused research. In the following paragraphs some suggestions for increased research in the area will be discussed.

1. Asthenia must be defined in a reproducible way by investigators and clinicians. There is an urgent need for valid and reliable tools for the assessment and staging of the intensity and associations of this symptom. These tools would help in the clinical and research areas and would allow scientists and clinicians to develop a common language.

2. Asthenia occurs in patients with a number of other frequent findings such as cachexia, anorexia, nausea, pain, cognitive failure, etc. Major efforts should take place in order to directly investigate tumour-induced asthenia by attempting to identify direct tumour effects or tumour-induced factors. This would require the co-operation between clinicians and tumour biologists and the development of adequate animal models for the assessment of cancer related asthenia.

3. The association between malnutrition and asthenia is well recognized in cancer and geriatric patients. However, aggressive nutrition has not been proven to significantly improve asthenia in cancer patients. Malnourished patients without cancer frequently benefit from substances such as vitamins and trace elements. Cancer patients frequently present with a number of nutritional deficiencies. The role of some of these specific nutrients on asthenia should be better established.

4. Prospective studies are needed in the area of activity–rest. How much rest is beneficial? Is the fear of causing increased dependency by deconditioning justified? At which level is physical activity leading to counter-productive exertion?

5. The role of drugs such as megestrol acetate, corticosteroids, and anabolic steroids should be better established. All these drugs have been suggested anecdotally to have effects on

asthenia in cancer patients. However, since these findings have consistently not been the main outcome measurement of the studies, it is difficult to establish a role for any of these pharmacological interventions in the management of asthenia.

References

1. Theologides A. Asthenia in cancer. *American Journal of Medicine*, 1982; 73:1–3.
2. Bruera E, MacDonald RN. Asthenia in patients with advanced cancer. *Journal of Pain and Symptom Management* 1988; 3: 9–14.
3. Smets EMA, Garssen B, Schuster-Uitterhoeve ALJ, de Haes JCJM. Fatigue in cancer patients. *British Journal of Cancer*, 1993; **68**: 220–4.
4. Morant R. Asthenia in cancer patients: a double-edged inflammatory response against the tumor? *Journal of Palliative Care*, 1991; **7**: 22–4.
5. Saunders C. *The Management of Terminal Malignant Disease*, (2nd edn). Edward Arnold: London, 1989.
6. Irvine DM, Vincent L, Bubela N, Thompson L, Graydon J. A critical appraisal of the research literature investigating fatigue in the individual with cancer. *Cancer Nursing*, 1991; **14**:188–99.
7. Lehman J, De Lisa J, Warren C, *et al.* Cancer rehabilitation: assessment of need, development and evaluation of a model care. *Archives of Physical and Medical Rehabilitation*, 1978; **59**: 410–9.
8. Walsh T, Saunders C. Hospice Care: the treatment of pain in advanced cancer. *Recent Results in Cancer Research*, 1984; **89**: 201–11.
9. Bruera E, MacDonald RN. Asthenia in patients with advanced cancer. *Journal of Pain and Symptom Management*, 1988; **3**: 9–14.
10. Bruera E, Brenneis C, Michaud M, Jackson F, MacDonald RN. Association between involuntary muscle function (IMF) and asthenia (AST), nutritional status (NS), lean body mass (LBM), psychometric assessment and tumor mass (TM) in patients (PTS) with advanced breast cancer. Presented at ASCO, Atlanta, Georgia May 17–19, 1987. *Proceedings of the American Society of Clinical Oncology*, 1987; **6** 1024: 261.
11. Theologides A. Asthenins and cachectins in cancer. *American Journal of Medicine*,1986; **81**: 696–8.
12. Beutler B, Cerami A. Cachectin: more than a tumor nercosis factor. *New England Journal of Medicine*, 1987; **316**: 379–85.
13. Bruera E, Brenneis C, Michaud M, Rafter J, Magnan A, Tennant A, Hanson J, MacDonald RN. Association between asthenia and nutritional status, lean body mass, anemia, psychometrical status and tumor mass in patients with advanced breast cancer. *Journal of Pain and Symptom Management*, 1989; **4**: 59–63.
14. Holroyde R, Axelrod RS, Skutchers CL, Haff AC, Paul P, Reichard SA. Lactate metabolism in patients with metastatic colorectal cancer. *Cancer Research*, 1979; **39**: 4900–4.
15. Warmolts JR, Re PK, Lewis RJ, Engel WK. Type II muscle fiber atrophy (II-Atrophy): an early systemic effect of cancer. *Neurology*, 1975; **2**: 374.
16. Bruera E, Jackson F, Michaud M, Jackson PI, MacDonald RN. Muscle electrophysiology in patients with advanced breast cancer. *Journal of the National Cancer Institute*, 1988; **80**: 282–6.
17. Grandjean EP. Fatigue: Yant Memorial Lecture 1970. *American Industrial Hygiene Association Journal*, 1970; **31**: 401–11.
18. Piper BF. *Fatigue, Pathophysiological Phenomena in Nursing, Human Responses to Illness.* In (ed. Carrieri VK, Lindsey AM, West CM). Philadelphia: WB Saunders Company, 1986: 219–34.
19. Proctor SJ, Kernahan J, Taylor P. Depression as a component of post-cranial irradiation somnolence syndrome. *Lancet*, 1981; **1**: 1215–6.
20. Bruera E. Current pharmacological management of anorexia in cancer patients. *Oncology*, 1992; **6**: 125–30.
21. Bruera E. Clinical management of cachexia and anorexia in patients with advanced cancer. *Oncology*, 1992; **49**(Suppl 2):35–42.
22. Beck S, Mulligan H, Tisdale M. Lipolytic factors associated with murine and human cancer cachexia. *Journal of the National Cancer Institute*, 1990; **82**: 1922–6.
23. Smith KL, Tisdale MJ. Mechanism of muscle protein degradation in cancer cachexia. *British Journal of Cancer*, 1993; **68**: 314–8.
24. Beck SA, Tisdale MJ. Production of lipolytic and proteolytic factors by a murine tumor producing cachexia in the host. *Cancer Research*, 1987; **47**: 5919–23.
25. Beck SA, Smith KL, Tisdale MJ. Anticachectic and antitumor effect of eicosapentaenolic acid and its effect on protein turnover. *Cancer Research*, 1991; **51**: 6089–93.
26. Jones J, Ray G, Minnich L. Evidence for active Epstein-Barr virus infection in patients with persistent, unexplained illnesses: Elevated anti-early antigen antibodies. *Annals of Internal Medicine*, 1985; **102**: 1–7.
27. Strauss S, Tosato G, Armstrong G, *et al.* Persistent illness and fatigue in adults with evident Epstein-Barr virus infection. *Annals of Internal Medicine*, 1985: **102**: 7–16.
28. Plum F. Asthenia, weakness and fatigue. In: *Cecil Textbook of Medicine.* (ed. J. Wyngaaarden and L. Smith), Philadelphia: WB Saunders Company, 1985: 2044.
29. Henrich W. Autonomic insufficiency. *Archives of Internal Medicine*, 1982: 9–44.
30. Bruera E, Chadwick S, MacDonald N, Fox R, Hanson J. Study of cardiovascular autonomic insufficiency in advanced cancer patients. *Cancer Treatment Reports*, 1986; **70**: 1383–7.
31. Adams R. Anxiety, depression, asthenia and personality disorders. In: *Harrison's Principles of Internal Medicine* (ed. Petersdorf R, Adams R, Brawnnald E), New York: McGraw-Hill, 1983: 68–75.
32. Derogatis L, Morow G, Fetting J, *et al.* The prevalence of psychiatric disorders among cancer patients. *Journal of the American Medical Association*, 1983; **249**: 751–7.
33. Breitbart W, Pasnik SD. Psychiatric aspects of palliatie care. In: *Oxford Textbook of Palliative Medicine* (ed. Doyle D,Hanks G, MacDonald N), London: Oxford University Press, 1993: 609–26.
34. Hayes JR. Depression and chronic fatigue in cancer patients. *Primary Care*, 1991; **18**: 327–39.
35. Piper BF. Fatigue. In: *Pathophysiological Phenomena in Nursing: Human Responses to Illness.* 2nd edn. (ed. Carrieri V, Lindsey A, West C). Philadelphia: Saunders, 1993: 279–302.
36. Burfoot A. The brain connection. *Runners World*, 1994; **29**: 70–5.
37. Warenius HM. Paraneoplastic neurological syndromes. In: *The Clinical Neurology of Old Age* (ed. R. Tallis), New York: John Wiley and Sons Ltd., 1989: 323–34.
38. Rhoten D. Fatigue and postsurgical patient. In: *Concept Clarification in Nursing* (ed. Norris CM), Rockvill, MD: Aspen Publisher Inc., 1982: 277–300.
39. Pearson PG, Byars GE. *The Development and Validation of a Checklist Measuring Subjective Fatigue.* Report no. H556115. School of Aviation, USAF, Randolf AFB, Texas, 1956.
40. Stanley K. Prognostic factors for survival in patients with inoperable lung cancer. *Journal of the National Cancer Institute*, 1980; **65**: 25–32.
41. Minna J, Higgins G, Glastein E. Cancer of the lung. In: *Cancer: Principles and Practice of Oncology* (ed. V De Vita, S Hellmann, S Rosenberg). New York: JB Lippincott, 1985.
42. Kobashi-Schoot JAM, Hanewald GJFP, van Dam FSAM, *et al.* Assessment of malaise in cancer treated with radiotherapy. *Cancer Nursing*, 1985; **8**: 306–14.
43. Piper BF, Lindsey AM, Dodd MJ, *et al.* The development of an instrument to measure the subjective dimension of fatigue. In: *Key Aspects of Comfort. Management of Pain, Fatigue and Nausea* (ed. Funk SG, Tornquist EM, Campagne MT, Aracher Gopp RA, Wiese). New York: Springer Publishing Company, 1989.
44. Kaasa T, Gillis K, Middleton E, Bruera E. The Edmonton Functional Assessment Tool (EFAT) for terminal cancer patients. Presented at the 9th Int'l Congress on Care of the Terminally Ill, Montreal, Nov. 1–2, 1992.
45. Love R, Leventhal H, Easterling M, Nerenz D. Side effects and emotional distress during cancer chemotherapy. *Cancer*, 1989; **63**: 604–12.
46. Lopes J, Russell D, Whitwell HJ, *et al.* Skeletal muscle function in malnutrition. *American Journal of Malnutrition*, 1983; **36**: 602–10.

47. Bruera E, Roca E, Cedaro L, Carraro S, Chacon R. Action of oral methylprednisolone in terminal cancer patients: a prospective randomized double-blind study. *Cancer Treatment Reports*, 1985; **69**: 751–4.
48. Della Cuna GR, Pellegrini A, Piazzi M. Effect of methylprednisolone sodium succinate on quality of life in preterminal cancer patients: a placebo-controlled, multicenter study. *European Journal of Cancer and Clinical Oncology*, 1989; **25**: 1817–21.
49. Popiela T, Lucchi R, Giongo F. Methylprednisolone as palliative therapy for femal terminal cancer patients. *European Journal of Cancer and Clinical Oncology*, 1989; **25**:1823–9.
50. Forrest W, Brown B, Brown C, *et al.* Dextroamphetamine with morphine for the treatment of post-operative pain. *New England Journal of Medicine*, 1977; **296**: 712–5.
51. Weiner N. Amphetamine. In: *The Pharmacological Basis for Therapeutics* (ed. Goodman L, Gilman A). New York: MacMillan, 1980: 159–62.
52. Bruera E, Carraro S, Roca E, Barugel M, Chacon R. Double-blind evaluation of the effects of mazindol on pain, depression, anxiety, appetite and activity in terminal cancer patients. *Cancer Treatment Reports*, 1986; **70**: 295–8.
53. Bruera E, Brenneis C, Chadwick S, Hanson J, MacDonald RN. Methylphenidate associated with narcotics for the treatment of cancer pain. *Cancer Treatment Reports*, 1987; **71**: 67–70.
54. Koretz R. Parenteral nutrition: is it oncologically logical? *Journal of Clinical Oncology*, 1984; **2**: 534–8.
55. Evans W, Nixon D, Daly J. A randomized study of standard or augmented oral nutritional support versus ad lib nutrition intake in patients with advanced cancer. *Clinical and Investigative Medicine*, 1986; **9**: A-127 (Abstract).
56. Bruera E, Macmillan K, Hanson J, Kuehn N, MacDonald RN. A controlled trial of megestrol acetate on appetite, caloric intake, nutritional status, and other symptoms in patients with advanced cancer. *Cancer*, 1990; **66**: 1279–82.

9.5 Palliation of respiratory symptoms

Sam Ahmedzai

Introduction

The palliation of respiratory symptoms is only a small part of the whole field of palliative care, but it embraces a surprisingly wide area of clinical practice. This is because respiratory symptoms are relatively common and tend to become more important to the patient and family as the terminal illness progresses. They are also one of the more poorly understood areas of palliative medical practice, and this raises the possibility of irrational, unhelpful, and occasionally harmful intervention. The understanding and management of pain in terminal disease, paricularly from cancer, has been central to the development of palliative care itself as a science and a humanistic health care discipline. In this chapter we attempt to unravel some of the complexities of respiratory symptoms, so that clinicians may better comprehend and more effectively palliate these in the same way that is now taken for granted in pain control.

The structure and function of the respiratory system will be examined first as a foundation on which to base the practice of good practical palliation. To continue the analogy with pain management, it would be like attempting to provide good pain control in terminal disease without knowing about neural pathways, opioid receptors, or the role of prostaglandins.

Sections on the major respiratory problems of dyspnoea, cough, and haemoptysis follow this theoretical introduction. These headings cover most of the clinical issues faced in practical palliative care, and include both oncological and non-oncological approaches. They also embrace most of the clinical syndromes to be met in palliative care, ranging from airflow obstruction due to tumour or asthma, to rarer but distressing conditions like lymphangitis carcinomatosa and terminal respiratory panic. Brief sections on pleural pain, pneumothorax, and pulmonary embolism are also included because they are relevant to the care of terminally ill patients, although they are covered more fully in other medical practice texts.

Finally, the psychosocial aspects of respiratory distress, particularly in the terminal stages, and how these impinge on the quality of life of patients and their families are discussed.

Structure and function of the respiratory system

In attempting to give good palliation of respiratory symptoms, it is essential to have some understanding of how the respiratory system is constructed and how it functions. It is possible here to give only a broad introduction to this rather difficult and growing field of medical science. More detailed reviews of these topics can be found in the reference list provided at the end of this chapter.

For the purposes of this discussion the respiratory system includes the thoracic cage (bony and muscular), the lungs, the airways, and the peripheral and central centres involved in regulating breathing. The condition of the nose, mouth, pharynx, and larynx are also relevant to airflow.

Airways

The role of the airways is particularly important in respiratory palliative care.[1,2] The maintenance of patency of the airways is one of the most vital homeostatic mechanisms in the body. Any obstruction to airflow, whether from tumour, mucus, foreign body, or airway narrowing, can lead to physical and psychological distress. The control of tracheal and bronchial smooth muscle is complex and has been the subject of considerable research, particularly with regard to asthma and chronic obstructive airways disease. As these are very common conditions in the population at large, and may be more prevalent in patients who have smoking-related malignancies such as lung cancer, it is worthwhile exploring the mechanisms in more detail.

Bronchial smooth muscle is innervated by adrenergic, cholinergic, and other non-adrenergic pathways in humans and other species. Cholinergic stimulation (or adrenergic blockade) causes bronchoconstriction, whereas adrenergic stimulation (or anticholinergic drugs) relaxes bronchial muscle and opens the airways. The role of the non-adrenergic pathways is not clear, but they probably modulate the other effects.

The surfaces of the bronchi and trachea are covered with cilia, which serve to move the constantly produced mucus, other fluid from the alveoli, and inhaled foreign bodies up towards the pharynx. The cilia and mucus glands are under cholinergic control; therefore anti-cholinergic drugs will both dry up mucus secretion and slow down ciliary passage.

The design of the air passages from nose to alveoli encourages the deposition of larger inhaled particles above the trachea, where they are easily expelled. Only particles (whether of solid or aerosolized fluid) of size less than 10 μm penetrate to a significant extent beyond the larger airways. To reach the alveoli, particles need to be smaller than 5 μm.

Opioid receptors have been found in the major airways in man.[3] It has been shown that the opioid antagonist naloxone can prevent the bronchial secretion of mucus in response to inhaled irritants, which can give rise to chronic cough in smokers.Thus opioids may be involved in the modulation the hypersecretion of mucus in chronic airways disease, but whether this affects the sensation of breathing has not been proven.

Changes due to ageing

It is important to appreciate that pulmonary ventilation, which is largely determined by airflow and chest wall dynamics, may be affected by chronic conditions which occur in older people. Nearly 90 per cent of patients with Parkinson's disease show a loss of lung volume that is related to the severity of the disease and is probably caused by rigidity and weakness of chest wall muscles rather than intrinsic lung or airways disease.[4] Age itself has a strong effect on lung capacity and ventilatory efficiency.[5] Lung volumes in normal elderly people can be expected to fall to a quarter of the values for healthy young adults. This change occurs as a result of the normal effects of ageing on the skeleton, respiratory muscles, and lung elasticity, as well as the long-term effects of chronic illness and smoking. There are gender differences; for example, the forced expiratory volume in 1 s (FEV_1) declines by approximately 30 ml per year in non-smoking men and by 23 ml per year in non-smoking females. Other respiratory parameters, including diffusing capacity and gas exchange, also reduce with age.

Control of respiration

The act of breathing is normally under involuntary control and may be influenced by a large number of factors, both physiological and psychological.[2,6] The major physiological influences are neural, muscular, and chemical.[7,8] Thankfully, we are not usually aware of the ever-changing frequency and pattern of breathing as we go from rest to exertion and back. For example, when a normal 70-kg man walks at a slow 2.5 miles/h his ventilatory rate has to increase substantially, since, if the normal resting ventilation were maintained, his alveolar oxygen level would rapidly drop to a point below that of someone breathing the thin air at the top of Mount Everest, i.e. below the level for survival.[9]

Measurement problems

The methodology of studying respiratory mechanisms has been well described.[10] Much of the earlier knowledge was based on animal and *in vitro* research. There are numerous pitfalls in the measurement of respiration in humans, not least of which are the placebo effect of any intervention and the intrusive nature of most measurements.[11] There is significant variability between individuals, and even within the same individual for some tests, which can seriously confound studies.

Neural mechanisms

The neural mechanisms which influence breathing are mediated through the innervation of the airways, the lungs, and the chest wall and diaphragmatic muscles.[7,8] Inputs from these sources are received and integrated in the so-called 'respiratory centre' of the medulla oblongata in the brainstem. In reality, there are several discrete centres with specific regulatory functions (Fig. 1).[6]

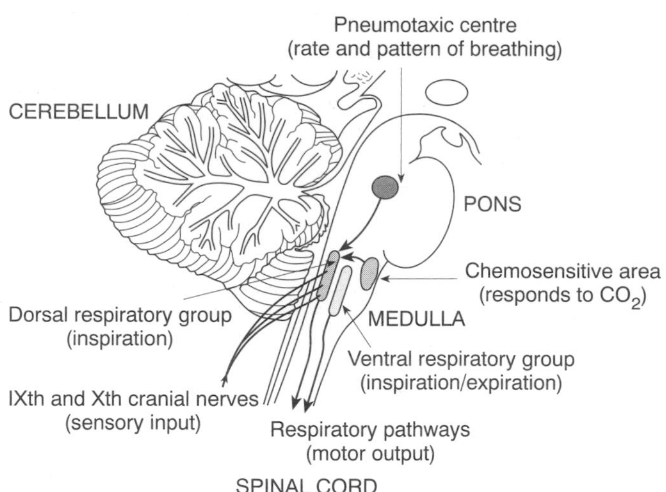

Fig. 1 Components of the central 'respiratory centre'.

Airway stretch receptors

The airways are heavily innervated with sensory nerves that end in a variety of receptors which respond to different forms of distortion. There is good experimental evidence that, through their central connections, they are responsible for controlling much of the normal breathing cycle.[2,7] It is not thought that they directly mediate the sensation of dyspnoea.

Lung parenchymal receptors

The juxtapulmonary capillary receptors (J-receptors), so called because they occur at the junction of the capillaries and alveoli deep in the lung parenchymal tissues, are of special interest. It is believed that they are primarily involved in the detection of any rise in pulmonary capillary pressure (e.g. caused by pulmonary congestion). J-receptors are responsible for rapid shallow breathing when stimulated experimentally by interstitial pulmonary oedema or microembolism. It is thought that, through their central connections with the brain via cholinergic nerve pathways, they may be involved in the sensation of breathlessness in these clinical situations.[7]

Respiratory muscles

The role of skeletal and diaphragm muscle receptors in the modulation of breathing is being increasingly recognized.[12,13] The stretching and, more importantly, the fatiguing of these muscles has significant effects on their efficiency and on the sensations perceived by the individual. The sensory receptors in these muscles may be significantly involved in the aetiology of the perception of breathlessness.[14] A wide range of acute or chronic disorders, including complications of malignancy, adversely affect respiratory muscle condition, and their importance is being increasingly recognized as a cause of respiratory distress.[15]

There is good evidence that the rib cage behaves differently from the diaphragm. Drugs which modify muscle and ventilatory activity also act differentially; for example, the benzodiazepine midazolam which is used frequently in palliative care reduces tidal volume and depresses ventilation predominantly by affecting the thoracoabdominal muscles, while opioids appear primarily to inhibit rib cage movement.[16]

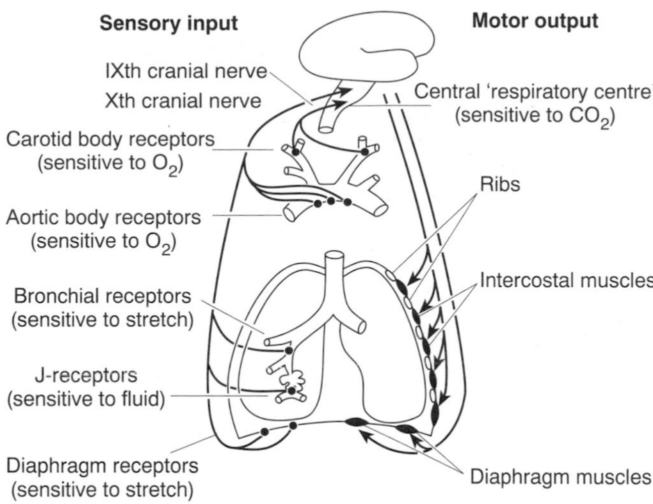

Fig. 2 Central and peripheral regulation of breathing.

Chemical control mechanisms

Chemical control mechanisms are extremely important in the regulation of breathing in health and disease. They are also among the main routes for modifying respiration and the sensation of breathlessness through drugs. There are two groups of chemical receptors—the peripheral receptors and the central receptors (Fig. 2).

Peripheral chemical receptors

The peripheral chemoreceptors are found in two locations: the aortic and the carotid bodies. The former are found at the arch of the aorta and the latter are highly vascular structures at the bifurcation of the common carotid arteries. They are innervated by cranial nerves IX and X which enter the brain at the medulla, near the site of the central chemoreceptors.

The peripheral chemoreceptors are sensitive to changes in the level of oxygen in the arterial blood. They are stimulated when the oxygen level in blood falls (hypoxaemia) and are involved in the stimulation of ventilation.[17] The mechanisms for regulating oxygenation of blood in the lungs are very complex, but increased ventilatory rate is one effective way of improving it.[18] The arterial chemoreceptors are only moderately sensitive, however, and fairly profound hypoxaemia has to arise before they significantly stimulate respiration and could give rise to abnormal perception of breathing.[6] When the carotid bodies have been removed or their innervation is interrupted, either experimentally or as a result of carotid artery surgery, there is not usually a profound or lasting effect on breathing pattern and respiratory sensation, except in conditions of reduced oxygen supply.[11] Similarly, it has also been found that the hypoxic drive to breathing remains unaffected in diabetic autonomic neuropathy, when many neurally mediated mechanisms are significantly impaired.[19]

Central chemical receptors

The central chemoreceptors are situated in the so-called respiratory centre within the medulla oblongata of the brain (Fig. 1). They are directly connected to the other neural centres present in this area that influence the pattern and rate of breathing.[6] The central receptors respond rapidly to extremely small changes in the acidity, or pH, of blood and cerebrospinal fluid. The pH is closely related to the pressure of carbon dioxide ($p\mathrm{CO}_2$) in the blood, which in turn reflects the level of ventilation of the lungs.[20] As CO_2 is very easily excreted through the alveolar walls, even a minute increase in blood $p\mathrm{CO}_2$ signifies a major reduction in ventilation. The response of the respiratory centre when it has detected a rise in $p\mathrm{CO}_2$ (via a fall in pH) is to stimulate ventilation in order to excrete more CO_2. Normally this is maintained automatically, but if $p\mathrm{CO}_2$ is allowed to rise artificially it causes a conscious unpleasant sensation of the need to breathe harder. Thus if the breath is held voluntarily for a prolonged time, it is the rising $p\mathrm{CO}_2$ (or hypercapnia) rather than the falling $p\mathrm{O}_2$ (hypoxaemia) that is the driving stimulus to take another breath.

Therefore the medullary centre is considered to be more important than the peripheral receptors in regulating the level and pattern of breathing in health and disease.[6] The degree of central chemical sensitivity is usually expressed in terms of the mathematical relationship between ventilation and $p\mathrm{CO}_2$. It is variously referred to as the hypercapnic drive to ventilation (or respiration) or the ventilatory response to hypercapnia.

The sensitivity of the central receptors may itself vary as a result of many internal and external influences in disease or after many drugs. A reduction in hypercapnic drive after drugs is often termed 'respiratory depression'. Hypercapnic drive falls off with increasing age.[21] It can be modified voluntarily through the chronic manipulation of respiration in certain yoga techniques.[22] Natural stimulation of the sympathetic autonomic nervous system, or administration of adrenergic drugs, will increase ventilatory drive and thus stimulate respiration.[11]

There has been considerable research on the role of endogenous and exogenous opioids on respiration, and most of this has focused on the well-established action of opioids on the medullary centre. For some time it has been known that opioids can attenuate the hypercapnic drive to ventilation, i.e. they render the medullary centre less sensitive to rising $p\mathrm{CO}_2$ levels.[10] All strong opioids are capable of this effect to varying degrees, depending on their receptor subtype affinity.[23] Studies of patients with chronic lung disease using the opioid antagonist naloxone have led to the concept that endogenous opioids (endorphins) could be involved in the regulation of respiration.[24]

The common observation that dyspnoea may abate when the CO_2 level rises above 75 mmHg could be due to the compensatory release of natural endorphins.[25] Indeed, patients with extreme hypercapnia are often somnolent, a condition that is referred to as 'CO_2 narcosis'. The sedation may occur directly due to the effect of hypercapnia on the brain or indirectly through the stimulation of endorphins.

The endorphin level has been found to rise after short-term induced hypercapnia in normal subjects, but only after pretreatment with naloxone.[26] It is known that alcohol also causes blunting of the ventilatory drive to hypercapnia, and this has been shown to be reversed by naloxone, suggesting that the respiratory sedative effect of alcohol may also be mediated by endorphins.[27] Because of the difficulty in studying the low levels of naturally occurring endorphins in humans, the evidence to support these hypotheses is mainly circumstantial so far and the results remain difficult to interpret.

In contrast with these depressant effects on ventilatory drive, the local anaesthetic agents lignocaine and bupivacaine are found, rather surprisingly, to increase ventilatory sensitivity.[28,29] The mechanism of this action is unclear and only emphasizes the complexity of the chemical control of respiration. The practical implications of these effects will be explored below with respect to the rationale of treatment.

Dyspnoea

Dyspnoea, or shortness of breath, is one of the most important challenges for clinical practice and research in palliative care. Like pain, it is a subjective sensation that is universally experienced by everyone at some time or other and has a useful function in limiting the indulgence in excessive exertion, but it can become pathological and restricting of normal activity. Again like pain, it has proved rather difficult to define.

Definitions

As with pain, it is perhaps inevitable that everyone will have his or her own personal favourite definition of dyspnoea. The derivation of the word 'dyspnoea' is from the Greek 'dys' meaning 'bad' or 'difficult' and 'pneo' meaning 'breathing'. Any clinical definition of dyspnoea should recognize that it is a subjective sensation of difficulty in breathing, not necessarily related to exertion, that compels the individual to increase his ventilation or reduce his activity. Although subjective, its effects on function and other activities of living may be objectively observable.

Other useful ways for looking at the 'meaning' of dyspnoea include the following.

1. Physiological: dyspnoea is the result of the demands on the lungs being out of proportion to their capacity to respond (adapted from ref. 2).

2. Aetiological: dyspnoea should be viewed first as a warning of disease — a call to investigate and treat the underlying medical condition (adapted from ref. 30).

3. Functional: dyspnoea is undue awareness of discomfort which is not commensurate with the level of physical activity (adapted from ref. 31).

4. Quality of life: dyspnoea is the suffering caused by difficulty in breathing which significantly impairs the individual's quality of life (adapted from ref. 32).

The concepts of 'distress' and 'total pain'[33] are well established in palliative care, and so it is helpful to think of dyspnoea as the major part of 'total respiratory distress' which would encompass the physical, psychological, and social manifestations. However, this must not be confused with 'respiratory distress syndrome' of either the adult or neonatal varieties. The psychological aspects of dyspnoea will be discussed further later in this section.

Terms sometimes confused with dyspnoea

Dyspnoea is sometimes used casually and wrongly to describe disturbed patterns of breathing. These include the following:

- tachypnoea (increased rate of breathing caused by elevated metabolic rate, e.g. with fever);

- hyperpnoea (increased ventilation through metabolic acidosis, e.g. with diabetic ketoacidosis);

- hyperventilation (psychologically induced increased respiration).

Patients describe dypsnoea in unique ways, ranging from tightness in the chest, or needing to gasp or pant, to extreme fear of suffocation or drowning. The different descriptors used may have aetiological or therapeutic significance.[34] For example, in the case of hyperventilation syndrome — a useful synonym is 'behavioural breathlessness' — subjects characteristically state that they find it more difficult to breathe in than out and that their breathlessness is episodic at rest, variable, and accompanied by feeling hot and sweaty and the well-known symptoms of hyperventilation-induced alkalosis.[35] However, it is fair to point out that this is also the pattern in many patients with advanced cancer with major airways obstruction, occult recurrent pulmonary embolism, or a functional overlay to another genuine cause of dyspnoea.

A functional aspect of breathlessness of great practical significance is exercise ability or tolerance, which may be taken (often inappropriately) as a proxy measure of dyspnoea. It should be appreciated that 'exercise' does not imply heavy physical exertion! To one person it can mean carrying a heavy shopping bag for a mile, to another it may mean walking to the front door, and to yet another it could represent being able to wash or dress. It is important to retain these unique interpretations of exercise when dealing with individuals, particularly in palliative care. However, standardized measures are necessary in controlled research studies, and these have usually adopted 'walking' as the model for exertion.

Prevalence

The published prevalence rates of dyspnoea in terminal disease show large variations between series, as they are reported to occur in 29 to 74 per cent of all patients.[30] This variation probably reflects as much the local definition and method of eliciting the symptom, and the selection of patients in the sample, as true differences between populations. Whereas some authors quote overall presence or absence of dyspnoea, others express the severity of the symptoms, but usually with different scoring systems. Of course, this problem is not unique to the documentation of dyspnoea, but is seen with other symptoms in palliative care.

In a small series of patients being cared for by a London hospital support team, dyspnoea was found in 18 out of 26 patients (69 per cent).[36] At St Christopher's Hospice, London, dyspnoea was noted in 41 per cent of 607 consecutively admitted patients, but a breakdown by gender showed a higher rate in men (50 per cent) than women (32 per cent).[37] It has been stated that 'dyspnoea is severe in 50 per cent of men but is distressing in only 25 per cent of women'.[38] At another English inpatient unit, dyspnoea was present in 55.5 per cent of all patients on admission, but the prevalence was 78.6 per cent in patients who died within 1 day.[39] In a report on 30 patients aged from a few months to 18 years who died in a children's hospice, dyspnoea was recorded as 'the most persistent' symptom in 32 per cent.[40]

In the National Hospice Study in the United States, which

Table 1 Causes of dyspnoea: relationship to time course of symptom

	Onset				
	Acute (hours)	**Subacute (days or weeks)**	**Chronic (months)**	**Recurrent episodes**	**Nocturnal attacks**
Pulmonary					
Asthma	+	+		++	++
Chronic obstructive airways disease		+	+	++	
Infection	+	+			
Pleural effusion		+		(+)	
Pneumothorax	+			(+)	
Bronchial obstruction		+	+		
Pulmonary embolism	+	+		(+)	
Cardiac					
Heart failure	+	+		+	+
Neuromuscular					
Motor neurone disease		+	++		(+)
Psychological					
Hyperventilation	+		++		

Adapted from ref. 49.

collected data from hundreds of patients receiving care in many different programmes including home care, dyspnoea was seen in 70 per cent in the final 6 weeks of life.[41] An Italian home care service recorded 'uncontrolled' levels of 'breathing difficulty' in 10 per cent of patients on entry to the programme; this figure rose to 17 per cent during care at the same time that uncontrolled pain fell from 59 to 35 per cent.[42] The same picture of increasing dyspnoea with falling pain scores was reported in a prospective study of a London home care team: towards death, 21 per cent of patients had dyspnoea as their main symptom.[43]

Patients and their carers may have different views about the severity of breathlessness. In one series from the north of England it was reported as occurring in 28 per cent by the general practitioner, in 35 per cent by the nurse, and in 43 per cent by the caring relative — all in the same patients.[44] In a series of 40 lung cancer patients who died while attending a Scottish chest clinic, the severity of dyspnoea as rated by spouses was significantly higher (mean 1.8 from a total score of 3) than the patients' self-rating (mean score 1.4).[45]

While the overall prevalence of dyspnoea for patients entering St Christopher's Hospice was 41 per cent, for lung cancer patients this figure rose to 61 per cent.[46] In a London home care study, at around the time of death dyspnoea was the main symptom for 78 per cent of patients with lung cancer, but only for 6 per cent of those with genitourinary cancers and in none with gastrointestinal cancers.[43] In the National Hospice Study in the United States, lung cancer again had the highest prevalence of dyspnoea.[41]

Pre-existing lung disease such as emphysema may influence the sensation of dyspnoea in cancer patients.[47] In a large postal survey of 'normal' adults, 9 per cent of male and 3 per cent of female respondents reported the occurrence of wheeze at least weekly, while other symptoms of chronic bronchitis occurred in 17 per cent and 7 per cent respectively.[48]

Causes

The causes of dyspnoea are as numerous and varied as the causes of pain, and, as with the latter symptom, in good palliative care it is important for the clinician to be familiar with these as therapeutic interventions are frequently best selected on the basis of aetiology. In the preceding section we focused on the physiological control of breathing in health and disease; the causes of dyspnoea often originate outside the respiratory system, but ultimately interfere with the control and perception of breathing in one or more ways.

Systematic classifications

A useful approach is to represent the causes with respect to time course of onset (acute = hours, subacute = days or weeks, and chronic = months to years) (Table 1).[50] Causes may also be differentiated on the basis of recurrence, previous occupational exposure, and the presence or absence of nocturnal attacks. Finally, the classification of dyspnoea may be based on associated features: wheeze, purulent sputum, haemoptysis, relation to smoking, chest pain, and peripheral oedema (Table 2).

A more theoretical way of looking at the causes of dyspnoea, pursuing the broader concept of 'respiratory distress', is a classification of aetiology based on anatomical–pathological correlations (Table 3).[32] Thus, for a given anatomical 'site' (or system), the pathological entities are described together with the symptoms to which they give rise. In this way it is possible to ascribe the main respiratory symptoms (dyspnoea, cough, haemoptysis, and pleural pain) to each anatomical–pathological group. This system emphasizes the previous observation that the same symptoms tend to arise from very different causes. Whichever of these classifications is used, a person's symptoms can be quickly checked against known or presumed clinical features to establish a better understanding of cause and hence a more rational treatment plan.

Table 2 Causes of dyspnoea: associated clinical features

	Wheeze	Purulent sputum	Cough	Haemoptysis	Chest pain	Oedema
Pulmonary						
Asthma	++	(+)	++			
Chronic obstructive airways disease	++	++	++	(+)		+ (Cor pulmonale)
Infection	+	++	++	(+)	(+)	
Pleural effusion			(+)		+	
Pneumothorax			(+)		++	
Bronchial obstruction	+	+	++	+	+	(+) (Superior vena cava obstruction)
Pulmonary embolism	(+)		+	+	++	+ (Deep vein thrombosis)
Cardiac						
Heart failure	+		+	+	(+)	++
Neuromuscular						
Motor neurone disease			(+)			
Psychological						
Hyperventilation					(+)	

Adapted from ref. 49.

Determining causation is useful for the doctor seeing a patient with a complaint of dyspnoea for the first time. It is also invaluable in reviewing such a patient who is well advanced in his disease, as it is all too easily assumed that the causes of the symptoms remain static within individuals. During the course of his or her illness, a 'typical' patient with lung cancer may be breathless as a result of any of the following problems: asthma (reversible airflow obstruction), chronic obstructive airways disease (non-reversible airflow obstruction), pulmonary collapse due to endobronchial occlusion by tumour, pleural effusion due to pleural extension, stridor due to tracheal tumour or mediastinal lymph nodes, respiratory infection (bronchitis or pneumonic consolidation), and pulmonary embolism from deep venous thrombosis caused by inactivity! If the patient is really unlucky, he or she could develop a pericardial effusion,

Table 3 Causes of respiratory distress: symptoms and their anatomical–pathological bases

Anatomical 'site'	Pathological change	Symptom
Pulmonary	Tracheal tumour	Dyspnoea, stridor, cough
	Lung collapse	Dyspnoea, cough
	Airway collapse	Dyspnoea, cough
	Tracheo-oesophageal fistula	Cough, haemoptysis
	Inhalation	Dyspnoea, cough, pain
	Consolidation	Dyspnoea, cough, pleurisy
	Infection	Dyspnoea, cough, pain, haemoptysis
	Fibrosis/vasculitis	Dyspnoea, cough
	Lymphangitis carcinomatosa	Dyspnoea, cough
	Thromboembolism	Dyspnoea, cough, pain
	Radiation damage	Dyspnoea, cough
Cardiac	Ischaemic heart disease	Dyspnoea, pain
	Cardiac failure	Dyspnoea, haemoptysis
	Pericardial disease	Dyspnoea
	Superior vena cava obstruction	Dyspnoea
Pleural	Effusion	Dyspnoea
	Thromboembolism	Dyspnoea, pain
	Tumour	Pain, pleurisy
	Pneumothorax	Dyspnoea, pain
Thoracic cage	Chest wall tumour	Pain, 'fungating' cancer
	Carcinoma en cuirasse	Dyspnoea, pain, 'fungating' cancer
	Diaphragmatic tumour	Dyspnoea, pain, hiccups
	Respiratory muscle fatigue	Dyspnoea

Reproduced from ref. 36.

lymphangitis carcinomatosa, or treatment-related acute pneumonitis. Each of these distinct problems could give rise to the same degree of subjective dyspnoea, albeit with different time courses and associated factors, but most would be palliated in distinct ways.

It should be readily apparent that dyspnoea can be caused by both intrathoracic and extrathoracic disease processes. Therefore it is important to look beyond the chest when taking a history, examining the patient, or ordering investigations. It is also important to consider chronic or other incidental diseases which are unrelated to the patient's main condition, whether this is malignancy, progressive neuromuscular illness such as motor neurone disease, or any other 'terminal' condition. It could be reassuring to the patient to appreciate that other, possibly readily treatable, causes for his or her dyspnoea are being considered.

Psychological factors in perception of dyspnoea

The sensation of breathlessness can itself be modified by the patient's own perception of the origin or the seriousness of the underlying cause. It is often impossible to extricate the 'physical' component from the frequently accompanying psychological, social, and spiritual dimensions of 'total dyspnoea'. The longer the duration of dyspnoea, the more likely it is that non-physical elements assume significance in its perception and expression in terms of behaviour. There is no published evidence on this aspect of 'breathless behaviour' in terminally ill cancer patients, unlike the situation with chronic 'pain behaviour'.

Some research has been conducted into how people interpret the cause of their dyspnoea. When normal subjects were made breathless by eight different stimuli, they tended to use different descriptions for different causes, suggesting that the term 'breathlessness' in fact encompasses several different sensations.[34] In contrast, when the perception of breathlessness was studied in asthmatic subjects, after challenge by antigen, exercise, or histamine, the perception of dyspnoea did not differ between types of challenge for the same degree of objective deterioration.[51] Other examples of the interaction of mood, expectation, dyspnoea, and objective markers are discussed later in this chapter.

Effect of ageing

The normal effect of ageing on ventilatory control and function has already been discussed. The subjective tolerance for exertion is also reduced with ageing, and older people have a higher level of ventilation than younger subjects at all levels of exercise. This appears to be due predominantly to less efficient gas exchange in the older individuals.[52] It is difficult to separate 'purely' respiratory from cardiovascular influences on exercise, and indeed it is artificial to regard these two systems as really distinct. It is noteworthy that the capacity for training to improve exercise tolerance and thereby reduce the perception of breathlessness is present in older as well as younger people.

The insidious effects of late-onset asthma in the elderly population are poorly recognized as a cause of dyspnoea.[53,54]

Muscle fatigue and dyspnoea

It is worth focusing more closely on the role of the respiratory muscles in the aetiology of dyspnoea. The classic concept described by Campbell and Howell [14] was that inappropriate stretching of neuromuscular receptors is a fundamental factor in the causation of the breathless sensation. The process and causation of respiratory muscle fatigue is now well understood, particularly with regard to patients with chronic obstructive airways disease.[49] (Indeed, the term 'chronic obstructive pulmonary disease' is perhaps preferable to chronic obstructive airways disease as much of the condition and its consequences are seen outside the airways themselves.) Three groups who are at risk of respiratory muscle fatigue have been identified:[49]

(1) patients with low respiratory muscle force, regardless of cause (this would include patients with motor neurone disease);

(2) patients with low lung or chest wall compliance (including patients with acquired deformities of chest wall, or extensive involvement from pleural tumour such as mesothelioma);

(3) patients with both factors.

Thoracotomy and malignant infiltration of the phrenic nerve are also potential causes of poor muscle action. Furthermore, undernourished and cachectic patients, who comprise much of palliative care practice, may have more than 40 per cent reduction in some parameters of respiratory muscle strength.[15]

There is considerable interplay between the factors affecting the rib cage and the diaphragm, although it is customary to regard them as separate functional units. Conditions which lead to diaphragmatic incapacity are thought particularly likely to lead to the sensation of dyspnoea.[55] It is not known from electrophysiological or ventilatory studies whether patients with chronically splinted diaphragms due to hepatic enlargement, direct tumour infiltration, or ascites are also at risk in this way.

Measurement of dyspnoea

In palliative care it is important to develop valid and reliable measures of symptoms, so that response to treatment in individuals as well as to therapeutic strategies in group studies can be scientifically assessed. The measurement of dyspnoea has been improved by a number of recent studies, but there is still no gold standard.

Symptom scoring

The reason for attempting to measure dyspnoea will in part determine the method used. If the purpose is to evaluate purely subjective symptom relief, then a 'simple' symptom scoring method will suffice. If the functional capability of the patient is also of interest, then objective markers such as exercise testing could be added. Only in studies of treatments which are likely to affect ventilatory abnormalities, such as asthmatic or tumour-related airflow obstruction, should tests of pulmonary function be carried out. Where the psychosocial consequences of dyspnoea on the patient and family are being studied, it would be inappropriate to perform dynamic breathing tests, but highly relevant to ask about physical and role functioning as well as posing the more conventional questions about mood and social restrictions. Finally, many new care programmes are inevitably expensive and cost–benefit analysis may play a part in the overall assessment.

Even at the level of the 'simple' scoring of physical symptoms, evaluations should do more than merely record the presence or absence of dyspnoea. Systems which grade the severity are numerous, and it is not within the scope of this chapter to describe their psychometric or methodological merits. Briefly, in palliative care the usual approaches are the verbal categorical scale (e.g. none,

Table 4 Investigation of dyspnoea

Recommended test	Useful for		
	Making diagnosis	Monitoring progress	Determining prognosis
Radiology			
Chest radiograph	++	+	(+)
Ultrasound (to localize pleural effusion)	+	(+)	
Ventilation–perfusion lung scan (for pulmonary embolism)	+	(+)	+
Blood			
Full blood count	++	(+)	
Skin oxygen saturation ($Sa\text{O}_2$)	++	+	
Pulmonary function			
Dynamic lung volumes (FEV_1, FVC) preferably with bronchodilator	++	+	

mild, moderate, or severe) or the linear analogue scale (usually a 10-cm line anchored with 'no dyspnoea' at one end and 'extreme dyspnoea' at the other). The former verbal approach is probably more intuitive for most older sicker patients (and often for staff!). For research purposes, the verbal scale usually yields less variance of data than the linear analogue scale, but in the description of patient groups it often makes more 'clinical sense' to talk of the proportion of patients with mild, moderate, or severe dyspnoea, than to talk of mean values from 0 to 100 mm.

In any verbal rating system it is important for all users to be familiar with the meaning of the categories used. For this reason, standardized and validated scales such as the EORTC Quality of Life Core Questionnaire (EORTC QL-30)[56] together with its Lung Module (QLQ-LC13)[57] are to be recommended. The EORTC questionnaires were designed as self-rating instruments, i.e. they are completed by patients. However, if patients are unable to fill in forms, they could be applied as a structured interview schedule.

The Chronic Respiratory Questionnaire has been tested against physical parameters and other symptom questionnaires in patients with chronic obstructive airways disease having walking tests.[58] While most workers have found generally poor correlation between dyspnoea and 'objective' indices such as lung volumes, the Chronic Respiratory Questionnaire correlated better with spirometry and walking test results than the other methods. The relatives of patients with chronic obstructive airways disease tended to report fewer problems than the patients themselves, but rated them more severely.[59]

Palliative care patients, like other groups, vary in their symptoms and capabilities from day to day and over longer periods of time. However, most study methods are not sensitive to these background variations. One questionnaire of physical functioning specifically asks the patient about the 'best' and 'worst' levels he achieves.[60] At face value, this approach would seem quite sensible to use in studies of terminally ill patients and may give more realistic results than questionnaires asking about the 'average' level of symptoms.

Exercise tests

Respiratory physiologists and clinicians are fond of exercise tests, particularly walking or bicycle ergometer tests.[61,62] These have obvious relevance for a patient population that is predominantly mobile and trying to remain functionally active. For typical palliative care cancer patients, they may not be so useful in the advanced stages of disease, but more appropriate standardized measures of function have yet to be proposed. The shorter walking tests (e.g. up to 100 m) may still be feasible.[63] When looking at 'objective' data of this sort, it is important to bear in mind that evidence of exercise capacity, at least in patients with chronic obstructive pulmonary disease, is more strongly related to inspiratory muscle strength and lung function than to dyspnoea and quality of life, which are useful parameters in palliative care.[62] Furthermore, the effect of practice and other artefacts should be considered when repeat testing is performed. Different diagnostic groups of patients behave differently in walking tests, but the tests themselves appear to be sensitive to either cardiac or respiratory impairment.

Investigations

Table 4 lists the investigations that may be found useful and appropriate in palliative care either to elucidate the cause or to follow the progress of respiratory symptoms. It is perhaps easier to state which diagnostic investigations are not helpful in palliative care!

Pulmonary function tests are not useful in palliative care unless proof of airflow obstruction, and in particular reversibility with a bronchodilator, is being sought. They are also strenuous for severely breathless patients. It is noteworthy that 49 per cent of a series of bronchial carcinoma patients attending a United Kingdom chest clinic were found to have unrecognized airflow obstruction on formal testing, and it was rated as moderate to severe in 69 per cent of these.[64] Less than a fifth of these had been prescribed a bronchodilator. The peak flow measurement, although appealingly simple to perform at the bedside or in the home with a portable handheld meter, is generally unhelpful in diagnosis. There are many limitations to its use which may give misleading results.[65] However, it may be a useful non-invasive way for motivated patients to monitor their progress after a new therapy has been instituted.

There is no place for 'routine' chest radiographs in the serial assessment of lung cancer patients in the advanced stages when active oncological interventions are not being pursued. However, chest radiographs may be invaluable in excluding pleural effusion or heart failure, which are eminently treatable conditions but which are not always diagnosed reliably by the history and clinical examination alone.

Other tests that are hardly ever needed or are difficult to justify because of patient burden include arterial blood gases, echocardiography, and pulmonary angiography (although isotope ventilation–perfusion scanning is quick and easy for most patients). It is important to note that, apart from the finding of pulmonary embolism on a lung scan, most of the tests included in Table 4 are not particularly helpful in determining the patient's prognosis. Regrettably there are no published studies to show the validity of these recommendations. Any research in this area should include a cost–benefit analysis, because of the economic implications of these tests.

Management

The management of breathlessness is now introduced in the light of the preceding discussion on regulation of normal respiration and the causes of dyspnoea.

General principles of palliation

The general principles of treating dyspnoea are the same as for any other aspect of intervention in palliative care:

(1) to determine and treat the underlying cause of dyspnoea wherever possible and reasonable for the patient (e.g. to drain a new pleural effusion rather than simply sedate);

(2) to relieve dyspnoea without adding other new problems (e.g. through side-effects, interactions, social or financial burden);

(3) to consider whether a treatment will be worthwhile for the patient and his or her family (bearing in mind the prognosis, adverse effects, social and financial cost, need for travel from home);

(4) to discuss all reasonable treatment options (which should always include 'no intervention') with the patient and the family, allowing them to make the final decision as far as possible.

Classification of treatments

A useful classification of management options is given in Table 5. There is no equivalent of the 'analgesic ladder' in the treatment of breathlessness, and so the order of choices in this system is not meant to represent priority of potency, ease of use, or any other preference.

In general, patients with malignancy should be considered for an oncological intervention unless this avenue has been previously tried and abandoned, or the patient is clearly too ill or unwilling. It is necessary for clinicians working in palliative care to be familiar with current anticancer treatments. The doctor's personal prejudices should not be allowed to prevail here. If he feels an oncological approach is feasible but is personally out of his depth, he should involve a local oncologist or trained palliative care specialist as soon as possible. Very often the 'expert' opinion will only confirm the initial suspicion that active antitumour therapy, although logical and potentially effective, is not justified in this particular instance.

Table 5 Management of dyspnoea: general approaches

Modality of treatment	Cause of dyspnoea
Oncological (including endobronchial therapy)	Malignancy
Drug therapy (particularly oral)	All
Inhaled therapy	Airways obstruction (all?)
Oxygen therapy	Hypoxaemia
Physiotherapy	All
Ventilatory support	Respiratory muscle fatigue or paralysis
Respiratory rehabilitation	Chronic obstructive airways disease, malignancy (all?)
Psychological methods	All?

Similarly, it is important for doctors to restrain those personal opinions which may be sceptical about the value of certain 'complementary' approaches for dyspnoea, such as relaxation therapy or massage. They should at least involve some colleagues, such as a specialist nurse or physiotherapist who is more knowledgeable about these treatments, in the decision-making. The final decision to embark on or reject a palliative treatment should come from the patient and his or her family, but they can only do this with adequate information, including some explanation of causes of the problem and the prognosis.

Oncological therapy

The majority of patients in palliative care programmes have an underlying diagnosis of malignancy. It cannot always be assumed that all oncological options have been exhausted by the time that the patient is considered as having 'advanced disease' or being 'terminally ill'. Therefore it is appropriate to bear these interventions in mind, unless the patient has already expressed a strong opinion about not having radiotherapy or chemotherapy.

General principles

The oncological options available for the relief of breathlessness (and other respiratory symptoms) are summarized in Table 6. In considering oncological treatments in palliative care, it is important to adjust the endpoints towards the quality, rather than the length, of the patient's life.[66] Issues about 'objective response' or increased survival, let alone curability, are not strictly relevant (but note that

Table 6 Oncological management of respiratory symptoms

Type of oncological intervention	Site applied
Radiotherapy	External beam Endobronchial
Laser therapy	Endobronchial
Cytotoxic chemotherapy	Systemic
Cryotherapy	Endobronchial
Stent	Endobronchial

prolonged survival, particularly to achieve some specific goal such as living up to an anniversary date, may be very important to some patients and relatives). The clinician needs to be familiar with the pattern of malignancy in the elderly population, as the behaviour of some cancers may be different in older compared with younger adults.

Few patients in specialist palliative care programmes are entered into clinical trials. If they are, it is essential that the full range of physical and psychosocial needs are addressed, and attempts should be made to measure these along with the more usual response rate and survival parameters.[67,68]

Radiotherapy (see Chapter 9.1.2)

Radiotherapy has a major role in relieving malignancy-related dyspnoea.[69] Breathlessness is more readily reversed if it is due to recent endobronchial obstruction, but the presence of a longer-standing lesion and pulmonary collapse should not preclude a trial of radiotherapy. There is increasing support for shorter radiotherapeutic protocols for lung cancer palliation. Very often a blocked bronchus can be reopened after just one treatment, or with two fractions given a week apart.[70] The burden to the patient, particularly if he or she wishes to remain at home, is minimal. This should be offered to all suitable patients, regardless of histological type; patients with small-cell lung cancer or bronchial obstruction due to lymphoma will respond more dramatically, but others may also gain good benefit with little upset. Tumours which are encroaching onto the carina or are causing tracheal obstruction should always be considered for early radiotherapy because of the unpleasant nature of dyspnoea accompanied by stridor in these conditions.

It is not always clear how radiotherapy relieves breathlessness. A radiograph may show re-expansion of a previously collapsed lobe or lung; however, the radiographic evidence is often not so clear, but the patient still seems to gain benefit. It should be appreciated that the balance between aeration (ventilation) and blood supply (perfusion) of an area of affected lung is probably more important than either component alone for optimal gas exchange to occur.[18] When there is an imbalance ('ventilation–perfusion mismatching'), improvement in either function may bring about an overall improvement in net gas exchange and, through more efficient respiratory muscular effort, in the sensation of dyspnoea.

It is possible that in some cases radiotherapy may work by relieving compression of pulmonary blood and lymphatic vessels, rather than just opening up blocked airways. Ventilation–perfusion lung scans show that this does indeed occur in parallel with symptomatic benefit after radiotherapy.[71] This would account for the noticeable subjective improvement in some patients after radiotherapy treatment which objectively is classed as unsuccessful because the appearance of the radiograph does not change.

Chemotherapy (see Chapter 9.11)

The place of cytotoxic chemotherapy in respiratory palliation is much more problematic than that of radiotherapy. In Europe there is, probably correctly, an in-built bias against the use of chemotherapy regimens in advanced cancer patients. However, the newer regimens of single agents or carefully selected combinations are worthy of consideration.

The best example of this approach is given by the modern management of small-cell (so-called 'oat cell') lung cancer. Although it accounts for only 25 per cent of all lung cancers, it is still sufficiently common to be a significant cause of mortality. Since it is a very aggressive malignancy, it also causes considerable morbidity in which respiratory symptoms predominate. However, the high growth rate of this tumour makes it more susceptible to most oncological interventions, and some of the highest response rates to chemotherapy for solid tumours are obtained in this condition. Earlier regimens, and those still used for younger fitter patients with early-stage disease in whom prolongation of survival is a major objective, used very potent and toxic combinations of cytotoxics. However, in recent years there has been great interest in the use of milder combinations or single agents in older advanced-stage patients. Some of these regimens are specifically designed for palliation, rather than to achieve impossible cure or unlikely life prolongation.[72] Unfortunately, most of these studies have not specifically documented details of symptom control, although toxicity is usually tolerable and global improvement in the patients' performance rating (which reflects physical functioning) may be observed.

The regimen that has now emerged as offering the best chance of palliation with minimal toxicity is single-agent oral etoposide.[73] Used on an outpatient basis, it is easily taken and is associated with useful relief of respiratory and other symptoms, although again oncologists have generally been less diligent about measuring these than more objective markers of response.

The case for chemotherapy in other cancers is much less well defined. The exceptions are the lymphomas, which are often chemosensitive even in the advanced stages, and breast cancer or gastrointestinal cancer, which cause dyspnoea due to bronchial obstruction or lymphangitis carcinomatosa. Breast cancer or prostate cancer with pulmonary involvement may also be treated, with fewer adverse effects, by means of hormonal manipulation.[74]

Superior vena cava obstruction

The oncological palliation of superior vena cava obstruction is worthy of special mention. The large majority (75 per cent) of cases are seen in lung cancer patients (3 per cent of all lung cancer cases are affected). It also arises in lymphoma patients (15 per cent of superior vena cava obstruction cases) and breast or other solid tumours (7 per cent of superior vena cava obstruction cases).[75]

The pathology in superior vena cava obstruction is extrinsic compression, sometimes accompanied by intravascular tumour or thrombosis, of the large central veins feeding into the heart; the superior vena cava is most usually affected, but occasionally the inferior vena cava is also blocked. The symptoms are dyspnoea associated with impaired venous return to the heart and possibly microembolism of the lungs, together with dilatation of veins and swelling of the soft tissues of the face, neck, and upper limbs. Headache and other cranial symptoms may occur as a result of cerebral congestion.

Superior vena cava obstruction often arises acutely and should be treated as an oncological (and palliative) emergency.[38] It is usually very responsive to a single dose of radiotherapy, regardless of tumour type. High-dose corticosteroids are also usually given to reduce oedema associated with the mediastinal tumour and to cover the possibility of radiotherapy-induced inflammatory reaction. Therefore active treatment should always be considered unless the patient is extremely ill, or is unable or unwilling to attend for radiotherapy. In such cases, the use of high-dose steroids alone may prove symptomatically beneficial, although for a shorter time. When the superior vena cava obstruction is caused by lymphoma, small cell lung cancer, or breast cancer, the patient should be considered for further oncological management.

Lymphangitis carcinomatosa

The diagnosis of lymphangitis carcinomatosa is difficult to make clinically and radiologically, and the condition probably exists more commonly than is recognized. It is characterized by severe and usually constant breathlessness, occurring even at rest and extremely limiting of any exertion, together with an unproductive cough.[2] Clinical examination of the patient may be unhelpful, but there may be basal crackles in the chest. The condition often arises insidiously in patients with known lung cancer and can be overlooked as merely 'progression' of disease. Other cases originate from metastatic breast, gastrointestinal, or prostate cancers.[74] Careful examination of the chest radiograph typically reveals widespread infiltration of the middle and lower zones with streaky markings originating from the lung roots (hila). The radiographic appearance is rather like that of acute left ventricular failure in the absence of an enlarged heart; small pleural effusions and Kerley's B lines may be seen in the peripheries, reflecting pulmonary congestion and interstitial oedema. Sometimes there is also hilar glandular enlargement which makes the diagnosis easier.

The pathology in lymphangitis carcinomatosa is blockage of the lymphatic drainage of the lungs. It is usually due to malignant obstruction of the hilar lymph glands and tends to occur bilaterally. The prognosis of such patients is extremely poor regardless of the tumour type, and they remain very disabled by the level of dyspnoea. The chronic congestion of the lung parenchyma in this condition and the severe distress is good circumstantial evidence to support the J-receptor theory of the cause of breathlessness.[7] Other factors include stiffening of the lungs leading to respiratory muscle fatigue, and a block to diffusion of oxygen through the alveoli caused by the interstitial fluid.

It is worth considering active oncological measures in lymphangitis carcinomatosa, as many cases arise from sensitive tumour types. Radiotherapy to the centre of the chest is most likely to help, but few patients are fit enough to receive chemotherapy. High-dose steroids may also be tried, but may add to the fluid retention. In most cases, opioid therapy and selective use of anxiolytics is indicated (with oxygen treatment as many patients are hypoxaemic) as the condition progresses.

Pleural effusion (see Chapter 9.1.3)

Pleural effusion is the collection of fluid in the space between the visceral and parietal pleura. Normally a small amount of fluid (10–20 ml) is always present to lubricate the surfaces. If pleural fluid is seen on a chest radiograph, at least 300 ml must be present, and must be it is not must be detectable by clinical examination until 500 ml have accumulated.[50] Both the radiograph and clinical signs may be misleading, particularly in the case of a right-sided effusion in the presence of an enlarged liver and where pleural tumour or thickening exists. If doubt exists, a lateral decubitus radiograph, in which the patient is positioned lying on the side of the supposed effusion, should confirm or refute the presence of free fluid. However, fluid may be present but not 'free' because of loculation, and thoracic ultrasound is a helpful localizing test.

Pleural effusion is a potent cause of dyspnoea, particularly if it arises rapidly. It is usually unilateral in association with malignancy, pulmonary embolism, or acute pneumonia, whereas bilateral effusions should raise the suspicion of heart failure or lymphangitis carcinomatosa.

Pleural aspiration is the definitive treatment for effusion, and most patients should be offered this treatment, even in hospices.[76] There is considerable literature on the most effective and least traumatic ways of draining pleural fluid.[77] In practice, many patients have had rather painful diagnostic pleural aspiration or biopsies taken, often in inexpert hands, and may be reluctant to have further therapeutic aspiration. Too rapid drainage or removal of a longstanding effusion may lead to increased dyspnoea and cough because of mediastinal shift and unilateral pulmonary oedema.

After aspiration, many clinicians feel that it is worth instilling an agent into the pleural space in order to prevent recurrence. These probably work by causing non-specific pleural inflammation which encourages the parietal and visceral surfaces to stick together, thus obliterating the potential space for reaccumulation. Although many drugs and materials have been used (e.g. talc, cytotoxics, and tetracycline with success rates of 93 per cent, 50–73 per cent, and 71 per cent respectively), there is considerable variation in clinical practice and many of these cause significant toxicity such as pleural pain or fever. There is also disagreement amongst chest physicians as to whether simple aspiration or the more elaborate intercostal tube and underwater seal drainage is better.[78]

Many patients in palliative care may not live long enough for significant reaccumulation of fluid to take place. Thus it seems reasonable simply to drain an effusion the first time. If it recurs quickly and causes further dyspnoea, it is then appropriate to use a sclerosing agent. At present the most frequently used agents are tetracycline and bleomycin—both cause painful pleural inflammation and therefore shoud be given with adequate oral analgesia or, alternatively, mixed with lignocaine. Another agent which has been used for chemical pleurodesis is mepacrine, which is an established anti-malaria antibiotic. In a recent Norwegian controlled trial, 40 patients with recurrent pleural effusions arising from variety of malignancies were randomly allocated to intrathoracic bleomycin or mepacrine.[79] In this study mepacrine was associated with a better response in terms of reduced volume of fluid and shorter times for drainage. Side-effects such as pain and fever were similar in both groups, and so it appears that mepacrine should also be considered in this situation.

Some patients who live longer may be subject to many recurrences of pleural effusion. An option for these is to have a Denver pleuroperitoneal shunt placed surgically.[80] However, the invasive nature of this approach precludes its use in many palliative care settings, and other non-specific drug approaches to the relief of dyspnoea would be more appropriate.

Pericardial involvement

Tumours occasionally invade or irritate the pericardial surface and cause pericarditis or a pericardial effusion. The symptoms from the latter are severe dyspnoea and limitation of exertion owing to reduced return of blood to the heart from the lungs. It usually arises in lung cancer, mediastinal lymphomas, breast cancer, and the rare cardiac tumours.

When pericardial involvement first develops or is suspected, pericardial aspiration may be undertaken in specialist centres with diagnostic and supportive facilities. In some situations with repeated pericardial effusions that are causing severe symptoms but are not necessarily life-threatening, the surgical creation of a 'window' to drain the fluid away continuously into the peritoneal cavity may be considered. However, more frequently this is a life-limiting condition and maximal drug treatment and other supportive care to control dyspnoea and fear should be given.

Endobronchial therapies

Recently there has been a surge of interest in the application of antitumour treatment directly at the site of disease by the endobronchial approach. The four types of endobronchial therapy currently available are local radiotherapy, laser treatment, cryotherapy, and stents.[81,82] While at first sight they may appear to be invasive and expensive and to require specialist knowledge and equipment, it is important to be aware of them for the occasional patients encountered in palliative care who have extremely resistant symptoms but are not nearing the end of life.

Endobronchial radiotherapy Localized radiotherapy (also known as brachytherapy) has long been a favoured approach in certain tumours (e.g. cancer of the cervix or uterus). There is now considerable experience in the application of radiation directly at the site of tracheal or bronchial tumours. Radio-active gold grains can be implanted into tumours via the bronchoscope after necrotic tissue has been cleared away by diathermy.[83] Relief of dyspnoea and objective improvement in airflow obstruction have been reported. This approach could be used after conventional external beam radiotherapy, as the dose to the tumour is very high but that to other nearby normal tissues is quite tolerable.

An alternative approach is the insertion, via a bronchoscope, of a catheter down which are passed radio-active particles of caesium or iridium. However, unlike implantation of gold grains, the particles and catheter are withdrawn after a short period of time. Sophisticated equipment is necessary for this form of application. The published results demonstrate relief of dyspnoea in 64 per cent of patients, and also relief of cough and particularly haemoptysis (50 per cent and 86 per cent of patients respectively).[84] In a German series, 79 per cent had palliation of dyspnoea and there was accompanying improvement in lung function and hypoxaemia.[85] A comprehensive assessment of physiological and symptomatic response was carried out in 20 patients who received endobronchial brachytherapy before treatment and after 6 weeks.[86] Patients improved after treatment in terms of subjective reports of symptoms (dyspnoea and haemoptysis improving more often than cough), radiographic appearances, ventilation–perfusion balance measured by isotope scanning, and various static and exercise pulmonary function tests.

A new technique has been described involving transtracheal placement of a catheter, via an minitracheostomy incision, which is then used to deliver caesium-137 to endobronchial lesions under bronchoscopic guidance.[87] This approach was apparently well tolerated, although the authors did not give details of symptomatic benefit. A potential advantage is that the equipment for delivering caesium-137 is widely available as it is used for the brachytherapy of uterine cervical cancer. Again, this form of intraluminal treatment is possible in patients who have received previous external radiotherapy as the radiation is very localized.

Endobronchial laser therapy Laser therapy has potential advantages over ionizing radiation treatment in terms of safety to patients and staff, but it is also limited because of cost and availability of facilities. Nevertheless there is now increasing evidence that endobronchial treatment using a neodymium-doped yttrium aluminium garnet (Nd:YAG) laser directly onto tracheal and proximal bronchial tumours can dramatically open up blocked airways, relieving breathlessness as well as haemoptysis.[88] Another advantage of laser treatment over radiotherapy is that it can be repeated many times without damage to healthy tissue. However, the need for bronchoscopy is a limiting factor, and the preference for general anaesthetic in some centres makes laser therapy less suitable for many older or frail patients.[89] A combined approach is to use an endobronchial laser first to recanalize an obstructed bronchus, followed quickly by conventional external-beam or intraluminal radiotherapy to give longer relief by necrosis deep within the tumour.[87,90]

A potentially useful development of endobronchial laser therapy is photodynamic therapy. In this technique, tumour tissue is highlighted by the systemic administration of a photosensitizing drug such as porfimer sodium (Photofrin); the laser is then guided to the malignant cells in a more specific way. However, the available evidence indicates that this method is better suited to early-stage bronchial cancers than to the palliation of large tumours.[91]

Unfortunately, the published data on laser treatment have not included good assessment of subjective symptoms such as dyspnoea, and evaluation is further complicated by the use of surgical resection during or after laser application.[92] However, there is impressive evidence of objective improvements after laser therapy on radiograph appearances, pulmonary function, and regional ventilation–perfusion scanning, all circumstantially suggesting that breathlessness may be helped.[93,94]

Endobronchial cryotherapy The endobronchial palliative reduction of major airways tumour by cryotherapy has been reported in a series of 81 patients.[95] Symptom relief was formally evaluated using verbal scales, with encouraging results for dyspnoea, stridor, and haemoptysis. Breathlessness improved significantly, and more than half showed improvement in at least one test of pulmonary function. The objective changes correlated with dyspnoea scores and exercise tolerance.[96] Unfortunately, experience with and availability of this treatment remains very limited.

Endobronchial stents Stents are mechanical splints used within a tubular organ to keep its lumen open. They do not directly cause necrosis or regression of tumour. In the management of respiratory symptoms there is now considerable experience in the use of stents for endobronchial stenosis.[81,82] Two types of stent are used: the expandable metal variety[97] and the moulded silicone variety.[98] The most frequently used stent in the United Kingdom is the Gianturco Z stent, which is of the expandable wire type.

The patient needs to tolerate a bronchoscopy for the placement of a thoracic stent; however, this can be done under local anaesthetic using a fibreoptic instrument. The silicone stents can be made to support even high tracheal occlusion, and can be designed to extend from the carina into a tracheostomy orifice. Unfortunately, there are few published data on the symptomatic value of endobronchial stents in relieving respiratory distress. In one series of 21 patients from Leicester, who had the Gianturco Z stent fitted for endobronchial occlusion from lung, tracheal, oesophageal and other metastatic malignancies, it was claimed that the clinical outcome was improved in all but four.[99] Persistent cough (due presumable to a 'foreign body' irritation) is surprisingly uncommon; only two of the 21 patients were troubled by this. More formal evaluation of subjective benefits needs to be performed.

Drug treatment

General principles

The management of breathlessness using palliative drug therapy, excluding the cytotoxic agents described above, is covered in this section. Many of the treatments discussed here will be familiar as examples of routine medical practice. This is not surprising; after all there are relatively few disease processes in the field of respiratory medicine, with the notable exceptions of pulmonary infections, that are definitely 'curable'.

The drug treatments that can be used for dyspnoea are listed in Table 7. The ordering within the list does not imply a priority of importance or potency, nor does it necessarily reflect the ease and frequency of use of these approaches. The very multiplicity of drug therapies may provoke the cynical reaction that no single treatment can be overwhelmingly helpful, and that is undoubtedly true.[100] Much of the practical information in this section can be usefully represented as flow diagrams.[101,102] The algorithmic approach to decision-making in palliative care is particularly suited to respiratory symptoms, where numerous factors have to be considered and multiple drug regimens may be unavoidable.

The management of obstructive airways disease is considered briefly at the begining of this section, as asthma and chronic obstructive airways disease are commonly found to coexist with advanced cancer or other terminal diseases. Non-malignant airflow obstruction can occur alongside other more intractable causes of respiratory distress and is often eminently treatable.

Table 7 Drug treatment of dyspnoea

Cause	Drug
Airways obstruction (asthma, chronic obstructive airways disease)	Bronchodilators Methylxanthines Corticosteroids
Chronic obstructive airways disease with hypoventilation	Respiratory stimulant
Chronic obstructive airways, disease, malignancy	Respiratory sedatives Non-opioids Opioids
Heart failure	Diuretics ACE inhibitors Digoxin
Superior vena cava obstruction	Corticosteroids
Lymphangitis carcinomatosa	Corticosteroids Respiratory sedative
Pulmonary embolism	Respiratory sedative

Inhaled local anaesthetics and cannabinoids are also used (see text).

Table 8 Indications for corticosteroids for respiratory distress

Airways obstruction (asthma, chronic obstructive airways disease)
Tracheal tumour (stridor)
Superior vena cava obstruction
Lymphangitis carcinomatosa
Pneumonitis (e.g. after radiotherapy)

Bronchodilators

Bronchodilators fall into three main categories: β-adrenergic stimulants (such as salbutamol, terbutaline, and numerous analogues), anticholinergics (such as ipratropium), and the methylxanthine drugs (such as theophylline).[103] The last group will be discussed separately as these drugs have other properties.

The bronchodilators are best given by aerosol inhalers, unless the patient is unable to co-ordinate the device or is too ill from airflow obstruction.[104] The newer breath-actuated devices and spacer attachments may make inhaler therapy easier for more people,[105,106] but nebulizer delivery should be considered whenever there is doubt about the patient's skill with an inhaler. Nebulized treatment is discussed in more detail below.

The adverse effects of chronic regular, as opposed to intermittent 'as required', use of inhaled bronchodilators have recently been highlighted.[107] Excessive use of the β-adrenergic agents may cause cardiac stimulation, which can be particularly harmful in the elderly.[108]

There is little to choose between the individual inhaled bronchodilators, but a combination of a β-adrenergic agent with an anticholinergic seems to be particularly helpful in older patients with chronic bronchitis.

Methylxanthines

The methylxanthine class of drugs — aminophylline and theophylline are the two in common usage — are more than just bronchodilators. Like the β-adrenergic agents they can stimulate the heart, which may lead to toxic arrhythmias, but they can also be usefully employed in heart failure. There is good evidence that the methylxanthines can stimulate respiration predominantly by a central effect on the medullary centre, i.e. they increase the hypercapnic (and also the hypoxic) drive to ventilation. This can be useful in acute respiratory failure, but the cerebral stimulation is non-specific in larger doses and may cause irritability and fits. Studies have shown that methylxanthine drugs can augment the failing respiratory muscles, particularly in the diaphragm. However, there is debate as to whether these potentially useful effects can be obtained with the conventional doses of oral methylxanthines like theophylline.[109]

Corticosteroids

Corticosteroids are a ubiquitous group of drugs in palliative care, and not surprisingly have acquired a number of indications in the palliation of respiratory symptoms (Table 8). A genuine indication for steroids is the failure to respond to bronchodilators and methylxanthines in airflow obstruction. This can arise in acute severe exacerbations of asthma or in chronic obstructive airways disease. It is justifiable to give almost all patients with troublesome chronic obstructive airways disease a trial of steroid. The dose should be high enough to work quickly without causing undue gastric toxicity or fluid retention (e.g. prednisolone 30–60 mg daily or dexamethasone 4–8 mg daily).

There is no evidence as to which drug is superior for respiratory symptoms, although respiratory physicians have traditionally used prednisolone. The oral route is probably more reliable than inhaled steroid for acute relief of symptoms,[110] although the inhaled route is preferable for maintenance.

Although many patients improve within a few days, at least 2 weeks should be allowed to assess the respiratory response to steroids in chronic obstructive airways disease.[111] This is considerably longer than is normally needed to obtain a response with steroids for, say, appetite stimulation or relief of inflammatory pain. Some patients fail to respond altogether to high-dose steroid, and it is important to recognize these so that the drug is stopped before long-term toxicity arises.

Among the other respiratory benefits of steroids, the most impressive are the acute relief of superior vena cava obstruction, relief of stridor due to tracheal obstruction, and as an adjunct in the management of lymphangitis carcinomatosa. However, steroids used without close individual monitoring can cause severe adverse effects. Therefore, apart from the specific indications given above, it is probably not justifiable to give steroids to all dyspnoeic patients on a 'try it and see' basis.

Treatment of heart failure

When trying to deal with major problems, such as lung cancer with pleural effusion, it is all too easy to forget that heart failure may be partly responsible for breathlessness and reduced exercise capability, particularly in older patients.

If anaemia is contributing to heart failure or is directly causing dyspnoea on exertion, blood transfusion may be considered. Diuretics are often helpful but may cause electrolyte disturbance and can precipitate urinary problems. Digoxin should be avoided unless there is definite atrial fibrillation. The angiotensin-converting enzyme inhibitors are very potent drugs for relieving the symptoms and clinical features of heart failure. Limiting factors with these are hypotension and an unproductive cough (see later in this chapter).

Respiratory stimulants

Although the hypoxic drive to respiration is relatively weak compared with the hypercapnic drive, the consequences of chronic hypoxaemia are clinically significant. They include pulmonary vasoconstriction, which ultimately leads to pulmonary hypertension, polycythaemia, inactivity, and the 'Pickwickian syndrome' of obesity and somnolence. Paradoxically, patients in this situation have disturbed nights because the natural oxygen desaturation that occurs in deep sleep is added to their resting hypoxaemia, and this in turn causes intermittent arousal and wakening.[7,11] The end result of these effects is cor pulmonale and heart failure, from which 60 per cent of patients die within 5 years.[2] Therefore there has been considerable research into ways of stimulating the ventilation in chronically hypoxaemic patients to improve symptoms and prevent or delay the fatal consequences. Several drugs have now been explored for their respiratory stimulant properties (Table 9).

It has long been recognized that the pattern of respiration in women varies during the menstrual cycle, and this is thought to be associated with the production of endogenous progesterone. Synthetic progestogen compounds have been shown to stimulate ventilation, probably by increasing the central sensitivity to CO_2, although they may also work at the peripheral chemoreceptors.[11] Studies of patients with chronic obstructive airways disease using medroxyprogesterone acetate at 60 to 100 mg/day have confirmed this action, but, despite small improvements in arterial blood gases, symptomatic benefit has not been shown.[112,113]

Table 9 Respiratory stimulant drugs (i.e. drugs that increase pulmonary ventilation)

Drug	Site of stimulation	
	Peripheral	Central
Progestogens	+?	+
Methylxanthines		+
Almitrine	+	
Doxapram	+	
Cannabinoids		+
Local anaesthetics		+?

The progestogen group of drugs is extensively used in the management of breast and other hormone-responsive cancers.[114] Medroxyprogesterone acetate and megestrol acetate are among the most common prescribed. Paradoxically, one of their recognized adverse effects at high doses is the causation of dyspnoea, which may be mediated by fluid retention leading to pulmonary congestion and by increased risk of venous thrombosis leading to pulmonary embolism. Fortunately, the stimulation of ventilation by progestogens is achieved at lower doses.[115]

Other classes of drugs that have been shown to stimulate ventilation include nebulized local anaesthetics,[28,29] doxapram,[116] almitrine,[113] and inhaled cannabis and the synthetic cannabinoid nabilone.[117,118] Nabilone may be helpful in sedating an anxious dyspnoeic patient in borderline respiratory failure without aggravating CO_2 retention.[32] However, none of the other drugs has found favour in routine palliative care because of serious cerebral or other toxic effects. They would probably only be useful in cases of advanced hypoxia or hypercapnia that were causing excessive somnolence by day or significant disturbance of sleep pattern by night because of oxygen desaturation.

Factors other than purely respiratory ones can influence the ease of breathing. Notably, chest pain due to rib fracture, pleurisy, or postoperative restriction of diaphragm movement can all impair respiration. Paradoxically, the relief of pain in these situations with a strong analgesic, which would normally depress respiration, may actually improve ventilation and blood gases as well as the sensation of breathing.[119]

Respiratory sedatives

In the palliation of dyspnoeic patients with advanced cancer, neurological disease, or cardiorespiratory disease, the main benefit comes from the suppression of respiratory awareness.

It should be noted that the reduction of ventilatory drive itself should not be confused with the relief of respiratory sensation. Ventilatory drive is the net result of the complex automatic and subconscious, peripheral and central, and neural and chemical mechanisms described above. Dyspnoea is the conscious perception

Table 10 Respiratory sedative drugs (i.e. drugs that reduce respiration sensation and may reduce pulmonary ventilation)

Phenothiazines
Benzodiazepines
Opioids
Alcohol
Cannabinoids

which has taken account of the net result of those mechanisms and integrated it with other cognitive and emotive factors that are also affecting the individual. Furthermore, while it is often reasonable to use exercise tolerance as a proxy measure of dyspnoea perception, it is usually misleading to regard the ventilatory drive in the same way. Another factor to consider is that some drugs, including opioids, may reduce the metabolic requirements of the body (e.g. by overall sedation) so that a lower level of ventilation is actually appropriate.

The complex interrelationship of pharmacological and psychological actions has led to the proposal of a classification of respiratory palliative drugs based on the link between their actions on subjective breathlessness and on objectively measured ventilation.[120] A type I response occurs when a drug affects both equally, and a type II response occurs when breathlessness is reduced with ventilation remaining the same. However, this classification seems rather arbitrary and is even incomplete, as it does not include drugs that reduce ventilation without affecting the sensation of breathlessness (such as general anaesthetics and muscle relaxants) or drugs that reduce dyspnoea but stimulate ventilation (such as local anaesthetics and nabilone). It appears that a comprehensive and rational classification has yet to be devised, and it is perhaps advisable to refer to these drugs simply as 'respiratory sedatives' (Table 10).

However, there is no doubt that most drugs which induce global cerebral sedation can also reduce dyspnoea and furthermore are potent depressors of ventilatory drive. This has been confirmed both clinically and experimentally with alcohol, barbiturates, benzodiazepines, phenothiazines, and opioids.[10,119] Even if we did not know that they had specific effects on the respiratory control mechanisms, we would still prescribe them in palliative care as empirically effective tranquillizing agents for breathlessness. (Barbiturates have not been formally evaluated, but the use of alcohol to relieve symptomatic distress is probably more frequently self-prescribed by our patients than we recognize.) However, to use these drugs more rationally requires an examination of how they may be working, and in what circumstances some may work better than others.

To call upon the analogy previously drawn with analgesia, palliative medicine has long progressed beyond the 'blanket' use of morphine for all patients with malignant pain without regard to the cause or severity. We now recognize different levels of potency and the existence of opioid-resistant pains, and can call upon a range of other drug classes that are sometimes used with morphine and sometimes replace opioids altogether. Similarly, there should be a move towards a more rational application of respiratory sedative drugs in palliative care. Once again the basis for present knowledge is rather lacking from the field of palliative care research, and most of what is known has come from studies of chronic obstructive airways disease. The non-opioid and opioid drugs will be discussed separately; this division is more for convenience but may also have a scientific basis, as will be seen.

Non-opioid respiratory sedatives Non-opioid drug classes investigated for the relief of breathlessness include the benzodiazepines and phenothiazines. In a controlled study of patients with chronic obstructive airways disease, promethazine was associated with reduction in dyspnoea.[121] In contrast, diazepam showed negative changes in terms of exercise tolerance and blood gases, but the dose used (25 mg) may be regarded as excessive. In another study, the effect of a single night-time dose of diazepam 5 mg on patients with chronic obstructive airways disease was studied.[122] This improved sleep duration without making nocturnal hypoxaemia worse. Interestingly, it did not increase the number of apnoeic episodes during the night. Since nocturnal hypoxaemia and apnoeic episodes are associated with arousal, which may disturb the quality of sleep, this is a beneficial result.[10]

Diazepam may have an even more potent depressant effect on the ventilatory response to CO_2 than many opioids (50 per cent reduction after diazepam 14 mg intramuscularly versus 30–40 per cent reduction after morphine 7.5–10 mg intramuscularly).[10] Until the recent introduction of the specific benzodiazepine antagonist flumazenil, there was an understandable reluctance to use this class of drug in patients with compromised respiratory function.

Many other benzodiazepines are now available which may have advantages over diazepam in terms of the duration of action, potency, and adverse effects. Lorazepam is a quick-acting oral drug which many patients prefer to diazepam. Midazolam has the major advantage of being injectable parenterally without causing irritation or phlebitis. A bolus of midazolam 5 to 10 mg by slow intravenous injection can be very helpful for the relief of acute severe dyspnoea in the absence of pain, particularly if there is a large anxiety reaction. Once the patient is relaxed (but preferably not unconscious), oral lorazepam can be started or the midazolam can be continued as a subcutaneous infusion if the stimulus for dyspnoea persists. No controlled studies using these newer agents for dyspnoea have been published, nor have benzodiazepines been specifically evaluated in advanced cancer or neurological patients. There is also a lack of controlled studies of phenothiazines in cancer patients with dyspnoea. Factors which may limit the use of phenothiazines include extrapyramidal effects and hypotension with chlorpromazine.

The butyrophenones comprise another major group of psychotropic agents that are used commonly in palliative care. Haloperidol is perhaps the most widely prescribed of these because of its antiemetic properties. It is surprising that the relief of respiratory sensation by this potent tranquillizing drug does not appear to have been studied.

Opioid respiratory sedatives Of all the centrally acting drugs, opioids have received most attention and are most widely used in the control of dyspnoea. However, frequency of use does not necessarily imply that opioids are properly understood, nor does it ensure that they may not be misused for the control of dyspnoea—a

Table 11 Effects of opioids on respiratory sensation

Effect	Unique to opioids*
Cerebral sedation	No
Reduced anxiety	No
Reduced sensitivity to hypercapnia	No
Improved cardiac function	Yes
Inhaled route—act on airways opioid receptors	Yes
Analgesia	Yes

* Compared with other 'respiratory sedative' drugs (see Table 10).

situation that is rather similar to the application of opioids in the field of pain control a few years ago. The rationale of opioid usage is examined in the following sections.

How do opioids reduce dyspnoea? Where and how do opioids work in controlling dyspnoea? It is relatively easy to answer the first part of the question with respect to the effect of opioids on ventilatory drive, since this is known to take place at the CO_2-sensitive medullary respiratory centre and not on the peripheral oxygen-sensitive chemoreceptors.[119] However, as opioid receptors are present in many other parts of the brain and peripheral tissues, it is not easy to be sure exactly where else morphine is working when it modifies the sensation of breathlessness. Drugs that stimulate the μ, δ, and κ opioid receptors are all known to depress respiration, while agonists of the σ receptor group that mediate some of the opioid adverse effects stimulate respiration.[23] It is not known how stimulation of the opioid receptors which are present in the human brainstem leads to changes in sensitivity of the medullary chemoreceptors. The actions of different opioids on these receptors, and at other central sites such as the limbic system or midbrain, may account for the confusing picture of respiratory versus cerebral sedation.[123] The role that opioid receptors in the airways may play in the sensation of dyspnoea (as opposed to the regulation of mucus secretion and sensation of cough) is also relevant and will be discussed below.

A further difficulty in understanding the respiratory effects of opioids is that, in human studies, the magnitude of the changes in ventilation and the sensitivity of the hypercapnic drive is not related to plasma morphine concentrations.[124]

How does morphine reduce breathlessness? It is clear that several mechanisms are probably involved (Table 11). The main function of the hypercapnic drive to ventilation is to maintain the excretion of CO_2 that would build up after exertion or when respiratory muscles become fatigued. Therefore it seems reasonable to postulate that if a drug reduces the sensitivity to $p\text{CO}_2$, the individual could tolerate a greater amount of 'respiratory fatigue' without becoming aware of it. Thus, although the afferent messages from the neural receptors in the airways, lung tissue, or respiratory muscles would indicate an abnormal state that called for an increase in ventilation, the central point where the control is integrated would become less 'aware' and less able to respond to them. This could lead to a resetting of the homeostatic control of $p\text{CO}_2$ to a new level and a temporary reduction of the abnormal respiratory sensation. Furthermore, a positive adaptive benefit may arise from this shift, as the same degree of ventilation with a higher $p\text{CO}_2$ will lead to a greater amount of CO_2 being excreted per breath. Supporting circumstantial evidence for this theory comes from the work previously described on the natural secretion of endorphins after induced hypercapnia.[26] This may also explain why some patients stop feeling breathless once the $p\text{CO}_2$ reaches a critical level.[25]

However, this proposed mechanism does not necessarily explain how exogenous opioids work. In the limited data on blood gases in cancer patients who are given morphine for pain control, $p\text{CO}_2$ has been found to remain static after morphine. Ironically, this observation is used to convince sceptical physicians not to deprive chronic respiratory patients of pain-relieving opioid analgesia![125] It is possible that patients with residual pain or anxiety may still be subject to a pain-led drive to ventilation, despite receiving clinically adequate doses of morphine.[119] Clearly, this is an area that could be investigated further in cancer patients who are breathless but do not have pain.

If the medullary sensitivity can actually be 'reset' by endorphins, this is probably only a short-lived phenomenon as the everyday experience is that in chronically hypercapnic individuals, say with advanced chronic obstructive airways disease or neuromuscular disease, the capacity for feeling breathless is still present and is just as strong.

Other possible sites of action for morphine within the respiratory system are the opioid receptors present in the airways.[3] Some evidence to support this comes from recent work on the nebulization of morphine in low doses to patients with chronically obstructive airways disease.[126] However, the same route has been used effectively to deliver morphine for postoperative analgesia,[127] and thus it is possible that the nebulized drug acts centrally after systemic absorption. (The local effect of opioids on the airways irritant receptors will be discussed later.)

The spinal delivery of opioids provides an opportunity for seeking respiratory effects via yet another route. Not surprisingly, the literature on this subject is concerned primarily with analgesia, and the respiratory effects recorded have been confined mainly to ventilatory depression and breathing rhythms during sleep. In general, it is probable that the epidural route for opioids is just as susceptible to respiratory complications as are more conventional routes. The delayed onset of respiratory depression which is associated with the rostral spread of opioid in the cerebrospinal fluid up to the medulla can be particularly problematic.[128] The observed differences in degrees of ventilatory depression between drugs are likely to be a function of their intrinsic potency as well as their lipophilicity which influences diffusibility and persistence in the cerebrospinal fluid.[129]

Morphine may relieve dyspnoea by actions that do not directly affect the respiratory system. It is well known that morphine is helpful for patients with established or incipient heart failure by virtue of its vasodilator action, which reduces the load on the heart. In the absence of heart failure, it is debatable whether reduction of peripheral vascular pressure is beneficial.

In concentrating on cardiorespiratory pharmacological actions, it is easy to overlook the fact that morphine has an important cortical sedative ('narcotic') action with measurable effects on cognitive function. Therefore opioids can be regarded as psychotropics or tranquillizers, reducing the perception of dyspnoea along with other psychosomatic sensations. It is possible to differentiate the cerebral sedative and respiratory sedative effects objectively.

For example, meptazinol, an opioid antagonist with analgesic properties, is associated with mild CO_2 retention due to cerebral sedation, but the ventilatory response to hypercapnia is unimpaired.[130] Similarly, the cannabinoid nabilone is also associated with drowsiness accompanied by a fall in po_2 , but at the same time hypercapnic sensitivity is increased.[118] However, even a high dose of oral diazepam (25 mg per day) which caused drowsiness was not associated with reduction in the sensation of breathlessness in patients with chronic obstructive airways disease.[121] These apparently conflicting results are in fact compatible with two distinct actions of the drugs in question — a cerebral tranquillizing effect and an effect on the control of ventilation.

Clearly, this dual effect is not unique to the opioids, and it is admittedly difficult to interpret how it may be relevant to clinical practice. What singles out opioid drugs from the other sedative agents discussed above is that so far only the opioids have been found to have natural endogenous equivalents (in the form of the endorphins) which may be responsible for mediating or modulating the normal responses to stimuli that induce dyspnoea.

Clinical studies of opioids for dyspnoea Once again it must be stressed that most of the controlled studies have been conducted in patients with chronic obstructive airways disease or normal controls, and it may not be strictly appropriate to transfer their results to patients with dyspnoea due to malignant or chronic neuromuscular diseases.

Codeine does not reduce breathlessness, but the more potent analogue dihydrocodeine is effective—interestingly, whether it is taken regularly or on an 'as required' basis.[131] Oral morphine solution significantly improves exercise tolerance in normocapnic patients with chronic obstructive airways disease, even though po_2 falls and pco_2 rises.[132]

Pharmacokinetic studies comparing nebulized with intramuscular morphine have shown a 1:6 difference in peak plasma levels.[126] The nebulization of 5 mg of morphine has been associated with an increase of 35 per cent in exercise endurance time in patients with chronic obstructive airways disease.[127] After accounting for the expected loss of drug during expiration, the dose absorbed would be approximately 1.7 mg. Even allowing for the sparing of first-pass metabolism in the liver by using the nebulized route, it is remarkable that such a small dose could be acting systemically. Therefore it has been postulated that nebulized opioids may have a direct pulmonary effect. Unfortunately, more recent controlled studies in patients with chronic obstructive airways disease have yielded either inconclusive or negative results.[133,134] In a double-blind randomized crossover trial of nebulized morphine (10 and 25 mg), equivalent intravenous doses (1 and 2.5 mg), and placebo, none of these interventions were found to alter breathlessness, ventilation, or gas exchange at rest or on exercise.[134]

Uncontrolled and retrospective chart reviews and personal series in cancer patients have been published which support the use of nebulized morphine for dyspnoea.[135] It is clearly more difficult to perform prospective controlled trials in severely dyspnoeic cancer patients than in subjects with stable chronic obstructive airways disease, but the true value of this treatment will not be known until these are done.

Nebulization of a respiratory sedative would seem to be a logical route of delivery, particularly if the drug has a local action on the airways or lung tissue. Even if it is mainly working by systemic absorption, there are two distinct advantages in pursuing this route.

1. The airways and lungs present a huge surface area, so that inhaled drugs can be absorbed efficiently and rapidly (nebulized opioid produces a mental effect of relaxation within 2–5 min).
2. Many patients with chronic respiratory disease are already accustomed to taking inhaled or nebulized drugs and may prefer to take a new antidyspnoea treatment by this route also.

Early experience with nebulized opioid has shown a further practical advantage over other parenteral routes: the patient and family can be taught to prepare a nebulizer at home within minutes of an attack of breathlessness, and this can give the patient symptomatic relief within a much shorter time than would be required for an emergency doctor or nurse to call and give an injection. For many patients with severely disabling bouts of breathlessness, this has been a major psychological crutch that has enabled them for the first time to contemplate the possibility of returning home from the hospice.

It would be remarkable if this route of opioid delivery were to be free of adverse effects. In United Kingdom palliative care units, doses of morphine up to and over 50 mg are used in nebulizers, and even in patients who are not taking oral morphine it is very difficult to assess whether they experience more or less constipation, nausea, tiredness, etc. than other patients with advanced cancer. However, many patients report that they prefer to take nebulized morphine 'as required' once or twice a day for exercise-related dyspnoea rather than suffer constant sedation all day by taking regular morphine.

However, a serious adverse effect to be aware of is that morphine can induce bronchospasm in some individuals. This has previously been recognized as a complication of heroin inhalation among drug addicts.[136] The mechanism in therapeutic morphine inhalation is probably the release of histamine by morphine in the airways. It is not known if this is more likely to occur in asthmatics. The recent finding of opioid receptors in the airways which *in vitro* actually reduced the effect of irritant stimuli on mucus production suggests that bronchospasm may be an idiosyncratic reaction. Therefore it is good practice to take the precaution, as with most other nebulized drugs, of giving the first test dose to patients in the inpatient unit or outpatient clinic where antiasthmatic treatment is immediately available.

Another opioid that has received much study in the last few years, particularly in the field of epidural analgesia, is fentanyl. This is more potent than morphine, more lipid soluble, and hence more readily absorbed and shorter acting. In postoperative patients fentanyl 300 μg nebulized for pain control produces a peak plasma level after 2 min and a mean duration of action of 305 min.[137] Unfortunately, respiratory sensation was not measured in this study.

As fentanyl is thought not to release histamine like morphine, it has a major theoretical advantage over it for the nebulized route. Although the equivalent doses have not been confirmed objectively for this route, in practice 50 to100 μg of fentanyl has an approximately equal effect to 25 to 50 mg of morphine. (The dose used and probable effect are strongly dependent on whether the patient is opioid naïve or is already taking oral opioids.) Bronchospasm following nebulized fentanyl has so far not been reported.

How is the use of opioids for dyspnoea different from their use in pain control? Clinical observation of the antidyspnoeic use of the opioid drugs in advanced cancer patients is confounded by their frequent prescription for analgesia in the same population. This is different from the management of asthma, chronic obstructive airways disease, progressive neuromuscular disease, or endstage cardiorespiratory failure, where opioids are not used to any great extent and therefore their prescription for dyspnoea is 'uncontaminated'. However, the background use of opioids in cancer patients has three major effects.

1. It is easier to justify starting an opioid-naïve patient on morphine for dyspnoea because it could be reasonably argued that ultimately he or she may need morphine for pain (or general 'distress').
2. It is easier in a patient already on morphine for pain control to increase the dose to accommodate a new symptom of dyspnoea than to start a new and possibly unfamiliar drug.
3. Because most cancer patients are asked to take analgesic medication for malignant pain on a regular basis, it is likely that opioids for dyspnoea will also be prescribed in this way.

These three factors, which are in themselves fairly reasonable, may sometimes result in the following inappropriate use of morphine in patients with breathlessness:

(1) use of morphine for dyspnoea when another drug (or even a non-drug therapy) would have been more successful;

(2) escalation of morphine dose to levels which result in excessive sedation that would not be considered reasonable in patients needing purely pain control;

(3) continuous use of morphine for dyspnoea when the breathlessness is intermittent, again resulting in unnecessary sedation at other times.

There is as yet no way of proving or rejecting these assertions, but they should serve to stimulate further discussion and research on alternative approaches.

How should opioids be used in dyspnoea management? A common clinical impression in the palliative care of cancer patients (as opposed to the care of patients with advanced chronic obstructive airways disease in conventional respiratory care) is that many patients are dyspnoeic only intermittently, usually in relation to exertion, blockage of airways with mucus, or psychological factors. Therefore the use of intermittent 'as required' opioids (or any other class of drug) would seem more logical for breathlessness than chronic regular dosing in these patients. This approach to malignant dyspnoea clearly contrasts with the situation of most patients with malignant pain, which tends to be constant and unremitting, albeit with exacerbations due to movement or mood. In these it is accepted as good palliative care practice to prescribe regular prophylactic pain medication.

In patients with intermittent dyspnoea, however, it may be more logical policy to offer them 'as required' treatment with opioids or any other class of drug, making sure of course that the treatment given is capable of working quickly in response to the stimulus. Some patients learn to take 'as required' medication of this sort before exercise, in the same way that patients with chronic obstructive airways disease find pre-exercise supplementary oxygen helpful. It is interesting to note again that in a controlled study 'as required' dihydrocodeine has been found to be as helpful for breathlessness as regular administration.[131] This regimen possibly results in less overall cerebral sedation for the same degree of relief of acute exacerbations compared with continuous opioid dosing.

Of course, if a patient has continuous dyspnoea (e.g. from lymphangitis carcinomatosa or a pericardial effusion), regular respiratory sedation should be prescribed. Similarly, if the patient has constant severe pain as well as unrelieved dyspnoea, the needs of the pain should prevail and therefore opioid should be offered continuously, with the facility for 'topping-up' for breakthrough dyspnoea. It has yet to be tested experimentally whether continuous, pulsed, or 'as required' morphine provides the best form of symptom control in dyspnoea.

The nebulized route of delivering opioids may prove to be a most fruitful line of research and development, as it offers the following:

(1) speed of effect;

(2) reduced systemic side-effects (and with fentanyl reduced risk of bronchospasm compared with morphine);

(3) most importantly, the patient has the opportunity to regulate his own medication on an 'as required' basis, so minimizing drug intake while bestowing more autonomy.

The British Thoracic Society has recently prepared guidelines for nebulizer usage in various clinical situations. The putative benefits as well as the disadvantages and lack of evidence are summarized in the section on nebulizers in palliative care.[138]

Cannabinoids

Marijuana or cannabis is the raw material obtained from the hemp plant *Cannabis sativa*. It has been used since antiquity as a drug of pleasure, but was also employed in medicine until the first half of this century. One of the indications for cannabis-containing medicinal cigarettes was bronchial asthma.

Natural cannabinoids Studies of the effects of smoking marijuana cigarettes have shown a bronchodilator effect together with either an increase in CO_2 sensitivity[117] or a slight respiratory depressant effect.[139] However, the potential benefits that could accrue from these actions are overshadowed by the finding that repeated smoking of cannabis is associated with a form of chronic bronchitis that is even more severe than that found in tobacco smokers.

The psychoactive ingredient of cannabis, tetrahydrocannabinol, is a moderate bronchodilator but depresses ventilation, and by inhalation can also cause an irritant effect.[140]

Nabilone The synthetic cannabinoid nabilone was developed as an antiemetic, but its use has been limited by troublesome psychotropic effects, sedation, and hypotension at the usual dose of 2 mg twice daily.[141] At this dose, it has significant bronchodilator activity in normal subjects and also increases ventilatory response to CO_2.[142] Interestingly, this respiratory stimulation occurs at the time of maximal cortical sedation. Both the bronchodilatation and the ventilatory enhancement may be a reflection of a widespread non-specific reflex sympathetic arousal. Therefore subjects taking nabilone can feel relaxed and sleepy, and may have demonstrable reduction in pO_2 as a result, but paradoxically sensitivity to CO_2 is increased.

This interesting combination of pharmacological effects has led to its occasional use in the relief of the endstages of dyspnoea in terminally ill patients.[32] Nabilone should be reserved for patients who are frequently or continuously breathless, who exhibit great anxiety, but who would be in danger of slipping into hypercapnic respiratory failure with other conventional respiratory sedatives. The doses for such patients are much lower than for antiemetic use, starting at 0.1 mg twice daily and increasing gradually up to 0.25 mg four times daily. Above this dose, most patients with advanced cancer find the sedation and occasional dysphoria unacceptable. Because of the significant hypotension and reflex tachycardia, nabilone is unsuitable for patients with atrial fibrillation or in heart failure.

Nabilone needs to be evaluated more formally in the context of palliative care, with controlled comparisons with the benzodiazepines or low-dose morphine being the logical areas for study.

Local anaesthetics

The elucidation of the neural mechanisms of breathing control has logically led to attempts to blockade those receptors which mediate increased ventilatory function. One line of study has been the delivery of local anaesthetic drugs to the J-receptors in the lung parenchyma. It was suggested that blocking the J-receptors could lead to reduced sensitivity to pulmonary congestion, a common and potent cause of dyspnoea.

The early results were encouraging; nebulizing bupivacaine into normal subjects enabled them to exercise with a reduced sensation of breathlessness compared with nebulized saline.[29] There were no significant differences in the actual level of exercise achieved or most other objective parameters. It has already been noted that, paradoxically, the sensitivity of the medulla to pCO_2 (hypercapnic ventilatory drive) was increased by nebulized bupivacaine at the same time as dyspnoea was decreased. The mechanism for this is unclear, but it also occurs after application of bupivacaine, although not lignocaine, by the spinal route.[128]

It has been proposed that the inhaled local anaesthetic exerts its antidyspnoeic effects by blocking airways stretch receptors rather than the deeper pulmonary receptors.[29] The aerosol particle sizes obtained with modern nebulizers driven by electric compressors are sufficiently small to penetrate down to terminal bronchiole and alveolar level, but it would still be difficult to know where the drug was actually working.

Surprisingly, there has been little follow-up to this approach and, until recently, subsequent studies using bupivacaine or the shorter-acting drug lignocaine have been inconclusive.[100]

A recent United Kingdom study of six cancer patients, who were given 100 and 200 mg of lignocaine and saline as placebo, failed to show any subjective benefit from the local anaesthetic.[143] Indeed, while effort of breathing, measured on a visual analogue scale, was unchanged by any agent, the distress of breathing was less after the saline!

One reason for the lack of enthusiasm for nebulized local anaesthetics is the known toxic effect of these agents on the upper airways: in asthmatics, and to a lesser extent in normal people, the local anaesthetics can provoke serious and occasionally fatal bronchospasm.[142] Therefore it is not advisable to use this method for the control of dyspnoea, but these agents still have a useful place in the palliation of cough (see below).

Oxygen therapy

Oxygen therapy is a rather poorly understood and often misused treatment in the palliation of breathlessness. It is sometimes seen by patients and professional staff as being less invasive than drug treatment because it does not involve the taking of medicines. However, it may be unhelpful, irrelevant, or even harmful in the same way that pharmacological interventions can be.

Measurement of hypoxia One of the problems in deciding when to use oxygen therapy is knowing when a patient is hypoxaemic. Clinical impression may be quite misleading here. The classic dusky blue appearance of cyanosis may be found in peripheral parts of the body when the patient is cold or has circulatory shutdown for a variety of reasons. Cyanosis may be difficult to discern in very anaemic or dark-skinned patients. The proper place to look for 'central' cyanosis, which is a more reliable sign of true hypoxaemia than peripheral cyanosis, is the tongue or lips; often, however, a dry, coated, or infected mouth makes even this difficult.

The definitive diagnostic tests are measurement of arterial blood gases or percutaneous oxygen saturation measurement (also called pulse oximetry). The former is invasive and usually painful; repeated measurements are traumatic and may require an indwelling arterial catheter. It also requires access to a laboratory for the estimation. In contrast, skin pulse oximetry is painless, gives bedside readings, and can be done continuously or intermittently even when the patient is resting, asleep, or exercising.[144] Measurements are made with a sensor attached to the finger or earlobe. Although there are potential problems of reliability and slow response times, in most palliative care situations these are outweighed by the benefits compared with arterial blood gas determination.

It is important to appreciate that oxygen saturation Sa_{O_2} initially remains high with falling blood oxygen tension Pa_{O_2}, but once Sa_{O_2} itself starts to fall it reflects serious hypoxaemia. In normal individuals Sa_{O_2} is around 100 per cent, but levels below 90 per cent are significantly low and levels below 80 per cent may be associated with considerable distress. With a skin probe fitted it is possible to measure the reduction in oxygenation with exercise and the degree of response to supplementary oxygen minute by minute. Oximetry can usefully feed back to the patient the lowest flow rates and the shortest period of time necessary for oxygen therapy.

If objective testing of oxygenation is not available, a purely subjective trial of oxygen may be given. It is essential to review this critically, taking into account the observed behaviour of the patient as well as his or her symptoms. Home oxygen therapy has been recommended as a part of American 'hospice symptom management', as it provides the family with 'something to do'.[145] However, the prevailing British view is that there is no case for providing oxygen purely as a 'preventive' measure or as a 'placebo' to reassure the patient that something is being done.

Causes of hypoxaemia The usual causes of hypoxaemia seen in palliative care are listed in Table 12. Most of these are also treatable

Table 12 Causes of hypoxaemia

Acute (hours–days)
Asthma
Cardiac failure
Pulmonary embolism
Pneumothorax
Infection
Chronic (weeks–months)
Trachael obstruction (tumour)
Lymphangitis carcinomatosa
Respiratory muscle fatigue/paralysis

by other interventions and so oxygen therapy alone is not usually indicated. For example, breathlessness due to anaemia may often be more appropriately relieved by blood transfusion than by supplementary oxygen.

Therapeutic uses of oxygen Oxygen therapy may be given either continuously or intermittently. The former is indicated for patients with chronic obstructive airways disease who have proven hypoxaemia and a tendency to develop pulmonary hypertension.[146] It is also necessary in some cancer patients with lymphangitis carcinomatosa, stridor due to central airway stenosis, pneumothorax, or other causes of continuous dyspnoea. Because of the inconvenience and cost of the frequent replacement of cylinders, the oxygen concentrator is better for long-term continuous use at home. This device increases the concentration of oxygen by filtering out nitrogen from the ambient air, but, as it has an electric motor, it has the disadvantage of being rather noisy. This could be a nuisance unless the concentrator is placed well away from the patient and connected by long tubing.

Intermittent oxygen therapy is more appropriate for the large majority of patients with breathlessness related to exertion. It can be given just prior to, during, or after exercise.[146] Short-burst oxygen therapy from small portable cylinders increases exercise endurance in patients with chronic obstructive airways disease, even when they have to carry the cylinder themselves,[147] but its effects on the sensation of dyspnoea are less convincing.

Connecting a patient up to a mask and piping has a strong placebo effect; in one study oxygen was associated with a median improvement in walking distance of 9.7 per cent, while a control application of air gave an 'improvement' of 6.1 per cent.[148] Therefore it has been suggested that a short trial of exercise should be carried out, with a documented improvement of at least 10 per cent in physical tolerance or breathlessness rating, before prescribing portable supplementary oxygen in chronic obstructive airways disease. In palliative care of cancer patients, the theoretical approach should not be lax but formal exercise testing would often be inappropriate.

Data on oxygen use in breathless cancer patients is relatively poor compared with the volume of published studies in chronic obstructive airways disease. However, a Canadian prospective double-blind crossover study of 14 patients has shown that oxygen was rated better by patients and the investigators than air.[149] These patients were all severely hypoxaemic (skin oximetry, >90 per cent saturation), and there is inconclusive evidence of the benefits of oxygen in less physiologically disturbed patients. For example, a British study of cancer patients who were not hypoxaemic at rest showed that when oxygen or air were offered in a double blind fashion, patients were unable to distinguish between them.[150]

The oxygen delivery route is important. Masks are traditionally preferred in United Kingdom hospitals, but with long-term use they can cause a dry mouth because of the flow of gas and the inhibition of free drinking. Speech and communication are also impaired, cutting off the dyspnoeic patient even more from his more able neighbours. Nasal cannulas are preferable as they avoid all these problems. Even so, the nasal mucosa should be protected with a simple cream to prevent dryness and physical irritation. Humidification of oxygen is not usually necessary unless it is being applied directly to a tracheostomy.

The rate of oxygen delivery is also relevant, particularly if the patient has chronic lung disease and borderline or established hypercapnia. In such individuals the hypercapnic drive can be attenuated, and therefore the hypoxic drive to ventilation plays a more important role. If too high a flow rate of oxygen is used or the mask allows too high an inspired oxygen concentration, the hypoxic drive can become fully 'satisfied'. The inability of hypercapnic drive to take over may then result in the patient ventilating less and less, to the point of respiratory arrest. If there is any doubt, the arterial blood gases (not just oxygen saturation) should be measured before starting oxygen.

Transtracheal oxygen delivery has been used in severely ill patients with chronic obstructive airways disease and found to be well tolerated and to improve functional ability compared with the traditional mask or nasal cannulas. It requires a lower flow rate of oxygen than other routes and so may reduce costs.[151] Its use has not been described in terminal cancer patients.

Helium–oxygen mixture

A mixture of helium and oxygen is sometimes used to help the laboured breathing in patients with severe stridor due to tracheal obstruction. It is thought to work because the helium–oxygen gas mixture is much lighter than air and therefore can be inspired with reduced respiratory muscle effort. It has the unfortunate side-effect of making the patient's speech sound strange and high-pitched, and there are no reports of its formal assessment.

Cough

Like dyspnoea, cough is a normal mechanism in the respiratory system designed to protect the individual from potential harm, but when it is mediated by disease and becomes chronic, it can be the cause of great suffering. Again like dyspnoea, it is often the reason why patients first seek medical help with conditions that turn out to be malignant. The cough is then often seen by patients and their families as a marker of disease activity. Any deterioration, particularly if accompanied by pain, breathlessness, or haemoptysis, can be very frightening.

Cough is often associated with other symptoms. In a survey of asthmatics, it was found to cause breathlessness in 39 per cent, wheezing in 34 per cent, and chest tightness in 25 per cent.[152] Conversely, 49 per cent of the same patients stated that coughing sometimes relieved their asthma, usually when it was associated with the expectoration of sputum. Prolonged bouts of coughing

Table 13 Cough: causes and management approaches

Cause	Management
Respiratory infection	Antibiotic (if purulent sputum) Suppressant Expectorant Physiotherapy Nebulized saline
Airways disease	
Asthma/chronic obstructive airways disease	Bronchodilator Corticosteroid Physiotherapy
Malignant obstruction	Corticosteroid Suppressant Nebulized local anaesthetic Physiotherapy
Drug-induced (e.g. ACE inhibitor)	Stop or change drug
Oesophageal reflux	Position patient upright Antireflux agent
Aspiration of saliva (e.g. motor neurone disease, multiple sclerosis)	Anticholinergic (to reduce saliva) Nebulized local anaesthetic (to reduce sensation)

may also sometimes lead to fainting ('cough syncope') or vomiting.

Prevalence

Cough is one of the most common symptoms in both normal and sick people, accounting for up to 50 per cent of consultations with general practitioners in winter months.[153] In the palliative care literature, its prevalence has been reported as ranging from 29 to 83 per cent of patients.[30,46]

Causes

In normal health, cough serves a useful function by maintaining the patency and cleanliness of the airways. It is important in helping the ciliated airways to bring mucus, fluid including blood, and inhaled foreign bodies up to the larynx where they can be expelled into the pharynx and either spat out or swallowed.[2] Cough can arise by the production of excessive amounts of these fluids, inhalation of too much foreign material, or abnormal stimulation of the irritant receptors in the airways (Table 13).[154]

Clearance of airways

In persistent cough it is important to exclude chronic production of excess sputum, which may or may not be infected (mucopurulent). By definition, chronic bronchitis patients produce sputum every day, but this is normally clear (mucoid). Nocturnal coughing can arise from inhalation of gastric contents which are regurgitated into the pharynx during sleep when the subject lies back. Patients with neuromuscular incoordination of the pharynx arising from disease of the bulbar cranial nerves (e.g. motor neurone disease or multiple sclerosis) may be unable to swallow saliva normally secreted in the mouth. If this trickles onto the larynx or into the trachea, it can produce very unpleasant coughing related to posture.

In order to generate sufficient intrathoracic pressure to expel the ball of sputum in the trachea, the glottis has to close briefly. If this is not possible because of paralysis of one vocal cord, as frequently arises in left upper-lobe lung cancers, coughing becomes less efficient and may be physically tiring for the patient.

Role of airways in cough receptors

The pharynx, larynx, and upper airways are richly supplied with sensory nerves which join the vagus nerve that enters the brain near the respiratory centre and end in the medullary 'cough centre'.[153,155] The receptors of these nerves can be stimulated by particles of inhaled matter, chemicals, cigarette smoke, and noxious gases. Cough can be induced experimentally by nebulization of water, capsaicin, and prostaglandins.[155] The opioid receptors produce mucus in response to irritation, and excessive mucus may in turn irritate the other sensory nerves in the airways.[3,156] They are blocked by opioids taken orally, which suggests that the well-known antitussive effect of opioids may be mediated both centrally at the cough centre and at the opioid receptors in the airways.[155]

Patients taking angiotensin-converting enzyme inhibitors such as captopril and enalapril for heart failure are prone to a dry cough, which is due to abnormal increase in the sensitivity of the irritant receptors.[157] Obviously, this should be distinguished from the cough of heart failure itself arising from pulmonary congestion leading to excess water in the lower airways.

Factors that cause airflow obstruction in diseases such as asthma may also induce a dry cough, presumably because of the distortion of the airway nerve endings by the bronchospasm. Ironically, some of the inhaled medications taken for asthma or chronic obstructive airways disease, such as sodium cromoglycate or ipratropium, may themselves cause cough by a direct irritant action on the upper airways.

In pulmonary cancers the chronic cough is usually associated with the production of excess mucus, infected sputum, or blood. Alternatively, endobronchial spread of tumour onto the carina or in the trachea, which are heavily innervated, may be associated with constant dry cough because of the distortion of the bronchial mucosa.

Treatment

The palliation of distressing cough should follow the same general principles as those suggested above with respect to management of dyspnoea. If possible, the main aim of the treatment should be to eliminate the underlying cause (Table 13). If cough is due to some iatrogenic factor, such as an angiotensin-converting enzyme inhibitor or inhaled drug, then the first step should be to remove this treatment.

In cases of respiratory infection, antibiotics may be valuable in reducing productive cough that is causing sleep disturbance, pain, or haemoptysis.[38] It is unlikely that oral antibiotics used symptomatically in this way will unduly prolong life that would otherwise have been threatened by pulmonary infection. Therefore the palliation of infective cough with antibiotics should not usually pose an ethical dilemma in advanced cancer.

In cases of stridor due to centrally encroaching airways tumour, the use of steroids may help not only cough but also dyspnoea by reducing local oedema and consequent endobronchial narrowing and distortion. Pleural effusion in some patients provokes an irritating dry cough, which resolves promptly on drainage; presumably distortion of the airways through mediastinal shift is responsible for this. It is important to remember that simple attention to the positioning of the patient (e.g. lying on the same side as a pleural effusion) may help to reduce cough.[38]

Cough suppressants

In most cases oral therapy should be sufficient for relief of cough. The most effective agents are the cough suppressants, of which opioid drugs are the best example.[153,155] No doubt part of the effectiveness of a cough linctus is the soothing nature of the liquid carrier for the active component. For this reason 'simple linctus' is probably the most appropriate first-line therapy in mild irritating cough. Obviously, the excessive use of sugar-containing syrups should be restrained in diabetic patients.

There is little experimental evidence as to which opioid is the most potent antitussive,[155] and it seems unnecessary to use morphine itself unless this drug is also indicated for another reason, such as pain or dyspnoea. Codeine, pholcodine, and dihydrocodeine, made up as sweet elixirs, should be the first line.[137] Methadone syrup may be particularly helpful taken as a single dose at night or twice daily because of its relatively longer duration of action. Dextromethorphan hydrobromide, which is often incorporated in proprietary cough mixtures, is structurally related to opioids and has a central cough suppressant action with few or no analgesic and sedative effects.

Local anaesthetics may be effective taken orally in the form of lozenges if cough is caused by an irritated pharynx usually due to infection or local malignancy. Nebulized local anaesthetics have long been used for reducing the severe cough produced by bronchoscopy. There is considerable anecdotal evidence that they are also very good for relieving cough associated with endobronchial malignancy. In a case report of unexplained chronic cough in a 52-year-old male, it was claimed that twice-daily nebulized lignocaine (3 ml of 1 per cent solution) gave good relief for over a year.[158] The practical aspects of using nebulizers are discussed later in this chapter.

Nebulized lignocaine (5 ml of 2 per cent solution), up to four times daily, seems to be as effective and, interestingly, may last as long in many patients as bupivacaine (5 ml of 0.25 per cent solution). As these agents reduce the sensitivity of the gag reflex, it is important to fast the patient immediately after nebulization to avoid the possibility of accidental inhalation of food or drink. The length of time to fast is not agreed; in palliative care it seems inhumane to fast too strictly, and so it seems reasonable to offer the patient a drink just before nebulizing local anaesthetic, and to restrict food or thick drinks for 1 h. Clear water may be taken within a few minutes, and may help to clear the mouth of the taste of the drug which some find unpleasant.

The potentially serious adverse effect of bronchospasm after nebulized local anaesthetics has been discussed above; the first dose should always be given in a place where medical attention and urgent antiasthma treatment are available.

A specific situation where nebulized local anaesthetics may be very helpful is when saliva pools in the hypopharynx of patients with swallowing difficulties. This occurs readily in motor neurone disease and multiple sclerosis, and can be particularly troublesome at night as the overflow of saliva into the trachea can induce prolonged bouts of severe coughing. A single dose of nebulized lignocaine or bupivacaine before retiring at night can abolish the hypopharyngeal and tracheal sensation sufficiently to allow better sleep. Of course, aspiration of saliva may still proceed and with greater ease, and the risks of this need to be weighed up and discussed with the patient and family.

Expectorants

Expectorants work by either stimulating the cough reflex or thinning the viscosity of mucus to make it easier to cough up. Most of the first type are based on agents such as ammonium chloride and ipecacuanha which work by stimulating the chemotactic trigger zone in the brain.[155] In high doses they may cause vomiting. They are unlikely to be helpful in palliative care.

Drugs which claim to reduce the viscosity of mucus have usually been found to be lacking in effectiveness.[155] Mucolytic or so-called expectorant agents are frequently unpleasant to take orally and are usually formulated in a sweet syrup; the soothing antitussive action of the latter may confound the claimed expectorant effect.

The nebulization of saline or an adrenergic bronchodilator such as terbutaline can improve the effectiveness of cough by loosening mucus or stimulating ciliary movement.[159] Expectoration may be further enhanced by physiotherapy following these agents. It should be noted that the inhalation of anticholinergic drugs, such as ipratropium and hyoscine compounds, or the use of oral nabilone may reduce ciliary motion and thicken mucus, thus making cough more troublesome.

Haemoptysis

Haemoptysis is the coughing up of blood. It is not a normal activity, although it may occur in patients with chronic lung disease and cough without indicating any new pathology. Usually haemoptysis is a sign of a significant disorder, and patients recognize this as it is one of the symptoms that lead them to consult a doctor early. However, with a new presentation the cause remains undiagnosed in up to 40 per cent of patients.[50]

Prevalence

Haemoptysis is best documented in reports of lung cancer, and the prevalence at diagnosis is reported as 47 to 70 per cent.[47,70] In palliative care, it has been found to occur in 24 per cent of lung cancer patients being admitted to St Christopher's Hospice.[46] There has been no formal attempt to grade severity of haemoptysis for the purposes of research, and the difficulties of undertaking this are considerable. In some patients it is the amount of blood that matters, in others it is the frequency of coughing blood up, and in yet others haemoptysis only causes distress if it occurs effortlessly, as opposed to the blood that they may regularly notice after chronic coughing.

Causes

Blood that has been coughed up may not have originated from the lungs, and it is particularly important to exclude bleeding from the

Table 14 Causes of haemoptysis: associated clinical features

Cause	Purulent sputum	Specks of blood	Pleural pain	Massive haemoptysis
Acute bronchitis	++			
Pneumonia	+		+	
Lung cancer		+		+
Pulmonary embolism		+	++	

Adapted from ref. 49.

nose or oropharynx in patients who have platelet deficiency or other types of bleeding tendency. It is not always reliable to judge the source of such bleeding on the freshness of blood—bright red blood may originate just as easily from a vessel in the bronchus as in the nose. However, old dark blood is more likely to have come from the lungs.

Common causes of haemoptysis are given in Table 14 (see also the anatomical–pathological classification of respiratory distress in Table 3). Haemoptysis has also been classified according to accompanying features such as purulent sputum, pleuritic pain, and the possibility of a massive bleed.[50] The latter is the symptom (and mode of death) that many patients (and their relatives) fear most. It is always worth asking patients about this point, as it is not a false reassurance to tell them that death from exsanguination is extremely rare (7 per cent of deaths due to haemorrhage of any kind in the series from one American cancer hospital).[145]

Treatment

Mild or moderate haemoptysis

Occasional specks of blood arising from the lungs need not be actively treated, but the patient should never be told to 'ignore it'. First it is unlikely that he will be able to, second he may think less of the doctor or nurse who gave such casual advice, and third he may be tempted not to report increasing amounts that do require treatment.

If haemoptysis persists or deteriorates despite cough suppressant therapy as described above, an oral haemostatic agent should be prescribed. There are no published trials of drugs such as ethamsylate or tranexamic acid for haemoptysis, but we have found both useful in controlling small streaks or moderate blobs of bleeding. These agents work mainly by reducing oozing from capillaries and would not be expected to cope with venous or arterial bleeding.

If oral haemostatics do not work within a few days, radiotherapy should be considered. Several series have reported the benefits of external beam radiotherapy for haemoptysis, with response rates of 83 to 90 per cent.[70] The histological type is not important, and it is worth offering palliative radiotherapy to all patients.

Endobronchial radiation with ionizing sources or by laser has been discussed earlier.[81,82] Laser therapy is particularly effective in controlling bleeding, and patients can have repeated sessions for recurring episodes.

The suspicion or proof of pulmonary embolism as the cause of recurrent small or moderate bleeds can lead to both clinical and ethical dilemmas. In general, the risks of anticoagulation frequently outweigh the benefits in patients with advanced malignancy, but each case should be taken on its own merits. If anticoagulation is felt to be worthwhile, the acute heparin stage can usually be dispensed with, and the patient started immediately on an oral drug such as warfarin.

Massive haemoptysis

'Massive haemoptysis' is defined as the expectoration of over 200 ml of blood in 24 h.[160] It is more likely to come from the higher-pressure arteries than the venous or capillary systems. It occurs predominantly in bronchiectasis, aspergilloma, lung abscess, and infection such as tuberculosis. Once again, it is truthfully reassuring to point out to patients that, in general hospital studies, malignancy is hardly ever the cause (7 per cent of 456 patients in one series).[161]

In palliative care, massive haemoptysis should be seen as an emergency, but the conventional life-saving interventions such as bronchoscopy, intubation, and bronchial artery embolization are almost never indicated. Usually, there will have been warning signs, and the possibility of a large bleed should have been discussed among the professional team and a decision made 'not to resuscitate'. Wherever possible, the family should be brought into this discussion, and in some cases the patient may personally give the directive.

If a massive bleed is expected, it is helpful to have a strong opioid such as diamorphine, syringe and needles, etc. readily available. If a doctor is present, he may wish to give the diamorphine by slow intravenous injection, titrating the rate to the patient's level of panic and consciousness. If available, a benzodiazepine such as midazolam or diazepam may be given intravenously as well as, or in place of, the opioid.[38] The aim should be to reduce awareness and fear, not necessarily to render the patient unconscious. If a doctor is not present or a suitable vein for injection is not found, diamorphine may be given by deep intramuscular injection (not subcutaneously, as the peripheral shutdown will impede absorption); diazepam may be given by the rectal route. The blood pressure may fall as a result of the bleeding or the opioid, and the bleeding may arrest temporarily; if the pressure then rises again, brisk bleeding could restart and so the patient should never be left alone.

If the patient does not immediately die as a result of the large haemorrhage, a continuous infusion of opioid, possibly with midazolam, should be instituted to maintain gentle sedation. It is most helpful, if the patient is at all conscious, for all signs of blood to be covered by coloured towels or bedding as soon as possible, as the sight of it will acutely heighten his or her fear.

Pleural pain

The subject of pleural pain will be dealt with only briefly, as analgesia is covered more fully elsewhere. The reason for including it here is that it often accompanies the other symptoms, particularly dyspnoea and cough, that are described in detail in this chapter.

Pain affecting the pleura is not intrinsically different from pain in other organs. Its distribution is anywhere in the chest wall, and by referral from the diaphragmatic surface it can include the shoulder tip. What sets pleural pain apart is its particular relationship to the act of breathing; the pain is often aggravated by respiratory movements and coughing. It is commonly known as 'pleuritic pain', although this implies that there is 'pleurisy', i.e. inflammation of the pleural surfaces, but this is not necessarily the case.

Prevalence

There is poor documentation of how commonly pleural pain occurs. The prevalence may be inferred from that of pains arising in lung cancer, but pleural pain probably comprises only a small part of these. In one hospice series 63 per cent of patients admitted with lung cancer had 'pain'.[46] In an oncology textbook 'chest pain' (which need not have been pleural) was said to occur in 40 per cent of lung cancer patients.[47]

Causes

Pleural pain arises when the surfaces of the pleura are irritated, inflamed, or infiltrated. Blood is extremely irritant and even a small amount, such as arises with a spontaneous pneumothorax, can cause severe unilateral chest wall and shoulder tip pain related to breathing. Inflammation is commonly due to infection, usually as pleural extension of lobar pneumonia, such as occurs with an obstructed bronchus. It can also arise after a segment of pulmonary infarction, i.e. necrosis of lung and pleura, which follows from a pulmonary embolus. Rib fractures due to trauma after surgery or metastasis cause severe limitation of breathing movements. Malignancy infiltrating the pleura (or pericardium) directly, such as in mesothelioma, peripheral extension of lung cancers, or deep penetration of chest wall tumours such as breast cancer, can all cause pleural pain.

It is important not to overlook shingles (herpes zoster) of a thoracic segment, which may cause severe pain mimicking pleurisy days before the characteristic rash appears on the skin in the distribution of a nerve.

Treatment

Since pleural pain can restrict the respiratory movements, it does not strictly cause the sensation of dyspnoea but may aggravate it. Cough that is coexisting or which arises from the same cause as the pleural disease will make the pain worse, and so is suppressed involuntarily. The result of these is that the patient is less mobile, and is at risk of sputum retention and consequent pulmonary infection. The importance of treating pleural pain after chest wall surgery has been well recognized by anaesthetists as contributing to postoperative recovery as well as the comfort of the patient.

For localized areas of pain (e.g. arising from a rib fracture or area of malignant chest wall infiltration), intercostal nerve block using a local anaesthetic may be obtained from nerve-destroying procedures such as alcohol or phenol injection, radiofrequency irradiation, or cryotherapy.

A recently described technique which may be beneficial for more extensive areas of pain is intrapleural instillation of bupivacaine.[162] This can be done as a single injection, or by continuous or intermittent infusion through a catheter placed in the pleural space.

Oral medication using an opioid may be useful as it could reduce the sensation of cough as well as pain when these two symptoms coexist and aggravate each other. If pleural inflammation is suspected, a non-steroidal anti-inflammatory drug could be added. Systemic corticosteroids are not helpful in most causes of pleural pain.

If persistent pain is arising from a rib metastasis, a single treatment of external-beam radiotherapy may be beneficial with little upset to the patient.

Pneumothorax

Pneumothorax is the presence of air in the pleural cavity, which leads to the compression (often misnamed 'collapse') of the underlying lung. In a tension pneumothorax, the pressure of air in the pleural cavity keeps rising so that not only is the underlying lung embarrassed, but the mediastinum is shifted away from the affected side and the function of the opposite lung is also hampered. Untreated tension pneumothorax is extremly distressing and potentially fatal.

Prevalence

The frequency of pneumothorax is not recorded in the palliative care or oncology literature. 'Spontaneous' pneumothorax arises infrequently in patients with chronic obstructive airways disease and emphysematous bullas, asthmatics, and normal individuals with asthenic build.[2]

Causes

A pneumothorax may arise from leakage of air either through the visceral pleura or the chest wall. The latter may occur inadvertently during paracentesis of a pleural effusion. The former may also occur iatrogenically by puncturing the lung during pleural aspiration or giving an intercostal nerve block.

In advanced cancer patients a pneumothorax can occur through malignant rupture of the visceral pleura, and will be accompanied by a pleural effusion (hydropneumothorax).

Treatment

In very sick patients with a small or moderate pneumothorax that is not under tension, it may be quite appropriate to take no specific action. With rest, adequate analgesia, and relief of cough, the air may be resorbed slowly through the pleura. In malignant cases the pneumothorax may become chronic and only partially impede the mobility of the patient.

With a tension pneumothorax, unless the patient's death is acknowledged to be imminent and active intervention would be inappropriate, an attempt should be made to aspirate the air. The least traumatic method is simple aspiration with a wide-bore needle or plastic intravenous cannula and a syringe, using a three-way tap. For larger collections of air, a wide-bore intercostal drain with an underwater seal to ensure one-way passage of air out of the chest cavity is usually necessary.[163] These techniques should only be carried out in units with adequate resources for monitoring and radiography, and the decision to treat symptomatically may be taken if the person is unwilling to leave home or the comfort of an inpatient hospice unit without these facilities. This would probably involve opioids to relieve dyspnoea, pain, and cough, as well as continuous or intermittent oxygen therapy if there is significant hypoxaemia.

Pulmonary embolism

Pulmonary embolism is included in this chapter because it is a potent cause of respiratory symptoms, even though it is largely undiagnosed and untreated. Pulmonary embolism is the passage of thrombotic emboli from distal veins into the pulmonary circulation, where the blood clots wedge and cause ischaemia and ultimately necrosis of the local lung tissue. Small emboli often go unnoticed clinically but may summate to produce insidious pulmonary hypertension. Wheezing may result, which can be mistaken for asthma.[164]

Large emboli are often dramatic, causing sudden severe breathlessness, cough, haemoptysis, hypotension, and loss of consciousness. Less violently, they may still be the cause of death in many slowly deteriorating cancer patients who expire during an apparently unremarkable exertion such as using the lavatory.

Prevalence

Pulmonary embolism is relatively easy to diagnose when acute or severe, and in patients with known predisposing factors such as recent surgery or immobilization. It is found in 10 to 15 per cent of post-mortem examinations of adults who die in hospital, but is regarded as the principal cause of death in only 3 per cent.[2] It is tempting to speculate on the morbidity associated with chronic, recurrent, and non-fatal pulmonary embolism in the older mainly sedentary or bedbound population, as there is no documentation in the literature.

Causes

Deep venous thrombosis, usually in the pelvic or leg veins, is the usual cause in chronically immobile patients. Malignancy predisposes to a thrombotic tendency. Some forms of hormonal therapy may predispose a patient to thrombosis. In some cases of superior vena cava obstruction, the stasis of blood in the large central vein leads to thrombosis there, which may become dislodged and pass into the heart and lungs.

The diagnosis of pulmonary embolism can often be made clinically, but definitive confirmation is best made with an isotope ventilation–perfusion scan of the lungs. It is important to be aware that 'false-positive' lung scans may occur, perhaps because of acute local vasculitis, soon after radiotherapy.[165] Occasionally the emboli are not thrombotic in nature, but actually arise from tumour tissue in the peripheral organs. The symptoms and other clinical features of tumour emboli may be indistinguishable from thrombotic pulmonary embolism, but of course the treatment would not include anticoagulation as described below.

Table 15 Inhaled and nebulized therapy

Clinical indication	Drug
Asthma/chronic obstructive airways disease	Inhaled/nebulized bronchodilator Inhalled/nebulized corticosteroid
Cough	
Tenacious sputum	Nebulized saline
Unproductive	Nebulized local anaesthetic
Pulmonary malignancy	
Cough	Nebulized local anaesthetic
Dyspnoea	Nebulized opioid
Pulmonary embolism	Nebulized opioid

Treatment

Prevention of pulmonary embolism is much easier than treatment, and involves keeping the patient well hydrated, as mobile as possible, and avoiding the obstruction of the leg veins by inappropriate positioning of the legs when the patient is seated in a chair. The use of compression 'antiembolism' stockings is uncomfortable and should be reserved for patients with a proven tendency to deep vein thrombosis in the legs.

Very often there is little to be done for acute severe pulmonary embolism other than offering an opioid (oral or parenteral) for immediate relief of breathlessness, pleural pain, and cough. With a large embolus there is considerable ventilation–perfusion mismatching which can lead to significant hypoxaemia; this is best treated with high-flow oxygen.

Lesser grades of pulmonary embolism could also be treated symptomatically, but the possibility of preventive anticoagulation should normally be considered. However, if the patient is elderly (e.g. over 70 years), if the prognosis is thought to be in terms of days or weeks, or if there is a definite recent history of bleeding from peptic ulcer, anticoagulation would often be ruled out. In most cases the acute phase of anticoagulation with heparin can be omitted and oral treatment started immediately with a loading dose of warfarin. The oral anticoagulation should be continued for at least 6 weeks after a suspected or proven episode of pulmonary embolism; after that, a trial period off warfarin with close observation for recurrence may be undertaken. It should be emphasized that this form of therapy needs regular monitoring, particularly in the early days, and should not be undertaken lightly.

Inhaled therapy

Inhaled therapy would seem to be a logical mode of administration of drugs for the relief of respiratory symptoms, and no doubt one of its psychological advantages is that many patients feel that it is treatment directed to the site of their problem. A number of agents may now be offered by this method (Table 15).

A traditional remedy is inhalation of 'steam' or hot water, often containing pleasant and soothing aromatic compounds, for cough and difficulty in breathing because of nasal congestion. There is no reason why these should not still be used, but the danger of scalding of elderly or weak patients should be recognized.

Aerosol and dry powder inhalers

Many patients with chronic asthma or chronic obstructive airways disease will be familiar with inhaled bronchodilators before they develop malignant or neuromuscular causes of dyspnoea or cough. The newer dry powder devices are more environmentally friendly because they do not release chlorofluorocarbons into the atmosphere. Breath-actuated devices and those which can be used with spacer attachments improve the efficiency of the drug delivery in many older or weak patients.[166] The use of bronchodilator drugs has been described above.

Nebulizers

Nebulizers are devices which produce an aerosol from water, saline, or a solution of drug. The smaller the size of particles produced in the aerosol, the better is the penetration into the lungs: optimal deposition in the airways and to the alveoli is achieved with particles of sizes 6 to 10 μm and 3 to 4 μm respectively.[167] There are two types in common use: the ultrasonic nebulizer achieves very small particle sizes but has not been as readily adopted as the jet nebulizer, which has also been the subject of more detailed study. Factors that are known to influence the size of particle include the design of nebulizer, the rate of flow of air (via cylinder or electric compressor), the temperature of the solution, and the lung function of the patient.[168] Easily portable combinations of an electric or battery-powered compressor and a jet nebulizer, which are suitable for home use with a little training of the patient and relatives, are now available. Nearly all United Kingdom hospices now offer nebulizer therapy.[76] Better results are obtained with a mouthpiece than with a full face mask, but the latter is preferred by some patients and may be necessary if they tend to nose breathe.

Uses of nebulizers

Bronchodilators are only one group of drugs that can be delivered by the nebulizer. Pure water should not be nebulized as it readily causes bronchospasm in asthmatic subjects.[169] However, nebulized saline can greatly help the expectoration of tenacious mucus, with or without chest physiotherapy.[159] Other agents which have been described in earlier sections of this chapter include local anaesthetics for the relief of cough and dyspnoea, and opioids for the control of breathlessness.

As with all treatments and routes, there are adverse effects with inhaled and nebulized drugs. The induction of bronchospasm with nebulized local anaesthetics,[142] morphine, and diamorphine[136] has already been discussed. Pulmonary infection with *Pneumocystis carinii* causes severe respiratory distress in patients with AIDS; nebulizing the antibiotic pentamidine has been shown to be helpful prophylactically, but the drug is associated with cough (33 per cent), excess salivation (35 per cent), and bronchospasm (4 per cent).[170] If a high concentration of oxygen is being used to drive the nebulizer, the possibility of precipitating dangerous hypercapnia in susceptible patients with chronic obstructive airways disease should be remembered.[171] The British Thoracic Society guidelines for nebulizer usage in palliative care summarize the known experience in their favour and draw attention to the disappointing lack of scientific evidence of effectiveness.[138]

Physiotherapy (see Chapter 12.2)

Physiotherapy (or 'physical therapy') is a form of treatment that has traditionally been closely allied to respiratory care and has also long been recognized as an integral part of the multidisciplinary approach typically used in palliative care. It has many useful roles in the management of respiratory symptoms.[172]

Manual techniques

Manual techniques, including postural drainage and chest percussion, have been regarded important examples of the techniques available to physiotherapists.[173] However, the traditional views about these methods, particularly in patients with advanced malignancy, have been called into question by recent studies. It has been proposed that percussion and vibration are now redundant, and should be replaced by the forced expiratory technique with postural drainage in patients with chronic sputum production.[174] Chest percussion and vibration have been shown to be useless, or indeed harmful, in patients who do not produce excessive sputum (defined as more than 30 ml daily).[175]

The benefit of the forced expiratory technique, which is also known as 'huffing', has been shown convincingly in studies. Patients can be taught to perform it alone, and it can improve the yield of postural drainage.[176] Although in many of these studies mucus was moved more efficiently, there were no objective benefits in terms of lung function. Unfortunately, subjective markers of respiratory symptoms have not been formally evaluated.

Another area where physiotherapists have traditionally been involved is the application of airways suction for the removal of tenacious mucus. This is relatively easily performed in the intensive care unit where patients are heavily sedated and may be intubated. In palliative care situations, the insertion of a tube into the trachea may be very distressing for the patient (and for relatives to watch). The adverse effects of airways suction include tracheobronchial trauma, bronchial obstruction, pneumothorax, and even cardiac arrhythmias.[177] For these reasons, and because it is generally felt to be 'invasive' for very sick patients, there is a strong resistance to using airways suction in palliative care units. It has been replaced, as described later in this chapter, by the use of anticholinergic agents to dry up mucus secretion. However, it should not be completely discarded, as even after anticholinergics there may be a ball of already secreted mucus present in the trachea just under the larynx which can only be removed by gentle suction.

Relaxation and massage

Another traditional role of physiotherapy is massage, which has now been supplemented by relaxation training, sometimes using prerecorded audiotapes. (Clearly, these techniques are not confined to the discipline of physiotherapy.) Although there have been no trials of these techniques for respiratory distress, relaxation training has become accepted in some areas of oncology as a valuable behavioural modification to help patients to cope with the stress of disease and treatment. The old instructions for 'breathing exercises' have now been supplanted by these approaches. In patients with severe airflow limitation, being taught to breathe with pursed lips can help prevent collapse of central airways during expiration.[173]

Ventilatory support

The importance of the respiratory muscles in maintaining normal ventilation and in the mediation of respiratory distress was stressed in the first section of this chapter, in which control of breathing was discussed. It may seem surprising to include a section on mechanical ventilation in a book on palliative medicine, as this initially sounds invasive and more associated with life-prolonging treatment. However, the use of ventilatory support techniques has recently expanded, and applications are being explored which may soon become extended into the terminal care of some patients.

Mechanical ventilation

Artificial ventilation by mechanical means is not new, but much of the present knowledge has arisen from the experience of the poliomyelitis epidemics of the 1950s. Mechanical ventilation is of two types: negative-pressure and positive-pressure. The former is exemplified by the old 'tank ventilators' and their descendants such as the jacket and cuirass ventilators. These are cumbersome and unappealing devices that would not usually be acceptable for patients in palliative care programmes.

Positive-pressure ventilation is a much more acceptable approach for patients with slowly advancing neuromuscular diseases leading to respiratory muscle fatigue.[178] The main techniques available are continuous positive-pressure ventilation or intermittent positive-pressure ventilation. The latter is becoming more established, but both can be applied by face or nasal masks and are feasible in the patient's home.

A typical patient who would benefit from nasal intermittent positive-pressure ventilation has motor neurone disease which has affected the respiratory muscles more than the muscles of locomotion, speech, or swallowing. This is not uncommon, and in such an individual the distress of respiratory restriction coupled with the knowledge that he or she is slowly suffocating can lead to great physical and emotional suffering. Although they have to be monitored frequently by respiratory specialists and may need additional equipment such as emergency back-up generators at home in the case of a power failure, the improvement in symptoms such as quality of sleep and daytime breathlessness may well justify the resources involved. As we have found, it is challenging but not impossible to maintain part of such a patient's management in a hospice where the psychosocial skills of staff may be additionally brought to bear on the anxious patients and their families.[172]

Continuous positive-pressure ventilation delivered via a facial mask has been used to support patients with AIDS who have acute respiratory distress due to intercurrent *Pneumocystis carinii* pneumonia.[179] As the prevalence of AIDS increases, the possibility that patients attending palliative care units will develop serious and life-threatening *Pneumocystis carinii* pneumonia may also rise. It may be considered entirely appropriate to offer 'active' interventions such as prophylactic nebulized pentamidine, as described earlier,[170] or continuous positive-pressure ventilation support to such patients during a *Pneumocystis carinii* pneumonia episode. The ethical position of when to withdraw such support has still to be debated and worked out, but it is important for physicians in palliative care to become familiar with such methods.

The aim of most forms of mechanical ventilation is to enable the patient to return home. Prospective studies have shown that domiciliary ventilatory support can improve quality of life by relieving sleep and daytime symptoms.[180] Both positive- and negative-pressure ventilation have been used at home. Patients who benefited symptomatically included those with rapidly progressive neuromuscular disease that caused death within months of initiating treatment.

Electrical stimulation

The role of the diaphragm in sustaining normal respiration, and in mediating the sensation of breathlessness when it becomes fatigued or paralysed, has been discussed earlier. The dyspnoea may be felt more acutely when the patient is lying down (orthopnoea) because the abdominal organs can compress the thoracic contents. When the diaphragmatic insufficiency is due to phrenic nerve disorder, it is possible to provide artificial transcutaneous stimulation of the muscle by electrodes placed at the neck.[181]

Even unilateral hemidiaphragm weakness may cause breathlessness in 10 to 24 per cent of patients.[182] This condition might arise from phrenic nerve paralysis due to mediastinal malignancy, as well as after thoracic surgery. The possibility of improving diaphragmatic function in such subjects using transcutaneous stimulation is an approach to non-invasive palliation that requires further study.

Patient and family support

The introduction of ventilatory support in patients with more chronic disorders and in their own homes could lead to the creation of new psychological and social stresses for them and their family carers.[183] The educational needs of the family when faced with the responsibilities of caring for such a patient are also important.

Respiratory rehabilitation

Respiratory rehabilitation is usually regarded as a subject of acute disease management and is associated with curable illnesses. However, most of the progress in this field has been in patients who have progressive and ultimately fatal chronic obstructive airways disease.[184] Although the aim of pulmonary rehabilitation is to prolong life, this has been only partly successful, but in many programmes the quality of life of individuals has improved because of better control of respiratory symptoms and increased participation by patients in their own care. In older patients with chronic lung disease the rehabilitative approach may be appropriate and consistent with other aspects of geriatric care.[108]

The aim of a rehabilitation programme is to educate and train the individual with respiratory impairment or disability to make most efficient use of his or her remaining lung function, to relieve the dyspnoea, and thereby to improve quality of life. This involves the following:

(1) discussion with the patient and family about modifications to lifestyle;

(2) reduction or cessation of work and household duties (of the patient or family carers);

(3) rearrangements within the house such as bringing the patient's bed downstairs or adding downstairs toilet facilities.

Therefore an important aspect of rehabilitating patients is to identify and preferably also measure the degree of impairment or disability.[185] Ideally, this should involve both the objective measures of exercise tolerance discussed above and the psychosocial measures to be described below.

Exercise training inevitably forms an important part of respiratory rehabilitation. Although improved tolerance is itself a reasonable endpoint, reduction of breathlessness has also been demonstrated in a programme aimed at cystic fibrosis patients.[186] Whether cancer patients with malignancy-related dyspnoea or coexisting chronic airways disease could also benefit from planned exercise training programmes has not been studied. The relatively more rapid deterioration in function in malignancy compared with chronic obstructive airways disease clearly needs to be considered, and the occurrence of other symptoms that restrict mobility, such as pain, weakness, or oedema, may mitigate against positive benefits in cancer subjects.

Patients with malignancy often have coexisting chronic lung disease, and these may be causally related, as in the case of lung cancer and some head and neck cancers. In the latter group it is important to recognize the aspiration of gastric contents because of disturbed swallowing control as another risk factor for respiratory problems.[187]

The ability to modify the ventilatory response to hypercapnia through yoga training has been described above.[22] A device which slows down respiratory movements in a manner similar to that of pranayama breathing methods was found to improve objective indicators of airflow obstruction and even airways reactivity in asthmatics.[188] The use of a control (which did not induce positive changes) in this interesting study was important as the psychological component of any response to a training programme should not be underestimated.

The role of specialist workers (e.g. mastectomy counsellors, stoma care advisers, palliative care nurse specialists) has become well accepted in oncological and palliative care. The place of the 'respiratory health worker' in chronic respiratory disease has been discussed.[189] Patients under the care of such an adviser live longer, but quality of life may not be improved directly. This may be because the measures used are insensitive, but the economic consequences of employing such staff have to be considered in establishing support for patients with respiratory disease.

Psychosocial and quality-of-life issues

The psychological component of respiratory distress has been referred to frequently in this chapter. In the following sections we shall briefly consider the range of psychosocial consequences of respiratory symptoms which may become significant in the delivery of holistic palliative care. Studies have also shown that pre-existing attitudes and beliefs may significantly affect patients' physical functioning in chronic disease.[190,191] The fear of inducing symptoms such as breathlessness or bouts of coughing, usually based on previous personal experience but sometimes arising from deep-seated feelings about dying, can severely restrict the motivation and mobility of some patients. Ironically, the negative physical changes caused by inactivity in a chair or bed further add to the risk of developing these symptoms.

General impact of cancer

Much has been written elsewhere about the psychosocial impact of having cancer from the patient's and family's point of view. The usual reactions include uncertainty, a feeling of helplessness, a sense of failure or guilt, and stigma leading to isolation. It is important to recognize that elderly subjects with malignancy sometimes exhibit different emotional and psychiatric forms of behaviour.[192]

Psychosocial effects of lung cancer

The reaction to lung cancer is essentially the same as that to other malignancies, but may be modified because many patients also have chronic pre-existing lung disease. Studies have shown incidences of anxiety and depression of 41 per cent and 16 per cent respectively in lung cancer patients.[193] Deteriorating physical capability is usually correlated with increasing psychological distress. The various treatments for lung cancer, such as radiotherapy and chemotherapy regimens, may have different degrees of impact on psychological well being, and this should be taken into consideration when a treatment plan is being formulated for an individual.

The social and financial consequences of having cancer, which may lead to loss of employment for the patient or a family carer and the cost of attending hospital for certain treatments, also have to be counted in the overall burden.

Psychosocial assessment

Assessment of psychosocial stability and problems is often made by 'clinical judgement', and if the physician or nurse knows the patient and family well this may be sufficient. The need to bring the relatives into the discussion has been stressed.[59,194] However, usually we do not know our patients well enough to make such assumptions about their emotional and social well being. In assessing the response to therapies in large groups (e.g. clinical trials), it is not feasible to use personal evaluations.

This is where the application of standardized quality-of-life instruments may be helpful. Those which have been developed for self-assessment by cancer patients are to be preferred, although staff-rated measures have also been shown to be reliable. The quality-of-life scales which may be used for cancer patients in palliative oncology trials or hospice care programmes have been reviewed.[66,195] The modular approach of the European Organization for Research and Teaching in Cancer (EORTC) quality-of-life assessment in different cancers has special merit, and it has also been validated in several European languages.[196]

A number of useful instruments have been devised for use in patients with advanced non-malignant diseases which are causing respiratory distress.[197] These include the Chronic Respiratory Questionnaire[58] and the St George's Respiratory Questionnaire.[198]

Psychosocial interventions

Psychosocial intervention should be considered an integral part of palliation of respiratory distress. All the symptoms discussed so far (dyspnoea, cough, haemoptysis, pleural pain) may be modified by the patient's anxiety, and conversely they may also contribute to mood disturbance.

It is not appropriate here to discuss details of psychosocial drug support; the respiratory sedative drugs described above, including opioids, benzodiazepines, phenothiazines, and cannabinoids, may all play a part. Antidepressants may be useful in chronic disability where depression is inextricably linked to the patient's functional restriction.[199]

Non-drug approaches to psychological support are also relevant. Behavioural techniques such as relaxation and biofeedback have been used in chronic obstructive airways disease,[200] and their use in cancer patients needs to be explored. Yoga training may also be useful in helping suitably motivated patients to control the sensation of breathlessness.[22] Recently a nurse-led initiative in London, UK, has stressed the importance of the non-pharmacological approaches to dyspnoea in lung cancer patients.[201] Acupuncture has also been tried and found to give short-term benefit for cancer-related dyspnoea.[202] It is important that all these interventions are formally evaluated against 'conventional' methods, althought admittedly some do not lend themselves to quantification using the biomedical model.

Respiratory terminal care

General principles

In the terminal stages of diseases such as cancer, progressive neuromuscular disorders, and some respiratory conditions, the emphasis of management changes recognizably from active forms of intervention to purely supportive and symptomatic measures. Thus radiotherapy may be ruled out because the patient is too frail to travel, and ventilatory support may be gradually withdrawn at the patient's or family's request because it is interfering with quality of life.

The drug treatments already described are mostly still applicable in this phase, except for the cytotoxic agents that are used earlier on to palliate endobronchial obstruction. In general, the fewer drugs that the patient has to take, the better. However, with multiple symptoms such as pain, breathlessness, haemoptysis, and constipation, multiple drug therapy may be unavoidable. If possible, drugs should be given by mouth, and sustained release preparations which reduce dosing to once or twice a day are preferred. Continuous subcutaneous infusions may replace the need for other drugs to be taken orally or by intermittent injection.

Nebulized therapy remains a helpful intervention that even very sick patients can continue until they are not able to sit upright enough to use them or have such shallow or laboured breathing that they would be inappropriate. Intermittent nebulization of opioid for paroxysmal dyspnoea, together with a local anaesthetic for distressing cough, may be used even into the last days or hours of life.

Oxygen therapy has already been discussed, and it is worth emphasizing again that there is no case for starting it just because a patient is breathless and thought to be dying. The use of a face mask in the last few days or hours may impede valuable opportunities for whispered words or affectionate contact, and therefore nasal cannulas are much preferred.

Nursing care

The contribution of good nursing care is as important at this time as anywhere else in palliative care. Simple measures, such as allowing a constant draught of air from an open window or a table fan, can be very helpful for patients who frequently feel that they are suffocating.[101] Those with oxygen being delivered for long periods by face mask should frequently be invited to take drinks or sips to keep the mouth moist. Face masks may also restrict conversation, and so special efforts are needed to prevent the patient from becoming isolated.

Many chronic lung disease patients prefer to sit out in a chair rather than lie in bed. This is because their hyperexpanded rib cages work more efficiently when maintained upright, even leaning slightly forward, with the arms supported on a table top so that the accessory muscles of inspiration in the neck and shoulders can be used.

If the patient is confined to bed, it is preferable to keep him or her propped up on pillows rather than lying flat. There is a significant loss of lung volume with the supine posture.[203] When the heart is enlarged, as in cardiac failure, lying flat has been shown to cause obstruction of the left lower-lobe bronchus, which can lead to increased breathlessness (orthopnoea), retention of mucus, and hypostatic pneumonia.[204] Keeping the patient on one side for too long may predispose to unilateral pulmonary oedema in the dependent lung. Finally, aspiration of gastric contents, particularly in those with neuromuscular problems of the swallowing mechanism, is more likely to occur with the recumbent patient and can lead to bouts of coughing and dyspnoea.

Respiratory panic

At the end of a long illness, patients are sometimes more readily subject to episodes of acute respiratory distress, which may be referred to as 'respiratory panic'. This term is used to emphasize the speed and distress of the paroxysm, and does not imply a hysterical component.[38] These episodes may also occur at any time earlier in the disease, for example as a result of pulmonary embolism, tracheal obstruction, or asthmatic attacks. The management of acute respiratory panic is similar whatever the cause or stage of disease (Table 16).

The quickest relief is undoubtedly obtained by parenteral administration of a benzodiazepine or opioid, perhaps with oxygen. However, if medical or nursing staff are not immediately available (e.g. when the patient is at home), teaching relatives to set up a nebulizer with an opioid, and possibly rectal diazepam, within a few minutes of the onset of panic can give great reassurance to the whole family.

The 'death rattle'

In the final hour, many patients in semiconscious or deeply unconscious states are unable to swallow saliva reflexly or to cough up mucus from the trachea. Breathing with a partial loose obstruction of this sort in the central airways or glottic area gives rise to noisy respiration, known starkly as the 'death rattle'. Mercifully, most patients are unaware of this noise, but it may give great distress to relatives or other patients nearby. It is readily prevented by an anticholinergic such as hyoscine, given either as a single parenteral dose or by continuous infusion.[38] Occasionally a ball of

Table 16 Respiratory panic: causes and management approaches

Causes	Management
Major malignant airways obstruction (stridor)	Opioid Benzodiazepine (Oxygen)
Superior vena cava obstruction	Opioid Benzodiazepine (Oxygen)
Pulmonary embolism	Oxygen Opioid
Left ventricular failure	Diuretics Opioid Oxygen
Gastric contents/saliva aspiration	Opioid Benzodiazepine Nebulized local anaesthetic

mucus is already lying in the trachea and hyoscine will not remove this; repositioning of the patient, or gentle suction using a soft catheter, may be necessary (see Section 17).

References

1. Empey D. Diseases of the respiratory system. *British Medical Journal*, 1978; 1:631–3.
2. Crofton J, Douglas A. The structures and function of the respiratory tract. *Respiratory Diseases*. Oxford: Blackwell, 1981: 14.
3. Rogers D, Barnes P. Opioid inhibition of neurally mediated mucus secretion in human bronchi. *Lancet*, 1989; **335**:930–2.
4. Mehta AD, Wright WB, Kirby BJ. Ventilatory function in Parkinson's disease. *British Medical Journal*, 1978; **280**:1456.
5. Sykes DA, Mohanaruban K, Finucane P, Sastry BSD. Assessment of the elderly with respiratory disease. *Geriatric Medicine*, 1989; **19**:49–54.
6. Guyton AC. *Textbook of Medical Physiology*. Philadelphia, PA: WB Saunders, 1986.
7. Paintal AS. Lung and airway receptors. In: Pallot DJ, ed. *Control of Respiration*. London: Croom Helm, 1983:78.
8. Petersen ES. The control of breathing pattern. In: Whipp BJ, ed. *The Control of Breathing in Man*. Manchester University Press, 1987.
9. Whipp BJ. The control of exercise hyperpnoea. In: Whipp BJ, ed. *The Control of Breathing in Man*. Manchester University Press, 1987.
10. Jordan C. Assessment of the effects of drugs on respiration. *British Journal of Anaesthesia*, 1982; **54**:763–82.
11. Patrick JM. Studies of respiratory control in man. In: Pallot DJ, ed. *Control of Respiration*. London: Croom Helm, 1983:203–20.
12. Estenne M. Respiratory muscle physiology with particular regard to rib cage muscles. In: Grassino A, Fracchia C, Rampulla C, Zocchi L, ed. *Respiratory Muscles in COPD*. London: Bi and Gi, 1988:35.
13. Macklem PT. Inspiratory muscle physiology, with particular regard to the diaphragm. In: Grassino A, Fracchia C, Rampulla C, Zocchi L, ed. *Respiratory Muscles in COPD*. London, Bi and Gi, 1988:23.
14. Campbell EJM, Howell JBL. The sensation of breathlessness. *British Medical Bulletin*, 1963; **19**:36–40.
15. Mier A. Respiratory muscle weakness. *Respiratory Medicine*, 1990; **84**:351–9.
16. Morel DR, Forster A, Bachmann M, Suter PM. Effect of intravenous midazolam on breathing pattern and chest wall mechanics in humans. *Journal of Applied Physiology*, 1984; **57**:1104–10.
17. Ward SA, Robbins PA. The ventilatory response to hypoxia. In: Whipp BJ, ed. *The Control of Breathing in Man*. Manchester University Press, 1987.
18. West JB. Oxygen transport from air to tissues. *Ventilation/Blood Flow and Gas Exchange*. Oxford: Blackwell, 1978.
19. Calverley PMA, *et al.* Preservation of the hypoxic drive to breathing in diabetic autonomic neuropathy. *Clinical Science*, 1982; **63**:17–22.
20. Loeschcke HH. Central chemoreceptors. In: Pallot BJ, ed. *Control of Respiration*. London: Croom Helm, 1983:41.
21. Brischetto M, Millman R, Peterson D, Silage D, Pack A. Effect of aging on ventilatory response to exercise and CO_2. *Journal of Applied Physiology*, 1984; **56**:1143–50.
22. Stanescu D, Nemery B, Veriter C, Marechal C. Pattern of breathing and ventilatory response to CO_2 in subjects practicing hatha-yoga. *Journal of Applied Physiology*, 1981; **51**:1625–9.
23. Thompson JW. Clinical pharmacology of opioid agonists and partial agonists. In: Doyle D, ed. *Opioids in the Treatment of Cancer Pain*. London: Royal Society of Medicine Services, 1990:17–38.
24. Santiago TV, Remolina C, Scoles V, Edelman NH. Endorphins and the control of breathing. *New England Journal of Medicine*, 1981; **304**:1190–5.
25. Petty TL. Dealing with final stages of disease. In: Hodgkin JE, Petty TL, ed. *Chronic Obstructive Pulmonary Disease: Current Concepts*. Philadelphia, PA: WB Saunders, 1987:279.
26. Weinberger SE, *et al.* Endogenous opioids and ventilatory responses to hypercapnia in normal humans. *Journal of Applied Physiology*, 1985; **58**:1415–20.
27. Michiels TM, Light RW, Mahutte CK. Effect of ethanol and naloxone on control of ventilation and load perception. *Journal of Applied Physiology*, 1983; **55**:929–34.
28. Labaille T, Clergue F, Samii K, Ecoffey C, Berdeaux A. Ventilatory response to CO_2 following intravenous and epidural lidocaine. *Anesthiology*, 1985; **63**:179–83.
29. Winning I, Hamilton RD, Shea SA, Knott C, Guz A. Effect of airway anaesthesia on the control of breathing and the sensation of breathlessness in man. *Clinical Science*, 1985; **68**:215–25.
30. Billings JA. The management of common symptoms. *Outpatient Management of Advanced Cancer*. Philadelphia. PA: JB Lippincott, 1985.
31. Ogilvie C. Dyspnoea. *British Medical Journal*, 1983; **287**:160–1.
32. Ahmedzai S. Respiratory distress in the terminally ill patient. *Respiratory Disease in Practice*, 1988; **5**:20–9.
33. Saunders C. What's in a name? *Palliative Medicine*, 1987; **1**:57–61.
34. Simon PM, *et al.* Distinguishable sensations of breathlessness induced in normal volunteers. *American Review of Respiratory Disease*, 1989; **140**(4):1021–7.
35. Howell JBL. Behavioural breathlessness. *Thorax*, 1990; **45**:287.
36. Hockley JM, Dunlop R, Davies RJ. Survey of distressing symptoms in dying patients and their families in hospital and the response to a symptom control team. *British Medical Journal*, 1988; **296**:1715–17.
37. Baines MJ. Control of other symptoms. In: Saunders CM, ed. *The Management of Terminal Disease*. London: Edward Arnold, 1983:99–118.
38. Doyle D. *Domiciliary Terminal Care*. Edinburgh: Churchill Livingstone, 1987.
39. Heyse-Moore LH, Ross V, Mullee MA. How much of a problem is dyspnoea in advanced cancer? *Palliative Medicine*, 1991; **5**:20–6.
40. Hunt AM. A survey of signs, symptoms and symptom control in 30 terminally ill children. *Developmental Medicine and Child Neurology*, 1990; **32**:341–6.
41. Reuben DB, Mor M. Dyspnoea in terminal cancer patients. *Chest*, 1986; **89**:234–6.
42. Ventafridda V, de Conno F, Ripamonti C, Gamba A, Tamburini M. Quality of life assessment during a palliative care programme. *Annals of Oncology*, 1990; **1**:415–20.
43. Higginson I and McCarthy M. Measuring symptoms in terminal cancer: are pain and dyspnoea controlled? *Journal of the Royal Society of Medicine*, 1989; **82**:264–7.
44. Wilkes E. *A Source Book of Terminal Care*. University of Sheffield Printing Unit.

45. Ahmedzai S, Morton A, Reid JT, Stevenson RD. Quality of death from lung cancer: patients' reports and relatives' retrospective opinions. In: Watson M, *et al.*, ed. *Psychosocial Oncology*. Oxford: Pergamon Press, 1988:187–92.
46. Twycross RG. The terminal care of patients with lung cancer. *Postgraduate Medical Journal*, 1973; **49**:732–7.
47. Spiro SG, Oroth M. Clinical Features. In: Hoogstraten B, *et al.*, ed. *Lung Tumors*. Berlin: Springer-Verlag, 1988:55–62.
48. Littlejohns P, Ebrahim S, Anderson R. Prevalence and diagnosis of chronic respiratory symptoms in adults. *British Medical Journal*, 1989; **298**: 1556–60.
49. Grassino A. Pathways leading to skeletal muscle fatigue. In: Grassino A, Fracchia C, Rampulla C, Zocchi L, ed. *Respiratory Muscles in COPD*. London: Springer-Verlag, 1988: 77.
50. Johnson N. *Respiratory Medicine*. Oxford: Blackwell, 1986:131.
51. Turcotte H, Corbeil F, Boulet LP. Perception of breathlessness during bronchoconstriction induced by antigen, exercise, and histamine challenges. *Thorax*, 1990; **45**:914–18.
52. Mahler DA, Cunningham LN, Curfman GD. Aging and exercise performance. *Respiratory Diseases*, 1986; **2**:433–52.
53. Banerjee DK, Lee GS, Malik SK, Daly S. Underdiagnosis of asthma in the elderly. *British Journal of Diseases of the Chest*, 1987; **81**:23–9.
54. Ayres JG. Late onset asthma. *British Medical Journal*, 1990; **300**:1602–3.
55. Fitting JW. Inspiratory muscles and dyspnoea. In: Grassino A, Fracchia C, Rampulla C, Zocchi L, ed. *Respiratory Muscles in COPD*. London: Springer-Verlag, 1988:125.
56. Aaronson N, Bullinger M, Ahmedzai S. A modular approach to quality of life assessment in cancer clinical trials. *Cancer Research*, 1988; **111**: 231–49.
57. Bergman B, Aaronson NK, Ahmedzai S, Kaasa S, Sullivan M. The EORTC QLQ-LC13: a modular supplement to the EORTC core quality of life questionnaire (QLQ-C30) for use in lung cancer clinical trials. *European Journal of Cancer*, 1994; **30A**(5):635–42.
58. Guyatt GH, Townsend M, Keller J, Singer J, Nogradi S. Measuring functional status in chronic lung disease: conclusions from a randomised control trial. *Respiratory Medicine*, 1991; **85** (Supplement B):17–21.
59. Guyatt G, Townsend M, Berman L, Pugsley S. Quality of life in patients with chronic airflow limitation. *British Journal of Diseases of the Chest*, 1987; **81**:45–54.
60. Peel ET, Soutar CA, Seaton A. Assessment of variability of exercise tolerance limited by breathlessness. *Thorax*, 1988; **43**:960–4.
61. Morgan A. Simple exercise testing. *Respiratory Medicine*, 1989; **83**:383–7.
62. Wijkstra PJ, *et al.* Relation of lung function, maximal inspiratory pressure, dyspnoea, and quality of life with exercise capacity in patients with chronic obstructive pulmonary disease. *Thorax*, 1994; **49**:468–72.
63. Morice A, Smithies T. The 100 m walk: a simple and reproducible exercise test. *British Journal of Diseases of the Chest*, 1989; **78**:392.
64. Congleton J, Muers MF. The incidence of airflow obstruction in bronchial carcinoma, its relation to breathlessness, and response to bronchodilator therapy. *Respiratory Medicine*, 1995; **89**:291–6.
65. Apps MCP. A guide to lung function tests. *British Journal of Hospital Medicine*, 1992; **48**(7):396–401.
66. Ahmedzai S. Palliative care in oncology: making quality the endpoint. *Annals of Oncology*, 1990; **1**:396–8.
67. Ahmedzai S. Palliative and terminal care of elderly cancer patients. In: Fentiman I, Monfardini S, ed. *Cancer in the Elderly—Treatment and Research*. Oxford University Press, 1992.
68. Fergusson RJ, Cull A. Quality of life measurement for patients undergoing treatment for lung cancer. *Thorax*, 1991; **46**:671–5.
69. Mosley JG. Intrathoracic malignancy. *Palliation in Malignant Disease*. Edinburgh: Churchill Livingstone, 1988:12.
70. Lung Cancer Working Party. Inoperable non-small-cell lung cancer (NSCLC): a Medical Research Council randomised trial of palliative radiotherapy with two fractions or ten fractions. *British Journal of Cancer*, 1991; **63**:265–70.
71. Fazio F, Pratt T, McKenzie C, Steiner R. Improvement in regional ventilation and perfusion after radiotherapy for unresectable carcinoma of the bronchus. *American Journal Review*, 1979; **133**:191–200.
72. Lung Cancer Working Party. Survival, adverse reactions and quality of life during combination chemotherapy compared with selective palliative treatment for small-cell lung cancer. *Respiratory Medicine*, 1989; **83**:51–8.
73. Smit EF, Carney DN, Harford P, Sleijfer DT, Postmus PE. A phase II study of oral etoposide in elderly patients with small cell lung cancer. *Thorax*, 1989; **44**:631–3.
74. Mestitz H, Pierce RJ, Holmes PW. Intrathoracic manifestations of disseminated prostatic adenocarcinoma. *Respiratory Medicine*, 1989; **83**:161–6.
75. Jones LA. Superior vena cava syndrome: an oncologic complication. *Seminars in Oncology Nursing*, 1987; **3**:211–15.
76. Johnson IS, Rogers C, Biswas B, Ahmedzai S. What do hospices do? A survey of hospices in the UK and Republic of Ireland. *British Medical Journal*, 1990; **300**:791–3.
77. Tattersall MHN, Boyer MJ. Management of malignant pleural effusions. *Thorax*, 1990; **45**:81–2.
78. McAlpine LG, Hulks G, Thomson NC. Management of recurrent malignant pleural effusion in the United Kingdom: survey of clinical practice. *Thorax*, 1990; **45**:699–701.
79. Koldsland S, Svennevig JL, Gustav L, Johnson E. Chemical pleurodesis in malignant pleural effusions: a randomised prospective study of mepacrine versus bleomycin. *Thorax*, 1993; **48**:790–3.
80. Ponn RB, Blancaflor J, D'Agostino RS, Kiernan ME, Toole AL, Stern H. Pleuroperitoneal shunting for intractable pleural effusions. *Annals of Thoracic Surgery*, 1991; **51**:605–9.
81. Pierce RJ. Lasers, brachytherapy and stents—keeping the airways open. *Respiratory Medicine*, 1991; **85**:263–5.
82. Hetzel MR, Smith SGT. Endoscopic palliation of tracheobronchial malignancies. *Thorax*, 1991; **46**:325–33.
83. Ledingham SJM, Goldstraw P. Diathermy resection and radioactive gold grains for palliation of obstruction due to recurrence of bronchial carcinoma after external irradiation. *Thorax*, 1991; **44**:48–51.
84. Burt PA, O'Driscoll BR, Notley HM, Barber PV, Stout R. Intraluminal irradiation for the palliation of lung cancer with the high dose rate micro-Selectron. *Thorax*, 1990; **45**:765–8.
85. Macha HN, Koch K, Stadler M, Schumacher W, Krumhaar D. New technique for treating occlusive and stenosing tumours of the trachea and main bronchi: endobronchial irradiation by high dose iridium-192 combined with laser canalisation. *Thorax*, 1987; **42**:511–15.
86. Goldman JM, Bulman AS, Rathmell AJ, Carey BM, Muers MF, Joslin CAF. Physiological effect of endobronchial radiotherapy in patients with major airway occlusion by carcinoma. *Thorax*, 1993; **48**:110–14.
87. George PJM, Hadley JM, Mantell BS, Rudd RM. Medium dose rate endobronchial radiotherapy with caesium-137. *Thorax*, 1992; **47**:474–7.
88. Colles MJ. What is a laser and how is it applied for therapy? *British Journal of Hospital Medicine*, 1988; **40**:111–14.
89. George PJM, Garrett CPO, Nixon C, Hetzel MR, Nanson EM, Millard FJC. Laser treatment for tracheobronchial tumours: local or general anaesthesia? *Thorax*, 1987; **42**:656–60.
90. Tobias JS, Bown SG. Palliation of malignant obstruction—use of lasers and radiotherapy in combination. *European Journal of Cancer*, 1991; **27**:1352–5.
91. Lam S. Photodynamic therapy of lung cancer. *Thorax*, 1993; **48**:469.
92. Shankar S, George PJM, Hetzel MR, Goldstraw P. Elective resection of tumours of the trachea and main carcinoma after endoscopic laser therapy. *Thorax*, 1990; **45**:493–5.
93. Gilmartin JJ, Veale D, Cooper BG, Keavey PM, Gibson GJ, Morritt GN. Effects of laser treatment on respiratory function in malignant narrowing of the central airways. *Thorax*, 1987; **42**:578–82.
94. George PJM, Clarke G, Tolfree S, Garrett CPO, Hetzel MR. Changes in regional ventilation and perfusion of the lung after endoscopic laser treatment. *Thorax*, 1990; **45**:248.

95. Walsh DA, Maiwand MO, Nath AR, Lockwood P, Lloyd MH, Saab M. Bronchoscopic cryotherapy for advanced bronchial carcinoma. *Thorax*, 1990; **45**:509–13.
96. Walsh DA, Nath AR, Maiwand M. Authors' reply. *Thorax*, 1990; **45**:150.
97. Simonds AK, Irving JD, Clarke SW, Dick R. Use of expandable metal stents in the treatment of bronchial obstruction. *Thorax*, 1989; **44**:680–1.
98. Cooper JD, Pearson FG, Patterson GA, Todd GR, Ginsberg RJ. Use of silicone stents in the management of airway problems. *Annals of Thoracic Surgery*, 1989; **47**:371–8.
99. de Souza AC, Keal R, Hudson NM, Leverment JN, Spyt TJ. Use of expandable wire stents for malignant airway obstruction. *Annals of Thoracic Surgery*, 1994; **57**:1573–8.
100. de Conno F, Spoldi E, Caraceni A, Ventafridda V. Does pharmacological treatment affect the sensation of breathlessness in terminal cancer patients? *Palliative Medicine*, 1991; **5**:237–43.
101. Regnard C, Ahmedzai S. Dyspnoea in advanced cancer—a flow diagram. *Palliative Medicine*, 1990; **4**:311–15.
102. Regnard C, Ahmedzai S. Dyspnoea in advanced nonmalignant disease—a flow diagram. *Palliative Medicine*, 1990; **5**:56–63.
103. Ziment I. Pharmacologic therapy of COPD. In: Hodgkin JE, Petty TL, ed. *Chronic Obstructive Pulmonary Disease: Current Concepts*. Philadelphia, PA: WB Saunders, 1987:75.
104. British Thoracic Society. Guidelines for management of asthma in adults: I—chronic persistent asthma. *British Medical Journal*, 1990; **301**:651–3.
105. Newman SP, Clark AR, Talaee N, Clarke SW. Pressurised aerosol deposition in the human lung with and without an 'open' spacer device. *Thorax*, 1989; **44**:706–10.
106. Newman SP, Weisz AWB, Talaee N, Clarke SW. Improvement of drug delivery with a breath actuated pressurised aerosol for patients with poor inhaler technique. *Thorax*, 1991; **46**:712–16.
107. Sears MR, *et al.* Regular inhaled beta-agonist treatment in bronchial asthma. *Lancet*, 1990; **336**:1391–6.
108. Morris J. Respiratory disease: a rehabilitative approach. *Geriatric Medicine*, 1987; **17**:33–35.
109. Rees PJ. Theophyllines in the treatment of asthma. *British Journal of Clinical Pharmacology*, 1991; **45**:9–10.
110. Weir DC, Gove RI, Robertson AS, Sherwood Burge P. Corticosteroid trials in non-asthmatic chronic air flow obstruction:a comparison of oral prednisolone and inhaled beclomethasone diproprionate. *Thorax*, 1991; **45**:112–17.
111. Weir DC, Robertson AS, Gove RI, Sherwood Burge P. Time course of response to oral and inhaled corticosteroids in non-asthmatic chronic airflow obstruction. *Thorax*, 1990; **45**:118–21.
112. Al-Damluji S. The effect of ventilatory stimulation with medroxyprogesterone on exercise performance and the sensation of dyspnoea in hypercapnic chronic bronchitis. *British Journal of Diseases of the Chest*, 1986; **80**:273.
113. Daskalopoulou E, Patakas D, Tsara V, Zoglopitis F, Maniki E. Comparison of almitrine bismesylate and medroxyprogesterone acetate on oxygenation during wakefulness and sleep in patients with chronic obstructive lung disease. *Thorax*, 1990; **45**:666–9.
114. Tchekmedyian NS, Tait N, Aisner J. High-dose megestrol acetate in the treatment of postmenopausal women with advanced breast cancer. *Seminars in Oncology*, 1986; **13**:20–5.
115. Mikami M, *et al.* Respiration effect of synthetic progestin in small doses in normal men. *Chest*, 1989; **96**(5):1073–5.
116. Burki N. Ventilatory effects of doxapram in conscious human subjects. *Chest*, 1984; **85**:600–4.
117. Vachon L, Fitzgerald MX, Solliday NH, Gould IA, Gaensler EA. Single-dose effect of marihuana smoke. *New England Journal of Medicine*, 1973; **288**:985–9.
118. Ahmedzai S, Carter R, Mills RJ, Moran F. Effects of nabilone on pulmonary function. *Marihuana '84. Proceedings of the Oxford Symposium on Cannabis*. Oxford:IRL Press, 1984:371–8.
119. Jennett S. Respiratory effects of strong analgesics. In: Harcus AW, Smith RB, Whittle BA, ed. *Pain—New Perspectives in Measurement and Management*. Edinburgh: Churchill Livingstone, 1977:34–40.
120. Stark RD. Dyspnoea: assessment and pharmacological manipulation. *European Respiratory Journal*, 1988; **1**:280–7.
121. Woodcock A, Gross E, Geddes D. Drug treatment of breathlessness: contrasting effects of diazepam and promethazine in pink puffers. *British Medical Journal*, 1981; **283**: 343–6.
122. Wedzicha JA, Wallis PJW, Ingram DA, Empey DW. Effect of diazepam on sleep in patients with chronic airflow obstruction. *Thorax*, 1988; **43**:729–30.
123. Morin-Surun MP, *et al.* Pharmacological identification of delta and mu opiate receptors on bulbar respiratory neurons. *European Journal of Pharmacology*, 1984; **98**:214–47.
124. Rigg JRA. Ventilatory effects and plasma concentration of morphine in man. *British Journal of Anaesthesia*, 1978; **50**:759–65.
125. Walsh TD. Opiates and respiratory function in advanced cancer. *Recent Results in Cancer Research*, 1984; **89**:115–17.
126. Young IH, Daviskas E, Keena VA. Effect of low dose nebulised morphine on exercise endurance in patients with chronic lung disease. *Thorax*, 1989; **44**:387–90.
127. Chrubasik J, Wust H, Friedrich G, Geller E. Absorption and bioavailability of nebulised morphine. *British Journal of Anaesthesia*, 1988; **61**:228–30.
128. Hall GM. Metabolic and respiratory effects of regional anaesthesia. *Current Opinion in Anaesthesiology*, 1989; **2**:614–16.
129. McQuay HJ, Sullivan AF, Smallman K, Dickenson AH. Intrathecal opioids, potency and lipophilicity. *Pain*, 1989; **36**:111–15.
130. Jordan C, Lehane JR, Robson PJ, Jones GJ. A comparison of the respiratory effects of meptazinol, pentazocine and morphine. *British Journal of Anaesthesia*, 1979; **51**:497.
131. Johnson MA, Woodcock AA, Geddes DM. Dihydrocodeine for breathlessness in "pink puffers". *British Medical Journal*, 1983; **286**:675.
132. Light RW, Muro JR, Sato RI, Stansbury DW, Fischer CE, Brown SE. Effects of oral morphine on breathlessness and exercise tolerance in patients with chronic obstructive pulmonary disease. *American Review of Respiratory Diseases*, 1989; **139**:126–33.
133. Davis CL, Hodder CA, Love S, Shah R, Slevin ML, Wedzicha JA. Effect of nebulised morphine and morphine 6-glucuronide on exercise edurance in patients with chronic obstructive airways disease. *Thorax*, 1994; **49**(4):393.
134. Masood AR, Reed JW, Thomas SHL. Lack of effect of inhaled morphine on exercise-induced breathlessness in chronic obstructive pulmonary disease. *Thorax*, 1995; **50**:629–34.
135. Farcombe M, Chater S, Gillis A. The use of nebulised opioids for breathlessness: a chart review. *Palliative Medicine*, 1994; **8**:306–12.
136. Hughes S, Calverley P. Heroin inhalation and asthma. *British Medical Journal*, 1988; **297**:1511–12.
137. Worsley MH, MacLeod AD, Brodie MJ, Asbury AJ, Clark C. Inhaled fentanyl as a method of analgesia. *Anaesthesia*, 1990; **45**:449–51.
138. Ahmedzai S, Davis CL. Nebuliser use in palliative care. In: Muers M, ed. Current Best Practice for Nebuliser Treatment. Nebuliser Project Group of British Thoracic Society Standards of Care Committee. *Thorax*, in press.
139. Bellville JW, Swanson GD, Aqleh KA. Respiratory effects of delta-9-tetrahydrocannabinol. *Clinical Pharmacology and Therapeutics*, 1975; **17**:541–8.
140. Tashkin DP, Reiss S, Shapiro BJ, Calvarese B, Olsen JL, Lodge JW. Bronchial effects of aerosolized 9-tetrahydrocannabinol in healthy and asthmatic subjects. *American Review of Respiratory Disease*, 1977; **115**:57–65.
141. Ahmedzai S, Carlyle D, Moran F. Short-term cardiovascular effects of nabilone. *Marihuana '84. Proceedings of the Oxford Symposium on Cannabis*. Oxford: IRL Press, 1984:365–9.
142. McAlpine LG, Thomson NC. Lidocaine-induced bronchoconstriction in asthmatic patients. Relation to histamine airway responsiveness and effect of preservative. *Chest*, 1989; **96**:1012–15.
143. Wilcock A, Corcoran R, Tattersfield AE. Safety and efficacy of nebulized

lignocaine in patients with cancer and breathlessness. *Palliative Medicine*, 1994; 8:35–8.

144. Anonymous. The trust in pulse oximeters. *Lancet*, 1990; **335**:1130–1.
145. White EJ. Home care of the patient with advanced lung cancer. *Seminars in Oncology Nursing*, 1987; 3:216–21.
146. Petty TL. Respiratory therapy techniques. In: Hodgkin JE, Petty TL, ed. *Chronic Obstructive Pulmonary Disease: Current Concepts*. Philadelphia, PA: WB Saunders, 1987:91.
147. Davidson AC, Leach R, George RJD, Geddes DM. Supplemental oxygen and exercise ability in chronic obstructive airways disease. *Thorax*, 1988; **43**:965–71.
148. Lock SH, Paul EA, Rudd RM, Wedzicha JA. Portable oxygen therapy: assessment and usage. *Respiratory Medicine*, 1991; **85**:407–12.
149. Bruera E, de Stoutz N, Velasco-Leiva A, Schoeller T, Hanson J. Effects of oxygen on dyspnoea in hypoxaemic terminal-cancer patients. *Lancet*. 1993; **342**:13–14.
150. Booth S, Kelly MJ, Cox MP, Adams L, Guz A. Does oxygen help dyspnoea in patients with cancer. *American Review of Respiratory and Critical Care Medcine*, 1996; **153**: 1515–18.
151. Walsh DA, Govan JR. Long term continuous domiciliary oxygen therapy by transtracheal catheter. *Thorax*, 1990; **45**:478–81.
152. Young S, Bitsakou H, Caric D, McHardy GJR. Coughing can relieve or exacerbate symptoms in asthmatic patients. *Respiratory Medicine*, 1991; **85**:7–12.
153. Lowry R, Higenbottam T. The causes, diagnosis and treatment of cough. *Prescriber*, 1991; **Issue 30**:39–50.
154. Fuller RW. Symptoms that puzzle doctors: cough. *British Journal of Hospital Medicine*, 1991; **45**:100–1.
155. Fuller RW, Jackson DM. Physiology and treatment of cough. *Thorax*, 1990; **45**:425–30.
156. Adcock JJ. Peripheral opioid receptors and the cough reflex. *Respiratory Medicine*, 1991; **85**: 43 6.
157. Fuller RW. Pharmacology of inhaled capsaicin in humans. *Respiratory Medicine*, 1991; **85**:1–4.
158. Trochtenberg S. Nebulized lidocaine in the treatment of refractory cough. *Chest*, 1994; **105**:1592–3.
159. Sutton P, *et al.* Use of nebulised saline and nebulised terbutaline as an adjunct to chest physiotherapy. *Thorax*, 1988; **43**:57–60.
160. Jones KDA, Davies RJ. Massive haemoptysis. *British Medical Journal*, 1990; **300**:889–90.
161. Wedzicha JA , Pearson MC. Management of massive haemoptysis. *Respiratory Medicine*, 1990; **84**:9–12.
162. Mozell EJ, Sabanathan S, Mearns AJ, Bickford-Smith PJ, Majid MR, Zografos G. Continuous extrapleural intercostal nerve block after pleurectomy. *Thorax*, 1991; **46**:21–4.
163. Harriss DR, Graham TR. Management of intercostal drains. *British Journal of Hospital Medicine*, 1991; **45**:383–6.
164. Windebank WJ, Boyd G, Moran F. Pulmonary thromboembolism presenting as asthma. *British Medical Journal*, 1973; **1**:90–4.
165. Bateman NT, Croft DN. False-positive lung scans and radiotherapy. *British Medical Journal*, 1976; **1**:807–8.
166. Newman SP, Clark AR, Talaee N, Clarke SW. Pressurised aerosol deposition in the human lung with and without an 'open' spacer device. *Thorax*, 1989; **44**:706–10.
167. Mitchell DM, Solomon MA, Tolfree SEJ, Short M, Spiro SG. Effect of particle size of bronchodilator aerosols on lung distribution and pulmonary function in patients with chronic asthma. *Thorax*, 1987; **42**:457–61.
168. Newman S, Woodman G, Clarke S. Deposition of carbenicillin aerosols in cystic fibrosis: effects of nebuliser system and breathing pattern. *Thorax*, 1988; **43**:318–22.
169. Schoeffel R, Anderson S, Altounyan R. Bronchial hyperreactivity in response to inhalation of ultrasonically nebulised solutions of distilled water and saline. *British Medical Journal*, 1981; **283**:1285–8.
170. McCarthy N. Nebulised pentamidine and AIDS. *Respiratory Disease in Practice*, 1988; **5**:15–18.
171. Doshi MK, Bhakri HL, Bowman CE. Dangers of nebulisers in nursing and residential homes. *Lancet*, 1990; **336**:113.
172. Allen D, Ahmedzai S. Palliative care in advanced respiratory disease. *Association of Chartered Physiotherapists in Respiratory Care (Newsletter)*, 1991; **19**:25–9.
173. Cherniack RM. Physical therapy techniques. In: Hodgkin JE, Petty TL, ed. *Chronic Obstructive Pulmonary Disease: Current Concepts*. Philadelphia, PA: WB Saunders, 1987: 113.
174. Sutton PS. Chest physiotherapy: time for reappraisal. *British Journal of Diseases of the Chest*, 1988; **82**:127–37.
175. Selsby DS. Chest physiotherapy. *British Medical Journal*, 1989; **298**:541–2.
176. Webber BA, Hofmeyr JL, Morgan L, Hodson ME. Effects of postural drainage. Incorporating the forced expiration technique on pulmonary function in cystic fibrosis. *British Journal of Diseases of the Chest*, 1986; **80**:353–9.
177. Young CS. A review of the adverse effects of airway suction. *Physiotherapy*, 1984; **70**:104–6.
178. Branthwaite MA. Non-invasive and domiciliary ventilation: positive pressure techniques. *Thorax*, 1991; **46**:208–12.
179. Miller RF. Continuous positive airways pressure ventilation as an alternative to mechanical ventilation for respiratory failure associated with *Pneumocystis carinii* pneumonia. *Thorax*, 1990; **45**:304.
180. Branthwaite MA. Mechanical ventilation at home. *British Medical Journal*, 1989; **298**:1409.
181. Mier A, Brophy C, Moxham J, Green M. Phrenic nerve stimulation in normal subjects and in patients with diaphragmatic weakness. *Thorax*, 1987; **42**:885–8.
182. Laroche CM, Mier AK, Moxham J, Green M. Diaphragm strength in patients with recent hemidiaphragm paralysis. *Thorax*, 1988; **43**:170–4.
183. Thompson CL, Richmond M. Teaching home care for ventilator-dependent patients: the patients' perception. *Heart and Lung*, 1990; **19**:79–83.
184. Hodgkin JE. Pulmonary rehabilitation. In: Hodgkin JE, Petty TL, ed. *Chronic Obstructive Pulmonary Disease: Current Concepts*. Philadelphia, PA: WB Saunders, 1987: 154–71.
185. Kanner RE. Impairment and disability evaluation and vocational rehabilitation. In: Hodgkin JE, Petty TL, ed. *Chronic Obstructive Pulmonary Disease: Current Concepts*. Philadelphia, PA: WB Saunders, 1987:172.
186. O'Neill PA, Dodds M, Phillips B, Poole J, Webb AK. Regular exercise and reduction of breathlessness in patients with cystic fibrosis. *British Journal of Diseases of the Chest*, 1987; **81**:62.
187. Fine R, Krell W, Ranella K, Sessions D, Williams M. Respiratory problems and rehabilitation in the head and neck cancer patient. *Head and Neck*, 1991; **13**(1):12–13.
188. Singh V, Wisniewski A, Britton J, Tattersfield A. Effect of yoga breathing exercises (pranayama) on airway reactivity in subjects with asthma. *Lancet*, 1990; **335**:1381–3.
189. Cockcroft A, *et al.* Controlled trial of respiratory health worker visiting patients with chronic respiratory disability. *British Medical Journal*, 1987; **294**:225–8.
190. Morgan AD, Peck DF, Buchanan DR, McHardy GJR. Effect of attitudes and beliefs on exercise tolerance in chronic bronchitis. *British Medical Journal*, 1983; **286**:171.
191. King B, Cotes JE. Relation of lung function and exercise capacity to mood and attitudes to health. *Thorax*, 1989; **44**:102–9.
192. Holland J, Massie M. Psychosocial aspects of cancer in the elderly. *Clinics in Geriatric Medicine*, 1987; **3**:533–9.
193. Specht RL. Lung cancer: psychosocial implications. *Seminars in Oncology Nursing*, 1987; **3**:222–7.
194. Partridge M. Lung cancer and communication. *Respiratory Medicine*, 1989; **83**:379–80.
195. Ahmedzai S. Measuring quality of life in hospice care. *Oncology*, 1990; **4**:115–19.
196. Aaronson N, *et al.* The EORTC core quality of life questionnaire: interim results of an international field study. In: Osoba D, ed. *Effect of Cancer on Quality of Life*. Boca Raton, FL: CRC Press, 1991:186–202.

197. Jones PW. Quality of life measurement for patients with diseases of the airways. *Thorax*, 1991; **46**:676–82.
198. Jones PW, Quirk FH, Baveystock CM. The St George's Respiratory Questionnaire. *Respiratory Medicine*, 1991; **85**:25–31.
199. Glaser EM, Dudley DL. Psychosocial rehabilitation and psycho-pharmacology. In: Hodgkin JE, Petty TL, ed. *Chronic Obstructive Pulmonary Disease: Current Concepts*. Philadelphia, PA: WB Saunders, 1987:128.
200. Sexton DL. Relaxation techniques and biofeedback. In: Hodgkin JE, Petty TL, ed. *Chronic Obstructive Pulmonary Disease: Current Concepts*. Philadelphia, PA: WB Saunders, 1987:99.
201. Corner J, Plant H, Warner L. Developing a nursing approach to managing dyspnoea in lung cancer. *International Journal of Palliative Nursing*, 1995; **1**: 5–11.
202. Filshie J, Penn K, Ashley S., Davis C. Acupuncture for the relief of cancer-related breathlessness. *Palliative Medicine*, 1996; **10**: 145–50.
203. Allen SM, Hunt B, Green M. Fall in vital capacity with posture. *British Journal of Diseases of the Chest*, 1985; **79**:267–71.
204. Alexander MSM, Arnot RN, Lavender JP. Left lower lobe ventilation and its relation to cardiomegaly and posture. *British Medical Journal*, 1989; **299**:94.

9.6 Management of skin problems

9.6.1 Medical aspects

P. S. Mortimer

Introduction

The skin is the largest and most exposed organ, and so it is not surprising that it rarely escapes problems in any chronically sick patient. Fortunately, these problems are generally minor; nevertheless they can be debilitating and uncomfortable, and are frequently distressing because of their visibility. The general condition and, in particular, the nutritional status of the patient will be reflected in their skin. Minor and usually reversible skin disorders may become a major problem in the chronically sick patient where healing powers are limited.

No branch of medicine is more dependent on clinical acumen and less dependent on the laboratory than dermatology. The skin can provide a window on general health, and any professional carer should be aware of the importance of recognizing signs of internal disease such as purpura due to thrombocytopenia or scurvy, excoriation due to itching from renal or liver disease, or pigmentation due to Addison's disease.

It must be remembered that the skin serves several important functions and it is when these fail that problems arise.

1. The skin is a barrier between the body and its environment 'to keep in what should be in', particularly water, electrolytes, and other body constituents, 'and to keep out what is out', namely noxious materials and biological hazards, including infection. The skin also has to be physically tough and resistant and so prevent the effects of mechanical injury, such as pressure, stretching, or scratching. The success of this barrier depends on the integrity of the epidermis through the close cohesion of the stratum corneum cells sealed by surface lipids. The ability to rebuff irritants, chemicals, and micro-organisms can be compared with the smooth resilient surface of a varnished table top, a polished floor, or a newly laid road. The dermis provides support to the epidermis, both nutritionally and physically, so that a decline in the quality of the blood supply as well as of the collagen and elastic fibres will limit the ability of the skin to resist injury from pressure and stretch, or to repair itself if critical damage occurs.

2. A second major function is the control of body temperature. The skin's blood supply far exceeds its metabolic needs because of its thermoregulatory role. Extensive cutaneous disease can result in the shunting of most of the cardiac output through the skin to the detriment of critical organs such as the kidney; at the same time it can place excessive demands on the heart, leading to high output failure. These events are more likely to occur in an elderly or chronically sick patient.

3. A third function is as a sense organ. Cutaneous sensation helps orientation in relation to the environment. This is particularly important in the cancer patient where nerve damage from cancer (e.g. paraplegia) or its therapy (e.g. drug-induced neuropathy) may expose the skin to unforeseen damage and so lead to a chronic wound. The use of sedating opioid drugs for pain relief only serves to compound this situation. For reasons that are not completely understood, anaesthetized skin is prone to ulceration. This can be observed following herpes zoster infection and is akin to circumstances arising in leprosy and diabetes.

4. The skin normally has excellent powers of regeneration in the form of wound and tissue repair. These are obviously necessary because of its 'exposed' position as part of the integument. This process of repair is efficient and quick compared with that in other tissues, and is due mainly to the blood supply. Ill health, particularly wasting states such as cancer cachexia, undermines this function.

5. The skin is responsible for vitamin D production. It is not known what happens to this function in the cancer patient who spends prolonged periods indoors, but it is possible that calcium homeostasis will become compromised.

All these functions are crucial for internal homeostasis, particularly adequate hydration and electrolyte balance. A weakened skin barrier, which is inevitable in a debilitated patient, predisposes to dehydration, dermatitis, infection, and ulceration.

In the same way that skin diseases become much more prevalent in poor communities of the world through water shortage, malnutrition, and poor hygiene, so they do in patients debilitated by neoplasia and chronic infections. Dryness and a mild ichthyosis lead to a stratum corneum that is non-supple and cracks easily (asteotosis). Dermatitis, which can be itchy and sore, then supervenes. The skin changes associated with chronic illness, particularly cancer, are similar to those seen with malnutrition. Anaemia, oedema, and sore tongue often feature. Pressure points are particularly vulnerable initially to dermatitis and then to ulceration, which is slow to recover. Therefore management of skin disorders in advanced cancer should first and foremost address aspects of general welfare such as hydration, nutrition, and hygiene. The likelihood of serious skin problems will then be greatly reduced.

Primary tumours

Primary skin cancer is rarely a problem in the patient with advanced cancer except perhaps as a visible reminder of the source of the spread. Melanoma may metastasize locally, producing unsightly nodules which may ulcerate or fungate. Skin nodules from melanoma do not kill the patient but may cause considerable morbidity. Simple excision of nodules as they appear may prevent problems later. If this is not possible, radiotherapy or laser treatment[1] may prove helpful.

Basal cell carcinoma

Basal cell carcinoma is common and may coexist by chance or as a secondary tumour within an irradiated field. It is usually possible to leave well alone unless symptomatic. If treatment should be necessary because of problems of bleeding, recurrent crusting, or even smell, excision under local anaesthetic or radiotherapy should be considered.

Cutaneous squamous cell carcinoma

Cutaneous squamous cell carcinoma may be the source of metastatic spread, particularly in the immunocompromised patient such as the renal transplant recipient. Usually the primary tumour has been satisfactorily treated, but occasionally recurrent local tumour may develop ulceration, bleeding, or infection. Radiotherapy will usually control symptoms.

Kaposi's sarcoma, cutaneous T-cell lymphoma, and angiosarcoma

Kaposi's sarcoma, cutaneous T-cell lymphoma, and angiosarcoma are all tumours arising in the skin and capable of producing extensive skin involvement. Although these tumours are incurable, the patient may remain well for a considerable period of time. In the case of T-cell lymphoma this can be in excess of 20 years.

Kaposi's sarcoma

Kaposi's sarcoma is a multifocal neoplastic process in which each tumour arises *de novo* and is not considered a metastasis. In the classic form lesions begin slowly and insidiously around the ankle and slowly spread up the leg. It is rarely responsible for the death of the patient. The endemic form, which arises mainly in Africa, can frequently affect children. Crops of vascular lesions associated with gross oedema develop in the skin. The prognosis is poor if there is extracutaneous involvement. Kaposi's sarcoma associated with non-HIV-induced immunosuppression such as renal transplantation or when associated with AIDS may produce widespread and unsightly lesions. Interestingly, Kaposi's sarcoma regresses if it is possible to remove the immunosuppression. Lesions are flat at first, but can become tumid and possibly painful over pressure points. Bleeding may be a problem and rarely lesions may ulcerate or fungate. Superficial radiotherapy is a rapid and effective treatment, although excision can be used for small areas. Extensive disease can be treated by cytotoxic drugs such as chlorambucil;[2] AIDS-related cases may respond temporarily to interleukin 2 or interferon.[3]

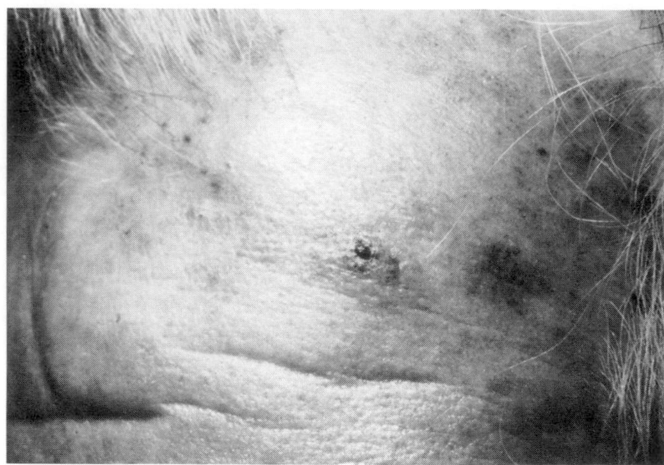

Fig. 1 Angiosarcoma: the bruised appearance with ill-defined borders is typical of this tumour.

Cutaneous T-cell lymphoma (mycosis fungoides)

Cutaneous T-cell lymphoma (mycosis fungoides) characteristically persists for years in the skin alone and systemic involvement occurs only in the terminal phase. Problems arise from tumour ulceration with secondary infection and bleeding. Death may occur from septicaemia, particularly as host immunity becomes compromised. In Europe there is a general trend towards a palliative approach to treatment from an early stage in the disease. A large proportion of patients with mycosis fungoides are frail, elderly, and likely to succumb to either general medical problems or overenthusiastic therapy. Photochemotherapy (PUVA) may keep the disease in check, but radiotherapy, either electron beam or conventional X-rays, is most effective in eradicating tumours. Chemotherapy is generally disappointing. A recent study reported no difference in survival or disease-free interval in patients receiving electron beam radiotherapy plus chemotherapy compared with topical therapy progressing to PUVA if required.[4] Pruritus may be troublesome, but some symptomatic relief may be provided by topical steroids and antihistamines.

Angiosarcoma

Angiosarcoma (Fig. 1) is rare and occurs most commonly around the scalp and face in the elderly as a slowly spreading bruise. Death occurs when the tumour invades a vital structure. Eradication of the tumour is extremely difficult and therefore prognosis is poor. Fortunately, symptoms are few until the terminal phase. Both radiotherapy and chemotherapy are disappointing.

Skin metastases and fungating wounds

Skin infiltration with the subsequent development of ulceration or a fungating wound can be a distressing problem for the cancer patient. At one extreme is the patient who is upset by the appearance of a metastatic nodule of melanoma as this is a visual reminder of disease progression, and at the other is the patient with extensive fungating carcinoma of the breast and consequent malodour, discharge, and bleeding. These symptoms add to the misery of advanced and uncontrolled malignant disease, so deepening the patients' sense of helplessness, embarrassment, and social isolation.

Metastatic malignant tumours

Most malignant tumours can produce cutaneous metastases. Hypernephroma is one of the less common malignancies but accounts for 9 per cent of skin metastases.[5] The skin is involved by metastases in 3 to 4 per cent of malignant tumours and occurrence suggests a poor outcome.

Direct invasion of the skin usually presents with ulceration or inflammation. The most frequent cause is carcinoma of the breast, which may manifest in a number of ways. Paget's disease of the nipple represents the most reliable sign of underlying malignancy, namely carcinoma of the breast. It is due to direct extension of cancer cells into the epidermis of the nipple and areola. In extramammary Paget's disease the relationship with malignancy is less clear. Nevertheless, a careful search for a primary adenocarcinoma of rectum, uterus, or appendageal glands should be undertaken.

Inflammatory carcinoma of the breast may suggest infection, 'carcinoma erysipeloides', with spreading sheets of erythema and oedema (Fig. 2). A failure to respond to antibiotics and a lack of constitutional upset should arouse suspicion, and a biopsy will invariably reveal carcinoma cells within the dermis or lymphatics associated with inflammation. This type of cancer is difficult to eradicate and exhibits a slowly progressive natural history during which time the patient remains remarkably well. The process tends to spread by contiguity until the whole of the upper trunk becomes enveloped. Induration ensues and the skin of the chest wall and subcutaneous tissues become hard (cancer *en cuirasse)*. Dermal lymph stasis results in elephantiasic skin changes with hyperkeratosis and papillomatosis. Occasionally, a scirrhous dermal reaction similar to localized scleroderma (morphoea) may occur or the skin may become crusted and itching due to a dermatitis.

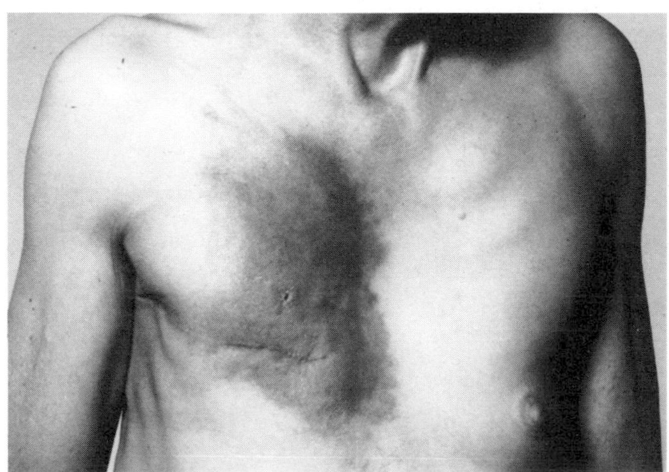

Fig. 2 Carcinoma erysipeloides: the fixed erythema resembling cellulitis/erysipelas is due to dermal infiltration with breast cancer.

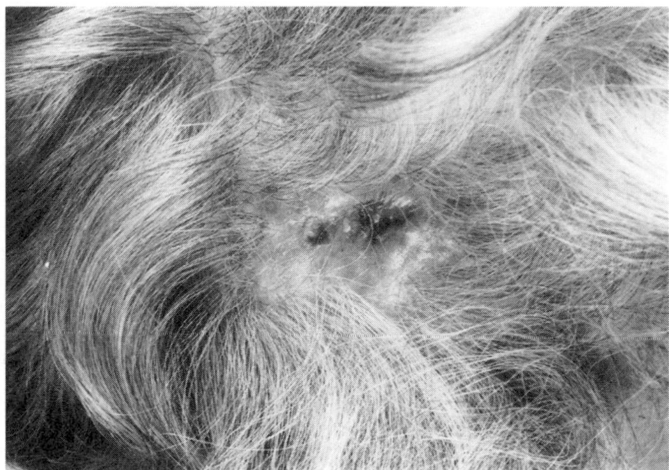

Fig. 3 Alopecia neoplastica: tumour infiltration of the scalp, in this case with breast cancer, gives rise to a scarring alopecia.

Unlike other forms of eczematous dermatitis, symptom control is difficult except with very potent topical steroids. A recent study has demonstrated some relief from a cream containing the vitamin D analogue calcipotriol.[6]

Specific cutaneous infiltrations of the skin may occur with myeloproliferative disorders. This is commonly observed with lymphoma but also with leukaemia, particularly the prolymphocytic type.

The scalp is a site where metastases may present (e.g. hypernephroma) and they may go unnoticed until hair loss is observed. Alopecia neoplastica (Fig. 3) produces scarring which is permanent even with tumour regression. Extensive scalp involvement may be very distressing because of this unsightly scarring. Advice from an appliance officer skilled in the provision of wigs or hairpieces may restore some self-esteem in the patient.

Although skin deposits almost always indicate wide dissemination of cancer, removal of lesions is recommended whenever possible. Excision of solitary metastases combined with treatment of the primary tumour may give worthwhile remissions. Equally, removal of cutaneous metastases when they are small may prevent later problems.

Malignant wounds

There is surprisingly little information on malignant wounds in the medical literature. Breast cancer is the most common neoplasm to fungate (a term which conveys a situation of combined ulceration and proliferation), but this process can also occur with cancers of the lung, stomach, head and neck, uterus, kidney, ovary, colon, and bladder, as well as with melanoma and lymphoma.[7] Local extension of malignancy or embolization by vascular or lymphatic spread results in a tumour mass which compromises tissue viability. This is achieved by compressing or invading local blood or lymphatic vessels, thus interfering with blood flow and the supply of oxygen and nutrients in the circulating extracellular fluids. In addition, tumour angiogenesis will lead to an inefficient and vulnerable microcirculation within the tumour as it replaces normal surrounding tissues. Capillary rupture and infarction of the tumour leads to necrosis. Anaerobic organisms flourish in the inaccessible necrotic

Table 1 Non-metastatic cutaneous manifestations of malignancy

Non-specific cutaneous markers	Paraneoplastic dermatoses	Genetic syndromes with a predisposition to cancer
Pallor	Acanthosis nigricans	Gardner's syndrome
Pigmentation	Erythema gyratum repens	Peutz–Jegher syndrome
Pruritus	Dermatomyositis	Neurofibromatosis
Acquired ichthyosis	Acquired hypertrichosis lanuginosa	Tuberous sclerosis
Exfoliative dermatitis	Migratory thrombophlebitis	Torre–Muir syndrome
Erythroderma	Pyoderma gangrenosum	Multiple endocrine neoplasia type III (MEN 3)
Erythema annulare centrifugum	Acute febrile neutrophilic dermatosis	Basal cell naevus syndrome (Gorlin's syndrome)
Erythema multiforme	Subcorneal pustular dermatosis	Palmoplantar keratoderma (Howel–Evans syndrome)
Erythema nodosum	Cutaneous amyloid	
Urticaria	Endocrine malignancies	
	Carcinoid flushing	
Panniculitis	Glucagonoma (necrolytic migratory erythema)	
Vasculitis		
Pemphigus	Unilateral lymphoedema	
Bullous pemphigoid	Leser–Trelat sign	
Dermatitis herpetiformis	Bowen's disease of covered skin	
Acquired epidermolysis bullosa	Arsenic keratoses/arsenic pigmentation	
Porphyria cutanea tarda	Pachydermoperiostosis	
Skin tags (?)	Follicular mucinosis	
	Multicentric reticulohistiocytosis	
	Paraneoplastic acrokeratosis (Bazex's syndrome)	

Reproduced with permission from ref. 9.

tissues, and the malodorous volatile fatty acids which are released as a metabolic end product are responsible for the characteristic offensive smell.

Ulcerated skin lesions can readily become colonized by aerobic pathogens, and therefore microbiological culture of skin swabs is advisable, particularly if a purulent discharge appears or pain supervenes. *Staphylococcus aureus* is a common cause of secondary infection which can be overcome with topical antibiotics (e.g. mupirocin cream). Gram-negative organisms may colonize wounds in anogenital sites and demand appropriate antibiotic treatment. Silver sulphadiazine may prove useful in the local control of infection, particularly with Pseudomonas spp. The use of potassium permanganate baths or wet dressings may be helpful in preventing reinfection.

Ulcerating malignant wounds usually indicate advanced disease and suggest an incurable condition, but this may be far from the case. For example, cutaneous T-cell lymphoma may present with ulcerating tumours, although prognosis is often excellent following therapy. Similarly, certain primary tumours such as melanoma and cancer of the breast are amenable to curative procedures. Therefore in those patients who present with fungating tumours, histopathological assessment is essential for correct planning of treatment. Even with very advanced disease conventional treatment (surgical resection and reconstruction, radiotherapy, chemotherapy, or biological therapy) may reduce symptoms by decreasing tumour bulk and can sometimes lead to healing. Local palliation is all that can be offered for tumours that are resistant to all therapeutic measures. Radiotherapy, if permitted, will reduce bleeding and discharge. The nursing management of fungating wounds[8] is discussed in Chapter 9.6.3.

Non-metastatic cutaneous manifestations of malignancy

There are many well-known examples of skin changes that are associated with internal malignancy but are not due to direct infiltration (Table 1); only a few are reliable markers of underlying disease. Their importance depends on their specificity in guiding the physician along the correct path of investigation. With paraneoplastic syndromes removal of the offending tumour usually results in clearance of skin manifestations, whereas recurrence of cutaneous signs indicates relapse of tumour. Often, however, the cancer is metastatic by the time that skin signs appear. Equally, cutaneous problems are likely to persist as the cancer progresses.

Cutaneous manifestations may present in three ways:

(1) a genetically determined syndrome with a cutaneous component in which there is also an inherent predisposition to neoplasia (e.g. the Peutz–Jegher syndrome, neurofibromatosis);

(2) a cutaneous marker of exposure to a carcinogen capable of inducing internal malignancy (e.g. nicotine staining of fingers, arsenical pigmentation and keratoses, radiation damage to the skin over the thyroid);

(3) a group of cutaneous syndromes which appear to represent a

response from the neoplasm itself—the paraneoplastic dermatoses.

Genetic syndromes

Progress in molecular biology has helped to identify family cancer syndromes. The familial atypical mole-malignant melanoma syndrome (FAMM syndrome or BK mole syndrome) has been described in which affected family members have large numbers of atypical moles (more than 2 cm in diameter), each with irregular markings (Fig. 4).[10,11] Those patients with dysplastic naevi and one first-degree relative who has had melanoma have a very high risk for development of melanoma. Therefore it is important to identify patients with advanced melanoma who have the FAMM syndrome so that family members can be screened and counselled. Controversy remains over whether or not patients with familial dysplastic naevi and melanoma are at risk of other malignancies.

The basal cell naevus syndrome is an autosomal dominant condition in which multiple basal cell carcinomas develop, often from a young age, in association with mandibular keratocysts, skeletal abnormalities, and abnormal calcification.[12] The most commonly reported internal malignancy is medulloblastoma, but astrocytoma and ameloblastoma have also been described.

Genetic syndromes with skin signs indicative of a predisposition to internal malignancy include Gardner's syndrome (epidermal cysts, fibromas, lipomas, and neurofibromas in association with malignant intestinal polyps) in which all untreated cases will eventually develop colonic cancer, neurofibromatosis (*café-au-lait* patches, axillary freckling, neurofibromas) in association with tumours of the central nervous system, palmoplantar keratoderma (tylosis) in association with oesophageal cancer,[13] and multiple hamartoma and neoplasia syndrome (Cowden's disease) in which there is a high risk of breast and thyroid cancer. The recognition of a genetic syndrome is important even in a dying patient because it may identify other family members at risk so that precautionary measures can be taken.

Exposure to carcinogens

Heavy nicotine staining is a simple but good example of one of the most common skin signs of exposure to a carcinogen. Others include X-ray damage to the skin, particularly if it occurred many years previously, because it suggests an increased risk of neoplasia in both the skin and underlying tissues such as the thyroid and bone marrow. Arsenic-induced keratoses on the sides and palmar aspects of the fingers (Fig. 5), associated with truncal Bowen's disease and superficial basal cell carcinomas, convey an increased risk of internal neoplasia, particularly bronchial. Vinyl-chloride-induced scleroderma-like skin changes are associated with angiosarcoma of the liver.[14]

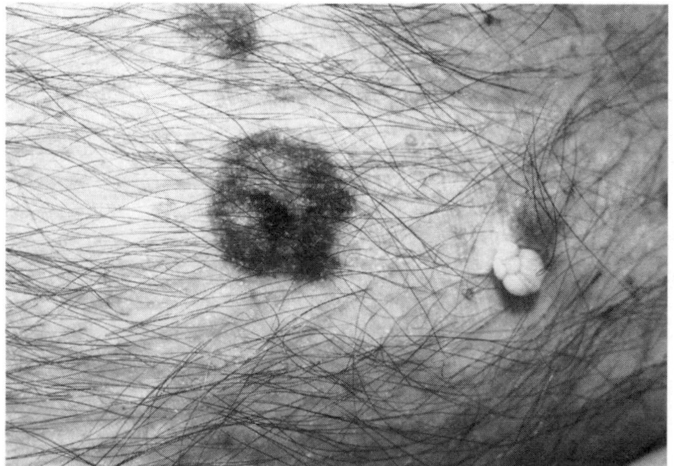

Fig. 4 Dysplastic naevus: a large atypical-looking naevus which characteristically occurs on the trunk and is usually multiple.

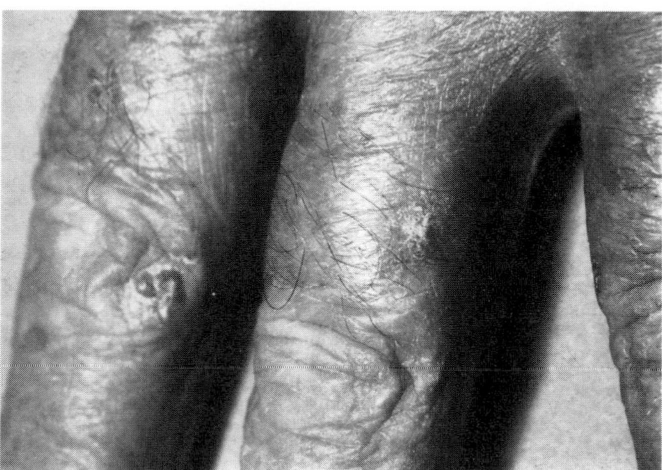

Fig. 5 Arsenical keratoses characteristically occur on the sides of the digits.

Paraneoplastic syndromes

Acanthosis nigricans

When acanthosis nigricans develops in adult life in the absence of obesity or endocrinopathy, there is invariably an associated internal neoplasm. Epidermal papillomatous thickening with hyperkeratosis leads to a velvety pigmented rash with a predilection for flexures of the neck, axillae, and groin. It may later become more extensive, involving periareola and periumbilical areas.[15] Other presentations include acanthosis palmaris ('tripe palms') and multiple cutaneous wart-like lesions. Irritation is common in the malignant form and may be severe. The mucous membranes and mucocutaneous junctions (Fig. 6) are involved in at least 50 per cent of cases. The hair may be shed. The vast majority of cases are associated with intra-abdominal adenocarcinoma, and in over 50 per cent the underlying tumour is a gastric carcinoma.[16] The prognosis is usually very poor, with a fatal outcome shortly after the rash appears; occasionally, however, acanthosis nigricans accompanies a slow-growing tumour and it may then precede detection of the associated tumour by a considerable period (even years).

Benign forms of acanthosis nigricans as seen in obesity and endocrine diseases are associated with insulin resistance. The hyperinsulinaemia appears to activate insulin-like growth factor receptors non-specifically through phosphorylation of tyrosine residues. Epidermal growth factor receptor activity occurs in a similar way. It is likely that tumour-derived factors such as epidermal growth factor provoke the skin changes via stimulation of insulin-like growth factor receptor pathways.

Erythema gyratum repens

This particular type of annular erythema has a frequent but not invariable association with malignancy, most commonly carcinoma of the breast or lung. The striking and characteristic appearance results from migrating whorls of annular erythema, giving a pattern resembling woodgrain. Resolution of the rash follows successful treatment of the neoplasm.

Glucagonoma syndrome

The glucagonoma syndrome (necrolytic migratory erythema) has a high specificity for islet cell carcinoma of the pancreas. Its distinctive appearance is due to the migrating epidermal necrosis which peels off. Diabetes results from the glucagon effect.[17] It tends to have a prolonged fluctuating course with migratory annular erythematous lesions which coalesce into a geographic serpiginous pattern. Removal of the tumour or treatment of hepatic metastases results in immediate resolution. Streptozocin[18] and dacarbazine[19] have proved helpful in cases with hepatic metastases.

Dermatomyositis

Dermatomyositis presents the most important challenge as the neoplasm may be curable.[20] When classical, the rash is very characteristic with erythema (often deep red or heliotrope in colour) and swelling of periorbital skin, cheeks, and forehead, together with linear violaceous plaques on the dorsal aspects of the fingers and hands. It is a photosensitive eruption, but may appear at any time of year and remains confined to sites exposed to light (Fig. 7). Periungual erythema, nail-fold telangiectasia, and ragged cuticles are also typical (Fig. 8). Proximal muscles are affected, but the degree of myositis is very variable and may be absent. An incidence of underlying neoplasia in 66 per cent of males over 40 was reported in one series.[21] In Chinese patients 75 per cent of associated cancers were nasopharyngeal,[22] but in Caucasians a much wider variety of cancers have been described, most commonly those of lung, breast, female genital tract, stomach, rectum, kidney, or testis. The condition may also be associated with lymphomas, lymphosarcoma, and myeloproliferative disorders. A possible relationship with tamoxifen therapy for carcinoma of the breast has been reported.[23] Serum from affected patients can be shown to contain complement-fixing antibodies to their own tumour. It may be that tumour antigens share common antigenic determinants with skin and muscle. The immune response triggered by a 'foreign' tumour will then inadvertently be directed against these tissues. However, dermatomyositis might result from the damaging action of cellular autoantibodies synthesized by forbidden mutant clones of immunologically competent cells such as lymphocytes.

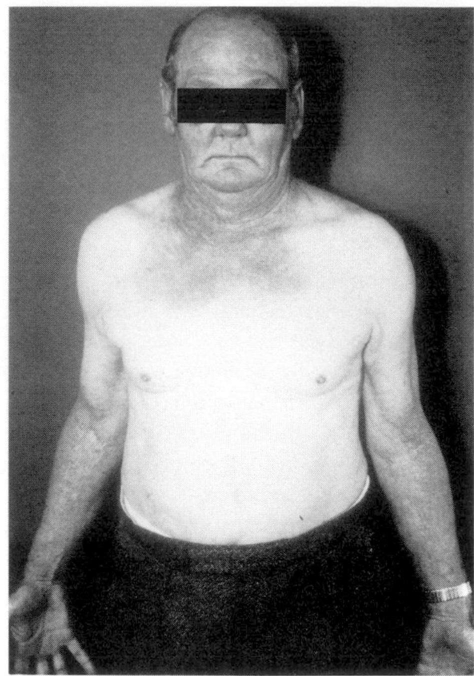

Fig. 7 The photosensitivity rash of dermatomyositis in a patient with carcinoma of the stomach.

The first line of treatment is removal of the cause, if possible. The course is variable. Two-thirds of deaths are due to carcinoma.[21] Adverse factors include pulmonary infiltrations, dysphagia, and increasing age. Rest is essential in the acute phase. Treatment with corticosteroids is required in almost all cases, with initial prednisolone doses as high as 60 to 120 mg. Dose reduction should be according to clinical response and serum muscle enzyme (creatine phosphokinase) levels. A maintenance dose of between 5 and 15 mg may be required for many months. Immunosuppression with antimetabolites such as azathioprine may be inadvisable in the presence of tumour.

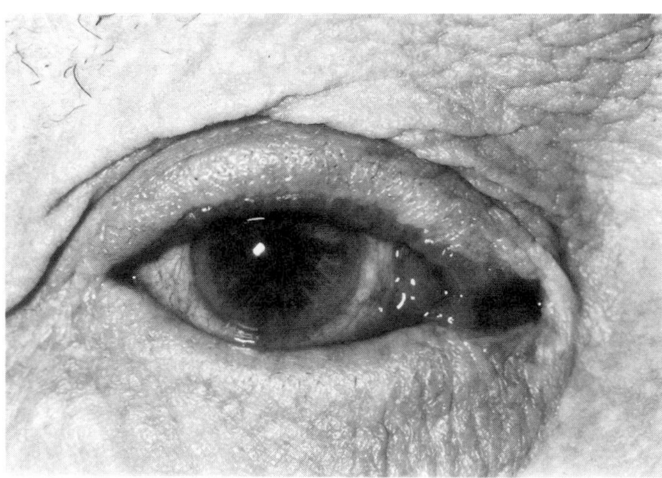

Fig. 6 Acanthosis nigricans of the conjunctiva is a rare but pathognomonic sign of underlying malignancy.

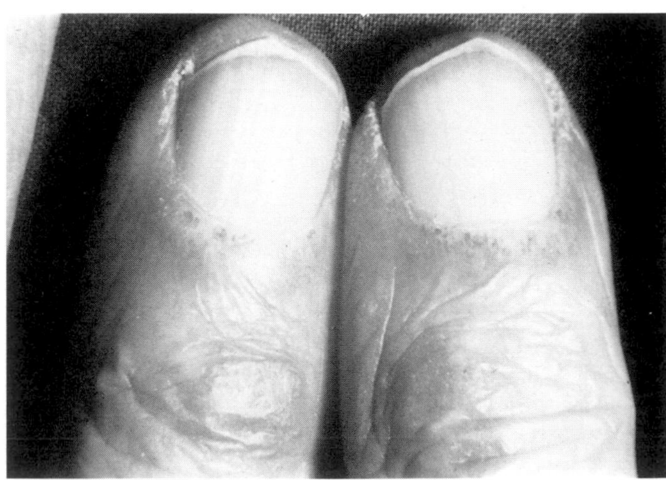

Fig. 8 Nail-fold telangiectasiae and ragged nail folds of dermatomyositis

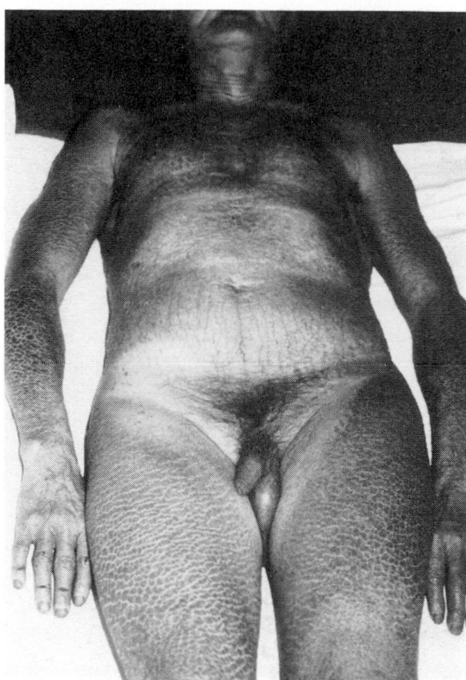

Fig. 9 Acquired ichthyosis associated with lymphoma.

Acquired ichthyosis

Acquired ichthyosis (Fig. 9) appears to be associated with internal malignancy, particularly lymphoproliferative disorder, but has also been described with solid tumours. The extremely dry flaky skin resembling fish scales (ichthos=fish) should not be confused with asteostosis which is a common problem, particularly on the lower legs. Ichthyosis due to underlying lymphoma may be indistinguishable from the ichthyosis associated with malnutrition, hypothyroidism, and drug reactions, or even that due to cancer cachexia.

Acquired hypertrichosis lanuginosa

Acquired hypertrichosis lanuginosa ('malignant down') presents with excessive growth of fine silky lanugo-like hair, first over the face but later over the entire body, and has a close association with malignancy, particularly carcinoma of the bronchus.

Pyoderma gangrenosum

Pyoderma gangrenosum (Fig. 10) is best known in association with inflammatory bowel disease and rheumatoid arthritis, but has been increasingly described with myeloproliferative disorders. It is often mistaken in the early stages for an abscess or septic lesion, but the manner in which a rim of blue-black inflammation spreads centrifugally, leaving central necrosis, is typical. Pain is often a feature. Lesions are usually solitary, but may be multiple, and are very sensitive to high-dose steroids.

Subcorneal pustular dermatosis

Subcorneal pustular dermatosis (Fig. 11) is frequently associated with IgA or IgG gammopathy. Multiple sterile pustules, with the larger ones containing a fluid level, occur particularly around the axillae and flanks. Waves of pustules are characteristic, as is the initial response to dapsone.

Other paraneoplastic dermatoses

Other paraneoplastic dermatoses exist but none are quite as specific and reliably identified as those discussed above. Reference to

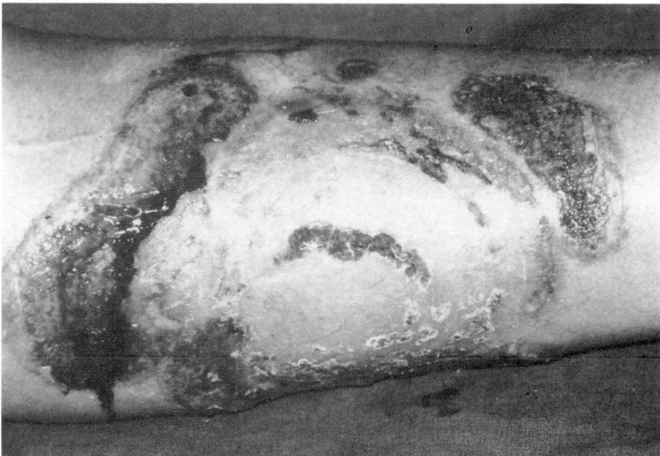

Fig. 10 Pyoderma gangrenosum is an inflammatory ulcer which usually develops on the lower limb and is associated with myeloproliferative disorders. The blue-black necrotic spreading edge is typical.

migratory thrombophlebitis (visceral carcinoma, usually pancreas or lung), cutaneous amyloid (myeloma), carcinoid syndrome, and follicular mucinosis (T-cell lymphoma) can be found elsewhere.[9]

Skin conditions

Pallor, pigmentation, pruritus, and purpura are common in advanced malignant disease. Immunoparesis and general debilitation predispose cancer patients to infections, particularly candidiasis, herpes simplex, and herpes zoster. Atypical manifestations of common infections, for example severe and protracted herpes simplex, may deceive.

Dry skin and ichthyosis

Xerosis or dry skin is a frequent accompaniment of advanced cancer. Chemotherapy tends to induce dryness, often permanently making a distinction from ichthyosis difficult in severe cases. Nutritional deficiencies, occurring because of underlying malignancy, give rise to a dry fine scaling resembling mild ichthyosis.

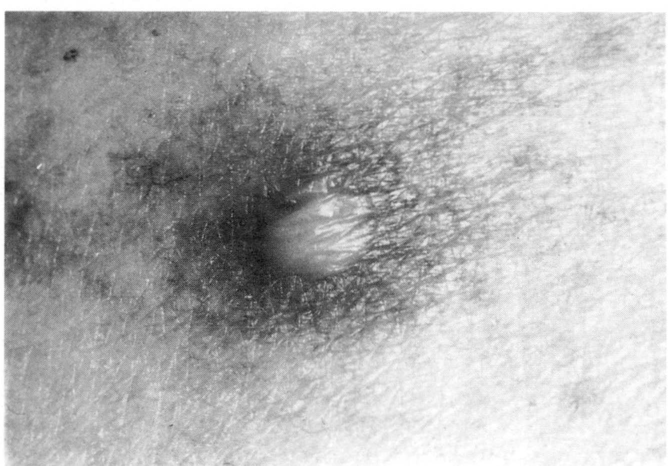

Fig. 11 The sterile pustules of subcorneal pustular dermatosis (Sneddon Wilkinson disease) are often flaccid and contain a fluid level (of pus).

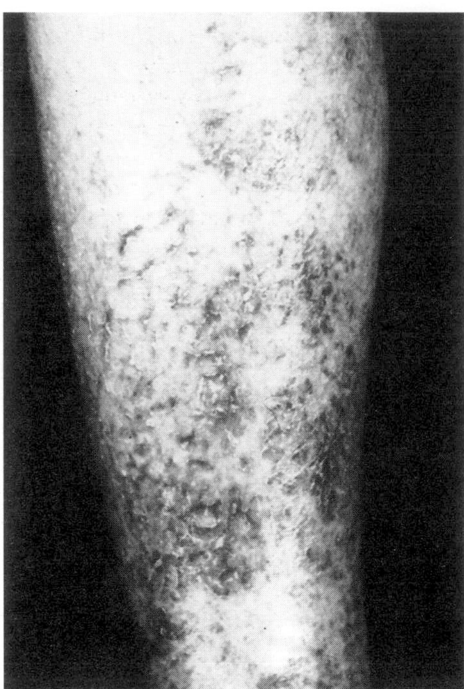

Fig. 12 Asteototic dermatitis: drying of the epidermis results in a loss of flexibility within the stratum corneum; splits develop and dermatitis is established.

When the superficial layer of the epidermis cracks, giving a 'crazy paving' appearance, inflammation and itching supervene, indicating dermatitis ('asteotosic dermatitis') (Fig. 12). If this is allowed to progress, profound dermatitis with weeping and oedema can ensue, particularly on the shins. The regular application of emollients should limit, if not prevent, most of these changes. Ointments are more effective but tend to be unpleasant to use. As patient compliance is important, a compromise may have to be reached. Recommendations include 50 per cent liquid paraffin in 50 per cent white soft paraffin or emulsifying ointment. Severe scaling may be helped by the addition of 2 per cent salicylic acid to the emollient. Critical drying of the skin may also exacerbate pre-existing disease such as atopic dermatitis (eczema) or allow it to re-emerge in those patients predisposed to it.

Erythroderma and exfoliative dermatitis

Erythroderma (red skin all over) reflects widespread skin inflammation and may result directly from underlying disease, for example Sézary syndrome (T-cell lymphoma/leukaemia), a drug eruption, or exacerbation of a pre-existing disease such as atopic dermatitis (eczema) or psoriasis. The patient is often systematically unwell, and attention to general medical considerations such as temperature control, fluid and electrolyte balance, and protein loss is of the utmost importance, particularly in the frail or elderly patient. Distinction from septicaemia may be difficult and, as there is a high risk of secondary infection even without any other factors such as neutropenia, prophylactic antibiotics may be advisable. Potassium permanganate baths are safe in exudative and/or infected dermatitis and are often very helpful. Apart from addressing the underlying cause, therapy should include emollients, topical or systemic corticosteroids if appropriate, and oral antihistamines for itch.

Exacerbation of skin diseases

The increasing use of biological therapies is likely to result in the emergence of new skin problems or reactivation of known diseases. Psoriasis, for example, is related to cytokine release and γ-interferon use can provoke an outbreak..

Equally, all the psychological and physical effects of cancer and its treatment can reveal latent skin disease such as psoriasis or atopic dermatitis. Often a delay of some 3 months is observed, making a relationship difficult to confirm.

Seborrhoeic dermatitis with red flaky skin over the central face, eyebrows, ears, scalp, and central chest can be particularly troublesome. Stress is a known contributing factor, but so is immunosuppression as witnessed in AIDS patients. Treatment can be difficult and containment may be the only realistic approach. Two per cent sulphur with 2 per cent salicylic acid in 1 per cent hydrocortisone cream may be helpful. In severe cases oral fluconazole or itraconazole may be necessary to control the yeast component.

Hair and nail changes

Nail changes may be associated with malignant disease, but the majority of nail changes are the result of therapy. Clubbing is one of the best-established signs of underlying disease such as primary or metastatic bronchopulmonary cancers, pleural and mediastinal tumours including lymphoma, and oesophageal, gastric, and colonic cancer. The nail may react to cytotoxic therapy in several ways. Beau's lines frequently occur after courses of cytotoxic administration. Arrested nail growth may result in a horizontal break in the nails (onychomadesis) and subsequent shedding.

Reference has already been made to patchy alopecia arising from tumour infiltration, but diffuse alopecia due to a generalized telogen or anagen loss is more common. Hair loss in patients with malignant disease is a 'telogen effluvium' and the mechanism is unexplained. Iron deficiency and hypoproteinaemia may contribute. Telogen effluvium simply represents an acute moult following some 'insult'. Shedding occurs 3 to 9 months after the 'insult', which may have been fever, haemorrhage, sudden starvation, accidental or surgical trauma, severe emotional stress, or drugs. Cytotoxic agents interfere with mitosis in the hair papilla, leading to weakness and subsequent fracturing of the hair shaft leading to complete failure of hair formation (anagen alopecia). Continued therapy with two or more cytostatic drugs has a greater effect than a larger dose of only one.

Alopecia mucinosa is associated with cutaneous T-cell lymphoma. The late stage of Sézary syndrome may give rise to diffuse alopecia. Alopecia associated with widespread pruritus, for example in Hodgkin's disease, may result from repeat rubbing and scratching.

Cutaneous aspects of cancer treatment

Cancer treatment frequently involves the skin for intravascular access or as a tissue through which radiotherapy is delivered. Extravasation of chemotherapeutic agents and radiation damage can both result in major skin problems including necrosis. Generally these complications can be avoided with care.

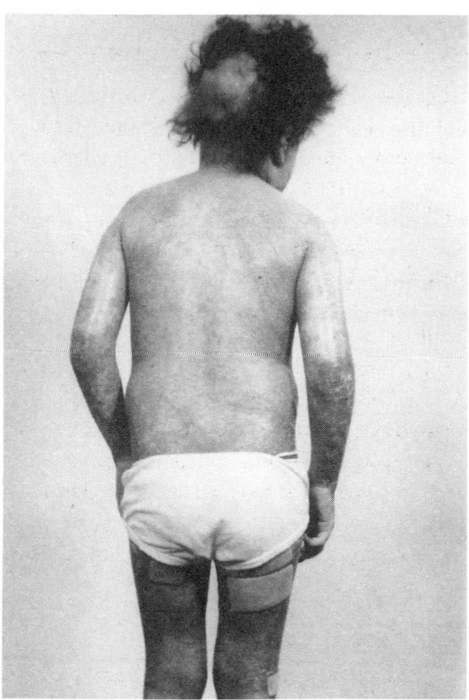

Fig. 13 Chronic graft-versus-host disease: progressive widespread sclerotic changes in the skin lead to joint contractures, alopecia, sores, and eventually death.

Graft-versus-host disease

Graft-versus-host disease particularly affects the skin, but also the liver and gastrointestinal tract, and follows allogeneic bone marrow transplantation. There are two forms of the disease, acute and chronic, although one can merge into the other. Problems arise when immunologically competent lymphoid cells which are histoincompatible are given to a recipient who is incapable of rejecting them. The acute form, which occurs 10 to 20 days post-transplantation is characterized by fever and a non-specific macular rash. Mucous membranes are often involved. Diarrhoea and liver dysfunction coexist. Chronic graft-versus-host disease, although less common, may be encountered more often in the palliative care setting. This form, which develops at least 3 months post-transplantation, may vary from resembling lichen planus to systemic sclerosis (scleroderma). Features of Sjögren's syndrome with dry eyes and mouth may be associated with widespread sclerotic skin changes and alopecia. A particularly disabling form (Fig. 13) results in cutaneous sclerosis, contractures, malabsorption, wasting, alopecia, skin ulceration, and death. Treatment for established disease can be disappointing, and there is little evidence that survival is improved. Pulsed methylprednisolone may be of value in the acute phase and azathioprine can be useful in chronic graft-versus-host disease. Cyclosporin is only of use in prevention and not in the treatment of established disease. Some 40 to 50 per cent of patients with the chronic disease are dead within 10 years from either the disease or superadded infection.

Drug reactions

Drug rashes are a common consequence of cancer therapy for two reasons. Firstly, the vast number of drugs prescribed, often in repeat courses, increases the risk of sensitization. Secondly, immunosuppression, while depressing some aspects of immunity, heightens others such as allergy. Few drug rashes are specific enough to permit identification of the culprit. By examining the time course from the first administration of the drug to the onset of rash (usually 7 to 10 days for sensitization, but within 48 h in somebody previously sensitized) plus selection of the most common offender, an intelligent guess at the cause can usually be made. Only by a process of elimination and rechallenge can the relationship between drug and rash be proven. This is rarely ethical in a patient with advanced cancer. Sometimes it can be the interaction between two drugs or between the drug and the underlying disease which prompts the rash (e.g. the severe morbilliform eruption from ampicillin if given to a patient with infectious mononucleosis or lymphatic leukaemia).

Not all drug reactions are allergic in origin.. Certain drugs such as opioids, amphetamines, atropine, pentamidine, and radiocontrast media may release mast cell mediators directly to produce urticaria. Certain drugs may exacerbate, or even induce, skin disease. Reference has already been made to γ-interferon-induced psoriasis. Other examples include withdrawal of high-dose corticosteroids, particularly dexamethasone, causing acneiform and pustular eruptions. Characteristically, steroid-induced acne produces sheets of monomorphic pustules over the back. Rosacea manifests with redness and pustules over the central face and cheeks. Natural resolution of acne or rosacea is slow under these circumstances, and a 6-week course of tetracycline or erythromycin 500 mg twice daily may prove helpful.

Cytotoxic agents may, through bone marrow suppression, produce signs such as pallor or purpura in the skin. Mucocutaneous surfaces are particularly vulnerable to the toxic effects of this group of drugs on rapidly dividing cells. Therefore common side-effects are stomatitis and alopecia. Skin or nail hyperpigmentation may occur with busulphan, doxorubicin, bleomycin, and cyclophosphamide.

Chemotherapy-induced acral erythema (chemotherapy associated palmar–plantar erythrodysaesthesia syndrome), which is a distinct localized cutaneous response to fluorouracil, doxorubicin, and particularly cytosine arabinoside, has recently been described. A progressive evolution from painful well-demarcated erythema to blistering and eventual desquamation occurs primarily on the palms and soles.[24] The mechanism is poorly understood, but the clinical and histopathological features resemble an acute graft-versus-host reaction.

Neutrophilic eccrine hidradenitis, a condition of necrotic sweat ducts,[25] and eccrine squamous syringometaplasia, which may be confused with squamous cell carcinoma histologically,[26] have also been described in chemotherapy patients.

Cutaneous manifestations of immunosuppressive therapy

Most published data on this topic relate to renal transplant patients, but the principles apply to patients with advanced cancer. Cutaneous manifestations may also develop with immune-modulating treatments which may share certain characteristics with immunosuppressive therapy.

The cutaneous complications of steroids include Cushing's syndrome, skin atrophy, striae, telangiectasiae, hirsutism, and acne.

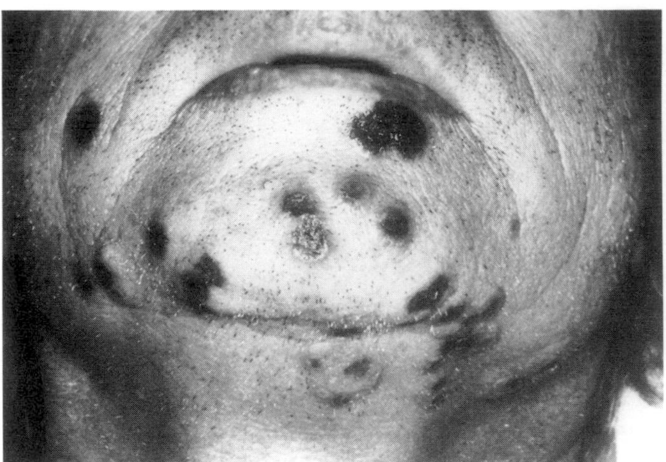

Fig. 14 Chronic recalcitrant herpes simplex in a patient with malignancy.

Immunosuppressive therapy, in general, results in a susceptibility to infection and an increased incidence of malignancy, particularly skin malignancy.

Reactivation and then persistence of varicella zoster, herpes simplex, and cytomegalovirus can be problematic. The atypical behaviour and appearance of common infections such as herpes simplex can provide considerable diagnostic difficulties (Fig. 14). Furunculosis, impetigo, and cellulitis of bacterial aetiology also occur more frequently. Tuberculosis or atypical mycobacterial infections may also become reactivated.

Candidiasis of the mouth and intertriginous areas of the skin is common and occurrence has increased as a result of the use of broad-spectrum antibiotics. More widespread cutaneous candidiasis results in numerous small pustules with a superficial scaling margin. Treatment with oral fluconazole or itraconazoic is recommended. Conventional pityriasis versicolor giving rise to patchy hypo- or hyperpigmentation over the upper trunk is also a frequent finding in the immunosuppressed.

True fungal infection with ringworm fungi may develop as subcutaneous nodules or simply extensive conventional infection with or without nail involvement. Treatment, if indicated, is best with oral terbinafine 250 mg daily.

Infestations such as scabies, sometimes of the Norwegian variety (very heavy mite infestation), can become a problem in the immunosuppressed as itching may not be present. Treatment with lindane painted on with a paintbrush over the entire skin surface and repeated after 3 days is required for eradication.

Skin and internal neoplasms can arise from immunosuppressive therapy, particularly if prolonged after bone marrow transplantation. The incidence of Kaposi's sarcoma and forms of skin cancer, particularly squamous cell carcinoma, is increased. The potential for aggressive behaviour of these lesions appears greater in the immunosuppressed.

Radiation reactions[27]

Radiotherapy necessarily treats the surface of the skin on the way to its target, and in breast cancer it may be pertinent to treat the skin in case of recurrence. X-rays produce acute and late radiation reactions and, as with ultraviolet light (non-ionizing radiation), there is great individual variation in tissue response. Therefore, despite careful dosimetry and fractionation, profound erythema, oedema, and consequently moist desquamation of skin may occur. Little influences the evolution of the reaction once it is set in motion, and thus the only treatment is symptomatic relief and good nursing care. In a randomized double-blind trial comparing clobetasone butyrate with 1 per cent hydrocortisone cream radiation reactions were found to be more severe with the stronger (0.05 per cent clobetasone butyrate) of the two topical steroids. It was concluded that neither cream should be used as first choice in the control of radiation dermatatitis.[28] A more recent trial showed that acute radiation reactions were significantly prevented by sulcralfate cream.[29]

Late radiation reactions manifest as atrophic telangiectatic skin with underlying fibrosis. The skin feels stiff and tethered to underlying structures. Resilience and compliance are greatly reduced and so radionecrotic ulceration may readily occur in areas of moisture and trauma. Late radiation changes leading to necrosis should not occur, but they do. The effects of normal ageing and sun exposure may add to the effects of ionizing radiation and produce accelerated changes of atrophy, necrosis, and secondary malignant change.

Radionecrotic ulceration may be difficult to distinguish from a malignant lesion, whether a recurrent tumour or an X-ray-induced neoplasm. Severe pain suggests radionecrosis. Breast cancer recurring within a previously irradiated skin field may ulcerate, fungate, enhance sclerosis (carcinoma *en cuirasse*), or produce papillomas which readily weep and bleed. Basal cell carcinoma is the most common X-ray-induced cutaneous tumour and may be multiple. Treatment is difficult as excision is required, but progress is slow and a 'wait and see' policy can usually be adopted. Postradiation sarcomas and atypical fibroxanthomas may rarely occur.

Occasionally radiation may induce or localize a particular skin disease which had previously not been manifest. This may be a source of confusion when combined with the effects of radiation damage. Bullous pemphigoid, lichen sclerosus et atrophicus, and localized scleroderma (morphoea)[30] have been reported in this context.

References

1. Waters RA, Clement RM, Thomas JM. Carbon dioxide laser ablation of cutaneous metastases from malignant melanoma. *British Journal of Surgery*, 1991; **78**:493–4.
2. Degos R, *et al.* Le traitement de la maladie de Kaposi par le chlorambucyl. *Dermatologica*, 1967; **135**:345–54.
3. Wit RD, *et al.* Anti retroviral effects of interferon in AIDS associated Kaposi's sarcoma. *Lancet*, 1988; **ii**:1218–22.
4. Kaye FJ, *et al.* A randomised trial comparing combination electron beam radiation and chemotherapy with topical therapy in the initial treatment of mycosis fungoides. *New England Journal of Medicine*, 1989; **321**:1784–90.
5. Beerman H. Some aspects of cutaneous malignancy. *American Journal of Medicine*, 1957; **233**:456–72.
6. Bower M, *et al.* Topical calcipotriol treatment in advanced breast cancer. *Lancet*, 1991; **337**:701–2.
7. Ivetic O, Lyne P. Fungating and ulcerating malignant lesions: a review of the literature. *Journal of Advances in Nursing*, 1990; **15**:83–8.
8. Anonymous. Management of smelly tumours. *Lancet*, 1990; **i**:141–2.
9. Proby CM, Mortimer PS, Badger C. Non-metastatic manifestations of malignancy. *Palliative Medicine*, 1989; **3**:167–80.

10. Clark WH, *et al.* Origins of familial malignant melanomas from heritable melanocytic lesions. *Archives of Dermatology*, 1978; **114**:732–5.
11. Lynch HT, Frichot BC, Lunch JF. Familial atypical multiple mole melanoma syndrome. *Journal of Medical Genetics*, 1978; **15**:352–60.
12. Gorlin RJ, *et al.* The multiple basal cell nevi syndrome. *Cancer*, 1965; **18**:89–103.
13. Harper PS, Harper RM, Howel-Evans AW. Carcinoma of the oesphagus with tylosis. *Quarterly Journal of Medicine*, 1970, **155**:317–33.
14. Anonymous. Vinyl chloride and cancer. *British Medical Journal*, 1974; **i**:590–1.
15. Mikhail GR, *et al.* Generalised malignant acanthosis nigricans. *Archives of Dermatology*, 1979; **115**:201–2.
16. Rigel DS, Jacobs MI. Malignant acanthosis nigricans: a review. *Journal of Dermatology and Surgical Oncology*, 1980; **6**:923–7.
17. Doll DC. Necrolytic migratory erythema. *Archives of Dermatology*, 1980; **116**:801–2.
18. Hashizumet T, *et al.* Glucagonoma syndrome. *Journal of the American Academy of Dermatology*, 1988, **19**:377–83.
19. van der Loos T, Lambrecht E, Lambers I. Successful treatment of glucagonoma related necrolytic migratory erythema with dacarbazine. *Journal of the American Academy of Dermatology*, 1987; **16**:468–72.
20. Barnes BE. Dermatomyositis and malignancy. *Annals of Internal Medicine*, 1976; **84**:68–76.
21. Devere R, Bradley WG. Polymyositis: its presentation, morbidity and mortality. *Brain*, 1975; **98**:637–66.
22. Wong KO. Dermatomyositis: a clinical investigation of 23 cases in Hong Kong. *British Journal of Dermatology*, 1969; 544–47.
23. Harris AL, Smith I, Snaith M. Tamoxifen-induced tumour regression associated with dermatomyositis. *British Medical Journal*, 1982; **284**: 1674–5.
24. Baack BR, Burgdorf WH. Chemotherapy-induced acral erythema. *Journal of the American Academy of Dermatology*, 1991; **24**:457–61.
25. Beutner KR, Packman CH, Markowitch W. Neutrophilic eccrine hidradenitis associated with Hodgkin's disease and chemotherapy. *Archives of Dermatology*, 1986; **122**:809–11.
26. Hurt MA, *et al.* Eccrine squamous syringometaplasia. *Archives of Dermatology*, 1990; **126**:73–7.
27. Spittle MF. Ionizing radiation. In: Rook A, Wilkinson D, Ebling, F, Champion R, Burton J, eds. *Textbook of Dermatology*, Oxford: Blackwell, 1986: 652–6.
28. Glees JP, Mameghan-Zadeh H, Sparkes CG. Effectiveness of topical steroids in the control of radiation dermatitis. *Clinical Radiology*, 1979; **30**:397–403.
29. Maiche A, Isokangas OP, Grohn P. Skin protection by sucralfate cream during electron beam therapy. *Acta Oncologica*, 1994; **33**:201–3.
30. Colver GB, *et al.* Post irradiation morphoea. *British Journal of Dermatology*, 1989; **120**:831–5.

9.6.2 Pruritus and sweating

Mark R. Pittelkow and Charles L. Loprinzi

Introduction

Itching (pruritus) and sweating (perspiration, diaphoresis) are physiological functions of the skin that normally serve human existence well. Itching is the sensory input arising from the skin and mucous membranes that alerts man to potentially harmful insults from physical, chemical, and biological sources. The reflex of scratching is closely linked to the perception of itch, and in most situations functions effectively as an aversive motor response to relieve the sensation and protect the skin. Similarly, sweating is a well-developed and finely coordinated sudomotor response designed to regulate body temperature and prevent hyperthermia.

However, both pruritus and sweating have the potential to function aberrantly and develop into pathological conditions that create significant suffering and morbidity. Since these skin responses encompass both normal and abnormal function, effective treatments to alleviate or eliminate the pathological component are challenging. In this chapter we provide a practical overview of the normal function and pathophysiology of pruritus and sweating, and offer a variety of therapeutic options and general comforting measures for patients experiencing these maladies.

Pruritus

Terminology

Itch and pruritus are terms used to described both physiological and pathological sensory perception. Itch is a distinctive and common cutaneous sensation that arises from the superficial layers of the skin and mucous membranes. It is often fleeting, and the sensation may pass relatively unnoticed since the reflex action of scratching is largely involuntary and typically relieves the temporary discomfort.

Itch (itching, itchy, or itchiness) and pruritus (from the Latin *prurire*, to itch) are generally considered to have equivalent meanings. Itch and related descriptions such as 'terrible itching' are terms commonly used by the patient to convey this distinctive symptom. However, subtle differences in the terminology of itch and pruritus have evolved in the medical literature. In this respect, the terms itch and pruritus have been used to characterize the spectrum of unique cutaneous sensations ranging from the physiological response to severe pathological symptoms.[1–5] Physiological itch is the short-lived cutaneous response to the usual events of living, while pruritus is more closely associated with pathological itch.[1,2] Use of the term pruritus represents the symptomatic level or quality of itch that is defined as an intense cutaneous discomfort occurring with pathological change in the skin or body and eliciting vigorous scratching.

The definition of pruritus or itch is subjective and not entirely precise. Although the general sensation is well known and implicitly understood, many patients with more severe symptoms assimilate itch with various other discomforting or unpleasant sensations. The term itch frequently encompasses a range of descriptive or qualifying terms such as tickle, prickle, pins and needles, burning, stinging, chafed, raw, aching, and even 'painful' sensations.[2]

To avoid confusion and to focus on the palliative medicine perspective, the terms itch and pruritus are used interchangeably to describe this pathological symptom. Patients experiencing pruritus may develop this symptom only mildly and transiently, or itching may be so severe and unrelenting that it preoccupies and completely disrupts their daily existence. It must be recognized that itch or pruritus is variable in its perceived quality and intensity. As with pain, the perception and tolerance of pruritus and the response to this sensation depends significantly on the individual's physical and emotional state, the functional level of activity, adaptive coping mechanisms, and the overall outlook.

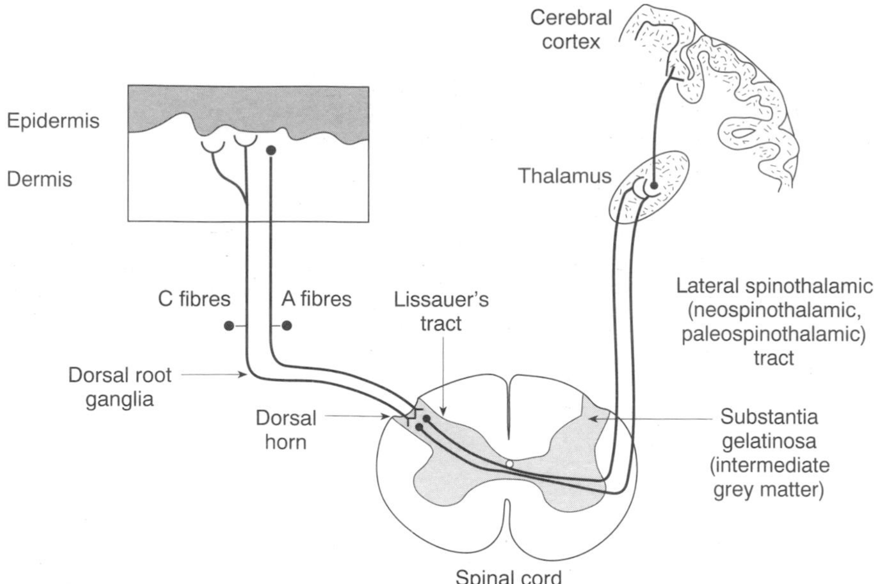

Fig. 1 Pathway for transmission of itch sensation. The C fibres terminate in substantia gelatinosa. Spinothalamic relay axons cross and ascend contralaterally at the spinal level of entering sensory neurones. Larger-diameter A fibres and other interneuronal and central pathways may modulate signalling information. (Modified with permission from refs. 2 and 7.)

Anatomy and physiology

Pruritus is a discrete sensation and a primary sensory modality arising from the activation and integration of cutaneous sensory neural receptors, afferent pathways, and central nervous system processing centres (Fig. 1). In the past itch was considered to be a low-threshold form or submodality of pain based on various clinical and experimental observations. Both pain and itch are induced by noxious stimuli and therefore are designated 'nociceptive'.

A prevailing theory was that itch and pain were related sensations that differed only in the strength of the stimulus, with itch being a response to a weak stimulus and pain being elicited by a stronger stimulus. Further investigation of pain and pruritus revealed similarities but also clearly demonstrated the distinctive differences between these two sensations. At present, itch and pain are regarded as separate entities.[2,6]

Many definitions of pruritus specifically include the reflex action of scratching. Scratching illustrates the distinctive sensation of pruritus, and the scratching reflex is routinely elicited and intimately coupled to itch. Scratching is regarded as a protective reflex, much as withdrawal (flexion) and guarding are comparable reflexes in response to painful stimuli.

Pruritogenic stimuli

Pruritus is induced in skin by various stimuli. Both exogenous and endogenous factors have the capacity to elicit itch.[7,8]. Most experimental and spontaneous triggering factors are mediated via the exogenous or external route. Cutaneous sensory nerves which convey the pruritic signal become activated through the application of either physical or chemical stimuli to the skin (Fig. 2). Many physical stimuli induce pruritus, including pressure, thermal stimulation, low-intensity electrical stimulation, formation of suction blisters, and epicutaneous application of caustic substances.

Chemical stimuli include histamine, proteases, prostaglandins, and neuropeptides. Delivery of histamine to the upper layers of skin by injection or iontophoresis has been a quantitative and reproducible method of examining pruritus experimentally. Histamine is also secreted in skin by mast cells. It acts directly on free nerve endings in skin.

Proteases such as trypsin, chymotrypsin, papain, and kallikrein have the ability to induce pruritus when injected into skin. For example, the spicules of the plant cowage (*Mucuna pruriens*) contain an endopeptidase. These fine spicules are an active ingredient of itching powder and induce an itching sensation when they penetrate into the epidermal layers or dermoepidermal junction of skin. Other natural proteases produced in cells and tissues of the body or by micro-organisms such as bacterial or fungal microflora of the skin also have the potential to induce pruritus.

Mediators of pruritus

The nerve fibres that conduct signals representing itch are located predominantly at the epidermal–dermal junction and have free endings extending into the epidermis.[7] Many of these nerve fibres contain neuropeptides such as substance P, neurokinin A, and calcitonin gene-related peptide (CGRP) (Fig. 2). Other neuropeptides contained in nerves deeper in the dermis and located around blood vessels include vasoactive intestinal peptide (VIP) and neuropeptide Y. Substance P, which is the best characterized pruritogenic neuropeptide, is a sensory transmitter of nociception. It is localized to sensory nerve endings in the skin and is abundant in the prevertebral ganglia, the dorsal roots of the spinal cord, and the brain. Administration of substance P intrathecally causes intense scratching that can be blocked by an antagonist. Nerve fibres containing substance P appear to transmit direct synaptic sensory impulses for the itch sensation.

Capsaicin, an alkaloid derived from the common pepper plant, is a well-known stimulant of erythema and pain when applied to mucous membrane or skin. It depletes substance P from the sensory nerves and excites the type C polymodal nerve fibres conveying pain and itch. However, after initial stimulation, capsai-

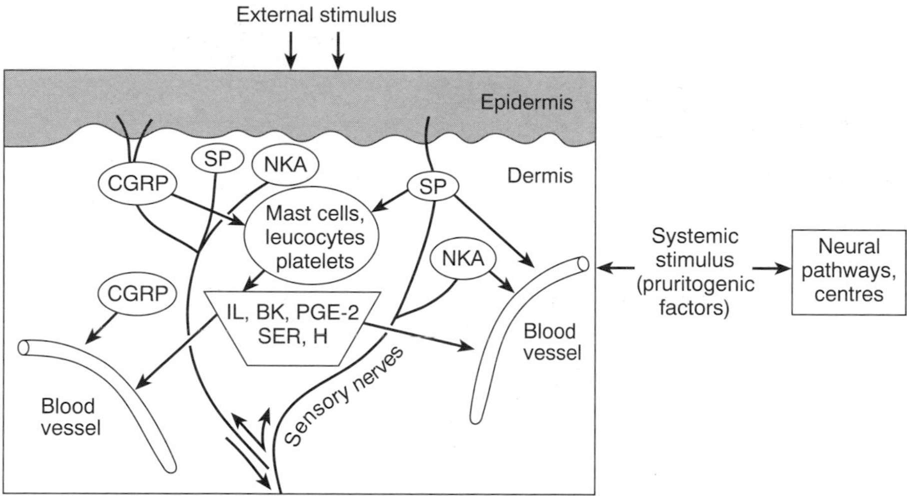

Fig. 2 Stimuli of itch in skin or at peripheral and central neural sites. External or endogenous (systemic) routes of activation trigger nerve fibre stimulation in the skin and the release of neuropeptides including substance P (SP), neurokinin A (NKA), and calcitonin gene-related peptide (CGRP). These mediators trigger inflammatory cells in the skin to release histamine (H), bradykinins (BK), serotonin (S), interleukins (IL), and prostaglandin E_2 (PGE-2). Vascular permeability, inflammatory cell infiltration, and nerve stimulation are evoked by stimuli. (Modified with permission from ref. 7.)

cin blocks C-fibre conduction and mediates neuronal toxicity which eventually decreases fibre density. These activities of capsaicin have stimulated the use of this agent for the treatment of pruritus.[9]

Neuromediators directly influence vascular permeability and erythema (Fig. 2). They also activate release of other mediators such as interleukins, prostaglandins, bradykinin, serotonin, and histamine from infiltrating leucocytes and tissue-localized mast cells. Together, these neural and cellular mediators induce the sensation of itch, augment local activation of inflammatory responses that often accompany itch, and create areas of hyper-responsiveness around the primary stimulus zone for itch. For example, the phenomenon of 'itchy skin' (alloknesis) may be due to regional hyper-responsiveness as well as a lowering of the threshold to itch stimuli at the level of the spinal cord. Additionally, neuromediator release is probably augmented through antidromic nerve stimulation.

Cutaneous neural input

Human skin is supplied principally by nerve fibre networks composed of A and D myelinated fibres and thin type C unmyelinated fibres.[10] Afferent type C fibres include C mechanoreceptors, cold thermoreceptors, and C polymodal nociceptors. Itch is primarily conveyed by the C polymodal fibres which represent 80 per cent of all afferent C fibres (Fig. 1). The exact location of the itch receptor is unknown, but it is generally believed to reside in free nerve endings.

Both itch and slow, aching, dull, or burning pain are conducted by type C polymodal fibres.[10,11] Myelinated A delta nociceptors conveying sharp pain have been identified, but specific receptors for itch and burning pain conveyed by C polymodal fibres have not been clearly delineated. None the less, physiological and pharmacological studies have shown that separate independent sensory channels conduct itch and pain stimuli. The latency between stimulation and onset of the sensation coincides with the relatively low rates of conduction (2 m/s) by the neurones that serve these sensory functions. Some investigators have suggested separating 'itch' into the 'pricking' sensation carried by myelinated fibres and the 'burning' sensation conveyed by unmyelinated fibres. This classification of sensations correlates with the two different systems of sensation described by Head[12] in 1905 as the epicritic or specific well-defined sensation that mediates spontaneous itch and the protopathic or diffuse poorly localized sensation that conveys the perception of itchy skin. However, on the basis of current scientific knowledge pain and itch are largely separable cutaneous sensations.

In addition to the external or exogenous pathway for initiation of the itch sensation, there is considerable clinical evidence for the endogenous activation of pruritus.[1-5] (Fig. 2). The endogenous route for stimulation of pruritus represents a major and clinically relevant pathway; however, it is poorly understood. The potential sites of stimulation (the peripheral nervous system, the spinal cord, and/or the central nervous system), the inciting agents and mediators, and the relative overlap of exogenous versus endogenous activation pathways remain to be clearly delineated and applied effectively in the clinical setting. The systemic or endogenous stimuli for itch have been only partially characterized, and the biochemical causes for pruritus associated with a spectrum of systemic illnesses, including metabolic disease, organ failure, and various malignancies, continue to be ill-defined and vexing problems.

Several substances have been shown to mediate different or opposing effects on itch when tested experimentally. Their activities depend on the route of administration and their specific responses at the peripheral, spinal cord, and/or central nervous system levels. These observations support the concept of itch as a neural message that is interpreted in the context of signal reception, transmission, and modulation at each level of the nervous system.

Opioid and serotonergic mediators

Opioids are one example of substances that exert separate and potentially disparate responses in modulating the transmission and perception of itch and pain at different levels of the nervous system.[2,13] Uncovering the existence of central opioid receptors led to the discovery of encephalins, endogenous pentapeptides that bind to these receptors. Opioids are powerful analgesics that mimic the effects of encephalins. However, opioids mediate both excitatory and modulatory effects on pruritus at several levels. At the spinal level, encephalins released from short spinal interneurones and opioids stimulate an inhibitory presynaptic signal transmitted to primary afferents that modulates secondary transmission of itch. However, within some regions of the central nervous system, opioids directly trigger itch. Clinically, intrathecal or epideral morphine has been known to induce localized or generalized itching. At the peripheral level within skin, opioids stimulate mast cell degranulation and release of histamine which produces itch.

Central activation of itch by opioids appears to play a dominant role in some diseases, since opioid antagonists have been shown to exert significant antipruritic effects.[13,14] The parenterally administered opioid antagonist naloxone inhibits induction of itch following histamine injection of skin. Pruritus of cholestatic liver disease (primary or secondary biliary cirrhosis) can be dramatically reduced with naloxone or the oral antagonist nalmephene.[14,15]

Serotonergic compounds are another group of agents that modulate effects on pruritus primarily at the peripheral level, although receptors for serotonin are present in the peripheral and central nervous systems.[13] Cutaneous injection but not intravenous infusion of a serotonergic agonist increases the scratching reflex in animals. Peripheral serotonin receptors in humans are presumed to play a role in the mediation of pruritus. Temperature-dependent pruritus experienced by patients with polycythemia vera may be stimulated by serotonin. Of potential clinical significance, generalized pruritus of hepatic cholestatic disease and chronic renal insufficiency have been relieved dramatically with intravenous administration of the type 3 serotonin (5-HT$_3$) receptor antagonist ondansetron.[16,17] Opioid and serotonin receptor antagonists have revealed the complex mechanisms involved in transmitting signals for pruritus at the peripheral and central nervous system levels.

Pathogenic correlates in management of pruritus

The similarity of the symptoms of exogenous and endogenous forms of pruritus has prompted empirical use of similar treatment measures for both types of conditions. Frequently, however, effective therapy for pruritus caused by one condition is not particularly beneficial for pruritis of another cause. Also, treatments that ameliorate or relieve pruritus induced by exogenous agents have limited or minimal effects on alleviating pruritus of endogenous cause. This is probably related to the site and mode of activity of these treatments and their limitations in targeting the receptors, mediators, or central neural pathways that control expression of endogenous versus exogenous pruritus.

The nuclei of the afferent C polymodal nerves reside in the dorsal root ganglia and axon extensions that synapse in the dorsal horn of the substantia gelatinosa (Fig. 1). Secondary neurones cross the spinal cord to the contralateral spinothalamic tract of the venterolateral quadrant before ascending to the thalamus. There is also evidence in animals that pathways in addition to the anterolateral system can transmit pruritogenic stimuli. The synaptic neurones within the thalamus project to the somatosensory cortex of the postcentral gyrus. Scratching is the spinal reflex in response to itching but also has input from higher neural centres.

Perception of itch has the potential to be modulated at the level of the spinal cord and, probably at other levels, by additional neural input as described for pain by Melzak and Wall.[18] The description of 'a gate control system that modulates sensory input from the skin before it evokes pain perception' can also be applied to the perception of itch.

A-fibre impulse conduction is self-regulated by a negative feedback pathway that tends to dampen continued firing. It also interrupts summation of sensations of itch and pain conveyed by the C polymodal fibres. The 'gate' has the ability to control neural transmission. Gate closure is envisaged to produce inhibition at the spinal cord level such that stimulation of A fibres by scratching would induce or enhance inhibition of conduction. Although the gate-control theory has been intensively evaluated and revised over the past three decades and its operational functionality has been challenged, practical application based on this theory appears to have been made in the control of pain and itch using transcutaneous electrical nerve stimulation.[19,20]

Table 1 Pruritus: causes and distribution

Aetiology
Primary
Idiopathic
Essential
Secondary
Dermatological
Systemic
Distribution
Localized
Generalized, diffuse

Clinical evaluation and treatment of pruritus

The clinical approach to pruritus can present a considerable diagnostic as well as therapeutic challenge. To formulate a simple clinical strategy for diagnosis and treatment of pruritus, pathological itch can be classified as primary or secondary (Table 1). Secondary pruritus is caused by either dermatological or systemic disease.[1-4] Pruritus can be further separated into localized and generalized forms based on the location and extent of body surface involvement. In most cases, localized pruritus is due to cutaneous infections or other regionalized expressions of dermatological disease.

Generalized or diffuse pruritus typically presents more troublesome symptoms for the patient and a greater challenge for the physician. Diffuse pruritus is usually related to a dermatological or systemic disorder affecting the entire skin surface. However, even pruritus which is generalized or diffuse exhibits symptoms that may be accentuated and localized to certain regions of the body, and these symptoms may fluctuate, migrate, or extend over time.

Primary pruritus

Primary or idiopathic pruritus is identified in the majority (more than 70 per cent) of patients where dermatological disease (secondary pruritus) has been excluded as a cause for itching.[21] Idiopathic pruritus may be fairly limited in extent and intensity. Symptoms can be reasonably controlled by conscientious skin care and topical soothing measures. However, other cases of primary pruritus prove to be quite extensive, severe, and chronic. The diagnosis of primary pruritus is established following a thorough medical and dermatological evaluation to exclude secondary causes of itching.

Evaluation and management of idiopathic pruritus is frequently a frustrating experience for the patient and physician as possible causes and beneficial treatments are sought. When no clear aetiology is delineated, both the patient and physician may experience disappointment. With severe idiopathic pruritus, there is also lingering uncertainty whether an occult disease, particularly malignancy, may eventually be uncovered. However, several clinical studies have shown that only a small percentage of patients referred to dermatologists for generalized pruritus will develop a malignancy during follow-up evaluation.[21,22] The majority manifest haematological malignancies, particularly lymphomas, and therefore periodic clinical surveillance is warranted. However, the duration and severity of chronic primary pruritus may be sufficiently debilitating for palliative intervention and the identification of effective therapies to become the principal goals.

Secondary pruritus—dermatological

Secondary pruritus is associated with a variety of disorders including both dermatological and systemic diseases (Tables 2 and 3). For example, contact dermatitis is a common characteristic skin disease that has itching and scratching as its hallmarks. Table 2 lists the major dermatological entities that are accompanied by pruritus. Some disorders, such as scabies, insect bites, folliculitis, and allergic contact dermatitis, are caused by exogenous agents that elicit pruritus. Other conditions, including atopic dermatitis, bullous pemphigoid, lichen planus, psoriasis, and urticaria, are endogenously mediated inflammatory skin conditions that exhibit variably intense symptoms of pruritus.

Table 2 Skin diseases associated with pruritus

- Aquagenic pruritus
- Atopic dermatitis (eczema)
- Bullous pemphigoid
- Contact dermatitis
- Cutaneous T-cell lymphoma (mycosis fungoides, Sézary's syndrome)
- Dermatitis herpetiformis
- Drugs (dermatitis medicamentosa)
- Folliculitis
- Grover's disease
- Insect bites
- Lichen planus
- Lichen simplex chronicus
- Mastocytosis
- Miliaria
- Pediculosis
- Pityriasis rosea
- Prurigo
- Prurigo nodularis
- Pruritus ani and vulvae
- Psoriasis
- Scabies
- Sunburn
- Systemic parasitic infection (onchocerciasis, trichinosis, echinococcosis)
- Urticaria, dermographism
- Xerosis

Table 3 Systemic disorders associated with pruritus

Biliary and Hepatic disease
- Biliary atresia
- Primary biliary cirrhosis
- Sclerosing cholangitis
- Extrahepatic biliary obstruction
- Cholestasis of pregnancy
- Drug-induced cholestasis

Chronic renal failure—Uraemia

Drugs
- Opioids
- Amphetamines
- Cocaine
- Acetylsalicylic acid
- Quinidine
- Niacinamide
- Etretinate
- Other medications
- Subclinical drug sensitivity

Endocrine diseases
- Diabetes insipidus
- Diabetes mellitus
- Parathyroid disease
- Thyroid disease (hypothyroidism, thyrotoxicosis)

Haematopoietic diseases
- Hodgkin's and non-Hodgkin's lymphoma
- Cutaneous T-cell lymphoma (mycosis fungoides, Sézary's syndrome)
- Systemic mastocytosis
- Multiple myeloma
- Polycythaemia vera
- Iron-deficiency anaemia

Infectious diseases
- Syphilis
- Parasitic
- HIV
- Fungal

Malignancy
- Breast, stomach, lung, etc.
- Carcinoid syndrome

Neurological disorders
- Distal small-fibre neuropathy
- Stroke
- Multiple sclerosis
- Tabes dorsalis
- Brain abscess/tumours
- Psychosis, psychogenic causes
- Delusions of parasitosis

The mechanisms that induce itching have been partially characterized for some of these disorders. Specific inflammatory cell types, such as mast cells, lymphocytes, and eosinophils, play important roles in the pathogenesis of specific diseases and the development of pruritus. Neuropeptides, cytokines, and proteases, among other mediators, are the main cellular products initiating

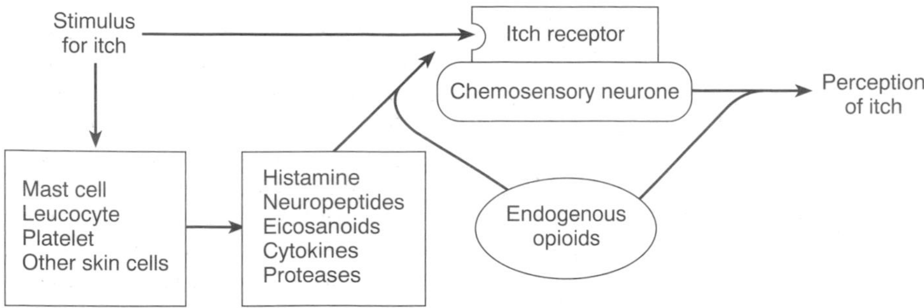

Fig. 3 Factors mediating itch: direct or indirect activation of itch receptor by specific pruritogens. The itch signal is transmitted to a chemosensory neurone which is activated and conveys perception centrally in the nervous sytem. Endogenous opioids, among other factors, modulate pruritogenic signals. (Modified with permission from ref. 2.)

pruritus (Fig. 3). These mediators probably act in addition to specific neurotransmitters which directly convey a pruritogenic signal to the itch receptor. Treatment of the specific skin condition and elimination of any offending exogenous agent(s) typically alleviate the symptoms of pruritus. When dealing with pruritus which may be skin related, it is crucial to identify and classify any primary skin lesions and obtain appropriate skin sample specimens or skin biopsies. This information is often very helpful in establishing a diagnosis. The correct diagnosis and appropriate therapy for dermatological disorders should be sought through specialist consultation and is well described in standard dermatology textbooks.

Cutaneous diseases which cause pruritus should not be overlooked. For example, unrelenting pruritus caused by scabies infestation, sometimes lasting for months to years, has been mistakenly attributed to concurrent malignancy (Fig. 4). Other cutaneous infections, irritant or allergic contact dermatitis (Fig. 5), or autoimmune blistering diseases such as bullous pemphigoid (Fig. 6) have been repeatedly observed to develop during the course of malignancies or other systemic illnesses. By recognizing that pruritus is due to a supervening dermatological condition, prompt and appropriate treatment can be instituted and the skin disease and pruritus both resolve. Therefore the periodic evaluation and re-evaluation of the causes of idiopathic or poorly controlled pruritus may uncover new information that will significantly benefit total patient care and improve overall comfort.

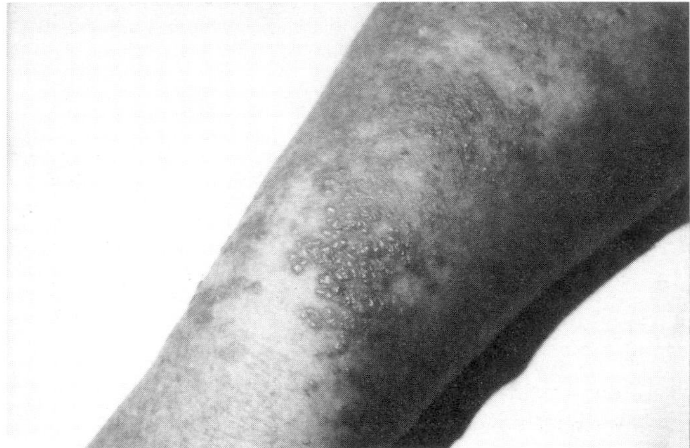

Fig. 5 Acute dermatitis: erythema, scaling, and blister formation due to allergy after application of triple antibiotic ointment containing neomycin.

Some dermatological conditions provide instructive lessons on the aetiology and limitations of managing pruritus. For example, prurigo nodularis is a distinctive pruritic dermatosis that can be chronic and is often recalcitrant to therapy.[23] The symptom of pruritus appears to play a more central role in the pathogenesis and propagation of this disease. The pruritus of prurigo nodularis largely localizes to the nodular lesions that appear to develop and become more prominent as a result of scratching (Fig. 7). Cutaneous nerve elements are accentuated within the lesions and are

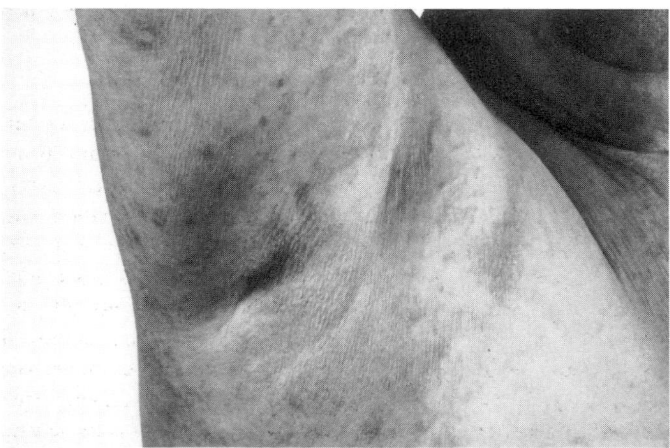

Fig. 4 Scabies: erythematous papules, crusts, and excoriations. Mite burrows can be identified under magnification.

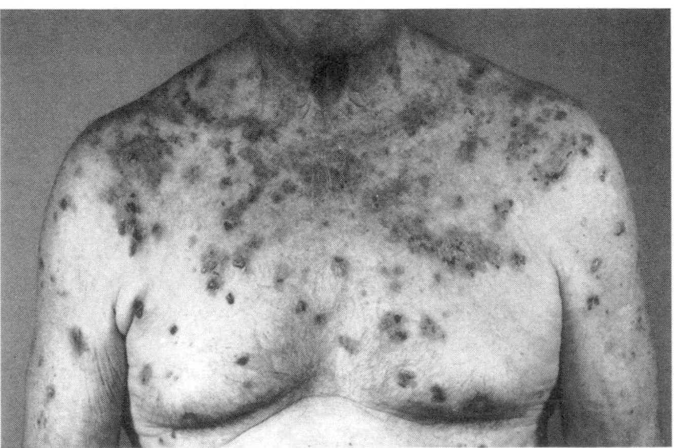

Fig. 6 Bullous pemphigoid: tense blisters on an erythematous and urticarial base with rupture of secondary blisters, erosions, and crust formation.

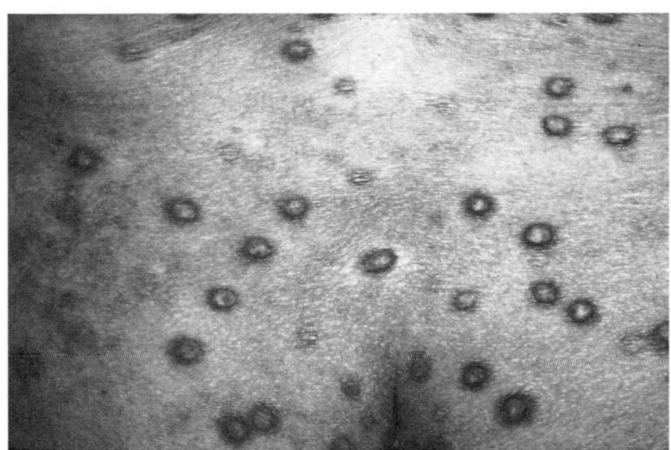

Fig. 7 Prurigo nodularis: discrete firm pruritic globular nodules over the sacral area which often have a verrucous crust and an excoriated surface.

often difficult to block effectively or eliminate. These factors probably account for the refractory nature of the condition to various treatments. Clinical and therapeutic observations on prurigo nodularis potentially have aetiological and practical relevance to non-dermatological disorders that are associated with pruritus since some of these conditions may also be quite refractory to many therapeutic measures directed at alleviating the itch.

Secondary pruritus—systemic

Pruritus is a feature of a broad range of systemic diseases (Table 3). For some diseases, specific medical or surgical treatment provides cure of the illness and pruritus. However, with many of the chronic systemic diseases, patients may survive for long periods with adequate control of the illness. Unfortunately, pruritus often continues to be a major symptom and may cause considerable morbidity.

Topical antipruritic agents

A variety of topical medications have been developed through the years to provide symptomatic relief of itching.[24,25] Many of the active ingredients have long been known to ease the symptoms of itch. A list of the common therapeutic antipruritic lotions, creams, and gels, together with their active ingredients, is given in Table 4. Topical medications are not convenient to apply to the entire body surface on a routine basis, but even patients with more generalized pruritus often have localized areas of accentuated itching that are more troublesome to control. Therefore topical agents have a role in treating both regionalized accentuation of generalized pruritus and localized itching.

Phenol in dilute solution (0.5–2 per cent) alleviates pruritus by anaesthetizing cutaneous nerve endings. Phenol is potentially neurotoxic and hepatotoxic, and should be avoided in pregnancy and in infants under 1 year of age. Menthol and camphor relieve itching by counter-irritant and anaesthetic properties. Menthol (typically 0.25–2 per cent, but can be as high as 16 per cent) produces a cool sensation, and camphor (typically 1–3 per cent, but can be as high as 9 per cent) exerts similar effects. Zinc oxide, coal tars, calamine, glycerine, and salicylates also have been used in many preparations with reported benefit, although their specific modes of action have not been elucidated.

Pramoxine hydrochloride is a topical anaesthetic similar to dyclonine that has been used as the sole ingredient or has been compounded with hydrocortisone or menthol and is available as an aerosol, foam, cream, gel ,or lotion. Newer anaesthetic prescription medications include EMLA cream, a combination of the caine drugs lignocaine (lidocaine) and prilocaine which are absorbed transcutaneously and produce anaesthesia as well as abolish itch. Doxepin has been demonstrated to be effective in relieving the itch of skin disease and may be useful for pruritus of various aetiologies. Capsaicin has been reported to be effective in localized neurogenic pruritus of various causes and has demonstrated benefit in other conditions accompanied by itch. Initial applications of the medication produce burning sensations and other discomfort. The patient must be alerted to these sensations and coaxed to continue if sustained use is planned and benefit is to be obtained.

Systemic therapies and other treatments

A plethora of systemic medications and various other modalities have been used in the treatment of pruritus.[1,4,5,25–27]). These agents are organized and listed in Table 5 according to their standard pharmacological activities. On examining this list, it becomes apparent that no drug has ever been successfully developed, tested, and produced exclusively or even primarily for pruritus. This fact alone reveals the potential difficulties that are encountered in the pharmacological treatment of chronic and severe cases of pruritus. All too frequently, patients requiring palliative relief from intractable itching are subjected to trials of various medicines in an attempt to discover which one 'works best' for them. With persistence and luck, a particular drug or modality can be identified that offers benefit and has tolerable side-effects. Combinations of systemic and topical agents often seem to provide the best relief. Clinical experience has also shown that certain medications or treatment modalities seem to provide more consistent benefit for specific types of secondary pruritus, as is the case for ultraviolet B (UVB) phototherapy and the pruritus of chronic renal failure. Unfortunately, few controlled clinical studies have ever been conducted on the palliative management of pruritus, and a well-developed and simple clinical management strategy does not exist. Therefore, as outlined above, the practical aspects of establishing the probable cause(s), selecting a treatment, and assessing its benefit, side-effects, and potential risks must all be addressed routinely as part of the process of providing palliative care for the patient with pruritus. In addition, several simple measures can be adopted to give patients and their skin some relief from the anguish of itching and the injury of scratching.

Pruritus of malignancy

Itching associated with malignancy presents special challenges and dilemmas. It can be among the most severe and recalcitrant forms of secondary pruritus. Patients with malignancy-associated pruritus represent a significant percentage of those requiring palliation, and many may manifest this symptom at some time during their illness. However, the frequency, chronicity, and severity of pruritus associated with malignancy and its response to treatment are difficult parameters to determine, and they have not been examined systematically and reported in the literature. For example, the percentage of patients for whom the symptoms of itching have been relieved by primary treatment of the malignancy versus those who have benefited from symptomatic therapies has not been defined in this population of patients. As a result, a single, specific, and

Table 4 Topical antipruritic agents

Preparation	Active ingredient
Dodd's lotion	Phenol, glycerine, zinc oxide
Lerner's lotion	Ethyl alcohol, glycerine, zinc oxide
Pamscol	Phenol, acetylsalicylic acid
Sarna	Menthol, camphor, phenol
Schamberg's lotion	Menthol, phenol, zinc oxide
Topic gel	Benzl alcohol, ethyl alcohol, methol, phenol
Wibi lotion	Menthol
Crude coal tar 3%–10% solution	Crude coal tar
Caladryl	Diphenhydramine, calamine, camphor
Pramosone, Prax	Pramoxine
Quotane	Dimethisoquin
EMLA	Lignocaine, prilocaine
Zonalon	Doxepin
Zostrix	Capsaicin

Modified from ref. 25.

effective treatment plan for pruritus of malignancy is not available.

Symptomatic skin care

Patients with itching of malignancy may manifest different types of pruritic skin lesions that warrant individualized therapies. Many patients will demonstrate excoriations due to scratching and injury of the skin from fingernails or other implements (brushes etc.) (Fig. 8). Other patients show discrete papular, crusted, or excoriated lesions more characteristic of prurigo (Fig. 9). As a routine, close trimming and filing of sharp edges of fingernails as well as wearing cotton gloves, if necessary, are initial steps to minimize further skin injury. Tepid (not too warm or too hot) baths are usually soothing and temporarily relieve the itch. Patients often relate that a hot bath or shower feels more relaxing and offers symptom relief, but the itch is worse afterwards due in part to vasodilation and the accentuated neural response of cutaneous heating. Immediately following the bath and a light towelling, the patient or caregiver should lubricate the skin with a fragrance-free cream-base emollient containing phenol or menthol if this is found to be beneficial. Applying a cream results in better maintenance of skin hydration and lessens the chance of further aggravation of pruritus from xerosis. Wearing clothing that is loose fitting, less irritating (e.g. avoid wools), and minimizes heat retention and sweating (e.g. avoid synthetics) can also be helpful in lessening the frequency and intensity of itch. Cotton fabric clothing usually meets these requirements.

For patients with numerous excoriations and crusting due to scratching, application of tap water wet dressings (or cotton long underwear soaked in water) to the affected areas several times daily for 1 to 2 h provides temporary relief and hastens healing of injured skin. A low- to medium-potency corticosteroid cream containing 1 to 2.5 per cent hydrocortisone can be applied to the skin prior to the wet dressings for topical anti-inflammatory action. A more potent corticosteroid such as triamcinolone 0.05 to 0.1 per cent in a cream base can be used for 7 to 10 days as needed on an intermittent basis, but prolonged use should be avoided to prevent atrophy and bruising of the skin, secondary skin infections, or hypothalamic–pituitary–adrenal suppression.

Oral corticosteroids

Various systemic anti-inflammatory agents are useful in the management of pruritus. Oral corticosteroids often improve the symptoms of itching for patients with primary or secondary pruritus. In many patients, the specific activity is unknown. The corticosteroid may inhibit release of pruritogens, inflammatory factors, or neuromediators, or it may block pruritogen activity or alter its metabolism. As with topical steroids, prolonged use has significant adverse side-effects. However, in cases where the duration of treatment is limited, an oral corticosteroid can provide much sought relief of itching.

Antihistamines

Antihistamines are another class of agent that offers benefit in treatment of itching. More than 30 different antihistaminic compounds of at least six different classes are available over the counter or by prescription. Although antihistamines provide minimal benefit for some patients with problematic itching such as that associated with Hodgkin's disease, obstructive jaundice, or uraemic pruritus, they have a good safety profile and should be used at full dose to attempt amelioration of pruritus. For example, pruritis is an early manifestation of HIV infection, and antihistamines, sometimes at high dosages, are used to control symptoms. Studies have shown superior efficacy of sedating over low-sedating antihistamines for relieving itch. Low-sedating antihistamines (e.g. terfenadine, astemizole, loratadine) should be reserved for the histamine-mediated whealing disorders that are accompanied by pruritus. Longer-acting antihistamines with central nervous system sedation are preferred for control of itch. These include chlorpheniramine, diphenhydramine, clemastine, hydroxyzine, and cyproheptadine. Agents of different classes should be tried if an antihistamine of one class is not effective. Sometimes, combination of agents from different classes is efficacious when a single agent is ineffective.

Other drug therapies

Cromones and thalidomide are anti-inflammatory agents that have been reported to be useful in pruritus associated with several different types of chronic or malignant disease. Disodium chromoglycate improves the flushing and pruritus of systemic mast cell disease.[36] It also has been reported to improve the pruritus of Hodgkin's disease when other therapies have failed.[37] Thalidomide has been found to relieve the intractable pruritus and development of skin lesions in prurigo nodularis.[38] More recently, thalidomide (100 mg/day) was found to produce significant relief of uraemic pruritus.[39] This drug is used primarily in the treatment of leprosy reactions and graft-versus-host disease. Because of its neuropathic and teratogenic side-effects, thalidomide is not routinely available for prescription. However, selected patients who require only a limited course of therapy and can be monitored regularly may be candidates for thalidomide when an alternative medication is sought .

Many drugs have effects on the peripheral or central nervous system, and some of these agents have been found to be very useful in the treatment of itching from many causes. Anaesthetic agents administered by the intradermal, intravenous, or intra-arterial routes have effects similar to topical anaesthetics in blocking sensory input and transmission, including the sensation of pruritus. Parenteral lignocaine (200 mg in 100 ml saline by an intra-arterial line) alleviates refractory pruritus in hepatic cholestasis and chronic renal failure.[40,41] Hypotension, cardiovascular effects, seizures and psychosis are possible side-effects. Recently, the anaesthetic sedative propofol, used at subhypnotic doses (15 mg) daily when itch was most severe or by continuous infusion at 1 to 1.5 mg/kg/h, produced significant reduction in pruritus due to cholestatic disease of pancreatic neoplasia, hepatic and bile duct metastasis, cholangitis, and primary biliary cirrhosis.[42,43] A rapid onset of action within 5 to 10 min was observed. Propofol also relieves pruritus from spinal morphine administration, and it is postulated that propofol blocks effects of opioid-like pruritogens at the spinal

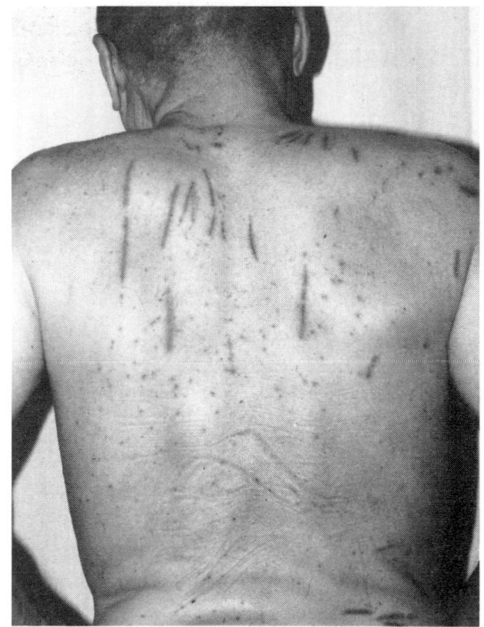

Fig. 8 Linear excoriations, erosions, and crusts resulting from unrelenting pruritus and scratching by a patient with small cell carcinoma of the lung.

Table 5 Pruritus therapies

Anti-inflammatory agents
Corticosteroids
H_1, H_2, H_3 blocking agents
Salicylates
Cromolyn
Thalidomide
Vasoactive drugs
α-Blockers
β-Blockers (e.g. propranolol)
Central and peripheral nervous system agents
Anaesthetic agents
Lignocaine etc.
Propofol
Antidepressant agents
Neuroleptic agents
Tranquillizing agents
Sedatives
Opioid antagonists (naloxone, naltrexone, nalmephene)
Serotonin antagonists (ondestranon)
Sequestrants
Cholestyramine
Charcoal
Heparin (IV)
Miscellaneous
Disease-specific drugs and therapies
Cholestatic disease: rifampicin, methyltestosterone ursodeoxycholic acid, partial external biliary diversion [25, 28-30]
Uraemia: erythropoietin, parathyroidectomy, ultraviolet B phototherapy[31-33]
Polycythaemia vera: (α-interferon)[34]
Neurofibromatosis (neurofibroma): ketotifen[35]
Phototherapy: ultraviolet A, ultraviolet B, photochemotherapy (PUVA)[25, 33]
Transcutaneous nerve stimulation [19, 20]
Plasma exchange, apheresis[25]
Acupuncture[25]
Psychotherapy, biofeedback, relaxation techniques[25]

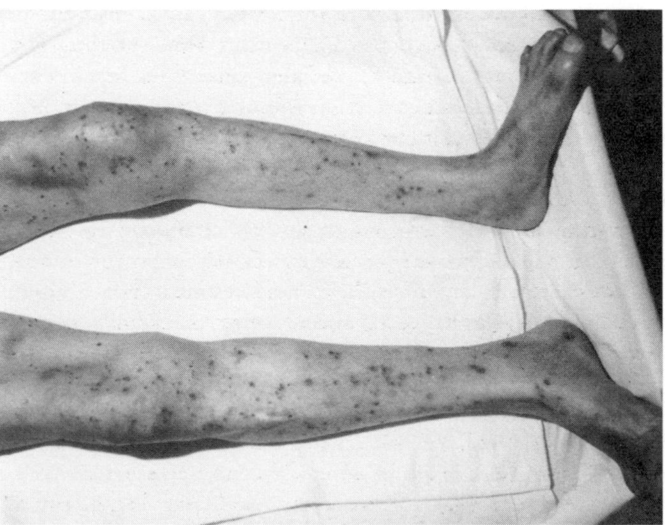

Fig. 9 Discrete, crusted, and haemorrhagic prurigo-like lesions accompanying generalized pruritus of chronic renal failure and diabetes mellitus.

level.[44] Parenterally administered agents such as lignocaine, propofol, and naloxone are of relatively limited use in chronic pruritus. However, if acute severe episodes of pruritus become incapacitating, these agents can often provide much sought relief and re-establish some measure of symptom control.

Antidepressant drugs including doxepin, amitriptyline, nortriptyline, and imipramine have antihistaminic effects as well as psychoactive and analgesic properties that make them useful in the management of various pain and itch states. Neuropathic pain with protopathic features of diffuse burning itch as well as the sensation of pain is improved by chronic antidepressant treatment.[45] These medications may also benefit patients with pruritus where depression appears to be playing a role in the prominence or severity of symptoms.[46] Neuroleptic medications include pimozide, a drug useful in the management of delusions of parasitosis, and haloperidol. Although not indicated for the primary treatment of organic pruritus, these agents may be useful when patients exhibit delusional ideation in conjunction with their disease process. Treatment improves the symptoms of psychosis and diminishes the mental fixation on pruritus.[46]

Sedative medications such as diazepam have been shown to be ineffective in reducing experimental itch, although mechanically induced pruritus was eliminated with this agent.[25,47] Sedatives in conjunction with other antipruritic agents appear to offer greater relief if the patient is experiencing anxiety as part of the chronic pruritic reaction. In addition to the sedative effects of antihistamines such as hydroxyzine, doxepin, and diphenhydramine, specific anxiolytic agents, including buspirone, clomipramine, and benzodiazepines such as alprazolam, can be used when anxiety appears to be playing a role in magnifying the symptoms of pruritus.[46] Long-term treatment with benzodiazapines should be avoided as there is a risk of habituation.

The opioid and serotonin antagonists, as reviewed earlier, have been found to be very effective in selected types of chronic pruritus. The opioid antagonists have been evaluated most extensively in the clinical setting of pruritus of cholestasis where they show significant benefit in symptom relief.[14,48] Naloxone must be administered parenterally. Naltrexone and nalmephene are orally active agents which may be useful as longer-term therapeutic agents for chronic pruritus. Serotonin (5-HT) antagonists are few in number and less well evaluated in pruritus. However, the 5-HT_3 receptor antagonist ondestranon shows promise as the first in a new class of agents to alleviate the symptoms of generalized pruritus in patients with cholestasis and chronic renal failure.[16,17]

Sequestrants such as cholestyramine or charcoal administered orally or heparin administered by intravenous infusion have been reported to be helpful in the treatment of obstructive biliary pruritus.[25] Cholestyramine was also observed to improve itching in polycythaemia vera and uraemia.[25] These treatments may be useful as adjuvant or alternative therapies during the management of chronic pruritus due to these diseases.

A variety of miscellaneous therapies are listed in Table 5, which also includes additional disease-specific medications reported to benefit chronic pruritus and other treatment modalities such as phototherapy, transcutaneous nerve stimulation, plasma exchange, and acupuncture. Pertinent references reporting the benefit of specific therapies are cited for each modality. For example, several medications and physical modalities have been found to relieve the pruritus of chronic renal failure. Despite our lack of knowledge regarding specific pruritogenic factors and their expression and activity in chronic renal failure, ultraviolet B phototherapy often provides symptomatic relief. Ultraviolet B phototherapy is well tolerated, has few side-effects, and can be administered at many dermatological practices or regional clinical phototherapy centres. Erythroprotein and thalidomide have been reported to improve uraemic pruritus. Newer agents such as ondansetron may prove to be clinically useful and routinely available for the pruritus of chronic renal failure. Parenteral lignocaine is typically reserved for severe recalcitrant episodes of pruritus in uraemic patients unresponsive to other measures.

The multitude and variety of medications and sundry other therapeutic modalities reviewed in this chapter attest to the magnitude, severity, and chronicity of pruritus. All these drugs and therapies have been successful, to some extent, in ameliorating or abolishing this troublesome symptom. In managing the symptom of pruritus as well as the disease, it behoves the physician to make the best possible assessment of the specific physical and emotional factors that may be contributing to the intensity and character of a patient's problem of itch. With reassurance, flexibility, creativity, persistence, and a demonstrated concern by the physician, most patients will find relief and comfort.

Sweating

Anatomy and physiology

Sweating is a physiological sudomotor response of skin that has pathological counterparts. Abnormalities of sweating can be classified in terms of quantitative or qualitative dysfunction. From the perspective of palliative care, the most troublesome sudomotor symptoms relate to inappropriate or excessive sweating which occurs as part of malignant disease or its treatment. To understand the aetiological factors contributing to abnormal sweating and its palliative management, the anatomy and physiology of the peripheral and central thermoregulatory system of the human are presented and reviewed.

Sweating or perspiration is a unique function of the skin of humans and apes that allows evaporative heat loss and regulation of body temperature in a hot environment or during physical exertion. Other mammals must pant, seek a cooler location, rest, or splash the skin with water to lower body temperature thermally. The crucial function and efficiency of sweat production is witnessed in individuals with the inherited disorder anhidrotic ectodermal hypoplasia who are unable to rely on evaporative heat loss through sweating. Physical inactivity, a cool ambient environment, or wetting the clothing or skin with water substitutes for sweating in order to achieve thermoregulation. Another group of persons particularly susceptible to the adverse consequences of thermal stress are young infants and the sedentary elderly who fail to sweat sufficiently and are also more likely to develop and succumb to hyperthermia.

Temperature regulation

Sweating is an important component of the elaborate thermoregulatory system of humans that is shown diagrammatically in Fig. 10.[49] The hypothalamus integrates inputs from central and peripheral thermoreceptors with the efferent response mechanisms,

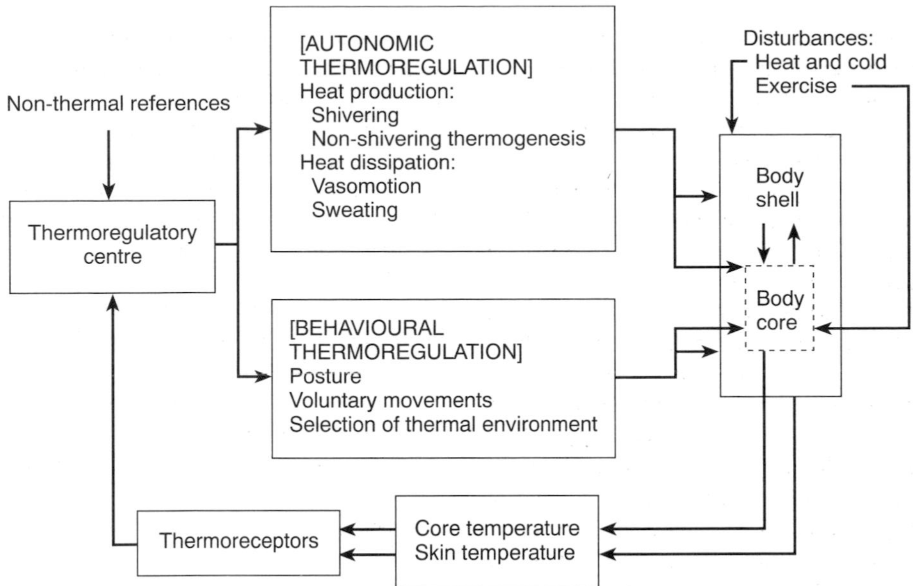

Fig. 10 The human thermoregulatory system. (Reproduced with permission from ref. 49.)

particularly sweating. The two types of thermosensitive neurones, warm-sensitive and cold-sensitive, are located in the preoptic and anterior hypothalamus (POAH). Warm-sensitive neurones respond to a rise in peripheral body temperature and are more abundant than cold-sensitive neurones which are activated by a decrease in peripheral temperature.

Body temperature is sensed at several crucial sites within the body, including specific thermoreceptors in the skin, spinal cord, and brainstem as well as thermal responses from the abdominal viscera. The POAH integrates thermal information from these sites and others in the body. Body temperature appears to be regulated to match a set-point. An abnormal upward shift of the set-point is believed to be the mechanism for production of fever. Additional control of the central thermoregulatory centre is mediated at several other sites in the brain with projections to the POAH, including the midbrain reticular formation, the raphe nucleus, the amygdala, the hippocampal formation, the sulcal prefrontal cortex, and the medial forebrain bundle. Thermoregulatory control of the hypothalamus can be modified by higher brain activity such as sleep, mental stress, and emotional excitement.

Hypercapnia, plasma osmolality, intravascular volume changes, and dehydration also alter the body temperature and set-point. Chemical mediators, including neurotransmitters such as catecholamines and acetylcholine and the eicosanoid prostaglandin E, play central roles in the control of normal thermoregulation as well as the expression of fever. Hypothalamic peptides including thyrotropin-releasing hormone, bombesin, neurotensin, ACTH, and vasopressin are also important in the modulation of central thermoregulation.

Autonomic control

The afferent input and efferent responses of thermoregulation are complex but are intimately coupled and controlled by both peripheral and central mechanisms (Fig. 11). The main thermoregulatory response affecting vasomotion and sweating is mediated through the autonomic system. The cutaneous vasculature is innervated mainly by adrenergic vasoconstrictor nerve fibres. Vasodilation and constriction are coordinated with sweating responses and interact to control blood flow and dissipate or preserve body heat. Sympathetic efferent pathways descend from the hypothalamus through the brainstem to the spinal cord and the preganglionic neurones. From here the fibres exit the cord and enter the sympathetic chain.

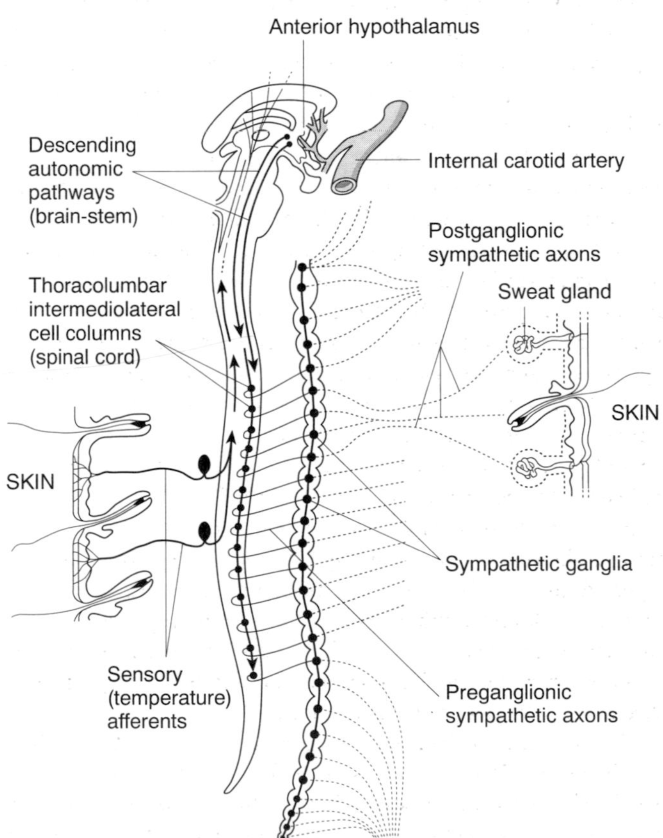

Fig. 11 Autonomic thermoregulatory sweat pathways: afferent and efferent limbs integrating temperature sensation and sudomotor response. (Reproduced with permission from ref. 50.)

Postganglionic sympathetic axons innervate sweat glands, blood vessels, and pilomotor muscles in skin. Eccrine glands are innervated by cholinergic fibres. Sweating is produced by both thermal and mental stimulation of eccrine glands, but the distribution and inciting factors causing the sudomotor response are different. Thermal sweating results from excess temperature that is perceived by the body. A local thermal stimulus will generate a uniform sweat response over the body surface while sparing the palms and soles.

The palms and soles show a baseline sweat pattern in the waking state, and mental excitement and stress will increase the rate. This response is called mental sweating. Mental sweating is controlled by the cerebral neocortex limbic system as well as by the hypothalamus. Thermal and mental sweating have some overlap in their central control but are also coordinated independently. General body surface sweating can be affected by various mental stresses. Mental sweating may augment or depress the thermal response of sweating over the body surface, but always increases sweating of the palms and soles. Axillary and, in some individuals, forehead sweating have a lower threshold to stimulation and are often active when there is no thermal sweating elsewhere.

Thermal sweating normally occurs uniformly over the body. Various factors, including body position, exercise, dehydration, sweat gland blood flow, ambient humidity, gender, and age, have also been shown to exert significant effects on the distribution, rate of production, activation thresholds, and other functional aspects of sweating. These factors must be taken into consideration in determining whether sweating responses are physiological or pathological.

Hyperhidrosis

In considering the palliative aspects of sweat dysfunction, most patients are typically bothered by hyperhidrosis (excessive sweating) or the distinctive symptom of nocturnal diaphoresis (night sweats).[51] A variety of underlying disorders contribute to localized or generalized hyperhidrosis (Table 6). Hyperhidrosis can be further classified as primary or secondary. It also should be appreciated that it may be a compensatory response to anhidrosis at other body sites (Fig. 12). Therefore the cause of hyperhidrosis should be determined if possible, and attempts should be made to alleviate underlying abnormalities that may induce pathological states of excessive or insufficient sweat production.

Table 6 Hyperhidrosis

Localized hyperhidrosis

Essential (primary)
Neurogenic
- Spinal cord disease
- Peripheral neuropathy
- Cerebrovascular disease (stroke)

Intrathoracic neoplasms or masses
Unilateral circumscribed
Cold-induced
Associated with cutaneous lesions
Gustatory

Generalized hyperhidrosis

Systemic illness
- Phaeochromocytoma
- Thyrotoxicosis
- Hypopituitarism
- Diabetes insipidus
- Diabetes mellitus
- Acromegaly
- Hypoglycaemia
- Carcinoid syndrome
- Menopause
- Tuberculosis
- Lymphoma
- Endocarditis
- Angina
- Malignancy

Nocturnal
Episodic
Medication-induced

Clinical evaluation

Determination of sweating abnormalities can be based on the clinical history and examination, or on more comprehensive evaluations such as thermoregulatory sweat testing or specific measurements such as quantitative sudomotor axon reflex tests (QSART).[50] QSART measures the pattern of sweat response and discriminates whether abnormalities in sweat production are pre- or postganglionic. Postganglionic abnormalities demonstrate alterations in the QSART while disturbances at the preganglionic level typically spare QSART function.

Thermoregulatory sweat testing assesses the integrity of the peripheral and central sympathetic sudomotor pathways.[50] Thermal stimulation is achieved by raising the skin temperature and the central or core body temperature. An environmentally controlled cabinet that warms the ambient air temperature to 45 to 50°C and also heats the skin with infrared lamps is used to raise central (oral or tympanic membrane) temperature and skin temperature to levels that stimulate sweating. Sweating on the skin surface is visualized with a special indicator powder containing iodinated corn starch,

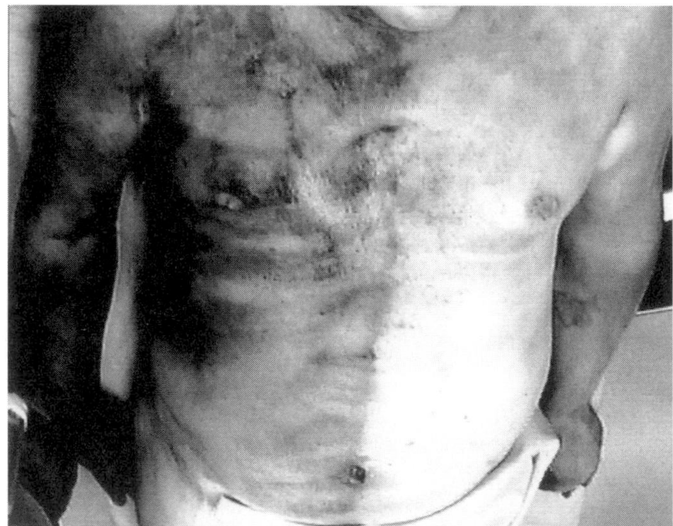

Fig. 12 Compensatory hyperhidrosis resulting from hemitruncal anhidrosis measured by thermoregulatory sweat testing (sweat indicated by dark areas). (By courtesy of Dr R. Fealey, Mayo Clinic.)

iodine solution, or alizarin-red-containing corn starch and sodium carbonate. Reduced or absent sweating can be delineated clearly (Fig. 12), and the distribution and extent of sweat loss is useful in further characterizing potential pathological abnormalities of the pre- or postganglionic pathways (Fig. 13) or the end organ, i.e. the sweat glands (Fig. 14).

Disruption of the sympathetic chain or white rami produces localized loss of sweating as can be seen with a Pancoast tumour involving the apical lung (Fig. 13). In contrast, irritation of the sympathetic chain by encroachment of a neoplasm such as bronchial carcinoma, mesothelioma, or osteoma may also produce ipsilateral hyperhidrosis.[52] Stroke rarely causes contralateral hyperhidrosis if large infarcts affect both the superficial and deep cerebral structures. Basilar artery strokes have been known to produce focal symmetrical sweating.

Generalized or regionalized hyperhidrosis

Generalized hyperhidrosis occurs with various systemic diseases including endocrine disorders, menopause, infections, lymphomas and other cancers, carcinoid syndrome, and drug withdrawal.[53] Endocrine disturbances observed to cause excessive sweating include acromegaly, diabetes mellitus, diabetes insipidus, hypopituitarism, hypoglycaemia thyrotoxicosis, and phaeochromocytoma. Drugs reported to cause hyperhidrosis include opioid analgesics such as morphine, diamorphine, methadone, butorphanol, and pentazocine, antidepressants such as fluoxetine, acyclovir and naproxen. If patients experience significant symptoms of sweat excess as a result of a particular medication, switching to an alternative drug may provide significant relief. Although the mechanism producing hyperhidrosis is not clearly understood and may be different for each of these causes, a downward shift of the set-point of the POAH could stimulate inappropriate sweating.

The patient may confuse excessive regionalized sweating with generalized hyperhidrosis. Compensatory hyperhidrosis may occur within normal sweat-producing areas of the skin in response to anhidrosis that involves other areas of the skin. The patient may not notice the loss of sweating, but, rather, experiences discomfort from the exaggerated sweating response. In this case, detection of the underlying cause of the loss of sweating would guide further treatment and appropriate management for symptomatic hyperhidrosis.

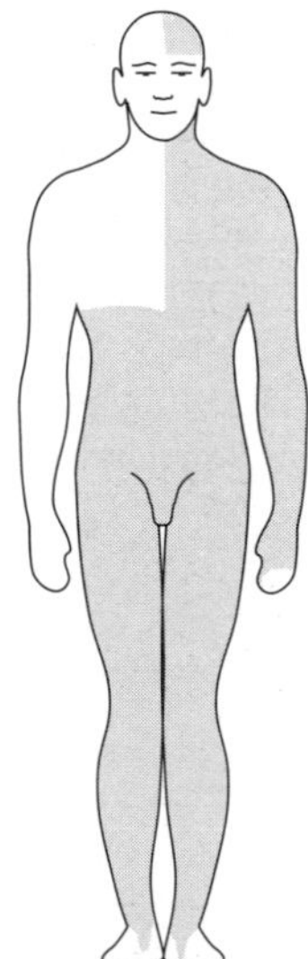

Fig. 13 Anhidrosis (light coloured areas) of the right head, upper trunk, and upper extremity due to a right-sided Pancoast tumour. Distal sweat loss is due to peripheral neuropathy. (Reproduced with permission from ref. 50.)

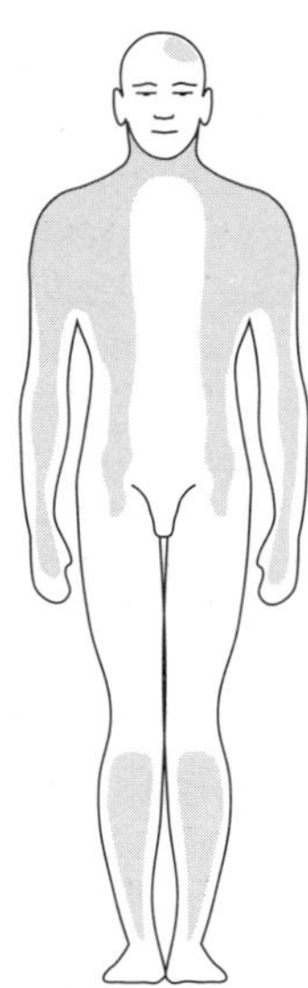

Fig. 14 Loss of sweating in the distribution of the truncal radiation port. Anhidrosis is caused by damage to the dermis and loss of sweat gland function. (Reproduced with permission from ref. 50.)

Treatment of sweating

The management of hyperhidrosis is based on identifying the primary cause underlying the abnormal sweat response as well as eliminating any potential aggravating factors that may further augment sweating. Primary hyperhidrosis will not be considered in the discussion of the palliative management of sweating. A variety of therapies offer benefit in treatment of primary hyperhidrosis but are not usually applicable to management of secondary hyperhidrosis.[54]

Hot flushes

Hot flushes are a prominent cause of excessive sweating in patients with cancer.[55-57] A detailed discussion of the proposed pathophysiological mechanisms for this problem is outside the scope of this chapter but can be found in ref.55. Hot flushes classically occur in menopausal women and are associated with oestrogen depletion. Breast cancer survivors are not exempt from this clinical problem; in fact, they are more at risk for several reasons. First, adjuvant chemotherapy given to premenopausal women can frequently result in premature ovarian failure with all the sequelae of oestrogen-depletion problems; second the commonly used anti-oestrogen, tamoxifen, causes hot flushes as its most common toxicity; third, general clinical practice has been to deny hormone replacement therapy to these women because of theoretical concerns that oestrogen replacement might harm them.

Given that breast cancer is a commonly diagnosed cancer whose incidence is rising, particularly among younger women, and that hot flushes are a very common clinical problem, what therapeutic options are available? Potential options can be grouped into two classes: hormonal and non-hormonal. Non-hormonal options are considered first. Drugs investigated in this category include Bellergal (a proprietary compound composed of ergotamine tartarate, laevorotatory alkaloids, and phenobarbital),[58] methyldopa,[59] and clonidine.[60] The beneficial effects from these medications are relatively small. To illustrate this effect, a double-blind placebo-controlled clinical trial demonstrated that clonidine produced a statistically significant decrease ($p<0.0001$) in hot flushes in breast cancer survivors , but only to a clinically moderate degree at best (17 per cent greater reduction in hot flush frequency from clonidine than from placebo).[60] In addition, the clonidine was blamed for significantly more mouth dryness ($p<0.0001$), constipation ($p<0.02$), and drowsiness ($p<0.05$) than was the placebo. Thus these non-hormonal therapies are not very helpful for patients with hot flushes.

Vitamin E (400–800 IU daily) has been recommended for treatment of hot flushes in women's health literature,[61,62] nursing journals,[63] and even an American National Breast Cancer Prevention Trial. Despite these recommendations, it is clearly stated in the United States Pharmacy Dispensing Drug Information Book that vitamin E has not been proved effective for treatment of menopausal syndromes.[64] In addition, a current Medline search revealed no support for the use of vitamin E to treat menopausal symptoms. However, literature published in the 1940s reported that vitamin E was efficacious in menopausal women who could not take oestrogen therapy.[65–67] A randomized placebo-controlled trial aimed at improving understanding of the efficacy of vitamin E for hot flushes is currently underway in the North Central Cancer Treatment Group.

Turning to hormonal therapeutic options, a number of pilot trials strongly suggested that progestational drugs could alleviate hot flushes in women.[68–73] A placebo-controlled randomized clinical trial reported recently definitively demonstrated that low-dose megestrol acetate (40 mg/day) can decrease hot flushes (by 74 per cent compared with a placebo reduction of 27 per cent) in breast cancer survivors.[74] The drug's full effect on hot flushes commonly takes 2 to 3 weeks to occur. Megestrol acetate was effective for patients whether or not they were receiving concomitant tamoxifen therapy. The only acute treatment-related side-effect noted in this trial was withdrawal menstrual bleeding, which commonly occurred 2 to 3 weeks after stopping megestrol acetate. We recommend a starting megestrol acetate dose of 40 mg/day for clinical practice. At 1-month intervals, the dose can be titrated by increments of 10 to 20 mg to establish the lowest dose that effectively controls hot flushes. We recommend warning breast cancer survivors that the effect of low-dose progesterones on breast cancer risk is not fully understood. It can be argued theoretically that this treatment might either increase or decrease the risk of subsequent breast cancer, but any effect is expected to be small.[74]

The use of oestrogen can sometimes be considered for treatment of hot flushes or other clinical problems associated with oestrogen depletion in breast cancer survivors. Although this may sound heretical to many, there is much uncertainty about the theoretical risks of oestrogen replacement therapy on breast cancer,[75] and many potential benefits are ascribed to oestrogen replacement therapy in women.[76,77] Instead of denying oestrogen therapy to all breast cancer survivors and thus being governed by the 'knee-jerk' response that 'oestrogen should never be used in a patient with a history of breast cancer', the pros and cons of the use of this therapy should be individualized in breast cancer survivors in the same manner as should be done in women in general. This topic is the focus of substantial research efforts at present, and it is hoped that new insights into this matter should become apparent in the near future.

Another group of cancer patients who suffer from hot flushes are men who have had androgen ablation therapy for prostate cancer. Hot flushes affect approximately 75 per cent of such men and can be a very substantial problem.[56,57,74,78] Recent placebo-controlled trials demonstrate that clonidine does not appear to decrease hot flushes in men.[78] However, low-dose megestrol acetate alleviates hot flushes in men as well as it does in women.[74] Low-dose megestrol acetate is without any apparent toxicity in prostate cancer patients who have undergone an orchidectomy.

Treatment of other causes of sweating

Another cause of sweating is related to fever. Sweating is a physiological response to fever, and documented fevers that elicit diaphoresis either during or following the episodes need to be investigated and treated appropriately. Sweating can be a prominent clinical problem in patients with advanced cancer who have tumour fever. Antipyretic agents such as aspirin and paracetamol (acetaminophen) appear to reduce fever by resetting the POAH set-point, and these agents improve symptoms, including sweating, that are associated with fever. At times, however, patients with tumour fever are relatively asymptomatic while they are febrile, but they may perspire and chill during defervescence. A simple solution to this problem is to discontinue antipyretic medications. Asymptomatic fever may continue but symptomatic periods of defervescence decrease. Another method of treating tumour fever is to use non-aspirin-containing non-steroidal anti-inflammatory drugs (NSAIDs) such as naproxen. These drugs can be remarkably successful in alleviating tumour fevers and associated sweating.[79–81] While the efficacy may cease after a period of weeks or months, switching to another NSAID may again induce defervescence.[79]

Sweating may be a chronic and prominent concern for many patients who do not have any malignancy or infectious aetiology. Even in patients with malignancy, where antipyretic therapies have either been instituted or discontinued to attempt symptom relief, diaphoresis may continue to be a major symptom. Various medications, including H_2-antagonists, have been tried empirically in attempts to provide relief. Although a specific mechanism of action is not well defined and documented clinical trials are lacking, clinical experience has indicated marked benefit from cimetidine (400–800 mg twice daily) in both idiopathic and malignancy-associated sweating. Whether other newer H_2-blockers exhibit a better or worse clinical response is not known. It is hoped that improved therapies will follow as the peripheral and central neural control of sweating becomes better understood.

References

1. Winkelmann RK, Muller SA. Pruritus. *Annual Reviews of Medicine*, 1964; **15**:53–64.
2. Bernhard JD. *Itch: Mechanisms and Management of Pruritus.* New York: McGraw-Hill, 1994.
3. Winkelmann RK. Dermatological clinics. 1. Comments on pruritus related to systemic disease. *Mayo Clinic Proceedings*, 1961; **36**:187–96.
4. Gilchrest BA. Pruritus: pathogenesis, therapy, and significance in systemic disease states. *Archives of Internal Medicine*, 1982; **142**:101–5.
5. Denman ST. A review of pruritus. *Journal of the American Academy of Dermatology*, 1986; **14**:375–92.

6. McMahon SB, Koltzenburg M. Itching for an explanation. *Trends in Neurological Sciences*, 1992; **15**:497–501.
7. Wallengren J. The pathophysiology of itch. *European Journal of Dermatology*, 1993; **3**:643–7.
8. Hägermark O. Peripheral and central mediators of itch. *Skin Pharmacology*, 1992; **5**:1–8.
9. Bernstein JE. Capsaicin and substance P. *Clinics in Dermatology*, 1992; **9**:497–503.
10. Winkelmann RK. Cutaneous sensory nerves. *Seminars in Dermatology*, 1988; **7**:236–68.
11. Handwerker HO, Forster C, Kirchhoff C. Discharge patterns of human C-fibres induced by itching and burning stimuli. *Journal of Neurophysiology*, 1991; **66**:307–15.
12. Head H. The afferent nervous system from a new aspect. *Brain*, 1905; **28**:99–115.
13. Lowitt MH, Bernhard JD. Pruritus. *Seminars in Neurology*, 1992; **12**:374–84.
14. Bergasa NV *et al.* Effects of naloxone infusions in patients with the pruritus of cholestasis. *Annals of Internal Medicine*, 1995; **123**:161–7.
15. Khandelwal M, Malet PF. Pruritis associated with cholestasis: a review of pathogenesis and management. *Digestive Diseases Sciences*, 1994; **39**:1–7.
16. Schworer H, Ramadori G. Treatment of pruritus: a new indication for serotonin type 3 receptor antagonists. *Clinical Investigation*, 1993; **71**:659–62.
17. Raderer M, Muller C, Scheithauer W. Ondansetron for pruritus due to cholestasis. *New England Journal of Medicine*, 1994; **330**:1540.
18. Melzack R and Wall PD. Pain mechanisms: a new theory. *Science*, 1965; **150**:971–9.
19. Carlsson C-A, Augustinsson L-E, Lund S, Roupe G. Electrical transcutaneous nerve stimulation for relief of itch. *Experientia*, 1975; **31**:191.
20. Monk BE. Transcutaneous electronic nerve stimulation in the treatment of generalized pruritus. *Clinical and Experimental Dermatology*, 1993; **18**:67–8.
21. Paul R, Paul R, Jansen CT. Itch and malignancy prognosis in generalized pruritus: A 6-year-follow-up of 125 patients. *Journal of the American Academy of Dermatology*, 1987; **16**:1179–82.
22. Kantor GR, Lookingbill DP. Generalized pruritus and systemic disease. *Journal of the American Academy of Dermatology*, 1983; **9**:375–8.
23. Doyle JA, Connolly SM, Hunziker N, Winkelmann RK. Prurigo nodularis: a reappraisal of the clinical and histological features. *Journal of Cutaneous Pathology*, 1979; **6**:392–403.
24. Arndt KA, Bowers KE, Chuttani AR. *Manual of Dermatological Therapeutics: With Essentials of Diagnosis.* 5th edn. New York: Little, Brown, 1995: 145–8, 317–22.
25. Fransway AF, Winkelmann RK. Treatment of pruritus. *Seminars in Dermatology*, 1988; **7**:310–25.
26. Winkelmann RK. Pharmacologic control of pruritus. *Medical Clinics of North America*, 1982; **66**:1119–33.
27. Lorette G, Vaillant L. Pruritus: current concepts in pathogenesis and treatment. *Drugs*, 1990; **39**:218–23.
28. Ghent CN, Carruthers SG. Treatment of pruritus in primary biliary cirrhosis with rifampin. *Gastroenterology*, 1988; **94**:488–93.
29. Gregorio GV, Ball CS, Mowat AP, Mieli-Vergani G. Effect of rifampicin in the treatment of pruritus in hepatic cholestasis. *Archives of Disease in Childhood*, 1993; **69**:141–3.
30. Whitington PF, Whitington GL. Partial external diversion of bile for the treatment of intractable pruritus associated with intrahepatic cholestasis. *Gastroenterology*, 1988; **95**:130–6.
31. Marchi S, Cechin E, Villalta D, Sepiacci G, Santini G, Bartoli E. Relief of pruritus and decreases in plasma histamine concentrations during erythropoietin therapy in patients with uremia. *New England Journal of Medicine*, 1992; **326**:969–74.
32. Hampers C, Katz A, Wilson R, Merril J. Disappearance of uraemic itching after subtotal parathyroidectomy. *New England Journal of Medicine*, 1986; **279**:695–700.
33. Gilchrist B, Rowe J, Brown R, Steinman T, Arndt K. Relief of uraemic pruritus with ultraviolet phototherapy. *New England Journal of Medicine*, 1977; **297**:136–8.
34. Finelli C, Gugliotta L, Gamberi B, Vianelli N, Visani G, Tura S. Relief of intractable pruritus in polycythemia vera with recombinant interferon alfa. *American Journal of Hematology*, 1993; **43**:316–18.
35. Riccardi VM. A controlled multiphase trial of ketotifen to minimize neurofibroma-associated pain and itching. *Archives of Dermatology*, 1993; **129**:577–81.
36. Soter NA, Austin KF, Wasserman SI. Oral disodium cromoglycate in the treatment of systemic mastocytosis. *New England Journal of Medicine*, 1979; **301**:465–9.
37. Leven A *et al.* Sodium cromoglycate and Hodgkin's pruritus. *British Medical Journal*, 1979; **2**:896.
38. Winkelmann RK *et al.* Thalidomide treatment of prurigo nodularis. *Acta Dermato-Venereologica*, 1984; **64**:412–17.
39. Silva SRB, Viana PCF, Lugon NV, Hoette M, Ruzany F, Lugon JR. Thalidomide for the treatment of uraemic pruritus: a crossover randomized double-blind trial. *Nephrology*, 1994; **67**:270–3.
40. Levy M, Catalano R. Control of common physical symptoms other than pain in patients with terminal disease. *Seminars in Oncology*, 1985; **12**:411–30.
41. Tapia L, Cheigh JS, Davis DS, Sullivan JF, Saal S, Reidenberg MM. Pruritus in dialysis patients treated with parenteral lidocaine. *New England Journal of Medicine*, 1977; **296**:261–2.
42. Borgeat A, Wilder-Smith OHG, Mentha G. Subhypnotic doses of propofol relieve pruritus associated with liver disease. *Gastroenterology*, 1993; **104**:244–7.
43. Borgeat A, Savioz D, Mentha G, Giostra E, Suter PM. Intractable cholestatic pruritus after liver transplantation–management with propofol. *Transplantation*, 1994; **58**:727–30.
44. Borgeat A, Wilder-Smith OHG, Saiah M, Rifat K. Subhypnotic doses of propofol relieve pruritus induced by epidural and intrathecal morphine. *Anesthiology*, 1992; **76**:510–12.
45. Willner C, Low PA. Pharmacologic approaches to neuropathic pain. In: Dyck P, Thomas PK, Griffin JW, Low PA, Poduslo JF, eds. *Peripheral Neuropathy.* 3rd edn. Philadelphia, PA: Saunders, 1993: 1700–20.
46. Fried RG. Evaluation and treatment of 'psychogenic' pruritus and self-excoriation. *Journal of the American Academy of Dermatology*, 1994; **30**:993–9.
47. Hagermark KO. Influence of antihistamines, sedatives and aspirin on experimental itch. *Acta Dermato-Venereologica*, 1973; **53**:363–8.
48. Jones EA, Bergasa NV. The pruritus of cholestasis: from bile acids to opiate agonists. *Hepatology*, 1990; **11**:884–7.
49. Ogawa T, Low P. Autonomic regulation of temperature and sweating. In: Low PA, ed. *Clinical Autonomic Disorders: Evaluation and Management.* Boston, MA: Little, Brown, 1992: 79–91.
50. Fealey RD. The thermoregulatory sweat test. In: Low PA, ed. *Clinical Autonomic Disorders: Evaluation and Management.* Boston, MA: Little, Brown, 1992: 217–29.
51. Lea MJ, Aber RC. Descriptive epidemiology of night sweats upon admission to a university hospital. *Southern Medical Journal*, 1985; **78**:1065–7.
52. Walsh JC, Low PA, Allsop JL. Localized sympathetic overactivity: an uncommon complication of lung cancer. *Journal of Neurology, Neurosurgery and Psychiatry*, 1976; **39**:93–5.
53. Freeman R, Waldorf HA, Dover JS. Autonomic neurodermatology (Part II): disorders of sweating and flushing. *Seminars in Neurology*, 1992; **12**:394–407.
54. White JW. Treatment of primary hyperhidrosis. *Mayo Clinic Proceedings*, 1986; **61**:951–6.
55. Casper RF, Yen SSC. Neuroendocrinology of menopausal flushes: an hypothesis of flush mechanism. *Clinical Endocrinology*, 1985; **22**:293–312.

56. Charig CR, Rundle JS. Flushing: Long-term side effect of orchiectomy in treatment of prostatic carcinoma. *Urology*, 1989; **33**:175–8.
57. Quella S, Loprinzi CL, Dose AM. A qualitative approach to defining 'hot flashes' in men. *Urological Nursing*, 1994; **14**:155–8.
58. Bergmans MGM, Merkus JMWM, Corbey RS, Schellekens LA, Ubachs JM. Effect of Bellergal retard on climacteric complaints: a double-blind, placebo-controlled study. *Maturitas*, 1987; **9**:227–34.
59. Young RL, Kumar NS, Goldzieher JW. Management of menopause when oestrogen cannot be used. *Drugs*, 1990; **40**:220–30.
60. Goldberg RM *et al*. Transdermal clonidine for ameliorating tamoxifen-induced hot flushes. *Journal of Clinical Oncology*, 1994; **12**:155–8.
61. Seaman B, Seaman G. *Women and the Crisis in Sex Hormones*, New York: Bantam, 1979.
62. Murray M. *Menopause*, Rocklin, CA: Prima, 1994.
63. Cutick R. Special needs of perimenopausal and menopausal women. *JOGN Nursing*, 1984; **13**:68s–73s.
64. United States Pharmacopeia Dispensing Information, Vitamin E. Drug information for the health care professional. *United States Pharmacopeial Convention*, 1991; **1**:2596.
65. Finkler RS. The effect of vitamin E in the menopause. *Journal of Clinical Endocrinology and Metabolism*; 1949; **9**:89–94.
66. Christy C. Vitamin E in menopause. *American Journal of Obstetrics and Gynecology*, 1945; **50**:84–7.
67. McLaren HC. Vitamin E in menopause. *British Medical Journal*, 1949; **2**:1378–82.
68. Erlik Y, Meldrum DR, Lagasse LD, Jidd HL. Effect of megestrol acetate on flushing and bone metabolism in post-menopausal women. *Maturitas*, 1981; **3**:167–72.
69. Bullock JL, Massey FM, Gambrell RD Jr. Use of medroxyprogesterone acetate to prevent menopausal symptoms. *Obstetrics and Gynecology*, 1975; **46**:165–8.
70. Morrison JC *et al*. The use of medroxyprogesterone acetate for relief of climacteric symptoms. *American Journal of Obstetrics and Gynecology*, 1980; **138**:99–104.
71. Albrecht BH, Schiff I, Tulchinsky D, Ryan KJ. Objective evidence that placebo and oral medroxyprogesterone acetate therapy diminish menopausal vasomotor flushes. *American Journal of Obstetrics and Gynecology*, 1981; **139**:631–5.
72. Young RL, Kumar NS, Goldzieher JW. Management of menopause when oestrogen cannot be used. *Drugs*, 1990; **40**:220–30.
73. Schiff I, Tulchinsky D, Cramer D, Ryan KJ. Oral medroxyprogesterone in the treatment of postmenopausal symptoms. *Journal of the American Medical Association*, 1980; **244**:1443–5.
74. Loprinzi CL *et al*. Megestrol acetate for the prevention of hot flushes. *New England Journal of Medicine*, 1994; **331**:347–52.
75. Cobleigh MA *et al*. Oestrogen replacement therapy in breast cancer survivors. *Journal of the American Medical Association*, 1994; **272**:540–5.
76. American College of Obstetricians and Gynecologists. *Hormone Replacement Therapy*. Washington, DC: American College of Obstetricians and Gynecologists, 1992: 166.
77. Wiklund I *et al*. A new methodological approach to the evaluation of quality of life in postmenopausal women. *Maturitas*, 1992; **14**:211–24.
78. Loprinzi CL *et al*. Transdermal clonidine for ameliorating post-orchiectomy hot flushes. *Journal of Urology*, 1994; **151**:634–6.
79. Tsavaris N *et al*. A randomized trial of the effect of three non-steroid anti-inflammatory agents in ameliorating cancer-induced fever. *Journal of Internal Medicine*, 1990; **228**:451–5.
80. Chang JC, Gross HM. Utility of naproxen in the differential diagnosis of fever of undetermined origin in patients with cancer. *American Journal of Medicine*, 1984; **76**:597–603.
81. Chang JC, Hawley HB. Neutropenic fever of undetermined origin (N-FUO): why not use the naproxen test? *Cancer Investigation*, 1995; **13**:448–50.

9.6.3 Nursing aspects

Catherine Miller

Introduction

The skin is the largest and most visible organ of the body. It weighs 6 to 8 lb (2.7–3.6 kg) and covers more than 20 square feet (1.86 m^2). This organ is often at risk of damage or subsequent breakdown in patients with advanced cancer. This may be directly or indirectly related to the underlying cancer. Direct causes are fungating breast lesions, sarcomas, malignant melanomas, and any solid tumour that erodes through the surface of the skin. Indirect causes include poor nutritional status, drug therapy, radiotherapy, and reduced mobility resulting in pressure ulcers.

In this chapter we concentrate on nursing assessment, the evaluation and management of patients with skin lesions, and in particular the nursing management of fungating and ulcerating malignant lesions, external fistulas causing skin excoriation, and pressure ulcers. When medical intervention (surgery, radiotherapy, chemotherapy, hormone therapy, or immunotherapy) is no longer appropriate, care is directed towards minimization of pain, infection, bleeding, and odour.[1] Awareness of, and sensitivity to, the psychological problems that the patient with a malignant lesion may be experiencing is equally as important as the control of physical symptoms.[2] This highlights the need to treat not only the wound, but the patient as a whole.

Fungating and ulcerating malignant lesions

The nature of the lesions

In most of the literature relating to fungating skin lesions they are assumed to be most commonly associated with carcinoma of the breast.[1,3–6] However, almost any internal malignancy can give rise to cutaneous metastases.[7] Ulcerating and fungating malignant lesions may appear at the site of the primary cancer or at a secondary site related to metatastic disease. Patients with such lesions invariably have a poor prognosis and suffer not only the physical symptoms of tissue breakdown and disfigurement but also the psychological effects of a lesion that may be impossible to heal. This will have an impact not only on the patient but also on his or her family, and the approach to intervention should encompass supportive family care.

Medical and surgical interventions

Of course, the treatment of choice for fungating lesions is eradication of the problem. This can sometimes be achieved by either local or systemic treatment. Local measures include surgical intervention by way of myocutaneous flaps or surgical debridement which can improve the appearance, exudate, and odour. Radiotherapy can reduce the size of the lesion and have a haemostatic effect, and chemotherapy and hormonal therapy can result in regression of the disease, depending on the tumour type.

When such treatments are no longer successful or appropriate, the care of the intractable wounds often comes within the role of the nurse. It is important that nurses caring for patients with malignant lesions have an up-to-date knowledge of the research-tested treatments available so that they can initiate appropriate nursing interventions which aim to improve the quality of life of these patients and their families.

The following case history illustrates the appropriate use of surgery to alleviate difficult symptoms and highlights the need for co-operation of disciplines in providing palliative care.

Case history

A 57-year-old woman with advanced carcinoma of the breast was referred for the control of pain, predominantly arising from the chest area and surrounding tissue. Figure 1 illustrates extensive recurrence following a left mastectomy for primary carcinoma of the breast some 18 months previously. The photograph shows bilateral cutaneous spread of tumour and extensive ulceration from the suprasternal area to the left lower border of her rib cage. The problems that the patient experienced were both physical and psychological.

1. The lesions were infected and extremely painful when dressings were changed.
2. The lesions bled profusely and this particularly distressed the patient.
3. The odour of and exudate from the wound had made this woman a virtual recluse at home, creating family difficulties.
4. The size and irregular shape of the cutaneous spread and the body contour of this woman made it difficult to find a dressing which was unobtrusive under normal clothing.
5. The number of dressing changes required each day severely curtailed the patient's independence and normal daily activity.

After reassessment as an inpatient and using conventional dressing techniques, it was apparent that her quality of life and independence were not improved. Palliative radiotherapy was not possible as she had already received a maximum dose to the chest wall following her mastectomy (Fig. 1 also shows the skin pigmentation on the chest wall resulting from radiotherapy). The option of surgery was discussed with the patient and her family, and the possibility of another mastectomy was raised. The patient and her family felt that if surgical intervention could restore some quality of life and reduce the pain and constant reminder of cancer and death, this treatment was appropriate. A right mastectomy was performed with a wide excision of the left chest wall and a rectus-abdominus flap was lifted to provide a good cosmetic appearance. Figure 2 shows the appearance a week postoperatively with the flap viable and the drains removed. The effect upon the patient was dramatic, not only because pain was alleviated but more importantly because she felt that her confidence and her ability to participate within the family unit had been restored. Figure 3 shows the patient 1 month after surgery. The return home was a great moment for both the patient and family, marking a period of re-evaluation and cohesiveness that allowed the family unit some 'prime' time together. This palliative intervention gave the family an extra 7 months of quality and normality that other conventional modes of intervention could not achieve. The patient died peacefully, returning to the palliative care unit only days before her death.

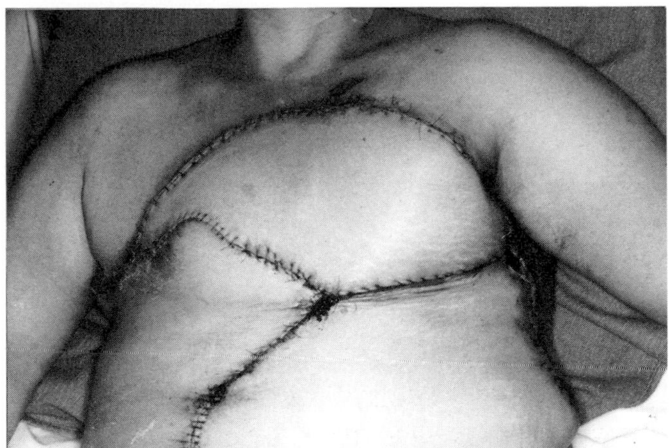

Fig. 2 Appearance of the wound 1 week after a right mastectomy in the patient illustrated in Fig. 1.

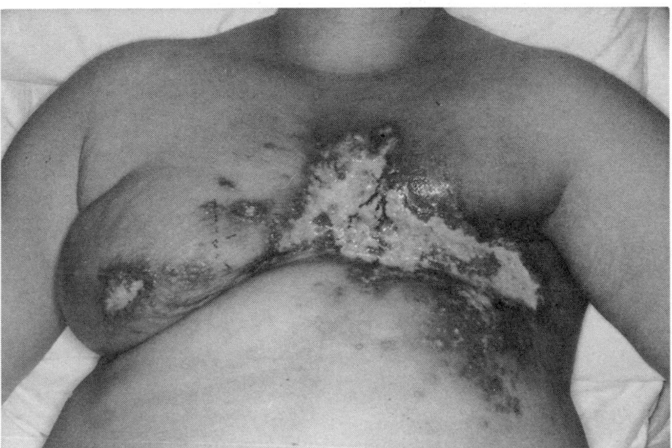

Fig. 1 Extensive recurrent disease following a left mastectomy for primary carcinoma of the breast some 18 months previously.

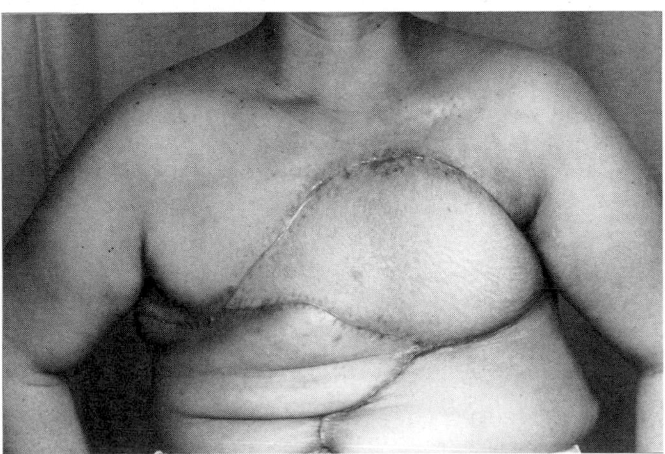

Fig. 3 The patient illustrated in Figs. 1 and 2 1 month after surgery.

Assessment

If a malignant wound is to be managed effectively, a comprehensive assessment of the patient must be carried out.[8] This assessment should address the following:

(1) the history of the lesion including how long it has been present, previous treatments received, and their effectiveness;

(2) the physical properties of the lesion including its diameter, depth, colour, and odour

(where appropriate, photography can be used as a baseline to assess subsequent progress);

(3) the bacteriological status of the wound and the presence of any exudate or bleeding;

(4) factors which may exacerbate the condition of the lesion (e.g. previous radiotherapy, poor nutritional status, drug therapies, and disease progression);

(5) pain associated with the lesion;

(6) the psychosocial impact of the lesion (e.g. depression, altered body image, anxiety, shame, embarrassment, and isolation);

(7) the patient's home situation, establishing the need for support in coping with the wound at home if necessary.

Further tools for the assessment of fungating malignant wounds are being developed.[9,10] One technique involves ultrasound examination. This technology was developed in the mid 1980s when a high-frequency ultrasound transducer (20 MHz) was incorporated into a portable handset which could be used as a diagnostic ultrasound scanner for skin lesions and fungating wounds. However, Grocott[10,11] found that there was insufficient penetration of thick layers of slough and necrosis so that the image quality was poor. This technique is not suitable as an assessment tool for the group of patients with this type of wound presentation. Patient discomfort was also a limiting factor as the need to hold one position for a long period of time during this procedure was difficult for some individuals.

Photographic recording of wounds using a special camera designed to take two-dimensional views of the surface characteristics of wounds has also been employed, but this technique also has limitations. It requires that the camera angle and patient position are consistent, and this is difficult to ensure in some patients because of the relative inaccessibility of the wound sites.

One must not underestimate the importance of continuity of assessment and intervention, realizing the effectiveness of the observations of patients themselves and carers as well as their goals and priorities. This aspect of wound management will continue to be a challenging area in the future.

Nursing management of fungating lesions (Fig. 4)

Wound cleansing

Physical management of these wounds is often governed by product availability in both hospitals and the community. Ease of treatment is particularly important; patients at home often rely on district nurses and therefore it is advisable to avoid labour-intensive dressings where possible. These wounds should be cleaned with normal saline, which does not have a detrimental effect on granulating tissue.[12]

A variety of cleansing solutions have been tested on various wounds. Antiseptics such as chlorhexidine, iodine, and cetrimide have been shown to be toxic to baby hamster kidney fibroblasts in culture.[13] This toxicity occurred even when low dilutions were used. Hypochlorites can cause irreparable damage to new capillary buds in the granulating wound and should not be used as desloughing agents.[12–15] Most antiseptics and hypochlorites are rapidly inactivated by body fluids and therefore their cleansing action is mostly mechanical.[16] This action could be achieved more safely by allowing patients to shower or bath with ordinary tapwater.[17,18]

Indications for wound cleansing are when excess exudate is profuse and causing discomfort, or when the wound is obviously infected. Irrigation with normal saline or water is preferable as mechanical cleansing with swabs can be painful and traumatic.[19]

Wound dressing

Criteria for ideal wound dressings

The tissue within a fungating ulcer is fragile. It tends to bleed easily to the touch, it may produce large amounts of exudate, and it may also be malodorous. In treating these ulcers, special attention should be directed towards haemostasis, odour restriction, absorption of exudate, comfort, and cosmetic appearance.

The characteristics of an ideal wound dressing are well documented.[20,21] For the management of malignant ulcers we suggest that the dressing should satisfy the following criteria.

1. It should allow the removal of excess wound exudate and toxic compounds. As exudate is drawn out of the wound, so too are toxins, dead cells, and micro-organisms. This process helps to relieve swelling and pain by reducing tissue oedema. The dressing should be capable of absorbing wound exudate.

2. It should not adhere to the wound surface as it will literally tear away epidermal cells and granulation tissue on removal, causing trauma and pain.

3. It should allow a high humidity to be maintained. Epithelial cells require a moist environment in order to migrate across the wound surface. If the wound is dry, healing is delayed and a dry painful eschar forms.

4. It should allow gaseous exchange. Varghese *et al.*[22] examined fluid collection beneath occlusive dressings and noted that the oxygen tension (Po_2) was zero or very low. The low pH underneath hydrocolloid dressings is believed to have an inhibiting effect on the growth of some bacteria, particularly Pseudomonas species. A low Po_2 beneath these dressings assists in a more rapid formation of capillaries, promoting granulation tissue in this anaerobic wound environment.[23] Capillary buds form, which develop into capillary loops. Thus the microcirculation of the wound site is restored, providing a supply of oxygen and nutrients.

5. It should be impermeable to bacteria. The dressing should not allow access to bacteria or allow the spread of pathogens from an infected wound.

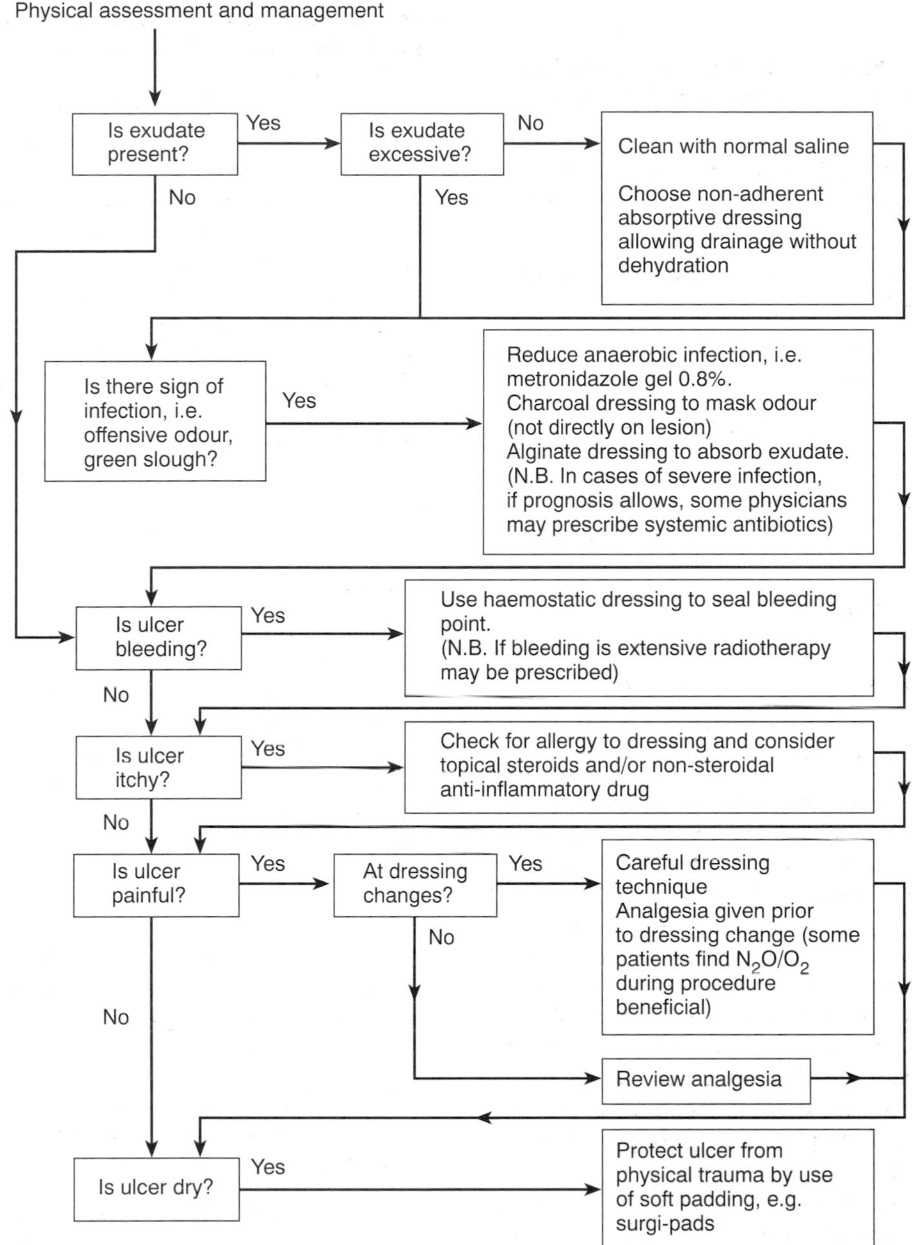

Fig. 4 An algorithm for managing fungating and malignant ulcers.

6. It should be thermally insulating. A constant temperature of 37°C is essential to maintain the biological processes of wound healing. This is important in treating malignant ulcers, as maintaining the temperature of the environment may reduce the amount of wound exudate.

7. It should be non-toxic and non-allergenic. The dressing should not produce toxic contaminants, i.e. it should be presented in a sterile form. Also, it should not thread or shed non-biodegradable fibres of any kind; these act as foreign bodies in the wound which can be a source of infection.

8. It should be comfortable and conforming. Where possible, the dressing should aim to conform to body symmetry. Bulky dressings can increase a patient's anxiety about his or her body image and cause social isolation. Any uncomfortable dressing can cause much distress as well as friction, and may also be constant reminder of its presence.

9. It should provide protection from further trauma. Any trauma to the lesion can cause further pain and/or haemorrhage. The wound should be covered with protective sterile padding as necessary for individual patients.

Many dressings are available and are designed to conform to these criteria in order to facilitate moist wound healing. Table 1 lists the composition and uses of the three main types of dressings.

Innovative practices in devising individually tailored wound support systems using a moulded foam latex have been described, providing a unique and comfortable system for a protruding or

Table 1 Wound management products

Type of dressing	Composition	Uses
Alginates	Mixed salts of alginic acid, derived from certain species of brown seaweed. Extraction of seaweed with dilute alkali produces sodium alginate, which is soluble in water and forms visual colloidal solution. The calcium in these dressings acts as a primary catalyst in the clotting process	Exuding wounds Haemostatic properties Bleeding lesions
Hydrogels	Insoluble polymers with hydrophilic sites which interact with aqueous solutions absorbing and retaining water	
Type 1	Fixed 3-dimensional macrostructure presented as a thin flexible sheet. This dressing absorbs fluid without changing its physical shape	Low exudate wounds
Type 2	Amorphous hydrogels do not possess a fixed macrostructure. As fluid is absorbed, viscosity decreases and the dressing can take up the shape of the wound that it covers	Leg ulcers Sloughy wounds Necrotic wounds
Hydrocolloid	Carboxymethylcellulose based; some contain other polysaccharides and proteins. Presented as a flexible foam or film sheet coated with a layer of the hydrocolloid base. The base may be available in the form of granules or paste, applied directly to the wound with an hydrocolloid sheet for added absorbency	Pressure area sites Exuding wounds Leg ulcers

eccentric-shaped wounds.[24] Figure 5 shows an example of moulded foam latex in a wound.

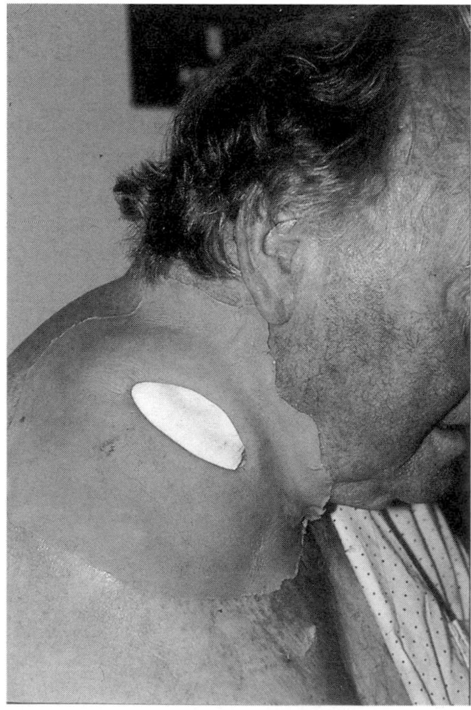

Fig. 5 A moulded foam latex filling a malignant ulcer.

Some creativity in individual wound management may achieve impressive results. In one patient the use of dental addition curing silicone rubber impression materials (a form of silicone rubber) creating a high viscosity putty to temporarily close an abdominal fistula was successfully employed, providing pain relief and independence for a young patient with advanced cancer.[25]

Managing malodorous wounds

The unique problem of unpleasant odour arising from malignant cutaneous manifestations and fistulas is due to two impact odours, putrescine (1,4-diaminopentane) and cadavarine (1,5-diaminopentane) which at their worst can cause a vomit or gag reflex in individuals. Habituation to these odours does not occur and individuals can constantly detect their presence. This can lead to grave psychological reactions which may lead to social withdrawal or depression, or to the patient's becoming a virtual social outcast.[26] This profound problem highlights a further area of research, fundamental-to-quality of life issues.

Activated charcoal dressings reduce the concentration of offensive odours to low levels.[27] Some dressings are said to absorb bacteria. It has been suggested that there could be an electrostatic or physicochemical affinity between the charcoal and the bacteria. During their preparation, charcoal fibres become microporous and develop thin slit-like pores; hence they have a high absorptive capacity.

Dressings alone are unable to control the odour of some fungating ulcers. In these circumstances a trial of metronidazole gel may be warranted. In a study involving 68 hospice patients, metronidazole gel 0.8 per cent was found to have an effective deodorizing action:[28] it was totally effective in 50 per cent of patients and reasonably effective in a further 46 per cent; it had no effect in only three patients. The gel is now commercially available and is a valuable treatment option for malodorous fungating lesions. If it fails, oral metronidazole may be necessary.[29]

Honey and icing sugar are two agents that have been used topically to treat malodorous ulcers.[30] It is thought that the sugar may exert its antibacterial effect by competing for the water present in the cells of bacteria. Yoghurt and buttermilk have also been used to prevent the growth of odour-forming micro-organisms. The efficacy of these treatments has not been properly evaluated in clinical studies.

Skin management of fistulas

A fistula is defined as an abnormal congenital or acquired communication between two hollow organs, or between a hollow organ and skin.[31] Enterocutaneous fistulas occur between the gut and the skin. In patients with advanced cancer this type of fistula is usually a complication of progressive intra-abdominal disease.

Radiation damage to the bowel may occur during radiotherapy to the pelvic region which can give rise to internal fistulas, often between the rectum and the vagina (rectovaginal) or between the rectum and bladder (rectovesical). Managing a patient with a fistula requires a systematic approach. Firstly the problems created by a fistula must be identified.

1. Damage to the skin: discharge of intestinal contents, particularly from the small bowel, will almost certainly cause skin deterioration.

2. Foul-smelling discharge, often of high output: odour from the discharge may provoke nausea and also make the patient feel a need to isolate him- or herself.

3. The site of the fistula (e.g. on an irregular body contour) and the nature of the output (e.g. highly acidic) often makes management difficult, leading to the need for more skin protection and increased dressing changes.

4. Malnourishment and loss of electrolytes: the higher the fistula the more severe this problem can be, leading to reduced healing powers and increased risks of infection.

5. Patient anxiety: long stays in hospital are frequently necessary for these patients. It can be a frightening and seemingly endless condition, reducing the morale of the patient, his or her family, and the staff.

Management of fistulas in patients with advanced cancer differs from that of patients in the intensive care unit. The aim is often not to eradicate the problem but to minimize symptoms and promote comfort. Most of the literature available today does not address the physical and psychological needs of patients with fistulas that are not going to heal spontaneously or be resolved with surgery.

Fistulas may be of two types: an internal fistula connects one hollow viscus to another, but without direct communication to the body surface (e.g. ileum to colon); an external or enterocutaneous fistula connects a hollow organ directly to the skin surface (e.g. ileum to skin). Patients with either of these types of fistula are likely to be in a poor nutritional state owing to their long illness and the treatment that they have received. Also, treatment such as long-term steroids, radiotherapy, and chemotherapy will result in poor wound healing. The aim in management of either type of fistula is the same. When surgery is no longer an option, nursing care should be directed toward the psychological support of the patient with this potentially devastating symptom of their disease. In an attempt to improve patients' morale the problem of odour, discharging bowel contents, and pain from skin excoriation should be dealt with as effectively as possible.

Aims of nursing care

Removal of odour

The smell from a fistula can be very offensive. Not only can this be very nauseating to the patient, but it also affects his or her self-esteem and is embarrassing if other patients and their families are aware of the smell. A well-fitted appliance should be odour proof, but there will always be a smell when the appliance is changed or emptied. One of the most effective ways to counteract this is to place a few drops of aromatherapy oil into a bowl and pour boiling water over it before the appliance is changed.[32] The resulting perfumed steam is much more effective and certainly more pleasant than many traditional stoma deodorants.

Collection of effluent

It is important that the appliance is suitable for the particular fistula, that it is comfortable, and that it has a leak-proof seal that will stay in situ for several days where possible. A guide to successful application of a drainage bag is given below.

1. Assess the fistula. Is the skin inflamed or excoriated? Is it close to a wound or any indentation in the skin? The size of the fistula opening, whether small and well defined, irregular in shape, or in the depths of a gaping wound, should be estimated.

2. How many openings are there? Are they close enough to be incorporated into one bag or do they require separate bags?

3. Assess the amount of drainage and its composition. Is it likely to be an irritant?

4. If the skin is intact, a plasticized skin dressing may prove a useful prophylactic measure. If it is sore and excoriated, application of calamine lotion is soothing and cooling, and dries weeping areas.

5. If the output of exudate is high, it will be necessary for an assistant to apply gentle suction to the mouth of the fistula to prevent spillage of discharge during the procedure.

6. Clean the fistula and surrounding skin with warm water and tissues. Do not use soap or antiseptics as they dry the skin and remove its protective oils, thereby reducing its water-repellent property.

7. The appliance must be attached to a flat surface to gain a proper seal. Therefore any creases or indentations in the skin must be filled until the surface is flat. Examples of 'fillers' are carmellose gelatin proprietary pastes for weeping sore areas and mucous membranes, cohesive ostomy seals, and skin protective wafers.

8. The skin surrounding the fistula must be completely protected, particularly if the output is a strong irritant. The hole in the adhesive of the bag or wafer should be cut as closely as possible to the shape of the fistula.

9. Applying stomahesive paste to the skin edges increases the protection and improves the seal.

10. The choice of appliance depends on the size of the fistula, the condition of the skin, and the output. Sore moist skin will need an appliance with a backing that absorbs a certain amount of moisture, for example those with a stomahesive or cohesive backing. Appliances with large areas of backing help adherence, particularly with high-output fistulas. Light pressure to the appliance for about a minute helps to ensure a good seal. 'Picture framing' the appliance with a hypoallergenic tape also helps to secure and support it.

11. The bag should be emptied frequently to prevent the weight of the effluent pulling it off the skin. Patients who are ambulant can be taught to empty their own bags. High-output fistulas which need emptying more frequently than every 2 h will need an extension tube and a collecting device, for example a urostomy appliance and night drainage system.

12. The appliance should be changed before, not after, it leaks in order to prevent skin excoriation. If a patient experiences burning or irritation beneath the appliance it should be removed and renewed as this is usually an indication of leakage. Very rarely a fistula is not 'baggable', for example if it is situated in a very large wound or the skin is so excoriated that a bag will not adhere. Suction tubes may need to be inserted and low-pressure suction applied. However, it is often difficult to obtain a complete seal and so the surrounding skin will still need to be protected, for example with a skin-protective wafer. An absorbent dressing placed around the suction tube insertion site will absorb any slight leakage, and should be changed as necessary.

Research is being initiated to evaluate the effectiveness of a lignocaine-releasing topical gel for the treatment of excoriating skin conditions which potentially could be extremely useful in reducing pain caused by excoriation, a frequent problem in fistula management.[33]

Patient morale

Ensuring that the patient and his family are kept informed when problems arise and explaining the avenues of care which will be followed can promote feelings of involvement and security in the caring team; this can stimulate a supportive environment for all concerned. It is very important to fit the patient with a leak-proof odour-proof appliance. This in itself will do much for morale, for there is nothing more demoralizing for the patient than to be continually reminded of the fistula by inadequate leaky dressings. Nursing staff will also find this situation demoralizing since they will have spent a considerable amount of time fitting appliances. In contrast, it is very rewarding to fit an appliance that stays in place and does not leak.

It is important to remember that small actions, such as ensuring good personal hygiene and keeping up appearances with visits from the hairdresser or barber, can have a very beneficial effect. Patients with fistulas tend to reduce their mobility considerably because they worry that movement will cause the appliance to leak. Ensuring that they have what they need close at hand in a microenvironment can be of considerable benefit. Caring for a patient with a fistula can be very demanding, but if well managed, the rewards to all, most importantly the patient, can be high.

Pressure sores

Healthy man is a dynamic person who does not develop decubitus ulcers or bed sores.[34] The term decubitus comes from the Latin root *decub* which means lying down. As numerous studies have shown that patients in chairs are more likely to have sores than patients in bed,[35-37] the term decubitus should not be synonymous with pressure sore. Pressure sores are reported in up to 9.4 per cent of all hospital patients.[36] The incidence of pressure sores in cancer patients is likely to be very much higher because of all the associated risk factors.

Pressure sores are not irremediable afflictions of long-stay patients but a sign of acute illness.[38] This point was established by the observation that 70 per cent of sores occurring in hospital appeared within the first 2 weeks, i.e. when patients are most ill.[39] Indeed, one study showed that the acute ischaemic episode which precipitated the necrosis frequently occurred in the accident and emergency department or on the operating table.[40]

Pressure sores are associated with a number of adverse outcomes including osteomyelitis, septicaemia, amyloidosis, and anaemia. In the cancer patient a pressure sore adds insult to injury, creating a further source of pain and degradation, increased hospital stay, and a need for greater medical resources with resulting costs.

Pathophysiology

The pressure sore represents localized tissue death and is the result of impairment of the vascular and lymphatic systems of the skin and deeper tissues caused by compression, tension, or shear forces above a critical value acting for a critical period of time.[34]

Intracellular metabolism survives even at very high pressures, indicating that the role of pressure in the formation of pressure sores is to restrict extracellular circulating fluid. Both intrinsic and extrinsic factors determine the formation of pressure sores. Intrinsic factors, including old age, neurological deficit, vascular disease, and nutritional deficiency, lower tissue resistance to pressure. Extrinsic factors include compression and shear forces as well as skin maceration from sweat or incontinence. Pressure sores are produced by both high pressure of short duration and low pressure of long duration.

When pressure is exerted upon normally innervated tissue, painful stimuli arise that are transmitted centrally. Discomfort produces the response of movement in order to redistribute pressure. It follows that injury to the nervous pathways leads to a lack of protecting movements and results in immobility of the patient (Table 2). When sufficient pressure is applied to the skin, the underlying blood vessels are occluded or partially occluded, and oxygen and other nutrients are no longer delivered at a rate sufficient to satisfy the metabolic requirements of the tissues.[41] In the absence of a blood or lymph circulation, the breakdown products of metabolism accumulate within the interstitial spaces and the cells. Arterial occlusion is usually short-lived and followed

Table 2 Conditions affecting spontaneous movement

Pain
Paralysis or weakness secondary to:
 Cord compression from spinal metastases
 Brain metastases
 Cerebrovascular
 Spinal cord trauma
 Neurological injury
Sedation from opioid analgesia
Massive ascites or oedema
Coma
Contractures
Dementia or severe depression

by a period of increased blood flow, known as reactive hyperaemia. Partial occlusion of the arterial supply to an area of tissue may occur temporarily as a result of compression. The vascular bed distal to the occlusion shows a compensatory reduction in vascular resistance. In this way it is possible to maintain the flow of nutrients to a tissue in the face of a falling perfusion pressure; this is the phenomenon of autoregulation of blood flow. Conversely, a rise in local venous pressure is accompanied by constriction of the arterioles, which reduces total blood flow and protects the capillary bed from damaging rises in microvascular pressure. This mechanism, the venoarteriolar response, is of considerable physiological importance for countering the effects of gravity (Table 3).

When an arterial obstruction is relieved after a prolonged period of ischaemia, the microcirculation may fail to reperfuse or perfusion may be at a level well below normal. Equally, reperfusion itself may promote tissue damage through the release of superoxides and oxygen free radicals, the so-called reperfusion injury.

Peripheral non-contractile small lymphatic vessels are almost entirely dependent on changes in local tissue hydrostatic pressure for lymph drainage. No other system is as sensitive to pressure and shearing strain. The structural integrity of the delicate initial lymphatic vessels can be damaged more readily than the blood capillaries during external mechanical force application. Impaired lymph flow will lead to a build-up of metabolic waste products which will compound any effects from ischaemia. Lymph flow appears to reduce to zero when external pressure exceeds 70 mmHg.[42]

It is likely that prolonged excessive mechanical stresses cause breakdown of skin and subcutaneous tissue by impairing blood flow, lymph circulation, and interstitial transport processes. When interstitial fluid is squeezed out of a tissue region, direct contact of the cells induces stresses on fibroblasts, interrupting collagen synthesis, and this persists after the load is removed. After squeezing and load release, the interstitial fluid suddenly becomes more negative, causing cavitation, capillary rupture, haemorrhage, and protein-rich oedema. At this point any loss in lymphatic function contributes to the poor tissue viability.

Table 3 Factors affecting tissue perfusion

Dehydration
Anaemia
Peripheral vascular disease
Surgical intervention
Massive ascites or oedema
Radiation fibrosis
Congestive heart failure related to:
 High doses of doxorubicin or daunorubicin
 Prior myocardial infarction
 Arrhythmias
Decreased lung perfusion related to:
 Bleomycin
 Radiation fibrosis
 Pleural effusion
 Chronic obstructive pulmonary disease
 Pulmonary oedema
Fever
Smoking
Emotional stress

Intrinsic factors predisposing to pressure sores

An understanding of tissue stiffness is necessary to appreciate what happens when pressure deforms the body surface of a healthy person. Normal tissue stiffness allows the body to resist deformation by damping the effects of pressure on underlying structures including blood vessels. When tissue stiffness is reduced the body begins to sag. This sagging is due to several factors including dehydration and ageing. A deterioration in the 'supporting framework' of collagen and elastic fibres reduces tissue stiffness and consequently tissue resilience.

Blood flow to a tissue may be compromised before the application of any pressure if the patient has a reduced cardiac output (heart failure, atrial fibrillation, myocardial infarction), peripheral vascular disease, or reduced oxygen transport capacity resulting from anaemia. Cardiac or pulmonary function can be reduced by the drug and radiation therapy regimens of the cancer patient. Radiotherapy to metastases in bony prominences can compromise the circulation and tissue quality in overlying soft tissues.

Therefore, in debilitated patients who have impaired tissue stiffness and perfusion, a low external compression of the vasculature has a more serious effect on tissue viability than application of a high pressure for short periods. Moreover, the development of low-pressure ischaemia gradually impairs nerve conduction and leads to local anaesthesia with abolition of protective reflexes which prompt movement. Equally, inappropriate sedation of the patient may produce critical immobility. Pain is a special concern to the patient with cancer. Pain from bony metastases may dominate discomfort from pressure points as well as discourage any movement. Achieving pain control that increases mobility with minimal sedation is difficult!

In a recent study[43] factors significantly associated with the presence of a pressure sore on admission were shown to be altered level of consciousness (odds ratio, 4.1), bed- or chair-bound (odds ratio, 2.4), impaired nutritional intake (odds ratio, 1.9), and hypoalbuminaemia (odds ratio, 1.8 for a decrease of 10 mg/ml). Of the 185 patients without a pressure sore on admission, 20 (10.8 per cent) subsequently developed a sore. Factors significantly associated with the development of a new pressure sore were a history of cerebrovascular accident (odds ratio, 5.0), bed- or chair-bound (odds ratio, 3.8), and impaired nutritional intake (odds ratio, 2.8).

The importance of nutritional intake is clear, but nutritional status is far more complicated than simply intake as it includes hypermetabolic states of prolonged fever and cancer cachexia. Negative nitrogen balance will result in tissue breakdown and poor tissue repair.

Extrinsic factors predisposing to pressure sores

Pressure sores can develop over any bony prominence, but 96 per cent present on the lower half of the body. In addition to direct pressure, the effect of shearing forces should not be underestimated. Shearing force occurs, for example, when the head of a bed is elevated by 30°. Gravity pulls the patient down and the shearing force is reversed when attendants heave the patient back up the bed. Gravity also produces a shearing force in a sitting patient who starts to slide towards the floor.

Skin maceration by sweat, urine, and faeces will predispose to pressure sores by interfering with barrier function. Moisture can accumulate from perspiration, incontinence, wound or fistula drainage, and food spills. Plastic sheets placed underneath the patient will serve to increase the moist environment. Moisture will also increase friction, and friction burns can result if the patient is dragged over a sheet to which he or she is adhering.

Risk assessment tools

If pressure sores are to be prevented, it is important that those patients at risk are identified. A valid and reliable method of assessing risk of pressure sores is needed. It should be accurate, comprehensive, and usable at the bedside. Several assessment tools have been developed. Most are based on the Norton scale which was designed in 1962 and validated in geriatric patients.[44] It uses five basic headings: physical condition, mental state, activity, mobility, and incontinence. The lower the score, the higher is the risk. The scale is well known but has been criticized because it was designed for patients over the age of 65; it tends to overpredict pressure sore risk in some patients[45] and is not effective in assessing patients who are only at risk for part of the day.[46] It has also been criticized because it does not include nutrition or pain.[47] However, a patient's nutritional status will be reflected to some extent in the 'physical condition' score, and the absence or presence of pain will affect the patient's mobility score.

As long as its limitations are borne in mind, the Norton scale has stood the test of time because of its simplicity and it remains a valuable adjunct to the direct observation and clinical judgement of the nursing staff. There have been several attempts to refine the scale by including other parameters.

A more recent assessment tool devised by Waterlow[48] includes nutritional factors, assessment of skin type, and a 'weighting' for predisposing diseases. This assessment scale has been updated and refined in the light of the findings of two large pressure sore surveys in the United Kingdom.[49] It has a wide applicability and is a useful aid for developing awareness of pressure sore risk.

The Braden scale,[50] which is an assessment tool commonly used in North America, incorporates a parameter not included in other tools. It assesses friction and shearing forces which are present for most patients in hospital. Each parameter of the scale is defined more descriptively than in the Norton scale.

No risk assessment scale is a substitute for sound clinical judgement, and any scale is of little use if the risk is not reassessed regularly as the patient's condition changes.[51]

Prevention strategy

The following strategy has been suggested for preventing pressure sores in hospice patients.[52]

1. Maintenance of skin integrity by keeping the skin clean and as free as possible from contamination with urine and faeces. Prevention of excessive dryness.
2. Pressure relief, particularly over all bony prominences.
3. Promotion of patient movement by providing active and passive motion as well as frequent turning.
4. Improvement of nutritional status by correcting nutritional deficiencies and promoting adequate hydration.
5. Education of the patient and his or her family regarding the need for a prevention programme and the family's role.

Aids to preventative management

The actual surface that a patient rests on is very important.[53] An ideal support system should satisfy the following criteria:

(1) distribute pressure evenly, or provide frequent relief of pressure;

(2) provide a comfortable well-ventilated patient support interface which does not restrict movement;

(3) minimize friction and shearing forces;

(4) be easy to maintain;

(5) be inexpensive;

(6) be acceptable to the patient;

(7) not impede nursing procedures.

Devices consisting of air cells which alternately deflate and inflate by means of an electric pump (e.g. a large-cell ripple mattress) change the area of the body under pressure. Devices such as air fluidized beds reduce and distribute pressure more evenly by using dry flotation to provide hydrostatic support. A low-air-loss bed consists of waterproof, but vapour-permeable, sacs arranged in groups with pressure valves controlling each group to suit body contours. Silicone padding mattresses are made up of horizontal filled tubes.

Most of these devices are expensive and are not always the correct choice for the patient. The value of inexpensive alternatives should not be underestimated. Natural sheepskin reduces friction and shear forces to some extent, and monkey poles and rope ladders relieve pressure from the sacral area. A variety of cushions, of variable effectiveness, are available. Cushion fillings can be of gel, air, foam, and fluid. Sorbo foam rings should not be used as they concentrate pressure in one area.

It should be remembered that the pressure-relieving aid used must be acceptable to the patient, and a full explanation of why and how the aid is being used will help promote patient comfort.

Pressure sore development

When early signs of pressure appear, or a pressure sore itself develops, it is important to prevent misperception of what is being seen. Classification of pressure sores into the following four grades improves patient assessment and subsequent intervention.

Grade I. This is not a pressure sore but the precursor phase. It is characterized by redness which blanches under even light finger pressure, indicating that the microcirculation is present and intact.

Grade II. Redness remains even when light finger pressure is applied. This stage can involve excoriation, vesiculation, or skin breakthrough at the epidermis. The tissues are firmer and warmer to the touch.

Grade III. Full-thickness loss of skin which does not include the subcutaneous tissue level and which produces serosanguineous exudate drainage.

Grade IV. The sore extends into subcutaneous fat and the deep fascia with destruction of muscle tissue, and there may even be bony involvement. This stage often includes eschar formation and/or infection.[54]

The shape of the wound should be drawn, and its measurements should be charted and periodically updated.

The Agency for Health Care Policy and Research was established in the United States in 1989 to 'enhance the quality, appropriateness, and effectiveness of health care services and access to these services'. Subsequently, the Agency has published a series of guidelines for assessment and management of common clinical problems. In the summer of 1992 guidelines on the prediction and prevention of pressure illness in adults were published.[55] These guidelines recommend a common assessment system and a management approach to grade I and grade II ulcers.

Guidelines for treatment

As discussed earlier in this chapter the criteria for the ideal wound dressing also apply here. Treatment should aim at removing the source of irritation, necrotic tissue, and infection, and protecting new healthy tissue.

Wounds that are neither necrotic or infected need only a moist environment to encourage healing. This can be achieved by using an occlusive hydrocolloid dressing or a semipermeable film. Cleansing and debriding are necessary to remove necrotic tissue, bacteria, and exudate. Cleansing by irrigation with normal saline solution is recommended. Enzymatic agents can be used to remove eschar, which can also be softened and lifted with occlusive wafers. Absorption of exudate and debriding can be achieved using alginates.

Table 4 provides a guide for treatment according to the grade of pressure sore. Maintenance of skin integrity and prevention and treatment of pressure sores begin with a systematic assessment of the patient and the risk factors involved. It must be recognized that a pressure sore is a serious problem and the whole multidisciplinary team should be involved in treatment and prevention. The most effective intervention is preventing the development of pressure sores: 'Where there is no pressure, there is no sore'.[56]

Therapeutic ultrasound

Ultrasound is a mechanical disturbance transmitted at a frequency above the normal limit of human hearing and has been used as an adjunctive physical therapy in a variety of disorders usually involving soft tissue injury. Ultrasound is widely used to stimulate wound healing.[57] The effects of ultrasound on wound healing are not fully understood, although it is known to facilitate repair to the dermis. This can be divided into three phases: the inflammatory phase, the proliferation phase, and remodelling.

In soft tissue injury platelet and mast cells are activated, releasing agents that initiate acute inflammation. Pain and swelling are symptoms of inflammation which is a normal response of tissues to injury and is part of the healing process. Ultrasound can accelerate the inflammatory phase of repair and thereby significantly accelerate wound healing.

The proliferation phase is a later part of the inflammatory process which begins about 3 days after injury. It is characterized by the appearance of a highly vascularized collagen-rich granulation tissue at the site of the injury. Fibroblast activity increases; these cells produce matrix materials and assist in reducing the size of the wound defect. Ultrasound stimulates fibroblasts to secrete more collagen and increase new blood capillary formation, thereby accelerating tissue repair.

In the remodelling phase granulation tissue is replaced with tissue identical with that existing before the injury. The application of therapeutic ultrasound is less useful during remodelling than in the other phases. Expedient use of ultrasound following an injury or wound will assist in dermal repair.

The use of therapeutic ultrasound is contraindicated in many circumstances including previously irradiated tissue, precancerous lesions, and malignancies. It may be beneficial in the treatment of some patients with pressure sores, provided that a proper assessment is undertaken by a suitably trained person. Since there are personal and financial costs associated with the management of pressure sores, it is essential to weigh benefits against risks. Reducing pain and discomfort and restoring independence to individuals with this complicated clinical problem cannot be underestimated.

Professional intervention

The complexity of the problem of maintaining skin integrity or combating symptoms associated with wounds in patients who are compromised by their underlying cancer cannot be underestimated. It is important that the doctor and nurse recognize the value of intervention by other members of the multidisciplinary team, family, and friends. Continual vigilance is required to prevent further skin problems and the patient is often too weary or immobile to sustain this effort. Thus the informal carer has a valuable contribution to make. However, it is important that undue pressure is not placed upon these informal carers to help in a situation where they may be too stressed, frightened, or repulsed by the change in the body image of their loved one. Insight is essential when using a 'family-centred' approach to care. A comprehensive assessment and understanding of the patient's social circumstances will avoid causing further stress in a crisis situation in a family where illness is present.[58] However, an enormous amount of practical and emotional support can be provided for both patient

Table 4 A guide for treatment according to the grade of pressure sore

Grade	Aims	Dressing	Action	Use
Grade I (skin intact) + Grade II (superficial break in skin)	Prevent contamination and shear forces	Polyurethane film	Prevents large molecules or bacteria from entering or leaving Allows small molecules of H_2O, O_2 to pass freely	Place completely over wound Leave 3–4 days Change only when necessary
Grade III (full-thickness loss of skin (infection not present))	Wound protection Promotion of healing	Hydrocolloid (low exudate)	Hydrocolloid fluidizes when in contact with wound exudate producing a gel which aids wound debridement	Clean with normal saline Extend wafer at least 3 cm beyond wound margin Can remain *in situ* until wafer changes to a transparent colour over wound site or leakage occurs
		Calcium alginate (high exudate)	Exudate absorption via strong hydrophillic gel formation Controls wound secretion levels and bacterial contamination	Clean only with normal saline Apply alginate Cover with semi-occlusive dressing Change when leakage occurs
Grade IV (full thickness with cavity; can include eschar formation and/or infection)	Remove necrotic tissue	(a) Hydrocolloid as above		
		(b) Hydrogel	(b) Rehydrates dry eschar and aids its removal	(b) Clean with normal saline. Apply directly to eschar and cover with a film dressing as this will further help the rehydration process
		(c) Enzymatic	(c) Loosens necrotic tissue Liquefies pus and wound exudate for rapid desloughing	(c) Inject under the eschar or score the surface of the eschar to aid penetration Apply occlusive dressing to reduce rate of evaporation of enzymatic dressing
	Eliminate/control infection	Polysaccharide dextranomers	On contact with wound exudate, beads absorb fluid and swell—moist gel-like mass. Larger molecules of bacteria and dead cells are drawn up between beads and away from wound	Do not use on dry wounds Clean with normal saline Pour granules into wound or mix with glycerol Cover with semi-occlusive dressing NB This dressing will not reduce odour and a charcoal dressing may be required

and family to encourage them to be involved in the caring process.

Many families have expressed fear and impotence when trying to identify their role in caring for their loved ones. More importantly, a 'release' avenue for these carers should be initiated to enable them to articulate their fears and problems, and even to withdraw from giving practical help without experiencing guilt or remorse. The role of the multidisciplinary team and community staff in preparing these patients and families for the experience of 'caring' and showing them the 'normality' of expressing their feelings in a supportive environment cannot be overestimated (see Section 16).

Wherever possible, the community staff, the patient, the family and the hospital staff should meet to discuss the practicalities of the specific home situation and to formulate a suitable plan to care for the patient, whether the problem is wound management, fistula care, or prevention of skin breakdown at home. These practicalities may well require the experience of the occupational therapist in ascertaining the modification and adaptation required to provide a safe and easy environment for both patient and family. This may be a simple procedure such as providing rails for a bath or installing a shower to help to cleanse wounds rather than using a time-consuming conventional dressing.[17,18] Thus family activities are not focused around a 'procedure', and this particular intervention can become accepted as normal (see Chapter 12.3).

The physiotherapist can also provide valuable help in the extent to which to patient and family are able to maintain an independent lifestyle. Adapting to a change in mobility due to either sickness or a functional problem caused by the disease can be both frightening and devastating for the patient. This can also have a direct effect on the intervention required to maintain skin integrity and prevent pressure sores and skin breakdown due to friction caused by poor lifting or lack of passive movement. The role of the physiotherapist as a teacher is of great significance; he or she provides the skills that the family will need to be able to allow the patient as much freedom of access as possible in his or her own home. This requires skills in lifting, in movement from bed to chairs, and in safe transfer to the toilet, and confidence to carry out these tasks without fear of causing pain or distress. Again, the task of trying to assist a person who may have an obvious wound can be quite daunting, and families require much support and advice to help minimize this potential distress for them. There is great satisfaction and comfort for the family who believe that they have made a contribution to the patient's welfare rather than feeling that they have aggravated his or her problems because of their perceived 'inept' care (see Chapter 12.2).

Any provision of facts or intervention for the family must be approached in a sensitive and realistic manner. The reality for some is that their actual home circumstances will not be suitable for modification or adaptation, or the social network is not there to provide this added care. In these circumstances, when the individual will remain in an inpatient setting, careful planning and a flexible approach to the patient's wishes should remain the priority of the staff. The overlap of disciplines is inevitable in this problem-solving approach, but the wealth of skill and information can result in true consumer participation and promotion of an individual's lifestyle in a hospital setting. With this in mind, the treatment, irrespective of prognosis, should be realistic and agreed by patient and carers. Doyle[59] pertinently summarizes the distressing nature of these skin conditions as follows: 'Can we begin to imagine what it must feel like for a patient to see part of his body rotting and to have to live with the offensive smell from it, see the reaction of his visitors (including doctors and nurses) and know that it signifies lingering death'. The application of a multidisciplinary approach in palliative care attempts to alleviate the devastating consequences of advanced cancer and promote self-esteem in this group of patients.

The following case history illustrates a multidisciplinary approach to care, and highlights the integration required to promote an individual lifestyle.

Case history

A 53-year-old woman with a sarcoma of the left buttock was referred for pain control and 'terminal care'. She had been in hospital on an acute surgical ward for about 5 months following two operative procedures to remove a sarcoma which had left a huge open wound following the breakdown of a rotational flap to the buttock. Both hips had open wounds which leaked copious amounts of exudate, and the dressings had to be changed every 2 to 4 hours. At the time of referral she was believed to be disease free, and the wound breakdown appeared to be due to infection rather than cutaneous spread. The patient presented as a demoralized withdrawn woman who felt 'disgusted'' and 'dirty' because of her wounds. Her very supportive family were despondent and upset at the dramatic change in the once vivacious and outgoing wife and mother. She felt trapped and totally dependent on others as she had little control over her daily routine. Sitting in a chair was possible for limited periods only, as this resulted in severe pain. Also, pressure caused exudate to leak through the dressings. She refused to dress in her own clothes, as she could not bear to remember how she looked when she was well.

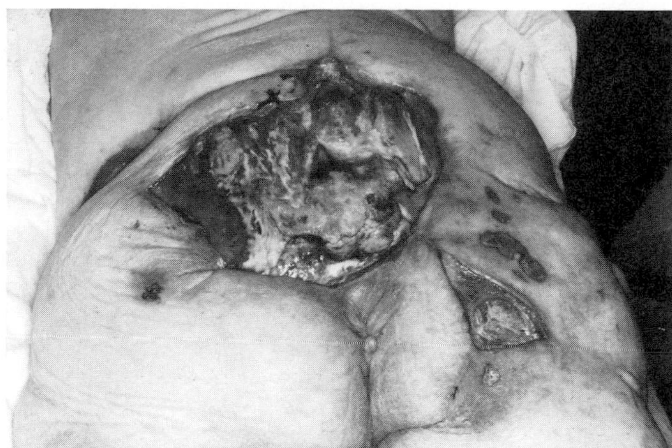

Fig. 6 A 53-year-old woman with sarcoma of the left buttock, showing wound breakdown following an unsuccesful rotational flap.

Figure 6 demonstrates the extent of the wound and the infected and necrotic areas within the wound surface itself. A plan of management to sort out this complicated problem included the following steps:

(1) the consideration of appropriate systemic antibiotic treatment for the infection;

(2) physiotherapy to maintain muscle tone in legs and upper arms with a view to walking with an aid;

(3) involvement of a dietician to design a programme of nutritional intake to sustain her and promote wound healing if possible;

(4) occupational therapy to create a modified cushion for a chair that would be more comfortable and to provide a suitable 'seat' for the toilet or commode;

(5) an agreed programme of activities to provide some focus and direction (in fact she became an adopted ward clerk, helping with filing and similar tasks);

(6) the need for the family to have a role in supporting her and an understanding of her emotional state.

Dressings were initially changed four times daily with the patient lying face down on the bed. Analgesia was given 30 min prior to dressings and she self-administered nitrous oxide throughout the dressing procedure. Systemic antibiotic therapy combined with regular dressings to clean the wound were successful in reducing exudate and relieving pain. Figure 7 shows the sacral wound after 1 month, and, although the wound diameter is larger (caused by the wound tracking under the skin to the right hip), the tissue is healthier with some signs of granulation. The exudate had diminished to such an extent that the patient was able to dress daily and could sit comfortably for longer periods in a chair, and the frequency of dressing change was reduced to three times daily. This small achievement enormously improved her self-esteem and she began to think about having her house decorated with a view to going home. This step had to have careful planning and co-operation from community staff and confidence from the family.

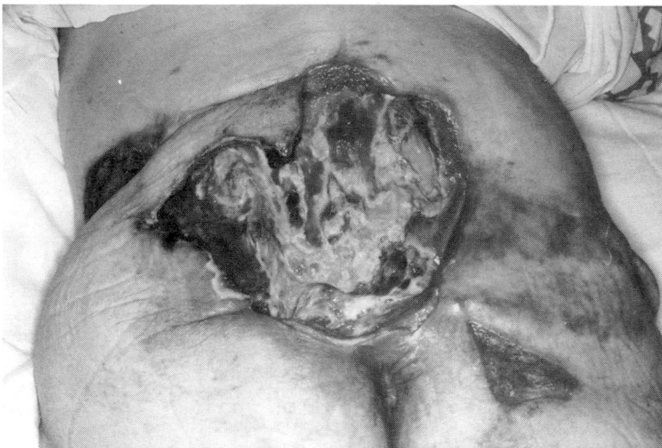

Fig. 7 The sacral wound after 1 month in the patient illustrated in Fig. 6.

Although further assessment of her clinical status revealed hepatic secondaries she remained determined to return home. This knowledge spurred the family to arrange for her to be cared for at home. The community staff became involved and the local district nurse visited the unit to watch a dressing being changed. The procedure was time consuming, but the district nurse was confident that if the dressing change was reduced to twice daily and the family were able to change the outer padding, if necessary, it would be realistic and manageable at home.

As arrangements were being made, the patient developed septicaemia which obviously impeded the progress she had made. The infection resolved with antibiotic treatment but this episode left her weary and weak. However, with stoic determination, she fought back to promote her independence and was able to walk short distances with the aid of a walking frame. Aware that her prognosis was poor, the patient and her husband arranged to have their wedding vows reaffirmed and this took place on the ward with family, friends, and staff present. This day marked a milestone for her and a time for the family to reflect and to prepare realistically for her limited future.

Figure 8 shows the wound 1 month further on. Although the target of twice daily dressings had been achieved, her condition had deteriorated further and she again became septicaemic. In view of her rapidly advancing liver disease and general condition, it was agreed by the patient, her family, and the caring team that antibiotic therapy would be inappropriate; the symptoms were controlled by drug therapy via a syringe driver and she died peacefully with her family present some days later.

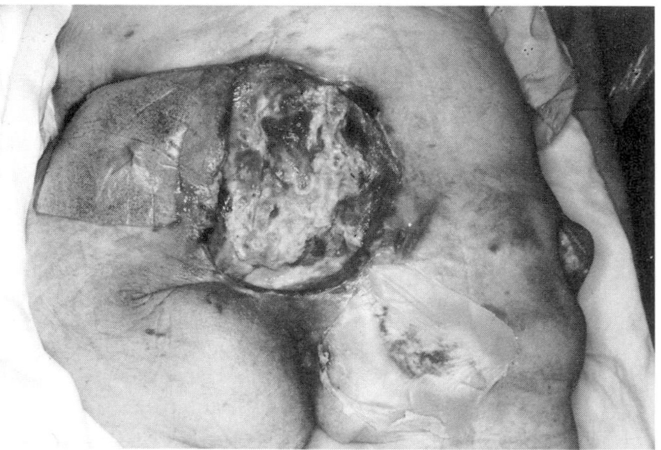

Fig. 8 The wound after 2 months in the patient illustrated in Fig. 6.

Community care

The changes taking place in the delivery of health care have implications for patients receiving care in hospitals, hospices, or the community.[60,61] Wound management is expensive, and an understanding of the availability and price of dressing materials is necessary. Historically, hospitals have had a distinct advantage in both choice and availability of modern dressings, while community nurses have worked with much more limited resources. Cost effectiveness and value for money have become synonymous with the National Health Service in the United Kingdom. This also impacts on our rationalization of wound products, so that there is less reliance on users' 'preferences' and more on skilled professional nursing assessment of particular wound management problems. However, in reality, the availability of resources can be somewhat inconsistent and access to them for community staff can be both complicated and time consuming. This is generally not understood by hospital nurses, many of whom are unaware of the limited availability of products in certain health districts. Indeed, this also has ramifications for other necessary services such as equipment loan and laundry services.

Within palliative care in the United Kingdom, a group sponsored by the Cancer Relief Macmillan Fund have developed guidelines to act as a resource, enabling purchasing authorities to draw service specifications for holistic care for the dying and bereaved. This information will enable purchasing authorities to buy a comprehensive and flexible service for local requirements based on need. The multi-agency provision should introduce choice for the patient and carer with an expectation of a high standard of service.[62]

Future trends

In this chapter we have attempted to draw attention to the complexity of the management of skin care in patients with cancer, highlighting preventative measures as well as assessment and intervention by nurses. A large proportion of the published literature concerning skin and wound management focuses on acute care. Information concerning metastatic skin disease is still limited, and to some degree anecdotal, as it is perceived as a small problem in caring for patients with cancer. However, every occurrence of cutaneous malignancy provides a challenge to the nurse in devising an agreed intervention that is acceptable to patient, doctor, and nurse alike. Therefore, unlike treating a primary wound, the emphasis and relationship are changed and the outcome is uncertain: 'Expert nurses know...definitive evaluation of a patient's condition requires more than vague hunches, but through experience they have learned to allow their perceptions to lead to confirming evidence'.[63] This is the case in the treatment of malignant wounds. Formal research is needed to confirm the rationale for 'popular' wound management approaches and the applicability of these approaches in both the hospital and the community.

There are recognized difficulties in initiating clinical trials in malignant wound management because of the great diversity of the lesions and because the important outcome measures are patient satisfaction and comfort rather than cure. Individual nurses have made their mark in the field of wound management, but formal research has been limited owing to lack of resources and funding.[64] Wound management in cancer patients has not been seen as a lucrative area by drug companies, and the perceived limitation of the palliative care field has kept formal research on the sidelines. It is obvious that there is a wealth of untapped knowledge and experience in dealing with difficult malignant wounds within the field of palliative care, and the aim should be to formalize and rationalize this information to ensure a standard of care than can be emulated thoughout the nursing profession.

References

1. Foltz AT. Nursing care of ulcerating metastatic lesions. *Oncology Nursing Forum* 1980; 7:8–13.
2. Bennet M. As normal a life as possible *Community Outlook*, 1985; **81**:35–8.
3. Charles-Edwards A. *The Nursing Care of the Dying Patient*. Beaconsfield: Beaconsfield Publishers, 1983.
4. Rosenberg FW. Cutaneous manifestations of internal malignancy. *Cutis*, 1977: **20**:227–34.
5. Saunders C M. *The Management of Terminal Disease*. London: Edward Arnold, 1978.
6. Sims R, Fitzgerald V. *Community Nursing Management of Patients with Ulcerating/Fungating Malignant Breast Disease.* London: RCN Oncology Nursing Society, 1985.
7. Rosen T. Cutaneous metastases. *Medical Clinics of North America*, 1980; **64**:885–900.
8. Gould D. Wound management. *Nursing Mirror*, 1984; **159**:3–4.
9. Thomas S, Fear M, Humphries J. Assessment of patients with chronic wounds. *Journal of Wound Care*, 1994; **3**(3):151–4.
10. Grocott P. Palliative management of fungating malignant wounds: the development of a wound assessment tool. *Proceedings of the 4th European Wound Management Association Meeting, Copenhagen 1994*. London: Macmillan Magazines, 1994.
11. Young SR, Dyson M. Principles of ultrasonography and skin ultrasonography. In: Christman R, ed. *Foot and Ankle Radiology.* Edinburgh: Churchill Livingstone, 1996.
12. Brennan S, Leaper D. Antiseptics and wound healing. *British Journal of Surgery*, 1985; **72**:780–2.
13. Dean J, Billings P, Brennan SS, Silver I, Leaper DS. The toxicity of commonly used antiseptics on fibroblasts in tissue culture. *Phlebology*, 1986; **1**:205–9.
14. Leaper D. Antiseptics and their effect on healing tissue. *Nursing Times*, 1986; **82**:45–7.
15. Thomas S. *Wound Management and Dressings*, Chapter II. London: Pharmaceutical Press, 1990.
16. Butler GA. Desloughing agents at work. *Nursing Mirror*, 1985; **160**:29.
17. Chrintz H, Vivits H, Cordtz TD, Harreby JS, Waaddegaard P, Larsen SD. Need for surgical wound dressing. *British Journal of Surgery*, 1989; **76**:204–5.
18. Harding KG, Hughes LE, Marks J. *A Guide to the Practical Management of Granulating Wounds.* Crewe: Wellcome Foundation, 1986.
19. Wood RAB. Disintegration of cellulose dressings in open granulating wounds. *British Medical Journal*, 1976; **i**:1444–5.
20. Turner TD. Which dressing and why? In: Westaby S, ed. *Wound Care.* London: Heinemann Medical, 1985.
21. Johnson A. Criteria for ideal wound dressings. *Professional Nurse*, 1988; 3:191–3.
22. Varghese MC, *et al.* Local environment of chronic wounds under synthetic dressings. *Archives of Dermatology*, 1986; **122**:52–7.
23. Piper SM. Effective use of occlusive wound dressings. *Professional Nurse*, 1989; **4**:402–4.
24. Grocott P. The latest on latex. *Nursing Times*, 1992; **88**(12):61–2.
25. Walls AWG, Regnard CFB, Mannix KA. The closure of an abdominal fistula using self-polymerizing silicone rubbers—case study. *Palliative Medicine*, 1994; **8**:59–62.
26. Van Tolter S. Invisible wounds: the effects of skin ulcer malodour. *Journal of Wound Care*, 1994; **3**(2):103–5.
27. Morgan D A. *Formulary of Wound Management Products.* 3rd edn. Aldershot: Britcair, 1989.
28. Newman V, Allwood M, Oakes R A. The use of metronidazole gel to control the smell of malodorous lesions. *Palliative Medicine*, 1989; 3:303–5.
29. Morgan D. Wound management: which dressing? *Pharmaceutical Journal*, 1993; **29 May**:738–43.
30. Thomlinson RH. Kitchen remedy for necrotic malignant breast ulcers. *Lancet*, 1980; **ii**:707.
31. Breckman B. *Stoma Care.* Beaconsfield: Beaconsfield Publishers, 1981.
32. Taylor I. Fistula management. *Nursing Standard*, 1988; 7: 30–1.
33. Grocott P. Unpublished research, 1995.
34. Scales JT. Pathogenesis of pressure sores. In: Bader DL, ed. *Pressure Sores.* London: Macmillan, 1990:15–26.
35. Barbenel JC, Jordan MM, Nichol SM, Clark MD. Incidence of pressure sores in the Greater Glasgow Health Board area. *Lancet*, 1977; **ii**:548–50.
36. David J. The size of the problem of pressure sores. *Care, Science and Practice*, 1981; **1**:10–13.
37. Nyquist R, Hawthorn PJ. The prevalence of pressure sores within an area health authority. *Journal of Advanced Nursing*, 1989; **12**:183–7.
38. Anonymous. Preventing pressure sores. *Lancet*, 1990; **i**:1311–12.
39. Norton D, McLaren R, Exton-Smith AN. *An Investigation of Geriatric Nursing Problems in Hospital.* Edinburgh: Churchill Livingstone, 1975.
40. Versluysen M. How elderly patients with femoral neck fracture develop pressure sores in hospital. *British Medical Journal*, 1986; **292**:1311–12.
41. Michel CG, Gillott H. Microvascular mechanisms in stasis and ischaemia. In Bader DL, ed. *Pressure Sores.* London: Macmillan, 1990:153–63.
42. Miller GE, Searle J. Lymphatic clearance during compressive loading. *Lymphology*, 1981; **14**:161–6.
43. Berlowitz DR, Wilking S van B. Risk factors for pressure sores. *Journal of the American Geriatrics Society*, 1989; **37**:1043–50.
44. Norton D, *et al. An Investigation of Geriatric Nursing Problems in Hospital.* London: National Corporation for the Care of Old People, 1962.
45. Goldstone LA, Goldstone J. The Norton Score: an early warning of pressure sores? *Journal of Advanced Nursing*, 1982; **7**:419–26.
46. Horsley JA, *et al. Preventing Decubitus Ulcers.* New York: Grune and Stratton, 1981.
47. Barratt E. A review of risk assessment methods. *Care, Science and Practice*, 1988; **6**:49–52.
48. Waterlow J. A risk assessment card. *Nursing Times*, 1985; **81**:49–55.
49. Waterlow J. The Waterlow card for the prevention and management of pressure sores: towards a pocket policy. *Care, Science and Practice*, 1988; **6**:8–12.
50. Bergstrom N, Bradden BJ, Laguzza A, Holman V. The Braden scale for predicting pressure sore risk. *Nursing Research*, 1987; **36**:205–10.
51. Morrison MJ. Early assessment of pressure sore risk. *Professional Nurse*, 1989; **4**:428–31.
52. Colburn L. Pressure ulcer prevention for hospice patients. *American Journal of Hospice Care*, 1987; **4**:22–6.
53. Morrison MJ. Pressure sores: removing the causes of the wound. *Professional Nurse*, 1989; **5**:97–8, 100–1, 103–4.
54. Low AW. Prevention of pressure sores in patients with cancer. *Oncology Nursing Forum*, 1990; **17**:179–84.

55. Agency for Health Care Policy and Research. *Clinical Practice Guidelines on 'Pressure Ulcers in Adults: Prediction and Prevention'.* Silver Spring, MD: AHCPR Publications, 1992.
56. Reuler JB, Cooney TG. The pressure sore: pathophysiology and principles of management. *Annals of Internal Medicine*, 1981; **94**:661–6.
57. Dyson M. The role of ultrasound in wound healing. In: *Clayton's Electrotherapy.* 10th edn, London: WB Saunders, 1996: 243–67.
58. Murgatroyd S, Woolfe R. *Helping Families in Distress. An Introduction to Family Focused Helping.* London: Harper 38; Row, 1985.
59. Doyle D. *Conference Proceedings in Symptom Control*, Edinburgh: St Columba's Hospice, 1980.
60. *Working for Patients: The Health Service* (CM555). London: HMSO, 1989.
61. *Caring for People. Community Care in the Next Decade and Beyond.* (CM849). London: HMSO, 1989.
62. Webb J, Doyle J, Terry Y, Webber J. One last chance to get it right. *Health Service Journal*, 1991: 22–3.
63. Benner P. *From Novice to Expert.* San Francisco, CA: Addison-Wesley, 1984.
64. Moody M, Grocott P. Let us extend our knowledge base. Assessment and management of fungating malignant wounds. *Professional Nurse.* 1993; **June**:586–90.

9.7 Lymphoedema

P. S. Mortimer, Caroline Badger, and Joseph G. Hall

The scope of the problem

Lymphoedema is best defined as tissue swelling due to a failure of lymph drainage.[1,2] It may be primary in type due to an inherent or congenitally determined problem of lymph drainage, or secondary to obliteration or obstruction of lymph channels from extrinsic factors such as infection, surgery, or radiation. Lymphoedema remains an enigma because its basic pathophysiology is poorly understood. It is difficult to induce experimentally, and the reason for the long latent period from lymphatic damage during cancer therapy to onset of swelling is unknown.

Lymphoedema is considered rare, but chronic swelling due to oedema, particularly of the lower extremities, is a common disorder. The chief function of the lymphatic system is the control of extracellular fluid volume and content. Therefore it is a safety valve for the prevention of oedema—any oedema—and it follows that all forms of oedema concern the lymphatic system.

Clinical teaching categorizes oedema into that associated with heart failure, with renal failure, or with venous obstruction, rather than considering it from a physiological standpoint, namely the balance between capillary filtration and lymph drainage. This latter approach not only simplifies understanding but indicates the pivotal role of lymph drainage in all forms of oedema. Oedema frequently develops from either an excess of capillary filtrate with normal but overloaded regional lymphatics, as occurs in heart failure, renal failure, hypoproteinaemia, and chronic venous disease, or from a defective lymphatic system with an unaltered lymph load (lymphoedema). Chronic oedema rarely arises solely from a failure of one system; usually several factors combine to disturb the fine balance of forces controlling extracellular fluid volume. For example, in advanced pelvic cancer, lymphatic obstruction may coexist with inferior vena caval obstruction to generate gross lower limb swelling, but additional hypoproteinaemia and obstructive uropathy may further fuel the oedematous state.

There is little information on the prevalence of chronic oedema in general or of lymphoedema (oedema caused primarily and predominantly from lymphatic obstruction) in cancer patients. There are two main explanations for this: first the diagnosis of lymphoedema is not as straightforward as would at first appear, and second the problem has been relatively neglected. During the era of the Halstead radical mastectomy, the incidence of lymphoedema was variously reported at between 6.7 and 62.5 per cent.[3,4] Since the extensive review by Hughes and Patel in 1966,[5] there has been one paper[6] which examined the risk of arm swelling in 200 breast cancer patients attending for regular review. Objective lymphoedema (a difference in limb volume of more than 200 ml) was present in 25.5 per cent overall, but the incidence after axillary clearance plus radiotherapy was significantly greater (38.3 per cent). When extrapolated to 20 000 new cases of breast cancer per year for a condition which is incurable, this indicates a sizeable clinical problem. No equivalent data exist for lower-limb swelling following cancer therapy.

Pathophysiology

Comparative physiology

Research on experimental animals has not provided an adequate explanation for the chronic postoperative lymphoedema that may follow either mastectomy or radical block dissection of the groin in humans. The latter procedure is a useful example because its effects are not usually complicated by later radiotherapy. Some lymphoedema of the leg occurs in about 10 per cent of patients, yet a similar procedure carried out in animals (usually dogs, rabbits, or sheep) does not cause such effects. In order to produce lymphoedema in the hind limbs of animals one must do much more than perform a simple lymphadenectomy; all tissues except the major artery, vein, and long bone must be divided and fibrogenic silica dust should be distributed throughout the wound for good measure.[7] Even then, despite these gross mutilations and later fibrosis, genuine lymphoedema will not occur in every case. A better method involves the total blockage of both the superficial and deep lymphatic networks by the direct instillation of Neoprene latex,[8] but this, too, is hardly relevant to the clinical situation.

What can account for this difference between animals and humans? There are several partial and unconvincing explanations. Perhaps the fact that man walks upright on two legs puts an additional burden on fluid return from these limbs which is not shared by quadrupeds. Also, surgeons carrying out a block dissection of the groin will deliberately strive to excise the lymph nodes with as wide a margin of normal subcuticulum as possible. Inevitably, this will lead to a gap of several inches between the cut ends of the afferent and efferent lymphatic vessels of the nodes. An equivalent operation in experimental animals (which are nearly all smaller than humans) leaves a gap of at most a few centimetres, which can be made good rapidly by the vigorous regeneration that proceeds from the cut ends of the lymphatic vessels.[9] *De facto,* the lymphatic vessels of humans seem to have less regenerative capacity than those of animals, but it is not known whether this is genuine intrinsic deficiency or merely reflects the greater absolute distances that may be involved. When such uncertainties exist about such a relatively simple situation, a real understanding of what happens after mastectomy, for example, must be even more elusive.

The surgical procedures used in the treatment of cancer of the breast are various and are often followed by radiotherapy. Sometimes radiotherapy is the only treatment. Obviously, patients with confirmed cancer of the breast who are treated by surgery alone usually undergo a procedure which includes the excision of many lymph nodes and lymphatic vessels. Any lymphoedema that occurs later is assumed to have an aetiology similar to that described above in relation to inguinal–iliac lymphadenectomy. However, the incidence of lymphoedema is greatest when the insult of radiotherapy is added to the injury of less radical surgery in the axilla. Although large doses of radiotherapy cause no immediate change in the structure or function of peripheral lymphatic vessels,[10] the irradiated lymph nodes of sheep soon begin to show unequivocal fibrosis[11] and later defects in the function of cutaneous lymphatic vessels have been detected in irradiated pigs.[12] These facts, together with the observation that radiotherapy for cancer of the breast can alone cause lymphoedema, leave no doubt that irradiation can damage the lymphatic system severely. Several factors probably operate: the postirradiation fibrosis of nodes may obstruct lymph flow directly, the irradiation may damage the mechanisms that control the intrinsic rhythmic contractility of lymphatic vessels, and, where lymphatic vessels have been cut or removed, the irradiation may inhibit the cell division necessary for their regeneration. In addition, irradiation may increase the general fibrosis in the mastectomy wound and thus create a mechanical barrier to those lymphatic vessels still capable of regeneration. In other words, the irradiation substitutes for the fibrogenic silica dust used to cause lymphoedema in experimental animals. Unfortunately, it is impossible to describe these effects in quantitative terms, and so there is no means of ranking them in order of importance.

A central difficulty is the very great variation in the amount of postirradiation fibrosis that occurs in different species of experimental animals or even between different inbred strains of the same species. In addition, it is often practically impossible to expose experimental animals to the accurate regional fractionated irradiation that is given to human patients in clinical radiotherapy protocols. It is also true that the anatomy of the regional lymphatic systems differs a great deal. Whereas the lymphatic vessels from the breast of the human female may drain into between 20 and 30 individual lymph nodes the (much larger) mammary glands of sheep and cattle often drain into only one. These difficulties and differences are not the only ones that preclude any accessible animal model from relating directly to the human situation.

Clinical lymphoedema may not appear in the affected limb for months or even years after the primary treatment. This may be explained partly by the so-called 'die-back' of lymphatic vessels. The basis of this phenomenon is the progressive centrifugal atrophy of those lymphatic vessels that remained intact after the original therapeutic onslaught. As usual, the cause of this is unknown. In some cases, no doubt, progressive fibrosis and contraction of irradiated tissues may be an important factor, but this cannot apply when the condition occurs in non-irradiated patients. It is a matter of common observation that frank lymphoedema may occur only after one or more episodes of inflammatory 'cellulitis' and lymphangitis in the affected limb, which seem to erode further the already parlous structure and function of the remaining lymphatic vessels.

Capillary dynamics

The flux of fluid from blood vessel (capillary) to interstitial space is determined by the balance of osmotic and hydrostatic forces across the capillary wall. In a steady state (where there is no swelling) there should be no net movement of fluid (plus protein and solutes), but in reality there is, and this net flow is counterbalanced by the lymph drainage. As lymph contains macromolecules, in particular protein, obstruction to lymph drainage will result in a gradual build-up of protein within the tissues. By attracting water, osmotic forces will lead to swelling. This represents traditional thinking with regard to the pathophysiology of clinical lymphoedema.

In reality the situation is probably far more complicated. Recent work in breast-cancer-related arm swelling has shown that lymphoedematous fluid does not possess the high concentration of protein previously supposed, although the total mass of protein trapped within the swollen limb is considerable.[13] The relative increase in interstitial water is not explained by lymphatic obstruction alone and suggests other haemodynamic disturbances. One unexpected finding which needs further confirmation is a lower plasma osmotic pressure in the lymphoedema patients compared with matched breast cancer patients without swelling. This would result in a reduced absorptive capacity of the vascular compartment for water, and oedema would be encouraged.

Other abnormalities discovered so far, which would tend to enhance capillary filtration and thus place extra demands on an already vulnerable lymph drainage, are increased limb blood flow and venous outflow obstruction. Over 50 patients with post-surgery/radiotherapy swollen arm were examined using pulsed and colour duplex ultrasound.[14,15] All had had total or partial mastectomy and 85 per cent had received radiotherapy. Arterial blood flow was increased by over 50 per cent in more than half the patients studied.[14] Fifty per cent had obstructed or narrowed subclavian or axillary veins, and colour duplex ultrasound clearly demonstrated collaterals which were not visualized on conventional grey-scale images. A further 25 per cent of patients had normal venous anatomy but abnormal venous flow patterns. Subclavian vein thrombosis, which was clinically unsuspected, was demonstrated in two cases.[15] Thus serious macrovascular abnormalities, which would further contribute to oedema formation, seem to exist in the majority of these patients.

Inflammation

If lymphatic obstruction is the sole cause of lymphoedema, then why does swelling not occur immediately following lymphadenectomy or radiotherapy in all patients undergoing cancer therapy? Following venous obstruction, venous collaterals develop readily to permit satisfactory venous drainage, and so there is no reason to believe that lymphatic vessels behave any differently provided that a sufficient incentive to lymph drainage, for example muscle pump activity, is maintained (see below). Mention has already been made of the difficulties in creating experimental lymphoedema, and so lymphatic vessel regeneration must be considered efficient on the whole. Extensive scar formation and tissue fibrosis following radiotherapy or wound infection are all known to discourage lymph vessel reanastomosis. Collateral lymph drainage routes may be damaged by X-rays even if they lie outside the field of irradiation.[12] Inflammatory processes may easily cause intraluminal obliteration of lymphatic vessels due to lymphangitis or lymphangiothrombosis. Infections such as bacterial lymphangitis and cellulitis are the major culprits and may herald the onset of lymphoedema.

Movement

Lymphatics rely almost entirely on local tissue movement for lymph propulsion. Lymph capillaries and precollectors possess no smooth muscle in the vessel wall. Lymph movement into and along these smallest peripheral vessels is largely a passive process dependent on changes in local hydrostatic and osmotic pressures; it is only the larger contractile lymphatic collectors and trunks which actively pump lymph. A common but poorly documented form of peripheral oedema results from a combination of immobility and dependency. Immobility leads to chronic lymph stasis[2] which is compounded by enhanced lymph formation from venous hypertension in a dependent lower limb. This clinical syndrome is most vividly seen in infirm patients who are confined to a chair, day and night, by heart and respiratory failure. The phrase 'armchair legs' has been coined to describe this syndrome, for which the clinical appearances are indistinguishable from lymphoedema.[1] An alternative term is lymphostasis verruciformis or verrucosis. Chronic oedema arises under similar circumstances in paralysed limbs and with severe arthritis where the combination of immobility and dependency prevail.

Tumour

Tumour rarely presents as lymphoedema except in circumstances of advanced cancer, for example cancer of the prostate. For this to occur, infiltration with carcinoma or lymphoma has to be extensive as lymph flow is maintained surprisingly well through malignant nodes. More commonly, lymphoedema is a manifestation of recurrent cancer when lymph transport capacity has already been compromised through previous cancer therapy. Skin infiltration with tumour, particularly carcinoma of the breast, frequently targets in and around dermal lymphatic vessels. Expansion of the lymphatic vessel permits bidirectional growth of tumour throughout the lymph network. Extensive infiltration of skin and subcutaneous lymphatic vessels produces profound obstruction and tense oedema, leading to a firm to hard consistency of the tissues, so-called carcinoma *en cuirasse*. Fibrosis and elephantiasis soon ensue.

Clinical manifestations

Lymphoedema most commonly affects an anatomical region drained by regional lymph glands. Less commonly, a more localized area may be affected owing to damage to smaller, more peripheral lymphatic collectors. Swelling tends to occur in those non-compartmentalized tissues where expansion is possible, such as the subcutis. The overlying skin tends to suffer secondarily as a result of back pressure from obstructed proximal lymphatic vessels 'downstream'—the so-called 'dermal backflow'. Limbs are affected most by lymphoedema simply because of the limited exit route.

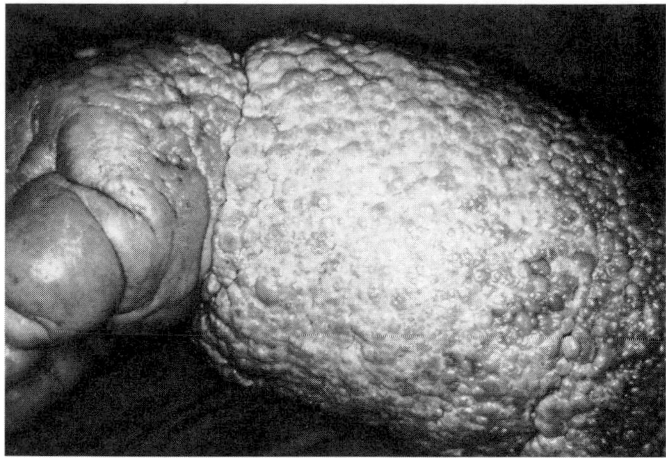

Fig. 1 'Elephantiasis' skin changes characteristic of lymphoedema.

Lymph drainage of the adjoining quadrant of the trunk is equally affected, but the possibilities for collateral drainage are that much greater. Nevertheless, close inspection of the upper trunk in any case of arm lymphoedema secondary to axillary intervention will reveal some truncal lymphoedema, usually in the anterior and posterior axillary folds.

Lymphoedema differs from all other forms of oedema in the changes that it generates in the skin and subcutaneous tissues. Enhanced skin creases, increased tissue turgor, hyperkeratosis, and papillomatosis are most obvious in circumstances where peripheral lymphatics are overloaded and severely obstructed (Fig. 1). This occurs most commonly in lower-limb lymphoedema and malignant infiltration of skin lymphatic vessels, and the clinical diagnosis of lymphoedema depends almost entirely on these changes in skin and subcutaneous tissue. Stemmer[16] described the useful sign of thickened skin folds of the toes which prevent pinching of the skin, particularly at the base of the second toe (Fig. 2).

Traditionally, lymphoedema is described as brawny oedema which does not readily pit. Whilst this may be generally true, pitting is a most unreliable sign as many cases of lymphoedema will exhibit easy displacement of tissue fluid on pressure. Most forms of oedema respond to elevation and diuretics, but lymphoedema does

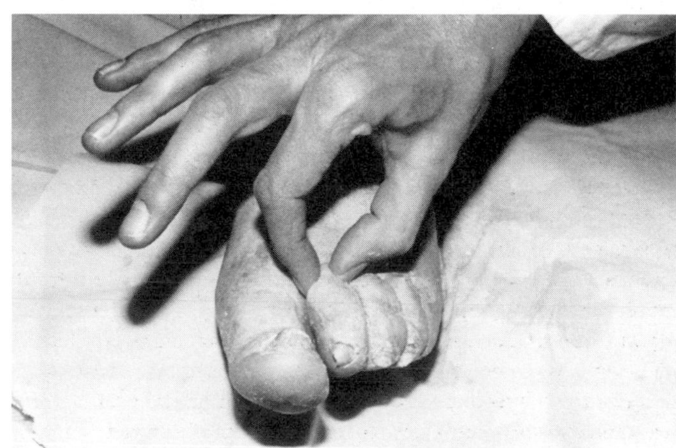

Fig. 2 Stemmer's sign: the thickened skin and subcutaneous tissues prevent pinching of a fold of skin at the base of the second toe.

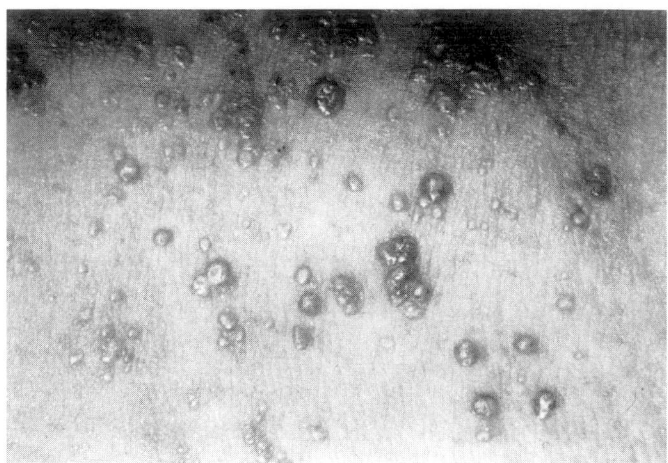

Fig. 3 Acquired lymphangiomas: lymph 'blisters' due to dilated superficial dermal lymphatic vessels.

not, except in the very early stages or when compounded by increased capillary filtration. Indeed, chronic swelling that does not reduce significantly after overnight elevation is likely to be lymphatic in origin.

Dilatation of upper dermal lymphatic vessels to the extent whereby they visibly bulge on the skin surface as lymph 'blisters' is referred to as lymphangioma. Such lesions can appear anywhere on a lymphoedematous limb, but occur more commonly in areas of subcutaneous fibrosis, perhaps within or close to radiation damage (Fig. 3). From time to time the lymphangiomas release lymph on to the skin surface and serve as a portal of entry for infection. With time, organization of lymphangiectatic or dilated surface lymphatic vessels results in papillomatosis.

There is one specific and characteristic complication of lymphoedema, and that is recurrent erysipelas or cellulitis. The patient feels constitutionally unwell, as if influenza is starting, and within 8 to 24 h redness and tenderness appear in the lymphoedematous area. Swelling invariably increases, and may remain even after the resolution of the attack. Because of the failure to isolate an organism in the majority of cases, the bacterial aetiology of all such cases has been brought into question. Under normal circumstances the lymphatic system contains and handles any infection regionally between the portal of entry and the lymph node. Presumably an impaired lymph drainage route permits more rapid dissemination of micro-organisms within the tissues and into the blood, leading to constitutional upset before any signs of inflammation are evident. All infections—viral, fungal, and bacterial—seem more common in lymphoedema, but data on true incidence are lacking. Indeed, fungal infection (*Tinea pedis*) is almost invariable at some time in lower-limb lymphoedema.

There is a small but significant risk of the development of a secondary malignancy within chronic lymphoedema. The most infamous is lymphangiosarcoma (Stewart–Treves syndrome), but other tumours including squamous cell carcinoma, lymphoma, melanoma, and malignant fibrous histiocytoma have been described. The favoured theory for the association of chronic lymphoedema and subsequent malignancy is altered immune surveillance in the affected region.[17] Kaposi's sarcoma is frequently associated with lymphoedema, but the tumour usually antedates the onset of the swelling. Lymphoedema may facilitate the local spread of the primary tumour, for example in melanoma. This is presumably because the obstructed and dilated lymphatics allow free bidirectional spread of tumour cells within the vessel lumen.

When the clinician is presented with chronic asymmetrical oedema, for example arm swelling in a breast cancer patient, there is a tendency to diagnose lymphoedema automatically. As discussed in the section on pathophysiology, there may be several underlying factors contributing to oedema. All breast cancer patients who have had axillary intervention, whether it be simple node sampling or full axillary clearance plus radiotherapy, will have lymph drainage impairment, albeit in different degrees of severity. Therefore the addition of hypoalbuminaemia, venous outflow obstruction, neurological deficit, or restricted joint movements may, in the face of compromised lymph drainage, tip the balance in favour of tissue oedema. Thus the development of lymphoedema depends upon the dynamic interplay of all these factors.

A full clinical assessment should bear all these possibilities in mind. Venous outflow obstruction may manifest with dilated collateral veins around the shoulder and on the chest wall (Fig. 4). In addition, the brachial vein may be distended permanently or perhaps only in certain arm positions. Sometimes the skin may appear rather cyanosed or mottled, further signs of compromised venous drainage.

Poor shoulder movements will not only lead to a limb that is held in a dependent position, but the lack of use will limit the activation of the muscle pump, which is so important for both lymph and venous drainage.

Neurological deficit usually results from brachial plexus neuropathy either from radiation damage or tumour compression/infiltration. The reduced mobility and dependency of the arm will encourage swelling, as seen so often in patients who are paralysed following a stroke. Therefore a careful neurological examination is important. Progressive neurological signs may be the first clue to axillary recurrence of tumour.

Similar problems occur in lower-limb lymphoedema, but venous hypertension with consequent increased capillary filtration coexists more frequently. Apart from the recurring theme of a dependent and immobile limb, the risk of silent deep vein thrombosis is much

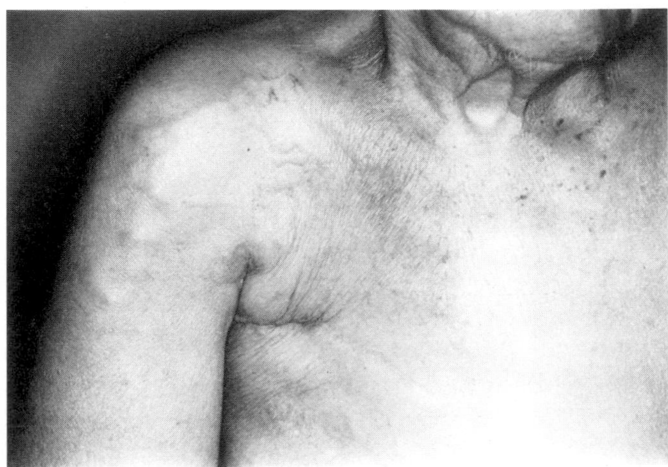

Fig. 4 Visibly dilated collateral veins around the shoulder indicative of venous outflow obstruction.

greater in the leg. In addition, pelvic tumours may compress or infiltrate the main collecting veins including the inferior vena cava. Thrombosis may then ensue. Venous outflow obstruction will manifest with dilated skin venules and a cyanotic congested look to the skin. Haemorrhage into the skin may occur and collateral veins may be evident on the abdomen or flanks.

Severe pain is never the result of lymphoedema alone, and usually indicates other problems such as bone metastases or nerve infiltration. Profound venous obstruction or deep vein thrombosis can also be painful. Lymphoedema usually causes symptoms of discomfort, heaviness, tightness, or bursting.

Diagnostic considerations

The diagnosis of lymphoedema is not always straightforward. *In vivo* visualization of lymphatic vessels (lymphangiography) and nodes (lymphography) using a radiographic contrast medium remains the gold standard for demonstrating lymphatic vessel abnormalities. However, the technique is invasive and difficult to perform in the presence of oedema. Only subcutaneous lymphatics as large as, or larger than, the collectors can be opacified, except in pathological circumstances when dermal backflow occurs and smaller skin lymphatics become visible. Lymphangiography is rarely if ever justified for the investigation of oedema in the cancer patient.

The need for more functional information rather than simply anatomical detail, as contrast lymphography provides, has seen the emergence of quantitative lymphoscintigraphy (isotope lymphography). The dynamics of lymph flow as depicted by radiocolloid uptake and transit via lymphatic vessels can be studied using a gamma camera with a large field of view. The tracer is administered by interstitial injection, which obviates the need for direct cannulation of peripheral lymphatic vessels. Transit times and time–activity curves calculated from regions of interest (e.g. over nodes) permit quantitative analysis. Quantitative lymphoscintigraphy (isotope lymphography) has proved useful in the differential diagnosis of chronic limb swelling by detecting lymphatic insufficiency.[18] The main lymph drainage routes can be identified. Lymphatic obstruction results in retrograde lymph flow to cutaneous lymphatics (dermal backflow). Thus various subgroups of lymphoedema can be identified without recourse to conventional lymphography, and in this way it is possible to identify subtle or incipient lymphoedema and lymphatic insufficiency in cases of chronic oedema of compound origin. Obviously, if total or partial lymphadenectomy has taken place, nodal radioactivity cannot be used as an index of lymph drainage function! In such cases the fractional removal rate of tracer from the injection site has to be used for functional assessment of lymph drainage.

The overriding consideration in the investigation of lymphoedema must be the quest for underlying malignancy, if not already known. Its exclusion is not always straightforward or guaranteed by negative results. Therefore the possibility must always be borne in mind.

Sometimes tumour may be present within the lymphoedema. This is not infrequently the case with inflammatory breast carcinoma, and a simple skin biopsy may put the clinical problem into context.

A major advance in the investigation of the venous system has been the development of colour duplex ultrasound.[15] The colour facility permits imaging of vessels not previously visible and indicates direction of flow. Consequently, flow disturbances indicative of venous obstruction and thrombi can be readily identified by non-invasive means. Unfortunately, not all centres have access to colour duplex facilities, and so conventional venography has to be performed if venous abnormalities are suspected. This procedure is not only invasive but is difficult to perform in the presence of oedema.

Management approaches

The same principles of treatment that apply to the active treatment of patients with no evidence of malignant disease can still be applied, in a modified form if necessary, in the palliative care setting.[19] In cases where the cause of oedema is not primarily the presence of tumour, much can be done to reduce and control swelling. Where uncontrolled tumour is the principal cause, it is less likely that the oedema will be responsive to treatment; palliating the symptoms associated with swelling becomes the priority in these situations and is a realistic aim.

Many of the factors that predispose to the onset of oedema in patients with advanced disease can be identified during the routine monitoring of such patients (Fig. 5). The onset of swelling in the feet and ankles of a patient with reduced mobility, for example, is rarely seen as a significant problem. Yet, if allowed to progress, this can have a devastating effect on what little mobility the patient already has, and can lead to great distress when complications such as lymphorrhoea and deterioration in the condition of the skin develop. If treatment is instigated promptly, as soon as swelling is evident, the quality of life for such patients is greatly enhanced. Preventive measures can even be taken where it is known that the risk of developing oedema is high.

Drug therapy

Drug therapy for uncomplicated lymphoedema is extremely disappointing. Diuretics achieve little more than relief of symptoms of tightness in a congested limb and do not improve swelling. Nevertheless, this indication may be justified in cases of very tense oedema where symptoms of tightness and congestion may be very uncomfortable. Care must be taken as fluid may be mobilized from everywhere but the offending limb, leaving the chronically ill patient with a reduced plasma volume, hypotension, and altered electrolyte status.

In circumstances of advanced cancer it is not unusual for both venous and lymphatic obstruction to occur, for example with extensive abdominal and pelvic tumour. In this situation potent diuretics may be necessary in order to achieve some symptom relief. High-dose steroids are also justifiable if, by reducing tumour bulk, venous and lymphatic channels can be reopened, albeit temporarily.

Claims[21] that benzopyrones are effective in the treatment of lymphoedema need further substantiation. Experimental work on the related hydroxy-rutosides has shown that they have vasoactive properties, and their action in helping lymphoedema may be through influencing capillary protein flux and filtration rather than lymph flow.[22]

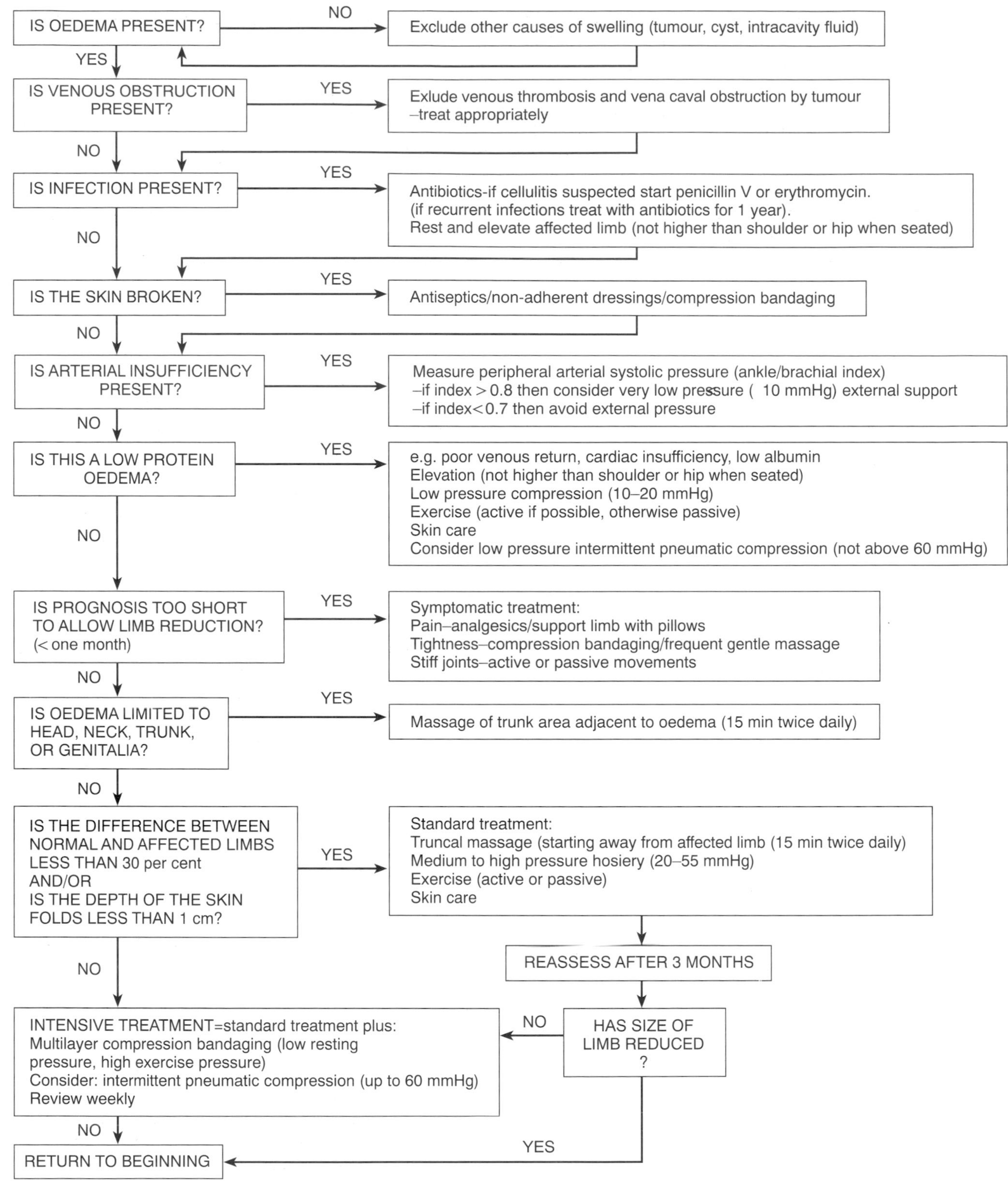

Fig. 5 Routine monitoring of patients with advanced disease. (Reproduced with permission from ref. 20.)

Physical therapy treatment: principles and rationale

The four main principles of treatment are care of the skin, external support or compression, movement, and massage.[23]

Care of the skin

One of the characteristic features of lymphoedema is an increased risk of local infections due to a locally compromised immune system. Since the skin in oedematous areas is particularly vulnerable to trauma, its care is an essential component of treatment.

Some patients are prone to recurrent acute inflammatory attacks (cellulitis) in the swollen limb. Antibiotics started at the peak of an attack are probably of little use and the emphasis is on prevention. Daily low-dose penicillin-V is recommended as a prophylactic for patients experiencing recurrent attacks. Treatment with compression should be postponed until an attack has resolved, and the patient should be advised to elevate and rest the affected limb.

External support and compression

'Support may be defined as the retention and control of tissue without the application of compression'.[24] Under support, pressure is achieved by the tissue pushing against the bandage: 'Compression implies the deliberate application of pressure ... in order to produce a desired clinical effect'.[24] In other words, the tension in the fabric of the bandage or stocking causes pressure to be exerted beneath it.

External compression, in the form of bandages or hosiery, is used when the aim of treatment is to reduce swelling or when trying to maintain the reduced limb size. Support, in contrast, is used when a reduction in limb size is not anticipated or perhaps not necessarily desirable. It can also be supplied by either a bandage or stocking, although in this case a lower degree of pressure is used.

Bandages

The technique used in the treatment of oedema is that of a system of layers.[25] Tubular stockinette is first applied to the limb to protect the skin from any chafing effects. Next, a layer of padding is applied to protect the joint flexures and to even out any distortion in the shape of the limb, thus providing a smooth profile on which to bandage. Finally, high-compression bandages are applied to give an evenly graduating pressure, high distally reducing to low proximally, up the length of the limb.

When the treatment objective is reduction of the oedema, the bandages are left in place around the clock and reapplied every 24 h to ensure the maintenance of adequate pressure. Treatment is carried out daily until the limb size has reached a satisfactory level, when compression hosiery can be fitted to maintain the improvement. In situations where the maintenance of high levels of pressure is not critical and where the principal aim is support and the alleviation of discomfort arising from the distension of the tissues, the bandages may be left in place for longer periods than this. However, bandaging should never result in trauma to the skin, and it is wise to check the condition of the skin regularly, particularly when bandaging patients with reduced sensation in the affected limb.

The indications for using bandages in place of hosiery include gross swelling, fragile or damaged skin, lymphorrhoea, and significant distortion in limb shape. In all other cases hosiery is to be preferred since it is less time consuming to apply, is less bulky, and involves less disturbance to the patient.

Hosiery

The availability of 'off-the-shelf' elastic hosiery in a wide range of sizes, designs, and compression classes means that most patients can be accommodated. Shaped Tubigrip has a useful role to play in containing soft pitting oedema, and layers can be added to increase pressure when this is desired. It is generally best used on arms or lower legs rather than full-length on the leg, since it has a tendency to roll over at the top causing constriction in the area of the groin. Antiembolism stockings have no part to play in either reducing or controlling swelling in the legs because they offer poor ungraduated external pressure.

Movement

The presence of oedema in a limb reduces mobility in the affected joints and often hampers free movement of the limb owing to the increased weight. There is usually an understandable tendency for the patient to be reluctant to move the affected limb, and to support a swollen arm, for instance, in a sling. This can result in the joints becoming fixed and encourages pooling of fluid and increased discomfort.

Emphasis on improving or simply preserving any residual movement in the swollen limb by regular gentle movement and exercise will help to promote the drainage of fluid[25] and to minimize joint stiffness. The use of slings should be discouraged and a collar and cuff substituted. This is preferable because the weight of the arm is distributed across the patient's back, not around the neck, and supports the arm at the wrist at a level just sufficient to relieve the weight from the affected shoulder. This avoids immobilizing the arm with the elbow flexed. When the patient is sitting or resting, the cuff should be removed and the arm supported outstretched on pillows high enough to relieve pressure on the shoulder. There is no need to elevate the limb beyond the horizontal, nor is there any advantage to be gained from doing so.

Massage

A very gentle form of massage is used to encourage the movement of lymph from congested oedematous areas to areas of the body where it can drain normally.[25,26] The amount of pressure used when massaging should only be enough to move the skin and tissues beneath the hand; it should not cause the skin to redden. The technique is more one of stroking the surface of the body. The skin should be free of oils, creams, or talcum powder when massaging.

Specific problems

A careful assessment of the patient is needed before treatment begins to determine the cause and type of oedema, since the appropriate approach is largely determined by this. An assessment will also highlight the patient's main symptomatic problems. The aim of treatment is to make the patient feel more comfortable, and regular reassessment is needed so that treatment can be adjusted as their condition progresses.

Lymphorrhoea

Lymphorrhoea is the term used to describe the leakage of lymph through a break in the skin. This may occur as a result of accidental trauma to the skin. It may also occur in an acute onset or exacerbation of oedema, when the skin is not able to stretch quickly enough to accommodate swelling, or if acquired lymph blisters (lymphangiomas) are present. Lymphorrhoea requires prompt treatment since it results in an increased risk of infection. Pressure applied to the affected limb and maintained over 24 to 48 h will usually resolve the leakage. Bandages are the most convenient and effective method of treatment. Ensure that the limb is clean and apply a thick sterile pad to the leaking area, with a layer of paraffin gauze beneath it to prevent the pad from adhering. Then bandage the limb in the usual way. Change the wet bandages as often as necessary and maintain the pressure around the clock. Once the leaking has resolved, compression hosiery will need to be applied to control the swelling and prevent further leakage.

Fragile skin

Acute onset or exacerbation of swelling, particularly in the legs of elderly or debilitated patients, often results in disruption of the capillaries, leading to bruising and small tears in the skin which appear as fine red streaks or cracks. The skin looks taut and shiny and is extremely fragile. In these cases support or compression bandages are the most suitable approach to treatment until the condition of the skin improves, since the application and removal of close-fitting hosiery carries the risk of further trauma.

Cutaneous tumour infiltration

Tumour involving the skin of an oedematous limb further impairs lymph drainage by obstructing collateral lymph drainage routes through the skin. Pressure in the limb is increased, and the tissues become tense and hard. The skin is often discoloured and inflamed in appearance. Breakdown of the skin is common and is often accompanied by weeping from areas of tumour or from lymph blisters that have formed. Most patients find relief from the intense feeling of pressure in the tissues when a counterpressure is applied to the limb. A support bandage is the simplest way of achieving this and has the added advantage of being easy to apply over any necessary dressings. Be guided by what the patient finds comfortable when choosing the amount of pressure to use, since the aim here is to alleviate discomfort and not necessarily to force fluid out of the limb.

Venous obstruction

Venous blood flow may be compromised by tumour or by thrombosis, or by a combination of the two. Swelling of a limb due to vein thrombosis generally eases as the clot resolves and is not usually an indication for the application of compression or support. However, if a blood clot develops in a lymphoedematous limb, an extra burden is placed on the already impaired lymph drainage routes and the subsequent increase in swelling may not resolve as easily. Compression can safely be applied if a thrombus develops in the upper limb, usually with considerable effect on the reduction of limb size. In the case of deep vein thrombosis in the lower limb or obstruction to blood flow by tumour, support to the limb will help the associated discomfort and is more appropriate than the use of compression. Once again either bandages or one of the lower classes of compression hosiery (i.e. class I stockings giving a pressure of 10-20 mmHg at the ankle) can be used. This reduces the risk of embolism.

Tumour in the abdomen or pelvis

Tumour in the abdomen or pelvis may result in compression or occlusion of venous blood flow and a resulting backlog of fluid in the lower limbs, the genitals, and the tissues of the lower trunk. Depending on the level and degree of obstruction, oedema can extend as far up the body as the level of the axillae. Obviously, any treatment that results in a reduction in the size of the tumour will lead to a corresponding improvement in the degree of oedema. If this is not possible, a trial of high-dose steroids and diuretics may bring some relief. In theory, reducing peritumour swelling and thereby relieving the compression of the blood vessels to some degree should allow some improvement in the drainage of fluid.

Although the oedema in the legs may be soft, pitting, and easily displaced, there is little to be gained from applying compression to reduce their size; fluid will be forced into the already congested tissues of the trunk, adding to the patient's discomfort. Low-class compression hosiery will give a feeling of support to the tissues; stockings that come in the form of tights are preferred since they also provide some support to the genital area. Maternity panty-hose are a particularly useful alternative since they are designed to accommodate large abdomens. Gentle massage can be used to encourage whatever drainage is possible. Massage should start above the level of the swelling, concentrating on areas such as the axillae and the supraclavicular fossae, and move gradually down the trunk. This can have the effect, albeit short-term, of easing the tightness in the oedematous tissues, and many patients find it soothing and comforting. Massage can be performed as often as the patient wishes, and it is something that can be taught to visiting relatives and friends who benefit from the feeling of involvement in the patient's care.

Midline oedema

Midline oedema refers to swelling affecting the head and neck and the genitals. Swelling of the head and neck is rarely seen, and its appearance suggests the presence of local tumour. Genital oedema is commonly seen in patients with abdominal or pelvic tumour. It can be precipitated if compression (either bandages or more commonly pneumatic compression pumps) is used to treat leg swelling in patients with obstructive lower-limb oedema. Treatment of both these sites is difficult, and regular gentle massage performed several times a day is the only feasible option.

Dependency/immobility oedema

Oedema due to dependency or immobility is common in elderly or very debilitated patients who often spend long periods sitting in a chair or wheelchair with their legs down. In the absence of movement there is no propulsion to the flow of lymph, and if the limb is positioned in a dependent position gravitational forces encourage pooling of fluid. Brachial plexus damage leading to weakness and disuse of the limb can also result in the formation of oedema in the dependent arm. This kind of oedema is often disregarded and left untreated, particularly when it affects the lower legs, until inevitably problems develop. The typical picture is one of grossly puffy feet and ankles with dry flaking skin. There are often bruises and small injuries to the skin from knocks on surrounding furniture; the weight of the swollen legs adds to the patient's immobility and they are often more clumsy and unstable on their feet. There is frequently copious weeping from these injuries as well as from the lymph blisters that can form, and consequently constant wetting of the skin. This, together with the fact that swelling makes it difficult to wear footwear, means that the feet and legs are often icy cold to the touch.

Bandages are used until any weeping has resolved and will usually result in a considerable reduction of the limb size. Low- to medium-compression hosiery (class 1 or 2) and elevation of the limbs when the patient is seated will help to control oedema formation. Regular movement of the limbs will bring the muscle pump into play and encourage lymph and blood flow.

Neurological deficit

If a neurological deficit is present in the limb, there is an additional problem besides that of dependency oedema. The reduction or absence of sensation in the limb greatly increases the risk of skin trauma. Great care must be taken when applying compression so as to avoid accidental trauma or constriction of blood flow; the fingers and joint flexures are particularly vulnerable. Since the patient will not be able to report feelings of pain or discomfort, regular checks must be made on the position of hosiery (it may be rolling over at the top or gathering in joint flexures) or the bandage. The temperature and colour of the tips of the fingers or toes must also be monitored regularly and the skin inspected for signs of friction or breakdown.

Future prospects

Chronic lymphoedema resulting from cancer therapy should be preventable, but it is always possible that lymphoedema will develop in the advanced stages of cancer. How can treatment-related lymphoedema be prevented? In the first place, any pre-existing or congenitally determined lymphatic insufficiency should be identified prior to cancer therapy. This can easily be done by quantitative lymphoscintigraphy, but whether cancer physicians and surgeons would want, or indeed be willing, to include yet another test in the staging protocol is doubtful. Even if incipient lymphoedema were identified prior to cancer therapy, would it change oncological practice? Probably not.

Changes in clinical practice, and in particular a move towards medical therapy rather than surgery or radiotherapy, will undoubtedly reduce the risk of lymphoedema. At present this is some way off and, considering that lymphoedema can develop many years after treatment and, once established, is incurable, the problem is likely to be with us for some time.

There is little doubt that the earlier lymphoedema treatment is introduced the more successful it is. Chronic swelling represents endstage lymph flow failure, and therefore, to avoid reaching this point, measures should be introduced the moment oedema occurs or better still beforehand! So often patients suffer a period of transient and intermittent swelling prior to the chronic stage, but are told: 'Don't worry, it will settle'. A different attitude should be adopted, namely 'This is a warning that the lymph system is about to fail, and preventive measures should be introduced without delay'.

References

1. Mortimer PS. Investigation and management of lymphoedema. *Vascular Medicine Review*, 1990; **1**:1–20.
2. Mortimer PS, Regnard CF. Lymphostatic disorders. *British Medical Journal*, 1986; **293**:347–8.
3. Handley WS. Lymphangioplasty: new method for relief of brawny arm of breast-cancer and for similar conditions of lymphatic origin. *Lancet*, 1908; **i**:783–5.
4. Lobb AW, Harkins HN. Postmastectomy swelling of the arm with note on the effect of segmental resection of axillary vein at time of radical mastectomy. *Western Journal of Surgery*, 1949; **57**:550–7.
5. Hughes JH, Patel AR. Swelling of the arm following mastectomy. *British Journal of Surgery*, 1966; **53**:4–15.
6. Kissin MW, Querci della Rovere G, Easton D, Westbury G. Risk of lymphoedema following the treatment of breast cancer. *British Journal of Surgery*, 1986; **73**:580–4.
7. Drinker CK, Field ME, Homans J. The experimental production of oedema and elephantiasis as a result of lymphatic destruction. *American Journal of Physiology*, 1934; **108**:509–20.
8. Calnan JS. Lymphatics in the swollen leg. In: Gilliland I, Francis J, eds. *The Scientific Basis of Medicine.* London: Athlone Press, 1971:349–64.
9. Gray JH. Studies of the regeneration of the lymphatic vessels. *Journal of Anatomy*, 1939–40; **74**:309–35.
10. Hall JG. Unpublished data.
11. Hall JG. The function of the lymphatic system in immunity. Ph.D. Thesis, Australian National University, 1964.
12. Mortimer PS, Simmonds R, Rezvani M, Robbins M, Ryan TJ, Hopewell JW. Time-related changes in lymphatic clearance in pig skin after a single dose of 18 Gy of X-rays. *British Journal of Radiology*, 1991; **64**:1140–6.
13. Bates DO, Levick JR, Mortimer PS. Starling pressures in the human arm and their alteration in postmastectomy oedema. *Journal of Physiology*, 1994; **477**(2):355–63.
14. Svensson WE, Mortimer PS, Tohno E, Cosgrove DO. Increased arterial inflow demonstrated by Doppler ultrasound in arm swelling following breast cancer treatment. *European Journal of Cancer*, 1994; **30**:661–4.
15. Svensson WE, Mortimer PS, Tohno E, Cosgrove D. Colour Doppler demonstrates venous flow abnormalities in breast cancer patients with chronic arm swelling. *European Journal of Cancer*, 1994; **30**:657–60.
16. Stemmer R. Ein klinisches Zeichen zur frühund differential Diagnose des Lymphodems. *VASA*, 1976; 5(3): 261–2.
17. Schreiber H. *et al.* Stewart-Treves syndrome: a lethal complication of post mastectomy lymphoedema and regional immune deficiency. *Archives of Surgery*, 1979; **114**:82–5.
18. Proby CM, Gane JN, Joseph AE, Mortimer PS. Investigation of the swollen limb with isotope lymphography. *British Journal of Dermatology*, 1990; **123**:29–37.
19. Badger C. Lymphoedema: management of patients with advanced cancer. *Professional Nurse*, 1987; **2**(4):100–2.
20. Badger C, Regnard C. Oedema in advanced disease: a flow diagram. *Palliative Medicine*, 1989; **3**:213-15.
21. Casley-Smith JR, Gwn Morgan R, Piller NB. Treatment of lymphoedema of the arms and legs with 5,6-benzo-[X]-pyrone. *New England Journal of Medicine*, 1993; **329**:1158–63.
22. Michel CC, Blumberg S, Clough G. Hydroxyethyl rutosides reduced the increased permeability which follows perfusion of frog capillaries with protein free solutions. *International Journal of Microcirculation: Clinical and Experimental*, 1988; Special Issue:544.
23. Foldi E, Foldi M, Weissleder H. Conservative treatment of lymphoedema of the limbs. *Angiology*, 1985; **36**:171–80.
24. Thomas S. Bandages and bandaging: the science behind the art. *Care Science and Practice*, 1990; **8**(2):56–60.
25. Badger C, Twycross RG. *Management of Lymphoedema—Guidelines.* Oxford: Sobell Study Centre, 1988.
26. Leduc O, Peeters A, Bourgeois P. Bandages: scintigraphic demonstration of its efficacy on colloidal protein reabsorbtion during muscle activity. In: Nishi M, Uchino S, Yabuki S, eds. *Progress in Lymphology*, Vol. 12. Amsterdam: Excerpta Medica, 1990:421–3.

9.8 Genitourinary disorders

Richard W. Norman

Introduction

The genitourinary system may produce a variety of disturbing symptoms or life-threatening dysfunction in patients in palliative care. Unilateral or bilateral ureteral obstructions occur commonly in association with primary or secondary malignancies involving the retroperitoneum and pelvis. This can lead to pain and/or impaired renal function. Lower-tract obstruction may be associated with benign or malignant conditions involving the bladder neck, prostate, or urethra. Anticholinergic drugs, frequently prescribed for patients in palliative care, may be responsible for voiding dysfunction and may need modification of type or dosage. Interaction between the bladder and other pelvic organs may be significant and can lead to fistula formation. Haematuria requires investigation to determine whether it is of upper- or lower-tract origin and, if severe, will need intervention.

This chapter is concerned with the practical aspects of symptom control in patients in palliative care suffering from urinary tract dysfunction. Emphasis is placed on less aggressive, non-invasive therapies, in keeping with the general condition of these patients. Decisions to recommend more complex, invasive procedures may be appropriate but should always be based on the quality of life anticipated, stage of the disease, and reasonable likelihood of symptomatic improvement.

Pathophysiology and factors governing voiding

The bladder wall is composed of a mesh of smooth muscle fibres which become organized in layers at the bladder neck (detrusor muscle). The outer layer extends throughout the length of the female urethra (Fig. 1) and to the distal aspect of the prostate in the male, where its arrangement (circular/spiral) is responsible for the major involuntary sphincter (Fig. 2). The middle circular layer ends at the bladder neck and contributes to sphincteric function. Internal fibres remain longitudinal and extend to the distal end of the urethra in the female and the distal prostate in the male. Converging, they form the muscle of the vesical neck, which contributes to urinary continence.

The bladder receives its principal nerve supply from one paired somatic and two paired autonomic nerves. The hypogastric nerves, arising from lumbar spinal segments, mediate sympathetic activity, while the pelvic nerves, derived from S2–S4 contain parasympathetic fibres. The pudendal nerves (S2–S4) primarily serve as a conduit for non-autonomic fibres. With distension of the bladder wall, stretch receptors trigger pelvic nerve fibres which, unless inhibited by higher centres, will lead to a parasympathetic motor response and bladder contraction (Fig. 3).

The voluntary external sphincter is made up of striated muscle, which is located between the layers of the urogenital diaphragm. In the male, these fibres are concentrated at the distal aspect of the prostate; in the female, they are found mainly in relation to the middle third of the urethra. Smooth muscle investing the vesical neck and posterior urethra is under sympathetic control, mediated through the hypogastric nerve with thoracolumbar origin (T11–L2). Noradrenaline is the neurotransmitter in this sympathetic release. The external sphincter is under pudendal nerve control (S2–S4) and influenced by autonomic as well as somatic innervation from the pelvic floor. All are co-ordinated by higher centres to initiate or inhibit bladder emptying.

Satisfactory voiding requires an unobstructed passage from the bladder to the urethral meatus, in addition to a functioning detrusor muscle, an intact bladder wall, and integrity of the nerves initiating and co-ordinating detrusor and sphincteric activity. Stimulation of the parasympathetic bladder nerves causes contraction of the detrusor muscle and relaxation of the bladder neck sphincter. Stimulation of the sympathetic system (T10–T12, L1) has the reverse effect.

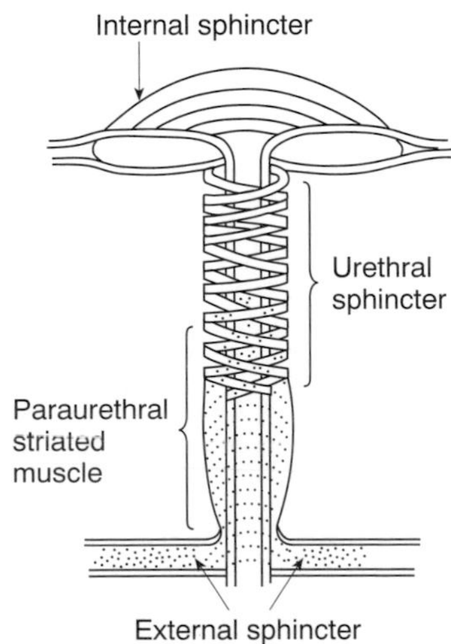

Fig. 1 Sphincter arrangement in the female (redrawn from ref 1. by courtesy of Williams and Wilkins Co.).

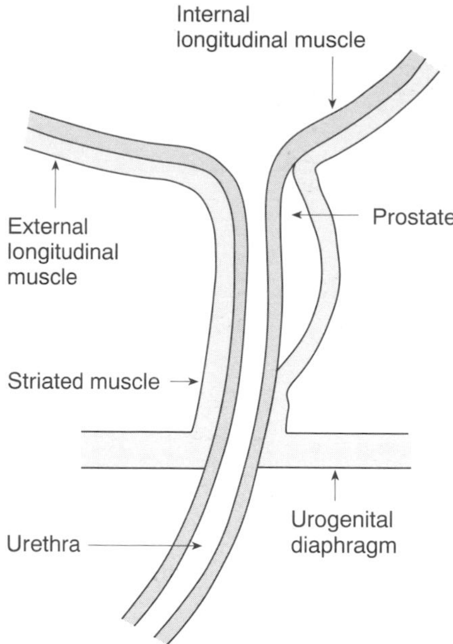

Fig. 2 Sagittal section of the male urethra (redrawn from ref 2. by courtesy of Williams and Wilkins Co.).

Neurological damage associated with metastases to the spine and epidural space causing spinal-cord compression or nerve-root injury secondary to tumour infiltration may interfere with voiding. Drugs required for control of pain and other symptoms in patients with advanced cancer also have an important impact on bladder function. Anticholinergic drugs can interfere by causing contraction of the bladder neck sphincter and relaxation of the detrusor muscle. Drugs with such effects which are frequently used in patients with advanced cancer include phenothiazines, haloperidol, antihistamines, and tricyclic antidepressants. Opioid drugs have little impact on bladder function unless combined with other problems, for example faecal impaction, which, when significant, adds an obstructive component by pressure on the urethra. Particular caution is indicated in the use of these drugs in the elderly and in patients who have pre-existing early bladder outlet obstruction.

Bladder outlet obstruction with distension produces great physical distress which may be masked in the elderly and in patients taking opioid drugs and neuroleptic agents. Confusion is a common presentation, particularly in the elderly. This may result from the physical discomfort or as a result of metabolic disturbance from impaired renal function.

In the evaluation of dysfunction, the anatomical and functional integrity of the bladder and urethra should be considered. Spinal-cord or nerve-root damage should be ruled out. The patient's drug profile must be reviewed. If possible, drugs with anticholinergic effects should be eliminated or the dosage reduced. Constipation should be considered. Biochemical abnormalities which may increase urinary flow must be remembered—hypercalcaemia, hyperglycaemia, and diabetes insipidus should be excluded.

Urinary incontinence

Involuntary loss of urine or urinary incontinence is described usually as total, overflow, urgency, or stress. In patients with advanced malignant disease, total urethral incontinence or extra-urethral loss from urinary fistulas are the most common and significant.

Total urethral incontinence

This is associated with sphincteric incompetence. Direct tumour invasion, surgical intervention, or loss of innervation from spinal cord or nerve root damage represent the usual responsible factors in patients in palliative care. Direct visualization confirms the urethral nature of the loss. Endoscopic examination or urodynamic evaluation may be necessary to establish a diagnosis. The presence of other motor or sensory abnormalities suggesting spinal cord or nerve root damage may provide the necessary evidence to implicate a neurological deficit. Management usually entails use of an indwelling Foley catheter in women and condom drainage or a penile clamp in men. If the condom or penile clamp are not well tolerated, a Foley catheter would be the next choice. Although artificial sphincters are being used with increasing frequency, their use in patients with active and advanced malignant disease is ordinarily inappropriate.

Overflow incontinence

This type of urinary incontinence is associated with bladder outlet or urethral obstruction. Initially associated with the acute distress of acute retention, voiding occurs in small amounts and without control. The bladder is distended and usually palpable except in the very obese or in patients with pelvic masses or extensive lymphoedema involving the lower abdominal wall.

Catheterization is indicated. Definitive treatment must be individualized and may include surgical or other interventional techniques to correct the obstruction, long-term dependence on an indwelling catheter, intermittent catheterization, or an intraurethral stent.

Urgency incontinence

Associated with an irritable but intact bladder musculature, the detrusor force is excessive in relation to urethral sphincter tone. The urge is sudden and urinary loss may be severe. The impaired mobility of patients in a palliative care setting may be an aggravating factor in preventing them from reaching the toilet in time. Causes include intrinsic and extrinsic tumours which produce irritation of the bladder wall, particularly in the region of the trigone and vesical neck. It may also be associated with inflammatory changes from physical agents (e.g. previous radiation), drugs (e.g. cyclophosphamide), or bacteria. An irritable bladder producing urgency incontinence may be of non-specific type or related to lack of inhibition from neural deficiency, as seen in association with cerebrovascular insufficiency. It usually responds to anticholinergic therapy, such as oxybutynin 2.5 to 5.0 mg orally two to three times per day. In the elderly, only one dose daily is recommended. If this is not tolerated other drugs can be considered to reduce detrusor over-activity (Table 1).

Stress incontinence

This does not usually represent a major problem in patients in palliative care. It consists of involuntary urethral loss of urine associated with increased intra-abdominal pressure from coughing,

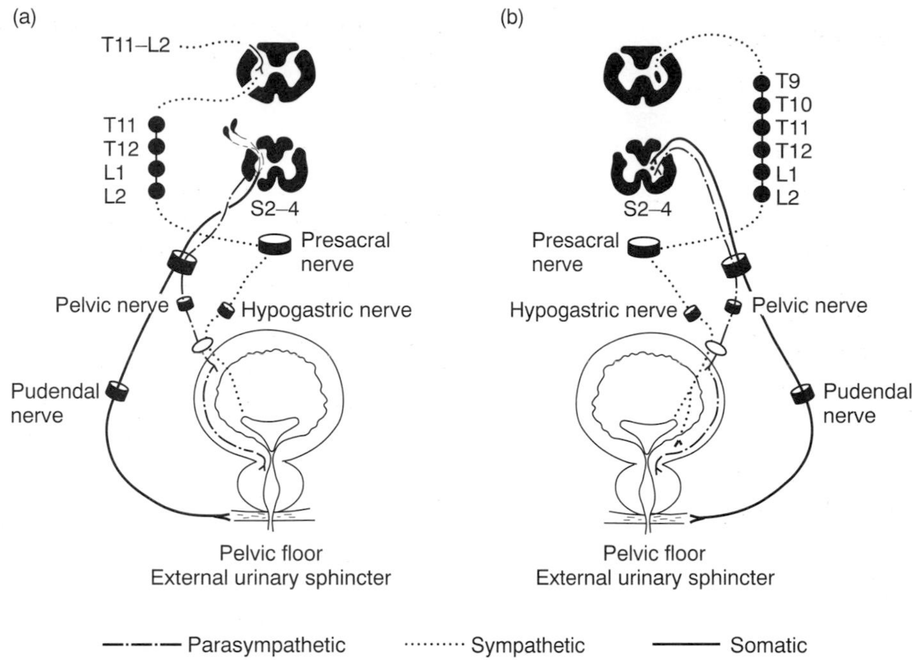

Fig. 3 Innervation of bladder and sites of drug activity.

sneezing, jumping, laughing, or, in severe cases, even walking. It is associated with faulty urethral support, wherein the increased intravesical pressure cannot be resisted. Surgery is the usual treatment but it is unlikely to be appropriate in patients with advanced cancer. A trial of sympathomimetic drugs, such as ephedrine, and tricyclic antidepressants, such as imipramine, may be appropriate. Palliative catheterization may be necessary in severe cases.

Extraurethral incontinence

Urinary fistulas are covered elsewhere in the chapter.

Investigation and management of sudden urinary stoppage

Sudden and marked decrease in urinary output can be both a distressing and potentially lethal problem for patients if it persists and is associated with the metabolic abnormalities characteristic of acute renal failure. Complete cessation of urinary output usually implies obstruction of either the lower urinary tract at the level of the bladder neck, prostate, or distal urethra or upper tract obstruction of both ureters. These will be discussed separately.

Lower tract obstruction as a cause of sudden urinary stoppage

Most patients who develop urinary retention will have had some milder, usually progressive, symptoms of obstruction. They may have noticed hesitancy, decreased urinary stream and inability to empty the bladder satisfactorily. There may also have been symptoms of urinary frequency, nocturia, incontinence, and urinary tract infection. Past history of urethral instrumentation, injury, or infection may point towards the development of a urethral stricture. A history of anticholinergic or α-adrenergic drug use may be a contributing factor. On physical examination, these patients are usually restless and uncomfortable due to a painfully overfilled bladder—usually one is able to see, palpate, and percuss the distended organ. Attention should be paid to the urethral meatus, to rule out significant meatal stenosis, and to the entire length of the urethra, to identify areas of scarring or induration which could imply stricture or tumour formation. Rectal examination is imperative in order to assess the size and consistency of the prostate gland. Firm irregularities may be indicative of cancer of the prostate.

The most appropriate treatment at this time is passage of a urethral catheter to drain the bladder. If this is impossible, insertion of a suprapubic catheter will permit satisfactory bladder drainage and allow relief of symptoms until further, definitive, endoscopic assessment of the lower urinary tract can be arranged. It is important that the subsequent urinary output of these patients be measured on an hourly basis for several hours to ensure that they do not develop a significant postobstructive diuresis. Although most of these patients with prostatic enlargement will benefit from a limited transurethral prostatectomy, some may be treated with an intraurethral stent.[3] Medical therapy, such as the use of 5-reductase inhibitors and α-blockers, has gained in popularity for the management of men with symptomatic benign prostatic hyperplasia but it is not indicated in men with refractory urinary retention.

Case history: A 79-year-old man presented with mild obstructive voiding symptoms and lower back discomfort. He underwent a digital rectal examination and cystoscopy which confirmed the presence of a large, necrotic, nodular prostatic tumour mass with invasion into the right side of the trigone. Biopsies confirmed poorly differentiated adenocarcinoma of the prostate. Renal ultrasound was consistent with right-sided hydronephrosis and a bone scan showed diffuse metastases. Serum prostate specific antigen measured 987 ng/ml. He was treated with total androgen blockade with some improvement in his voiding symptoms and back

Table 1

Action	Dosage	Comments
For detrusor overactivity		
Flavoxate hydrochloride (Urispas) is a papaverine-like antispasmodic with some anticholinergic and anesthetic properties.	200 mg by mouth three or four times daily but up to 1200 mg/day may be used.	Low incidence of side-effects. Recommended for elderly patients and patients who have trouble tolerating other drugs.
Dicyclomine chlorhydrate (Bentylol) has both a musculotropic and anticholinergic effect on smooth muscles.	The Dospan formulation provides continuous-release medication. Up to 80 mg by mouth per day in three or four doses.	
Oxybutynin chloride (Ditropan) has anticholinergic, antispasmodic and anesthetic properties.	2.5 mg by mouth once daily to 5 mg four times a day. For elderly patients stick to 5 mg once a day by mouth	
Propantheline bromide (Pro-Banthine) is a cholinergic receptor competitor.	From 7.5 mg by mouth once daily to 15 mg by mouth four times a day. Where absorption in the digestive tract is incomplete up to 30 mg by mouth four times a day can be advised.	
Imipramine chlorhydrate (Tofranil, Apo-Imipramine) is a tricyclic antidepressant with anxiolytic, anticholinergic, direct musculotropic, and adrenergic properties. It also has mild anesthetic and antihistamine effects. Inhibits the nomdienaline reuptake at presynaptic nerve terminals. Common indications include enuresis and voiding dysfunctions arising from supraspinal lesions.	Increase gradually to about 25 mg twice daily, but up to a maximum of 200 mg/day can be used if necessary.	Imipramine should not be given along with MAO inhibitors.
Belladonna/opium suppositories have analgesic, anticholinergic, and antispasmodic properties. Because of their potential addictiveness, they should only be used over the short term, for example to control pain and bladder spasm after bladder or prostate surgery.	One suppository every 3-4 hours as required	

discomfort. Three months later, he suffered a myocardial infarction. Two weeks following discharge he went into urinary retention and, despite attempts at catheter removal, was unable to void spontaneously. He found the catheter very uncomfortable, but because of his recent cardiovascular problem, he was not felt to be a suitable candidate for a transurethral resection of the prostate. He was treated by placement of an intraurethral stent (Fig. 4) under local anaesthesia and subsequently voided normally.

Comment: There are an increasing number of alternatives for the management of bladder outlet obstruction and it is important to individualize therapy for a specific patient. In this particular case, it was possible to treat this man's problem in a palliative fashion and improve his quality of life without the catheter, despite his serious underlying malignant and cardiovascular diseases.

Bilateral ureteric obstruction as a cause of sudden urinary stoppage

Acute renal failure secondary to bilateral ureteric obstruction is a common problem in palliative care. In 75 per cent of patients within this group, an underlying malignant disorder will be diagnosed. In almost one-half, the development of bilateral ureteric obstruction is the initial manifestation of the underlying cancer. About three-quarters of the tumours are pelvic in origin; the most common in women is carcinoma of the cervix, and in men, carcinoma of the prostate. The most frequent benign diagnosis is retroperitoneal fibrosis.[4]

Common symptoms are a lack of urinary output and abdominal pain. Physical examination may reveal evidence of flank masses or tenderness. The bladder will not be distended and the urethra should be unremarkable. The importance of an adequate rectal and pelvic examination is emphasized in view of the anticipated causes of obstruction.

Because the obstruction may have been progressing over several days prior to causing complete urinary stoppage, most of these patients will reveal laboratory evidence of acute renal failure with elevated levels of serum creatinine and potassium and as a result, investigation and treatment become urgent. Intravenous pyelography is unsuccessful and contraindicated in acute renal failure, but renal ultrasonography can be extremely useful in identifying both kidneys and the degree of obstruction. Occasionally, it may show obstructing stones in the upper ureter or renal pelvis. In the presence of bilateral ureteric obstruction, cystoscopy and bilateral retrograde pyelograms are usually done next. These studies can

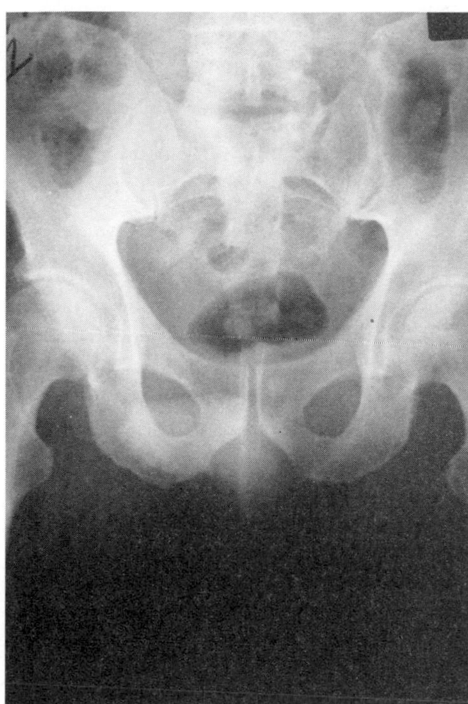

Fig. 4 Urethral stent bridging prostatic urethra.

reveal abnormalities within the urinary bladder such as a primary or secondary tumour involving the trigone, and will outline the ureters to define the level, and often the cause, of the ureteric obstruction. Once this has been accomplished, an indwelling ureteric stent can be passed, under cystoscopic control, up the ureter such that one end lies within the renal pelvis and the other within the bladder.[5] This would usually be attempted on both sides if feasible and if both kidneys appear to have reasonable potential for regaining function. In circumstances in which it is impossible to endoscopically position ureteric stents, one would proceed to percutaneous placement of a nephrostomy tube under ultrasound guidance. These can sometimes be replaced by antegrade insertion of ureteric stents and eliminate the need for an external drainage device.

These patients must be watched for changes in their potassium and creatinine levels, as well as the volume of urinary output, following relief of obstruction. If fluid and electrolyte abnormalities are severe, it may be necessary to arrange early, temporary haemodialysis to correct life-threatening problems.

In situations where this scenario is the result of long-term progression of an underlying malignancy, active intervention at this stage may not be warranted. This option should be discussed with the patient and family. In cases where this is the initial manifestation of underlying cancer, therapy is usually tailored towards the underlying malignancy in the hope of relieving the obstruction. Ordinarily, definitive surgical intervention would be entertained only in this situation.

Unilateral ureteric involvement by underlying malignancy

Because of their long length through either side of the retroperitoneum, the ureters are susceptible to involvement by a wide variety of primary and secondary malignancies. In many cases this can be insidious and asymptomatic; in other instances the effect can be sudden and associated with significant discomfort. In either case, the presence of ureteric obstruction is usually established by either intravenous pyelography, renal ultrasonography, or computerized tomography of the abdomen. These studies may also give further clues to the possible underlying cause of obstruction.

Physical examination of the abdomen, pelvis, and rectum is critical and may provide important information that will assist in determining the underlying problem. Because of the presence of obstruction and the associated decrease in renal function, intravenous pyelography may fail to demonstrate the site of blockage. Many patients, therefore, will require cystourethroscopy and a retrograde study. This will provide important information in terms of the site, degree, and cause of obstruction.

If the involved side is symptomatic, or if the contralateral side is absent or non-functioning, cystoscopic placement of an indwelling ureteric stent is useful in providing temporary relief of the obstruction while further investigation and treatment can be established. When this is impossible, percutaneous placement of an indwelling nephrostomy tube can be a useful means of drainage and can permit injection of dye into the upper tract to define further the site and degree of obstruction. In general, the ultimate outcome in these circumstances will be dictated by the underlying disease. Specific surgical therapy to divert the urine or to lyse the ureters is not usually indicated in the face of advanced underlying malignancy, except in the rare circumstance where the opposite kidney is absent or non-functional. Assuming the contralateral kidney to be functioning reasonably well, it is sometimes necessary to remove the involved, obstructed kidney if it continues to be symptomatic, despite satisfactory internal or external drainage. This is often better tolerated than a heroic attempt at reconstruction. In circumstances where the obstructed kidney is completely asymptomatic and the contralateral kidney is functioning well, intervention is usually not required.

Case history: A 57-year-old man complained of some very minimal fullness and discomfort in the right flank for six weeks. Past history revealed that he had undergone an abdominoperineal resection for carcinoma of the rectum two years previously. At that time, the surgical margins were clear and the lymph nodes were negative. Current investigations included a renal ultrasound which showed high grade ureteric obstruction on the right side with a normal left kidney. Cystoscopy and a right retrograde pyelogram confirmed the presence of marked obstruction of the lower end of the right ureter, secondary to an extrinsic mass. An abdominal and pelvic computerized tomography scan were consistent with liver metastases, right hydroureteronephrosis, and a large, right pelvic mass encasing the lower end of the ureter (Fig. 5(a) and 5(b)). Attempts at insertion of a ureteric stent were unsuccessful and in view of the fact that the patient was coping well, it was decided to perform no further interventions to the right kidney or ureter.

Comment: There are a number of endoscopic and percutaneous approaches to the obstructed ureter, but when a patient has a variety of other underlying problems it is not always appropriate to intervene unless there are significant symptoms. In this situation, the patient was reasonably comfortable and it was decided not to get involved in any more complicated interventional procedures.

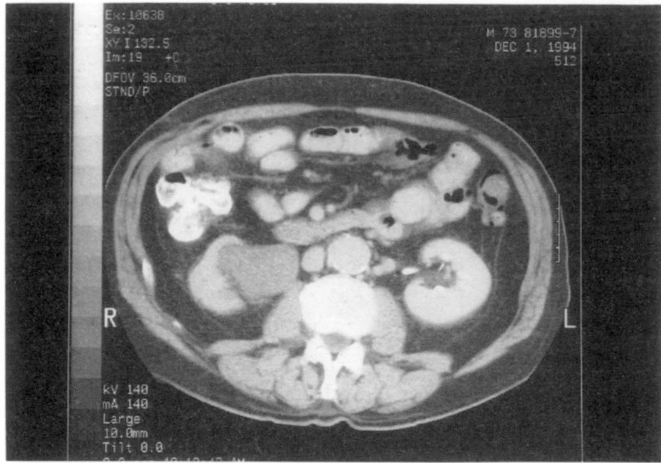

(a)

(b)

Fig. 5 (a) CT scan showing obstructed and dilated right renal pelvis. (b) CT scan showing large tumour mass behind the bladder and obstructing the right ureter.

Haematuria

Haematuria is a frequent symptom and sign of underlying urological disease but the degree of bleeding does not always correlate with the seriousness of the underlying condition.[6] Although a specific cause for asymptomatic microscopic haematuria can often not be determined, it may signal the presence of an underlying malignancy. It is important, therefore, that all degrees of newly diagnosed haematuria be assessed. A key feature in the history relates to whether the urine has been previously examined and whether the presence of blood is a new and persistent finding. Other symptoms, such as dysuria and urinary frequency and urgency, may point toward a urinary tract infection which can be diagnosed with an adequate urinalysis and urine culture. The use of non-steroidal anti-inflammatory drugs and aspirin have been associated with microhaematuria. Danthron, a common component of laxatives used in palliative care, may tint alkaline urine a harmless pink or orange and be confusing. Lower abdominal or flank discomfort may point towards abnormalities in the bladder, ureter, or kidney as the cause. Unfortunately, physical examination often fails to provide satisfactory clues. In these patients, an intravenous pyelogram will allow assessment of the upper tracts in terms of presence, function, and drainage. Although the bladder is also seen, small lesions within it can be missed radiographically and complete cystourethroscopy is indicated when upper tract radiological procedures do not establish a diagnosis. Specific therapy will be directed towards individual abnormalities.

One of the most frightening symptoms is the sudden onset of gross haematuria. This may simply mean the passage of brown- or red-coloured urine, or it could involve the passage of large clots or the development of clot retention or colic. Either will require prompt urological consultation. In the palliative care setting, knowledge of the site of an underlying malignancy, possibility of a major coagulation disorder, history of cyclophosphamide use, or prior pelvic irradiation may be significant. In less urgent cases, investigations as described above would be necessary.

Lower tract

Patients with clot retention require immediate intervention and management prior to the initiation of specific studies. Most of these patients will be frightened and uncomfortable due to bladder distension from blood clots and urine. Usually they are extremely restless and unable to remain still because of discomfort, but in rare cases bleeding may have been sufficient to cause hypotension and shock. On physical examination the distended bladder can be seen, palpated, and percussed. Tenderness or a mass in either flank may hint at an upper-tract cause for the bleeding. Rectal examination is important in men to assess the size and consistency of the prostate and pelvic and rectal examination are important in women to try to identify a pelvic abnormality.

Adequate initial management requires complete evacuation of clots from the bladder. This is best achieved with urethral placement of a 24 or 26F multi-eyed Robinson catheter. Percutaneous insertion of a suprapubic catheter is contraindicated in the presence of clot retention because of the inability to place a catheter of satisfactory size to provide adequate irrigation and the potential for seeding of the percutaneous tract by an unsuspected bladder carcinoma. Once the urethral catheter has been passed into the bladder, vigorous irrigation with water or saline, using a Toomey syringe, will usually permit removal of all clots. This manual irrigation should be continued until no further clots are obtained and the backflow becomes relatively clear. At this stage the Robinson catheter should be replaced with a 22 or 24F three-way indwelling catheter and continuous bladder irrigation (CBI) should be established using cold water or saline.

Unsuccessful attempts at initial placement of a satisfactory urethral catheter, or continued bleeding and recurrent obstruction of the irrigating catheter, are specific indications for early endoscopic evaluation. Recurrent obstruction of the urethral catheter is usually related either to the persistence of clots or significant continuous bleeding. Cystourethroscopy permits complete evaluation of the entire penile and prostatic urethra as well as the bladder. In these circumstances it is important to rule out other causes of obstruction and to identify sites of bleeding. The larger and more rigid cystoscope or resectoscope sheath (compared with the urethral catheter) allows improved evacuation of bladder clots. In the majority of instances, this type of bleeding will be caused by local disease involving either the bladder or prostate. Depending upon the specific circumstances, small and isolated bleeding sites can be cauterized or fulgurated at this time, but usually there is a requirement for transurethral resection of specific lesions to stop the bleeding and to obtain tissue for histological diagnosis. When these procedures have been completed, continuous bladder irrigation is established using an indwelling three-way Foley catheter.

If the bleeding is refractory to these conservative measures, bladder instillations with formalin,[7] silver nitrate (0.5–1.0 per cent), alum (1 per cent),[8] or epsilon aminocaproic acid[9] may be tried. Haemorrhagic cystitis secondary to cyclophosphamide responds to intravesical instillation of carboprost tromethane, an F_2-prostaglandin, in more than 50 per cent of cases.[10] Bleeding from established radiation cystitis may respond to hyperbaric oxygen.[11] On the other hand, local irradiation of the bladder can be palliative in the presence of unresectable cancer and oral tranexamic acid may be helpful, but can cause clot formation and retention. Rarely, it is necessary to resort to surgical intervention, such as hypogastric artery ligation or proximal urinary diversion with or without cystectomy.

Upper tract

Occasionally gross haematuria is not due to local bladder pathology but to upper-tract bleeding. Cystoscopy under these circumstances is again useful in confirming the side from which the blood is coming, and in permitting removal of bladder clots. Retrograde pyelography is occasionally useful under these circumstances, but it should be remembered that many apparent filling defects within the ureter or renal pelvis at these times may simply represent blood clots.

The next investigation would be an intravenous pyelogram, if renal function is satisfactory, or a renal ultrasound if not. The most likely causes of upper-tract bleeding, under these circumstances, would be the presence of renal tumour, such as a renal cell carcinoma or transitional cell carcinoma of the renal pelvis or ureter, or a stone. Rarely, a specific cause will not be identified with these studies and it may be necessary to progress to renal arteriography. Selective injections permit optimal visualization of the intrarenal vasculature and can identify small arteriovenous malformations, small neoplasms, or renal vein varices. Occasionally, even the renal arteriogram will be normal, despite continued gross haematuria, and in these circumstances ureteroscopy can be helpful to identify the specific site of haemorrhage, which can be biopsied and/or cauterized.

In the event that a renal tumour is identified, appropriate management requires metastatic work-up and, if this is negative, a radical nephrectomy is performed. Radical nephroureterectomy with removal of a bladder cuff is usually indicated if it is a transitional cell lesion of the upper tract.

Occasionally the chest radiograph, abdominal computerized tomography scan, or bone scan will confirm the presence of metastases which would obviate the need for radical surgery. In these circumstances, therapeutic arteriography with the injection of pharmacodynamic agents and/or clot or gelfoam can be used to control bleeding. In persistent cases, palliative nephrectomy may be required despite the presence of metastases.[12]

Urinary fistulas

In patients with underlying malignancy, the symptoms associated with urinary tract fistulas, such as abnormal interorgan connections, can be devastating. The psychological distress and physical afflictions associated with these problems can make patients, their families, and their caregivers distraught and give them a sense of hopelessness. The four most common urinary fistulas are vesicoenteric, vesicovaginal, urethrocutaneous, and rectourethral. These will be dealt with individually.

Vesicoenteric fistulas

Fistulization between the bladder and the alimentary tract can involve any segment of bowel. Usually the problem is secondary to colonic malignancy, diverticulitis, or small bowel inflammatory disease. Rarely, the primary problem originates from the bladder. The most characteristic symptom associated with vesicoenteric fistulas is pneumaturia, i.e. the passage of gas or froth in the urine. Because of a connection between the bowel and urinary tract, many patients will suffer from persistent urinary tract infections, particularly when the colon is involved. The urine usually has a foul odour. In circumstances where the connection is large, patients may be aware of passing particulate faecal matter in the urine. Physical examination may reveal the presence of an associated, bowel-related mass from underlying disease, but it is often non-contributory. Cystoscopy usually reveals a localized area of erythema and bullous inflammation at the fistulous site, which is frequently high on the posterior wall. Small amounts of stool may be seen extruding from the involved area. The remainder of the bladder may or may not appear inflamed. Occasionally, the fistulous site may be so small that it cannot be appreciated at the time of endoscopy, and in these circumstances a variety of other tests, including cystography, intestinal barium studies from above or below, computerized scanning tomography,[13] visible contrast media, or oral ^{51}Cr-labelled sodium chromate[14] may be required to identify the abnormal communication.

Management of vesicoenteric fistulas is usually dictated by the underlying bowel disease. Ideally, the segment of bowel and bladder are removed together and bowel and bladder integrity are re-established. If this is not technically feasible, intestinal diversion may redirect enough of the faecal stream to reduce the urinary symptoms to a tolerable level. In rare circumstances when massive bladder involvement is present, a total cystectomy, with or without complete pelvic exenteration, and ileal conduit urinary diversion may be necessary. Placement of bilateral percutaneous nephrostomy tubes would be a poor alternative because such external drainage devices are awkward for a patient to manage and often become displaced.

Case history: An 83-year-old woman with severe, chronic obstructive lung disease was admitted to hospital with pneumonia. She deteriorated rapidly and required endotracheal intubation and ventilation. She was treated with antibiotics, bronchodilators, and steroids and eventually required a tracheostomy. Although she remained alert and was able to communicate with sign language, mouthing of words and writing, it was impossible to wean her from the respirator. As a result she had difficulty mobilizing. Three weeks later, her urine developed a foul smell and was noted to contain large particles of faeces. Cystoscopic evaluation revealed a large fistula arising from the posterior aspect of the bladder in the midline, above the trigone. Barium enema confirmed a large colovesical fistula (Fig. 6). She was not felt to be a candidate for a major

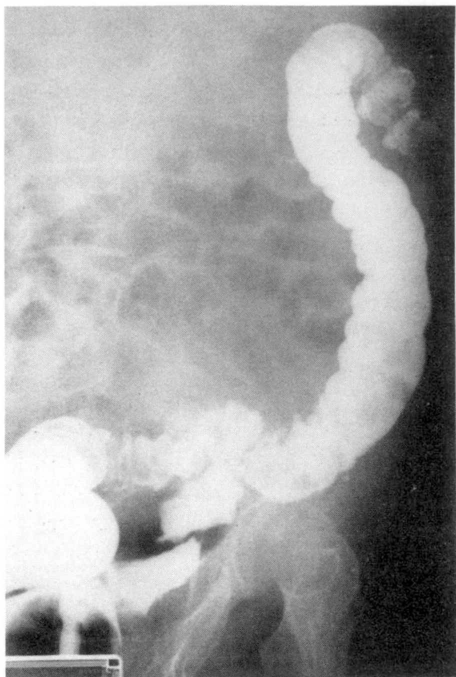

Fig. 6 Barium enema showing large vesicoenteric fistula originating in sigmoid colon.

surgical procedure because of her underlying respiratory difficulties and she was therefore treated with a defunctioning colostomy.

Comment: In a healthy patient, a vesicoenteric fistula would be treated with bowel resection and closure of the bladder. In the palliative care setting, the optimal therapy is often not possible because of underlying restrictions on choices due to the idiosyncrasies of the patients. In this case, it was felt that the patient would not tolerate any further insult to her tenuous respiratory status and the minimal procedure of faecal diversion was carried out to eliminate the fecaluria and associated symptomatology.

Vesicovaginal urinary fistulas

Most vesicovaginal fistulas are the result of gynaecological surgery or local trauma. The characteristic symptom is leakage of urine from the bladder into the vagina. Routine physical examination is usually unrewarding, although occasionally one may be able to identify a large fistulous site on pelvic examination. Intravenous pyelography is necessary to exclude the presence of ureteric involvement in the fistula. The latter is usually heralded by evidence of associated obstruction or significant displacement of the ureter. Cystoscopy will allow characterization of the vesicovaginal fistula in terms of size, site, and multiplicity. It is usually present low on the posterior wall, but the demonstration of proximity to a ureteric orifice is crucial to planning corrective surgery. Escape of irrigating fluid from the vagina while filling the bladder confirms the diagnosis. When the fistula is small it is occasionally helpful to place a vaginal pack and then fill the bladder with methylene blue to demonstrate the connection. In circumstances where the cause of the fistula is not obvious, a biopsy of the involved area at the time of cystoscopy is imperative to establish a specific diagnosis.

In the absence of underlying malignancy or other significant pathology, small fistulas occasionally close spontaneously following 4 to 6 weeks of urethral or suprapubic catheter drainage. Usually it will be necessary to proceed with a surgical repair and this can be accomplished vaginally or transabdominally, with interposition of an omental pedicle graft. Success of surgical management is dependent upon gentle and selective tissue handling, layered closure, lack of tension along suture lines, use of absorbable sutures, use of suprapubic catheter drainage of the bladder postoperatively, and administration of appropriate antibiotics perioperatively.[15]

In circumstances where there is extensive pelvic disease, which is not manageable by surgical reconstruction or requiring anterior or pelvic exenteration, urinary diversion may be required.

When the patient has diffuse metastases or is unable to tolerate major surgery, placement of bilateral percutaneous nephrostomy tubes may be indicated as a means of diverting the urine and restoring continence.

Urethrocutaneous fistulas

Urethrocutaneous urinary fistulas are most frequently a complication of hypospadias repair, but may be the result of primary or secondary urethral or penile malignancies. Patients complain of a localized penile mass and drainage of urine through the fistulous site. Ultimate management usually requires a proximal, total or partial penectomy with subsequent adjuvant surgical or pharmacological therapy as necessary. In those patients who are not candidates for definitive therapy, a percutaneous suprapubic cystostomy would be the ideal form of urinary diversion.

Rectourethral fistulas

Rectourethral fistulas occur most often as a complication of radical prostatectomy, but they are seen occasionally in association with locally invasive prostatic or rectal cancer. Most patients will complain of the passage of urine per rectum and/or pneumaturia and the passage of faecal material per urethram. The diagnosis is usually confirmed at the time of cystourethroscopy and/or proctoscopy. If the fistulous site is small, it may occasionally close spontaneously following a temporary diverting colostomy and bladder catheterization. If this is unsuccessful and there is no obvious persisting local malignancy, surgical repair is indicated. If persistent malignancy is present, the optimal treatment for the underlying malignancy should be determined.

Urethral catheters

The indwelling urethral catheter remains one of the most useful and commonly used urological instruments. Its primary uses are to provide continuous drainage of urine from the bladder in patients who are unable to void spontaneously or who suffer from marked urinary incontinence not amenable to condom drainage. Occasionally, urethral catheters are used as a means of assessing the degree of bladder emptying, irrigating blood clots from the bladder, and measuring hourly urine output.

The most frequently used urethral catheters are made from latex rubber and are blunt-tipped. These have one channel for draining the urine and another smaller channel for inflating the balloon which prevents displacement of the catheter. Because of a tendency towards encrustation, irritation, and infection, a variety of new hydrophilic polymers have been developed to improve catheter biocompatibility. These lubricious coatings provide protection against irritation of urethral mucosa, help to minimize encrustation, and enhance patient comfort. Their effectiveness has reduced the need for more expensive silicone catheters.

A critical factor to be considered when choosing the catheter is the size. Most are labelled with respect to the measurement of the outer circumference of the catheter. The most frequently used system is the F-scale and conversion to the diameter of the catheter is possible by remembering that each number of the F-scale equals 0.33 mm. In the usual situation of using an indwelling urethral catheter, one would use a 16 or 18F. Catheters smaller than this are less useful because of their tendency to coil up in the urethra during passage and to obstruct.

In patients for whom urethral catheterization is difficult, it is useful to fill the urethra with 10 ml of 2 per cent lignocaine (lidocaine) jelly; one should allow 5 minutes for this to take effect. This lubricates the urethra, allows the external sphincter to relax, and decreases some of the discomfort. Occasionally, a curved or Coudé catheter can be used to simplify passage through the external sphincter and prostatic urethra or bladder neck.

When it is impossible to pass a urethral catheter to drain a distended bladder, a suprapubic drainage system can be used. There are many kits to permit placement of a suprapubic catheter, but the principles of the technique involve placing the patient in a slight Trendelenburg position, treating the suprapubic area with an appropriate antiseptic, infiltrating a small area of skin 5 cm above the pubis in the midline with a local anaesthetic, and using a syringe and needle to aspirate urine through this area to confirm the position of the distended bladder. Once this had been accomplished, a plastic trocar and sheath can be passed through the same tract into the bladder. The trocar is then removed and the indwelling catheter passed through the sheath, which is then withdrawn or peeled away. The catheter is sutured in place and left indwelling. This can be an extremely important technique in patients with extensive urethral stricture disease.

The incidence of urinary-tract infections in patients with indwelling urinary catheters is related to the duration of catheterization. This acquired bacteriuria occurs at a rate of about 5 per cent per day of catheterization.[16] Since it is impossible to eliminate catheter-associated infections, and the bacterial flora changes rapidly[17] in patients with chronic indwelling urethral catheters, treatment of asymptomatic bladder bacteriuria or funguria is not recommended. Because of the risk of blockage and encrustation and formation of stones on the catheter, it is recommended that it be changed every 4 weeks. Patients whose catheters block are metabolically different from patients without blocked catheters and should receive fresh catheters at 7 to 10 days to avoid obstruction.[18] It would be appropriate to use a short course of antibiotics around the time of manipulation; the author uses oral norfloxacin for 24 h when changing a catheter, especially if the catheterization has been difficult or traumatic. In some instances, if patients are physically able to or if they have assistance, it can be beneficial to initiate a programme of regular intermittent clean catheterization to maintain low urinary residuals. This technique is useful in both males and females.[19] The frequency may be individualized, depending on bladder capacity. This type of protocol is associated with fewer urinary-tract infections and obviates the problems of a long-term indwelling catheter.

Having an intravesical balloon inflated with 5 ml of water as the mechanism of preventing displacement, these self-retaining catheters may produce considerable bladder irritation and discomfort in some patients. Bladder spasms are described as intermittent episodes of excruciating, suprapubic discomfort, often associated with leakage of small amounts of urine through the urethra alongside the catheter when the bladder contracts. These can often be reduced by using a catheter with a smaller balloon or evacuating some of the fluid within the balloon. These tips are especially useful if a 30 ml balloon had been used initially. In patients in whom this does not provide symptomatic improvement, the use of belladonna and opium (B and O) suppositories per rectum every 4 h, low-dose oxybutynin 2.5 to 5.0 mg orally two times per day, or hyoscine butylbromide 10 mg orally once or twice per day can be helpful.

Failure of the catheter balloon to decompress after aspiration of its contents has been attempted, is not uncommon and can make removal of the catheter difficult or impossible. Gentle passage of a ureteric wire stylet along the inflation channel will puncture the balloon and correct the problem.[20]

Pain

Renal colic

Pain associated with urinary dysfunction represents one of the most distressing types of acute pain. In the absence of personal experience as sufferer or observer, it is unlikely that the distress of severe ureteric colic can be appreciated fully. Induced by acute ureteric obstruction, usually a stone or blood clot, pain in renal distribution is thought to be due to capsular distension. The severe, colicky-type pain, which is probably due to ureteric muscle spasm, extends from the costovertebral angle, along the course of the ureter, and radiates to the ipsilateral testis or labium. The associated autonomic outpouring is reflected in a characteristic response associated with severe restlessness, pallor, and diaphoresis. An intramuscular injection of a non-steroidal anti-inflammatory drug such as ketorolac or diclofenac is effective in relieving this discomfort.[21] In patients with active bleeding, an opioid such as morphine would be preferable.

Bladder pain

This may be identified as obstructive or irritative.

Obstructive

Chronic distension of the bladder, developing over a period of weeks or months, is usually associated with little more than a sense of fullness in addition to the symptoms of chronic urinary retention. Overflow incontinence may be associated. On the other hand, acute retention of sudden onset will produce agonizing lower abdominal pain, severe restlessness, and a constant and compelling urge to void. If the obstruction is not relieved spontaneously or by passage of a catheter, the acute urge will gradually subside but bladder distension will persist. Symptoms, particularly in the elderly and those on opioid drugs, may be masked. Confusion may be the major presenting symptom.

Irritative symptoms

Inflammation of the bladder is most often due to infection and symptoms consist of excessive urinary frequency, dysuria, and urgency incontinence. Dysuria at the end of voiding suggests prostatic origin in the male and trigone in the female.

Irritative bladder symptoms are frequently associated with external radiation and with certain chemotherapeutic agents, such as cyclophosphamide. Idiopathic detrusor instability and central neurological disease may also be responsible. Metabolic abnormalities producing polyuria should be excluded. Intravesical or extravesical tumours may produce irritative bladder symptoms and, along with other agents, may be responsible for the development of bladder spasms, which comprise an exquisitely painful sensation felt mainly in the bladder region. These spasms are due to severe contraction of the detrusor muscle responding to some irritation, usually on the trigone. In addition to tumour, infection, radiation, and calculi may be responsible. Irritation is often associated with an indwelling catheter, particularly with encrustation. Treatment of this condition is covered under the section on catheters, above.

References

1. Hutch JA. A new theory of the anatomy of the internal urinary sphincter and the physiology of micturition: IV The urinary sphincteric mechanism. *Journal of Urology*, 1967; **97**: 705.
2. Hutch JA, Rambo OA. A new theory of the anatomy of the internal urinary sphincter and the physiology of micturition: III. Anatomy of the urethra. *Journal of Urology*, 1967; **97**: 696.
3. Vincente J, Salvador J, Chechile G. Spiral urethral prosthesis as an alternative to surgery in high risk patients with benign prostatic hyperplasia: prospective study. *Journal of Urology*, 1989; **142**: 1504–6.
4. Norman RW, Mack FG, Awad SA, Belitsky P, Schwarz RD, Lannon SG. Acute renal failure secondary to bilateral ureteric obstruction: review of 50 cases. *Canadian Medical Association Journal*, 1982; **127**: 601–4.
5. Androile GL, Bettmann MA, Garnick MB, Richie JP. Indwelling double-J ureteral stents for temporary and permanent urinary drainage: experience with 87 patients. *Journal of Urology*, 1984; **131**: 239–41.
6. Mariani AJ, Mariani MC, Macchioni C, Stams UK, Hariharan A, Moriera A. The significance of adult hematuria: 1,000 hematuria evaluations including a risk-benefit and cost-effectiveness analysis. *Journal of Urology*, 1989; **141**: 350–5.
7. Donahue LA, Frank IN. Intravesical formalin for hemorrhagic cystitis: analysis of therapy. *Journal of Urology*, 1989; **141**: 809–12.
8. DeVries CR, Freiha FS. Hemorrhagic cystitis: a review. *Journal of Urology*, 1990; **143**: 1–9.
9. Singh I, Laungani GB. Intravesical epsilon aminocaproic acid in management of intractable bladder hemorrhage. *Urology*, 1992; **40**: 227–9.
10. Levine LA, Jarrard DF. Treatment of cyclophosphamide-induced hemorrhagic cystitis with intravesical carboprost tromehamine. *Journal of Urology*, 1993; **149**: 719–23.
11. Norkool DM, Hampson NB, Gibbons RP, Weissman RM. Hyperbaric oxygen therapy for radiation-induced hemorrhagic cystitis. *Journal of Urology*, 1993; **150**: 332–4.
12. Flanigan RC. The failure of infarction and/or nephrectomy in stage IV renal cell cancer to influence survival or metastatic regression. *Urology Clinics of North America*, 1987; **14**: 757–62.
13. Sarr MG, Fishman EK, Goldman SM, Siegelman SS, Cameron JL. Enterovesical fistula. *Surgery, Gynecology and Obstetrics*, 1987; **164**: 41–8.
14. Lippert MC, Teates CD, Howards SS. Detection of enteric-urinary fistulas with a non-invasive quantitative method. *Journal of Urology*, 1984; **132**: 1134–6.
15. Turner-Warwick R. Urinary fistulae in the female. In: Walsh PC, Gittes RF, Perlmutter AD, Stanley TA, eds. *Campbell's Urology*. 5th edn. Philadelphia: W.B. Saunders, 1986: 2718–38.
16. Warren JW, *et al.* Antibiotic irrigation and catheter-associated urinary-tract infections. *New England Journal of Medicine*, 1978; **299**: 570–3.
17. Breitenbucher RB. Bacterial changes in the urine samples of patients with long-term indwelling catheters. *Archives of Internal Medicine*, 1984; **144**: 1585–8.
18. Kunin CM, Chin QF, Chambers S. Indwelling urinary catheters in the elderly: relation of 'catheter life' to formation of encrustations in patients with and without blocked catheters. *American Journal of Medicine*, 1987; **82**: 405–11.
19. Lapides J, Diokno AC, Silber S, Lowe BS. Clean intermittent self-catheterization in the treatment of urinary tract disease. *Journal of Urology*, 1972; **107**: 458–61.
20. Browning GPP, Barr L, Horsburgh AG. Management of obstructed balloon catheters. *British Medical Journal*, 1984; **144**: 1585–8.
21. Oosterlink W, Philip NH, Charig C, Gillies G, Hetherington JW, Lloyd J. A double-blind single dose comparison of intramuscular ketorolac tromethamine and pethidine in the treatment of renal colic. *Journal of Clinical Pharmacology*, 1990; **30**:336–41.

9.9 Palliation in head and neck cancer

R. H. MacDougall, A. J. Munro, and Janet A. Wilson

Scope of the problem

Although head and neck tumours form only a minority of the total cancer problem (2 per cent of all cancer in the United Kingdom) they are more common in many Third World countries. Demographic variations in the incidence of subtypes of head and neck cancers are caused by varying environmental and other cultural factors.[1] For example betel-nut chewing in the Indian subcontinent causes a high incidence of field changes in the buccal mucosa with consequent carcinoma of the oral cavity.

The clinical importance of head and neck tumours reflects the anatomical importance of the structures affected in the head and neck—the aerodigestive tract and most of the vital senses—and also the manifest disfiguring consequences of both the primary tumour and ablative treatment. Head and neck cancers are heterogeneous both anatomically and histologically. Apart from cancers of the larynx which produce the symptom of hoarseness early in their natural history, most head and neck cancers are silent and present late and at a stage of doubtful curability. Cigarette smoking accounts for the male preponderance in head and neck cancer. Alcohol appears to be a cocarcinogen in the susceptible, cigarette smoking individual.

Because of the diversity and variety of individual tumour variants in the head and neck, definitive clinical trials are uncommon. Palliative therapy of advanced disease has not been subject to systematic analysis. This chapter therefore describes the principal distressing symptoms and introduces decision analysis as a possible aid to therapeutic decision-making.

Pathophysiology and clinical manifestations of disease

Tumours of the head and neck produce problems by obstructing hollow organs, by causing neurological impairment (both sensory and motor), and, perhaps most crucially of all to the patient, by the destruction of communication—both expressive and, where there is external disfigurement, receptive.[2-6]

Obstructive symptoms, haemorrhage, and fistulas

Uncontrolled malignant disease of the upper aerodigestive tract can lead to obstruction of the airway, the food passages, or both.

Airway obstruction

Upper airway obstruction produces dyspnoea, fatigue, and, if in the laryngotracheal segment, stridor which is inspiratory in laryngeal obstruction and biphasic (expiratory and inspiratory) in tracheal obstruction. A large tracheostomal recurrence can cause obstruction to the distal trachea, while external compression by uncontrolled nodal disease can also compromise the airway. As with any upper airway obstruction, it is vital to remember that the blood gas concentrations are maintained within normal limits until the late stages. Cyanosis may not develop until respiratory failure is imminent.

Pharyngeal obstruction

Oropharyngeal obstruction results most commonly from tumours of the base of the tongue, tonsil, or retromolar trigone. Hypopharyngeal obstruction is most frequently due to pyriform fossa carcinoma or external compression by nodes in the thyrohyoid area. Primary hypopharyngeal tumours on the posterior pharyngeal wall or in the postcricoid area are relatively rare.

Nasal obstruction

Nasal obstruction gives rise to troublesome symptoms of anosmia, headache, and secondary sinusitis with facial pain. Tumours of the anterior nasal fossa or postnasal space can also give rise to an unpleasant smell (cacosmia), hyponasal speech, and xerostomia secondary to mouth breathing.

Vascular obstruction

Obstruction of the internal jugular veins (or vein, if one has already been removed during radical neck dissection) by thrombosis or external compression gives rise to headache, facial congestion, and ultimately blurred vision, papilloedema, and confusion. Carotid obstruction is rare because of the resistance of the vessel wall to tumour invasion but light-headedness, transient ischaemic attacks, and, occasionally, cerebrovascular accident are recognized complications of malignant disease of the neck.

Haemorrhage

Erosion of the walls of the carotid results in so-called 'carotid blow-out' where the patient exsanguinates dramatically in 2 to 3 min. Carotid blow-out is more likely in patients who have undergone combination therapy with surgical removal of soft tissue cover combined with radiotherapy.[7] Changes in the vasa vasorum affect the integrity of the vessel wall. Fatal haemorrhage is sometimes presaged by a herald bleed which may be mucosal, stomal, or from a skin ulcer. When minor vessels are involved, epistaxis, oral bleeding, or haemoptysis may also prove distressing.

Fistulas

The most common neoplastic fistula in the head and neck is a pharyngocutaneous communication. Others include oroantral and tracheo-oesophageal fistulae.

Dysphagia

Dysphagia is one of the most common symptoms requiring palliation in head and neck cancer. Diverse mechanisms including compression by local or nodal masses, neurological dysfunction, aspiration, and postsurgical complications can all result in dysphagia.[8,9]

Muscular dysfunction

Reduction in tongue mobility, due to mechanical fixation by tumour or surgery, lymphoedema, or hypoglossal nerve paralysis, severely compromises the oral preparatory phase of swallowing, as does failure of good lip closure which results in oral incompetence and unpleasant drooling. Conversely, trismus, due to fibrosis or tumour involvement of the muscles of mastication, may prevent patients from managing to eat a normal diet. Pharyngeal paralysis, if unilateral, is said not greatly to compromise swallowing but, in practice, compensatory strategies may be required to ensure adequate bolus passage past the glottic aperture. Following laryngectomy there is loss of the normal radial and axial asymmetry of the upper oesophageal sphincter[10, 11] and of the forward pull of the laryngeal cartilages by the suprahyoid musculature which causes opening of the relaxed upper sphincter during swallowing.[12] Severe dysphagia, however, usually indicates the presence of a postoperative pharyngeal stricture.

Xerostomia following irradiation of the major salivary glands, as in nasopharyngeal carcinoma, may exacerbate dysphagia. Dysmotility or a defect in the soft palate can produce nasopharyngeal regurgitation of food (especially liquids), but aspiration into the tracheobronchial tree is a much more common problem.

Aspiration

The larynx is usually protected against the entry of food by at least five mechanisms—a natural redundancy which reflects the importance of the prevention of the ingress of food into the airway. The series of three sphincters—aryepiglottic folds, false cords, and vocal cords—is supplemented by the flap-like action of the epiglottis which tilts posteriorly during bolus passage, and the dense sensory innervation of the supraglottis (the internal branch of the superior laryngeal nerve) which provides the protective cough reflex. The supraglottic sphincters are more important in preventing entry while closure of the true glottis will prevent air escape during a Valsalva manoeuvre or when lifting. (Therefore a laryngectomee cannot fill his lungs with a fixed volume of air and lift a heavy weight.)

Although unilateral vocal cord palsy does not usually result in significant aspiration, the presence of a bilateral palsy of the adductor muscles or bilateral superior laryngeal nerve palsy can produce copious aspiration due to glottic incompetence. The presence of a side tracheostomy may cause dysphagia for a variety of reasons. The presence of the stoma may prevent build-up of an adequate subglottic pressure for swallowing. The loss of laryngeal elevation because of tethering by the prosthesis to the skin, the presence of aspiration if there is overspill with an uncuffed tube, or cervical oesophageal compression by an overinflated cuff can all contribute, as will the original problem for which the tracheostomy was fashioned in the first place. Cervical anastomosis following total or subtotal oesophagectomy has also been shown to cause pharyngeal dysfunction and aspiration, particularly where the anastomosis is less than 1.5 cm below the cricopharyngeal sphincter.[13]

Loss of special sensory functions

Vision

Visual disturbance secondary to ear, nose, and throat disease is most frequently caused by direct orbital involvement by antroethmoid or, more rarely, sphenoid neoplasms.

Smell and taste

Anosmia may result from failure of the smell-bearing, and therefore taste-bearing, air to penetrate the area of the anterior nasal fossa above the superior turbinate where the olfactory nerve endings are located. The nerve endings are extremely sensitive and can be destroyed by even a simple polypectomy. A major craniofacial resection with *en bloc* removal of the cribriform plate always results in anosmia, as does involvement of the area by ethmoid malignancy or a frontal lobe tumour or sphenoid ridge meningioma.

Hearing

Deafness is rarely a direct result of cancer. Tumours of the external auditory canal or mastoid are extremely rare. Acoustic neuroma—a benign but steadily expanding nerve sheath tumour of the eighth cranial nerve—arises most often from its superior vestibular division, but in the early stages causes deafness and tinnitus rather than loss of balance. Nasopharyngeal tumours obstruct the medial end of the eustachian tube, giving secondary serous otitis media with a mild conductive hearing loss. Deafness may also arise from the ototoxic effects of cisplatinum, to which brown-eyed individuals have recently been shown to have an increased susceptibility.[14]

Balance

Dizziness is much more common than deafness in advanced cancer. A wide variety of cancer-related problems and treatments give rise to unsteadiness or light-headedness. Poor nutrition, anaemia, anxiety, and postural hypotension are among general causes, as are treatments such as antiemetics, tranquillizers, opioids, vestibulotoxic antibiotics (notably the aminoglycosides but also drugs such as cotrimoxazole and metronidazole), and hormonal and diuretic therapy. Endocrine disorders, including thyroid, adrenal, and pituitary imbalance or postural hypotension, also cause light-headedness, as does transient cerebral ischaemia. This may be caused by carotid compression or associated atheroma, a frequent concomitant of head and neck squamous carcinoma because of the common risk factor—smoking.

Vertigo is a term covering a more severe abnormality in balance. Commonly expressed by the patient as a sense of spinning, it is a sensation of movement of the patient relative to his surroundings. It may be caused by either peripheral vestibular or central disorders.

Tumours rarely involve the inner ear directly, but pressure on the vestibulocochlear nerve or inner ear vasculature gives rise to the triad of vertigo, deafness, and tinnitus.

The principal differential diagnoses of central vertigo are vertebrobasilar ischaemia and multiple sclerosis. Central causes of vertigo may evoke dysarthria, double vision, or symptoms arising from abnormalities in the long spinal tracts. Other cerebellar signs—ataxia, past pointing, dysdiadochokinesis, pendular reflexes, scanning speech—may also be present. Papilloedema is found in only about 50 per cent of posterior fossa lesions.

Nystagmus is commonly associated with both peripheral vestibular and central vertigo. Vestibular nystagmus is a horizontal jerk–fine-amplitude oscillation which can be abolished by optic fixation. Its detection may therefore require an electronystagmography examination. In contrast, the horizontal nystagmus which accompanies posterior cranial fossa tumours is enhanced by eye opening and is of a coarser amplitude than vestibular nystagmus. Midbrain compression can also result in a variety of other patterns, for example pendular nystagmus.[15]

Communication disorders

The patient with advanced head and neck cancer frequently has a psychological barrier to communication, irrespective of any physical barrier, due to a visible orofacial deformity. Foetor, a cervical mass, a surgical scar, or an offensive ulcer reduce personal confidence, self-esteem, and the desire for contact with the outside world. There may be a receptive communication disorder (see the discussion of deafness above), but an expressive problem is more common. Dysarthria in patients with restricted mobility in the oral cavity due to tumour, surgery, or oedema is particularly common. Dysphonia or aphasia from laryngeal disease or resection is also common.

Vagal palsy affecting the motor supply to the pharyngeal plexus results in hypernasal speech (rhinolalia aperta). More common are the breathy voice and bovine cough of unilateral or bilateral adductor paralysis due to recurrent laryngeal or vagal trunk compression or division. A unilateral paralysis of the abductors associated with recurrent laryngeal nerve paralysis rarely produces marked dysphonia, while bilateral abductor paralysis results in stridor as the dominant symptom.

Facial nerve palsy

Facial nerve palsy has both functional and cosmetic implications. Loss of lip occlusion during swallowing leads to drooling and dysphagia. Corneal exposure and facial ache are equally unpleasant. Patients may have an almost symmetrical appearance at rest but feel extremely self-conscious during facial animation.

The investigation of advanced head and neck cancer

Diagnostic imaging

The planning of radical and palliative management of head and neck disease has been revolutionized by the advent of computerized tomography (CT) and magnetic resonance imaging (MRI). In particular, the delineation of inoperable disease has spared many patients fruitless resections, although the differentiation of necrosis or oedema from neoplasm may be difficult. Gadolinium contrast improves MRI resolution, providing a clear picture of the extent of intracranial neurogenic tumours such as acoustic neuromas. Coronal reformating of CT scans is particularly useful for the examination of orbital or antral disease, for example when deciding whether resection of a maxillary tumour could be possible with preservation of the orbital floor. Most radiologists prefer to use CT for evaluation of pathology in the infrahyoid portion of the neck.

In the posterior cranial fossa, MRI is superior to CT in the demonstration of axial and extra-axial structures.[16] In some centres, ultrasound has also proved useful in the detection of nodes in the clinically negative neck. Duplex ultrasound scanning of the carotid and vertebral arteries is a useful non-invasive method for investigating dizziness.[17] Intravenous digital subtraction angiography for the investigation of pulsatile neck masses is easier and more pleasant than conventional angiography.[18]

Advances in endoscopy

Until the twentieth century, examination of the postnasal space, hypopharynx, and larynx relied on the use of indirect mirror examination. In 1901, a modified cystoscope was used as a nasendoscope. Since then, rigid fibreoptic endoscopy has come to play an increasingly important role in the visualization of the nose and paranasal sinuses. Antroscopic inspection under local or general anaesthesia is now a routine ear, nose, and throat investigation, and the techniques of functional endoscopic sinus surgery have led increasingly to examination of the ethmoid and even the sphenoid by this method. Miniature light sources and chip cameras allow a permanent record to be obtained and disease progress to be assessed. An endoscope 2.7 mm in diameter is available to examine the most distant recesses of the sphenoethmoid complex, and biopsies can readily be taken. Rigid endoscopy is useful for laryngeal examination, but the transnasal passage of a fine-bore flexible fibreoptic instrument allows the patient to breathe and phonate more naturally. Projection of the image on to a video screen allows simultaneous observation by the patient, the speech therapist, and trainee staff.

Assessment of dizziness

The mainstay of the diagnostic approach to dizziness remains a careful history, despite the recent advances of computerized electronystagmography programmes and dynamic moving platform posturography.[19] The latter is unique among tests of balance as it incorporates visual and proprioceptive information. Manipulation of the platform supporting the subject and of the surrounding visual frame of reference allows separate analysis of sensory organization and movement co-ordination. Proprioception can also be tested in isolation by a force platform, but all types of posturography are, of course, useless in the severely dizzy patient who cannot maintain an upright position during the test.

Evaluation of swallowing pathophysiology

In the head and neck conventional contrast radiography is of limited value in the study of dysphagia because of the speed of bolus passage through the oropharyngeal segment and the risk of aspiration. A modified barium swallow technique has been developed combining the technique of video-recording of the barium swallows for later frame-by-frame analysis with the use of small boluses of liquid, semisolid, and solid consistency.[8] The subsequent digitization of the radiographs allows some quantification. Manometric study of the pharyngo-oesophageal segment was of little value before the advent of intraluminal strain gauges[20] because of the rapid upstroke of the pharyngeal contraction wave and the sensitivity of the pharynx to water from perfused catheters.[21] The introduction of fine-bore strain gauge assemblies now allows reliable manometric evaluation of the hypopharynx and upper oesophagus. Synchronous manofluorometry yields both pressure and bolus transit information.[22] The most recent development in this field is the use of ultrasound[23] to study movements of the tongue, the floor of the mouth, and the hyoid, and to assess bolus propulsion, initiation of the swallow reflex, and hyoid elevation.

Fine-needle aspiration cytology

Fine-needle aspiration cytology is a particularly useful diagnostic tool in patients with gross or recurrent disease and avoids the need for open biopsy under general anaesthesia. Fine-needle aspiration cytology of head and neck lesions can achieve high diagnostic accuracy.[24] The technique causes very little discomfort and can give the answer in a few hours, although the cytological distinction between a necrotic and a neoplastic lesion can be difficult.

Management approaches

Decision analysis—theory and practice

The illnesses of two American Presidents illustrate two extremes in the management of head and neck cancer.[25] General Ulysses S. Grant, hero of the Civil War, ex-President, was found in October 1884 to have squamous carcinoma of the tonsil. His doctors decided that his illness was fatal and that all that they could do was attempt to relieve his suffering. Opioids and cocaine were prescribed. In his lucid moments the General dictated his memoirs, the income from which would be essential for the financial security of his family. In one sitting alone he dictated 10 000 words. When they were eventually published his memoirs earned his widow nearly $500 000. General Ulysses S. Grant died on the morning of 23 July 1885.

In 1893, President Grover Cleveland was found to have carcinoma of the maxilla. On 1 July, in secret, on a yacht sailing slowly off the coast, surgeons performed a partial maxillectomy. A second operation followed 12 days later and a rubber prosthesis was constructed. On 7 August the President was able to give a reassuring speech to Congress on the state of the economy—no one suspected that he had recently had surgery for cancer. Grover Cleveland died in 1917, from heart disease.

The treatment of Sigmund Freud exemplifies a clinical course for head and neck cancer intermediate between the strictly palliative approach used for Grant and the successful cure enjoyed by Cleveland.[26] Freud, a heavy smoker of cigars, was first found to have a carcinoma of the palate in 1923. This was treated initially with surgery. He had further operations in 1931 and 1938. He had a course of radium treatment in 1936 and again in 1939. On 23 September 1939, Sigmund Freud died with uncontrolled carcinoma fungating through his cheek.

It would be comforting to think that the management of head and neck cancer had made great progress since the time of Grant, Cleveland, and Freud. Techniques of surgery and radiotherapy have improved and cytotoxic drugs are now available, yet only a minority of patients can be cured. The majority of patients are, or should be, candidates for palliative treatment. Patients for whom cure is impossible must be identified and potentially curative treatment must not be denied to those who might benefit from it.

Tumours of the head and neck are extremely heterogeneous in site, histology, macroscopic appearance, and biological behaviour. There are no simple prognostic rules, though complex indices have been constructed. Unfortunately, even the simplest radical treatments for head and neck cancer, for example radiotherapy for early laryngeal tumours, entail significant distress and discomfort. Radical treatment for some tumours of the head and neck—particularly where surgery and radiotherapy have to be combined—come close to the limits of acceptability even if cure could be guaranteed.

It is an axiom of palliative radiotherapy that, since cure is deemed impossible and the sole aim of treatment is relief of symptoms, it should not incur significant morbidity. There is no real problem with this at many sites in the body: five fractions, or even a single fraction, of radiotherapy are sufficient to control pain from bony metastases or to control haemoptysis from lung cancer. However, this is not the case with cancer of the head and neck. It is extremely difficult to devise a schedule of radiotherapy that will produce sufficient regression of tumour to alleviate symptoms from head and neck cancer without producing significant unpleasant local side-effects—in particular painful mucositis and xerostomia.

These considerations have led many experienced radiotherapists to conclude that there can be no such thing as palliative radiotherapy for head and neck cancer, and that to achieve adequate control of symptoms, radical doses, with all that is thereby implied in terms of morbidity to the normal tissues, are required. A similar argument applies to surgery. A conservative palliative excision is usually promptly succeeded by local recurrence, and the spread of this recurrence is often facilitated by the surgical violation of fascial boundaries.

Decision analysis offers a repertoire of techniques which may be useful for the evaluation of complex choices in clinical medicine.[27] The crude approximations involved in decision analysis make it unsuitable for decision-making for individual patients. However, it may have a role in providing guidelines for managing groups of patients—in formulating management policies.

A decision tree for the management of head and neck cancer can be sketched in a general highly schematic form (Fig. 1). The possible outcomes of the original decision—radical versus palliative therapy—are as follows.

Live1 Patient is cured, survives to normal life expectancy, and has no complications from treatment.

Live2 Patient is cured, but has minimal complications from treatment.

Live3 Patient is cured, but has moderate complications from treatment.

Live4 Patient is cured, but has severe complications from treatment.

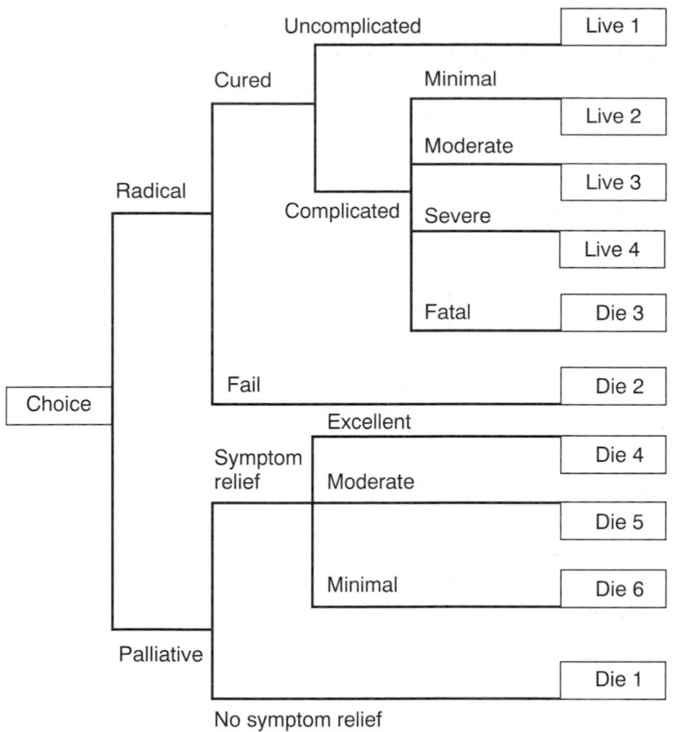

Fig. 1 A decision tree for the management (radical versus palliative) of a patient with a stage III carcinoma. The calculation of the expected values for the choice, radical versus palliative, is outlined in the text. Baseline data for radiotherapy or for surgery as the radical option are summarized in Tables 2 and 3 respectively. The outcome states, Live1 etc., Die1 etc. are defined in the text.

Die1 Patient is treated palliatively, has no relief from symptoms, and dies.

Die2 Patient has radical treatment which fails to control the tumour and dies.

Die3 Patient has radical treatment which does control the tumour but patient dies from fatal complications of treatment.

Die4 Patient is treated palliatively, has excellent relief of symptoms, but then dies.

Die5 Patient is treated palliatively, has fair relief of symptoms, and dies.

Die6 Patient is treated palliatively but has minimal symptomatic benefit.

Quality-adjusted survival can be estimated by multiplying the duration of survival by a quality factor. The quality factor is introduced to take account of any morbidity experienced by the patient. Ideally, this quality factor should be provided by the patients themselves. A variety of techniques are available for eliciting such information, but all tend to be cumbersome and somewhat impractical. A more pragmatic approach is simply to choose a range of realistic values and then see whether the consequent variation in results affects the preferred decision a technique called sensitivity analysis.

Quality-adjusted survival can be used as a measure of utility for each of the defined outcomes in an analysis. By taking the value of an outcome state and calculating its overall probability, that is the product of all the probabilities encountered on the route to that outcome, the overall expected utility (utility of outcome multiplied by overall probability) of any given branch of a decision tree can be calculated. This can be applied iteratively as far back as the original decision, in this example radical versus palliative, and rational decision-makers can base their decisions upon which of the choices produces the highest utility. For a simple utility assessment this would be the greatest number of quality-adjusted life-years.

For patients treated unsuccessfully or left untreated, the quality-adjusted survival must include the impairment of quality produced by symptoms from the primary tumour. One of the main problems in palliative management is identified immediately. By virtue of the complex anatomy and physiology of the head and neck, these tumours almost always produce symptoms. In contrast with lung cancer, asymptomatic occult tumours are rare. The exceptions would be silent primary tumours of the nasopharynx or pyriform fossa presenting as painless cervical lymphadenopathy. In such cases, as with radical therapy, the trade-off is simply between the toxicity of treatment, its severity and incidence, and the probability of cure. When, as in palliative therapy, cancer is already producing symptoms, when treatment itself will inevitably produce further morbidity, and when the probability of success is low, the issue becomes almost intolerably complex.

When making decisions in medicine it is often forgotten that treatment may deny patients the opportunity to use their time in the ways they might wish. This phenomenon is known to economists as opportunity cost.[28] Given finite resources, it may be impossible to have both a holiday abroad and a new car. Either alone can be afforded but not both. A choice has to be made and, if the holiday abroad is chosen, then the opportunity cost is the loss of the new car. By using up limited time and energy, attempts to treat patients when cure is impossible will incur their own opportunity costs. The concept is cognate with, but in some respects distinct from, Feinstein's chagrin factor.[29] Feinstein pointed out that doctors, in attempts to avoid the chagrin associated with failing to diagnose and treat a potentially curable condition, were sometimes overzealous in investigation and treatment. Physicians' underlying personalities and subsequent training emphasize intervention as the means to improve patients' well-being: there is less concentration on the more difficult art of being able to judge when not to intervene. Radiotherapists have long been accused of this particular trait: 'radiotherapy suffers more or less from men who meddle with it . . . '.[30] Pressures from relatives ('there must be something you can do doctor'), from peers ('this new trial I am running shows very exciting early results'), and from the threat of malpractice ('if you knew this treatment was available, doctor, why did you not prescribe it?') all favour intervention. The patient's own voice is small and often lost in the clamour. Would Grant have been able to die knowing his dependents were financially secure had the writing of his memoirs been disrupted by vain attempts to extirpate his tumour? Could Puccini have completed Turandot himself had he not made the trip to Brussels in a futile attempt to find a cure for his throat cancer? The issue of the opportunity costs of treatment applies to all, not just to the famous. It is a quite specific problem: it is related to overall quality of life but is in danger of being swamped if only global quality of life measures are used to assess outcome. Such measures make no formal provision for what might have been.

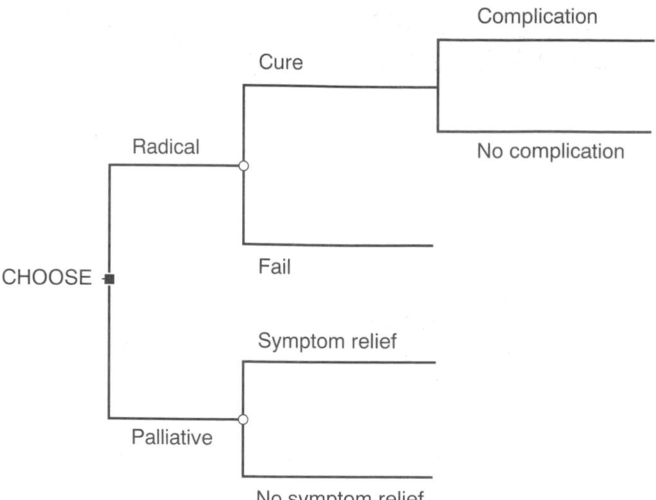

Fig. 2 A short version of a decision tree for the management (radical versus palliative treatment) of a patient with a T_3 carcinoma of the pyriform fossa. The probabilities and utilities used in the baseline analysis are summarized in Table 1. The calculation of the expected values for the choice — radical versus palliative — is outlined in the text.

Table 1

Parameter	Value
Probability of cure from radical treatment	0.1
Survival time for untreated patients	30 weeks
Duration of palliative treatment	0 weeks
Duration of radical treatment	8 weeks
Latent period before complications develop	0 weeks
Life expectancy for cured patients	465 weeks
Quality factors	
complications	0.7
for tumour-related symptoms	0.3
during radical treatment	0.5
with palliation	0.7
Survival increments (cf. untreated patients)	
for radical treatment (no cure)	x1.0
for palliative treatment	x1.0

Patients' attitudes to survival, and the quality thereof, may differ widely and may be at variance with their doctors' opinions. The studies in laryngeal cancer and lung cancer by McNeil and her colleagues[31,32] show that some people would be prepared to accept decreased survival if this meant that they could avoid the loss of voice associated with laryngectomy or the immediate risks arising from surgery for lung cancer. It may be difficult to incorporate such subtle factors into a decision analysis directly. Sensitivity analyses may be useful, however, in determining the bounds within which such factors might affect the balance of the decision.

Decision analysis can be used to study a fairly typical clinical problem in head and neck cancer—the management of American Joint Committee Stage III (T3NOMO, T1–3NIMO) carcinoma of the pyriform sinus. The options for radical treatment have been modelled previously.[33] The options analysed suggested that the best radical treatment for this tumour would be combined surgery and radiotherapy, and that the worst would be radiotherapy alone. However, the most compelling feature of the analysis is just how poor the results of radical treatment are shown to be. Even the best result produces only 108 weeks of quality-adjusted survival. Given the mediocrity of the results from radical therapy in this example, the question then becomes: should radical treatment be offered to all and, if so, under what circumstances?

The decision tree shown in Fig. 1 can be simplified as shown in Fig. 2. This slightly artificial approach makes several assumptions compared with the unpruned version: all cures are complicated; there are no gradations in either treatment-related morbidity or degree of palliation; all patients treated palliatively achieve benefit; there is no prolongation of survival, compared with patients treated palliatively, for patients who fail radical therapy. The values for the other variables are shown in Table 1.

Figure 3 shows the results of a sensitivity analysis for three variables using the pruned tree. It shows the critical interdependence of cure rate, the life expectancy for cured patients, and the length of survival for patients treated palliatively. Given the underlying assumptions, this basic analysis will overestimate the utility of palliative therapy. If the survival of patients treated palliatively is set at 30 weeks, then the relative quality of life for patients treated radically, as opposed to palliatively, can be plotted against the life expectancy of radically treated patients for a range of cure rates (Fig. 4). There is little impact on the decision for cure rates between 15 and 30 per cent, but if cure rates fall below 15 per cent then a palliative approach may be more appropriate, particularly if patients treated radically have an inferior quality of life compared with those treated palliatively. Even this oversimplified analysis is able to show that palliative therapy can sometimes be a better policy than treating all patients radically.

Figure 5 shows a sensitivity analysis performed using the unpruned tree (Fig. 1). The baseline values for the variables are shown in Table 2. The values were chosen to be consistent with radiotherapy alone as the radical treatment. Figure 6 shows a

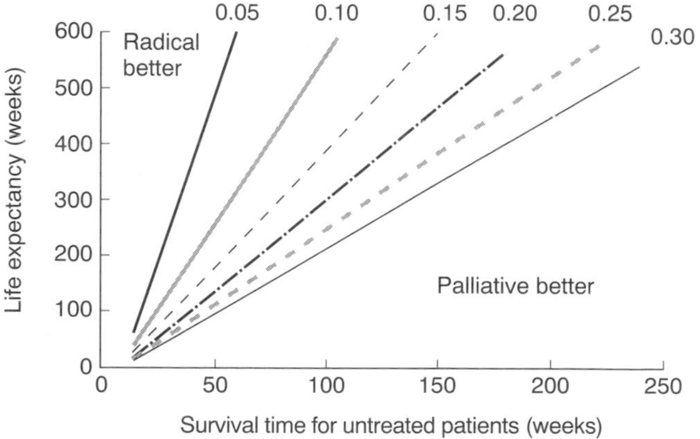

Fig. 3 A sensitivity analysis for the decision tree shown in Fig. 2. Life expectancy and survival times are in weeks. The lines indicate thresholds for a range of cure rates from radical treatment (0.05–0.3). For points above and to the left of a line, radical treatment is preferable. For points below and to the right of a line, palliative treatment is preferable. For example when the cure rate with radical treatment is 20 per cent, the life expectancy of a cured patient is 10 years, and the survival time for an untreated patient is 6 months then radical treatment provides better results. When the life expectancy of a cured patient is less than 5 years, the cure rate is 5 per cent, and the survival time for an untreated patient is greater than 6 months then palliative treatment would be the better choice.

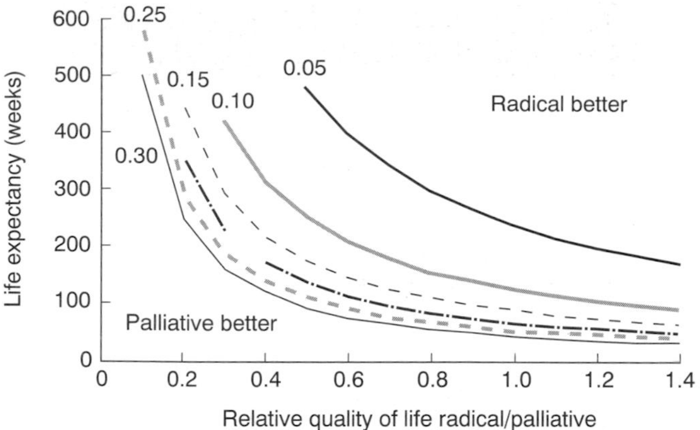

Fig. 4 The tree from Fig. 2 is used and it is assumed that all patients treated palliatively will survive for 30 weeks. As quality of life after radical treatment, relative to that after palliative treatment, falls there is an increasingly abrupt change in favour of palliative treatment.

similar analysis, but with surgery as the radical treatment option; the baseline values are shown in Table 3. These further analyses, based on the more complex decision tree, demonstrate once again the crucial relationship between the life expectancy of cured patients and the cure rate in determining the optimal choice of treatment. Obviously, the life expectancy for cured patients will depend upon age at the start of treatment, and the data suggest that very elderly patients, with life expectancies of less than 2 years, might best be treated palliatively under almost all circumstances. This argument is based purely on assessment of utility and is not influenced by the tyranny of youth that applies when cost-effectiveness or cost–utility analyses are used to set priorities for medical expenditure.

The decision analyses have been used purely for illustration. They fall a long way short of the specific, exhaustive analyses that are required for a rigorous approach to decision-making. However, they do draw attention to some important points and, by virtue of their non-restricted structure, might have some general relevance.

The most important point to be made is that palliative treatment may be an appropriate option for some patients with advanced cancer of the head and neck. It is no longer justifiable simply to treat all patients radically on the 'damned if I do, damned if I don't' principle. The challenge for the future is to devise palliative regimens with minimal intrinsic morbidity that not only relieve symptoms but also produce modest prolongation of life. Even when cure is impossible, increased survival, provided that from the patient's point of view the time is spent usefully, is a goal worth achieving. The recent demonstration[34] that a simple non-toxic regimen of chemotherapy can significantly improve results in patients treated with radical radiotherapy is, in this respect, both intriguing and promising.

Table 2

Parameter	Value
Probability of	
relief of symptoms by palliative treatment	0.5
cure from radical treatment	0.2
uncomplicated cure	0.7
minimal complications	0.59
moderate complications	0.3
severe complications	0.1
fatal complications	0.01
excellent symptom relief	0.2
fair symptom relief	0.6
minimal symptom relief	0.2
Survival time for untreated patients	30 weeks
Duration of palliative treatment	4 weeks
Survival time with complications (fatal only)	12 weeks
Duration of radical treatment	8 weeks
Latent period before complications develop	50 weeks
Life expectancy for cured patients	250 weeks
Quality factors	
minimal complications	0.8
moderate complications	0.6
severe complications	0.4
for tumour-related symptoms	0.35
during radical treatment	0.35
during palliative treatment	0.5
with excellent palliation	0.9
with fair palliation	0.7
with minimal palliation	0.6
Survival increments (cf. untreated patients)	
for radical treatment (no cure)	x1.25
for palliative treatment	x1.0

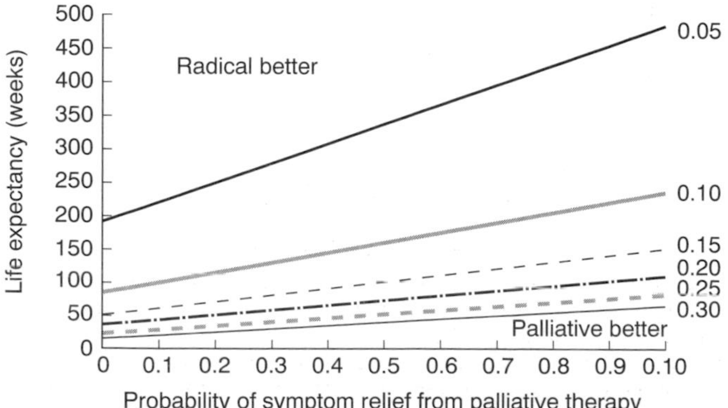

Fig. 5 Sensitivity analysis based upon the fuller form of the decision tree (Fig. 1). Life expectancy for cured patients (weeks) is plotted against the probability of symptom relief from palliative therapy. The baseline values (Table 2) have been chosen to be consistent with radiotherapy as the radical treatment.

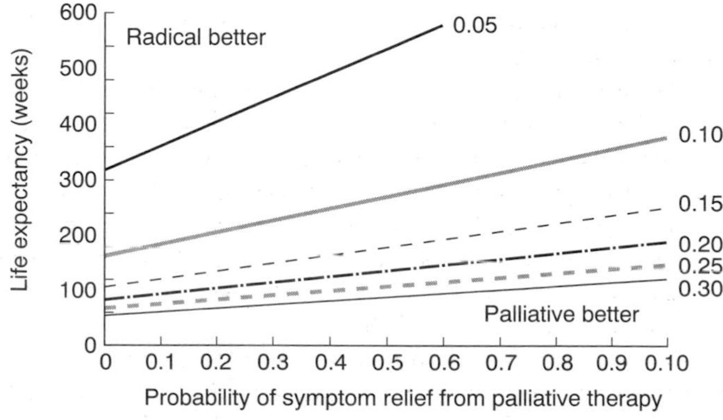

Fig. 6 A similar analysis to that shown in Fig. 5 except that the baseline values (Table 3) are consistent with surgery as the radical treatment.

Table 3

Parameter	Value
Probability of	
relief of symptoms by palliative treatment	0.5
cure from radical treatment	0.2
uncomplicated cure	0
minimal complications	0
moderate complications	0.7
severe complications	0.2
fatal complications	0.1
excellent symptom relief	0.2
fair symptom relief	0.6
minimal symptom relief	0.2
Survival time for untreated patients	30 weeks
Duration of palliative treatment	4 weeks
Survival time with complications (fatal only)	12 weeks
Duration of radical treatment	8 weeks
Latent period before complications develop	0 weeks
Life expectancy for cured patients	250 weeks
Quality factors	
minimal complications	NA
moderate complications	0.6
severe complications	0.4
for tumour-related symptoms	0.35
during radical treatment	0.35
during palliative treatment	0.5
with excellent palliation	0.9
with fair palliation	0.7
with minimal palliation	0.6
Survival increments (cf. untreated patients)	
for radical treatment (no cure)	x1.25
for palliative treatment	x1.0

NA, not available

Treatment options

General

Not much has been written about the palliation of head and neck cancer. This probably reflects the doctors' dilemma that all too often it is unclear at the outset of treatment whether the aim should be curative or palliative. For advanced squamous carcinoma, the survival rate is under 40 per cent but, unlike other sites, the detection of early or micrometastatic disease is no guide to prognosis as head and neck cancer remains a local disease until the late stages. More than 50 per cent of patients with head and neck cancer die from local disease progression, although the majority will have evidence of distant metastases at autopsy. Some of the functional symptoms of large tumours, given their location close to the major sensory organs, are so immediate for the patient that major surgery—even massive surgery, particularly in North America—is considered by some to be a justifiable method of palliation.

Many European head and neck cancer patients are managed in general ear, nose, and throat departments, most of whose patients have minor rhinological and otological problems. Therefore terminal care skills are exercised only sporadically.

In one study of 150 patients with head and neck cancer[3] the eight major complaints were pain (50 per cent), dysphagia (38 per cent), airway obstruction (28 per cent), fungating wound (14 per cent), nausea and vomiting (12 per cent), mucosal dryness (10 per cent), conductive deafness (< 5 per cent), and bleeding (< 1 per cent). A smaller North American study[4] reported a higher incidence of pain (85 per cent), feeding problems (62 per cent), and respiratory difficulties (43 per cent). The average duration of the final hospital stay was 68 days in the 86 per cent of patients whose deaths occurred in hospital, perhaps reflecting the difficulties encountered in managing the head and neck patients' specific problems in the home. Most patients underwent 'definitive cancer therapy' during their last admission. Interestingly a comparison of the progress of the 18 per cent of patients who failed to comply with therapy with the compliant majority showed that non-compliers lived an average 4 months longer and with 90 days fewer in hospital.

Pain can be an intractable concomitant of certain types of tumours—notably adenoid cystic salivary gland tumours, with their capacity for perineural invasion, and middle ear carcinoma invading the base of skull and petrous temporal bone. Other symptoms, less feared by the patient, can at times be equally refractory.

Xerostomia

Oral candidiasis is a frequent finding in all types of cancer,[35,36] and is dealt with in detail elsewhere (Chapter 9.10). One study of 46 admissions for terminal care found clinical evidence of candidiasis in 87 per cent of the patients and more than one-half complained of xerostomia.[37] It must be remembered that patients with poorly fitting dentures secondary to weight loss or with a loose oromaxillary prosthesis will not be cured of the subsequent candidiasis unless the prosthesis is also rinsed in antifungal solution each time topical treatment is administered.

Severe xerostomia leads not only to candida colonization but also to secondary parotid or submandibular sialadenitis unless good oral hygiene is maintained. Suppuration within a major salivary gland is nowadays usually a preterminal development.

Where xerostomia has been associated with radiotherapy to the head and neck this can now be treated effectively with oral pilocarpine.

Pain control

Where pain control by regular oral or subcutaneous opioids is inadequate, cranial nerve section may have to be considered. In the United Kingdom, trigeminal nerve section is usually performed by a neurosurgeon, but it is possible to divide both the trigeminal and glossopharyngeal nerves by using a transmastoid retrolabyrinthine approach to the posterior cranial fossa dura. A simpler method of ablating trigeminal pain is to use percutaneous radio-frequency rhizotomy. The most direct route to the glossopharyngeal nerve is via the tonsillar fossa,[38] but this may not be possible in cases of oropharyngeal malignancy. It is easiest to locate as it winds round stylopharyngeus deep to the angle of the jaw. Transcutaneous electrical nerve stimulation is used infrequently for head and neck cancer, but is an effective therapy for temporomandibular joint dysfunction and probably warrants further attention. In intractable pain caused by head and neck cancer,[39–41] neuraxial surgical approaches (e.g. high cervical or pontine spinothalamic tractotomy, mesencephalic tractotomy, or thalamotomy) may be considered.

Malodorous growths

Antibiotic therapy (e.g. metronidazole) can be useful in malodorous growths and superficial cleansing with a 'water-pik' irrigator or topical antibiotic can be useful. Overuse of peroxide leads to sloughing, however, and adequate ventilation, deodorizers, and frequent dressing and bed changes are the mainstay of local symptom control.

Management of speech and communication disorders

Speech problems are almost universal in advanced oral cancer and follow most major head and neck resections. In addition, in one study airway obstruction and conductive deafness alone accounted for communication deficiency in 30 per cent of patients. The speech therapist can help the patient to develop compensatory movements, particularly after partial glossectomy for consonants requiring a high degree of lingual mobility (t, d, and s). There are also general strategies to help communication such as slowing the speed of speech, breaking words into syllables, maintaining face-to-face contact, and reducing background noise (see Chapter 12.5).

Artificial speech

Conventional speech therapy (see Chapter 12.5) has much to offer those with severe dysarthria, but rehabilitation after laryngectomy requires special techniques. The larynx functions as a vibrator, creating a vibrating column of air of a given fundamental frequency upon which the oropharyngeal articulators and resonators then impose a pattern of speech.[42] Laryngeal function can therefore be simulated either by use of the repaired pharyngeal segment as a resonator (oesophageal speech) or by the application of a battery-operated external vibrator to the cervical skin or oral cavity. The patient then articulates on this new column of vibrating air. The probable success of oesophageal speech can be assessed post-operatively by insufflating the segment from an external source of air and asking the patient to phonate.[43] Patients with less powerful speech may find a tracheo-oesophageal fistula and valve a useful adjunct.

Paralysed larynx

Glottic competence is important not only for speech but also for successful swallowing. In patients with an anatomically normal but paralysed larynx, it is possible to return an abducted cord to the midline using cricoarytenoid reinnervation with a branch of the phrenic nerve.[44] It has been argued that reinnervation of the paralysed muscle or surgical medialization (thyroplasty) are superior to the traditional injection of Teflon paste, which is at least quick and cheap.[45] In expert hands, thyroplasty and ansa cervicalis–recurrent laryngeal anastomosis will give excellent functional results. The use of a combination of a silastic implant–laryngeal framework medialization with the transfer of a nerve/muscle pedicle from the anterior omohyoid is also reported to give good results.[46] The chief disadvantage of Teflon injection is, however, its irreversibility. A patient developing postoperative stridor may require a tracheostomy. None the less, the use of a simple injection has obvious appeal in a patient with extensive disease for whom palliation of aspiration and dysphonia rather than restoration of optimum phonatory quality is the primary aim. Over the past few years, a variety of collagen injections suitable for use in the vocal cords have become available. Collagen appears more suitable for patients with any residual vocal cord movement and is also better tolerated than Teflon by the host tissue.[47]

Management of swallowing disorders

Swallowing exercises and compensatory strategies

Patients who have an immobile hemipharynx, due to either neurological paralysis or surgical repair, can be advised to tilt or turn the head towards the paralysed side to open the contralateral normally functioning lateral food channel.[48] Reduced tongue control can be treated by postural compensation techniques or by exercises (see Chapter 12.5).

Aspiration

Aspiration caused by reduced adduction of the vocal cords can be treated by the methods discussed under speech rehabilitation. The aspiration of liquids may be a problem, for example following supraglottic laryngectomy, and in this situation dietary modification to include foods of a pasty consistency may be of great benefit (see Logemann, Chapter 4, Table 4[8]). Treatment of the tracheotomized patient with aspiration involves both non-surgical and surgical considerations. The use of a vertical neck incision and avoidance of the Bjork flap may lessen the chance of aspiration. Postoperatively the tracheostomy cuff should be minimally inflated. The area above the cuff should be suctioned carefully before regular deflations and suctioning should also be carried out after any oral intake.

Artificial feeding

Patients with head and neck cancers who cannot swallow rarely require parenteral nutrition. Usually, feeding on a long-term basis with a fine-bore nasogastric tube is possible if swallowing function cannot be restored. However, the use of tube feeding in dying patients does raise a variety of ethical issues.[49] Failure to provide nutrition at the end of illness may prove distressing for relatives. Symptomatically, xerostomia will probably dominate the clinical picture and can be troublesome even in the presence of adequate fluid replacement.

Palliative radiotherapy

The traditional opinion regarding radiotherapy for locally advanced head and neck cancer has been that radical doses, given in 20 to 30 fractions, are necessary to produce adequate relief of symptoms. These schedules produce significant morbidity, particularly mucositis, and are disruptive to normal life. They are difficult to justify for patients whose life expectancy is limited; the cost of treatment should not be forgotten.[28]

A recent study of palliative radiotherapy for head and neck cancer has demonstrated that a schedule using 14.8 Gy in four fractions, given over 2 days, and repeated every 3 weeks to a maximum of three courses, is both well tolerated and effective.[50] Mucositis is unusual with this regimen but xerostomia may be troublesome. This latter symptom can now be effectively managed by oral pilocarpine at a dose of 5 mg three times per day.[51–53]

Specific clinical problems amenable to radiotherapy include the following:

Recurrent single inoperable neck metastases

These can often be treated effectively with a single plane iridium wire implant. This involves the insertion of fine polythene tubing into the metastasis in a regular arrangement either with direct surgical exposure or blindly. Iridium wire is afterloaded along the tubes and dose calculations carried out to achieve 60 to 70 Gy in 6 to 7 days. The tubes are removed at the end of treatment.

Tracheostomal recurrence
Palliative doses of radiotherapy may prevent ulceration and bleeding. The tracheostomy may also be kept patent.

Orbital metastases
Short palliative courses of radiotherapy (e.g. 20 Gy in five fractions or 10 Gy in a single fraction) may achieve excellent resolution of proptosis associated with retro-orbital tumour. This is particularly successful in the rapidly growing anaplastic tumours.

Recurrent inoperable parotid tumours
Neutron therapy has not upheld its early promise in the treatment of cancers at most sites. However, the use of neutrons to treat advanced, recurrent salivary gland tumours remains popular in some centres with this facility. Others suggest that adequate external beam dosages will achieve the same control rates.

Haemorrhage
Haemorrhage is common only in the heavily pretreated patient where surgery, radiotherapy, and chemotherapy may all have been used previously. Further palliative radiotherapy is not usually indicated.

The role of chemotherapy in head and neck cancer

Several fundamental points must be considered before raising the question of whether chemotherapy does indeed have any palliative function in head and neck cancer.

1. Untreated patients with advanced squamous carcinoma of the head and neck have a median survival of 88 days.[54] Survival time is significantly related to T stage and the patient's general condition.
2. In the neoadjuvant situation chemotherapy has been shown in many studies to be ineffective in prolonging life despite the fact that it is highly successful in shrinking tumours.[55-58] This may be due to the presence of drug-resistant subpopulations so that even patients with a complete clinical response may have a considerable number of surviving cells.
3. It has been shown recently that patients with cancer are much more likely to opt for radical treatment with minimal chance of benefit than are their carers and others without cancer.[59]
4. It has been said that not only is our ability to assess palliation and quality of life rudimentary but also the current 'proliferation of trial results that cannot be properly evaluated may lead both oncologists and non-oncologists to overestimate the role of chemotherapy and, at the same time, to undervalue the impact of toxicity related to treatment'.[60]

A prospective randomized trial comparing cisplatinum, vincristine, and bleomycin with weekly methotrexate in patients with previously treated advanced squamous cell carcinoma of the head and neck[55] showed that the combination chemotherapy was no more effective in producing response or prolonging survival then weekly methotrexate. A subsequent study[57] from the same group indicated that the combination of cisplatinum with 5-fluorouracil in patients with recurrent disease gave a 27 per cent complete response and a 43 per cent partial response. A contemporary review of United Kingdom practice in respect of chemotherapy suggested that 70 per cent of head and neck oncologists used palliative chemotherapy for head and neck cancer—bleomycin in 80 per cent and cisplatinum in 35 per cent.[61] A trial carried out in Liverpool comparing the benefits of cisplatinum and bleomycin indicated that cisplatinum resulted in prolonged survival and time spent at home in contrast with bleomycin which did not. There also appeared to be a synergistic effect between cisplatinum and bleomycin.

Despite the proliferation of such small studies using cytotoxic chemotherapy in the palliative situation its true role remains unclear. There is no doubt of the chemoresponsiveness of many head and neck tumours. With some combinations the response rates approach those of lymphoma or small-cell lung cancer. Survival benefits appear doubtful and morbidity of treatment is significant. Despite these clear facts, most oncologists continue to use cytotoxic drugs probably partly due to patient demand and also because of the real difficulties in doing nothing when an active agent remains untried in the individual patient. However, many clinicians have anecdotal experience that partial responders in this situation die a more unpleasant death with further recurrent or metastatic disease at other sites.

In the absence of good data on the costs and benefits of chemotherapy for patients with advanced head and neck cancer, the use of such treatment can neither be adequately defended nor criticized.

Surgery

The importance of one-stage reconstruction
Advances in plastic surgery have increased the surgical options in the palliation of head and neck malignancy.[62-64] Now that many procedures can be completed in one stage with a relatively short hospital stay, many large lesions are amenable to surgical palliation. Also, in carefully selected patients with advanced carcinoma of the hypopharynx, partial, as opposed to total, oesophagectomy may not only be adequate oncologically but also allow more speedy swallowing rehabilitation and discharge from hospital.[65]

Until recently, the principal flaps for head and neck reconstruction were the latissimus dorsi and pectoralis major myocutaneous pedicle flaps.[66] These have now been superseded by free flaps such as the jejunal autograft and the free radial forearm flap.[67,68] This has been shown to be extremely reliable when used in intraoral reconstruction, allowing oral intake to be established between 6 and 30 days. Osseomyocutaneous pedicle grafts have transformed mandibular reconstruction.

Examples of surgical palliation
Some patients with extensive T_3 or T_4 squamous carcinomas of the oropharynx can now be treated palliatively with a radical resection and immediate repair with a myocutaneous or free-flap technique. Total glossectomy with a myocutaneous flap for a diffuse tongue tumour with no obvious metastasis is reported to be a good example of the grey area between surgical palliation and cure. Following pharyngolaryngo-oesophagectomy, the use of a stomach pull-up procedure carries such morbidity that it is hard to view this reconstruction as palliative. However, a jejunal interposition has less morbidity and may reasonably be considered a palliative procedure in the motivated patient. In patients with orbital space-occupying lesions not responsive to radiotherapy, orbital decompression by the transfrontal or antroethmoid routes gives prompt symptomatic relief.[69]

Finally, the use of radical neck dissection for cervical metastasis from an unknown primary site is a classic case of surgical palliation and occasional cure. The relevance of surgery to the palliation of head and neck cancer is discussed in greater detail elsewhere (Chapter 9.1.3).

Laser therapy, photodynamic therapy, and cryotherapy

Laser therapy

Several types of laser can be used to palliate head and neck disease. CO_2 laser energy is absorbed primarily by water and soft tissue and has the capacity to coagulate blood vessels up to 0.5 mm in diameter. These properties make the CO_2 laser ideally suited for the excision or vaporization of cutaneous and mucosal lesions. The neodymium: yttrium aluminium garnet (Nd:YAG) laser has the ability to photocoagulate large amounts of tissue and also promotes an intense thermal reaction that can penetrate deeply into tissue. It is extremely useful endoscopically or on mucosal surfaces.

The CO_2 laser is useful within the oral cavity although it is not suitable for the excision of large lesions. It coagulates the microcirculation and allows for precise visualization of the operative field with less tissue manipulation and less postoperative oedema. Therefore, it is possible that in future some patients who at present require to have a tracheostomy to cover either a debulking or biopsy procedure for an obstructive upper airway lesion may be spared the necessity for tracheostomy for airway protection. The small amount of tissue oedema and haemorrhage caused by laser debulking or biopsy suggests that this may be possible, and this may be a great help in the palliation of malignancy, particularly in elderly subjects.

The Nd:YAG laser is also used in the tracheobronchial tree.[70,71] Its energy is absorbed by dark colours, such as haemoglobin and melanin, and is transmitted through clear liquids with very little loss of energy. Therefore, the hallmark of its tissue interaction is the scattering of the laser energy within the tissue. Opening a closed bronchus or an obstructed trachea often relieves the patient's cough, dyspnoea, and fever. The Nd:YAG can coagulate a large volume of tissue. The distal end of the rigid bronchoscope can then be used to shear the tumour away from the tracheobronchial tree or, alternatively, the CO_2 laser can be used to vaporize the coagulated tumour bulk. A review of the use of the CO_2 rigid bronchoscope system in 34 patients with primary tracheal and lung cancers or metastases from different sites identified contraindications as being extrinsic tracheobronchial compression, widespread distant metastases, rapidly progressing tumours, and highly vascular neoplasms.[72] The best palliation was achieved in proximal, that is tracheal or main stem bronchial, slower-growing tumours. Clearly, the use of the laser requires the purchase of expensive equipment and considerable expertise in order to render the procedure safe. A more readily available approach to treatment of tracheal stenosis uses a bifurcated silicone stent.

Photodynamic therapy

Photodynamic therapy is the use of light to activate an exogenous photosensitizer based on the relatively selective retention of photosensitizers in malignant tissues. Radiation with visible red light (628 nm) excites a molecule of photosensitizer which returns to its ground state through the emission of photons, an increase in surrounding temperature, and the cytotoxic release of oxygen which causes thrombosis of tumour microcirculation.[73] The most commonly used photosensitizer is a haematoporphyrin derivative. The therapy is curative only in superficial tumours, as light penetrates only to a depth of under 10 mm, and the response rate in head and neck skin lesions is reported to be around 30 per cent. Initial clinical studies suggest that the tumour response is rather variable, but in future there may be applications for intraoperative phototherapy. Photodynamic therapy also provides useful palliation for obstructive lesions of the lower trachea or main bronchus.[74]

Cryotherapy

Cryotherapy, using multiple freezes, can also be very useful in debulking recurrent lesions within the oral cavity. Cryotherapy induces a thermal sensory neuropraxia with good pain reduction and a beneficial cleaning of debris which helps reduce odour.

Pharmacological treatments

These aspects are dealt with elsewhere in this textbook.

Conclusion

Effective palliative management of the patient with head and neck cancer poses a considerable challenge to clinicians. In this context, there can be no clear-cut rules and guidelines. In this chapter we can only indicate some of the underlying principles as well as the practical approaches to the problem. Perhaps the most important conclusion is that until there has been much more work on patients' attitudes to, and experiences of, treatment, it is virtually impossible to place the palliative management of head and neck cancer on a rational basis.

References

1. Kleinsasser O. In: Stell PM, ed. *Tumours of the Larynx and Hypopharynx*. Stuttgart: Thieme Verlag, 1988: 2–24.
2. Shaw H. Palliation in head and neck cancer. *Journal of Laryngology and Otology*, 1985; **99**: 1131–42.
3. Aird DW, Bihari J, Smith C. Clinical problems in the continuing care of head and neck cancer patients. *Ear, Nose and Throat Journal*, 1983; **62**: 10–30.
4. Shedd DP, Carl A, Shedd C. Problems of terminal head and neck cancer patients. *Head and Neck Surgery*, 1980; **2**: 476–82.
5. Pashley NRT. Practical palliative care for the patient with terminal head and neck cancer. *Journal of Otolarngology*, 1980; **9**: 405–11.
6. Herzon FS, Boshier M. Head and neck cancer emotional management. *Head and Neck Surgery*, 1979; **2**: 112–18.
7. Francfort JW, Gallagher JF, Penman Fairman RM. Surgery for radiation-induced carotid atherosclerosis. *Annals of Vascular Surgery*, 1989; 3:14–19.
8. Logemann, J. *Evaluation and Treatment of Swallowing Disorders*. San Diego: College Hill Press, 1983.
9. Edelman G. Speech and swallowing difficulties and their management. In: Stafford N, Waldron J, eds. *Management of Oral Cancer*. Oxford: Oxford University Press, 1989: 183–94.
10. Welch RW, Luckmann K, Ricks PM, Drake ST, Gates GA. Manometry of the normal upper esophageal sphincter and its alteration in laryngectomy. *Journal of Clinical Investigation*, 1979; **63**: 1036–41.
11. Hanks JB, Fisher SR, Meyers WC, Christian KC, Postlethwait RW, Jones RS. Effect of total laryngectomy on esophageal motility. *Annals of Otology, Rhinology and Laryngology*, 1981; **90**: 331–4.
12. Jacob P, Kahrilas PJ, Logemann JA, Shah V, Ha T. Upper esophageal sphincter opening and modulation during swallowing. *Gastroenterology*, 1989; **97**: 1469–78.

13. Hambreus GM, Ekberg O, Fletcher R. Pharyngeal dyfunction after total and subtotal oesophagectomy. *Acta Radiologica*, 1987; **28**: 409–13.
14. Barr-Hamilton RM, Matheson LM, Keay DG. Ototoxicity of cis-platinum and its relationship to eye colour. *Journal of Laryngology and Otology*, 1991; **105**: 7–11.
15. Bronstein AM, Miller DH, Rudge P, Kendall BE. Down-beating nystagmus: magnetic resonance imaging and neuro-otological findings. *Journal of the Neurological Sciences*, 1987; **81**: 173–81.
16. Mafee MF, Capos M, Raju S. Head and neck: high field magnetic resonance imaging versus computed tomography. *Otolaryngology Clinics of North America*, 1988; **21**: 513–46.
17. Bluth EI, Merritt CRB, Sullivan MA, Bernhardt S, Darnell B. Usefulness of duplex ultrasound in evaluating vertebral arteries. *Journal of Ultrasound Medicine*, 1989; **8**: 229–35.
18. Platts AD, Valentine AR. The use of intravenous digital subtraction angiography in the evaluation of neck masses. *Annals of the Royal College of Surgeons of England*, 1986; **68**: 249–51.
19. Stockwell CW. Vestibular function testing: 4 year update. In: Cummings CW, Frederickson JM, Harker LA, Krause CJ, Schuller DE, eds. *Otolaryngology—Head and Neck Surgery Update II*. St Louis: Mosby, 1990: 39–53.
20. Dodds WJ, Hogan WJ, Reid DP, Stewart ET, Stef JJ, Arndorfer RC. Evaluation of pharyngeal peristalsis using a strain sensitive recording system. *Gastroenterology*, 1972; **62**: 743.
21. Wilson JA, Pryde A, MacIntyre CCA, Heading R. Normal pharyngo-oesophageal motility: a study of 50 healthy subjects. *Digestive Diseases and Sciences*, 1989; **34**: 1590–9.
22. McConnel FMS, Cerenko D, Hersh T, Weil LJ. Evaluation of pharyngeal dysphagia with manofluorography. *Dysphagia*, 1988; **2**: 187–95.
23. Stone M, Shawker JH. An ultrasound examination of tongue movement during swallowing. *Dysphagia*, 1986; **1**: 78–83.
24. Wilson JA, McIntvre MA, von Haake NP, Maran AGD. Fine needle aspiration biopsy and the otolaryngologist. *Journal of Laryngology and Otology*, 1987; **101**: 595–600.
25. Patterson JT. *The Dread Disease. Cancer and Modern American Culture*. Cambridge, MA: Harvard University Press, 1987.
26. Jones E. *The Life and Work of Sigmund Freud*. Harmondsworth: Penguin, 1964.
27. Weinstein MC, Fineberg HV, Elstein AS. *Clinical Decision Analysis*. Philadelphia: WB Saunders, 1980.
28. Munro AJ, Sebag-Montefiore D. Opportunity cost—a neglected aspect of cancer treatment. *British Journal of Cancer*, 1992; **65**: 309–10.
29. Feinstein AR. The 'chagrin factor' and quantitative decision analysis. *Archives of Internal Medicine*, 1985; **145**: 1257–9.
30. *Journal of the American Medical Association*, 1906.
31. McNeil BJ, Pauker SG, Sox HC, Tversky A. On the elicitation of preferences for alternative therapies. *New England Journal of Medicine*, 1982; **306**: 1259–62.
32. McNeil BJ, Weichselbaum R, Pauker SG. Speech and survival. Tradeoffs between quantity and quality of life in lung cancer. *New England Journal of Medicine*, 1981; **305**: 982–7.
33. Plante DA, Piccirillo JF, Sofferman RA. Decision analysis of treatment options in pyriform sinus carcinoma. *Medical Decision Making*, 1987; **7**: 74–83.
34. Gupta NK, Pointon RCS, Wilkinson PM. A randomised clinical trial to contrast radiotherapy with radiotherapy and methotrexate given synchronously in head and neck cancer. *Clinical Radiology*, 1987; **38**: 575–81.
35. De Conno F, Ripamonti C, Sbanotto A, Ventafridda V. Oral complications in patients with advanced cancer. *Journal of Palliative Care*, 1989; **5**: 7–15.
36. Calman FMB, Langdon J. Oral complications of cancer. *British Medical Journal*, 1991; **302**: 484–5.
37. Clarke JMG, Wilson JA, von Haake NP, Milne NJR. Oral candidiasis in terminal illness. *Health Bulletin*, 1987; **45**: 268–71.
38. Neil JF. Glossopharyngeal nerve section in malignant disease of the oropharynx. *Ear, Nose and Throat Journal*, 1983; **62**: 255–7.
39. Malyan Wilson PJE. Neurosurgery and relief of pain associated with head and neck cancer. *Ear, Nose and Throat Journal*, 1983; **62**: 250–4.
40. Kelly J, Arena S. Pain control in recurrent head and neck cancer. *Archives of Otolaryngology*, 1985; **101**: 26–8.
41. Boop WC. Methods of pain control. In: Myers EN, Suen JY, eds. *Cancer of the Head and Neck*. New York: Churchill Livingstone, 1990: 1005–20.
42. Singer MI. The upper oesophageal sphincter: role in alaryngeal speech acquisition. *Head and Neck Surgery*, 1988; Suppl.II: S118–23.
43. Blom ED, Singer MI, Hamaker RC. An improved esophageal insufflation test. *Archives of Otolaryngology*, 1985; **111**: 211–15.
44. Baldissera F, Cantarella G, Marini G, Ottaviani F, Tredici G. Recovery of inspiratory abduction of the paralysed vocal cords after bilateral reinnervation of the cricoarytenoid muscles by one single branch of the phrenic nerve. *Laryngoscope*, 1989; **99**: 1286–92.
45. Crumley RL. Teflon versus thyroplasty versus nerve transfer: a comparison. *Annals of Otology, Rhinology and Laryngology*, 1990; **99**: 759–63.
46. Tucker HM. Combined laryngeal framework medialization and reinnervation for unilateral vocal fold paralysis. *Annals of Otology, Rhinology and Laryngology*, 1990; **99**: 778–81.
47. Remacle H, Marbaix E, Hamoir M, Bertrand B, Beckhaut J. Correction of glottic insufficiency by collagen injection. *Annals of Otology, Rhinology, and Laryngology*, 1990; **99**: 438–44.
48. Logemann JA, Bytell DE. Swallowing disorders in three types of head and neck surgical patients. *Cancer*, 1979; **44**: 1095–105.
49. Campbell-Taylor I, Fisher RH. The clinical case against tube feeding in palliative care of the elderly. *Journal of the American Geriatric Society*, 1987; **35**: 1100–4.
50. Paris KJ, Spanos WJJ, Lindberg RD, Jose B, Albrink F. Phase i–ii study of multiple daily fractions for palliation of advanced head and neck malignancies. *International Journal of Radiation Oncology Biology Physics*, 1993; **25**: 657–60.
51. Greenspan D, Daniels TE. Effectiveness of pilocarprine in postirradiation xerostomia. *Cancer* 1987; **59**: 1123–5.
52. LeVeque FG, Montgomery M, Potter D, Zimmer MB, Rieke JW, Steiger BW, Gallagher SC, Muscoplat CC. A multicenter, randomised, double-blind, placebo-controlled, dose-titration study of oral pilocarpine for treatment of radiation-induced xerostomia in head and neck cancer patients. *Journal of Clinical Oncology*, 1993; **11**: 1124–31.
53. Rieke JW, Hafermann MD, Johnson JT, LeVeque FG, Iwamoto R, Steiger BW, Muscoplat C, Gallagher SC. Oral pilocarpine for radiation-induced xerostomia: integrated efficacy and safety results from two prospective randomised clinical trials. *International Journal of Radiation Oncology Biology Physics*, 1995; **31**: 661–9.
54. Stell PM, Morton RP, Singh SD. Squamous carcinoma of the head and neck: the untreated patient. *Clinical Otolaryngology*, 1983; **8**: 7–13.
55. Drelichman A, Cummings G, Al-Sarraf M. A randomised trial of the combination of cis-platinum, oncovin and bleomycin versus methotrexate in patients with advanced squamous carcinoma of the head and neck. *Cancer*, 1983; **52**: 399–403.
56. Snow GB, Vermorken JB. Neoadjuvant chemotherapy in head and neck cancer: state of the art. *Clinical Otolaryngology*, 1989; **14**: 371–5.
57. Kish JA, Weaver A, Jacobs J, Cummings G, Al-Sarraf M. Cisplatin and 5-fluorouracil infusion in patients with recurrent and disseminated epidermoid cancer of the head and neck. *Cancer*, 1984; **53**: 1819–24.
58. Siodlak MZ, *et al.* Alternating cisplatinum and VAC ineffective in end stage squamous carincoma of the head and neck. *Journal of Laryngology and Otology*, 1990; **104**: 631–3.
59. Slevin MI, *et al.* Attitudes to chemotherapy: comparing views of patients with cancer with those of doctors, nurses, and the general public. *British Medical Journal*, 1990; **300**: 1458–60.
60. Kearsley JH. Cytotoxic chemotherapy for common adult malignancies: 'the emperor's new clothes' revisited? *British Medical Journal*, 1986; **293**: 871–5.
61. Morton RP, Benjamin CS. Elderly patients with head and neck cancer. *Lancet*, 1990; **335**: 1597.

62. Tucker H, Rabuzzi DD, Reed GF. Massive surgery for palliation in malignancy of the head and neck. *Laryngoscope*, 1973; **83**: 1635–43.
63. McConnel FMS, Teichgraeber JF, Adler RK. A comparison of three methods of oral reconstruction. *Archives of Otolaryngology*, 1987; **113**: 496–500.
64. Gullane PJ, Grace A. Developments in oral and pharyngeal reconstruction. In: Gray RF, Rutka JA, eds. *Recent Advaces in Otolaryngology*. Edinburgh: Churchill Livingstone, 1988: 125–42.
65. Gluckman JL, *et al.* Partial vs total esophagectomy for advanced carcinoma of the hypopharynx. *Archives of Otolaryngology*, 1987; **113**: 69–72.
66. Leonard AG. Musculocutaneous flaps in head and neck reconstruction. *Annals of the Royal College of Surgeons of England*, 1989; **71**: 160–8.
67. Soutar DS. Free flaps in reconstructive surgery. *Annals of the Royal College of Surgeons of England*, 1989; **71**: 169–74.
68. Coleman JJ, *et al.* Ten years' experience with the free jejunal autograft. *American Journal of Surgery*, 1987; **154**: 394–8.
69. Wilson JA, von Haake NP, Adams GGW, Dale BAB. Surgical decompression of the orbit. *Journal of the Royal College of Surgeons of Edinburgh*, 1986; **31**: 22–6.
70. Duncavage JA, Ossoff RH. Laser application in the trachcobronchial tree. *Otolaryngology Clinics of North America*, 1990; **23**: 67–75.
71. Schwartz MR, Povalski Aj, Sills C. Palliation of airway obstruction with endoscopic laser photocoagulation. *New Jersey Medicine*, 1987; **84**: 585–8.
72. Shapshay SM, Davis RK, Vaughan CW, Norton M, Strong MS, Simpson GT. Palliation of airway obstruction from trachcobronchial malignancy: use of the CO_2 laser bronchoscope. *Otolaryngology and Head and Neck Surgery*, 1983; **91**: 615–19.
73. Davis RK. Photodynamic therapy in otolaryngology—head and neck surgery. *Otolaryngology Clinics of North America*, 1990; **23**: 107–19.
74. Veldhiuzen JA, Annyas AA, Overbeek JJM, von Wit HP. Photodynamic therapy: a new method of treatment of malignant tumours; preliminary results in 21 patients with malignant tumours in the head and neck and bronchus. *Clinical Otolaryngology*, 1990; **15**.

9.10 Mouth care

Vittorio Ventafridda, Carla Ripamonte, Alberto Sbanotto, and Franco De Conno

Introduction

Lesions of the oral cavity have a great impact on the quality of life of patients with advanced cancer. Such lesions have a considerable morbidity and interfere a great deal with both physical and psychological function. Perhaps most importantly, these complications impair oral nutrition with a variety of consequences, including malnutrition, anorexia, and cachexia. In addition, psychological disturbances relate to the role that the oral cavity plays in communication, social life, and pleasures associated with eating.

Oral hygiene

Good oral hygiene is fundamental to the well-being of cancer patients. Its purpose is to:

(1) keep lips and oral mucosa clean, soft, and intact, as far as is possible;

(2) remove plaque and debris;

(3) prevent oral infection, decay, periodontal disease, and halitosis;

(4) relieve oral pain and discomfort and increase or maintain oral intake;

(5) prevent further damage to oral mucosa in patients undergoing antineoplastic and pharmacological treatments;

(6) minimize psychological distress and social isolation and increase family involvement;

(7) maintain the patient's dignity even as death is approaching.

Oral cavity examination (Table 1), should be carried out routinely during the patient's stay in hospital or hospice or at home and should follow a fixed schedule of at least twice a week (Table 2). Daily brushing with a soft-bristle toothbrush, use of unwaxed dental floss, and rinsing with a mild solution of sodium bicarbonate (1 teaspoonful per large cup of water), form the basis of correct oral hygiene. A thick paste of sodium bicarbonate and a few drops of warm water can be applied by the patient with a soft toothbrush in a 'pat and push' manner into the gingival sulcus and around the teeth. This technique is an effective complementary regimen to mechanical plaque debridement for reducing sulcus/pocket organisms and improving periodontal health.[1,2] Commercial mouthwashes may be helpful, but patients affected by stomatitis may have to avoid products containing alcohol, lemon, and glycerine as well as dentifrices with an abrasive action.

Many patients wear partial or complete dentures. Cachectic patients may note that their dentures are loose and ill-fitting, with consequent abrasions and ulcerations of soft tissue, and pain. Some principles for the care of dentures are presented in Table 3. An accurate oral examination is important for correct hygiene.

Importance of saliva for oral health

Saliva is a major protector of the tissues and organs of the mouth. In its absence both the hard and soft tissues of the oral cavity may be severely damaged, with an increase in ulcerations, infections such as candidiasis,[3] and dental decay.[4,5]

About 1000 to 1500 ml of saliva are produced daily by the parotid, submaxillary, and sublingual glands and by small, minor salivary glands of the oral cavity. Salivary pH is about 6 to 7, favouring the digestive action of a salivary enzyme, α-amylase. Saliva is composed of a serous part (α-amylase), devoted to starch

Table 1 Factors to be considered before oral cavity examination

Local
Oral hygiene (methods, products used)
Previous/actual dental diseases (periodontopathy, decay)
Dentures (type, cleaning methods)
Local pain
Haemorrhages
Ulceration (infections, trauma, tumour)
Xerostomia
Taste alterations
Dysphagia
Local tumour
Previous/current chemotherapy/local radiotherapy and/or surgery
Oxygen therapy, breathing by mouth
Previous/current infections (viral, bacterial, mycotic)
Systemic
Drugs (steroids, antibiotics, anticholinergic, chemotherapy)
Dehydration
Cachexia syndrome
Diabetes, hypothyroidism
Immunological diseases
Nutritional status

Table 2 Oral cavity: routine examination

Equipment: examination gloves, light, tongue depressor, hand mirror

1. External examination of the lips, degree of mouth opening
2. Remove dentures (if present)
3. Observe the state of the following structures:
   The hard and soft palate
   The pillars of the fauces and pharynx
   The internal side of the cheeks
   The oral vestibule and outer part of the gums
   The upper side of the tongue
   The lower part of the tongue, the floor of the mouth, and of inner part of the gums
   The state of the teeth
   The state of any denture

digestion, and a mucous component which acts as a lubricant. It is saturated with calcium and phosphate and is necessary for maintaining healthy teeth. The bicarbonate content of saliva enables it to buffer and produces the conditions necessary for the digestion of plaque which holds acids in contact with teeth.[6] Moreover, saliva helps with bolus formation and lubricates the throat for the easy passage of food. The organic and inorganic components of the salivary secretions have a protective potential. They act as a barrier to irritants and a means of removing cellular and bacterial debris. Saliva contains various components involved in defence against bacterial and viral invasion, including mucins, lipids, secretory immunoglobulin, lysozymes, lactoferrin, salivary peroxidase, and myeloperoxidase.

Amylase originates from the salivary glands; its production is reduced by gland damage, as occurs following radiotherapy.[7] Lysozyme, lactoferrin, and myeloperoxidase are all present in polymorphonuclear leukocytes, which may release these molecules into the saliva. Lysozyme and lactoferrin are also synthesized in acinar cells. The activity of these molecules is increased following oral inflammation[8,9]. Although the minor glands only produce approximately 10 per cent of the total salivary output, they account for 70 per cent of the total mucin in saliva.[10] This substance protects the oral tissues from chemical and mechanical trauma, infections, and lubricates the oral membranes[11]. serum and salivary immunoglobulin concentrations have been found in patients with

Table 3 Care of dentures

Reline dentures if they are loose
Brush and clean well after meals
Remove dentures overnight and leave them (non-metal) in an antiseptic solution (1% sodium hypochlorite)
Brush metal dentures with povidone–iodine solution
If dentures are stained, soak in warm water with a commercial denture cleaner* (brushing and rinsing before reinserting)
If oropharyngeal candidiasis is present, leave dentures in nystatin suspension

* Many disinfectant solutions can also promote certain microbial growth if left to stagnate for more than 24 h.

oral cancer.[12,13] These may result from the production of soluble immunostimulatory tumour-associated antigens by such patients.

Numerous other factors are also important in the preservation of oral mucosa.[14] In frogs, the presence of magainins, intrinsic protective components of the skin, has been described recently. According to Zasloff, similar substances may have a protective role for mammalian mucosa.[15]

Xerostomia

Xerostomia is the subjective feeling of mouth dryness, not always accompanied by a detectable decrease in salivation flow.[16,17] In general, unstimulated whole salivary flow rates of less than 0.1 ml/min are considered low and indicative of xerostomia.[18] It is a symptom that receives little attention and so its prevalence may be underestimated. In a study of 529 adults in a primary care setting, Sreebny *et al.*[17] found the prevalence of xerostomia to be 29 per cent. Women were more frequently affected and there was a positive correlation with age. Few data are available on the frequency of xerostomia in patients with advanced cancer, although 30 per cent of the patients at the beginning of a palliative care programme describe it as 'a lot' and 'awful'.[19] It was a specific complaint in 40 per cent of the patients at the time of admission to a hospice, but probably all patients suffer from a dry mouth at some point during the terminal stage of cancer.[20] Causes of xerostomia are listed in Table 4.

A variety of symptoms may be associated with the feeling of oral dryness. In the study of Sreebny *et al.*[17] the symptoms most frequently present (in 48 per cent or more of the xerostomic subjects) were: the need to do something to keep the mouth moist; the need to get up at night to drink water; and difficulty with speech. Other problems included:

(1) having to keep fluids at the bedside;

(2) a loss in taste acuity;

(3) difficulty with chewing dry foods;

(4) burning and tingling sensations on the tongue;

(5) the presence of cracks or fissures at the corners of the lips;

(6) difficulty in swallowing.

These symptoms contribute to anorexia, loss of weight, and cachexia. Dental prostheses will frequently traumatize the vulnerable mucosa, with further difficulty in mastication and reduced intake of food.[21]

Xerostomia due to radiotherapy

Patients treated with radiotherapy for oral or head and neck cancer often suffer from xerostomia from the beginning of treatment. Radiation can affect one or both parotid glands and the submandibular salivary glands, resulting in a marked diminution in the normal salivary flow [22–28] as a consequence of inflammation and degeneration of the acini and ducts,[23,29] connective tissue,[30] and

Table 4 Causes of xerostomia

1. Reduced salivary secretion caused by
   - Radiotherapy of the head and neck regions
   - Surgery in the buccal and submandibular regions
   - Drugs
   - Obstruction, infection, aplasia, malignant destruction of salivary glands
   - Encephalitis, brain tumours, neurosurgical operations, autonomic pathways destruction
   - Hypothyroidism
   - Autoimmune diseases
   - Sarcoidosis
2. Widespread erosion of buccal mucosa caused by
   - Cancer
   - Chemotherapy, radiotherapy, immunodeficiency
   - Stomatitis
   - Viral, bacterial, and fungal oral infections
3. Dehydration caused by
   - Anorexia
   - Diarrhoea
   - Fever
   - O_2 therapy
   - Breathing by mouth
   - Large bedsores and/or ulcers
   - Vomiting
   - Polyuria
   - Haemorrhage
   - Diabetes insipidus
   - Difficulty in swallowing
4. Depression, anxiety

vascular components of the salivary glands. The most important factor affecting the salivary flow after a curative dose of radiotherapy seems to be the volume of the major salivary glands irradiated,[22] particularly the parotid gland as it is more radiosensitive than other major salivary glands.[31-33] The flow rate of an irradiated parotid gland is almost negligible after only two irraditions of 2.25 Gy each.[34] When 100 per cent of the parotid gland is irradiated, no salivary flow at all can be produced; however, exclusion of 10 to 20 per cent of the gland from the radiation field allows the production of saliva.[31] A sharp decrease in the salivary flow usually occurs after the first week of radiotherapy with a dose of about 10 Gy.[28,32,35] The decrease in the flow rate continues throughout the treatment, which may lead to persistent xerostomia.[28,32] While one study noted a partial return of salivary flow 8 months after the end of radiotherapy,[27] others found minimal, if any, improvement some years after radiotherapy.[36,37]

Irradiation of the salivary glands causes saliva to become more viscous,[7,24,29,38] and to undergo a reduction in pH,[26,35] with a loss of organic and inorganic components.[39,40] Production of the aqueous component of whole saliva is much more sharply depressed than that of the protein component during xerostomia. Therefore, the capacity of saliva to act as a barrier against irritating substances or to remove bacterial and cellular debris is reduced. The bicarbonate content also diminishes,[7,24,29] further impairing the cleansing action of saliva and there is an increase in the salivary content of Na^+, Cl^-, Mg^{2+} and protein.[24,29,33] The reduction in the salivary flow,[29,41] together with these qualitative changes, can alter the oral microbial flora and result in increased growth of streptococcus, lactobacillus, and candida. These often irreversible alterations can rapidly damage dental structures and increase tooth decay.[25,39]

In patients undergoing radiotherapy, tooth decay can be rapid and lesions can be manifest within 3 to 6 months.[24] The process of decay may cause pain in the oral cavity, adding to the suffering of the patient. Loss of already decaying teeth causes further difficulty in mastication, which, when added to xerostomia, may cause difficulty in swallowing and digestion. Saving the minor oral glands may play an important role in protection against new colonization by micro-organisms[7,33,42,43] or against tooth decay.[44,45]

Apart from flow rate measurements, the level of α-amylase seems to be the best indicator of salivary gland function during radiotherapy, whereas albumin and lactoferrin are good indicators of the inflammatory reactions often related to irradiation.[7]

Drug-induced xerostomia

A large number of drugs with xerostomic side-effects are known including tricyclic antidepressants, antihistamines, anticholinergic drugs, anticonvulsants, antipsychotics, hypnotics, β-blockers, and diuretics.[7,46-50] They may reduce the flow of saliva directly or indirectly and initiate the feeling of oral dryness. Some of these drugs induce xerostomia through parasympatholytic effects. In the study of Sreebny *et al.*,[49] almost 60 per cent of those patients with a dry mouth took xerogenic drugs.

The intake of xerostomia-inducing medications is positively correlated with age and with the total number of drugs taken daily[48,49] and it is highest among institutionalized patients.[48] Reductions in salivation in the elderly may be related to drug use rather than to age.

Xerostomia is not generally recognized as a side-effect of morphine[51] but clinical experience suggests that it is a common problem in cancer patients treated with morphine. Ventafridda *et al.*[52] observed a significantly higher incidence of dry mouth following treatment with oral aqueous morphine than with methadone or controlled-release morphine tablets.[53] Another study, carried out for a 2-month period after initial treatment, noted that dry mouth was present 35 per cent of the time during treatment with an anti-inflammatory and/or adjuvant drugs, 36 per cent of the time during treatment with weak opioids and/or adjuvants, and 51 per cent of the time during treatment with strong opioids and/or adjuvants.[54] White *et al.*[51] also describe a highly significant association between the use of morphine and xerostomia.

Possible contributing factors to xerostomia

Dehydration

Advanced cancer patients are often dehydrated (Table 4), with consequent thirst and dry mouth.[55] There have been no controlled clinical trials which have demonstrated any relief of xerostomia following hydration, and the use of parenteral hydration in the palliative care setting remains controversial. A recent study[56] did not show any association between the severity of thirst and fluid intake in palliative care patients. When present, symptoms related

Table 5 Specific therapies for oral complications

Xerostomia

- 2% citric acid solution[16]
- 75–100 mg nicotinic acid more than once per day[20]
- Dihydroergotamine[189]
- Pilocarpine[65-68]
- Antholetrithione ANTT[69]
- ANTT + pilocarpine[30]

Xerostomia caused by drugs

- Reduce the dosage and/or change the drug if possible
- Application of fluoride gel to avoid dental damage

Xerostomia caused by systemic dehydration

- Correct the cause
- Increase the liquid intake by mouth
- Hypodermoclysis (not endstage patients)
- Make use of intravenous hydration in selected patients

Decay

- Good dental hygiene
- Gargle with saline, peroxide, or solutions of baking soda[41,190,191]
- Daily application of fluoride gel[41,190,191]
- Dental treatment

to dehydration seem to be manageable with simple measures, such as oral fluids or ice chips and lubrication of the lips.[57] The therapy of dehydration-induced xerostomia can be specific (Table 5) or exclusively palliative (Table 6).

Decreased mastication

Mastication plays an important role in the regulation of salivary secretion, its effects being mediated through somatic afferent nerves of the oral mucosa and in the periodontal tissues. Patients taking a liquid diet or with immobilized jaws following oral surgery show a significant decrease in salivary flow.[18] No data are available concerning decreased salivation in enterally fed patients or those with gastrostomy or affected by trismus.

Table 6 Palliative therapy for xerostomia

Oral hygiene every 2 h
Humidified air
Suck: ice cubes, vitamin C tablets, frozen tonic water[20]
Chew: sugarless chewing gum, lemon sugar candy, acid substances, pieces of pineapple[20]
Artifical saliva:
* glycerin, cologel, normal saline (1:1:8)
* carboxymethylcellulose, sorbitol, water, sodium fluoride, menthol, minerals and chlorhexidine
* methylcellulose + lemon essence + water[20]
* hydrophilic chewing gum which releases artifical saliva with a remineralizing effect[192]
* mucin-containing artificial saliva based on bovine salivary gland extract[193]

Dentures which include a reservoir for the release of artificial saliva[194]

Psychological factors

Psychological factors, including anxiety, are known to reduce salivary flow. Hyposalivation and xerostomia may be observed in patients suffering from depression.[58]

Prevention and treatment of xerostomia

The regimen currently used by the authors involves good oral hygiene, the treatment of infections such as candidiasis by administration of clotrimazole or fluconazole (especially in high risk patients such as those undergoing high-dose corticosteroid therapy or radiotherapy for head and neck cancer), and a review of the drug regimen to avoid the use of drugs that may induce xerostomia.

Xerostomia after radiation therapy may be the most difficult to treat since irreversible damage to the salivary glands may occur. Current therapy for chronic xerostomia includes the use of salivary substitutes or salivary stimulants. Water, glycerine preparations, and artificial saliva are used as substitutes for saliva, while sialogogues, sugarless candies, and chewing gum stimulate the production of saliva.[59] Many commercial products are available for use primarily as a gargle to relieve the symptoms of xerostomia. Rarely do they improve the problem but only a small number of controlled clinical studies have been performed. Artificial preparations of saliva that contain mucin provide substantially more symptomatic relief to patients with xerostomia than do conventional, non-mucin substitutes.[60-64]

Currently available therapies for xerostomia are listed in Table 5. Pilocarpine, an alkaloid, functions primarily as a muscarinic–cholinergic agonist, and has potent effects on both smooth muscle and exocrine tissues. It has been shown to stimulate salivary flow and increase salivation in patients treated by radiotherapy and in those with Sjögren's syndrome.[65-69] The peak secretory effects of pilocarpine are assumed to occur within 1 h after its intake.[66] Controlled studies have been carried out on the use of oral pilocarpine for radiation-induced xerostomia.[66-68,70-72] All these studies show that pilocarpine produces clinically significant benefits with acceptable side-effects. Best results are obtained with continuous treatment for more than 8 weeks with doses greater than 2.5 mg three times a day. A 5.0 mg three times a day regimen produces the best clinical results when both efficacy and side-effects are considered. Higher doses (10 mg three times a day) can increase clinical benefits; however, an increase in side-effects (mainly moderate sweating) can be present. Pilocarpine treated patients require lesser amounts of artificial saliva; furthermore, patients treated with pilocarpine reported that improvements in xerostomia, comfort, and speaking occurred immediately. It is contraindicated in patients subject to bronchospasm or who have pre-existing bradycardia.

Anethole-trithione (Sialor, Sulfarlem) seems to act directly on the secretory cells of the salivary glands. Some studies found it to improve salivary flow, while others did not.[73] Epstein and Schubert reported a phase I–II trial of the combined use of pilocarpine and anethole-trithione in patients who had not responded with increased saliva production to either agent alone.[30] A statistically significant increase in salivary volume and improved symptoms were reported. Seemingly the anethole-trithione prepared the salivary glands cells for the stimulation provided by pilocarpine.

Dietary advice includes the ingestion of foods with a high

moisture content and the drinking of plenty of liquids with meals to facilitate mastication.

Infections

In comparison to normal subjects, the oral flora of patients with advanced cancer more often includes yeasts (83 per cent), coliforms (49 per cent), and coagulase-positive staphylococci (28 per cent).[74] Such data indicate a loss of colonization resistance of the oral mucosa in terminal cancer patients. Many predisposing factors for candidiasis may be present, including antibiotics and immunosuppressive agents,[75] nutritional factors,[76] and low salivary rates.[77,78] Increased oral coliforms has been reported in several groups of compromized patients, including those on cytotoxic therapy for malignant disease,[79] patients who have received radiotherapy for oral and laryngeal cancer,[80] and those with acute leukaemia.[81] Perhaps the release of endotoxin by Gram-negative bacilli may be responsible for oral soreness and clinical inflammation of the oral mucosa.[82] Microbial factors such as adhesion and interbacterial interference, exogenous factors including antimicrobial chemotherapy, and miscellaneous host factors, such as xerostomia,[74] seem to play an important part in the loss of resistance to bacterial colonization.

Fungal infections

Candidiasis is the most common fungal infection seen in cancer patients.[83] Candida species are reported to be present in the normal oral flora of 40 to 60 per cent of the population.[84] In healthy asymptomatic subjects candida is usually present in the vegetative form (blastospore); when pathogenic it can also exist in a hyphal form. Positive cultures are obtained from about 75 per cent of asymptomatic hospital patients; this proportion can reach 89 per cent if repeated cultures are obtained over a period of time.[55,78]

Clinically evident candidiasis developed in up to 27 per cent of patients admitted to an oncological ward.[85] Oropharyngeal candidiasis can be the source of regional and systemic dissemination, particularly in granulocytopenic and immunosuppressed patients.[86]

The primary pathogen is *Candida albicans*, but other Candida species and other fungi, including Aspergillus, may be involved. The development of clinically evident oral candidiasis depends on local and/or systemic factors commonly involved in other oral infections and symptoms (Table 7). The role of xerostomia and drugs (such as steroids) should to be emphasized; about 40 per cent of patients receiving adrenal corticosteroid therapy and about 30 per cent of those receiving antibiotics, develop oropharyngeal candidiasis.[87] Oral Candida infection usually presents as acute pseudo-membranous candidiasis (thrush), acute atrophic candidiasis (or acute erythematous candidiasis), chronic atrophic (or chronic erythematous) candidiasis, chronic hyperplastic candidiasis, or candidal cheilosis (Table 8).

Other clinical pictures are seen more rarely.[88,89] Thrush appears as a white–yellowish plaque, which is easily wiped off, leaving a bleeding, painful surface. The acute atrophic form is often related to broad-spectrum antibiotics; white plaques are minimal and painful lesions of the oral mucosa and depapillation of the dorsum of the tongue are present. Chronic atrophic candidiasis is characterized by erythema and oedema, usually localized to the part of the palatal mucosa in contact with dentures. This particular form of candidiasis occurs in up to 65 per cent of elderly individuals who wear complete maxillary dentures and is more common in women. Individuals with denture-related chronic atrophic candidiasis often also have angular cheilitis characterized by soreness, redness, and cracks at the corners of the mouth. It can be either erosive or granular in type; habitual licking of the corners of the mouth and reduction in the vertical dimensions of lower third of face, due to edentia, play a major role in this clinical form. Chronic candidal infections are also capable of producing a hyperplastic clinical picture which can resemble leucoplakia, especially when occurring in the retrocommissural area; its role as a precancerous lesion is currently a matter of discussion.[90]

Table 7 Main factors involved in fungal infections of oral cavity

1. Local factors
   - Wearing dentures
   - Xerostomia
   - Saliva composition alterations*
   - Oral mucosa disruption**
   - Microbial alterations
   - Reduced mechanical debridement***
   - Previous infections
   - Poor oral hygiene
2. Systemic factors
   - Diabetes
   - Immunosuppression
   - Medical therapies (e.g. steroids)
   - Nutritional status alterations

* Mainly proteins and electrolytes.
** Radiotherapy, chemotherapy, surgery, cancer.
*** Comatose patients, enterally/parenterally fed patients, trismus, etc.

Table 8 Common clinical pictures of oral candidiasis

Type	Signs/symptoms (see text for more details)
Thrush (acute pseudomembranous form)	Typical white–yellowish plaques. Usually accompained by tenderness, burning, dysphagia, dysgeusia
Acute atrophic	More generalized red lesions, tongue depapillation. Dysgeusia usually present
Chronic atrophic	Bright red surface (denture print); often accompanied by angular cheilitis, which can be moderately painful and bleeding. Dysgeusia usually present
Chronic hyperplastic	Usually resembles leukoplakia. Symptoms are usually absent

In patients with advanced cancer a cytological diagnosis is not generally necessary; when indicated, wet-mounted potassium hydroxide preparation or Gram stain may be performed. Immunofluorescent techniques are less useful.[91]

Both topical and systemic treatments are available, and they can be used together in more severe cases. Nystatin suspension (100 000 U/ml, 4–6 ml every 6 h) is the classic, topical treatment of oral candidiasis but results can sometimes be disappointing.[92,93] Its action is limited to the time of contact with the mucosal surface; consequently ice lollies made of nystatin diluted with water are a soothing and effective alternative. Any combination with chlorhexidine reduces its activity.[94] Clotrimazole lozenges (10 mg five times a day) have good antimycotic activity, even in nystatin-resistant patients.[95,96] Clotrimazole is well tolerated and less expensive[97] and seems to be an effective drug for the prevention of oropharyngeal candidiasis.[98] Miconazole, an imidazole derivative, is another suggested topical treatment, and is very effective in the form of lozenges (250 mg four times daily) or gel (two–four times daily),[99,100] although the taste of lozenges may be found unpleasant. Amphotericin B lozenges can also be used for oral candidiasis, but are not as effective as clotrimazole and miconazole.[101] Intravenous amphotericin is not indicated in the treatment of oral candidal infection, due to the low concentrations that are achieved in saliva.[102]

Among systemic treatments, ketoconazole (200 mg once daily)[103,104] has largely been replaced by the new triazole derivatives, such as fluconazole (50–150 mg once daily) and itraconazole (100–200 mg once daily), which have fewer side-effects. These are well absorbed by the gastrointestinal tract, and have a long half-life, allowing once daily administration. Their spectrum of action is wide; they are active against many different fungi, and hence are useful in the treatment of oropharyngeal candidiasis and systemic and deep fungal infections.[105-110] Side-effects are minimal. Fluconazole treatment of oropharyngeal candidiasis (50 g once daily for 7–14 days) is possibly more effective than traditional treatments such as nystatin and ketoconazole,[109] and its once-a-day schedule makes it an attractive alternative for patients with advanced cancer. A recent controlled trial, comparing fluconazole versus clotrimazole troche, showed a superior capacity of fluconazole in preventing oesophageal and oropharyngeal candidiasis in patients with advanced HIV infection;[111] the presence of breakthrough episodes of infections in 10.6 per cent of patients taking fluconazole, raises the possibility of the development of a resistance to this antifungal agent.[112] Table 9 shows the relative costs for a 1-week course of the different antifungal drugs.

Specific treatment must be accompanied by good oral hygiene.

Table 9 Weekly costs of some antifungal drugs

Drug	Daily dosage	Cost ($)
Nystatin suspension (100000 U/ml)	2400000 U	8.00
Miconazole (oral gel 2%)	12 ml	19.00
Ketoconazole (capsules 200 mg)	200 mg	9.00
Fluconazole (capsules 50 mg)	50 mg	40.00

Bacterial infections

Few data are available concerning bacterial infections in advanced or terminal cancer patients.[113] Periodontal disease is very common in the healthy population: about 70 to 80 per cent of adults are affected by minor periodontatis. About 15 per cent of those between the ages of 60 and 64 are affected by more severe levels of periodontal destruction.[114] Studies in patients with acute leukaemia suggest that periodontal disease may be an important cause of death during myelosuppression.[115-117] While the common oral flora is characterized by a prevalence of Gram-positive bacteria, xerostomia, chemotherapy, radiotherapy, and immunosuppression cause a shift of oral flora toward Gram-negative colonization.[118] The presence of heterogeneous flora, including Candida and other species, makes bacterial cultures difficult to interpret, and interactions between bacteria and fungi contribute to the adherence and colonization of host tissues by micro-organisms.[119] Small haemorrhages, pain localized to the peridontium, and fever can be present, especially during chemotherapy. Secondary infection can be present in nearby [116,117]structures and radiographic signs of periapical abscess may exist.

The treatment of bacterial infections depends first on adequate hygiene[120-122] (Table 10, Fig. 1). Periodontal probing and scaling could possibly reduce postchemotherapy oral complications:[123-125] the exact role of these treatments in advanced cancer patients has to be evaluated. In acute periodontal infection, broad-spectrum antibiotic therapy is usually initiated, followed by a more precise therapy based on the bacterial cultures, if possible and if indicated. Teeth debridement with 2 per cent hydrogen peroxide and frequent rinsing are helpful. Povidone iodine and chlorhexidine 0.2 per cent mouthwashes can be added to the oral hygiene schedule, especially in the presence of fungating cancer lesions. In a palliative setting the pain treatment, usually with common non-steroidal anti-inflammatory drugs and topical treatments may play an important role.

Viral infections

Herpes simplex virus, cytomegalovirus, varicella zoster virus, and Epstein–Barr virus are the main causes of viral infections of the oral cavity.[126] Herpes simplex virus type 1 is the most common in patients receiving cancer chemotherapy; the reported incidence of infections ranges from about 11 to about 65 per cent[127-129] and different studies suggest a strong correlation of oral mucositis with isolation of herpes simplex virus.[130,131] Oral lesions due to herpes simplex appear to represent recurrent rather than primary infection. There are no data on the incidence of this infection in patients with advanced disease.

Herpetic infections appear as yellowish lesions, which are easily removed from the mucosa and are extremely painful; vesicles can also appear on the lips (cold sores) and fever, anorexia, and malaise may coexist. In severe infections, pain can be so intense as to produce complete dysphagia. The diagnosis of herpes simplex virus infection is mainly clinical: some difficulties can arise from the

Table 10 Causes of poor oral hygiene and treatment

Pain

If possible, treat the basic cause
Good titration of systemic analgesic drugs
Analgesic gargles with:
* benzydamine hydrochloride 0.15%, 15 ml every 2 h
* Xylocaine viscous 2%, 5–15 ml every 4 h
* Xylocaine spray 10%, every 4 hr
* diphenhydramine hydrochloride elixir 12.5 mg/5 ml and aluminum hydroxide in equal parts up to 30 ml every 2 hr
* choline salicylate dental paste 8.7%, every 3–4 h on the oral and perioral lesions
* aluminum hydroxide and lignoeaine 2% in equal parts
* dyclonine hydrochloride
* cetacaine (benzocaine) 20% solution
* systemic analgesics
* avoid alcohol and lemon containing mouthwashes

Haemorrhage

Treat the basic cause (e.g. thrombocytopenia)
Avoid using toothbrush and dental floss
Use a low-pressure dental jet and/or a gauze pad wrapped around a finger or a disposable sponge (toothette) moistened in a mild solution of baking soda and water
Gargles with:
* saline solution
* hexetidine 0.1%
* sodium perborate
* chlorhexidine 0.2%
* povidone–iodine 1%
* bicarbonate of soda
* cetylpyridinium
* H_2O_2 3–6% in water 1:4
Gargles or soaked gauzes with antihaemorrhagic drugs:
* thrombin 1–2 g/day
* tranexamic acid 2–4 g/day

Debility or unconsciousness

Assisted oral hygiene by using a brush, gargles, spray, dental jet, cotton swabs moistened with mouthwash, gauze
Lips cracking prevention (petroleum jelly)
Room humidifier

presence of other oral infections. When needed, exfoliative cytology permits an accurate diagnosis (95 per cent) in a short time.[132] The infection should be differentiated from aphthous ulcers: a history of vesicles preceding ulcers, a location on hard gingiva and hard palate, and crops of lesions are indicative of herpetic infection rather than aphthous ulcers.

Specific treatment of the herpes infection is provided by acyclovir, which can be administered intravenously, with few side-effects, although patients must be hydrated and creatinine clearance monitored.[127, 133–135] Venous extravasation must be avoided. Lymphocyte counts greater than 600/mm^3 and monocyte counts greater than 250/mm^3 have been shown to be necessary for infection to resolve in patients with haematological malignancy.[136] Acyclovir can be employed also for prophylaxis in patients undergoing antineoplastic chemotherapy: a screening for anti-HSV antibodies might be useful in order to identify patients at high risk for herpes simplex virus infection.[137] In patients with advanced cancer, the oral and topical route (5 per cent acyclovir ointment) are better employed (Table 10, Fig. 1). Control of associated infections and oral hygiene are necessary. Chlorhexidine (0.2 per cent twice daily rinsing) may be beneficial with herpes simplex virus type 1 infection.[138] Extraoral lesions may become secondarily infected: topical antibiotics are then indicated.

Neutropenic ulcers

Severe neutropenia (neutrophil count less than 100 mm/3) is very often complicated by mouth ulcers:[139] up to 50 per cent of admissions to hospital with acute leukaemia suffer from this complication.[140] The epidemiology of neutropenic ulcers in patients with advanced solid tumours is unknown. In about one-third of cases neutropenic ulcers can be traced to some local factors—drug toxicity, herpes simplex virus infection, leukaemia infiltration, trauma, or haemorrhage—but the remainder have no identifiable cause.[139,140] Ulcers appear as one or more lesions, characterized by few signs of inflammation, regular margins, and a yellowish appearance; they are not easily removed.[130,140]

Recovery of the neutrophil count is essential for healing.[115] Topical symptomatic measures, such as hydrocortisone pellets or other corticosteroid preparations, and oral hygiene are necessary. Concurrent oral infections have to be specifically treated and prevented. The role of granulocyte colony-stimulating factor is still a matter of study: the high cost is an important limiting factor for a palliative care setting. Thalidomide, a sedative drug withdrawn from the market 30 years ago because of its teratogenic and neurotoxic effects, has been recently used for the treatment of a variety of ulcerative and immunological conditions, especially for recurrent aphthous stomatitis in HIV patients.[141,142] Its role in the treatment of neutropenic ulcers in cancer patients is not known.

Drug- and radiotherapy-induced stomatitis

The epidemiology of these conditions is complicated by the scarcity of data and the fact that other pathogenetic factors may coexist, complicating the exact diagnosis.[113,127,128]

Drug-induced stomatitis

Mucositis induced by chemotherapy is a common side-effect of cancer treatment: approximately 40 per cent of patients receiving chemotherapy develop an oral problem related to treatment and patients with haematological malignancies develop oral problems at two or three times the rate of patients with solid tumours.[143] Patients with poor oral health have a higher risk of oral infections following chemotherapy.[144,145]

Stomatotoxicity generally results from the non-specific inhibitory effect of the chemotherapeutic agents on mitosis of the rapidly dividing cells of the oral epithelium (direct toxicity). The reduction of the renewal rate of the mucosa results in atrophic changes and ulcerations.[146] Mucositis most often affects the non-keratinized oral mucosa, including the cheek, soft palate, lips, ventral surface of the tongue, and the floor of the mouth. It occurs about 5 to 7 days after drug administration, often a few days before the patient's haematological nadir. Thus, the mucosal disruption provides a portal of entry for micro-organisms at the time of maximum myelosuppression, and may be accompanied by haemorrhages.

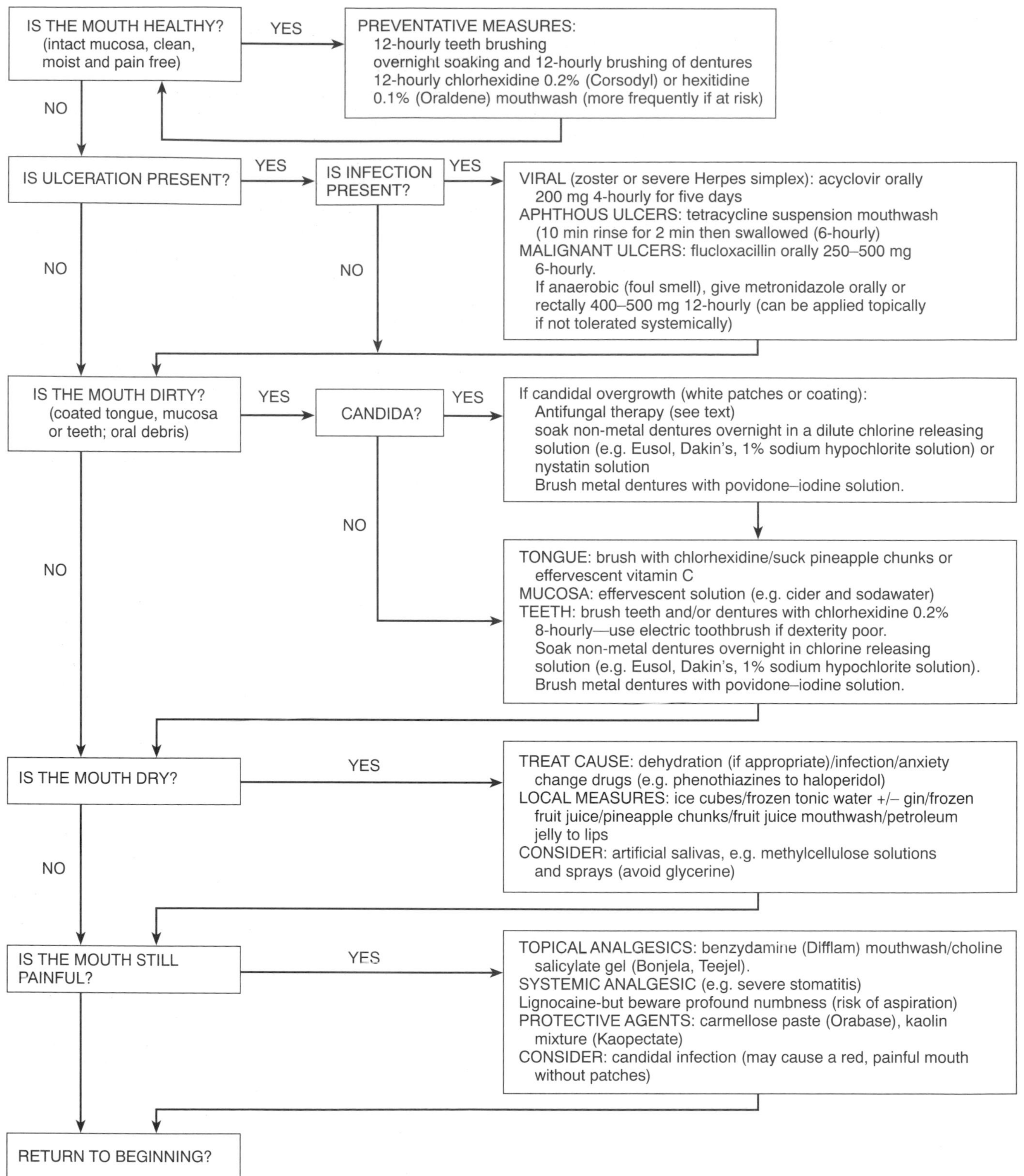

Fig. 1 A mouth care flow diagram. (Modified from reference 122.)

A wide variety of agents may product direct toxicity: notable examples include 5-fluorouracil, methotrexate, and doxorubicin.[143] In general, mucositis is dose-related: drug administration in divided doses, rather than a bolus, can reduce this problem.

Specific treatment of the oral lesions induced by chemotherapy is almost non-existent:[113] early pilot studies suggested that allopurinol mouthwash could be an effective antidote to 5-fluorouracil-induced mucositis;[147,148] recent results from controlled clinical studies have been controversial.[149,150] Due to the very short serum half-life of 5-fluorouracil, mouth cryotherapy around the time of administration of the intravenous bolus has been proposed. This would agree with data demonstrating that scalp cooling decreases chemotherapy-induced alopecia. Controlled clinical trial data demonstrate the importance of sucking ice chips during chemotherapy administration in patients receiving short half-life drugs, such as 5-fluorouracil.[151] Prevention of secondary infection, oral hygiene (Table 10, Fig.1), and supportive therapy are most important. Spontaneous gingival bleeding occurs when the platelet count falls below 10 000 cells/mm^3 : topical thrombin-soaked gauze held under pressure or microcrystalline collagen may be helpful. When local measures fail, platelet transfusion should be considered: in patients with advanced disease its role seems to be very limited.

Radiotherapy-induced stomatitis

Virtually all patients who receive radiation therapy to the head and neck develop oral side-effects.[40] Radiation-induced oral mucositis (characterized by xerostomia, taste alterations, diffuse erythema, pseudomembrane formation, and ulceration) [152] usually develop about 2 weeks after initiation of the therapy (due to the 2 weeks renewal rate of oral mucosa). Oral soreness may result from treatment with as little as 10 Gy; about 20 Gy are usually necessary to cause diffuse erythema. Generally, non- keratinized oral epithelium is affected. Mucositis can be very painful and can markedly reduce oral intake. However, it is self-limiting and heals by about 2 to 3 weeks after the end of radiation treatment.

Palliative treatment of mucositis

Minimizing mucosal trauma and controlling oral pain are the main principles of the palliative treatment of mucositis. The therapeutic schedules currently used are mainly empirical and no controlled clinical studies are available.[153]

Ice chips or popsicles are soothing. Anaesthetic rinses containing lignocaine hydrochloride may allow simple oral intake; analgesic treatment is usually necessary. Hydrogen peroxide rinsing seems helpful for removing debris and mucus from the teeth.[135] Spicy or acidic food should be avoided; soft, low salt foods should be given[154]. Oral hygiene should be stressed: mouth care protocols, including toothbrushing, flossing, mouth rinsing, and fluoride applications, can significantly decrease the frequency of oral complications (Table 10, Fig.1).[155-157] Concurrent oral infections, especially candidiasis, should be energetically treated.

Severe oral pain may require systemically administered medications. Morphine or methadone can be administered orally or parenterally[158]. In bone-marrow transplant recipients, where severe mucositis is often present, intravenous continuous morphine is used routinely with good results.[159] Patient controlled analgesia seems to obtain the same results as continuous infusion, with less morphine consumption and less sedation and difficulty in concentrating.[160] Results of prostaglandin E_2 administration for treatment of mucositis in patients undergoing chemotherapy and/or radiotherapy or bone marrow transplantation are controversial.[161,162] In a randomized double blind clinical trial, patients undergoing bone marrow transplantation, treated with prostaglandin E_2 prophylactically, had no significant benefit in comparison with placebo administration. Importantly, the incidence of herpes simplex virus infection was significantly higher in patients receiving prostaglandin E_2.[163]

Local complications of oral tumours

Facial trismus

Facial trismus is the consequence of tumour invasion of masticatory muscles, usually the pterygoid. It is common in retromolar trigone lesions, in very advanced anterior tonsillar pillar and tonsillar fossa tumours, and in soft palate lesions.[164] It is often accompanied by local pain or by pain felt in the external ear, in the preauricular, or the temporal area. Occasionally, the cranial nerves may be involved. More rarely a neoplasm originating in the pharingotympanic tube region can present sharp, neuralgic pain in the distribution of the third division of the trigeminal nerve, associated with trismus (sinus of Morgagni syndrome).

Radiotherapy, when possible, produces good results in alleviating facial trismus and chemotherapy can also be helpful.[164] Systemic analgesics, steroids, anticonvulsants (such as carbamazepine), muscle relaxants such as diazepam, and local anaesthetic infiltration may help when trismus develops in response to a painful stimulus. Oral hygiene presents many problems due to reduced access to the oral cavity. Cotton swabs soaked with antiseptics, sprays, and dental jet can help. Liquid or semisolid feeding is not always possible: whenever indicated a nasogastric or a gastrostomy tube should be inserted.

Abscesses, fistulas

Infections are very common in head and neck cancer patients, reported to contribute to 44 to 46 per cent of causes of death in this population.[165]

Cellulitis, tumour infections, and orocutaneous fistulas make up about 22 per cent of febrile episodes in patients with head and neck cancers.[165] This group of patients is very often malnourished, with a previous history of alcoholism and of chronic lung disease and with decreased salivary flow and secretory IgA levels.[143] Moreover surgery, radiotherapy, and chemotherapy often seriously damage head and neck structures of these patients.

Shifting of oral flora, towards a Gram-negative population, including aerobic Enterobacteriaceae and *Pseudomonas aeruginosa*, is particularly important. Anaerobic Gram-negative bacteria also play an important role in head and neck infection.[166] All of these aspects must be considered when approaching the management of abscesses and orocutaneous fistulas. A simple povidone–iodine solution is a sufficient preventive measure in patients at risk for developing secondary bacterial infections. The same antiseptics can be used as oral medication when an abscess is already present. In presence of signs of sepsis or of local pain or discharge, broad spectrum antibiotics, including metronidazole, should be administered.[166] Patient's relatives should be carefully instructed about medication and possible emergencies, such as massive haemorrhages (Table 10).

Tumour discharge

Many oral cavity tumours discharge, causing problems in swallowing and dysphagia and creating a chronic bad taste in the mouth. Radiotherapy may help this symptom, reducing the tumour mass and its secretions, but if this is not possible, local measures must be applied. Frequent rinsing with hydrogen peroxide can help removing by tumour debris. Benzydamine hydrochloride rinse can reduce the colonization of the oral cavity and help patients to cleanse the mouth[167]. Prevention and treatment of other oral problems such as candidiasis is very important (Table 10, Fig.1).

Taste alteration

Taste alteration occurs as a reduction in taste sensitivity (hypogeusia), an absence of taste sensation (ageusia), or a distortion of normal taste (dysgeusia). The incidence of these symptoms is unknown, but according to Twycross between 25 and 50 per cent of cancer patients have a diminished taste sensation.[168] Our clinical experience suggests that taste alterations are hardly ever reported spontaneously by the patients, but many will report it as a reason for loss of appetite if specifically questioned. Patients typically report that 'the food is tasteless', or 'the food is bitter'.

Taste is mediated through the taste buds, each of which contain about 50 cells and are continuously renewed. The number of taste buds decreases with age. They are found on the tongue, soft palate, pharynx, larynx, epiglottis and uvula, lips and cheeks, and in the upper third of the oesophagus. The tongue is most sensitive to sweetness on the anterior surface and tip, to salt and sour tastes on the two lateral sides, and to bitter tastes on the circumvillate papillae on the posterior surface. Sour and bitter taste are perceived most acutely on the palate; salt and sweet are most sensitive on the tongue. The pharynx has decreased sensitivity to all four tastes.

The cells of the taste buds are provided with microvilli in direct communication with the oral cavity through an apical pore. A protein (the gate-keeper) regulates the quantity of stimuli that pass through the pore per unit of time. Changes in these protein molecules are controlled by the equilibrium of metals and zinc in particular is associated with hypogeusia and anorexia.[169-171]

Taste information is sent by way of the fifth, seventh, ninth, and tenth cranial nerves to the medulla (nucleus of the tractus solitarius), and from there through the pons and thalamus to the cortical area subserving taste. Information in this pathway is also projected to the lateral hypothalamus. A lesion in any one of these areas can alter taste perception.[172]

The effect of cancer on taste is unknown. Potential causes of taste alteration are listed in Table 11. Taste abnormalities in cancer patients may be correlated with the site or extent of the tumour, independent of the histological type. A positive correlation exists between weight loss and the presence of abnormal taste sensation.[173] Disturbances in taste can also alter digestion because stimulation of taste organs can increase salivary and pancreatic flow, gastric contractions, and bowel motility.[172] There is also an association between advanced disease and an abnormality in the recognition of sugar and urea. A higher concentration of sweetness is needed for the solution to be recognized.[173]

Williams and Cohen [174] demonstrated elevated thresholds for recognition of sour (HCl), but not bitter (urea), sweet (sucrose), or salt (NaCl) in a group of patients with lung cancer who were tested before receiving chemotherapy or radiotherapy. An elevated threshold of detection for all four basic tastes was reported in a group of patients with laryngeal cancer who were examined before laryngectomy.[175]

Taste alterations have been reported as a consequence of radiotherapy for tumours in the head and neck regions. This effect may be due to damage to the microvilli of the taste cells or to reduced salivation. Taste loss is not observed until radiation doses of 20 Gy have been administered.[176,177] At doses of 20 to 40 Gy taste loss increased rapidly and a dose of 60 Gy causes a relative taste loss of over 90 per cent.[176] Mossman *et al.*[37] demonstrated that curative courses of radiotherapy for tumours of the head and neck resulted in long-term changes in taste and salivary function; the maximum tolerance doses resulting in a 50 per cent complication rate 5 years after treatment were estimated to be 40 to 65 Gy for xerostomia and 50 to 65 Gy for taste loss.

Table 11 Causes of taste alteration

Local disease of the mouth and tongue caused by cancer
Partial glossectomy
Tobacco usage
Elimination of the olfactory component of taste after laryngectomy
Surgical removal of the palate
Damage to the nervous system following surgery or cerebral lesions
Alteration of the cell renewing, or cell regenerating cycle
* malnutrition
* radiotherapy
* drugs
* metabolic disturbances
* xerostomia
* stomatitis and oral infections
* endocrine factors (thyroidectomy, hypophysectomy, adrenalectomy)
Modification in the receptor cells due to alteration of saliva by metabolic agents, drugs, radiation
Dental pathology
Bad dental hygiene

In most instances, taste acuity is partially restored between 20 and 60 days after radiotherapy and is fully restored within 2 to 4 months. Three weeks after initiation of radiotherapy, detection of bitter and salty tastes show the earliest and greatest impairment, with sensitivity to sweet tastes being least affected.[178]

Drugs administered to cancer patients may also alter the taste. Although about 80 different drugs have been associated with taste alterations,[179] many of these have been reported as a cause only once.

Zinc deficiency has been noted as a potential cause of anorexia, dysgeusia, or hypogeusia. Plasma zinc levels have been found to be reduced in patients with bronchial carcinoma compared to the healthy population, and the zinc level in leukaemic cells appears to be lower than that in normal white blood cells.[180] The administration of zinc has been reported to correct abnormalities of taste in some patients (176), and copper and nickel have also been used with good result in clinical trials. Patients treated prophylactically with 25 mg of oral zinc four times a day prior to radiotherapy developed less severe hypogeusia than those given radiotherapy without zinc treatment.[181-183] Zinc must be administered in the middle of a meal to reduce potential gastrointestinal symptoms.[183] Controlled clinical trials need to be carried out to document the potential for zinc administration in cancer patients.

Patients suffering from taste alterations need correct oral hygiene, treatment to increase salivation, and the suspension of the drugs that can induce or increase the symptoms. Patients can sometimes take hot food with a strong smell, the addition of lemon, pineapple, or vinegar being useful if stomatitis or mouth ulcers are not present.

Sialorrhoea

Sialorrhoea (excessive salivation) is uncommon in advanced cancer patients but can cause discomfort, inconvenience, and social embarrassment as well as irritation of lips, commissure, and chin. The most frequent causes are:

(1) oral pain (apthous ulcers);

(2) local irritants (ill-fitting dentures);

(3) drugs (lithium, cholinesterase inhibitors, cholinergic agonists);

(4) psychosis;

(5) epilepsy;

(6) radical mandibular resection procedures;

(7) recurrent oral cancer which suspends the mouth in an open position.[184-187]

In a controlled clinical trial, a single dose of 0.02 mg/kg of hyoscine (scopolamine) hydrobromide solution, rinsed in the mouth for 5 min before swallowing, reduced non-stimulated and paraffin-stimulated salivation at 60 min by 81 per cent and 80 per cent respectively. The heart rate of these patients increased significantly when compared with those given placebo and subjective sedation and relaxation were experienced by most of the volunteers.[185] Clinically useful sedative and antisialogogue effects can be produced by gastrointestinal and transdermal absorption of hyoscine (scopolamine) hydrobromide solution.[188] No data are available about the long-term use of this drug in patients suffering from sialorrhoea.

Table 12 Causes of halitosis

Diseases of the oral cavity
Poor oral hygiene, xerostomia, periodontal disease
Dental plaque, decay, cancer, bleeding gums
Tongue coating
Acute necrotizing ulcerative gingivitis
Gingivostomatitis (herpes virus, candidosis)
Inflammatory-suppurative phenomena
Diseases of the respiratory tract
Infection of the nose, tongue, nasal sinuses, pharynx, lungs
Tonsillar abscess, necrotic ulcers
Chronic rhinitis and rhinopharyngitis
Pharyngeal-laryngeal cancer with superinfection
Bronchiectasis, lung abscess
Abscess-forming lung cancer
Diseases of the digestive tract
Oesophageal diverticula, hiatal hernia, gastric stasis
Gastric stagnation due to pyloric stenosis and/or cancer with/without regurgitation, dyspepsia
Altered secretion or bile-composition, colon stasis
Metabolic failure
Diabetic ketoacidosis (sweet acetone breath)
Uraemia (ammoniacal smell)
Severe hepatic insufficiency (foetor hepaticus)
Drugs
Causing xerostomia and/or taste alteration
Anticancer drugs causing oral complications
Dimethylsulphoxide, antibiotics
Amyl nitrite, chloral hydrate, or iodine-based drugs
Foods
Garlic, onions, leeks, radishes
Meat, fish

Halitosis

Halitosis (unpleasant or bad breath), occurs when exhaled air is combined with foul-smelling substances coming from various sections of the respiratory tract or from the upper digestive tract.[189] No epidemiological data are available about the incidence and prevalence of this symptom in cancer patients. Table 12 shows the most important causes of halitosis.

Between 56 and 85 per cent of the cases of halitosis are a consequence of diseases of the oral cavity.[190,191] A careful history and an accurate examination of the oral cavity, sinuses, and the upper respiratory tract must be carried out to exclude inflammatory, infective, or neoplastic conditions. If the examination of this tract is negative, the physician should investigate one of the other causes.[192,193]

When the sensation of halitosis is subjective, without objective evidence, it is necessary to investigate neurological or psychiatric illness. Sometime, dysgeusia or dysosmia can cause these disturbances. Hygiene measures, mainly use of toothbrush and dental floss, are extremely important.[191] The diet plays an important role in the genesis of halitosis. Some substances, such as garlic, leek, onions, and alcohol contain volatile products which are absorbed by the intestinal wall and then excreted through the lungs. Alcohol also causes a decrease in salivary flow. The sulphur-containing amino acids in meat and fish can cause halitosis. A decreased intake of food can deplete body fat stores, with acidosis and ketosis giving an acetone odour. The role of smoking is controversial, but may modify the oral environment, exerting a local effect upon the oral mucosa. Oral rinses, such as 0.2 per cent aqueous chlorhexidine gluconate, are helpful.[194]

The treatment of halitosis is summarized in Table 13. It is necessary to give individual drug treatment according to the causes and the general condition of the patient.

Educational and prevention programmes

Health professionals involved in cancer management should be trained in the prevention, assessment, and treatment of oral problems.

An oral disease prevention programme for patients receiving radiation and chemotherapy should be available at every institution involved in cancer care: oral hygiene should not be a matter for only advanced or terminally ill patients. A dental team involved in early dental referral (before treatment) and long-term maintenance, as well as family-oriented education and motivation programmes, are necessary to enhance patient understanding and compliance.

In 1985, the National Institute of Dental Research (National Institutes of Health, Bethesda, USA) developed a programme for

Table 13 Treatment of halitosis

General measures
- Oral hygiene:
  - Toothbrushing, tongue scraping, and dental flossing
- Dietary advice
- Reduce alcohol intake and smoking
- Denture care

Specific measures
- Oral and upper airway
  - – systemic and/or topical antibiotics and local antiseptics (e.g povidone–iodine mouthwash, chlohexidine 0.2%, hydrogen peroxide 1%)
- Xerostomia
  - – see Tables 5, 6
- Oral bleeding
  - – see Table 10
- Gastric stasis
  - – prokinetic drugs (metoclopramide, domperidone)
- Dyspepsia
  - – reduce fat intake and administer enzymatic products specific for lipid digestion (e.g. ursodeoxycholic acid 50–150 mg before meals)
- Pulmonary infection
  - – cultured sputum examination
  - – start broad-spectrum antibiotic and/or antifungal drugs while waiting for culture results (metronidazole)
- Drugs
  - – discontinue use of drugs causing the symptom, if possible.

enhancing the oral health care of cancer patients undergoing therapy.[158] Four topics were presented during an orientation slide programme:

(1) deleterious effects of medical treatment;

(2) oral preparation by the dental team;

(3) patient oral health regimens;

(4) points to review and emphasize.

Table 14 Family education programme

- The importance of oral hygiene in advanced and terminal cancer
- Family-oriented oral cavity examination
- The correct use of toothbrushes, dental floss, gauzes, toothette, gloves
- Different mouthwashes: preparation, indication, and uses
- The main oral complications of advanced cancer patients
  - General
  - Specific to their relative
- Personalized oral care programme (centred on the patient and his family)
- Dietary and behavioural advice (e.g if mucositis, dysgeusia, xerostomia)
- Oral care in the unconscious patient

Table 15 Future research

- Perform epidemiological studies, evaluating the incidence and prevalence of oral cavity problem in patients with advanced cancer, including the role of pre-existing infections (e.g. HSV).
- Define the impact of oral complications on the quality of life of patients with advanced and terminal cancer.
- Develop quantifiable and reproducible criteria for assessing and classifying oral cavity pathologies in patients with advanced and terminal cancer.
- Define the importance of long-term oral side-effects of anticancer therapies and their optimal planning, according to these aspects (e.g. radio therapy-fractionation schedules, different kinds of destructive and/or reconstructive surgery).
- Study the interactions between oral cavity problems and different systemic conditions present in advanced cancer (e.g. cachexia, anorexia, malnutrition).
- Develop controlled studies in patients with advanced cancer, completely integrated with antineoplastic therapies.
- Develop appropriate evaluation methods for xerostomia and its treatment.
- Define and develop appropriate diagnostic tools for oral care in patients with advanced cancer.
- Develop and determine the role of oral care protocols in the palliative care setting.
- Develop adequate education tools to get the family involved in their relative's oral care.
- Determine the preventive and therapeutic role of the different antifungal drugs according to their administration schedules, to their compliance, their side-effects, and costs.
- Perform clinical studies evaluting the oral complications of drugs currently used in palliative care (e.g. steroids, morphine, anticholinergic drugs).
- Evaluate the role of biological response modifiers in preventing oral complications due to antineoplastic treatment performed in patients with advanced cancer.
- Evaluate the topical and systemic treatments for the prevention and cure of taste alterations.
- Evaluate the role of systemic hydration in the management of xerostomia.
- Conduct controlled studies to define and select topical and systemic analgesics for mucositis.
- Evaluate the different treatments for the management of fistulas, abscesses, and fungating tumours, in head and neck cancers.
- Develop prevention and treatment strategies for oral problems feasible within developing countries.
- Develop new specific treatments for oral cavity problems.

In a retrospective study conducted on 440 patients with malignancies other than those of the head and neck, Sonis and Kunz *et al.*[155] showed that the frequency of oral problems was reduced from 38.7 per cent to 10.5 per cent after the introduction of a dental team referral system.

The family must be involved in the patient's oral care, especially in a palliative care setting, when patients are often unable to take care of themselves. The palliative care team should have a teaching programme for oral care: this can be applied during hospice and/or hospital admissions and continued during home care (Table 14). It is essential to involve relatives actively in this programme, training them in the main oral hygiene measures, in the presence of the team. A range of different teaching aids is useful: videos, booklets, group sessions, and slides (see Section 6).

Conclusions

Many aspects of oral care need to be better defined. A greater effort has to be made in both the oncological and the palliative care settings. The main areas of research should include the epidemiology of oral complications, their impact on the quality of life, the evaluation tools, and controlled clinical studies. Table 15 reports the main directions for future research. Only a close collaboration between the oncologists and palliative care teams will help to give an answer to the many open and debatable questions that remain.

References

1. Daeffler R. Oral hygiene measueres for patients with cancer III. *Cancer Nursing*, 1981; **2**: 29–35.
2. Rosling BG, *et al.* Microbiological and clinical effects of topical subgingival antimicrobial treatment on human periodontal disease. *Journal of Clinical Periodontology*, 1983; **10**: 487–514.
3. Tapper-Jones L, Aldred M, Walker DM. Prevalence and intraoral distribution of Candida albicans in Sjögren's syndrome. *Journal of Clinical Pathology*, 1980; **33**: 282–7.
4. Markitziu A, Gedalia I, Stabholz A, Shuval J. Prevention of caries progress in xerostomic patients by topical fluoride applications: a study in vivo and in vitro. *Journal of Dentistry*, 1982; **10**: 248–53.
5. Grad H, Grushka M, Yanover L. Drug-induced xerostomia—the effect and treatment. *Canadian Dentistry Association Journal*, 1985; **4**: 296–301.
6. Bahn SL. Drug-related dental destruction. *Oral Surgery*, 1972; **33**: 49–54.
7. Makkonen TA, Tenovuo J, Vilja P, Heimdahl A. Changes in the protein composition of whole saliva during radiotherapy in patients with oral or pharyngeal cancer. *Oral Surgery*, 1986; **62**: 270–5.
8. Mandel ID. Sialochemistry in diseases and clinical situations affecting salivary glands. *CRC Critical Reviews in Clinical and Laboratory Science*, 1980; **11**: 321–66.
9. Tenovuo J, Lehtonen OP, Altonen AS, Vilja P, Tuohimaa P. Antimicrobial factors in whole saliva of human infants. *Infection and Immunity*, 1986; **51**: 49–53.
10. Milne RW, Dawes C. The relative contributions of different salivary glands to the blood group activity of whole saliva in humans. *Vox Sanguinis*, 1973; **25**: 298–307.
11. Tabak LA, *et al.* Role of salivary mucins in the protection of the oral cavity. *Journal of Oral Pathology*, 1982; **11**: 1–17.
12. Mandel MA, Dvorak K, DeCosse JJ. Salivary Immunoglobulins in patients with oropharyngeal and bronchopulmonary carcinoma. *Cancer*, 1973; **31**: 1408–13.
13. Brown AM, Lally ET, Frankel A, Harwick R, Davis LW, Rominger CJ. The association of the IgA levels of serum and whole saliva with the progression of oral cancer. *Cancer*, 1975; **35**: 1154–62.
14. Wolff A, Fox PC, Ship JA, Atkinson JC, Macynski AA, Baum BJ. Oral mucosal status and major salivary gland function. *Oral Surgery, Oral Medicine, Oral Pathology*, 1990; **70**: 49–54.
15. Zasloff M. Magainins, a class of antimicrobial peptides from Xenopus skin: isolation, characterization of two active forms, and partial cDNA sequence of a precursor. *Proceedings of the National Academy of Sciences of the USA*, 1987; **84**: 5449–53.
16. Spielman A, Ben-Aryed H, Gutman D, Szargel R, Deutsch E. Xerostomia—diagnosis and treatment. *Oral Medicine*, 1981; **51**: 144–7.
17. Sreebny LM, Valdini A. Xerostomia. Part I: relationship to other oral symptoms and salivary gland hypofunction. *Oral Surgery, Oral Medicine, Oral Pathology*, 1988; **66**: 451–8.
18. Sreebny LM, Valdini A. Xerostomia. A neglected Symptom. *Archives of Internal Medicine*, 1987; **147**: 1333–7.
19. Ventafridda V, De Conno F, Ripamonti C, Gamba A, Tamburini M. Quality-of-life assessment during a palliative care programme. *Annals of Oncology*, 1990; **1**: 415–20.
20. Twycross RG, Lack SA, comps. *Control of Alimentary Symptoms in far Advanced Cancer.* The mouth. Edinburgh: Churchill Livingstone, 1986; **2**: 12–39.
21. Chen MS, Daly TE. Xerostomia and complete denture retention. *Oral Health*, 1980; **70**: 27–9.
22. Makkonen TA, Nordman E. Estimation of long-term salivary gland damage induced by radiotherapy. *Acta Oncologica*, 1987; **26**: 307–12.
23. Anderson MW, Izutsu KT, Rice JC. Parotid gland pathophysiology after mixed gamma and neutron irradiation of cancer patients. *Oral Surgery*, 1981; **52**: 495–500.
24. Brown LR, Dreizen S, Rider I. The effect of radiation- induced xerostomia on saliva and serum lysozyme and immunoglobulin levels. *Oral Surgery*, 1976; **41**: 83–92.
25. Carl W, Schaff NG, Chen TY. Oral care of patients irradiated for cancer of the head and neck. *Cancer*, 1972; **30**: 448–53.
26. Dreizen S, Brown LR, Daly TE, Drane JB. Prevention of xerostomia-related dental caries in irradiated cancer patients. *Journal of Dental Research*, 1977; **56**: 99–104.
27. Eneroth CM, Henrikson CO, Jakobsson PA. Effect of fractionated radiotherapy on salivary gland function. *Cancer*, 1972; **30**: 1147–53.
28. Wescott WB, Mira JG, Starcke EN, Shannon IL, Thoruby JI. Alterations in whole saliva flow rate induced by fractionated radiotherapy. *American Journal of Roentgenology*, 1978; **130**: 145–9.
29. Dreizen S, Brown LR, Handler S, Levy BM. Radiation-induced xerostomia in cancer patients. Effect on salivary and serum electrolytes. *Cancer*, 1976; **38**: 273–8.
30. Epstein JB, Schubert MM. Synergistic effect of sialagogoues in management of xerostomia after radiation therapy. *Oral Surgery, Oral Medicine, Oral Pathology*, 1987; **64**: 179–82.
31. Cheng VST, Downs J, Herbert D, Aramany M. The function of the parotid gland following radiation therapy for head and neck cancer. *International Journal of Radiation Oncology, Biology, Physics*, 1981; **7**: 253–8.
32. Wescott WB, Starcke EN, Shannon IL. Some factors influencing salivary function when treating with radiotherapy. *International Journal of Radiation Oncology Biology Physics*, 1981; **7**: 535–41.
33. Kuten A, *et al.* Oral side effects of head and neck irradiation: correlation between clinical manifestations and laboratory data. *International Journal of Radiation Oncology, Biology, Physics*, 1986; **12**: 401–5.
34. Shannon IL, Trodhal JN, Starcke EN. Radiosensitivity of the human parotid gland. *Proceedings of the Society of Experimental Biology and Medicine*, 1978; **157**: 50–3.
35. Shannon IL. Management of head and neck irradiated patients. In: Zelles T, ed. *Saliva and Salivation*. Oxford: Pergamon Press, 1981: 313–20.
36. Liu RP, Fleming TJ, Toth BB, Keene HJ. Salivary flow rates in patients with head and neck cancer 0.5 to 25 years after radiotherapy. *Oral Surgery, Oral Medicine, Oral Pathology*, 1990; **70**: 724–9.
37. Mossman K, Shatzman A, Checharick J. Long-term effects of radiotherapy on taste and salivary function in man. *International Journal of Radiation Oncology, Biology, Physics*, 1982; **8**: 991–7.
38. Dudiak LA. Mouth care for mucositis due to radiation therapy. *Cancer Nursing*, 1987; **10**: 131–40.
39. Carl W. Dental management of head and neck cancer patients. *Journal of Surgical Oncology*, 1980; **15**: 265–81.
40. Beumer J, Curtis T, Harrison RE. Radiation therapy of the oral cavity: sequelae and management. *Head and Neck Surgery*, 1979; **1**: 301–2.
41. Wescott WB, Starcke EN, Shannon IL. Chemical protection against postirradiation dental caries. *Oral Surgery*, 1975; **40**: 709–19.
42. Heimdahl A, Nord CE. Colonization of oropharynx with pathogenic micro-organisms—a potential risk factor for infection in compromized patients. *Chemotherapia*, 1985; **4**: 186–91.
43. Marks JE, Davis CC, Gottsman VL, Purdy JE, Lee F. The effects of radiation on parotid salivary function. *International Journal of Radiation Oncology, Biology, Physics*, 1981; **7**: 1013–9.
44. Crawford JM, Taubman MA, Smith DJ. Minor salivary glands as a major source of secretory immunoglobulin A in the human oral cavity. *Science*, 1975; **190**: 1206–9.

45. Hensten-Petersen A. Biological activities in human labial and palatine secretions. *Archives of Oral Biology*, 1975; **20**: 107–9.
46. Bennett DR, McVeigh S, Rodgers B, comps. *AMA Drug Evaluations*. 5th edn. Chicago: American Medical Association, 1983.
47. Goodman Gilman A, Rall TW, Nies AS, Tylor P, eds. *The Pharmacological Basis of Therapeutics*. 8th edn. New York: Pergamon Press, 1990.
48. Handelman SL, Baric JM, Espeland MA, Berglund KL. Prevalence of drugs causing hyposalivation in an institutionalized geriatric population. *Oral Surgery, Oral Medicine, Oral Pathology*, 1986; **62**: 26–31.
49. Sreebny LM, Valdini A, Yu A. Xerostomia. Part II: Relationship to nonoral symptoms, drugs, and diseases. *Oral Surgery, Oral Medicine, Oral Pathology*, 1989; **68**: 419–27.
50. Sreebny LM, Schwartz SS. Reference guide to drugs and dry mouth. *Gerodontology*, 1986; **5**: 75–99.
51. White ID, Hoskin PJ, Hanks GW, Bliss JM. Morphine and dryness of the mouth. *British Medical Journal*, 1989; **298**:1222–3.
52. Ventafridda V, Ripamonti C, Bianchi M, Sbanotto A, De Conno F. A randomized study on oral morphine and methadone in the treatment of cancer pain. *Journal Pain and Symptom Management*, 1986;1: 203–7.
53. Ventafridda V, Saita L, Barletta L, Sbanotto A, De Conno F. Clinical observations on controlled-release morphine in cancer pain. *Journal of Pain and Symptom Management*, 1989; **4**: 124–9.
54. Ventafridda V, Tamburini M, Caraceni A, De Conno F, Naldi F. A validation study of the WHO method for cancer pain relief. *Cancer*, 1987; **59**: 850–6.
55. Baines MJ. Control of other symptoms. In: Saunders C, ed. *The Management of Terminal Disease*. 2nd edn. London: Edward Arnold, 1984.
56. Burge FI. Dehydration symptoms of palliative care cancer patients. *Journal of Pain and Symptom Management*, 1993; **8**: 454–64.
57. McCann RM , Hall WJ, Groth-Juncker A. Comfort care for terminally ill patients. The appropriate use of nutrition and hydration. *Journal of the American Medical Association*, 1994; **272**: 1263–6.
58. Mathew RJ, Weinman M, Claghorn JL. Xerostomia and sialorrhea in depression. *American Journal of Psychiatry*, 1979; **136**: 1476–7.
59. Levine MJ, Aguirre A, Hatton MN, *et al*. Artificial salivas: present and future. *Journal of Dental Research*, 1987; **66**: 693–8.
60. 'S-Gravenmade EJ, Roukema PA, Panders AK. The effect of mucin-containing artificial saliva on severe xerostomia. *International Journal of Oral Surgery*, 1974; **3**: 435–9.
61. Duxbury AJ, Thakker NS, Wastell DG. A double-blind cross-over trial of a mucin-containing artificial saliva. *British Dental Journal*, 1989; **166**: 115–20.
62. Vissink A, De Jong HP, Busscher HJ, 'S-Gravenmade EJ. Wetting properties of human saliva and saliva substitutes. *Journal of Dental Research*, 1986; **65**: 1121–4.
63. Vissink A, *et al*. The efficacy of mucin-containing artificial saliva in alleviating symptoms of xerostomia. *Gerodontology*, 1987; **6**: 95–101.
64. Visch LL, 'S-Gravenmade EJ, Schaub RM, van Putten WLJ, Vissink A. A double-blind crossover trial of CMC- and mucin-containing saliva substitutes. *International Journal of Oral and Maxillofacial Surgery*, 1986; **15**: 395–400.
65. Greenspan D. The use of pilocarpine in irradiation-induced xerostomia. *Journal of Dental Research*, 1979; **58**: 420–3.
66. Fox PC, Van Der Ven PF, Baum BJ, Mandel ID. Pilocarpine for the treatment of xerostomia associated with salivary gland dysfunction. *Oral Surgery*, 1986; **61**: 243–8.
67. Schuller DE, Stevens P, Clausen KP, Olsen J, Gahbauer R, Martin M. Treatment of radiation side effects with oral pilocarpine. *Journal of Surgical Oncology*, 1989; **42**: 272–6.
68. Greenspan D, Daniels TE. Effectiveness of pilocarpine in postradiation xerostomia. *Cancer*, 1987; **59**: 1123–5.
69. Epstein JB, Decoteau WE, Wilkinson A. Effect of sialor in treatment of xerostomia in Sjögren's syndrome. *Oral Surgery*, 1983; **56**: 495–9.
70. LeVeque FG, *et al*. A multicenter, randomized, double-blind, placebo-controlled, dose-titration study of oral pilocarpine for treatment of radiation-induced xerostomia in head and neck cancer patients. *Journal of Clinical Oncology*, 1993; **11**: 1124–31.
71. Johnson JT, *et al*. Oral pilocarpine for post-irradiation xerostomia in patients with head and neck cancer. *New England Journal of Medicine*, 1993; **329**: 390–5.
72. Rieke JW, *et al*. Oral pilocarpine for radiation-induced xerostomia: integrated efficacy and safety results from two prospective randomized clinical trials. *International Journal of Radiation Oncology, Biology, Physics*, 1995; **31**: 661–9.
73. Greenspan D. Management of salivary dysfunction. *National Cancer Institute Monographs*, 1990; **9**: 159–61.
74. Jobbins J, Bagg J, Parsons K, Finlay I, Addy M, Newcombe RG. Oral carriage of yeasts, coliforms and staphylococci in patients with advanced malignant disease. *Journal of Oral Pathology and Medicine*, 1992; **21**: 305–8.
75. Macfarlane TW, Samaranayake LP. Systemic infections. In: Jones JH, Mason DK, eds. *Oral Manifestations of Systemic Disease*. 2nd edn. London: Ballière Tindall, 1990: 339–86.
76. Samaranayake LP. Nutritional factors and oral candidosis. *Journal of Oral Pathology*, 1986; **15**: 61–5.
77. Aldred MJ, Addy M, Bagg J, Finlay I. Oral health in the terminally ill: a cross sectional pilot survey. *Specialist Care in Dentistry*, 1991; **11**: 59–62.
78. Finlay IG. Oral symptoms and candida in the terminally ill. *British Medical Journal*, 1986; **292**: 592–3.
79. Samaranayake LP, *et al*. The oral carriage of yeasts and coliforms in patients on cytotoxic therapy. *Journal of Oral Pathology*, 1984; **13**: 390–3.
80. Martin MV, Al-Tikriti U, Bramley P. Yeasts flora of the mouth and skin during and after irradiation for oral and laryngeal cancer. *Journal of Medical Microbiology*, 1981; **14**: 457–61.
81. Wahlin YB, Holm AK. Changes in the oral microflora in patients with acute leukaemia and related disorders during the period of induction therapy. *Oral Surgery, Oral Medcine, Oral Pathology*, 1988; **65**: 411–17.
82. Spijkervet FKL, van Saene HKF, Van Saene JJM, Panders AK, Vermey A, Mehta DM. Mucositis prevention by selective elimination of oral flora in irradiated head and neck cancer patients. *Journal of Oral Pathology and Medicine*, 1990; **19**: 486–9.
83. Bodey GP. Candidiasis in cancer patients. *American Journal of Medicine*, 1984; **77D**: 13–19.
84. Epstein JB, Truelove EL, Izutzu KT. Oral candidiasis: pathogenesis and host defense. *Reviews of the Infectious Diseases*, 1984; **6**: 96–106.
85. Yeo E, Alvarado T, Fainstein V, Bodey GP. Prophylaxis of oropharingeal candidiasis with clotrimazole. *Journal of Clinical Oncology*, 1985; 3:1668–71.
86. De Gregorio MW, Lee WMF, Linker CA, *et al*. Fungal infections in patients with acute leukemia. *American Journal of Medicine*, 1984; **73**: 543–8.
87. Bodey GP, Samonis G, Rolston K. Prophylaxis of candidiasis in cancer patients. *Seminars in Oncology*, 1990; **17**: 24–8.
88. Dreizen S. Oral candidiasis. *American Journal of Medicine*, 1984; **77D**: 28–33.
89. Samaranayake LP, Yacob HB. The classificaion of oral candidosis. In: Samaranayake LP, MacFarlane TW, eds. *Oral Candidosis*, London: Wright, 1990: 124–131.
90. Regezi JA, Sciubba JJ, comps. White lesions. *Oral pathology: Clinical-Pathologic Correlations.*. Philadelphia: WB Saunders Company, 1989; **3**: 84–124.
91. Lynch DP, Gibson DK. The use of Calcofluor white in the histopathologic diagnosis of oral candidiasis. *Oral Surgery, Oral Medicine, Oral Pathology*, 1987; **63**: 698–703.
92. Barret AP. Evaluation of nystatin in prevention and elimination of oropharingeal candida in immunosuppressed patients. *Oral Surgery*, 1984; **58**: 148–51.
93. DeGregorio MW, Lee MW, Ries CA. Candida infections in patients with acute leukemia: ineffectiviness of nystatin prophylaxis and relationship between oropharyngeal and systemic candidiasis. *Cancer*, 1982; **50**: 2780–4.

94. Barkvoll P, Attramadal A. Effect of nystatin and chlorexidine digluconate on Candida Albicans. *Oral Surgery, Oral Medicine, Oral Pathology*, 1989; **67**: 279–81.
95. Kirkpatrick CH, Alling DW. Treatment of chronic oral candidiasis with clotrimazole troches: a controlled clinical trial. *New England Journal of Medicine*, 1978; **299**: 1201–3.
96. Yeo BS, Bodey GP. Oropharyngeal candidiasis treated with a troche form of clotrimazole. *Archives of Internal Medicine*, 1979; **139**: 656–7.
97. Quintiliani R, Owens NJ, Quercia RA, *et al*. Treatment and prevention of oropharyngeal candidiasis. *American Journal of Medicine*, 1984; **10**: 44–8.
98. Meunier F, Paesmans M, Autier P. Value of antifungal prophylaxis with antifungal drugs against oropharyngeal candidiasis in cancer patients. *Oral Oncology, European Journal of Cancer*, 1994; **30B**: 196–9.
99. Roed-Petersen B. Miconazole in the treatment of oral candidiasis. *Internatioal Journal of Oral Surgery*, 1978; **7**: 558–63.
100. Brincker H. Treatment of oral candidiasis in debilitated patients with miconazole—a new potent antifungal drug. *Scandinavian Journal of Infectious Diseases*, 1976; **8**: 117–20.
101. de Vries-Hospers GH, van der Waaij D. Salivary concentrations of amphotericin B following its use as an oral lozenges. *Infection*, 1980; **8**: 63–5.
102. Holbrook WP. Sensitivity of Candida Albicans from patients with chronic oral candidiasis. *Postgraduate Medical Journal*, 1979; **55**: 692–4.
103. Symoens J, Moens M, Dom J, *et al*. An evaluation of two years of clinical experience with ketoconazole. *Reviews of the Infectious Diseases*, 1980; **2**: 674–82.
104. Hughes WT, Bartley DL, Patterson GG, Tufenkeji H. Ketoconazole and candidiasis: a controlled study. *Journal of Infectious Diseases*, 1983; **147**: 1060–3.
105. Saag MS, Dismukes WE. Azole antifungal agents: emphasis on new triazoles. *Antimicrobial Agents and Chemotherapy*, 1988; **32**: 1–8.
106. Heykants J, Michiels M, Meuldermans W, *et al*. The pharmacokinetics of itraconazole in animals and man: an overview. In: Fromtling RA, ed. *Recent Trends in the Discovery, Development and Evaluation of Antifungal Agents*. Barcelona: JR Prou Science Publ, 1987: 223–4.
107. Cauwenbergh G, DeDoncker P, Stoops K, *et al*. Itraconazole in the treatment of human mycoses: Review of three years of clinical experience. *Reviews of the Infectious Diseases*, 1987; **9**: S146–52.
108. Humphrey MJ, Jevenson S, Tarbit MH. Pharmacokinetic evaluation of UK-49858, a metabolically stable triazole antifungal drug, in animals and humans. *Antimicrobial Agents and Chemotherapy*, 1985; **28**: 648–53.
109. DeWit S, Weerts D, Goossens H, Clumeck N. Comparison of fluconazole and ketoconazole for oropharingeal candidiasis in AIDS. *Lancet*, 1989; **1**: 746–8.
110. Dupont B, Drouhet E. Fluconazole for the treatment of fungal diseases in immunosuppressed patients. *Annals of the New York Academy of Sciences*, 1988; **544**: 564–70.
111. Powderly WG, *et al*. A randomized trial comparing fluconazole with clotrimazole troches for the prevention of fungal infections in patients with advanced human immunodeficency virus infection. *New England Journal of Medicine*, 1995; **332**: 700–5.
112. Cameron ML, Schell WA, Bruch S, Bartlett JA, Waskin HA, Perfect JR. Correlation of in vitro fluconazole resistance of Candida isolates in relation to therapy and symptoms of individual seropositive for human immunodeficency virus type 1. *Antimicrobial Agents and Chemotherapy*, 1993; **37**: 2449–253.
113. Poland JM. Stomatitis and specific oral infections of the oncologic patients. *American Journal of Hospice Care*, 1987; **Sep/Oct**: 30–2.
114. Epidemiology and Oral Disease Prevention Program, National Institute of Dental Research. *Oral Health of United States Adults: the National Survey of Oral Health in US Employed Adults and Seniors, 1985–86: National Findings*. Bethesda, Md.: Department of Health and Human Services, Public Health Service, National Institutes of Health, 1987 (NIH publication no. 87–2868).
115. Lockart PB, Sonis ST. Relationship of oral complications to peripheral blood leukocyte and platelets count in patients receiving cancer chemotherapy. *Oral Surgery, Oral Medicine, Oral Pathology*, 1979; **48**: 21–8.
116. Overholsen CD, Peterson DE, Williams LT, *et al*. Periodontal infections in patients with acute non lymphocytic leukemia: prevalence of acute exacerbations. *Archives of Internal Medicine*, 1982; **142**: 551–4.
117. Peterson DE, Overholsen CD. Increased morbidity associated with oral infections in patients with non acute lymphocytic leukemia. *Oral Surgery, Oral Medicine, Oral Pathology*, 1981; **51**: 390–3.
118. Minah GE, Rednor JL, Peterson DE, *et al*. Oral succession of gram-negative bacilli in myelosuppressed cancer patients. *Journal of Clinical Microbiology*, 1986; **24**: 210–13.
119. Peterson DE, Minah GE, Reynolds MA, *et al*. Effect of granulocytopenia on oral microbial relationships in patients with acute leukemia. *Oral Surgery, Oral Medicine, Oral Pathology*, 1990; **70**: 720–3.
120. Daeffler R. Oral hygiene measures for patients with cancer I. *Cancer Nursing*, 1980; **Oct**: 347–56.
121. Daeffler R. Oral hygiene measures for patients with cancer II. *Cancer Nursing*, 1980; **Dec**: 427–32.
122. Regnard C, Fitton S. Mouth care: a flow diagram. *Palliative Medicine*, 1989; 3: 67–9.
123. Slots J, Mashimo P, Levine MJ, Genco RJ. Periodonthal therapy in humans. *Journal of Periodontology*, 1979; **50**: 495–509.
124. Weikel DS, Peterson DE, Rubinstein LE, Metzeger-Samuels C, Overholser CD. Incidence of fever following invasive oral interventions in the myelosuppressed cancer patient. *Cancer Nursing*, 1989;**12**: 265–70.
125. Peterson DE. Dental Care. In: Wiernik PH, ed. *Supportive Care of the Cancer Patient*. New York: Futura Publishing Co., 1983; 145–71.
126. Barret AP. A long term prospective clinical study of orofacial herpes simplex virus infection in acute leukemia. *Oral Surgery, Oral Medicine, Oral Pathology*, 1986; **61**: 149–52.
127. Rand HR, Kramer B, Johnson AC. Cancer chemotherapy and associated symptomatic stomatitis and the role of herpes simplex virus. *Cancer*, 1986; **50**: 1262.
128. Barret AP. A long term prospective clinical study of oral complications during conventional chemotherapy for acute leukemia. *Oral Surgery, Oral Medicine, Oral Pathology*, 1987; **63**: 313–16.
129. Montgomery RT, Redding SW, Le Maistre CF. The incidence of oral herpes simplex virus infection in patients undergoing cancer chemotherapy. *Oral Surgery, Oral Medicine, Oral Pathology*, 1986; **61**: 238–42.
130. Beattie G, Whelan J, Cassidy J, Milne L, Burns S, Leonard R. Herpes simplex virus, Candida Albicans and mouth ulcers in neutropenic patients with non-haemathological malignancy. *Cancer Chemotherapy and Pharmacology*, 1989; **25**: 75–6.
131. Bergmann OJ, Mogensen SC, Ellegard J. Herpes simplex virus and intraoral ulcers in immunocompromised patients with haematological malignancies. *European Journal of Clinical Microbiology and Infectious Disease*, 1990; **9**: 184–90.
132. Barret AP, Buckley DJ, Greenberg ML, *et al*. The value of exfoliative cytology in diagnosing of oral herpes infection in immunosoppressed patients. *Oral Surgery, Oral Medicine, Oral Pathology*, 1986; **62**: 175–8.
133. Dreizen S, Mc Credie KB, Keating MJ, Bodey GP. Oral infections associated with chemotherapy in adults with acute leukemia. *Postgraduate Medical Journal*, 1982; **71**: 133–46.
134. Harm JM, Prentice HG, Blacklock HA, *et al*. Acyclovir profilaxis against herpes virus infections in severely immunocompromised patients: a randomised double blind study. *British Medical Journal*, 1983; **287**: 384–8.
135. Sheperd IP. The management of the oral complications of leukemia. *Oral Surgery, Oral Medicine, Oral Pathology*, 1978; **45**: 543–8.
136. Epstein JB, Sherlock C, Page JL, Spinelli J, Phillips G. Clinical study of herpes simplex virus infection in leukemia. *Oral Surgery, Oral Medicine, Oral Pathology*, 1990; **70**: 38–43.
137. Carrega G, *et al*. Herpes simplex virus and oral mucositis in children with cancer. *Support Care-Cancer*, 1994; **2**: 266–9.
138. Park JB, Park NH. Effect of chlorexidine on the in vitro and in vivo herpes simplex virus infection. *Oral Surgery, Oral Medicine, Oral Pathology*, 1989; **67**: 149–53.

139. Barret AP. Neutropenic ulceration—a distinctive clinical entity. *Journal of Periodontology*, 1987; **58**: 51–5.
140. Barret AP. Long term prospective clinical study of neutropenic ulceration in acute leukemia. *Journal of Oral Medicine*, 1987; **42**:102–5.
141. Revuz J, Guillaume JC, Janier M, *et al.* Crossover study of thalidomide vs placebo in severe recurrent aphtous stomatitis. *Archives of Dermatology*, 1990; **126**: 923–7.
142. Paterson DL, Geoghiou PR, Allworth AM, Kemp RJ. Thalidomide as treatment of refractory aphtous ulceration related to human immunodeficiency virus infection. *Clinical Infectious Diseases*, 1995; **20**: 250–4.
143. Sonis ST. Oral complications of cancer therapy. In: De Vita VT Jr, Hellman S, Rosenberg SA, eds. *Cancer—Principles and Practice of Oncology.* 3rd edn. Philadelphia: JB Lippincott Co. 1989: 2144–52, 1989.
144. Beck S. Impact of a systematic oral care protocol on stomatitis after chemotherapy. *Cancer News*, 1979; **2**: 185–99.
145. Greenberg MS, Cohen SG, Mckifrick JC, *et al.* The orak flora as a source of septicemia in patients with acute leukemia. *Oral Surgery, Oral Medicine, Oral Pathology*, 1982; **53**: 32–6.
146. Guggenheimer J, Verbhin RS, Appel BN, *et al.* Clinico-pathologic effects of cancer chemotherapeutic agents on human buccal mucosa. *Oral Surgery, Oral Medicine, Oral Pathology*, 1977; **44**: 58–63.
147. Lynch MA, Ship II. Initial oral manifestations of leukemia. *Journal of the American Dental Association*, 1977; **75**: 932–40.
148. Clark PI, Slevin ML. Allopurinol mouthwash and 5-fluoruracil-induced oral toxicity. *European Journal of Surgical Oncology*, 1985; **11**: 267–8.
149. Dose AM, Loprinzi CL, Cianflone S, *et al.* A controlled evaluation of an allopurinol mouthwash as prophylaxis against 5-fluoruracil (5-FU)-induced stomatitis: a North Central Treatment Group and Mayo Clinic Study. *Proceedings of the American Society of Clinical Oncology*, 1989; **8**: 341.
150. Porta C, Moroni M, Nastasi G. Allopurinol mouthwashes in the treatment of 5-Fluorouracil-induced stomatitis. *American Journal of Clinical Oncology*, 1994; **17**: 246–7.
151. Mahood DJ, Dose AM, Loprinzi CL *et al.* Inhibition of fluorouracil-induced stomatitis by oral cryotherapy. *Journal of Clinical Oncology*, 1991; **9**: 449–52.
152. Reynolds WR, Hickey AJ, Feldman MI. Dental management of the cancer patient receiving radiation therapy. *Clinical and Preventive Dentistry*, 1980; **2**: 5–9.
153. De Conno F, Ripamonti C, Sbanotto A, Ventafridda V. Oral complications in patients with advanced cancer. *Journal of Palliative Care*, 1989; **5**: 7–15.
154. Bruya MA, Maderia NP. Stomatitis after chemotherapy. *American Journal of Nursing*, 1975; **75**: 1349–52.
155. Sonis ST, Kunz A. Impact of improved dental services on the frequency of oral complications of cancer therapy for patients with non-head-and-neck malignancies. *Oral Surgery, Oral Medicine, Oral Pathology*, 1988; **65**: 19–22.
156. Dudjak LA. Mouth care for mucositis due to radiation therapy. *Cancer Nursing*, 1987; **10**: 131–40.
157. Borowsky B, Benhamou E, Pico JL, Laplanche A, Margainaud JP, Hayat M. Prevention of oral mucositis in patients treated with high-dose chemotherapy and bone marrow transplantation: a randomised controlled trial comparing two protocols of dental care. *Oral Oncology, European Journal of Cancer*, 1994; **30B**: 93–107.
158. Wright WE, Haller JM, Harlow SA, Pizzo PA. An oral disease prevention program for patients receiving radiation and chemotherapy. *Journal of the American Dental Association*, 1985; **110**: 43–7.
159. Hill HF, Chapman CR, Kornell J, Sullivan K, Saeger L , Benedetti C. Self-administration of morphine in bone-marrow transplant patients reduces drug requirements. *Pain*, 1990; **40**: 121–9.
160. Mackie AM, Coda BC, Hill HF. Adolescents use patient-controlled analgesia effectively for relief from prolonged oropharyngeal mucositis pain. *Pain*, 1991; **46**: 265–9.
161. Kuhrer I, Kuzmits R, Linkesch W, Ludwig H. Topical PGE_2 enhances healing of chemotherapy-associated mucosal lesions. *Lancet*, 1986; **1**: 623.
162. Porteder H, Rausch E, Kment G, Watzek G, Matejka M, Sinzinger H. Local prostaglandin E_2 in patients with oral malignancies undergoing chemo-and radiotherapy. *Journal of Cranio-Maxillo-Facial Surgery*, 1988; **16**: 371–4.
163. Labar B *et al.* Prostaglandin E_2 for prophylaxis of oral mucositis following BMT. *Bone Marrow Transplant*, 1993; **11**: 379–82.
164. Million RR, Cassini NJ, Clark JR. Cancer of the head and neck. In: De Vita VTJr, Hellman S, Rosenberg SA, eds. *Cancer—Principles and Practice of Oncology.* 3rd edn. Philadelphia: JB Lippincott, 1989: 488–590.
165. Hussain M, Kish JA, Crane L, *et al.* The role of infection in the morbidity and mortality of patients with head and neck cancer undergoing multimodality therapy. *Cancer*, 1991; **67**: 716–21.
166. Barret AP. Metronidazole in the management of anaerobic neck infection on acute leukemia. *Oral Surgery, Oral Medicine, Oral Pathology*, 1988; **66**: 287–9.
167. Epstein JB, Stevenson-Moore P. Benzydamine Hydrochloride in prevention and management of pain in oral mucositis associated with radiation therapy. *Oral Surgery, Oral Medicine, Oral Pathology*, 1988; **62**: 145–8.
168. Twycross RG and Lack SA, comps. Taste change. *Control of Alimentary Symptoms in Far Advanced Cancer.*Edinburgh: Churchill Livingstone, 1986; **4**: 57–65.
169. Gray H. *Anatomy, Descriptive and Surgical*, 15th edn. New York: Bounty Books, 1977.
170. Guyton AC. *Textbook of Medical Physiology*, 5th edn. Philadelphia: WB Saunders Co, 1976.
171. Murray RG. Ultrastructure of taste receptors. In: Beidler LM, ed. *Handbook of Sensory Physiology.* New York: Springer-Verlag, 1971: 31–5.
172. Schiffman SS. Taste and smell in disease. *New England Journal of Medicine*, 1983; **308**: 1275–9.
173. DeWys WD, Walters K. Abnormalities of taste sensation in cancer patients. *Cancer*, 1975; **36**: 1888–96.
174. Williams LR, Cohen MH. Altered taste thresholds in lung cancer. *American Journal of Clinical Nutrition*, 1978; **31**: 122–5.
175. Kashima HK, Kalinowski B. Taste impairment following laryngectomy. *Ear, Nose, and Throat Journal*, 1979; **58**: 88–92.
176. Mossman KL. Gustatory tissue injury in man: Radiation dose response relationship and mechanisms of taste loss. *British Journal of Cancer*, 1986; **53**: 9–11.
177. Herrmann Th, Adamski K, Stefan M. Storungen von Speichelproduktion und Geschmacksempfindung nach Bestrahlung intramuscular oropharyngeal Bereich. *Radiobiology Radiotherapy*, 1984; **25**: 621–9.
178. Mossman KL, Henkin RI. Radiation-induced changes in taste acuity in cancer patients. *International Journal of Radiation Oncology, Biology, Physics*, 1978; **4**: 663–70.
179. Willonghby JM. Drug-induced abnormalities of taste sensation. *Adverse Drug Reaction Bulletin*, 1983; **100**: 368–71.
180. Davies KJT, Musa M, Dormandy TL. Measurements of plasma zinc in malignant disease. *Journal of Clinical Pathology*, 1986; **21**: 359–65.
181. Henkin RI, Brandley DF. Hypogeusia corrected by Ni++ and Zn++. *Life Science*, 1970; **9**: 701–9.
182. Henkin RI, Schecter PJ, Hoye R, Mattern C. Idiopathic hypogeusia with dysgeusia, hyposmia and dysosmia: a new syndrome. *Journal of the American Medical Association*, 1971; **217**: 434–40.
183. Henkin RI. Prevention and treatment of hypogeusia due to head and neck irradiation. *Journal of the American Medical Association*, 1972; **220**: 870–1.
184. Mullins WM, Gross CW, Moore JM. Long-term follow-up of tympanic neurectomy for sialorrhea. *Laryngoscope*, 1979; **89**: 1219–23.
185. Lieblich S. Episodic supersalivation (idiopathic paroxysmal sialorrhea): Description of a new clinical syndrome. *Oral Surgery, Oral Medicine, Oral Pathology*, 1989; **68**:159–61.
186. Donaldson SR. Sialorrhea as a side effect of lithium: a case report. *American Journal of Psychiatry*, 1982; **139**: 1350–1.
187. Markkanen YJ, Pihlajamaki K. Oral scopolamine Hydrobromide solution

as an antisialagogic agent in dentistry. *Oral Surgery, Oral Medicine, Oral Pathology*, 1987; **63**: 417–20.

188. Markkanem YJ, Lauren L, Peltomaki T. Serum antimuscarinic activity after a single dose of oral scopolamine hydrobromide solution measured by radioreceptor assay. *Oral Surgery, Oral Medicine, Oral Pathology*, 1987; **63**: 534–8.
189. Molinari F. Notes on gastroenterology from symptom to therapy. In: *Halitosis*. Cheli R, ed. Florence: Boehringer Ingelheim, 1987: 25–8
190. Attia EL, Marshall GL. Halitosis. *Canadian Medical Assocation Journal*, 1982; **126**: 1281.
191. Scully C, Porter S, Greenman J. What to do about halitosis. *British Medical Journal*, 1994; **308**: 217–8.
192. Richardson HC, Prichard AJN. Managing halitosis (letter). *British Medical Journal*, 1994; **308**: 652.
193. Parmar SC, Naik PC. Remember the tongue (letter). *British Medical Journal*, 1994; **308**: 652.
194. Rosenberg M. Halitosis—the need for further research and education. *Journal of Dental Research*, 1992; **71**: 424.

Bibliography

National Cancer Institute. *Consensus Development Conference on Oral Complications of Cancer Therapies: Diagnosis, Prevention, and Treatment*. Bethesda, Md.: U.S. Department of health and human services, 1990 (Monographs 9).

Twycross RG, Lack SA, comps. *Control of Alimentary Symptoms in Far Advanced Cancer*. Edinburgh: Churchill Livingstone, 1986.

9.11 Endocrine and metabolic complications of advanced cancer

Mark Bower, Lucy Brazil, and R.C. Coombes

Introduction

Advanced malignancy causes endocrine and metabolic complications in two ways. Firstly, the primary tumour or its metastases may interfere with the function of endocrine glands, kidneys, or liver by invasion or obstruction. Secondly, tumours may give rise to remote effects without local spread. Many of these paraneoplastic syndromes arise due to secretion of products by tumours, including hormones, cytokines, and growth factors. Paraneoplastic syndromes also arise when normal cells secrete products in response to the presence of tumour cells. Antibodies secreted in this way are responsible for many paraneoplastic neurological syndromes including cerebellar degeneration, Lambert–Eaton myasthenic syndrome, and paraneoplastic retinopathy.

This chapter discusses the pathogenesis, epidemiology, and management of the commonest paraneoplastic endocrinopathies and concludes with a brief discussion of the management of diabetes mellitus, renal failure, and liver failure in the context of advanced malignancy.

Paraneoplastic complications

Hypercalcaemia

Hypercalcaemia is the commonest life-threatening metabolic disorder associated with cancer. It usually occurs in those with advanced, disseminated malignancy and produces a number of distressing symptoms. The treatment of hypercalcaemia of malignancy frequently ameliorates these symptoms, and for this reason the diagnosis should always be sought and corrected.

Pathogenesis

Three related mechanisms may contribute to hypercalcaemia:

(1) increased osteoclastic bone resorption;

(2) decreased renal clearance of calcium;

(3) enhanced calcium absorption from the gut.

All three processes occur in malignancy and in different circumstances each plays a different role. Bone resorption in malignant hypercalcaemia is universal and may be related to local cytokine and prostaglandin production in response to metastases, or to humoral factors produced by tumours. It is undertaken by osteoclasts which are macrophage derived multinucleate giant cells derived from bone marrow stem cells. They act as cellular proton pumps secreting hydrogen ions into the extracellular space which dissolve hydroxyapatite and liberate bicarbonate and calcium phosphate into the blood stream. Decreased renal calcium excretion occurs with low glomerular filtration rates or increased tubular reabsorption of calcium in response to parathyroid hormone or its relatives. Increased gastrointestinal absorption of calcium in response to elevated levels of 1,25-dihydroxycholecalciferol (**1,25(OH)$_2$D$_3$**, calcitriol) occurs rarely with ectopic production of this vitamin by haematological tumours.

Cytokines

Hypercalcaemia in the context of bone metastases occurs due to osteoclastic bone resorption mediated by locally produced osteoclast-activating factors and osteoclast-recruiting factors which promote proliferation and maturation of osteoclast progenitors. Several cytokines with osteoclast-activating activity have been identified including transforming growth factor alpha (**TGF-a**), interleukin-1 (**IL-1**), interleukin-6 (IL-6), lymphotoxin (**TNF-b**), tumour necrosis factor alpha (TNF-α), and epidermal growth factor (**EGF**). All these cytokines cause bone resorption *in vitro* in organ cultures of fetal rat long bones or neonatal mouse calvariae. Interleukin-6 (IL-6), granulocyte colony stimulating factor (**G-CSF**), and granulocyte macrophage colony stimulating factor (**GM-CSF**) recruit osteoclasts. IL-6 is probably the dominant cytokine in bone reabsorption and has been implicated in autocrine myeloma cell growth.[1] In addition, it stimulates osteoclast growth in Paget's disease[2] and is suppressed by oestrogens which may explain their antiosteoporotic actions.[3,4] Mice bearing colon tumour xenografts develop hypercalcaemia and raised IL-6 levels. Treatment with chemotherapy reduces tumours, hypercalcaemia, and serum IL-6 levels, whist therapy with monoclonal antibodies to IL-6 prevents hypercalcaemia in these mice.[5] Cytokines may act indirectly to cause bone resorption by stimulating osteoblasts to secrete osteoclast recruiting factors[6] or by stimulating parathyroid hormone-related protein expression.[7]

Prostaglandins

Prostaglandin E$_2$ causes osteoclastic bone resorption *in vitro* and directly stimulates osteoclasts. Although some tumours produce large quantities of prostaglandins, levels do not correlate with hypercalcaemia, and prostaglandin synthesis inhibitors rarely lower serum calcium in malignant hypercalcaemia.[8] Prostaglandins may play a part in local osteolysis but appear to have only a limited role in hypercalcaemia of malignancy.

Parathyroid hormone

In most cases of malignancy associated hypercalcaemia cytokine mediated osteoclastic bone resorption appears to be the dominant factor; however, in up to 20 per cent of cases no bone metastases are present. In such cases of humoral hypercalcaemia of malignancy ectopic secretion of factors by the tumour accounts for the disturbance of calcium homeostasis. Humoral hypercalcaemia of malignancy resembles primary hyperparathyroidism biochemically with hypercalcaemia, hypophosphataemia, renal phosphate wasting, increased tubular reabsorption of calcium, and enhanced osteoclastic bone resorption. Early suggestions of ectopic parathyroid hormone (**PTH**) secretion by tumours have been invalidated by radioimmunoassay and gene expression studies; although very occasional cases of true ectopic secretion of PTH have been described in non-parathyroid tumours.

Parathyroid hormone related protein

Parathyroid hormone-related protein (**PTHrP**) is a 16-kDa peptide which resembles PTH in bioactivity but has different immunoreactivity. PTHrP (1–141) has four times the bioactivity of PTH and competitive binding studies show that it acts via the same PTH receptor; this is a G-protein coupled receptor which binds PTH and PTHrP with equal affinity. Antisera to PTH cross-reacts poorly with PTHrP except when polyclonal (as in the earliest radioimmunoassays) or in high concentrations (as in immunocytochemical stains). In addition to the actions on calcium metabolism, PTHrP acts as a mitogen in rat carcinoma models[9] and the expression of PRHrP is increased by Ha-*ras* and v-*src* oncogenes.[10] PTHrP gene expression is present in several normal tissues including skin keratinocytes, placenta, breast tissue, parathyroid glands, fetal liver, and brain. The physiological role of PTHrP is obscure but several hypotheses exist including a role in calcium homeostasis in the suckling neonate, keratinocyte differentiation, and smooth muscle relaxation.

PTHrP immunoperoxidase-staining was strongly positive in human squamous cell carcinomas from various sites.[11] In another study, the expression of PTHrP mRNA was detected in all tumours obtained from patients with humoral hypercalcaemia of malignancy but not in any of those obtained from normocalcaemic control patients with cancer,[12] and serum levels of PTHrP measured by radioimmunoassay have demonstrated elevated levels (>2.5 pg/ml) in cancer patients with hypercalcaemia.[13] Thus PTHrP assays may facilitate the diagnosis of hypercalcaemia.[14] PTHrP may also have a limited role as a tumour marker, although PTHrP levels do not necessarily reflect disease activity.[15] Levels of PTHrP expression in normocalcaemic breast cancer patients may predict the subsequent development of bone metastases.[16]

Antibodies to PTHrP alleviate hypercalcaemia in animal models of humoral hypercalcaemia of malignancy,[17] and serum levels of PTHrP fell in parallel with serum calcium in three patients with humoral hypercalcaemia of malignancy cured by surgery.[18] PTHrP has been shown to stimulate prostaglandin E_2 release from human osteoblast cell lines *in vitro*.[19] Nevertheless, PTHrP cannot explain all the biochemical changes seen in humoral hypercalcaemia of malignancy. In humoral hypercalcaemia of malignancy, unlike primary hyperparathyroidism, there is impaired intestinal calcium absorption, low $1,25(OH)_2D_3$ levels, and the osteoclastic bone resorption is far more prominent. These features suggest that other factors (probably cytokines) have an important role in humoral hypercalcaemia of malignancy even in the absence of bone metastases.

Vitamin D

The majority of cases of humoral hypercalcaemia of malignancy are associated with impaired gut absorption of calcium and low levels of ($1,25(OH)_2D_3$). However, there are a number of cases in the literature of humoral hypercalcaemia of malignancy in Hodgkin's disease associated with ectopic production of $1,25(OH)_2D_3$ by the tumour.[20] Elevated levels of $1,25(OH)_2D_3$ have been reported in other lymphoproliferative disorders and the mechanism is thought to involve extra-renal hydroxylation of $25(OH)D_3$.[21] The significance of tumour-related vitamin D excess causing increased gut absorption lies in the implications for therapy. Hypercalcaemia of malignancy is usually associated with low absorption and dietary calcium restriction is unnecessary; however, with elevated $1,25(OH)_2D_3$ levels, a low calcium diet is needed to control hypercalcaemia.

Epidemiology

Ten per cent of cancer patients develop hypercalcaemia and malignancy accounts for half the cases of hypercalcaemia amongst hospital inpatients. Hypercalcaemia occurs most frequently with myeloma (up to 50 per cent patients), breast, lung, and renal cancers, and up to 20 per cent of cases occur in the absence of bone metastases. Most patients with hypercalcaemia of malignancy have disseminated disease, and 80 per cent die within a year. Thus, hypercalcaemia is usually a complication of advanced disease and its treatment should be directed at symptom palliation.

Clinical features

The clinical manifestations of hypercalcaemia are myriad and many symptoms attributed to the underlying malignancy may resolve on correction of hypercalcaemia. Although severity of symptoms is not correlated with degree of elevation of serum calcium, most patients initially develop lethargy and malaise followed by thirst nausea and constipation before neurological and cardiological features appear (Table 1). A diagnosis of hypercalcaemia can only be made by biochemical investigation and so all symptomatic patients with malignancy considered candidates for treatment of hypercalcaemia should have their serum calcium measured.

Treatment

In parallel with the advances in the understanding of the pathogenesis of hypercalcaemia of malignancy have come improvements in therapy. These new therapies are more effective, less toxic, and easier to administer and represent a major advance in palliative therapy for cancer patients. The treatment of hypercalcaemia should be made on the basis of clinical features and the serum calcium level, and should consist of rehydration and calcium lowering agents. Low calcium diets are unpalatable, impractical, and exacerbate malnutrition; they have no place in palliative therapy. Drugs promoting hypercalcaemia (thiazides, vitamins A and D) should be withdrawn.

Table 1 Clinical features of hypercalcaemia of malignancy

General	Gastrointestinal	Neurological	Cardiological
Dehydration	Anorexia	Fatigue	Bradycardia
Polydipsia	Weight loss	Lethargy	Atrial arrhythmias
Polyuria	Nausea	Confusion	Ventricular arrhythmias
Pruritus	Vomiting	Myopathy	P–R interval prolonged
	Constipation	Hyporeflexia	Q–T interval reduced
	Ileus	Seizures	Wide T waves
		Psychosis	
		Coma	

Intravenous fluids

Dehydration due to polyuria and vomiting is a prominent feature of hypercalcaemia and intravenous hydration is the mainstay of acute therapy for severe or symptomatic hypercalcaemia. Although large volumes of fluid will lower serum calcium, patients rarely achieve normocalcaemia and careful monitoring to avoid fluid overloading is necessary. In view of this, 2 to 3 l/day of fluid is now the accepted practice with daily serum electrolyte measurement to prevent hypokalaemia and hyponatraemia. Loop diuretics are often prescribed as an adjunct to intravenous fluids and cause calciuresis. However, there is little evidence of any benefit and they may exacerbate hypovolaemia, hypokalaemia, and hypomagnesaemia.

Corticosteroids

Glucocorticoids have been widely used in cancer-related hypercalcaemia and rapidly inhibit osteoclastic bone resorption *in vitro* as well as reducing calcium absorption from the gut. However, their limited benefit to patients is chiefly due to tumour responsiveness to the cytostatic effects of steroids. They are most effective in myeloma, lymphoma, leukaemia, and in breast cancer when hypercalcaemia occurs as a 'flare' effect caused by endocrine therapy. The role of steroids in severe hypercalcaemia is limited to the haematological malignancies and oral prednisolone 40 to 100 mg/day is usually effective in these circumstances.

Bisphosphonates

Bisphosphonates are synthetic pyrophosphate analogues characterized by a phosphorus-carbon-phosphorus bond, making them resistant to enzymatic hydrolysis. They inhibit bone resorption although the mechanism is unclear. Bisphosphonates bind hydroxyapatite crystals with a high affinity and effects on osteoclast recruitment and activity have been demonstrated. They are highly effective in controlling hypercalcaemia of malignancy causing a gradual fall in serum calcium over a few days. There are three bisphosphonates commonly marketed—disodium etidronate and sodium clodronate are first generation bisphosphonates and disodium pamidronate is a second generation compound. All three drugs administered as intravenous infusions will control hypercalcaemia, although disodium pamidronate requires only a single infusion of 30 to 60 mg over 2 to 4 h and is more effective than disodium etidronate.[22] Lower (30 mg) dosages have been shown to be equally effective but higher doses (60–90 mg) have a longer duration of control lasting up to 4 weeks and so some clinicians prefer to prescribe dosages according to the serum calcium level. Disodium etidronate requires repeated infusions over 3 days and is therefore less suitable for palliative care. Sodium clodronate as a single 1.5 g infusion over 4 h is a suitable alternative to pamidronate. Maintenance therapy with oral bisphosphonates, to prevent recurrent hypercalcaemia, has been described for disodium etidronate and sodium clodronate; however, their low oral bioavailability and considerable gastrointestinal toxicity limit their value in this context. Bisphosphonates do not alter PTHrP levels or renal calcium reabsorption and so they may fail to control humoral hypercalcaemia of malignancy without bone metastases.[23] Indeed, there is a correlation between the responsiveness to disodium pamidronate in humoral hypercalcaemia of malignancy and the plasma PTHrP level. Non-responders had levels greater than 75 pg/ml and so PTHrP measurement may allow the identification of patients requiring higher doses of bisphosphonates and increased dose frequency.[24]

A further benefit of bisphosphonate therapy is the reduction of bone pain from metastatic deposits[25] (see Chapter 9.2.5). A number of new bisphosphonates are under development including alendronate, a second generation product which has been extensively studied in humoral hypercalcaemia of malignancy but is unavailable in the United Kingdom. Neridronate and residronate are at earlier stages of development, whilst tiludronate has been abandoned on account of the high risk of nephrotoxicity.

Calcitonin

Calcitonin is secreted by the parafollicular cells of the thyroid gland although its physiological role in calcium homeostasis remains undefined. In pharmacological doses calcitonin reduces bone resorption and increases calciuresis, thereby reducing serum calcium. It is effective in around a third of patients and usually causes a fall in serum calcium within 4 h (compared to 48 h for bisphosphonates) but normocalcaemia is rare. Doses of up to 8 IU/kg salmon calcitonin may be injected subcutaneously or intramuscularly every 6 h and this therapy has minimal toxicity (nausea and hypersensitivity only).

Calcitonin and calcitonin gene-related peptide are produced by alternative splicing from the same gene on chromosome 11p15.5 close to the PTH gene. Both may be produced by tumours but no clinical syndrome has been attributed to their production and conversely athymic patients who produce no calcitonin have no disturbance of calcium metabolism. Although production of calcitonin and calcitonin gene-related peptide is common in many tumours, its main value to oncologists is as a tumour marker for medullary cell carcinoma of the thyroid and multiple endocrine neoplasia type II.

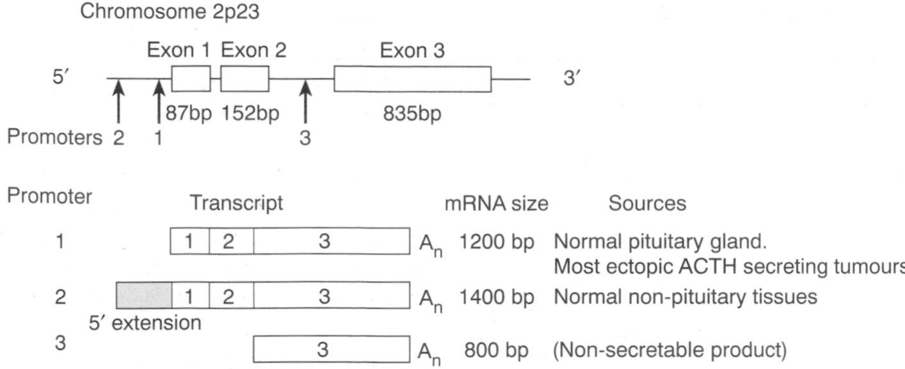

Fig. 1 The molecular biology of pro-opiomelanocortin gene expression.

Plicamycin

Plicamycin (formerly mithramycin), a cytotoxic antibiotic, is toxic to osteoclasts by blocking RNA synthesis and hence reduces bone resorption, producing prompt and effective lowering of serum calcium. It is administered as an intravenous bolus or 2 h infusion at a dosage of 25 mcg/kg. It produces normocalcaemia within 3 days in 80 per cent of patients and is usually repeated weekly. The disadvantage of this highly effective treatment is the toxicity; cumulative nephrotoxicity and hepatotoxicity are reported, and thrombocytopenia is common; nausea is frequent and may be reduced when given by infusion.

Phosphates

Oral phosphates may be effective in mild hypercalcaemia by a combination of effects on calcium metabolism. The usual recommended dose is 0.5 to 3 g/day phosphate (as sodium cellulose phosphate powder) and this frequently causes nausea and diarrhoea. Intravenous phosphate is a highly effective therapy for acute life-threatening hypercalcaemia and its onset of hypocalcaemic action is more rapid than any other agent. However, the severe toxicity of parenteral phosphate has lead to the abandoning of this therapy in all but exceptional circumstances. Recommended dosing is 1.5 g (50 mmol) elemental phosphate diluted in 1 litre of saline over 6 to8 h and should be given preferably in intensive care where the patient's cardiac and renal function can be monitored closely.

Gallium nitrate

Gallium nitrate is incorporated into bone rendering hydroxyapatite less soluble.[26] It directly inhibits bone resorption without killing osteoclasts and is not associated with the nausea or myelosuppression caused by plicamycin. Gallium is highly effective, producing normocalcaemia in 80 per cent of patients with hypercalcaemia of malignancy. Two randomized double-blind trials have demonstrated the superiority of gallium compared to calcitonin[27] and disodium etidronate.[28] The main drawback of gallium is that it requires continuous intravenous infusion (100–200 mg/m^2 per day) for 5 days, and it may cause nephrotoxicity. Gallium nitrate has no product licence in the United Kingdom.

Future approaches

Passive immunization with murine monoclonal antibody against PTHrP decreased serum calcium in nude mice bearing human tumour xenografts secreting PTHrP.[29] Herbimycin A, an antibiotic which inhibits pp60c-*src* tyrosine kinase, reduced osteoclastic bone resorption *in vitro* and hypercalcaemia in mouse model systems.[30] Osteoclasts bind proteins *in vitro* via integrins which recognize the Arginine-Glycine-Aspartate tripeptide sequence. Kistrin is a snake venom protein containing Arginine-Glycine-Aspartate which inhibits bone resorption *in vitro* and osteoclast activity *in vivo*. Kistrin infusion restored normocalcaemia in hypercalcaemic mice.[31] All these and other approaches may yield clinical advances in the management of hypercalcaemia.

Treatment summary

Symptomatic or severe hypercalcaemia requires intravenous rehydration with 2 to 3 l/day followed by a single infusion of disodium pamidronate 60 mg in 250 ml crystalloid over 4 h or according to calcium level. This combination will control hypercalcaemia in most patients simply, promptly, and with minimal toxicity. The majority of patients will remain normocalcaemic for 2 to 4 weeks with encouragement of oral hydration and maintenance disodium pamidronate infusions over 2 to 4 h and can be managed on an outpatient basis. Second line management of humoral hypercalcaemia of malignancy resistant to bisphosphonate should probably be with gallium nitrate.

Cushing's syndrome

Clinically, overt Cushing's syndrome caused by ectopic secretion of adrenocorticotrophic hormone (**ACTH**) by non-endocrine derived tumours is rare. However, the production of pro-opiomelanocortin (**POMC**) derived peptides by tumours is not uncommon and the rarity of clinical signs and symptoms reflects the subtle and complex control of hormone production from this gene. Usually, symptoms arise as a consequence of excessive ACTH production by tumours through uncontrolled gene expression following promoter switches or transcription activation. The mRNA transcripts may be of altered lengths and give rise to different POMC peptides by variations in protein cleavage and glycosylation.

Pathogenesis

The POMC gene is located at p23 on the short arm of chromosome 2 and includes three exons and three putative promoter sites which are active to different extents in different tissues (Fig. 1). The expression of the POMC gene is influenced by glucocorticoids which suppress transcription and corticotrophin which stimulates transcription via cAMP. Glucocorticoids act by binding to a steroid hormone receptor which in turn binds a glucocorticoid inhibitory element sequence of POMC gene. In this way steroids suppress POMC transcription only when it is driven by promoter 1, yielding

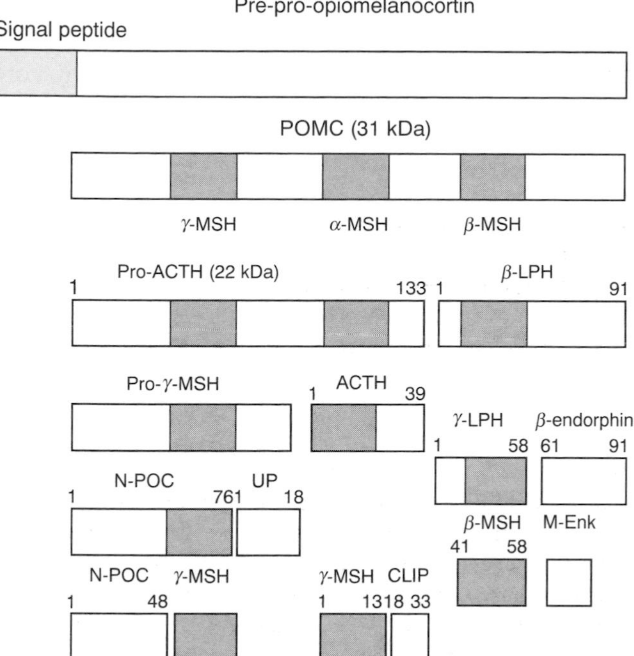

Fig. 2 Pro-opiomelanocortin (POMC) derived peptides.

a 1200 base transcript, and this may account for the lack of steroid suppression of ectopic ACTH production by some tumours where alternative promoters are active.

Post translational processing of POMC peptide gives rise to a large number of different peptides, many of which have been detected in tumour extracts and cell lines. Some of these peptides have also been identified in patient's plasma and are biologically active (Fig. 2). Until recently radioimmunoassay (**RIA**) was the sole method used to detect these peptides; this technique requires pre-extraction and long incubation with antisera and there is a high degree of cross-reactivity between peptides sharing some amino acid sequences. The introduction of immunoradiometric assay (**IRMA**) has improved sensitivity by using monoclonal antibodies, so that pre-extraction is no longer necessary, and by using two-site directed IRMA, specificity has improved. IRMA is able to discriminate between ACTH and its larger precursors (pro-ACTH and POMC) (Fig. 2). This methodology has been used to show that most patients with ectopic ACTH secrete proACTH, which has only 5 per cent of the steroidogenic activity of ACTH 1–39, whilst patients with pituitary adenomas produce normal 1200 base POMC transcripts and the peptide product undergoes normal glycosylation and proteolysis culminating in the secretion of ACTH 1–39. Thus, two-site directed IRMA may help in the differential diagnosis of Cushing's disease and ectopic ACTH. However, occasionally large aggressive pituitary adenomas secrete pro-ACTH and these patients often show behaviour more indicative of ectopic ACTH in the biochemical tests aimed at differentiating Cushing's disease and ectopic ACTH secretion.[32]

Elevated plasma levels and tumour extract concentrations of various other POMC derived peptides have been described. Although melanocyte-stimulating hormone (**MSH**) production is not light-sensitive (unlike melatonin) it regulates skin pigmentation by directly affecting dermal melanocyte growth and melanin production. Hence, ectopic secretion of MSH containing peptides (α-MSH, ACTH, pro-ACTH, β-MSH, γ-LPH, β-LPH, γ-MSH, N-POC, pro γ-MSH) may lead to generalized hyperpigmentation but this symptom is rarely distressing. Whilst other physiological roles for α-, β- and γ-MSH have been described, no other clinical correlates in the setting of ectopic MSH secretion are reported.

The secretion of endorphins and enkephalins derived from the POMC gene occurs frequently in conjunction with ectopic ACTH secretion.[33,34] Numerous clinical effects within the central nervous system have been postulated for these endogenous opioids that bind G-protein coupled receptors, inhibiting net cAMP synthesis by antagonizing adenyl cyclase and activating phosphodiesterase. However, these opioid molecules cross the blood–brain barrier with difficulty and although one-third of patients with Cushing's syndrome have psychiatric disturbances, the proportion is lower in Nelson's syndrome which suggests that these symptoms are related to excess steroids rather than opioids.[35]

Epidemiology

In up to 20 per cent of cases of Cushing's syndrome the cause is ectopic ACTH secretion by a tumour which is frequently occult at presentation.[36] For this reason the differential diagnosis between pituitary adenoma and ectopic ACTH is important clinically but biochemical overlap often makes this difficult. More than half the cases of ectopic ACTH syndrome are due to small cell lung cancer, with carcinoid tumours and neural crest tumours (phaeochromocytoma, neuroblastoma, medullary cell carcinoma of thyroid) accounting for a further 15 per cent each. Bronchial carcinoids and thymomas make up most of the remaining cases.

In small cell lung cancer, ectopic secretion of ACTH is generally not thought to be correlated with either stage or survival, although one recent retrospective analysis suggests an association with poor outcome and a high incidence of infectious complications.[37] The levels of ACTH may decline in response to chemotherapy or radiotherapy,[38] but any correlation between declining ACTH levels and tumour response is anecdotal only, and elevation of ACTH may persist in long-term survivors following chemotherapy.[39]

Clinical features

The typical presentation is a middle-aged smoking man with features of severe hypercortisolism and hypokalaemic metabolic alkalosis. Patients have muscle weakness or atrophy, oedema, hypertension, mental changes, glucose intolerance, and weight loss. When ectopic ACTH production arises from a more benign tumour (e.g. bronchial carcinoid or thymoma) the other classical features of Cushing's syndrome may be present including truncal obesity, moon facies, and cutaneous striae often making clinical distinction from pituitary dependent Cushing's disease impossible. Furthermore, biochemical tests do not always reliably differentiate a pituitary from an ectopic tumour as the source of ACTH.

Diagnosis

In addition to the clinical features, the diagnosis of Cushing's syndrome may be confirmed by elevated urinary free cortisol, loss of diurnal variation of plasma cortisol, and failure of cortisol suppression in the low-dose dexamethasone (2 mg) test. After confirming Cushing's syndrome, an elevated plasma ACTH supports a diagnosis of pituitary adenoma or ectopic ACTH syndrome. Failure of cortisol to suppress following high-dose dexamethasone (2 mg four times daily for 2 days, or 8 mg overnight) and very high levels of ACTH (>200 pg/ml) suggest an ectopic source of ACTH. However, half the cases of ectopic ACTH production from carcinoid tumours suppress with dexamethasone and in these cases ACTH levels may be in the lower range, and circadian rhythms of secretion may even be maintained. In difficult cases corticotrophin-releasing hormone stimulation tests,[40] selective venous catheterization of inferior petrosal sinus with ACTH estimations,[41] and two-site directed IRMA for pro-ACTH and ACTH measurements may be necessary to determine the source of ACTH.[42] Recently, both somatostatin analogue scintigraphy[43] and technetium-99 methoxyisobutylisonitrile (MIBI) imaging[44] have been used for localization of ectopic ACTH producing tumours.

Further difficulties in differential diagnosis have arisen with the description of ectopic corticotrophin releasing hormone secretion by tumours giving rise to Cushing's syndrome.[45] In these circumstances ectopically secreted corticotrophin releasing hormone stimulates the normal pituitary corticotrophs to secrete excesses of ACTH giving rise to Cushing's syndrome. Another diagnostic complication arises with the description in a patient with medullary carcinoma of the thyroid of Cushing's syndrome due to ectopic production of a bombesin-like peptide which is thought to stimulate ACTH secretion by pituitary corticotrophs.

Treatment

The mainstay of palliative therapy for Cushing's syndrome due to ectopic ACTH production is inhibition of steroid synthesis, although inhibition of ACTH release and blocking glucocorticoid receptors have also been attempted. Several steroid synthesis inhibitors are available and successful use in these circumstances has been reported for aminoglutethimide, metyrapone, mitotane, ketoconazole, and octreotide. In rare circumstances, bilateral adrenalectomy or adrenal artery embolization may be necessary to control symptoms.

Aminoglutethimide inhibits 20,22-desmolase enzyme which catalyses the cholesterol side-chain cleavage which gives rise to Δ5-pregnenolone. In this way the production of glucocorticoids, mineralocorticoids, and androgens is inhibited at higher doses (1.5–3 g/day), whilst at lower doses (125 mg twice daily) aminoglutethimide inhibits aromatase which converts androgens to oestrogens. The latter is responsible for the efficacy of aminoglutethimide in post-menopausal breast cancer. The high doses used to treat Cushing's syndrome are associated with considerable toxicity, in particular sedation, ataxia, and rashes.

Metyrapone inhibits 11-β-hydroxylase, the final step in cortisol and corticosterone synthesis and has been demonstrated to be effective in ectopic ACTH syndrome at doses of 250 to 750 mg four times daily. The short half-life of metyrapone and gastrointestinal toxicity (chiefly nausea) are drawbacks, and very high levels of ACTH secretion may over-ride the effects of metyrapone. For these reasons it has been suggested that metyrapone should be used in conjunction with low dose aminoglutethimide (250 mg twice daily) to reduce toxicities of both compounds.[46]

Mitotane is an adrenal cytotoxic, structurally related to the insecticide DDT, which irreversibly inhibits 11-β-hydroxylase and 18-hydroxylase thus reducing glucocorticoid, mineralocorticoid, and androgen production. It produces focal atrophy and necrosis of the zona fasiculata and zona reticularis. Doses of 1 to 12 g/day in four divided doses have been used and it is also active against primary adrenal tumours. Mitotane is a toxic drug with gastrointestinal side-effects (anorexia, nausea, vomiting, diarrhoea) reported in 80 per cent of patients and lethargy and somnolence in 40 per cent.

The imidazole antifungal ketoconazole inhibits cytochrome P450 dependent steroid hydroxylases and case reports document its successful use in Cushing's syndrome due to ectopic ACTH.[47] The potential side-effects include nausea, headaches, pruritic rashes, and liver failure. Bromocriptine has also been advocated for use in these circumstances. Bromocriptine acts on dopamine-2 receptors, inhibiting cAMP production, and decreasing POMC expression *in vitro* but it is only rarely successful *in vivo*.[48]

The suppression of ectopic ACTH secretion by the administration of octreotide, a long acting somatostatin analogue, has been documented. The mechanism of this action is unknown but may reflect the wide distribution of somatostatin receptors on tumours and the diverse endocrine actions of somatostatin. However, somatostatin analogues occasionally cause a paradoxical rise in plasma ACTH and cortisol levels in patients with ectopic ACTH production and so a preliminary evaluation of their therapeutic efficacy is suggested.[49]

Mifepristone (RU-486) is a partial progesterone agonist which inhibits the separation of heat shock protein (hsp 90) from the progesterone receptor. Case reports describe symptomatic improvement in Cushing's syndrome patients although it has yet to be used in ectopic ACTH secretion.[50] Antisense oligonucleotide complementary to a region of β-endorphin reduced the synthesis of POMC derived peptides *in vitro* and this approach may prove fruitful in the future.[51]

Treatment summary

The first line therapy in these patients should be aminoglutethimide 250 mg twice daily and metyrapone 250 mg four times daily used together. The efficacy of treatment should be monitored and this is most easily achieved by measuring 24-h urinary cortisol secretion. As levels return to normal in these patients hormone replacement therapy is frequently necessary. Regimens similar to those used in Addison's disease should be used (e.g. hydrocortisone 20 mg at 0800 hours and 10 mg at 1800 hours, fludrocortisone 0.05–0.15 mg daily).

Syndrome of inappropriate antidiuresis

Hyponatraemia is a common finding in association with advanced malignancy, and many factors may contribute including cardiac and hepatic failure, hyperglycaemia, diuretics, and the sick cell syndrome. However, the detection of concentrated urine in conjunction with hypo-osmolar plasma suggests abnormal renal free water excretion and the presence of the syndrome of inappropriate antidiuresis (**SIAD**). This acronym is more suitable than 'SIADH' since there is no detectable vasopressin secretion in approximately 15 per cent of cases.[52]

Pathogenesis

The vasopressin gene lies on human chromosome 20 and comprises three exons encoding a transcript of 700 base pairs. The peptide product includes the nine amino acid arginine vasopressin (**AVP**) and a 90 amino acid peptide—vasopressin-specific neurophysin II (**NP II**). This peptide complex is flanked by an N-terminal signal peptide and a C-terminal glycoprotein (absent in the oxytocin-NP

Table 2 Diagnosis of syndrome of inappropriate diuresis (SIAD)

Essential criteria
1. Plasma hypo-osmolality (plasma osmolality <275 mosmol/kg H_2O) (plasma Na^+ <135 mmol/l)
2. Concentrated urine (urine osmolality >100 mosmol/kg H_2O)
3. Normal plasma/extracellular fluid volume
4. High urine sodium on a normal salt and water intake (urine Na^+ >20 mEq/l)
5. Exclude i) hypothyroidism
   ii) hypoadrenalism
   iii) diuretics

Supportive criteria
6. Abnormal water load test (unable to excrete ≥90% of a 20 ml/kg water load in 4 h, and/or failure to dilute urine to osmolality ≤100 mosmol/kg H_2O)
7. Elevated plasma AVP

I peptide). The AVP-NP II polypeptide is transported by axonal streaming from its site of synthesis, in the supraoptic and paraventricular nuclei of the hypothalamus, to the posterior pituitary gland. The peptide is cleaved and secreted by the posterior pituitary to produce a nonapeptide (arginine vasopressin) and the 10-kDa transport peptide (NP II). This molecular mechanism is mimicked by oxytocin-neurophysin I whose gene is adjacent on chromosome 20p13 but in mirror-image orientation. Mutations in NP II are linked to autosomal dominant neurohypophyseal diabetes insipidus.

Epidemiology

In most cases of SIAD there is either stimulation of hypothalamic–pituitary secretion of AVP or a direct effect on the distal nephron. However, in malignancy-related SIAD, tumours secrete ectopic AVP or vasopressin-like peptides.[53] This has been demonstrated *in vitro,* in cell lines and tumour extracts and *in vivo* in plasma. SIAD is most commonly associated with small cell lung cancer or carcinoid tumours but has also been described in pancreatic, oesophageal, prostatic, and haematological malignancies. Collected data on 523 patients with small cell lung cancer showed 9 per cent had clinically evident SIAD, 32 to 44 per cent elevated plasma AVP detectable by radioimmunoassay, and 53 to 68 per cent had abnormal renal handling of water loads.[54,55] In another study 58 per cent of small cell lung cancer patients had raised plasma neurophysins (NP-1, 14 per cent; NP-2, 44 per cent),[56] although the high incidence of vasopressin/oxytocin gene expression in lung cancer is confined to neuroendocrine tumours[57] and both normal and abnormal gene products are found.[58] Prognosis, stage at diagnosis, and response to chemotherapy are similar in small cell lung cancer patients with or without SIAD.[59] Furthermore, although correction of hyponatraemia correlates with tumour response to chemotherapy[60] complete restoration of normal renal water handling is rare even when complete remissions are achieved.[61]

Clinical features

Significant symptoms of hyponatraemia appear at plasma sodium levels below 125 mmol/l with confusion progressing to stupor, coma, and seizures as levels fall. Nausea, vomiting, and focal neurological deficits may also occur. The clinical features depend on both the level of plasma sodium and the rate of decline; with gradual falls in sodium the brain cells are able to compensate against cerebral oedema by secreting potassium and other intracellular solutes. Asymptomatic hyponatraemia therefore suggests chronic SIAD rather than acute SIAD. The division into chronic and acute SIAD is of therapeutic importance as their management differs.[62]

Diagnosis

The diagnosis of SIAD requires the demonstration of plasma hyponatraemia and hypo-osmolality in the presence of concentrated urine and normal extracellular fluid volume (Table 2).

There are a large number of causes of SIAD, including ectopic AVP production by tumours, and several may play a role in hyponatraemia in patients with advanced malignancy. Pulmonary, meningeal, and cerebral infections are common causes and drug-induced SIAD may also present in patients with cancer. Most drugs which cause SIAD stimulate hypophygeal secretion of AVP, although the prostaglandin synthesis inhibitors directly inhibit renal tubular excretion of free water. The list of drugs implicated is long and includes morphine, phenothiazines, tricyclic antidepressants, non-steroidal anti-inflammatory drugs, and nicotine, all (except nicotine) frequently used in palliative care, as well as the cytotoxic drugs vincristine and cyclophosphamide. The possibility of drug related SIAD should always be considered before invoking ectopic AVP secretion by tumours, and in most circumstances the hyponatraemia resolves when the drug is stopped. When SIAD presents with no identifiable cause, a thorough search for occult malignancy (especially small cell lung cancer) should be undertaken, as SIAD may be the presenting symptom and may precede radiological evidence by up to 1 year.[63]

Treatment

The management of SIAD depends upon the rate of onset of hyponatraemia and the presence of neurological complications. Acute SIAD with an onset over 2 to 3 days and rates of fall of serum sodium in excess of 0.5 mmol/l per day are associated with neurological sequelae and require prompt correction by intravenous hypertonic saline. In contrast, the mainstay of therapy for chronic asymptomatic SIAD is fluid restriction and inhibition of tubular reabsorption of water.

Acute hyponatraemia with neurological symptoms has a mortality of 5 to 8 per cent, partly reflecting underlying pathology. Rapid correction of hyponatraemia by intravenous hypertonic saline causes central pontine myelinosis often with additional extra-pontine myelinosis. Central pontine myelinosis usually presents 1 to 2 days after correcting hyponatraemia with quadriparesis and bulbar palsy and is related to the rapidity of correction of hyponatraemia. A safe balance between overzealous correction of hyponatraemia causing irreversible central pontine myelinosis, and the considerable mortality of uncorrected SIAD is necessary.[64,65] Hypertonic saline infusions should correct serum sodium at a rate of 0.5 mmol/l per hour[66] although a correction rate of 2 mmol/l per hour is said to be safe.[67] The total rise in serum sodium should not exceed 25 mmol/l, and correction should stop once serum sodium exceeds 120 mmol/l and symptoms have resolved. To achieve a correction rate of 0.5 mmol/l per hour requires 0.3 × body weight (mmol Na^+/h). Hypertonic (twice normal) saline solution of 1.8 per cent contains 0.3 mmol/l Na^+. So the correct rate of infusion is 1 ml/kg body weight per hour of 1.8 per cent sodium chloride.

The mainstay of treatment for chronic asymptomatic SIAD is fluid restriction. It is suggested that intake is restricted to 500 ml/day or the daily urine output less 500 ml/day. This should include all fluids and takes several days to influence the hyponatraemia. In the context of palliative care, fluid restriction is frequently undesirable, as it is unpleasant for patients and onerous on their carers. Alternative strategies for chronic SIAD include the use of distal nephron inhibitors preventing water reabsorption, and osmotic diuretics.

The tetracycline analogue demeclocycline (desmethylchlortetracycline) causes nephrogenic diabetes insipidus by inhibiting vasopressin-induced cAMP formation in distal tubules and is used in the treatment of chronic SIAD. Demeclocycline administered orally in two divided doses equivalent to 900 to 1200 mg/day will reverse chronic SIAD gradually over 3 to 4 days and should be followed by a maintenance dosage of 600 to 900 mg/day. The main side-effects of demeclocycline are gastrointestinal disturbances and hypersensitivity reactions, although reversible nephrotoxicity may occur with prolonged use, especially when hepatic function is impaired. Lithium carbonate, which has similar effects on tubular water reabsorption, has also been used in the treatment of SIAD but is not recommended as its efficacy is less consistent and its toxicity is greater.

Urea acts as an osmotic diuretic increasing free water excretion and in addition reduces natriuresis by increasing intramedullary urea levels. It is effective in controlling SIAD when given both intravenously and orally. Oral urea should be given once daily at a dose of 30 g dissolved in 100 ml orange juice to mask the taste. On account of its diuretic properties there is no need to fluid restrict patients treated with oral urea.[68]

The development of vasopressin analogues which may act as specific antagonists is underway and these may hold the key to the control of SIAD in the future. One non-peptide antagonist, 5-dimethylamino-1- [4-(2-methylbenzoylamino)benzoyl]-2, 3, 4, 5-tetrahydro-1H-benzazepine, restored normonatraemia to rats with experimentally induced SIAD.[69]

Atrial natriuretic peptide

Atrial natriuretic peptide (**ANP**) is secreted by atrial monocytes and acts to regulate natriuresis and diuresis via the kidneys and adrenals. A role for ectopic or inappropriate ANP secretion had been proposed to account for cases of SIAD when vasopressin is undetectable.[70] Elevated serum levels of ANP in small cell lung cancer patients with SIAD have been demonstrated in conjunction with raised AVP, where ANP may be contributing to the hyponatraemia. A patient with small cell lung cancer and hyponatraemia with elevated plasma ANP, but undetectable AVP, has been described and it was proposed that inappropriate ANP was the cause of SIAD; however the source of ANP was not demonstrated.[71] More recently, ectopic production of ANP has been identified in various neuroendocrine tumours by radioimmunoassay.[72] The exact role of ANP in SIAD remains to be established and ANP inhibitors may in the future have a place in treating SIAD.

Non-islet cell tumour hypoglycaemia

Tumour related hypoglycaemia is a frequent complication of beta islet cell tumours of the pancreas which secrete insulin but occurs uncommonly with non-islet cell tumours. Although ectopic insulin production has been documented in a woman with cervical cancer,[73] most non-islet cell tumours produce hypoglycaemia by increased glucose use by the tumours, secretion of insulin-like factors, and failure of normal compensatory mechanisms.[74]

Pathogenesis

Increased glucose utilization by tumours has been documented in association with anaerobic metabolism by measuring arteriovenous differences in glucose concentrations. Daily glucose consumption by tumours may reach 200 g/kg per day. In addition, hepatic glucose production falls despite normal glycogen stores, producing an acquired glycogen storage disease which may contribute to hypoglycaemia. Furthermore, suppression of other compensatory mechanisms, including growth hormone and glucagon secretion, is believed to play a role.

Insulin-like growth factors (formerly called somatomedins) are a family of peptides involved in cellular growth, differentiation, and metabolism which cross-react with insulin in both bioassay and radioreceptor assay but may be differentiated from insulin by radioimmunoassay. Two insulin-like growth factors (**IGFs**) have been characterized and both have sequence homology with insulin but act via separate receptors. High levels of expression of IGF-II have been detected in tumours (including its precursor pro-IGF-II) and elevated plasma IGF-II levels are found in 40 per cent of non-islet cell tumours associated with hypoglycaemia. IGF-II (formerly somatomedin A) binds at least two receptors; an insulin-receptor-like tyrosine kinase which also binds IGF-I and the mannose-6-phosphate receptor. IGF-II expression is induced by human placental lactogen especially during fetal life where the expression of IGF-II and its type II receptor are reciprocally modulated by genomic imprinting. Unlike insulin, the IGFs are bound to several plasma IGF-binding proteins. At high levels of IGF-II there is specificity spill-over so that lower affinity binding to the insulin receptor occurs and this may mediate hypoglycaemia. IGF-II suppresses growth hormone secretion and thus suppresses production of IGF binding proteins by the liver; the levels of growth hormone and IGF binding proteins are lowered in many patients with tumour associated hypoglycaemia. Decreased IGF binding protein levels permit free IGF-II levels to rise, leading to the inhibition of hepatic glucose release and stimulation of peripheral glucose uptake. The role of IGFs, their binding proteins, and their receptors in the pathogenesis of cell transformation is under close examination.

Epidemiology

Non-islet cell tumours associated with hypoglycaemia are usually large (average 2.4 kg), retroperitoneal, or intrathoracic tumours, often with liver invasion, and follow a protracted time-course over several years. Histologically these tumours are 45 to 65 per cent mesenchymal (mesothelioma, neurofibroma, fibrosarcoma, leiomyosarcoma, rhabdomyosarcoma, neurofibrosarcoma, haemangiopericytoma, and spindle cell carcinoma), 20 per cent hepatoma, 5 to 10 per cent adrenal carcinoma (chiefly androgen-secreting), and 5 to 10 per cent gastrointestinal tumours. Unlike other endocrine complications of malignancy, lung cancer is very rarely associated with hypoglycaemia.

Clinical features

Hypoglycaemia may be a presenting symptom but more commonly occurs in the terminal stages of the disease. Clinical manifestations relate to cerebral hypoglycaemia and secondary secretion of catecholamines. Neurological features include agitation, stupor, coma, and seizures usually following exercise or fasting, and occur most often in the early morning and late afternoon. Focal neurological deficit may occur especially when cerebral circulation is poor.

Tumour related hypoglycaemia should be differentiated from other causes of hypoglycaemia including drugs (e.g. sulphonylureas), hypoadrenalism, hypopituitarism, liver failure, and antibodies directed against insulin or its receptor. In advanced malignancy the most common cause of hypoglycaemia is continued oral hypoglycaemic medication in long-standing diabetics who have developed tumours.

Treatment

The reversal of life-threatening or symptomatic hypoglycaemia initially requires intravenous glucose infusion. Hyperosmolar glucose solutions in excess of 10 per cent should be administered via central lines; serum glucose levels require frequent monitoring to ensure optimal correction of hypoglycaemia. Up to 2000 g/day may be required to control tumour-related hypoglycaemia. Debulking surgery and effective chemotherapy frequently improve paraneoplastic hypoglycaemia and should therefore be considered even in a palliative context. Dietary supplementation with frequent feeding, including during the night, may control symptoms of mild paraneoplastic hypoglycaemia. Corticosteroids in high doses, parenteral glucagon, and human growth hormone have been of benefit in some patients, whilst diazoxide, which inhibits insulin secretion, and somatostatin have been ineffective. Arterial embolization of tumours may also be used to palliate paraneoplastic hypoglycaemia.

Future approaches

The discovery of the possible role of IGFs in the pathogenesis of paraneoplastic hypoglycaemia suggests that antagonists of these peptides may become useful as therapy and may reduce the dependence on continuous glucose infusions to control hypoglycaemia in this context.

Enteropancreatic hormone syndromes

Enteropancreatic hormone production is relatively uncommon in malignant disease. A variety of clinical syndromes occur associated with hormone secretion by endocrine tumours of the pancreas and less frequently tumours arising in other organs. The majority of pancreatic islet cell tumours are malignant (with the exception of most insulinomas) and metastases are usually present at diagnosis. Surgical excision of small localized tumours is the optimal treatment and unresectable malignant secretory tumours may respond to chemotherapy. However, in many patients the distressing clinical manifestations arising from excessive secretion of gastrointestinal peptides require palliation and this may be difficult to achieve. These tumours often secrete more than one polypeptide hormone and may switch their hormone secretion during follow-up. Furthermore, many molecular species of the hormones, including precursor peptides with varying bioactivity, may be found in the circulation.

Therapy

The clinical manifestations listed according to the major hormone product of secretory endocrine tumours are shown in Table 3 along with the palliative endocrine manoeuvres that may control them. The control of insulinoma related hypoglycaemia is similar to paraneoplastic hypoglycaemia (see above) except that diazoxide may be a valuable additional agent in insulinoma. Diazoxide inhibits insulin release from beta islet cells but may cause salt and water retention and so is usually prescribed with chlorothiazide. Palliation of acid hypersecretion in Zollinger–Ellison syndrome is most effectively achieved by the proton pump inhibitor omeprazole, although other drugs including high-dose histamine H_2 receptor antagonists may be useful. The symptomatic control of other secretory tumours has been revolutionized by the introduction of long-acting somatostatin analogues.

Somatostatin is a widely distributed 14 amino acid cyclic neuroendocrine peptide which plays an inhibitory role in homeostatic mechanisms of the nervous system, gastrointestinal tract, and both endocrine and exocrine pancreas. A single gene on chromosome 3 encodes somatostatin which is translated as the 116 amino acid pre-pro-somatostatin, including a signal peptide, and extensive post-translational processing yields SOM-14, the biologically active form. SOM-14 acts via a number of somatostatin receptors activating G-proteins which in turn reduce adenyl cyclase activity and cAMP levels. Somatostatin has a short duration of action, requires intravenous administration and following infusion, rebound hypersecretion of hormones may occur. These shortcomings have been overcome by the use of the synthetic analogue octreotide which is given by subcutaneous injection.

The control of clinical symptoms associated with enteropancreatic hormone hypersecretion including profuse diarrhoea, hypokalaemia, attacks of hypoglycaemia, peptic ulceration, necrolytic skin lesions, and even Cushing's syndrome can be achieved by 100–450 mcg octreotide subcutaneously daily in many patients with endocrine pancreatic tumours. The response to octreotide seems to depend upon the presence of somatostatin receptors on the tumours and this has been exploited for tumour localization using *in vivo* scintigraphy with labelled octreotide.[75] Somatostatin analogues are valuable in symptomatic palliation in insulinomas, glucagonomas, gastrinomas, VIPomas, and GRFomas but there is

Table 3 Clinical manifestations of secretory endocrine tumours

Tumour	Clinical features: Major	Clinical features: Minor	Common sites	Malignant (%)	MEN-associated (%)	Palliative therapies
Insulinoma	Neuroglycopenia (confusion, fits)	Permanent neurological deficits	Pancreas (β cells)	10	10	Frequent feeding Glucose Glycogen Diazoxide & chlorothiazide Octreotide
Gastrinoma (Zollinger–Ellison syndrome)	Peptic ulceration	Diarrhoea Weight loss Malabsorption Dumping	Pancreas Duodenum	40–60	25	Gastrectomy Omeprazole H_2 receptor antagonists Octreotide
VIPoma (WDHA or Werner–Morrison syndrome)	*W*atery *d*iarrhoea *H*ypokalaemia *A*chlorhydria	Hypercalcaemia Hyperglycaemia Hypomagnesaemia	Pancreas Neuroblastoma SCLC Phaeochromocytoma	40	<5	Octreotide Glucocorticoids
Glucagonoma	Migratory necrolytic erythema Mild diabetes mellitus Muscle wasting Anaemia	Diarrhoea Thromboembolism Stomatitis Hypoaminoacidaemia Encephalitis	Pancreas (α cell)	60	<5	Octreotide Oral hypoglycaemics
Somatostatinoma	Diabetes mellitus Cholelithiasis Steatorrhoea Malabsorption	Anaemia Diarrhoea Weight loss Hypoglycaemia	Pancreas (β cells)	66	Case reports only	–
GRFoma	Acromegaly	–	Pancreas	?	Case reports only	Octreotide
PPoma	None	Diarrhoea Hypokalaemia Achlorhydria Weight loss	Pancreas	40	25	–

Abbreviations: SCLC, small cell lung cancer. VIP, vasoactive intestinal polypeptide. GRF, growth hormone releasing factor. PP, pancreatic polypeptide. MEN, multiple endocrine neoplasia. H_2, histamine type 2. WDHA, watery diarrhoea, hypokalaemia, achlorhydria.

little evidence to suggest that they control tumour growth. Resistance may develop with chronic use of octreotide and this is thought to occur due to the emergence of tumour cells lacking somatostatin receptors.

Octreotide therapy is well-tolerated; although initially abdominal cramps and diarrhoea may occur, significant steatorrhoea and malabsorption have not been observed.

Carcinoid syndrome

Carcinoid tumours arise from enterochromaffin cells principally in the gastrointestinal tract, pancreas, and lungs, but occasionally in the thymus and gonads. The incidence of these uncommon neoplasms is 1.5 per 100 000. The carcinoid syndrome develops in 6 to18 per cent of patients with these tumours[76] and these patients almost invariably have hepatic metastases.

The cardinal feature of carcinoid syndrome is the combination of diarrhoea and flushing, which occurs in at least 75 per cent, and may be associated with asthma, endomyocardial fibrosis, and pellagra. One-third of patients develop cardiac manifestations which are late complications, typically involve the right side of the heart, and lead to pulmonary valve stenosis and tricuspid valve regurgitation. Asthma and pellagra are less common. The pellagroid rash is thought to arise secondary to the diversion of tryptophan for 5-hydroxytryptamine (**5HT**) synthesis rather than nicotinamide production.[77] The clinical features are mediated by several potentially active substances secreted by the tumours including 5HT, 5-hydroxytryptophan, kallikrein, tachykinins (substance P, neuropeptide K), prostaglandins, catecholamines, and histamine.[78] The diagnosis is usually established by measuring the urinary excretion of 5-hydroxyindolacetic acid, a metabolite of 5HT. However, platelet 5HT levels are a more sensitive diagnostic test and are unaffected by diet.[79]

The pharmacological control of carcinoid syndrome is primarily directed at inhibiting the synthesis, release, and peripheral actions of circulating tumour products, principally 5HT (Fig. 3). The use of these agents remains empirical in view of the varied profiles of active substances released by different tumours. Parachlorophenyl-

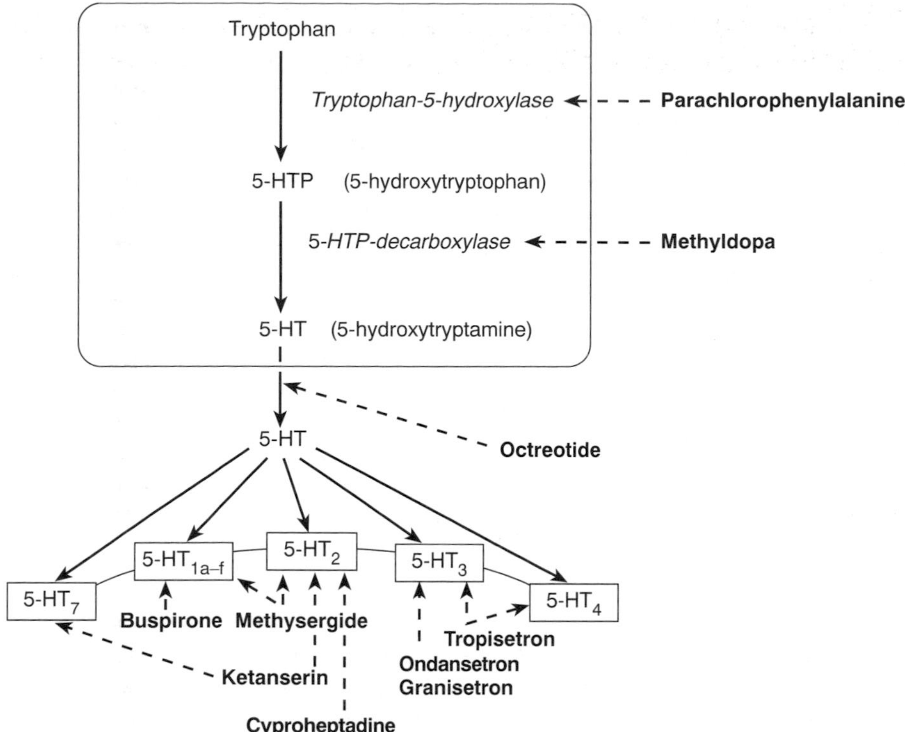

Fig. 3 Sites of action of drugs used to control carcinoid syndrome. Antagonists are in bold face type and their sites of action are marked by bold dashed arrows. Receptors are boxed.

alanine and methyldopa block 5HT synthesis but are poorly tolerated and, therefore, now rarely used. At least 16 5HT receptors have been cloned and most have been found to be G-protein coupled, although the $5HT_3$ receptor is a ligand-gated ion channel. The development of selective 5HT receptor ligands and antagonists will allow the investigation of the physiological roles of each receptor. However, the relevance of the different receptors in the clinical manifestations of the carcinoid syndrome remains uncertain and is obscured by the secretion of multiple products by these tumours. Of the drugs which block 5HT type 2 receptors, cyproheptadine (4–7 mg thrice daily) improves diarrhoea in 60 per cent of patients and flushing in 47 per cent. The mean duration of response to cyproheptadine is 8 months. In contrast, ketanserin (40–160 mg once daily) ameliorates flushing in 50 per cent but only 20 per cent find relief from diarrhoea. Selective $5HT_3$ receptor inhibitors has been shown to reduce diarrhoea in carcinoid syndrome. Metoclopramide and cisapride are believed to stimulate gastric motility via the $5HT_4$ receptor and antagonists of this receptor, which are in development, may prove useful in the palliation of carcinoid syndrome.

Octreotide is considered by most physicians to be the first line treatment of choice for patients with carcinoid syndrome. Doses of 50 to 150 mcg two or three times daily, subcutaneously reduces 5HT secretion and its peripheral action and is valuable in controlling both flushing and diarrhoea in the carcinoid syndrome. It produces initial relief of symptoms in 80 per cent.[80] A reduction in tumour rarely occurs, however, and the effects of treatment diminish with time.

Palliative debulking surgery may be offered to selected patients with metastatic disease as it can delay the development of the carcinoid syndrome. Hepatic artery embolization similarly can be employed and may produce good symptom palliation.[81] Alpha interferon has also been used successfully to palliate symptoms in carcinoid syndrome.[78] Finally, ^{131}I-*m*-iodobenzylguanidine has been used in patients with disabling symptoms in whom other therapeutic options have failed.[82]

Palliation of the clinical manifestations of carcinoid syndrome includes symptomatic therapy of diarrhoea (codeine phosphate, loperamide or diphenoxylate), β_2 adrenergic agonists for wheezing, and avoiding precipitating factors to reduce flushing (including alcohol and some foods).

Phaeochromocytoma

Phaeochromocytomas secrete catecholamines producing intermittent, episodic, or sustained hypertension and other clinical manifestations including anxiety, tremor, palpitations, sweating, flushing, headaches, gastrointestinal disturbances, and polyuria. These symptoms are all attributable to excessive adrenergic stimulation, and when surgery and chemotherapy are unable to control the disease, palliative treatment is usually achieved by α and β adrenergic receptor blockade. However, these tumours may elaborate and secrete other peptide hormones which may cause symptoms refractory to adrenergic inhibition, but this is rare. Initial treatment should be α blockade to control hypertension (e.g. phenoxybenzamine 10 mg twice daily) followed by β blockade to control tachycardia (e.g. propranolol 40 mg three times daily). This combination will control symptoms in most patients with malignant phaeochromocytoma. If palliation is not achieved despite full adrenergic receptor blockade, α-methylparatyrosine (metirosine) (250 mg twice daily increasing up to 4 g/day) may be used.

α-methyltyrosine is a competitive inhibitor of tyrosine hydroxylase, the rate limiting enzyme in catecholamine synthesis, and reduces catecholamine production by up to 75 per cent but it is poorly tolerated due to sedation, extrapyramidal effects, and diarrhoea. The noradrenaline analogue metiodobenzylguanidine is taken up by catecholamine synthesising tissues and ^{131}I- metiodobenzylguanidine is useful for imaging phaeochromocytomas. At higher doses ^{131}I-metiodobenzylguanidine may be used as therapy for phaeochromocytoma and neuroblastoma and it reduces catecholamine synthesis in patients with malignant phaeochromocytoma.[83]

Gonadotrophin secretion

Follicle stimulating hormone, luteinizing hormone, and human chorionic gonadotrophin (**hCG**) may be secreted by pituitary, trophoblastic, or germ cell tumours and ectopically by tumours arising in other organs. All three gonadotrophins are dimeric glycoproteins sharing the same β subunit with thyroid stimulating hormone but each has a unique α subunit which confers biological activity. The overproduction by tumours of gonadotrophins may result in precocious puberty in children, secondary amenorrhoea in women, gynaecomastia in men, and, rarely, hyperthyroidism. hCG is a valuable tumour marker for detecting and maintaining therapy in trophoblastic and germ cell tumours.

Precocious puberty

Central precocious puberty occurs with central nervous system tumours secreting gonadotrophins which activate the hypothalamic–pituitary axis. Incomplete or peripheral precocious puberty may result from hCG secretion by germinomas, teratomas, chorioepitheliomas, and hepatomas; and oestrogen or testosterone production by adrenal, testicular (Leydig cell), and ovarian (granulosa thecal cell) tumours. The treatment of precocious puberty includes psychological counselling for boys with increased aggression and excessive masturbation. Medical therapy is required to control both the psychosocial aspects and sustained effects on skeletal maturation. Central precocious puberty is amenable to gonadotrophin releasing hormone analogues which, following an initial phase of stimulation, lead to pituitary gonadotrophin receptor desensitization resulting in suppressed luteinizing hormone and follicle stimulating hormone secretion. The management of incomplete precocious puberty is more difficult and requires the use of antiandrogens (e.g. cyproterone acetate and spironolactone) and inhibitors of androgen synthesis (e.g. ketoconazole and finasteride).

Amenorrhoea

Secondary amenorrhoea in women with cancer may occasionally be a consequence of gonadotrophin, prolactin, oestrogen, or androgen secreting tumours although iatrogenic causes are far commoner. The vasomotor symptoms associated with menopause may be palliated by hormone replacement therapy and dyspareunia caused by vaginal atrophy may be alleviated by topical oestrogen preparations.

Gynaecomastia

Gynaecomastia in men with advanced cancer may be a consequence of drug therapy or tumour secretion of oestrogens or gonadotrophins. Alkylating agents, vinca alkaloids, nitrosureas, and antiemetics (including metoclopramide and phenothiazines) all cause gynaecomastia and should be considered as likely causes in patients with advanced cancer.

Oestrogens may be produced by adrenal or testicular tumours or may be synthesized from steroid precursors by hepatomas with high aromatase activity. The elevated, circulating oestrogen levels induce ductal, lobular, and alveolar growth of the breast leading to gynaecomastia. hCG secreting tumours (including testicular tumours, trophoblastic tumours, non-small cell lung cancers, hepatoma, and islet cell tumours of the pancreas) stimulate oestradiol production by interstitial and Sertoli cells of testes resulting in gynaecomastia. Symptomatic therapy for gynaecomastia should include cessation of any incriminated drugs and treatment of the primary tumour. Tamoxifen, clomiphene, topical dihydrotestosterone, and danazol have all been used with some success, as have liposuction,[84] subcutaneous mastectomy, and low dosage radiotherapy for palliation of painful gynaecomastia.[85]

Hyperthyroidism

On account of the structural similarities to thyroid stimulating hormone, hCG has intrinsic thyrotropic action via α thyroid stimulating hormone receptor spill-over effect.[86] Clinically overt hyperthyroidism caused by this mechanism only occurs with tumours secreting very large quantities of hCG, usually trophoblastic tumours.[87] The hyperthyroidism resolves after surgical removal of the tumour, and so palliation of the hyperthyroidism should be with drugs (e.g. carbimazole) rather than radioactive iodine or thyroidectomy.

Prolactin

Ectopic prolactin secretion from non-pituitary tumours is very rare and uncommonly causes galactorrhoea. Small cell lung cancer and renal cell adenocarcinoma have been described associated with elevated prolactin levels although the mechanism remains uncertain. Elevated serum prolactin levels are a poor prognostic indicator in women with breast cancer[88] and prolactin promotes the growth *in vitro* of human breast cancer cells. Galactorrhoea due to ectopic prolactin production may be treated by the dopaminergic agonist bromocriptine.

Oxytocin

The molecular biology of oxytocin resembles that of AVP with similar genes, precursor proteins, and transport by axonal streaming. Furthermore, ectopic secretion of both oxytocin and its carrier protein neurophysin I have been demonstrated in small cell lung cancer, usually in conjunction with ectopic AVP production. Although water intoxication and hyponatraemia may follow oxytocin infusions in women with obstetric problems, ectopic oxytocin secretion is not thought to contribute to SIAD nor any other clinical symptoms.

Pyrexia

Pyrexia is a common feature of terminal cancer and is usually attributable to infection or drugs. In only 5 per cent of cases is the fever related only to the cancer.[89] Malignancy accounted for only 7 per cent of cases in a series of 199 patients with pyrexias of unknown origin studied between 1980 and 1989.[90] This contribution is lower than found in previous studies and presumably reflects improvements in diagnostic techniques. Paraneoplastic pyrexia is a diagnosis of exclusion established after other causes of fever have been ruled out. Hodgkin's disease, renal cell adenocarcinoma, lymphoma, leukaemia, hepatoma, myxoma, and osteogenic sarcoma account for most cases of paraneoplastic fever.

Pathogenesis

Pyrexia is a consequence of endogenous pyrogens (including TNF, IL-1, and IL-6) stimulating the hypothalamic release of prostaglandin E_2 which mediates thermal homeostasis. Tumour related pyrexia is thought to be a consequence of cytokine production by neoplastic cells or by normal cells in response to tumour presence. Evidence for the former includes TNF-α production in Hodgkin's disease, which may be localized by *in vitro* hybridization to the Reed Sternberg cell.[91] Furthermore, the abnormal lymphocytes in Castleman's disease (an angiofollicular lymph node hyperplasia related to lymphoma and associated with fever) produce IL-6. After complete surgical excision of these tumours circulating plasma IL-6 is no longer detectable and symptoms resolve. In addition, mice transgenic for IL-6 develop a Castleman's disease-like condition with pyrexias[92] and monoclonal antibodies to IL-6 alleviate the systemic manifestations.[93] A similar mechanism has been elucidated in phaeochromocytoma where tumour cells produce IL-6 resulting in paraneoplastic pyrexia which resolves with tumour resection.[94] In addition, raised serum levels of TNF-α, IL-1, and IL-6 are found in patients with renal cell carcinoma and serum IL-6 may be used as a tumour marker in these patients.[95]

Therapy

Definitive therapy of the tumour will resolve paraneoplastic pyrexias in most cases of Hodgkin's disease and many lymphomas. Palliation of fever may be attempted by physical modalities such as sponging, ice-packs, and fans which often relieve discomfort. Pharmacological agents such as paracetamol, aspirin, non-steroidal anti-inflammatory drugs, and steroids are effective antipyretics.[96] The advances in understanding of the pathogenesis of paraneoplastic pyrexia propose a role for cytokine antagonists in therapy. The development of IL-1 false receptors is an attractive approach that has already been usurped by vaccinia virus; this virus secretes virally encoded IL-1β receptors which compete with endogenous receptor on T-lymphocytes thus attenuating the host response to infection.[97] Similarly strategies based upon IL-1 receptor antagonists including IL-1ra, which is structurally related to IL-1,[98] have been explored.[99]

Non-paraneoplastic complications

Hyperglycaemia

The prevalence of hyperglycaemia in cancer patients is higher than in the general population. It has repeatedly been claimed that diabetes mellitus is a risk factor for the development of pancreatic cancer. However, a recent multicentre study involving 720 patients failed to confirm this.[100] Several mechanisms may contribute to hyperglycaemia in advanced cancers including increased gluconeogenesis and Cori cycle activity, diminished glucose tolerance and turnover, and insulin resistance.[101] These changes may arise as a consequence of hepatic dysfunction, altered glucose metabolism by tumour cells, and the secretion of insulin antagonists. Furthermore, the frequent usage of corticosteroids in palliative medicine may contribute since one in five patients on high-dose steroids will develop steroid-induced diabetes mellitus.

The conventional treatment of diabetes advocates tight control of blood sugars to delay the onset of diabetic complications including neuropathy, retinopathy, and nephropathy. In contrast the aims of therapy in palliative care are to minimize symptoms associated with hypoglycaemia or marked hyperglycaemia. For this reason a wider range of blood sugars is acceptable and close blood glucose monitoring is unnecessary.

Weight loss and anorexia reduce the need for hypoglycaemic agents as cancer progresses, and strict dietary restrictions are neither kind nor valuable. Oral hypoglycaemic drugs can usually be reduced or stopped in non-insulin dependent diabetics without symptomatic hyperglycaemia ensuing. Similarly, insulin requirements of insulin dependent diabetics with advanced malignancy reduce and insulin regimens can usually be simplified to once daily, long-acting insulin injections (e.g. Ultratard, Insulatard). Blood sugars may be run on the high side to prevent the distressing symptoms of hypoglycaemia. Where possible, monitoring should be performed by urinalysis rather than blood sampling. Steroid-induced diabetes, which occurs frequently in advanced cancer, is usually asymptomatic and requires no therapy; however, if polyuria and polydipsia develop a short acting sulphonylurea may be useful (e.g. gliclazide 40–80 mg once daily).

Renal failure

Renal failure is a common feature of advanced malignancy and many aetiological factors play a role in its pathogenesis (Table 4). In the context of incurable malignant disease few of the conventional therapies for renal failure are applicable.

Metabolic causes of acute renal failure include urate nephropathy and tumour lysis syndrome which are usually features of early malignancy, requiring specific treatment. Hypercalcaemic nephropathy should also be treated actively to alleviate symptoms as discussed above. The remaining causes of renal failure including metabolic, iatrogenic, paraneoplastic, and infiltration are not amenable to specific measures. Prerenal and obstructive renal failure should be considered as potentially reversible, although treatment is frequently not appropriate. All patients with malignant disease and symptomatic renal failure should be investigated to exclude hypercalcaemia, prerenal, and obstructive causes as these require different treatments.[102]

The mainstay of palliation in renal failure is correction of fluid imbalance although this should not be pursued overzealously. Dehydration in this context need not be uncomfortable and the reduced urinary output may be welcomed by patients and their carers. The dry mouth, nausea, uraemic itching, and anorexia which accompany renal failure should be treated as mentioned elsewhere (Chapters 9.3.1 and 9.10). In patients with a better prognosis reduction in the dietary protein content reduces the symptoms of anorexia, nausea, and vomiting. If this approach is employed for adult patients a diet of no less than 0.6 g protein per kg of body weight is advocated and essential keto amino acid supplements should be given. Obstructive nephropathy may cause colicky pain in addition to the non-specific symptoms of renal failure. Although analgesics and antispasmodics may ameliorate the pain, prompt relief of symptoms is best achieved by percutaneous nephrostomy. This procedure may be performed under sedation

Table 4 Causes of renal failure in malignancy

1. Infiltration by tumour
2. Fluid imbalance
3. Electrolyte imbalance
    - Uric acid (tumour lysis syndrome)
    - Hypercalcaemia
    - Paraprotein (e.g. myeloma)
    - Amyloid (e.g. myeloma)
    - Lysozyme (e.g. acute myelomonocytic leukaemia)
    - Mucoprotein (e.g. pancreatic adenocarcinoma)
    - Nephrogenic diabetes insipidus (e.g. leiomyosarcoma)
4. Urinary tract obstruction
5 Iatrogenic
    - Chemotherapy
    - Radiotherapy
6 Paraneoplastic
    - Membranous glomerulonephritis (e.g. carcinomas)
    - Minimal change glomerulonephritis (e.g. Hodgkin's disease)
    - Membranoproliferative glomerulonephritis (e.g. non-Hodgkin's lymphoma)

and subsequent dilation of the obstruction by antegrade passage of catheters via the percutaneous tract may be undertaken. Nephrostomy tube insertion provides rapid effective palliation for urinary obstruction, but this procedure requires hospitalization and is an invasive procedure which should, therefore, not be undertaken without careful consideration. Renal support with diuretics, renovasodilators, and dialysis is inappropriate management in these patients.

Liver failure

Liver failure in cancer patients is usually a consequence of extensive hepatic metastases, biliary obstruction, or drug therapy, although a paraneoplastic hepatopathy has been described in patients with renal cell adenocarcinoma.[103] After excluding the latter causes, it is important to differentiate obstructive and parenchymal causes as the approach to palliation differs.

Obstructive jaundice may be differentiated from other causes by the detection of urinary bilirubin in the absence of urobilinogen. Biliary obstruction may be confirmed by ultrasonography and drainage may be undertaken to relieve jaundice and associated symptoms (anorexia, nausea, pruritus) (see Chapter 9.6.2). Biliary drainage may be obtained by percutaneous transhepatic biliary drainage or endoscopic retrograde biliary drainage, and both techniques provide good palliation.

Hepatic failure due to metastases may produce jaundice, pruritis, anorexia, liver capsular pain, ascites, disturbances of haemostasis, malabsorption, and electrolyte disturbances, culminating in hepatic encephalopathy.

The palliative treatment of hepatic metastases needs to be tailored to the particular symptoms of each patient. Anorexia and malaise may be relieved by corticosteroids which may also alleviate capsular pain. Prednisolone (20–30 mg daily) is usually adequate; however, muscle wasting will develop within a few weeks on this dosage and may be profound (see Chapter 9.3.1). Phenothiazines and metoclopramide may reduce nausea especially when administered preprandium. Pruritus may be reduced by cholestyramine (4 g four times daily) which binds dihydroxy bile salts in the bowel preventing their reabsorption. It is unpleasant to take and is ineffective in total biliary obstruction where no bile salts reach the gut (see Chapter 9.6.2).

Hepatic encephalopathy is thought to arise due to an excess of γ-aminobutyric acid (GABA) activity, ammonia, and other toxins in the central nervous system. Conventional therapies for hepatic encephalopathy include dietary protein and sodium restriction, bowel clearance with magnesium sulphate enemas and lactulose, as well as bowel sterilization with neomycin in an attempt to reduce ammonia production by gut microflora. Since hepatic encephalopathy is a terminal event in the context of advanced malignancy, these unpleasant treatments are rarely appropriate. The main symptom of encephalopathy is confusion, and after establishing the cause of confusion, familiar company, a light and quiet environment, and a regular routine should be provided. Explanation, reassurance, and reorientation are essential and it should always be assumed that the patient understands. Sedation is only necessary if patients are agitated and should not be routinely used. Under these circumstances, haloperidol (0.5–5 mg) may be given orally, subcutaneously, or intravenously, hourly until the patient settles.

The combination of portal hypertension and abnormal coagulation in liver failure predisposes to gastrointestinal haemorrhage which is a frequent cause of death in these patients. Major haemorrhage should not be managed aggressively; if the patient remains conscious, intravenous diamorphine (5–10 mg), diazepam (5–10 mg), and midazolam (5–10 mg) ease fear and distress.

Lactic acidosis

Type B lactic acidosis is a rare complication of malignancy which presents clinically with hyperventilation and hypotension. In most cases the underlying malignancy is haematological. Increased lactate production by tumour cells owing to uncoupled oxidative phosphorylation and glycolysis, and reduced lactate clearance due to liver dysfunction have both been implicated in the pathogenesis of malignancy-associated lactic acidosis. The diagnosis is established biochemically by the combination of wide anion gap acidosis and raised plasma lactate (>2 mEq/l). Intravenous isotonic (1.26 per cent) sodium bicarbonate may be used to correct the metabolic acidosis but should only be used if effective anticancer therapy is to be attempted.[104]

References

1. Suematsu S, Matsusaka T, Matsuda T, Ohno S, Miyazaki J, Yamamura K. Generation of plasmacytomas with the chromosomal translocation t(12;15) in Interleukin-6 transgenic mice. *Proceedings of the National Academy of Sciences USA*, 1992; **89**: 232–5.
2. Roodman GD, Kurihara N, Ohsaki Y, Kukita A, Hosking D, Demulder A. Interleukin-6: A potential autocrine/paracrine factor in Paget's disease of bone. *Journal of Clinical Investigation*, 1992; **89**: 46–52.
3. Jilka RL, *et al.* Increased osteoclast development after estrogen loss: mediation by interleukin-6. *Science*, 1992; **257**: 88–91.
4. Girasole G, *et al.* 17β-estradiol inhibits interleukin-6 production by bone marrow-derived stromal cells and osteoblasts in vitro: a potential mechanism for the antiosteoporotic effect of estrogens. *Journal of Clinical Investigation*, 1992; **89**: 883–91.
5. Strassmann G, Jacob C, Fong M, Bertolini D. Mechanisms of paraneoplastic syndromes of colon-26; involvement of interleukin 6 in hypercalcaemia. *Cytokine*, 1993; **5**: 463–8.
6. Felix R, Fleisch H, Elford P. Bone resobing cytokines enhance release of macrophage colony-stimulating activity by the osteoblastic cell line MC3T3-E1. *Calciferous Tissue International.*, 1989; **44**: 356.
7. Merryman J, DeWille J, Werkmeister J, Capen C, Rosol T. Effects of transforming growth factor beta on parathyroid hormone-related protein production and ribonucleic acid expression by a squamous carcinoma cell line in vitro. *Endocrinology*, 1994; **134**: 2424–30.
8. Laforga J, Vierna J, Aranda F. Hypercalcaemia in Hodgkin's disease related to prostaglandin synthesis. *Journal of Clinical Pathology*, 1994; **47**: 567–8.
9. Benitez-Verguizas J, Esbrit P. Proliferative effect of parathyroid hormone-related protein on the hypercalcaemic Walker 256 carcinoma cell line. *Biochemical and Biophysical Research Communication.*, 1994; **198**: 1281–9.
10. Li X, Drucker D. Parathyroid hormone-related peptide is a downstream target for ras and src activation. *Journal of Biological Chemistry*, 1994; **269**: 6263–6.
11. Danks J, *et al.* Parathyroid hormone-related protein of cancer: immunohistochemical localisation in cancers and in normal skin. *Journal of Bone and Mineral Research*, 1989; **4**: 273–8.
12. Honda S, *et al.* Expression of parathyroid hormone-related protein mRNA in tumours obtained from patients with humoral hypercalcaemia of malignancy. *Japanese Journal of Cancer Research*, 1988; **79**: 677–83.
13. Budayr A, *et al.* Increased serum levels of a parathyroid hormone-like protein in malignancy-associated hypercalcaemia. *Annals of Internal Medicine*, 1989; **111**: 807–12.
14. Hutchesson AC, Dunne F, Bundred NJ, Gee H, Ratcliffe WA. Parathyroid hormone-related protein as a tumour marker in humoral hypercalcaemia associated with occult malignancy. *Postgraduate Medical Journal*, 1993; **69**: 640–2.
15. Savage M, *et al.* Hypercalcaemia due to parathyroid hormone-related protein: long-term circulating levels may not reflect tumour activity. *Clinical Endocrinology (Oxford)*, 1993; **39**: 695–8.
16. Bouizar Z, Spyratos F, Deytieux S, de Vennejoul M, Jullienne A. Polymerase chain reaction analysis of parathyroid hormone-related protein gene expression in breast cancer patients and occurence of bone metastases. *Cancer Research*, 1993; **53**: 5076–8.
17. Kukreja S, *et al.* Antibodies to parathyroid hormone-related protein lower serum calcium in athymic mouse models of malignancy associated hypercalcaemia of cancer. *Journal of Clinical Investigation*, 1988; **82**: 1798–802.
18. Burtis W, *et al.* Immunocytochemical characterisation of circulating parathyroid hormone-related protein in patients with humoral hypercalcaemia of malignancy. *New England Journal of Medicine*, 1990; **322**: 1106–12.
19. Mitnick M, Isales C, Paliwal I, Insogna K. Parathyroid hormone-related protein stimulates prostaglandin E_2 release from osteoblast-like cells: modulating effect of peptide length. *Journal of Bone and Mineral Research*, 1992; **7**: 887–96.
20. Jacobsen J, Bringhurst F, Harris N, Weitzman S, Aisenberg A. Humoral hypercalcaemia in Hodgkin's disease. Clinical and laboratory evaluation. *Cancer*, 1989; **63**: 917–23.
21. Davies M, Hayes M, Yin J, Berry J, Mawer E. Abnormal synthesis of 1,25-dihydroxyvitamin D in patients with malignant lymphoma. *Journal of Clinical Endocrinology and Metabolism*, 1994; **78**: 1202–7.
22. Gucalp R, *et al.* Comparative study of pamidronate disodium and etidronate disodium in the treatment of cancer-related hypercalcaemia. *Journal of Clinical Oncology*, 1992; **10**: 134–42.
23. Walls J, Ratcliffe W, Howell A, Bundred N. Response to intravenous bisphosphonate therapy in hypercalcaemic patients with and without bone metastases: the role of parathyroid hormone-related protein. *British Journal of Cancer*, 1994; **70**: 169–72.
24. Wimalwansa S. Significance of plasma PTH-rp in patients with hypercalcaemia of malignancy treated with bisphosphonate. *Cancer*, 1994; **73**: 2223–30.
25. Morton A, Howell A. Bisphosphonates and bone metastases. *British Journal of Cancer*, 1988; **58**: 556–7.
26. Bockman R, *et al.* Distribution of trace levels of therapeutic gallium in bone as mapped by synchrotron x-ray microscopy. *Proceedings of the National Academy of Sciences USA*, 1990; **87**: 4149–53.
27. Warrell R, Israel R, Frisone M, Snyder T, Gaynor J, Bockman R. A randomised double-blind study of gallium nitrate versus calcitonin for acute treatment of cancer-related hypercalcaemia. *Annals of Internal Medicine*, 1988; **108**: 669–74.
28. Warrell R, Heller G, Murphy W, Schulman P, O'Dwyer P. A randomised double-blind study of gallium nitrate compared to etidronate for acute control of cancer related hypercalcemia. *Journal of Clinical Oncology*, 1991; **9**: 1467–75.
29. Sato K, *et al.* Passive immunisation with anti-parathyroid hormone-related protein monoclonal antibody markedly prolongs survival time of hypercalcemic nude mice bearing transplanted human PTHrP-producing tumors. *Journal of Bone and Mineral Research*, 1993; **8**: 849–60.
30. Yoneda T, *et al.* Herbimycin A, a pp60c-src tyrosine kinase inhibitor, inhibits osteoclastic bone resorbtion in vitro and hypercalcemia in vivo. *Journal of Clinical Investigation*, 1993; **91**: 2791–5.
31. King K, *et al.* Effects of kistrin on bone resorption in vitro and serum calcium in vivo. *Journal of Bone and Mineral Research*, 1994; **9**: 381–7.
32. Hale A, *et al.* A case of pituitary-dependent Cushing's disease with clinical and biochemical features of ectopic ACTH syndrome. *Clinical Endocrinology*, 1985; **22**: 479–88.
33. Pullan P, *et al.* Ectopic production of methionine enkephalin and beta endorphin. *British Medical Journal*, 1980; **280**: 758–9.
34. Chatikhine VA, *et al.* Expression of opioid peptides in cells and stroma of human breast cancer and adenofibromas. *Cancer Letter*, 1994; **77**: 51–6.
35. Jeffcoate W, Silverstone J, Edwards C, Besser G. Psychiatric mainfestations of Cushing's syndrome:response to lowering of plasma cortisol. *Quarterly Journal of Medicine*, 1979; **48**: 465–72.
36. Howlett T, Drury P, Perry L, Doniach I, Rees L, Besser G. Diagnosis and management of ACTH-dependent Cushing's syndrome: a comparison of the features in ectopic and pituitary ACTH production. *Clinical Endocrinology (Oxford)*, 1986; **24**: 699–713.
37. Delisle L, *et al.* Ectopic corticotropin syndrome and small-cell carcinoma of the lung. Clinical features, outcome, and complications. *Archives of Internal Medicine*, 1993; **153**: 746–52.
38. Abeloff M, Trump D, Baylin S. Ectopic adrenocorticotrophin (ACTH) syndrome and small cell carcinoma of the lung: assessment of clinical implications in patients on combination chemotherapy. *Cancer*, 1981; **48**: 1082–7.

39. Hansen M, Hammer M, Hammer L. ACTH, ADH and calcitonin concentrations as markers of response and relapse in small cell carcinoma of lung. *Cancer*, 1980; **46**: 2062–7.
40. Chrousos G, Schulte H, Oldfield E, Gold P, Cutler G, Loriaux D. The corticotropin-releasing factor stimulation test. An aid in the evaluation of patients with Cushing's syndrome. *New England Journal of Medicine*, 1984; **310**: 622–6.
41. Oldfield E, *et al.* Preoperative lateralisation of ACTH-secreting pituitary microadenomas by bilateral and simultaneous inferior petrosal venous sinus sampling. *New England Journal of Medicine*, 1985; **312**: 100–3.
42. Kaye T, Crapo L. The Cushing syndrome: an update on diagnostic tests. *Annals of Internal Medicine*, 1990; **112**: 434–44.
43. de Herder W, *et al.* Somatostatin receptor scintigraphy: its value in tumor localization in patients with Cushing's syndrome caused by ectopic corticotropin or corticotropin-releasing hormone secretion. *American Journal of Medicine*, 1994; **96**: 305–12.
44. Jacobsson H, Wallin G, Werner S, Larsson SA. Technetium-99m methoxyisobutylisonitrile localizes an ectopic ACTH-producing tumour: case report and review of the literature. *European Journal of Nuclear Medicine*, 1994; **21**: 582–6.
45. Carey R, *et al.* Ectopic secretion of corticotrophin-releasing factor as a cause of Cushing's syndrome: a clinical, morphologic and biochemical study. *New England Journal of Medicine*, 1984; **311**: 13–20.
46. Child D, Burke C, Burley D, Rees L, Fraser T. Drug control of Cushing's syndrome. Combined aminoglutethamide metyrapone therapy. *Acta Endocrinology*, 1976; **82**: 330–41.
47. Hoffman D, Boigham B. The use of ketoconazole in ectopic adrenocorticotropic hormone syndrome. *Cancer*, 1991; **67**: 1447–9.
48. Farrell W, Clark A, Stewart M, Crosby S, White A. Bromocriptine inhibits pro-opiomelancortin mRNA and ACTH precursor secretion in small cell lung cancer cell lines. *Journal of Clinical Investigation*, 1992; **90**: 705–10.
49. Rieu M, Rosilio M, Richard A, Vannetzel JM, Kuhn JM. Paradoxical effect of somatostatin analogues on the ectopic secretion of corticotropin in two cases of small cell lung carcinoma. *Hormone Research*, 1993; **39**: 207–12.
50. Miller JW, Crapo L. The medical treatment of Cushing's syndrome. *Endocrinology Review*, 1993; **14**: 443–58.
51. Spampinato S, Canossa M, Carboni L, Campana G, Leanza G, Ferri S. Inhibition of proopiomelanocortin expression by an oligodeoxynucleotide complementary to beta-endorphin mRNA. *Proceedings of the National Academy of Sciences USA*, 1994; **91**: 8072–6.
52. Verbalis J. Hyponatraemia. *Baillière's Clinical Endocrinology and Metabolism*, 1989; **3**: 499–530.
53. Smitz S, Legros J, Franchimont P, Le Maire M. Identification of vasopressin-like peptides in the plasma of a patient with the syndrome of inappropriate secretion of antidiuretic hormone and an oat cell carcinoma. *Acta Endocrinology (Copenhagen)*, 1988; **119**: 567–74.
54. Hansen M, Hammer M, Hummer L. Diagnostic and therapeutic implications of ectopic hormone production in small cell lung cancer. *Thorax*, 1980; **35**: 101–6.
55. Comis R, Miller M, Ginsberg S. Abnormalities in water homeostasis in small cell anaplastic lung cancer. *Cancer*, 1980; **45**: 2414–21.
56. North W, Ware J, Maurer L, Chatrinian A, Perry M. Neurophysins as tumour markers for small cell carcinoma of the lung. A cancer and leukemia group B evaluation. *Cancer*, 1988; **62**: 1343–7.
57. Friedmann AS, Memoli VA, North WG. Vasopressin and oxytocin production by non-neuroendocrine lung carcinomas: an apparent low incidence of gene expression. *Cancer Letter*, 1993; **75**: 79–85.
58. Friedmann AS, Malott KA, Memoli VA, Pai SI, Yu XM, North WG. Products of vasopressin gene expression in small-cell carcinoma of the lung. *British Journal of Cancer*, 1994; **69**: 260–3.
59. List A, *et al.* The syndrome of inappropriate secretion of anti-diuretic hormone in small cell lung cancer. *Journal of Clinical Oncology*, 1986; **4**: 1191–8.
60. Cohen M, *et al.* Chemotherapy rather than demeclocycline for inappropriate secretion of antidiuretic hormone. *New England Journal of Medicine*, 1978; **298**: 1423.
61. Srensen J, Kristjansen P, Osterlind K, Hammer M, Hansen M. Syndrome of inappropriate antidiuresis in small cell lung cancer. Classification and effect of tumour regression. *Acta Medica Scandanavica*, 1987; **222**: 155–61.
62. Hojer J. Management of symptomatic hyponatraemia: dependence on the duration of development. *Journal of Internal Medicine*, 1994; **235**: 497–501.
63. Cohen I, Warren S, Skowsky W. Occult pulmonary malignancy in syndrome of inappropriate ADH secretion with normal ADH levels. *Chest*, 1984; **86**: 929–31.
64. Sterns R. The treatment of hyponatremia: first, do no harm. *American Journal of Medicine*, 1990; **88**: 557–60.
65. Chitmans F, Meinders A. Management of severe hyponatremia: rapid or slow correction. *American Journal of Medicine*, 1990; **88**: 161–6.
66. Sterns R. Severe symptomatic hyponatremia: treatment and outcome. *Annals of Internal Medicine*, 1987; **107**: 656–64.
67. Ayus J, Olivero J, Frommer J. Rapid correction of severe hyponatremia with intravenous hypertonic saline solution. *American Journal of Medicine*, 1982; **72**: 43–8.
68. Decaux G, Prospert F, Penninckx R, Namias B, Soupart A. 5-year treatment of the chronic syndrome of inappropriate secretion of ADH with oral urea. *Nephron*, 1993; **63**: 468–70.
69. Fujisawa G, Ishikawa S, Tsuboi Y, Okada K, Saito T. Therapeutic efficacy of non-peptide ADH antagonist OPC-31260 in SIADH rats. *Kidney International*, 1993; **44**: 19–23.
70. Cogan E, *et al.* High levels of atrial natriuretic factor in SIADH. *Lancet*, 1986; **ii**: 1258–9.
71. Kamoi K, *et al.* Hyponatraemia in small cell lung cancer. Mechanisms not involving inappropriate ADH secretion. *Cancer*, 1987; **60**: 1089–93.
72. Yoshinaga K, Yamaguchi K, Abe K, Inoue T, Mishima Y. Production of immunoreactive atrial natriuretic polypeptide in neuroendocrine tumors. *Cancer*, 1994; **73**: 1292–6.
73. Kiang D, Baner G, Kennedy B. Immunoassayable insulin in carcinoma of the cervix associated with hypoglycaemia. *Cancer*, 1973; **31**: 801–5.
74. Gorden P, *et al.* Hypoglycemia associated with non-islet cell tumor and insulin-like growth factors. *New England Journal of Medicine*, 1981; **305**: 1452–5.
75. Lamberts S, *et al.* Parallel in vivo and in vitro detection of functional somatostatin receptors in human endocrine pancreatic tumors: consequences with regard to diagnosis, localization, and therapy. *Journal of Clinical Investigation*, 1990; **71**: 566–74.
76. Feldman J. Carcinoid tumours and syndrome. *Seminars in Oncology*, 1987; **14**: 237–46.
77. Vinik A, McLeod M, Fig L, Shapiro B, Lloyd R, Cho K. Clinical features, diagnosis and localization of carcinoid tumors and their management. *Gastroenterology Clinics of North America*, 1989; **18**: 865–96.
78. de Vries E, *et al.* Recent developments in the diagnosis and treatment of metastatic carcinoid tumours. *Scandanavian Journal of Gastroenterology*, 1993; **28**: 87–93.
79. Kema I, Schellings A, Meiborg G, Hoppenbrouwers C, Muskiet F. Influence of a serotonin and dopamine rich diet on platelet serotonin content and urinary excretion of biogenic amines and their metabolites. *Clinical Chemistry*, 1992; **38**: 1730–6.
80. Kvols L, Reub J. Metastatic carcinoid tumours and the malignant carcinoid syndrome. *Acta Oncologica*, 1993; **32**: 197–201.
81. Moertel C, *et al.* Hepatic arterial occlusion alone and sequenced with chemotherapy in the management of patients with advanced carcinoid tumors and islet cell carcinomas. *Annals of Internal Medicine*, 1993; **120**: 302–9.
82. Shapiro B. Summary, conclusions and future directions of ^{131}I-metaiodobenzylguanidine therapy in the treatment of neural crest tumors. *Journal of Nuclear Biological Medicine*, 1991; **35**: 357.
83. Shapiro B. Uses of MIBG in catecholamine-secreting tumours. *Ballière's Clinical Endocrinology and Metabolism*, 1993; **7**: 500–7.

84. Dolsky R. Gynaecomastia. Treatment by liposuction subcutaneous mastectomy. *Dermatological Clinics*, 1990; **8**: 469–78.
85. Wilson J. Gynecomastia-a continuing dilemma. *New England Journal of Medicine*, 1991; **324**: 334–5.
86. Fradkin J, Eastman R, Lesniak M, Roth J. Specificity spillover at the hormone receptor-exploring its role in human disease. *New England Journal of Medicine*, 1989; **320**: 640–5.
87. Giralt SA, Dexeus F, Amato R, Sella A, Logothetis C. Hyperthyroidism in men with germ cell tumors and high levels of beta-human chorionic gonadotrophin. *Cancer*, 1992; **69**: 1286–90.
88. Dowsett M, McGarrick G, Harris A, Coombes R, Smith I, Jeffcoate S. Prognostic significance of serum prolactin levels in advanced breast cancer. *British Journal of Cancer*, 1983; **47**: 763–9.
89. Petersdorf R. Fever and cancer. *Hospital Medicine*, 1965; **1**: 2–10.
90. Knockaert D, Vanneste L, Vanneste S, Bobbaers H. Fever of unknown origin in the 1980s. *Archives of Internal Medicine*, 1992; **152**: 51–5.
91. Kretschmer C, *et al.* Tumor necrosis factor alpha and lymphotoxin production in Hodgkin's disease. *American Journal of Pathology*, 1990; **137**: 341–51.
92. Brand S, Bodine D, Duncar C, Nienhuis A. Dysregulated interleukin 6 expression produces a syndrome resembling Castleman's disease in mice. *Journal of Clinical Investigation*, 1990; **86**: 592–9.
93. Beck JT, *et al.* Alleviation of systemic manifestations of Castleman's disease by monoclonal anti-interleukin-6 antibody. *New England Journal of Medicine*, 1994; **330**: 602–4.
94. Fukumoto S, Matsumo T, Harada S, Fujisaki J, Kawano M, Ogata E. Phaeochromocytoma with pyrexia and marked inflammatory signs: a paraneoplastic syndrome with possible relation to interleukin 6 production. *Journal of Clinical Endocrinology and Metabolism*, 1991; **73**: 871–81.
95. Dosquet C, *et al.* Tumour necrosis factor a, interleukin 1b and interleukin 6 in patients with renal cell carcinoma. *European Journal of Cancer*, 1994; **30**: 162–7.
96. Styrt B, Sugarman B. Antipyresis and fever. *Archives of Internal Medicine*, 1990; **150**: 1589–97.
97. Alcami A, Smith GL. A soluble receptor for interleukin-1β encoded by vaccinia virus: a novel mechanism of virus modulation of the host response to infection. *Cell*, 1992; **71**: 153–67.
98. Eisenberg SP, Brewer MT, Verderber E, Heimdal P, Brandhuber BJ, Thompson RC. Interleukin 1 receptor antagonist is a member of the interleukin 1 gene family: evolution of a cytokine control mechanism. *Proceedings of the National Academy of Sciences USA*, 1991; **88**: 5232–6.
99. Coceani F, Lees J, Redford J, Bishai I. Interleukin-1 receptor antagonist: effectiveness against interleukin-1 fever. *Canadian Journal of Physiology and Pharmacology*, 1992; **70**: 1590–6.
100. Gullo L, Pezzilli R, Morselli-Labate A, and the Italian Pancreatic Study Group. Diabetes and the risk of pancreatic cancer. *New England Journal of Medicine*, 1994; **331**: 81–4.
101. Nelson K, Walsh D, Sheehan F. The cancer anorexia-cachexia syndrome. *Journal of Clinical Oncology*, 1994; **12**: 213–25.
102. Garrick M, Mayer R. Acute renal failure associated with neoplastic disease and its treatment. *Seminars in Oncology*, 1978; **5**: 155–65.
103. Cronin R, *et al.* Renal cell carcinoma: unusual systemic manifestations. *Medicine*, 1976; **55**: 291–311.
104. Doolittle G, Wurster M, Rosenfeld C, Bodensteiner D. Malignancy-induced lactic acidosis. *Southern Medical Journal*, 1988; **81**: 533–6.

9.12 Neurological problems

Augusto Caraceni and Cinzia Martini

Introduction

Neurological complications in advanced progressive diseases, such as cancer and AIDS, occur frequently and therefore an adequate neurological assessment must always be part of patient evaluation in palliative medicine. Chronic debilitating neurological disease with a poor prognosis needs adequate palliative treatment to control physical symptoms and suffering.

Pain, a frequent occurrence in AIDS and cancer, is a traditional focus of palliative medicine. It always requires neurological evaluation to clarify the pathophysiology and cause. Correct diagnosis of the pain syndrome is necessary in order to achieve successful treatment and anticipate complications

Neurological complications of cancer

Neurological complications are estimated to occur in up to 20 per cent of patients with cancer.[1] In a large consultation survey conducted at a comprehensive cancer centre the most frequent complaints were pain and altered mental status (Table 1).[2]

Table 1 Cancer and cancer treatment related neurological diagnoses in 851 patients with cancer*

Diagnosis	Percentage
Brain metastasis	15.9
Metabolic or drug related encephalopathy	10.2
Pain associated with bone metastasis	9.9
Epidural tumour	8.5
Tumour plexopathy	5.8
Leptomeningeal metastasis	5.1
Chemotherapy peripheral neuropathy	3.2
Radiculopathy	2.7
Base-of-skull metastasis	2.7
Seizures due to metastasis	2.7
Seizures not due to metastasis	1.8
Paraneoplastic syndromes	1.2
Intracranial haemorrhage related to thrombocytopenia	1.3
Radiation myelopathy	1.2
Radiation plexopathy	1.1
Intracranial haemorrhage from tumour	0.6

* Modified from Clouston *et al.*, 1992.[2] A total of 1042 diagnoses were given with up to three per patient. Among the non-cancer related diagnoses cerebrovascular disease, headache, and degenerative spine disease were the most common diagnoses.

Brain metastases

Pathology

Intracranial metastases are found at autopsy in about 25 per cent of patients who died of cancer.[3] Other common intracranial lesions involve the skull and meninges. The choroid plexus and the pituitary are less commonly affected. There is evidence that the incidence of brain metastases and leptomeningeal metastases is increasing, because of better control of systemic disease and longer survival allowing 'sanctuary' cells in the central nervous system to grow and cause symptoms.[4] Lung cancer, melanoma, and breast cancer are the primary tumours most frequently associated with metastatic spread to the brain parenchyma. Tumours such as melanoma usually cause multiple lesions, while breast cancer more often causes single lesions (some 50 per cent of breast cancer patients have a single lesion and 20 per cent two lesions). It is important to bear this in mind when planning surgery or focal radiation treatment.

Brain metastases usually originate from tumours via neoplastic emboli. Tumour emboli lodge in the white matter at the grey/white matter junction where they grow as spherical masses displacing, rather than infiltrating, the brain and causing symptoms by various mechanisms. They usually involve the watershed territories at the end of the arterial supply. In general, their distribution in the brain relates to the cerebral vasculature and thus the supratentorial regions are more often affected (85 per cent of all central nervous system metastases). However, vasculature is not the only factor to influence the metastatic process. For example some pelvic tumours tend to metastasize to the posterior fossa and the cerebellum (53 per cent of central nervous system metastases from pelvic tumours, excluding gastrointestinal tumours).

The most common effect of a metastatic lesion on the surrounding brain tissue is oedema associated with disruption of the blood–brain barrier. Intracranial pressure may be increased and may contribute to symptoms by compression of brain structures remote from the lesion itself. Symptoms can, therefore, be caused by the lesion destroying or compressing the brain tissue locally, by the surrounding oedema, or by cerebral herniation.

Metastases from melanoma, choriocarcinoma, and cancer of the testis are more often associated with seizures, possibly because these lesions are often haemorrhagic and, in the case of melanoma, tend to invade the grey matter.

Table 2 Symptoms and signs due to cerebral metastases in 162 patients

Symptoms	Percentage	Signs	Percentage
Headache	53	Hemiparesis	66
Focal weakness	40	Impaired cognition	77
Mental change	31	Unilateral sensory loss	27
Seizures	15	Papilloedema	26
Ataxia	20	Ataxia	24
Aphasia	10	Aphasia	19

From Posner (1980).[7]

Clinical course

Median survival is about 2 months from diagnosis if no treatment is given, depending on tumour type.[5,6] Brain metastases are often the direct cause of death (a common situation in breast cancer patients)[6] but patients responding to brain radiotherapy usually die of their systemic disease.

Signs and symptoms at presentation are listed in Table 2. Symptoms can present progressively and deceptively or alternatively can be sudden and 'stroke-like'. It should be remembered that in many patients formal neurological tests of strength and mental function will reveal signs of changes in the central nervous system that are not otherwise apparent.[7]

Headache is an important symptom—usually of a dull aching quality and moderate intensity. It is caused by compression or traction of intracranial pain-sensitive structures. With supratentorial lesions it is often bifrontal, although it can occur on one side—always that of the tumour. Headache occurs more frequently and is more severe with infratentorial lesions and in this case is referred to the nuchal region and the neck.

Intracranial pressure is not always elevated but when it is clinical features are distinctive. They include severe headache, nausea and vomiting, and resistance to common analgesics. Raised intracranial pressure is more common with lesions of the posterior fossa and can be associated with neck pain. Sudden exacerbations of headache are characteristic of transitory rises in intracranial pressure ('plateau waves') and respond to immediate administration of bolus injection dexamethasone.[8]

Treatment

Options should include the provision of supportive treatment only.[9] Decisions should be taken after considering:

(1) the type of cancer and its sensitivity to radiation and chemotherapy;

(2) the neurological status of the patient;

(3) the extent of systemic disease and its associated symptoms and the expected quality of life.

Surgery is indicated only for single metastases with limited or no systemic disease, especially with radioresistant tumours.[6,9–11] Whole brain irradiation produces neurological improvement in the majority of patients but survival after treatment is only 4 to 6 months (see Chapter 9.1.2).[12] Metastases from breast and lung cancers usually have a better response to radiotherapy, showing both clinical and radiological improvement. Metastases from melanoma and colonic and renal carcinomas often do not show radiological changes even where clinical improvement occurs. Treatment should never be withheld solely on the basis of histology, however, because, on occasion, lesions from radioresistant tumours do respond.

Newer techniques for focal radiation may benefit selected cases.[13] Focal brain irradiation or 'radiosurgery' can have a role in treating single, or occasionally two, brain metastases in combination with whole brain irradiation; the aim being eradication of disease from the brain. Radiosurgery is suggested as a substitute for surgery in this strategy.[14] Radioresistant histology was not found to affect outcome.[14] In advanced cases where a shorter course of treatment and a shorter expected latency for improvement of symptoms are greatly preferred, radiosurgery can be used for palliation of single or double lesions in the brain. It can also be used in cases where there is recurrence in the brain after whole brain irradiation. The indications for and role of focal brain irradiation remain to be clearly defined.[15]

Steroids

Treatment with steroids is recommended for all symptomatic patients with brain metastases or tumour. Their main therapeutic effect is probably related to partial restoration of the blood–brain barrier which is disrupted by the tumour, thus reducing oedema.[16] Steroids are also recommended for all patients undergoing brain irradiation. Treatment should start 48 h before radiation. A traditional regimen is dexamethasone 16 mg/day in four divided doses,[17] although a recent study demonstrated that a regimen of 4 mg daily throughout the duration of radiation therapy (28 days) with subsequent discontinuation works as well and has fewer side-effects.[18] We recommend starting with a 16 mg daily dose in stable patients undergoing radiation and to commence tapering the steroid dose during the second week of radiation. Tapering should be gradual (2 to 4 mg every fifth day).[15]

Higher doses can be given acutely if symptoms recur (16 mg/day) or if there are signs of increased intracranial pressure or cerebral herniation (10 to 100 mg intravenously). The dose should always be tapered to the minimum required for symptom control. Dexamethasone taper and discontinuation should always be attempted after completion of radiation treatment since in most patients steroids are not necessary to preserve neurological function.[19]

Corticosteroids may have considerable side-effects (Table 3). Acute complications (which may be dose related) include gastrointestinal perforation, hypomania, and delirium. Administration of non-steroidal anti-inflammatory drugs can enhance gastrointestinal toxicity of corticosteroids.[20–23] The most troublesome, chronic side-effects are diabetes and steroid myopathy, which can be seen in most patients after 2 to 3 weeks of dexamethasone in doses of 8 to16 mg/day. Fluorinated steroids are associated with a higher risk of myopathy.[15] Methylprednisolone is a possible alternative; doses of 80 mg/day are equivalent to dexamethasone 16 mg/day. Dexamethasone has no mineralocorticoid (salt and water retaining) adverse effects and has been studied more extensively than other corticosteroids. Thus it has become the most commonly used corticosteroid for brain metastases.

Withdrawal of steroids may produce pseudorheumatism[24] or a neurological syndrome with headache, lethargy, and low-grade

Table 3 Steroid toxicity

Neurological side-effects
Myopathy
Insomnia
Behavioural changes
Hiccup
Tremor
Psychosis
Epidural lipomatosis
Non-neurological side-effects
Gastrointestinal perforation (usually bowel)
Gastrointestinal bleeding
Oedema
Perineal discomfort (after intravenous bolus injection)
Osteoporosis
Avascular necrosis of the hip or humeral head
Oral candidiasis and other opportunistic infections
Hyperglycaemia

fever[25] which can be confused with symptoms from recurrent cerebral tumour. Adrenal insufficiency may result if steroids are withdrawn too quickly.

In some centres, immunocompetent patients with brain tumour being treated with long-term steroids receive prophylactic therapy for *Pneumocystis carinii* pneumonia (one double strength tablet of trimethoprim–sulphamethoxazole three consecutive days each week).[15,26,27]

It is common for steroids to be continued indefinitely for no good reason.[28] Continuation of steroid therapy of any type must always be under constant review. While the benefits of rotating steroids in long-term treatment remain unclear, in view of the reduced risk of steroid myopathy with non-fluorinated corticosteroids (e.g. methylprednisolone) their use should be considered in patients requiring long-term steroids.

Cerebral herniation

Patients with brain tumours may experience sudden marked increase of intracranial pressure leading to the herniation of vital cerebral structures through existing cranial spaces, with immediate worsening of the level of consciousness and neurological and respiratory function.[29] If reversal is in the patient's interest, the condition can be treated with assisted ventilation (usually with an endotracheal tube if unconscious), hyperosmolar agents, and steroids. Steroids are usually given in high doses (dexamethasone 100 mg intravenous bolus). Mannitol solution (20 per cent) is given intravenously over 15 to 20 min at a dose of 1.5 to 2 g/kg.

Spinal cord compression

Pathology

This complication is usually due to extrinsic compression of the cord from the epidural space secondary to extension of adjacent bony or soft tissue lesions. Less commonly, spinal cord compression can be due to intradural and intramedullary metastases. Intradural spinal cord compression arises from meningeal metastases presenting as a single mass compressing the cord[30] instead of the more frequent diffuse pattern of leptomeningeal disease (see below). Intramedullary metastases are rare and are due to direct haematogenous dissemination to the cord or to invasion from meningeal disease.

Other causes of epidural compression include epidural abscess or haemorrhage, herniated disc and other rare epidural masses (such as epidural lipomatosis), and extramedullary haematopoiesis. Cauda equina and conus medullaris lesions have similar pathophysiology and clinical implications and are therefore considered here.

Most cases of epidural spinal cord compression in cancer are caused by a vertebral body metastasis invading the epidural space posteriorly and compressing the spinal cord or cauda equina structures. Another common cause is the invasion of the epidural space, through the intervertebral foramina, by a paraspinal lesion. This mechanism occurs typically in lymphoma and neuroblastoma,[31] and in these cases the absence of a bony lesion on radiography can be misleading. Very rarely spinal cord syndromes are due to epidural or cord metastases. Metastases from breast, lung, and prostate cancers more often affect the thoracic spine whereas the lumbar spine is more often affected by metastases from colorectal and other pelvic tumours.

Clinical course

Spinal cord compression occurs in 5 to 10 per cent of cases of cancer.[31,32] It is a neurological emergency as functional outcome is dependent on the degree of neurological impairment at diagnosis and initial response to therapy. Other factors important in prognosis are tumour histology and rate of progression of the neurological symptoms.[33,34] The importance of early diagnosis cannot be over emphasized; symptoms are usually present for some weeks before neurological emergency occurs. Pain precedes other neurological symptoms in almost every case but diagnosis is often delayed until the onset of symptoms and signs of myelopathy . In one series there was an interval of more than 1 week between the onset of neurological symptoms and surgery in 52 per cent of patients.[35,36]

Pain of long duration which suddenly changes its characteristics should prompt re-evaluation and spine imaging. Pain in a crescendo pattern is particularly worrying, as is Lhermitte's sign (a tingling shock-like sensation passing down the arms or trunk when the neck is flexed),[37] pain aggravated by lying down and the Valsalva manoeuvre, and radiculopathy.

Lhermitte's sign, also described as 'barber's chair sign' in the British literature, can also be precipitated by sudden limb movements, coughing, sneezing, or occur spontaneously. It is due to demyelination or compression of the posterior column of the spinal cord in the cervical or upper thoracic regions. Lhermitte's sign is frequent in multiple sclerosis but it is not uncommon in cancer and its differential diagnosis should include benign or relatively benign conditions such as transient radiation myelopathy, cisplatin polyneuropathy, or severe complications such as cord compression and progressive radiation myelopathy.[38]

Diagnosis

Signs of myelopathy usually begin in the lower extremities with weakness, paraesthesiae, and sensory loss starting in the feet and moving proximally. They are helpful in defining the level of the compression (Table 4). Emergency imaging of the spinal cord and

Table 4 Localizing signs in epidural spinal cord compression

Sign	Clinical level		
	Cord	Conus medullaris	Cauda equina
Motor	Paraparesis usually flaccid Pyramidal signs can be present	Same as cord	Never pyramidal signs Often asymmetrical weakness
Reflex	Absent or hyperactive	Patellar hyperactive Ankle hypoactive	Hypoactive Asymmetrical
Babinski	Usually present	Usually present	Never present
Sensory	Symmetrical level of dermatomal level sensory loss (locates compression within two dermatomes above the sensory level)	Same as cord (level usually at L1)	Asymmetrical findings in the lower extremities and perineum
Sphincter control	Can be initially preserved	Early involved sometimes selectively	Can be preserved

canal should be carried out in patients with cancer and back pain who have symptoms of myelopathy. Ideally this should be done when the characteristic back pain is noted.[39–42]

Other clinical and radiological characteristics are often associated with epidural invasion. In patients with back pain and bone changes on spine radiograph, epidural invasion has occurred in 60 to 70 per cent of cases,[39,40,42] and in 80 per cent of cases where there is vertebral collapse of more than 50 per cent.[43] In patients with radiculopathy there is epidural invasion in 60 per cent of cases. Ninety per cent of patients with radiculopathy and bone changes on radiograph have epidural invasion.[39,40,42] However, in cases of lymphoma, radiographs which show no bony changes may be seriously misleading and false-negative results can be as high as 70 per cent.[45] A positive bone scan without clinical changes is associated with epidural invasion in only 17 per cent of patients.[42]

Figure 1 summarizes the clinical and radiological findings which should prompt either immediate treatment or spinal cord imaging with magnetic resonance imaging (**MRI**), the results of which will dictate the treatment modality.[15,39–41,44] Although MRI is the best imaging procedure in these patients myelography or computerized tomography (**CT**) myelography still has a place when MRI is unavailable.[46–48] There may be multiple lesions and the whole spine should be evaluated.

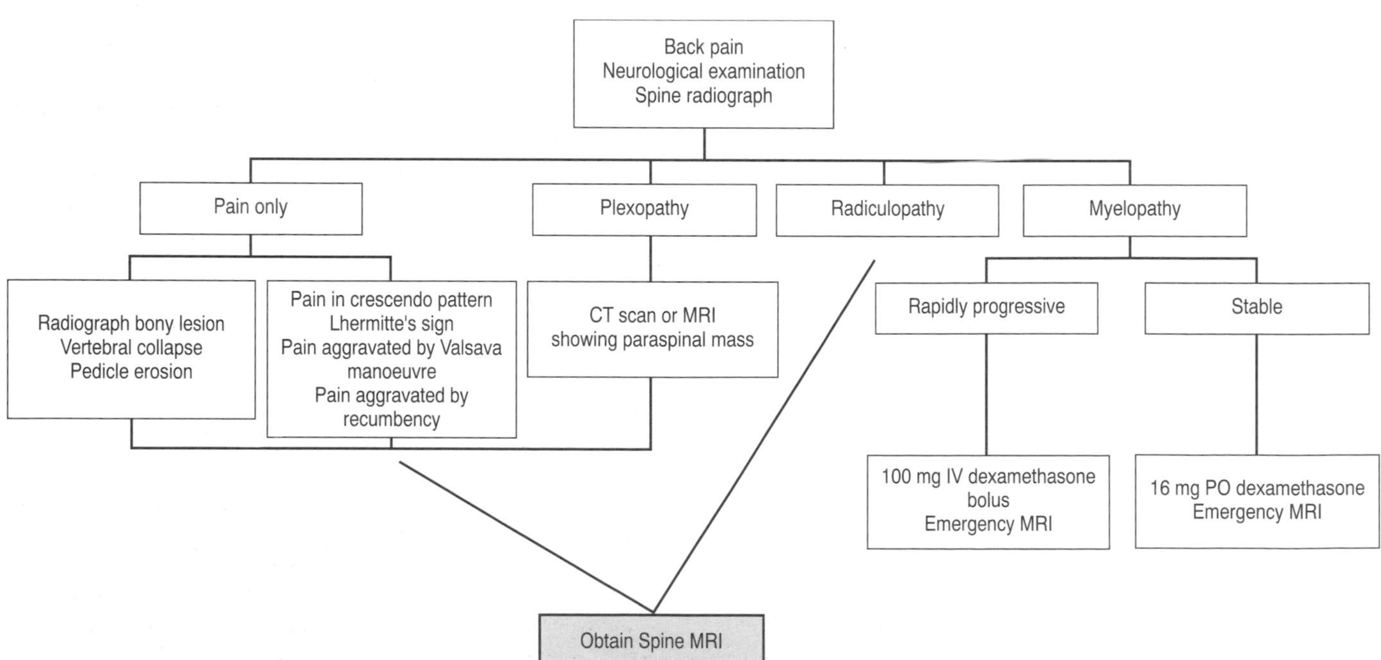

Fig. 1 Algorithm for the evaluation of back pain in the patient with cancer.

Treatment (see also Chapter 9.1.2)

High-dose steroids should be offered to all patients where feasible.[49,50] Steroids can reduce pain, preserve neurological function, and improve functional outcome after definitive treatment.[51] Dexamethasone in high doses is recommended for high-degree lesions as shown by MRI or myelographic block (80 per cent or more) or with rapidly progressing myelopathy. A low-dose regimen should be used for low-degree lesions as shown by MRI or myelography or with stable or slowly progressing myelopathy. The high-dose regimen includes an initial intravenous bolus of 100 mg followed by a tapering schedule of 96 mg orally for 3 days and subsequent halving of the dose every third day until the end of radiation treatment.[52] The use of high doses for epidural spinal cord compression has been questioned[53] but experimental data favour this method.[15]

In the past, posterior laminectomy and radiation were the most used treatment modalities. Review of the literature and one randomized trial shows no advantage for posterior laminectomy plus radiation over the use of radiation alone[15,54,55] and indeed posterior laminectomy can aggravate spine instability and neurological compromise.[56] A more rational surgical approach for anteriorly compressing lesions is vertebral body resection,[57,58] but the procedure requires intact vertebral elements above and below the affected level to stabilize the spine after surgery. Surgery is the first choice where the site of the primary tumour is unknown, where there is relapse after radiation treatment, and in cases of spinal instability or vertebral displacement. It should also be considered when neurological symptoms progress during radiotherapy, in plegia of rapid onset, or where tumours are not radiosensitive.[15]

An evaluation of overall results of radiation and posterior laminectomy showed that ambulatory patients retained ambulation, and about half of paraparetic patients regained ambulation, while paraplegic patients rarely recovered.[15] Some series showed impressive results with vertebral resection. In one series, 13 of 36 paraplegic patients regained ambulation.[59] However, the numbers of patients are still too small to assess the benefits of this type of surgery. Prognosis and expected quality of life should influence the decision, the indication is that it is certainly worthwhile in some individual cases.

Leptomeningeal metastases

Pathology

Leptomeningeal metastases (also known as carcinomatous meningitis or meningeal carcinomatosis) are caused by the dissemination of cancerous cells throughout the subarachnoid space. Such cells can reach the meninges through the general circulation or the perineural spaces along nerve roots, by direct invasion from epidural lesions, or by direct seeding from existing brain tumours.[60] Meningeal involvement can be multifocal or diffuse and visible nodes or microscopic infiltration may result.

Clinical course

Leptomeningeal metastases were once considered an unusual complication of systemic cancer (1–8 per cent of cases at autopsy)[3,61] but these are increasingly seen nowadays, usually as a result of breast or lung cancer, lymphoma, leukaemia, or melanoma. Life expectancy is usually short, ranging from 3 to 6 months in patients who have received intensive treatment. Many patients are not offered treatment and their survival is shorter.[62,63]

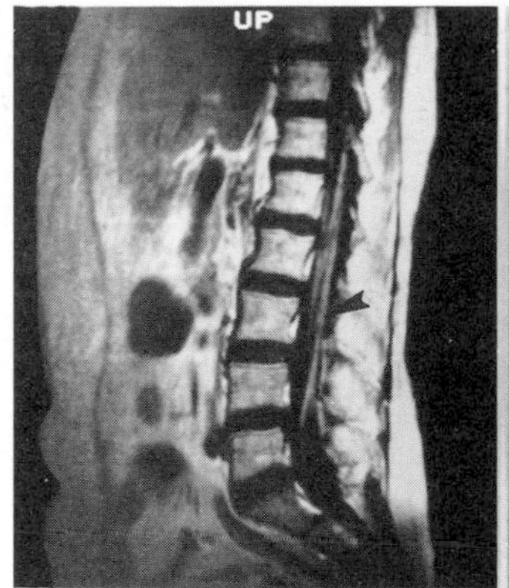

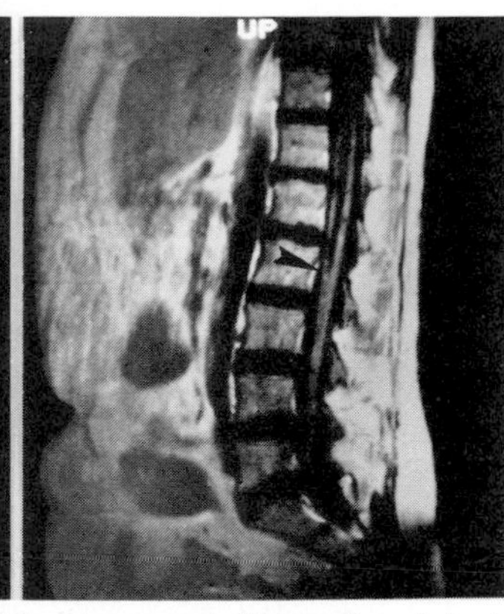

Fig. 2 MRI, gadolium enhanced. The white enhancement of the meningeal sheets around the cauda equina (left side, arrow) and the thecal sac (right side, arrow) is due to meningeal infiltration.

The central and peripheral nervous systems are usually both involved and exhibit variable clinical syndromes. The pathophysiology includes abnormality in the flow and absorption of cerebrospinal fluid which can result in hydrocephalus,[64] direct involvement of the cranial and peripheral nerve meningeal sheets, competition with brain metabolism, invasion of the brain parenchyma, and ischaemia.

The most common symptoms are headache, change in mental status, and radicular-type pain[65,66] but cranial nerve involvement, seizure, polyradiculopathy, and cauda equina syndrome also occur in varying combination. Meningismus is uncommon, unlike infectious meningitis. Multiple symptoms, from involvement of different levels of the neuraxis, are often seen.

Diagnosis

Diagnosis is usually made from examination of the cerebrospinal fluid;[65,67] contrast-enhanced MRI can also be useful (Fig. 2), as the only sign of leptomeningeal metastases may be slight enhancement of the meninges with paramagnetic contrast due to blood–brain barrier disruption. In these circumstances repeated spinal taps are required to identify malignant cells.

While malignant cells may not be apparent in the first sample of cerebrospinal fluid, other abnormalities are usually found such as high opening pressure, high protein content, increased white cell count, or low glucose content. In one series, only 3 per cent of the first samples were completely normal.[65] Other markers and immunocytochemical techniques have not been found to have clinical value.[15]

Therapy

Traditionally, treatment modalities have been based on a combination of corticosteroids, radiotherapy, and intrathecal chemotherapy. Systemic chemotherapy may also be helpful in some cases with appropriate tumour histology. In one series, only 23 per cent of treated patients could be regarded as long-term survivors. Intrathecal chemotherapy did not achieve better results than systemic chemotherapy (median survival 23 months),[63] and caused a treatment-related leucoencephalopathy in 58 per cent of cases. The role of intrathecal chemotherapy therefore requires prospective study.

Base of the skull and cranial nerve syndromes

Lesions at the base of the skull are commonly caused by metastasis of breast, prostate, and other tumours[68] and also result from local invasion by advanced head and neck tumours.[69] Symptoms secondary to bone lesions are commonly associated with alterations of cranial nerve function. Headache at the site of the lesion or referred to the vertex or to the entire affected side of the head is also frequent.[68,70,71] The best imaging procedure for all these syndromes is CT scan with bone window studies. Treatment with radiation is indicated, to control pain and neurological dysfunction.

Orbital syndrome

Progressive retro-orbital and supraorbital pain characterizes this syndrome, which may also be associated with blurred vision and diplopia. Chemosis, proptosis, external ophthalmoplegia, ipsilateral papilloedema, and sensory loss (in a trigeminal distribution) are common.

Parasellar and cavernous sinus syndrome

In this syndrome unilateral supraorbital and frontal headache is associated with ocular palsies, diplopia, and unilateral papilloedema. There may be hemianopsia or quadrantanopsia, secondary to optic chiasm compression.

Middle cranial fossa syndrome

The common symptom is facial pain associated with numbness along the distribution of the second or third trigeminal nerves. The pain can be continuous and dull, be referred to the affected side of the head, and be associated with paroxysmal episodes of lancinating pain in a trigeminal distribution. There may be ocular palsies, caused by contiguous extension to the cavernous sinus.

Jugular foramen syndrome

This syndrome usually presents with hoarseness and dysphagia. Pain is referred to the mastoid region, the neck, or the shoulder, with an associated diffuse, unilateral headache. Horner's syndrome and IXth, Xth, XIth, and sometimes XIIth, nerve palsy can occur.

Occipital condyle syndrome

Unilateral nuchal pain, aggravated by neck flexion, with neck stiffness and a characteristic tilt of the head, occur in this syndrome. There is limited movement of the head and tenderness on the occipitocervical junction. The XIth and XIIth nerves are often affected.

Clivus syndrome

While vertex headache may occur the pain can often be referred behind the eye, radiating posteriorly to the occiput. XIth and XIIth nerve dysfunction is the most common finding but other lower cranial nerves (VI–IX) can be affected. Symptoms can occur on one or both sides.

Sphenoid and ethmoid sinus syndromes

These usually present with bilateral frontal headaches, nasal congestion and discharge, and diplopia secondary to VIth nerve involvement.

Other cranial neuropathy syndromes

Glossopharyngeal nerve

The typical patient has throat and neck pain which radiates to the ear and is aggravated by swallowing. Pharyngeal and other carcinomas of the neck can present with odynophagia with reflex otalgia. Severe pain may be associated with syncope.[72] Although it has been described with leptomeningeal disease,[73] it commonly results from local nerve infiltration in the neck or base of the skull.

Trigeminal nerve

The most common presentation is a constant dull, well-localized pain related to the underlying disease of bone and other somatic structures, and associated with paroxysmal episodes of lancinating or throbbing pain. Lesions of the middle and posterior fossa can present with classical trigeminal neuralgia.[74] However, metastases at the base of the skull or leptomeningeal metastases can both produce atypical facial pain.[75] Atypical trigeminal pain and sensory abnormalities in the peripheral distribution of the Vth nerve, occasionally associated with incomplete lesions of the VIIth nerve, have been reported with different facial neoplasms.[76–78]

Involvement of the mental nerve does not usually produce pain but can cause the 'numb chin syndrome'. This is a sign of bony disease of jaw or foramen ovale, but can also be found with tumours of the base of the skull or leptomeninges and local perineural spread of lip carcinoma. The symptom can occur months before the discovery of a bony lesion.[79]

Radiculopathy

Radiculopathy is usually caused by leptomeningeal metastases, or by the compression of nerve roots by vertebral or paraspinal lesions. The pain of a root lesion is usually focal and radiates in the distribution of the affected root. It is sometimes difficult to distinguish a polyradiculopathy from a plexus lesion and in these cases the neurological assessment can be expanded to include electrical studies of the paraspinal muscles, thus identifying the level of the lesion. CT and MRI are useful for imaging non-bony paraspinal lesions. MRI is necessary for imaging the epidural space.

Herpes zoster and postherpetic neuralgia are common in patients with cancer[80] and should always be considered in the differential diagnosis of painful radiculopathies.

Cervical plexopathy

Infiltration of the cervical plexus by tumour can be a result of compression by head and neck neoplasms or can occur from metastasis to cervical nodes. Symptoms usually include local lancinating or dysaesthetic pain referred to the retroauricular and nuchal areas, the shoulder, and the jaw. Sensory abnormalities define the affected (greater auricular and greater occipital) nerves.[69] The differential diagnosis should include postradical neck dissection syndrome. The diagnosis may be difficult because of the major postoperative and postradiation changes often found in these patients.

CT or MRI scans are appropriate, and imaging of the cervical spine and paraspinal structures is very important in distinguishing

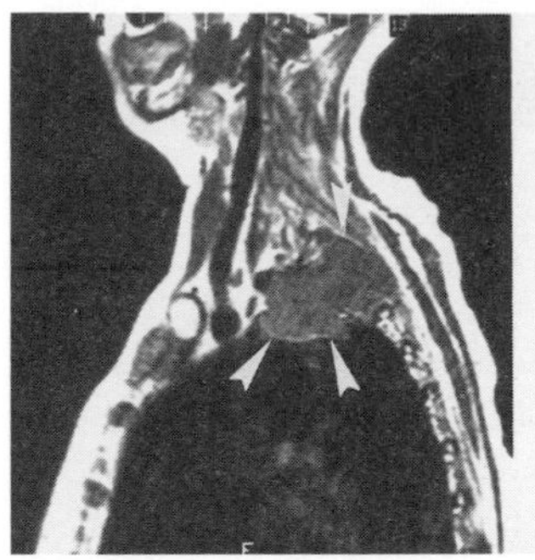
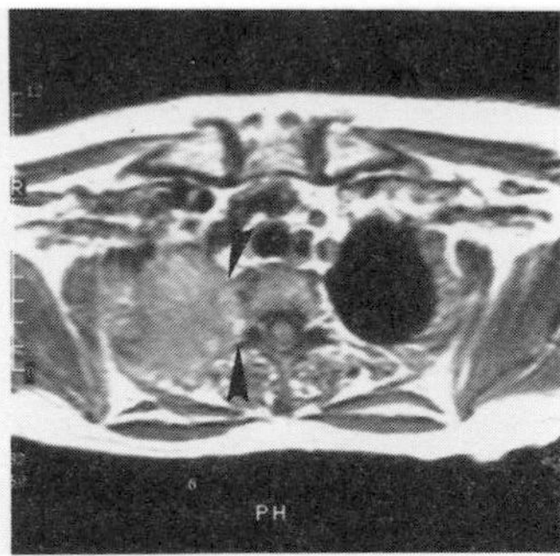

Fig. 3 MRI image. Lung tumour in the upper lobe compressing the lower trunk of the brachial plexus. Pain was reported in the inner aspect of the arm and paraesthesiae in the 5th and 4th finger. Left side: the arrows show the tumour mass invading the tissue planes in the area of the brachial plexus. Right side: the tumour is invading the left upper lobe, the arrows show the tumour invading one thoracic vertebral body. Reproduced with permission from Caraceni A. Clinicopathologic correlates of common cancer pain syndromes. *Hematology and Oncology Clinics of North America,* 1996; **10**: 57–78.

between bony lesions, cervical radiculopathy, and epidural spinal cord compression.

Brachial plexopathy

Five per cent of the neurological consultations at a comprehensive cancer centre were found to be initiated by brachial plexopathy.[2] It occurs most often with breast and lung carcinoma and with lymphoma. The plexus can be compressed or infiltrated by tumour lying in contiguous structures, such as axillary or supraclavicular nodes or apex of the lung. Pain is the first symptom in 85 per cent of patients,[81] preceding other neurological symptoms or signs by weeks or months.

Breast and lung malignancies typically affect the lower plexus (C7-T1) (Fig. 3) and cause pain in the shoulder, elbow, hand, and the fourth and fifth finger. Lung tumours can affect the intercostobrachial nerve, giving rise to a pain syndrome and associated sensory disturbances in the axilla (C8-T1-T2).[82] The upper brachial plexus (C5-C6) can also be affected, especially by breast cancer, when pain is usually referred to the paraspinal region, shoulder, biceps region, elbow, and hand; burning dysaesthesia in the index finger or thumb is common. The hallmark of the syndrome is the neuropathic nature of the pain with numbness, paraesthesia, allodynia, and hyperaesthesia.

CT scan with narrow sections and contrast enhancement is effective in imaging soft tissue and bony structures in the plexus area. All patients with symptoms of brachial plexopathy should have a scan of the contiguous paravertebral region before radiation therapy, since extension of disease in this region is common (13/41 cases in one series). MRI is particularly useful in imaging of the contiguous epidural space. While use of both techniques can give helpful complementary information in doubtful cases, sometimes neither is helpful even in cases of proven metastatic plexopathy.[83,84] Comparative data on specificity and sensitivity of the two techniques is lacking.

Epidural invasion will eventually occur in some patients with brachial plexopathy—6 out of 41 in one series (Fig. 4).[85] Imaging of the epidural space is essential when patients develop Horner's syndrome, panplexopathy, vertebral body erosion, or a paraspinal mass detected on CT scan. These are often hallmark symptoms of tumour progression into the epidural space.[85]

Radiation fibrosis is important in the differential diagnosis of brachial plexopathy in cancer (Table 5), particularly in patients who have had radiotherapy and who present with upper plexus signs. Pain is often less prominent in patients with radiation-induced plexopathy.

Electrodiagnostic studies are helpful in distinguishing radiation-induced plexopathies from malignant invasion.[86] Sometimes this differential diagnosis is difficult. MRI and CT scans may fail to distinguish fibrosis from tumour—in this case surgical exploration of the plexus is necessary to rule out fibrosis, a new primary tumour, a radiation-induced tumour, or recurrent cancer.[81]

Lumbosacral plexopathy

Lumbosacral plexopathy is one of the most disabling complications of cancer. Although it is commonly associated with colorectal, cervical, and other pelvic malignancies (bladder, uterus, prostate, sarcoma, lymphoma) it can also be caused by breast or lung cancer or melanoma. Retroperitoneal tumours (e.g. sarcoma, metastatic nodal tumours) may affect the lumbosacral plexus or its roots more proximally.

The presenting symptom in almost all cases (93 per cent)[87] is pain in the buttocks or the legs; it often precedes other symptoms by weeks or months. It is usually followed by numbness, paraesthesia, weakness, and, later, leg oedema. The pain is usually aching or pressure-like in quality, and is rarely burning or dysaesthetic. In Jaeckle's series[88] an upper plexopathy (L1–L4) was found in about one-third of cases, a lower plexopathy (L4–S1) in one-half of cases, and panplexopathy (L1–S3) in about 20 per cent (Table 6).

Other structures can be involved. These include roots of the plexus or contiguous structures, the sympathetic chain,[89] and psoas

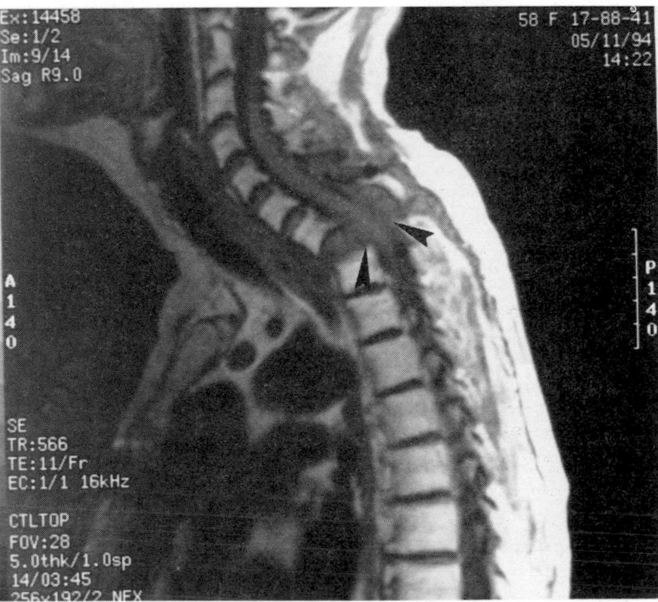

Fig. 4 MRI image in the same case as shown in Fig. 3. The tumour is invading the epidural canal and compressing the spinal cord. Reproduced with permission from Caraceni A. Clinicopathologic correlates of common cancer pain syndromes. *Hematology and Oncology Clinics of North America,* 1996; **10**, 57–78.

Table 5 Differential diagnosis of brachial plexopathy

	Tumour infiltration	Radiation fibrosis
Incidence of pain	89%	18%
Severity of pain	Severe in 98%	Mild to moderate
Dose of radiotherapy	–	> 6000 cGy large fractions (> 1900 cGy/day)
Latency	Not indicative	> 6 months < 5 years
Course	Progressive neurological dysfunction Pain progression with dysaesthetic quality C7-T1 distribution[a]	Progressive weakness Pain stabilizing with onset of weakness C5-C6 distribution
Horner	Can be present	Absent
CT scan findings[b]	Mass with tissue infiltration	Diffuse infiltration of tissue planes
MRI scan findings[b]	High signal intensity mass on T2-weighted images	Low signal intensity lesion on T_2-weighted images
Electromyography findings	Denervation no myochimia	Myochimia

[a] The distribution of the neurological findings can be helpful in some cases but it is not always indicative (see text for more details).

[b] The use of both techniques may provide complementary information. No method is totally credible in differentiating fibrosis from tumour (Krol 1993[84]).

muscle.[90] Selective involvement of the L1, iliohypogastric, ilioinguinal, or genitofemoral nerves can produce pain and paraesthesia in the inguinal and scrotal region.

A sacral plexopathy, often overlapping a sacral polyradiculopathy, can be produced from direct extension of a presacral mass invading the sacrum, as sometimes occurs with rectosigmoid and bladder carcinomas. The coccygeal plexus is usually affected in patients with sphincter dysfunction and perineal 'saddle' sensory loss.

Tumour is often found in the lumbar vertebrae, sacrum, or pelvis of patients with lumbosacral plexopathy (45/76 patients) and epidural extension is also common, especially with retroperitoneal tumours. Hydroureter or hydronephrosis is extremely common at diagnosis.[87,88]

Lumbosacral plexopathy can occur after pelvic irradiation. Thomas *et al.*[87] reported that radiation-induced lumbosacral plexopathy very rarely presents with pain and has a median latency of 5 years from radiotherapy. Motor involvement is bilateral in 80 per cent of cases and electromyography can be a useful diagnostic tool. Other differential diagnoses include leptomeningeal carcinomatosis, cauda equina compression, and non-cancer-related causes of lumbar plexopathy—for example iliopsoas muscle haemorrhage or abscess, aortic aneurysm, idiopathic acute lumbosacral neuritis, and postsurgical compressive lesions, which often present as mononeuropathies.

MRI and CT scanning both image the lumbosacral plexus effectively. CT gives more information on the bony structures, while MRI is more accurate for soft tissues. The assessment should extend from L1 through the true pelvis,[84] and should include the spine and adjacent pelvic soft tissues.

Table 6 Clinical findings in lumbosacral plexopathy due to cancer

	Upper plexopathy	Lower plexopathy	Panplexopathy
Local pain	Lower abdomen	Buttock, perineum	Lumbosacral
Referred pain	Flank, iliac crest	Hip and ankle	Variable
Radicular pain	Anterolateral thigh	Posterolateral thigh, leg	Variable
Paraesthesiae	Anterior thigh	Perineum, thigh sole	Anterior thigh, leg, foot
Motor and reflex changes	L2-L4 proximal leg weakness patella reflex	L5-S1 distal leg weakness ankle reflex	L2-S2 weakness can affect different muscle groups and reflexes
Sensory loss	Anterolateral thigh	Posterior thigh, sole	Anterior thigh, leg
Tenderness	Lumbar	Sciatic notch, sacrum	Lumbosacral
Positive SLRT			
direct	50%	50%	83%
reverse	15%	50%	83%
Leg oedema	41%	37%	83%
Rectal mass	25%	43%	15%
Anal sphincter weakness	0	50%	0

SLRT = straight leg raising test or Lasegue manoeuvre

Modified from Jaeckle *et al.* (1985),[88] with permission.

Mononeuropathy

Mononeuropathy is less common than plexopathy or radicular lesions. It is caused by compression or infiltration of a nerve by bony lesions or by soft tissue masses in the limbs. Obturator,[91] femoral, and sciatic neuropathies are seen when tumour involves the soft tissue along the nerve distribution in the pelvis and thigh. Peroneal mononeuropathy can occur with bony lesions of the head of the fibula and sarcoma of the popliteal fossa. Ulnar and radial neuropathies result from bony lesions in the elbow or humerus.[92] These mononeuropathies must be distinguished from traumatic or compressive lesions, or from nutritional–metabolic lesions of nerves. Intercostal nerve neuropathy from invasion of the chest wall is the most common of the mononeuropathies caused by cancer.

Treatment of peripheral nerve compression

Radiation is indicated for all cases of plexopathy, neuropathy, and radiculopathy caused by tumour compression. Lesions caused by radioresistant tumours, such as sarcomas, are unlikely to respond. However, the results of radiotherapy in brachial plexopathy have been disappointing with only 46 per cent of patients reporting relief from pain in a retrospective series.[81]

Management of pain is often difficult in these syndromes; opioids are indicated and adjuvants for neuropathic pain should be used for specific indications. Clinical experience suggests that dexamethasone can be particularly effective for pain due to compression and oedema of peripheral nerves.

Peripheral neurolytic blocks, with alcohol or phenol, can be considered for severe arm and leg pain in patients with advanced plexus lesions. These blocks are sometimes associated with significant side-effects such as paresis and incontinence.[93] Sacral root blockade with phenol for perineal pain caused by root invasion is more acceptable when patients already have established urinary and rectal sphincter dysfunction. Late onset dysaesthesia may occur in long-term survivors (see Chapter 9.2.6).

Percutaneous cordotomy is feasible for the pain of lumbosacral plexopathy. Brachial plexopathy is more difficult to treat with cordotomy because the cervical dermatomes up to C4 must be included. This is technically difficult and increases the risk of respiratory depression and neurological sequelae. A short prognosis (6 months to 1 year) is required to avoid long-term postcordotomy dysaesthetic pain (see Chapter 9.2.7).[94–96]

Peripheral polyneuropathy

Polyneuropathy in cancer patients can be caused by neurotoxicity of chemotherapy, metabolic nutritional deficiency, or paraneoplastic syndromes; the aetiology of the condition is summarized in Table 7.[97,98] Subclinical dysfunction of small and large sensory fibres can be demonstrated with quantitative sensory testing in 30 to 40 per cent of cancer patients.[99]

Peripheral neuropathy is characterized by a stocking–glove distribution of negative sensory (hypoaesthesia) and positive sensory symptoms, including painless paraesthesia or distressing burning dysaesthesia, allodynia, and hyperalgesia. Early sensory loss and later motor signs (weakness) are characteristic of some drug-induced sensorimotor neuropathies (vincristine, paclitaxel).

Table 7 Polyneuropathies and peripheral neuropathies

Related to cancer

Myeloma associated neuropathies
Paraneoplastic sensory neuronopathy (Denny–Brown)
Sensory–motor peripheral neuropathy
Nutritional factors (cachexia-associated neuromyopathy[a])
Cancer related metabolic dysfunction: hepatic, renal
Infiltration of peripheral nerves (lymphomas, leukaemias)[b]
Vascular (haemorragic or ischaemic) peripheral nerve lesion[b]

Related to chemotherapy and radiation

Vincristine
Vinblastine
Vinorelbine
Cisplatin
Paclitaxel
Suramin

Radiation to limbs with worsening of vincristine neuropathy

Non-cancer related

Metabolic dysfunction: diabetes

[a] Very frequent
[b] Mononeuritis multiplex

Sensory involvement can be selective in neuropathies associated with cisplatin or paraneoplastic syndromes. Often the only early sign of polyneuropathy is reduction or loss of the ankle reflex. Muscle cramps may be associated with neuropathy and can sometimes be prominent symptoms in vincristine neuropathy.[100] Muscle cramps are relatively frequent in cancer (see Table 8 for different aetiologies).

Paraneoplastic sensory neuropathy and sensory neuropathy caused by vincristine or paclitaxel is often more painful than that caused by cisplatin. Cisplatin induces a sensory neuronopathy mainly affecting the cells of the dorsal root ganglia with predominant involvement of the large fibre functions (proprioception) which causes sensory ataxia rather than pain. Vinca alkaloids and paclitaxel produce a mostly sensory axonopathy with some motor component.

Clinical examination is usually sufficient for diagnosis although nerve conduction studies and electromyography can be used.[101] Treatment is palliative, with analgesics and adjuvants (see Chapter 9.2.5).

Table 8 Muscle cramps in cancer

Aetiology	Number of patients
Peripheral neuropathy	22
Root and plexus pathology	17
Polymyositis	2
Hypomagnesaemia	1
Unknown	9

Modified from Steiner I, Siegal T., Muscle cramps in cancer patients. *Cancer*, 1989; **63**: 574–7, with permission.

Table 9 Cerebrovascular complications of cancer

Central nervous system complication	Mechanism
Cerebral haemorrhage	Intratumoural bleeding[a] Disseminated intravascular coagulation[b] Coagulopathy[b] Leukostasis[c]
Subdural haematoma	Dural metastases[d] Coagulopathy[d]
Embolic infarct	Non-bacterial thrombotic endocarditis[d] Tumour embolism[d] Fungal embolism[b]
Sinus thrombosis	Dural, bony tumour[d] Coagulopathy[d] L-asparaginase[b]
Thrombotic microinfarcts	Disseminated intravascular coagulation[b,d]

[a] Associated with cerebral and leptomeningeal tumour
[b] Associated with leukaemia/lymphoma
[c] Only found with leucocytes ≥ 100 000
[d] Associated with solid tumours

Cerebrovascular disorders in patients with cancer

Cerebrovascular disease in patients with cancer is not uncommon. It is often tumour related, either as a direct effect of the tumour or its treatment or as an indirect effect of coagulation changes. Coronary and cerebral arteriosclerosis is less common in patients dying of cancer than in the general population.[15] In one study, cerebrovascular lesions were found at autopsy in 15 per cent of cases[102] and half of these patients had clinical symptoms related to the pathological findings. There were 500 vascular lesions, of which 244 were haemorrhagic and 256 ischaemic. Only 72 of the ischaemic lesions were related to atherosclerosis and 9 haemorrhages were hypertensive, the remaining lesions being related to tumour-associated conditions. Haemorrhagic diatheses (thrombocytopenia, disseminated intravascular coagulation) or hypercoagulability states are common causes.

Cerebral haematoma is more common than subarachnoid haemorrhage and is the complication most frequently seen in leukaemia.[102] Ischaemic complications caused by thrombotic emboli due to non-bacterial thrombotic endocarditis are a frequent finding at autopsy in patients with advanced cancer but are difficult to demonstrate *in vivo* since transoesophageal echocardiography is required.[103,104] Treatment with heparin is recommended.[15]

Multiple microinfarcts can produce a global encephalopathy associated with mild disseminated intravascular coagulation, but with no laboratory abnormalities, in patients with leukaemia, lymphoma, or breast cancer.[105] Other syndromes are listed in Table 9.[106-111]

Paraneoplastic syndromes

The pathogenesis of remote effects of systemic cancer on the nervous system is unknown, although autoimmune processes are seen in many syndromes and autoantibody determinations are sometimes helpful in diagnosis.[61,112,113] Paraneoplastic syndromes are rare, probably affecting less than 1 per cent of patients with cancer (see also Table 1), even if the most commonly associated neoplasms, such as small-cell lung cancer and ovarian cancer are considered.[98] Some classic paraneoplastic syndromes can be recognized and diagnosed with confidence (Table 10). Cerebellar degeneration associated with ovarian and lung cancer, or peripheral neuronopathy and limbic encephalitis associated with small-cell tumours of the lung are relatively stereotyped clinicopathological entities associated with the presence of specific autoantibodies (anti-Yo for cerebellar degeneration and anti-Hu for neuronopathy with encephalomyelitis).[15] Opsoclonus–myoclonus and Lambert–Eaton myasthenic syndrome occurring in children with neuroblastomas and in small-cell lung cancer respectively are also classic in their presentation. However, many syndromes present with varying symptoms, affecting the brain and cranial nerves, spinal cord and dorsal root ganglia, and peripheral nerves and muscles, and pose a difficult diagnostic problem.[15] There is little in the literature on these syndromes, although the term encephalomyelitis is reserved by some authors for those patients with evidence of widespread neurological dysfunction without findings predominantly in one particular area.[112,113]

In general, neurological symptoms develop acutely and are severe. Subtle, long-lasting symptoms are not usually caused by paraneoplastic syndrome. Examination of cerebrospinal fluid and immunofluorescence techniques for testing circulating autoantibodies can aid diagnosis. MRI scans are usually normal.[114]

The clinical course is independent of that of the original

Table 10 Paraneoplastic neurological syndromes

Lambert–Eaton myasthenic syndrome
Subacute cerebellar degeneration
Subacute sensory neuronopathy
Opsoclonus–myoclonus
Motor neuronopathy (with lymphoma)
Limbic encephalitis

tumour, which in 50 per cent of cases is found after the onset of neurological symptoms, and is often small and slow growing with a relatively benign course.[15] Remission of the neurological symptoms only occasionally follows treatment of the tumour. Spontaneous remissions have been seen but the syndrome is usually irreversible.[15] The results of treatment are poor; steroids and plasmapheresis are not effective except in the Lambert–Eaton syndrome, where plasmapheresis is indicated.

Lambert–Eaton myasthenic syndrome presents with muscle weakness and fatiguability. Proximal muscles are affected and bulbar musculature usually spared. Strength initially improves with exercise and examination can therefore be ambiguous since power can improve during testing, although weakness recurs after continuous effort. Fifty per cent of patients have dry mouth and impotence. The diagnosis is made by electromyography, with a classic finding of small compound action potentials which increase with exercise. Repetitive stimulation at a low and high rate produces a decrease and increase in the compound action potential respectively.

The syndrome is caused by a reduced release of acetylcholine from presynaptic membranes. Most patients have autoantibodies which react with the calcium channels at the cholinergic synapse level. The Lambert–Eaton syndrome is the only paraneoplastic syndrome for which an autoimmune pathogenesis has been proved with animal models. It often responds to immunosuppression and plasmapheresis.

Adverse neurological effects of anticancer therapy

Surgery, chemotherapy, or radiation can cause neurological syndromes.[15,115] They are discussed in greater detail elsewhere in this textbook (Section 9.1). In particular, irradiation of the brain can produce multiple acute and chronic adverse effects;[116] acute effects include worsening of neurological symptoms, somnolence, and Lhermitte's sign, and the main chronic effect is dementia caused by radiation necrosis and leucoencephalopathy.

Change in mental status

Change in mental status is one of the most common neurological symptoms seen in palliative medicine (see also Table 1). A standardized approach to the examination of cognitive function is given in Section 15. Table 11 outlines the laboratory tests useful in evaluating a patient with an acute change in mental status.

Most cases of acute encephalopathy are caused by drugs (Table 12). A large number of drugs have such effects and many are used, often in combination, in palliative medicine.

Management of seizures

Seizures are often encountered in palliative medicine. They may be caused by metastatic cerebral lesions in advanced cancer, by AIDS, or as a consequence of metabolic derangement or of therapy.

Seizures may occur in 25 per cent of patients with brain metastases.[4] Prophylactic anticonvulsant treatment is controversial. All anticonvulsants have potentially serious side-effects and many interact with chemotherapeutic drugs and steroids. They also sedate and produce cognitive impairment.[4,117-119] The usefulness of prophylactic treatment has been demonstrated only in patients with brain metastases from melanoma.[120] Prophylaxis is therefore only

Table 11 Diagnostic work up for acute change in mental status

Abnormal mental state examination
Focal signs or symptoms at neurological examination
- CT to rule out haemorrhage
- MRI to rule out space occupying lesion or cerebrovascular disease

Absence of focal signs or symptoms at neurological examination
- Serum glucose, Na^+, Ca^{2+}, K^+, Cl^-, Mg^{2+}, blood urea nitrogen, pH, $P\text{CO}_2$, $P\text{O}_2$
- Disseminated intravascular coagulation profile
- Liver function tests
- Cerebrospinal fluid examination for blood or infection
- Electroencephalography can confirm diffuse cerebral dysfunction
- CT scan

Table 12 Drugs which have been associated with delirium or encephalopathy

Anticholinergics
- Antihistamines (diphenhydramine, hydroxyzine)
- Antispasmodics (hyoscine)
- Tricyclic antidepressants (amitriptyline)
- Phenothiazines (thorazine, thioridazine, chlorpromazine)
- Antiparkinsonian (trihexyphenidyl)
- Antiarrhythmics (quinidine)

Hypnotics–anxiolytics
- Benzodiazepines (lorazepam, triazolam, diazepam, flurazepam)
- Barbiturates

Opioids
Cardiac (digitalis)
Antihypertensives (propranolol, methyldopa)
Antibiotics (aminoglycosides, penicillins, cephalosporins, sulphonamides, ciprofloxacin)
Chemotherapy agents
- Ifosfamide (high dose, 20–40% of cases)
- Methotrexate (high dose)
- Cytarabine (ARA-C, high dose)
- 5-Fluorouracil (rare, cerebellar syndrome more common)
- Vincristine (rare)
- L-Asparaginase
- Busulphan (high dose)
- Thiotepa (high dose)
- Procarbazine (intravenous)
- Carmustine (intracarotid, high dose)

Other known associations
- Anticonvulsants
- Cimetidine
- Ranitidine
- Famotidine
- Non-steroidal anti-inflammatories
- Lithium
- Interferons
- Interleukins
- Levodopa
- Cyclosporin
- Acyclovir

recommended in patients who have already had a seizure or in patients with melanomas.[4] It is not recommended in other patients who have not had seizures.

Carbamazepine can induce bone marrow depression and is, therefore, less suitable for patients undergoing chemotherapy. Dexamethasone interferes with the hepatic metabolism of phenytoin and phenobarbitone, enhancing their elimination and thus possibly decreasing their anticonvulsant efficacy. Conversely, phenytoin can decrease dexamethasone bioavailability, eventually reducing its therapeutic effect.[121] Bioavailability of oral dexamethasone can be decreased by 20 per cent after starting phenytoin. Patients on stable doses of phenytoin can develop toxicity if dexamethasone is decreased, or start seizures when dexamethasone is increased and phenytoin levels become subtherapeutic.[15] It is, therefore, important when using combination therapy to be particularly sensitive to changes in clinical symptoms and to be ready to modify doses accordingly.

Personal experience and local practice must guide the choice between phenytoin, carbamazepine, valproate, and phenobarbitone; there is no reported evidence that any one of these drugs is superior in treating seizures in patients with systemic cancer. In the United States, phenytoin is the drug of choice, followed by carbamazepine, valproate, and phenobarbitone respectively.[15,119]

Seizures, often idiopathic, occur in 10 to 15 per cent of AIDS patients. Once present, recurrence is common and continuing antiepileptic therapy is therefore recommended. As phenytoin has been associated with frequent reactions in these patients, carbamazepine is a reasonable first choice.[122]

Blood levels of anticonvulsants must be monitored because of the unpredictability of metabolic changes and drug interactions, although it must be remembered that clinical response and not blood levels should guide dosage. The role of newer anticonvulsants, such as vigabatrin, felbamate, or lamotrigine, is not clearly established in this clinical situation.

Table 13 Management of status epilepticus

Restore homeostasis

Airway, blood pressure, nasal O_2, electrocardiography, intubate only if necessary
Administer 50 ml of 50% glucose and 100 mg of thiamine IV
Start isotonic saline slow drip
Send blood for laboratory analysis

Stop convulsive seizures

Diazepam 0.25 mg/kg IV up to 20 mg (< 5 mg/min) followed immediately by phenytoin 15 mg/kg (< 50 mg/min)
Monitor blood pressure and electrocardiography; repeat phenytoin 7 mg/kg if necessary

or

Lorazepam 0.1 mg/kg IV (< 2 mg/min); phenytoin as above

If seizures persist

Intubate, electroencephalography monitoring
Phenobarbitone 20 mg/kg IV (< 100 mg/min)

or

Midazolam 200 µg/kg IV bolus followed by 0.75–11µg/kg per min IV infusion

If seizures persist

General anaesthesia with short-acting barbiturates (e.g. pentobarbitone 5 mg/kg, then 1–3 mg/kg per hour), adjust dose to obtain burst suppression pattern on electroencephalography and titrate to keep patient seizure-free
Use additional anticonvulsants as necessary

IV = intravenous
Modified from Posner (1995),[15] with permission.

Other seizure-related conditions

The condition where seizures last for more than 30 min or recur after brief intervals during which the patient does not fully recover consciousness is termed status epilepticus. Tonic–clonic convulsions are life-threatening and require emergency treatment (Table 13).[123,124]

Toxic metabolic encephalopathies complicating advanced terminal illness can be associated with seizures. Side-effects of high-dose opioids and phenothiazines have also been implicated;[125,126] midazolam infusion has been beneficial.[125] Multifocal myoclonus is increasingly seen with high-dose opioids and can respond to opioid rotation, and to careful assessment and treatment of renal failure. Symptomatic treatment is feasible with clonazepam (see Chapter 9.2.10).[127]

Non-convulsive status epilepticus can be clinically indistinct from acute confusional state or delirium. It is characterized by impaired consciousness without involuntary movements; sometimes myoclonus can be present, with seizure-like electroencephalography findings. It can be seen in the course of high-dose ifosfamide administration. The diagnosis can be made with electroencephalography; anticonvulsant treatment or diazepam can improve consciousness, as shown in the case of ifosfamide toxicity.[128]

Neuropathic pain syndromes

Neuropathic pain syndromes include those in which the pain process is thought to be sustained by a lesion in the peripheral or central nervous system. Abnormal processing of the somatosensory signal at peripheral and/or central level is thought to play a major role in the pathogenesis of the pain.[129] The pathophysiology of neuropathic pain conditions has been widely studied and various experimental mechanisms have clinical relevance. All suggest an abnormal function in the periphery (mainly the nociceptor) and in the central component of the pain pathways (the spinothalamic neurones in the dorsal horn and the spinothalamic tract).[130-132] These mechanisms may not be totally specific for the known neuropathic syndromes; they may also be involved in non-neuropathic chronic pain conditions (see Chapters 9.2.1 and 9.2.2).[129,133]

Table 14 lists the most clearly defined neuropathic pain syndromes. In cancer patients many treatment-related syndromes can produce neuropathic pain and many cases of compression or infiltration by tumour have the same neuropathic mechanism and clinical features. Some authors report that pain caused by compression is more often aching and severe (nociceptive nerve pain), but with less neurological dysfunction, while invasive lesions cause more dysaesthetic sensation, burning pain, paraesthesia, or neuralgic pain (neuropathic pain).[134]

Table 14 Neuropathic pain syndromes

Painful peripheral neuropathies
Painful mononeuropathies
Plexopathies
Phantom limb pain
Postherpetic neuralgia
Avulsion of the brachial plexus
Injury to the spinal cord
Cerebrovascular lesion to the thalamus, subcortical, or cortical structures
Syringomyelia
Sympathetically maintained pain syndromes, reflex sympathetic dystrophy

All neuropathic syndromes have some factors in common, albeit variably so (Table 15). Symptoms caused by the neurological lesion will depend on its location and will affect function accordingly, but the lesion will always involve the sensory system (sometimes selectively) when there is neuropathic pain. The sensory systems most affected are pain and temperature; less commonly vibratory and two-point discrimination are affected. This is consistent with the observation that in painful peripheral neuropathies small fibres, which subserve pain and temperature sensation, are more often involved, whereas in central lesions associated with pain the spinothalamic system is more often affected.[135-139]

Manifestations vary with the underlying cause. Allodynia, for example, is typical of postherpetic neuralgia (87 per cent of cases in one study)[137] but is not always present in central pain after stroke (57 per cent)[136,140] and is rarely present in central pain caused by multiple sclerosis.[139]

Table 15 Common sensory neurological findings in neuropathic pain

Spontaneous pain
Burning, shooting, lancinating
Negative findings
Hypoaesthesia to touch and vibratory stimulation
Hypoalgesia to pinprick
Hypoaesthesia to thermal (warm and cold) stimuli
Enhanced thermal pain threshold to quantitative sensory testing
Positive findings
Paraesthesiae
Abnormal non-painful sensations
Dysaesthesias
Abnormal uncomfortable sensations
Allodynia
Painful sensation evoked by a non-noxious stimulus
Hyperalgesia
Exaggerated response to a noxious stimulus
Hyperpathia
Exaggerated painful response to a noxious or non-noxious stimulus
for example when the burning pain evoked by light touching (= allodynia) outlasts for seconds or minutes the duration of the stimulus

Painful polyneuropathies

A number of polyneuropathies can be painful. Many are characterized by axonal damage of the sensory fibres, particularly small diameter fibres important for temperature and pain sensation. They include diabetic neuropathy, AIDS-related neuropathy, alcohol–nutritional neuropathy, toxic neuropathies caused by thallium and arsenic, and some rare hereditary neuropathies.[141] Paraneoplastic sensory neuronopathy, in which all sensory modalities are affected, is also painful. Other peripheral nerve lesions which produce pain are more heterogeneous. This group includes leprous neuritis, Guillain–Barré syndrome, compression of spinal roots, and brachial neuritis.

Postherpetic neuralgia

Postherpetic neuralgia is a common cause of neuropathic pain, occurring in the dermatomal distribution of previous herpes zoster infection; the condition is usually defined as pain persisting 1 month after herpes zoster. It is more common in the elderly patient and in patients with cancer, particularly those with disease of the midthoracic dermatomes and of the ophthalmic branch of the trigeminal nerve. Pain is referred to the affected dermatomes; common symptoms are constant burning or aching pain, intermittent paroxysmal spontaneous episodes of lancinating pain, and pain induced by otherwise innocuous tactile and thermal stimulation (allodynia). Pathological examination shows pronounced lesions in the dorsal root ganglia sometimes extending into the spinal cord.[142] Clinical and quantitative sensory testing shows hypalgesia and hypaesthesia to touch, vibration, pinprick, and thermal stimulation in the affected dermatomes in all cases. Often pain is most severe where hypaesthesia is most marked. Allodynia and hyperaesthesia are also commonly present.[137,143] After 12 months or more spontaneous resolution of the pain will occur in many patients.[144] A comprehensive review of available treatment can be found in the literature.[145]

The treatment of neuropathic pain is also reviewed elsewhere in this textbook (Chapter 9.2.10). Tricyclic antidepressants have an established role in the treatment of this difficult pain syndrome but recent researches suggest that opioids are also effective analgesics in postherpetic neuralgia;[146] topical capsaicin can be helpful in some cases, but is often poorly tolerated,[147] and topical lignocaine (lidocaine) proved effective in a recent double-blind controlled trial.[148] Local anaesthetic blockade is temporarily effective while sympathetic block proved totally ineffective.[149] *N*-methyl-D-aspartate receptor antagonists are the subject of ongoing experimental trials.[150]

Sympathetically-maintained pain

Reflex sympathetic dystrophy (RDS or complex regional pain syndrome type 1 according to the new taxonomy)[151] and causalgia (or complex regional pain syndrome type 2)[151] are terms defining pain with associated dysautonomic and trophic changes following a soft tissue injury (RDS) or injury to a major mixed or sensory nerve (causalgia). It has been observed that patients with these syndromes benefit, sometimes, from sympathetic blockade, thus supporting the hypothesis that the sympathetic nervous system adversely mediates them.[152] However, the pathogenesis of sympathetically-

Table 16 Central and peripheral nervous system complications in the acute phase of HIV infection

Central nervous system	Peripheral nervous system
Aseptic meningitis	Acute demyelinating polyneuropathy (Guillain-Barré syndrome)
Acute encephalitis	Mononeuritis, mononeuritis multiplex, and acute plexopathy
	Facial palsy

mediated neuropathic pain syndromes remains unclear.[151-155] In controlled clinical experience the efficacy of sympathetic blockade in neuropathic pain is unpredictable and disappointing,[149,156,157] as is regional sympathetic blockade with guanethidine.[158] It is difficult, therefore, to identify patients who might benefit from a sympathetic block, and it has been suggested that a test block be used in those patients showing signs of vasomotor and/or trophic changes in the affected area (see Chapters 9.2.6 and 9.2.7).[131]

Neurological complications of AIDS (see also Section 20)

Disorders of both the central and peripheral nervous systems may complicate all stages of systemic infection by the human immunodeficiency virus type 1 (**HIV-1**).[159] The nervous system may be affected either directly by the virus or indirectly as a consequence of the immunosuppression it causes. HIV is a neurotropic as well as a lymphotropic virus and facilitates the development of opportunistic infections and tumours of the central nervous system.[160-162]

Disorders of the central and peripheral nervous systems occurring in the context of acute HIV-1 infection and seroconversion are listed in Table 16. These disorders are underestimated because they are indistinguishable from other acute viral encephalitides and usually resolve in weeks.

Forty to 60 per cent of AIDS patients have neurological complications and nervous system involvement is seen at autopsy in over 90 per cent.[163] Overall, neurological disorders make up about 10 per cent of index diagnoses in this disease.[164] One-third of adult and one-half of paediatric AIDS patients present neurological complications directly caused by the virus infecting the brain.[165] This is an evolving field and nomenclature is continually being updated and refined.[158,166] The differential diagnosis of central nervous system complications in HIV-1 infection is summarized in Table 17.

Aseptic meningitis

Aseptic meningitis in HIV infection can be either acute or chronic. Headache and cranial nerve palsies (usually of the Vth, VIIth, and VIIIth nerves) are clinical features. There are meningeal signs only in the acute form. Headache may be severe and intractable; when it is the only symptom the diagnosis can be difficult. There is no relationship between this syndrome and the subsequent development of AIDS dementia complex.[160]

AIDS dementia complex

AIDS dementia complex is one of the most important complications of HIV-1 infection. It may develop early without any systemic symptoms, although most patients have laboratory evidence of immunosuppression at the time they develop AIDS dementia complex.

Clinical features include cognitive, motor, and behavioural abnormalities. Cognitive disturbances usually appear earlier than motor involvement; the earliest symptoms are difficulties with concentration, attention, and memory. Initial motor symptoms are slowing of rapid eye and alternating hand movements, incoordinate gait, and a clumsiness of fine hand movements. Change in reflexes is frequently observed. Depression can be mild or absent; it may be difficult to separate depression or fatigue from early AIDS dementia complex. An agitated organic psychosis is rare, although psychological distress is common. It has been reported that two-thirds of patients had an adjustment disorder with depressed or anxious mood and one-quarter had major depression.[167] In the late stages of the disease the patients become nearly vegetative, incontinent, and unable to talk or communicate, although the level of arousal is not usually affected.[160,168] The clinical staging of AIDS dementia complex proposed by Price and Brew is a useful classification tool.[169]

Pathological examination of the brain reveals a variable degree of atrophy with ventricle enlargement. The major histological abnormalities are found in the subcortical structures—central white matter, deep grey structures, brainstem, and spinal cord. The characteristic histological features are white matter pallor and reactive astrocytosis, multinucleated giant cells, infiltration by macrophages, and vacuolar myelopathy. Whether the cortex can be involved is controversial.[170,171]

AIDS dementia complex is a direct consequence of viral seeding into the central nervous system due to transportation by monocytes through the blood–brain barrier. Early involvement of the central nervous system is confirmed by clinical leptomeningeal invasion (aseptic meningitis) and by laboratory abnormalities of cerebrospinal fluid. The pathogenesis is not well understood. There are two stages in the infection of brain macrophages: in the first, the virus binds to a receptor on the surface of the macrophage and is internalized; in the second, the viral genome is integrated in the macrophage genome and active viral replication follows. In the second phase, macrophages are stimulated to release large amounts of neurotoxic substances. There may be neuronal injury by an excessive influx of calcium ions into neurones in response to these neurotoxins.[165]

AIDS dementia complex may be the only manifestation of AIDS in 10 per cent of cases. Clinical diagnosis is made by excluding other central nervous system disease and definitive diagnosis by histopathological examination. Neuroimaging studies may show typical findings and are useful in distinguishing AIDS dementia complex from other neurological conditions complicating AIDS, especially treatable, opportunistic central nervous system infections. Both CT and MRI show cerebral atrophy while white matter abnormalities are better seen on MRI scans.

To date, results of treatment have been discouraging. Zidovudine may improve symptoms and prolong survival but this observation needs further confirmation.[172]

Table 17 CNS Complications in AIDS

Clinical presentation	Diagnosis	Aetiology	
Headache Delirium Fever	Cranial nerve palsy Meningeal signs Seizure Cerebrospinal fluid	Acute meningitis	Opportunistic bacterial infection
	Cranial nerve palsy Slight meningeal signs Cerebrospinal fluid diagnostic	Subacute meningitis	HIV-1 Cryptococcus neoformans Mycobacterium tuberculosis Others
	Seizures Focal signs Coma MRI diagnostic	Acute encephalitis	Toxoplasma Cytomegatovirus HSV-I, HSV-II Others
Delirium	Focal signs Seizures MRI diagnostic	Subacute or chronic encephalitis	HIV-1 (AIDS dementia complex) Toxoplasma Papova virus Others
Focal signs	Acute onset	Vascular complications (ischaemia, haemorrhage, vasculitis)	
	Subacute onset	Abscess	Toxoplasma Candida Aspergillus
		Neoplasia	Primary central nervous system lymphoma Metastatic lymphoma Metastatic Kaposi's sarcoma

Vacuolar myelopathy

Vacuolar myelopathy is the pathological definition of the most important complication of HIV-1 infection involving the spinal cord. The aetiopathogenesis of this condition is unknown. The involvement of the posterior and lateral columns of the spinal cord resembles subacute combined degeneration caused by vitamin B_{12} deficiency.

Early symptoms are weakness of the lower extremities and unsteadiness. Clinical examination shows hyperactive deep tendon reflexes, Babinski sign, and sensory loss to proprioception and vibration. Spastic paraparesis, sensory ataxia, and sphincter disturbances develop. More than half the cases also have AIDS dementia complex. Myelography, MRI, and cerebrospinal fluid are normal.

Opportunistic infections of the central nervous system

Opportunistic infections come second only to AIDS dementia complex in producing central nervous system symptoms in AIDS. Agents most frequently involved are *Toxoplasma gondii*, *Cryptococcus neoformans*, JC virus, and cytomegalovirus.

Cerebral toxoplasmosis

Cerebral toxoplasmosis is the most frequent of the central nervous system infections in AIDS, occurring in 3 to 40 per cent of patients;[173] it is more common in advanced stages of the disease. The onset is usually subacute over several days. Common presenting symptoms are persistent headache (55 per cent), confusion (52 per cent), and fever (47 per cent). Focal neurological deficits are present in 69 per cent of patients and seizures are also common.[173]

The infection causes single or multiple cerebral abscesses or encephalitis. Diagnosis can be assisted by CT or MRI; the latter is superior in revealing location and number of lesions. Cerebral lymphoma is the main differential diagnosis. The absence of antitoxoplasma antibodies on immunofluorescence assay does not exclude the diagnosis. Patients who do not respond to treatment should have a brain biopsy.[174]

A combination of pyrimethamine and sulphadiazine is effective. Improvement is usually rapid, both clinically and on MRI, but treatment is often complicated by adverse drug effects.[173]

Cryptococcal meningitis

Cryptococcal meningitis is a common fungal infection in AIDS, usually acquired by haematogenous spread from the lung. The patient presents with meningeal symptoms such as headache, nausea, vomiting, neck stiffness, and fever. Signs of encephalopathy may also be seen with confusion, behavioural alteration, lethargy, and psychosis. Cranial nerve palsies are very suggestive of cryptococcosis. Diagnosis relies on identification of cryptococcal antigen in fungal cultures of cerebrospinal fluid. Treatment with amphotericin B is effective.[175,176]

Progressive multifocal leucoencephalitis

Progressive multifocal leucoencephalitis is caused by JC virus, one of the papovaviruses. The first case of AIDS-associated disease was described in 1982.[177] It occurs in 2 to 7 per cent of patients and is characterized by infection of oligodendrocytes followed by central demyelination.

Patients present with focal neurological deficit (hemiparesis, hemianopsia, aphasia, and ataxia) while consciousness is initially spared. There is progressive deterioration of cognitive function and a worsening of focal deficits resulting in death. Definite diagnosis can only be made by brain biopsy or at autopsy. There is no effective treatment.[178,179]

Cytomegalovirus infection

Systemic infection with cytomegalovirus is common in patients with AIDS. The brain becomes affected in advanced stages of immunosuppression and retinopathy often occurs. Symptoms and signs may overlap those of the AIDS dementia complex; they usually develop subacutely over days and include fever, alterations of consciousness, seizures, and focal signs. Ganciclovir may be useful.[159]

Neoplasms

Primary lymphoma and metastatic systemic lymphoma affecting the central nervous system have been described in patients with AIDS. Metastatic Kaposi's sarcoma has been described only rarely.

Primary lymphoma of the central nervous system

In the general population, primary lymphoma of the central nervous system is a rare brain tumour but it may occur in up to 5 per cent of patients with AIDS. It usually occurs late in the course of the infection. Unlike systemic lymphomas which tend to affect the leptomeninges, primary lymphomas of the central nervous system present as intraparenchymal multicentric masses. Histologically they are usually of B-cell origin.

Headache, confusion and memory loss, seizures, and focal symptoms occur.[180] Toxoplasmosis and progressive multifocal leucoencephalitis should be considered in the differential diagnosis. When lethargy is a prominent symptom it is difficult to distinguish central nervous system lymphoma from AIDS dementia complex. MRI is the most effective of the scans but definite diagnosis must be from brain biopsy. Standard treatment is with whole brain irradiation and corticosteroids. Lymphoma in patients with AIDS is usually aggressive and prognosis is extremely poor, with an average survival of less than 2 months.[181]

Metastatic lymphoma

Systemic lymphoma can occur early in the course of infection with HIV-1 and metastasizes to the central nervous system in up to 40 per cent of cases, usually to the meninges, causing cranial nerve palsies and epidural spinal cord compression. Chemotherapy and whole brain irradiation are indicated.

Peripheral neuropathies

Peripheral neuropathies often complicate HIV-1 infections (occurring in 15 to 20 per cent of patients).[182,183] In the early stage (category 1, see Section 20) mononeuritides, polyneuropathy, and brachial plexopathy may occur but are benign with spontaneous recovery.

In the asymptomatic phase of HIV-1 infection (category 2) a demyelinating neuropathy is common. There is an acute form resembling Guillain–Barré syndrome but the more common form is a chronic inflammatory demyelinating polyneuropathy.[184] Both forms can evolve acutely and can be self limiting or respond to plasma exchange. Rapid, fatal evolution is rare.

In patients with AIDS the most common form is a distal, predominantly sensory, axonal neuropathy, often associated with AIDS dementia complex.[185] Painful paraesthesiae in the lower extremities and burning pain are typical symptoms, and are caused by direct infection of the dorsal root ganglia by HIV-1.

Other common neuropathies of the advanced stage of infection are the infectious neuropathies caused by varicella zoster virus and cytomegalovirus.[186,187] The latter causes a distinct lumbosacral polyradiculopathy characterized by sphincter involvement.[188] Polyneuropathy can also be a complication of treatment by several nucleoside antiretroviral agents,[189] of chemotherapy (particularly by vincristine), or of treatment by phenytoin and isoniazide. Autonomic neuropathy with severe postural hypotension is rare.[190]

Myopathy

A typical polymyositis occurs in patients infected with HIV-1, characterized by a subacute onset with proximal weakness, increasing serum creatophosphokinase, and inflammatory changes seen on muscle biopsy.[191,192] Myopathy can complicate prolonged treatment with zidovudine, producing wasting of the gluteal and thigh muscles. Serum creatinophosphokinase is useful for monitoring treatment.[193,194]

Pain

The lives of patients infected with HIV-1 can now be prolonged by early antiretroviral therapy and prophylaxis of opportunistic infection, and quality of life is increasingly important. The need for control of pain is underestimated and fear of addiction is an important barrier in this patient population.

Pain is a significant problem for patients infected with HIV-1.[195,196] Reported prevalence varies from 40 to 60 per cent depending on the stage of disease and the care setting.[197–199] Pain becomes more common as the disease progresses.[200] Among ambulatory HIV-1 patients, 28 per cent of asymptomatic seropositive patients, 55 per cent of those with AIDS related complex, and 80 per cent of those with AIDS reported one or more pain symptoms over a 6-month period.[201]

Common pain syndromes are headache, pharyngeal and abdominal pain, back pain, arthralgia, herpes zoster, and skin lesions.[201,202] Rheumatological manifestations are important causes of pain, producing Reiter's syndrome, reactive arthritis and polymyositis, and psoriatic arthritis; the musculoskeletal system is involved in 72 per cent of patients.[203,204] Oesophageal and oropharyngeal mucositis, gastroenteritis, and rectal lesions are common painful conditions related to infections, tumours, or treatment.[202]

Neurologists will be particularly concerned with headache, and painful neuropathies and myopathies. Headache is a symptom of most central nervous system complications associated with HIV-1 infection and AIDS and identifiable causes are found in 82 per cent of cases.[202] It can be treatment related; 50 per cent of patients on zidovudine develop headache.

Multiple sclerosis

Multiple sclerosis is a disease characterized by the dissemination of plaques of demyelination in the white matter of the central nervous system. Histologically the disease is inflammatory, with destruction of the myelin sheets, perivascular infiltrates of inflammatory cells (mainly lymphocytes), oedema, and gliosis. Onset is usually between 20 and 40 years of age. The prevalence shows regional variation, increasing from equatorial areas towards the northern hemisphere (from less than 1/100 000 to between 30 and 80/100 000 in northern Europe and Canada). Environmental and genetic factors are important.

Pathogenetic mechanisms are now thought to involve two phases. The first phase, entailing damage to the myelin of the central nervous system and occurring in childhood, has been linked to a viral or viral-like infection which sensitizes the immune system. The second phase, operating later in life, involves an autoimmune attack against myelin components.

Clinically the disease is protean with focal involvement of the optic nerve, the brain, and the spinal cord. The patient presents with a sudden onset of neurological symptoms which may recover after the acute phase. Remissions of varying extent and progressions occur over many years; the extent of these varies with the clinical subtype. The clinical subtypes are identified by differing courses; the primary chronic progressing subtype is characterized by progressive deterioration from the onset whereas the other types (relapsing–remitting, relapsing–progressive, and secondary chronic progressive) are typified initially by relapses, followed by variable degrees of remission.

The disease is characterized by motor impairment of pyramidal type with hyperreflexia and spasticity, sensory disturbances with paraesthesiae, loss of proprioception and ataxia, loss of vision due to optic neuritis, sphincter and sexual dysfunction, vertigo and cerebellar signs, seizures, and cognitive deterioration.

Different subtypes have differing life expectancies; in the more benign forms it is not reduced. Overall, 5 per cent of patents are dead 10 years after onset and median survival is 30 years from the first clinical episode. Death is rarely due to neurological lesions; it is usually the result of infectious complications or of unrelated illness.[205,206]

Diagnosis is made with MRI and study of evoked potentials (abnormal in 80 per cent of cases) and with the demonstration of oligoclonal bands in the cerebrospinal fluid (90 per cent of cases). At the time of writing, there is no cure and treatment of acute episodes with corticosteroids was the only therapy available until recently, when long-term administration of interferon-β was found effective in reducing relapses in the remitting–relapsing form; this treatment may also improve function in the long term.[207]

Symptoms that require specific evaluation and treatment are pain, spasticity, fatigue, depression, and sexual and bladder dysfunction.

Pain

Fifty to 60 per cent of patients suffer pain[139,208,209] and pain has a specific impact on quality of mental and social health.[209] Acute pain, characterized by paroxysmal attacks, occurs in 4 to 9 per cent of patients and is due to trigeminal neuralgia, Lhermitte's sign, paroxysmal dysaesthetic pain, and painful tonic seizures. Trigeminal neuralgia is more often bilateral but is otherwise indistinguishable from the idiopathic form of tic doloureux. In Lhermitte's sign paroxysms of dysaesthetic pain can be spontaneous or can occur in response to movement, tactile stimuli, or hypoventilation. Painful tonic seizures can affect the upper or lower extremities and can be associated with paroxysmal dysaesthetic pain which may be contralateral to the distribution of the tonic seizures. These paroxysmal manifestations respond well to anticonvulsant treatment.[208,210]

Headache is frequent in multiple sclerosis and migraine and tension headache may be more common than in the general population.[211] Optic neuritis can produce periorbital pain aggravated by eye movement.

The most disabling chronic pain, however, is dysaesthetic central pain, low back pain, and painful leg spasms. Dysaesthetic pain is part of the central pain syndrome and is due to myelopathy. It presents with continuous dysaesthetic discomfort, described as a burning pain in the lower extremities, although on occasion it can affect the trunk and arms. It may also be aching, stabbing, or squeezing.[139] All patients with multiple sclerosis-related central pain have sensory abnormalities and abnormal thresholds to thermal and painful stimuli, supporting the modern view that central pain in multiple sclerosis only occurs in patients with lesions affecting the spinothalamic tract.[139]

Low back pain is related to scoliosis and degenerative changes in the lumbosacral spine. It is posture related and is aggravated by prolonged sitting. It tends to overlap spasticity-related pain.

Spasticity due to lesions of the pyramidal tract produces cramping and pulling pain, mainly in the legs. Flexor spasms can be precipitated by external stimuli such as touch, movement, or irritating lesions. The pain responds to muscle relaxants (baclofen, tizanidine). However, use of these agents is limited by the onset of weakness which can reduce function and they should be used within a framework of comprehensive rehabilitation. Neurolysis or the administration of spinal baclofen can also be useful in the treatment of spastic pain.

Visceral pain in multiple sclerosis can be due to chronic constipation, bladder spasms, and bladder distension.

Bladder dysfunction

Urgency or urge incontinence are due to detrusor hyperreflexia and can be managed with regular bladder voiding (every 3 h) using suprapubic percussion and anticholinergics. As the disease progresses urinary retention develops, due to bladder areflexia, requiring intermittent catheterization. Adequate management of bladder function should prevent complications such as infections and stone formation. Rehabilitation has a major role in helping with functional disabilities.[212]

Fatigue

Fatigue is a major and often presenting symptom in multiple sclerosis. The pathogenesis is obscure; the fatigue has motor, cognitive, and psychological components, tends to occur in the late afternoon or evening, and can be exacerbated by physical activity, stress, and heat. Amantidine and pemoline are effective against fatigue.[213,214] Treatment should be carried out in conjunction with psychological rehabilitation and nursing care.[215]

Amyotrophic lateral sclerosis

Amyotrophic lateral sclerosis is a progressive, degenerative disease of motor neurones in the cerebral cortex, brainstem, and spinal cord. The upper and lower motor neurones are affected simultaneously and there is currently no cure.[216] The term 'motor neurone disease' is used in the British literature to include amyotrophic lateral sclerosis and related diseases such as primary lateral sclerosis. The prevalence is between 4 and 6/100 000 population and the annual average death rate world-wide is 1/100 000 population. Mean age at onset is 56 years and mean disease duration is 2.5 years.

Amyotrophic lateral sclerosis is predominantly a neuronopathy; large myelinated fibres are lost from the ventral roots and from all levels of the nerves, and the motor neurone pool in the cervical and lumbosacral enlargements of the spinal cord is reduced, resulting in depletion of pyramidal neurones in the motor cortex and, therefore, in the corticospinal tracts. Pathological evidence of non-motor system involvement is also well established and there is associated dementia in 5 per cent of cases.

Muscle cramps are very often the initial symptom. In about one-third of cases muscular atrophy begins in one hand and in one-quarter weakness begins in the mouth and throat. Muscle weakness presents in a segmental pattern, rather than in the distribution of a peripheral nerve. Onset is usually in adult life and spreads in months or years to affect all the striated muscles, except the extraocular muscles and sphincters. Motor symptoms include cramps (72 per cent), atrophy of one or more extremities (98 per cent), fasciculations (89 per cent), hyper-reflexia (87 per cent), dysphagia (44 per cent), dysarthria (57 per cent), and dyspnoea (35 per cent).[217] Strength is lost more rapidly in the upper extremities. Death is usually secondary to involvement of the respiratory muscles[218] and occurs by 3 years in 50 per cent of patients. The presence of dyspnoea, dysphagia, dysarthria, and four-limb fasciculation gives a poorer prognosis.[218] When onset is in an older patient survival tends to be shorter.[218]

Care should be taken in diagnosis. Cramps and fasciculation occur in several conditions such as recovered poliomyelitis, myelitis, and the muscle pain–fasciculation syndrome. Abnormal fatigue occurs in myasthenia gravis and the Lambert–Eaton syndrome.

There is no effective specific treatment. There should be a careful rehabilitation programme to optimize residual function and encourage the use of orthotic devices. Speech therapy can help patients with mild dysarthria and specific interventions are useful for more severe cases. Dysphagia may require corrective surgery and feeding by gastrostomy or jejunostomy,[219] although improving nutrition may not prevent the cachexia seen with disease progression. Respiratory failure can be helped by inspiratory muscle training. Home care ventilation and nursing require early discussion with patients and relatives. Patients must have the opportunity to make active decisions about respiratory support and when it is requested emergency treatment must be efficient and long-term care carefully planned.[220]

Symptom control is important in these patients. In one study, pain, constipation, dyspnoea, pressure sore, anxiety, depression, and insomnia were among the symptoms assessed and treated during respite hospice admission.[221,222] Opioids, benzodiazepines, muscle relaxants, and night sedation were given in 40 to 50 per cent of the patients. In another study, 64 per cent of patients reported pain, mainly aching and cramping, but also burning and shock-like.[223] Pain is caused by spasticity, joint immobility, malpositioning, and skin pressure. In some cases a neuropathic cause, associated with sensory abnormalities and burning pain, was noted.[223]

References

1. Gilbert MR, Grossman SA. Incidence and nature of neurologic problems in patients with solid tumors. *American Journal of Medicine*, 1986; **81**: 951–4.
2. Clouston PD, De Angelis L, Posner JB. The spectrum of neurological disease in patients with systemic cancer. *Annals of Neurology*, 1992; **31**: 268–73.
3. Posner JB, Chernik NL. Intracranial metastases from systemic cancer. *Advances in Neurology*, 1978; **19**: 575–87.
4. Posner JB. Management of brain metastases. *Revue Neurologique*, 1992; **148**: 477–87.
5. Chang DB, Yang PC, Luh KT, Kuo SH, Lee LN. Late survival off non-small cell lung cancer patients with brain metastases. *Chest*, 1992; **101**: 1293–7.
6. Boogerd W, Vos VW, Hart AAM, Baris G. Brain metastases in breast cancer; natural history, prognostic factors and outcome. *Journal of Neuro-Oncology*, 1993; **15**: 165–74.
7. Posner JB. Clinical manifestations of brain metastasis. In: Weiss L, Gilbert H, Posner J, ed. *Brain Metastasis*. The Hague: Martinus Nijhoff, 1980.
8. Forsyth PA, Posner JB. Intracranial neoplasm. In: Olesen J, Tfelt-Hansen P, Welch KMA, ed. *The Headaches*. New York: Raven Press, 1993: 705–14.
9. Hoang-Xuan K, Delattre J. Treatment of brain metastases. In: Hildebrand J, ed. *Management in Neuro-oncology*. Berlin: Springer Verlag, 1992: 23–39.
10. Patchel RA, Tibbs PA, Walsh JW, *et al.* A randomized trial of surgery in the treatment of single metastases to the brain. *New England Journal of Medicine*, 1990; **322**: 494–500.
11. Haaxma-Reiche H, Vecht C, Padberg G, *et al.* The outcome of single brain metastasis after treatment with irradiation alone or combined with neurosurgery. *Annals of Neurology*, 1992; **32**: 286–7.
12. DeAngelis LM. Management of brain metastases. *Cancer Investigation*, 1994; **12**: 156–65.
13. Phillips MH, Stelzer KJ, Griffin TW, Mayberg MR, Winn HR. Stereotactic radiosurgery: a review and comparison of methods. *Journal of Clinical Oncology*, 1994; **12**: 1085–99.
14. Alexander EI, Moriarty TM, Davis RB, *et al.* Stereotactic radiosurgery for the definitive treatment of brain metastases. *Journal of the National Cancer Institute*, 1995; **87**: 34–40.
15. Posner JB. *Neurologic Complications of Cancer*. Contemporary Neurology Series vol 45. Philadelphia: FA Davis, 1995.
16. Andersen C, Astrup J, Gyldensted C. Quantitative MR analysis of glucocorticoid effects on peritumoral edema associated with intracranial meningiomas and metastases. *Journal of Computer Assisted Tomography*, 1994; **18**: 509–18.
17. Galicich JH, French LA. Use of dexamethasone in the treatment of cerebral edema resulting from brain tumors and surgery. *American Practitioner and Digest of Treatment*, 1961; **12**: 169–74.
18. Vecht CJ, Hovestadt A, Verbiest HBC, van Vliet JJ, van Putten WLJ. Dose-effect relationship of dexamethasone on Karnofsky performance in metastatic brain tumor: a randomized study of doses of 4, 8, 16 mg per day. *Neurology*, 1994; **44**: 675–80.
19. Cairncross JG, Kim JH, Posner JB. Radiation therapy for brain metastases. *Annals of Neurology*, 1980; **7**: 529–41.
20. Ingham JM, Portenoy RK. Drugs in the treatment of pain: NSAIDS and Opioids. *Current Opinion in Anaethesiology*, 1993; **6**: 838–44.
21. Fadul CE, Lemann WT, Posner JB. Perforation of the gastrointestinal

tract in patients receiving steroids for neurologic disease. *Neurology*, 1988; **38**: 348–52.
22. Heimdal K, Hirschberg H, Slettebo H, Watne K, Nolme O. High incidence of serious side effects of high-dose dexamethasone treatment in patients with epidural spinal cord compression. *Journal of Neuro-Oncology*, 1992; **12**: 141–4.
23. Breitbart W, Stiefel F, Kornblith AB, Pannullo S. Neuropsychiatric disturbance in cancer patients with epidural spinal cord compression receiving high dose corticosteroids: a prospective comparison study. *Psychooncology*, 1993; **2**: 233–45.
24. Rotstein J, Good RA. Steroid pseudorheumatism. *Archives of Internal Medicine*. 1957; **99**: 545–55.
25. Dixon RA, Christy NP. On the various forms of corticosteroid withdrawal syndrome. *American Journal of Medicine*, 1980; **68**: 224–30.
26. Sepkowitz KA, Brown AE, Telzak EE, Gottlieb S, Armstrong D. *Pneumocystis carinii* pneumonia among patients without AIDS at a cancer hospital. *Journal of the American Medical Association*, 1992; **267**: 832.
27. Slivka A, Wen PY, Shea WM, *et al*. *Pneumocystis carinii* pneumonia during steroid taper in patients with primary brain tumors. *American Journal of Medicine*, 1993; **94**: 216–9.
28. Twycross R. Corticosteroids in advanced cancer (editorial; comment). *British Medical Journal*, 1992; **305**: 969–70.
29. Plum F, Posner JB. *The Diagnosis of Stupor and Coma*, vol. 19. Philadelphia: FA Davis, 1980.
30. Perrin RG, Livingston KE, Aarabi B. Intradural extramedullary spinal metastasis. A report of 10 cases. *Journal of Neurosurgery*, 1982; **56**: 835–7.
31. Lewis DW, Packer RJ, Raney B. Incidence, presentation and outcome of spinal cord disease in children with systemic cancer. *Pediatrics*, 1986; **78**: 438.
32. Barron KD, Hirano A, Araki S, *et al*. Experience with metastatic neoplasms involving the spinal cord. *Neurology*, 1959; **9**: 91–100.
33. Barcena A, Lobato RD, Rivas JJ, *et al*. Spinal metastatic disease: analysis of factors determining functional prognosis and choice of treatment. *Neurosurgery*, 1984; **15**: 820–7.
34. Hacking HG, Van AH, Lankhorst GJ. Factors related to the outcome of inpatient rehabilitation in patients with neoplastic epidural spinal cord compression. *Paraplegia*, 1993; **31**: 367–74.
35. Shaw MDM, Rose JE, Paterson A. Metastatic extradural malignancy of the spine. *Acta Neurochirurgica*, 1980; **52**: 113–20.
36. Gilbert RW, Kim JH, Posner JB. Epidural spinal cord compression from metastatic tumor: diagnosis and treatment. *Annals of Neurology*, 1978; **3**: 40–51.
37. Kanchandani R, Howe JG. Lhermitte's sign in multiple sclerosis: a clinical survey and review of the literature. 1982; **45**: 308–12.
38. Ventafridda V, Caraceni A, Martini C, Sbanotto A, De CF. On the significance of Lhermitte's sign in oncology. *Journal of Neuro-Oncology*, 1991; **10**: 133–7.
39. Rodichok LD, Harper GR, Ruckdeschel JC, *et al*. Early diagnosis of spinal epidural metastases. *American Journal of Medicine*, 1981; **70**: 1181–8.
40. Rodichok LD, Ruckdeschel JC, Harper GR, *et al*. Early detection and treatment of spinal epidural metastases: the role of myelography. *Annals of Neurology*, 1986; **20**: 696.
41. Portenoy RK, Lipton RB, Foley KM. Back pain in the cancer patient: an algorithm for evaluation and management. *Neurology*, 1987; **37**: 134–8.
42. Portenoy RK, Galer BS, Salamon O, *et al*. Identification of epidural neoplasm. Radiography and bone scintigraphy in the symptomatic and asymptomatic spine. *Cancer*, 1989; **64**: 2207–13.
43. Graus F, Krol G, Foley KM. Early diagnosis of spinal epidural metastasis: Correlation with clinical and radiological findings (abstract). *Proceedings of the American Society of Clinical Oncology*, 1986; **5**: 1047.
44. Caraceni A. Compressioni midollari metastatiche: diagnosi e terapia. *Argomenti di Oncologia*, 1988; **9**: 45–52.
45. Haddad P, Thaell JF, Kiely JM, Harrison EG, Miller RH. Lymphoma of the spinal epidural space. *Cancer*, 1976; **38**: 1862–6.
46. Carmody RF, Yang PJ, Seeley GW, Seeger JF, Unger EC, Johnson JE. Spinal cord compression due to metastatic disease: diagnosis with MR imaging versus myelography. *Radiology*, 1989; **173**: 225–9.
47. Hagen N, Stulman J, Krol G, Foley KM, Portenoy RK. The role of myelography and magnetic resonance imaging in cancer patients with symptomatic and asymptomatic epidural disease. *Neurology*, 1989; **39**: 309.
48. Hagenau C, Grosh W, Currie W, *et al*. Comparison of spinal magnetic resonance imaging and myelography in cancer patients. *Journal of Clinical Oncology*, 1987; **5**: 1663–9.
49. Ingham J, Beveridge A, Cooney NJ. The management of spinal cord compression in patients with advanced malignancy. *Journal of Pain and Symptom Management*, 1993; **8**: 1–6.
50. Boogerd W, van der Sande JJ. Diagnosis and treatment of spinal cord compression in malignant disease. *Cancer Treatment Reviews*, 1993; **19**: 129–50.
51. Sorensen PS, Helweg-Larsen S, Mouridsen H, *et al*. Effect of high-dose dexamethasone in carcinomatous metastatic spinal cord compression treated with radiotherapy. A randomized trial. *European Journal of Cancer*, 1994; **30A**: 22–7.
52. Greenberg HS, Kim J, Posner JB. Epidural spinal cord compression from metastatic tumor: results with a new treatment protocol. *Annals of Neurology*, 1980; **8**: 361–6.
53. Vecht CJ, Haaxma-Reiche H, van Putten WLJ, de Visser M, Vries EP, Twijnstra A. Initial bolus of conventional versus high-dose dexamethasone in metastatic spinal cord compression. *Neurology*, 1989; **39**: 1255–7.
54. Young RF, Post EM, King GA. Treatment of spinal epidural metastases. Randomized prospective comparison of laminectomy and radiotherapy. *Journal of Neurosurgery*, 1980; **53**:741–8.
55. Findlay GF. Adverse effects of the management of malignant spinal cord compression. *Journal of Neurology, Neurosurgery and Psychiatry*, 1984; **47**: 761–8.
56. Findlay GF. The role of vertebral body collapse in the management of malignant spinal cord compression. *Journal of Neurology, Neurosurgery and Psychiatry*, 1987; **50**: 151–4.
57. Harrington KD. Anterior cord decompression and spinal stabilization for patients with metastatic lesions of the spine. *Journal of Neurosurgery*, 1984; **61**: 107–17.
58. Cooper PR, Errico TJ, Martin R, Crawford B, Di BT. A systematic approach to spinal reconstruction after anterior decompression for neoplastic disease of the thoracic and lumbar spine. *Neurosurgery*, 1993; **32**: 1–8.
59. Harrington KD. Anterior decompression and stabilization of the spine as treatment for vertebral collapse and spinal cord compression from metastatic cancer. *Clinical Orthopaedics*, 1988; **233**: 177–97.
60. Kokkoris CP. Leptomeningeall carcinomatosis. How does cancer reach the pia-arachnoid ? *Cancer*, 1983; **51**: 154–60.
61. Henson RA, Urich H. *Cancer and the Nervous System*. Boston: Blackwell Scientific Publications, 1982: 100–19, 368–405.
62. Sause WT, Crowley J, Eyre HJ, *et al*. Whole brain radiation and intrathecal methotrexate in the treatment of solid tumor leptomeningeal metastases—a southwest oncology group study. *Journal of Neuro-Oncology*, 1988; **6**: 107–12.
63. Siegal T, Lossos A, Pfeffer MR. Leptomeningeal metastases. Analysis of 31 patients with sustained off-therapy response following combined-modality therapy. *Neurology*, 1994; **44**: 1463–9.
64. Chamberlain MC. Comparative spine imaging in leptomeningeal metastases. *Journal of Neuro-Oncology*, 1995; **23**: 233–8.
65. Wasserstrom WR, Glass JP, Posner JB. Diagnosis and treatment of leptomeningeal metastasis from solid tumors: experience with 90 patients. *Cancer*, 1982; **49**: 759–72.
66. Kaplan JG, DeSouza TG, Farkash A, *et al*. Leptomeningeal metastases: comparison of clinical features and laboratory data of solid tumors, lymphomas and leukemias. *Journal of Neuro-Oncology*, 1990; **9**: 225–9.
67. Fleisher M, Wasserstrom WR, Schold SC, Schwartz MK, Melamed MR, Posner JB. Lactic dehydrogenase isoenzymes in cerebrospinal fluid in patients with systemic cancer. *Cancer*, 1981; **47**: 2654–9.

68. Greenberg HS, Deck MDF, Vikram B, *et al.* Metastasis to the base of the skull: clinical findings in 43 patients. *Neurology*, 1981; **31**: 530–7.
69. Vecht CJ, Hoff AM, Kansen PJ, de Boer HF, Bosch DA. Types and causes of pain in cancer of the head and neck. *Cancer*, 1992; **70**: 178–84.
70. Foley KM. Pain syndromes in patients with cancer. In: Bonica JJ, Ventafridda V, eds. *Advances in Pain Research and Therapy*, vol.2. New York: Raven Press, 1979: 59–75.
71. Foley KM. The management of pain of malignant origin. In: Tyler HD, Dawson PM, eds. *Current Neurology*, vol.2. New York: Raven Press, 1979: 279–302.
72. Weinstein RE, Herec D, Friedman JH. Hypotension due to glossopharyngeal neuralgia. *Archives of Neurology*, 1986; **40**: 90–2.
73. Sozzi C, Marotta P, Piatti L. Vagoglossopharyngeal neuralgia with syncope in the course of carcinomatous meningitis. *Italian Journal of Neurological Science*, 1987; **8**: 271–6.
74. Cheng TM, Cascino TL, Onofrio BM. Comprehensive study of diagnosis and treatment of trigeminal neuralgia secondary to tumors. *Neurology*, 1993; **43**: 2298–302.
75. DeAngelis LM, Payne R. Lymphomatous meningitis presenting as atypical cluster headache. *Pain*, 1987; **30**: 211–6.
76. Carter RL, Pittam MR, Tanner NSB. Pain and dysphagia in patients with squamous carcinomas of the head and neck: the role of perineural spread. *Journal of the Royal Society of Medicine*, 1982; **75**: 598–606.
77. Clouston PD, Sharpe DM, Corbett AJ, Kos S, Kennedy PJ. Perineural spread of cutaneous head and neck cancer. Its orbital and central neurologic complications. *Archives of Neurology*, 1990; **47**: 73–7.
78. Brazis PW, Vogler JB, Shaw KE. The 'numb cheek-limb lower lid' syndrome. *Neurology*, 1991; **41**: 327–8.
79. Burt RK, Sharfam WH, Karp BI, Wilson WH. Mental neuropathy (numb chin syndrome). A harbinger of tumor progression or relapse. *Cancer*, 1992; **70**: 877–81.
80. Rusthoven JJ, Ahlgren P, Elhakim T, *et al.* Risk factors for varicella zoster disseminated infection among adult cancer patients with localized zoster. *Cancer*, 1988; **62**: 1641–6.
81. Kori SH, Foley KM, Posner JB, *et al.* Brachial plexus lesions in patients with cancer 100 cases. *Neurology*, 1981; **31**: 45–50.
82. Marangoni C, Lacerenza M, Formaglio F, Smirne S, Marchettini P. Sensory disorder of the chest as presentig symptom of lung cancer. *Journal of Neurology, Neurosurgery and Psychiatry*, 1993; **56**: 1033–4.
83. Castagno AA, Shuman WP. MR imaging in clinically suspected brachial plexus tumor. *American Journal of Roentgenology*, 1987; **149**: 1219–22.
84. Krol G. Evaluation of neoplastic involvement of brachial and lumbar plexus: imaging aspects. *Journal of Back and Musculoskeltal Rehabilitation*, 1993; **3**: 35–43.
85. Cascino TL, Kori S, Krol G, Foley KM. CT scan of brachial plexus in patients with cancer. *Neurology*, 1983; **33**: 1553–7.
86. Harper CM, Thomas JE, Cascino TL, Litchy WJ. Distinction between neoplastic and radiation-induced brachial plexopathy, with emphasis on EMG. *Neurology*, 1989; **39**: 502–6.
87. Thomas JE, Cascino TL, Earl JD. Differential diagnosis between radiation and tumor plexopathy of the pelvis. *Neurology*, 1985; **35**: 1–7.
88. Jaeckle KA, Young DF, Foley KM. The natural history of lumbosacral plexopathy in cancer. *Neurology*, 1985; **35**: 8–15.
89. Dalmau J, Graus F, Marco M. 'Hot and dry foot' as initial manifestation of neoplastic lumbosacral plexopathy. *Neurology*, 1989; **39**: 871–2.
90. Stevens MJ, Gonet YM. Malignant psoas syndrome: recognition of an oncologic entity. *Australasian Radiology*, 1990; **34**: 150–4.
91. Rogers LR, Borkowski GP, Albers JW, Levin KH, Barohn RJ, Mitsumoto H. Obturator mononeuropathy caused by pelvic cancer: six cases. *Neurology*, 1993; **43**: 1489–92.
92. Martini C. *Sindromi Dolorose da Cancro.* (Oncology specialty thesis). Univerita' degli Studi di Milano, Facolta' di Medicina a Chirurgia, Scuola di Specializzazione in Oncologia, 1991.
93. Ventafridda V, Martino G. Clinical evaluation of subarachnoid neurolytic blocks in intractable cancer pain. In: Bonica JJ, *et al*, eds. *Advances in Pain Research and Therapy.* New York: Raven Press, 1976: 699–703.
94. Ischia S, Ischia A, Luzzani A, Toscano D, Steele A. Results up to death in the treatment of persistent cervico-thoracic (Pancoast) and thoracic malignant pain by unilateral percutaneous cervical cordotomy. *Pain*, 1985; **21**: 339–55.
95. Sanders M, Zuurmond W. Safety of unilateral and bilateral percutaneous cervical cordotomy in 80 terminally ill cancer patients. *Journal of Clinical Oncology*, 1995; **13**: 1509–12.
96. Ventafridda V, Caraceni A. Cancer pain. In: Prithvi RP, ed. *Current Review of Pain.* Philadelphia: Current Medicine, 1994: 156–78.
97. Posner JB. Paraneoplastic syndromes. *Neurologic Clinics*, 1991; **9**: 919–36.
98. Delattre JY, Posner JB. Neurological complications of chemotherapy and radiation therapy. In: Aminoff MJ, ed. *Neurology and General Medicine.* New York: Churchill Livingstone, 1989: 365–87.
99. Lipton RB, Galer BS, Dutcher JP, *et al.* Large and small fibre type sensory dysfunction in patients with cancer. *Journal of Neurology, Neurosurgery and Psychiatry*, 1991; **54**: 706–9.
100. Siegal T. Muscle cramps in the cancer patient: causes and treatment. *Journal of Pain and Symptom Management*, 1991; **6**: 84–91.
101. Chaudhry V, Rowinsky EK, Sartorius SE, Donehower RC, Cornblath DR. Peripheral neuropathy from taxol and cisplatin combination chemotherapy. Clinical and electrophysiological studies. *Annals of Neurology*, 1994; **35**: 304–11.
102. Graus F, Rogers L, Posner JB. Cerebrovascular complications in patients with cancer. *Medicine*, 1985; **64**: 16.
103. Barrow KD, Sigueira E, Hirano A. Cerebral embolism caused by nonbacterial thrombotic endocarditis. *Neurology*, 1960; **10**: 391.
104. Rogers LH, Cho ES, Kempin S, Posner JB. Cerebral infarction from nonbacterial thrombotic endocarditis. A clinical and pathological study including the effects of anticoagulation. *American Journal of Medicine*, 1987; **83**: 746.
105. Collins RC, Al-Mondhiry H, Chernik NL, Posner JB. Neurologic manifestations of intravascular coagulation in patients with cancer. A clinicopathological analysis of 12 cases. *Neurology*, 1975; **25**: 795.
106. Frits RD, Forkner CE, Freirich EJ, Frei E, Thomas LB. The association of fatal intracranial hemorrhage and 'blastic crisis' in patients with acute leukemia. *New England Journal of Medicine*, 1959; **261**: 59.
107. Lossos A, Siegal T. Spinal subarachnoid hemorrage associated with leptomeningeal metastases. *Journal of Neuro-Oncology*, 1992; **12**: 167–71.
108. Sigsbee B, Deck MDF, Posner JB. Non-metastastatic superior sagittal sinus thombosis complicating systemic cancer. *Neurology*, 1979; **29**: 139.
109. Mandybur TI. Intracranial hemorrhage caused by metastatic tumors. *Neurology*, 1977; **27**: 650.
110. Shimamura K, Oka K, Nakazawa M, Kkojima M. Distribution patterns of microtrombi in disseminated intravascular coagulation. *Archives of Pathology and Laboratory Medicine*, 1983; **107**: 543–7.
111. Posner JB. Cerebrovascular disorders in patients with cancer. In: *Neuro-oncology V: Recent Advances in Diagnosis and Treatment.* Syllabus of the postgraduate course Memorial Sloan Kettering Cancer Center. New York: Memorial Sloan Kettering Cancer Center, 1992.
112. Graus F, Rene R. Clinical and pathological advances of central nervous system paraneoplastic syndromes. *Review of Neurology*, 1992; **148**: 496–501.
113. Posner JB. Pathogenesis of central nervous system paraneoplastic syndromes. *Review of Neurology*, 1992; **148**: 502–12.
114. Glantz MJ, Biran H, Myers ME, Gockerman JP, Friedberg MH. The radiographic diagnosis and treatment of paraneoplastic central nervous system disease. *Cancer*, 1994; **73**: 168–75.
115. Tuxen MK, Werner Hansen S. Neurotoxicity secondary to antineoplastic drugs. *Cancer Treatment Reviews*, 1994; **20**: 191–214.
116. Crossen JR, Garwood D, Glatsein E, Neuwelt EA. Neurobehavioral sequelae of cranial irradiation in adults: a review of radiation-induced encephalopathy. *Journal of Clinical Oncology*, 1994; **12**: 627–42.
117. Delattre J, Safai B, Posner JB. Erythema multiforme and Stevens-Johnson syndrome in patients receiving cranial irradiation and phenythoin. *Neurology*, 1988; **38**: 194–8.
118. Taylor LP, Posner JB. Phenobarbital rheumatism in patients with brain tumor. *Annals of Neurology*, 1989; **25**: 92–4.

119. Posner JB. Supportive care in the neuro-oncology patient. In: Hildebrand J, ed. *Management in Neuro-oncology*. Berlin: Springer-Verlag, 1992: 89–103.
120. Hagen NA, Cirrincione C, Thaler HT, DeAngelis L. The role of radiation therapy following resection of single brain metastasis from melanoma. *Neurology*, 1990; **40**: 158–60.
121. McLellan J, Jack W. Phenytoin/dexamethasone interaction: a clinical problem. *Lancet*, 1978; **1**: 1096–7.
122. Wong MC, Suite NDA, Labar DR. Seizures in HIV infection. *Archives of Neurology*, 1990; **47**: 640–2.
123. Engel J. *Seizures and Epilepsy*. Philadelphia: FA Davis, 1989
124. Parent JM, Lowenstein DH. Treatment of refractory generalized status epilepticus with continuous infusion of midazolam. *Neurology*, 1994; **44**: 1837–40.
125. Burke AL, Diamond PL, Hulbert J, Yeatman J, Farr EA. Terminal restlessness—its management and the role of midazolam. *Medical Journal of Australia*, 1991; **155**: 485–7.
126. Gregory RE, Grossman S, Sheidler VR. Grand mal seizures associated with high-dose intravenous morphine: incidence and possible etiologies. *Pain*, 1992; **51**: 255–8.
127. Eisele JH, Grigsby EJ, Dea G. Clonazepam treatment of myoclonic contractions associated with high dose opioids: a case report. *Pain*, 1992; **49**: 231–2.
128. Wengs WJ, Talwar D, Bernard J. Ifosfamide-induced nonconvulsive status epilepticus. *Archives of Neurology*, 1993; **50**: 1104–5.
129. Elliot KJ. Taxonomy and mechanisms of neuropathic pain. *Seminars in Neurology*, 1994; **14**: 195–205.
130. Devor M, Rappaport H. Pain and pathophysiology of damaged nerve. In: Fields H, ed. *Pain Syndromes in Neurology*. London: Butterwoths, 1990: 47–83.
131. Fields HL, Rowbotham MC. Multiple mechanisms of neuropathic pain: a clinical perspective. In: Gebhart GF, Hammond DL, Jensen TS, eds. *Proceendings of the 7th World Congress on Pain, Progress in Pain Research and Management*, vol 2. Seattle: IASP Press, 1994: 437–54.
132. Gonzales GR. Central pain. *Seminars in Neurology*, 1994; **14**: 255–62.
133. Devor M, Basbaum AI, Bennett GJ, *et al.* Group report: mechanisms of neuropathic pain following peripheral injury. In: Basbaum A, Besson J-M, eds. *Towards a New Pharmacotherapy of Pain*. New York: John Wiley and Sons, 1991: 417–40.
134. Asbury AK, Fields HL. Pain due to peripheral nerve damage: an hypothesis. *Neurology*, 1984; **34**: 1587–90.
135. Boivie J, Leijon G, Johanson I. Central poststroke pain—a study of the mechanisms through analyses of the sensory abnormalities. *Pain*, 1989; **37**: 173–85.
136. Leijon G, Boivie J, Johanson I. Central post-stroke pain—neurological symptoms and pain characteristics. *Pain*, 1989; **36**: 13–25.
137. Nurmikko T, Bowsher D. Somatosensory findings in postherpetic neuralgia. *Journal of Neurology, Neurosurgery and Psychiatry*, 1990; **53**: 135–41.
138. Asbury AK. Pain in generalized neuropathies. In: Fields H, ed. *Pain Syndromes in Neurology*. London: Butterwoths, 1990: 131–41.
139. Osterberg A, Boivie J, Holmgren H, Thuomas K, Johanson I. The clinical characteristics and sensory abnormalities of patients with central pain caused by multiple sclerosis. In: Gebhart GF, Hammond DL, Jensen TS, eds. *Proceedings of the 7th World Congress on Pain, Progress in Pain Research and Management*, vol 2. Seattle: IASP Press, 1994: 789–96.
140. Boivie J. Hyperalgesia and allodynia in patients with CNS lesions. In: Willis W, ed. *Hyperalgesia and Allodynia*. New York: Raven Press, 1992: 363–73.
141. Dyck PJ, Low PA, Stevens JC. 'Burning feet' as the only manifestation of dominantly inherited sensory neuropathy. *Mayo Clinic Proceedings*, 1983; **58**: 426–9.
142. Watson CP, Deck JP. The neuropathology of herpes zoster with particular reference to postherpetic neuralgia and its pathogenesis. In: Watson CPN, ed. *Herpes Zoster and Postherpetic Neuralgia. Pain Reseach and Clinical Management*, vol. 8. Amsterdam: Elsevier, 1993: 139–57.
143. Watson CPN, Evans RJ, Watt VR, Birkett N. Postherpetic neuralgia: 208 cases. *Pain*, 1988; **35**: 289–97.
144. Watson CPD. Postherpetic neuralgia: clinical features. In: Fields HL, ed. *Pain Syndromes in Neurology*. London: Butterwoths, 1990: 223–38.
145. Rowbotham MC. Postherpetic neuralgia. *Sem Neurol*, 1994; **14**: 247–54.
146. Rowbotham MC, Reisner L, Fields HL. Both intravenous lidocaine and morphine reduce the pain of postherpetic neuralgia. *Neurology*, 1991; **41**: 1024–8.
147. Watson CPN, Evans RJ, Watt VR. Postherpetic neuralgia and topical capsaicin. *Pain*, 1988; **33**: 333–40.
148. Rowbotham MC, Davies PM, Fields HL. Topical lidocaine gel relieves postherpetic neuralgia. *Annals of Neurology*, 1995; **37**: 246–53.
149. Nurmikko T, Wells C, Bowsher D. Pain and allodynia in postherpetic neuralgia: role of somatic and sympathetic nervous systems. *Acta Neurologica Scandinavica*, 1991; **84**: 146–52.
150. Eide PK, Jorum E, Stubhaug A, Bremnes J, Breivik H. Relief of post-herpetic neuralgia with the n-methyl-d-aspartic acid antagonist ketamine: a double-blind cross-over comparison with morphine and placebo. *Pain*, 1994; **58**: 347–54.
151. Stanton-Hicks M, Janig W, Hassenbusch S, Haddox JD, Boas R, Wilson P. Reflex sympathetic dystrophy: changing concepts and taxonomy. *Pain*, 1995; **63**: 127–33.
152. Backonia M. Reflex sympathetic dystrophy/sympathetically mantained pain/ causalgia: the syndrome of neuropathic pain with dysautonomia. *Seminars in Neurology*, 1994; **14**: 563–71.
153. Perl ER. Causalgia and reflex sympathetic dystrophy revisited. In: Boivie J, Hansson P, Lindblom U, eds. *Touch, Temperature and Pain in Health and Disease: Mechanisms and Assessment. Progress in Pain Research and Management*, vol 3. Seattle: IASP Press, 1994: 231–48.
154. Campbel JN, Meyer RA, Davis KD, Raja SN. Sympathetically mantained pain. A unifying hypothesis. In: Willis W, ed. *Hyperalgesia and Allodynia*. New York: Raven Press, 1991: 141–9.
155. Schott GD. Visceral afferents: their contribution to 'sympathetic dependent' pain. *Brain*, 1994; **117**: 397–413.
156. Verdugo RJ, Ochoa JL. 'Sympathetically mantained pain.' I Phentolamine block questions the concept. *Neurology*, 1994; **44**: 1003–10.
157. Verdugo RJ, Campero M, Ochoa JL. Phentolamine sympathetic block in painful neuropathies. II. Further questioning of the concept of 'sympathetically maintained pain'. *Neurology*, 1994; **44**: 1010–14.
158. Jadad AR, Carroll D, Glynn CJ, McQuay HJ. Intravenous regional sympathetic blockade for pain relief in reflex sympathetic dystrophy: a systematic review of the literature and a randomized double-blind crossover study. *Journal of Pain and Symptom Management*, 1995; **10**: 13–20.
159. Price RW, Brew BJ, Roke M. Central and peripheral nervous system complications of HIV-1 infection and AIDS. In: DeVita VT, Hellman S, Rosenberg SA, Curran J, Essex M, Fauci AS, eds. *AIDS. Etiology, Diagnosis, Treatment, and Prevention*, 3rd edn. Philadelphia: Lippincott, 1992.
160. Price RW, Brew B, Sidtis J, Rosenblum M, Scheck AC, Cleary P. The brain in AIDS: central nervous system HIV-1 infection and AIDS dementia complex. *Science*, 1988; **239**: 586–92.
161. Ho DD, Rota TR, Schooley RT, *et al.* Isolation of HTLV-III from cerebrospinal fluid and neural tissues of patients with neurologic syndromes related to the acquired immunodeficiency syndrome. *New England Journal of Medicine*, 1985; **313**: 1493–7.
162. Levy RM, Bredesen DE, Rosenblum ML. Neurological manifestations of the acquired immunodeficiency syndrome (AIDS): Experience at UCSF and review of the literature. *Journal of Neurosurgery*, 1985; **62**: 475–95.
163. Bacellar H, Munoz A, Miller EN, *et al.* Temporal trends in the incidence of HIV-1-related neurologic diseases: Multicenter AIDS Cohort Study, 1985–1992. *Neurology*, 1994; **44**: 1892–900.
164. Wang F, So Y, Vittinghoff E, *et al.* Incidence proportion of and risk factors for AIDS patients diagnosed with HIV dementia, central nervous system toxoplasmosis, and cryptococcal meningitis. *Journal of Acquired Immune Deficiency Syndrome*, 1995; **8**: 75–82.

165. Lipton SA, Gendelman HE. Dementia associated with the acquired immunodeficiency syndrome. *New England Journal of Medicine*, 1995; **332**: 934–40.
166. Nomenclature and research case definitions for neurologic manifestations of human immunodeficiency virus-type 1 (HIV-1) infection. *Neurology*, 1991; **41**: 778–5.
167. Tross S, Hirsch DA. Psychological distress and neuropasychological complications of HIV infection and AIDS. *American Psychologist*, 1988; **43**: 929–34.
168. Sidtis JJ, Price RW. Early HIV-1 infection and the AIDS dementia complex. *Neurology*, 1990; **40**: 323–6.
169. Price RW, Brew BJ. The AIDS dementia complex. *Journal of Infectious Diseases*, 1988; **158**: 1079–83.
170. Everall IP, Luthert PJ, Lantos PL. Neuronal loss in the frontal cortex in HIV infection. *Lancet*, 1991; **337**: 1119–21.
171. Seilhean D, Duyckaerts C, Vazeux R, *et al.* HIV-1-associated cognitive/motor complex: absence of neuronal loss in the cerebral neocortex. *Neurology*, 1993; **43**: 1492–9.
172. Portegies P, Enting RH, de Gans J, *et al.* Presentation and course of AIDS dementia complex: 10 years of follow-up in Amsterdam, The Netherlands. *AIDS*, 1993; **7**: 669–75.
173. Porter SB, Sande MA. Toxoplasmosis of the central nervous system in the acquired immunodeficiency syndrome. *New England Journal of Medicine*, 1992; **327**: 1643–8.
174. Editorial. Brain biopsy for intracranial mass lesions in AIDS. *Lancet*, 1992; **340**: 1135.
175. Chuck SL, Sande MA. Infections with *Cryptococcus neoformans* in the acquired immunodeficiency syndrome. *New England Journal of Medicine*, 1989; **321**: 794–9.
176. Dismukes WE. Cryptococcal meningitis in patients with AIDS. *Journal of Infectious Diseases*, 1988; **157**: 624–8.
177. Miller JR, Barrett RE, Britton CB, *et al.* Progressive multifocal leukoencephalopathy in a male homosexual with T-cell immune deficiency. *New England Journal of Medicine*, 1982; **307**: 1436–8.
178. Berger JR, Kaszovits B, Donovan Post MJ, Dickinson G. Progressive multifocal leukoencephalopathy in association with human deficiency virus infection: a review of the literature with a report of sixteen cases. *Annals of Internal Medicine*, 1987; **107**: 78–87.
179. Major EO, Amemiya K, Tornatore CS, Houff SA, Berger JR. Pathogenesis and molecular biology of progressive multifocal leukoencephalopathy, the JC virus-induced demyelinating disease of the human brain. *Clinical Microbiology Reviews*, 1992; **5**: 49–73.
180. So YT, Beckstead JH, Davis RL. Primary central nervous system lymphoma in acquired immune deficiency syndrome: a clinical and pathological study. *Annals of Neurology*, 1986; **20**: 566–72.
181. Northfelt DW, Kaplan LD. Clinical manifestations and treatment of HIV related non-Hodgkins lymphoma. *Cancer Surveys*, 1991; **10**: 121–33.
182. Parry GJ. Peripheral neuropathies associated with HIV infection. *Annals of Neurology*, 1988; **23**: S49–53.
183. Cornblath DR. Treatment of neuromuscular complications of human immunodeficiency virus infection. *Annals of Neurology*, 1988; **23**(suppl): S88–91.
184. Vendrell J, Heredia C, Pujol M. Guillan-Barre' syndrome associated with seroconversion for anti-HTLV III. *Neurology*, 1987; **35**: 544.
185. Cornblath DR, McArthur JC. Predominantly sensory neuropathy in patients with AIDS and AIDS-related complex. *Neurology*, 1988; **38**: 794–6.
186. Behar R, Wiley C, McCutchan A. Cytomegalovirus polyradiculopathy in AIDS. *Neurology*, 1987; **37**: 557–61.
187. Grafe MR, Wiley C. Spinal cord and perpheral nerve pathology in AIDS: the roles of cytomegalovirus and HIV. *Annals of Neurology*, 1989; **25**: 561–6.
188. Eidelberg D, Sotrel A, Vogel H, Walker P, Kleefield J, Crumpacker CS. Progressive polyradiculopathy in acquired immune defiency syndrome. *Neurology*, 1986; **36**: 912–6.
189. Lambert JS, Seidlin M, Reichman RC. 2',3'-dideoxyinosine (ddI) in patients with the acquired immunodeficiency syndrome or AIDS-related complex. *New England Journal of Medicine*, 1990; **322**: 1333–40.
190. Freeman R, Roberts MS, Friedman LS. Autonomic function and HIV infection. *Neurology*, 1990; **40**: 575–80.
191. Dalakas MC, Pezeshkpour GH. Neuromuscular diseases associated with human immunodeficiency virus infection. *Annals of Neurology*, 1988; **23**: S38–48.
192. Simpson DM, Bender AN. Human immunodeficiency virus-associated myopathy: analysis of 11 patients. *Annals of Neurology*, 1988; **24**: 79–84.
193. Dalakas MC, Illa I, Pezeshkpour GH, Laukaitis JP, Cohen B, Griffin J. Mitochondrial myopathy caused by long term zidovudine therapy. *New England Journal of Medicine*, 1990; **322**: 1098–105.
194. Arnaudo E, Dalakas M, Shanske S, Moraes CT, Dimauro S, Schon EA. Depletion of muscle mitochondrial DNA in AIDS patients with zidovudine-induced myopathy. *Lancet*, 1991; **1**: 508–10.
195. O'Neill WM, Sherrard JS. Pain in human immunodeficiency virus disease: a review. *Pain*, 1993; **54**: 3–14.
196. Penfold J, Clark AJ. Pain syndromes in HIV infection. *Canadian Journal of Anaesthesia*, 1992; **39**: 724–30.
197. Schofferman J. Pain: diagnosis and management in the palliative care of AIDS. *Journal of Palliative Care*, 1988; **4**: 46–9.
198. Lebovits AH, Lefkowits M, McCarthy D, Simon R, Wilpon H, *et al.* The prevalence and management of pain in patients with AIDS: A review of 134 cases. *Clinical Journal of Pain*, 1989; **5**: 245–8.
199. Moss V. Patient characteristics, presentation and problems encountered in advanced AIDS in a hospice setting—a review. *Palliative Medicine*, 1991; **5**: 112–6.
200. Schofferman J, Brody R. Pain in far advanced AIDS. In: Foley KM, *et al*, eds. *Advances in Pain Research and Therapy.* New York: Raven Press, 1990: 379–86.
201. Singer EJ, Zorilla C, Fahy-Chandon B, Chi S, Syndulko K, Tourtellotte WW. Painful symptoms reported by ambulatory HIV-infected men in a longitudinal study. *Pain*, 1993; **54**: 15–19.
202. Lipton RB, Feraru ER, Weiss G, *et al.* Headache in HIV-1-related disorders. *Headache*, 1991; **31**: 518–22.
203. Kaye BR. Rheumatologic manifestations of infection with human immunodeficiency virus (HIV). *Annals of Internal Medicine*, 1989; **111**: 158–67.
204. Espinoza LR, Aguilar JL, Berman A, Gutierrez F, Vasey FB, Germain BF. Rheumatic manifestation associated with human immunodeficiency virus infection. *Arthritis and Rheumatism*, 1989; **32**: 1615–21.
205. Confavreux C, Aimard G, Devic M. Course and prognosis of multiple sclerosis assessed by the computerized data processing of 349 patients. *Brain*, 1980; **103**: 281–300.
206. McAlpine D, Lumsden CE, Acheson ED. *Multiple Sclerosis. A Reapraisal.* Edinburgh: Churchill Livingstone, 1972.
207. Weinstock-Guttman B, Ransohohoff RM, Kinkel RP, Rudick RA. The interferon: biological effects, mechanisms of action, and use in multiple sclerosis. *Annals of Neurology*, 1995; **37**: 7–15.
208. Moulin DE, Foley KM, Ebers GC. Pain syndromes in multiple sclerosis. *Neurology*, 1988; **38**: 1830–4.
209. Archibald CJ, McGrath PJ, Ritvo PG, *et al.* Pain prevalence, severity and impact in a clinic sample of multiple sclerosis patients. *Pain*, 1993; **58**: 89–93.
210. Espir MLE, Millac P. Treatment of paroxysmal disorders in multiple sclerosis with carbamazepine (Tegretol). *Journal of Neurology, Neurosurgery and Psychiatry*, 1970; **33**: 528–31.
211. Watkins SM, Espir MLE. Migraine and multiple sclerosis. *Journal of Neurology, Neurosurgery and Psychiatry*, 1969; **32**: 35–7.
212. Pearson CL. The bladder in multiple sclerosis. In: Hallpike JF, Adams CWM, Tourtelotte WW, eds. *Multiple Sclerosis.* London: Chapman and Hall, 1983:
213. Rosemberg GA, Appenzeller O. Amantadine, fatigue and multiple sclerosis. *Archives of Neurology*, 1988; **45**: 1104–6.

214. Wenshenker BG, Penman M, Bass B, *et al.* A double blind randomized cross-over trial of pemoline in fatigue associated with multiple sclerosis. *Neurology*, 1992; **42**: 1468–71.
215. Hubsky EP, Sears JH. Fatigue in multiple sclerosis: guidelines for nursing care. *Rehabilation Nursing*, 1992; **17**: 176–80.
216. Mulder DW, ed. *The Diagnosis and Treatment of Amyotrophic Lateral Sclerosis.* Boston: Houghton Mifflin, 1980.
217. Ringel SP, Murphy JR, Alderson MK, *et al.* The natural history of amyotrophic lateral sclerosis. *Neurology*, 1993; **43**: 1316–22.
218. Norris F, Shepherd R, Denys E, *et al.* Onset, natural history and outcome in idiopathic adult motor neuron disease. *Journal of Neurological Sciences*, 1993; **118**: 48–55.
219. Hillel AD, Miller RM. Management of bulbar symptoms in amyotrophic lateral sclerosis. *Advances in Experimental Medical Biolology*, 1987; **209**: 201–21.
220. Tandan R, Bradley WG. Amyotrophic lateral sclerosis: Part 1. Clinical features, pathology, and ethical issues in management. *Annals of Neurology*, 1985; **18**: 271–80.
221. O'Brien T, Kelly M, Saunders C. Motor neurone disease: a hospice perspective (see comments). *British Medical Journal*, 1992; **304**: 471–3.
222. Hicks F, Corcoran G. Should hospices offer respite admissions to patients with motor neurone disease? *Palliative Medicine*, 1993; **7**: 145–50.
223. Newrick PG, Langton-Hewer R. Pain in motor neuron disease. *Journal of Neurology, Neurosurgery and Psychiatry*, 1985; **48**: 838–40.

9.13 Sleep

Michael J. Sateia and Peter M. Silberfarb

Introduction

Sleep disorders have been recognized for centuries as a frequent complication of medical illness. The last few decades have produced an explosive growth in our knowledge and understanding of sleep physiology and pathophysiology. Unfortunately, the practical application of this knowledge has been slow in reaching the majority of health care providers, including those in palliative medicine. However, examination of the literature on this subject does suggest a growing recognition on the part of clinicians that attention to patients' sleep is a necessary and important aspect of care in this population. A good night's sleep may provide a patient receiving palliative care with an invaluable respite from the worries and pain of the day, and may allow him to meet the next day with renewed energy and motivation. In this chapter, we review basic aspects of sleep and sleep disorders, particularly as they apply to palliative care, and discuss strategies for the evaluation and treatment of these conditions.

Sleep physiology

Human sleep is a complex and dynamic physiological function, the nature of which we have only begun to unravel. Contrary to the historical view of sleep as a passive state of little medical interest or relevance, it has become increasingly clear that sleep is an active condition which is affected by waking physiological and psychological states and which, in turn, has significant effects on those waking conditions. This is particularly true in the case of major medical illnesses in which marked perturbations in somatic and psychological function may result in severe disruption of sleep and concomitant waking complications.

Normal sleep consists of two distinct states: non-rapid eye movement (NREM) sleep (stages 1–4) comprises approximately 75 per cent of the night; the remainder consists of rapid eye movement (REM) or 'dreaming' sleep. In the NREM sleep of the healthy young adult, stage 1 (light sleep) normally represents only 5 to 10 per cent of total sleep, stage 2 (medium sleep) represents approximately 50 per cent, and stages 3 and 4 (deep sleep) represent about 20 per cent. These stages, along with the REM stage of sleep, repeat themselves in cyclical fashion through the night. The deepest stages of sleep occur predominantly during the first half of the night, while REM periods are significantly longer and more intense during the second half of the night. NREM sleep is a period of relative physiological and cognitive quiescence, quite distinct from REM sleep which is characterized by muscle atonia, dreaming, and autonomic variability. The last mentioned characteristic includes periodic increases in pulse, blood pressure, and respiration, as well as increased cerebral blood flow, decreased temperature regulation, and erection activity in males. The sleep–wake cycle is a component of the body's overall circadian rhythm. As such, its timing is synchronized with other biological rhythms including temperature oscillation and secretion of cortisol and growth hormone. The onset and maintenance of normal sleep patterns are dependent on the satisfaction of a number of conditions. These include appropriate timing of sleep within the 24-h circadian rhythm, an adequate level of physical comfort, an acceptable sleeping environment, an intact central nervous system function, and relative absence of psychological distress.

The restorative functions of sleep are dependent on a well-organized and reasonably uninterrupted structure or 'sleep architecture'. In many medical conditions, as well as with advancing age, there is a tendency towards lighter sleep, with an increase in stage 1 and a decrease in stages 3 and 4. The percentage of REM sleep remains relatively constant in a healthy elderly population but is typically decreased when cognitive impairment disorder or certain other medical conditions are present. Sleep often becomes more fragmented, with increased awakening through the night. Disturbances of this nature result in complaints of poor sleep from affected patients.

Classification of sleep disorders

Sleep disorders are classified according to the International Classification of Sleep Disorders of the American Sleep Disorders Association.[1] This system categorizes sleep disorders into three primary groups: (1) dyssomnias, (2) parasomnias, and (3) sleep disorders secondary to medical or psychiatric conditions. Dyssomnias include primary disorders which result in disturbance of the quantity, quality, or timing of nocturnal sleep, as well as those conditions which are associated with excessive daytime sleepiness. Dyssomnias may be related to intrinsic factors (e.g. obstructive sleep apnoea, narcolepsy, or 'primary' insomnias) or extrinsic factors (drugs, medications, or environmental conditions). Parasomnias are events or conditions which are caused or exacerbated by sleep, such as nightmares, sleep terrors, or enuresis. For the purposes of this chapter, we shall focus on primary patient complaints—most often insomnia or excessive sleepiness.

Table 1 Common causes of insomnia in the terminally ill

Depression	Major depressive illness related to loss, chronic pain, effects of tumour on central nervous system
Anxiety	Adjustment disorder or generalized anxiety related to fears of illness, procedures, pain, or death; medication; direct effects on central nervous system
Cognitive impairment disorder	Delirium secondary to medication, metabolic derangement, direct involvement of central nervous system, or non-specific deliriogenic factors
Pain	Related to direct tumour effects, diagnostic or treatment interventions, non-specific causes
Nausea and vomiting	Associated with chemotherapy, medication or primary gastrointestinal disturbance
Respiratory distress	Dyspnoea due to hypoxia and/or anxiety; obstructive sleep apnoea
Medications	Stimulants, bronchodilators, steroids, some antihypertensives, activating antidepressants; withdrawal or rebound from sedative hypnotics or analgesics
Psychophysiological insomnia	Caused by conditioned arousal response and poor sleep hygiene
Sleep–wake schedule disorder	Associated with disruption of normal schedule, excessive time in bed or napping, disturbed nocturnal sleep
Periodic limb movement	Secondary to sedative hypnotic withdrawal, tricyclic medication, anaemia, uraemia, leukaemia, diabetes mellitus, peripheral neuropathy

Insomnia

In clinical practice, insomnia can be defined as a subjective complaint by the patient of poor sleep. This definition encompasses complaints of insufficient sleep, difficulty in initiating or maintaining sleep, interrupted sleep, poor-quality or 'non-restorative' sleep, or sleep which occurs at the wrong time in the day–night cycle. Insomnia is a symptom, not a diagnosis. It is incumbent upon the clinician to clarify the nature of the complaint and to consider potential aetiologies. In the case of insomnia associated with medical conditions there are often a number of contributing factors which give rise to a patient's sleep disturbance. These include physiological, psychological, and environmental factors. Among the most common physiological determinants are pain, toxic and metabolic disturbance, medications, sleep-disordered breathing, movement disorders, and diseases of the central nervous system. Depression and anxiety are leading psychological causes of insomnia. Environmental circumstances, such as unfamiliar surroundings, frequent interruptions, or noise, are particularly important factors for patients in hospital. The most frequent causes of insomnia among terminally ill patients are outlined in Table 1.

Sleep deprivation may result in a broad spectrum of physiological and psychological changes, which vary according to the degree and type of deprivation. The changes most frequently described include progressive fatigue, sleepiness, impairment of concentration, and irritability.[2],[3] Individuals who are chronically sleepy as a result of physiological disruption of night-time sleep frequently become depressed.[4] Sleep, particularly the deepest stages of non-REM sleep, may play a critical role in tissue restoration.[5] This observation is supported by the finding that a musculoskeletal pain syndrome may be experimentally induced by specific sleep deprivation.[6] Of particular interest in cancer or AIDS patients is the observation that sleep deprivation results in alterations of immune system function.[7] Morley *et al.*[8] noted that immune activation has a stimulating effect on slow-wave sleep and, conversely, that slow-wave sleep enhances immune function. They speculated that sleep may be a factor in recuperative processes, including recuperation from infection.

Excessive daytime sleepiness

Excessive sleepiness is a common and frequently overlooked symptom, particularly among patients with serious medical illness. Because sleepiness renders many individuals quieter and more 'compliant', medical staff and other caregivers are often not motivated to identify sleepiness as a problem. As Kubler-Ross[9] points out, daytime sedation may actually be encouraged by health professionals as a means of dealing with their own discomfort with the dying patient. While some degree of daytime sedation can be desirable in certain cases, this is by no means uniformly the case. Excessive somnolence is a potentially quite disabling symptom which may further compromise already tenuous function in the terminally ill. The sleepy patient is inactive, poorly motivated, and less capable of participating in treatment. The ability to attend to and thereby retain information is compromised. Social interactions, which may be of great importance in the final weeks or months of life, become seriously impaired. Depression, irritability, and withdrawal are also potential complications of pathological sleepiness.

Sleepiness must be distinguished from more general and vague complaints of 'tiredness' and 'fatigue' which are very common among patients receiving palliative care. Specifically, it must be determined to what extent an individual experiences drowsiness or episodes of irresistible sleepiness, particularly under circumstances of physical inactivity, or takes naps during normal waking hours. The Multiple Sleep Latency Test,[10] which is an objective measure of pathological sleepiness, can be utilized when appropriate. Diagnostic difficulty may arise in the final stages of disease when the distinction between excessive somnolence and alteration of consciousness associated with delirium becomes blurred.

There is very little documentation of sleepiness as a symptom in patients with terminal malignancies or other endstage disease. Munro *et al.*[11] noted 'sleeping more than usual' as one of the most troublesome symptoms of patients undergoing radiation therapy. Excessive sedation is described in association with opioid analgesics[12],[13] and some forms of chemotherapy.[14],[15]

There are many potential causes of excessive sleepiness in this population. They include insufficient or disturbed night-time sleep, medication (analgesic, sedative hypnotic, antidepressant, and chemotherapeutic), metabolic disorders, and disruption of the sleep–wake schedule. In some cases, sleepiness may occur as a form of psychological withdrawal or as an atypical symptom of depressive illness. For many patients, the aetiology is multifactorial. A careful review of potential causes must be conducted in order to identify the source(s) of the complaint. Most importantly, it is essential that the clinician does not dismiss excessive sleepiness as an inevitable part of terminal illness but rather approaches it as a treatable symptom.

Disorders of the sleep–wake schedule

Maintenance of a normal sleep pattern is dependent on adherence to a well-established schedule of sleep and wakefulness. Because of frequent disruptions of night-time sleep, an absence of usual daytime schedule demands, and relative inactivity during normal waking hours, terminally ill individuals are particularly prone to disturbances of the sleep–wake schedule. When night sleep has been poor, there is an inclination to delay the hour of rising and/or to engage in lengthy daytime naps. While these practices are understandable, they pose a problem in that the onset of sleep may be significantly delayed on the subsequent night. This, in turn, results in further delays in rising and increased napping. Ultimately, there is a pronounced difficulty in falling asleep until the early morning hours, with subsequent sleep often stretching into the early afternoon. This cycle is referred to as delayed sleep phase syndrome. In other cases, the fatigue and sedation so often associated with major medical illness may result in advancement of the normal sleep–wake schedule, resulting in early morning awakening (advanced sleep phase syndrome). For some, the normal circadian rhythm disappears altogether and is replaced by a pattern of multiple shorter sleep periods which are interspersed with wakefulness throughout the 24-h cycle.

These disorders may result in complaints of insomnia or excessive sleepiness, depending on the nature of the schedule disturbance and the particular focus of the patient. In addition to the dysfunction and frustration which these disorders engender for the patient, the burden imposed on caregivers can be substantial in that they are required to respond to the needs of a patient who is awake at all hours.

Circadian rhythm disorders of the type described may respond to straightforward efforts at regularization of the sleep–wake schedule and adherence to proper sleep hygiene, as described later in this chapter. Short-term treatment with hypnotic medications can be helpful in regularizing the circadian rhythm in certain patients. However, the more formal behavioural approach of 'chronotherapy' is required in some cases.[16]

Sleep in cancer and AIDS

Patients with malignant disease consider sleep disturbance to be an important and troubling symptom. Women with metastatic breast cancer rated sleep in the highest quartile of quality-of-life items.[17] Patients undergoing radiation therapy ranked sleep disturbance as one of the 10 most troubling difficulties associated with their illness.[11] Current data suggest that sleep may be disturbed in 50 per cent or more of those with advanced cancer, particularly when pain is a complicating factor.[18–20] Patients with cancer sleep less at night and are more likely to sit, lie down, and sleep during the day than normal subjects.[21] The nocturnal disturbance may be associated with any of the factors listed in Table 1, although pain is of particular importance in cancer patients. Daytime fatigue and sleepiness may occur as a result of tumour effects (e.g. cytokines), treatment, or disturbance of quantity or quality of nocturnal sleep.

Greater insight into the magnitude of this problem can be gained by analysing the prescribing practices of physicians who treat these patients. In two large surveys of psychotropic drug utilization by patients with neoplastic disease, hypnotic medication accounted for 48 to 55 per cent of all psychotropic medication prescriptions. Derogatis *et al.*[22] reported that 44 per cent of all psychotropic prescriptions written for cancer patients were for sleep disturbance, while Jaeger *et al.*,[23] in a survey of prescribing practices in terminally ill cancer patients, found that 34 per cent of psychotropic drugs were prescribed for sleep. These findings clearly suggest that, at the very least, physicians perceive that a high percentage of patients with neoplastic disease require treatment for sleep disturbance.

In one of the few direct investigations of insomnia in cancer patients, Beszterczey and Lipowski[24] found that 45 per cent of a mixed group of cancer patients referred for radiotherapy had a total sleep time of less than 50 h per week, while 23 per cent slept for less than 40 h per week. A comparison of sleep in their patients with that in an independent group of mixed medical and surgical patients revealed less sleep in the group with neoplastic disease. Other comparisons between cancer patients and those with non-malignant disease or normal controls have yielded mixed results. Lamb[25] found no difference between the sleep of newly diagnosed cancer patients and a group with benign medical illness. Another survey[26] which compared patients with cancer with cardiac patients and normal controls indicated that the cancer group had no less difficulty falling asleep than cardiac patients, but they reported significantly more problems in maintaining sleep than either of the two comparison groups. Approximately 30 per cent of the cancer patients with sleep maintenance complaints described pain as a cause of awakening. Interpretation of this study is complicated by the use of hypnotics or analgesics in a higher percentage (33 per cent) of the cancer group.

The only laboratory-based study of sleep in cancer patients to date is that of Silberfarb *et al.*[27] who provided a preliminary report on a group of 14 patients with unresectable lung cancer. Nine patients were self-described 'good sleepers' and five were 'poor sleepers'. All patients were studied for three consecutive nights in a sleep laboratory. The groups did not differ with respect to sleep efficiency, sleep latency, or distribution of sleep stages, with the exception that good sleepers spent a significantly greater amount of time in stages 3 and 4 (delta sleep). The authors suggest that, for cancer patients, the subjective appraisal of quality of sleep may relate to the amount of time spent in delta sleep, although both groups spent so little time in deep sleep that this explanation should be considered preliminary.

In a continuation of the aforementioned study, the sleep of 17 patients with unresectable lung cancer and 15 with breast cancer (in various stages of their disease) was compared with that of 32 insomniacs without medical illness and an equal number of normal controls.[28] All cancer patients were ambulatory and, for the most part, only mildly impaired by their illness, with mean Karnofsky ratings of 85.4 and 92.8 for the lung and breast cancer groups respectively. Overall, cancer patients slept as long as the controls and significantly longer than the insomniacs. Patients with breast cancer were not distinguishable from controls on polysomnographic variables. Lung cancer patients achieved total sleep times which were comparable with those of the controls by spending significantly more time in bed. However, their sleep was clearly more disturbed, with prolonged latency to stage 2 sleep, lower sleep efficiency, increased stage 1 sleep, and increased awakening through the night. Curiously, and in contrast with the usual reports of insomniacs, the lung cancer group under-reported the sleep disturbance, denying the presence of sleep problems despite polysomnographic evidence to the contrary. Psychological questionnaires and interviews suggested that the differences observed were not a function of psychological disturbance which, in fact, was not evident in this group of cancer patients.

Sleep disorders are common in HIV-infected patients. Fatigue, daytime sleepiness, and difficulties initiating and maintaining sleep have been described.[29,30] The severity of sleep disturbance and associated daytime dysfunction is correlated with progression of the disease. Darko *et al.*[29] postulate that the debilitating fatigue of these patients may be related to elevated levels of somnogenic humoral factors such as interferon, tumour necrosis factor, and interleukin 1.

Sleep has been studied in a limited number of HIV-infected patients, including some with clinical manifestations of AIDS. St Kubicki *et al.*[31] described disturbance of sleep, including decreased percentages of slow-wave sleep, in patients with diagnosed cerebral disease. Norman *et al.*[32] reported alterations in the sleep of 10 asymptomatic HIV-infected males. These patients demonstrated an increase in total slow-wave sleep, particularly as a result of increased slow-wave sleep in the second half of the night, when compared with normal controls. Seven of the patients complained of excessive sleepiness, although daytime nap studies yielded objective evidence of pathological sleepiness in only one. Norman *et al.* speculated that sleep changes may represent early changes in the central nervous system associated with the infection or an adaptation to bolster immune response.

Sleep disturbance has also been described in association with treatment for AIDS. Insomnia has been reported as a side-effect of azidothymine (AZT).[33,34] Severe sleepiness in patients receiving a combination of AZT and acyclovir[35] has also been observed. As noted, the sleep changes in HIV-infected individuals may vary widely according to the stage of disease and its complications. The sleep of asymptomatic infected persons as described by Norman *et al.*[32] is probably quite different from that in late-stage AIDS with attendant neoplastic or infectious manifestations. Likewise, the presence of depression, anxiety, and cerebral involvement, particularly AIDS dementia complex, is likely to have a major impact on the sleep of these patients, although this issue has not been fully clarified. Hintz *et al.*,[36] noting estimates of a 10 to 20 per cent incidence of depression in HIV-positive patients, reported on the response to antidepressant treatment in 90 such patients. Their investigation revealed that decreased sleep was a particularly prominent finding which distinguished this population from a depressed HIV-negative group.

Factors contributing to sleep disorder

Depression

Sleep disturbance is a hallmark of major depression. It is generally held that 90 per cent or more of depressed patients exhibit abnormal sleep patterns. Although early morning awakening is most commonly associated with depression, difficulty initiating sleep and repeated awakenings are not uncommon, particularly in a population in which the depression is associated with medical illness and its attendant complications. Current evidence indicates that specific abnormalities can be identified in the sleep electroencephalograms of primary depressive patients. These include disturbances in the continuity of sleep, decreased latency to the first REM sleep period, and diminished slow-wave sleep (stages 3 and 4).[37] The extent to which these findings are valid in depression associated with or secondary to medical disorders, particularly those of palliative care patients, is not clear. What is certain is that the sleep disturbance experienced by depressed terminally-ill patients is a major source of concern, frustration, and added disability.

Studies to date indicate that depression is common among cancer patients. The manner in which the presence of 'depression' has been assessed varies widely from one investigator to another, making comparisons of prevalence difficult. Depressive illness accounts for approximately 50 per cent of psychiatric consultations in cancer patients.[38] Studies of self-reported depressive symptoms indicate 'moderate' to 'severe' symptoms in 25 to 50 per cent of cancer patients.[39,40] Derogatis *et al.*[41] reported a prevalence of approximately 6 per cent for major depressive disorder assessed by DSM III criteria, with an additional 25 per cent diagnosed as having adjustment disorder with depressed or mixed features. Bukberg *et al.*[42] found a prevalence rate of 42 per cent for moderate to severe depression in cancer patients in hospital.

These prevalence statistics suggest that depression is a very significant cause of sleep pathology in the terminally ill. In the light of this, it is surprising to find that, according to some estimates, antidepressant medication is administered to a relatively small percentage of cancer patients. A multicentre study of psychotropic drug utilization by the Psychosocial Collaborative Oncology Group found that antidepressant medications accounted for only 1 per cent of all psychotropic prescriptions.[22] In the study of Bukberg *et al.*,[42] in which 42 per cent of patients met criteria for depression, only 6 per cent were receiving an antidepressant. In contrast, Jaeger *et al.*[23] found that 10 per cent of patients with advanced neoplastic disease (life expectancy less than 3 months) received antidepressants. This higher rate of administration may reflect a greater degree of overt psychological distress among the terminally ill.

To some extent the underusage of antidepressant medication may be a function of the complications of establishing a diagnosis of depression in palliative care patients. There is ample room for debate regarding the distinction between appropriate grief and clinical depression. In addition, uncertainty exists regarding the use of somatic symptoms (including sleep) in establishing the diagnosis of depression, inasmuch as such symptoms may be a function of the medical disorder. There is some preliminary evidence which suggests that sleep-related symptoms may be of particular importance in identifying depressive illness in cancer patients. One analysis of the association between insomnia, depression, anxiety, and pain revealed that insomnia was closely correlated with depression and anxiety.[24] In an effort to address the issue of specificity of somatic symptoms in the diagnosis of depression in cancer patients, Bukberg *et al.*[42] found that, with the exception of insomnia, somatic symptoms did not distinguish the patients with depression from the non-depressed cancer population. Although no statistical analysis is offered, the data strongly suggest that early, middle, and late insomnia were significantly more diagnostic of depression. In contrast with the above findings, Plumb and Holland[40] found that depressed patients with malignant disease did not manifest significantly greater insomnia than their next of kin and reported less insomnia than a psychiatric group with depression and suicide attempt. Unfortunately, these results do not make clear whether these findings are indicative of little insomnia among the cancer patients or a relatively high degree of insomnia in the next of kin.

There is no specific evidence regarding the efficacy of antidepressant medications in the treatment of insomnia associated with depression in the terminally ill. Antidepressant medications, particularly the more sedating compounds such as amitriptyline, doxepin, and trazodone, have been effective in the treatment of chronic pain syndromes which are frequently accompanied by depression and insomnia.[43–45] Patients with combined pain, depression, and insomnia may benefit not only from the sedative and antidepressant effects of tricyclic medication, but also from the analgesic activity of these compounds.[46]

The available literature makes it clear that depression is a common cause of insomnia among patients with advanced malignancies and that this aspect of their condition frequently goes unrecognized or untreated. Insomnia is an important diagnostic marker for depressive illness which must not be overlooked, particularly in view of the fact that highly efficacious treatment is available.

Anxiety

Although there has been little specific investigation of the relationship between terminal illness, specifically cancer, and anxiety symptoms, the available literature supports the common-sense conclusion that anxiety is a frequent complication among these patients.[25,39,41] Anxiety symptoms may be directly related to aspects of the patient's medical condition or treatment. Pain is frequently associated with increased anxiety. Early delirium, withdrawal from analgesics or sedative hypnotics, and shortness of breath can frequently result in anxiety symptoms. Sleep disturbance is common among patients with significant anxiety. Battelli *et al.*[47] reported that 63 per cent of cancer patients with anxiety had insomnia.

Fears which are masked by distractions during the daylight hours may rapidly come to the fore once the patient is left with nothing but the stillness of night. Anxieties regarding the illness itself, concerns about forthcoming procedures, and worries regarding family or financial matters are just a few of the tensions which can disrupt the onset or maintenance of sleep. Pain may be exacerbated during the night (owing to inadequate medication and lack of distraction), giving rise to further anxiety about the meaning of the pain as a possible sign of advancing disease. For patients in the final stages of their illness, the prospect of sleep may provoke anxieties about the possibility that they will never awaken.

As sleeplessness ensues, additional anxiety often arises over the inability to fall asleep. A vicious circle is set in motion in which the patient with an initially transient insomnia disturbance develops a negative expectation regarding sleep and begins to dread the prospect of another tension- and frustration-laden night in bed. Thus the bed becomes a powerful conditioned stimulus for escalating anxiety and arousal which prevents the onset of sleep. This dilemma may be particularly difficult for patients who are not ambulatory and are unable to 'escape'. The combination of heightened internal arousal and conditioned anxiety gives rise to a chronic condition of self-propagating sleep disturbance which is referred to as psychophysiological insomnia. The disturbance may be accompanied by an increase in muscle tension, sympathetic arousal, and unrelenting cognitive activity. As sleep steadily becomes more difficult, daytime anxiety and rumination regarding the inability to obtain a restful night may intervene.

The sleep of patients with diagnosed anxiety disorders has not been studied in great detail. Laboratory studies have revealed prolonged sleep latency, decreased sleep efficiency (the percentage of time in bed which is spent asleep), increased time awake during the night, decreased deep sleep, and higher percentages of light sleep.[48,49] In addition to the alteration of sleep architecture, specific anxiety-related disturbances such as nocturnal anxiety attacks or nightmares may occur.[50] The latter are dream anxiety episodes which ordinarily arise from REM sleep. They are accompanied by awakening from sleep with a sense of dread or terror and a moderate level of autonomic arousal. The frightening dream content is recalled in detail upon awakening. Nightmares may occur as a complication of severe anxiety or other psychiatric illness, or use of certain medications such as β-blockers, L-dopa, or reserpine.

Non-pharmacological measures, including support, reassurance, proper sleep hygiene, and behavioural techniques such as relaxation training, may help to ameliorate the sleep disturbance associated with anxiety. Benzodiazepines have been effective in treating anxiety-related insomnia. Battelli *et al.*[47] found that 80 per cent of patients with insomnia were sleeping normally after 2 weeks of treatment with lorazepam. Diazepam suppositories have also been used with similar beneficial effects, although many patients experienced daytime sedation. Psychotherapy, benzodiazepines, and tricyclic medication have all been employed with some success in the treatment of recurrent nightmares.

Cognitive impairment disorders

Numerous investigations have revealed that cognitive dysfunction, particularly delirium, is common among cancer patients.[38,51] The incidence of delirium is particularly high among those in the terminal stages of illness.[52] Disturbance of the sleep–wake schedule is an intrinsic component of delirium. As described by Lipowski,[53] wakefulness during the daytime is typically reduced, while night-time often brings increased alertness and agitation. As a result, the normal circadian rhythm may be reversed or severely disrupted in this population. The multiple aetiologies of delirium in patients with terminal malignancies have been reviewed elsewhere.[54,55] Sleep deprivation itself may predispose to the development of delirium.[56] Polysomnographic studies of delirium have been limited to withdrawal states,[57] and the applicability of these findings to the sleep of patients with delirium due to other causes is uncertain.

Dementia, while less commonly a direct result of cancer, may be encountered in terminally ill patients,[41] particularly in the geriatric population. This disorder is often associated with nocturnal delirium ('sundowning'). Sleep studies of dementia patients reveal increased sleep latencies, lighter sleep, reduced REM sleep, and increased awakening after sleep onset.[58,59]

The sleep disturbance associated with cognitive impairment disorders can be exceedingly difficult to manage. Accurate diagnosis is the first step. Delirium often goes unrecognized, particularly in its early stages, and may be mistaken for depression or anxiety in some patients. Attempts to treat or control the deliriogenic factors, particularly with medication, constitute the primary approach. Efforts to prevent excessive sleep during the daytime are advisable. Patients with cognitive dysfunction may sleep better in a lit room, where disorientation and agitation are minimized. Conventional hypnotic medications have typically been avoided because they may aggravate delirium. The usual pharmacological treatment for patients with non-drug-related delirium and disruptive behaviour is haloperidol which may be given in low starting dosages of 0.5 to 2.0 mg (orally or intramuscularly) and gradually increased. In patients whose agitation is largely limited to the night-time, it is often helpful to begin administration of the medication in the late afternoon before agitation begins to escalate. Subcutaneous midazolam has been used effectively in terminal patients with delirium or agitation when other agents were not helpful.[60,61]

Pain

A number of issues must be taken into consideration in assessing the relationship between pain and sleep in terminally ill patients. What are the effects of pain on sleep? How does sleep deprivation affect pain threshold and perception? What intervening variables, such as psychiatric disorders, influence the relationship between pain and sleep?

Numerous studies of cancer patients indicate that up to 50 per cent experience significant pain. In individuals with advanced cancer, estimates rise to 60 to 90 per cent.[62-64] These data, combined with observations regarding the effects of pain on sleep in other conditions and indications that pain is often inadequately treated, suggest that pain plays an important role in sleep disturbance among cancer patients. Dorrepaal *et al.*[65] evaluated pain experience and management in a group of 240 cancer patients in hospital. They found that, upon admission, 37 per cent of patients with pain reported that it interfered with sleep onset, while 65 per cent complained of difficulty in maintaining sleep through the night because of pain. An investigation of the influence of cancer-related pain on various quality-of-life indicators revealed that 58 per cent of cancer patients woke during the night because of pain.[66] Pain intensity has also been demonstrated to correlate inversely with the total hours of sleep in patients with advanced cancer.[67]

Donovan *et al.*[68] examined the issue of pain in hospital patients and the effects of inadequate analgesia. In this mixed group, which consisted of predominantly non-cancer patients with acute or chronic pain, 61 per cent reported that they were awakened by pain. The patients were receiving an average of less than 25 per cent of the total analgesic dosage ordered. It should be noted that the cancer patients in this population did not differ from the non-cancer patients with respect to incidence or severity of pain.

Pain models and related variables

Further insight can be gained by addressing the issue of sleep in chronic pain states. In assessing peak pain-related symptoms, Kinsman *et al.*[69] reported that 60 per cent of the group complained of frequent sleep disturbance. Sleep was characterized as 'poor' by 70 per cent of a group of patients attending a pain clinic.[70] The poor sleepers reported greater pain intensity, less total sleep time, and a tendency towards greater disability. Pain intensity and depression were the only significant predictors of sleep disturbance, leading the investigators to speculate that degree of insomnia may serve as a useful marker for pain intensity.

Animal models of chronic pain demonstrate an increase in wakefulness, a shift to lighter stages of NREM sleep, a reduction in paradoxical (REM) sleep, and fragmentation of sleep.[71,72] A loss of the normal diurnal variation of the sleep–wake cycle was also noted. Similar polysomnographic findings have also been described in humans with rheumatic and other pain conditions.[73,74]

The observation of increased sleep disturbance in patients with pain does not, in itself, establish a direct cause and effect relationship between these variables. It is quite possible that intervening factors, particularly psychological distress, may play an important role. For example, it has been reported that the incidence of pain among cancer patients with psychiatric disorder is twice that of those without such disorder.[75] This may reflect the fact that patients with pain are also likely to have more advanced illness and therefore to be more susceptible to depression or organic mental disorders. Nevertheless, it is apparent that comorbidity of this nature (i.e. psychiatric illness) may have as much responsibility for the sleep disturbance as the pain *per se*. This issue has not been examined in great detail. Beszterczey and Lipowski[24] described decreased total sleep time in a group of cancer patients referred for radiation therapy. Analysis revealed that the insomnia correlated far better with the degree of depression and anxiety than with pain. Thus, while pain itself may be an important determinant of sleep disturbance, other factors which covary with pain may be of equal importance.

Sleep deprivation and pain

In order to understand fully the relationship between sleep and pain, it is necessary to address the question of how sleep deprivation affects pain perception and, in turn, to what extent improvement in sleep might produce a beneficial response with respect to pain. Hicks *et al.*[76] reported that pain threshold in rats is decreased in response to deprivation of REM sleep, and that the effect persisted for up to 96 h following the deprivation. This may be related to the fact that opioid receptor binding decreases after sleep deprivation.[77] It has been shown that sleep deprivation lowers the pain threshold in humans.[3] Repeated interruptions of sleep induced experimentally result in a pain syndrome which is akin to fibromyalgia.[6] The work of Moldofsky and others related to fibromyalgia syndrome suggests that sleep may play an important role in pain modulation and that disturbance of sleep might predispose to the development of rheumatic pain disorder by interference with the tissue-restorative functions of NREM sleep in particular. The relationship of these findings to pain of other origins is uncertain.

Clinical experience suggests that patients whose coping skills are enhanced by improved sleep are in a far better position to maintain optimal function despite their pain and, perhaps, to perceive the pain as less severe. This supposition is supported by reports from hospital patients with acute and chronic pain that sleep helped to reduce their pain.[68] This perspective is strengthened by the evidence that administration of delta-sleep-inducing peptide to chronic pain patients resulted in reduction of pain and associated symptoms of depression.[78]

Effects of pain treatment

It is clear that improved control of pain results in better sleep. One notable advance in this area has been the use of controlled-release opioids for pain control. Hanks *et al.*[13] describe improved sleep in a group of advanced cancer patients in response to crossover from aqueous morphine sulphate administered every 4 h to controlled-release morphine. Ventafridda *et al.*[79] reported that mean total sleep time was doubled in patients with cancer pain treated by the World Health Organization (WHO) three-step pain relief method. Similar observations have been described by other investigators.[12,80]

Significant improvements in sleep have been reported with the use of the non-steroidal anti-inflammatory drugs (NSAIDs) nimesulide and diclofenac in advanced cancer pain.[81] Carrol *et al.*[82] demonstrated that a combined regimen of methadone, an NSAID, a tricyclic, and hydroxyzine produced marked improvement in pain and sleep in patients not responsive to single-drug therapy. For patients refractory to all other routes of opioid administration, combined long-term intrathecal morphine and bupivacaine have produced prolonged improvement in sleep and pain.[83] A multidisciplinary approach which included various combinations of oral and epidural opioids, non-opioid analgesics, antidepressants, benzodiazepines, anticonvulsants, and nerve blocks produced an almost 80 per cent reduction in the number of cancer patients whose sleep was interrupted by pain.[84] In appropriate circumstances, continuous infusion and/or patient-controlled analgesia will be superior to immediate-release oral opioids in fostering sustained sleep. A comparison of the effects of a mild sedative with those of a mild analgesic on sleep in non-cancer patients demonstrated that the analgesic was most important in improving sleep for those with pain.[85] The pharmacological effects of opioids on sleep physiology and wakefulness are discussed below.

In summary, pain is a frequent and often inadequately treated symptom of cancer which is an important factor contributing to the development and maintenance of sleep disturbance. Sleep deprivation, in turn, may exacerbate pain problems and compromise the already tenuous function of patients receiving palliative care. Intervening variables such as depression and anxiety play a contributory role. Improved control of pain can result in marked improvement in sleep disturbance and thereby greatly improve the quality of life.

Medication

Discussion of the effects of medication on sleep in palliative care must include attention to those medications which interfere with normal sleep, as well as those which result in excessive or undesirable sedation. The effects of specific hypnotic medication are discussed later in this chapter.

Very little attention has been paid to the effects of chemotherapy agents on sleep. Shapiro[86] has pointed out that certain chemotherapeutic agents may produce insomnia as a result of their potential for inducing nausea or cognitive dysfunction. Clinical experience suggests that corticosteroids produce sleep disturbance, although this has not been well documented. Steroids do appear to decrease REM sleep,[87] but the clinical implications of this are uncertain. Methylxanthine derivatives (bronchodilators) are well known for their stimulant properties and may disturb sleep severely. Certain antihypertensives, such as methyldopa and propranolol, have been reported to cause insomnia; the latter is also associated with nightmare activity in some patients. Central nervous system stimulants, sometimes advocated for their energizing effect in gravely ill individuals, have clear potential for disrupting sleep when given too close to bedtime, as do certain types of 'stimulating' antidepressants (monoamine oxidase inhibitors, fluoxetine, protriptyline, or bupropion). Withdrawal from sedative-hypnotic medication is an important cause of insomnia.

Psychotropic agents

Excessive sleepiness and associated daytime impairment may severely compromise the function of patients already adversely affected by other aspects of their disease. The most common offending agents are psychotropic medications prescribed for anxiety, sleep, depression, or control of nausea. Older patients with medical illness are particularly vulnerable to excess sedation due to drug accumulation as a result of delayed metabolism and excretion. Sedating antidepressants such as amitriptyline, doxepin, or trazodone may result in daytime sleepiness, even when given at bedtime. Phenothiazines and other dopamine antagonists used in the treatment of nausea due to chemotherapy may be very sedating. This is particularly true for aliphatic and piperidine compounds, but less so for piperazine derivatives and butyrophenones. H_1 antagonists are common sources of daytime sleepiness, but this does not appear to be true for H_2 antagonists which have less effect on the central nervous system.

Opioids

The effects of opioids on sleep and wakefulness are complex and appear to include both stimulant and sedative properties.[88] Initial doses of morphine administered to non-dependent addicts decrease total sleep but increase drowsiness. With chronic usage, sleep latency is decreased but the total time awake after sleep onset is somewhat increased. Although drowsiness is a feature of acute morphine administration, this appears to abate with chronic usage. The effects of opioids on sleep structure vary with duration of usage. The most prominent initial effect is suppression of REM activity. However, this is less evident with longer-term administration. The effects on NREM sleep vary according to type of drug, length of usage, and specific sleep stage. There is evidence to suggest that cognitive performance may be slowed as a result of opioid administration.[89] Although these data are of some use in understanding the effects of opioid analgesics on sleep, it should be noted that they are based largely on studies of subjects who were not medically ill or in pain. As already discussed, effective analgesia clearly results in improved sleep for patients in pain, and any alterations of 'normal' sleep which may be induced by medication are surely outweighed by the benefits attributable to relief of pain.

Likewise, while opioids can produce some degree of daytime drowsiness, particularly in the earlier phases of administration, this must be considered a potentially unavoidable sequela of adequate pain relief. While the clinician should attempt to strike an appropriate balance in this regard, sufficient analgesia must take precedence.

Respiratory disorders

Respiratory disturbance is a common cause of sleep disorder. Obstructive sleep apnoea is associated primarily with heavy snoring and excessive daytime sleepiness, although some patients report frequent nocturnal wakening. The syndrome is observed more commonly in older patients and those who are obese. There is no clear connection between obstructive sleep apnoea and malignancy, although it should be noted that patients whose upper airway structure or function is compromised directly as a result of tumour mass or indirectly through treatment may be predisposed to the development of obstruction during sleep. This has been described in patients with parapharyngeal tumour mass[90,91] and those who have undergone mandibulectomy without reconstruction.[92] Perhaps of greater importance for the majority of cancer patients is the fact that medications that depress respiratory function, particularly opioid analgesics, worsen this condition. Etches[93] described severe respiratory depression associated with patient-controlled opioid analgesia. Pre-existing sleep apnoea and concomitant use of sedative hypnotics were associated with the development of respiratory compromise. Central sleep apnoea has also been reported to occur with malignancy.[94] Sleep apnoea frequently goes unrecognized and may be a source of major compromise of function (due to sleepiness and attendant neuropsychological factors) in terminally-ill patients.

Dyspnoea is a disturbing symptom for some palliative care patients, particularly those with primary lung cancer or pulmonary metastases. Pulmonary involvement may give rise to complaints of insomnia through two primary mechanisms. Patients describe the sensation of breathlessness as psychologically disturbing, and they have difficulty initiating or maintaining sleep as a result of heightened arousal associated with this anxiety. Studies of patients with chronic obstructive pulmonary disease also suggest that severe hypoxia and/or hypercapnoea, as well as chronic cough, may play a role in determining sleep disturbance. Decreased total sleep time, increased light sleep, multiple arousals, and decreased REM sleep have been reported in such patients.[95] Non-pharmacological treatment (e.g. relaxation training) for heightened arousal associated with breathlessness may aid sleep. Nocturnal oxygen supplementation is indicated for hypoxic patients. Pharmacological treatment with benzodiazepines may be used cautiously in patients without major blood gas alterations, but is contraindicated in more severely hypoxic or hypercapnoeic patients.

Gastrointestinal disorders

Nausea and vomiting following certain forms of chemotherapy can severely disrupt sleep. Some terminally ill patients report nocturnal diarrhoea or discomfort associated with chronic constipation as a cause of repeated sleep disruption. These occur as a result of autonomic dysfunction, medication, or other forms of treatment. Peptic ulcer and gastro-oesophageal reflux are commonly aggravated during sleep, giving rise to epigastric pain, heartburn, and cough, with repeated disruption of sleep.

Hospital admission

It is well known that admission to hospital can be associated with marked disruption of sleep.[96,97] Although most studies of this issue have been performed with patients in surgical and intensive care units, it stands to reason that other seriously ill patients also experience frequent interruptions of sleep as a direct result of the hospital environment. Potential interruptions include intrusions by staff to monitor vital signs, check lines and equipment, or administer medications, excessive noise or light, or difficulties experienced by other patients occupying the same room. Under these circumstances sleep may become highly fragmented and total sleep time markedly reduced, giving rise to increased napping and disturbance of the sleep–wake cycle. Efforts by staff to minimize such disrupting factors are likely to result in improved sleep.[98]

Other conditions affecting sleep and wakefulness

Numerous other disorders may contribute to poor sleep in the terminally ill. Nutritional deficiency has not been well studied, although investigations of patients with anorexia nervosa suggest that a strong link exists between starvation and sleep disturbance.[99] Thus nutritional deficiency may contribute to sleep disturbance in terminal cancer patients. Endocrine disturbance can give rise to sleep disorder,[100] although this has not been described specifically in cancer patients. Nocturia is a common source of repetitive awakening in patients receiving diuretics. Similarly, many patients suffer from frequent nocturnal headaches which disrupt sleep.

There is limited, and largely anecdotal, information relating specific cancers to sleep disorders. Symptoms of narcolepsy and cataplexy have been described in association with midbrain or brainstem tumours, including those in the region of the third ventricle.[101,102] Centrally mediated respiratory disorders which disrupt sleep have been described in patients with brainstem tumours.[103] It seems certain that other primary malignancies or metastases of the central nervous system may affect sleep indirectly through cerebral oedema or directly through structures subserving sleep. An understanding of such effects awaits further investigation.

Other primary sleep disorders may occur in terminally ill patients. The most notable of those not mentioned elsewhere in this chapter is periodic limb movement in sleep. This disorder consists of repetitive stereotyped leg and/or arm movements which occur at intervals of 20 to 40 s, typically in clusters throughout the night. Potential aetiologies of the disorder are noted in Table 1, although the disturbance is frequently idiopathic. The repetitive movements result in frequent arousals during sleep, leading to complaints of sleep maintenance disturbance, daytime sleepiness, or both. In some cases, there may be an associated restless legs syndrome which interferes with sleep onset. This complaint is characterized by an uncomfortable sensation, usually localized to the lower legs, which is most often described as an irresistible urge to move the lower extremities. These disorders will respond to correction of the underlying causative factor, when one can be identified. In idiopathic cases, clonazepam or L-dopa may be efficacious. Opioids have also been successful in the treatment of refractory cases.

Evaluation

The most serious and fundamental problem in the identification of sleep disorders is that patients are frequently not asked about their sleep. When complaints are offered by the patient, they are too often dismissed by clinicians out of ignorance or therapeutic nihilism. It is essential that health care practitioners recognize the importance of adequate sleep and alertness to the psychological, social, and physical well being of their patients. The following two basic questions should be asked of all patients as a component of the general systems review: How are you sleeping at night? Are you excessively sleepy during the day? When sleep-related complaints are elicited, a more detailed history is required. As previously emphasized, insomnia and hypersomnolence are not diagnoses—they are symptoms. The aetiology of these complaints must be established before any reasonable treatment approach can be constructed. The basic principles of evaluation are outlined in Table 2.

A complaint of 'insomnia' may arise as a result of several different types of sleep-related disturbance. Although reports of difficulty in initiating or maintaining sleep are most often associated with insomnia, other factors such as the perceived quality of sleep, timing of the sleep–wake cycle, or total duration of sleep may also give rise to a complaint of poor sleep. Since these varied presentations may suggest different causative factors, an effort must be made to clarify these components of the disorder. It is helpful to identify the context in which the sleep disturbance began, with consideration of possible precipitating factors. Elucidation of the influence of intervening variables, including treatment efforts, may also yield useful information regarding aetiology. The patient's 24-h schedule must be determined. Sleep disorder clinicians frequently employ sleep logs for this purpose. Such logs typically include information regarding bedtime, sleep latency (time to onset of sleep), number of awakenings, length of awakenings, time of final awakening, estimated total sleep time, and perceived quality of sleep. Entries concerning daytime naps, unusual daytime activities, medications, drugs, and alcohol are also included. Some patients report that the mere process of completing such a log helps them to identify conditions unfavourable to sleep.

Table 2 Evaluation of sleep disorders

Identify the primary complaint: insomnia, excessive sleepiness, parasomnia (abnormal event), sleep–wake schedule disturbance

Characterize the complaint: difficulty initiating sleep, recurrent nocturnal awakening, insufficient total sleep, non-restorative sleep, advanced or delayed sleep onset, excessively long sleep, chronic drowsiness, sleep attacks

Document the sleep–wake cycle: sleep logs including night-time sleep schedule, naps, activities, medications

Identify possible precipitants of disturbance: information from patient and spouse or family members (see Table 1)

Consider the particular sleep requirements of the patient: short/average/long sleepers, variation in sleep habits with age and situation

Medical and neuropsychiatric history

Substance use: medications, alcohol, drugs, caffeine, nicotine

Physical examination and laboratory data

Polysomnography, particularly in elderly medically ill patients with excessive sleepiness or those with histories suggesting underlying physiological disturbance

Multiple Sleep Latency Test: evaluation of excessive daytime sleepiness

Difficulty in falling asleep is often associated with negative expectations regarding sleep, specific anxieties, ruminations, and, in some cases, heightened physiological arousal (increased heart rate, respiratory rate, or muscle tension). In a medically ill population, physical factors, most notably pain, may interfere with the onset of sleep. In order to gain an understanding of associated patterns of cognition, affect, and behaviour which may further contribute to delayed sleep onset, it is necessary to determine what the patient thinks, feels, and does during the time in bed prior to sleep initiation. Identification of anxieties regarding the course of their illness, upcoming procedures, family matters, and death is of particular importance in terminally ill patients.

When patients have difficulty in maintaining sleep, an effort must be made to identify possible precipitants for the awakenings. Although psychological factors, particularly depression, may contribute to awakening and difficulty in returning to sleep, mid-cycle awakening should increase the clinician's suspicion of an underlying physiological cause. Failure to provide analgesia of sufficient dosage and duration often results in awakening due to pain. Other readily identifiable causes such as nocturia, respiratory disturbance (sleep apnoea, congestive heart failure, primary or metastatic pulmonary disease), headache, or non-specific musculoskeletal discomfort must be sought. Repeated awakenings may be associated with specific sleep-related conditions such as periodic movements in sleep, sleep apnoea, nightmares, or sleep terrors. Disease of the central nervous system can result in severe disruption of the normal sleep–wake architecture and inability to maintain sound sleep for any length of time.

Some patients report that they do not feel rested despite what seems to be a normal amount of sleep. This 'non-restorative' pattern of sleep has been associated with repeated intrusion of alpha activity (7–12 Hz) in the sleep electroencephalogram, particularly during NREM sleep. Steady state disturbance (such as pain) or frequent episodic abnormalities (such as movement disorder) may give rise to such sleep disturbance and concomitant daytime complaints of fatigue, poor concentration, and sleepiness in the absence of overt difficulty initiating or maintaining sleep.

In evaluating complaints of insomnia, the clinician must keep in mind that the duration of normal sleep varies significantly from person to person. The 'normal' amount of sleep for a given individual is best defined as that amount which is required to achieve adequate daytime alertness, concentration, and energy. This may be difficult to assess in terminally ill patients, and therefore it is necessary to rely on the patient's premorbid sleep history to determine how many hours of sleep that individual can reasonably expect. A complaint of insomnia should include evidence of impairment of daytime function which is attributable to insufficient or poor-quality sleep. If such evidence is absent, the patient may be a 'short-sleeper', i.e. someone who requires less than the average amount of sleep for a person of that age. Likewise, there are some individuals who may complain of fatigue and sleepiness despite having what the clinician assumes to be a normal amount of sleep. These patients may be 'long-sleepers' whose sleep need is greater than average. Although no systematic investigation has been conducted, it seems plausible that a need for extra sleep may arise in conditions of systemic illness.

For some patients, the complaint of insomnia may be more related to the timing of sleep in the 24-h cycle. Specifically, patients may complain of difficulty in falling asleep, although, once asleep, they are capable of achieving an appropriate amount of sleep. This and other sleep–wake rhythm disorders are discussed elsewhere in this chapter.

A careful review of medication, drugs, and alcohol usage is a crucial component in assessing complaints of insomnia and excessive sleepiness. The role of medication has been discussed already. Patients who are experiencing difficulty in sleeping may resort to alcohol in an effort to alleviate their symptoms. Although sufficient amounts of alcohol will ultimately induce sleep onset, sleep during later stages of the night is often light and marked by frequent awakenings and increased autonomic arousal. Caffeine is an obvious, but surprisingly overlooked, cause of sleep disturbance. In assessing its role, one must be aware of the fact that some individuals experience marked and prolonged arousal in response to even small quantities of caffeine. Nicotine has also been demonstrated to have similar disruptive effects on sleep.

The physical examination and laboratory data must also be considered an essential part of the evaluation of patients with sleep disorder. Particular attention must be paid to the evaluation of pain and to the neurological, endocrine, and cardiopulmonary examinations. General laboratory screening should include blood count and general chemistries as well as screening for nutritional deficiency, endocrine disturbance, and medication levels.

Electrophysiological evaluation (polysomnography) is an important element in the assessment of sleep disorders. However, such studies should clearly be used in a judicious manner for patients receiving palliative care. Nevertheless, when proper indications exist, the information gained from such studies may allow dramatic improvements in the quality of life. Standard polysomnography typically includes monitoring of sleep electroencephalography, submental electromyography, eye movement, airflow, respiratory effort, oxygen saturation, ECG, and leg movements, with additional parameters as indicated. An adequate diagnostic study can usually be accomplished in one night with minimum discomfort or inconvenience for the patient. Such studies are most useful when an underlying physiological disturbance, such as periodic limb movement or sleep-disordered breathing, is suspected. Further characterization of abnormal events (parasomnias) or medical conditions in sleep may also be productive. When complaints of daytime fatigue or sleepiness are present, daytime nap studies (Multiple Sleep Latency Test) can provide an objective determination of the degree of true sleepiness, as well as shedding light on certain specific diagnoses such as narcolepsy.

Treatment

The treatment of sleep disorders must be carefully tailored according to the aetiology of the condition and the particular needs and situation of the patient. As there are usually a number of contributing factors in the genesis and maintenance of a sleep disorder, treatment must also be multifactorial. When insomnia or excessive sleepiness is secondary to another medical or psychiatric condition, the primary condition must be accurately identified and treated before there can be any reasonable expectation of improvement in sleep. However, it must also be recognized that secondary psychophysiological complications may forestall amelioration of the disorder even when the primary condition has been adequately addressed. These conditioned factors must also be treated. By definition, it is not possible to abolish the primary disease process for palliative care patients, but it is usually feasible to control aspects of the process in a manner that will have a positive impact on sleep.

Sleep hygiene

Most people are aware of the common-sense rules and behaviours for promoting good sleep. Nevertheless, failure to adhere to these guidelines is an almost ubiquitous component of many sleep disorders. The problems in this area are so common that the Internation Classification of Sleep Disorders nosology now includes a separate diagnosis for 'Inadequate Sleep Hygiene', although it should be understood that disturbances in this area frequently exist as a complication of some other primary sleep disorder. Adequate sleep is dependent on the proper internal (psychophysiological) and external (environmental) circumstances. In effect, the rules of sleep hygiene attempt to operationalize these conditions. Suggestions for sleep hygiene in palliative care patients are summarized in Table 3.

Excessive arousal in bed is a frequent cause and effect of insomnia. The level of arousal may be quite pronounced for the terminally ill patient who carries multiple concerns to bed. Lying in bed, with mind racing, agitated and tense, there is little possibility that the patient will soon fall asleep. Remaining in bed at this point becomes distinctly frustrating and most certainly counterproductive. However, this is often what patients with insomnia do, either by choice or, in the case of non-ambulatory patients, because they have no option. Under the mistaken impression that they are 'resting' (which is seldom the case) or because getting out of bed is a sign of defeat, they remain in bed fully awake, sometimes for hours. When this occurs on a regular basis for weeks or months, the bed becomes associated not with relaxation and sleep but, rather, with frustration and tension. In time, the mere sight of the bed evokes increased arousal. At this point, the patient's worst fear has become a self-fulfilling prophecy.

An individual who is unable to fall asleep within a reasonable period (best defined by the sleeper, but typically within 30 min), should get out of bed and engage in some relaxing activity until he or she feels ready to sleep. This presents a problem for patients who require assistance to get out of bed. In such cases, some provision should be made to allow for some relaxing activity (e.g. reading, music, television, or handwork) in bed. It is most important that the focus be diverted from a pressure to fall asleep. Other stimuli may

Table 3 Sleep hygiene for palliative care patients

Maintain as regular a sleep–wake schedule as possible, particularly with respect to the hour of morning awakening
Avoid unnecessary time in bed during the day; for bedridden patients, provide as much cognitive and physical stimulation during daytime hours as conditions permit
Nap only as necessary and avoid napping in the late afternoon and evening whenever possible
Keep as active a daytime schedule as possible; this should include social contacts and, when able, light exercise
Minimize night-time sleep interruptions due to medication, noise, or other environmental conditions
Avoid lying in bed for prolonged periods at night in an alert and frustrated or tense state; read or engage in other relaxing activity (out of bed, when appropriate) until drowsiness ensues
Remove unpleasant conditioned stimuli, such as clocks, from sight or sound
Identify problems and concerns of the day before trying to sleep, and address these issues with an active problem-solving approach
Avoid stimulating medication and other substances (e.g. caffeine, nicotine), particularly in the hours before bedtime
Maintain adequate pain relief through the night, preferably with long-acting analgesics
Use sleep medication as indicated after proper evaluation of the sleep problem and avoid overusage

also come to evoke a response of wakefulness. One of the most common is the clock. When unable to fall asleep, or following an awakening, patients often stare at the clock. In time, the clock becomes a very powerful reminder of their inability to fall asleep. This, and other such conditioned stimuli, must be identified and removed from sight or sound.

Palliative care patients are particularly susceptible to alterations of their normal schedules. Because of fatigue, immobility, discomfort, or lack of motivation, the daytime level of activity is often severely curtailed. When this occurs, the division between day and night becomes blurred. This is particularly true if napping and periods in bed are a significant part of the daily routine. In the absence of many of the usual environmental cues (*zeitgebers*) which serve to strengthen basic circadian rhythms, the affected individual is no longer well adjusted to an organized sleep–wake rhythm. As a result, the sleep pattern may become chaotic and unpredictable. The solution to this problem is to take steps to reinforce the basic rest–activity sleep–wake cycle. A regular hour for bedtime and rising is the most essential part of this. Complete avoidance of daytime napping and recumbent rest are not realistic for very sick patients, but these periods should be as short as possible and scheduled such that there is a prolonged 'up time' prior to bedtime. A programme of physical activity and cognitive and social stimulation will emphasize day–night differences and strengthen biological rhythms. Although vigorous physical exercise is not usually possible in this population, mild exercise, even in a sitting or recumbent position, may be helpful. However, physical stimulation should be avoided immediately before bedtime as this may interfere with sleep onset.

Patients frequently manage to avoid anxieties during the day by means of distraction, only to be inundated by them in bed. Therefore it is important to address anxieties, concerns, and disappointments in a direct fashion during the waking hours, thus allowing the person to put these feelings to rest prior to bedtime. Identifying these issues, considering what they themselves can do about problems, seeking information, assistance and support from others, and, finally, accepting those aspects of a situation which cannot be changed must all be a part of this process.

The sleeping environment cannot be overlooked as a potential source of sleep disturbance. Medically ill patients who are receiving some type of institutional care often experience frequent interruptions of sleep as a result of staff activities, background noise, lighting, or other factors. It is necessary to identify environmental circumstances of this nature and to seek solutions in conjuction with the patient. For example, some patients prefer a darker sleeping environment while others, particularly those with some degree of cognitive disturbance, find a partially lit room to be orienting and reassuring. Hospital beds may assist some patients in attaining comfortable positions not possible in standard beds. Individuals who are not ambulatory and require special assistance in meeting minimal needs will be reassured to have access to necessary articles at the bedside as well as a reliable means of calling for assistance.

Substances such as caffeine, nicotine, and alcohol which may interfere with sleep have been discussed. The relationship between sleep and food intake is not clear. Some patients find a snack at bedtime comforting, while others insist that food before bedtime promotes wakefulness. L-Tryptophan, which is found in higher concentrations in certain foodstuffs, has been promoted as a potential sleep aid, although laboratory studies indicate only modest results.[104]

Non-pharmacological treatment of insomnia

Cognitive-behavioural treatment has emerged as a mainstay of the treatment of insomnia which is due wholly or partially to heightened cognitive or physiological arousal and poor sleep hygiene. Numerous reviews of this subject are available[105,106] There is no single most effective behavioural approach. Successful application depends most on appropriate matching of treatment modality and patient characteristics.

Successful applications of behavioural techniques for control of sleep disturbance in cancer patients have been reported. Cannici *et al.*[107] described the use of muscle relaxation training in 15 patients with insomnia 'secondary to cancer'. They reported a significant reduction in sleep latency and increase in total sleep time for the treatment group following 3 days of relaxation training. Anecdotal reports indicate that other behavioural approaches, including hypnosis[108] and somatic focus/imagery training,[109] have been effective for insomnia in cancer patients. In a related vein, behavioural interventions are frequently employed for patients with cancer pain and chronic pain syndromes.[110,111]

Progressive muscle relaxation therapy has been used widely in the treatment of insomnia. This approach is based largely on the assumption that excessive muscle tension is an important component of sleep disturbance. This assumption appears to be true for some, but not all, insomniacs. Relaxation exercises may accomplish more than simple alleviation of muscle tension. The process of focusing on relaxation may, in effect, block the cognitive factors such as worry, apprehension, and rumination which serve to maintain wakefulness. Relaxation training can be accomplished by means of a bedside tape-recorded training session, although patients with more severe chronic insomnia may require the intervention of a skilled behavioural therapist.

Biofeedback is a potentially useful technique in the treatment of insomnia. The specific focus of the feedback may be muscle tension, skin conductance, or vasomotor tone, with the ultimate aim being to teach the patient how to recognize and achieve a state of relaxation. Psychophysiological assessment prior to biofeedback may help to direct the training at the most appropriate function. Biofeedback training has also been directed at specific sleep-related brain physiology such as sensorimotor rhythms, a particular manifestation of stage 2 sleep. Other behavioural approaches such as hypnosis, autogenic training, systematic desensitization, or meditation may be helpful for some patients.

The previously noted observation that many patients with insomnia spend excessive time in bed in a waking and aroused state, thus establishing an undesirable association between bed and inability to sleep, has given rise to two behavioural interventions with demonstrated effectiveness. Sleep restriction, described by Spielman *et al.*,[112] is designed to limit the amount of time that a person spends in bed in a waking state. The patient is instructed to determine the average total sleep time per night at baseline by means of sleep logs. That amount of time then becomes the maximum allowable time in bed. Once subjects are able to sleep for 90 per cent or more of the time in bed on five consecutive nights, sleep time is increased by 15 min and the same trial is repeated. In stimulus control therapy[113] the patient is, in effect, instructed to use the bed only for sleeping. If unable to sleep, the patient must get out of bed and do something else until sleepy, at which time a return to the bed is permitted. This same procedure is repeated as often as necessary through the night. Both these approaches can be quite stressful on patients in their early phases and may result in substantial initial sleep deprivation. Therefore they are of limited practicality in very sick patients.

Finally, brief supportive psychotherapy contacts which allow the patient to ventilate hopes and fears can be most helpful. Although some of the therapeutic time may be spent in discussion of the sleep problem *per se*, it is unwise to allow this to become the sole focus. It is advisable for the therapist to turn the patient's attention toward anxieties, conflicts, or disappointments which inevitably arise during the terminal period of illness. A practical problem-solving approach to these matters is particularly appropriate at this stage of the disease.

Pharmacological treatment of insomnia

The conventional wisdom regarding the use of hypnotic medications for the treatment of insomnia is that they should be largely limited to short-term use. This approach is predicated on concern regarding tolerance, dosage escalation, psychological addiction, and physical dependency. While such concerns are valid under any circumstance, they are of less importance in the population of palliative care patients for whom life expectancy is limited and symptom relief is the primary aim. It is clear from data previously cited that hypnotic medications are used very frequently in cancer patients. Unfortunately, these data do not provide information about the specific medications used, their effectiveness, their appropriateness, or their side effects. Depending on which medications are prescribed, their dosage, and their indications, hypnotic drugs may greatly enhance the quality of remaining life in the terminally ill or may further complicate an already difficult period.

Benzodiazepines

Benzodiazepine and imidazopyridine hypnotics are currently the medications of choice in the treatment of transient or short-term insomnia. Before such drugs are prescribed, however, the clinician must carefully consider the differential diagnosis in an effort to rule out other treatable aetiologies for the sleep disturbance. When this has been done, it is reasonable to consider use of a hypnotic drug as one component of a comprehensive treatment approach to insomnia. Such an approach should also incorporate non-pharmacological elements, as previously described.

Several factors must be considered in employing hypnotic medication. These include the short- and long-term effectiveness of the drug, its rate of absorption and metabolism, and the potential risks or side-effects. Characteristics of selected hypnotic drugs, and other benzodiazepiness often employed as hypnotics, are summarized in Table 4. This group of medications has a reasonably well-established record of effectiveness in the short-term treatment of insomnia. Studies report reductions in sleep latency and wake time after sleep onset.[114,115] However, there has been substantial controversy over the issue of long-term effectiveness of these medications, and at present they are recommended primarily for short-term usage.

Many benzodiazepines, as well as the imidazopyridine zolpidem, are absorbed rather quickly, reaching peak concentrations within approximately 1 h or less. Temazepam, in the hard capsule form, has delayed absorption, although the soft gelatin capsule is more rapidly absorbed. Lorazepam and oxazepam have not been extensively studied as hypnotic medications, but are frequently used as such. Their rate of absorption is also somewhat slower. Delayed absorption suggests that these drugs may be more suitable for treatment of sleep maintenance problems or should be given somewhat ahead of bedtime if used for sleep initiation difficulty. The half-life of flurazepam's major active metabolite (*n*-desalkyl flurazepam) is in excess of 50 h, resulting in significant accumulation when the compound is used on a nightly basis. Zolpidem and triazolam (triazolam has now been removed from the market in certain countries) are rapidly metabolized to inactive compounds. Temazepam, lorazepam, and oxazepam have intermediate half-lives ranging from about 8 to 15 h. These figures have been established for healthy adults. It is essential to recognize that the rate of metabolism may be substantially slower in medically ill and geriatric patients, predisposing to greater accumulation of the drug and daytime carry-over effects.

The benefits which may be achieved through the use of hypnotic medication in palliative care patients must be weighed against the potential for complications and side-effects associated with their

Table 4 Characteristics of benzodiazepines and other hypnotic drugs

Medication	Dosage[a] (mg)	Elimination half-life[b]	T_{ma}[b] (h)	Active Metabolites	Comments[c]
Rapid elimination					
Triazolam[d]	0.125	2–4	1.0	No	Promote rapid sleep onset with minimal accumulation of drug over time; may be less effective for sleep maintenance problems; rebound insomnia, anterograde amnesia, untoward drug reactions described with triazolam
Zolpidem	5	1.5–4	1.0	No	
Intermediate elimination					
Temazepam[e]	15	8–13	1.5	No	Promote sleep onset/maintenance; slower absorption a factor in treating sleep onset difficulty; minimal accumulation
Lorazepam	1	12–15	2.0	No	
Oxazepam	10	6–11	2.5	No	
Slow elimination					
Flurazepam	15 mg	47–100 (*n*-desalkyl-flurazepam)	1.0	Yes	Effective for sleep onset and maintence; may be effective over 2 nights or more after single dosage; daytime sedation; performance decrements; drug accumulation, especially in elderly or those with delayed metabolism
Quazepam	7.5[f]	29–73 *n*-desalkyl-flurazepam)	2.0	Yes	

[a] Recommended starting dosage in elderly and medically ill patients.
[b] Elimination half-life and T_{ma} represent estimated averages for healthy adults.
[c] All benzodiazepines carry potential for dosage escalation and for psychological and physical dependence.
[d] Not available in Norway and the United Kingdom.
[e] Elimination rate partially dependent on capsule form.
[f] Manufacturer recommends initial dosage of 15 mg with reduction to 7.5 mg after 1 to 2 nights.

use. Perhaps the most common undesirable effect is that of daytime sedation and performance decrement. In populations of otherwise healthy insomnia patients, there is clear evidence that longer-acting benzodiazepines, such as flurazepam, are associated with significant deficits in daytime performance. However, there are some questions regarding the relevance of the psychomotor tasks on which these findings are based to the population of palliative care patients. Long-acting hypnotics may have daytime carry-over antianxiety effects which may be beneficial for some patients. Performance decrement and daytime sedation are not prominent characteristics of shorter-acting hypnotics. Benzodiazepines may also predispose to nocturnal confusion, particularly in individuals with baseline cognitive dysfunction. Likewise, respiratory disturbance in sleep, which is most prominent in geriatric patients, may be exacerbated by hypnotic medication, and cognitive impairment, [117–119] a particular concern in patients who may have metastatic bone disease.

In prescribing hypnotic medication, the clinician must consider the complication of rebound insomnia. Extensive data suggest that the shorter-acting benzodiazepines predispose to transient insomnia following abrupt withdrawal of the medication, even after short-term use.[116] It has also been suggested that these medications may result in increased daytime anxiety and morning insomnia. These phenomena do not appear to be present with flurazepam or other long-acting benzodiazepines, for which daytime sedation is the more likely complication. The clinical safety of the benzodiazepines has been well established. The lethality of these medications in the absence of other central nervous system depressants is very low. When any of these medications are discontinued after regular usage, clinicians must be mindful of the possibility of withdrawal symptoms and taper dosage appropriately.

Other sleep medications

A number of non-benzodiazepine medications have been employed in the treatment of insomnia. Barbiturates, although effective in short-term treatment, result in rapid development of tolerance and are more lethal in overdose situations. These medications and similar barbiturate-like compounds play a minor role in the treatment of sleep disturbance. Chloral hydrate appears to have moderate short-term efficacy but is more toxic than benzodiazepines. Sedating antidepressant drugs have assumed a more important role in the treatment of various forms of insomnia and non-restorative sleep in the past decade. These medications have the advantage that they can be administered over long periods of time without concern regarding addiction. Sedating tricyclics such as amitriptyline or doxepin, administered in lower dosages than are typically required for treatment of major depression, may be helpful adjuncts. Anticholinergic side-effects and daytime sedation can cause problems, particularly in the medically ill. Delirium due to central anticholinergic activity is a potential complicating factor, as is lethality in overdose situations. Secondary amine tricyclics such as desipramine or nortriptyline, although less sedating, may be beneficial and produce fewer anticholinergic complications. Trazodone is a sedating non-tricyclic antidepressant which has milder anticholinergic effects. Antidepressant medications have also been employed for the treatment of non-restorative sleep.

Melatonin has received recent widespread attention as a treatment for insomnia and other sleep disorders. The popularity of melatonin, at the time of writing, far exceeds the amount of scientific evidence to support its use. Current data suggest that melatonin has substantial potential as a treatment for disorders of the sleep–wake schedule, as one might expect in light of its role in circadian rhythm regulation.[117–119] There is also preliminary evidence which indicates that there may be some benefit from melatonin in the treatment of insomnia in elderly individuals, in whom melatonin secretion may be impaired as a result of ageing.[120–121] To date, no large scale, controlled trials of melatonin in the treatment of insomnia have been published. It must be recognized that the current 'off the shelf' preparations of melatonin are not regulated as a drug in many countries and, as a result, the contents and source of the preparation cannot be clearly identified by the consumer. Finally, consumers should be aware that melatonin is a potent hormone with widespread effects, including those on the reproductive and cardiovascular systems. While the ultimate clinical significance of those effects in patients taking exogenous melatonin is not known, some degree of caution is advisable.

The choice of a particular pharmacological treatment for insomnia must be based on the specific situation in which it will be used. Considerations include the nature of the insomnia, the expected duration of treatment, potential side-effects, including daytime sedation and performance decrement, and patient tolerance. Once initiated, it is most important to determine efficacy and complications and to adjust dosage or type of medication accordingly.

Choice of hypnotics in the elderly and infirm

The choice of a hypnotic medication in the elderly or the infirm must be predicated on achieving a careful balance between therapeutic efficacy and adverse consequences, for which this population is particularly at risk. A number of studies suggest that the use of sedative hypnotics in the elderly is associated with increased risk of falls, hip fracture, and cognitive impairment.[122–124]

Alterations in drug sensitivity and pharmacokinetics among the elderly and sick must be taken into account in prescribing. Older patients may have heightened sensitivity to hypnotic medications compared with younger age groups, even at comparable plasma levels. In addition, drug clearance of at least some benzodiazepines is decreased in the elderly.

Benzodiazepines and their active metabolites which undergo oxidative metabolism in the liver (e.g. diazepam, quazepam-flurazepam/desalkyl-flurazepam, alprazolam, and triazolam) are cleared more slowly in the elderly, whereas those drugs which are directly conjugated (e.g. temazepam, oxazepam, and lorazepam) show little change in rate of clearance in the elderly compared with younger age groups.[125] Furthermore, epidemiological evidence suggests a relationship between longer-acting benzodiazepine hypnotics and risk of injury.[126] These data appear to suggest that the optimal choice of hypnotic in the elderly and debilitated would be a shorter-acting drug which undergoes direct glucuronide conjugation.

Concerns about sensitivity and drug accumulation have prompted manufacturers and clinicians to recommend lower dosages of these medication in geriatric patients and those with severe medical illness. Recommended starting dosages for these populations are included in Table 4. Although nightly use of benzodiazepines or other hypnotics may be appropriate for patients in the terminal phase of illness, short-term intermittent use may suffice and will minimize the possibility of drug accumulation. Aggravation of existing cognitive impairment, risk of fall and injury, worsening of nocturnal respiratory disturbance, and unwanted daytime sedation with its attendant impact on mood and behaviour are particular concerns in the elderly and infirm.

The metabolism of heterocyclic antidepressants may be substantially slowed in medically ill and older patients. Low starting dosages should be utilized and the potential for accumulation must be recognized. Development of excessive sedation, orthostatic hypotension, cardiotoxicity, and anticholinergic side-effects are the major risks associated with elevated plasma levels of these agents.

Sleep in family and caregivers

It has been recognized for some time that good palliative care includes attention to the needs and difficulties of the patient's family and other caregivers. This is certainly true with respect to sleep disturbances, which are common in this group. Focus on these issues is particularly important because sleep disruption and fatigue may contribute to loss of hope among family caregivers.[127] Grief, anxiety, and depression are frequently cited psychological disturbances which may cause insomnia among relatives.[128] For those providing direct care, frequent night-time interruptions to attend to the patient fragment sleep and, in time, can result in psychophysiological insomnia. Caregivers may feel compelled to 'keep one eye open' through the night so as not to miss a call for assistance.

Inquiries about the sleep patterns of the family should be a component in assessing how well the palliative care system is succeeding. Discussion of sleep hygiene issues, practical problem-solving approaches to reducing night-time interruptions, and consideration of short-term use of a benzodiazepine hypnotic may be appropriate. Antidepressant medication is indicated for some. While it is clearly not advisable to employ sedating medication or antidepressants as a means of inhibiting normal grief, it must also be recognized that sleep deprivation and its sequelae may significantly interfere with the quality of relationships in the palliative care period and complicate bereavement following the patient's death.

References

1. Diagnostic Classification Steering Committee, Thorpy MJ, Chairman. *International Classification of Sleep Disorders: Diagnostic and Coding Manual.* Rochester, MN: American Sleep Disorders Association, 1990.
2. Roth T, Kramer M, Leston W, Lutz T. The effects of sleep deprivation on mood. *Sleep Research*, 1974; 3:154.
3. Johnson LC. Psychological and physiological changes following total sleep deprivation. In: Kales A, ed. *Sleep: Physiology and Pathology.* Philadelphia, PA: Lippincott, 1969; 206–20.
4. Millman RP, Fogel BS, McNamara ME, Carlisle CC. Depression as a manifestation of obstructive sleep apnea: reversal with nasal continuous positive airway pressure. *Journal of Clinical Psychiatry*, 1989; **50**(9):348–51.

5. Oswald I. Sleep as a restorative process. *Progress in Brain Research*, 1980; **53**:279–88.
6. Moldofsky H, Scarisbrick P. Induction of neurasthenic musculoskeletal pain syndrome by selective sleep stage deprivation. *Psychosomatic Medicine*, 1976; **38**:35–44.
7. Moldofsky H, Lue FA, Davidson JR, Gorezynski R. Effects of sleep deprivation on immune function. *Federation of American Societies for Experimental Biology Journal*, 1989; **3**:1972–7.
8. Morley JE, Kay NE, Solomon GF, Plotnikoff NP. Neuropeptides: conductors of the immune orchestra. *Life Sciences*, 1987; **41**(5):527–44.
9. Kubler-Ross E. On the use of psychopharmacologic agents for the dying patient and the bereaved. In: Goldberg IK, Malitz S, Kutscher AH, eds. *Psychopharmacological Agents for the Terminally Ill and Bereaved*. New York: Columbia University Press, 1973: 3–6.
10. Carskadon MA, Dement WC, Mitler MM, Roth T, Westbrook PR, Keenan S. Guidelines for the Multiple Sleep Latency Test (MSLT): A standard measure of sleepiness. *Sleep*, 1986; **9**:519–24.
11. Munro AJ, Biruls R, Griffin AV, Thomas H, Vallis KA. Distress associated with radiotherapy for malignant disease: a quantitative analysis based on patient's perceptions. *British Journal of Cancer*, 1989; **60**(3):370–4.
12. Lapin J, Portenoy RK, Coyle N, Houde RW, Foley KM. Guidelines for use of controlled-release oral morphine in cancer pain management. *Cancer Nursing*, 1989; **12**(4):202–8.
13. Hanks GW, Twycross RG, Bliss JM. Controlled release morphine tablets: a double-blind trial in patients with advanced cancer. *Anaesthesia*, 1987; **42**(8):840–4.
14. Smedley H, Katrak M, Sikora K, Wheeler T. Neurological effects of recombinant human interferon. *British Medical Journal*, 1983; **286**(6361):262–4.
15. Harris AL, Powles TJ, Smith IE. Aminoglutethimide in the treatment of advanced post menopausal breast cancer. *Cancer Research*, 1982; **42**(Supplement 8):3405S–8S.
16. Czeisler CA *et al.* Chronotherapy: resetting the circadian clocks of patients with delayed sleep phase insomnia. *Sleep*, 1981; 4:1–21.
17. Sutherland HJ, Lockwood GA, Boyd NF. Ratings of the importance of quality of life variables: therapeutic implications for patients with metastatic breast cancer. *Journal of Clinical Epidemiology*, 1990; **43**(7):661–6.
18. Krech RL, Walsh D. Symptoms of pancreatic cancer. *Journal of Pain and Symptom Management*, 1991; **6**(6):360–7.
19. Portenoy RK *et al.* Symptoms prevalence, characteristics and distress in a cancer population. *Quality of Life Research*, 1994; **3**(3):183–9.
20. Grond S, Zech D, Diefenbach C, Bischoff A. Prevalence and pattern of symptoms in patients with cancer pain: a prospective evaluation of 1635 cancer patients referred to a pain clinic. *Journal of Pain and Symptom Management*, 1994; **9**(6):372–82.
21. Malone M, Harris AL, Luscombe DK. Assessment of the impact of cancer on work, recreation, home management and sleep using a general health status measure. *Journal of the Royal Society of Medicine*, 1994; **87**:386–9.
22. Derogatis LR *et al.* A survey of psychotropic drug prescriptions in an oncology population. *Cancer*, 1979; **44**(5):1919–29.
23. Jaeger H. Morrow GR, Carpenter DJ, Brescia F. A survey of psychotropic drug utilization by patients with advanced neoplastic disease. *General Hospital Psychiatry*, 1985; **7**:353–60.
24. Beszterczey A, Lipowski ZJ. Insomnia in cancer patients. *Canadian Medical Association Journal*, 1977; **116**:355.
25. Lamb MA. The sleeping patterns of patients with malignant and nonmalignant diseases. *Cancer Nursing*, 1982; **5**:389–96.
26. Kaye J, Kaye K, Madow L. Sleep patterns in patients with cancer and patients with cardiac disease. *Journal of Psychology*, 1983; **114**:107–13.
27. Silberfarb PM, Hauri, PJ, Oxman TE, Lash S. Insomnia in cancer patients. *Social Science and Medicine*, 1985; **20**(8):849–50.
28. Silberfarb PM, Hauri PJ, Oxman TE, Schnurr P. Assessment of sleep in patients with lung cancer and breast cancer. *Journal of Clinical Oncology*, 1993; **11**(5):997–1004.
29. Darko DF, McCutchan JA, Kripke DF, Gillin JC, Golshan S. Fatigue, sleep disturbance, disability, indices of progression of HIV infection. *American Journal of Psychiatry*, 1992; **149**(4):514–20.
30. Moeller AA, Oechsner M, Backmund HC, Popescu M, Emminger C, Holsboer F. Self-reported sleep quality in HIV infection: correlation of the stage of infection and zidovudine therapy. *Journal of Acquired Immunodeficiency Syndrome*, 1991; **4**(10):1000–3.
31. St Kubicki H, Henkes H, Terstegge K, Ruf B. AIDS-related sleep disturbances—a preliminary report. In: St Kubicki H, Henkes H, Bienzle H, Pokle HD, eds. *HIV and Nervous System*. Stuttgart: Fischer, 1988: 97–105.
32. Norman SE, Chediak AD, Kiel M, Cohn MA. Sleep disturbances in HIV-infected homosexual men. *AIDS*, 1990; **4**(8):775–81.
33. Harris PF, Careres CA. Azidothymidine in the treatment of AIDS. *New England Journal of Medicine*, 1988; **318**:250.
34. Richman DD *et al.* The toxicity of azidothymidine (AZT) in the treatment of patients with AIDS and AIDS-related complex. A double-blind, placebo-controlled trial. *New England Journal of Medicine*, 1987; **317**:192–7.
35. Bach MC. Possible drug interaction during therapy with azidothymidine and acyclovir for AIDS. *New England Journal of Medicine*, 1987; **316**:547.
36. Hintz S, Kuck J, Peterkin JJ, Volk DM, Zisook S. Depression in the context of human immunodeficiency virus infection: implications for treatment. *Journal of Clinical Psychiatry*, 1990; **51**(12):497–501.
37. Reynolds CF. Sleep in affective disorders. In: Kryger MH, Roth T, Dement WC, eds. *Principles and Practice of Sleep Medicine*. Philadelphia, PA: Saunders,1989: 413–15.
38. Levine P, Silberfarb PM, Lipowski ZJ. Mental disorders in cancer patients. *Cancer*, 1978; **42**:1385–91.
39. Craig TJ, Abeloff MD. Psychiatric symptomatology among hospitalized cancer patients. *American Journal of Psychiatry*, 1974; **131**(12):1323–27.
40. Plumb MM, Holland J. Comparative studies of psychological function in patients with advanced cancer-I. Self-reported depressive symptoms. *Psychosomatic Medicine*, 1977; **39**(4):264–76.
41. Derogatis LR *et al.* The prevalence of psychiatric disorders among cancer patients. *Journal of the American Medical Association*, 1983; **249**(6):751–7.
42. Bukberg J, Penman D, Holland JC. Depression in hospitalized cancer patients. *Psychosomatic Medicine*, 1984; **46**(3):199–212.
43. Walsh TD. Antidepressants in chronic pain. *Clinical Neuropharmacology*, 1983; **6**:271–95.
44. Hameroff SR *et al.* Doxepin's effects on chronic pain and depression: a controlled study. *Journal of Clinical Psychiatry*, 1984; **45**(3 Part 2):47–53.
45. Hameroff SR *et al.* Doxepin effects on chronic pain, depression and plasma opioids. *Journal of Clinical Psychiatry*, 1982; **43**(8 Part 2):22–7.
46. Spiegel K, Kalb R, Pasternak GW. Analgesic activity of tricyclic antidepressants. *Annals of Neurology*, 1983; **13**:462–5.
47. Battelli T, Bonsignori M, Manocchi P, Rossi G. Anxiety therapy in the neoplastic patient. *Current Medical Research and Opinion*, 1976; **4**(3):185–8.
48. Reynolds CF, Shaw DH, Newton DF, Cable PA, Kupfer DJ. EEG sleep in outpatients with generalized anxiety: a preliminary comparison with depressed outpatients. *Psychiatry Research*, 1983; **8**:81–9.
49. Rosa RR, Bonnet MH, Kramer M. The relationship of sleep and anxiety in anxious subjects. *Biological Psychology*, 1983; **16**:119–26.
50. Neuhas W, Lanij B, Ahr A, Bolte A. Psychological disease adjustment in breast cancer patients. *Geburtshilfe und Frauenheilkunde*, 1994; **54**(10):564–8.
51. Massie MJ, Holland J, Glass E. Delirium in terminally ill cancer patients. *American Journal of Psychiatry*, 1983; **140**(8):1048–50.
52. Fasinsinger R, Miller MJ, Bruera E, Hanson J, Maceachern T. Symptom control during the last week of life on a pallative care unit. *Journal of Palliative Care*, 1991; **7**(1):5–11.
53. Lipowski ZJ. Delirium (acute confusional state). *Journal of the American Medical Association*, 1987; **258**(13):1789–92.

54. Posner JB. Neurological complications of systemic cancer. *Medical Clinics of North America*, 1979; **63**:783–800.
55. Silberfarb PM. Psychiatric treatment of the patient during cancer therapy. *CA: A Cancer Journal for Clinicians*, 1988; **38**(3):133–7.
56. Sofer DJ. The concomitant effects of mild sleep loss and an anticholinergic drug. *Psychopharmacologia (Berlin)*, 1970; **17**:425–33.
57. Evans JI, Lewis SA. Sleep studies in early delirium and during drug withdrawal in normal subjects and the effect of phenothiazines on such states. *Electroencephalography and Clinical Neurophysiology*, 1968; **25**:508–9.
58. Prinz PN *et al.* Sleep EEG and mental function changes in senile dementia of the Alzheimer's type. *Neurobiology of Aging*, 1983; 3:361–70.
59. Reynolds CF *et al.* EEG sleep in elderly depressed, demented and healthy subjects. *Biological Psychiatry*, 1985; **20**:431–42.
60. Stiefel F, Fainsinger R, Breura E. Acute confusional states in patients with advanced cancer. *Journal of Pain and Symptom Management*, 1992; 7(2):94–8.
61. Burke AL, Diamond PL, Hulbert J, Yeatman J, Farr EA. Terminal restlessness—its management and the role of midazolam. *Medical Journal of Australia*, 1991; **155**(7):485–7.
62. Panutti F, Martoni A, Rossi AP, Piana E. The role of endocrine therapy for the relief of pain due to cancer. In: Bonica JJ, Ventafridda V, eds. *Advances in Pain Research and Therapy*, Vol. 2. New York: Raven Press, 1979: 59–77.
63. Twycross RG, Fairfields S. Pain in far advanced cancer. *Pain*, 1982; **14**:303–10.
64. Bonica JJ. Importance of the problem. In: Bonica JJ, Ventafridda V, eds. *Advances in Pain Research and Therapy*, Vol. 2. New York: Raven Press, 1979: 1–12.
65. Dorrepaal KL, Aaronson NK, van Dam FS. Pain experience and pain management among hospitalized cancer patients. *Cancer*, 1989; **63**:593–8.
66. Strang P, Quarner H. Cancer-related pain and its influence on quality of life. *Anticancer Research*, 1990; **10**:109–12.
67. Tamburini M, Selmi S, DeConno F, Ventafridda V. Semantic descriptors of pain. *Pain*, 1987; **29**(2):187–93.
68. Donovan M, Dillon P, McGuire L. Incidence and characteristics of pain in a sample of medical-surgical inpatients. *Pain*, 1987; **30**(1):69–78.
69. Kinsman R, Dirks JF, Wunder J, Carbaugh R, Stieg R. Multidimensional analysis of peak pain symptoms and experiences. *Psychotherapy and Psychosomatics*, 1989; **51**(2):101–12.
70. Pilowsky I, Crettenden I, Townley M. Sleep disturbance in pain clinic patients. *Pain*, 1985; **23**(1):27–33.
71. Landis CA, Levine JD, Robinson CR. Decreased slow-wave and paradoxical sleep in a rat chronic pain model. *Sleep*, 1989; **12**(2):167–77.
72. Carli G, Montesano A, Rapezzi S, Paluffi G. Differential effects of persistent nociceptive stimulation on sleep stages. *Behavioural Brain Research*, 1987; **26**:89–98.
73. Wittig RM, Zorick FJ, Blumer D, Heilbronn M, Roth T. Disturbed sleep in patients complaining of chronic pain. *Journal of Nervous and Mental Disease*, 1982; **170**(7):429–31.
74. Moldofsky H, Lue FA, Smythe HA. Alpha EEG and morning symptoms in rheumatoid arthritis. *Journal of Rheumatology*, 1983; **10**:373–9.
75. Breitbart W. Psychiatric management of cancer pain. *Cancer*, 1989; **63**:2336–42.
76. Hicks RA, Coleman DD, Ferrante F, Sahatjian M, Hawkins J. Pain thresholds in rats during recovery from REM sleep deprivation. *Perceptual and Motor Skills*, 1979; **48**:687–90.
77. Fadda P, Tortorella A, Fratha W. Sleep deprivation decreases μ and ∂ opioid receptor binding in the rat limbic system. *Neuroscience Letters*, 1991; **129**:315–17.
78. Larbig W, Gerber WD, Kluck M, Schoenenberger GA. Therapeutic effects of delta-sleep-inducing peptide (DSIP) in patients with chronic, pronounced pain episodes. A clinical pilot study. *European Neurology*, 1984; **23**(5):372–85.
79. Ventafridda V, Tamburini M, Caraceni A, DeConno F, Naldi F. A validation study of the WHO method for cancer pain relief. *Cancer*, 1987; **59**(4):850–6.
80. Goughnour BR, Arkinstall WW, Steward JH. Analgesic response to single and multiple doses of controlled-release morphine tablets and morphine oral solution in cancer patients. *Cancer*, 1989; **63**(Supplement 11):2294–7.
81. Corli O, Cozzolino A, Scaricabarozzi I. Nimesulide and diclofenac in the control of cancer-related pain. Comparison between oral and rectal administration. *Drugs*, 1993; **46**(Supplement 1):152–5.
82. Carrol EN, Fine E, Ruff RL, Stepnick D. A four-drug regimen for head and neck cancers. *Laryngoscope*, 1994; **104**:694–700.
83. Sjoberg M, Nitescu P, Appelgren L, Curelaru I. Long-term intrathecal morphine and bupivacaine in patients with refractory cancer pain. *Anesthesiology*, 1994; **80**(2):284–97.
84. Banning A, Sjogren P, Henriksen H. Treatment outcome in a multidisciplinary cancer pain clinic. *Pain*, 1991; **47**:129–34.
85. Smith GM, Smith RH. Effects of doxylamine and acetaminophen on post-operative sleep. *Clinical Pharmacology and Therapeutics*, 1985; **37**(5):549–57.
86. Shapiro W. Sleep behaviour among narcoleptics and cancer patients. *Behavioural Medicine*, 1980; **7**:14–21.
87. Gillin JC, Jacobs LS, Fram DH, Snyder F. Acute effect of a glucocorticoid on normal human sleep. *Nature, London*, 1972; **237**:398–9.
88. Kay DC, Samiuddin Z. Sleep disorders associated with drug abuse and drugs of abuse. In: Williams RL, Karacan I, Moore CA, eds. *Sleep Disorders: Diagnosis and Treatment*. New York: Wiley, 1988:315–71.
89. Nicholson AN, Bradley CM, Pascoe PA. Medications: effect on sleep and wakefulness. In: Kryger MH, Roth T, Dement WC, eds. *Principles and Practice of Sleep Medicine*. Philadelphia, PA: Saunders, 1989:228–36.
90. Veitch D, Rogers M. Blanshard J. Pharyngeal mass presenting with sleep apnea. *Journal of Laryngology and Otology*, 1989; **103**(10):961–3.
91. Zorick F, Roth T, Kramer M, Flessa H. Exacerbation of upper airway sleep apnea by lymphocytic lymphoma. *Chest*, 1980; **77**:689–90.
92. Panje WR , Holmes DK. Mandibulectomy without reconstruction can cause sleep apnea. *Laryngoscope*, 1984; **94**(12 Part 1):1591–4.
93. Etches RC. Respiratory depression associated with patient-controlled analgesia: a review of eight cases. *Canadian Journal of Anaesthesia*, 1994; **4**(2):125–32.
94. Thomas M, von Eiff M, van de Loo J. Central sleep apnea syndrome as a cause of impaired wakefulness in multiple myeloma. *Deutshe Medizinische Wochenschrift*, 1993; **118**(51–52):1884–8.
95. Flenley DC. Chronic obstructive pulmonary disease. In: Kryger MH, Roth T, Dement WC, eds. *Principles and Practice of Sleep Medicine*. Philadelphia, PA: Saunders, 1989:601–10.
96. Dlin BM, Rosen H, Lyons JW, Fischer HK. The problems of sleep and rest in the intensive care unit. *Psychosomatics*, 1971; **12**:155–63.
97. Broughton R, Baron R. Sleep of acute coronary patients in an open ward type intensive care unit. *Sleep Research*, 1973; **2**:144.
98. Fabizan L, Gosselin MD. How to recognize sleep deprivation in your ICU patient and what to do about it. *Canadian Nurse*, 1982; **78**(4):20–3.
99. Crisp AH. Sleep, activity, nutrition and mood. *British Journal of Psychiatry*, 1980; **137**:1–7.
100. Regestein QR. Sleep disorders in the medically ill. In: Stoudemire A and Fogel BS, eds. *Principles of Medical Psychiatry*. New York: Grune and Stratton, 1987: 271–305.
101. Anderson M, Salmon MV. Symptomatic cataplexy. *Journal of Neurology, Neurosurgery and Psychiatry*, 1977; **40**:186–91.
102. Stashl SM, Layzer RB, Aminoff MJ, Townsend JJ, Feldon S. Continuous cataplexy in a patient with a midbrain tumour: the limp man syndrome. *Neurology*, 1980; **30**: 1115–18.
103. Jaeckle KA, Digre KB, Jones CR, Bailey PL, McMahill PC. Central neurogenic hyperventilation: pharmacological intervention with morphine sulfate and correlative analysis of respiratory, sleep, and ocular motor dysfunction. *Neurology*, 1990; **40**:1715–20.
104. Hartmann E. L-Tryptophan: a rational hypnotic with clinical potential. *American Journal of Psychiatry*, 1977; **134**:366–70.
105. Hauri PJ, Sateia MJ. Nonpharmacological treatment of sleep disorders. In:

Hales RE, Frances AJ, eds. *American Psychiatric Association Annual Review*, Vol. 4. Washington, DC: American Psychiatric Press, 1985: 361–78.

106. Morin CM, Kwentus JA. Behavioural and pharmacological treatments for insomnia. *Annals of Behavioural Medicine*, 1988; **10**(3):91–100.
107. Cannici J, Malcolm R, Peck LA. Treatment of insomnia in cancer patients using muscle relaxation training. *Journal of Behaviour Therapy and Experimental Psychiatry*, 1983; **14**(3):251–6.
108. LaClave LJ, Blix S. Hypnosis in the management of symptoms in a young girl with malignant astrocytoma: a challenge to the therapist. *International Journal of Clinical and Experimental Hypnosis*, 1989; **37**(1):6–14.
109. Stam HJ, Bultz BD. The treatment of severe insomnia in a cancer patient. *Journal of Behaviour Therapy and Experimental Psychiatry*, 1986; **17**(1):33–7.
110. Fishman B, Loscalzo M. Cognitive-behavioural interventions in management of cancer pain: principles and applications. *Cancer Pain*, 1987; **71**(2):271–87.
111. Morin CM, Kowatch RA, Wade JB. Behavioural management of sleep disturbances secondary to chronic pain. *Journal of Behaviour Therapy and Experimental Psychiatry*, 1989; **2**(4):295–302.
112. Spielman AJ, Saskin P, Thorpy MJ. Sleep restriction: a new treatment of insomnia. *Sleep Research*, 1983; **12**:286.
113. Bootzin RR, Nicassio PN. Behavioural treatments of insomnia. In: Hersen M, Eisler R, Miller P, eds. *Progress in Behaviour Modification*, Vol. 6. New York: Academic Press, 1978: 1–45.
114. Dement WC, Carskadon MA, Mitler MM, Phillips RL, Zarcone VP. Prolonged use of flurazepam: a sleep laboratory study. *Behavioural Medicine*, 1978; **5**:25–31.
115. Spinweber CL, Johnson LC. Effects of triazolam (0.5 mg) on sleep, performance, memory and arousal threshold. *Psychopharmacology*, 1982; **76**:5–12.
116. Vogel G, Thurmond A, Gibbons P, Edwards K, Sloan KB, Sexton K. The effect of triazolam on the sleep of insomniacs. *Psychopharmacology*, 1975; **41**:69–9.
117. Dawson D, Encel N, Lushington K. Improving adaptation to simulated night shift: time exposure to bright light versus daytime melatonin administration. *Sleep*, 1995; **18**:11–21.
118. Attenburrow ME, Dowling BA, Sargent PA, Sharpley AL, Cowen PJ. Melatonin phase advances circadian rhythm. *Psychopharmacology*, 1995; **121**:503–5.
119. Lewy AJ, Sack RL, Blood M, Bauer VK, Cutler NL, Thomas KH. Melatonin marks circadian phase position and resets the endogenous circadian pacemaker in humans. *Ciba Foundation Symposium*, 1995; **183**:303–17.
120. Garfinkel D, Laudon M, Nof D, Zisapel N. Improvement of sleep quality in elderly people by controlled-release melatonin. *Lancet*, 1995; **346**:541–4.
121. Haimov I, Lavie P, Laudon M, Herer P, Vigder C, Zisapel N. Melatonin replacement therapy of elderly insomniacs. *Sleep*, 1995; **18**:598–603.
122. Robbins AS, Rubenstein LZ, Josephson KR, Schulman BL, Osterweil D, Fine G. Predictors of falls among elderly people. *Archives of Internal Medicine*, 1989; **149**:1628–33.
123. Ray WA, Griffin MR, Schaffer W, Baugh DK, Melton LJ. Psychotropic drug use and the risk of hip fracture. *New England Journal of Medicine*, 1987; **316**:363–9.
124. Larson EB, Kukull WA, Buchner D, Reifler BV. Adverse drug reactions associated with global cognitive impairment in elderly persons. *Annals of Internal Medicine*, 1987; **107**:169–73.
125. Greenblatt DJ, Harmatz JS, Shader RI. Clinical pharmacokinetics of anxiety and hypnotics in the elderly. *Clinical Pharmacokinetics*, 1991; **21**:165–77.
126. Ray WA, Griffin MR, Downey W. Benzodiazepines of long and short elimination half-life and the risk of hip fracture. *Journal of the American Medical Association*, 1989; **262**:3303–7.
127. Herth K. Hope in the family caregiver of terminally ill people. *Journal of Advanced Nursing*, 1993; **18**:538–48.
128. Sawyer MG, Antoniou G, Toogood I, Rice M, Baghurst PA. A prospective study of the psychological adjustment of parents and families of children with cancer. *Journal of Paediatrics and Child Health*, 1993; **23**(5):352–6.

9.14 Haematological aspects

A. Robert Turner

Anaemia

Anaemia is a common problem in patients receiving palliative care and can produce significant symptoms. They include:

easy fatiguability, reduced mental acuity

dyspnoea

postural hypotension

oedema

anorexia

headache

exacerbation of angina.

To the extent that these symptoms are caused by anaemia, correction to a more normal haemoglobin will result in dramatic relief. Fortunately, several therapeutic options exist but, first, the cause of the anaemia must be determined. This may be challenging since the aetiology of anaemia is often multifactorial.

The differential diagnosis of the cause of anaemia in a patient seen in a palliative care setting is different from the differential diagnosis of patients with anaemia in a general medical context. Six major entities should be considered and it should be remembered that several of these causes of anaemia may be occurring in an individual patient. These six major causes are:

(1) anaemia of chronic disorders;

(2) acute and chronic haemorrhage;

(3) marrow failure;

(4) malnutrition;

(5) haemolysis;

(6) underlying chronic or congenital anaemia.

Anaemia of chronic disorders[1-4]

This is a hypoproliferative anaemia which is unresponsive to haematinic therapy. Severe anaemia is unusual but transfusions are often required to maintain the patient's activity levels. The anaemia of chronic disorders is caused by a reaction to the presence of a malignancy or inflammation. Several cytokines are released in this reaction. Interleukin 1 is one of a large family of glycoprotein hormones which carry signals from various types of leucocytes to other types of white cells. Interleukin 1 (IL-1), previously known as endogenous pyrogen, is released by macrophages stimulated by neoplasms or inflammation. It interacts with other cytokines such as tumour necrosis factor (TNFα) and gamma interferon (γIF) to initiate an immune response. IL-1 affects the haematological system in many ways. One of these is to impede the transfer of iron molecules from storage sites in the reticuloendothelial system to developing red cell precursors. This results in the paradoxical situation of iron deficient erythropoiesis occurring in a marrow replete with iron. IL-1 also causes stimulation of splenic macrophages which leads to hypersplenism and a shortened red cell survival. TNFα and γIF both impair red cell proliferation. Antagonists may be developed to counteract their effects.

The diagnosis of anaemia of chronic disorders is often based on the exclusion of other forms of anaemia. However, this diagnosis should always be considered in the palliative care setting. The anaemia will be slightly microcytic or near the lower limits of the mean corpuscular volume (MCV). The reticulocyte count will be low, reflecting a reduced marrow output. The serum ferritin is normal as the patient's iron stores are not reduced. Serum iron studies should be interpreted carefully. The serum iron may be low but the total iron binding capacity (transferrin) is also low. (In iron deficiency, the total iron binding capacity would be elevated.) Modest elevations of indirect bilirubin and lactate dehydrogenase (LDH) and slight reduction of serum haptoglobin are the result of the mild haemolysis and ineffective erythropoiesis which is occasionally noted. Red cell survival is shortened but this test should not be part of routine investigations.

These patients do not respond to conventional marrow stimulation with agents such as iron, vitamins, or steroids. Transfusion of packed red cells may be needed from time to time in order to avoid symptoms of anaemia. Recently, the use of erythropoietin has been advocated as a means to improve red cell production and avoid transfusions—150 to 300 U/kg, three times weekly subcutaneously are needed. After 2 weeks of therapy, an increase in haemoglobin of greater than 5 g/l in the presence of a serum erythropoietin of less than 100 U/l is highly predictive of response to this treatment. Erythropoietin is expensive and the cost factor may become important in deciding how to support the haemoglobin concentration.

Acute and chronic haemorrhage[5-8]

Haemorrhage can occur in palliative care patients due to bleeding from neoplastic lesions within the gastrointestinal tract, the upper and lower respiratory tract, or the genitourinary system. Less commonly, haemorrhage can occur within tumour masses or around a pathological fracture. This bleeding can be acute and massive, resulting in a rapid depletion of intravascular volume and consequent shock. More commonly, the bleeding is of a chronic nature with a loss of a few millilitres of blood daily. This chronic loss of blood can lead to iron deficiency and to chronic congestive heart failure. In most cases, the chronic blood loss is obvious from the presence of blood in bodily fluids but occasionally tests for occult blood or endoscopic examinations are necessary to determine the presence and site of the bleeding.

Therapy for chronic haemorrhage can be divided into three components. The first, and most important, is to control the bleeding lesion if practicable. This may be accomplished surgically, endoscopically, or by radiation of the bleeding lesion. Medical therapy is helpful for some patients with chronic haemorrhage who are bleeding from non-neoplastic lesions within the gastrointestinal tract. H_2 antagonists such as cimetidine or ranitidine are of use in treating chronic peptic ulcer bleeding. Other agents which have been utilized in such patients are omeprazole, misoprostol, and sucralfate. Patients whose chronic bleeding has led to iron deficiency can be treated with an orally administered simple iron salt such as ferrous sulphate or ferrous gluconate (300 mg two to three times daily). In some patients, intravenous administration of 1 to 2 g parenteral iron is a very useful way to provide a reserve of iron when oral iron preparations can not be tolerated or are poorly absorbed. The third modality, transfusion therapy, will be discussed in a separate section below.

Chronic haemorrhage can also be seen in patients with thrombocytopenia secondary to marrow failure or coagulation factor deficiencies due to liver failure. Extensive ecchymoses are often evident in patients whose platelet count is less than 50 000 or whose prothrombin time or activated partial thromboplastin time is prolonged. These patients tend to have a gradual drop in their haemoglobin levels without gross evidence of blood in the stool or other body fluids.

An important cause of anaemia due to chronic haemorrhage in patients in any type of institutional setting is chronic bloodletting for laboratory testing purposes. Each vial of blood that is drawn represents 7 to 10 ml of whole blood. Routine, repetitive laboratory testing should be limited.

Marrow failure[9]

Many patients being seen in the palliative care setting have had extensive previous treatment with myelotoxic chemotherapy and/or radiation treatments. In general, the more extensive the past treatments, the more likely that marrow failure is present. Marrow failure can present as an isolated cytopenia, such as a reduced platelet count, reduced total white cell count, or an anaemia, but it more commonly is associated with modest reductions of all three lineages of haematopoiesis. These patients cannot respond to haemorrhage or haemolysis by increasing their marrow output, producing a reticulocytosis, and often require transfusion therapy.

Other important causes of marrow failure are the presence of metastases or fibrosis within the bone marrow or the chronic effects of haematological malignancies. These direct effects of cancer on the bone marrow can produce a variety of changes. Many of these patients will have changes in the morphology of the peripheral blood cells (teardrop-shaped red cells and immature white cells and red cells) which suggest the presence of metastases or fibrosis. The documentation of metastatic disease within the bone marrow or of myelofibrosis is the only indication for doing a bone marrow aspirate and biopsy in a patient with anaemia in a palliative care setting. The need to know the diagnosis should be balanced against the discomfort induced by this test and the lack of therapeutic options for metastatic disease within the bone marrow.

Malnutrition[10]

Many patients receiving palliative care have protein and/or calorie malnutrition. Along with protein/calorie malnutrition, there will be deficiencies in the dietary intake of haematologically important nutrients such as iron or folic acid. Iron deficiency usually results from chronic haemorrhage and not from malnutrition alone, but patients can readily become deficient in folic acid if they have not had it in their diet for 4 to 6 weeks. Patients with chronic anaemias, rapidly growing tumours, and prior treatment with folic antagonists such as methotrexate are at especially high risk for this easily correctable deficiency. Folic acid, 5 mg daily, can be administered orally or subcutaneously.

Deficiencies of iron should be suspected when the mean corpuscular volume is reduced. Serum iron/transferrin or serum ferritin tests should be done to establish the diagnosis as the anaemia of chronic disorders often causes a very similar microcytic picture. Folic acid deficiency should be suspected in a patient who has a macrocytic anaemia. It can be confirmed by doing a serum or red cell folate assay. Other important causes of macrocytic anaemia in palliative care patients include liver disease and B_{12} deficiency.

Chronic protein malnutrition can lead to a generalized hypoproteinaemia that is often accompanied by a normocytic anaemia and marrow failure. The anaemia in these patients may respond to improvement in overall nutrition if the cachexia–anorexia syndrome is not present.

Chronic haemolysis[11-13]

Haemolysis is seen rarely in patients in the palliative care setting. Some neoplasms are associated with haemolysis such as chronic lymphocytic leukaemia, non-Hodgkin's lymphomas and adenocarcinomas of diverse origins. Haemolysis should be suspected in the patient who has a progressive anaemia and in whom chronic haemorrhage cannot be documented. The laboratory evaluation of these patients usually shows an elevation of lactate dehydrogenase, indirect bilirubin, and a reduction in serum haptoglobin. Because of the effects of the anaemia of chronic disorders and/or marrow failure, a reticulocytosis may not be seen despite active haemolysis.

Three general types of haemolysis can be seen in these patients. They are:

(1) immune haemolysis (Coombs' positive);

(2) microangiopathic haemolytic anaemia;

(3) hypersplenism.

Immune haemolysis is due to the presence of an immunoglobulin or complement on the surface of red cells. The Coombs' test, or direct antiglobulin test, detects the immunoglobulin or complement. If active haemolysis is occurring, there will be evidence of red cell breakdown (including elevation of red cell derived lactate dehydrogenase) and evidence of increased haemoglobin release (that is, an increase in unconjugated bilirubin and decreased haptoglobin). An examination of peripheral blood may show spherocytes present.

Immune haemolysis may be treated with corticosteroids (prednisolone, 0.5 to 1.0 mg/kg). Other forms of treatment include splenectomy or the use of immunosuppressive drugs, such as cyclophosphamide or azathioprine, but they are not often utilized in the palliative care setting.

Microangiopathic haemolytic anaemia may be seen when there is destruction of the red cell membrane as it passes through abnormal vasculature within a tumour or in a disorder sometimes associated with neoplasms or chemotherapy called thrombotic thrombocytopenic purpura. There are striking changes noted in the peripheral blood of these patients. Their red cells are very misshapen with prominent fragmentation seen. The therapy of these disorders has been unrewarding if the malignancy could not be removed.

Hypersplenism is a disorder in which an enlarged spleen causes an increased rate of destruction of red blood cells or other blood elements. This disorder can be treated with splenectomy or by radiation to the spleen. The latter approach may be attractive in palliative care when the general condition of the patient would make surgery difficult.

Table 1 Approach to the diagnosis of anaemia in a palliative care setting

Anaemias	Diagnosis	Therapy
Anaemia of chronic disorders	exclude other causes, iron deficiency or thalassaemia	transfusion, erythropoietin
Haemorrhage	determine site	control haemorrhage, block H_2 receptor, treat iron deficiency
Marrow failure	marrow examination	
Malnutrition	iron, folate levels	increase calories, iron or folate supplementation
Haemolysis	Coombs' test, lactate dehydrogenase, indirect bilirubin, haptoglobin, peripheral blood smear (fragmentation indicates microangiopathy)	prednisolone

Chronic or congenital haematological disorders[1,14]

Patients receiving palliative care bring with them a variety of medical disorders. Some of these can be associated with anaemia and should not be disregarded in the differential diagnosis of the cause of anaemia in the palliative care patient. Examples of chronic disorders include rheumatological diseases, inflammatory bowel disorders, or chronic infections. Perhaps the most common cause of chronic anaemia in the world is the presence of α- or β-thalassaemia trait. Thalassaemia trait will cause a chronic anaemia marked by the presence of severe microcytosis and target cells in the peripheral blood. It can easily be confused with iron deficiency or anaemia of chronic disorder. Many patients with thalassaemia trait will have a positive family history. β-thalassaemia trait can be diagnosed by demonstrating an elevation in the proportion of haemoglobin A_2 on haemoglobin electrophoresis.

General approach to the diagnosis of anaemia

In the palliative care setting, anaemia is very common and is almost always multifactorial in aetiology (Table 1). Any patient who has a neoplasm or chronic infection will have some degree of anaemia of chronic disorders. Many of these patients will also have chronic haemorrhage and marrow failure. Haemolysis and malnutrition occur in a minority of patients but need to be recognized since the therapeutic options will be influenced. Laboratory investigation needs to be individualized to each patient depending upon their prognosis and the likelihood of remediable causes of the anaemia. The peripheral blood smear often gives very valuable clues as to the diagnosis and the cause of anaemia. A bone marrow examination is done infrequently. Estimates of iron stores using a serum ferritin, the demonstration of immune hemolysis with the direct antiglobulin test (Coombs'), and the estimation of serum or red cell folate are other commonly used tests.

Transfusion therapy in the palliative care setting

In the past, for many patients, transfusion therapy represented the extent of palliation. Transfusion of packed red cells remains a very important part of the comprehensive care of palliative care patients. In addition to red cells, platelets and plasma components can also be administered.

Indications for transfusion of red blood cells[15-19]

Red blood cells provide two important factors to patients—oxygen transport to tissues from the lung is augmented and intravascular volume expansion is provided. Other blood products provide superior means to produce plasma volume expansion and will be discussed later. Oxygen carrying capacity can only be provided by red cell concentrates.

This discussion will deal exclusively with the provision of red cell concentrates in the chronically anaemic patient. The management of acute haemorrhage will not be dealt with here.

The most important factor in determining the need for red cell transfusion in the patient with chronic anaemia is the presence or absence of symptoms attributable to the anaemia. Patients who have developed their anaemia chronically will tolerate levels of haemoglobin much lower than that tolerated by patients suffering an acute haemorrhage. Therefore, no specific guidelines can be given as to the degree of anaemia which necessitates transfusion. If the patient is symptomatic from dyspnoea, angina, postural hypotension, headache, or peripheral oedema and there are no other medical explanations for these symptoms, a trial of transfusion is indicated.

One can anticipate the progression of anaemia in many patients in the palliative care setting. Patients who have marrow failure develop anaemia at the rate of approximately 10 g/l per week. It is common to transfuse these patients at a rate of 3 to 4 units of red cells every 3 to 4 weeks.

In estimating the number of units required it is convenient to aim for a post-transfusion haemoglobin of 110 to 120 g/l. Each unit of packed red cells administered to an adult will result in a rise in haemoglobin concentration of 10 g/l. In a patient with a haemoglobin of 80 g, a transfusion of 3 to 4 units will raise the haemoglobin concentration to 110 to 120 g/l.

Three major types of complications can be seen with red blood cell transfusion. They are:

(1) volume overloading;

(2) febrile/urticarial reactions;

(3) iron overloading.

Many patients receiving palliative care have a compromised cardiovascular system which will not tolerate the rapid addition of several hundred millilitres of fluid. Each red cell unit provides the equivalent of approximately 450 ml of fluid. Three units therefore have in excess of 1200 ml and this can not be tolerated over a short period by many palliative care patients. Volume overload problems can be avoided by administering a small amount of frusemide (furosemide) (20 mg) with alternate units and by administering the blood slowly. Each unit can be administered over a period of 4 to 6 h. It is advisable to administer no more than 2 units per day.

Febrile and urticarial reactions can occur in patients receiving blood products because of the presence of white blood cells in the transfused product carrying HLA antigens to which the patient has become immunized. These febrile or urticarial reactions can be quite disabling. They can be attenuated by the use of premedication with antihistamines such as diphenhydramine (50 mg). If the patient has more than one of these reactions, the blood bank should be asked to provide leucodepleted blood products. This can be accomplished by the use of white cell filters or by having the red cells washed.

Iron overload is not often a concern in the palliative care setting since it does not become evident until between 50 and 75 units of red cells have been transfused to the patient. Each unit of blood adds 250 mg of iron to the patient's iron stores. Patients with more than 20 g of iron in their stores are at risk for haemosiderosis. Haemosiderosis can cause heart failure or arrhythmias, liver dysfunction, or failure of pancreatic endocrine function. The best way to avoid the problem of haemosiderosis is to transfuse red blood cells only when the patient's symptoms demand it. Iron chelation therapy (desferrioxamine) can remove iron from the patient's stores but is very rarely indicated in the palliative care setting.

Infectious complications of blood transfusion have been minimized by recent improvements in the screening of blood donations. AIDS, hepatitis B, hepatitis C, HTLV-1/2, and syphilis can be screened for and the risk of these infections arising from a blood transfusion prepared in a blood bank with these procedures in place are minimal. In most situations, the benefit of improved quality of life with the transfusion of red blood cells would outweigh the potential risk from infectious complications. Although there is some experimental evidence that transfusion might induce immunosuppression and enhance the growth of neoplasms, this complication of transfusion is not of practical importance in the palliative care setting and patients should not be denied the benefit of red cell transfusion because of this theoretical disadvantage.

Transfusion of other blood products

Platelets[20]

Thrombocytopenia may be seen in the palliative care setting when the patient has extensive marrow involvement with their neoplasm, has a disseminated coagulopathy (DIC), has an enlarged spleen, or has received extensive myelotoxic therapy. Platelet counts of less than $50 \times 10/^9$l be associated with bleeding problems. If the patient has a platelet count of less than 50 and is bleeding, transfusion of 6 to 8 units of platelet concentrate may be helpful in curtailing the bleeding for a short period of time. In most patients in the palliative care setting, the thrombocytopenia is a chronic problem and chronic platelet transfusion can be very difficult. Nevertheless, platelet transfusions can be given on a regular basis to some patients with good results.

Platelet transfusions are sometimes associated with febrile and urticarial reactions due to HLA antibodies which can be attenuated by premedication as noted with red cell transfusion or by leucodepletion of the platelets.

Albumin[21]

Many palliative care patients are hypoalbuminaemic. This is not an indication for the transfusion of albumin. Albumin should be administered only when there is a need for an acute expansion of plasma volume such as when acute diuresis is necessary. There is no use in transfusing albumin to the patient with chronic hypoalbuminaemia for 'nutritional' purposes. In most cases, hypoalbuminaemia is a feature of the cachexia–anorexia syndrome (see Chapters 9.3.5, 9.3.6).

Other plasma components[22]

Fresh plasma and cryoprecipitate should be used only when specific and documented bleeding diatheses remediable by plasma or cyroprecipitate are present. Examples of this would be the correction of a prolonged prothrombin time due to liver failure, or warfarin anticoagulation by frozen plasma, or the correction of an abnormal bleeding time due to a deficiency of von Willebrand's factor by cryoprecipitate. DDAVP, 20 µg intravenously, is a useful way to raise von Willebrand's factor activity if required.

Thrombosis

Venous thrombosis is commonly seen in patients with disseminated malignancies and is therefore a frequent problem in the palliative care setting. Immobility caused by pain and hormonal effects of therapy of various cancers can exacerbate the thrombotic tendency.

Acute deep venous thrombosis[23-27]

Acute deep venous thrombosis can produce painful swelling of the lower limbs, or less commonly, an upper limb. Extension and embolization of these clots can occur if the clotting is present above the popliteal fossae. An important complication is pulmonary embolization. This may be a common cause of death in the palliative care setting.

The diagnostic and therapeutic approach has to be individualized to each patient's circumstances. If the decision to treat has been made, the deep venous thrombosis should be documented by venography, plethmysography, or Doppler studies. The presence or absence of pulmonary embolism can be difficult to establish with certainty and the diagnostic imaging tests available for this condition are not very specific. Nevertheless, a ventilation perfusion scan of the lung is often done. The results of lung scanning have to be integrated with the clinical findings to make a diagnosis of pulmonary embolism.

The therapy of acute deep venous thrombosis usually involves the administration of a bolus of 5000 units of heparin followed by an initial continuous intravenous infusion of 800 to 1000 units of heparin hourly. Sufficient heparin should be infused to raise the activated partial thromboplastin time to between 60 and 90 s. Oral warfarin should be started at a dose of 5 to 10 mg and continued daily until the prothrombin INR is between 2 and 3. Once a therapeutic prothrombin INR is achieved, the heparin can be discontinued and the warfarin continued indefinitely.

The decision to use heparin in the patient in the palliative care setting is often a complex one. Many of these patients have major or minor contraindications to the use of heparin. Major contraindications include active gastrointestinal haemorrhage, active bleeding from any other site, an intracranial neoplasm, and uncontrolled hypertension. Minor contraindications include a past history of gastrointestinal haemorrhage, retinopathy, and a history of prior coagulation problems now quiescent. It is the author's approach to recommend full anticoagulation in most patients without major contraindications whose prognosis exceeds a few days and who are having significant symptoms from the deep venous thrombosis.

Low molecular weight heparins are now available which have the advantage of requiring much less monitoring than warfarin or whole heparin. These expensive agents may be useful in the palliative setting where blood testing should be minimized for patient comfort.

Chronic venous thrombosis[28-31]

Patients with neoplastic lesions obstructing veins or with a hypercoagulability related to disseminated malignancy can have chronic venous thrombosis. Two therapeutic approaches are suggested for these patients:

(1) chronic warfarin;

(2) subcutaneous whole heparin or low molecular weight heparin.

Chronic warfarin therapy can be administered quite safely if the prothrombin time is monitored closely. The prothrombin INR should be checked every 1 to 2 weeks after establishment of the initial therapeutic dose. The INR should be kept within 2 to 3. Some patients will have continued thrombosis despite maintenance therapy with coumarins and an INR between 2 and 3. In some of these patients, increasing the warfarin dose so that the INR is between 3 and 4 will be successful in controlling the thrombotic tendency but many of these patients will have bleeding complications. If warfarin therapy has to be reversed rapidly, the administration of 3 to 4 units of fresh plasma and 10 mg of vitamin K will bring the PT INR back to baseline rapidly.

In those patients who continue to have thrombotic problems despite warfarin therapy, subcutaneous whole heparin or low molecular weight heparin should be considered. This approach involves subcutaneous injection of heparin twice daily and therefore is more troublesome to the patient. Many patients can self-administer heparin and it does not necessarily involve increased use of medical personnel. An adjusted dose of whole heparin or a standard dose of low molecular weight heparin should be utilized. In this approach, a starting dose of 10 000 to 15 000 units of heparin is given every 12 h and adjusted such that the activated partial thromboplastin time is prolonged to approximately 50 s at 6 h after the subcutaneous injection is given. If the patient has been receiving intravenous heparin therapy, the total dose administered over a 24-h period can be used as a guide to selecting the initial subcutaneous dose. Half of the total 24-h dose is administered each 12 h.

Trousseau's syndrome is a migratory polyphlebitis affecting superficial veins primarily. It is seen in some patients with disseminated bronchogenic tumours or adenocarcinomas. It can be very bothersome and may not be adequately treated with either warfarin or subcutaneous heparin. Indomethacin at a dose of 25 mg, 3 to 4 times daily, is a useful adjunct in these patients, but gastrointestinal side-effects must be monitored.

Chronic disseminated intravascular coagulopathy (DIC) may be seen in patients with metastatic prostatic carcinoma as well as some other solid tumours and haematological neoplasms. Chronic DIC is produced by an activation of the clotting process but the result is the consumption of the components of the clotting system. Thrombocytopenia, hypofibrinogenaemia, and prolongation of the prothrombin time and activated partial thromboplastin time are commonly present. Chronic DIC can lead to troublesome bleeding. Effective therapy is difficult when the underlying neoplasm can not be eradicated. If therapeutic measures are to be utilized, emphasis should be placed upon augmenting the fibrinogen levels with cryoprecipitate and transfusing platelets when there is thrombocytopenic bleeding. ε-aminocaproic acid has occasionally been helpful in controlling the fibrinolysis commonly seen in this disorder.

References

1. Ludwig H, Fritz E, Leitgeb C, Pecherstorfer M, Samonigg H, Schuster J. Prediction of response to erythropoeitin treatment in chronic anemia of cancer. *Blood*, 1994; **84**: 1056–63.
2. Fuchs D, Zangerle R, Denz H, Wachter H. Inhibitory cytokines in patients with anemia of chronic disorders. *Annals of the New York Academy of Sciences*, 1994; **718**: 344–6.
3. Keown PA. Quality of life in end-stage renal disease patients during recombinant human erythropoietin therapy. The Canadian Erythropoietin Study Group. *Contributions to Nephrology*, 1991; **88**: 81–6.
4. Spivak JL. Recombinant human erythropoietin and the anemia of cancer. *Blood*, 1994; **84**: 997–1004.

5. Hillman RS. Acute blood loss anemia. In: Beutler E, Lichtman MA, Coller BS, Kipps TJ, eds. *Williams Hematology* (5th edn). New York: McGraw-Hill, 1994: 704–8.
6. Fairbanks VF, Beutler E. Iron deficiency. In: Beutler E, Lichtman MA, Coller BS, Kipps TJ, eds. *Williams Hematology* (5th edn). New York: McGraw-Hill, 1994: 490–510.
7. Schwartzberg LS, Holbert JM. Hemorrhagic and thrombotic abnormalities of cancer. *Critical Care Clinics*, 1988; **4**: 107–28.
8. Smoller BR, Kruskall MS. Phlebotomy for diagnostic laboratory tests in adults. Pattern of use and effect on transfusion requirements. *New England Journal of Medicine*, 1986; **314**: 1233–5.
9. Erslev AJ. Anemia associated with marrow infiltration. In: Beutler E, Lichtman MA, Coller BS, Kipps TJ, eds. *Williams Hematology* (5th edn). New York: McGraw-Hill, 1994: 516–17.
10. Daly JM, Torosion MH. Nutritional Support. In: DeVita VT Jr, Hellman S, Rosenberg SA, eds. *Cancer, Principles and Practice of Oncology* (4th edn). Philadelphia: J. B. Lippincott, 1993: 2480–501.
11. Pirofsky B. Clinical aspects of autoimmune hemolytic anemia. *Seminars in Hematology*, 1976; **13**: 251–65.
12. Ruggenenti P, Remuzzi G. Thrombotic microangiopathies. *Critical Reviews of Oncology and Hematology*, 1991; **11**: 243–65.
13. Weatherall DJ. Molecular biology at the bedside. *British Medical Journal*, 1986; **292**: 1505–8.
14. Aster RH. Pooling of platelets in the spleen: role in the pathogenesis of 'hypersplenic' thrombocytopenia. *Journal of Clinical Investigation*, 1966; **45**: 645–57.
15. Menitove JE. Transfusion in the hypoproliferative anemias. In: Rossi EC, Simon TL and Moss GS, eds. *Principles of Transfusion Medicine*. Baltimore: Williams and Wilkins, 1991:151–6.
16. Office of Medical Applications of Research. National Institute of Health Consensus Development Conference on Red Blood Cell Transfusion. Perioperative red blood cell transfusion. *Journal of the American Medical Association*, 1988; **260**: 2700–3.
17. Snyder EL, Stack G. Febrile and nonimmune transfusion reactions. In: Rossi EC, Simon TL, Moss GS, eds. *Principles of Transfusion Medicine*. Baltimore: Williams and Wilkins, 1991: 641–8.
18. Bordin JO, Heddle NM, Blajchman MA. Biologic effects of leukocytes present in transfused cellular blood products. *Blood*, 1994; **257**: 1703–21.
19. Pippard MJ, Callender ST, Finch CA. Ferrioxamine excretion in iron-loaded man. *Blood*, 1982; **60**: 288–94.
20. Consensus Development Conference. Platelet transfusions. *Journal of the American Medical Association*, 1987; **257**: 1777–80.
21. Alexander MR, Alexander B, Mustion AL, Spector R, Wright C. Therapeutic use of albumin. *Journal of the American Medical Association*, 1982; **247**: 831–3.
22. Braunstein AH, Oberman HA. Transfusion of plasma components. *Transfusion*, 1984; **24**: 281–6.
23. Lensing AWA, Hirsh J, Buller HR. Diagnosis of venous thrombosis. In: Colman RW, Hirsh J, Marder VJ, Salzman EW eds. *Hemostasis and Thrombosis, Basic Principles and Clinical Practice* (3rd edn). Philadelphia: J. B. Lippincott, 1994: 1297–321.
24. Hirsh J, Bettman M, Coates G, Hull RD. Diagnosis of pulmonary embolism. In: Colman RW, Hirsh J, Marder VJ, Salzman EW, eds. *Hemostasis and Thrombosis, Basic Principles and Clinical Practice* (3rd edn). Philadelphia: J. B. Lippincott, 1994: 1321–30.
25. Hirsch J, Prim MH, Samama M. Therapeutic agents and their practical use in thrombotic disorders. In: Colman RW, Hirsh J, Marder VJ, Salzman EW, eds. *Hemostasis and Thrombosis, Basic Principles and Clinical Practice* (3rd edn). Philadelphia: J.B. Lippincott, 1994: 1543–61.
26. Patterson WP and Ringenberg QS. The pathophysiology of thrombosis in cancer. *Seminars in Oncology*, 1990; **17**: 40–6.
27. Wolf H. Low-molecular-weight heparin. *Medical Clinics of North America*, 1994; **78**: 733–43.
28. Loberman JS, Borrero J, Urdaneta E, Wright IS. Thromboembolism associated with neoplasm: review of seventy-seven cases. *Journal of the American Medical Association*, 1961; **177**: 542–5.
29. Sack GH, Levin J, Bell WR. Trousseau's syndrome and other manifestations of chronic disseminated coagulopathy in patients with neoplasms: clinical, pathophysiologic and therapeutic features. *Medicine*, 1977; **56**: 1–37.
30. Hull R, Hirsh J, Jay R, Carter C, England C, Gent M, Turpie AGG, McLoughlin D, Dodd P, Thomas M, Raskob G, Ockelford P. Different intensities of oral anticoagulant therapy in the treatment of proximal vein thrombosis. *New England Journal of Medicine*, 1982; **307**: 1676–81.
31. Colman RW, Rubin RN. Disseminated intravascular coagulation due to malignancy. *Seminars in Oncology*, 1990;**17**: 172–86.

10

Cultural issues in palliative care

10.1 Introduction

Julia Neuberger

Introduction

There is considerable variation between people of different faiths, ethnic backgrounds, and national origins in their approach to terminal illness. Those who have settled in a society where there is a dominant faith or culture other than their own increasingly adopt that dominant culture in many ways. However, they retain, almost deliberately to emphasize differences, their different practices at times of birth, marriage, and death.

This is hardly surprising. Any anthropologist would argue that in most societies, but particularly perhaps those of the Middle East and the Indian subcontinent, people define themselves by their religious grouping, even when their personal faith is limited or non-existent. Their definition of their religious grouping is very often demonstrated by how they deal with the major lifecycle events of birth, marriage, and death.

This must obviously be born in mind when dealing with cultural differences in the palliative care of the terminally ill. Attitudes will vary considerably according to whether a Muslim is living in a Muslim country or a country with a significant Muslim population, such as the United Kingdom or France, or in a country with a relatively small Muslim population, such as Scandinavia or parts of Latin America. Similarly, Jews will vary considerably in their practices according to whether they are living in a country with a large Jewish population, such as the United States, or somewhere where the Jewish population is diminishing rapidly, such as Ireland.

This is further complicated by the attitude of government authorities, both local and central, to various religious practices. For instance, it is difficult to ensure cremation for a Hindu or a Sikh in a country where cremation is not allowed, such as Israel. The issue is further complicated when individuals of a particular cultural or religious group decide that they are not personally going to observe the tenets of their faith with respect to their needs at the time of a death. A classic example of this is where Jews or Muslims, usually but not always of a more liberal or lapsed disposition, opt for cremation rather than burial, which is normally demanded by their faith. (In fact, this is extremely rare for Muslims, and much frowned upon by the Muslim community.) The complications in dealing with religious authorities, national or local authorities, and family members are legion!

These are just some of the examples of the issues that must be faced when looking at cultural differences in palliative care. The overriding rule is that there are no absolute hard and fast rules; there is always considerable personal variation except in those very few countries which are truly monocultural and monolithic in the power of their religious authorities, and where personal preferences on the part of the dying person are disregarded in favour of community interests.

Such disregard does happen, of course, and not only in those countries which are often described as 'developing'. It is all too common to hear on hospital wards in the Western world members of families, in conjunction with medical and nursing staff, discussing the preferences expressed by a gravely ill person, and discounting those views as being the product of a disordered mind or a brief aberration. This is particularly common when the dying person is asking for something that goes against the common practice, or common code, of his or her own religious or ethnic or social group, and where other members of that group, and those caring staff who have read the appropriate textbooks, cannot believe that the person concerned wishes to be a nonconformist at this stage of his or her life.

For this reason it is essential to stress that the following sections, which look at cultural and religious variations in attitudes to terminal illness and at how individuals might wish to be treated, can only be used as the roughest of guides. The best thing to do is to ask the individual concerned, for two powerful reasons. The first is that few of us are whole-hearted in our absolute acceptance of the ways of our religious or cultural group, or so confident that we do not wish to have our own input in some way, even if it is only about which clergyman should officiate at the funeral. Therefore personal preference is a factor which must be taken into account in almost all circumstances, and is as powerful a force in determining behaviour amongst those of different cultures and religions from one's own as it is amongst those whose cultural and religious patterns are deeply familiar.

The second point is even more important. The desire to put those people who are different from oneself into categories, because somehow their differences are easier to deal with if they seem to belong to a group with clearly defined norms, leads to depersonalization. The individual, whether Jew, Christian, Muslim, Taoist, Sikh, Hindu, or Buddhist, will usually be delighted, and even feel honoured, at being asked to explain to caring staff something of the nature of his or her religious beliefs and cultural traditions. It can provide an opportunity for people in that situation to explore some of their own attitudes to their own tradition, and it certainly provides a moment when the patient is fully in control since he or she has valuable information that the carer does not have. Therefore it is imperative that, however much the carers know about other cultures and religions and their attitudes to palliative care and to expressing the details of death, they ask the patient for his or her preferences and encourage him or her to talk about the different patterns of observance within that religious and cultural grouping, as well as about broad principles and practices.

This requires a different kind of relationship from the usual one between carer and patient, but it is an extraordinary opportunity for both sides to learn about other traditions, other interpretations, and other acceptances; it can lead to a level of human understanding that is hard to reach when carers and patients come from the same broad religious and cultural group, where the traditions are already assumed to be a given.

Religious variations

Although not all adherents of the religious communities listed below necessarily stick to all the rules and customs described, it is nevertheless essential to consider briefly each of the main faiths of the world. Such a discussion cannot be more than cursory, but in each case it is essential to realize that the factors of concern are attitudes to the afterlife, attitudes to death itself, which may be too complicated to go into here, attitudes to pain relief and to pain itself, attitudes to food and religious observance in the last stages of life, and last rites, if they exist.

Many of the world's religions have very strict rules about food and modesty, which it is essential for carers to understand. It is impossible to prescribe pain-controlling drugs for certain more observant Muslims during Ramadan, for instance, despite the fact that Muslim law (the Shari'a) requires that the very sick do not observe the fast. Nevertheless, even where the pain relief is not given by mouth but by syringe driver, there are Muslims who would prefer to endure the pain. Similarly, in some Hindu and Sikh groups, there are individuals, particularly women, whose attitudes to modesty are so pronounced that, despite extreme pain and the need, for instance, to be helped with manual evacuation of faeces because of severe constipation, they will not consent to receiving that help. These two areas of food and modesty probably have the most profound effect on the physical aspects of palliative care, whilst theological, philosophical, and ritual views affect the psychological approach to those of different faiths and cultures.

Islam

Islam is one of the world's fastest growing religions. There are Muslims in almost all countries, and Europe, hitherto thought to have a small Muslim population, has over 30 million Muslims, excluding those in Turkey. Muslims are divided into four main categories. There are Sunni (approximately 90 per cent of the world's Muslims), Shi'a (just under 10 per cent), Ismaili, and Ahmediyya, although most other Muslims dispute the Islamic status of the last group. Sunni and Shi'a groupings are very large, and there are often major disputes between them, particularly when one group holds sway in a country with a predominantly Muslim population drawn largely from the other group. The Ismailis are followers of the Aga Khan and, although numerically a very small group, they tend to be very successful in international affairs and often play a major role in explaining Islam to non-Muslims around the world.

Islam is closely related to Judaism and Christianity, and Muslim rulers have traditionally recognized members of the other two faiths as being 'people of the Book'. The faith could be described as militantly monotheistic ('I bear witness that there is no god but Allah and the Muhammad is his messenger') and, although it regards Moses and Jesus as important messengers, leaders, and prophets, Muhammad is the final and true interpreter.

The ritual requirements of Islam, i.e. the five main religious duties which very ill Muslims will wish to carry out, are faith, prayer, giving alms, fasting, and the pilgrimage to Mecca. Indeed, anecdotal evidence (conversations with nurses and doctors at two large London teaching hospitals with a large Muslim population in the catchment area, with hospice staff in London, and with Muslim friends) suggests that there are those Muslims who, while being terminally ill, have a little time left and still wish to make the gruelling pilgrimage to Mecca. Muslims regard the Qur'an (Koran) as their holy book and accept its teachings, along with later Islamic law and legal interpretation, although there are variations not only between Muslim teachers but between schools of Islamic thought, between countries of origin where customs vary whatever the law, and between people from the Sunni and Shi'a communities.

Modesty

There is an almost universal concern for modesty. Women are traditionally clothed from head to foot except for their faces, and in stricter societies women in the street wear a veil (the chadur) so that only their eyes can be seen. Even at night, Muslim women of relatively strict observance will remain fully clothed, although in looser clothes than their daytime garb, and require a similar degree of modesty at the end stage of their lives. Men also have strict rules for modesty, which include being covered from waist to knee at all times, with nudity being perceived as offensive.

Older men often want to keep their heads covered at all times, although younger men tend to cover their heads only for prayer. Muslims of both genders will usually prefer to be treated by a doctor or nurse of their own gender, particularly if it means uncovering any part of the body, a situation which can cause some difficulties in a terminal care setting but is absolutely essential to understand. The distress caused to Muslims, and others with strict rules about modesty, when those views are disregarded by people who have no similar tradition is unimaginable. Nudity is associated with prostitution and sexual licence, and a woman who is naked in the presence of a man other than her husband is thought to have dropped almost all her standards of decency. For this reason, it is extremely important to check with Muslim patients (and with Sikhs, Hindus, and any others whose origin is in the Indian subcontinent, as well as observant Catholics and orthodox Jews) about their attitude to baring arms for drips, if they are female, and to being washed.

Food

Almost all Muslims follow the prescribed dietary laws, at least to some extent. This means that no pork or pig products must be consumed, and that all meat should be halal (killed according to Islamic law). Muslims sometimes eat meat killed according to Jewish law (kosher) if no halal meat is available. No shellfish except prawns is consumed. Alcohol is expressly forbidden, and although many Muslims will drink alcohol despite the prohibition, the majority do not, and those hospitals and hospices that offer a 'cocktail' on a regular basis to terminally ill patients must realise just what offence this can cause. It must always be assumed that a Muslim will not drink alcohol, and this is an area which should be discussed with the patient and the family.

The most difficult thing for many institutions is the extent to which strict Muslims cannot eat food which has been prepared in utensils that have been used for cooking forbidden foods in the past. Degrees of observance vary considerably and staff will always need to check, but it is often helpful to enquire whether separate food needs to be brought in from home. Once again, this is an area where staff awareness of possible areas of difficulty will make life much easier.

Fasting

Problems are caused by fasting. Often patients who are being given continuous pain relief will refuse it during Ramadan, the major month-long fast which moves around the year since the Muslim calendar is lunar (360 days). They will refuse pain relief even though Islamic law does not require the sick to fast and to endure pain. The period just before Ramadan is used as a time for settling disputes and ill feeling, so that for the terminally ill it can be of particular significance as a last chance to solve the problems of this life with people in this life, whoever they might be. Even if the terminally ill person does not fast, she or he may wish to make donations to charity in lieu of fasting and will certainly wish to be provided with a glass of water and a bowl for washing out the mouth before prayers, if trying to fast to any extent at all.

Rituals

Most Muslims say their prayers five times a day, particularly when they are terminally ill. Hospice and hospital routines may need to be altered to accommodate this. Prayers are offered at dawn, at noon, at mid-afternoon, just after sunset, and at night. Prayer times vary according to the number of hours of daylight, and Muslims will not wish to disturb other patients, so that in summer, when daylight hours are at their longest, there may be some value in giving a terminally ill Muslim patient his or her own room, or a room with another Muslim.

A Muslim will want to wash before praying, and this needs to be arranged within the terminal care setting. Ideally, the patient should be standing, which can sometimes be achieved with the help of caring staff, or a wheelchair can be provided. Muslims face Mecca, remove their shoes, and cover their heads. The greatest difficulty within the terminal care setting is in ensuring that washing can be done effectively and in privacy before prayer, and this requires great sensitivity on the part of nursing and medical staff. The Qur'an demands that the face, ears, forehead, feet, hands, and arms are washed in running water before prayer, that the nose is cleaned out by sniffing up water, and that the mouth is rinsed out.

Muslims also wash their genitals with running water after urinating or defaecating, and cannot pray unless this has been done. Therefore, bedridden Muslim using a bedpan may wish for a jug of water immediately afterwards, and again staff must be sensitive to this, for the psychological need to be fit to pray, in a ritual sense, when terminally ill, is very strong.

Festivals

An awareness of the festivals is very helpful when caring for a terminally ill Muslim patient. If there is a significant Muslim population in the area, most staff will know when Ramadan occurs, but it is also helpful to be aware of 'Id al-Adha, the feast of the sacrifice, Islam's most important feast, and of 'Id al-Fitr, the breaking of the fast after the end of Ramadan. For Shi'ites, 'Ashura marks the anniversary of the martyrdom of Hussein in AD 680, and there is also the Lailat al-Qadr, the night of destiny, on one of the last 10 nights of Ramadan, when the Qur'an descended into the soul of the prophet Muhammad. Although, apart from Ramadan, there is little that caring staff need to do about these festivals, there is value in expecting celebratory food to be available and brought in, and in saying 'Happy 'Id' (pronounced 'eed'), thus making it clear that Muslim festivals are as important as anyone else's, and that the ability to observe religious festivals is seen as an important part of caring for the comfort of the terminally ill patient.

Attitudes to life and death

Devout and pious Muslims believe that death is a part of Allah's plan and that to struggle against it is wrong. Such fatalism is very disturbing for many doctors reared in the Western tradition. Yet the acceptance of terminal illness, and the desire to use it as a time of surrendering to the will of Allah, means that the Muslim patient will often want less in the way of pain relief and more in the way of opportunity for prayer and contemplation. This is not to suggest that Muslims will reject pain relief—there is a strong anti-pain tradition within the religion—but Muslims will often accept less treatment for pain and its associated discomforts in order to keep awake, and use the time for seeing family and surrendering.

The dying Muslim might well want to sit or lie with his or her face turned towards Mecca, whilst another Muslim whispers the call to prayer. There are no official last rites, so that the family, who often stay by the bedside praying, will say the statement of faith and encourage the dying person to say as his or her last words, 'There is no God but Allah and Muhammad is his prophet'.

After death, many Muslims require that only other Muslims touch the body. If it is necessary for non-Muslims to do so, they should wear rubber gloves, straighten the limbs, turn the head towards the right shoulder (so that the body may be buried with the face turned towards Mecca), and wrap the unwashed body in a plain sheet. When Muslims perform these rituals for their own people, they usually straighten the body with the eyes closed, the feet tied together with a thread around the toes, and the face bandaged to keep the mouth closed. The body is usually washed by the family, at home or at the mosque, and camphor is frequently put under the armpits and into the orifices. The body is clothed in clean white cotton garments and the arms are placed across the chest. Those who have been to Mecca may have brought back a white cotton shroud for themselves. Muslims are always buried, never cremated, and this is carried out as soon as possible. Because of the requirement for instant burial, it can be a source of considerable distress to a terminally ill Muslim to find that there may need to be an autopsy after a death.

Judaism

In some ways, it is more complicated to talk about Jews than about Muslims, despite considerable similarities, partly because the history of the Jewish people, who have lived in exile amongst other people over such a long period, means that they have adopted many customs and habits of these other communities. Nevertheless, there are some universal ways in which Jews will vary from others in their attitudes to palliative care.

Jews are a very small group in terms of world religions (an estimated 13 million). Large communities are only found in the United States, Israel, France, the United Kingdom, some South American states, and some of the countries of the former Soviet Union. However, there are many small communities elsewhere—from countries as surprising as India, Japan, and New Zealand to less surprising countries such as Germany, to which some Jews have returned, the Netherlands, and Sweden. Large numbers of Jews everywhere regard themselves as Jewish by peoplehood rather than by religion; nevertheless, they may well want Jewish rituals at their deathbeds, and may well want to discuss attitudes to life and death with those who are caring for them.

In addition, the life-affirming strand in Judaism is very strong, even amongst those who are disaffected from the religion itself, and therefore a fight against death, a desire to survive no matter what, and an unwillingness on the part of many Jewish doctors to admit to their patients that they are dying are all common features of coping with the terminally ill in the Jewish community. The complications that lead on from all this for palliative care are obvious. Although honesty is a prerequisite for enabling people to cope with pain and its consequences, there are still Jewish doctors who feel that a Jew who knows that he is going to die will give up hope, so that his life will thereby be shortened. The strength of feeling for life in Judaism is so great that even to lose a few minutes of it is thought to be a terrible thing; indeed, all laws except three, the prohibitions against murder, idolatry, and incest, may be broken to save a human life even for a few minutes (Talmud Yoma 85a).

Various traditional practices have been used, particularly in the medieval period, to avert the dread decree of death, and these may still be encountered. Among them is the changing of the person's name, which is something that those who are concerned with the psychological welfare of the dying person should appreciate. It is thought that changing one's name averts death, since God makes up the Book of Life at every High Holy Days (the Jewish New Year, culminating 10 days later in the Day of Atonement, Yom Kippur). Those whose names are written in the Book of Life will survive for another year. Those whose names are absent will die in the course of the coming year unless, during the 10 days between New Year and the Day of Atonement, they can avert the dread decree by good actions and putting things right between man and man and God and man.

Although relatively few modern Jews believe that this is a way of deciding who is to live and who to die, nevertheless it illustrates the strength of feeling about preserving human life. If, for European Jews, this is taken together with the meaninglessness of the massive numbers of deaths in the Holocaust, it can be seen why terminally ill Jews can be difficult patients when approaching death and why the instinct to stay alive is so strong.

There is considerable feeling against the consumption of any drugs which could be argued to be life-shortening, a criticism often made by Jewish doctors in the early days of palliative care, although heard less frequently in recent years. Rabbi Dr Maurice Lamm in the United States has done much to dispel this fear, and Jews have now become involved in the hospice movement the world over.

Modesty

Like Muslims, very orthodox Jews are extremely modest, although, since they are a very small group, this affects a relatively small section of the community. Many orthodox men will wish to keep their heads covered, and orthodox women will continue to wear a wig (a sheitl) so that none but their husbands can see their crowning glory.

Food restrictions

Food restrictions are many and complex, and their observance can cause considerable difficulty. Most Jews will not eat pork or shellfish, and many will require fully kosher or vegetarian food. In addition, the mixing of meat and milk at the same time is prohibited. This goes back to the prohibition against 'seething the kid in its mother's milk' (Exodus. 23:19), and the exact time lapse from eating meat to eating milk products varies from community to community.

Further complications exist at Passover, the spring festival commemorating the journey from slavery in Egypt to freedom in the Promised Land, when no leaven may be eaten; any Jew who is trying to observe Passover strictly will need to have food brought from home. They may also ask about the methods of preparation of some drugs, and the use of beer or wine or gin as a cocktail will not be possible during that week.

Food plays a very large part in the folk religion of Judaism. The jokes about the cure-all potential of chicken soup are legion, and less amazing when it is brought into the ward or hospice room day after day! Neither is the dependence on feeding the sick as a method of cure or alleviation surprising; the experience of starvation, of real poverty in the ghettoes of eastern Europe, and of starving in the concentration camps of the Nazis has meant an unusual dependence on food and a belief in its healing properties.

All minority groups in any society have their own food and wish to feed their own people with their specialities, and Jews are no exception. However, for the reasons stated above, it is often even more marked with Jews, and quite often families will continue to bring in food when there is no chance at all that the terminally ill person will eat.

Festivals

Terminally ill Jews may well want to have the Sabbath and festivals marked in some way. Families will usually do this, but staff can help. For instance, it is helpful if staff assist terminally ill Jews in lighting the sabbath candles on a Friday night and do not try to blow them out because of the fire risk. It helps for staff to say 'Shabbat shalom', meaning Sabbath Peace. It encourages Jewish patients to know that staff are aware that the Jewish special day, the Sabbath, is sundown on Friday night to sundown on Saturday night, following the night and stars like the Muslim system, and that Sunday is just an ordinary day of the week for them. It is good for Jewish patients to know that the staff have realized that the High Holy Days, the most solemn days of the year, are occurring and that they have a particular relevance to the terminally ill Jew facing his or her death, with the picture of his or her life coming to the front of the mind. These 10 days of penitence (which occur in

September or October) often encourage terminally ill Jews to make their peace with the world and their God, making for an easier death.

It also helps if Passover is noted, and if staff realize that in other years the patients would have been with their families and friends celebrating the seder (Passover meal), recounting the story of the Exodus from Egypt. Sometimes,if the patient is in an institution, it can be helpful to encourage friends or family to come in and conduct a very short seder at the bedside; there are several anecdotal accounts of how helpful this has been to some individuals and, indeed, how fascinating staff have found it.

Attitudes to death

There are no last rites in Judaism, although a dying Jew, or the family, often ask to see a rabbi. Staff need to be aware that there are various kinds of Jews of different denominations, from the most orthodox to the most liberal, with differences between Ashkenazi (originating in Europe) and Sephardi (originating in Spain, Portugal, or North Africa) as well, and that it helps to ask for the right kind of rabbi. This is no different from the different kinds of Christian or Muslim denominations, and it is usually helpful to ask the family for guidance.

When death is very near, Psalms are read and the dying person is encouraged to say the first line of a prayer called the Shema ('Hear, O Israel, the Lord is our God, the Lord is one') as his or her dying words. There is also an opportunity for private confession, not spoken, and for all assembled to gather together for Psalms. After the death, there is much to be done. Jews, like Muslims, want no delay in the funeral, preferring to have the burial conducted within 24 hours of the death if possible, or 48 hours at most. (Jews and Muslims often feel disgusted at the week-long delays before funerals they see for Christians amongst whom they live. They also argue that it is impossible to begin to grieve properly if one is still waiting for the funeral.) For this reason, there is considerable resistance to postmortem examinations (and others) and it is preferred that the body remains intact without the removal of vital organs, although some less orthodox Jews are committed organ donors. The usual insistence on burial does not always apply, since non-orthodox Jews (Reform and Liberal, commonly grouped together as Progressive) allow cremation, although the preference still tends to be for burial.

When the death occurs, people stay by the body for 8 min whilst a feather is left over the nose and mouth to check that breathing has completely stopped. The eyes and mouth are then closed by the son or nearest relative, the arms are extended down by the sides of the body, and the jaw is bound up before rigor mortis sets in. Traditionally, the body is then placed on the floor with its feet towards the door, covered with a sheet, with a candle beside it, and is not left alone until burial. This cannot fit in with the routine of most hospitals and hospices, but the body may be removed to a side-room where it can remain until the sexton comes to collect it. It should be made clear that, unless the family has given express permission, the staff should not attempt to lay out the body.

In general, Jews do not leave a body alone, and there is a system of watchers (called wachers) staying by the body, reciting Psalms. Many congregations also have a group called the chevra kaddisha (holy assembly) of men and women who wash and prepare the bodies for the funeral, an act considered to be a great honour.

Traditionally, orthodox Jews believe in an afterlife, a world to come, although on the whole Jewish tradition has left the precise nature of this afterlife unclear. Orthodox Jews assert in their daily prayers that they believe in such an afterlife and in the coming of a personal Messiah, but the extent to which Jews genuinely believe this is unclear. The experience of the Holocaust has rocked the faith of many Jews in a dramatic fashion, and little research has been done on the precise nature of modern Jewish belief. Suffice it to say that non-orthodox Jews do not tend to believe in a physical afterlife, and many do not believe in an afterlife at all; the extent to which they believe in a personal God is also unclear.

It is essential to understand that many Jews will want to go through the rituals, observing Sabbaths and festivals that they have not noticed for years, at the time of terminal illness even though their belief system may be very weak. This tends to be done as a sign of belonging, of showing a form of group loyalty, more than as an act of faith. Nevertheless, it will be very much appreciated if note is taken of festivals and Sabbaths, as it will be for staff to recognize the extraordinary grip on life that many Jews show *in extremis*, which can make them difficult patients but also allows them to be survivors against the odds.

Sikhism

There is a great deal of dispute between academics and historians as to the exact definition of Sikhism. Some argue that it is an offshoot of Islam, whilst others claim that it is an Islamic-influenced breakaway from Hinduism. Whatever the truth of these assertions, it is a religion of increasing international importance, and its adherents are usually easily recognized by their wearing of the turban and the other four signs of Sikhism.

A Sikh is a follower or disciple of Guru Nanak, who founded the religion in the sixteenth century and whose nine successors consolidated his work. The book of Sikhism is the Guru Granth Sahib, which is often read aloud to dying Sikhs.

Community action is the mode by which Sikhism operates; there is no priesthood. The gurdwara is a centre of learning and of prayer, of eating together and hospitality. It is also the source of help for any Sikh in distress, and where once travellers and the homeless stayed, and indeed can still sometimes stay.

Sikhism has no clear belief in an afterlife. Like Judaism, it is very much oriented towards a this-life approach and to this world. It has a disciplined approach to life, and Sikhs are supposed to be involved with family, friends, and community rather than following the sometimes ascetic, and very often other-worldly, disciplines of Hinduism. There is also a strong military strand to Sikhism, and it is thought of, on one level at least, as a military fellowship. The last of Guru Nanak's disciples, Guru Gobind Singh (late seventeenth century), instituted five symbols which all initiated Sikhs were to wear.

The symbols

The first symbol is the kesh, the uncut hair left long and worn in a bun by men and women alike, covered with a turban by men and by some older women. The kesh has enormous ramifications for palliative care, because palliative radiotherapy and chemotherapy can often cause hair loss. This can be extremely distressing for Sikhs, and must be discussed in detail before being undertaken and before the final decision is made. There are many Sikhs who would prefer not to have the treatment at all if it is palliative and not curative (although it is often hard to give a hard and fast prognosis) and who resent their hair loss more than anything. (The offer of a hairnet, or a series of nets of different meshes, to save hair and keep it near the head can often be very useful.)

The kesh requires the kangha, the comb which keeps the bun in place. The kangha should be left close to the sick person even if all the hair has been lost, and its significance must be respected, along with that of the kara, the steel bangle that all Sikhs wear. If surgery is ever required, the kara should be taped to the body and not removed like other jewellery. The same is true for the kirpan, the ceremonial dagger which has, anecdotally, been the cause of some horror on the part of caring staff. It is usually a very small weapon, worn traditionally under the clothes, including in bed for many Sikhs, in a cloth sheath (the gatra) over the right shoulder and under the left arm at waist level. Some Sikhs wear a dagger-shaped brooch or pendant, rather than the actual weapon. It is worn everywhere, in the shower, in bed, and in hospital; its existence must be respected and Sikhs should be encouraged to wear it with pride.

The last of the five symbols is the kaccha, the underpants or shorts worn at all times by all Sikhs. These garments are part of the modesty requirement of Sikhs, who feel very strongly about these matters. Those caring for Sikhs often find it difficult to believe that a Sikh will require to have one leg in a pair of underpants at all times, even when in the shower or giving birth. Sikh women give birth with one foot in a pair of pants. Sikh men shower wearing one pair of pants and then change them afterwards, one leg into the clean pair and one leg still in the old. The implications for washing, and bathing, of terminally ill Sikh patients is obvious, and this is an additional illustration of the modesty requirements of religions which have their origins, or much of their practice, in the Indian subcontinent.

Food

There are some food restrictions for Sikhs; these include never eating halal meat, as killed for Muslims (and therefore, to avoid any offence, never being offered it), and a tendency, particularly among women, towards vegetarianism, as for Hindus. Of those Sikhs who are not vegetarian, some follow Muslim customs and do not eat pork, whilst others follow Hindu custom and will not eat beef. Alcohol is forbidden to Sikhs, and would be regarded as deeply distasteful if offered in a terminal care setting. The other substance expressly forbidden is tobacco; this was proscribed by Guru Gobind Singh and is found disgusting by many Sikhs. Every effort should be made to keep terminally ill Sikhs away from those who smoke, even in the last days of life. This is a fact which can cause some difficulty in some hospices, since the rules for those terminally ill patients who wish to smoke are often relatively relaxed as there is little point in worrying about the health implications at this stage. However, for the benefit of Sikh patients, tobacco should not be allowed anywhere near them.

Death and the afterlife

Like Hindus, Sikhs tend to believe in a series of reincarnations, which means that they often have very little difficulty in accepting forthcoming death. Each soul goes through cycles of rebirth, so that death causes no fear. The ultimate objective is for each soul to reach perfection, to be reunited with God, and not to have to re-enter this world. Despite the concentration on this world and this life in much of Sikh thought, the doctrine of the karma remains, so that each person's present life is influenced by his actions in the last life, and the actions of this life set the scene for what will happen in the next life, and so on.

The major difference between Sikhs and Hindus, which has important psychological and social consequences, is that, unlike Hindus, Sikhs believe that the cycle can be altered by exceptionally virtuous actions. They believe in the power of the individual and in the extension of God's grace. Therefore they will not be particularly frightened at the time of the death and will welcome readings from the Guru Granth Sahib, organized by the local gurdwara or the family, as well as opportunities for private prayer.

When death comes, the family will usually take charge. In all Asian traditions (and most others) last rites are a family affair, and nurses will merely be asked to close the eyes (if a member of the family does not do it), straighten the limbs, and wrap the body in a plain sheet. Sikhs are cremated, wearing their five signs, with men wrapped in a white cotton shroud and women wrapped in red, if young, or white if they are older. Cremation is required within 24 hours of the death where possible, similar to the speed required for Muslims and Jews, and there is usually the desire for the eldest son to light the funeral pyre, which is often difficult to arrange in the United Kingdom. Nevertheless, arrangements can often be made for a family member to push the button at the crematorium which starts off the process. The ashes are collected, to be scattered in a river or in the sea, ideally in the River Sutlej at Anandpur in the Punjab, where Sikhism was founded.

The combined fatalism and essential practicality and this-worldliness of Sikhs make it difficult to forecast their reactions to their impending deaths. It is important that they are given a chance to express their feelings, both within their own community and sometimes outside it, because of the varying views within Sikhism itself and the different attitudes to the extent to which an individual can affect his or her fate.

Hinduism

There are Hindus all over the world, with different groupings among them and different castes within the Hindu system. Although the caste system has theoretically been abolished in India, it still seems to have an extraordinary presence in some Hindu families and communities.

Food

Hindu food laws indicate that the cow is sacred, and no beef is eaten. The further south in India the origin of the family concerned, the more likely it is that they will be vegetarian, and the more strict they are likely to be about the consumption of food which has touched beef or, in some instances, meat at all. However, these restrictions are less likely to affect the greater part of palliative care (except for a concern about the use of animals in the making and sometimes testing of drugs) than is the prevalence of fasting, particularly amongst elderly and widowed women. This can lead to an unwillingness, at the end of life, to take drugs of any kind on a fast day, and to prolonged periods of fasting. This is relatively common amongst some Hindu groups, and can have a considerable effect on fluid balance and on the titration of drug dosage.

Modesty

As with other religions of the Indian subcontinent, Hindus have strong requirements for modesty and need total privacy for bedbaths, examinations, and almost any procedure, as well as requiring treatments to be given by health care workers of the same gender. A further problem can be caused by an unwillingness to discuss any problem in the genitourinary area, so that constipation can be a major undeclared problem. These areas will not be mentioned, particularly if a spouse is present, but traditional Hindu law regards it as improper for a woman to be attended by a doctor if her husband is not present. This can present considerable problems and can complicate treatment and caring for Hindu patients unless watched for quite carefully.

There is also a strong emphasis on physical purity. Hindus try to bathe daily in running water, and require help to do this when very ill, particularly if they are older. They also prefer to bathe before saying their prayers. Hindus believe that bathing renders one both physically and spiritually clean, so that the desire to bathe can be very strong amongst those who are terminally ill and they must be assured that help is available.

Hindu thought

There is considerable confusion in the West as to the nature of Hinduism. Some regard it as polytheistic, whilst other commentators regard it as monotheistic, with God's various guises and attributes being expressed in and by the various deities in the Hindu pantheon.

Whichever is the case, it is clear that Hindus pray to several different figures, and many terminally ill Hindus may well have a small figurine or picture of a god beside their bed. Often this will be of Vishnu, the preserver, in his incarnations as Rama or Krishna; sometimes it will be Brahma or one of the many others in the pantheon. The literature of Hinduism, dating from 3000 to 2000 BC, is enormous, and much of it can be recited by learned Hindus.

Most Hindus welcome hearing one of the Vedas or the Bhagavad Gita being read aloud by another Hindu, but prayer and spiritual life for Hindus varies considerably. Some pray, meditate, and take their physical exercise all at once by means of Hatha Yoga. Others rarely go to a Temple. Yet others go through the four stages of life which most Hindus share as a basic approach to life, and go to a Temple only occasionally, but pray and meditate frequently. These stages of life are the brahmacharya, the period of education, the garhasthya, the period of working in this world, the vanapastha, the time when worldly ties and worries are gradually loosened, and the pravrajya or yati, the time of waiting for death. This must be seen in the context of a religion that believes in reincarnation where, according to the karma (frequently misinterpreted in the West as a kind of mindless fatalism, which it is not), the individual is reincarnated either better or worse off than in the previous life. Actions in this world affect status in the next. The status in this world is likely to be the result of actions in the last existence, and so on. The period of loosening ties and preparing for death, which is not the end, very considerably affect the way that many Hindus face their mortality in this life, in the here and now.

Treatment may be combined with the use of traditional Hindu Ayurvedic medicine, which requires physical moderation in all things, from food and sex and physical exercise to a regular routine of sleep, defecation, and bodily cleanliness. Part of the thinking of Ayurvedic medicine, often challenged by Hindus themselves, is the idea that good health is the reward for living by religious and moral laws. Hindus are by no means alone in this, and Judaism, Christianity, and Islam all have the idea somewhere in their literature that, to some extent, length of days is a reflection of virtue, and that sickness can be, but is not always, a punishment. Nevertheless, there is a particularly strong strand of this type of thinking amongst some Hindus, combined with a fatalism that may make it easier to treat them in practical terms but which makes psychological support very difficult indeed.

Rituals at death

There are no actual last rites in Hinduism, but the pandit (the Brahmin priest) can be called in and can be very helpful. He may talk with the dying person about the philosophical attitudes to death in Hinduism, and he may also be able to help with the puja, the act of worship. He may also bring Ganges water as a comfort for the dying person, and may read from Hindu texts.

After death, there is a ceremony known as Sreda, when food is brought for the Brahmins and rites are performed for the dead. The chief mourners often go into retirement, but grief is expressed openly and warmly.

Hindus are always cremated, and where possible this is done in such a way that the ashes can be scattered on the River Ganges at Varanasi (Benares) in India. This custom has its origin in the burning ghats floating down the Ganges, and suburban crematoria have no such magnificence. Nevertheless, even in the suburbs, Ganges water is usually present, often in a brass or bronze container, and the pandit will conduct a moving and beautiful service, often at the express wish of the deceased, who may have made stringent requirements about the kind of funeral that he or she wanted.

Buddhism

Buddhism is growing rapidly in the West, and has a huge number of adherents throughout the world. However, their practices are very varied. Many Western Buddhists have their origin in the 'hippy' culture of the 1960s and early 1970s; their world view is very different from that of Tibetan or Nepali Buddhists. Although they all centre themselves on the discipline of Siddhartha Gautama and his revelation of four truths, after which he was called Buddha, their similarities are limited to the absence of a godhead and a search for a disciplined life.

There is a doctrine of rebirth in Buddhism, which is somewhat different from that in Hinduism and Sikhism, for everything changes as the individual progresses from one life to the next. It is possible to observe the teachings of the Buddha and to live such a good life that one gradually approaches nirvana, perfection, where selfishness is gone and separate identity is no more.

Although these ideas make it easy in some ways to care for dying Buddhists, most Western Buddhists are singularly influenced by their original culture. Nevertheless, there is a rigorous discipline which recognizes that human existence and suffering are inextricably linked, and demands of its adherents a gradual heightening of the awareness of the spirit, where physical realities matter less and less, leading to a state of perfect freedom and peace.The search for this awareness may mean that the Buddhist will not wish to take any drugs which could blunt perception in any way. A Buddhist will require time and peace for meditation, and can find the hospital or even hospice setting too busy to allow the kind of meditation desired. The refusal of pain relief is not uncommon, and makes caring for and treating the patient quite difficult. This is combined with quite strict requirements for diet, often including a vegan or strictly vegetarian diet. A considerable section of the Buddhist community also requires strict attention to modesty, similar to that of Sikhs and Hindus.

The difficulty in providing palliative care for Buddhists is that the desire for palliation may simply not be there. The main request may be for information and peace in order to prepare for death and the next life, as well as to try to achieve a sense of equanimity. This may cause an extreme reaction in staff who cannot bear to see the suffering of a person who has refused pain relief, particularly if they are in a hospice setting where pain relief is an aspect of care so much at the heart of staff pride. All the training of staff in palliative care is directed towards treating and alleviating pain. That task may still be there with Buddhists, but the pain concerned is more likely to be psychological and emotional, where peace to meditate is unavailable, rather than physical pain from the disease, although that may of course be present.

Most Buddhists are cremated, and the ceremony is conducted by a bhikku (monk) or sister, or a member of the family. Buddhists often like to be visited by their teachers, or by a bhikku or sister, and to have Buddhist texts read to them. So much variation exists in patterns of dealing with terminal illness in Buddhism that the only sensible thing to do is ask the person concerned or the family.

Christianity

The spiritual aspects of Christianity are dealt with elsewhere in this volume, but the cultural variations are important. They can be summarized quite briefly at this stage and divided into two main groups. The first is belief-based variation. These variations depend on the extent to which belief in an afterlife, such as heaven or hell, means that attitudes to death include fear and hope, more than anger and acceptance. To some extent, this is dealt with elsewhere, but some manifestations in the way that some dying Christians of a more fundamentalist persuasion conduct themselves should be mentioned. These people tend to seek bedside confessions and reconciliations, so that scenes of 'the good death', much admired in earlier times, occur. There is almost a sentimentalization of death to be found in some of these encounters, which may have their origin partly in a fashion for the glorification of death in Europe in the late eighteenth and early nineteenth centuries, leading to magnificent funerals and stately clothes for mourning.

Other variations lie in the countries of origin. For instance, there is a remarkable similarity in practice between a south Indian Christian and his Hindu neighbour with respect to diet, hygiene, and fatalism. Muslims who have lived close to Hindus are also more likely to take on part of that fatalism than if they have lived outside an area of such influence. Meanwhile, Jews who live in the broadly Christian West find themselves, for instance, increasingly abandoning the prescribed 7 days of official mourning after the death, in favour of just 1 or 2 days, even though psychologists are united in regarding a mourning period as having a greater effect than just the day of the funeral with no proper follow-up.

There are also purely cultural differences, such as the way that Irish people look at death. Protestants and Roman Catholics in Ireland, north and south, make much more of dying than do their co-religionists in Britain. The custom of the wake is not confined to Catholics, and the signs of respect for the removal of a body occur on both sides of the border between north and south and in both communities. Death is not a taboo subject among Christians in Ireland, as it is in English Christian circles, and on the whole Catholics are more open about it than Protestants, perhaps because of the insistence on last rites and the use of the final confession. However, Christians in Ireland will tend to be as speedy about the funeral as Muslims, Jews, and Sikhs, very different from the tolerance of, and even demand for, delays commonplace in the United States and England.

Interesting questions lie in attitudes and fear of death among Christians: some Christian circles have the most well-developed pictures of hellfire and damnation of any religious group. The fear of death can be very considerable, not because of pain or loss, but because of a fear of what is to follow. This is not a common phenomenon in other religious groups, and may affect some Christians extremely strongly.

Cultural trends

There are those who argue that views about death and the emotions that it causes have gradually become more and more alike in different cultures and religions. However, the evidence does not point in this direction. Attitudes to 'stiff upper lips' and to reincarnation, to a heightened awareness and to the desire to be physically and spiritually clean, to fast and to desist from pain relief, are all found among those of different cultures and religions, but each is by no means widely held. The most common feature is to see similarities between people whose families originate from the same area, and the most striking phenomenon is that few people, however apparently rigorous and orthodox they appear to be, adhere wholly to the attitudes that the textbooks say that they are supposed to hold. In the end, the most accurate information will come from the individual or his or her family. All that can be given here is a picture painted with broad brush-strokes, which suggests what is likely to be the case.

Bibliography

Burkhardt VR. *Chinese Creeds and Customs.* Hong Kong: South China Morning Post, 1982.

Dinnage R. *The Ruffian on the Stair.* London: Viking, 1990.

Enright DJ. *The Oxford Book of Death.* Oxford University Press, 1983.

Henley A. *Asians in Britain.* Vol. 1. *Caring for Sikhs and their Families: Religious Aspects of Care.* Vol. 2. *Caring for Muslims and their Families: Religious Aspects of Care.*Vol. 3. *Caring for Hindus and their Families: Religious Aspects of Care.* London: DHSS and King Edward's Hospital Fund for London, National Extension College, 1982–1984.

Iqbal M. *East meets West.* 3rd edn. London: Commission for Racial Equality, 1981.

Locke DC. *Increasing Multicultural Understanding—A Comprehensive Model.* Newbury Park, CA: Sage, 1992.

Lothian Community Relations Council. *Religions and Cultures: A Guide to Patients' Beliefs and Customs for Health Service Staff.* Edinburgh: Lothian Community Relations Council, 1984.

McGilloway O, Myco F, eds. *Nursing and Spiritual Care.* London: Harper and Row, 1985.

Neuberger, J. *Caring for Dying Patients of Different Faiths.* St Louis, MO: Mosby, 1994.

Neuberger J, White, J, eds. *A Necessary End.* London: Macmillan, 1991.

Sampson C. *The Neglected Ethic: Religious and Cultural Factors in the Care of Patients.* Maidenhead: McGraw-Hill.

10.2 Cultural issues in sub-Saharan Africa

Charles L.M. Olweny

Definition

The classic definition of culture was provided by the nineteenth-century English anthropologist Edward Burnett Tylor in the first paragraph of his treatise *Primitive Culture* published in 1871. In it Tylor described culture as that complex whole which includes knowledge, beliefs, art, morals, law, customs, and any other capabilities and habits acquired by man as a member of society. Tylor subsequently stressed that culture so defined is a behaviour peculiar to *homo sapiens.* Culture is now regarded as referring to ideas, beliefs, ceremonies, codes, customs, language, rituals, taboos, techniques, tools, works of art, and institutions such as marriage. Human infants are born culture-less and culture-free, but the environment in which the infant finds itself will mould and create a culture that the infant will grow into, develop, and accept as its own. Benjamin Paul[1] indicates that man lives in a double environment: an outer layer of climate, terrain, and natural resources, and an inner layer of culture that mediates between man and the world around him.

Cultural differences between the Western world and sub-Saharan Africa

There are major differences between the perception of cultural issues in the Western world and in sub-Saharan Africa (Table 1).[2] In the Western context, discussion of culture often centres on films, music, sport, and the theatre. Death, dying, and bereavement rarely feature in public discussions. In Western culture death, like marriage, is a private affair, but in sub-Saharan Africa birth, marriage, and death are major social events.

There is no such thing as an African culture. There are many subcultures, and even within these there is considerable variability

Table 1 Differences between Western and sub-Saharan cultures

	Western	Sub-Saharan
Personhood	Emphasis on: individualism; autonomy; privacy	Emphasis on: familial self; extended family; family togetherness
Family values	Focus on nuclear family, equality is stressed	Extended family, respect for elders, communal upbringing of children are key elements
Love and affection	Expressed openly, even in public	Private affair, Public expression loathed
Disease and illness	Technology based Due to invasion by bacteria, viruses, parasites	No natural explanation Supernatural carries more weight Influence of ancestral spirits
Pain	Physiology gone wrong Different pill for every level of pain	Stoicism cherished Endurance training encouraged
Death	Funeral a private family affair	Funeral a major social event
Bereavement	Counselling by professionals	Extended family support in abundance
Palliative care team	Narrow base (volunteers and health professionals)	Broad base (family, extended family, village community, traditional healers)

and heterogeneity. However, in matters appertaining to illness, death, bereavement, and life after death there appears to be some commonality and uniformity of purpose and practice across sub-Saharan Africa.

Unlike in the West, there is no extensive record of beliefs and practices. Most cultural practices in sub-Saharan Africa are handed down from generation to generation by word of mouth. Africans generally are not in the habit of keeping diaries. The existing recorded cultural practices have mostly been written by foreigners, and these are suspect as the locals tend not to reveal their feelings, beliefs, private lives, and actions to strangers.

Concepts of wellness, illness, and death

In sub-Saharan Africa wellness or good health is equated with strength. Good health is believed to be inherited, and it is maintained by eating well, avoiding exposure to cold, heat, exhaustion, and grief. Illness is said to result from one's departure from the code of conduct (unwritten) and behaviour. The ancestors are expected to provide a blanket protection over the people. However, if the ancestors are unhappy (because the clan has failed to perform certain rituals), they will allow evil forces to penetrate the protective cover. In other words, persons who have misbehaved are not deserving of ancestral protection. Guilt weakens one's ability to ward off evil, and a guilty person becomes vulnerable to evil forces. Generally there are no natural explanations for illness and there are no accidents. Disfiguring diseases such as leprosy or unsightly conditions such as hernia or the deformity of poliomyelitis are considered to have arisen from misconduct—the ancestors withdrew protection from evil forces and intercession to the supreme god. Thus disease and illness are due to direct divine intervention and are a retribution for past misdeeds.

There is general acceptance that illness, if not treated, leads to death. Death is accepted as part of life. Among the Zulu and Xhosa of South Africa a child who dies is believed to represent an ancestor who has revisited the world for a brief period and then returned. Another child is expected to replace the lost one, and the newborn child is given a special name, i.e. 'Buyile' meaning one who has returned. Since death is part of life people are not afraid of it except in instances when it is considered to be a bad death. A bad death is one which occurs prematurely before accomplishments, and where there is no formal burial and the remains are consumed by vultures, hyenas, or other beasts of prey. Suicide is also classified as a bad death; anyone committing suicide is not accorded a solemn burial, his or her name is not perpetuated, and the community does not mourn such a death.

The concept of the 'living dead' is universal in sub-Saharan Africa, and refers to dead relatives who are no longer with the community physically but remain spiritually connected. Among the Igbo in Nigeria, the head of the family is buried in his living room as a symbol of his continued presence in the household. Some Yoruba families in Nigeria have ceremonies on the anniversary date of death in which they symbolically 'turn the dead person' from side to side as they might have done in life.

Death is generally considered an occasion for joy if it is a good death, i.e. one occurring at a ripe old age, the death of a good person, or the death of an achiever. A good death is celebrated by singing, dancing, and drinking.

Generally the dead are accorded great respect. Even today in Zambia, city traffic comes to a halt when a funeral procession passes. All persons, whether on foot or bicycle, must stop to pay their respect to the dead person. Radios in nearby houses are turned off as a sign of honour.

Palliative care

Palliative care is particularly important to the practice of medicine in sub-Saharan Africa for a variety of reasons, prominent among which are the following.[3]

1. Patients with a variety of diseases, including malignancies, present at a very advanced stage of their illness when cure is no longer possible.
2. A number of patients will seek to consult the traditional healers first and thus further delay their entry into established care.
3. Modern management, particularly of cancer, is a high-technology venture, and few sub-Saharan countries can afford the capital outlay for diagnostic and therapeutic facilities.
4. Currently, the highest prevalence globally of the acquired immunodeficiency syndrome (AIDS) is in sub-Saharan Africa. Since AIDS is an incurable condition at present, the need to develop and expand palliative care services in the continent is further emphasized.

It is worth remembering that cultural differences in approaches to palliation are evident even within the Western world. For example, although American and Canadian physicians agree that the probability of cure for non-small-cell lung cancer is less than 10 per cent, they differ in their treatment goals for the same disease, with 85 per cent of Americans aiming at cure as opposed to 40 per cent of Canadians.[4]

Pain

Treating pain successfully requires an understanding of its physiology and the pharmacology of pain-relieving drugs as well as the psychology and attitudes of the person(s) being treated. In most sub-Saharan cultures, pain is regarded as a manifestation of illness and patients are encouraged to bear it as part of their illness. Stoicism is encouraged from a very young age. Circumcision without anaesthesia in adolescent boys is common practice in some African cultures and is viewed as the rite of passage to manhood. Training in endurance is an accepted protocol in adolescents and young adults. Prominent parallel scarification marks observed on the cheeks of many in Northern Uganda and some parts of Nigeria and Zaire are examples of such endurance practices. Beauty marks on the faces, chests, and abdomens of girls are another example. Painful labour is believed to enhance bonding between mother and child. There are no specific herbs or medications for pain relief. Individuals with severe pain are given 'hypnotics' and 'tranquillizers', including alcohol, to relax them and help them to sleep.

Experiences, beliefs, attitudes, and meanings derived from growing up may affect and colour one's perception of pain intensity. Although this has not been studied specifically in the context of sub-Saharan Africa, there are suggestions that Africans do endure more pain than their Caucasian counterparts. African-Americans are related ethnoculturally to sub-Saharan Africans. In one study of ethnocultural influences on variation in chronic pain perception in a large multicultural community, only seven African-Americans were encountered at a pain clinic when at least 50 were expected on the basis of population demographics.[5] Although the most likely explanation was the underutilization of health care resources by the African-Americans, it is tempting to speculate that they chose to bear their pain in silence rather than complain about it. In the study alluded to above,[5] ethnic identity was one of the independent variables that was significantly related to the perception of intense pain. Hispanics had a significantly higher mean pain intensity score than the Old American, French Canadian, or Polish ethnic groups.

Familial self and palliative care

In sub-Saharan cultures personhood is perceived in the context of 'familial self', characterized by togetherness and interdependence among members of a close-knit extended family. A person perceives himself or herself as an intermediary between the ancestors and the future generations.[6] In this context, life and death are regarded as being part of the same continuum. A sick person will be visited not only by his family and extended family but also by the entire village community. Failure to visit the sick may be viewed with suspicion, as it might suggest being responsible for the patient's illness by invoking the powers of the evil spirits. One reason why traditional Africans may not feel comfortable in a Western-style hospital is related partly to the restrictions imposed on the number of visitors and the arbitrary determination of visiting hours intended to suit the hospital staff. An adult African at his or her deathbed would like to be surrounded by his children and grandchildren. Dying in isolation suggests poverty and implies lack of love by the family. A person surrounded by 15 to 20 family members may be in pain, but the suffering may be greatly alleviated. Traditional Africans tend to have spiritual and moral preoccupations and are not concerned with material matters as death approaches.[7] These concerns may relate to family relationships and the fulfilment of requests made by deceased relatives. Such preoccupations are often resolved through rites and rituals performed by the patients and their families.

Bereavement

As previously indicated, death is a major social event and brings together not just the immediate and extended family members, but the entire village community and beyond. The Igbos believe that when you mourn the dead you are mourning yourself and that enmity does not go beyond death. In their culture, a bereaved family will not lack company, food or material requirements, and support.

Generally, non-attendance at a funeral is viewed with suspicion and the non-attendee is considered somehow responsible for the death. During the funeral ceremony, which may last up to a week, emotions run high, relatives cry out loud and sing songs in praise of the deceased, and special funeral dances are performed.

Among some Ugandan communities (true of most East African communities) the bereaved is not left alone until it is reckoned that he or she has come to terms with his or her loss. This period of support may last for weeks, months, or up to a whole year. At the end of the mourning period a special ceremony, referred to in Uganda as the 'last funeral rites', is held and those in attendance implore the ancestors to welcome the deceased into their community.

Among the Zulu and Xhosa of South Africa, bereavement lasts for a year. Soon after burial the bereaved go into seclusion. During that time they wear heavy blankets, paint their faces white, and spend their day dreaming about the deceased. In their retreat they listen carefully to what the deceased and the other ancestors have to say. The retreat period lasts for 3 months, after which the bereaved come out of their seclusion to report the experience of their ancestral contact to a special medicine person (Itola) who endeavours to interpret the meaning of the dreams and messages. At the end of the year, a ceremony is held to 'see off the deceased'. After 18 months another ceremony is held, this time to 'welcome the deceased back into the family'.

Traditional healers

One aspect of palliative care recommended by most authorities in the field is the team approach. In Western-style palliative and hospice care, this refers to collaboration between lay persons, mostly volunteers and the health care professionals (nurses, physicians, social workers). In sub-Saharan culture, this team must embrace a wider circle of collaborators. It must include the family (first-generation volunteers) and the traditional healers, in addition to the other health-care professionals. In sub-Saharan Africa, a dying person will almost invariably have one or more traditional healers to attend them and, if they are on medication, they may be taking the supply concocted by the traditional healer as well as hospital drugs.

Traditional healers in sub-Saharan Africa represent a resource that is untapped and underutilized.[8] With minimal training they could revolutionize palliative care delivery in Africa and elsewhere. In Zimbabwe the traditional healers (N'angas) have formed a national association, the Zimbabwe National Traditional Healers Association (Zinatha). It has a membership of about 1000 and is chaired by highly influential and well-educated Zimbabweans. Increasing recourse to traditional healers in Zimbabwe and elsewhere is attributed to economic reforms. The slashing of state subsidies has made services like health that were free become unaffordable for many people.

Good traditional healers attribute their powers to the ancestors and to the superior god. If they perform their healing function during the day, they may invoke the sun; at night they may invoke the stars and the moon. Good healers are detached from materialism and will seek payment in kind rather than cash, or may merely request a symbolic gesture (coffee beans or cola nut). Such healers are humble about their art and are humane. In addition, their holistic approach makes their services particularly appealing.

Conflict between the old and the new

The modernization process leads to the passing away of traditional practices and values. Among the key elements that have contributed to cultural change in sub-Saharan Africa are education, urbanization, and foreign religions. Urbanization is spawning a new generation of Africans less tied to the land, the clan, and ethnic identities. Reduced access to the land has enhanced the value of education as a viable alternative to land ownership as a strategy for self-improvement. Africans are by nature a very religious and god-fearing people. There is a god of rain, a god of harvest, a god of war, a god of plenty, a god of famine, etc. At all times the ancestors intercede with these various gods to maintain balance and provide protection. The traditional religions emphasized animism. This explains the feeling of togetherness and oneness with nature, and the totem practice whereby an animal or a plant is taken by a clan or community as one of them. The unity of man and nature is taken for granted and is the basis of the sub-Saharan philosophy of life and death.

Both Christianity and Islam, although originating outside sub-Saharan Africa, have principles that support animism, and this may be the reason why both religions have found favour with Africans and have such a strong foothold in the continent. Christians and traditionalists ask the saints and the ancestors respectively to intercede on their behalf with God.

However, there are some conflicts between these foreign religious beliefs and traditional practices that deserve mention.

1. Islam accepts illness as part of God's plan.[9] This clearly contradicts the widely held notion of evil forces causing illness. Among some Ugandan tribes, it is believed that nobody ever dies without being bewitched. In Islam neither magic nor sorcery are allowed. Islam encourages burial soon after death (same day), while in sub-Saharan Africa funerals traditionally last for several days. The family is urged not to engage in wailing and crying, and not to question God's plans. The creator takes away what he created. The 'last funeral rites' are forbidden if they are not in accordance with Islamic teaching. All these contradict traditional beliefs and practices.

2. Christian churches have taught and continue to teach that consulting the traditional healer is sinful, and have branded some funeral practices as pagan and evil. The use of traditional instruments like drums were at one time prohibited as they were regarded as accessories of the spirits!

3. The Judaeo-Christian belief of hell fire as punishment for sins is another point of departure. Hell is a foreign concept in sub-Saharan Africa; when a person dies, he or she automatically joins the communion of saints (the ancestors).

Hospitals

Although hospitals are increasingly gaining acceptance, most traditional Africans still view them as places where people die and which therefore ought to be avoided unless one is seriously ill. Most traditionalists will consult with the traditional healer first and will accept admission to hospital only if the illness progresses. However, if they perceive that death is imminent, they will discharge themselves, preferring to die at home. Also, if they die in a hospital, they do not want their body to be stored in a mortuary. Some believe that storage in a mortuary does not allow the spirit of the deceased to find its appropriate resting place. Finally, every traditional African society has a family burial ground. Burial in a cemetery is treated with considerable disdain. The Luo in East Africa will go to great lengths to ensure burial in the traditional family burial ground, and to them burial in a public cemetery is taboo. The Kikuyu, in contrast, have no qualms about such practices. Those setting up hospices in Africa should bear these issues in mind.

Impact of AIDS

The emergence of the AIDS epidemic in sub-Saharan Africa has emphasized the urgent need to develop palliative care facilities. Sub-Saharan Africa has the highest prevalence rate with 8 to10 million adults currently infected with the human immunodeficiency virus (HIV), the putative agent for AIDS. The disease is incurable at present and manifests with symptoms calling for compassion and care.

AIDS has undermined the African extended family system. Families have been eroded and torn apart. Orphans, who would normally be looked after by relatives, are now institutionalized. In some instances 20 to 30 orphans may be cared for by one grandmother.

Friends find it difficult to visit individuals with AIDS as they do not know what to say to them. Do you wish the patient speedy recovery when everyone knows that he or she will not recover? Far fewer people attend funerals than was the case before the emergence of the AIDS epidemic, and those who do attend may leave early to be at two or three other funerals in the same village.

AIDS has disrupted the traditional support structure that existed. Upon the death of a husband, the widow was 'inherited' by one of the brothers of the deceased. This ensured that the widow and her children remained within the family and thus were adequately supported. If the cause of death is AIDS, the probability of the bereaved spouse being infected with HIV is high. Thus many cultural practices may have to be abandoned.

Summary

Sub-Saharan cultural practices differ substantially from those of the Western world, particularly in the areas of wellness, illness, and death. Life and death are seen as a continuum. Stoicisms and endurance training are encouraged in adolescents. Palliative care is important in sub-Saharan Africa because of the advanced stage of disease at presentation, the emergence of the AIDS epidemic, and the high cost of medical technology. Bereavement support is provided by family members and relatives as long as it is needed. Traditional healers arc an important resource waiting to be tapped. Old traditions die hard, but education, urbanization, and foreign religions are having a major impact on long-held beliefs and practices.

References

1. Paul B. *Health, Culture and Community.* New York: Russell Sage Foundation, 1990:467.
2. Olweny C. Quality of life in developing countries. *Journal of Palliative Care*, 1992; **8**(3):25–30.
3. Olweny C. Ethics of palliative care medicine: palliative care for the rich nations only! *Journal of Palliative Care*, 1994; **10**(3):17–22.
4. Porzsolt F, Tannock I. Goals of palliative cancer therapy. *Journal of Clinical Oncology*, 1993; **11**(2):378–81.
5. Bates MS, Edward WT, Anderson KO. Ethnocultural influences on variations in chronic pain perception. *Pain*, 1993; **52**:101–12.
6. Durojaiye MDA. Ethics of cross cultural research viewed from a Third World perspective. *International Journal of Psychology*, 1979; **14**:137–41.

7. Ngu VA. Dying with dignity: spiritual considerations are all important. *World Health Forum*, 1991; **12**:394–5.
8. Olweny C. The ethics and conduct of cross-cultural research in developing countries. *Psycho-Oncology*, 1994; **3**:11–20.
9. Baider L, De-Nour AK. The meaning of disease: an exploratory study of Moslem Aram women after mastectomy. *Journal of Psycho-Social Oncology*, 1986; **4**:1–13.

10.3 Chinese patients with terminal cancer

K. S. Chan, Zarina C. L. Lam, Roxco P. K. Chun, David L. K. Dai, and Antony C.T. Leung

Chinese attitudes towards death and dying

Confucianism, Taoism, and Buddhism are the three classical beliefs in Chinese culture. Confucianism centres on the moral development of people and Li (appropriate social conduct) in interpersonal relationships. It has had a tremendous impact on familial relationships among the Chinese. The search for Tao (truth) is the core of Taoism. It adopts a strong naturalistic view and has a strong tradition of nourishment of life. Buddhism holds that there is a cycle of reincarnation. Life is a result of Yin (previous deed) and Yuan (chance of nature).[1,2]

Communism, which espouses dialectic materialism and has dominated contemporary China, has enforced naturalistic beliefs about death.[3] In addition, the Chinese communities in Taiwan, Hong Kong and Singapore have undergone rapid socio-economical change in recent decades. These processes have inevitably made an impact on the attitudes of the Chinese people to death.[4] Nevertheless, folk religion still persists among the Chinese and ethnic minorities, and ancestor worship is still widely practised as an act of respect to and seeking of blessing from the deceased. Among Chinese, the line of descendants is treated as an extension of self and a form of immortality.[5]

With regard to the timing of death, 'let nature take its course' and 'old age' are the two most acceptable attitudes.[3] The former reflects the ability and readiness of the Chinese people to accept the course of nature even if death is the result. Yuan is a significant cultural concept acknowledging the inevitability and chance element in every event.[6] The external attribution of causes of the event promotes its acceptance.[7] Nevertheless, because of this cultural characteristic, people may attribute the cause of death to quite innocent individuals such as the newborn baby or the wife married into the family. It is believed that good deeds and a clear conscience make peace for the dying if death means a new cycle of reincarnation with reward for the 'good'. Dying in old age is regarded as the most natural way of dying; a funeral for an old person is called a 'happy' funeral.[8] A good death is regarded as one in old age, passing away in the presence of family members with no unfulfilled family responsibility, with pain well controlled, and with a clear conscience.

Family interaction and communication during the dying phase

Traditional Confucian beliefs encourage an enmeshed family system to perform multiple functions for ideological, social, and economic reasons. For instance, the Law of Kinships, involving five cardinal relations (emperor–people, parent–child, spouses, siblings, and friends), classifies family members according to age, gender, and status into a hierarchical structure and determines interactional patterns[9,10] during important family occasions such as weddings, death, or the serious illness of a family member.

Filial piety or hsiao, which is a highly meritorious and ideal representation of Chinese culture, implies strong devotion to the dying parent. As the father–son relationship is the key to the family structure, the eldest child (preferably the son) is expected to accompany the patient passing through the final stage of life as an expression of filial piety. Reconciliation of old unresolved conflicts and avoidance of over-expression of emotions, such as quarrels with the dying, are some examples of maintaining this filial reputation. Filial duty is further reinforced by the Buddhist concepts of Yin and Yuan. Blessings from the dying guarantee future prosperity and success. Thus the dying patient expects physical caring and emotional concern from children or other relatives.[11,12]

Symbolic interactions amongst family members, which provide psychosocial support, are often expressed in delicate, subtle, and sometimes paradoxical ways. A direct request for help from a senior member of the family may mean 'losing face'. To avoid this, actions such as preparing and offering food are commonly used as non-verbal ways of showing care and concern.[13] Soups which require many hours of preparation and involve multiple ingredients are more than just for nutritional purposes. The symbols of family hope, concerns, and traditional beliefs on balanced body–mind or man–nature relationships are significant. Ginseng or medicated herbal soup for supplementing Ying (female part) or Yang (male part) in order to promote longevity may be employed for similar reasons.[14]

Death remains a taboo subject for many Chinese.[3,15] Talking about death is believed to speed it up or even bring it about. Very often any discussion of death is avoided by family members to protect the dying person or the young.

Management and care of the cancer patient

Breaking bad news to the patient and the family is often a delicate and complex process. It involves the identification of the key family members and clarification of particular people's roles within the enmeshed Chinese family. The patient often requests the doctor not to reveal the diagnosis to the other family members, and vice versa, so as not to arouse extremes of emotion.[16] As the family is often more highly valued than the individual in Chinese culture, the degree of truth-telling has to be individualized and family wishes respected as much as possible.[17] An 'evasive stage' has been described as a common psychological reaction among patients, family members, and health-care workers,[18] in addition to the five psychological reactions described by Kubler Ross.[19] Although a permissive approach to 'evasiveness' is adopted in traditional Chinese society,[20] more open communication is usually encouraged in Westernized Chinese society and particularly with the development of hospice care concepts in various Chinese communities.[21-23]

Chinese patients and members of their families often express their emotions in subtle and non-verbal ways.[24,25] Somatization is a common presentation of underlying depression.[26] As Chinese health belief regards body and emotion as one,[24] patients often have difficulty in expressing their emotions which makes counselling an arduous and difficult process.

Traditional Chinese medicine

The traditional Chinese medical techniques of Qigong, and acupuncture are frequently employed in the treatment of cancer either as the principal approach or complementary to Western medicine. They are based on the theory of balancing Ying and Yang, Qi (vital energy), and five elements, namely metal:lung, water:kidney, wood: liver, fire:heart, and earth:spleen,[27] and are used mainly for symptom control and general health promotion, particularly in the augmentation of the immune defence system of the body. Qigong, a breathing exercise for progressive muscular relaxation, has proved to be effective for some patients and families.[28] Different Chinese communities have different predilections for these treatments.[29,30]

Fulfilling familial obligations is the most common death wish among most Chinese.[31] As frank expression of emotions is often avoided to conserve energy during the dying period, a longer period of mourning is needed for the family to get over the fear of having the same illness, for queries about fulfilment of expectations, and for acceptance of the death that has occurred. A Chinese family will gather on successive occasions, over a period of 7 weeks to 100 days, which serve as an after-death ritual for the bereaved.[32-35]

References

1. Meng Xian Wu. A study on Chinese traditional thinking on terminal care. In: *Proceedings of the First East–West International Conference on Hospice Care, Tianjin, 1992*: 454–61. Tianjin: Tianjin Medical College. (In Chinese.)
2. Koo LC. A journey into the cultural aspects of health and ill-health in Chinese society in Hong Kong—the importance of health and preventive medicine in Chinese society. *Hong Kong Practitioner*, 1989; **11**:51–8.
3. Tsuei YT, Hwang MTC. *Hospice Theory and Practice.* Taipei, Taiwan: Chinese Medicine Technology, 1992: 202–15. (In Chinese.)
4. Hui CH. Death cognition among Chinese teenagers: beliefs about consequences of death. *Journal of Research in Personality*, 1989: **23**:99–117.
5. Yang Mao Chun. Chinese familism and Chinese national character. In: Li Yi Yuan,Yang Kuo Shu, eds. *Chinese Personality.* Taipei, Taiwan: Chuan Kuo, 1972. (In Chinese.)
6. Yang Kuo Shu. *The Metamorphosis of the Chinese.* Taipei, Taiwan: Kwai Kuan, 1989. (In Chinese.)
7. Cheung FMC. Psychopathology among Chinese people. In: Bond MH, ed. *The Psychology of the Chinese People.* Oxford University Press, 1986: 119–203.
8. Qiao Ji He. *Chinese Customs in their Life Span.* Taipei, Taiwan: Bai Guan, 1992. (In Chinese.)
9. Yang CK. The communist revolution and the change of Chinese social institutions. In: Yang CK, ed. *The Chinese Family in the Communist Revolution.* Cambridge, MA: Harvard University Press, 1959: 4–21.
10. Leung A. Assessment of family needs and the choice of treatment approach. *Hong Kong Association for the Promotion of Family Therapy Newsletter,* Spring 1993.
11. Tang MC. *Life and Family Structure in a Chinese City.* Ann Arbor: UMI, 1994:254–61.
12. Yu JS. The preliminary psychologic study of the senile cancer patients. In: *Proceedings of the First East–West International Conference on Hospice Care, Tianjin, 1992*: 161–3.
13. Pietroni PC. Complementary medicine—its place in the care of dying people. In: Dickenson D, Johnson M, eds. *Death, Dying and Bereavement.* London: Sage, 1993: 208–14.
14. Zhuo DH. Preventive geriatrics: an overview from traditional Chinese rnedicine. *American Journal of Chinese Medicine*, 1982; **10**:32–9.
15. Hwang MTC. Comparative study on death attitude between Chinese and American University students. In: Tsuei YT, Hwang MTC, eds. *Hospice Theory and Practice.* Tianjin: Chinese Medical Technology, 1992: 170–201. (In Chinese.)
16. Kerr D, Lin Zhang Guan Hwai. Terminal care in China. *American Journal of Hospice and Palliative Care*, 1993; **10**(4):18–27.
17. Shi Li Hua. Ethics of nursing terminally ill patients and their countermeasures. In: *Proceedings of the First East–West International Conference on Hospice Care, Tianjin, 1992*: 371–3. Tianjin: Tianjin Medical College. (In Chinese.)
18. Jiao Die Ying. The psychological stages of dying patient and countermeasures of hospice care. In: *Proceedings of the First East–West International Conference on Hospice Care, Tianjin, 1992*: 94–8. Tianjin: Tianjin Medical College. (In Chinese.)
19. Kubler Ross E. *On Death and Dying.* New York; MacMillan, 1969.
20. Wang De-Shang. Talking about Chinese death bed care. In: *Proceedings of the First East–West International Conference on Hospice Care, Tianjin, 1992*: 427–9. Tianjin: Tianjin Medical College. (In Chinese.)
21. Tseui YT, Hwang MTC, eds. *Hospice Theory and Practice*, 1992: 85–90, 93–105, 268–78..
22. Tsao SY, Leung ACT. Palliative care in Hong Kong. *Palliative Medicine*, 1991; **5**:262–6.
23. Merrimann A, Lau TC, Thompson M. Terminal care—what the carers think. *Singapore Medical Journal*, 1986; **27**(4):288–92.
24. Wu DYH. Psychotherapy and emotions in traditional Chinese medicine. In: Marsella AJ, White GM, eds. *Cultural Conceptions of Mental Health and Therapy.* Dordrecht: Reidel, 1982: 285–301.
25. Guo Lih-Yea. The measurement of traditional Chinese health beliefs, a cultural prism. In: Cheng LY, Cheng F, Chen CN, eds. *Psychotherapy for the Chinese.* Chinese University of Hong Kong, 1993: 69–80.
26. Kleineman A. *Patients and Healers in the Context of Culture.* University of California Press, 1981: 119–77.
27. Bridgman RF. Traditional Chinese medicine. In: Bowers JZ, Purcell EF,

eds. *Medicine and Society in China*. Philadelphia: Josiah Macy Foundation, 1974: 1–24.

28. Koh TC. Qigong—Chinese breathing exercise. *American Journal of Chinese Medicine*, 1992; **10**:86–91.
29. Lee RPL. Perception and use of Chinese medicine among the Chinese in Hong Kong. *Culture, Medicine and Psychiatry*, 1980; **4**:345–75.
30. Ho SMY, Leung SF. Attitude of Hong Kong medical students toward different modalities of cancer treatment. *Psychological Reports*, 1995; **76**: 1291–6. Tianjin: Tianjin Medical College. (In Chinese.)
31. Tseui YT. The Chinese attitudes towards death and dying. In: *Proceedings of the First East–West International Conference on Hospice Care Tianjin, 1992*: 3–15. Tianjin: Tianjin Medical College. (In Chinese.)
32. Sun S L. The psychological nursing of the patients and their family members in hospice care. In: *Proceedings of the First East–West International Conference on Hospice Care, Tianjin, 1992*: 335–6. Tianjin: Tianjin Medical College. (In Chinese.)
33. Tan G. Analysis on the mood and care of terminal patients' family members. In: *Proceedings of First East–West International Conference on Hospice Care, Tianjin, 1992*: 325–8. Tianjin: Tianjin Medical College. (In Chinese.)
34. Lam ZCL. *Enhancing quality care for frail and vulnerable clients: case management approach and applications.* Hong Kong: Hong Kong Christian Service, 1996. (In Chinese.)
35. Lam ZCL, Chan KS, Chun RPK, Leung ACT. *Study on cultural and psychosocial aspects of terminal Chinese patients in Hong Kong*. Proceedings of 5th Asia/Oceania Conference in Gerontology, Hong Kong, 1995.

10.4 Palliative care in Japan

Tetsuo Kashiwagi

Attitudes to dying and death

There is a strong negative image of death, a subject which has typically been taboo in the twentieth century. Thus physicians, patients, and families are strongly oriented towards cure. In general, people prefer to receive curative treatment even during the terminal phase of their illness. However, since 1977 the work of St Christopher's Hospice in London has been introduced to Japan through the media, and as a result public interest in palliative care has intensified. During the past 10 years the topics of death and dying have been discussed openly in many meetings of physicians and nurses.[1]

The preferred place of death

People in Japan, particularly older people, want to die at home. However, statistics show that in 1992 76.6 per cent of all deaths occurred in institutions, mainly hospitals. Only 23.4 per cent of deaths took place outside an institution, most frequently at home. However, 93.7 per cent of all cancer deaths occurred in an institution with only 6.3 per cent in other places. Clearly, it is very difficult for Japanese cancer patients to be able to choose to die at home.

Attitudes to honesty and truth-telling

The patient

A questionnaire carried out in 1992 by the Japanese Ministry of Health and Welfare[2] revealed that 18.2 per cent of patients who died of cancer had been told the diagnosis, 42.5 per cent appeared to know it, and 25.1 per cent did not know it. Doctors may reveal the diagnosis to the family but they are reluctant to disclose the truth to the patients themselves, particularly if they are terminally ill. Families are also very reluctant to divulge the diagnosis, mainly because they do not want to distress the patient. The approach of conventional Japanese medical ethics is that physicians should not tell their patients of the terminal nature of their disease. Doctors may also lack the confidence to reveal such bad news and, as in other countries, they are often uncertain about their own ability to help and support the patient after the disclosure. Nevertheless there is a gradually increasing trend for doctors to tell the truth.

The family

The 1992 survey[2] showed that 98.1 per cent of families were told the diagnosis. Of the family members who were informed, 83 per cent were spouses and 34.6 per cent were siblings. Of the siblings, sons were informed much more frequently than daughters. Usually the family member who is told the diagnosis does not share this information with young children, particularly those under 10 years of age, nor with older people, particularly if they are over 80.

Psychological experiences of the dying patient in Japan

The psychological processes of the dying patient are influenced by the prevailing customs of medical practice (e.g. whether truth-telling is the usual practice or not). Furthermore, the nationality of the patient dictates the manner of communication, which is a very important factor in the psychological coping strategy.[3]

Because truth-telling or revealing the diagnosis is not the usual custom in Japan, dying patients often continue to receive aggressive treatment until the end of life. The Japanese way of thinking and communicating is different from that of Western cultures. Therefore, in any comparison of Western and Japanese cultures, it will be found that some psychological processes are similar and some are quite different.[4]

The psychological experiences through which the dying patient progresses in Japan are shown in Fig. 1.

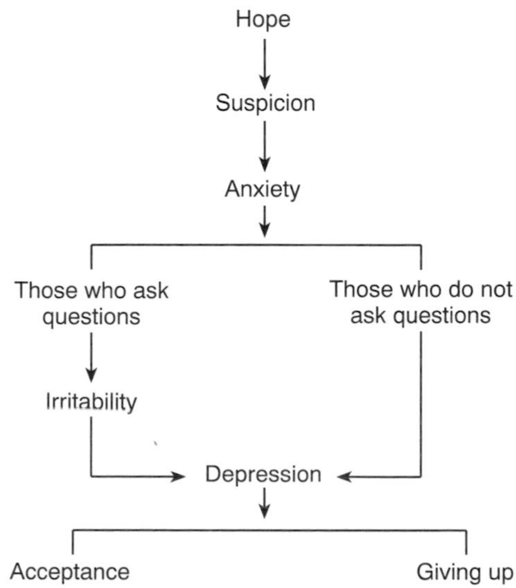

Fig. 1 Psychological process of a dying patient.

- Hope: many patients do not know that they are dying and therefore maintain some hope of recovery. Up to a certain point this hope supports the desire of the patient who would like to live longer. However, as the disease progresses, suspicion begins to creep in.
- Suspicion: even if they still have some hope of recovery, patients become suspicious when, for example, they have pain and a general increase in fatigue and other symptoms. This is usually followed by anxiety.
- Irritability: for many reasons 80 per cent of patients still do not ask questions even when experiencing suspicion and anxiety. The 20 per cent who ask questions usually do not receive satisfactory answers, and this induces a stage of irritability followed by depression. In 80 per cent of patients, death usually follows the stage of giving up; a much smaller number of patients die after denial or after trying to fight the illness. Approximately 20 per cent of people die after having come to some form of acceptance.

Reasons for not asking about the diagnosis

As already mentioned, 80 per cent of Japanese patients, even when suspicious about the diagnosis, do not ask questions. The reasons include the following.

- Fear: many people apparently fear the possibility of malignancy and are frightened of asking questions because they are unsure if they will be able to cope with the physician's answer if it confirms their suspicion.
- Denial: it seems that if the patient inwardly denies the possibility of malignancy, he or she will not ask about the diagnosis. Others exercise self-discipline or have a strong sense of reserve which holds them back.
- Distrust: some patients do not ask questions because they have no trust in the staff and others do not ask because of consideration for family and friends.

An awareness of some of these differences in thinking and in culture may enable non-Japanese caregivers to respond to Japanese patients and families with better sensitivity and understanding.

References

1. Kashiwagi T. Hospice care in Japan. *Postgraduate Medical Journal*,1991; **67** (Supplement 2):95–9.
2. Ishikawa Y, *et al*. *Cancer Death in Middle Age*. Report of the Statistics Bureau of the Ministry of Health and Welfare of Japan, 1992.
3. Kashiwagi T. Palliative care in Japan. *Palliative Medicine*, 1991; 5:165–70.
4. Kashiwagi T. Psychosocial and spiritual issues in terminal care. *Psychiatry and Clinical Neurosciences*, 1995; **49** (Supplement.1): 5123–7.

10.5 Cultural issues in indigenous Australian peoples

Nikki Blackwell

This account, which describes the experience of establishing a palliative care service for Indigenous people in a remote part of Northwestern Queensland, is written from the perspective of a white English woman. I am very grateful to my Indigenous colleagues and patients for all that they have taught me, and what follows is written with their permission. 'Aborigine' is not a word that Indigenous Australians use to describe themselves, but rather one which was coined by British colonizers to describe 'first occupants'. In addition, as a term it fails to convey the great diversity of different tribal groups in Australia, spread out across its vast land mass. Each group has different practices and therefore the term is a generalization.

There is very little in any of the medical, palliative care, anthropological, or indeed 'Aboriginal' literature about death and dying in these groups. This reflects the importance and secrecy attached to death and dying within Indigenous cultures.

The time of death may reflect the culmination of acquisition of 'The Law' (or secret tribal knowledge). As such this cannot be shared with lesser initiates or with people of the opposite sex (a distinction is drawn between 'women's business' and 'men's business'). It may be necessary for the dying person to pass on stories and knowledge about their land and its sacred sites to the next keeper of the land.

A great fear is attached to the process of becoming ill. Illness is thought to reflect an individual's being 'sung' by a medicine man (or Kadaitcha), usually for some slight or wrong-doing. This can only be undone by a healer whose strength is equal to or greater than that of the person who initially pointed the bone or cast the spell. Death may be followed by considerable 'payback' activities between clan groups if it is thought to have occurred as a result of sorcery.

Following the death important ritual activities must be observed. The place of death must be 'smoked' to allow the spirit of the deceased to return to the land (in 'Aboriginal' Dreamtime stories the Ancestors roamed the land and created life from it) and to protect the living from the actions of disaffected spirits. Funerals are generally a mixture of Christian tradition (following the missionary influence) and traditional tribal keening and wailing. It is considered imperative for all members of the clan to attend the funeral and it is a cause of great 'shame' should they fail to do so. For this reason funerals may be delayed for many weeks after death until all the relevant clan members are able to assemble.

How should palliative care workers take account of these cultural differences? The ideal would be for Indigenous health workers to provide palliative care to their people, therefore avoiding the need for others to be involved at this secret and sacred time. While to a certain extent this is possible, it is not practical in many areas of Australia while there is such a shortage of Indigenous doctors and nurses. Therefore the challenge is to allow the cultures to interface for the benefit of terminally ill Indigenous patients and their family.

Just as traditional healers have high status and respect within their communities which allows them to be involved with issues of death and dying, our experience suggests that it is possible for Caucasian workers to acquire the necessary respect for this to happen. There seem to be some fundamental principles which will allow this to happen. The workers should already be involved and highly visible in other aspects of the community's health, for example as the providers of primary health care, and should have demonstrated that they appreciate the best methods for communication with Indigenous people in these situations. Health care workers should make allowance at all times for the fact that they are dealing with a silent people (traditional writers suggest that this is because communication between Australia's Indigenous people can occur without words, i.e. through telepathy) and should not rush or hurry them into speech, expecting answers, when they come, to be very brief and spoken quietly. Workers must also be aware that there are still areas of Australia where people speak their own language and do not understand English. Of course, the use of an interpreter is crucial in this situation, and there will usually be a member of the clan who can translate. Direct eye contact should be avoided at all costs as this is regarded as a blatant act of aggression.

Workers should expect their patients and families to be very frightened of white medicine—it is only used when someone is very sick, and they will almost certainly have tried traditional methods first.

Men will prefer to be seen by another man and, particularly for an initiated tribal man, seeing a female health worker may be interpreted as insulting. It is possible for women health-care workers to be accepted because of their honoured role as healer, but they are still expected to show appropriate respect—for example a female doctor caring for a male tribal elder should kneel keeping her head below that of the patient and the front of her body turned away in deference. Patients do not volunteer this information; it must be actively sought out and sensitivity to these hierarchical issues of respect is greatly valued.

Gynaecological issues may be too 'rude' to be discussed directly with a young female patient, and the patient will be 'shamed' (i.e.

lose face) by such a consultation. However, the woman may nominate her 'Aunty' or 'Granny', who will be a respected clan female elder but not necessarily a relative according to Caucasian kinship systems. She can act as an intermediary allowing discussions to take place frankly. Gynaecological issues are strictly 'women's business' and it is very shaming to discuss them with a man present.

In our experience an important clan elder will be the 'index' patient, and this person will usually present with intolerable physical symptoms due to advanced disease. This person acts as a 'test case', and if the care provided is perceived as helpful, other Indigenous patients will follow.

Workers must be aware of 'parallel issues'; for example, although seeking 'white medicine', traditional patients will almost certainly believe that they have been cursed or sung, and they and their families will be involved in a process to try and undo this or at least understand the reason for it. This can cause great terror and impact significantly on patients' physical symptoms.

The Indigenous people of Australia have a profound relationship with the land, and while they are able they prefer to remain in close contact with it—living outdoors, eating traditional food ('bush tucker'), and making visits to sacred sites. They may need to be told explicitly that such things are not harmful and are in fact encouraged.

In contrast with the Caucasian palliative care view that death at home is a good thing, this is not perceived as so by Indigenous people, as it is necessary for the family to move away completely from the place where the person has died. Whilst this was practical when the family lived a traditional nomadic lifestyle, it is not easily achieved when they live in a conventional house. However, death at home may still be achieved in some of the remotest parts of Australia, where there has been a return to camp settlements and a shelter can be built specifically for the person to die in. For the majority, however, there will be a strongly expressed need by the patient and his or her relatives for the death to occur in hospital. This should be acknowledged, and reassurance should be given at an early stage that admission to hospital will be provided at the time of death if so desired

As the time of death approaches, it is often necessary to provide absolute privacy—to the extent of giving the relatives a key to lock the door of the room, to keep out the intrusion of hospital life in order for tribal secrets to be passed on and rituals to take place. It must be emphasized that it is not at all necessary or desirable for Caucasian health workers to know what takes place during these sessions in order to provide appropriate palliative care for their patients. One woman elder memorably told me, 'We lie to anthropologists anyway', and so it is unlikely that 'secrets' shared with workers would hold any real truth, given that they are often not shared with many clan members.

There is a tradition of sharing medication amongst Indigenous people—'if it helps me, it will help you'. This has serious implications when treating people with medications such as opioids and corticosteroids. It must be strongly emphasized to patients that their medicines are very powerful and meant for them alone. In general, however, dying Indigenous patients are extremely trusting and compliant with 'white medicine'. Therefore the initiation of morphine treatment is not usually met with reluctance or concerns about 'addiction'. Unfortunately, the side-effects of opioids, including constipation, appear to be as common in Indigenous people as they are in Caucasians.

For patients who wish to maintain their traditional lifestyle and 'go bush' but who require parenteral pain relief, the syringe-driver is an unwanted impractical encumbrance which is viewed with considerable fear and suspicion. In contrast, transdermal delivery systems (e.g. fentanyl) are highly prized and regarded as of great value, freeing the patient from technology and considered to be too 'special' to be shared with family members.

Experience suggests that the best approach to breaking bad news to Indigenous people is to begin with the patient. The news of terminal illness is usually met with expressions of fear. However, it is not the process of dying or death itself which is frightening, but rather the sorcery which the patient perceives as having caused their illness. The patient will then nominate others in the clan who should be told. In the case of a man this will often be older men, who will assemble to meet with the palliative care team and take on the role of visiting the patient. Female family members, including wives, may stay away from the hospital, keeping vigil in a 'sorry camp'. The 'sorry camp' will be established, traditionally out of doors, at a place where the extended clan can assemble and await the death. Likewise with a woman, sharing of the news and caring for the patient may be regarded as strictly 'women's business', and the men will make the 'sorry camp' where they will remain. When the dying person is a child, both parents will usually remain in attendance with close clan members, while the extended family will gather at the 'sorry camp'.

After the death relatives should be offered the opportunity to 'smoke' the hospital room to release the spirit of the deceased. This is a private ceremony from which Caucasian health workers are expected to be absent. Health workers should be aware of the impact of a death within the community. Violent episodes of 'payback' clan fighting may occur, other clan members may present to health facilities suffering from the consequences of 'sorry markings' (ritual wounds which are self-inflicted with a sharp blade across the arms and chest), and other patients will abscond from hospital to attend the funeral, often despite serious illness themselves. Patients may not be able to make their reasoning clear to health care workers as it is considered forbidden for the deceased's name to be mentioned after their death—they are referred to as 'our brother/our friend'. This can make delayed presentations of grieving difficult to disentangle. In contrast with 'smoking out', the funeral is a public affair; Caucasian workers are welcome to attend and it is a great honour to be invited to do so. Many groups of Indigenous people will have further mortuary rituals, approximately 3 months after the death, to conclude the reuniting of the deceased's spirit with the land, but these do not usually involve health care workers.

In conclusion, it is possible to offer excellent palliative care to Australia's Indigenous people in a way which is acceptable to them. This does not require a knowledge of Indigenous practice regarding death and dying, but rather the sensitivity and empathy to be guided by the patient and his or her family, as with all good palliative care.

Bibliography

Australian InFo International. *Aboriginal Australian Culture*. Canberra: Australian Government Publishing Service, 1989

Berndt RM, Berndt CH. *The World of the First Australians.* Canberra: Aboriginal Studies Press, 1992.

Campbell J. *The Power of Myth.* London: Transworld, 1989.

Cawte J. *The Universe of the Warramirri.* Kensington: New South Wales University Press, 1993.

Ginibi RL. *My Bundjalung People.* St Lucia: University of Queensland Press, 1994

Muecke S. *Textual Spaces.* Kensington: New South Wales University Press, 1992.

Myers FR. *Pintupi Country, Pintupi Self.* Los Angeles, CA: University of California Press, 1991.

Parker KL. *Wise Women of the Dreamtime.* Vermont: Inner Traditions International, 1993.

Pilger JA. *Secret Country.* London: Jonathan Cape, 1989.

Roughsey D. *The Rainbow Serpent.* London: Harper Collins, 1975.

Watson S. *The Kadaitcha Sung.* Ringwood, Victoria: Penguin Books Australia, 1990.

11

Spiritual issues in palliative care

11 Spiritual issues in palliative care

Peter Speck

Annette had just celebrated her 57th birthday when she was diagnosed as having breast cancer. She had seen her family doctor for a routine examination when the lump was discovered and had been referred to the local hospital for further investigation. A biopsy had revealed a malignancy and she had had a lumpectomy followed by treatment with tamoxifen. Now, four years later, Annette had metastatic disease and was experiencing a certain amount of physical pain which varied in intensity from day to day and for which she was receiving palliative treatment. She had had frank discussions with the medical team and was aware of her prognosis.

Annette was married with two grown-up children who lived quite near to her and her husband. She originally came from Poland and she and her sister had been the sole survivors of a family wiped out as a result of the holocaust and concentration camps during the Second World War. Her sister died quite suddenly, six months ago, as a result of heart disease. For some years Annette felt that she was the only one who seemed to be concerned about her origins and what had happened to the other members of her family. Her sister had never wanted to talk about it and Annette's husband and children had very mixed feelings about trips to Poland and to museums to trace the events of fifty years ago. However, as her illness progressed so Annette developed a growing sense of determination to document her family history which was so important in establishing her sense of identity.

The family's unwillingness to be too involved in the holocaust documentation also carried over to a reluctance in acknowledging how seriously ill Annette was. There were times when Annette would express anger at a God who seemed to be silent and who allowed such things to happen. At the same time she searched for some understanding, for some existential meaning to all that she was experiencing. During her period in hospital Annette talked with the hospital chaplain. She made it clear that she did not want any formal 'religious' ministry, but she did want someone who could be with her while she explored some of these issues. For Annette there was a clear need to share with someone else, in an accepting relationship, her own inner exploration for meaning within the current experience of illness and impending death. She also needed to find answers to important questions such as 'Who am I now?' and 'What has been the purpose of my life?' Because she had abandoned the practice of any orthodox faith (she had been brought up a Roman Catholic) this discussion needed to take place in a way that did not impose a religious framework upon her exploration.

It is only very recently that people have begun to make a distinction between the two words religious and spiritual. For a long time these words were used interchangeably. This has led to a measure of confusion over what needs one is seeking to meet in people who profess no religious belief yet still want to explore the cause of their illness and distress. The *Concise Oxford Dictionary*[1] defines a religion as a 'particular system of faith and worship' which is frequently interpreted in terms of the particular rules, regulations, customs, and practices as well as the beliefs of any named religion. When talking about religion one would not separate religion from spirituality since the spiritual refers to 'spirit as opposed to matter, of the soul, especially as acted upon by God; of or proceeding from God, holy, divine, inspired, concerned with sacred or religious things'.[1] For some people spirituality is described in terms of the ability to transcend the material, while for others it is described as the 'dimension of a person that is concerned with ultimate ends and values'.[2] The wider understanding of the word spiritual as relating to the search for existential meaning within any given life experience,[3] allows us to consider spiritual needs and issues in the absence of any clear practice of a religion or faith.

Death, for Annette as for many people, brought together the past, the present, and the future, and generated an anguish which contributed to her experience of pain—which was both spiritual and physical. The reality of her own situation rekindled the feelings of grief which she had earlier expressed in respect of the death of her parents and siblings, and the uncertainty as to how they died. There was also the quite recent death of her sister and her unresolved grief and feelings of being 'orphaned' now that her sole surviving relative had died. At times she found the sense of loss almost unbearable and felt that she could not 'let go' of her own life until she had attended to this unresolved grief and to the compilation of her family story which was so integral to her being reconciled with the past and establishing her own identity and worth.

To exhort Annette to accept a religious ministry at this time would have created a further obstacle for her since she first of all needed to establish a trusting relationship within which she could explore the various aspects of her situation. Assessing the spiritual needs of those who are terminally ill relies greatly on such a relationship being formed. In Annette's case that relationship was with a hospital chaplain, but it could equally have been with her local priest in the community, a lay (non-ordained) member of a church, a member of the medical or nursing staff, a volunteer visitor, a family friend, or a fellow patient. What is important is that the sick person is able to choose who they talk to and share with, rather than have someone imposed on them. If the person chosen to share with feels 'out of their depth' it may be possible for the 'professional' spiritual advisor to act as a backup for that individual and thus work indirectly with the patient.

Discerning the spiritual needs

To ask people to assess where someone has reached in the personal search for existential meaning is quite daunting. Not surprisingly, nurses and others have asked for help in making such assessments and in clarifying the inter-relatedness between spirituality, coping strategies, and health.[4] Several of the more recent studies concerning religion and health comment on the paucity of quality research in this area despite the high profile given to spiritual needs in nursing textbooks and journals.[5]

Reed in 1986[5] compared terminally ill and healthy adults in terms of 'religiousness and sense of well-being'. Religiousness was defined as 'the perception of one's beliefs and behaviours that express a sense of relatedness to spiritual dimensions or to something greater than the self. Well-being was defined as a sense of satisfaction with one's current life'. Fifty-seven adults were each matched for age; gender; education, and religious affiliation. The 114 participants completed two questionnaires: the Religious Perspective Scale (adapted from King and Hunt[6] and which measures the extent to which people hold certain religious beliefs and engage in religious practices) and the Index of Well-Being (constructed by Campbell, Converse, and Rodgers[7] which measures satisfaction with life as it is currently experienced). The results showed that women, particularly in the terminally ill group, showed greater religiousness than did the men. This finding has also been borne out in a recent study by King and Speck in a prospective study of the influence of spiritual/religious beliefs on physical and psychological recovery from acute illness.[8] Reed found that there was no difference between the two groups studied in their sense of well-being, in that both indicated moderately high levels of well-being, and there was no significant relationship between religiousness and well-being in the terminally ill group. Well-being in this study was found to be related less to medical condition than the ability to engage in activities which give life meaning. Reed, therefore, emphasised that 'individuals who are dying welcomed the opportunity to talk about and reflect upon their personal views.' In a later study[9] Reed looked at spirituality and well-being in terminally ill adult inpatients, again matching for age, gender, education, and religion. A weakness of the previous study was a confusion between the terms religious, spiritual, and well-being. In this later study some of this confusion is addressed in that spirituality is defined in terms of transcendence and as 'a broader concept than religion or religiosity'. However, the study still seems to struggle with problems of definition and clarity of the concepts being examined. The results (for 300 participants) show that a significant number of terminally ill adults showed an increased spirituality over non-terminally ill or healthy adults. Terminally ill adult inpatients also showed a greater spiritual perspective than non-terminally ill inpatents or healthy adults. There was also a low but significant positive correlation between spirituality and well-being for the terminally ill inpatient adult group.

The possible effect of religion on morbidity and mortality was investigated in 1987 in relation to Protestant, Catholic, Jewish, Muslim, Seventh-Day Adventists, Latter-Day Saints, Parsees, and Jehovah Witness followers and clergy.[10] The study sought to broaden from a study of health practices or health-related behaviour, to include social support, religious participation, and health-related attitudes.

Measuring subjective religiosity has been fraught with difficulty but a key development was the Religious Orientation Scale (ROS) developed by Allport and Ross which distinguished intrinsic from extrinsic orientation, and became known as I-E scales.[11] The intrinsic saw religion as an all pervasive, organizing principle while the extrinsic saw religion as an instrument or tool used to supply needs such as status and security.

Watson, Morris, and Hood later used the Allport and Ross scales in relation to mental health.[12] They showed that an intrinsic religious orientation was associated with healthy psychological characteristics, while an extrinsic orientation was associated with greater levels of anxiety and depression. Kirkpatrick and Hood later reviewed several decades of work using the Allport and Ross I-E scales and found them to be theoretically impoverished, not least because they are only really relevant to religious populations.[13] They recommended that each dimension of the scale be defined as a continuum from 'not at all' to 'very' with the former category representing the non-religious. A shorter version (14 items) has been developed by Gorsuch and McPherson which goes some way towards answering the critics of the I-E scales.[14]

These studies, however, illustrate the point made in a valuable review article by Levin and Vanderpool in which they critically examine the use of 'religious attendance' as a measure of religiosity in epidemiological studies.[15] In this paper they show how the lack of good quality work in this area of study is related, in no small part, to a lack of understanding of the language, research methods, and concepts being used by epidemiologists, medical sociologists, theologians, and various pastoral workers. It is argued that there needs to be a greater interdisciplinary co-operation in undertaking such studies so that a more productive alliance can result. The papers referred to by King, Speck, and Thomas[8]—a psychiatrist, a chaplain, and a researcher; and that by Jones, Johnson, and Speck[23]—a nurse, a clinical psychologist, and a chaplain are illustrative of a more collaborative approach.

There have been several attempts in recent years to develop a systematic approach to the discernment of spiritual needs which would be of value to caregivers. Hay[16] provides a useful example in which he seeks to offer a way for staff to achieve a spiritual diagnosis in terms of:

spiritual suffering—interpersonal and/or intrapsychic anguish of unspecified origin;

inner resource deficiency—diminished spiritual capacity;

belief system problem—lack of conscious awareness of personal meaning system;

religious request—specifically expressed religious request.

Hay's approach is very much in keeping with the 'medical model' and he adds the word pathology to his use of the term diagnosis. He acknowledges that it is difficult to distinguish between psychological and spiritual issues and that addressing these issues within the hospice context can be 'fraught with its own spiritual traps'. A 'Spiritual Well-being Scale' was devised by Paloutzian and Ellison in 1982.[17] The scale distinguishes between the religious and existential dimensions of spirituality and the 20-item-measure yields three scores: spiritual well-being, existential well-being, and religious well-being. In a recent American methodological study, however, Kirschling and Pittman found there was insufficient evidence to support the validity and reliability of the proposed scale.[18] Another study sought to use the scale in connection with anxiety in cancer patients and concluded that persons with high levels of spiritual well-being have lower levels of anxiety.[19] The study then invited the hospice community to undertake further exploration of the spiritual dimension and its healing potential. These studies still need to be done and it is to be hoped that they can be undertaken in the multidisciplinary and collaborative way outlined earlier.

Although it is not easy to examine a person's spiritual state systematically, I believe that it is helpful to approach the subject from the perspective of past, present, and future.

The past

Like Annette, many people approach a terminal illness with a history and a story to tell. It is beneficial if there is someone to listen to that story and the memories, and who can then help them come to terms with the painful episodes whether that be within or outside of a religious framework.

Feelings of guilt or shame

In the course of the story the person may experience and share feelings of guilt or shame which might be in relation to a specific event or person, or it may be in a very general and non-specific way. For some people who have undergone disfiguring surgery, or chemotherapy leading to hair-loss, there can be a great sense of shame for the altered appearance. This may be reflected in comments such as 'I don't want my visitors to come. They mustn't see me like this' or 'If people know my secret (a stoma) they won't want to eat with me'. The fear of loss of control over bodily functions can leave people feeling 'unclean' and therefore unacceptable to others as well as to themselves. To demonstrate pastorally that the person is acceptable, by regular and sensitive visiting, can be very important.

Sometimes there are very specific things that people have done which they later regret—usually at a time when they cannot undo any imagined or actual harm done. It is important to give due attention to the need for forgiveness. 'Forget it, it is all in the past' does not address the issue at the level it is being felt. The resolution of personal or family conflicts can contribute to a peaceful death and ease the consequent bereavement for others. In an interesting discussion of forgiveness in the setting of a hospice, Clark describes the importance of 'Naming and feeling the hurt; recognizing and feeling the anger; seeing the incident more fully; and then reaching out with love and concern to the person who has been hurt'.[20] Reminiscing can be very helpful for some people and may be triggered by the use of photographs or an invitation to tell or write their 'story'. This approach taps into a natural tendency for many people to review their life in order to identify what 'they have done to deserve this' and can make it a more therapeutic activity. Reminiscence can, therefore, be a useful way of integrating the past with the present.

Sometimes the hurt that is experienced is a feeling of being 'let down' by God and may be especially painful to someone who has always been an ardent believer but now finds that their faith has been severely shaken, if not broken. The religious person who has been known and respected for their faith and strong conviction in the face of difficulty can be under great pressure not to let any doubt show, not to let God down, if they now find that faith no longer seems sufficient. To seemingly lose one's faith in the midst of a crisis is a great loss and leads to a real sense of guilt and bereavement. In the *Courage to Be,* Paul Tillich describes the courage needed to 'accept that we are accepted though unacceptable', complete with all our doubts and questioning. Those who experience doubt need reassurance that they are still acceptable to God in spite of the doubts and questions that they are experiencing. In Christian terms the example of the apostle Thomas can be helpful to explore since he needed and sought physical, tangible, proof before he could acknowledge the truth of Christ's resurrection (John 20: 26–29). In spite of his initial scepticism Thomas was not sent away but was accepted by Jesus and his needs were met at the level they were being experienced. In this example Jesus is flexible in the way he responds to the differing needs of his disciples. Similarly we may need to be flexible in our responses. Remarks such as 'You shouldn't talk like that, especially you being a Vicar' can put a great constraint on the individual who is expressing doubt or conflict. Loss of faith can leave one feeling terribly isolated and alone and so it is important to feel that people with whom you share the loss express a continuing loving acceptance and that they are perhaps able to pray on your behalf the prayers you are no longer able to utter.

Because of the attendant guilt and shame for some religious people when they seem to lose their faith it may be appropriate for the relevant religious leader to formally pronounce forgiveness, and also to counsel the person as to the need to continue to put themselves in the presence of God in whatever way is possible. The person may feel that prayer and reading the scripture has lost all meaning and so they may need 'permission' to let go of this way of approaching God and to explore other ways of connecting with God, for example by focusing on an image or object such as an icon or a small plain olive-wood cross which can be held quietly. Sometimes it is not so much a lack of belief that blocks prayer but an anxiety that the prayer may indeed be answered. 'Not my way but thine O Lord' is much easier to pray at some points in one's life than at others. What people want as an answer to prayer and what they fear they may receive may be quite different. The pastor may therefore find he or she is expecting the sick person to say 'Amen' to something about which they feel very ambivalent. Once again it is necessary to take time to explore together what is being assumed in order that the communication with God (as well as between people) is in tune with what is being experienced. This is often the best way of ensuring that one is not imposing on to someone a ritual which has ceased to have any meaning. The traditional writers on spirituality describe periods of doubt and uncertainty as arid, desert, episodes which are nearly always seen as important opportunities for growth; as for example in the 'dark night of the soul' referred to by the Christian spiritual writer St John of the Cross. However it is experienced, to have one's beliefs destroyed by questioning and doubt can be very painful and have a profound effect on the person's understanding of themselves and of their identity. The resultant feeling of alienation can easily lead to despair and the enhancement of any physical pain already present. The reassurance and gentle pastoral exploration described above can enable the pain, guilt, and hurt to be transformed, or even absorbed, by the sufferer.

'The pain was not less. Or perhaps it must have become less since he could behave normally, eat meals, and go back to the office. It was as if the pain remained there but he had grown larger all round it and could contain it more easily. It no longer bent and racked his body. He carried it inside himself gently, almost gingerly, as if it were a precious egg.'[21]

Issues of trust

For some the guilt is non-specific and relates to a general feeling that they must have done something wrong at some time for this illness to have happened. This feeling gives rise to the many 'Why me, why now, what have I done to deserve this, If only . . . ?' questions. Although they may not lead to a complete loss of belief, behind these questions is a feeling of unfairness and, even in those without a religious faith, there is a sense that their body, or someone else, or God, has let them down. This can give rise to a difficulty in trusting people since their life history has shown them that believing in God has not given them (or others known to them) an immunity from things going wrong. The argument seem to be:

'I believed in God. God never lets you down or allows harm. Harm has happened to me. Therefore, God has let me down. If I can longer trust God (who has let me down) how can I possibly trust a human being? Thus, how can I trust the doctor to give me the truth etc.?'

This sort of argument may not always be expressed openly but it can be seen to be influential in patients who are finding it difficult to trust staff. For those who have had a religious belief it can be helpful to suggest that, as humans, we are frail and imperfect and that our bodies do let us down and succumb to illness. However, God is still involved and cares and can make His grace and strength available to us so that we can be strengthened to reconcile past and present and so face the future with renewed hope.

For all groups, religious and non-religious, it is important to seek to establish trust by giving clear and accurate information, coupled with appropriate reassurance of the help and/or treatment that is available, and ensuring consistency of care so that the person does not receive conflicting information from different people. Past experiences of doctors, nurses, and clergy may also reinforce some of the difficulties encountered with trust and the assumption that one should be trusted because of one's role may need to be 'checked out' with the patient and family.

Sometimes it is the break with religious practice that is presented as the main barrier and source of guilt. The sense of God being absent and therefore the possibility of everything being out of control can lead to fear, powerlessness, and a feeling of emptiness—'If only I'd gone to Church more often' etc.

Like Annette, therefore, there is a deep need to explore the past, to be integrated with it, and achieve some reconciliation with the more painful episodes. Where possible, the person may attempt to reconnect with old patterns and customs that helped in the past. Alternatively he or she may abandon old patterns since they are no longer relevant and will then search around for some other way of connecting past and present. As Annette was able to achieve this so her ability to trust began to grow in respect of herself, her doctors, and other people.

The present

In the present there may be various indications of spiritual searching.

Expression of anger

Closely linked to the previous comments there may be an anger with God, the illness, and the medical personnel who seem so ineffective. Since people sometimes perceive life-threatening illness as a violent assault they contain some of the violence within themselves. When the opportunity presents itself the sick person will off-load some of that violence by projecting hurt and anger on to others. In particular, people who seek to relate to the sick person from a position of power and health may seem not to understand what the sick person is feeling inside. Therefore, they may cause hurt to the carer in order to make them feel something of what the sick person is feeling. Whilst this is not pleasant for the carer it is helpful if the carer can receive this anger and not reject the sick person. Rejection confirms that the sick person is bad and deserves to be ill. Frequently the anger is thrown at representative people rather than the specific individual—though it may not feel that way! Behind much of this anger is a desperate need to understand the nature and cause of the illness, together with any part they may have played in bringing it about.

Suffering

Frankl wrote that 'Man is not destroyed by suffering, he is destroyed by suffering without meaning'.[22] There is a subtle change in language which is often an indicator of spiritual anguish. In the early stages of an illness people may talk about 'pain'. However, in later stages I notice that those with bone metastases, for example, talk more about 'suffering'. It would seem that the word pain is used when it is easier to understand the message being given by that pain, and when there is hope of relief from that pain. Suffering, however, seems to relate to pain indicating decay and a growing sense of hopelessness. Many of the requests to 'end it all' by some means seem to be related to this meaningless suffering, often compounded by loneliness and isolation and fears of what may yet be experienced. Being able to focus on 'one day at a time' does help some people feel a little more in control of their environment.[23]

Spiritual health

Not all spiritual issues are to do with problems since there are many who have been able to discover a way of understanding their illness which enables them to cope from day to day. It may be that this is a religious understanding that has always been of positive benefit, or a philosophical belief system which provides answers to many of the questions they ask. Some people are able to grow in their understanding and relationship with God through the experience of illness. This process may be backed up by a supportive group of people who share the same belief system either by praying for or visiting the person who is ill. Such supportive people may be officially appointed chaplains to a hospital or hospice, or they may be local ministers of religion visiting people from their own neighbourhood. The fact that someone is ill and unable to attend their usual place of worship should not lead to their being denied the opportunity to continue to practice their faith while in hospital, hospice, or their own home. This may range from an act of worship at the bedside, to attending a chapel or other place for corporate worship, or having time undisturbed while they undertake their own private meditation or prayer. Hoy provides a useful model for measuring the degree of personal commitment and the amount of religious support that can be expected or desired, with the clearest needs being expressed by those already committed to a faith and who are furthest away from home and their usual spiritual support group.[24] His model also enables us to identify those with a high degree of ambivalence who might especially benefit from chaplaincy or other appropriate involvement, by either a chaplain or staff member willing to explore and share spiritual issues in an open way.

There may well be people whose belief system is not a religious one but who may have a well thought out philosophical understanding which answers many of the questions confronting them. Thus, the practising Humanist may not be too worried about the thought of being dead, though he or she may have anxieties about the process of dying and how it will happen. There may be an appraisal of the person's life and achievements, together with the planning of a secular (non-religious) funeral. This may be supplemented by an expression of wishes in relation to an appropriate memorial and assurance that the person who is dying has made their mark on life and will not be forgotten either. The various caregivers should ensure that they do not assume that the non-religious person will not need similar support and opportunity to explore the meaning of what is happening to them.

The carer may sometimes find that the belief system expressed by the patient makes no links, or clashes very strongly, with that of the carer. For example a black woman married a white man and after many years of marriage, without children, she was found to have a uterine carcinoma. There was a history of interference within the marriage by members of the woman's family. They had never been happy with a mixed marriage and felt that the absence of children was a sign that it was not blessed by God. When the woman was admitted to hospital for investigation she was convinced that the witch-doctor had put a spell on her and that the discharge she was having was evidence of the evil within her. Pastorally, it was difficult to distinguish religious belief from cultural influence. The woman was, ostensibly, a practising Christian but clearly very much in the grip of her culture. It was hard for the carers to appreciate the powerfulness of this belief though the effect was quite clear. It was important that the carers acknowledged their recognition of the woman's belief, even if they could not fully understand it, and then to invite her to share with them her understanding of the witch-doctor's power. Only then could they begin to talk, in Christian terms, of the belief that Christ had conquered evil and therefore the devil or magical powers could not ultimately win! There was a great feeling of going out into uncharted waters together with doubt and anxiety (because one was outside of the culture) as to what powers the witch-doctor might actually have. The key seemed to lie in exploring the belief system together and valuing the other's understanding, even if quite alien to one's own.

Pastoral work is not the sole prerogative of the clergy but may also be undertaken by non-ordained people. It is, however, important that those who seek to work in this way are carefully selected, trained, and supported. Pastoral assistants fulfil a very important role and can often work in a way which is less encumbered by the image or stereotype of the 'institutional church'. If these people visit a hospital or hospice in a voluntary capacity they should be registered with the Voluntary Service Organizer or equivalent. Many hospitals and hospices are staffed by people from a variety of different cultural and religious backgrounds and those who already have a belief system of their own may not feel diffident about sharing that with the patients. It can be very reassuring and helpful to some patients to find that the staff also struggle to make sense of some of the experiences which they and the patients share. Although they may not have it all 'wrapped up' neatly in a parcel of faith, being willing to explore together in a way which doesn't induce guilt for not having a faith which is strong enough, can be very supportive. Similarly, if it feels appropriate to pray together this can be very affirming for both concerned. If this happens at the invitation of the patient and in a sensitive way, such a relationship can be very fruitful and supportive.

A sick person can, however, be a 'captive audience' and may need protecting from the zealous person (staff member or not) who feels they have a mission to bring people to a faith before they die. This 'mission' may manifest itself in many ways but is frequently linked to activity rather than stillness. The introduction of a 'healer' can either bring great peace and comfort or may become a source of pressure and stress in contradiction to the title. One source of pressure is the result of comments such as 'Well, if your faith is strong enough you will be healed'. Failure to make a full physical recovery can be interpreted as evidence to everyone that you just don't have sufficient faith. This amounts to a form of emotional blackmail. Bringing in more people to pray with, or over, one can increase the pressure to comply. It is difficult if the original request for such people has come from the patient, but carers do need to monitor what is happening in order to intervene if the patient is becoming distressed. The term 'healer' may either be ascribed to someone by a group such as a church or recognized healing centre, or it may be assumed by someone on their own authority. Because of the difficulty of deciding who to contact when a patient requests a healer, contact should be made with the chaplain, local church, or centre for alternative therapy for guidance.* Healers who belong to a nationally accredited healing organization (whether religious or not) will have an ethical code of practice which will usually exclude payment and emotional pressure and encourage the sick person to continue with orthodox treatment. In the absence of faith, or request for a non-religious healer, the same accepting relationship between the patient and carer may still allow for a mutual exploration of ways of understanding, and coping with, the illness without reference to religion.[23]

The future

Feelings about the future may vary according to how the previous day has been experienced.

* In the United Kingdom people can contact The Churches' Council for Health and Healing at St. Marylebone's Parish Church, London NW1 5LT or the National Federation of Spiritual Healers, Old Manor Farm Studio, Church Street, Sunbury on Thames, Middx. The Christian Medical Commission of the World Council of Churches, 150 route de Fernay, 1211 Geneva, Switzerland can also provide further help on an international basis.

The importance of hope

There is a need to express and develop a hope in respect of the future, whether that be for oneself or for one's family and others who are left behind after death.

1. There is the hope that perhaps there may be some new drug or treatment which will cure or prolong life—the hope of physical restoration.
2. Then there is the hope for the ability to love and be loved—which may result from being reconciled with one's past.
3. Finally there is the hope that, just as one might find meaning in life, so one might find a meaning in the mystery of death—which may lead to exploration of views and beliefs regarding life after death.

The hope for a cure is a natural one and may require a careful discussion of the treatment options open to the patient and a clear explanation of the nature of palliative care so that hope is not unrealistic. Becoming more loving and lovable is central to the needs of many dying people and to those who continue to live with a life-threatening illness and the uncertainty as to when it will become terminal. Continuing to relate to the patient or sick person, as a person, is fundamental to fostering healthy and loving relationships. Being ignored by a team of visiting doctors can imply that you are as good as dead now and that there is nothing new to say. Some patients are aware of this and can become demanding as a way of saying 'I won't let you forget me, I'm not dead yet'. Paternalistic approaches from any quarter serve to diminish not only the autonomy but also the personhood, and can so easily extinguish hope. If you have to fight to be heard you can so easily give up.

The mystery of death

This is a key area of concern for many. It can be helpful to some people to talk about beliefs in an after-life as well as the process of dying. Many people are fearful of what may precede death and may seek reassurance about symptom control and what help will be available to them and their family. Making a will and discussing funeral arrangements can be an important way of talking about the reality of death as well as giving reassurance as to how the farewells will take place. However, time and place are important for such discussions. For example an elderly, terminally ill man invited the chaplain to come and pray with him. The chaplain arrived at the bedside to find the man seemingly asleep or unconscious. His wife was seated at the side of the bed and the man's two sons (who did not want to take part in the prayers) were standing at the foot of the bed—discussing the merits of different coffins and whether they needed to waste good money on a fancy coffin when a basic cheap one would do perfectly well. After the prayers the old man opened his eyes slightly and winked at the chaplain who said, 'I think you're enjoying this'. The old man replied 'You bet!' and lived for a further two years.

Care may be needed in some cases to protect families from strict embargoes or extracted promises that may be impossible to keep. Such wishes may vary from 'Look after my tomato plants' to 'Don't ever remarry!' This can greatly add to the grief of the family later if they feel they are not complying with the 'last wishes' of the deceased person.

For Annette, planning her funeral was very important. Although she was not a practising Catholic, nevertheless, she wished for a Christian burial and for certain items to be buried with her: a crucifix which she had had since childhood and a ring given to her by her sister before she died. She also asked that a priest be contacted when it was known that she was dying so that she might receive the Sacrament of the Sick, which would consist of Holy Communion, appropriate prayers and anointing with holy oil. 'When the time comes for me to die, I want to do it well' she said.

Religious responses

Annette's requests for help at a later stage included a religious ministry and illustrates the way in which, sometimes, attending to the spiritual issues can lead to a desire for a more formal religious response. The form which this takes will vary from faith to faith and person to person. Broadly speaking, it will be a means whereby the individual can renew the relationship between themselves and God or whatever higher power they put their trust in. This might be through prayer as a focus of communication, through meditation, through study of the religious writings or scriptures, or the availability of a pastoral counsellor as distinct from a counsellor. Most schools of counselling, in keeping with the guidelines of the British Association of Counselling, would see their main aim as 'providing an opportunity for the client to work towards living in a more satisfying and resourceful way'. However, pastoral counselling would also have an existential focus in the counselling relationship in that it would provide an opportunity for the client to work towards living in a more satisfying and resourceful way in the context of a living relationship with God. An old, but still valid, definition is that provided by Clebsch and Jaekle who describe it in terms of 'helping acts, done by representative Christian persons, directed towards the healing, sustaining, guiding, and reconciling of troubled persons whose troubles arise in the context of ultimate meanings and concerns'.[25] To this end each major religious faith has provided a variety of rituals or religious acts which seek to be healing, sustaining, guiding, and reconciling within the context of the individual and the faith practised. An important aspect of training of ministers of any religion should be the proper use of such acts and actions, in conjunction with the appropriate use of counselling skills (see Chapter 21.5). In this way, perhaps, people can be encouraged to maintain a balance between doing things to and being with the person who is dying.

In addition to prayer and reading of the scriptures, some faiths have special means of focusing the relationship between people and God. Within Christianity, as well as the Word of God, the communication and strengthening can also be through the sacraments. A sacrament is a symbolic act which conveys, through the symbolism, not only an inner meaning but also a source of inner strength to the recipient. One of these is Holy Communion in which the believer receives a small portion of bread and wine, specially blessed by a priest or minister, and in doing so partakes mystically of the body and blood of Jesus Christ. In this way the believer receives spiritual strength from God and also shares in the victory of Jesus over death. For some Christians it might be important to make an act of confession to God, formally or informally, and to seek forgiveness as mentioned earlier. There are also formal prayers which can be offered at the time, and following, the death which are essentially designed to commend the dying person to God and to reassure them that they are already loved and accepted by God and so have nothing to fear in letting go of life. These prayers are really a special form of 'permission giving' and can be helpful both to the dying person and to the family, especially in those situations where either the patient or the family seem to be withholding permission to die because of fears about the future.

Such rituals and actions, as indicated, have their parallels in most of the major world religions. I am conscious of writing from within the Christian tradition and that many people, as mentioned above, will be searching for meaning outside of an orthodox religious belief system. Although the format and the words may be different an appropriate 'rite of passage' which seeks to facilitate the transition for family and sick person can be equally important for the religious and the non-religious person.[26]

Such rites of passage need to contain the three elements of separation, transition, and incorporation. Thus Annette, and other dying people, need to be able to separate from their attachments in life, from family and friends and ultimately their own bodies. In that death is a process rather than a single point in time, there is a need to be given permission to undergo the transition from life to death and be incorporated into that group of people described as 'the dead' or, in certain belief systems, those who have entered eternal life, heaven, their next incarnation, Nirvana, etc.

For the bereaved a similar process happens, in that they also need to separate and let go of the deceased in a physical sense and later to let go of the emotional attachment. The bereaved undergo a transition in relation to status (a 'wife' becomes a 'widow'; 'parents' become a 'childless couple') and since the association with death is stigmatizing they later need to be incorporated back into their family or social grouping with that new status. The process of grief is an important part of the management of this transition and religious and/or secular rituals can be effective ways of facilitating or blocking this process.[27]

It is important that people are given every opportunity to see, touch, talk to, and say goodbye in their own way to the person who has died. While any member of staff may arrange for such viewing, many families do appreciate the presence of the appropriate chaplain at such a time. A lot of the 'unfinished business' in a relationship can be expressed at this time and if this is prevented by family or hospice/hospital staff the bereaved can be left with a very heavy load to bear. In a similar way the funeral (religious or secular) needs to speak about the real person who has died so that, for example, there is no collusion with the desire to idealize the deceased to an extent that one is left wondering who one is saying 'goodbye' to. In a similar way the embalming and cosmetic presentation of the person who has died, as they were some years prior to their illness, can present a family with a vision of someone whom they have not known for many years—and perhaps said 'goodbye' to years before. The time of death, the viewing of the body, and the funeral all leave very graphic pictures in the mind and memory of relatives. They can recall in great detail things that they have seen and words spoken to them or overheard at the time. These occasions present opportunity for relevant pastoral and spiritual ministry by clergy and others. A belief system provides a useful context in which many bereaved people are able to work through the grieving process and feel supported and enabled to face the pain of physical separation.[28] In their study of a sample of elderly widowed people in England, Bowling and Cartwright[29] found that 47 per cent of the widowed claimed to have a belief, philosophy, or practice which had helped them to adjust to widowhood. A higher proportion (96 per cent) said that they had a religion: 65 per cent said they were Church of England (Episcopal), 19 per cent were 'other Protestant', 10 per cent were Catholic and 4 per cent said they had no religion (though some of this 4 per cent felt they had a philosophy which had helped). However, the results showed that 'Those who felt they had a helpful philosophy, however, had a similar score on our adjustment scale to those without one and there was no difference in the extent of the loneliness reported by the two groups'.[30] Parkes and Weiss in their return to the Harvard Bereavement Study found that it was difficult to look at religion or non-religion as predictive variables for outcome and the data they had collected only enabled them to distinguish between Catholic and other faiths and to comment that there was no difference in outcome for these two groups.[31] What is clear from these three studies, and others, is that a belief system helps to define what it is the bereaved have to accept and adjust to, and may help to answer the question concerning the deceased 'Where are they now?', but it does not provide a means of short-cutting the grief process. A key factor in making any pastoral response in bereavement is spending time listening to what this particular death means for the family, and being flexible in our response, rather than assuming the we know what is best for them, and ensuring that the local church community maintains contact with the bereaved during the mourning period.

Spiritual needs of professional carers

Those who care for the dying in any setting frequently find that the nature of the work confronts them with their own unresolved feelings about future personal death and their past experience of other losses. It is often the unexpected which throws us off balance and makes it difficult to function in the way we wish. The unresolved feelings and grief that carers have in their own lives can easily 'get in the way' and lead to a protective way of relating, designed to ensure that the patient or family do not affect us too deeply. In staff training it can be helpful to distinguish between the professional agenda and the personal agenda. The professional may be more concerned with an understanding of the psychological processes of adjusting to death and dying and of acquiring appropriate helping skills to make this process easier for patient and family. However, we each have our own personal agenda, even when we are in our professional role. From time to time we may find that the personal presents itself and makes it difficult to remain within the professional role. Time needs to be given, therefore, to identifying and understanding those parts of our personal agenda which make us especially vulnerable.

One way of doing this is to create a personal life-line along which one marks off all the losses (significant or not) that have happened during that person's life. The most significant loss is then selected and an atempt is made to recall the feelings and reactions that we experienced at the time, and subsequent to the loss. It is best if this exercise is shared since it can lead to the person getting in touch with quite deep feelings which they were not hitherto aware of—sadness, anger, guilt, isolation, etc. The feelings generated by such an exercise are an indication of areas of unresolved grief and the need for the person to continue sharing and working through the grief around that and perhaps other events. The control of personal emotions lies not in turning away from them and denying them, but in having the courage to face them so that we can recognize and understand where they belong and what they are about. This is a very important aspect of personal growth and of our own search for meaning and integration of the past.

Alongside the exploration of our psychological and emotional makeup, therefore, we may find that working with the dying also challenges us to search for meaning in all that we experience. The questions asked by the dying and their families may echo questions in our own minds. The carer may, therefore, also welcome an opportunity to explore these issues with someone else, whether that be a chaplain, local church minister, colleague, or group. The presence of some form of support network or group within a hospital or hospice may provide an opportunity for some of these concerns to be addressed. However, defensiveness may dictate that these are the very topics which are not explored since each member may feel a great pressure to be seen to be coping at all times and therefore such issues would be seen as inappropriate.[32]

The chaplain's role

The appointment and presence within a hospice or hospital of a chaplain is an indication that the institution recognizes that the patients they care for (and perhaps also the staff) have needs other than the purely physical, emotional, and psychological. If the need to search for existential meaning in the face of illness or death is understood by the organization then the chaplain may become an integral part of the life and work and not an odd appendage tacked on at the end. This has implications for methods of working which chaplain and institution need to sort out together. There will be as many styles of chaplaincy as there are chaplains but the core of this ministry would seem to be twofold:

Firstly, the ability of the pastor to try to understand the existential/spiritual meaning of all that is experienced by those involved within palliative care, in terms of the pastor's own relationship and understanding of God.

Secondly, the ability to explore and share that understanding with others through dialogue in order to discern the spiritual needs. Then, as and when appropriate, to offer a ministry of word and sacrament or pastoral counselling to patients, carers, and the organization as a whole. Above all there should be a willingness to 'be there' and to stay alongside those who are approaching death or grief in whatever capacity.

As more hospices and hospitals produce a 'Patient's Charter', which usually includes the spiritual needs in its terms, so consideration needs to be given as to how those needs will *best* be met. They can be met by an *ad hoc* arrangement reliant upon goodwill from local pastors, clergy, or interested staff members, and in a very small unit this might be very effective. But I would wish to argue that a chaplaincy/pastoral service needs to be properly budgeted for, consideration given to the inter-relationship of chaplain to other carers, and an official appointment made of the best person for the envisaged work—whether part-time or whole-time. The chaplain needs to have free access to all parts of the organization in order to develop appropriate links and networks so that support and good communication may occur. There has to develop a relationship of trust and credibility so that information about patients can be easily shared with or by the chaplain and confidentiality maintained. Facilities for worship also need to be budgeted for, whether in the form of a 'quiet room' or a chapel suitably furnished. An office needs to be provided, both as a base and also as a place where private interviews and counselling can take place. Opportunity also needs to be provided for appropriate study leave and a spiritual retreat so that the chaplain can continue to be a relevant resource to the institution.

In a paper entitled 'Where is the pastoral counsellor in the hospice movement?',[33] Gates reports on a survey conducted in 1987 of 153 hospice programmes in America which showed that pastoral counsellors needed to demonstrate their competence and contribution to the work of the hospice and that the American Association of Pastoral Counselors needed to foster and nurture pastors to equip them to participate in hospice programmes. In the United Kingdom the Association of Hospice Chaplains and the College of Health Care Chaplains seek to fulfil a similar supportive and educational role towards those entering such ministries, and to the establishment of professional standards. There would, therefore, seem to be a real need for pastors not to be shy or apologetic for entering the field of palliative care since the evidence to date (sparse though it may be) does still indicate the great importance of spiritual issues to patients, families, and staff involved with terminal illness. There is a recognition of the pastor/pastoral counsellor as a valuable resource to those trying to make sense of the experience of illness, and as a specialized professional person who is capable of being caring and competent in the face of grief and death.

Because of the inter-related nature of caring, the other staff can greatly facilitate the work of the chaplain and support the person in post. For example nurses spend a great deal more time with the patient than most other staff. They are, therefore, in a very good position to be able to identify when patients are showing signs of spiritual need. They may be able to meet some of these needs themselves, but they can also effect a referral to the chaplain and make the chaplain's visit much easier by the way they introduce him or her. It takes time to get around a unit on a one-to-one basis and so this sort of referral ensures that the chaplain does not miss those with an identified need.

A recent American study of the value of hospital chaplains showed that patients in hospital placed a high value on pastoral services and chaplaincy visits. They were more highly valued than social workers or patient's advocates. The families of patients also highly valued chaplaincy time, especially for those patients who were acutely ill, had frequent re-admissions, or were the subject of ethical debate about treatment decisions. Four spiritual needs were identified in relation to patient satisfaction: the patient's need for support and counselling; the family's need for support and counselling; the need for prayer; the need for sacraments. In respect of these needs it emerged that they were most effectively met in respect of Catholic patients. Overall, the study shows that chaplains were especially valued for their ability to provide support and counselling—'While providing prayer and sacraments are important aspects of the pastoral role, it is the chaplain's performance as a skilled professional which more clearly determines the patient's preference for a hospital'.[34] In addition, frequent visits were related to patient satisfaction and to a friendly image of the hospital, implying that effective chaplaincy can be an important factor in the total impression gained of the hospital by patient and family.

Referrals from, and co-operation with, medical staff is also crucial to effectively taking up the chaplaincy role. Doctors who are imparting 'bad news' might appreciate having a chaplain to accompany them, or to be available to see the patient afterwards. However, if the patient is not to react to the stereotype of 'clergy = funeral = death' the doctor needs a working relationship with the chaplain so that the introduction can be positive and clear regarding both the person and the task that might be addressed. In a recent and interesting British study of the attitudes of a group of general practitioners (family doctors) to involving clergy in patient care, Ward Jones shows that knowing the 'right' clergyman was important across each of the referral groups. (30.6 per cent thought referrals were more possible if the 'right' clergyperson was available) In this context 'right' seemed to relate more to a personal relationship than to any judgement about professional competence. Ward Jones states that the phrase 'Would like to meet local clergy' sums up a number of comments and indicates a need for a practical means of identifying clergy with whom doctors could work co-operatively'.[35]

If a chaplain is working long-term with a patient and family there needs to be some way of being regularly updated so that the chaplain is aware of any major decision or change regarding treatment, prognosis, or death. It can be very painful for a chaplain who has been working for some time with a patient and family to come back into a unit and find that the patient has died and no one has thought to inform him or her. Staff need to recognize that, while 'the Lord may provide' the chaplaincy, on a personal level, also needs support!

Wherever clergy seek to exercise a ministry in the field of palliative care they are going to meet up with a variety of charismatic figures who may be perceived as powerful people with a tendency to overshadow or compete with the person who is trying to take up and develop the role of chaplain. If the foundation of that hospice institution is a religious one then it can create even more tensions for the pastor as he or she seeks to work out what is their role alongside not only expert deliverers of palliative care, but also expert Christians! If the chaplain/pastor is appointed on a part-time basis then he or she may usually be in a situation where their role and authority are clearer when they occupy a focal position in the life of the worshipping community. When entering the hospital or hospice the pastor can initially feel stripped of that role, authority, and identity. This can be a great point of meeting with the patient, who may also feel quite vulnerable, but it can also have a 'de-skilling' effect on the pastor making it difficult to offer him or herself as the professional resource they are capable of being to patient, carer, or institution. Therefore, if the right sort of relationship is to develop, the chaplain must become involved in the non-patient aspects of the hospital/hospice or home care team. It is a great help if those already familiar with the environment, treatments, and procedures can 'induct' the pastor and create openings (both formal and informal) into the staff group. This may range from joining the staff for coffee in the office or canteen to attending case discussions, seminars, or staff support meetings.

Clearly, co-operative ways of working together take time to develop but there needs to be a commitment on the part of the institution and chaplain to nurture such links, in the best interests of the patients they care for. There is a great difference between multidisciplinary and interdisciplinary working. The chaplain needs to convey to the organization the special expertise and representative role that he or she has to bring to the interdisciplinary life of the unit, where each member is valued both personally and for the professional contribution they bring to the life of the whole. There is a risk that a chaplain can become a marginal member of a hospice or hospital, become the recipient of many negative projections, and as a result become a scapegoat. An effective staff support scheme in a palliative care programme, in which the chaplain is included, can be an important way of addressing this dynamic and of helping the chaplain to become known and integrated into the life of the unit.

The recognition that carers can have parallel needs to those of the people they care for is a vital part of enabling carers to feel that they are valued as people. It can be extremely difficult for carers to remain sensitive to the personal and spiritual needs of those in their care if they (including the chaplain) do not feel that their personal as well as professional needs are recognized. Sullivan wrote that 'One can respect others only to the extent that one respects oneself'.[36] Perhaps one can add 'and feels oneself to be valued by other significant people in one's own life'.

References

1. *Concise Oxford Dictionary.* 7th edn. Oxford: Oxford University Press, 1982
2. O'Brien ME. The need for spiritual integrity. In: Yura H, Walsh M, eds. *Human Needs (2) and the Nursing Process.* USA: Appleton-Century-Crofts, 1982.
3. Speck PW. *Being There—Pastoral Care in Times of Illness.* London: SPCK, 1988.
4. Piles CL. Providing spiritual care. *Nurse Education*, 1990; **15**: 36–41.
5. Reed PG. Religiousness among terminally ill and healthy adults. *Research in Nursing and Health*, 1986; **9**: 35–41.
6. King MB, Hunt RA. Measuring the religious variable: national replication. *Journal for the Scientific Study of Religion*, 1975; **14**: 13–22.
7. Campbell A, Converse PE, Rodgers WL. *The Quality of American Life: Perceptions, Evaluations and Satisfactions.* New York: Russell Sage Foundation, 1976.
8. King M, Speck P, Thomas A. Spiritual and religious beliefs in acute illness—is this a feasible area for study? *Social Science and Medicine*, 1994; **38**: 631–6.
9. Reed PG. Spirituality and well-being in terminally ill hospitalized adults. *Research in Nursing and Health*, 1987; **10**: 335–44.
10. Jarvis GK, Northcott HC. Religion and differences in morbidity and mortality. *Social Science and Medicine*, 1987; **25**: 813–24.
11. Allport GW, Ross JM. Personal religious orientation and prejudice. *Journal of Personality and Social Psychology*, 1967; **5**: 432–43.
12. Watson PJ, Morris RJ, Hood RW. Sin and self functioning part 2: Grace, guilt and psychological adjustment. *Journal of Psychology and Theology*, 1988; **16**: 270–81.
13. Kirkpatrick LA, Hood RW. Intrinsic-extrinsic religious orientation: The boon or bane of contemporary psychology or religion? *Journal for the Scientific Study of Religion.* 1990; **29**: 442–62.
14. Gorsuch RL, McPherson SE. Intrinsic/extrinsic measurement: I/E-revised and single item scales. *Journal for the Scientific Study of Religion*, 1989; **28**: 348–54.
15. Levin JS, Vanderpool HY. Is frequent religious attendance really conducive to better health?: Toward an epidemiology of religion. *Social Science and Medicine*, 1987; **24**: 589–600.
16. Hay MW. Principles in building spiritual assessment tools. *American Journal of Hospice Care*, 1989; **6**: 25–31.

17. Paloutzian RF, Ellison CW. Loneliness, spiritual well-being and quality of life. In: Peplau LA, Perlman D. eds. *Loneliness: A Source-book of Current Theory, Research, and Therapy.* New York: John Wiley and Sons, 1982.
18. Kirschling JM, Pittman JF. Measurement of spiritual well-being in a hospice caregiver sample. *Hospice Journal*, 1989; **5**: 1–11.
19. Kaczorowski JM. Spiritual well-being and anxiety in adults diagnosed with cancer. *Hospice Journal*, 1989; **5**: 105–16.
20. Clark R. Forgiveness in the hospice setting. *Palliative Medicine*, 1990; **4**: 305–10.
21. Murdoch I. *Bruno's Dream.* Harmondsworth: Penguin, 1970: p.238.
22. Frankl VE. *Man's Search for Meaning.* London: Hodder and Stoughton, 1987.
23. Jones K, Johnston M, Speck PW. Despair felt by the patient and the professional carer: a case study of the use of cognitive behavioural methods. *Palliative Medicine*, 1989; **3**: 39–46.
24. Hoy T. Hospice chaplaincy in the caregiving team. In: Corr CA, Corr DM, eds. *Hospice Care: Principles and Practice.* London: Faber and Faber, 1983.
25. Clebsch WA, Jaekle CR. *Pastoral Care in Historical Context.* New York: Harper, 1967.
26. Speck PW, Ainsworth-Smith I. *Letting Go: Caring for the Dying and the Bereaved.* London: SPCK, 1982.
27. Speck PW, Ainsworth-Smith I. *Letting Go: Caring for the Dying and the Bereaved.* London: SPCK, 1982: Chapter 5.
28. Flatt B. Some stages of grief. *Journal of Religion and Health,* 1987; **26**: 143–8.
29. Bowling A, Cartwright A. *Life after a Death—A Study of the Elderly Widowed.* London: Tavistock, 1982.
30. Bowling A, Cartwright A. *Life after a Death—A Study of the Elderly Widowed.* London: Tavistock, 1982: 156–7.
31. Parkes CM, Weiss RS. *Recovery from Bereavement.* New York: Basic Books, 1983.
32. Speck PW. *Being There—Pastoral Care in Times of Illness.* London: SPCK, 1988: Chapter 10.
33. Gates GN. Where is the pastoral counsellor in the hospice movement? *Journal of Pastoral Care,* 1987; **41**: 32–8.
34. Gibbons JL, Thomas J, VandeCreek L, Jessen AK. The value of hospital chaplains: patient perspectives. *Journal of Pastoral Care,* 1991; 45: 117–25.
35. Ward Jones A. A survey of general practitioners' attitudes to the involvement of clergy in patient care. *British Journal of General Practice,* 1990; **40**: 280–3.
36. Sullivan HS. *The Interpersonal Theory of Psychiatry.* London: Tavistock, 1955.

12

Rehabilitation in palliative care

12.1 Introduction

Derek Doyle

Rehabilitation is not the first word that comes to mind when speaking of palliative care. No-one would dispute the centrality of symptom relief or the importance of psychological and pastoral care, and all would agree that good palliative care is holistic in nature, but rehabilitation sounds like a contradiction in terms. In this section we shall seek to demonstrate that rehabilitation is actually a central key feature of all palliative care wherever it is practised, whatever the patient's underlying pathology.[1]

Once again we are reminded of the definitions of palliative care discussed in Section 1. They each speak of the incurable fatal nature of the illness, the predictably short prognosis, and that the focus of palliative care is the quality of life. The restoration and nurture of that quality of life is true rehabilitation. It is a reminder that palliative care is not about prolongation of life any more than it is about the abbreviation of life. It is exclusively concerned with maintaining as good a quality of life as possible, given the complex disabling problems that each patient faces.

As Kearney[2] has warned us, palliative care is not merely an exercise in pain and symptom control, with its practitioners being, in effect, 'symptomatologists'. Such symptom control is relatively simple, but what does it mean for someone to be free from pain only to remain bedbound or bored? What quality of life is there if every physical distress is relieved but the person regains no independence or continues to suffer embarrassment from an ostomy, dysphasia, ataxia, or social isolation. Rehabilitation has been described as 'making a patient into a person again', someone who feels not only wanted and respected but once again useful and creative. This is the heart of palliative care.

Perhaps in recent years too much attention has been focused on pain and symptom control, with the assumption being that freedom from pain in someone with a mortal illness inevitably leads to contentment. Anyone experienced in this field of care knows that an even more challenging problem is that of boredom. No longer spending every minute coping with pain, the patient wants not diversional therapy but a return to some semblance of usefulness and less dependence on others, once again able to function as a person. One of the most distressful aspects of terminal illness is no longer having one's opinion sought, no longer feeling needed and valued. Rehabilitation seeks to address this basic human need.

Quality of life, however it is defined or measured, always involves a sense of dignity, which is not an easy thing to define but is acknowledged as important by everyone with a mortal illness. For one person it might mean something as simple as being able to wear daywear rather than nightwear, for another being able to use a lavatory rather than a commode, and for most the ability to return to simple daily activities once taken for granted. For some, dignity will mean being addressed with respect, for another being able to change his own colostomy; the painter able to return to the easel, the writer back at the word-processor, the musician once again making music, each feeling useful, needed, and creative, as nearly whole people as their illness and frailty will permit. This is also rehabilitation—never easy, often challenging, always rewarding.

Palliative care always calls for teamwork, with no one discipline possessing all the skills and insights, and each subtly dependent on others. The rehabilitation component of palliative care also necessitates teamwork, and every team must learn about goals.[3–6] Such goals are not usually self-evident but require skilled definition, regular reviewing, and wholehearted acceptance by each member of the palliative care team. They may initially be very modest, for example relief of pain and gradual mobilization. As one goal is achieved, so the team members each work together to define new attainable goals, realistically tailored to the patient's changing abilities and expectations. Setting the sights too high can bring disappointment if they are unattainable; setting them too low can appear condescending and patronizing. Throughout this complex collaborative process, different specialists must confer regularly, learning from each other and deferring to each other, with the key worker today becoming less important tomorrow. This is never easy. The physician may start by helping to ease pain but soon the key worker may be the physiotherapist or occupational therapist, whilst only a day or two later all stand back as the stoma therapist or music therapist takes the lead. Sharing in every decision, every redefinition of goals, is each member of the team and the patient himself. This is rehabilitation as described in the section which follows.

Underpinning this whole dynamic process is hope, which is immensely important but as difficult to define as dignity or quality of life.[7]

To those inexperienced in palliative care, hope may appear as strange a concept as rehabilitation itself. How can one speak of hope when caring for someone whose days are numbered, their dreams shattered, and their body malfunctioning as a result of an advanced mortal illness? However, experience suggests that, for these people, hope is not related to cure or long-term remission. Rather, it describes a quality of personhood—of being loved, accepted, and valued despite, not because of, all that is happening.

Hope changes day by day, is a personal thing unique to each patient, is usually difficult to articulate, but is always worth speaking about. The professional carers who can work together, set and regularly define goals, and always know what today's hopes are for their patient—they are a true rehabilitation team.

Like so many things in palliative care, the principles of rehabilitation described here are equally relevant to all types of care, whatever the illness and whatever the life expectancy of patients. That is one reason why so many are described in this chapter, which brings together the principles of physiotherapy, occupational therapy, music therapy, ostomy care, and the myriad possibilities of creative art and writing. Blended together and taken with all the other principles in this textbook, they remind us that palliative care, ostensibly dedicated to the care of the dying, is more accurately described as a reaffirmation of living with dignity and hope.

References

1. Twycross, RG. Rehabilitation in terminal cancer patients. *International Rehabilitation Medicine*, 1981; 3:135–44.
2. Kearney M. Palliative medicine—just another speciality? *Palliative Medicine*, 1992; 6:39–46.
3. Hillier ER, Lunt BJ. Goal setting in terminal cancer. In: Twycross RG, Ventafridda, V, eds. *The Continuing Care of Terminal Cancer Patients*. Oxford: Pergamon, 1980.
4. Lunt BJ, Neale C. A comparison of hospice and hospital: care goals set by staff. *Palliative Medicine*, 1987; 1:136–48.
5. Lunt BJ, Jenkins J. Goal setting in terminal care: a method of recording treatment aims and priorities. *Journal of Advanced Nursing*, 1983; 8:495–505.
6. Lunt BJ. Terminal care: goal-setting—hospice philosophy in practice. In: Karas E, ed. *Current Issues in Clinical Psychology*, Vol.3. New York: Plenum, 1986.
7. Hockley J. Rehabilitation in palliative care—are we asking the impossible? *Palliative Medicine*, 1993; 7(Supplement 1):9–15.

12.2 Physiotherapy

Colette L. Fulton and Rhona Else

Introduction

Physiotherapy in palliative care is a relatively new development, coinciding with the development of the hospice palliative care movement. This chapter will explore the role of the physiotherapist within the context of rehabilitation in palliative care. The process of physiotherapy and the therapeutic techniques adopted in palliative care are described, with an overview of common functional impairments. The key theme of this chapter is that the physiotherapist is required to demonstrate a high level of problem solving, clinical skills, and communication ability in order to be a valuable member of the multidisciplinary team that is aiming to optimize the patient's quality of life.

The implementation of rehabilitation strategies in the palliative care setting can appear, at first glance, as paradoxical as many people believe that rehabilitation is most appropriate with patients who will make a full recovery. It will become clear, as is said in the Introduction, that rehabilitation in palliative care is highly appropriate given the ethos of palliative care as life affirming.

Rehabilitation in palliative care: definition and general strategies

Rehabilitation has been defined as 'the dynamic process directed towards the goal of enabling persons to function at their maximum level within the limit of their disease or disability in terms of their physical, mental, emotional, social, and economic potential'.[1] The key points of this quotation is that rehabilitation enables the person to function at their maximum level and that rehabilitation is appropriate throughout all the phases of the disease process; initial diagnosis, primary treatment, secondary recurrence, and palliation. Rehabilitation of the patient in the palliative phase of their disease involves the combined expertise of members of the multidisciplinary team and does not focus solely on the physical consequences of the disease. Habeck and colleagues[2] offered seven principles of rehabilitation:

1. Comprehensive care is provided to address the needs of the whole person; each person's life possesses a unique blend of psychological, social, vocational, economic, and physical factors.
2. A team approach is used to achieve co-ordinated interdisciplinary care.
3. Goals for rehabilitation are derived from the effects of medical problems in accordance with prognostic expectations.
4. Education is a major component of the rehabilitation process.
5. Intervention occurs as soon as the likelihood of disability is anticipated.
6. The unit of care includes both the patient and the family.
7. Rehabilitation needs must be reassessed on a continuing basis and met throughout all phases of care.

Most authors advocate a goal-oriented method of rehabilitation. Dietz[3] outlined the goals of rehabilitation during the various phases of the disease process. These rehabilitation goals are: preventative (when disability can be anticipated); restorative (when the patient can be expected to return to premorbid status without significant handicap); supportive (when the patient has ongoing, controlled disease but appropriate rehabilitation strategies can prevent complications which might occur); and palliative (when the patient has progressive disease and appropriate rehabilitation can minimize the effects of complications). These goals must be 'appropriate and obtainable, towards which treatment is directed', and the 'goal for each patient is determined by an aggregate of factors relevant to the individual'—age, type and stage of disease, other concomitant disease, inherent physical ability, social background, basic education, and job or work experience.[4]

The role of physiotherapy during the palliative care phase of the disease process

Palliative care occurs not only in the hospice or palliative care unit but more often in the general hospital and the home. In each of these work settings, the physiotherapist is involved in the rehabilitation of patients in the palliative stage of their disease. Physiotherapy of patients in the palliative phase of their disease adopts a rehabilitative model of practice in terms of the physical domain of function.[5] Physiotherapy aims to optimize the patient's level of physical function and takes into consideration the interplay between the physical, psychological, social, and vocational domains of function. In the palliative care setting, the physiotherapist is involved in the treatment of patients with active and progressive disease from the time its advancing nature is recognized until, and

Table 1 Stages in the process of physiotherapy in palliative care and the skills required

Stages in physiotherapy treatment	Skills required
Patient's needs identified through assessment (subjective and objective)	Communication and assessment skills
Identification of the patient's needs	Communication and problem-solving skills
Treatment plan developed with the patient	Communication and problem-solving skills
Implementation of treatment plan	Clinical skills
Evaluation of treatment plan	Communication, problem-solving, and clinical skills

including, the final phase of carcinoma, chronic respiratory, neurological, cardiac, rheumatological, and endocrine diseases.[6] The physiotherapist understands the patient's underlying pathological condition but this is not the focus of treatment. The focus of physiotherapy intervention is, instead, the physical and functional sequelae of the disease and/ or its treatment on the patient. An additional and important role of physiotherapy is to enable patients to gain control over their situation. Often patients in the palliative phase of their disease have a feeling of hopelessness and helplessness as a result of many months or years of treatment, in which they have invested much hope and faith. Patients do not feel in control of their destiny. General rehabilitation strategies and physiotherapy can, however, attempt to redress the balance by enabling patients to take an active role in the decision making process of setting rehabilitation goals and also to enable them to see how their own behaviour and functional routines can ameliorate troublesome side-effects and symptoms.

Physiotherapy treatment of patients in the palliative phase of their disease utilizes a problem-solving approach where the patient's needs are identified, a treatment plan is developed in negotiation with the patient and their carer, the treatment plan is implemented, and then evaluated. From Table 1 it is clear that communication and problem-solving skills are just as essential as clinical skills.

Physiotherapeutic approach to patient assessment and goal setting

Thorough and systematic assessment is the linchpin for the physiotherapist working in palliative care, given the possible range of symptoms and problems a patient in the palliative phase of their disease may have. It is important to note that the assessment may be carried out over several days as the patient may have a low exercise tolerance or may be generally weak and debilitated. Modification of assessment style and technique may, therefore, be necessary. A widely adopted system of patient management and assessment is based on the problem-oriented medical system (POMS) first proposed by Weed.[7] Problem-oriented medical records enable detailed assessment and planning of treatment and is compatible with the problem solving process involved in patient care.

Problem-oriented medical records are divided into five sections:

1. The database details information concerning the subjective and objective examination carried out by the physiotherapist to determine the patient's needs and level of function. The aim of subjective examination is to determine the patient's symptoms, their distribution, and their behaviour. The history of the present complaint, the social history, and the previous medical history are included in the subjective examination. The aim of the objective examination is to measure accurately the patient's level of function through observation, palpation, measurement, and testing.

2. The problem list is a concise list of the patient's rehabilitation problems. These problems relate to all the domains of rehabilitation and are not necessarily listed in order of priority.

3. The initial physiotherapy treatment plan and goals are based on the patient's rehabilitation needs identified from the subjective and objective assessment. The time scale for long- and short-term goals may vary between patients depending on their prognosis. It is important, however, that irrespective of life expectancy, there is a longer-term view of realistic rehabilitation goals in order to give incentive and purpose. The physiotherapist needs to identify the therapeutic approaches which meet the goals of rehabilitation most appropriately. The goals of treatment are planned jointly by the patient and the physiotherapist, who then informs the multidisciplinary team to ensure a co-ordinated approach.

4. Progress notes document systematically the patient's functional status and progress. These notes can be documented in the SOAP format (subjective, objective, analysis, and plan) in relation to each problem. The treatment plan is frequently evaluated and reassessed to monitor the effectiveness or appropriateness of the physiotherapy treatment and modified whenever indicated. The physiotherapist should identify goals of treatment which have been met, or those which need modification, and identify new goals according to changes in physical, psychological, disease, or social status.

5. A discharge summary is written when the patient completes treatment or is transferred to another service provider. The discharge summary may document current status and any remaining problems, home exercise programmes, and previous treatment undertaken.

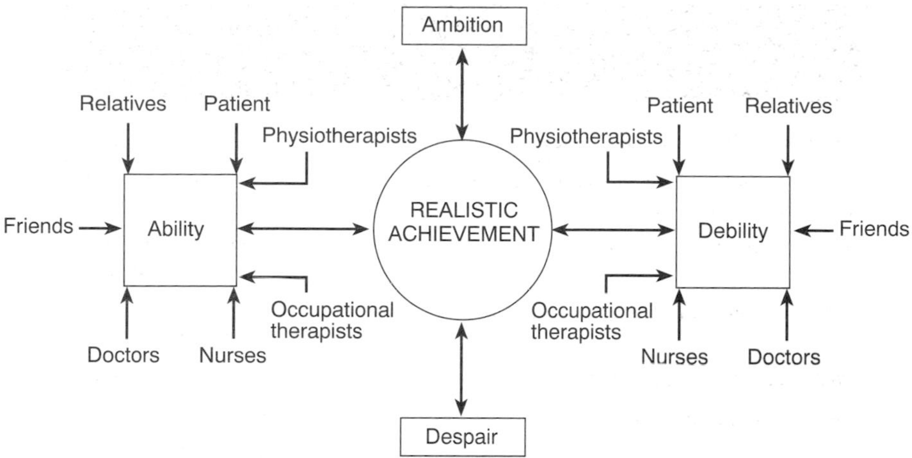

Fig. 1 Factors influencing patients' achievement.

Factors influencing patients' achievement in response to physiotherapy

One of the difficulties facing the physiotherapist treating patients receiving palliative care is that the patient can either be over ambitious as to what physiotherapy can offer or feel it is not worthwhile having any physiotherapy at all. When the patient is over ambitious they may think the harder they exercise, the fitter they will become, overcoming the disease and returning to their previous fitness level and lifestyle. Physiotherapy can be seen as a passport to 'getting better' and patients accept every treatment possible believing they will be fully rehabilitated. When the patient is in despair and has no hope of being restored to their former health they 'turn their face to the wall'. These patients do not want to accept any physiotherapy as they feel it is not worthwhile if they cannot be guaranteed full fitness.

The reality of the situation is that each patient has to balance what they are able to do ('ability') and what they can not do ('debility'). This is an ever changing equation which will vary as the disease progresses and it can alter from day to day (Fig. 1).

All the people surrounding the patient can influence how the patient shifts from his original attitude of despair or over ambition to realistic achievement. The ability of the patient is supported by the relatives, friends, doctors, nurses, occupational therapists, and physiotherapists. Ability can be nurtured by setting realistic goals and focusing on what is achievable. Reassurance of the importance of the patient being in control gives self-confidence in their ability. Debility can also be encouraged by these same people, for example if they do too much for the patient and do not plan a co-ordinated strategy of care.

General principles of physiotherapy treatment/ intervention in the palliative care setting

1. 'Little and often principle': the patient's stamina may be reduced and therefore physiotherapy intervention should be given on a regular basis for short periods of time.

2. Consideration of multipathology and effects of treatment: the assessment of the patient by the physiotherapist should identify the presence of metastatic deposits and other pathologies such as osteoarthritis, chronic obstructive pulmonary disease, etc. The goals of treatment should, therefore, address the functional sequelae of all pathologies.

3. Modification of general principles: in the palliative care setting, the physiotherapist often modifies techniques. For example the patient who has cerebral metastases may present with the signs and symptoms of a cerebral vascular accident. The techniques and principles of treatment adopted in the care of the patient following a cerebral vascular accident may be modified so as to optimize independence and function. Similarly, with the patient in the palliative care phase of chronic obstructive pulmonary disease or lung cancer, the physiotherapist may wish to modify chest physiotherapy techniques.

Physiotherapeutic techniques in the palliative care setting

Therapeutic exercise

Therapeutic exercise is often adopted with patients in the palliative care phase of their disease. Therapeutic exercise prevents dysfunction and develops, improves, restores, or maintains the following:[8]

(1) strength

(2) endurance and cardiovascular fitness

(3) mobility and flexibility

(4) co-ordination and skill

(5) relaxation.

Common therapeutic exercise techniques adopted by physiotherapists in the palliative care setting are as follows.

Passive movements

In passive movements, a joint is moved through its range with no voluntary contraction of muscles surrounding that joint. Movement is achieved through the application of an external force by the physiotherapist, the patient (autoassisted), or a continuous passive

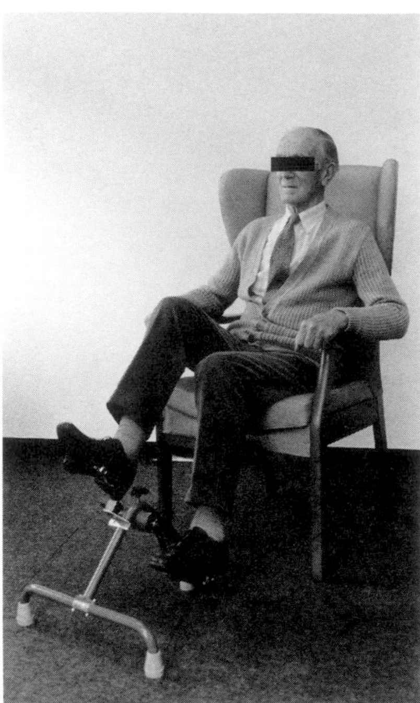

Fig. 2 Patient using a static bicycle.

movement machine. The rationale for passive movements is that they maintain and increase the joint range of movement, prevent contractures,[9] facilitate proprioceptive feedback,[10] and maintain and increase circulation.[11] Care needs to be taken to avoid overstretching the joint and damage to soft tissues. The joint should only be passively mobilized within the range that pain and spasm permit.

Active assisted exercises

The aim of active assisted exercises is to augment, but not substitute, active muscle forces. This is particularly useful in the palliative care setting, where patients may have muscle weakness but can actively contract the muscle. Assistance to movement can be provided by the physiotherapist, the patient, or equipment such as a pulley. Passive and active assisted movements are particularly appropriate for patients with motor neurone disease.

Active exercise

Active exercise is where the patient carries out a movement under their own voluntary control. The benefits of active and active assisted exercises are similar to those of passive movements with the added advantage of active muscular contraction, thereby maintaining elasticity and contractility of muscles, and bone integrity. In the palliative care setting, active exercises are usually performed as free exercises. Younger and relatively able patients may use equipment such as a static bicycle (Fig. 2) and light weight resistance, the emphasis being on number of repetitions rather than the force applied. Friction free boards are often used in the palliative care setting to aid, maintain, and improve mobility and muscle power in the lower limb.

Gait re-education

Normal gait results from a complicated process involving the brain, spinal cord, peripheral nerves, muscles, bones, and joints. The normal gait pattern will be affected by disease in any of these systems. Physiotherapists are, therefore, often involved in the re-education of gait. In order that a person can walk unaided, the locomotor system must be able to:[12]

(1) support the body weight without collapsing on either leg;

(2) balance on the supporting leg;

(3) swing each leg through to the advanced position in order to take over the supporting role;

(4) provide sufficient power to make the necessary limb and trunk movements.

The main aims of gait re-education training in the palliative care setting are:

(1) to enable the patient to remain independent;

(2) to prevent injury or discomfort through abnormal gait patterns;

(3) to minimize muscular effort required to walk thereby conserving energy.

As a result of these modified aims, the use of walking aids is common (Fig. 3(a) and (b)) Walking aids can be classified into three basic types; walking sticks (canes), crutches, and walking frames. All three forms operate by supporting part of the body weight through the arm rather than the leg. In addition, a walking aid may be advised when the patient can walk without support but requires an aid for a different purpose. For example patients with dyspnoea may use a walking frame to enable them to stabilize their shoulder girdle to alleviate dyspnoea, and patients with metastatic bone disease may use a stick to reduce the weight placed through the affected leg.

Hydrotherapy

Water has physical properties which have a direct bearing on pain relief—buoyancy, hydrostatic pressure, turbulence, and temperature.[13] Relaxation techniques, passive and active assisted movements, and breathing exercises can all be carried out in the pool. Patients who have metastatic bone disease resulting in chronic pain can gain confidence from painfree mobility with hydrotherapy and their rehabilitation can be facilitated.

Respiratory physiotherapy techniques

In the palliative care setting, the physiotherapist is often involved in the care of the patient who is breathless and has excess secretions. The skills of the physiotherapist as an assessor, problem solver, and communicator can be severely put to the test. Hough stated that:

> Chest physiotherapy is not the tip, tap, and cough sequence that commonly passes as its definition. It incorporates education, pain management, controlled activity, use of mechanical aids, and listening to patients in distress. It is ineffective to intervene with a process as personal as breathing without attention to the person as a whole.[14]

Breathing control and the forced expiration technique

Breathing control is a term used to describe normal tidal breathing using the lower chest with relaxation of the upper chest and shoulders.[15] When a patient is being taught breathing control, the patient should be sitting up comfortably and be well supported with pillows to encourage relaxation of the shoulder girdle and upper chest. The physiotherapist or the patient places a hand on

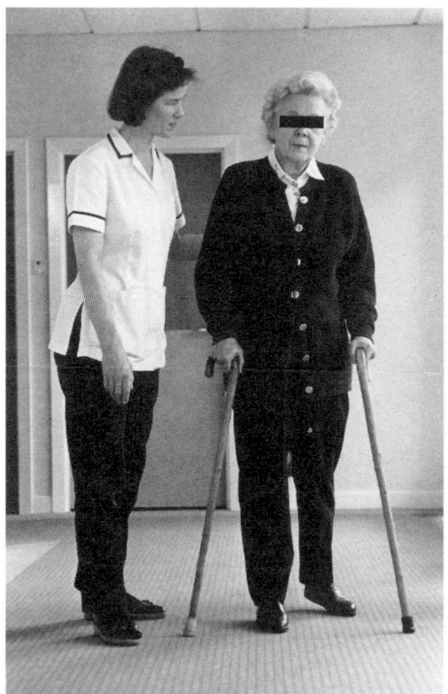

(a)

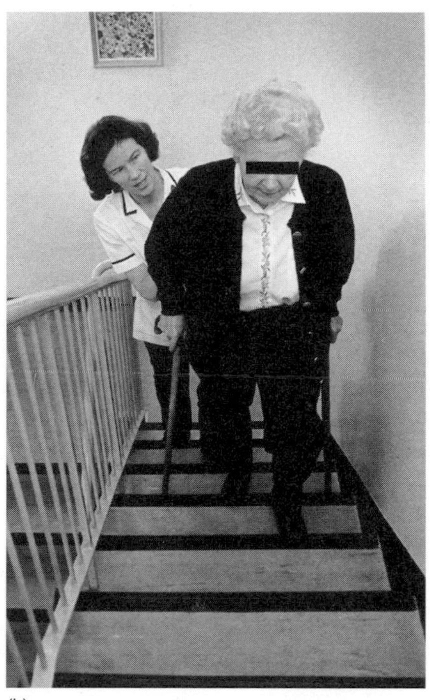

(b)

Fig. 3 (a) and (b) Re-education of patient's gait.

the upper abdomen to monitor movement of the abdomen. When the patient breathes in, the abdomen should be felt to move outwards and upwards. When the patient breathes out, the abdomen should be felt to move downwards and inwards (Figs 4, 5 (a) and (b)). Inspiration is the active movement, whereas expiration should be relaxed. Some patients in the palliative care phase of their disease who are breathless may use pursed lip breathing to maintain a small positive pressure during expiration, which may prevent collapse of small airways. The major disadvantage of pursed lip breathing is that is increases the work of breathing.

Patients who have excess secretions may benefit from the forced expiration technique (also known as 'huffing'). The forced expiration technique forms a crucial part of the active cycle of breathing technique.[16] The active cycle of breathing technique is a combination of one or two forced expirations, thoracic expansion exercises interspersed with periods of breathing control.[17] Patients take a half breath in and then force the air out. This manoeuvre mobilizes secretions from distal airways (Fig. 6). Care needs to be taken to ensure that the patient does not become exhausted by checking that they intersperse forced expiration with breathing control in a relaxed position.

Positioning

The physiotherapist can play a role in instructing the patient in methods to decrease the work of breathing. Positioning of the breathless patient can prevent recourse to more dramatic measures and whatever the physiotherapy treatment (for example administration of a nebulizer), consideration of the patient's position is vital. Jenkins and colleagues[18] demonstrated that the functional residual capacity is correlated with the patient's position; it is highest in standing and upright sitting and lowest in supine lying and slumped sitting. Patients can be instructed in positions which may

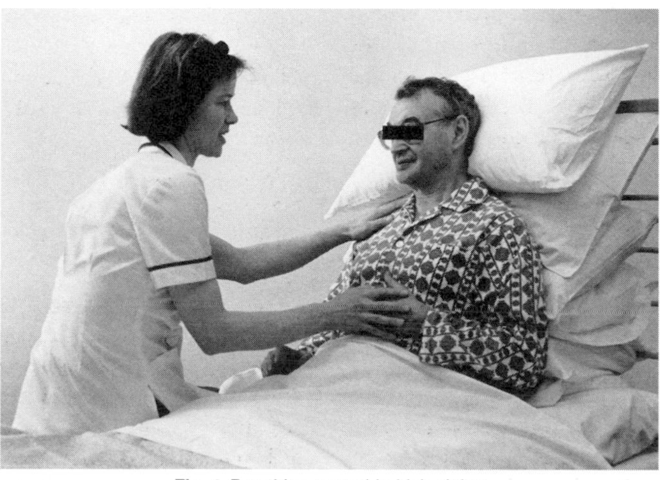

Fig. 4 Breathing control in high sitting.

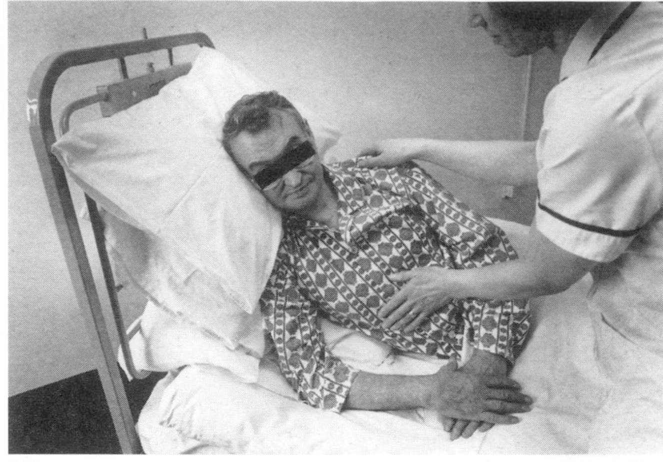

(a)

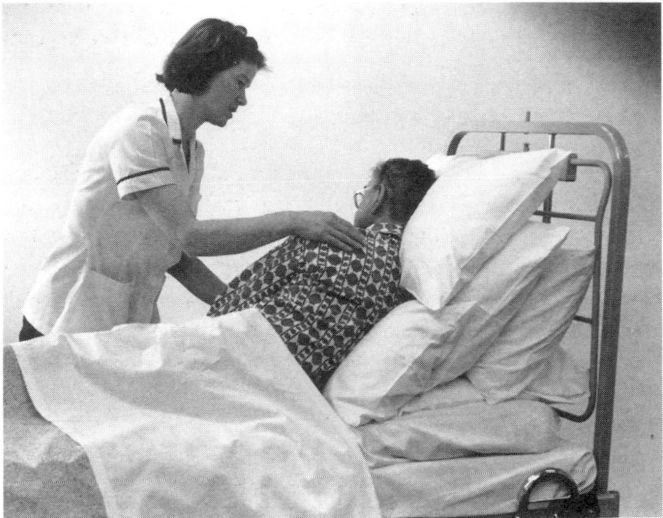

(b)

Fig. 5 (a) and (b) Breathing control in high side lying.

help alleviate breathlessness (Figs 7 and 8). These positions can be adopted if the patient is receiving nebulized salbutamol, etc.

Exercise

The most effective way of increasing lung volume is general mobility, for example walking,[19] as the patient is in the upright position and natural deep breathing is encouraged. General mobility should be controlled so as to increase the rate of breathing slightly, and the patient should have a period of rest by leaning against the wall to get their breath back (Fig. 8). Those patients who are unable to walk can undertake bed mobility exercises or transfer from their bed to a chair. Patients should be educated about the beneficial effects of controlled mobility and encouraged to plan a programme of activity for themselves.

Postural drainage

Postural drainage is the use of gravity to assist the clearance and promote drainage of bronchial secretions and it can be used when the patient has a defective clearance mechanism and has excess secretions. This technique is often used in tandem with the forced expiratory technique. Modification of postural drainage positions for the patient in the palliative phase of their disease is often adopted due to the distress caused by tipping the patient (for example alternate side lying is often used). In previous years, manual techniques such as percussion (also known as clapping) and vibrations were adopted in conjunction with postural drainage in patients of all ages with varied pathology. In recent years, however, the effectiveness of such manual techniques in respiratory physiotherapy has not been substantiated and their use is now redundant

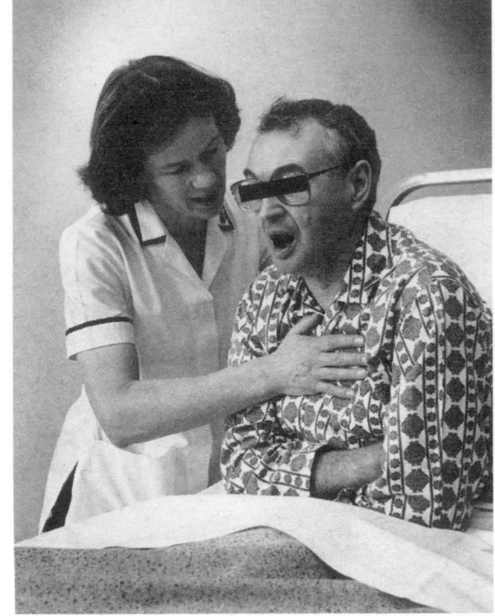

Fig. 6 The forced expiration technique.

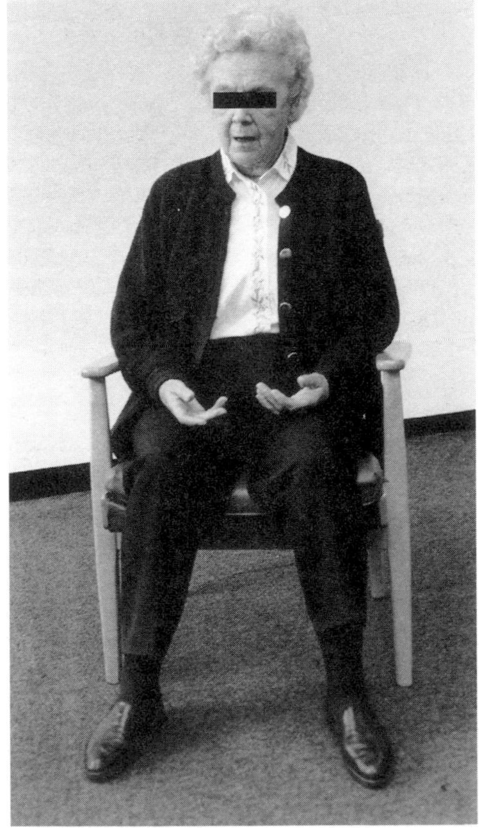

Fig. 7 Relaxed sitting in a chair to relieve breathlessness.

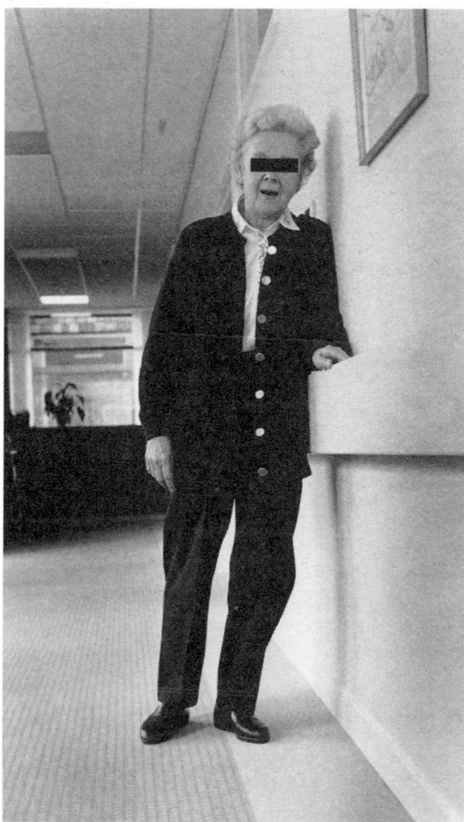

Fig. 8 Leaning against a wall to relieve breathlessness.

with adult patients,[20] especially in the palliative care setting (percussion is still used in younger patients with cystic fibrosis).

Nasopharyngeal suction

Nasopharyngeal suction is used rarely in the palliative care setting due to possible damage to the trachea and bronchus and the distress caused to patients. An exception to this, however, is with patients who have endstage motor neurone disease. The choice of catheter and technique can minimize the trauma to the tracheal epithelium. The catheter should have a terminal eye and two small cylindrical side holes which prevent adherence of the catheter to the airway walls.[21] The catheter size for an adult is commonly 12 or 14 French Gauge and for children sizes 4, 6, and 8 French Gauge. The suction pressure should be kept as low as possible (within the range 60–150 mmHg or 8–20 kPa) and varies with the viscosity of the mucus. Humidification may be given prior to treatment if the mucus is viscous, and oxygenation of the patient should precede and follow suction to avoid hypoxia.

Relaxation

In the last two decades, there has been an increased interest in relaxation procedures to relieve pain, muscle tension, and psychological distress. There are several types of relaxation techniques: progressive muscle relaxation; active inhibition techniques such as contract-relax; and guided imagery. Progressive muscle relaxation is the simplest and most popular relaxation technique. The patient is instructed to close their eyes and concentrate on relaxing one part of their body at a time. After initial instruction by the physiotherapist, patients can be given an audiotape recording which can be used by the patient on their own. The goal of relaxation is the attainment of a state of muscle relaxation that is as profound as possible.[22] The contract-relax technique is seldom used in the palliative care setting as it is believed that the repeated phases of muscular contraction can exacerbate pain.

Manual therapy

The laying on of hands is probably the oldest means of relieving pain and discomfort. Therapeutic massage may be used in the palliative care setting in the treatment of lymphoedema (manual lymphatic drainage techniques are discussed in Chapter 9.7), and the relief of pain and muscle spasm. The most commonly used techniques to relieve pain and muscle spasm are stroking (or effleurage) and gentle kneading. Deeper techniques, such as frictions and deep massage, are used rarely as they can exacerbate pain. Manual therapy techniques can complement relaxation and should be performed with the patient fully supported in a comfortable and warm position.

Electrotherapy modalities

Electrotherapy is defined as 'the treatment of patients by electrical means'.[23] There is a lack of research monitoring the objective risks and benefits of electrotherapy in the palliative care setting. To date, the majority of authors of electrotherapy textbooks warn against the use of therapeutic ultrasound, ice, interferential continuous shortwave diathermy, and pulsed shortwave diathermy over tumour sites and potential metastatic sites due to the possibility of encouraging neoplastic growth.[23,24,25] The contraindications of applying these modalities over neoplastic sites has not been formally substantiated. The use of such modalities, however, can be beneficial for patients in the palliative phase of their disease when they are applied over normal tissue. Pain and muscle spasm can be relieved by the application of heat, TENS (described in Chapter 9.2.8) interferential or pulsed shortwave diathermy.

Common functional impairments in palliative care: physiotherapy management and treatment

Functional and physiological impairments resulting from prolonged immobility

Patients in the palliative care phase of their disease may have spent many weeks in bed and, as a result, have a low level of functional status and mobility. The physiological and metabolic effects of prolonged bed rest have been well documented.[26,27]

1. Bone loss and hypercalcaemia may result from immobilization, or may lead to pathological fractures in those patients who have bone metastases or osteoporosis. Normal bone accretion and absorption are maintained by weightbearing and muscular contraction. Within 10 to 15 days of immobilization the rate of bone turnover changes and the mineral content of the bone decreases.[28]

2. Muscle atrophy and shortening occur as a result of immobilization.[29] The extent of muscle atrophy is dependent on factors such as fibre composition of the muscle, length of time

immobilized, and the position in which a joint has been immobilized. Slow twitch postural muscles, such as the soleus, have been found to atrophy more rapidly than fast contracting muscles. Muscles which have been in a shortened position adapt by losing sarcomeres in series so as to maintain the optimal overlap of actin and myosin. In contrast, those muscles which have been fixed in a lengthened position gain sarcomeres.

3. Joint contractures may result due to muscles shortening and connective tissue changes.[28]

4. Respiratory function changes occur as a result of immobility. Decreased respiratory movement due to increased intra-abdominal pressure prevents the normal descent of the diaphragm, thereby limiting inspiration. Prolonged immobility also causes stasis of bronchial secretions. The combined effects of a decrease in respiratory movement and stasis of bronchial secretions can result in deficient ventilation and, in turn, limited diffusion of oxygen and carbon dioxide.

5. Peripheral mononeuropathy occurs as a result of prolonged pressure on a peripheral nerve. In particular, pressure on the peroneal nerve as it runs over the head of the fibula results in the classic 'dropped foot'.

6. Circulatory changes due to immobility can lead to the development of deep venous thrombosis.

Many of these problems can be prevented and reduced by early intervention.

The aims of physiotherapy during prolonged bedrest are:

(1) to maintain optimum respiratory function;

(2) to maintain optimum circulatory function;

(3) to prevent muscle atrophy;

(4) to prevent muscle shortening;

(5) to prevent joint contractures;

(6) to optimize independence and function.

Physiotherapeutic approaches commonly used are:

(1) maintenance exercises (isometric exercises for quadriceps, glutei, ankle dorsi, and plantar flexion);

(2) bed mobility exercises;

(3) active exercises, active assisted exercises, passive movements;

(4) breathing control and forced expiratory technique;

(5) education and participation of the carer in treatment.

Dyspnoea

Hough[14] stated that 'physiotherapists themselves may feel helpless when faced with someone who has uncontrolled breathlessness, lungs like tissue paper, a pessimistic outlook, an unglamorous disease, and no straightforward problem like excess sputum, which can be dealt with by time-honoured techniques'. From the patient's perspective, however, the effect of dyspnoea can be devastating. DeVito wrote 'it's the worst feeling in the world, the worst way to die, it's like smothering to death . . . to lose control of your breathing.'[30]

There is usually a physiological basis for breathlessness in patients in the palliative care phase of their disease. Dyspnoea is associated with:

(1) increased drive to breathe, as in pulmonary oedema, pneumonia, or lung carcinoma;

(2) decreased power, as in inspiratory muscle weakness (e.g. motor neurone disease) or neuromuscular deficiency possibly, due to poor nutrition;

(3) increased work of breathing, as with barrel chest or distended abdomen (e.g. ascites);

(4) anxiety, which can be either a cause or an effect.

Physiotherapy assessment of the dyspnoeic patient should pay particular attention to:

(1) the patient's current drug history (β-blockers, bronchodilators);

(2) questions in the subjective assessment such as 'What is your main problem?', 'What does your breathlessness feel like?', 'What makes it better or worse?';

(3) levels of anxiety ascertained in the subjective and objective assessment by observation and questioning.

Physiotherapeutic approaches commonly used for dyspnoea are:

(1) education in positioning, relaxation, and breathing control, if dyspnoea is anticipated (for example at the diagnosis of lung cancer and before dyspnoea becomes a clinical problem);

(2) positioning;

(3) relaxation;

(4) breathing control;

(5) increasing exercise tolerance through graded exercise;

(6) education and participation of the carer.

It is important that the patient assumes the most comfortable and optimal respiratory position whilst they receive a nebulizer. For a detailed discussion on the use of nebulizers, see Chapter 9.5.

Physiotherapeutic approaches commonly used for excess bronchial secretions are:

(1) modified postural drainage;

(2) breathing control;

(3) forced expiratory technique;

(4) humidification (if the mucus is tenacious);

(5) education and participation of the carer.

Neurological impairment and disability

Patients in the palliative care phase of their disease may have damage to the central and/or peripheral nervous system, resulting in disorders of movement, sensation, and co-ordination. The most common sequelae of damage to the nervous system are disorders of movement, ranging from focal paralysis of one or selective muscle groups to generalized difficulties in instigating or co-ordinating movement.[31]

The aims of physiotherapy with the neurologically impaired patient are:

(1) promotion of independence;

(2) maintenance of voluntary movement;

(3) return to normal of muscle tone;

(4) prevention of deformity;

(5) re-education of posture and balance reactions;

(6) education and participation of carers in the treatment.

Physiotherapeutic approaches commonly used are:

(1) promotion of independence by mobility exercises;

(2) positioning to bring about normal tone;

(3) passive movements to prevent contractures;

(4) active and active-assisted exercise patterns to promote sensorimotor feedback, thereby facilitating normal movement;

(5) balance re-education;

(6) transfers;

(7) gait re-education.

Musculoskeletal impairment and disability

Many patients with breast, prostate, lung, kidney, or colon cancer have bone metastatic lesions: the axial skeleton and proximal long bones are commonly affected. The most frequent symptom of bone metastases is pain which is usually localized and worse at night. Patients are at risk of pathological fracture where the site of the bone lesion exceeds 60 per cent of the total bone width[32] and therefore prevention of fracture is important. Pain on weight bearing suggests a need to reduce the weight-bearing load and this can be achieved by instructing the patient to partially bear weight using a walking stick (cane) or a walking frame. The patient must also be advised against rotating the affected leg as this can often lead to fracture exacerbated by weight bearing. When pathological fractures do occur, they are often difficult to stabilize and can lead to significant morbidity and mortality.

Control of lymphoedema

A detailed description of lymphoedema and its treatment is given in Chapter 9.7.

The needs of the physiotherapist in palliative care

Emotional support

In the last two decades, there has been formal recognition of the psychological and emotional needs of staff working with patients in the palliative phase of their disease. Kubler-Ross's book *On Death and Dying*[33] highlighted the needs of the caregivers. Since then, Vachon[34,35] has monitored staff stress in cancer wards, and an increasing interest in staff 'burnout' or 'battle fatigue' has led to a steady interest in staff support groups.

The lack of formal education systems in palliative care physiotherapy may exacerbate the stress on the individual physiotherapist resulting in 'deskilling' and uncertainty. Lederberg wrote that 'the spectrum of staff responses can be divided into the categories of normal adaptation and coping, coping accompanied by reactive anxiety and depression, and frank psychiatric symptoms'.[36] Normal adaptation and coping with working in palliative care can be facilitated by ensuring professional competence. If the individual can meet the intellectual and organizational demands of the job, normal adaptation and coping are facilitated. A consequence of this statement, therefore, is to ensure that physiotherapy staff are sufficiently qualified and competent for the job. Environmental and organizational considerations are also important as these can ameliorate coping responses. The rehabilitation philosophy described earlier can enable the process of coping as the physiotherapist is part of a team which has a goal orientated approach to the patient's care and engages in regular team meetings. In addition, normal adaptation and coping are facilitated by ensuring that there is adequate support (formal and informal) for the physiotherapist. This is an important factor because in the majority of palliative care settings the physiotherapist is working on his/ her own. For a detailed discussion on the emotional needs of patients and staff, see Chapter 14.3.

Educational needs

The importance of education for physiotherapists in palliative care has not been formally recognized to date. Greater emphasis is needed at undergraduate and postgraduate level. Most learning occurs in an *ad hoc* fashion, driven by the personal needs of the physiotherapist to enhance their skills and expertise. A recent survey of postbasic education in Europe highlighted the fact that only the United Kingdom has a special interest group for physiotherapists working in palliative care and oncology.[37] Further development in the area of education in palliative care is therefore crucial.

Good communication skills underpin effective physiotherapy intervention. Working closely with patients and their carers in the palliative care setting can test the physiotherapist's communication skills and therefore education in communication skills training is essential (see Section 4).

Education on the role of other members of the multidisciplinary team should also be encouraged (see Chapter 21.1). Awareness of the exact roles and skills of other team members enables the physiotherapist to detect the patient's problems in the other areas of function and refer the patient to the appropriate member of the team, thereby facilitating the patient's rehabilitation.

There are few published studies monitoring the effectiveness of physiotherapy in palliative care. For many years, in the physiotherapy profession there was an emphasis on the need to acquire new clinical skills. Recently, however, the emphasis has shifted towards evaluation of these clinical skills thereby enabling the growth of the theoretical base of the physiotherapy profession. Many physiotherapists, however, have not been formally educated in research and there is an obvious need to educate physiotherapists in research methods appropriate in palliative care, such as single case studies, qualitative methods, etc.

References

1. Dudas S. Rehabilitation concepts of nursing. *Journal of Endostomal Therapy*, 1984; **11**: 6–18.

2. Habeck RV, Romsaas EP, Olsen SJ. Cancer rehabilitation and continuing care: a case study. *Cancer Nursing*, 1984; **7**: 315–19.
3. Dietz JH Jr. Rehabilitation of the cancer patient: its role in the scheme of comprehensive care. *Clinical Bulletin*, 1974; **4**: 104–7.
4. Dietz JH Jr. Rehabilitation of the patient with cancer. In: Calabresi P, Schein PS, Rosenberg SA, eds. *Medical Oncology: Basic Principles and Clinical Management of Cancer.* New York: Macmillan, 1985: 1501–22.
5. Hagedorn R. *Occupational Therapy: Foundations for Practice: Models, Frames of Reference and Core Skills.* Edinburgh: Churchill Livingstone, 1991.
6. Marcant D, Rapin CH. Role of the physiotherapist in palliative care. *Journal of Pain and Symptom Management*, 1993; **8**: 68–71.
7. Weed L. Medical records that guide and teach. *New England Journal of Medicine*, 1968; **278**: 593–600.
8. Kisner C, Colby LA. *Therapeutic Exercise: Foundations and Techniques.* Philadelphia: FA Davis, 1990: 10.
9. Swenson JR. Therapeutic exercise in hemiplegia. In: Basmajian JV, ed. *Therapeutic Exercise*, 4th edn. Baltimore: William and Wilkins, 1984.
10. Carr JH, Shepherd R. *Physiotherapy in Disorders of the Brain.* London: Heinemann Medical Books, 1980.
11. Ebel A. Exercise in peripheral vascular diseases. In: Basmajian JV, ed. *Therapeutic Exercise.* 3rd edn. Baltimore: William and Wilkins, 1978.
12. Whittle M. *Gait Analysis: an Introduction.* Oxford: Butterworth Heinemann, 1991: 91.
13. Skinner AT, Thomson AM. Hydrotherapy. In: Wells PE, Frampton V, Bowsher D, eds. *Pain: Management and Control in Physiotherapy.* Oxford: Butterworth Heinemann, 1988: 239.
14. Hough A. *Physiotherapy in Respiratory Care: a Problem Solving Approach.* London: Chapman and Hall, 1991: 97.
15. Webber BA, Pryor JA .Physiotherapy skills: techniques and adjuncts. In: Webber BA, Pryor JA, eds. *Physiotherapy for Respiratory and Cardiac Problems.* London: Churchill Livingstone, 1993: 113.
16. Webber BA. *The Brompton Hospital Guide to Chest Physiotherapy.* 5th edn. Oxford: Blackwell Scientific, 1988: 43.
17. Pryor JA. The forced expiration technique. In: Pryor JA, ed. *International Perspectives in Physical Therapy. 7, Respiratory Care.* Edinburgh: Churchill Livingstone, 1991: 79–100.
18. Jenkins SC, Soutar SA, Moxham J. The effects of posture on lung volumes in normal subjects and inpatients pre- and post- coronary artery surgery. *Physiotherapy*, 1988; **74**: 492–6.
19. Dull JL, Dull WL. Are maximal inspiratory breathing exercises or incentive spirometry better than early mobilization after cardiopulmonary bypass? *Physical Therapy*, 1983; **63**: 655–9.
20. Sutton PS. Chest physiotherapy: time for reappraisal. *British Journal of Diseases of the Chest*, 1988; **82**: 353–9.
21. Uno Plast Endotracheal suctioning. 1991.
22. Ferguson JM, Marquis JN, Barr Taylor C. A script for deep muscle relaxation. *American Journal of Psychotherapy*, 1977; **28**: 282–7.
23. Low J, Reed A. *Electrotherapy Explained.* London: Butterworth Heinemann, 1990.
24. Ward AR. *Electricity Fields and Waves in Therapy.* Marrickville: Science Press, 1980.
25. Forster A, Palastanga N. *Clayton's Electrotherapy: Theory and Practice.* Eastbourne: Bailliere Tindall, 1985.
26. Booth FW. Physiologic and biochemical effects of immobilization on muscle. *Clinical Orthopaedics and Related Research*; 1987: **219**: 15
27. Haggmark T, Eriksson E, Jansson E. Muscle fiber type changes in human skeletal muscle after injuries and immobilization. *Orthopedics*, 1986; **9**: 181.
28. Akeson WH, Ameil D, Woo SL-Y. Immobility effects of synovial joints: the pathomechanics of joint contracture. *Biorheology*, 1980; **17**: 95.
29. St-Pierre D, Gardiner P. The effect of immobilization and exercise on muscle function: a review. *Physiotherapy Canada*, 1987; **39**: 24–32.
30. De Vito A J. Dyspnea during hospitalization for acute phase of illness as recalled by patients with COPD. *Heart Lung*, 1990; **18**: 583–9.
31. Gordon J. Disorders of motor control. In: Ada L, Canning C, eds. *Key Issues in Neurological Physiotherapy.* Oxford: Butterworth Heinemann, 1990: 25.
32. Menck H, Schultze S, Larsen E. Metastasis size in pathologic femoral fractures. *Acta Orthopaedica Scandinavica*, 1988; **59**: 151.
33. Kubler-Ross E. *On Death and Dying.* New York: Macmillan, 1969.
34. Vachon MLS. Motivation and stress experienced by staff working with the terminally ill. *Death Education*, 1978; **2**: 113–22.
35. Vachon MLS, Lyall WAL, Freeman SJJ. Measurement and management of stress in health professionals working with advanced cancer patients. *Death Education*, 1978; **1**: 365–75.
36. Lederberg M. Psychological problems of staff and their management. In: Holland JC Rowland JH, eds. *Handbook of Psychooncology.* New York: Oxford University Press, 1990: 631–646.
37. Standing Liaison Committee of Physiotherapists Within the E.C. *Post-basic Physiotherapy Education in the European Community*, September 1993.

12.3 Occupational therapy

Kent Nelson Tigges

Introduction

Occupational therapy is perhaps the most misunderstood and, thus, the least valued profession in health care. Many professionals have the perception that occupational therapists are individuals who are little more than well meaning citizens trained in crafts, hand work, games, and the like thereof. It is often perceived that these 'lay people' can offer little more than diversional activities (bingo sessions, raffia pot plant holders, ceramic figurines) that will occupy the vacant hour between the real and essential health-care services.

There are those professionals that acknowledge that occupational therapists hold legitimate academic degrees enabling them to understand the direct relationship between purposeful engagement in familiar life activities and the pursuit of happiness and satisfaction. A useful service, but not a necessary service in palliative medicine, particularly when budgetary matters are pressing issues.

The following chapter is presented to dispel existing misperceptions and, it is hoped, to convey the true nature and essential contribution of occupational therapy.

Background philosophy

Many people with the diagnosis of cancer have experienced years of knowing that they have cancer and have undergone numerous medical procedures. Their illness and subsequent treatments have either slowly or rapidly eroded their ability to maintain their familiar and preferred roles in self-care, work, and leisure.

People are creatures of habit and, therefore, creatures of expectations—expectations that they will be capable of providing for their basic needs, and of making a magnificent and hopefully valued contribution during their lifetime—a lifetime of many years to come. Not to be able to carry on with life as a 'capable, productive, valued, and respected person' can, and does, cause an immense erosion in one's perception and realization of quality of life and, thus, one's self-esteem. This is perhaps the most damaging insult to a person's personal integrity.

When the final 'insult-to-injury' comes—the prognosis of less than 6 months to live is learned—health-care practitioners should not be surprised to see their patients express feelings of helplessness, hopelessness, or uselessness (Fig. 1), no matter what their effectiveness in everyday situations before becoming ill may have been (locus of control[1] profile).

These very real and justifiable feelings occur as a result of progressive or rapid loss of physical strength and endurance, and discomfort and pain. Typically, advanced cancer patients come to the painful realization that they will no longer be able to do the things they could in the past, and that they will not be able to achieve all of their life goals.

The occupational behaviour model

Although there are many substantiated models of practice in the discipline[2] it has been determined[3] that the generic model of occupational behaviour[4] is the most appropriate, economic, and efficient model to stabilize and/or maximize the terminally ill person's occupational roles and, thus, promote and improve their perception of competence and achievement, generating a feeling of well-being and quality of life.

The occupational behaviour model of practice has been developed on the principles of general systems theory, which is a valued and widely used method for model building and problem solving.[5] General systems theory states that a single system cannot adequately be addressed unless the systems below and above it are

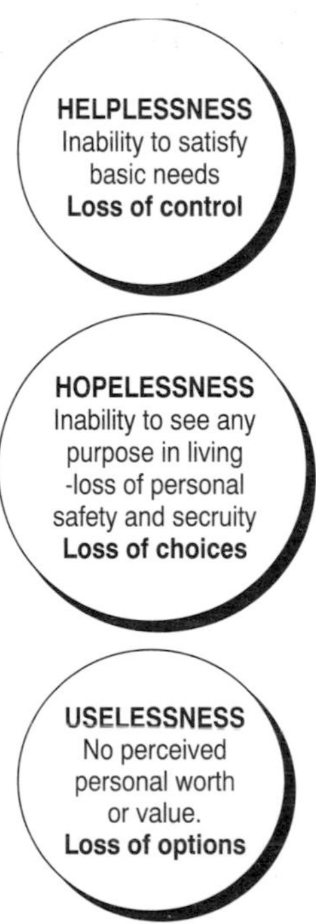

Fig. 1 Feelings expressed.

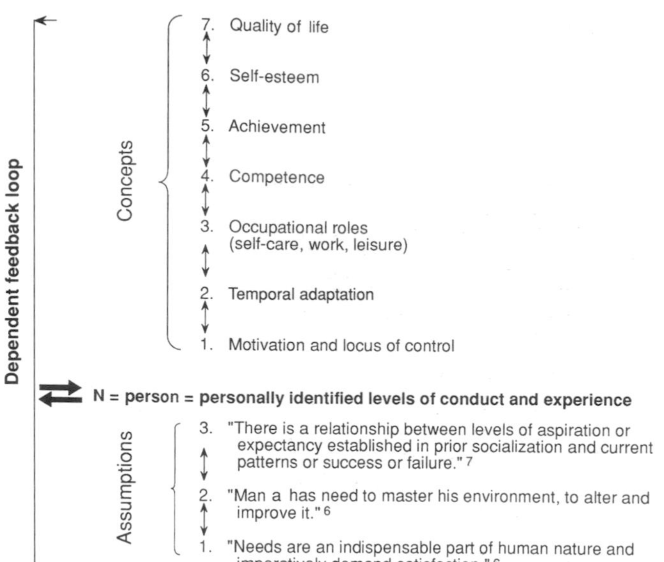

Fig. 2 Selected assumptions and concepts of occupational behaviour.

given equal and appropriate attention. General systems theory counteracts the reductionist's view of disease and illness. Therefore, the constant formulae in the occupational behaviour model is:

N + 1 = family (values, expectations, role responsibilities)

N = person = levels of conduct and experience

N – 1 = systems (muscle strength and endurance, joint mobility)

N = person = levels of conduct and experience is defined by occupational behaviour as:

(1) that to which one's time is devoted, or in which one regularly or habitually engaged;

(2) what one does in the company of others;

(3) one's regular business or occupation.

The occupational behaviour model embraces three basic assumptions and seven fundamental concepts that reflect the behaviour of adults (Fig. 2).

Assessment protocol

The assessment protocol involves five steps. In these steps, data relating to the seven concepts are obtained, although not in the order in which they appear in Fig. 2.

Step 1. Occupational history

N = person is the departure reference for the occupational therapist. This is supported by the principle, 'The patient is the pivotal initiative in assessment, treatment planning, and in the determination of the expected outcomes'.[8],[9] The first assessment, therefore, is the occupational history[10] (Fig. 3), a formal interview instrument, which was designed to yield a profile of persons based on family history, past self-care abilities, work experience, and leisure and recreational patterns—key elements in the development of personality. Following the formal interview, the patient is asked to describe his or her functional ability and/or lack of ability to perform self-care activities, as the self-care activities are the prerequisite skills for work and leisure. The therapist then does a functional mobility (ambulation) assessment, as ambulation is the prerequisite skill for self-care.

As all adults are accustomed to, and take for granted, carrying out their self-care roles completely independently, the loss of sufficient physical strength and endurance forces them out of their independent position and into an unacceptable position, to themselves, of either interdependence or dependence (Fig. 4). That is, there is a loss of control over the ability to take care of basic and private needs. It is during this part of the assessment that the occupational therapist is most likely to encounter feelings of helplessness, anger, and/or resentment.

Following the self-care assessment, the therapist assesses the work and leisure roles. It has been said that work is one of the most significant indices of a person's worth and value to society.[11] This is true for those individuals who have a regular job or career. For those individuals who do not have a regular job or career, and those who have retired, the connotation and value of work is restated. 'It is through the making of a contribution that people have a feeling of self-worth, and engender respect from others.'[12] Irrespective of the nature of a given person's 'work', 'work is the arena in which individuals endeavour to validate themselves'.[13] One's work is the impetus for a person to get up in the morning and face life and its responsibilities. Not to be able to attend to one's life responsibilities leads to insulted self-esteem.

Step 2. Self-esteem

An individual's self-concept and their soul are philosophically one and the same. A person's soul is very fragile, and, as such, must be ministered to with great care and concern. Self-esteem is the evaluative component of self-concept. Self-concept could be said to be 'my perception of who I am—my real or relative worth and value in life'.[14,15] An effective way to assess self-esteem is to examine the three progressive degrees of loss of self-esteem. This is accomplished by observing behaviours and examining probable causes (Fig. 5).[3]

People's feelings, and thus their reactions to these feelings, are expressions of their state of personal and emotional, physical, and social equilibrium and homeostasis. When there is a disruption in any one or more of these systems, individuals are going to 'react' because they have been assaulted. These reactions can range from anger, resentment, bitterness, and hostility, to withdrawal, apathy, and/or depression. These reactions (feelings) are defensive mechanisms that are employed to 'protect' one's damaged self-esteem.

These defensive reactions require a great deal of energy and serve no useful or constructive purpose. At the same time, these feelings can and do strain, stress, and often sever interpersonal relationships with significant others. The self-esteem diagnosis (helplessness, hopelessness, uselessness) helps the person to identify the cause(s) of his or her feelings and thus, more constructively, direct feelings and energies towards more positive ends. For example 'From what you have told me you must be feeling helpless because you have to depend on other people to help you take care of so many of your basic needs. It's humiliating, isn't it, to have to ask someone to help you on and off the toilet, to help you bathe and

Occupational history

Patient's name:
Date of history:
Time of history:

Occupational enquiries

A. Work history (employment)
1. I understand that before you became ill you were a ________________ . What an interesting job. How did you get started/ interested in that line of work?
2. What sort of training/education was involved?
3. Where did you get your training?
4. What was the first job you had (and subsequent jobs)?
5. What was the last job you had before you became ill?
6. Did you work up until you became sick?
7. (if retired) How long have you been retired?
8. What have you been doing with your time since you retired?

B. Work history (home-maker)
1. I understand that you have been a housewife/ mother for many years. That is more than a full-time job isn't it
2. What was the most challenging part of being a housewife, wife, mother?
3. What was the most frustrating part of being a housewife, wife, mother?
4. Apart from being a full-time housewife, were you ever interested or involved in community or religious activities?
5. Were you still active in these activities up until the time you became sick?
6. Since you became ill, what jobs have been the most difficult to give up?
7. What bothers you the most about the jobs you have had to give up?
8. What type of work is/was your husband involved in?

C. Family history
1. Have you always lived in __________ (city)? If no, where did you live before you moved here?
2. What did your parents do for a living?
3. Do you have brothers and sisters? Where do they live? Do you see/talk to them often?
4. I understand that you have children/ grandchildren. Where do they live? Are they married? Do you see/talk to them frequently?
5 (husband as patient) Before you got sick, what were your duties/responsibilities around the house?
6. Before you got sick which did you do with your spouse, children, grandchildren, friends for fun or relaxation?

Occupational enquiries

C. Family history (continued)
7. What are the most important things that your illness has prevented you from doing?
8. At the present time, what brings you the greatest pleasure?
9. What are the things that you would like to do now?

D. Leisure, sport, recreation
1. When you were finished with your day's work what did you do for relaxation or fun?
2. How often did you engage in these activities?
3. Who did you do them with?
4. When was the last time you enjoyed these activities?
5. If you could would you like to do them again?

E. Temporal adaptation
1. Before you got sick was it important for you to have a daily schedule? (in what way was it/was it not important to you?)
2. How did you organize your day? Start from the time you got up each morning and tell me everything you did before you went to bed.
3. What is your daily schedule like now?
4. If you had your choice, how would you like to spend tomorrow?

Therapist's comments:

Functional evaluation
Ask patient to demonstrate or describe problems in the following areas.

1. Bathing/dressing
2. Ambulation
3. Object manipulation
4. Home-making/home management
5. Child care/parenting/grandparenting
6. Leisure/sport/recreation

Fig. 3 Occupational history (a formal interview instrument).

dress yourself, and not to be able to get out of bed by yourself? You have lost control over the very tasks that we all take so much for granted and have always expected to do independently on our own. You are entitled to feel angry and resentful. If you are interested, there is self-help equipment available and techniques that I can teach you to use so that you can get out of bed, toilet, bathe, and dress yourself more independently. You can then have more control of how and when you want to do these activities.'

Step 3. Physical systems

The specific physical systems to be assessed will depend entirely on the individual patient's diagnosis, course of illness, and prognosis. Depending on the case, the following assessments may be performed in part or full.

Biological

Sensorimotor, neuromuscular, reflex integration, range of motion, gross and fine co-ordination, strength and endurance, sensory integration, sensory awareness, and body integration. Situational coping, cognition, orientation, concentualization, comprehension, cognitive integration.

The nature and intent of the above assessments are determined by the individual patient's lack of ability and/or dysfunction in the preferred occupational roles—namely self-care, work and leisure, and/or recreational.

The standard (basic) physical assessment

The purpose of the physical examination is twofold—not only to determine dysfunction resulting from the patient's diagnosis, but

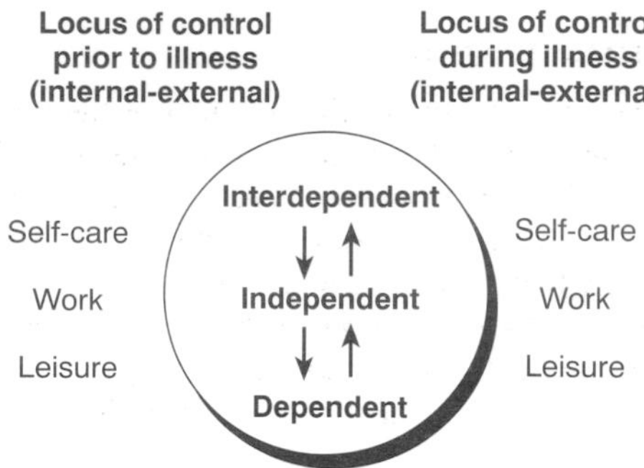

Fig. 4 A diagram illustrating the interdependence or dependence of adults after loss of physical strength. Interdependent = a state of action/acceptance of interacting with significant other individuals to initiate and accomplish aspects of roles. Independent = a state of action/acceptance of self initiated and completed aspects of roles. Dependent = a state of action/acceptance of relying on others for initiation and completion of roles.

also to determine the dysfunctions resulting from decreased physical activity (prolonged wheelchair sitting and/or bed rest), secondary to the diagnosis. These secondary dysfunctions are in many cases as significant as, if not more significant than, the primary diagnosis. For example, decreased muscle strength and endurance, decreased blood supply, venous retrograde pooling leading to orthostatic hypotension, poor appetite leading to decreased muscle bulk, poor skin and muscle nutrition, increased skin breakdown, muscle cramps, spasms and contractures, disuse of antigravity muscles leading to altered proprioceptive and vestibular apparatus responses and functions, and finally to problems of ambulation. These secondary dysfunctions occur after 3 to 7 days of bed rest or wheelchair sitting.

The basic physical examination of every patient begins with a muscle test and range of motion assessment of lower extremities, the trunk, upper extremities, and the head and neck. This assessment is then followed by a pain assessment. As with secondary physical dysfunction, there may be significant secondary pain not associated entirely with the primary diagnosis. It should be remembered that the degree of health of a given individual depends largely on the biological equilibrium of the body systems and their dynamic interaction.[16] The human body operates at its optimal level of efficiency when there are proportional periods of biomechanical activity, rest, and appropriate nutrition.

With acute or chronic pain, biomechanical activity, rest, and nutrition become disproportionate. Rest and inactivity become predominant because of such problems as; discomfort, loss of physical strength and endurance (muscle wasting, atrophy, contractures), decreased motor planning ability, vestibular and/or sensory dysfunction, fear of increasing pain, fear of falling and sustaining further injury. Another important factor to be considered is learned helplessness, that is, the patient's acceptance of, or resignation to the 'invalid' or 'disabled' role. Learned helplessness (be it initiated by patient, family, or professional staff) involves complex secondary gains that frequently complicate assessment of pain. Although the pain that the patient is experiencing is, in the patient's mind, a singular phenomenon, the professionals assessing the patient's pain must examine all systems separately, and then, as a team, integrate all assessment data and set appropriate courses of treatment.

Pain intensity must be determined on a patient-to-patient,

Probable causes

1. Loss of physical strength and endurance
2. Loss of preferred performance in self care, work, leisure
3. Bedbound/enforced dependence
4. Dependence on medications, catheters, colostomies, nasogastric tubes

Feelings expressed

HELPLESSNESS
Inability to satisfy basic needs
Loss of control

Observable behaviours

1. Withdrawal from active activity due to fear of additional physical injury
2. Excessively demanding
3. Diminished ability to control emotions

Probable causes

1. Loss of primary life roles
2. Recognition of declining physical health
3. Presence of nausea, vomiting, diarrhoea, constipation, loss of appetite
4. Recognition of impending death

Feelings expressed

HOPELESSNESS
Inability to see any purpose in living –loss of personal safety and security
Loss of choices

Observable behaviours

1. Anger, resentment, bitterness
2. Inability to identify goals
3. Strained interpersonal communications with family/friends
4. Increased anxiety/restlessness
5. Excessive psychosomatic/physical/emotional symptoms

Probable causes

1. Inability to have any direct/positive influence on immediate situation
2. Threatened personal safety and security
3. Loss of direction, goals
4. Loss of purposeful productivity
5. Feelings of being a burden on family

Feelings expressed

USELESSNESS
No perceived personal worth or value.
Loss of options

Observable behaviours

1. Withdrawal from active activity due to fear of additional physical injury
2. Excessively demanding
3. Diminished ability to control emotions

Fig. 5 Loss of positive self-esteem.

subjective basis. A standard patient-perception scale must be agreed upon by the interdisciplinary team, so that there will be an improved interrater reliability not only within disciplines, but also between disciplines. It must also be appreciated that, in home care, patients' reporting of their pain intensity may vary throughout the day, and, therefore, they may report different pain intensities to different professionals. Regular, longitudinal records need to be kept and entered on the patient's medication sheet. In this way, a patient's pain profile can be regularly monitored and treated for the appropriate level of activity, and not only at bed rest, which is, unfortunately, all too often the case in pain management[17, 18] (see Sections 6 and 16).

Step 4. Locus of control

This assessment[19] is a standardized interview that provides an insight into the person's effectiveness in everyday- life situations. There are two general profiles: internal and external. The external profile is characterized by the person not seeking out opportunities, not paying attention to feedback as a means of correcting performance, not engaging in a moderate amount of risk taking. These persons generally do not believe in their skills or ability to control what happens to them in daily life situations. Life events occur by fate, luck, and/or by chance.[20,21]

The internal profile is characterized by the person who does seek out opportunities in the environment, and pays attention to feedback as a means of correcting performance. This person engages in a moderate amount of risk taking. These are persons who have a basic belief in their skills, and a measure of expectancy of success and/or failure.[20,21]

This assessment will afford the occupational therapist a relative profile of how the person may respond to current and future interdependent, independent, and dependent life situations.

Step 5. Quality of life

Quality of life is the paramount concept of the hospice and palliative medicine movement. No other concept has been so fervently advocated as the single purpose of caring for people with terminal disease. Although much has been written about the relationship of active engagement in life activities and life satisfaction, health-care professionals and family members must be cautioned to not impose either professional or personal values on to the individual with terminal illness. For some, the opportunity for, and guidance into, a more active and engaged life may be highly desirable. For others, withdrawing and disengagement may be just as desirable. In the final analysis, it is the patient's ultimate choice. Their personal choice must be respected and valued.

Throughout this text there are numerous references to the issue of quality of life. Each discipline will, no doubt, make claims to providing patients with increased quality of life—and this is rightfully so. As with pain assessment, quality of life assessment and treatment must be a collaborative, team issue. For the occupational therapist, the quality of life assessment is the cumulative end of the general systems theory occupational behaviour model. In light of all the data obtained from step 1 to step 4, the quality of life assessment is administered by interview. This assessment has been developed by utilizing two subconcepts, namely subjective satisfaction and objective achievement[22] and correlating them with the occupational behaviour concepts of competence[23] and achievement[24] (Fig. 6; see also Chapter 5.6).

The evaluative process

The evaluative process requires the very best of the occupational therapist's academic and clinical skills. The evaluation of the data obtained from all the assessments requires not only attention to detail, but also a sensitive attention to the very real personal, medical, and rehabilitation needs of each patient. Sensitive evaluation also includes close discussions with the patient to set short- and long-term goals. In the evaluative process, the occupational therapist takes into account the following principles:

1. All patients, irrespective of their age, illness, disability, or any other circumstances, must always be considered as people first, and ill, diseased, or disabled second.
2. All patients must be considered as people whose lives are at risk.
3. All patients have the right to self-determined quality of life:
   (a) the patient is always the pivotal initiative in assessment, treatment planning, and treatment implementation;
   (b) each patient has the right to specific and detailed ideographic (personal) and nomothetic (disability-related) evaluation;[25]
   (c) patients' rights must be aligned with their respective responsibilities within their personal, economic, and social environment.

Treatment planning

Assessment and treatment planning must be considered a continuous and ongoing process. If complete compliance between the theoretical model of practice, assessment, and treatment planning does not exist, there will be inconsistency and fragmentation in the treatment process.[26]

Terminally ill people and their family members or caregivers are more than likely to feel frightened and vulnerable in regard to their situation. Furthermore, they are fearful of an uncertain future. Personal feelings frequently vacillate between the objective and logical, and the subjective and emotional. The first order of business for the occupational therapist is to raise the patient's level of function, and assist the caregivers in their task of augmenting the patient's level of independence, thus returning the patient and caregivers to a semblance of order, structure, control, and purpose.

Because of the urgency of the situation, the occupational therapist cannot afford the luxury of taking time to meditate over the accumulated data and development of a treatment plan. If possible, a treatment plan and intervention strategy should be formulated and carried out during the first assessment visit. In doing this, three important issues are addressed and set into place.

1. The patient can clearly realize that he or she can move from a present state of dysfunction to an increased state of function.
2. The caregivers can realize that specific help can be offered to facilitate their care of the patient, thus reducing unnecessary fears and apprehensions they may have in regard to how they

COMPETENCY

As measured against competency components: sufficient or adequate behaviours to meet demands of occupational roles; attempts to contact and master the environment.

1. **Intellectual ability**
   (a) Prior to present condition
   (b) Presently
   (c) Projected future potential
   (d) Patient's current perception (subjective satisfaction)

2. **Emotional stability**
   (a) Prior to present condition
   (b) Presently
   (c) Projected future potential
   (d) Patient's current perception (subjective satisfaction)

3. **Physical capacity**
   (a) Prior to present condition
   (b) Presently
   (c) Projected future potential
   (d) Patient's current perception (subjective satisfaction)

4. **Artistic, technical, educational/ professional skills**
   (a) Prior to present condition
   (b) Presently
   (c) Projected future potential
   (d) Patient's current perception (subjective satisfaction)

5. **Capacity to form, enjoy and maintain social relationships**
   (a) Prior to present condition
   (b) Presently
   (c) Projected future potential
   (d) Patient's current perception (subjective satisfaction)

ACHIEVEMENT

As measured against achievement components: a specified level of success, attainment, or proficiency; ability to solve situations in occupational roles with success/excellence

1. **Intellectual ability**
   (a) Prior to present condition
   (b) Presently
   (c) Projected future potential
   (d) Patient's current perception (subjective satisfaction)

2. **Emotional stability**
   (a) Prior to present condition
   (b) Presently
   (c) Projected future potential
   (d) Patient's current perception (subjective satisfaction)

3. **Physical capacity**
   (a) Prior to present condition
   (b) Presently
   (c) Projected future potential
   (d) Patient's current perception (subjective satisfaction)

4. **Artistic, technical, educational/ professional skills**
   (a) Prior to present condition
   (b) Presently
   (c) Projected future potential
   (d) Patient's current perception (subjective satisfaction)

5. **Capacity to form, enjoy and maintain social relationships**
   (a) Prior to present condition
   (b) Presently
   (c) Projected future potential
   (d) Patient's current perception (subjective satisfaction)

Key for competency, Achievement and Quality of Life Assessment and Evaluation

Prior to present condition:
If premorbid rules, skills and roles were appropriate as measured against the person's family, community and sub-cultural norms and values in regard to competency and achievement, put INTACT. If competency and achievement were not intact, state rules, skills and roles that are affected and give reasons. (Refer to UniformTerminology for Reporting Occupational Therapy Services. AOTA,1979)

Presently
Intact: (see above description)
Faulty: insufficient/inappropriate behaviour/s to meet the demands of the situation.
At risk: state roles and reasons.
A. Situational: difficulties/problems. Will resolve as conditions improve; patient requires/does not require therapeutic intervention.
B. In jeopardy: requires immediated and acute intervention.

Projected future outcome:
Based on objective and subjective data state therapeutic potential for:
1. No change/deterioration with intervention.
2. Maintenance with intervention.
3. Improvement with acute/ long-term intervention.
4. Restoration of function with acute or long-term intervention.

Patient's current perception:
With direct conversation with the patient state the patient's feelings (subjective/objective) about their quality of life prior to present condition, presently, and how they see their future.

Fig. 6 Quality of life assessment.

are going to manage caring for their disabled family member.

3. The therapist, patient, and caregivers develop a mutual sense of trust and regard for each other.

Developing and prioritizing goals

Having mapped out and established the patient's past and present positions in life (in regard to occupational roles, locus of control, self-esteem, and physical capabilities) the occupational therapist should state clearly and realistically his predictions of what he thinks the patient is capable of accomplishing; for example 'With the strength you have in your legs and arms, I believe that with the help of a walking frame you would be able to walk around with very little assistance. With some self-help equipment in the bathroom, I feel that you would be able to get into the bathtub and have a bath and shampoo. With instruction on how to transfer from your wheelchair into your car, you will be able to get out of the house, go for a ride, visit friends, or whatever else you feel that you would like to do. Getting out in the fresh air, and away from the confines of your home, can have a remarkably positive effect on your sense of well being.'

Then the patient should be asked to identify three or four goals that he would like to achieve. While some patients will be quick and eager to set goals, others may have difficulty and/or decline the offer to set goals. This type of response could be the result of several circumstances.

1. Due to an extended period of bed rest, the patient has 'accepted' the position of learned helplessness and does not have the energy and/or desire to confront a well-meaning but powerful environment.
2. The patient is a reluctant risk taker and avoids new and unfamiliar situations for fear of failure.
3. The patient is content with the present situation.
4. The patient is aware that caregivers are obtaining secondary gains by being overprotective and does not want to confront the situation for fear of alienation.
5. The patient is content or enjoys being dependent on others. The patient is actively disengaging from life.

The sensitive therapist will recognize these situations and gently attempt to pursue the 'true nature' of their situation in life. In some cases patients will alter their position and accept and set goals. However, there will be cases when patients will not alter their position. In these cases their position must be honoured and respected by the team.

As goals are agreed upon, the feasibility of the goals being accomplished independently, interdependently, or dependently should be discussed with the patient, team members, and caregivers. It is easy, for all concerned, to forget the patient's position and think that the patient will accept any level of performance. Goals requiring dependency and/or interdependency must be approached with sensitivity and caution, especially for patients who are strongly independent and internally motivated. After a lifetime of being independent and in control of most of life's situations, it could be a significant blow to one's personhood to hear others say that 'you'll just have to accept help with this goal'. Although this may not have been what was actually said, it is how the patient interpreted the statement. Assisting the patient to accept new and different methods of performance, and still maintain a sense of pride and dignity, is a challenge for the occupational therapist.

Obtaining family and caregiver compliance

Many palliative care programmes have home care programmes, because many patients express a desire to be at home rather than in an inpatient facility. Wherever patients are, caregivers frequently express feelings of anxiety and apprehension about the physical care of their family members. Some of these concerns are as follows:

(1) fear of hurting the patients physically by moving them;

(2) fear of hurting themselves when moving the patients in bed and/or during transfers out of bed;

(3) being overprotective in order to 'protect' the patients from any further injury or discomfort.

Although the majority of caregivers are sincerely interested in wanting to do whatever they can for their family members, many have not had previous experience in caring for an acutely ill and/or dying person and therefore do not have the necessary skills. The occupational therapist must assure caregivers that:

(1) they will not be asked or required to do any more than they are either physically or emotionally capable of doing;

(2) that they will be taught how to care safely for the patient in bed (pulling the person up in bed, bed positioning, range of motion exercises) and in the transferring of the patient from the bed to wheelchair, wheelchair to toilet/bathtub, into and out of the car (see Chapter 12.2).

Developing the treatment plan

When the patient and the caregivers have been assessed, and a degree of compliance is agreed upon regarding goals, the therapist gives a clear and precise overview of what the actual occupational therapy intervention process will look like, including what the patient will be taught to do, what caregivers will be taught to do, and how frequently the therapist will be seeing the patient. Two of the most important features of an effective treatment plan are clarity and structure. With a clear understanding of structure and expectations, both the patient and caregivers are more likely to put a sense of order into their lives. People, no matter what their circumstances may be, are more likely to cope and perform when they know what the plan of action is, particularly when the plan clearly states how they will be helped to improve their situation and achieve their goals.

Although each and every patient's and respective family member's needs and requests vary substantially, the following basic principle and interventions of occupational therapy are common to the majority.

Principle

New and/or altered options, choices, and controls for increased independence and/or interdependence in self-care, work, and leisure activities should be negotiated or renegotiated collaboratively, with the patient and family members.

Interventions

(1) recommending proper hospital bed and mattresses or floatation devices;

(2) assessing primary or secondary neuromuscular pain associated with either primary or secondary diagnosis, treat such pain with transcutaneous electrical nerve stimulation in conjunction with graded activity and/or positioning;

(3) teaching proper bed positioning and range of motion exercises to prevent or reduce contractures, maintain good joint mobility, and muscle flexibility;

(4) reducing muscle contractures with the use of splinting techniques;

(5) teaching appropriate and safe bed to wheelchair, cane, or walker transfers;

(6) prescribing proper wheelchair type, size, features, and appropriate seat cushions or floatation devices for proper posture, comfort, and skin protection;

(7) teaching wheelchair mobility in and out of the house or apartment, wheelchair to car transfers, and ways to access community resources for wheelchair-bound people;

(8) developing daily occupational routines to facilitate a sense of purpose and accomplishment;

(9) teaching and monitoring energy conservation techniques and procedures;

(10) teaching modified one-handed dressing and undressing techniques, including the use of assistive devices;

(11) recommending bath or shower seats, bath transfer benches, tub- and wall-mounted grab bars, hand-held showers, raised toilet sets, toilet-assist grab bars, and the proper and safe use of such equipment.

Discontinuation of therapy

Discontinuation of occupational therapy may occur due to one or more of the following reasons:

1. The patient and caregivers have accomplished their goals and are able to meet the day-to-day challenges without further intervention.

2. The patient and/or the caregivers request discontinuation due to interpersonal difficulties or problems.

3. The patient physically and/or mentally deteriorates to the point where intervention is inappropriate.

4. The patient dies.

Measuring success

It is a recognized fact that patients will die. Therefore, it should come as no surprise when they begin to deteriorate and ultimately die. No matter how well-educated or experienced occupational therapists may be, they are likely to experience feelings of loss when their patients die. These very real feelings can be comforted by reviewing the criteria for success.

1. The patients' functional abilities were increased and directed towards competence and achievement in their occupational roles.

2. Family and caregivers were given instruction and guidance in providing the necessary assistance and support to the patients.

3. The patients were given the opportunity to set and accomplish their goals.

4. The patients lived well, free from pain and symptoms, and even though life was not as long as they had hoped for, it was completed with a sense of strength, purpose, and dignity which would not have been possible without the skills and abilities of each and every member of the palliative care team. In the eyes of all there was hope without a future, a future without time.

References

1. Rotter J. *Ceneralized Epectancies for Internal versus External Control of Reinforcement*. Washington: American Psychological Association, 1966.
2. Reed K. *Models of Practice in Occupational Therapy*. Baltimore/London: Williams and Wilkins, 1984.
3. Tigges KN, Marcil WM. *Terminal and Life Threatening Illness: An Occupational Behavior Perspective*. Thorofare: Slack, 1988.
4. Tigges KN, Sherman LM. The treatment of the hospice patient: from occupational history to occupational role. *American Journal of Occupational Therapy*, 1983; **37**: 235–8.
5. Boulding K. General systems theory—the skeleton of science. *Management Science*, 1956; **2**: 197–208.
6. Reilly M. Occupational therapy can be one of the greatest ideas in 20th century medicine. *American Journal of Occupational Therapy*, 1962; **16**: 1–9.
7. Reilly M. The educational process. *American Journal of Occupational Therapy*, 1969; **23**: 299–307.
8. Marcil WM, Tigges KN. *The Person with AIDS: A Personal and Professional Perspective*. Thorofare: Slack, 1992: 105–122.
9. Pollock N. Client-centered assessment. *American Journal of Occupational Therapy*, 1993; **49**: 298–301.
10. American Occupational Therapy Association. *Guidelines for Occupational Therapy Services in Hospice Care*. Rockville, MD: American Occupational Therapy Association, 1987.
11. Gregory I, Smeltzer D. *Psychiatry*. Boston: Little, Brown and Co., 1983.
12. Tigges KN. The hospice movement—a time for professional action and commitment. *British Journal of Occupational Therapy*, 1980; **44**: 373–6.
13. Shannon PD. Work adjustment in the adolescent soldier. *American Journal of Occupational Therapy*, 1970; **24**: 112–18.
14. Gage M, Polatajko H. Enhancing occupational performance through an understanding of perceived self-efficacy. *American Journal of Occupational Therapy*, 1994; **48**: 452–61.
15. Gage M, Noh Samuel Polatajko H, Kasper V. Measuring perceived self-efficacy in occupational therapy. *American Journal of Occupational Therapy*, 1994; **48**: 783–90.
16. Sarno J. *Mind Over Back Pain*. New York: Berkley Books, 1982.
17. Vendenbosch TM. How to use a pain flow sheet effectively. *Nursing*, 1988; **18**: 50–1.
18. Tigges KN, Marcil WM. Pain assessment: An interdisciplinary perspective. *Home Healthcare Nurse*, 1989; **7**: 18–23.
19. Reid D, Zeigler M. Desired control measure. In: Lefcourt H. (ed.) *Research with the Locus of Control Construct*. New York: Academic Press, 1981.

20. Kielhofner G. *A Model of Human Occupation*. Baltimore: Williams and Wilkins, 1985.
21. Gage M. The appraisal model of coping: an assessment and intervention model for occupational therapy. *American Journal of Occupational Therapy*, 1992; **46**: 353–62.
22. Jonson AR, Siegler M, Winslade WJ. *Clinical Ethics: A Practical Approach to Ethical Decisions in Clinical Medicine*. London: Baillière Tindall, 1982.
23. White R. The urge towards competency. *American Journal of Occupational Therapy*, 1973; **25**: 273–7.
24. Chaplin JP. *Dictionary of Psychology*. New York: Dell, 1975.
25. Twycross RG. Quality before quantity—a note of caution. *Palliative Medicine*, 1987; **1**: 65–72.
26. Ottenbacher K, Cusick A. Discriminative versus evaluative assessment: Some observations on goal attainment scaling. *American Journal of Occupational Therapy*, 1993; **47**: 349–54.

12.4 Stoma management

Brigid Breckman

Stoma management

A stoma is an artificial opening created surgically for patients to allow their urine or faeces to leave their body by a new route through a spout or outlet on their abdomen. The management of stoma patients in palliative care involves three linked processes:

(1) the application of knowledge of the different operations and types of stoma in order to assess patients' condition and to plan, provide, and evaluate their treatment and its effects;

(2) management of the stoma and stomal appliances;

(3) provision of the physical and psychological care which patients need in their particular situation.

The four main contexts in which patients require stoma care are as follows:

- they are undergoing stoma surgery as a palliative strategy;
- they have an established stoma whose action and management are now being affected by other palliative interventions;
- they are in a preterminal or terminal condition;
- they have a fistula or a nephrostomy.

In this chapter information required to enable the first two major processes to take place will be considered in general terms. The third process will then be considered with reference to the four different contexts.

Application of knowledge of different operations and types of stoma

The after-effects of stoma surgery experienced by patients and the advice and care that they require will largely arise from three elements of their situation: the extent of their surgery, the type and site of their stoma, and the degree to which their disease and/or its effects have been removed or reduced. Identifying the third element accurately may be difficult, but knowledge of the more common stomas and stomal operations can be used in conjunction with patients' individual operation details to reach an informed opinion on each patient's probable situation and the care that is likely to be required.

Continent bowel and urinary stomas are not discussed here. They remain few in number compared with conventional stomas, and are usually created in younger patients with non-malignant conditions. Currently, they are rare in patients requiring palliative care. Descriptions of their formation and care are available.[1-4]

Bowel stomas

These are generally created from the ileum (ileostomy) or the colon (colostomy). The point at which diversion of faeces via the stoma occurs is important because the normal functions of the bowel before the diversion continue to take place but any functions which would normally take place further along the bowel are largely lost (Fig. 1). Elcoat[1] provides a useful summary of the different bowel operations and resultant types of stoma, and more detailed descriptions of the surgery are available.[5-7]

Temporary stomas

These include loop colostomies or ileostomies which are usually created to protect an anastomosis or facilitate decompression or healing in the distal bowel segment. A loop of bowel is brought out onto the abdominal wall and supported by a temporary rod or bridge so that it does not retract. The stoma has two openings: a

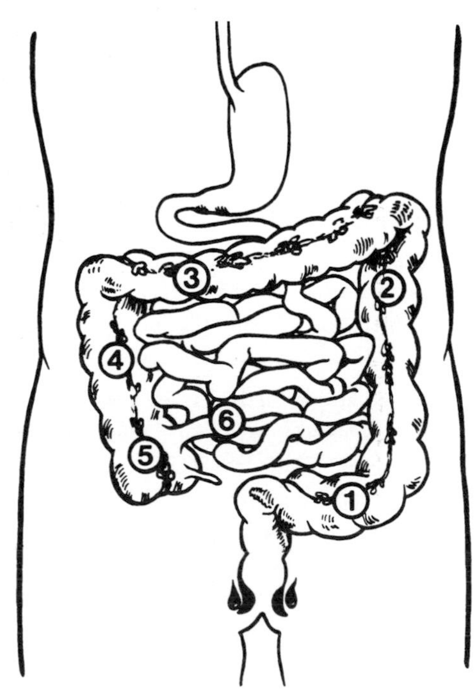

Fig. 1 Types of stoma and typical sites. (Reproduced with permission from ref. 27.)

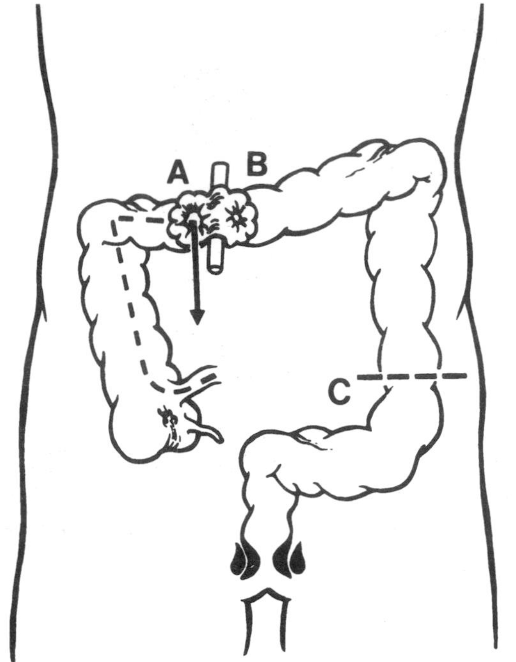

Fig. 2 Temporary loop colostomy with rod *in situ*: A, proximal opening; B. distal opening; C. anastomosis site. (Reproduced with permission from ref. 27.)

proximal opening through which faeces from the digestive tract will pass, and a distal opening which leads to the redundant bowel (Fig. 2).[1] The redundant section of bowel may continue to make mucus. Patients can find it confusing and distressing to have faeces coming out of a stoma and mucus (and sometimes old faeces) also coming from their rectum, and should be advised that this may occur and the reason for it. When bowel is to be reassessed for healing of an anastomosis, the distal segment will need to be emptied to allow assessment. Some oral laxatives will only aid clearance of the proximal section of bowel, and cannot clear a distal bowel segment which is not connected to the functioning digestive tract. Laxatives which are absorbed and therefore should act on all sections of the bowel do not always effectively clear the distal segment and washouts may also be required.

Bowel operations

Panproctocolectomy

The whole colon, rectum, and anal canal are excised and a permanent ileostomy is created from the terminal ileum.

Total colectomy

The colon is removed and an ileostomy is created, but the rectal stump is retained and may be brought out onto the abdominal wall as a mucous fistula.

Abdominoperineal excision of rectum

The rectum and anus are removed, often with a wide excision and removal of the upper third of the posterior wall of the vagina if the patient has cancer. The patient is left with a permanent (usually sigmoid) colostomy.

Formation of diversionary stoma only

Sometimes a colostomy or, more rarely, an ileostomy may be created without more extensive surgery, for example to enable distal bowel decompression to take place or to divert faeces prior to extensive tumour blockage.

Pelvic exenteration

This radical operation leaves the patient with both a colostomy and urostomy following removal of the pelvic organs. Women will also have their vagina removed, and may have an artificial vagina created. Men will be impotent. Any patient acquiring a stoma will take time to come to terms with the various changes in body image that their operation brings about. However, the major changes in body image and function created through this extensive operation can be particularly difficult for patients to accept, and a recurrence of their disease despite such surgery can be devastating.

Implications and results of the above surgery

Appliances and skin care

The position of the stoma along the bowel pathway and the nature of the faecal material that is therefore passed from it will largely determine which types of appliance are suitable for the patient, and the degree of skin protection which will be required. Surgery which removes all or most of the colon will generally mean that a patient has sizeable fluid to semisolid stomal action several times a day and will therefore require a standard capacity drainable bag.

A substantial degree of skin protection will be required if the effluent contains digestive enzymes likely to damage the skin (e.g. from an ileostomy) or if it is fluid enough to warrant a more watertight seal. A semiformed stomal action once or twice daily will generally warrant a lighter form of skin protection (see Fig. 1 and the section on principles of stoma care).

Diet

Most ostomists can eat most foods most of the time, including moderate amounts of fruit, vegetables, and alcohol. Unless a particular food is prohibited for medical reasons, patients who experience flatus, increased odour, or a more active stoma after certain foods can decide whether this creates too many problems and hence avoid such foods, or whether they gain sufficient pleasure to make the after-effects worthwhile. People with ileostomies need to take adequate fluids, particularly in hot weather, and may also require extra salt and fluids if they lose these from excess stomal action.[1]

Sexual activities

The degree to which sexual activities may be physically impaired will depend largely on the extent of the surgery. Men who only have a diversionary stoma raised should not experience erectile dysfunction, as the surgeon is unlikely to be operating in an area where pelvic nerve damage could take place. Likewise, women should not experience vaginal or perineal problems because the surgery has not taken place in those areas. However, cancer may cause problems, depending upon its location. These factors should be considered before information and advice is given pre- and postoperatively.[8]

Some patients have problems following removal of the rectum and anus. Kolodny *et al.*[9] suggest that 15 per cent of men are impotent following panproctocolectomy compared with 40 per cent following abdominoperineal excision of the rectum, with a 10 per cent and 40 per cent inability to ejaculate following these respective operations. Genital sensations and sexual desires continue to be present. Women having either operation tend to experience reduced vaginal secretions and therefore intercourse may be painful. Perineal scarring or (following abdominoperineal excision of rectum) vaginal shortening after removal of the posterior upper third of the vagina, and/or scarring along the area where the rectum was removed, can all result in a less elastic and accomodating vagina and hence dyspareunia.[10]

Urinary stomas

Diversion of the urinary tract is usually a permanent procedure involving either the formation of an intestinal conduit or, occasionally, a ureterostomy. Both ileal and colonic conduits and ureterostomies may also be called a urostomy. The term ileostomy should be reserved for faecal stomas.

Ileal and colonic conduits

These diversions provide a pathway for urine to leave the body via a stoma which protrudes sufficiently to enable a leakproof seal between a urostomy bag and the peristomal skin to be readily obtained. An ileal conduit entails separating a segment of ileum from the rest of the bowel, which is rejoined and thus continues to function as a separate digestive system. The ureters are anastomosed to the proximal end of the segment of ileum and the distal end is brought out on to the patient's abdominal wall as a urinary stoma.[11,12] The colon is similarly used to create a colonic conduit. The bowel segment acts as a conducting tube, or conduit, and is not a storage receptacle.

Ureterostomy

These stomas, formed from one or both ureters, are occasionally created if the patient is too ill for more major surgery. Formation of a good ureteric spout is difficult, and therefore it is not easy to achieve a leakproof seal with stomal equipment. Ureterostomies are more prone than conduits to stomal stenosis.[13]

Urinary operations

Total cystectomy

This operation is generally carried out to remove bladder cancer. The urethra is likely to be removed as well as the bladder to ensure tumour clearance. The patient is left with a permanent urostomy, usually an ileal conduit.[14]

Urinary diversion without bladder removal

The advent of self-catheterization techniques has led to this operation's being performed much less frequently. Generally an ileal conduit is created.

Implications and results of the above surgery

Appliances and skin care

Urine drips from a urinary diversion every few seconds and, if left on the skin, can cause considerable damage. A water-tight seal and adequate skin protection are necessary so that urine collects in the urostomy bag and not on the skin. The appliance should have an outlet/tap which allows easy emptying and connection to a larger drainage bag at night.

Diet

The removal of a segment of bowel to form a conduit usually creates a fair amount of flatulence and irregular bowel activity in the early postoperative period. As this decreases patients can resume a full range of foods. Fluid intake which is sufficient to ensure a urinary output of 1600 to1800 ml a day should be encouraged. Extra fluids should be taken in hot weather, if the urine appears concentrated, or if the patient's conduit produces large amounts of mucus which require flushing out.

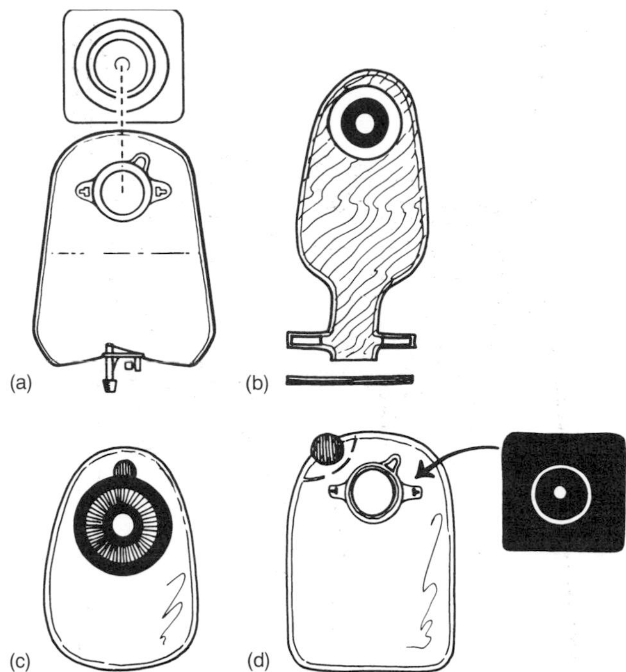

Fig. 3 (a) Urostomy appliance; (b) ilestomy or drainable appliance; (c) one-piece colostomy appliance; (d) two-piece colostomy appliance. (Reproduced from reference 16, with permission.)

Sexual activities

Urinary diversion alone should not impair physical activities. Radical cystectomy usually affects sexual function because there is pelvic nerve damage. In men, this generally leads to impotence although genital sensations and sexual desires should still be present . Women tend to experience reduced vaginal secretions. Removal of the anterior upper third of the vagina and scarring along the area where the bladder was removed can result in a less elastic and accomodating vagina and hence dyspareunia.[10,15]

Management of the stoma and stomal appliances

Effective stoma management entails:

- choosing a suitable appliance and skin care regime for each individual patient (Fig. 3);
- establishing a system of changing/emptying the appliance which follows the principles of good stoma care and can be carried out by the patient and/or other caregivers as necessary.[16]

The criteria used to aid skin care and appliance selection are established at the time of surgery and if the patient's situation changes, for example if his body contours, stomal effluent, or abilities to manage equipment alter. Likewise, the particular steps in an appliance change may need to be revised, but the basic principles should still be followed.

The choice of stomal equipment is a three-stage process.

1. Assess the following:
   - the stoma;
   - stomal effluent;
   - the patient's abdomen, skin protective needs, capabilities for using different styles of equipment, lifestyle, and preferences for different types of equipment.
2. Use this information to identify the criteria which the equipment should fulfill:
   - the stomabag—capacity, shape, outlet facility, ability to be used with other equipment (e.g. a convex insert, belt, or bag cover), one- or two-piece style;
   - the flange/gasket—size of gasket, adhesive area, style, flexibility/rigidity, level of skin protection, adhesiveness, degree of convexity (if this is required, see below);
   - skin protection—style and level required, compatibility with patient's skin type, level of adhesion required;
   - manageability of equipment—ease of preparation, application, removal, emptying by patient and relevant others.
3. Assess available stomal equipment to identify items meeting all or most of the above criteria, and choose the equipment (preferably, the patient should make the choice).

Stomas which are flush with the abdomen, or lie in creases, gulleys, or scars, create major difficulties if effluent pools at skin level or tracks along these channels, creating leakage; skin damage, and often a demoralized patient. These situations can be managed effectively by flattening the peristomal area either by using equipment with an integral convex flange or by adding a convex ring to the flange.[17,18] Therefore it is important to consider the need for convexity when responding to reports of leakage problems or noting stomas which are flush with the skin. This may occur if the patient's body contours alter with progression of the disease.

Principles of appliance and skin care management

Stomal equipment should provide sufficient adherence and skin protection to prevent leakage and skin damage. Changes should be frequent enough to prevent leakage and skin damage from stomal effluent, but not so frequent that their removal itself damages the skin. Patients can have quite excoriated skin before they experience discomfort. They should be taught to recognize signs that their bag is lifting and/or their skin protective is disintegrating and use these cues, as well as any irritation or pain in the stomal area, to decide when to change their equipment. The basic procedures of emptying and changing stomal appliances are well documented;[1,16,19,20] only key principles are outlined here.

Handwashing should take place before and after emptying or changing appliances. Patients do not need to wear gloves; faeces or urine passed through a stoma are no more infectious than when passed via a rectum or bladder. However, the advent of AIDs and HIV means that all staff should now wear gloves when handling urine or faeces from any patient, and when examining a stoma.

At each appliance change the condition of the stoma, peristomal skin, and effluent should be assessed. The stoma will usually shrink in size during the first 3 months but should retain the bright red colour which indicates that it has an adequate blood supply. The peristomal skin should be intact with no signs of excoriation or sogginess, which could indicate a reaction to the equipment or pooling of effluent on the skin. Assessment of the colour, odour, consistency, and amount of stomal effluent being passed should also take place routinely when equipment is being emptied or changed.

Skin protection is best achieved by ensuring that the gasket size of the appliance is about 3 mm larger than the stoma, and that peristomal wafers (if used) are cut to fit snugly around the base of the stoma. In situations where a stoma size may vary it is wise to measure it to identify the correct gasket size before preparing new equipment. Likewise, checking the patient's current abdominal state at the time of appliance change enables an up-to-date template to be prepared and used to ensure that the wafer covers all the skin right up to the stoma. Once a stable situation is achieved, patients can prepare their new equipment before removing the used equipment. This is particularly useful if the stoma is very active and speedy application of the new equipment is desirable. Where a separate appliance and peristomal wafer/flange are used it can be helpful to stick the bag and cut-out wafer together before removing the wafer backing and applying them all in one.

Teaching patients appliance and skin care management should include giving reasons for the various steps in the procedure so that they know what outcome they should be achieving and adapt their technique as necessary. Patients should also be taught how to dispose of used equipment and how to store new equipment wherever they live. Where household refuse is collected, appliances can be rinsed out before being wrapped up and placed with the rest of the refuse for collection. This system is also acceptable in most places of work, hotels, and public toilets. Appliances should not be flushed down the toilet as they are likely to cause blockage. Burning used appliances is inadvisable: remnants of melted plastic can be a fire hazard in enclosed stoves and create noxious fumes if open fires in the home are used. Some patients do burn equipment on outdoor fires. Non-disposable equipment will require washing, drying, and airing after use, and replacing about every 3 months.

New equipment should be stored in a cool dry environment and rotated so that old stock is used before new. Sufficient stock should be held to ensure that the patient does not run out of equipment. In countries where equipment has to be imported for individual patients, it may to be necessary to hold sufficient stock for 3 to 6 months usage. Where equipment is readily available, patients generally start off with enough equipment for 1 month and reorder when half of this has been used.

Provision of physical and psychological care

A stoma affects, and is affected by, its owner's physical and psychological well being, capabilities, and lifestyle.[21-24] The aim of staff providing palliative care must be to help patients continue as much of their normal way of life as possible with enjoyment, comfort, and satisfaction, using their curtailed lifespan resourcefully to gain the experiences that they want and to complete important tasks and goals. Therefore the components of stoma care and the way in which they are provided should support this overall aim and be responsive to the needs, concerns, and activities of other people (e.g. family, friends, neighbours) who may be involved in stoma care provision as well as those of the patient.[16,25] The general principles and goals of palliative care described in other chapters are also relevant in the care of ostomists and their families. The components of care described below will be required in addition to the overall physical and psychological care needed by all patients.

When stoma surgery is being provided as a palliative strategy

These patients are in a situation where their surgery is not going to cure their disease, but aims to alleviate difficulties (e.g. incontinence, obstruction, pain). As a result these patients:

- lose their normal physical appearance, style of eliminating urine or faeces, and control over when and where they eliminate, and may also lose various parts of the body and sexual functioning depending on the type of operation;
- will either have to learn to manage their own stoma care or allow other people to provide some or all of it.

Patients will need both physical and psychological care in order to gain the information and skills that they require and be helped to cope emotionally and socially with the losses and changes that they experience. Many patients take up to 2 years to come to terms with the effects of stoma surgery, experiencing the stages of loss described by Parkes.[26] Patients whose surgery is palliative may not have time to complete this process before having to contend with further disease or dying. Therefore it is essential that doctors and nurses in regular contact with these patients and their families facilitate the expression of concerns, issues, and feelings appropriately, so that these can be speedily and supportively responded to with the blend of psychological and physical care that is needed.[16,25]

When other palliative interventions are affecting stomal action and management

These patients may be receiving palliative interventions because the same disease which necessitated stoma surgery has advanced or recurred (e.g. cancer, multiple sclerosis), or they may have a stoma because of a previous disease (e.g. ulcerative colitis) and now require treatment for a different disease. In both situations provision of palliative interventions such as radiotherapy; chemotherapy; or analgesics can affect stomal activity and require changes in stoma management. The three most common difficulties are as follows:

- a bowel stoma becomes overactive, often with a more fluid faecal output;
- constipation occurs;
- patients are less able to manage their own stoma care because of the effects of their treatment.

In the first two situations the strategy will partly depend upon the cause, and whether this is likely to be temporary, during provision of treatment, or relatively permanent such as when regular analgesics are required. Other factors to consider are the patient's ability to eat, drink, and take medication; the level of bowel function available after previous surgery; and any constraints or requirements in the style of appliances and skin protectives that the patient can use (see above). An accurate history and examination are essential in order to differentiate constipation with overflow from either constipation or diarrhoea.

The goals in managing an overactive bowel stoma are to reduce the frequency and fluidity of stomal action and to contain the effluent without leakage or skin damage. Reducing stomal activity can take time, and so patients and staff should identify the kind of equipment needed and make any necessary changes. Generally, a drainable standard-sized bag and substantial skin protection will be required to enable the increased volume of effluent to be contained and discarded without frequent changes of equipment which can damage the skin. Increased activity due to chemotherapy may lead patients to wear a drainable appliance at the time of treatments, using their closed colostomy bag in between. Where abdominal or pelvic radiotherapy increases bowel activity, patients may prefer to wear a drainable bag throughout the treatment. If the stoma lies within the radiotherapy field, appliances should not contain metal and should be of minimal depth to avoid interference with skin-sparing techniques.[16,25]

Information about patients' abilities to eat, drink, and take medication should be used to develop appropriate strategies for reducing bowel activity. These include dealing with problems such as nausea or sore mouths as well as directly treating the bowel. Many patients find bran, granules, and high-fibre foods unpalatable in these circumstances, but may manage small tablets or liquid medication. Both patients and their families may need help to plan nutritious and palatable meals.

When constipation occurs, the goals are to relieve the immediate situation and prevent its recurrence. It is important to establish what patients mean by 'constipation' as well as their current patterns of bowel activity, eating, and drinking and whether these differ from normal. Patients taking regular analgesics are likely to require regular laxatives. It is important that patients realize that freedom from pain and constipation can be achieved, and that their treatment achieves this goal.

If faeces have become too hard and will not pass readily through the bowel, patients will require treatment to resolve this problem before establishing a preventative regime. Abdominal and stomal examination should establish whether constipated faeces lie near the stoma only or whether there is faecal material lodged further up the bowel. In the first situation instillation of oil into the stoma may resolve it. In the latter situation patients may also require a laxative which will encourage faeces to move along the bowel, although the presence of recurrent cancer may impede adequate bowel clearance.

As a stoma has no means of retaining suppositories, it is generally best to use a Foley catheter with the balloon inflated to aid retention of an enema. The following procedure is particularly helpful if oil is being given, as once it seeps on to the skin it makes bag adherence difficult.

1. Examine the stoma digitally to identify the direction of the colon and rule out the presence of local tumour. Clean the stoma and peristomal skin as usual.
2. Insert a medium-sized Foley catheter well into the stoma and inflate the balloon to 5 ml.

3. Apply a drainable bag over the stoma and pass the catheter into the bag so it can be reached through its outlet. Make sure a clamp for the catheter and a bag clip are readily available.

4. Instill the warmed oil retention enema gently, and then clamp the catheter, tuck it into the stomabag, and apply its clip.

5. After 10 min (if only the oil is being given) let down the Foley balloon, withdraw the catheter, reclamp the bag, and make the patient comfortable.

If an enema which will attract fluid by osmosis is also to be given (e.g. a phosphate or a Microlax micro-enema), this should be given after the initial 10 min for the oil and the reclamped catheter should be left *in situ* for a further 10 min before removal.

Patients may report constipation when in fact extensive disease is causing obstruction. The number of temporary stomas created for obstruction appear to be decreasing as alternative strategies of symptom control are used.[28] Pharmacological regimens and other measures used in such situations may also aid symptom control in patients with stomas.

Either because of their condition or their palliative treatment, many patients experience tiredness; anxiety; pain, or nausea. In addition, they may be having to learn to manage different equipment for the reasons described above. In these circumstances help from family or staff may be required. Sometimes patients will allow others to empty or change equipment for them. Some patients may insist on changing their own bags, but allow others to prepare new equipment and collect everything needed for their appliance change, thus conserving their own energy for carrying out the change itself. Patients can also be helped to plan the timing of activities efficiently. Firstly, new appliances and skin-protective wafers can be prepared for future use at times when patients have more energy, thus reducing the amount that they have to do when actually changing the appliance. Secondly, patients can schedule appliance changes to coincide with times when they have maximum freedom from pain.

Patients who are easily nauseated should be discouraged from changing appliances just before meal times. Although odour from stomal effluent is rarely a problem when contained in modern appliances, some odour will be present when appliances are emptied or changed. Use of odour-containing sprays at such times may be helpful. Putting a couple of drops of vanilla essence in a bowel stomabag or vinegar in a urostomy bag often reduces odour as effectively as using proprietary powders and liquids. When drainable bags have been emptied, the outlet should be cleaned before replacing the clip, and many patients also like to rinse out drainable bags with warm water after emptying them. Attractive polycotton bag covers hide the contents and also reduce sweating from the plastic. This can be particularly helpful if the bag lies against skin which may be more fragile from radiotherapy to that area.

When the patient is in a preterminal or terminal condition

Ostomists in these situations require all the normal components of terminal care described in other chapters together with the relevant components of the stoma care described above to meet their specific needs and those of their families. Increased nursing care is often provided at such times, giving staff the opportunity to respond to difficulties which occur because of the presence of the stoma. Emptying or changing appliances can be distressing as it brings the patient or relative face to face with signs of his deteriorating condition. For example, stomal output may be minimal due to blockage of bowel or urinary pathways, or the inability of the patient to eat or drink. Changes in body shape and skin condition may make it difficult to obtain good bag adherence and freedom from leakage or skin damage. Patients and their families often welcome invitations to express their fears and feelings following the intimacy of a bag change, and should also have their questions answered with honesty and compassion.

Health care staff often have a compulsion to 'do something' to make such situations better. One of the most helpful activities is for staff to listen to patients' and relatives' accounts of their experiences and needs and seek to really understand them. The experience of being understood and having the burden of their distress shared through its uncurbed expression is cited by many patients and relatives as being a valuable and lasting source of comfort and support.[29,30]

When the patient has a fistula or a nephrostomy

An enterocutaneous fistula is a connection from a hollow viscus directly to the body surface. Patients with either urinary or faecal fistulas can benefit from using stomal equipment and principles of management to contain the fistula output and protect the skin. This makes patients more comfortable and enables the amount and content of fistula output to be accurately estimated and used to aid prescription of suitable nutritional replacements.[1,31] The strategy for choosing stomal equipment and the principles of stoma care outlined earlier should be used in fistula management. There are three particular characteristics which also have to be considered with fistulas:

- the opening is flush with the skin, and so effluent pools in the appliance flange/gasket rather than draining into the bag;
- they often occur in difficult positions such as abdominal creases or in a wound or scar which have to be filled in to create a flat surface before an appliance or protective wafer can adhere without leakages tracking beneath them;
- the output tends to be constant and of considerable volume, so that there is minimal time to clean and dry the surrounding skin and apply new equipment.

Appliances specifically designed for use with bowel fistulas are available. These provide a skin-protective wafer as an integral part of the flange, thus creating a gasket with little depth for the effluent to have to surmount to enter the bag. They also have an outlet which can be used to drain the bag frequently or connect it to a larger drainage bag. Bowel and urinary stomabags of a similar style can also be used. Where the fistula size is reasonably constant, a template can be used to prepare new equipment before the old appliance is removed, but this must be regularly checked for accuracy as the protective wafer must fit really closely around the fistula opening or skin damage will occur. Where a crease or dip needs filling in, it is sometimes possible to apply the paste to the relevant position on the prepared flange/wafer so that it fills in the crease as the new equipment is smoothed into place. It is also extremely useful to have a second person available to use a suction machine to keep the perifistula area free of effluent for long enough to clean and dry it and apply new equipment.

A nephrostomy is a surgically established fistula from the pelvis of the kidney to the body surface. A nephrostomy tube, or fine catheter, is used to channel urine, and its distal end can be inserted into a urostomy bag which is applied over the point where the tube leaves the body. Skin protection around this exit point is advisable as seepage of urine around the nephrostomy tube is common. As the exit point normally lies over the patient's rib cage, ensuring that protective wafers adhere this mobile ridged curved surface can be difficult. A plastic-type film barrier can be applied to the skin and allowed to dry, creating a flexible protective 'extra skin' onto which bags stick well. A soft flexible flanged style of urostomy bag is preferable as this will be reasonably comfortable when the patient lies on it.

Some authorities suggest that the amount of handling needed to insert nephrostomy tubes into urostomy bags has the potential for dislodging them. An alternative management strategy is to protect the skin as above but connect the nephrostomy tube directly to a larger drainage bag. The nephrostomy and bag tubing will need to be anchored lightly to the patient's body to prevent them being pulled on as he or she moves, and special supportive tube holders are available.

Finally, in any situation where care is being given, both the providers and receivers will have goals that they hope will be achieved as a result of this process. In much of this chapter the focus has been on the activities which health care staff should pursue as part of their clinical practice. It is essential to remember that the purpose of these activities is not just to provide elements of care, but is primarily to enable patients and their families to achieve their goals. Unfortunately, some staff identify successful goal achievement as completion of their tasks rather than in terms of whether the effects that task fulfilment has on the patient are what that person required. For example, 'provision of analgesics as prescribed' may be a staff goal but does not necessarily mean that patients achieve their goal of freedom from pain. When goals are identified as above, staff are much less likely to enquire about the patient's experience, yet that is where the focus should be. Accurate and empathetic understanding of each patient's situation and requirements is vital if care is to focus on meeting their needs. Staff must also learn to identify and evaluate goals in terms of the outcome for patients.[16,29] This includes patients being satisfied with the amount of information they have been given and understood, having acquired sufficient skills to manage their stoma care competently and confidently; and being able to understand and cope with their situation in ways that they find helpful.

References

1. Elcoat C. *Stoma Care Nursing.* London: Ballière Tindall, 1986.
2. Hampton BG, Bryant RA, eds. *Ostomies and Continent Diversions: Nursing Management.* St Louis, MO: Mosby, 1992.
3. Hohenfellner R, Wammack R, eds. *Continent Urinary Diversion. Societé Internationale d'Urologie Reports.* Edinburgh: Churchill Livingstone, 1992.
4. Lever, RB. Reconstructive surgery for promotion of continence. In: Laker C, ed. *Urological Nursing.* Harrow: Scutari Press, 1994.
5. Hawley PR, Thompson JPS. Colon. In: Kirk, RM. ed. *General Surgical Operations.* 3rd edn. Edinburgh: Churchill Livingstone, 1994:271–95.
6. Schofield PF, Jones DJ. Colorectal neoplasia III: treatment and prevention. In: Jones DJ, Irving MH, eds. *ABC of Colorectal Diseases.* London: BMJ, 1993:61–4.
7. Calne R, Pollard S, eds. *Operative Surgery.* London: Gower Medical, 1992.
8. Young CH, Shipes E. Sexual implications of stoma surgery. In: Brooke BN, Jeter KF, Todd IP, eds. *Clinics in Gastroenterology. Stomas.* London: WB Saunders, 1982:383–96.
9. Kolodny RC, Masters WH, Johnson VE, Biggs MA. *Textbook of Human Sexuality for Nurses.* Boston, MA: Little, Brown, 1979.
10. Topping A. Sexual activity and the stoma patient. *Nursing Standard,* 1990; 4(41):24–6..
11. Bensimon H. *Urologic Surgery.* New York: McGraw-Hill, 1991.
12. Pontes JE. *Surgery of Genito-urinary Pelvic Tumours: An Anatomic Atlas.* New York: Wiley, 1993.
13. Lawson AL. Urinary stomas and their management. In: Breckman B, ed. *Stoma Care.* Beaconsfield: Beaconsfield Publishers, 1981: 95–111.
14. Paulson DE. Radical cystectomy. In: Glenn JF, ed. *Urologic Surgery.* 4th edn. Philadelphia, PA: JB Lippincott, 1991:439–54.
15. Nordstrom GM, Nyman CR. Living with a urostomy: a follow-up with special regard to the peristomal skin complications, psychosocial and sexual life. *World Council of Enterostomal Therapists. Proceedings of the 9th Biennial Congress, Lyon, 6–10 July 1992.* Libertyville,Illinois: Hollister, 1992:49–53.
16. Breckman B, ed. *Stoma Care.* 2nd edn. Beaconsfield, UK: Beaconsfield Publishers, in preparation.
17. Turnbull GB. The tri-laminate hydrocolloid wafer: a new approach to convexity. *World Council of Enterostomal Therapists. Proceedings of the 9th Biennial Congress, Lyon, 6–10 July 1992.* Libertyville, Illinois: Hollister, 1992: 56–61.
18. Tappe AT. Integral convexity in a two-piece bodyside wafer. *World Council of Enterostomal Therapists. Proceedings of the 9th Biennial Congress, Lyon, 6–10 July 1992.* Libertyville, Illinois: Hollister, 1992:62–5.
19. Royle JA, Walsh M, eds. *Watson's Medical–Surgical Nursing and Related Physiology.* 4th edn. London: Ballière Tindall, 1992:502–14; 675–8.
20. Reilly NJ. Cancer of the bladder. In: Karlowicz KA, ed. *Urologic Nursing: Principles and Practice.* Philadelphia, PA: WB Saunders, 1995: 262–70.
21. Wade B. *A Stoma Is For Life.* Harrow: Scutari Press, 1989.
22. Breckman B. Success by stages. *Senior Nurse,* 1986; 5(3): 14–16.
23. Salter M, ed. *Altered Body Image—The Nurse's Role.* Chichester: Wiley, 1988.
24. Hanson EJ. *The Cancer Nurse's Perspective: Stress and the Person with Cancer.* Lancaster: Quay Publishing, 1994.
25. Topping A. Nursing patients with tumours of the gastrointestinal tract. In: Tiffany R, Borley D, eds. *Oncology for Nurses and Health Care Professionals.* Vol. 3, *Cancer nursing.* 2nd edn. London: Harper Collins, 1991:281–308.
26. Parkes CM. *Bereavement.* 2nd edn. Harmondsworth: Penguin, 1986.
27. Breckman B. *Stoma Care.* Beaconsfield: Beaconsfield Publishers, 1981.
28. Baines M. The pathophysiology and management of malignant intestinal obstruction. In: Doyle D, Hanks GWC, Macdonald N, eds. *Oxford Textbook of Palliative Medicine.* Oxford University Press, 1993: 311–16.
29. Nichols KA. *Psychological Care in Physical illness.* 2nd edn. London: Chapman and Hall, 1993.
30. Buckman R. Communication in palliative care: a practical guide. In: Doyle D, Hanks GWC, Macdonald N, eds. *Oxford Textbook of Palliative Medicine.* Oxford University Press, 1993: 47–61.
31. Frost S. Managing high-output fistulae. *Nursing Standard,* 1991: 5(51):25–7.

12.5 Speech therapy

Susan D. Clark

In this chapter the role of the speech and language therapist is considered under two headings, communication disorders and swallowing disorders.

Communication disorders

Inability to communicate is not a loss of life but a loss of access to life. If patients cannot convey their thoughts, they are isolated. A multidisciplinary approach is essential, and it must be carefully coordinated to ensure the minimum of overlap. The aim of all team members involved in palliative care is to improve the quality of remaining life. The specific role of the speech therapist is to maintain that access to life through communication for as long as possible.

Additional aims are as follows:

(1) to ensure that patients are using all communication modalities including gesture and writing to supplement speech;

(2) to introduce communication aids at the correct time, bearing in mind that each aid may be superseded by a different aid or switching device to match the patient's changing physical condition;

(3) to educate carers to change their communication strategies in order to optimize communication at home;

(4) to provide ongoing counselling to enable families to discuss the impact of the disorder on their family dynamics and to accept subsequent change.

Maintaining communication

In some conditions encountered in palliative care, for example progressive neuromuscular disorders, speech disorders are common, whereas in others dysarthria (articulatory disorders) and dysphonia (loss of voice) are the main barriers to verbal communication. Scott *et al.*[1] state that half of patients with Parkinson's disease develop dysarthria and/or dysphonia during the course of the disease. More than 90 per cent of patients with motor neurone disease become dysarthric, and 80 per cent of these will become unintelligible prior to death. Whether patients develop communication problems in multiple sclerosis depends on the area of the brain affected by the disease, but at least 50 per cent will have some degree of speech or language deficit. Communication disorders may also occur in patients with Huntington's chorea, cerebral and cerebellar atrophy, or myasthenia gravis. Patients with cerebral tumours may suffer dysphasia (loss of language) if the tumour is sited in the dominant hemisphere.

Another major group comprises patients with local malignant disease affecting, in particular, the tongue, pharynx, and larynx. The treatment itself (surgery, chemotherapy, radiotherapy, or combinations of these) may compound problems of verbal communication, and where laryngectomy is performed the patient has no choice but to learn alternative methods of speech and communication.

It is important that patients should be referred to the therapist in the early stages of the disease so that they can be given advice on speech conservation and begin a relationship before speech is lost.

Assessment

Dysarthria and dysphonia

Intelligibility of speech needs to be assessed not only in hospital, but also in the various environments in which patients need to make themselves understood. Specific assessment must be made at each level of the vocal tract: respiration affecting volume, laryngeal function affecting resonance, and efficacy of facial musculature and articulators.

How well patients communicate, particularly through eye contact, gesture, and facial expression, must be assessed as the listener gains important imformation in these ways. Patients are at a great disadvantage if facial muscles become immobile, as the ability to show feelings is lost.

Emotional lability may be present, and it should be emphasized to carers that if patients cry suddenly and uncontrollably they are not as distressed as may appear. Changing the subject can ease the tension. Uncontrolled laughter is easier to cope with! Depression is common in patients with speech disorders; Gotham *et al.*[2] reported that 30 per cent of patients with Parkinson's disease show signs of depression, and they suggest that antidepressant medication should be given to this group of patients if therapy is to be successful.

Receptive and expressive dysphasia

Receptive and expressive dysphasia are uncommon in progressive neuromuscular disease. Some patients with Parkinson's disease complain of mild word-finding difficulty and/or 'thought freezing'. High-level comprehension deficits, where the subtleties of meaning conveyed by complex intonation patterns, for example appreciation of irony, sarcasm, or a play on words, may be associated with dementia. A minority of patients with multiple sclerosis have difficulty in understanding what is said, and in recalling the vocabulary and grammar necessary to produce a sentence.

Patients, particularly those with cerebral tumours in the dominant hemisphere, may suffer a severe reduction in their ability to understand speech and/or the written word. Speaking and writing may be similarly affected. A language assessment by a speech and language therapist is essential to determine the degree of impairment and advice to be given to carers and medical staff. Common problems are confusion over semantically related words: 'yes' may be said when 'no' is the appropriate answer. Patients may be able to sing hymns or songs but not be able to converse, or may talk in jargon words which are unfamiliar to the listener.

Dyspraxia

Dyspraxia may be experienced by a few patients. This is an inability to programme the positioning and sequencing of muscle movements for articulation, causing difficulty in converting the remembered word into the physical representation needed for sound production.

Therapy

The speech and language therapist aims to achieve the best use of the damaged vocal mechanism for as long as possible. It is essential that patients and their carers are aware of the diagnosis and prognosis so that they do not have unrealistic expectations of their therapy programme. Realistic alternative ways of communication need to be established before speech is lost altogether.

In the early stages of the disease the mechanics of speaking, the specific problems of the patient, and proposed therapy to conserve speech should be explained, and appropriate leaflets should be made available (see Appendix 1) Although speech will continue to deteriorate, speech therapy intervention will maintain intelligibility, maximize speaking potential, and help patients to identify their communication problems and monitor their own speech.

Breathing

Many patients have decreased pulmonary function. Deep-breathing exercises using the diaphragm will help them avoid running out of breath at the end of a phrase. If the patient is only able to take shallow breaths, these should be combined with the use of shorter sentences or phrases. Patients need to be aware of increased difficulty of being understood against background noise or when fatigued.

Phonation

Linked with poor breath support are phonatory problems. The voice may be difficult to initiate, or may be weak, breathy, strained, or intermittent. Exercises may be required for patients to synchronize respiration and phonation. A patient who has difficulty in sustaining his or her voice throughout the length of a sentence will be able to improve auditory awareness by using audio tapes or a laryngograph which demonstrates the voice visually. Electrodes are placed on both sides of the thyroid cartilage at the level of the vocal cords. When the vocal cords adduct, the electric current increases and a waveform will be shown on the monitor. Patients with these problems often speak in a monotone with reduced pitch levels in conversation. The laryngograph will produce a histogram of pitch change for single words or sentences. This tracing on a bar chart can act as a visual guide which patients can use to improve their intonation. To extend pitch range they should concentrate on achieving different pitches (low, middle, or high). Subtle changes in inflexion can be introduced by varying pitch, such as changing a statement into a question: for example the statement 'It is hot today' can be changed to the question 'It is *hot* today?'. Putting stress on a different word in a sentence to alter its meaning will heighten the patient's awareness of the importance of stress.

Prosody

Some patients find it difficult to control the rhythm of speech, and conversation becomes faster and faster until it becomes unintelligible. A metronome or pace board can help to develop syllabic speech and slow conversation into an easy steady rate. A pace board is a small wooden tray with raised slats, similar to the rungs of a ladder, and patients move their fingers using each rung for a syllable. Either aid can be used for practising polysyllabic words to slow down conversation.

Articulation

Patients should be made aware of the positioning of tongue and lips for speech sounds; for example the consonants 't' and 'd' are made by using the front of the tongue, 'k' and 'g' are made by using the back of the tongue, and 'p', 'b', and 'm' involve firm lip closure. Therapy may involve improving the clarity of individual consonants or consonant blends (e.g. 'str', 'scr', etc.), and clarity may also be improved by changing the rate of speech, emphasizing stress and pauses. Phrases and short sentences can be used to conserve energy.[3] Patients need to be taught to monitor their own intelligibility and deterioration when fatigued, so that they give themselves a rest period. Patients who mumble need to exaggerate jaw, lip, and facial movement; this can be done by using the exaggerated vowel movements 'aa', 'ee', 'oo'. These exercises help to compensate for muscular rigidity.

Dentures

As disease progresses and patients lose weight, facial muscle tone will alter and dentures may become loose, affecting speech and eating. Relining or a dental fixative may maintain denture use for a longer period.

Palatal weakness

Patients with palatal incompetence need to be made aware of hypernasality. This can be done by improving auditory awareness with the use of a tape recorder, or with a nasal anemometer (Fig. 1) which visually displays nasal escape of air during speech. The nasopharynx is open for the production of 'n', 'm', and 'ng', and these consonants can be used to help the patient to gain contrast between oral and nasal resonance, for example 'may' and 'bay'. If palatal incompetence is the overriding problem and articulation is adequate, a palatal lift or loop (Fig. 2) fitted by an orthodontist will help alleviate nasal escape.

Tension

If speech musculature is hypertonic, tension will be increased. If the patient concentrates on beginning a sentence in an easy relaxed manner, spasticity in affected muscles will be reduced. Relaxation tapes and exercises, including awareness of general body posture, are important.

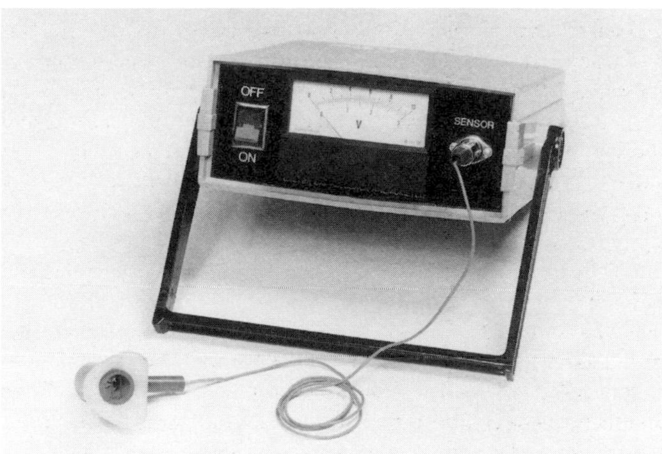

Fig. 1 Nasal anemometer.

General considerations

Patients and carers should be aware that speech will deteriorate if patients are tired, such as in the evening, or if demands to communicate have been increased. This can happen over very short periods of time, for example after a conversation lasting for only 5 min. It should also be remembered that listening is tiring for carers because they invest a lot of energy in compensating for poor communication from the patients. In fact it may be more emotionally tiring for carers and listeners than for the patient.

Listeners should allow patients time to communicate, they should not interrupt or finish sentences for them, and they should not shout, for the patients are not deaf. If the listener has not understood what the patient has said, the patient should be asked to repeat or rephrase the sentence and encouraged to talk slowly. Patient and listener should sit in a quiet room rather than talk over noise. Listeners should watch the patient's face for extra clues when he or she is talking, and observe the general body posture and language.

Communication aids

The possibility of needing a communication aid should be discussed before speech is lost. Patients are frequently resistant to the idea of an alternative means of communication, but it is important to raise this issue as it helps them to become accustomed to the idea of communicating without speech and gives them and their carers time to learn how to use the device.

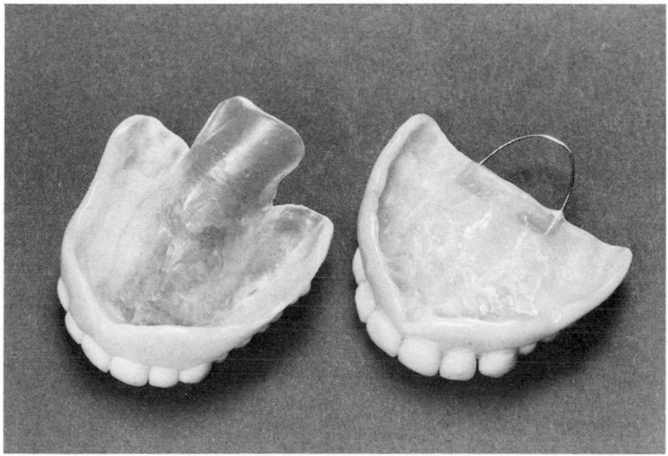

Fig. 2 (a) Palatal lift and (b) palatal loop.

Where possible, equipment should be adaptable to cope with the patient's changing abilities. A non-electric communication aid need only be provided as a back-up if powerful battery packs or rechargeable batteries are not supplied. Initially an aid may augment verbal or written communication, for instance at the end of the day when the patient is tired. Writing is the obvious alternative to speech if the muscles of the hand are strong enough to control a pen and coordination is adequate. As dexterity declines, clipboards can be used to keep the paper in place and foam-rubber pads around pens provide a larger diameter which requires less effort to grip and control. A pencil will give better friction than a ballpoint pen which tends to slip across the paper.

Before providing a communication aid a number of factors need to be considered:

(1) the patient's communication needs in various environments;

(2) the patient's environment;

(3) the patient's motivation and ability to use the aid;

(4) the patient's ability to understand the spoken and written word;

(5) the patient's physical ability to operate a communication aid;

(6) the needs of the main listener (for instance if the carer is deaf, an aid with a speech synthesizer may be inappropriate).

Electronic communication aids

Bearing in mind the above points, a variety of equipment is available on loan from communication aids centres or associations representing a particular disease (see Appendix 1). Speech and language therapists attached to the centres are able to assess patients for appropriate equipment. The assessment team frequently includes an occupational therapist and a rehabilitation engineer to give advice on adapting equipment to meet the patient's needs. Common adaptations may involve changing the angle of a table on which the aid stands, or fixing a microphone to a movable stand if the patient's arms are too weak to hold it up to the mouth.

All the communication aids described in this chapter are available world-wide.

Canon Communicator

The Canon Communicator (see Appendix 2) is a light-weight portable communication aid for keyboard and/or switch users. The user types the message on a QWERTY or ABCDE keyboard and it is then printed out on a ticker-tape printer. Alternatively, a row of scanning red lights on the right and bottom edges of the keyboard enables switch users to operate the Communicator via a single switch.

The CC-7S model has recording and playback features capable of up to 240 s of average quality recorded speech. The CC-7S/CC-7P Communicator is equipped with a message memory function which stores a total of up to 7000 characters under the 26 alphabet keys. This function allows rapid print-outs of frequently used phrases. With the CC-7S, it is possible to program the

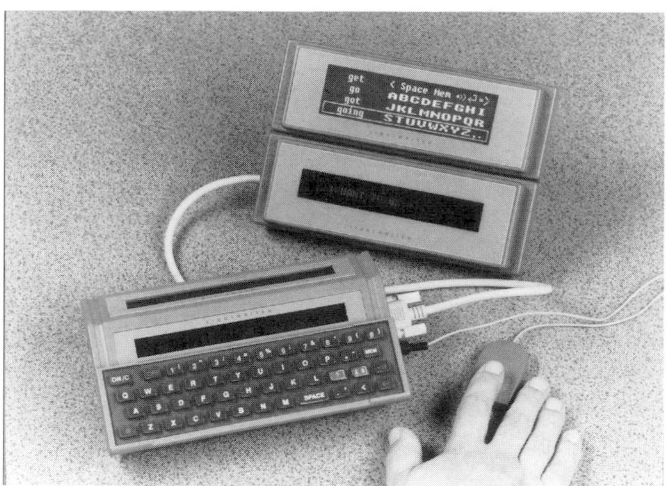

Fig. 3 Lightwriter SL35 with plug-in scan module.

message memory for simultaneous playback and print-out. Characters can be printed out in double width for easy viewing. Additional features are a waterproof saliva guard, a wheelchair mounting kit, a print window magnifier, a spare battery pack, an interface cable, a single-line display and plug-in, and armbelt or extension belts for attaching the Communicator to the arm or other parts of the body. The Communicator has an integral calculator function.

Memowriter

The Memowriter (see Appendix 2) has a till-roll printer for written output as well as a visual display window. A memory display facility can store 26 messages, which can be recalled by pressing two keys.

Lightwriter SL35

The Lightwriter SL35 (Fig. 3) (see Appendix 2) is an enhanced version of the SL30. The user types in a message on the keyboard which is then displayed on a two-way display, with one side facing the user and the other facing the communication partner. The speech output can reinforce the visual display if the communication partner has a visual impairment. For users with visual impairment or physical difficulties, a keyguard can be fitted with reference points and the speech system can be set to speak each letter as it is selected. The back-to-back message displays are available in vacuum fluorescent display, an option which is preferable to the standard liquid crystal display in some light conditions, particularly for people with impaired eyesight.

The SL35 has three speech synthesizers: Articulate, EuroTalk, and DECtalk. The DECtalk synthesizer is advisable if the Lightwriter is to be used in conjunction with the telephone, and has a range of four male voices, four female voices, and one child's voice.

The word prediction facility includes the 4000 most frequently used English words. This facility may benefit keyboard users who are slow around the keyboard, are poor spellers, or who have difficulty finishing words. Two types of keyboard are available, one with a rubberized 'calculator' feel and the other with a flat membrane which is easier to wipe clean. The QWERTY layout is standard, but an alphabetical layout is also available. The SL35 will store up to 8000 characters and up to 36 direct memories. Letter combinations can be stored to represent phrases. For example 'H H' could be defined as 'Hello how are you'; when the user enters 'H H' the expanded phrase is substituted.

The Lightwriter SL35 will connect to Macintosh or IBM-compatible computers to copy and/or program user memories and abbreviation expansions, and can also be used as an alternative keyboard for input to a computer. It has a built-in rechargeable battery, a mains adaptor, a wheelchair mounting kit, and a wrist strap. It is offered with a full range of European languages either internally or with a speech synthesizer. Operating instructions and a Help section are built into the SL35 so that the user can refer to them without reference to the handbook.

The Lightwriter is a light-weight easily portable communication aid, and is the first of its size to house the DECtalk synthesizer internally.

Lightwriter SL4b

The Lightwriter SL4b has replaced the SL4a and has all the SL35 facilities. The larger keys and wider key spacing are preferred by some users, and the brightness of the vacuum fluorescent displays can be controlled by the user. The inclusion of the extra facilities means that the integral printer is no longer available.

Giant Lightwriter

The Giant Lightwriter (Fig. 4) is an oversize communication aid which is specifically designed for people with ataxia or poor motor control who cannot access a standard size keyboard. A variety of scanning lightwriters are available for people who are unable to use a keyboard.

Lightwriter SL85

The Lightwriter SL85 is a small portable scanning communication aid for switch users. It replaces the SL8 lightwriter. The back-lit display can be set up with a QWERTY, alphabetical, or frequency layout. It has large bold letters on Scan Screen, which can be backlit for greater legibility. Word prediction increases typing speed and reduces fatigue. The same speech options are available as with the SL35. A plug-in keyboard is supplied to allow faster entry of memories and change of set-ups by the therapist or carer. There are three choices of scanning method: automatic scanning with a single switch, step scanning with two switches, and a mouse or other pointing device. Switching can be performed by suck–puff,

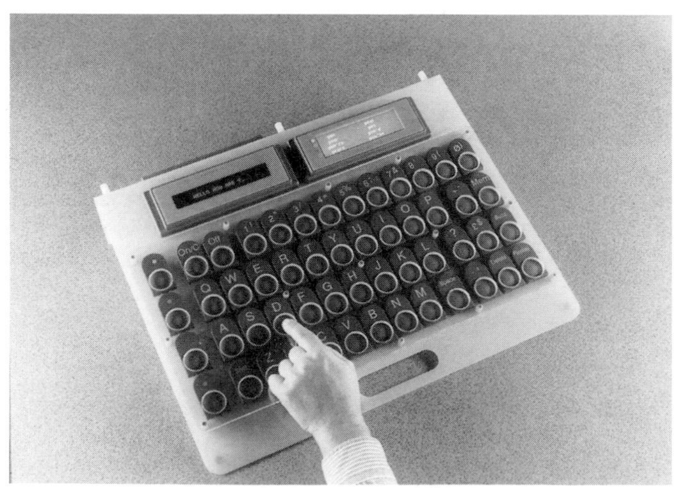

Fig. 4 Giant Lightwriter.

air pad, button, touch, click, squeeze, foot, or eyeblink, depending on the disability of the user. Adjustable antitremor delay is built in to prevent inadvertent operation by users with poor hand control.

SL35 Scan module

An add-on scan screen is an option for users with progressive conditions who become unable to use the keyboard of the SL35 model (Fig. 3) It plugs into the SL35 serial port and allows the user to scan with a switch. This allows the user to continue with the same machine, and the transition from keyboard to scanning is at the user's own pace. The keyboard is available to therapists and carers for faster entry of memories and change of set-ups, avoiding the need to transfer user memories from a keyboard aid to a scanning aid.

The Cameleon

The Cameleon is custom-built, flexible, and easy to use. It is based around an IBM-compatible laptop computer and is available with a choice of four voice synthesizers: Speech Plus, DECtalk, Smoothtalker and Apollo. The Cameleon can be mounted on a wheelchair and consists of a medium-sized box with a small computer screen. Any words and software can be incorporated in the Cameleon, providing spoken output, word processing, and total computer access for switch, touchscreen, or limited keyboard users. The EZ Keys for Windows package offers facilities such as dual word prediction (predicting the six most likely words to follow the word just finished), Abbreviation Expansion (allowing use of abbreviations to represent longer sentences), and Instant Phrases (allowing speedy access to groups of up to 1000 prestored phrases). These can be used in conjunction with word-processing packages and the Side Talk screen aimed at producing spontaneous speech. The word-prediction box can be enlarged to help those with visual impairment. EZ Keys also allows extensive environmental control capabilities (when used in conjunction with additional equipment) and access to telecommunication facilities via a modem.

Mini-Commac

Even when combined with the Gateway 486 subnotebook computer, this system weighs only 6 lb (2.7 kg), so that it is easily portable. It comes with a voice synthesizer and will run all the software available with the Cameleon.

General considerations

The therapist must ensure that patients are able to use equipment efficiently and that carers know how to maintain it. Trained volunteers working with the speech and language therapist and the patients can provide the extra help necessary for patients to become proficient with the aids.

Regular involvement with the speech and language therapist is essential as the type of communication aid required will change as the patient deteriorates. Patients often revert to a communication board or E Tran frame (see below) towards the end of their life. These aids demand less effort on the part of the patient, but maximum concentration and patience on the part of the listener.

Non-electronic communication aids

Communication board

The simplest form of aid is a communication board produced jointly by the patient, carer, and therapist. It may include commonly used phrases, words, pictures, and numbers in addition, or as an alternative, to the alphabet.

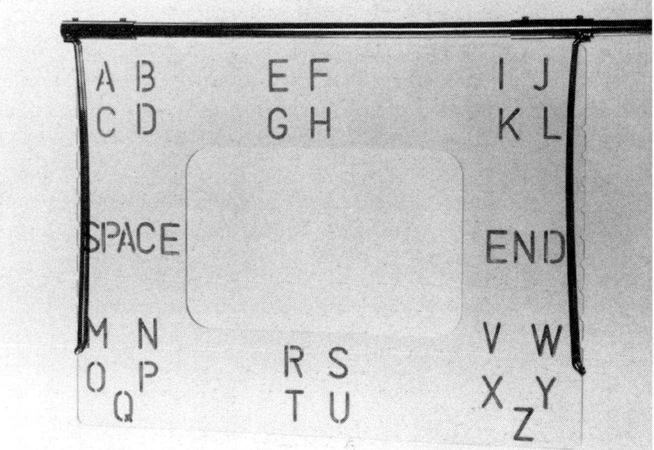

Fig. 5 E-Tran frame.

Communication booklet

A communication booklet is similar to a small Filofax with sections of blank sheets separated by pages containing thumb-tabs on which symbols are printed. The symbols designate particular categories about which the user may wish to communicate, for example food, clothes, feelings, etc. Pictures, words, symbols, etc., can be drawn or stuck onto blank pages within the appropriate category. When wishing to convey a message the user turns to the appropriate section and points to a picture, word, symbol or letter. The communication board or communication booklet can augment or replace speech using the patient's most reliable movement.

E-Tran frame

An E-Tran frame (Fig. 5) can be a lifeline to patients who are cognitively intact but have lost all limb movement as well as speech. The frame has a colour-coded alphabet to spell out words, using eye pointing only. It consists of a Perspex rectangle with the centre cut out which is placed between the user and the listener and allows face-to-face communication. The basic principle is that letters of the alphabet are drawn in groups around the frame and are colour coded. Each corner represents a colour. To indicate a letter the user looks to the group of letters and then to the appropriate coloured corner. If a patient has difficulty with spelling, symbols can replace letters. The advantages of the E-Tran frame are that it is very easy to use, requires very little physical movement, is portable, can be quicker than scanning or switch-operated system, and is relatively inexpensive. The disadvantages are that it has no speech, written, or printed output, and that the user is dependent on the communicative partner to pick up the 'messages'.

Amplifiers

Any disorder that reduces the volume of the voice to a whisper can be helped by an amplifier. A variety of pocket-size amplifiers are available. They come with a choice of hand-held, lapel, or headset microphones, with the option of an extension speaker. A special clip can be used to attach the microphone to the side-piece of spectacles. Amplifiers will not help patients with marked dysarthria as only the slurred articulation will be amplified (see Appendix 2).

Use of the telephone

Patients often wish to remain in their own homes and to be independent for as long as possible. Converse telephones amplify incoming and outgoing speech, and have on-hook dialling. Claudius II can be connected to any modern telephone, and can speak up to 52 recorded messages by pressing buttons on the keypad. It can also be used for face-to-face conversations without a telephone. Literature is available from telephone companies.

Communication aids for the visually impaired

A number of the communication aids already mentioned have adaptations for the visually impaired. Talking books (See Appendix 1) are available when large-print books are no longer appropriate.

Communication following oral or laryngeal cancer

Preoperative counselling

Therapy with patients suffering from oral or laryngeal cancer begins with preoperative counselling. Murrils[5] suggests that such counselling has five major aims:

(1) to establish a relationship and to provide support and reassurance for both patient and carer;

(2) to take a detailed case history and to assess present communication skills;

(3) to provide information regarding normal speech production;

(4) to assist the patient to prepare for subsequent complete or partial voice loss;

(5) to discuss alternative methods of communication.

Following a laryngectomy, most patients develop pseudo-voice either via oesophageal voice or by insertion of a voice prosthesis.

Communication aids

Communication aids may be used immediately following surgery or with patients who fail to achieve a pseudo-voice. The intra-oral type of electronic speech aid (e.g. the Cooper–Rand (see Appendix 2)) can be used soon after surgery as the mouthpiece does not interfere with the surgically affected neck area. The Servox artificial larynx (see Appendix 2) is held in the hand with the vibrating head placed firmly against the neck, allowing sound vibrations to be introduced through the skin into the vocal tract to be articulated into speech.

Swallowing disorders

The physiology, incidence, and treatment of dysphagia are discussed in Chapter 9.3.2. Speech and language therapists are involved in swallowing disorders because of their specialized knowledge of the structure, muscles, and nerves associated with swallowing. The role of the speech therapist is as follows.

1. Assessment of the dysphagic problem; the most common problems are a weak cough reflex, difficulty with feeding at the oral or pharyngeal stage of the swallow, and risk of aspiration.
2. Maximizing residual function and anticipating future decline in swallowing.
3. Recommending alternative feeding options if eating should become unsafe or undesirable.

The timing and degree of intervention is determined in consultation with patients, carers, and staff.[5] Management of dysphagia always involves teamwork, ideally in conjunction with some or all of the following: medical and nursing staff, dietitian, physiotherapist, occupational therapist, radiologist, and social worker.

Assessment

Following examination, the therapist will be able to assess the following:

(1) the best position to place food in the mouth;

(2) the best food consistency for the patient;

(3) the posture that will result in the most proficient swallow;

(4) the patient's awareness of secretions, general alertness, affect, motivation, and ability to understand verbal or written instructions;

(5) the efficiency of tongue, lip, palate, and laryngeal function.

Therapy

Lip and tongue exercises

Lip seal and tongue exercises may be appropriate in the early stages of progressive disease. Patients should be encouraged to search for food with the tongue, stretch the tongue, bite firmly, and form better lip closure. Oral motor control of the bolus can be improved by dipping an oral sponge into liquid and sucking the liquid from the sponge using the back of the tongue, holding the liquid in the mouth, and controlling the swallow using the preferred head posture.

Thermal stimulation

The swallow reflex can be achieved by stimulating the base of the anterior faucial arch on each side using a long-handled laryngeal mirror which has been held in iced water; light contact is repeated five to ten times on each side.[6] If a dry swallow appears normal, iced water can be administered from a syringe starting with 2 ml of liquid. If this is successful, amounts may be increased.

Voluntary protection of the airway

With this technique the patient is asked to take a breath, hold it, place food in the mouth, tilt the head forward, and swallow. A cough is essential after each swallow to rid the pharynx of any residue. In this sequence voluntary protection of the airway prevents any aspiration that may occur before the swallow reflex is triggered.

Vocal cord closure

Protection of the airway can be improved by increasing the efficiency of vocal cord adduction if the patient has an ineffectual cough. Patients should hold their breath while pushing down on a chair for 5 to 10 seconds.

Palatal appliances

Where there is reduced palatal competency, a palatal loop may assist stimulation of movement or, later in the disease, a palatal lift may lessen nasal escape (Fig. 2).[3,7] Assessment by an orthodontist is advisable. Such appliances can be added to existing dentures.

Oral feeding

Tremor, spasticity, or loss of upper-limb movement may make it difficult or impossible to get food or drink to the mouth. Adapted cutlery and crockery, Pat Saunders straws which have a one-way valve, an Autosip machine (Appendix 1) which can be activated by any reliable movement, syringes, and mobile arm supports can be invaluable. Occupational therapy, physiotherapy, and medical physics departments can adapt equipment for the particular needs of the patient. Liquidizers and thickening agents can be used to obtain the safest texture for the patient. It is important to remember that chemotherapy and radiotherapy may alter the flavour of food. Dairy produce may cause excessive mucus, resulting in distressing drooling. The first indication of dysphagia in progressive disease is often an inability to chew salads. Attention should be paid to the environmental aspects of eating, such as calmness on the part of the feeder, privacy, and freedom from distractions. Consideration of the sensory aspects of fluid and food is important (e.g. taste, smell, appearance, texture, temperature), as is remembering to include only food that the patient enjoys.[8]

Initiation of the swallow may be helped by the following:

(1) giving food which has a strong flavour;

(2) sips of iced water between mouthfuls;

(3) talking the patient through the swallowing routine;

(4) altering the head position.

Head posture alters the way that gravity carries food through the pharynx. i.e. the head-forward position helps to trigger the swallow and increases the epiglottic protection of the airway if there is reduced laryngeal closure.[6] The swallowing routine should be written down for patient, carer, nursing staff, and medical staff to follow.

Non-oral feeding

Patients who are not helped by alternative swallowing strategies or different food textures, or who aspirate more than 10 per cent of swallowed material, may require non-oral feeding.[9] This is indicated when patients become dehydrated and malnourished through inadequate oral intake of food, although otherwise the quality of life remains good. A gastrostomy is generally preferred to nasogastric feeding as it can be concealed and it is easier for the patient to obtain adequate nourishment. Croghan *et al.*[10] found that patients with nasogastric tubes had a higher death rate (7/9) than patients with gastrostomy tubes (2/80; $p < 0.05$).

Tube feeding may improve the quality of life and maintain weight and functional status in some patients receiving surgery and radiotherapy for head and neck malignancies.[11]

Conclusion

The aim of this chapter has been to show the role of the speech and language therapist in enhancing and maintaining the quality of life of patients for whom there is no cure, and also to offer better control of symptoms, thus giving patients happy and useful lives for as long as possible. As C.S.Lewis wrote in *A Grief Observed*, 'It is incredible how much happiness, even gaiety, we sometimes had together after all hope of recovery was gone'.

Appendix 1

Relevant associations and societies

The Royal College of Speech and Language Therapists, 7 Bath Place, Rivington Street, London NW11 8ER, UK. Tel. +44–0171–613–3855

Parkinson's Disease Association, 2 Upper Woburn Place, London WC1H ORA, UK. Tel. + 44-0171-383-3513

Parkinson's Disease Association, PO Box 2408, North Parramatta, Sydney 2151, NSW, Australia

International Alliance of ALS/MND Associations, PO Box 246, Northampton NN1 1PR, UK. Tel. +44-01604-250505

International Federation of Multiple Sclerosis Societies, 10 Heddon Street, London W1R 7LJ, UK. Tel. +44-0171-734-9120

Multiple Sclerosis Society, 25 Effie Street, London SW6 1EE, UK. Tel. +44-0171-736-6267. Professionals' helpline +44-0171-371-8000

Huntington's Chorea Association, 108 Battersea High Street, London SW11 3HP, UK. Tel. +44-0171-223-7000

National Association of Laryngectomee Clubs, Ground Floor, 6 Pickett Street, London SW1 1RU, UK. Tel. +44-0171-381-9993

Chattanooga Choo Choo Lost Cord Club, PO Box 1011, Dalton, GA 30722, USA

Talking books

National Listening Library, 12 Lant Street, London SE1 1QH, UK. Tel. +44-0171-4079417

Autosip

Brunel Institute for Bioengineering, Brunel University, Uxbridge, Middx UB8 3PH, UK

Pat Saunders drinking straw

Nottingham Rehab Ltd, 17 Ludlow Hill Road, West Bridgford, Nottingham NG2 6HD, UK. Tel. +44-01159-452345

Appendix 2

Communication aids

Communication Aids List

Disabled Living Foundation, 380–384 Harrow Road, London W9 2HU, UK. Tel. +44-0171-289-6111

Canon Communicator

Canon UK Ltd, Canon House, Manor Road, Wallington, Surrey SM6 0AJ, UK.

Canon USA. Inc., One Canon Plaza, Lake Success, NY 11042, USA.

Memowriter

Easiaids Ltd, 5 Woodcote Park Avenue, Purley, Surrey CR8 3NH, UK. Tel. +44-0181-763-0203

Lightwriter

Toby Churchill Ltd, 20 Panton Street, Cambridge CB2 1HP, UK. Tel. +44-0223-462037

Campac

Cambridge Adaptive Communication, The Mount, Toft, Cambridge CB3 7RL, UK. Tel. +44-0223-264244

Amplifiers

Kapitex Healthcare Ltd, Kapitex House, 1 Sandbeck House, Wetherby, West Yorks LS22 4GH, UK. Tel. +44-0191-580211

Lions Club International, c/o 3 Campbell Close, Linden Village, Buckingham MK18 7HP, UK. Tel. +44-01280-813747

References

1. Scott S, Caird FI, Williams BO. *Communication in Parkinson's Disease*. London: Croom Helm, 1985.
2. Gotham AM, Brown RG, Marsden CD. Depression in Parkinson's Disease; a quantatative and qualitative analysis. *Journal of Neurology, Neursurgery and Psychiatry*, 1986; **46**:381–9.
3. Enderby PM, Langton Hewer W. Communication and swallowing: problems and aids. In: Cochrane GM, ed. *The Management of Motor Neurone Disease*. Edinburgh: Churchill Livingstone, 1987.
4. Murrils G. Pre- and early post-operative care of the laryngectomee and spouse. In: Edels Y, ed. *Laryngectomy: Diagnosis to Rehabilitation*. London: Croom Helm, 1983.
5. Serrandura A, Hill P. *Transitional Feeding—The Team Approach*. Fullarton, Australia: Julia Farr Centre, 1989.
6. Logemann J. *Evaluation and Treatment of Swallowing Disorders*. Boston, MA: College Hill Press, 1983.
7. Enderby PM, Hawthorne I, Servant S. The use of intra-oral appliances in the management of velopharyngeal disorders. *British Dental Journal*, 1984; **157**:157–60.
8. Scott A, Austin HNG. Feeding in the management of severe dysphagia in M.N.D. *Palliative Medicine*, 1994; **8**:45–9.
9. Reynard CFB. Managing dysphagia in advanced cancer—a flow diagram. *Palliative Medicine*, 1990; **4**:215–18.
10. Croghan JE, Burke EM, Caplan S, Denman S. Pilot study of 12-month outcome of nursing home patients with aspiration on videofluoroscopy. *Dysphagia*, 1994; **9**:141–6.
11. Boyd K. Tube feeding in palliative care: benefits and problems. *Palliative Medicine*, 1994; **8**:156–8.

12.6 Music therapy

Susan Porchet-Munro

Introduction

In 1978, the first publication about music therapy in palliative care appeared in the *Canadian Medical Journal*.[1] Since then, many hospice and palliative care programmes around the world have hired the services of professionally trained music therapists. An international group of these therapists met in New York in 1988 to review the state of the art and to begin networking in terms of the development of intervention techniques as well as the preliminary formulation of feasible research modalities.[2] A second, similar gathering in Oxford in 1994 provided evidence of the continuing development in this particular field of music therapy.[3]

Music therapy in palliative care: definition

Music therapy is the intentional use of the properties and the potential of music and their impact on the human being, either as a form of psychosocial and spiritual support or as an adjunct intervention strategy to symptom management, nursing, and medical care.

Interventions are tailored to the individual needs of patients and may include the following modalities:

(1) listening to music (recorded or live);

(2) musical improvisation and expression;

(3) traditional music making;

(4) verbal communication.

Music therapy is based on the interplay of relationships between the patient, the music, and the therapist, and, therefore, cannot be compared to a standardized treatment intervention but should be considered as a supportive intervention strategy which complements other medical and supportive measures.

The scope of music

The nature of music itself differentiates music therapy from all other forms of therapy. Elements of the nature of music are:

(1) the intrusive and reaching qualities of sound, certain melodies, and songs;

(2) the expression of thought, experience, hopes, and dreams;

(3) the elements of music—frequency, intensity, tone colour, intervals, harmony, rhythm, tempo;

(4) the physiological impact on the body;

(5) the intricate connection to human experience throughout time;

(6) the potential to stimulate creativity and to provide aesthetic experience;

(7) the representation of diverse cultures and beliefs;

(8) the reflection of spirituality;

(9) the ability to stimulate memories;

(10) the ability to unite people;

(11) the ability to express ideas and feelings symbolically.

Human beings can connect with music at any level appropriate to their personality, intellect, or need at any given moment regardless of age, race, or creed. They can connect with music either superficially, emotionally, cerebrally, or at innermost depth. Yet, music has the potential and power to reach, move, disturb, comfort, or relax people beyond their cognitive control.

The music therapist

While it has been recognized since the days of David and Saul that any motivated person, irrespective of training, may effectively use music in ministering to the sick, the term 'music therapist' refers to a specially trained, professionally accredited individual whose intervention is based on a thorough knowledge of all facets of music, the behavioural sciences, current treatment, educational and medical models, and accepted therapeutic approaches.

The scope of music is the *raison d'être* of the music therapist but, while music itself plays a key role in the therapeutic intervention and process, it is in the exchange between patient and the music therapist that processes such as the changing of awareness, the sharpening of perceptions, and the altering of perspectives are nurtured, facilitated, and made conscious. Competently trained music therapists are at ease in the intuitive and emotional spheres of interaction and use this ease within their professional mandate. They can relate relevant patient information in a meaningful way to other staff.

Table 1 Indications that warrant music therapy

Coping difficulties, withdrawal
Depression, anger
Complex pain problems
Persistent unexplained nausea and vomiting
Anxiety, fear, anguish
Insomnia
Extreme physical tension
Disorientation, confusion
Dyspnoea
Dysphasia, aphasia
Cultural and language barriers
Difficult family relationships
Boredom, loneliness
Patient's search for meaning
Difficult medical and nursing interventions
Need for an aesthetically pleasing life interest

The context

Progression of disease, despite treatment, entails a renewed confrontation not only with troublesome symptoms, but also with the life-threatening nature of the disease. The individual is facing multiple existential losses, invariably increasing dependence, and menacing uncertainty. Therefore, in the face of suffering, the thought of music remains for many individuals puzzling, unless the subject is broached gently and in consideration of their particular circumstances.

While music therapy, as described below, may contribute to and enhance patient care in significant ways, one needs to consider that people are defenceless against the emotional and physiological impact of sound and music. The intentional use of music, therefore, has to occur with utmost respect for the potency of this medium and the wishes of the individual patient at the given time. Useful questions to ask are: 'Whose need is it to have music, the patient's, the family's, or the caregiver's?' 'Do prolonged and persistent sadness, withdrawal, and complex symptom control make us, the interveners, helpless and long for a lift in mood and ambience?'

Indications

Indications for considering music therapy are listed in Table 1.

Methods

Active music making

Music therapists will play their instruments according to given situations and the needs and requests of the patients at the time. The emphasis here is not on performance but rather on non-verbal communication and expression through music. The content of meaning of particular melodies and songs or the timbre of the instrument or voice, will have a specific relationship with patients and their situation at the time. By requesting particular music, patients may express issues which they are unable or unwilling to state verbally. Music's power of association can provide an impulse for life review, expression of longing for lost health and mobility, or be a catalyst to touch on deep rooted psychological wounds and unfinished business.

Improvisation—here defined as the unpractised, spontaneous playing of instruments or use of voice, offers an avenue for expression and communication and encourages mobility and motivation. The availability of good quality instruments which do not necessarily require previous musical or instrumental skills is essential (see below). In improvisation, sound 'pictures' may be spontaneously searched for and created. Their content may express non-verbally what cannot easily be put in words, or repeat and reinforce what has been said before in other ways. Improvisation allows the possibility of experiencing and accepting 'imperfect' music, just as emotions and thoughts are often 'imperfect'. However, improvisations are often experienced as beautiful and meaningful.[4] This method holds a potent key to unconscious issues which are not easily addressed verbally such as anger, jealousy, existential loneliness, or fear and should only be used by a therapist with astute psychotherapeutic skills.

Music making invites participation. Patients may impulsively join the music therapist in singing familiar songs. If suitable, the therapist can encourage improvised accompaniments on appropriate instruments, according to the patient's capabilities.

How far patients are able to begin to play an instrument of their choice or can continue to play one they played previously, will have to be considered in relationship to their physical status, and their psychological frame of mind. Progressing disease often infringes on physical mobility and well being and, thus, the loss of musicianship skills may represent another major loss to be dealt with. If the issue is addressed skilfully, this may be a form of significant support for the patient. Should individuals be capable of continuing to use their skills regardless of the disease, they can benefit from the enjoyment of music making and have the opportunity to give pleasure to others.

Song writing

Throughout the centuries, people have expressed their thoughts, feelings, and experiences through song. If feasible, the music therapist will assist and encourage patients to enunciate their thoughts and trials through song, or personally improvise or write a melody to the words of the patient. The song itself, thus, functions as a container for thoughts and feelings which might otherwise not be put into words.

Song writing is a creative process of self-expression which leaves room for reflection, introspection, or diversion. The product, the song, brings gratification and may subsequently remain a memento in the grieving process of those who are left behind.[5]

Listening to music

Listening to music, live or recorded, is often carelessly labelled as a passive venture or passive music therapy. Referring to the previously described scope of music, we see that music influences man despite his defence mechanisms on a physical level (see below) and on a psychological and emotional level. Much of the power of music lies in its intricate and intimate connection to the uniqueness of one's being.[6] Music has the potential to reach, comfort, and heal in terms of nurturing the feeling of being understood or of stimulating personal growth. Music thus 'heals' frequently far better than the most skilled therapist. Listening to music, therefore, implies by no means merely a passive endeavour.

Given the context of palliative medicine, the matter of music should not be an additional demand on the patient. The use of recorded music, therefore, allows the patients unconditional access to their personally preferred music, day and night, regardless of the environmental constraints. This gives them autonomy and is therapeutic in itself.

Recorded music offers a broader and individual choice, since no music therapist or musician is capable of performing all types of music. However, recorded music lacks the intimate presence of the performer.[7]

In the therapeutic intervention, music therapists assess together with the patient, and on rare occasions with the care team or the family, if and what recorded music is meaningful. Subsequently, they will judge carefully to what extent they should question the impact of the music. If music 'speaks' to the individual, the content of that non-verbal message loses in the translation into words. On the other hand, listening to music may become the potent element to be integrated into the overall therapeutic process.

Guided imagery and music

For the purpose of relaxation, listening to music may be enhanced by the use of imagery. The term 'guided imagery' refers to the practice of encouraging a person to think of a particular image that may match the music, for instance a place in nature or a positive past experience.

The music therapist may also use 'The Bonny method of guided imagery and music' (GIM), which focuses on the conscious use of spontaneous imagery which arises in a formalized programme of relaxation and classical music to effect self-understanding and personal growth processes in the person.[8,9] This technique requires specific training.

Verbal communication

Because music often elicits deep emotions, the music therapist must have both verbal and non-verbal skills, to work meaningfully with that which arises in music therapy sessions. Processes, such as the changing of awareness, the sharpening of perceptions, or the altering of perspectives, are nurtured, facilitated, and made conscious in the exchange between patient and music therapist.[10] Much of this process involves verbal communication in relationship to the music, the individual, his/her illness, circumstances, concerns, hopes, and fears. Therefore, astute, verbal communication skills (including active listening) are required to inter-relate all these dimensions appropriately.

In an introductory conversation the therapist tunes in to the patient's relationship to music. In the context of life-threatening illness this first encounter can provide a previously unseen profile of the person within, it can be crucial for the development of trust between therapist and patient, and caution the therapist not to push music on to the patient too eagerly. Occasionally, music may never even be introduced and heard but, like a theme, remain the connecting thread of known experience between therapist and patient, and a particular basis for trust. In the ensuing conversations, the therapist will know how to use this silent connection, the symbolism of musical messages, music's links to historical, emotional, social, and spiritual issues, or the situation at hand, in order to support the patient at a given time. While not being able to introduce music challenges the therapist's *raison d'être* and patience, it respects the patient's wishes and may pay off much later in terms of gained understanding and trust.

Symptom management

Issues of symptom control are delineated extensively in this textbook. It may seem far-fetched to consider the topic in relationship to music therapy but experience in palliative care has shown that the scope of music can hold unmatched potential in the complexity of this area.[11] Music therapy does not replace other treatment modalities, it complements them.

Pain

Music, as auditory stimulation, may play a part in controlling pain. 'Auditory stimulation has pronounced physiological effect on the body that may be related to the gate control theory of pain. Intense stimuli through the thalamus, midbrain, and brainstem cause production of modulating substances (i.e. endorphins and serontonin) that inhibit the release of neurotransmitters, therefore stimulating the closure of the gate'.[12] Furthermore, the diversional and associative qualities of music may distract the attention from the adverse nature of the stimulus, thus inducing relaxation of muscle guarding at the site of the pain. Music therapy may also have a powerful impact on reducing the emotional component of pain, for example fear or anxiety, thus mediating the very perception of pain.[13]

Just as the threshold of pain is an individual matter which is influenced by many variables, the threshold of tolerance of music in the presence of pain may be affected. The choice as to when and how to use music has to be made in collaboration with the wishes of the patient. Patients know best what type of music distracts them or what they experience as relaxing while they experience pain. The therapist can, where appropriate, expand on these preferences according to music-related or physiology-related theories and make the suggestion that music may decrease pain. Music therapists play and improvise or may put together a particular tape with or for a particular patient, and use tapes developed by practising music therapists[6,14] or appropriate commercially produced relaxation tapes. They are responsible for introducing such tapes to the patient and for observing and monitoring their impact. Carelessly introduced music may aggravate the experience of pain. Attention has to be paid to sound intensity, the use of headphones where needed, patient control over equipment wherever possible, and adverse effects.

Nausea and vomiting

Occasionally, music may be helpful in diverting a patient's attention from nausea or in interrupting a retching reflex. Given the complex nature of these symptoms in palliative care, the same careful considerations mentioned with regard to pain control apply.

Insomnia, anxiety, fear, dyspnoea, and restlessness

The therapeutic effect of lullabies seems to be widely accepted. For this reason, patients are rather open to the idea of using music to facilitate sleep and relaxation, even in critical situations.

The most remarkable attribute of music in this domain is its ability to influence the heart, respiration rate, and the brain on a physiological and psychological level simultaneously. While rhythmic pulse and musical sound waves affect pulse rate and brain functions,[15] the transcendent quality of music reaches the person beyond reason and analysis. If we consider the complex symptom picture of some patients, it is exactly this combination of effects which breaks through irrationality, anxiety, or the intangible and inexplicable resistance to medication and other supportive measures.[16]

Here, music must be chosen carefully, particularly with regard to rhythm. Melodic and harmonic elements which elicit associations must be of non-threatening significance for the patient. Again, the type of sound source (live or taped), its volume, and location are vital details to consider.

The music therapist may tailor music specifically to promote relaxation. The spontaneous use of the voice (humming or quiet singing) or a suitable instrument allows a particular choice of melody or harmonic intervals and an adjustment of rhythm to the breathing of the patient. Close observation of the impact of such endeavour is required. These interventions with live music allow great flexibility but they demand an extended presence of the therapist. Therefore, the music therapist may introduce the use of specific music on tape, monitor and titrate its effectiveness, and then teach the patient and or caregivers how to use the tapes. Thus, music can be available day and night, in the hospital setting or at home.

Confusional states

The relaxation strategies described above may, with careful consideration of the given circumstances, be useful in the care of the disorientated or confused patient. Occasionally, however, reorientation through the use of familiar tunes or songs, as well as the use of other music therapy approaches described, may be the method of choice with brain-impaired individuals.[17]

Dysphasia, aphasia

The 'singing aphasic' is not uncommon with patients who have dominant hemisphere damage. The patient with an astrocytoma, for example, may be expressively as well as receptively dysphasic. Supportive communication may be possible when patients are able to indicate their musical preferences and join in familiar songs.

Difficult treatment and nursing interventions

In addition to symptom control, music induced relaxation may be considered to support patient and caregiver in difficult treatment or nursing interventions such as a paracentesis or a painful change of a dressing.

Family involvement

So far, music therapy interventions have been described in terms of the individual patient in order to underline the highly personal nature of the relationship between music and people, and the highly individual experience of coping with life-threatening disease. However, as in other care situations, the music therapist considers the patients and their loved ones as the unit of care, and will readily involve family and friends during interventions. Once initiated, certain activities (singing, making and playing tapes, and searching for songs etc.) can be continued by persons close to the patient. This may reduce their feelings of helplessness and may turn the focus away from illness to life-confirming activity.

Since music has often played a significant role in relationships or during particular periods in life, it may facilitate life review or rekindle dormant feelings of closeness and affection. In the face of approaching death, issues that may be difficult to express between partners, parent and child, or friends occasionally find expression through particular songs or musical selections associated with memories. As the person who encourages the use of music in such ways, the music therapist is aware of the inhibitions, difficulties, and manifold emotions underlying such sharing and will support the individuals involved appropriately. The music, thus experienced, often plays a significant role in subsequent grieving. Some music therapists are actively involved in memorial and funeral services and bereavement follow-up.[18,19]

Group activities

The nature of music favours social interaction, nurtures feelings of community, and tends to be able, in unique ways, to draw individuals out of isolation and withdrawal into shared musical experience. Thoughtfully prepared group interventions can, therefore, add a very valuable dimension to patient care.[20] However, careful assessment must be made as to when and how to use music in a given or predetermined group setting with patients. Diverse needs, tastes, and physical and emotional states of the patients involved should be considered.

It is important to reflect on the intentions and goals of such activities, that is diversion, interaction, fun and games, celebration, sharing feelings, spiritual, support, or other. Each goal has its own merits at a given time. Some may be complementary, others contradictory, to the needs of members of the group. The same reflective questions, raised earlier with regard to the appropriateness of music, are of vital importance in group activities.

The visits of choirs and musicians to a palliative care unit are a fairly common and appreciated practice and generally bring much joy to the patients. However, care teams should be alert to the individual reactions of patients who, at this time, may be particularly vulnerable and may need additional support to work through the evoked feelings (see above).

Music, music therapy, and volunteers

Just as in other areas of palliative care, volunteers can be of invaluable assistance in terms of music and music therapy. The competently trained volunteer will be aware of the complexity of issues in this work as well as the temptation for, and the danger of, imposing things on patients. They usually have access to a volunteer coordinator and other members of the care team for information and support. A volunteer needs to be familiar and at ease with the patients and the multifaceted issues involved in patient care before attempting to integrate music into this work. This does not preclude the spontaneous sharing of the love for music, a familiar song or melody, or a past musical experience during interactions. However, should volunteers use music intentionally, where the services of a trained music therapist are not available, the potency of music should not be underestimated and its use must be guided by the considerations outlined above. Music therapy, as defined at the beginning of this paper, should be the domain of a professionally trained and accredited therapist.

Volunteers with interests and skills in music are of invaluable assistance.[21] Variety in the musical and cultural background of the volunteers increases the ability to tune in to diverse cultural and religious practices with music and widen the spectrum of live music making. The music therapist can match and channel the skills of a volunteer to the particular needs of patients, and support patient and volunteer when warranted. Furthermore, the additional help from volunteers in creating and monitoring a tape collection, and in the maintenance and control of audio equipment is valuable.

Instruments and equipment

Music therapists use a wide variety of instruments in their work. Their professional training demands accomplished skills on two instruments (one generally being the piano or the guitar) as well as ease in the use of the singing voice. They will also choose other instruments that can encourage patient participation such as the autoharp, the omnichord, the electronic keyboard or piano, small harps, various percussion instruments, chimes, and bells, if funds are available. It is essential that instruments are of good quality if the experience of music making is to be therapeutic. The handling of an instrument is a multisensory sensation: the eyes behold it, the hands touch and feel it, and the ear receives its sound. Subsequently, every one of these avenues may play a key role in particular instances.

The quality of audio equipment is equally important. Portable tape recorders and comfortable headphones should be available. Tape recorders need to be easy to handle for the weak and bedridden patient who, with staff and volunteers, requires instruction in their use. Audio tapes must be of good sound quality and include selections from diverse musical styles and possibly diverse cultures.

Education

The music therapist working in palliative care will need to be familiar with the care philosophy as well as the principal diagnostic and treatment modalities in this field. Over the last few years, some music therapy training programmes have begun to include courses on the subject. It is recommended that the therapists who will be working extensively with palliative care patients should be given the opportunity for a thorough introduction to this area of care before they are expected to function as therapists. Adequate training, the possibility for continuing education, as well as regular staff support, are essential for this work.

It is important that other health-care professionals and volunteers in the care team have an understanding of music therapy principles and methods in order to recognize the indications for referral or consultation and the potential for collaboration with the therapist. Music therapists can introduce their work through workshops and lectures. Their services may also be valuable in terms of staff support. The scope of music as a means of expression, communication, and relaxation can offer an avenue for dealing with the caregiver's burden of witnessing continual suffering, death, and the demands of the job. Furthermore, the experiential nature of music therapy methods are particularly suitable to enhance educational programmes in palliative rehabilitation and care since they provide a non-threatening approach to emotional and intangible issues.[22]

Research

Research documenting the impact of music therapy in palliative care is limited. Given the multifaceted nature of music therapy and of terminal illness, the pursuit of meaningful clinical research in this area is of great concern to all music therapists working in this field. One of the main difficulties is the definition of appropriate outcome measures. The pertinent questions are whether they should address:

(1) the impact of music in terms of physiological, psychological, or musical parameters;

(2) the psychological impact of music in terms of physical parameters or emotional adjustment and change;

(3) musical preferences or responses;

(4) the creative response to non-verbal communication through music;

(5) the effectiveness of the music therapist compared to a psychologist.

Such questions raise issues of suitable research modalities, meaningful, possibly validated, research instruments, and, in terms of the patient population, clinical feasibility.

Academic palliative care programmes continue to press for quantitative research, whereas many practising music therapists plead for more understanding of qualitative research, its problems, limitations and merits, particularly with regard to music therapy.[23,24,25]

Music therapists are relative newcomers on the health-care team. They are often the sole professionals of their kind and are frequently expected to practise music therapy, and like many colleagues, provide in-service education, write, publish, and possibly research.

To date, the initial research projects in palliative care document some of the impact of music therapy. However, further research in this field will require medical directors, interdisciplinary teams and experienced researchers, who are willing to tackle the complexity of the issues, to work in collaboration with music therapists. In addition, a suitable infrastructure and adequate support from care teams are indispensable for clinical music therapy research projects.

Conclusions

The diversity of music therapy can contribute to the effective alleviation of palliative care problems and challenges. For optimum benefit, interventions need to be carefully elaborated and integrated into the overall treatment approaches. At the same time, they are equally essential and autonomous in their effectiveness.

The significant and distinguishing element in this therapeutic endeavour is the contribution of music itself, with its intricate connections to human experience. Music invokes the realm of emotional and aesthetic experience, imagination, creativity, and the intangible. While the effect of music on physiological parameters can be an important asset in particular interventions, it is far more the power of music to add to the meaningfulness of life that makes it invaluable for music therapy in palliative medicine.

References

1. Munro S, Mount B. Music therapy in palliative care. *Canadian Medical Association Journal*, 1978; **119**: 1029–34.
2. Martin JA (ed.). *The Next Step Forward: Music Therapy with the Terminally Ill.* New York: Calvary Hospital, 1989.
3. Lee C (ed.). Lonely Waters. Proceedings of the International Conference, *Music Therapy in Palliative Care*, Oxford 1994. Oxford: Sobell Publications, 1995.
4. Lee C. The analysis of therapeutic improvisatory music. In: Gilroy and Lee, eds. *Art and Music: Therapy and Research*. London: Routledge, 1995: 35–50.
5. O'Callaghan C. Song Writing in Palliative Care. M.Mus. Thesis, University of Melbourne, 1994.
6. Munro S. *Music Therapy in Palliative/Hospice Care.* St Louis: Magnamusic-Baton, 1984. (German Translation: Stuttgart: Fischer 1986).
7. Bailey L. The effects of live music versus tape-recorded music on hospitalized cancer patients. *Music Therapy*, 1983; **3**: 17–28.
8. Summer L. The Bonny method of guided imagery (GIM). *Bonny Foundation Newsletter*, 1990; **2**: 1–2.
9. Bruscia K, Embracing life with AIDS: psychotherapy through guided imagery and music. In: Bruscia K, ed. *Case Studies in Music Therapy.* Phoenixville: Barcelona, 1991: 581–602.
10. Salmon D. Music and emotion. *Journal of Palliative Care*, 1993; **9**: 48–52.
11. Porchet-Munro S. Music therapy in support of cancer patients. In: Senn HJ, Glaus A, Schmid L, eds. *Recent Results in Cancer Research*. Heidelberg: Springer, 1988; **108**: 289–94.
12. Zimmerman L, Pozehl B, Duncan K, Schmitz R. Effects of music in patients who had chronic cancer pain. *Western Journal of Nursing Research*, 1989; **11**: 298–309.
13. Magill-Levreault L. Music therapy in pain and symptom management. *Journal of Palliative Care*, 1993; **9**: 4,42–8.
14. Bonny HL. *Music Rx Tape Series.* Salina, KS 67401: The Bonny Foundation.
15. Clynes M (ed.). *Music, Mind and Brain: the Neuropsychology of Music.* London: Plenum Press, 1982.
16. Boisvert M. In: Munro S, ed. *Music Therapy in Palliative/Hospice Care.* St Louis: Magnamusic-Baton, 1984: 50–1.
17. O'Callaghan C. Communicating with brain-impaired palliative care patients through music. *Journal of Palliative Care*, 1993; **9**: 53–5.
18. Loyst D. A time to remember: music therapy in bereavement follow-up. In: Martin JA, ed. *The Next Step Forward: Music Therapy with The Terminally Ill.* New York: Calvary Hospital, 1989: 53–60.
19. Ryan K. Access to music in paediatric bereavement support groups. In Lee C, ed. Proceedings of the International Conference. *Music Therapy in Palliative Care*, Oxford 1994. Oxford: Sobell Publications, 1995.
20. Salmon D. Partage: group-work in palliative care. In: Martin JA, ed. *The Next Step Forward: Music Therapy with the Terminally Ill.* New York: Calvary Hospital, 1989: 47–51.
21. Mandel S. Music therapy in hospice: 'musicalive'. *Palliative Medicine,* 1991; **5**: 155–60.
22. Munro S. Music therapy perspectives in palliative care education. Music therapy in pain and symptom management. *Journal of Palliative Care*, 1993; **9**: 39–42.
23. Forinash M, Gonzalez D. A phenomenological perspective of music therapy. *Music Therapy*, 1989; **8**: 35–46.
24. Kenny C. *The Field of Play, A Guide for the Theory and Practice of Music Therapy.* Atascadero: Ridgeview, 1989.
25. Aldridge D. Music therapy II. Research methods suitable for music therapy. *Arts in Psychotherapy*, 1991; **20**: 117–31.

Further reading

Beggs C. Life review with a palliative care patient. In: Bruscia K, ed. *Case Studies in Music Therapy.* Phoenixville: Barcelona, 1991: 611–16.

Curtis S. The effect of music on pain relief and relaxation of the terminally ill. *Journal of Music Therapy*, 1986; **23**: 10–24.

Forinash M. Research in Music Therapy with the Terminally Ill: A Phenomenological Approach. D.A. Dissertation, Ann Arbor, University Microfilms 91–02617, 1990.

Frank J. The effects of music therapy and guided visual imagery on chemotherapy-induced nausea and vomiting. *Oncology Nurses Forum*, 1985; **12**: 47–52.

Kenny C. Music therapy: A whole system approach. *Music Therapy*, 1985; 5.

Martin J. Music therapy at the end of a life. In: Bruscia K, ed. *Case Studies in Music Therapy.* Phoenixville: Barcelona, 1991: 617–32.

O'Callaghan C. Musical profiles of dying patients. *Australian Music Therapy Association Bulletin*, 1984; **7**: 5–11.

O'Callaghan C. Music therapy skills used in songwriting within a palliative care setting. *Australian Journal of Music Therapy*, 1990; **1**: 15–22.

Whittal J. *A Handbook of Music Therpy in Palliative/Hospice Care.* Montreal: Palliative Care Service, Royal Victoria Hospital, 1990.

Whittal J. Songs in palliative care: a spouse's last gift. In: Bruscia K, ed. *Case Studies in Music Therapy.* Phoenixville: Barcelona, 1991: 603–10.

12.7 Creative arts and literature

David R. Frampton

Amongst the many strands of our efforts to keep terminally ill patients comfortable, mobile, mentally active, and involved, their fundamental need for an ongoing purpose in living is easily overlooked. The multiple losses of job, status, mobility, and independence slowly unmask another—the loss of purpose—which can be the most destructive of all. 'There's no point in living any more'; 'I'm no use to anybody now', are deep cries from the well of spiritual pain, and they sometimes culminate in the more or less specific request, 'Can't you put an end to it for me, doctor?' Is our aim simply to help our patients die comfortably, or does it include the further aim of helping them live until they die?

Creative arts and literature are tools through which fresh purpose and self-worth can be found by at least some patients. A number of them have within themselves a well of self-worth and a creativity of outlook which enables them to adjust to their new circumstances and maximize their opportunities.[1] A little encouragement, and sometimes the provision of resources, catalyse living to the full. There are also those who seem steadfastly to turn themselves away from all help, overcome by the tragedy that has overtaken them. However, the majority of patients fall between these extremes, and with imaginative, skilled help can surprise themselves with their achievements and begin to come alive again in their whole demeanour.

Creativity and therapy

Activity is not an end in itself. Bailey examines the energizing effect of creativity for both patients and staff and its potential for spiritual nourishment at a time of conflict and potential disintegration.[2] Breslow describes her goals for the use of creative arts as, 'to reduce anxiety, depression and stress in cancer patients, enhancing their self-control and reducing dependence on families, friends and health care team and to develop new skills or reinforce existing ones'.[3] Eisenhauer and Frampton specified their objectives (Table 1) and Moss has examined the healing role of the arts.[4],[5] Patients with advanced disease are often easily tired, their attention span is short, and strength is fading. It is acceptable to 'sit and think and sometimes just to sit'. There is a lot to be worked through and come to terms with, but points of focus, episodes of new interest, opportunities for fun, and the thrill of producing something good help to retain or recover perspective in what can be a dismal landscape. In short they build hope.[6]

Table 1 Aims of a palliative care arts programme

- To occupy time creatively, not just passively
- To improve feelings of personal worth and purpose at a time when life seems worthless and pointless
- To leave behind something of oneself — one's own creation
- To share tasks with a close relative (or friend) producing a joint result
- To open up recreational and refreshment opportunities for the staff

Thus, the use of creative arts is something other than therapy.[7] It is coming from another direction—a resource available to the patient rather than a treatment prescribed in appropriate situations. Occupational therapy has to do with maintaining and restoring function—important in its own right. Arts therapies are concerned with the exploration and resolution of emotions.[8,9] These therapeutic disciplines employ trained personnel in the professions allied to medicine and lie within the spectrum of medical treatment.

Creative arts and literature are not primarily diversional or recreational, although they may be both of these, nor are they concerned with improving the aesthetic quality of the environment of the hospital or hospice, although that is important too. An experimental project in a British hospice using sculpture students in residence for a 3-month period was limited in its effectiveness because it was not truly patient orientated. Patients had no say in its initiation or participation in its development.[10] Whatever else it achieved, it was not able to empower dispirited and struggling patients.

Research

The sculpture project was one of the few in health care where evaluation was attempted. Most publications have been of a descriptive nature, and evidence of the value, or otherwise, of arts activities needs to be sought and documented carefully.[11,12] Responses to the arts do not lend themselves readily to the kind of clinical analysis favoured by the medical profession.

The introduction of artists, professional or amateur, into a hospice clearly raises anxieties. The artist is in an unfamiliar, and perhaps personally threatening, environment. The hospice staff may feel anxious about giving medically untrained persons direct access to vulnerable patients. However, hospices use lay volunteers in many areas of their work, usually with suitable training, supervision, and support, and therefore should be experienced in facilitating such an interaction. Indeed, many patients seem to find the presence of suitable, non-medical personnel amongst the caring team positively supportive, contributing towards a less clinical and intimidating environment.

Literature

Writing

In many ways the use of writing as a creative medium is the easiest place to begin. Writing is a natural process to most people, the idiom is familiar and the resources are to hand and clean. However, there needs to be some purpose to motivate the patient. Some have a need to write down their life story,[13] perhaps for their children or grandchildren, or perhaps in the usually vain hope that it will be published. They will probably soon be submerged in the sheer volume of this task and give it up if not helped to be selective, focusing on a few carefully chosen incidents.

Case histories: A 36-year-old unmarried teacher had four children under the age of 12 whose future seemed very uncertain as her life was approaching its end. She wanted to leave them an explanation of why life had turned out as it had for them, which they could read when they were older. However, she was drawn into long descriptions of her early life and deteriorated and died before the task was completed.

A 37-year-old man with two small children was dying of advanced malignancy. He wanted to leave something of himself for his children to know him by. Photographs show the outer man. He chose to give them an inside view by writing and illustrating short stories and incidents.

Some hospices have a writer in residence[14] who may encourage patients to tell stories of their early life. These have been recorded on tape or in note form and transcribed for the patient and his family, and sometimes for local archives when the story is told of a past life-style or historically interesting location.[15]

Poetry

The medium of poetry can also be used, with poetry readings and poetry writing by individuals or in groups. Eisenhauer, a poet at St Joseph's Hospice, London, encouraged patients to write of their experiences of their illness and its treatments.[16,17] The motivation to do this can be generated by explaining that although the medical and nursing staff constantly work with patients like themselves they usually lack personal experience of life-threatening disease.

Afraid
I am afraid of death
death rather than dying
fear of the unknown
Nothing is worse than death.
Life is terribly important.
Any sort of life
—just being alive . . .
Life is important even
the importance of life
is sometimes hidden . . .
Life is important because
I am afraid of death.

Fred Julian[18]

Crystallizing his own experience in simple poetry created a teaching tool which then brought home to the professional in a powerful way the battleground within his patient.

Often the idea of writing poetry is paralysing. Shared authorship is one solution,[19] but it may help to get the patient to write down or dictate a series of thoughts. These can be abbreviated into a set of short, perhaps truncated, phrases and set under each other in a verse format. When typed-up the quality of the result often amazes the author. Poetry writing can also be used with some patients to help them to express what they cannot say.

Case history: A middle-aged couple had had a difficult marriage. The husband, now dying from cancer, felt that he had not been able to express what he really felt for his wife beneath the tangles of their relationship. In poems he began to express how much he really cared for her, and after his death his grieving wife said, 'If he wrote all those things he must have meant at least some of them.' Perhaps they went some way towards easing what was inevitably a difficult bereavement.

Some of these poems have been published together with poems by some of the professionals.[18,20] One palliative medicine physician resorted to poetry to communicate with his own mother when she was dying from cancer[21] and many bereaved relatives have written articles, poems, and books as a part of their way of dealing with their grief about their loved one.[22] This illustrates how the arts can draw carer and cared-for together in their common humanity as their life journeys intertwine.

Basic facilities

Of course, even a resident writer or poet can only be available for short periods of time. However, he or she can be instrumental in setting-up or improving the infrastructure, which should include a mobile library for patients—available on most days as patients may not be around long enough to 'wait until next week'. Large print books, although heavy, are a real help to many patients who find their eyesight deteriorating rapidly. Book rests and page turners are available for the more seriously disabled.

Books on tape, full-length and abridged, provide another important medium. A portable tape recorder with lightweight earphones can transport a patient, too weary or too weak to cope with a book, into another world of his choice. A good relationship with the local library will facilitate the availability of a wide selection of books and tapes.

Small crafts

Many palliative care units use crafts, most often in the context of a Day Care Unit, as a way of giving patients something to do with their time and perhaps encouraging some social interaction. Unfortunately, some of these activities can seem rather like a return to junior school and are unlikely to build self-respect and a sense of achievement. It is vital that anything the patient makes is of a quality to be proud of, and good enough to be displayed as an achievement or given away as a gift. Quality artefacts made by ill or dying patients are often precious mementoes for grieving friends or relatives, bridges that may ease the parting. For the patient, being able to give is very important as most of the time he finds that he is on the receiving end.

The craftsperson, therefore, needs to be well prepared. With time and energy in short supply, results need to be achieved quickly. A metalsmith can help patients to make silver jewellery using miniature tools and soldering, even on the bed table.[23] Fabric painting with prepared stencils on plain T-shirts, cloths, and handkerchiefs, can produce impressive results in 20 to 30 min. Hobby ceramic glazing of a variety of precast bisque-fired pottery is a gentle and peaceful craft and, as a group activity, is usually associated with much excitement and fun. When the items are returned a week later after the second firing, patients are amazed at what they have made. When it is impossible to get out to the shops, these artefacts frequently solve the problems of birthday and Christmas presents. Tiny tapestries, decoupage gift cards, patchwork, dried and fresh flower arranging, and silk flower and doll making tempt patients from the inertia of their illness into new adventures.[6]

Previous hobbies

It is sometimes more successful to introduce new ideas than to revive old skills. Advancing illness may have adversely affected the patients' ability to do well what they once did expertly, which may simply serve to emphasize disability and lower morale. With ingenuity, familiar materials can be put to new uses.

If patients are still able to enjoy old skills, they may be willing to teach them to a family member, another patient or a member of staff, so producing a welcome role reversal. Other skilled crafts persons may be enlisted to visit and demonstrate a craft too complex to be learnt in a short time.

Painting

Talking about paintings can be a particularly effective way of facilitating communication on difficult topics. As one nurse tutor described in her own experience with a patient, specific art therapy skills, although useful, are not essential.[24] A sensitivity to the patient, a seizing of opportunities, and good communication skills go a long way. Artists working with cancer patients find ways of talking about things that matter, either as they help a patient paint a subject of their choice, or perhaps as they themselves paint at the patient's direction. Concentration on the job in hand allows sensitive subjects to be alluded to, followed up, or dropped as the patient dictates.[7] Another way of beginning with a group is to get members to paint significant episodes from their lives and the artist, while helping them individually, can draw out further discussion. Like writing of past events, this can be part of surveying one's life, which seems to become important as the end approaches.

Of course, unless patients already have painting skills, such pictures are unlikely to be of the quality referred to earlier. Many people feel inhibited at the sight of a paintbrush, so ways of simplifying things may be appropriate.

Fun art

Abstract painting can be fun and also effective and practical. A random design with water-colours, where patches of the paper have been previously waxed, and marbling with oil colours floated on water can make attractive gift cards, especially if the most interesting areas of the design are cut out and mounted separately. The use of music during a session with paints may enhance the benefits at all levels.

Venues and personnel

Almost all of these activities can be undertaken in a variety of places. The Day Centre is the most usual venue, where people can work singly but usually work as a group (Chapter 2.4). The latter has its own benefit, but also its limitations on privacy and individual attention. Some hospices include the availability of arts experiences in their provisions for care in patients' homes,[7] where possibly the greatest deprivation exists.[2]

Case history: A 56-year-old man was seen at home, partly paralysed from cancer, withdrawn, and difficult to manage. A potter was asked to visit to try to help awaken some interest in living. She discovered he had been a budgerigar fancier who had given away his prize-winning birds when his cancer was diagnosed. Although he had never painted a picture before, he sketched out a prize bird he had bred and then painted it in full-colour glazes on a bisque-fired plate. The fine end-result, with its caption 'Webbs Wonder', brought one of the joys of his life alive again as a final celebration and left a significant memorial for his family.[25]

A third focus would be at the bedside of an inpatient, perhaps best exemplified by the work of the arts team at the Connecticut Hospice, where the artist carries a holdall of materials to the bedridden patient and offers to engage with him in one of a variety of projects.

Drawing relatives, staff, and volunteers into these arts activities is invaluable in eroding barriers and creating common areas of experience. They also have a place in helping bereaved relatives, both adults[26] and children,[27] move on with their grief work. Consideration should also be given to specific opportunities for creativity for staff as part of their support and growth.

More important than the skills the artist brings is the person himself. Warmth and openness, gentleness with directness, an easy manner, and a clear way of giving explanations make for good relationships. Adaptability and ingenuity are vital to make the skill concerned available to novices. Whether the artist is a paid professional artist in residence, a sessional paid art teacher, an art therapist with an interest in this broad approach, or a volunteer with a hobby which he can share depends on the circumstances and finances available. Ideally, there needs to be a team of available experts with a wide variety of skills.[3,7] Their co-ordinator can then construct a programme to suit the needs of the current patients and call on appropriate individuals for one-to-one work in home or inpatient settings.

In the same way that all volunteers need to be both carefully selected and properly trained to work with dying patients, so do those who will contribute to the creative arts and literature.

Being fully alive includes creative fulfilment, and making this available turns waiting to die into living to the end.

References

1. Gordon R. *Dying and Creating—a Research for Meaning.* United Kingdom Society of Analytical Psychology, 1978.
2. Bailey. The arts as an avenue to the spirit. In: Wald F, ed. *In Quest of the Spiritual Component of Care for the Terminally Ill.* Yale University Press, 1987: 67–73.

3. Breslow DM. The role of the arts in US cancer centres. In: *The Healing Arts*. Carnegie UK Trust/Rockerfeller Foundation Conference report, 1978: 30–43.
4. Moss LM. The arts as healing agents: a critical review. *Theoretical Surgery*, 1986; **1**: 96–102.
5. Moss LM. *Art for Health's Sake*. Manchester: Carnegie United Kingdom Trust, 1987.
6. Herth K. Fostering hope in terminally ill people. *Journal of Advanced Nursing*, 1990;**15**:1250–9.
7. Frampton DR. Arts activities in United Kingdom hospices: a report. *Journal of Palliative Care*, 1989; **5**:**4**: 25–32.
8. Kern-Pilch K. Art therapy with a terminally ill patient. *American Journal of Art Therapy*, 1980; **20**: 3–11.
9. Connell C. Art therapy as part of a palliative care programme. *Palliative Medicine* 1992; **6**: 18–25.
10. Crimmin M, Shand WS, Thomas JA. *Sculptors in Residence at St John's Hospice, Lancaster*. London: Kings Fund, 1989 (14 Palace Court, London W2 4HT, UK).
11. Harper R, Faulkner A. *Creative in a Practical Way*. Hospice Arts, 1993. (c/o 9 Artillery Lane, London E1 7LP.)
12. Higginson I. *A Description and Preliminary Evaluation of the Chelmsford Hospice Arts Project*. Hospice Arts, 1991. (c/o 9 Artillery Lane, London E1 7LP.)
13. Lichter I, Mooney J, Boyd M. Biography as therapy. *Palliative Medicine*, 1993; **7**: 133–7.
14. Hawes C. Writing in residence. *British Medical Journal*, 1991; **303**: 527.
15. Gittins C. Somebody said that word. *Littlewood*, 1991
16. Frampton DR. Restoring creativity to the dying patient. *British Medical Journal*, 1986; **293**: 1593–5.
17. Eisenhauer J. Poetry within hospice. *St Joseph's Hospice, Hackney*, 1987. (London, E8 4SA, UK.)
18. Eisenhauer J (ed.). *Travellers Tales: Poetry from Hospice*. London: Marshall Pickering, 1989.
19. Alexander L. *Throwaway Lines*. Oxford: Sobell Publications, 1991.
20. Gloag D. Death is no longer a stranger. *British Medical Journal*, 1990; **300**: 1214–15.
21. Mount B. *Sightings in the Valley of the Shadow*. Illinois: Inter Varsity Press, 1983.
22. Zorza V, Zorza R. *A Way to Die*. Deutsch Sphere, 1980 (out of print).
23. Bridgeman M. Artistic creation and the power to heal. *Metalsmith*,1986 (summer edn): 22–3.
24. Ames B. Art and a dying patient. *American Journal of Nursing*, 1980; **80**: 1094–6.
25. Gloag D. Hospice arts. *British Medical Journal*, 1990: **300**: 1609.
26. Simon R. Bereavement art. *American Journal of Art Therapy*, 1981; **20**: 135–43.
27. Burroughs A, Tyler J. Grief work with children, workshop days at Pilgrims Hospice in Canterbury. *Palliative Medicine*, 1992: **6**; 6–33.

Further reading

Bailey S. *Creativity and the Close of Life*. Connecticut: Connecticut Hospice Inc., 1991.

Hague I, Barnett J. *Celebration—the Arts and Terminal Care: First Steps for Managers*. Dewsbury: Yorkshire and Humberside Arts,1992. (WF13 1AX.)

Senior P, Croall J. *Helping to Heal: Arts in Health Care*. London: Calouste Gulbenkian Foundation, 1993.

13

Social work in palliative care

13 Social work in palliative care

Barbara Monroe

Introduction

Social work is a necessary and appropriate part of palliative care. Palliative care starts with specific physical symptoms but it can only be completed by consideration of the patient's feelings, family, and social circumstances. This requires a variety of skills and roles, including the social work skills and roles considered in this chapter. The chapter describes the forces that shape the social work role in palliative care, examines the social work task, provides a practical illustration, looks at the work that social workers do, and considers the social worker's contribution to extending the resources and values of palliative care.

Shaping the social work role

Three forces shape the social work role: the non-medical social goals that palliative care teams set themselves; the teamwork and multidisciplinary skills required to meet these social goals; and the expectations of patients, relatives, and the various palliative care professionals of social work and social workers.

Non-medical social goals

Relieving a patient's physical symptoms reveals their and their families' emotional, spiritual, and practical needs. Because doctors can often release patients from the horror of a physically painful and unpleasant death, palliative care teams are able to set themselves non-medical social goals aimed at these non-medical needs.

The patient's first non-medical need is to express emotional pain. Terminal illness frightens people, makes them angry, and distances them from those to whom they are close. Helping patients to express their feelings, and convincing them that this expression is acceptable and appropriate, can reduce their fear and anger and put them back in touch with their partners, families, and friends.[1] It allows patients to say a proper good-bye and gives them the opportunity to heal rifts and complete unfinished business.

The second need is the exploration of spiritual pain.[2,3] Dying people want to explore 'why'; why me, why now, for what purpose? Helping them in this journey will alleviate their isolation and give them the comfort of knowing that their concerns, even if unanswered, are real, important, and valid.

The third need is for practical help. Dying people are often reduced to passive patienthood; however, they need to make decisions and exercise choice, both for practical reasons and in order to maintain their own sense of dignity and worth. For instance they may need to make a will or to discuss and influence a child's future care. They may need the most basic assistance in order to pay a bill or get a telephone at home.

Patients' partners, families, and friends will experience the same three needs and ensuring that their needs are also met is a proper goal for palliative care. They may also feel frightened and angry. They too will ask 'why', and they too may have practical needs, such as some relief from a 24-hour caring role. They will need to feel involved in the processes of dying and that they did what they could to help the patient. Whether or not these needs are met can have a profound impact on their health in bereavement and their ability to cope with future crises.

Teamwork

The non-medical goals permitted by good symptom control require different and extra skills beyond those traditionally accruing to the doctor and nurse. In addition, patients may want to discuss emotional, spiritual, or practical problems with someone who is not involved in their physical care, or someone wearing a different label, such as a minister of religion or a social worker. As a result good palliative care is delivered by multidisciplinary teams.[4] Each member of the team will have a range of overlapping roles, some medical and some non-medical, each focused on a specific set of patient needs. Whilst medical needs will be met from the medical disciplines, no one discipline has the monopoly in fulfilling the non-medical roles. Patients' other needs do not come in neat boxes with discreet professional labels. Doctors, nurses, social workers, and ministers will all have to respond to patients' emotional, spiritual, and practical concerns. What matters is the definition and delivery of the social work task, and not the allocation of a role or task to the social worker or any other non-medical discipline. All disciplines will do some social work, and the patient will expect a consistent, careful, and effective approach to be adopted by all of them.

The social work profession does, however, bring its own perspective and approaches, and the exposition and demonstration of these is an important part of the contribution that a social worker should make within a palliative care team. These perspectives come in three forms. The first reflects what social workers cannot do. They cannot cure pain, dress wounds, or offer the appropriate religious rituals. Their professional starting point has to be that defined by the patient and his or her family, not that defined by their professional role.

The second perspective is that of the patient as part of a family with a past and a future and a social and cultural context. For the social worker, the patient is not just an individual with problems but part of a social network which has a variety of strengths and resources which can be marshalled to cope with the consequences of the individual's illness and death.

Lastly, the social worker will have a perspective of how the patient and their family will be affected by the law and other social institutions. For instance the social worker will understand the implications of family and mental health legislation in particular cases. He or she will know what community services might be applicable and what social welfare provision may be available.

Expectations and attitudes

The role of the social worker is also shaped by expectations and attitudes of society, of colleagues, and of patients and families.

People expect the welfare state to provide a safety net when things go wrong; a residential home for the elderly handicapped widow whose carer has died or foster parents for the children of a dying single parent. Society sees the social worker as an agent for the welfare state, able to manipulate its institutions to the patient's advantage. For example social workers are expected to negotiate financial benefits from government agencies, organize child care from a local authority, and find charitable finance for a holiday. Palliative care colleagues expect social workers to provide them with a safety net for managing difficult social work tasks. Palliative care teams will frequently meet situations which are emotionally exhausting and difficult to deal with. A young dying mother or a suicidal relative may need both extra time and specialist social work skills that are best provided by a separate resource, rather than by stretching—both physically and emotionally—the team responsible for the day-to-day care of a group of patients.

Patients and their families will also have specific expectations from organizations which provide palliative care. They increasingly expect access to professional counselling services in order to help them manage emotional problems. They will expect expert advice on personal family matters, such as how much should a young child know about and be involved with a parent's death and how they should be told what they need to know.[5]

In summary, the social work task arises from the non-medical goals that palliative care teams set themselves. The task exists within the context of a multidisciplinary team and is not unique to social workers. Patients need to be seen in the context of their family and friends and as belonging to a community within society. As part of the task social workers themselves are expected to act as the patient's agent with the state, the long-stop for difficult or time-consuming problems, and the provider of counselling and social work expertise.

The core social work task

The core social work task concerns the social and psychological health of the patient and family before and after death; it has two parts, assessment and intervention.

Assessment

The normal assessment of the patient will start with the medical 'clerking-in' procedure and the formulation of a care plan by a nurse. This assessment should identify any need for further assessment, for co-ordination between disciplines, and for specialist help. Sometimes the process by which the patient has arrived will have already identified problems which require a more detailed psychosocial assessment. For instance, in admitting the mother of a dependent adult with severe learning difficulties the normal admission routine might be expanded to involve the social worker as well as the doctor and the nurse. There may be immediate care needs and the patient's adult child may need particular help to become involved in and to understand his mother's impending death.[6]

An assessment requires four perspectives: the individual; the family; physical resources; and social resources.

The individual

In assessing the individual we need to establish what changes their illness has wrought, as well as who they are. We need to know how their life has changed since the illness and who or what currently supports them. We need to understand their reaction to the illness and its implications for them. We need to identify any practical or emotional unfinished business they may have. Assessing practical issues will lead us on to values and beliefs.[7] Does the individual see their illness as a punishment? How have they dealt with crises in the past? What are their aims now that they have entered palliative care; do they, for instance, want to die at home or in a hospital or hospice?

The family

The individual must be placed in the context of his family. In order to assess the strengths and difficulties of a family and its members, we need to understand how it works.[8] We must discover the normal patterns of communication, support, and conflict in the family, and the extent to which they have been disrupted by the illness.[9] For example is an argumentative family style usual and therefore acceptable and comfortable to the family, or does it represent a new and frightening response to the tensions of serious illness? Roles and shifts in role are important. For example what gaps will be left in the family when the patient dies; is he perhaps the peacemaker or the decision taker?

The history of the current family and their individual experiences within their previous families will be significant factors in their ability to cope with the present crisis. For example a wife who watched her own mother nurse her father through a protracted, exhausting, and painful terminal illness will in consequence approach her husband's death with reduced confidence. We need to understand the family's methods of coping with crisis and whether they are facing any additional change at the moment such as a house move, a redundancy, or a pregnancy.

Lastly, it is vital that we enquire about the existence of other vulnerable individuals within the family such as children, dependent elderly, or handicapped relatives. The terminal illness of a family member can be the final burden that topples a delicately balanced system of nurture and support and it may be necessary to provide additional external help.

Physical resources

The assessment should cover the family's physical resources, such as money and housing. We need to know about unmet physical needs because they may become the patient's biggest concern, and our expertise may be able to unlock money from charities or the state to relieve the problem. For instance a washing machine for the exhausted carer of a patient with night sweats and incontinence may be of more value than extra counselling or nursing support. A patient's physical resources may also affect how we care for them. Adaptations to their home, the provision of domestic help or meals on wheels may avoid or delay the need for inpatient care.

Social resources

Finally, the family themselves must be placed within the context of their community and social network. The team must understand their ethnic, cultural,[10] and religious[11] background and the potential impact of these influences on the individual and his illness. We must enquire about informal and formal helping systems available to the family within their community such as churches, social groups, and schools.[12]

An assessment of the individual, their family, and the physical and social resources available to them will lead to decisions. At one end of the spectrum the decision will be to do nothing. Assessment may reveal adequate coping mechanisms in the patient and their family and community. For instance, the family's priest may visit regularly and provide the support that they and the patient need; the palliative care team only need to maintain the appropriate communications.

Doing nothing may also be the right decision in less satisfactory cases. Withdrawn and lonely patients may need their defences, and the sensitive provision of physical care may be sufficient to ensure their dignity, whereas an attempt to solve their isolation may be resented. The result of the assessment may, however, be a decision to intervene in order to help the patient and family cope with their situation.

Interventions

Interventions will be aimed at patients and families who need help in order to cope with their situation.[13] They will typically need help because: they do not have the information they need; they cannot communicate sufficiently with each other to reach a solution; they lack the confidence to act; or they do not have the resources they need. In addition, an intervention may be addressed at the needs of bereaved individuals or families after the patient has died.

Information

Sometimes patients or families cannot cope simply because they lack information, leaving them at the mercy of their fears and fantasies. For instance many patients and their relatives will be very frightened of the moment of death because they do not know how it will happen; children sometimes imagine that death involves quantities of blood. Patients and families need information about what normally happens and what their options are. Patients will want to know how their illness will progress to death and how difficult symptoms will be treated. The patient with motor neurone disease will need reassurance about what exactly will be done if he chokes. Parents will want to know what to expect from their child in bereavement and what options they should consider for involving their child in the death.[14] Patients and relatives may want to understand the bereavement process they are going through; for example bereaved relatives may not know that it is normal to hear a dead person's key in the door.[15] They may also want information about arranging funerals and registering the death.

The way information is delivered is vital to its accurate reception. The style must be appropriate to the recipient both in terms of vocabulary and venue. Some people, for example, can discuss 'bad news' better in their own homes, others prefer the professional anonymity of a clinic. Pace is the other important component. Information must be offered when requested and at a speed that allows absorption.[16] Too much information delivered too quickly can paralyse and frighten; giving information is a two-way process that involves as much listening as talking.

The person who delivers the information may also be important; one of the advantages of the multidisciplinary team is the flexibility it provides. For example an elderly wife may be frightened to ask how her husband will die for fear of wasting the doctor's time. The social worker may be seen as less daunting. People often make their own choices about who to ask. A teenager with cancer, fearing medical jargon, may first discuss the options for further radiotherapy with the social worker. Conversely, an anxious dying mother, frightened of a social worker's potential judgement, may first express her worries about her son's shoplifting to the nurse.

Communication

The second objective for intervention is to help patients and their families communicate.[17] Communication is particularly difficult at the time of a bereavement, and a family that cannot share information and feelings cannot easily resolve the problems that death brings. Intervention is needed to restore the family's communications by reducing the barriers that impending bereavement may have raised.

The immediate barrier to communication is likely to be the strong, unfamiliar, and often conflicting feelings that each family member may experience in relation to the forthcoming death. These will disrupt their normal approach to communicating with each other. In addition, death and crisis often encourage people to protect one another. Loyalty and a conventional dislike of emotional display and upset may inhibit discussion of what is going on both emotionally and practically.

More specific barriers to communication may reflect the redistribution of roles within the family; a husband may be assuming unfamiliar parenting roles and responsibilities just as his dying wife is experiencing their loss. Communicating both the practical and emotional material within this transaction will be difficult. Similarly, the different perspectives of family members will reduce their ability to communicate; the husband's experience of his wife's impending death may be very different from his father-in-law's pain in losing a much loved daughter and this new difference may not be understood by the daughter, the husband, or the father.

Intervention will be aimed at overcoming these barriers and ensuring that the family and patient can communicate effectively. The intervention will work because a skilled outsider can provide the security and control which family members feel they need to release their emotions. The outsider will ensure that every member of the family hears a complete and shared story and that all understand properly how each one reacts to it. The shared information and the shared perceptions make possible a shared plan for the future and provide a powerful example which builds confidence for resolving problems in the future.

Improving a family's communication can be a very powerful tool, releasing the existing strengths within the family and allowing them to solve their own problems. Family members can begin to help rather than protect each other and new roles and relationships can be established. For some families a bereavement may provide the only opportunity for resolving historic arguments; exploiting the shared love of a dying parent to restore communication between family members who have not spoken for many years may allow the parent to see some meaning in his or her death, as well as releasing resources to deal with the immediate problems.

Intervention in a family's communication can also achieve very rapid results. The Hollywood cliché of the deathbed reconciliation is a real image. The crisis of impending bereavement can loosen the glue surrounding gummed-up communication patterns. Even in the final twenty-four hours of life it is possible to reopen communication and this can have a profound effect on the survivor's future emotional health.

The confidence to act

The dying patient and their family will often believe that they have no influence on events and may lack the confidence to take decisions for themselves. They will have emerged from medicine's final attempt to cure them; they will not know how long they have before they die; they will have been confused by the changing series of professionals they met as active treatment ended and palliative care began. Medical staff may have become the only key to hope and salvation, with their friends and family apparently as helpless as they themselves are. Often they will adopt a passive role, helpless at the mercy of forces they do not understand. Physical disability may be reinforcing their emotional conclusion. Patients need to be convinced that they have the scope to control events and that they can set themselves aims and objectives that can be met before they die.

For patients to have the confidence to act they must be reminded of the resources available to them and of how they have coped with crises in the past. They may need help to segment their problems in order to identify each element and its individual solution, and to focus on one or two difficulties that can be tackled out of a chaos that threatens to overwhelm. They may simply want the comforting presence of a concerned outsider as they think each stage through. For instance, the individual will often already know who or what can help them; the sympathetic teacher who can assist their child, the local church group who can mobilize a rota of supplementary carers. Sometimes the patient may only need to be asked in order to provide their own answers and solutions.

The confidence to act depends on setting realistic goals. Dying patients and their families will have experienced a dramatic change in what is achievable. They may need to be encouraged to plan for what is left and to decide what is important to them; some things may not be possible, but much will be. For instance, a dying mother can go for a few hours to her daughter's birthday party but may not be able to spend the weekend at home preparing party games and food. Her daughter can have a birthday cake but her husband will have to purchase it.

The resource to act

Patients and families may have the information they require, the ability to discuss and resolve their problems, and the confidence to do what is needed. Ultimately, however, they may simply not have the resources to do what needs to be done. If you are threatened with eviction for rent arrears because your dying husband cannot work, it may be difficult to focus on other needs. More prosaically, patients may not have access to the resources they need; what aids to daily living or housing adaptations are available and who will supply them? A raised toilet seat may help the patient to continue using the lavatory rather than a commode, a ramp may allow access to the garden for a wheelchair user.

Families need information about financial resources and sources of social support. These services should not be imposed but must be provided in a way that allows families to obtain the kind of help that they decide they need. Effectiveness in this role requires advocacy and influence with social services departments, government agencies, and charities.

Helping patients with resources can usefully be separated from counselling work even though both carry the social work label. Knowledge of available physical resources and welfare rights may be acquired by a member of staff without a specific social work qualification, who may be trained to help patients in these areas. Intimate and frequent contact with local resources is as important as the theoretical knowledge of institutions and welfare legislation that should underpin it.

Checklists can help many palliative care professionals to screen for a potential requirement for practical assistance. For example the recording form for the home care nurse's initial assessment could include boxes to tick about financial benefits, the necessity for a day centre place, the need for any aids to daily living.

Table 1 shows the kind of practical issues that may need to be addressed in the United Kingdom. Clearly, these will vary both according to the role of the palliative care institution and according to the characteristics of the community and country in which it operates. It is important to recognize that the task of the palliative care institution is to manipulate whatever is already available in society, rather than rushing to set up specialist services, expending time and energy that should be devoted to direct patient and family care. One of the most important components of the social work task is to act on behalf of the patient in order to get other agencies to do their job properly.

After the death

Further interventions may be necessary following the death of the patient. The normal process of providing palliative care should include efforts to identify those individuals at special risk in bereavement.[18] Loss and the grief that follows it are normal human experiences, but some people may need help to express their grief either because of their previous experiences and relationships or because of the particular circumstances of their bereavement. Unexpressed grief can result in physical symptoms, obsessive behaviours, and can precipitate individual or family breakdown.[19]

Bereavement services to solve these problems can take many forms. A brief and possibly routine intervention following the bereavement can offer relatives, including children, the opportunity to view the body, to say a final farewell, to ask questions about the illness and death, and to be given permission to start the necessary but painful process of remembering.[20] It may be important to offer longer-term help, perhaps from a volunteer bereavement counsellor who represents the community from which the patient came and to which the relative is returning. Specialist help may be required when circumstances are more extreme.[21] Examples are the child who firmly believes Mummy has gone on a journey

Table 1 Practical issues in social work

Need	Agency	Examples
Money	Government	Standard allowances for subsistence and rent. Special allowances for poor mobility, additional personal care, free prescriptions, fares for visiting, grants for funerals etc.
	Charitable (e.g Cancer Relief Macmillan Fund* Motor Neurone Disease Association)	Against specific needs; e.g. high heating bills, bedding, holidays, washing machine, food liquidizer, extra nursing help
Assistance in the home and for daily living	Local Authority Social Services Social Workers	Personal assistance Home help (Homemaker in N. America) Meals on wheels Childminding Family aides Fostering
	Occupational therapists Domiciliary physiotherapists Health Centres General practitioners District nurses Health visitors Charities (e.g. Red Cross)	Physical aids Telephone installation Personal alarm system Bathing aids Incontinence equipment Commodes Wheelchairs Stair rails etc.
		Concessions Disabled car badges Taxi concession cards Dial-a-ride transport for disabled
Housing and adaptations to housing	Local Authority Housing Department Charitable (e.g. Housing Association)	Transfer to more suitable accommodation adaptations (e.g. downstairs toilet) Sheltered housing Rent arrears
Relief and support to carers	Local Authority Social Services Department Charities (e.g. Age Concern, Help the Aged, Counsel and Care for the Elderly) Community institutions	Nursing homes Residential homes for the elderly Day Centres Luncheon clubs Schools Nurseries Playgroups Churches
Legal and financial advice and information	Solicitor	Preparing a will Appointing someone to act on your behalf in financial matters
	Citizens' Advice Bureau Funeral Directors	Debt counselling Advice about particular arrangements, e.g. sending a body abroad to be buried
	Local Authority Social Work Department Health centres	Child abuse
	Social workers Community psychiatric nurses	Mental illness

* United Kingdom charities.

and will return; the adult son who insists that he has caused his father's death by refusing to pursue an approved career.

Social work methods

Interventions can provide information, increase communication, give confidence, provide resources, or help the bereaved. There are three traditional methods for making these interventions; one-to-one meetings, family meetings, or groups involving unrelated individuals with shared circumstances or problems. For all forms of intervention adolescents and young children often represent the most challenging and draining group, and palliative care teams will typically want to take extra care in these cases. Finally, all interventions will be made by listening and talking and here too there are particular skills and particular responsibilities.

One-to-one help

Any member of the team may find themselves talking to the patient or a family member with therapeutic intent. There are no answers or solutions to the emotional anguish experienced by dying people but they can be helped by being heard. Sharing the problem is sometimes enough to provide relief; knowing yourself to be heard and understood is a vital human need. It is not necessary to approve what the patient says or does; it is important to show understanding of the feeling behind his words and actions.

Staff may fear being overwhelmed by the intensity of emotion they release in the patient and more particularly that in talking about things they may have made them worse. We must often allow people to cry, to express and feel their anger, and to become worse; they may thus become more aware of the nature and origin of their pain and more able to decide how to cope with it.[22]

Meeting the patient or members of the family on a one-to-one basis may be an important precursor to work with the whole family. It ensures that we understand individual perspectives and problems. For example the loving wife of a dying patient may need privacy to begin acknowledging her resentment at the exhausting task of caring. She may want to rehearse the exposure of her conflicting feelings with a sympathetic outsider before seeking a reconciliation between her resentment and grief with her husband.

Family meetings

Meeting with a family group can be a powerful tool for change and the resolution of problems. Some professionals fear that such groups will get out of control.[23] A common fear is that the family will simply shout at one another, as indeed they sometimes will. However, the initial conflicts are the data from which understanding and reconciliation may come. An argument about which of the adult children should provide Christmas lunch for their dying mother may reveal that the cause of the shouting is that one child believes that the other has always been mother's favourite.

It is important to prepare properly for such meetings, and to decide, often with the patient, who should be there and which members of staff will be the most appropriate facilitators. It is helpful for the team to work in pairs; for example a doctor and a social worker. The doctor might begin with an overview of the illness and its history, to be followed by the social worker exploring the family's reaction to it. The family should do most of the talking, as the aim is to help them solve the problem, not to solve it for them. The family may need to experience new ways of relating to one another. For example they may need to be told to allow each other to talk without interruption; a child may need to be invited to speak for himself. They may need help to address painful issues: 'I think everyone in this family is wondering what will happen when Mum isn't here to look after you all.'

Groups

Group work will normally involve people who share similar problems or experiences, but who are otherwise strangers to each other. For instance bereaved fathers may meet to share the practical and emotional problems of bring up their children alone.[24,25] Patients may use a group to explore feelings about the stigmatizing nature of their illness, anger at loss of control and dependence, and thoughts of hopelessness and suicide.[26] Bereaved children[27–29] and adults[30] may gain increased confidence from the normalization of grief that group work permits in contrast to their social communities where they may feel excluded or misunderstood.

Such groups have many benefits. Members will hear others express the difficulties they felt too embarrassed, guilty, or frightened to share. Individuals within the group will increase their self esteem by giving support as well as receiving it. Group work does not represent a 'cheap' alternative in terms of manpower or time. Groups are usually more effectively run by two leaders who will need time for preparation before a session and time for assessment and discussion after it. The leaders themselves will need supervision, training, and support.

Working with children

Children facing bereavement have similar needs and emotions to adults. However, they may be expressed differently, for example through behaviour rather than words.[31] The quiet child who becomes aggressive and demanding at school or the child who refuses to eat or wets the bed, has a problem similar to that of an adult, even if we cannot recognize it as readily. Research indicates that a child's later development may be powerfully and adversely affected by the early loss of an important family member, particularly a parent.[32,33] Palliative care professionals have a responsibility to ensure that such potential damage is minimized and social workers possess specialist skills in this area.

It is impossible not to communicate with children.[34] Terminal illness causes enormous changes within the family and children quickly sense when something so serious is happening. They pick up the emotions around them, read body language, overhear conversations, piece together chance remarks by neighbours and school friends, and see the evidence of physical deterioration. However, children's apparent vulnerability often evokes an impulse in both parents and professionals to protect children from the truth. The difficulties of deciding what level of information is appropriate and what words to use, added to the fear that saying the wrong thing will make matters worse, often lead to an excluding silence. Exclusion leads to isolation, leaving children unprotected from their fantasies and unsupported in their feelings.

Like adults, children need an opportunity to ask questions, to receive information and reassurance, and a chance to express and share their feelings in safety.[35] This help needs to be delivered in ways that are appropriate to their age and individual level of understanding and this can only be determined by asking them about their experiences.[36,37] Four-year-old Jack asked immediately after his mother's death, as he sat by her body, 'Is she completely dead?' He then asked, 'What does 'completely' mean? He then wanted to know, 'Will she still be dead when I'm fifteen?' I have seen Jack and his brother every 3 weeks since their mother's death 6 months ago. Jack still greets me by saying, 'Mummy is completely dead', checking out that something so awful is still true. When I agree, he accepts the fact quietly.

Help for children has to start with their parents and families who will be around long after the professionals have disappeared. The task of professionals is to help parents to help their children. Parents may have good reasons for their reluctance to share information about illness and death with their children. They will be struggling to maintain some control in an uncertain situation. They, themselves, will be grieving and they may want to protect their children from this pain. The child may also want to protect its parents by trying to pretend that nothing is happening. It is often necessary to work with parents on their own before children's needs can be addressed. For example a couple who cannot openly acknowledge impending death between themselves are not well placed to help their children.

We do not help parents by taking over from them—they know their children best, but we can offer them support, encouragement, and practical help. We can begin by creating environments that release parents from the expectation that children should not be involved. We must invite their presence, perhaps with a designated area with small chairs and a toy box. Equipment, such as dolls in beds, puppets, toy medical kits, and telephones, can help children to act out their concerns and to ask questions. Drawing can help them to express and control powerful emotions that they lack the vocabulary to voice. There are a number of specially designed drawing and creative workbooks available for this purpose.[38–41] Parents may appreciate advice about their child's likely understanding of death, their needs as they face bereavement, and the kinds of explanation and vocabulary appropriate to their age. Professionals must, of course, always respect the family's own belief system. Lists of books and leaflets for parents to read for themselves[42,43] or to read with their children[44,45] will often be appreciated. For many parents this will be sufficient and they will then want to speak to their children alone. Others may welcome sharing the task with a professional.

Parents want to do what is best for their children and they learn very fast. They may be reassured by the suggestion that a professional meet them and their children to discuss changes in the family and to answer questions about the illness. Just being part of one such direct conversation can help parents to feel confident enough to continue for themselves.[46] Children facing the death of a parent need reassurance about their own continuing care and assistance in managing their inevitable separation anxieties.[47] Whether we raise it or not they will be wondering who will look after them and perform the familiar activities such as taking them to school. It is an enormous relief to them and their parents when these painful issues are addressed. Children also need explicit reassurance about the illness itself, for example whether it is contagious, and to know that their own thoughts or behaviour could not have caused the death. Parents may need encouragement to widen their child's support network by involving other adults close to them such as teachers, clergy, or friends and relatives. Parents sometimes need assistance to anticipate, understand, and accept altered or difficult behaviour in their grieving children.

Children learn to mourn and to grieve healthily by observing others and families can be encouraged to understand that sharing feelings often helps, as does involvement in important rituals such as viewing the body, attending the funeral,[48] or being given something that belonged to the dead person.[49] Such activities help children to feel included and act as tangible reminders of the existence of the dead person and their importance. Professionals help parents by giving them information so that they and their children can decide together about what they feel comfortable with. An important piece of recent research is the finding that children's emotional well being after the death of a parent appears to be linked to their ability to remain connected to the deceased in some way after the death—to find an appropriate way to keep them in their lives.[50] Discovering ways of helping families to facilitate this is a challenge for professionals in palliative care.

Listening and talking

Listening and talking to patients is one of the key tasks in palliative care. Most dying patients are not looking to carers, professional, or family for solutions to their situation. They want someone to share the problems with; what helps people who are grieving is someone trustworthy who will listen to their experiences and help them explore the depths of their pain without offering false reassurance.

People facing loss awaken powerful feelings in the professionals who meet them.[51,52] We cannot listen properly to the loss of others if our own losses, actual or feared, are unexplored and unresolved. Work with the dying often makes us worry about not coping or about becoming over involved. We do not know what to say; we do not know how to 'make things better'. We have to learn how to share what we do not know as well as our knowledge, and above all, how to listen accurately.

Silence is an important part of listening. Professionals often misinterpret and feel uncomfortable with silence. They may interrupt too readily rather than allowing the patient to express his concern for himself. Silence is a necessary part of the patient's exploration of his thoughts and feelings. Prompts should be gentle and open—'You have been quiet for a long time now. I wonder if it would help you to share some of your thoughts.'

The professional must use language sensitively. Questioning should be direct but unassertive: 'What is the worst thing for you at the moment?' We need to help people to clarify their feelings for themselves: 'Can you give me an example of that . . . can you help me to understand a bit better?' The use of clear, simple, feeling words such as 'sad, angry, death, guilty' helps the patient to express their emotions.

Body language should be both observed and used. 'You say you are feeling fine, but you look so very tense and anxious'. Team members should be aware of the power of touch to convey understanding and comfort when words seems inadequate.

For some people and some circumstances talking and listening may be ineffective.[53] Ritual is an alternative way of reaching feelings. Familiar rituals can offer great comfort, such as a cup of tea or the rites of prayer and religious observance.[54] New rituals can be created to meet new needs. A team member may encourage a whole family to hold hands or to spend a moment in silence remembering their love for one another. A bereaved daughter may finally be able to express her ambivalent feelings towards her dead mother and to forgive her, by writing a letter to her and burying it at the grave.

Sharing information

Personal information received from patients and families places particular responsibilities on team members.[55] All palliative care professionals will operate within a professional framework requiring respect for the individual's privacy and autonomy and underlining the ethic of confidentiality. However, confidentiality can sometimes suffer unnecessarily in the particular atmosphere of the multidisciplinary team. The need to pass on personal information must always be questioned; it is neither right nor necessary that every team member should know everything a patient or relative shares with an individual within that team. Patients choose who they talk to. Wherever possible the permission of the patient or family member should be sought explicitly: 'Thank you for telling me such an important and difficult thing. Would you mind if I tell other members of the team looking after you?' No one needs to know more than will enable them to fulfil their own role in caring for the patient. A volunteer car driver, for example, does not need to know details of the patient's diagnosis but will need to know that he uses a walking frame.

Within teams we must be clear about why we want information. Often, in the rapidly developing environment engendered by terminal illness, the emotional truth perceived and expressed by patient or family is more important than amassing painstaking details about the past. The desire for more and more information can represent power, confirmation of inclusion in the 'inner circle' or just plain inquisitiveness. A test of the trust necessary for teams to function well is the willingness of members to accept that another may hold confidential information and use it appropriately.

Recording of information also demands great care. What is written, particularly if it is subjective, can easily assume the status of objective truth. Recording should always be undertaken with regard to the possibility of patient and family access. Entire detailed conversations should never be recorded, rather, general issues and guidelines for future staff conduct. It would not, for example, be appropriate for every nurse in a team to know that a patient had told the social worker about past convictions for violent crime or that they had been sexually abused as a child.

Case study

Introduction

This case study is intended to illustrate the most demanding form that the social work task takes. Janet Skinner (no real names are used here) and her family faced a series of difficult and interconnected medical and social problems associated with Janet's death. These concerned her attempted suicide, her marriage, her children, and the threat of breast cancer in succeeding generations. The scale and breadth of her problems are untypical but they illustrate clearly the sequence of assessment and intervention, and the value of a competent and thoughtful professional approach.

Janet was 36 when she was admitted to St Christopher's Hospice. She had been married to her husband Rob for 12 years and they both knew she could no longer be cured. She had two children, Susan aged seven and Paul aged five. Her breast cancer had been diagnosed 5 years previously and was at that time treated with surgery, radiotherapy, and chemotherapy. She remained well and disease free for two and half years when evidence of metastatic disease in the lung and liver was discovered. She received further chemotherapy which she tolerated very poorly.

Three months later she presented with multiple brain metastases and an enlarged liver, and was again treated with chemotherapy and cranial irradiation, despite her previous low tolerance of the treatment and her poor prognosis. She developed a left sided weakness, walking became increasingly difficult, and she began to

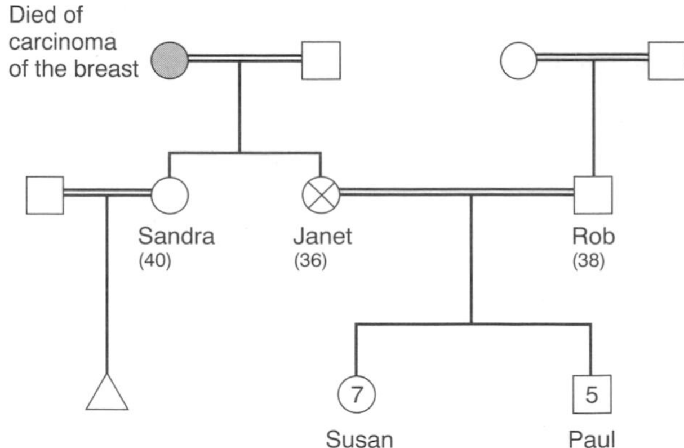

Fig. 1 Family structure.[56]

use a wheelchair. She was cushingoid. She became depressed and cancelled a hospital appointment. On the evening before her rescheduled appointment she took an overdose of drugs and cut her wrists whilst her husband was busy getting tea for the children. Janet was admitted to the hospice from the local hospital who had treated her following the suicide attempt.

The assessment

Individual

Janet expressed sadness and anger about the many losses she was facing; she had lost her role as mother, involvement in and a sense of security about her children's future, her physical attractiveness, a normal family life, and her faith in a caring God. She was also angry about the treatment she had endured, given its eventual futility. She felt she had been trapped into continuing with active treatment and on the day of her admission said that she 'just wanted to die'.

Janet experienced her pain as total and unendurable but she also desperately wanted to live to be a mother for her children. She described them being shunted between friends and neighbours and told us that it was her son's birthday next week and that she would be useless to him. Janet felt very guilty about her suicide attempt and asked about the possibility of having further chemotherapy at the hospice. Above all, she felt completely powerless.

Family

Everyone in the family was affected by Janet's illness. It emerged that Janet's mother had also died of breast cancer when Janet was the same age as her own daughter was now (Fig. 1). Her father was reliving the loss of his wife in the loss of his daughter.

Janet's older sister, Sandra, was pregnant. She had been trying to conceive for many years. Amniocentesis the previous week had confirmed that the fetus was both healthy and female. Sandra and Janet knew what it was like to lose a mother. Sandra felt that giving birth while her sister was dying was 'obscene'.

Janet's husband, Rob, concerned the team by his noticeable reticence. He was silent throughout the procedures of his wife's admission, merely expressing concern that he might be late collecting the children from school.

The team was informed that the children had not been told about their mother's specific illness or prognosis, just that she was 'ill'. The family said that they had become clinging and difficult to get to bed at night.

Physical

Money was not a problem for this family. However, concerns were expressed about how Janet could manage at home, even on a visit, in her wheelchair with increasing weakness making transfers difficult. How would she get to the lavatory, could she negotiate the stairs, what would happen if she fell?

Social

Janet and Rob had had a wide circle of friends and an active social life. However, the stresses and upheaval of her illness and treatment had caused them to become isolated. The consequences of this isolation were that Janet and Rob were no longer getting emotional support or sufficient practical help from their friends, family, and community network. Janet was refusing visitors and had stopped attending the local church or seeing the vicar. The children's teachers were not fully informed about Janet's illness. Rob was relying on a series of temporary arrangements with neighbours to care for his children while he tried to continue with his job. Janet's and Rob's parents wanted to help but they were uncertain both about how to offer help, and what help they could best give.

Intervention

This family were perceived to be in emotional crisis, unable to cope with the problems facing them. Just as the scream of pain demands a response from the palliative care team, so does the scream of emotional anguish. The family did not appear to be able to communicate with one another. They were all stunned by Janet's suicide attempt. The team thought that if this pain and guilt was not addressed, Janet's wider family, and in particular her husband, would be unable to offer both Janet and her children the support and care they needed so badly. However, at this stage it was impossible to assess the problem fully and it was clear that there were many potentially conflicting individual needs. The team therefore decided to see the family individually, both to allow them to express their emotional pain and in order to understand what was going on.

Individual meetings

Rob and Janet both individually revealed that a major source of anguish and anger was a love affair of Rob's which had resulted in a child. The love affair had ended but Rob knew that Janet had not forgiven him for his betrayal of her, particularly whilst she was ill. Rob felt guilty and wanted to repair his relationship with Janet, yet felt trapped by his past. Janet feared that once she was dead he would create a new family for his daughters by marrying his former girlfriend.

Janet's sister was uncertain about continuing her pregnancy. Both she and Janet had lost their mother; Janet's children were now losing theirs. Sandra was wondering whether the same would happen to her unborn child. Janet and Sandra both feared that their daughters would repeat the same cycle of events.

Although the team had decided that the social worker needed to have a prominent and co-ordinating role in these meetings, the variety of team members involved allowed significant later interventions. For example an early meeting with the chaplain paved the way for a later service in the hospice chapel focusing on peace and forgiveness with the laying on of hands. This ritual was profoundly helpful to Janet.

The data from these initial, individual meetings seemed to predict an even more hopeless future. It did, however, pinpoint some important issues for joint meetings. The team began to create a series of specific objectives against known problems.

Having met Janet and Rob individually we were aware of their conflict and the source of the distance between them. We needed to try to achieve a sufficient reconciliation between them for them at least to address their children's needs together. Sandra needed to talk to her husband about her fears and her pregnancy. The children needed information and support.

Joint meetings

Rob and Janet voiced a wish to be seen together, although neither of them was hopeful about the outcome. They expressed enormous and vociferous anger towards one another. It was necessary to confront them very directly: 'Is this really how you want things to end?' The turning point was Rob's open expression of anguish at his inadequacies as a father. He wept at his inability to iron his daughter's dress for her brother's birthday party. He and Janet began to share their pain as well as their anger, and their common purpose in loving and caring for their children.

Sandra, Janet's sister, was seen with her husband and told him for the first time of her anxieties. He had felt excluded and he had not known why. Sharing their fears enabled him to support Sandra and together they decided that the pregnancy should continue.

Family meetings and the children

Susan and Paul joined their parents in a series of meetings with the social worker and the doctor. They were encouraged to ask questions: 'What is wrong with Mummy?' 'Why hasn't Mummy got any hair?' 'Why does her breathing sound funny?' They expressed their feelings: 'I try hard not to cry because I'm scared I'll upset Daddy'. They gradually came to a realization of the gravity of their mother's illness and it was Rob who Susan finally asked: 'Is Mummy going to die?'. He was able to answer her directly and began to express more confidence in his role of father. Janet was very upset by these meetings but also reassured and moved by the children's expression of love for her: 'I love you Mummy, I want you to come home'.

These meetings and meetings with other family groupings succeeded in creating a calmer and more positive atmosphere in which Janet and her husband could set goals for the future. The couple began to request and share appropriate information and take control. During the family meetings, and subsequently, they took a number of decisions and actions.

1. Janet decided against further active treatment.

2. Janet's family and her sister's family had a meeting with a consultant who specialized in genetic cancer counselling.

3. Janet planned her own funeral and had special watches engraved for the children to keep after her death. She had not been given any proper explanation of her mother's death nor attended the funeral, and wanted things to be different for her children.

4. The family as a whole discussed the approach they would take towards the children's needs as they faced bereavement. With Janet's help they planned an advertisement for a nanny.

5. The headmaster of the children's school came to the hospice to discuss future options for their education with Janet and Rob.

6. Janet and Rob's parents and friends arranged a rota for visiting and helped Janet to get home most weekends and to go out to the theatre and restaurants.

7. With the help of a nurse escort from the hospice Janet and Rob planned and successfully completed a short holiday abroad with the children. It was important to Janet that the children had one last family memory involving her that was fun.

After death

The social worker saw Rob and the children on three occasions. Together they discussed the impact of the death, the funeral, the children's behaviour at school and home, and the family's grief. With Rob's permission the social worker again contacted the children's class teachers to discuss the help that might be offered in school. A volunteer bereavement counsellor was in touch with the parents of Janet and Rob.

Difficulties

Helping this family posed many difficulties for the team. It was difficult not to become personally involved with the intensity of their pain. We certainly neglected this area for the nurse who accompanied them on holiday. As the social worker I can remember how difficult it was to say good-bye to Janet when I went on annual leave knowing she might well be dead on my return. Janet herself solved this for me: 'I want to say good-bye. I probably won't be here when you get back'.

We had to grapple with setting boundaries for Janet and her family, boundaries that they could not be expected to set for themselves. Rob needed us to tell Janet when he and she could no longer cope with the visits home. However, we also needed to remember that we were not part of the family and that they needed to make their own decisions and to experience their own pain. Janet died peacefully 8 weeks after her admission to the hospice. Rob and her father were present.

The wider role

So far we have examined the social work task to which all members of a palliative care team will contribute, including the social worker. Next we examine the wider and more specific roles of the social worker within palliative care.

The balance of the social worker's work will depend on the circumstances of the institution in which they work and on the other skills that are available within the team. For instance a part-time worker, whose colleagues are experienced at counselling patients, might focus on bereavement services; a social worker at a day centre might specialize in group work. The consultative and educational aspects of the role may be more pronounced in hospital support and home-care teams or in those hospices with study centres. However, the components of the social worker's task are likely to include internal consultancy, community liaison, equality of access, training and the development of social work practice, and staff support and management.

Internal consultancy

The basic component of a typical social worker's role will be the support of nurses and doctors in carrying out the social work task. At one extreme the support will be simple advice; at the other it will be taking a leadership role in the management of a specific patient and their family. In effect the social worker will operate as an internal consultant.

In fulfilling this role the social worker should be involved in the day-to-day decisions about how best to manage individual patients. He or she will not be an effective resource if they are only summoned from their office when someone thinks they are needed. Thus, the social worker should participate in ward meetings and rounds, should contribute to medical notes, and should understand the major concerns of the other disciplines in palliative care, such as medicine and nursing.

Social workers will also contribute to policy advice within the palliative care team: how to deal with drunken relatives; how to respond to suicide threats; what facilities should be provided for children; what guidelines should be available on the issue of confidentiality.

Community liaison

Social workers will normally assume responsibility within the palliative care team for liaison with the community and its non-medical resources. This task requires both routine general contact and specific action on behalf of individual patients and their families.

The specific action will be to create a 'package of care' for the patient in question perhaps involving both the resources of the social worker's institution and those of the wider community. For example these might include domestic help, adaptations to the home, meals on wheels, childminders, and nightsitters. The community resources which may be available for tapping include money from government agencies or charities, or the time and attention of community social workers or local voluntary groups. Help may also be available from or through school teachers, community nurses, and family doctors.

Equality of access

The training and community experience of social workers means that they should be in the vanguard of the important moves to examine and respond to the challenges of equal access and opportunity in palliative care. Many palliative care services operate in multicultural communities and are increasingly seeking to improve access to their services. If services are to become truly available, thought needs to be given to the different groups in any given population and the different ways in which they may use health services.[57] This process operates at every level, from the experiments to extend primarily cancer centred palliative care services to those patients with progressive non-malignant disorders,[58] to the consideration of ways of improving knowledge of palliative care services and access to them by people from ethnic minority communities. Issues of disability, gender, race, and sexual orientation[59] represent challenges to develop antidiscriminatory practice both for staff responding to patients and families and for institutions in their plans for training and recruitment of those staff, both paid and voluntary. For example do the volunteer counsellors in a bereavement service represent a cross section of the communities they seek to serve? The clear standards for service delivery set by purchasers of HIV/AIDS services[60,61] merely define and reiterate those that ought to be in place for all users of health-care services.

Social workers should assist their services to develop equal opportunity strategies including clear and well publicized codes of conduct and complaints procedures. They can be expected to be active in the development of links between local voluntary groups in the community and palliative care services. They should also be available to help with the training needs of other staff.

Culture affects us all. The crisis of death may make an individual's relationship with his or her culture and spiritual roots deeper and closer, or may reveal conflicts with generations in transition between their family's culture and local cultural practices.[62] The dying who have experienced previous persecution as a result of political, racial, or religious differences will often have special needs as they re-experience traumatic losses.[63] Everyone deserves respect for their individual cultural values and expectations. It is important, therefore, to clarify individual preferences about cultural and religious practices (for example not every Jewish person keeps kosher) as well as improving general knowledge about the likely needs of specific groups.[64,65] Such needs may include diet, methods of medical treatment, personal care and clothing, religious and mourning rituals, access to trained and supported interpreters and religious leaders of all faiths, and literature and signposts in languages that users can understand.[66]

In 1995, the National Council for Hospice and Specialist Palliative Care Services in the United Kingdom published a report on access to services by members of black and ethnic minority communities in which the need to monitor take-up of services was emphasized.[67] We cannot assess whether our services are accessible until we are aware of how much potential users known about the services, and until we have accurate and detailed data on who is actually using our services and the reason why those who choose not to do so, decline.[68]

Training and the development of social work practice

Social workers should lead the development of social work practice within their institutions. This should include both the development of the service provided and the development of the skills required to support the service. Service development activities might include setting up a multidisciplinary group to examine, for instance, potential improvements in the care offered to relatives immediately after the death. It will also include individual activity; for example social workers should ensure that their colleagues have access to good written material such as booklists for a bereaved child or leaflets explaining how to claim state benefits for widows. Social workers will want to develop and write their own publications, particularly where these need to be tailored to their institutions or their local community. An example might be a leaflet for bereaved adolescents.[69]

Development of social work practice within the institution should extend naturally into skills training and development. Sharing and passing on skills should also flow from the internal consultancy role; all joint work with patients is an opportunity to learn new skills and understand new perspectives, both for the social worker and his or her colleague.

More formal contributions to the development of skills might include, for example, training sessions for nurses, preferably integrated into the nursing profession's own training and development programmes. Training is also a way of changing practice within the team; for example informal training sessions for multidisciplinary teams on subjects such as 'coping with anger' or 'talking about sex'[70] can be used to improve the whole team's performance and confidence in dealing with specific problems.

Staff support and management

Social workers who successfully involve themselves in service and skill development are likely to find themselves also involved in staff support. Palliative care makes difficult and personal demands on the individuals who provide it. Any professional discussion on providing a better service will also need to focus on the emotional reactions of members of the team, and these reactions will frequently relate to the individual's own experience. Palliative care workers can enrich their work from their experience of the death of their own friends or relatives; however, the commonality between their own experience and those for whom they care is also a possible problem with which they may need help. For instance, the ethics of sedation and the proper response to relatives' questions such as 'Why can't you put Dad out of his misery?' are likely to arise both as practice issues and as personal issues for those involved. Social workers who take some leadership in the service development of their institution will, in setting policy on ethical questions, also need to take some leadership on ethical questions in training and in response to the personal concerns raised by staff.

Staff support may be provided to a team or to individuals. At St Christopher's Hospice in the United Kingdom, individual help, offered on a confidential basis, by the Social Work Department, is restricted to two or three meetings, aimed primarily at examining options and identifying, where necessary, an appropriate further referral for additional help. It is not usually appropriate for long-term individual counselling to be provided to staff within their workplace, particularly in a palliative care institution where personal and institutional objectives are likely to be all too readily confused.

Social workers should also have a role in managing the wider issues within their institution. They should be involved in setting policy on patient care, as well as decisions on individual patients. They are likely to be involved in admissions, staff recruitment, quality control, and education and training services, both internal and external. They will specifically manage their own responsibilities such as welfare services and volunteer bereavement services. They may be called upon to initiate and manage innovative interdisciplinary practice. For example the director of social work at St Christopher's Hospice in the United Kingdom has recently assumed managerial responsibility for developing and running two new services. The first is a formal, advertized, multidisciplinary telephone advisory service for health-care professionals that took over 500 calls in its first year of operation, ranging from a family doctor wanting advice about the management of secretions not controlled by hyoscine, to a headmistress requesting advice about helping a seven-year-old whose mother had been killed in a road traffic accident. The second is a consultancy service intended to help patients and families for whom the usual range of hospice services is inappropriate. It is a short-term service offering the patient or family between one to five contacts from a variety of professionals. Ideally, social workers will also be able to influence and take part in the management process of the institution itself.

Extending the service

The wider values and goals of palliative care are, at least in Western economies, under resourced and poorly acknowledged. Support is improving; for instance in the United Kingdom specific bereavement services are now normally established after major disasters such as the Bradford Football Stadium fire.[71] However, the extent to which the community provides resources or acknowledges the need for such services depends on how those in the field spread their message and how they demonstrate their effectiveness and value. Social workers have a particular duty in this area as they are the professional group in palliative care which claims to have the strongest links into the community. The social worker's response to under-resourcing and poor acknowledgement should take two forms: the use of volunteers and spreading the word.

The use of volunteers

Used properly, volunteers can extend enormously the variety and scope of services offered to patients and families. Volunteers also have the advantage of representing the community from which patients come and therefore have the ability to educate and influence that community about loss, bereavement, and palliative care values. Volunteers can be used in many areas, for example as nursing aides, hairdressers, car drivers, or bereavement counsellors. Social workers in palliative care will frequently want to provide counselling for bereaved relatives. One social worker can supervise a team of six volunteers, each carrying a caseload of six people, thus providing a considerable volume of service at reasonable cost.[72] The use of volunteers should not be a reason for reduced quality; an effective volunteer bereavement service should select its volunteers rigorously and provide appropriate training. It will have a programme for extending and maintaining skills through group events and individual supervision and will certainly aim to be a genuinely professional service and not an untutored or unfocused provision of 'tea and sympathy'.

Volunteers can be organized internally or externally. Some social workers, for example, might choose to work with an external voluntary organization to provide bereavement counselling, rather than personally organizing a group of volunteers. The relationship with the external agency may include some elements of training and individual supervision. Volunteers' activities will also be complementary; the social worker might run a regular bereavement session for all the institution's clients, followed up by individual support where appropriate from volunteer counsellors.

Spreading the word

The message of palliative care is relevant in many settings within the wider community, and the resources that the community devotes to palliative care depend upon effective advocacy of both our work and our message. Social workers within palliative care should be involved in a broad spectrum of activities which serve to spread the message. At one end of the spectrum these will be an extension of the normal liaison with other local organizations concerned with the care of patients, at the other it may include political lobbying and direct attempts to influence decisions in favour of palliative care.

The direct task of liaising with other local caring organizations for the benefit of individual patients may broaden in a number of ways. For example a social worker may become involved in lecturing to staff in a general hospital about the care of dying patients, or in helping a local health centre to develop its approach to terminal care in the community. Other contacts, such as with school teachers,[73] funeral directors, community social workers, or welfare workers in large public or commercial organizations, may turn into opportunities to offer training or support to other professionals who have to deal with the consequences of death. For example the Social Work Department at St Christopher's Hospice in the United Kingdom recently ran a series of training sessions for the Metropolitan Police Force on breaking bad news, in particular informing relatives of a sudden death. Such help and assistance may be particularly relevant in special cases such as the death of a child. For instance a social worker in palliative care may be the most experienced resource within the community to advise a school on how to cope after the murder of a pupil.

In addition to influencing attitudes locally, social workers should participate in the development of palliative care regionally, nationally, and internationally. By the nature of their work, social workers in palliative care are widely dispersed, and it is important that this fragmentation does not cause the social workers' perspective to be lost. Social workers should seek roles on advisory committees and offer their expertise and advice both to specialist groups, such as the specialist disease charities, and to government.

When appropriate social workers should be prepared to lobby actively for change. For instance in the United Kingdom the Association of Hospice Social Workers spearheaded a successful campaign to change welfare benefit rules so that terminally ill patients could claim a special attendance allowance more quickly. They are now carefully monitoring the impact of new legislation on the financing and provision of care in the community.[74]

Finally, social workers must be involved in defining the future of palliative care. We have come to understand more and more of the medical aspects of palliative care, but we know little about the long term impact of terminal illness on family members and even less about what helps them.[75] Social workers will increasingly be involved in developing a better understanding of the psychosocial aspects of palliative care, and in the implementation of new ways of caring for patients and their families.[76]

References

1. Earnshaw-Smith E. Emotional pain in dying patients and their families. *Nursing Times*, 1982; **78**: 865–7.
2. Lunn L. Spiritual concerns in palliation. In: Saunders C, Sykes N, eds.

The Management of Terminal Malignant Disease. 3rd edn. London: Edward Arnold, 1993: 213–25.

3. Speck PW. *Being There—Pastoral Care in Times of Illness*. London: SPCK, 1988.
4. Firth P, Anderson P. Teamwork with families facing bereavement. *European Journal of Palliative Care*, 1994; **1**: 157–61.
5. Monroe B. Children and bereavement. In: Open University Department of Health and Social Welfare. *Death and Dying*. Student Pack Workbook 4 Pack K260S. Milton Keynes: Open University, 1992: 74–84.
6. Oswin M. *Am I Allowed to Cry?* London: Souvenir Press, 1991.
7. Barkwell DP. Ascribed meaning: a critical factor in coping and pain attenuation in patients with cancer-related pain. *Journal of Palliative Care*, 1991; **7**: 5–14.
8. Kirschling J.M. ed. *Family-Based Palliative Care*. New York: Howarth Press, 1990.
9. Smith N. The impact of terminal illness on the family. *Palliative Medicine*, 1990; **4**: 127–35.
10. Oliviere D. Cross-cultural principles of care. In: Saunders C, Sykes N, eds. *The Management of Terminal Malignant Disease*. 3rd edn. London: Edward Arnold, 1993: 202–12.
11. Abeles M. Features of Judaism for carers when looking after Jewish patients. *Palliative Medicine*, 1991; **5**: 201–5.
12. Capewell E. Responding to children in trauma: a systems approach for schools. *Bereavement Care*, 1994; **13**: 2–7.
13. Carter B, McGoldrick M. *The Changing Family Life Cycle*. London: Allyn and Bacon, 1989.
14. Sheldon F. Children and bereavement—what are the issues? *European Journal of Palliative Care*, 1994; **1**: 42–4.
15. Worden JW. *Grief Counselling and Grief Therapy*. London: Routledge, 1991.
16. Buckman R. *How to Break Bad News*. London: Papermac, 1992.
17. Sheldon F. Communication. In: Saunders C, Sykes N, eds. *The Management of Terminal Malignant Disease*. 3rd edn. London: Edward Arnold, 1993: 15–32.
18. Sanders C. Risk factors in bereavement outcome In: Stroebe M, Stroebe W, Hansson R. eds. *Handbook of Bereavement: Theory Research and Intervention*. New York: Cambridge University Press, 1993: 255–67.
19. Middleton W, Raphael B, Martinek N, Misso V. Pathological grief reactions. In: Stroebe M, Stroebe W, Hansson R, eds. *Handbook of Bereavement: Theory Research and Intervention*. New York: Cambridge Unversity Press, 1993: 44–61.
20. O'Brien T, Monroe B. Twenty four hours before and after death. In: Saunders C, ed. *Hospice and Palliative Care: An Interdisciplinary Approach*. London: Edward Arnold, 1990: 46–53.
21. Pincus L. *Death and the Family*. London: Faber, 1976.
22. Stedeford A. *Facing Death: Patients, Families and Professionals*. Oxford: Sobell Publications, 1994.
23. Monroe B. Psychosocial dimensions of palliation. In: Saunders C, Sykes N, eds. *The Management of Terminal Malignant Disease*. 3rd edn. London: Edward Arnold, 1993: 174–201.
24. Burnell A, Goodchild J. Working with bereaved fathers. *Bereavement Care*, 1994: **13**: 28–30.
25. O'Dowd T. The needs of fathers. *British Medical Journal*, 1993; **306**: 1484.
26. Carter P. The Thursday Group Hospice Bulletin. *St Christopher's Hospice Information Service*, 1994; **24**: 5.
27. Fleming S, Balmer L. Group intervention with bereaved children. In: Papadatos C, Papadatou D, eds. *Children and Death*. New York: Hemisphere, 1991: 105–24.
28. Baulkwill J, Wood C. Groupwork with bereaved children. *European Journal of Palliative Care*, 1994; **1**: 113–15.
29. Kitchener S, Pennells M. A bereavement group for children. *Bereavement Care*, 1990; **9**: 30–1.
30. Broadbent M, Horwood P, Sparkes J, De Whalley G. Bereavement groups. *Bereavement Care*, 1990; **9**: 14–16.
31. Jewett C. *Helping Children Cope with Separation and Loss*. London: Batsford, 1984.
32. Black D. The bereaved child. *Journal of Child Psychology and Psychiatry*, 1978; **19**: 287–92.
33. Brown G, Harris T. *The Social Origins of Depression*. London: Tavistock, 1978.
34. Monroe B. Psychosocial dimensions of palliation In: Saunders C, Sykes N, eds. *The Management of Terminal Malignant Disease*. 3rd edn. London: Edward Arnold, 1993: 174–201.
35. Dyregov A. *Grief in Children*. London: Jessica Kingsley, 1991.
36. Kane B. Children's concepts of death. *Journal of Genetic Psychology*, 1979; **134**: 141–53.
37. Lansdown R. The development of the concept of death in childhood. *Bereavement Care*, 1985; **4**: 15–17.
38. Social Work Department. *My Book About.....* London: St Christopher's Hospice, 1989.
39. Heegard M. *When Someone has a Very Serious Illness*. Minneapolis, Minnesota: Woodland Press, 1991.
40. Capacchione L. *The Creative Journal for Children*. Boston: Shambhala, 1989.
41. Machin L. *Working With Young People in Loss Situations*. Harlow, England: Longman, 1993.
42. Couldrick A. *Grief and Bereavement: Understanding Children*. Oxford: Sobell Publications, 1988.
43. Cancerlink. *Talking to Children When an Adult Has Cancer*. London: Cancerlink, 1993.
44. Social Work Department. *Someone Special Has Died*. London: St Christopher's Hospice, 1989.
45. Couldrick A. *When your Mum or Dad has Cancer*. Oxford: Sobell Publications, 1991.
46. Hildebrand J. Working with a bereaved family. *Palliative Medicine*, 1989; **3**: 105–11.
47. Hemmings P. Working with children facing bereavement as individuals. *European Journal of Palliative Care*, 1994; **1**: 72–7.
48. Silverman PR, Worden JW. Children's understanding of funeral ritual. *Omega*, 1992; **25**: 319–31.
49. Blackburn M. Bereaved children and their teachers. *Bereavement Care*, 1991; **10**: 19–21.
50. Silverman PR, Worden JW. Children's reactions to the death of a parent. In: Stroebe M, Stroebe W, Hansson R, eds. *Handbook of Bereavement: Theory Research and Intervention*. New York: Cambridge University Press, 1993: 300–16.
51. Vachon M. *Occupational Stress in the Care of the Critically Ill, the Dying and the Bereaved*. Washington: Hemisphere, 1987.
52. Homer LE. Organisation defences against the anxiety of terminal illness—a case study. *Death Education*, 1984; **8**: 137–54.
53. Kearney M. Image work in a case of intractable pain. *Palliative Medicine*, 1992; **6**: 152–7.
54. Ainsworth-Smith I, Speck P. *Letting Go*. London: SPCK, 1982.
55. *A Code of Ethics and Practice for Counsellors*. Rugby: British Association for Counsellors, 1993.
56. McGoldrick M, Gerson R. *Genograms in Family Assessment*. New York: Norton, 1985.
57. O'Neill J. Ethnic minorities—neglected by palliative care providers? *Journal of Cancer Care*, 1994; **3**: 215–20.
58. Dunlop R. Wider applications of palliative care. In: Saunders C, Sykes N, eds. *The Management of Terminal Malignant Disease*. 3rd edn. London: Edward Arnold, 1993: 287 96.
59. Cave D. Gay and Lesbian Bereavement. In: Dickenson D, Johnson M, eds. *Death, Dying and Bereavement*. London: Sage, 1993: 293–5.
60. South East Thames Regional Health Authority. *Standards for HIV Prevention and Care Services: A Discussion Document*. Bexhill: South East Thames Regional Health Authority, 1994.
61. Miller R, Bor R. *Aids: A Guide to Clinical Counselling*. London: Science Press, 1988.

62. Cook A, Dworkin D. *Helping the Bereaved*. United States: Basic Books, 1992.
63. Balder L, Sarell M. Coping with cancer among holocaust survivors in Israel: an explanatory study. *Journal of Human Stress*, 1994; **10**: 121–7.
64. Neuberger J. *Caring for Dying People of Different Faiths*. London: Mosby, 1994.
65. Green J. *Death with Dignity—Meeting the Spiritual Needs of Patients in a Multiracial Society*. London: A Nursing Times Publication, 1993.
66. Gunaratum Y. *Health and Race Check List*. London: Kings Fund Centre, 1993.
67. Hill D, Penso D. *Opening Doors: Improving Access to Hospice and Specialist Palliative Care Services By Members of the Black and Ethnic Minority Communities*. London: National Council for Hospice and Specialist Palliative Care Services; 1995.
68. Addington Hall J, McCarthy M. Regional study of care for the dying: Methods and sample characteristics. *Palliative Medicine*, 1995; **9**: 27–35.
69. Social Work Department. *Your Parent Has Died*. London: St Christopher's Hospice, 1991.
70. Cancerlink. *Body Image and Sexuality and Cancer*. London, 1993.
71. Newburn T. *Disaster and After*. London: Jessica Kingsley, 1993.
72. Earnshaw-Smith E, Yorkstone P. *Setting Up and Running a Bereravement Service*. London: St Christopher's Hospice, 1986.
73. Urbanowicz M. Teaching about grief and loss—a whole school approach. *Bereavement Care*, 1994; **13**: 8.
74. Brodribb C. Quality Control. *Community Care*, 1995; **26 Jan–1 Feb**: 2–3.
75. MacCabee J. The effect of transfer from a palliative care unit to nursing homes—are patients' and relatives' needs met? *Palliative Medicine*, 1994; 8: 211–14.
76. Payne S, Relf M. The assessment of need for bereavement follow up in palliative and hospice care. *Palliative Medicine*, 1994; **8**: 291–7.

14

Emotional problems in palliative care

14.1 The emotional problems of the patient

Mary L.S. Vachon

Emotional problems and psychosocial distress are common as individuals confront the terminal phase of illness and their impending death.[1-5] Appropriate intervention at this critical point may decrease the immediate emotional suffering for all concerned.[6,7] In addition intervention can also ease the family bereavement period.[7-9] Some controversy still exists about the concept of anticipatory grief, both as a phenomenon[10,11] and whether it has a positive or negative impact on grief.[12,13]

The assessment and treatment of the psychosocial distress associated with terminal illness involve distinguishing between the normal symptoms of adjustment to the illness and the symptoms of a major psychiatric disorder. The skilled practitioner must be able to identify, assess, and when possible treat the physical symptoms of the disease together with the increasing debility and changes in social roles and social isolation associated with the disease and the dying process. At the same time he or she must be able to distinguish when the social isolation or change in social roles are signs of a major depression and when the pain and symptoms of the disease have a strong psychological overlay requiring psychiatric or psychological referral.

Overview of the chapter

Focus of the chapter

First, the underlying assumptions on which this chapter is based are outlined. Next, the epidemiological data on the psychosocial distress and clinical depression experienced by persons with terminal cancer are reviewed and some of the factors associated with increased risk of psychosocial distress are reviewed. This is followed by a clinical discussion of the emotional and psychosocial problems confronting dying persons. The primary focus of the chapter is on psychosocial variables, issues, and concerns as well as psychosocial symptoms involved in the process of adjusting to terminal illness and caring for those with a terminal illness. Finally, normal adjustment, situational adjustment reactions, depressive symptoms, and anxiety symptoms in patients are reviewed.

The format adopted in this chapter is to discuss issues of adaptation in general, to highlight specific symptoms to alert the clinician to problems that must be addressed, and then to give some specific intervention strategies. Clinical examples of dying trajectories (processes or patterns) taken from the author's research and clinical practice will be used throughout the chapter to give the reader better insight into the experience of the dying person.

Underlying assumptions of the chapter

- Cancer does not occur in a vacuum
- The illness trajectory may affect adaptation
- Early intervention may affect later distress
- Intervention should meet patient and family needs
- Good palliative care involves options
- Titrate information to patient needs
- There is no one right way

Cancer does not occur in a vacuum

Sir William Osler has been quoted as saying, 'Ask not what disease the person has, but rather what person the disease has'.[14] The underlying premise of this chapter is that cancer, like any other disease, does not occur in a vacuum. The individual has a personal history, personality characteristics, and coping mechanisms that may prove to be helpful or unhelpful in dealing with the present situation.

In addition, most individuals are members of a social network. The manner in which an individual's significant others respond to him or her and the illness may in part determine the individual's response to the disease. An individual's process of adaptation to the disease will also be determined in part by a number of other variables including the following:[15]

- age and stage of family development
- the nature of the disease
- the trajectory or pattern of the illness
- the individual's and family's previous experience with illness and death
- socio-economic status
- cultural variables.

A young woman with dependent children living in rural Africa who is diagnosed with widely disseminated breast cancer will obviously have a different disease experience requiring a different

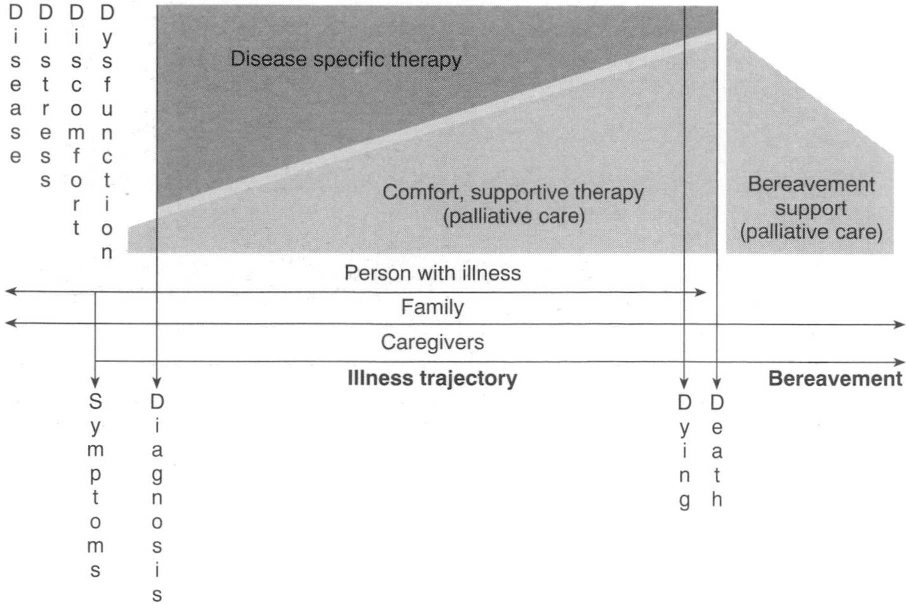

Fig. 1 The continuum of palliative care. (Reproduced with permission from ref. 17.)

response from that of a woman of the same age living in a Western society who carefully assesses her options, chooses to have a bone marrow transplant, and then relapses.

The illness trajectory may affect adaptation

Both the person with cancer and the support network will respond differently depending on whether the illness was initially perceived as having been 'cured' and has now relapsed, whether the cancer was perceived to be a chronic disease which was expected to go on 'for ever' and is now at the point where treatment aimed at prolonging survival is no longer appropriate, or whether the disease has had a fairly rapid trajectory to death.[15,16]

Early intervention may decrease later distress

It is assumed that, if the needs of the person with cancer and the significant others are handled reasonably well from the time of diagnosis, then even if the final outcome is death, the problems associated with this will be fewer and less complicated than would be the case if there were numerous unresolved problems during the early stages of the illness.[15] Figure 1 shows a model of palliative care integrated into the continuum of care.[17] Comfort and supportive treatment are initiated from the time of the presentation with the initial symptoms and continue with greater or lesser intensity until the final phase of life, at which time the intensity increases. In this model bereavement support is seen as being an integral part of palliative care.

Intervention should meet patient and family needs

It is not appropriate simply to intervene. Intervention must be done carefully and at a pace best matched to patient and family needs rather than caregiver expectations and agendas about what 'should' be done.

A 40-year-old man was diagnosed with metastatic cancer of the kidney and was expected to die within a few months. He was urged to put his business affairs in order, to make a will, and to speak to his 6-year-old daughter about his disease. He refused to take any of these actions and made it clear that he would do what he wished to do in his own time. His wife expressed great concern that he was not dealing with his will. One day on the spur of the moment and in his own time, he went to his lawyer's office and made out his will, telling his wife that it was completed after the fact. He continued to work and to be involved with his daughter's sports events. He told his daughter that he had cancer, but when she asked if he was going to die he assured her that he was not. He received palliative home care for pain relief but continued to work. He worked on Monday, attended his daughter's softball game, was admitted to hospital on Tuesday with a haemorrhage, and said 'I think this is the last bus stop'. He died peacefully on Friday.

While caregivers sometimes inappropriately make the decision not to tell patients and family members what is likely to happen, at other times they may inappropriately err on the side of giving too much negative information too soon and too often, allowing for no possibility of hope.

A man whose 39-year-old fiancée was diagnosed with a brain tumour said, 'I'll never forgive the residents who spoke with Sue soon after her diagnosis. They said "You might just as well go to Florida. There is nothing that we can do to change things. You are going to die soon". We barely had time to adjust to the news and they were writing her off. They gave us no hope. The surgeon let us know that things were serious, but she at least gave us some hope that they could do something to help us to have some quality time as we began to adjust to what was happening'.

Good palliative care involves options

People should have some choice with regard to where and how they choose to spend their final days. In order to do this, they will need to be aware of the extent of their disease and its expected prognosis. Given this knowledge and the available resources, they should be able to choose to continue active treatment, albeit possibly within some limits, to choose palliative treatment; to choose to be at home with or without a support programme, or to choose to be in a hospital or hospice setting.

Figure 2 shows three models of the continuum of palliative care programs. Programme 1 focuses on the comparatively brief period

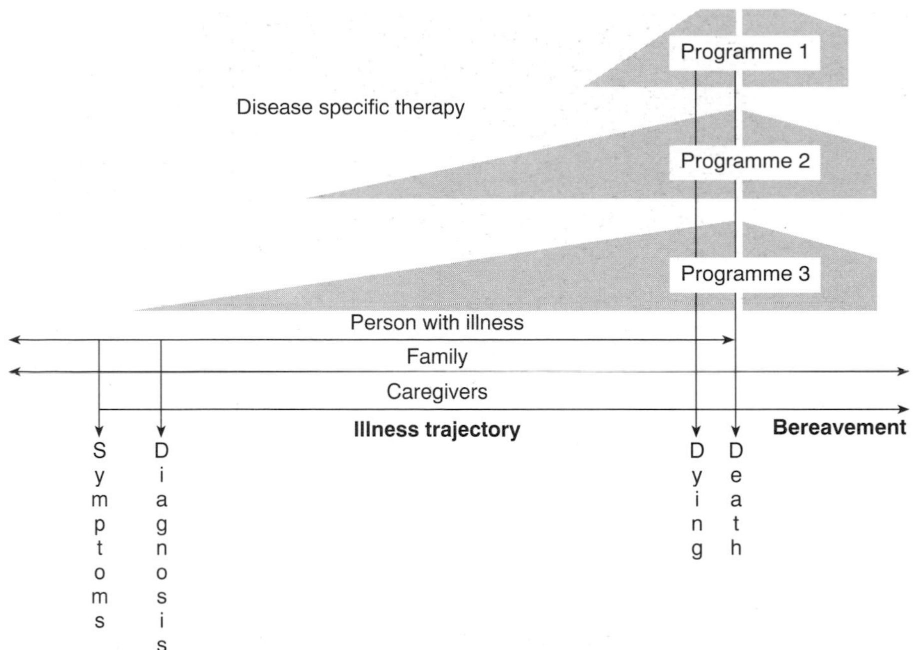

Fig. 2 Palliative care programmes. (Reproduced with permission from ref. 17.

surrounding death and bereavement. Programme 2 begins at an earlier point in the illness trajectory, at the time of recurrence or at the point at which it becomes clear to the caregivers, but may not yet be acknowledged by the patient, that it will not be possible to cure the disease but treatment aimed at prolonging life will be utilized. Programme 3 integrates comfort and supportive treatment at the same time as disease-specific treatment begins early in the disease trajectory.

Obviously not everyone has the ideal options and choices available to them because of a variety of social beliefs, economic constraints, and other issues. These variables range from cultural beliefs that people should not be told that they have cancer or that they are going to die, to settings that strongly encourage terminally ill patients to transfer to a hospice because of the economic problems associated with expensive 'active treatment' which will not cure the patient, to cultures in which there is not enough money for even the very basic necessities of health care. Here, people die at home or even on the streets, not because they choose to do so but because no other options are available.

The provision of treatment options can be difficult. In some settings, it is sometimes easier for the oncologist to proceede with chemotherapy rather than acknowledge that current antineoplastic treatments are inadequate and may cause morbidity greater than that due to the underlying cancer.[18,19] In addition, some patients may have great difficulty in accepting that there are limits to the current treatments for their particular cancer, and they may push or demand to continue with current or experimental treatment.

The issue of patient choice in the face of terminal illness is a cause of some controversy in the 1990s 'as clinicians cannot continue to argue for the primacy of individual need and ignore the communal cost implications of their prescriptions; they must be prepared also to address the ethics of resource allocations'.[20] In addition, although advances in the area of antiemetics and growth factors have allowed the use of increasingly aggressive regimens in many solid tumours, many of these have yet to have a demonstrated benefit.[18,19]

However, there is a role for palliative chemotherapy in the care of the terminally ill. There is 'suggestive evidence that, possibly because of the impact of chemotherapy on the host response and the tumor milieu, chemotherapy and radiotherapy may influence cancer pain even in the absence of objective tumor response'.[21]

When chemotherapy or radiation is being prescribed primarily for symptom control, it is imperative for the treatment team to be able to communicate clearly with both the patient and family regarding the specific purpose of the therapy, for example for symptom control and not for prolongation of life.

> The ideal informing process beomes one of shared learning. Patients learn about the medical facts, and the potential benefits and burdens of treatment, in the context of a realistic appraisal of their overall medical condition. Physicians, in turn, must learn of their patient's personal experiences and perceptions about the diagnosis, their current quality of life, and the amount of suffering they are willing to tolerate... .[22]

These conversations are difficult. Caregivers must be prepared to give this information in a caring and sensitive manner, being ready to deal with the difficulty patients and families have in accepting this information. Caregivers must also be aware that patients and families may sometimes deny the reality of what is being said. Conversations to clarify the purposes of palliative therapies may have to take place periodically over the course of treatment.

Titrate information to patient needs

Given that, under ideal circumstances, people should have the choice of where and how to spend their final days, they should also have the option of choosing how much information they want about their illness including choosing not to know their prognosis. The medical practitioner must be aware that, much as there is a 'right to know', there is also a corresponding 'right not to know' provided that the patient has given the health care provider the clear message that this is his or her choice.

However, problems arise in this situation if the patient chooses 'not-to-know' that the treatment he or she is demanding has almost no likelihood of success and refuses to acknowledge the possiblity that death may result from this disease episode.

A young mother of two daughters, aged 6 and 8, refused to acknowledge that she might die of her colon cancer and that her children should be prepared for the possiblity of her death. She kept repeating that she would search the world for treatments and would eventually manage to cure her disease, and so her children did not need to be upset by discussing the possiblity that she might die. She refused to speak to her children about her illness, even when their behaviour indicated that they were having considerable difficulty in dealing with her obvious deterioration while they were being reassured that all was well. However, when it became clear that she was dying, she and her husband spoke openly with their children on their own initiative, prepared them for the fact that she might die, after which they were open to talking as a family with the staff about what was happening. At the time of her funeral the children read a poem describing their mother's struggle with illness and their coming to terms as a family with the need to let her go as her condition deteriorated and she slipped into unconsciousness.

The choice not to tell a person of his or her prognosis should not be a decision that the health-care provider makes for the patient in order to increase the provider's comfort level. Rather, it should be an acknowledgement that the caregiver is available to 'walk with' the patient along the path that has been chosen. When the patient chooses not to know that he or she is dying, the provider should always be open to talking about the illness and prognosis when the patient is prepared to do so. The care provider should also be willing to speak to the person in 'symbolic' language as this is appropriate. However, if the caregiver initiates discussions in symbolic language he or she must be certain that the patient understands what is being said.

One woman spoke of being told by her minister that there 'was someone inside me guiding me and telling me what to do about dying'. The woman did not understand what was meant by this comment and was afraid to ask for fear that she would appear to be 'stupid'. The concept of 'letting go' and trusting in God was explained. Her face glowed as she understood what was meant. When she was asked what insights she might like to share with people reading this chapter, she replied: 'Keep it simple. Make sure that people understand what you are saying.'

There is no one right way

Clinical examples illustrating communication with dying people will be given throughout this chapter in order to provide clarity and the understanding that there is no one 'right way' to handle the problems confronting the dying person and his or her family.

Epidemiology of psychosocial distress

Psychosocial distress

Prevalence estimates of psychological distress in terminally ill patients are higher than those in a general cancer population.[23-28] From 61 to 79 per cent of the palliative care subgroup (N=69) in a stratified randomized registry-based Canadian community cancer sample of 1319 people living with cancer currently registered high distress on the General Health Questionnaire[29] compared with 18 to 34 per cent of the general cancer population.[3-5] In a replication

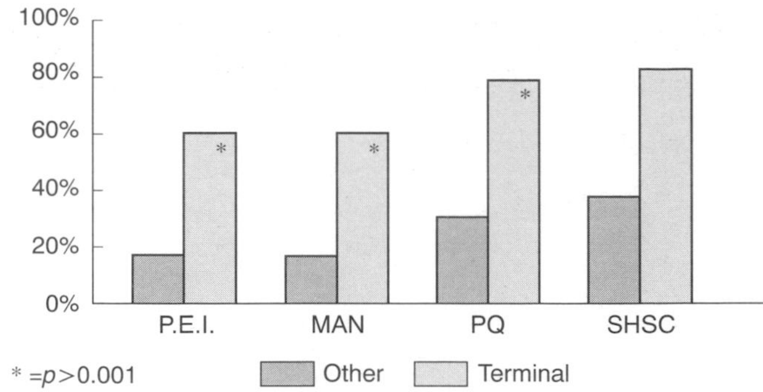

Fig. 3 Prevalence of psychological distress.

of the original study,[30] 79 per cent of both terminally ill inpatients (N=31) and terminally ill outpatients (N=14) registered high distress compared with 66 per cent of the total inpatient population (N=97) and 30 per cent of the outpatient population (N=346). Thirty-eight per cent of the total population (N=443) registered high distress (Fig. 3).

In the original study, pain, other symptoms, treatment side-effects, and cancer-related fears were seen to have direct and indirect effects on the psychological symptoms of distress (Tables 1, 2). Impaired role performance was a central mediator for the indirect effects. The model explained 34 per cent of the variance in General Health Questionnaire scores (see Fig. 4 for the standardized regression coefficients (e.g. β)[24]) and was equally applicable to all three study sites, male and female subjects, rural and urban settings, and all stages of illness. Pain was the single most important

Table 1 Determinants of distress in cancer patients

Pain

Having had a pain-related problem since diagnosis

Impaired role performance

Problems performing one's normal activities in the following areas

- Caring for elderly parents or other relatives
- Household activities
- Activities at work
- Social activities
- Relationships with friends
- Relationships with partner
- Role as a partner
- Role as a parent
- Inability to participate in usual religious practices

Illness-related fears

- Fears about dying
- Fears about recurrenc of disease

Other symptoms and side-effects

- Problems with seeing/hearing
- Lack of energy
- Feeling tired
- Loss of interest in food
- Cognitive impairment
- Gastrointestinal symptoms

Table 2 Variables associated with high distress

Physical functioning: difficulty with walking/climbing stairs, ability to sleep/sleeping habits, interest in food/appetite, ability to eat, ability to see/hear/speak, ability to care for personal needs, decreased energy, inability to perform normal household activities and fatigue
Physical integrity: nausea, breathing problems, pain, sore mouth, physical appearance, constipation
Emotional wellbeing: thoughts and concerns regarding one's eventual death; feelings of depression, anxiety and frustration; outlook on life; ability to relax and happiness with life
Social relationships: time spent at social and leisure activities and inability to perform one's normal activities as a marital partner, such as going out and doing things together
Illness adaptation: fear of recurrence or getting worse and coming to terms with the various stages of one's disease
Economic/occupational: feeling that one will not have enough money for the future
Cognitive ability: difficulty with ability to concentrate or remember

explanatory variable, but other symptoms, including fatigue, had an impact on impaired role performance.[24,31] However, impaired role performance also had a negative effect on distress over and above the effect of pain.

Clinical depression

Five to 15 per cent of the general cancer population experience a major depression.[32] The incidence of depression increases with the severity of the illness,[23-28,33,34] with active disease and inpatient status,[35] with physical discomfort or limitations related to its symptomatology or treatment,[34,36,37] and with younger age[34,38] as well as older age.[39] Clinical depression amongst the terminally ill ranges from 6 per cent in a United Kingdom sample[40] to 21.4 to 22.6 per cent in the much larger American National Hospice study[41] and 25 per cent in a Canadian sample of hospital inpatients.[42] However, the prevalence of depression in the terminally ill is related to the diagnostic approach and the instruments used to assess both minor and major depressive episodes and is dependent on whether or not somatic symptoms are replaced with non-somatic alternatives.[33] At least 25 per cent of hospital inpatients with significant levels of physical impairment meet the criteria for major depression or adjustment disorder with depressed mood.[43] The prevalence of depression in those with advanced cancer is probably not significantly different from that found in patients with other major physical illnesses. Similar rates (25 per cent) were found in a study of endstage renal disease patients awaiting cadaveric transplants.[44]

More detailed information on depression and anxiety is given in the section on risk assessment for emotional distress.

The patient's experience with cancer

Psychosocial variables and the initiation and development of cancer

At least since the second century, there has been speculation about the effect of the psyche on cancer initiation. Galen stated that 'cancer was much more frequent in melancholic than in sanguine women'.[45]. During the eighteenth and nineteenth centuries it was suggested that women who were prone to develop cancer were sedentary and melancholic and that they suffered from depression and/or deep anxiety. In addition, such women were thought to have experienced numerous disasters, losses, or reversals of fortune in their lives.

In the twentieth century, the focus has gradually shifted from an emphasis on the psychosocial factors which were hypothesized to be associated with the development of the disease,[46-52] to the psychosocial factors that may or may not be associated with the experience of the disease and its progression,[53-64] to programmes of intervention designed to alter the distress associated with the disease or even the course of the disease.[65-73] Research on programmes that purport to alter the course of the disease may include biased samples; thus results must be viewed with caution.[68,73] Therefore more recent work with more carefully controlled samples is seen to be very important.[60,70-72]

In this section we review some of the current controversies in the field in an attempt to synthesize some of the findings on psychosocial factors that are believed to be associated with the

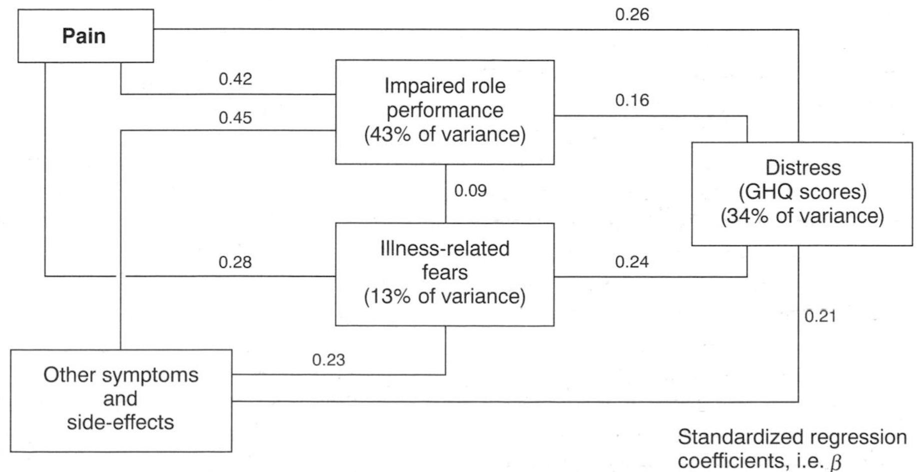

Fig. 4 Model for determinants of distress in cancer patients. (Reproduced with permission from Ref. 24.)

disease or its progression. The reader who wishes a more detailed overview is referred to a number of other sources.[15,45,55,60,65,67-74]

Do psychological factors play a role in the initiation and/or development of cancer?

The interaction between biological and psychological factors

In giving an overview of the psychosocial factors that may have a part to play in the initiation and/or development of cancer, the first point to be made is that cancer is first and foremost a biological disease that would continue to exist even if it were possible to remove stressful life events, transform personalities, and create ideal social support systems.[15]

The length of time between the initiation of a tumour and its development into clinically recognized disease may take a decade or more. Therefore, if one is looking for a connection between psychosocial variables and tumour development, one must look at events and traits from at least a decade earlier.[15,75]

Psychosocial variables and the promotion of cancer

The argument that psychosocial factors, such as stress, could play a part in the aetiology of breast cancer is based on the observation that there is a much higher incidence of mammary neoplastic cells than ever becomes evident. Autopsy results have shown that between 25 and 30 per cent of all women have either *in situ* or invasive cancer at autopsy.[75] The findings in men are also striking. Autopsies show that 10 per cent of men aged 50 and 70 per cent aged 80 have small prostate cancers that have not spread or caused problems.[76] The release of metastatic cells does not necessarily lead to the development of metastatic disease. Presumably, there are body conditions that may be more or less conducive to the growth of breast cancer. It is reasonable to assume that psychological factors could have a role to play in this situation.[75]

Some of the psychosocial variables that have been implicated in the development of cancer include chronic stressors, such as loneliness, loss, and problems in living and/or an inability to cope with stressful life situations,[77] parental rejection or rejection in the early family environment,[47,77-81] bereavement,[82] and personality factors.[55,62-64,79,80,83-86] It is hypothesized that early deprivation and loss may lead to early immunological malfunction due to abnormal neurohormonal regulation. The body's normal host resistance might then be weakened 'so as to favour the neoplastic transformation of normal cells or to lower antitumour resistance...[and] weaken their defences against oncogenesis'.[77]

Three psychosocial factors that have been associated with an increased biological risk of developing cancer include 'inadequate social support, cognitively generated helplessness, and inadequate expression of negative emotion'.[87] Levy and Wise suggest that in attempting to understand the role of psychosocial variables in the course of cancer, it makes sense to study cancers in which psychosocial variables might account for a fair amount of the variance, for example those in which biological factors do not assume a primary role such as occurs in the more virulent malignancies (e.g. pancreatic or lung cancer). In their own work they have focused on melanoma and breast cancer which have a more unpredictable course in their intermediate stages.[87]

Cancer relapse has been associated with severe social stress,[88] and decreased survival has been found to be associated with poor coping styles [89] and low quality or quantity of social support.[90-92] Married cancer patients have been found to survive longer than those who are unmarried.[91]

Personality and cancer

A type C cancer personality,[55,63,83-86] in contrast with the type A personality that has been associated with cardiac disease, has been suggested. The type C personality has been hypothesized to be '...cooperative and appeasing, unassertive, patient, unexpressive of negative emotion (particularly anger) and compliant with external authorities, in contrast to the hostile, aggressive, tense and controlling type A individual'.[55] The type C personality has been associated with more prognostically unfavourable lesions in cutaneous melanoma and breast cancer.[55]

When subjects with breast cancer (N=37) were compared with those with coronary heart disease (N=37), anxiety disorders (N=35), and normal control subjects (N=72), the cancer group was strongly predicted by loss and illness events, while the coronary group was more associated with work events. There was also a strong relationship between depressive reactions in the cancer group in contrast with the anger–anxiety variable found in the infarct group.[93]

Other authors [53,60,61] have found no association between personality factors and disease progression in patients with advanced cancer. This may be because by the time that the disease is far advanced, whatever psychosocial factors might have been operative play a secondary role to the biology of the disease.

It is important to note at this point that when so much work is being done on psychosocial variables and disease outcome, there is the potential to 'blame the victim' inappropriately.[94] The patient can come to be seen as being consciously or unconsciously responsible for the development of the disease and for the success or failure of efforts made to alter its course.[15]

Psychosocial variables and the course of disease

The effect of psychosocial variables on the length of survival of those with terminal illness has also been studied. Patients with greater depression and low self-esteem anticipated and experienced greater stress during the first few months in a nursing home.[95] In a well-designed study of 90 elderly patients (average age 78) with advanced cancer, newly admitted to 10 Florida nursing homes, age, sex, marital status, and years of education did not distinguish between survivors and non-survivors.[96] In addition, none of the cancer and treatment-related variables differed significantly. However, psychosocial variables did predict early death. Those patients who died within 3 months of admission (28 per cent) more often acknowledged their condition as being terminal, anticipated greater environmental stress and adjustment problems, expected fewer visitors, and had poorer self-esteem. The authors concluded that for cancer patients undergoing the stress of nursing home placement, feelings of hopelessness and helplessness were associated with earlier death.

In other studies of persons with advanced lung and breast cancer,[97,98] patient-rated well being was associated with longer survival time. This finding was often, but not always, independent of initial performance status, stage of advanced disease, and type of treatment. Ganz and colleagues[97] also found that, while patient-rated quality of life was a statistically significant predictor of longevity in both married and unmarried patients, those who were

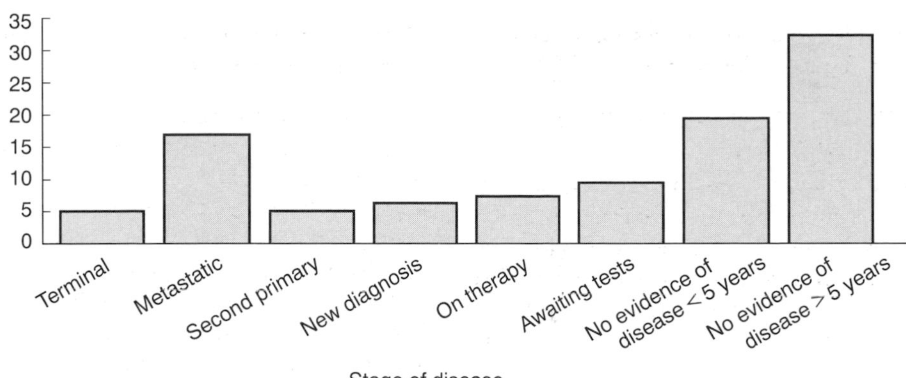

Fig. 5 CCS sample.

married still had an increased length of survival compared with the unmarried.

Psychosocial intervention to affect survival in cancer

As psychosocial variables may have an impact on survival, there is growing interest in assessing whether it is possible to alter the expected outcome of the disease by manipulating them. Spiegel and colleagues[70] designed a 10-year follow-up study on women with metastatic breast cancer who had participated in a 1-year programme of supportive group therapy and self-hypnosis for pain.[99] Those in the experimental group lived twice as long as those in the control group (36.6 months for the intervention group versus 18.9 months for the control group).[70]

Fawzy and coworkers[71,72] studied the effects of a 6-week structured group intervention on a group of 38 newly diagnosed melanoma patients and compared them with 28 control subjects. The structured psychoeducational intervention consisted of health education, stress management, and coping skills. The intervention took place in a supportive group format consisting of six weekly sessions, each lasting approximately 1.5 h. At the end of 6 weeks the experimental group reported significantly lower levels of confusion, depression, fatigue, and total mood disturbance and higher levels of vigour on the Profile of Mood States.[100] In addition, they were more likely to use active behavioural coping techniques (defined as helping one to solve problems and/or to make one feel better in both the short and the long term) as well as active cognitive coping methods (defined as mental thoughts and techniques that one can use that help to solve problems and/or make oneself feel better in both the short and the long term).[72]. At 1-year follow-up the experimental group continued to show significantly lower confusion and higher vigour. On immunological tests the experimental group had an increase in their percentage of large granular lymphocytes (LGLs) defined as CD57 with Leu7: 'Six months following the intervention, there continued to be an increase in the percentage of LGLs (defined as CD57 with Leu7) as well as increases in NK cells (defined as CD16 with Leu11 and CD56 with Leu19) and interferon alpha augmented NK cell cytotoxicity'.[101] At the end of 6 years there was a statistically significant greater rate of death (10/34) in the control group compared with the experimental group (3/34). Being male and having a greater Breslow depth predicted greater recurrence and poorer survival. Analysis of multiple covariants showed that only Breslow depth and the group intervention were significant. Even after adjusting for Breslow depth, the treatment effect remained significant. Higher levels of baseline distress as well as baseline coping and enhancement of active behavioural coping over time were predictive of lower rates of recurrence and death.[72]

Numerous investigators are currently attempting to replicate these exciting findings. It is anticipated that research focusing on relaxation, social support, and disease-specific components could be fruitful in providing answers to questions about immunity and disease endpoints.[74]

The patient's experience with terminal cancer

The Canadian studies of the needs of persons living with cancer

This section is based on the data obtained in two Canadian studies: the Needs of Persons Living with Cancer in Three Canadian Provinces (CCS study) and the Needs of Cancer Patients and Their Families Attending Toronto-Sunnybrook Regional Cancer Centre (T-SRCC study).

The CCS study involved a stratified randomized registry-based sample of 1319 people living with cancer in three Canadian provinces who were interviewed in order to assess their unmet needs.[3-5] People were interviewed in the provinces of Prince Edward Island (PEI), Manitoba, and Quebec (Fig. 5). This study represented population-based experience which provided a contrast with existing institutional or programme-based reports.

The study was then replicated at Toronto-Sunnybrook Regional Cancer Centre (T-SRCC), a tertiary care cancer centre located in Toronto. T-SRCC treats 5000 new cancer patients yearly. Patients are referred from the greater Metropolitan Toronto area as well as from other cities, towns, and villages in Ontario. T-SRCC consists of an outpatient facility and an 89-bed inpatient oncology patient service unit. T-SRCC is located on the campus of Sunnybrook Health Science Centre, a 1300-bed University of Toronto teaching hospital with 649 acute and 670 chronic care beds. An eight-bed palliative care unit is located in the continuing care wing.

The eligible sample included all outpatients who attended the T-SRCC outpatient clinic during a period of 3 weeks and all inpatients in the oncology patient service unit during a period of 1 month. Patients in the palliative care unit were interviewed over a period of several months in order to accrue a larger sample. The T-SRCC sample consisted of 105 inpatients and 354 outpatients.

Table 3 Canadian studies of the needs of persons living with cancer: demographic variables

	PEI (*N* = 364)	Manitoba (*N* = 526)	Quebec (*N* = 429)	T-SRCC (*N* = 459)
Gender				
Male (%)	34	37	37	38
Female (%)	66	63	63	62
Age				
Range (years)	20–92	23–88	25–83	20–91
Mean (years)	59	63.5	57.4	59.4
Under 45 (%)	17	11	17	25
45–54 (%)	16	12	19	18
55–64 (%)	26	20	30	19
65–74 (%)	28	38	28	26
75+ (%)	14	19	6	12
Diagnosis				
Breast (%)	33	28	26	26
Genitourinary (%)	19	28	22	33
Digestive (%)	15	15	17	10
Haematological (%)	13	7	12	14
Lung (%)	5	5	8	5
Other (%)	15	17	15	12
Length of time since initial diagnosis				
Mean (months)	57.7	57.6	48.9	48.3
Median (months)	44.5	48	43.0	25.6

Sample

Table 3 shows that the two samples are similar, although the patients in the Manitoba sample were on average older than those in the T-SRCC sample. Two-thirds of those studied were females. All major cancer diagnoses were represented. Both studies were representative of persons at various stages of their cancer trajectory. The mean time since diagnosis was 57 months for the Prince Edward Island and Manitoba samples and 48 months for the Quebec and Toronto samples. The median time since diagnosis for the T-SRCC sample was 25.6 months compared with 43 to 48 months for CCS sample. The reason for this difference is the length of time that it takes for patients to be placed on the registries from which the provincial samples were derived.

The definition of the person's stage of illness in the CCS study was a combination of self-report and author interpretation. In the T-SRCC study the stage of the illness was taken from medical charts, although the same self-reported data for staging were obtained from subjects. Figures 5 and 6 show the stage of disease trajectory for both samples. The T-SRCC sample has double the percentage of terminally ill patients because of the inclusion of the inpatients in the acute and palliative care units. The T-SRCC sample also contains more patients receiving active treatment, both

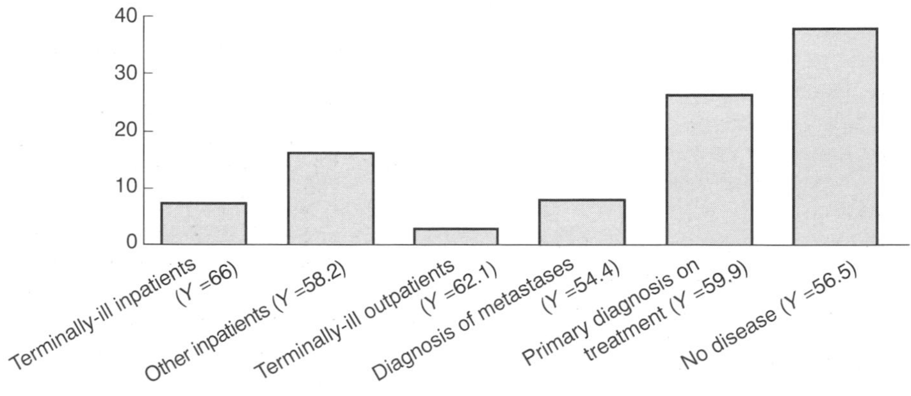

Fig. 6 T-SRCC sample.

Table 4 Variables associated with terminal disease

	PEI	Manitoba	Quebec	T-SRCC inpatients	T-SRCC outpatients
N	22/364 (6%)	21/526 (4%)	26/429 (6%)	34/459 (7%)	14/459 (3%)
Diagnosis*					
Breast (%)	3	4	4	2	2
Lung (%)	17	22	17	49	13
Digestive (%)	9	4	4	4	0
Genitourinary (%)	3	2	5	6	2
Haematological (%)	2	5	4	5	3
Other (%)	11	0	8	11	5
	CCS sample				
Age range (years)	33–87			39–88	
Mean age (years)	60			65.95	62.1
Median age (years)	61			66.24	63.89
SD	12.7			12.06	13.71

* Presented as a percentage of persons with this diagnosis who currently had terminal disease.

as inpatients and outpatients. This difference is due to the difficulty in obtaining the names of recently diagnosed persons in the CCS study and to the fact that inpatients in the T-SRCC sample could be interviewed. Similar patients might have been screened out of the previous studies by physicians or the patients might not have had the energy to respond to the request for an interview.

One-third of the CCS sample had been free of disease for 1 to 5 years, and 16 per cent had been free of disease for 5 years or more. Over 60 per cent of the T-SRCC sample were receiving either active or palliative treatment compared with 35 per cent of the CCS sample.

The CCS cancer population was found to have a lower income and educational level than the provincial average.[102] The T-SRCC sample had a lower income than the average for the population of Metropolitan Toronto and was less likely to have received post-secondary education.[103,104] These findings are reflective of the higher incidence and mortality rate of certain cancers (stomach, lung, cervical, mouth, pharynx, larynx, and oesophagus) in the economically disadvantaged.[105–110] Moreover, the sample is older than the general population and therefore less likely to have completed secondary school, and younger people with cancer were found to have their economic potential decreased.

The terminally ill subgroup

In the three provinces studied, 5 per cent of terminally ill persons were willing to participate. The study was registry based so that inpatients were eligible for inclusion; however, few inpatients consented to be interviewed. The percentage of terminally ill patients in the T-SRCC study (10.5 per cent) is presumed to reflect the percentage of terminally ill in this setting fairly accurately. Because Sunnybrook Health Science Centre is a community hospital as well as the host hospital for the tertiary referral cancer centre, the patients interviewed included both those who received chemotherapy and radiation for their disease and those who would not have been referred to the cancer centre. The latter group consisted of patients who might be considered to be 'surgical cures' (e.g. some breast, colon, and prostate cancers) as well as patients diagnosed with cancers that would not be expected to respond to chemotherapy or radiation.

Table 4 shows a comparison of the two terminally ill samples. In all cases those with lung cancer are the most likely to be in the terminal phase of disease.

Distress in terminally ill patients

The unmet needs of terminally ill patients were correlated with level of distress as measured on the 30-item Goldberg General Health Questionnaire.[29] The General Health Questionnaire was chosen as a measure of distress because it allowed comparison with a large 'normal' Canadian population in which 21 per cent of those surveyed were found to have high distress.[111] Not surprisingly, the terminally ill patients had much higher distress (61–79 per cent in the three provinces). Of patients who reported distressing to excruciating pain in the previous week in the CCS study, 90 to 100 per cent had high distress.[3–5] In the T-SRCC study 69 per cent of those with distressing to excruciating pain in the previous week (31 per cent of those with pain) had high distress.[30]

The variables associated with high distress are shown in Table 1. These include problems with physical functioning, physical integrity, emotional well being, social relationships, illness adaptation, economic/occupational roles, and cognitive ability. Table 5 shows the physical and psychological symptoms of distress reported in the CCS and T-SRCC studies in comparison with similar studies.[1,112–114] Although there are differences between the studies, the most commonly reported problems are pain, decreased energy or weakness, fatigue, appetite disturbances, psychological disturbance, breathing problems, sleep disturbances, nausea, and constipation. Confusion and problems with walking and climbing stairs were more common in the CCS and T-SRCC studies.

Variables associated with high distress are as follows.

- Physical functioning: difficulty with walking/climbing stairs, ability to sleep/sleeping habits, interest in food/appetite, ability to eat, ability to see/hear/speak, ability to care for

Table 5 Symptoms associated with terminal cancer

Symptom	Ref. 112[a]	Ref. 113[b]	Refs. 3–5	Ref. 30		Ref. 114[c]
	(*N* = 203)	(*N* = 90)	(*N* = 69)	**Inpatients** (*N* = 31)	**Outpatients** (*N* = 14)	(*N* = 77)
In pain (%)	55–56	100	68	53	71	92
Decreased energy/weakness (%)		43	80	71	93	79
Tiredness/fatigue (%)		58	70	64	86	
Appetite disturbances (%)	49–54		56	61	79	31
Psychological distress	50%–56% Depression	21% Anxiety	46% Feelings of depression, anxiety, frustration	56% Feelings of depression, anxiety, frustration	57%	32%
	32%–43% Anxiety	20% Suicidal ideation plus 4% suicidal intent	67% High distress on 30-item GHQ	79% on 30-item GHQ	79%	17%
Breathing problems (%)	61	17	35–47	36	39	32
Nausea (%)	19–20	12	44	39	57	56
Ability to walk/climb stairs (%)	–	18	55	58	64	
Sleep (%)	35–37	24	49	52	43	
Constipation (%)	31–36		36	42	50	36
Confusion/concentration (%)		24	32	52	50	10

* GHQ, General Health Questionnaire.
[a] Addinton-Hall *et al.* reported on 203 terminally ill cancer patients in the United Kingdom who were interviewed at least twice for a study to determine the efficacy of a co-ordination program. There were minimal differences between the experimental and control groups.
[b] Coyle *et al.* studied 90 consecutive terminally ill cancer patients, living at home, referred to the Supportive Care Team of the Pain Service of Memorial Sloan-Kettering Cancer Center. The author recorded only the symptoms reported by patients and therefore, may, be under-reporting them.
[c] Hinton studied 77 adults and their relatives in St Christopher's Hospice Home Care Service. These patients had 90 per cent of their care at home.
Adapted from ref. 1

personal needs, decreased energy, inability to perform normal household activities and fatigue.

- Physical integrity: nausea, breathing problems, pain, sore mouth, physical appearance, constipation.
- Emotional well being: thoughts and concerns regarding one's eventual death; feelings of depression, anxiety and frustration; outlook on life; ability to relax and happiness with life.
- Social relationships: time spent at social and leisure activities and inability to perform one's normal activities as a marital partner, such as going out and doing things together.
- Illness adaptation: fear of recurrence or getting worse and coming to terms with the various stages of one's disease.
- Economic/occupational: feeling that one will not have enough money for the future.
- Cognitive ability: difficulty with ability to concentrate or remember.

In Hinton's study of patients on the St Christopher's Home Care programme,[114] during the final 8 weeks of life, a mean of 63 per cent of patients each week reported physical symptoms and 17 per cent reported psychological symptoms. Some distress was felt by 11 per cent of the patients; this was usually due to pain, depression, weakness, dypsnoea, or anxiety. In the T-SRCC study terminally ill inpatients reported a mean of 17.6 problems in the previous month (median 15) and terminally ill outpatients had a mean of 20.92 problems (median 19.5). Ninety-four per cent of the terminally ill group reported a current major problem compared with 73 per cent of the total sample. The most commonly reported major problems were as follows:

- physical side-effects of disease and treatment—23 per cent
- changes in lifestyle—14 per cent
- pain—10 per cent
- dealing with recurrent disease or death—8 per cent

Pain was the current major problem most likely to be associated with high distress (88 per cent) for the total sample. This was followed by dealing with recurrent disease or death (70 per cent), physical side-effects of the disease and illness (54 per cent),and changes in lifestyle (38 per cent).

In a group of 196 patient–caregiver dyads dealing with solid tumours or lymphomas, patient immobility, symptom distress, and number of dependences in activities of daily living were all moderately to highly correlated with the reported levels of depression of both the patients and their caregivers.[36] Kaasa *et al.*[25] found that patients who had impaired role performance in addition to pain were the most distressed and that their distress varied with the severity of the pain and role impairment. In the CCS study, pain had the greatest direct impact on distress scores, followed by other symptoms and side-effects. Impaired role performance was a central mediator for the indirect effects on the level of distress.[24]

Having documented the connection between physical symptoms and impairment and psychological distress, we shall now focus on the psychosocial issues associated with high distress.

Coping and adaptation in terminal cancer

Having some understanding of the psychosocial problems confronting terminal patients is crucial to being able to recognize the need for, to initiate, or to conduct appropriate and helpful interventions for patients and/or their family members.

In this section we focus on the process of coping and adaptation in terminal illness and discuss issues such as accepting or denying the disease, distress in response to terminal cancer, and factors which might alter the response of the patient or the family to the disease.

The meaning of the illness

The nature and extent of psychosocial vulnerability to cancer is specific to individuals and depends on the personal meaning of the disease. Meaning is defined as an 'individual's perception of the potential significance of an event, such as the occurrence of serious illness, for the self and one's plan of action'.[115]. Meaning encompasses the individual's perception of the ability that he or she has to accomplish future goals and to maintain the viablilty of interpersonal actions. The meaning of cancer comprises the set of physical, social, and intrapsychic changes that are associated with the illness. The changes associated with cancer include loss of personal control, loss of self-esteem and self-worth, changes in body image, reduced social status, and disruption of interpersonal relationships.[115]

The meaning of cancer pain for individuals has been defined as challenge (36 per cent), punishment (23 per cent), and enemy (20 per cent).[116] Those patients who saw their pain as a challenge had significantly lower depression scores, lower pain scores, and higher coping scores than those who defined their pain as an enemy or punishment. It was concluded that the perceived meaning of cancer pain was the most important determinant of effective coping with it.

Accepting the disease and prognosis

Patients in the CCS and T-SRCC studies[3-5,30] were asked to identify the three greatest problems that they had confronted since their diagnosis. Difficulty in accepting the illness was the first or second most commonly mentioned problem, but by the time of the interview about two-thirds of those in the CCS study and three-quarters of those in the T-SRCC study who had identified this as a major problem said that they had managed to resolve it. People said that they relied upon themselves, their spouse, physicians, and family members for help in learning to accept their illness. Their primary coping methods were to share their concern about the problem and to confront the situation in a practical way, for example making plans for their family in the event of their death, making a will, and taking treatment. Only 4 to 8 per cent of the total sample mentioned that accepting the disease *per se* was their current greatest problem.

Terminally ill patients did not feel that they were having difficulty in accepting the thought of their illness, but they did acknowledge having difficulty in coming to terms with its different stages and in dealing with the physical symptoms and with thoughts of their illness returning or becoming worse.

At the initial interview of patients referred to the St Christopher's Hospice Home Care Service 78 per cent of patients and 74 per cent of their carers at least partly accepted the possibility of impending death but 9 per cent were clearly troubled: 'Acceptance grew more positive and, at the last interview, 50 per cent of patients and 68 per cent of relatives appeared fully accepting or nearly so...but 4 per cent of patients and 9 per cent of carers were troubled and unaccepting. . .'.[114]

Awareness of dying and the coping attitudes of these patients at their first visit by the home care team were better predictors of which patients were likely to die at home than the symptoms they presented at that time.[117] Patients who stayed at home for death showed more awareness of dying than those who later became inpatients. Only two of the 22 patients (out of 77) who died at home initially denied or partly suppressed their prognosis compared with 30 of the 55 patients subsequently admitted to the hospice for death: 'At first the inpatient death group were more optimistic and declared stronger intention to fight the illness, although they later came closer to the home death patients in attitude'[114].

Denial of the disease

Difficulty in accepting the illness may be a problem for some people as they are dying. Patients may tend to deny the diagnosis and the implications of the disease: 'Denial is how one simplifies the complexity of life... While downright denial can be harmful, denying itself is a phase of the coping process. It revises or reinterprets a portion of a painful reality avoiding what it threatens to be, and holding fast to the image of what has been'.[118]

In the St Chrisopher's study,[114] on average 26 per cent (standard deviation 9 per cent) of respondents partially suppressed awareness of impending death and 8 per cent (standard deviation 5 per cent) showed clear denial in each of the last eight weeks of life. Those rated as being more optimistic and mentally avoiding the true prognosis at the first interview more often became inpatients: 'Before admission some appeared to suffer a collapse of psychological defences and needed help; some quietly re-evaluated their situation while a few continued in denial and took inpatient treatment to be curative'.[117]

The term 'extreme denial' is used to refer to individuals 'whose denial of their symptoms or aspects of their illness is so pervasive and persistent that it may jeopardize aspects of their physical well-being, intimate social attachments, and ultimate prognosis'.[119] In these cases, the defence mechanism does not serve to assist in helping the patient's overall adaptation, although immediate anxiety may be decreased.

Caregivers must be aware that, for some people, denial of the expected prognosis may be associated with a life expectancy that is longer than anticipated.

A 35-year-old university professor was diagnosed with a brain tumour. His neurosurgeon replied 'In your type of cancer we don't talk about years, we talk about months'. He said that he thought to himself that when one heard of a film star with cancer they always had 5 to 6 years to live, and so he decided that he would live that long as well. He lived for 5 years. Although he had many side-effects of his disease, he continued to work productively and felt that he had a very good quality of life.

Denial as a social process Denial is a part of a social process and may be encouraged with the collusion of others, sometimes in order to preserve a relationship or to maintain self-esteem.[118] Such denial may take place within the context of familial relationships, and caregivers may be asked to collude with the patient or the family member to pretend that all is well.

Mutual pretence awareness Patients and their professional caregivers sometimes become involved in 'mutual pretence awareness'[120] in which all concerned know that the person is going to die but all agree non-verbally to pretend that the person will live. This phenomenon may look like denial but it operates at a more conscious level of awareness. Mutual pretence awareness may involve patients and family members being hesitant to report symptoms to caregivers because they fear that the caregiver will withdraw physically or emotionally or transfer the patient elsewhere if he or she is officially apprised of the fact that the person has symptoms that indicate deterioration and the possibility of impending death.

Risk assessment and intervention with denial Denial is sometimes seen as the most primitive of the defence mechanisms.[121] It is the one that is used when no other coping mechanism is readily available. Caregivers must carefully assess when it is appropriate to intervene to break down denial.

Whose need is it to break down denial? 'Awareness and denying often run together, crossing over as one emotion or perception gains ascendance and blurs another'.[118] Caregivers who decide to intervene when patients or family members are denying must be sure that they are motivated by appropriate consideration for the persons involved and not just because they have set as their goal that the patient and family must accept the disease.

Thoughtless intervention shows little regard for the needs of the patient and reflects unrealistic goals that caregivers often set for themselves. Unrealistic goals may lead to caregivers assuming responsibility that does not belong to them and can lead to feelings of burnout.

Intervention should be guided by assessment of the nature of denial Clinical intervention in cases of denial should be guided by an assessment of the specific nature of the denial: its severity, persistence, and effect on coping.[119] In assessing denial it is first important to exclude any underlying organic mental disorder or major psychiatric disorder. Next it must be established what the patient has been told about the illness.[119] If the person has never been given the diagnosis in a way that is clearly understandable, he or she cannot be assessed as utilizing denial.

Avoidance and denial can appear quite similar and must be distinguished. Denial is unconscious and aimed against an external or internal threat which is perceived as being intolerable. One cannot infer that a person is denying simply because he or she does not volunteer information about his or her illness.[119]

Avoidance is a conscious defence mechanism and reflects an effort to shun circumstances that bring stressful material, such as conversation about one's illness, to the forefront.

Mrs P was aware that she had a very aggressive breast cancer. She wished to live as long as it was possible to have a reasonably good quality of life. At a fairly early point in her illness trajectory she revised her will and met a new minister for the purpose of organizing her funeral. She and her husband discussed the implications of her possible death and the dreams that she had for their children. She decided in advance that she would like to be admitted to the acute care oncology unit where she had previously been treated when the time for her death came. She tried a variety of chemotherapy and alternative treatments in the hope of prolonging her life and improving her symptoms. Psychotherapy interviews with Mrs P and her husband focused almost entirely on possible treatments because that was her stated wish. She was at home, actively involved with her husband and three children, until a few days before her death.

Mrs P had consistently refused to discuss her illness with her children, stating that until it interferred with their lives she was not going to upset them by talking about it. She gave them information as she felt that they needed it. When she and her husband were told that death could occur quite precipitously they were quite shocked. She discussed the fact that her disease was getting worse and that there was a possiblity that she might die with each of her children individually. She was admitted to the hospital for the final few days of her life to be treated with one final course of chemotherapy in the hope of buying a little more time. She maintained her positive attitude until a couple of days prior to her death, at which point she briefly referred to her impending death. She then lapsed into a coma for the final day of her life. Her husband and children have done well during bereavement with no obvious unresolved issues. Her 9-year-old daughter has made it clear since her mother's death that she that she was aware that her mother was more ill than she acknowledged, but she realized that this information was being kept from her out of love and she accepted this. Mrs P's behaviour reflects avoidance, rather than denial.

The author's clinical experience has repeatedly shown that if patients are helped to have the information they want at the pace at which they want it, acknowledging that there will be episodes of 'denial' along the way, then they often have a very peaceful death.

Assessment of the impact of denial In making the decision on whether or not to intervene when denial has been diagnosed, it may be helpful to ask the following questions.[119]

- Is denial affecting help-seeking behaviour and compliance?
- Is denying reducing emotional distress?

It is also helpful to remember that adaptive functioning primarily seeks to enable the person to attain or maintain emotional stability, social support, and compliance with necessary medical treatment. Whether or not the disease is explicitly acknowledged is secondary to these broader issues. When an attempt is made to modify extreme denial, the goal may need to be realistically set to enable the person to comply with treatment or to experience a reduction in emotional distress, but not necessarily to be able to say, 'I have terminal cancer'.[119]

Intervening to break down denial When denial is diagnosed intervention strategies should be tailored to a level that is appropriate for the individual person.[119] It may not be helpful to try to break down a person's denial unless there is something else to put in its place (e.g. a promise to stand by the patient no matter what, appropriate reassurance regarding the hospice to which the person will be transferred, etc.).

When extreme denial breaks down, either if the patient is confronted by disease progression that cannot be ignored any longer or when participation in treatment requires confrontation by caregivers, patients may feel flooded by emotion and experience a reactive psychosis or severe depression or anxiety.[119] Expert psychiatric intervention is indicated at this point.

An example of a situation in which denial was present and careful intervention was required over a period of a few weeks is described below. The intervention had to acknowledge the patient's need to maintain as much control as possible and to deny the implications of her long-term prognosis until the circumstances were such that she was ready to do so.

Mrs L. was a 45-year-old widowed mother of three adult children who was paraplegic from spinal metastasis as a result of breast cancer. She was referred in the very advanced stage of her disease because she cried constantly and the staff were very concerned that she was suicidal. Initially, Mrs L was quite hesitant to talk. She required a relationship with some degree of reciprocity and a recognition that in the past she had been able to cope better.

After several weeks Mrs L mentioned that she became very upset whenever a physician entered her room because she was concerned that something would be done to cause her pain. It was explained that this was one of the reasons for which transfer to a palliative care facility had been suggested. She was assured that on the palliative care unit the staff would focus primarily on her symptoms and would not be doing any more investigative work-ups. She agreed to the transfer.

At the palliative care facility Mrs L. became agitated because she felt that the staff were not doing anything to cure her disease. She said that when she spoke to the staff about walking out of the hospital, one of the nurses told her that this would never happen as she had come there to die. Mrs L said that she found this unnecessarily cruel as she still had hope of a cure. By this time she was on antidepressants and was more able to speak about her illness. She was gently reminded that she had been transferred to a palliative care setting because nothing more could be done to cure her disease, no matter how hard anyone tried. Despite having been told this numerous times before, she was now ready to accept the reality of her illness and to face the fact that she would never again be able to walk and be self-sufficient. She finally acknowledged this situation and made a decision to deal with some legal issues. Within a couple of days she went into a coma and died peacefully.

Emotional distress in response to terminal illness

The emotional response to terminal disease can range from little apparent response, to feelings of dysphoria and some anxiety, to major psychiatric disturbance.[122] Robert Shepherd, a Canadian psychiatrist, published a series of articles chronicling his personal experience with terminal cancer. He summed up the emotional response of many people as follows: '. . . everybody with life-threatening sickness is depressed. It is loss, you understand, catastrophic loss; you will never be the same again...Then...imperceptibly at first, the light starts to come back. There is less pain, less despair, longer periods of rest at night. . .'.[123]

The entire range of psychiatric syndromes are encountered in the care of dying people. These may be accentuated by the terminal illness because of the maladaptive use of defence mechanisms or the onset of organic brain syndrome or a combination of the two.[122]

Coping patterns in terminal illness Good copers differ from poor copers in that the former seem to have a special skill that helps them to overcome many of the problems associated with cancer. Weisman[124] has found that good copers were generally optimistic and self-confident, even during very difficult times. While they were aware of the possible consequences and threats implied by their disease, they were nevertheless diligent about their care and able to maintain their composure throughout adverse circumstances. Good copers were generally pragmatic about their future and seemed to exude an inner confidence that whatever happened they would be able to cope. They were generally able to confront issues directly, even if little could be done about their problems.

Poor copers were able to cope reasonably well in some situations but not at all well in others. The worst copers 'complained of having been *deserted, depressed, defeated and disappointed*. Self pity was a signal trait. Expectation of the future was usually excessive and absolute, permitting no compromise'.[124]

What determines a good or bad coping outcome is a question of viewpoint. Patients, family members, and health care professionals may have different perspectives: 'the patient's subjective priority is to keep up an acceptable intrapsychic and interpersonal psychosocial equilibrium; the family wants to see the patient as a functioning member of the social network at large, whereas doctors and other healthcare providers expect optimal compliance, in view of difficult and sometimes even harmful medical procedures'.[125] In the case of terminal illness the adaptive goals of the patient might be as follows:

- overcoming insecurity and loss of control in view of self-image and orientation toward the future;
- mastering existential threat (e.g. in view of terminal illness);
- preserving a meaningful quality of life under whatever circumstances.

The family and social network expectations might be as follows:

- preserving or regaining an acceptable relationship with the spouse;
- securing the family's financial and social resources;
- sustaining social relationships with friends and acquaintances.

The health professional's expectations might be as follows:

- Preserving emotional stability despite long-term illness or progressive impairment, including terminal outcome.[125]

In Heim's longitudinal study of 72 women with breast cancer,[125] 'good' coping included seeking and perceiving social and emotional support and an attitude of stoical acceptance of cancer. Poor psychosocial adjustment involved a pattern of resignation–fatalism, combined with a passive–avoiding attitude. High distress was associated with resignation, withdrawal, rumination, and emotional release. Distress was low and well being was high when emotions were denied, isolated, and suppressed.

Prevalence of emotional distress in terminal cancer A number of studies have shown an increased incidence of psychological distress in patients with advanced cancer.[23-28,32-34,39-43] In one study over 400 bereaved survivors responded to questioning about the deceased's experience with depression, anxiety, anger, feeling dependent or alone, difficulty in thinking, or needing someone to talk to.[126] Almost a quarter of the sample (21 per cent) had unmet emotional needs.

In the CCS and T-SRCC studies [3-5,30] terminally ill patients were significantly more likely to rate themselves as having difficulty with self-reported feelings of depression, anxiety, and frustration. Forty-six per cent of the terminally ill patients in the CCS study reported a problem with feelings of depression, anxiety, and frustration in the previous month, as did 56 to 57 per cent of the T-SRCC sample.

Risk assessment for emotional distress The clinician must be able to distinguish between the psychological symptoms which are a common response to terminal cancer and are amenable to supportive interventions from staff members, and those syndromes which require a more aggressive approach from skilled mental health practitioners or psychiatrists.[127] It is also important to identify the psychological symptoms associated with drugs such as corticosteroids, vincristine, interferon, and cimetidine,[128] and metabolic alterations such as hypercalcaemia or damage to the central nervous system by either the tumour or its treatment.[128-130]

In this chapter we focus on symptoms of depression and anxiety, distinguishing those cases which will require intervention from those with which the primary clinician may be able to deal without the use of psychiatric professionals. Much more detailed information about psychiatric diagnosis and pharmacological intervention in the care of people with psychiatric disturbance in response to advanced disease is given elsewhere in this text (Section 15).

Dying may precipitate people into psychiatric illness if they are unduly vulnerable as a result of previous unresolved separation or loss experiences; a lack of support from at least one loved person, or inappropriate discussions of prognosis which do not allow the natural process of adjustment and assimilation to take place.[122] A history of early parental death, loss, or strained interpersonal relationships may also leave adults susceptible to depressive episodes when confronted with later adult loss, such as a diagnosis of cancer or the awareness that the disease is becoming worse.[78,131]

Cancer patients at greatest risk for psychological problems are young (age 40 and younger), female, receiving palliative or active treatment as opposed to follow-up care, and symptomatic or not fully ambulatory.[53] Problems with the family's adaptation to illness were found to be key risk factors for patient mood disturbance, role conflicts, and self-care in a group of homebound patients.[132]

Depressive symptoms and depression (see Section 15) A review of 20 studies of depression in cancer patients found that the prevalence varied by site and ranged from 1.5 to 50 per cent (mean 24 per cent; median 22 per cent).[133] Studies of symptom severity were also reviewed and showed that 1 to 38 per cent of cancer patients had major depression. Caution must be exercised in evaluating these studies because they have a number of complicating variables, such as hospitalization status and site of tumour.[133]

Mor[134] analysed large data sets from three previous studies of cancer patients and found that terminally ill patients scored significantly higher on most depression items, including 'lonely', 'blue', and 'hopeless', than did newly diagnosed patients. Not surprisingly, depression was strongly correlated with decreased quality of life.

The assessment of depression in the terminally ill can be difficult because there is no agreement on how to classify patients with depression associated with physical illness.[42] Many of the vegetative symptoms associated with depression, such as anorexia, weight loss, insomnia, reduced energy, and reduced concentration, are features of debilitating disease including malignant cachexia.[134]

A diagnosis of major depression can be made if the person has symptoms of dysphoria and/or anhedonia (loss of interest or pleasure) pervasively for at least a 2-week period. In addition, the person must have at least four of the following symptoms (at least three if the person has both dysphoria and anhedonia): sleep disorder, appetite change, fatigue, psychomotor retardation and/or agitation, low self-esteem and/or guilt, poor concentration and/or indecisiveness, and thoughts of suicide and/or suicidal ideation.[133,135] Fearfulness, depressed appearance, social withdrawal, decreased talkativeness, brooding, self-pity and pessimism may also be indicative of depression.[128] Mermelstein and Lesko[136] suggest focusing on the psychological symptoms of persistent dysphoria, feelings of helplessness and hopelessness, loss of self-esteem, feelings of worthlessness, and wishing to die as reliable diagnostic indicators. When these symptoms interfere with functioning or overwhelm the patient, treatment is indicated.[133]

Additional indicators of depression in this group might include chronic pain, lack of response to therapy, physical disability out of proportion to physiological impairment, failure to engage in a rehabilitative measure, somatic preoccupation, and the wish to discontinue treatment.[39,137] Pain must always be addressed as the potential primary problem in patients with depressive symptoms. The presence of chronic pain in and of itself may be sufficient to produce depression.[32] The prevalence of depressive disorders of all types was found to be higher in a group of cancer patients reporting high pain compared with a group with low pain. Patients with high pain were found to be significantly more anxious and emotionally distressed than those with low pain. In a second study of women with metastatic breast cancer, pain intensity correlated significantly with fatigue, vigour, and total mood disturbance, and pain frequency correlated significantly with fatigue, vigour, and depression.[37]

Social support and quality of life have also been found to be associated with depression in a group of older males with cancer. Quality of life accounted for more of the variance in Beck Depression Inventory scores than did social support.[138]

It may be difficult to distinguish the withdrawal that many consider to be the final stage of a terminal illness from the picture of pathological depression. Attempts must be made to analyse the source of depression before treating it with counselling or psychotherapy.[39,137]

Patients with a family or personal history of depression are at greater risk of developing depression during cancer,[128] as are those with a history of alcohol abuse. The latter finding is associated with the increased incidence of depression in patients with head and neck cancers.[128,139] Those with pancreatic cancer are also at higher risk of depression.[128,140] The cause is unknown but a paraneoplastic syndrome is suspected.[132,141]

The use of biological markers in depression Current work is suggesting the use of biological markers to help to distinguish cancer patients in whom neurovegetative symptoms are associated with major depression from those whose symptoms are a result of their cancer. Certain markers may reflect and even portend treatment response in patients with depression. The rates of dexamethasone suppression in the dexamethasone suppression test and of thyrotropin blunting in a significant number of depressed cancer patients have been found to be similar to those of depressed psychiatric outpatients without cancer.[133] The work of McDaniel and colleagues[133] suggests that many cancer patients have a dysregulation of the hypothalamic–pituitary–adrenal axis. The impact of diminished immune functioning in depressed patients with cancer is also under investigation.[133]

Suicide There is still some controversy as to whether suicide is more common in cancer patients, but it has been established that it is more common among the physically ill than in the healthy population.[142] In a Swedish study, cancer patients were found to have an increased risk of suicide compared with the normal population. That rate was highest in the first year of diagnosis when the rate was multiplied by 15.[143]

Ideas of suicide in a terminally ill person might not be so much a sign of depression as of wanting to retain control over one's life to the end, and of wanting to shorten the period of dying and thus relieve others of the burden of care:[122] 'Maintaining a sense of control is an important issue for the patient who expresses the wish to die. The wish for control may focus on uncontrolled pain or other symptoms; on the diminished sense of one's self and one's life; or even on family, friends, and caregivers'.[144] Not only is the patient at risk for suicide, so too are the spouse and other family members.[144]

In a study of 200 terminally ill inpatients, the desire for early death was associated with ratings of pain and low family support, but most significantly with measures of depression. The prevalence of diagnosed depressive syndromes was 58.8 per cent among patients with a desire to die and 7.7 per cent in patients without such a desire. This study showed that the desire for death was closely associated with clinical depression which is a potentially treatable illness.[145]

Suicide in terminal illness is discussed in detail elsewhere in this text (see Sections 3 and 15).

Anxiety Not surprisingly, anxiety is common in terminally ill patients.[26,146] Symptoms of anxiety in the latter stages of cancer may be part of a generalized response to the disease or reflective of an adjustment disorder with anxious mood (DSM IV).[135] Anxiety disorders, such as generalized anxiety, phobia, or panic disorder, are rare in cancer patients and are often pre-existent[147]

Generalized anxiety disorders have the following characteristics.[135]

1. Excessive anxiety and worry (apprehensive expectation), occurring more days than not for at least 6 months, about a number of events or activities (such as work or school performance).
2. The person finds it difficult to control the worry.
3. The anxiety and worry are associated with three (or more) of the following six symptoms (with at least some symptoms present more days than not for the previous 6 months):
    - restlessness or feeling keyed up or on edge
    - easily fatigued
    - difficulty in concentrating or mind going blank
    - irritability
    - muscle tension
    - sleep disturbance (difficulty falling or staying asleep, or restless unsatisfying sleep)
4. The anxiety, worry, or physical symptoms cause clinically significant distress or impairment in social, occupational, or other important areas of functioning.
5. The disturbance is not due to the direct physiological effects of a substance (e.g. a drug of abuse, a medication) or a general medical condition (e.g. hyperthyroidism).

Panic attacks may occur in stressful situations and are defined as follows:[135] a discrete period of intense fear or discomfort, in which four (or more) of the following symptoms develop abruptly and reach a peak within 10 min:

- palpitations, pounding heart, or accelerated heart rate
- sweating
- trembling or shaking
- sensations of shortness of breath or smothering
- feelings of choking
- chest pain or discomfort
- nausea or abdominal distress
- feeling dizzy, unsteady, lightheaded, or faint
- derealization (feelings of unreality) or depersonalization (being detached from oneself)
- fear of losing control or going crazy
- fear of dying
- paraesthesia (numbness or tingling sensations)
- chills or hot flushes.

The clinical symptoms of anxiety, including anxious mood, increased attention, fearfulness, inability to concentrate, and restlessness, are easy to observe. Associated symptoms, such as dypsnoea, tremor, palpitations, or sweat can be due to the cancer or its treatment. Therefore these are less reliable for diagnosis.[147]

Anxiety has been classified[146] as follows.

Situational anxiety: while some anxiety is normal in adjusting to cancer, a prolonged feeling of anxiety of an unusual intensity that interferes with the person's ability to cope with the disease or to engage in normal social activities is not normal. Situational anxiety can be intensified by unrealistic thoughts about the aetiology and course of cancer or the side-effects of the proposed treatment. Imminent death is often not the most frequent source of anxiety which may be due more to concerns about pain, isolation, anxiety, dependence, cachexia, and shortness of breath.

Psychiatric anxiety: in addition to adjustment disorders with anxiety symptoms, anxiety may arise in the form of phobias about some aspect of medical care, panic, and generalized anxiety disorders. Anxiety is also a prominent symptom in up to 50 per cent of delerious patients. Withdrawal from drugs or alcohol can also cause symptoms of anxiety.

Organic anxiety may be caused by acute pain. It may also be associated with asthenia, nausea, shortness of breath, metabolic disturbances, such as hypercalcaemia and hypoglycaemia, structural changes in the brain, and drugs such as corticosteroids and morphine.

Existential anxiety may have a spiritual dimension. This anxiety may be associated with thoughts about a wasted life, fear of the current illness situation, and thoughts of the future, including the possibility of death.[147]

A more detailed review of the symptoms and treatment of anxiety is given in Section 15.

Depression and anxiety While anxiety and depression may be seen as separate and distinct symptoms, they may well occur together.[27,35] A high concordance between the two symptoms in cancer patients suggests that both will need to be attended to in many situations.

Intervention for emotional problems There are several ways of approaching an assessment of what causes most concern in a terminally ill person. One approach would be to conduct an open-minded open-ended interview on potential concerns. A second approach would be to address the issue of what the patient wants and is worried about not getting.[124]

The first approach involves inquiring into ' (1) health and well being of every kind; (2) family and marital attitudes; (3) housing and money worries; (4) sexual and social activities; (5) job and daily life; (6) self image; and (7) existential issues about illness, invalidism, and death'.[124]

The second approach involves assessing what patients want and should include '(1) relief of symptoms; (2) better support; (3) firmer security: (4) sustained relationships, both personal and professional; and (5) stronger morale to face the future'.[124]

Patients who have difficulty in defining their mental status and do not necessarily want to speak about personal matters, may be quite willing to discuss issues such as the following.[118]

1. What has been the major problem you've had to face since this illness started, and that maybe still bothers you?
2. How is your morale these days, considering what has happened?
3. What can you tell me about how discouraged you ordinarily get?
4. If you had some advice for someone else who was just starting out on what you've already been through, what would that advice be?

Using these approaches the interviewer can begin to assess the areas in which patients will be able to use practical assistance to help them to cope more effectively. This will also allow the clinician to decide in which areas he or she is comfortable about intervening and which will require some outside assistance.

Sometimes it is possible to begin to intervene to decrease the possibility of later distress during the time of the initial interview. Simply offering the opportunity to discuss issues at the time they arise may provide a useful intervention. Caregivers may make comments such as: 'It must have been very difficult to have your father die in respiratory distress. What impact do you think that has on your concerns regarding your own impending death?' or 'It must have been quite a shock finding out that you had cancer of the pancreas when you were expecting to hear that you had gallstones' or 'It sounds as if you and your wife have not been able to talk about what your diagnosis means in your life. Do you think it might be helpful to do some talking now?' At other times it might be helpful to offer the services of a social worker or mental health professional.

Caregivers sometimes express concern that by bringing up difficult issues, they will cause patients to think about unhappy or troublesome problems. Generally, if the caregiver acts in a warm non-judgemental professional manner, giving the impression that such issues are a part of normal life and not particularly shocking, the patient will be willing to discuss these and other difficult issues. If the caregiver avoids asking such questions, important information might be overlooked.

Intervention is indicated with an identifiable psychiatric disorder and may be indicated in situations of depression where there is poor social support and other concurrent stressors.[127] Even those without a diagnosable psychiatric illness have need for some type of support.[148] Psychotherapy for the medically ill is often conducted in conjunction with appropriate psychopharmacological treatment and consists of emotional support, social support, cognitive restructuring, and coping skills training.

Spiegel[148] concludes that group psychotherapeutic intervention has been found to improve mood, adjustment, fatigue, and pain. It has been shown to help patients to cope better with their disease and to live more fully. Individual and group psychotherapy have been shown to be effective in reducing depression and anxiety as well as fatigue, nausea, and pain. As already noted, such intervention may also increase the quantity and quality of life. In addition, such interventions have been shown in numerous studies to reduce total medical costs by reducing costly and unneeded medical interventions.[148]

Referral for psychosocial intervention When is it appropriate to refer? Although it has been estimated that 47 per cent of cancer patients suffer from psychiatric disorders, the majority of which are situational adjustment reactions,[23] few receive psychiatric consultations.[27] The reasons for the low referral rate seem to be twofold: the inability of primary care physicians to identify psychiatric problems, and the belief that psychiatric intervention is not helpful.[27] It has been estimated that about half of the total group of cancer patients will not need any intervention, about 35 to 40 per cent can have intervention through social workers, psychologists, or counsellors, and about 10 to 15 per cent should receive psychiatric intervention.[127]

In the Canadian needs studies the percentage of people receiving intervention from social workers, psychologists, psychotherapists, counsellors, and psychiatrists ranged from 9 to 13 per cent in the CCS study to 22.6 per cent in the T-SRCC study. Almost all of those who had mental health intervention found it to be useful. Of the group as a whole, another 4 to 7 per cent in all the samples said that they would have found it helpful to have had access to some type of mental health counselling.[3-5,30] In the CCS study those with advanced disease were more likely to have received psychosocial intervention (15–22 per cent).[3-5] In the T-SRCC study the inpatients with terminal illness were the most likely (55.9 per cent) and the terminally ill outpatients were the least likely (2/14 (14 per cent)) to have received mental health counselling. However, the size of this sample is so low as not to be generalizable. Given that the terminally ill outpatient group had more symptoms than the terminally ill inpatients and that they were less likely to have received any type of assistance, future research will need to assess whether this group is 'falling through the cracks' or whether they have rejected services offered.

Since at least some of those not currently being referred for psychological support feel that it might be helpful, some guidelines regarding when the caregiver might be able to help and when outside referral might be indicated will be given below.

Intervention for depression The research database on the treatment of depression in patients with cancer is limited. However, there is evidence that the treatment of depression improves dysphoria and other signs and symptoms of depression, improves quality of life, and may improve immune function and survival time.[133] Current research is investigating the possiblity of using biological markers as diagnostic adjuncts in the treatment of patients with cancer.[133] Until this method becomes more readily available, the best that can be done is carefully to elicit the symptoms that the patient is currently experiencing and to make a judgement based on 'the person's past history of reacting to stress and on his or her hereditary predisposition to mood disorder, whether any present stress accounts for the mood disorder or, alternatively, whether a biogenic state is present'.[149]

Referral to a psychiatrist or highly skilled mental health practitioner is indicated if a difficult diagnostic problem is present, if there is evidence of a major depression, or there is a question of suicidal ideation. Anhedonia (lack of pleasure or interest in life) is useful in distinguishing biogenic from psychogenic depression. If a person is not able to look forward to events that previously gave pleasure, such as the visit of family or friends or a planned trip, or if the person's sense of humour has gone, antidepressants anti-depressants may well be effective.[149] Depressed patients with cancer are usually treated by a combination of supportive psychotherapy and antidepressants.[144] Depressed terminally ill patients may or may not be open to intervention that allows them to reflect on the meaning of their current situation within the context of their life, to deal with unresolved issues, and to deal with issues of loss and impending death.

More specific information on the treatment of depression is given in Section 15.

Intervention for suicidal risk If there is a question of a suicidal risk, a skilled psychiatrist or mental health practitioner should be involved. Allowing cancer patients to speak about suicidal thoughts does not increase the individual's risk of committing suicide. Rather, it allows the patient to feel a sense of control by allowing him or her to express feelings, fears, and misconceptions. Exploring the meaning of suicidal thinking can allow the clinician to address the covert issues and to tailor interventions.[144] Despite expert care it is not always possible to prevent suicide in terminal illness.

Mr and Mrs Smith were a couple in their late thirties, childless by choice, who had been actively involved in caring for her mother, Mrs Williams, who had died of lung cancer 6 weeks prior to Mr Smith's diagnosis of inoperable gastric cancer. Mrs Williams' final illness had been marked by extreme pain and communication problems with the treating physician. Two days prior to her death another physician referred them to a home palliative care team who were able to achieve good pain relief for her final days. The Smiths had been married for 10 years and had chosen to lead a socially restricted life, feeling very satisifed with just themselves and Mrs Williams as their primary group. Mrs Williams was concerned with how they would cope at the time of her death. They assured her that they would survive because they had each other.

Mr Smith had had gastric problems for years and had frequently seen physicians without ever receiving a diagnosis. At the time of his diagnosis he was in extreme pain. It was immediately recognized that this couple could be at risk of a joint suicide attempt, and the issue was addressed then and 2 weeks later. They insisted that they would not consider this option and Mrs Smith was able to discuss how she would handle her grief after her husband's death. When asked specifically about the availability of drugs from Mrs Williams final illness, they said these were still around but were in packing boxes which they had just moved from Mrs Williams apartment across the hall. They maintained that they would not be able to find the pills even if they wanted to.

Very high doses of opioids and neuroablative procedures were required to allow Mr Smith finally to achieve pain relief. He was in good pain control for only the second time in his 4-week hospital stay when he was told that he would probably die of a gastric haemorrhage within the next few days. The couple asked to go home for an overnight pass. They said that they did not want to be discharged yet, but would want to be discharged to the care of the palliative home care team closer to the time of his death. They openly spoke of the plans that they had for his being at home during his final days and of the confidence they had in the palliative care team they had used previously.

During their first night at home the couple made a joint suicide attempt. Mr Smith died and his wife survived, although she was almost moribund when she was discovered. Mrs Smith was initially seen in twice weekly and then weekly grief therapy and was able to develop a good relationship with the therapist. She also had a good relationship with her family physician who prescribed antidepressants. Mrs Smith refused to see a psychiatrist because of anger at the way she felt she had been treated at the time of her initial suicide attempt when she felt threatened by the possibility of being committed.

During her initial phase of grief she purchased a new apartment which she totally redecorated. She resisted attempts to encourage her to enlarge her social circle, but was gradually seeking out new employment possibilities when she unexpectedly committed suicide on the anniversary of her mother's death. In her will she expressed gratitude to the caregivers who had worked with her and her husband and left them some of her significant belongings.

Intervention into anxiety The following psychiatric techniques may be helpful in alleviating the anxiety and distress of cancer patients.[150]

- See patients at regular intervals.
- Listen to what the patient is saying; avoid premature reassurance.
- Correct misconceptions about the disease, its treatment, and its pathophysiology.
- Be realistic and straightforward with both patient and family, but allow them to maintain hope.
- Assess the family's needs and offer preventive treatment
- Allow denial and regression within reasonable bounds.
- Be aggressive in attempting to relieve physical discomfort
- Treat anxiety, depression and insomnia pharmacologically if necessary.
- Keep staff conflict away from patients.

Other non-pharmacological approaches to dealing with anxiety include deep muscle relaxation, visualization, and guided imagery. The same concepts can also be applied to relieve anxiety. Psychologists can teach other health-care professionals to use these techniques, thus expanding the psychosocial resources available within a programme.

Issues of personal control in terminal cancer

In addition to anxiety and depression, patients may experience a number of other emotional responses to their disease. A review of the literature on cancer and communication[151] concluded that loss of control was the single most important problem confronting cancer patients. This may involve the feeling that one no longer has the ability to make choices which will affect the outcome of events that impinge one's life, and this may lead to feelings of powerlessness and helplessness.

The process of dying involves giving up various aspects of control over one's life as it becomes necessary to relinquish control over one's future plans, relationships with other people, social roles, and even various aspects of one's bodily functions. People cope with this threat of loss of control in a variety of ways:

- by quietly relinquishing control;
- by struggling to maintain control through seeking alternative treatments; [152]
- by trying to maintain as much control is possible under difficult circumstances;
- by attempting to inconvenience others as little as possible through one's dying process;
- by trying to maintain as much control as possible, even if this imposes considerable hardship on other people;
- sometimes through suicide.

A model of control for cancer patients has been hypothesized.[153] The greater the expectation of control at the time of diagnosis or recurrence, the more one is motivated to try to find every possible way of controlling the disease and the more likely it is that one will become frustrated when the disease becomes uncontrollable. When the patient realizes that things may be beyond his or her control, the expectation of control gradually decreases often leading to decreased motivation, passivity, helplessness, and depression. The greater the individual's initial expectation of control, the more controlling the person is before giving up and the greater is the depression when the individual does finally give up.

Most ambulatory terminally ill cancer patients will continue to do their best to manage and structure their lives through the use of a variety of behavioural and cognitive coping strategies. These include the following:[154]

- carefully monitoring the progress of their disease;
- 'waiting out' the cancer, i.e. holding things in abeyance waiting for normality to return and selectively using coping strategies to maintain a state of perseverance;
- refocusing on areas over which they could maintain control;
- turning it over (actively relinquishing control over the disease).

Dying persons often attempt to normalize selected aspects of their lives through trying to bring routine, order, and control to their lives despite the disease.[154]

Risk assessment and intervention with patients with a strong need for control Patients with a strong need for control can threaten professional caregivers who may have a similar need. The caregiver can be helped by reflecting that this way of coping often covers up real feelings of panic at the thought of losing control. Often this underlying panic is due to a basic fear of trusting people in positions of authority. This may be due to early childhood difficulty and a lack of ability to trust parent figures.

The caregiver who frequently gets into power struggles with patients or families with a strong need for control might do well to consider whether he or she has some 'unfinished business' from the past that might well be dealt with in personal therapy. Caregivers must be aware that the time of terminal illness is not the time to try to resolve all old unresolved personality conflicts in patients and family members. When dealing with a patient or family with a strong need for control, allow them to have as much control as possible, particularly in the early stages of the disease. When this is done, the caregiver will often find that a sense of trust in the caregiver and/or the caregiving team is built up, and over time patients, families, and caregivers may all become more willing to share control.

Information exchange and decision-making

Part of the issue of control during the final illness involves access to information—both how much and how little information may be desired. The patient's need to maintain a sense of control is closely related to a need to seek information. Information can reduce uncertainty and thus provide patients with a sense of control over the circumstances of their illness.[151]

Factors affecting information exchange and decision-making The amount of information given and the amount desired may be influenced by a number of variables including the age of the patient,[4,154,155] social class variables,[156] the type of disease,[4,156] and the country of residence.[4,156-158] There is some evidence that American patients may have a greater desire for information about their disease than patients in other countries.[155,157] Another factor affecting information exchange and the possibility of informed decision-making is the patient's relationship with medical staff and other health care professionals.

In a Scottish survey[156] 120 general practitioners were interviewed and postal questionnaires were answered by a further 627 general practitioners. The physicians were questioned about a patient who had recently died of cancer. They were asked whether the patient was aware of the diagnosis and whether the physician had discussed the future with the patient. The questions were asked in a slightly different way in each study so that the results needed to be reported separately.

The interview sample of general practitioners felt that less than half (42 per cent) of patients were fully aware of their diagnosis. Of the other 58 per cent, the general practitioners felt that about one quarter (23.7 per cent) were aware of the diagnosis, at least at the end, and another 15.3 per cent might know the diagnosis. The findings of the study give some insight into the process that occurs between patients, family members, and physicians involving information exchange. Physicians acknowledged that in at least one-third of the cases they did not even try to discuss the situation with patients. In 12.2 per cent of the cases they tried but were unsuccessful. The authors found no significant differences between the sexes, whether of patient or of physician, with regard to information exchange. In addition, there were no differences in age in patient awareness. However, there was a non-significant trend towards physicians choosing not to discuss the illness with older patients. Similar findings have been noted elsewhere.[4]

Whether or not the physician tried to discuss the situation with patients was related to the physician's estimate of the patient's social class (as opposed to the patient's actual social class). Physicians were more likely to have tried to have, and actually had, success with discussing diagnoses with those whom they perceived to be of a higher social class.

A somewhat surprising finding in the above study was that patients who died in hospice were not significantly more likely to be aware of their diagnosis or to have discussed the diagnosis with their physician than were people who died at home or in the hospital.

Although less than half of the patients in the physician interview study were fully aware of their diagnosis, more than four-fifths of their main caregivers were aware (83.3 per cent), although even here caregivers did not always appreciate what was happening.

In the postal study, almost three-quarters (73.5 per cent) of the patients were aware that they were dying. Again, there was no sex difference between patients or physicians and whether or not the patient knew that he or she was dying. There was a significant difference by age, with younger patients being more aware than older patients. Social class differences were also observed in this group, with patient awareness and physician discussion decreasing as the patient's social class decreased. Again, there was not a significant difference between patients who died in hospice and elsewhere with regard to whether or not they were aware that they were dying. In the postal survey there was very little difference in awareness between those dying in hospices (77.8 per cent), in a relative's home (77.5 per cent), in their own home (74.3 per cent), or in a teaching hospital (72.5 per cent).

The authors expressed surprise at finding that in the 1980s, when there was an emphasis on truth-telling and respect for personal autonomy, only about two-thirds of the general practitioners had discussed the diagnosis with the dying patient. Physician–patient–family communication is still a complicated issue, however, with patient/family/physician preferences, demographic variables, and cultural attitudes all having a substantial impact.

Age and information exchange In the CCS and T-SRCC studies, we investigated health care communication and information exchange from the perspective of the patient. Patients[4,5,30] were asked a number of questions about communication with health-care professionals and their preferences for information exchange. Data analysis showed that communication between the patient and the health-care provider is by no means a simple issue. In Manitoba[4] there was a significant association between communication with physicians and other health-care providers (nurses, radiotherapy technologists, social workers, etc.) and age of patients. The younger that patients were, the more likely they were to have had a frank and open discussion about their disease with their physician as well as with other health-care providers.[158]

However, in Quebec, where over 90 per cent of the sample was French Canadian, there was not a significant difference between age and communication. Each of the Quebec age cohorts was more likely to have discussed their illness than were their counterparts in Manitoba.

Patients were asked how much information that they wanted compared with other patients. Younger patients felt that they wanted more information than other patients. In Manitoba this finding held true for those under 30 and in Quebec for those aged 30 to 45.

Information preferences in patients with terminal and advanced disease Patients in the Canadian study with more advanced disease had difficulty with information exchange.

A 37-year-old woman with such severe financial problems that she did not have enough money for food had been diagnosed as having lung cancer 4 months before the interview. She was being followed by several doctors and claimed that, while her surgeon said that she had localized disease, another doctor said that she had 'disease all over'. She said that her doctors would not answer the questions that she asked about her disease. She had a great fear of dying and said that she wished that if her physicians did not have time to answer her questions, that they would refer her to someone who could help her.

Not all terminal patients wanted information, however. The data showed no clear information preference pattern amongst the terminally ill. Some wanted to know and others did not. Cassileth *et al.*[158] noted that, in an American sample, 'Not knowing about one's clinical reality is often associated with uncertainty and unrealistic fears, a condition that patients describe as "worse than knowing the facts". Becoming well informed may enable patients to maintain hope by freeing them from anxiety and fear'.

However, the Canadian sample showed that when Canadian patients are in the advanced or palliative phase of their disease, there may be much more variety in how much information they want than when they are healthier and say that they want to know everything.

Communication problems between patients in the palliative phase of their disease, their family members, and medical staff can obviously be a significant problem. Houts *et al.*[126], who conducted interviews with bereaved survivors, found that 20 per cent reported communication problems with medical staff in the last month of their family member's life. Three-quarters of those who reported problems with medical staff said that it was associated with difficulty in obtaining information about the dying person's medi cal condition, treatment, or prognosis. Typical comments reported in that study were: 'staff were not available' or 'staff tried to avoid us and so we didn't know what was going on'. Bereaved family members also reported difficulty with nursing care and insensitive behaviour on the part of medical staff.

Intervention and information exchange in terminal illness (see Section 4) Dealing appropriately with dying people requires a variety of skills including the ability to break news gently, often in the presence of supportive family members, friends, or helpful caregivers who will stay with the patient as the information is absorbed. Breaking news abruptly can precipitate patients into a major state of crisis or disequilibrium. The key to breaking bad news is to do it in a manner that 'facilitates acceptance and understanding, while minimizing the risk of provoking denial, ambivalence, unrealistic expectations, overwhelming distress or collusion'.[159]

The author's 'rule of thumb' is to give the information that the patient wants and needs while maintaining a note of guarded hope and optimism. This type of conversation usually starts with an assessment of what the person understands the current situation to be, to ask if the person has as much information as he or she wants, to ask if the person would want to know if things were worse than the person thinks that they are, and to let the person know that at any time the interviewer is prepared to answer questions, to help the person formulate the questions for the physician, or to arrange for the physician to speak directly to the person. The interviewer also lets patients know they can change their mind about the amount of information that they want that at any time.

When caregivers have allowed the patient to take the lead in determining how much information the person might want but the situation has changed and the patient does not indicate that he or she is aware of the change, the caregiver must reassess what the patient wants and needs. Such conversations should be held in a comparatively quiet private place with the caregiver sitting physically close to the patient, ready to reach out to give physical comfort by holding a hand or putting a hand on the patient's arm or shoulder if that seems to be appropriate. The caregiver might then say:

'Things aren't looking very good at this point.' [pause] 'Do you want to talk about it?'[pause]

'It looks as if there may not be much time left/time is getting short.' [pause and wait for the patient's response]'We're still going to do whatever we can to make you comfortable [pause] and we'll stick by you, no matter what happens.' [pause]

'We thought that you should know this in case there are things that you want to do or problems that you need to resolve.' [pause]

'The thing to remember is that we aren't God. One can always hope and pray that things will turn out differently.' (In a person without religious beliefs, 'but sometimes people prove us wrong and we're never offended/we're always pleased if that happens'.) [pause]

'This type of news is always difficult. Do you have any questions you might want to ask me at this time?' [pause]

'Is there anything particular you would like me/the staff to do?'

This type of conversation, which allows adequate time for the caregiver constantly to assess and reassess how much further to go with the patient and for the patient to ask questions or give clues as to which direction he or she wishes to go, can be quite helpful and rewarding for both patient and caregiver. Unexpected issues may often arise in this type of conversation, and the caregiver can facilitate helping to resolve some unfinished business.

Some patients make it quite clear that they do not want to know when their situation has deteriorated.

One 42-year-old mother of two young children said to the author, 'If you think there is something that I don't want to hear and don't want to talk about, but that you think my children should know about in order to make things easier for them, then I give you permission to speak with them about this thing that I don't want to talk about'. This woman spoke about her death only once a few days before she died, but the author met with her 11- and 14-year-old children and husband to work through their feelings prior to her death.

While open communication is often the preferred mode of communicating with people at most stages of their disease, ideally it should be given in a manner that encourages feedback and questions from patients. Some patients in the CCS and T-SRCC studies said that they were given 'bad news' in what they regarded as a very abrupt fashion. They felt unable to initiate discussion of the impact of this news and this caused them considerable distress.

The response to bad news can include acceptance, overwhelmed distress, denial, ambivalence, unrealistic expectations, and collusion.[159] Faulkner *et al.*[159] have provided a very useful flowchart for breaking bad news. Section 4 of this textbook also provides important guidelines.

There is no easy way to break bad news and it is painful for both patients and their caregivers. This painful process might well be more difficult if the patient and physician have developed a close professional/personal relationship over the years and both have come to care for and understand one another. Nevertheless, avoiding the discussion is not good for either the patient or the caregiver unless the patient has given the physician the message that he or she does not want to discuss the issue.

Tom, a 24-year-old man with leukaemia, was having a difficult time but was unaware that he was in a life-threatening situation. A young physician came into his room and asked, 'When you have to be moved to the intensive care unit, do you want to be put on a respirator?' Tom was quite shocked and asked if this would be a temporary measure or if it would be permanent. The physician said that he would be permanently on a respirator. Tom was quite upset but said that if that was the situation then he would rather not add to his family's stress by prolonging his life when there was no hope of quality time.

When he felt better the next day Tom tried to continue the discussion with the physician to clarify the situation, but the physician said that he was much better now so it would not be necessary to have such a conversation. Tom was left wondering what the implications were of his previous decision and if that would be regarded as his final statement on the artificial prolongation of his life in all situations.

The author asked Tom's permission to use this anecdote, saying that it could be used to illustrate the fact that young physicians might tend to identify with young patients and find it hard to discuss such difficult topics. Tom's response was that it would be fine to use the anecdote, but that his experience was that most physicians, regardless of their seniority, found it difficult to break bad news. Given his frequent relapses, Tom has heard negative information from a number of physicians.

At a later point in Tom's illness he was aware that there was only one experimental treatment that had any possibility of prolonging his life. He had an open, honest, and mutual conversation with the same physician about the serious possibility that the treatment would have such severe side-effects that he would die. He was in a new marriage and the couple had recently purchased their first home. He made the informed decision to take the treatment and was aware that he had developed the side-effects that had been explained to him. The physician had some difficulty with the fact that Tom was going to die of treatment complications, but Tom accepted his fate, he felt that he had tried his best, he said his goodbyes to his family, and he died very peacefully.

The role of social support in cancer

Social support has been found to be a critical variable in adaptation to cancer and other stressful life events. Lack of a confidant relationship (defined as someone with whom one can discuss difficulties, who is available, with whom one exchanges mutual confidences, and to whom one can talk about one's cancer) was associated with a lower quality of life, more distress directly attributable to cancer, and high distress as measured on the Goldberg General Health Questionnaire.[5]

Components of social support Because social support is a crucial component in adaptation to life-threatening illness, it is important to understand its various components. Social support can be seen as a transactional process requiring a fit between the donor, the recipient, and the individual circumstances for its appropriate provision.[160,161] It comprises emotional support, appraisal support, informational support, and instrumental support.[162] Emotional support involves actions which enhance self-esteem. Appraisal support provides feedback on one's views or behaviour. Informational support entails giving advice or information that promotes problem solving. Finally, instrumental support is the provision of tangible assistance.

Social support is a process with multiple components. The 'goodness of fit' between donor activities and the needs of recipients is governed by the amount, timing, source, structure, and function of social support. There must be an adequate balance between the amount of support offered and the perceived threat engendered by a particular situation. In addition, the type and amount of support most useful to distressed individuals may change over time. The support which is offered may not correspond to the circumstances of the individual.[8,15,160,161]

The amount of support needed may vary not only with individuals but also with the stage of the disease. In a study of patients with either breast or colon cancer[163] it was found that the greater the amount of social support amongst those with a good prognosis, the more positive was their affect and the higher was their self-esteem. This was not necessarily the case among those with a poor prognosis. Individuals in the fairly passive role associated with advanced disease might feel that by receiving extra support they incurred debts that they would never be able to repay. This could be threatening to some individuals who are not used to being in the role of receiver. In addition, when one's well being is threatened in multiple ways by a poor prognosis, social support cannot ward off all threats.

In Hinton's study[117] of patients dying at home, perceived support from family and friends was initially regarded as being 'very satisfactory' by 72 per cent of those who later died at home. Sixty-three per cent of those who died in the hospice initially rated their perceived support as being 'very high'. Preceding admission only 53 per cent felt that their perceived support was 'very satisfactory', which was significantly less than the 78 per cent of 'matched' patients who died at home. Some patients felt less perceived support because they were aware that the relative was begining to show signs of strain. Relatives generally felt less support than patients, but those whose relatives died at home had an increased perception of support (from 46 per cent initially to 65 per cent prior to death) as others rallied to help.

The value of religious faith

Social support can also come from religious beliefs. A consistent inverse relationship has been found between spiritual well being and state-trait anxiety.[164] This finding held true despite differences in gender, age, marital status, diagnosis, and a number of other variables. Stressors characterized as losses or threats provoke more coping by putting faith in God than stressors categorized as challenges.[165]

In the CCS study there were significant differences in the degree of religious belief that patients reported. Respondents in Prince Edward Island (56 per cent of the sample were Protestant and 41 per cent Catholic) were the most likely to rate themselves as being very religious (70 per cent). This compared with 45 per cent rating themselves as very religious in Manitoba (45 per cent Protestant, 22 per cent Catholic, 3 per cent Jewish, 6 per cent other, 25 per cent no religion), and 42 per cent rating themselves as very religious in Quebec (90 per cent Catholic, 6 per cent Jewish, 4 per cent Protestant, 5 per cent no religion). Although those in Manitoba and Quebec did not consider themselves to be very religious, 61 per cent of the Manitoba respondents and 44 per cent of the Quebec respondents turned to prayer as a way of coping with their illness (the question was not asked in Prince Edward Island). Almost everyone who used prayer (96–98 per cent) found it to be helpful. When asked to describe their three major problems confronted since the diagnosis of cancer and how they coped with them, turning to religion/prayer/God was specifically mentioned in Prince Edward Island as a coping mechanism to deal with major problems.[3]

In Manitoba and Quebec, turning to religion was mentioned as a coping mechanism only when the situation was fairly serious: dealing with one's prognosis or thoughts of death in Manitoba, and dealing with recurrence and thoughts of death in Quebec.[4,5] Given the difference in degree of religious belief amongst those in the three provinces, it was not surprising that there was also a difference in the percentage of people who had spoken with a member of the clergy about their illness. In the CCS sample 75 per cent of those in Prince Edward Island compared with 39 per cent in Manitoba and only 14 per cent in Quebec had discussed their cancer with a member of the clergy; in the T-SRCC sample 27 per cent had done so.

The impact of religious belief might well have contributed to the way that Canadian respondents dealt with their illness. In Prince Edward Island, the most religious of the provinces, there was less self-reported depression, anxiety, and frustration (although the General Health Questionnaire score was no lower than the Canadian norms).

Suffering in the face of terminal illness

Suffering goes beyond the physical and impacts on every aspect of a person's life. Cassel[165] stresses that suffering is experienced by people, not merely by bodies. Suffering has its source in challenges that threaten the intactness of the person as a complex social and psychological entity. Such threats exist at multiple levels including one's own past, the family's lived past, culture and society, one's social roles, the instrumental dimension (i.e. one's ability to do things), one's associations and relationships with others, one's unconscious mind, one's self as a political being, one's secret life, the perceived future, and the transcendent dimension.

Cassel[165] states that the relief of suffering as well as the care of disease must be seen as twin obligations of a medical profession that is truly dedicated to the care of the sick. The failure to understand the nature of suffering can result in intervention which, although technically adequate, not only fails to relieve suffering but becomes a source of suffering itself. More recently,[166] he has stated that, while one can never truly experience another's distress, caregivers can 'learn to recognize the particular purposes, values, and aesthetic responses that shape the sense of self whose integrity is threatened by pain, disease, and the mischances of life'.

Mrs L., who was referred to above in the section on denial, could be defined as suffering. Through her current experience, she felt that the sense of self that she had been able to attain in the past was threatened. The thought of the future and her inability ever to walk and be self-sufficient again was a source of great suffering in the present.

Intervention in suffering involves recognition by the caregiver that suffering is occurring. The easiest way to discover this is to ask. However, people may not be aware of the suffering that they are experiencing. Understanding the suffering of another involves an exhaustive understanding of who they are as individuals: 'an awareness of when they feel themselves whole, threatened or disintegrated'.[166] Obviously, this will require taking the time to know what an individual feels about being whole, threatened, or disintegrated, who they are, their ideas of the past, present, and future, their relationships with others and their environment, their aims, and their anticipated actions.

Fear of death

Closely aligned to the issue of suffering for the palliative care patient is fear of death. Patients' acceptance of death has been studied by Hinton[40] who found that 26 per cent of dying patients had untroubled acceptance of death, while 53 per cent had some concern, and 21 per cent were troubled by thoughts of dying. In another study [81] half of patients in psychotherapy at the time that they were dying had difficulty in believing that death was really imminent. In that study many patients, who might have been thought to have been using denial, did indeed live longer than was expected.

In the CCS study a third to more than half of the terminal patients interviewed (33–58 per cent) were able to acknowledge thoughts and concerns regarding their eventual death.[3-5] Those in Prince Edward Island were the least likely to acknowledge such concerns, which might have reflected their reliance on and comfort derived from their greater religious faith.

Intervention with dying persons In assisting dying persons who acknowledge a fear of death, it is often helpful to ask them to consider which aspect of death concerns them most: thoughts of the dying process with its possible loss of control, pain, etc., the moment of death and how this will occur (will there be respiratory difficulty, haemorrhage, etc.?), or concerns about what will happen after death. If the caregiver understands the person's concerns, then it is possible to target the intervention appropriately. Often this will involve helping the patient to look at the underlying major concern; then he or she may handle the situation with minimal intervention.

The issue of increasing debility and dependence is the major problem for some people.

A 42-year-old nurse with metastatic breast cancer and bony and lung metastasis was most afraid of the debilitation and loss of independence which she might experience if she could not walk. While intellectually she knew that the lung metastases were the more serious problem, she feared the bony metastases and being crippled more than she feared dying.

Mrs Q., an 83-year-old widow, was most concerned about the moment of dying—specifically she worried about dying in respiratory distress. She spoke to her family about her concerns. When it was clear that she was dying in respiratory distress at a hospital far from home and her caring family physician, her daughter was able to intervene to tell the treating physician that this was her mother's greatest worry. It was possible to medicate Mrs. Q. so that her distress was alleviated.

Mrs B. was concerned about what was going to happen after her death. She was a 40-year-old divorcée with a long-standing alcohol problem who was living in a common-law relationship. For many years her mother had been urging her to make her peace with God. One day she decided to do this and then announced that she would die that night. When asked why she should die now, she said: 'When I made my promise to God I said that I wouldn't drink anymore and I would stop living with men. Now you know dear, and I know dear, that there is no way that I can keep that promise. You know dear, and I know dear, that if you make a promise to God on your deathbed and you don't keep it, then the next time you make a deathbed promise God won't believe it. That's why I'm going to die tonight.' Mrs. B. completely surprised the staff by dying that night.

Future research agenda

A number of issues that will require future research have been identified in this chapter. In the author's opinion, the continued work on the immunological changes associated with psychosocial intervention and their possible impact on survivorship is most important. So too is the work on biological markers which might be helpful in identifying which patients can profit most from anti-depressants. More work needs to be done on decision-making at points in the illness trajectory when patients could choose to continue active treatment aimed, realistically or not, at prolonging life rather than palliative care. Who chooses which options? How much are decisions dictated by third-party payers and what are the results? What is the impact of patients being transferred to palliative care programmes because of economic issues on the patient, on family members, and on the programme? More work also needs to be done on matching caregiver and patient communication styles in the area of breaking bad news.

References

1. Vachon MLS, Kristjanson L, Higginson I. Psychosocial issues in palliative care: the patient, the family, and the process and outcome of care. *Journal of Pain and Symptom Management*, 1995; **10**:142–50.
2. Houts PS, Yasko JM, Kahn SB, Schelzel GW, Marconi KM. Unmet psychological, social, and economic needs of persons with cancer in Pennsylvania. *Cancer*, 1986; **58**:2355–61.
3. Vachon MLS, Conway B, Lancee WJ, Adair WK. *Report on the Needs of Persons Living with Cancer in Prince Edward Island*. Toronto: Canadian Cancer Society, 1989.
4. Vachon MLS, Lancee WJ, Conway B, Adair WK. *Final Report on the Needs of Persons Living with Cancer in Manitoba*. Toronto: Canadian Cancer Society, 1990.
5. Vachon MLS, Lancee WJ, Ghadirian P, Adair WK, Conway B. *Final Report on the Needs of Persons Living with Cancer in Quebec*. Toronto: Canadian Cancer Society, 1991.
6. Linn MW, Linn BS, Harris R. Effects of counseling for late stage cancer patients. *Cancer*, 1982; **49**:1048–55.
7. Haggmark C, Theorell T, Ek B. Coping and social activity patterns among relatives of cancer patients. *Social Science and Medicine*, 1987; **25**:1021–5.
8. Vachon MLS, Stylianos SK. The role of social support in bereavement. *Journal of Social Issues*, 1988; **44**:175–90.
9. Steele LL. The death surround: factors influencing the grief experience of survivors. *Oncology Nursing Forum*, 1990; **17**:235–41.
10. Sweeting HN, Gilhooly MLM. Anticipatory grief: a review. *Social Science and Medicine*, 1990; **30**:1073–80.
11. Rolland JS. Anticipatory loss: a family systems developmental framework. *Family Process*, 1990; **29**:229–44.
12. Levy LH. Anticipatory grief: its measurement and proposed reconceptualization. *Hospice Journal*, 1991; **7**(4):1–28.
13. Elison JCK. *Reactions to Spousal Death from Cancer*. Unpublished Doctoral Dissertation, College of William and Mary, Williamsburg, VA, 1991.
14. Sachs O. *An Anthropologist on Mars*. New York: Knopf, 1995.
15. Vachon, MLS. Psychosocial variables: cancer morbidity and mortality. In Corless I, Germino B, Pittman-Lindeman M, eds. *A Challenge for Living: Death, Dying and Bereavement*. Boston, MA: Jones and Bartlett, 1994:135–55.
16. Vachon MLS, Freedman K, Formo A, Rogers J, Lyall WAL, Freeman SJJ. The final illness in cancer: the widow's perspective. *Canadian Medical Association Journal*, 1977; **117**:1151–4.
17. Ferris FD, Flannery JS, McNeal HB, Morissette MR (eds.). *A Compre-*

hensive Guide for the Care of Persons with HIV Disease. Toronto:Mount Sinai Hospital and Casey House Hospice, 1995.

18. Weissmann DE, O'Donnell J, Brady A. A cry from the fringe. *Journal of Clinical Oncology,* 1993; **11**:1006.
19. Kearsley JH. Wanted: guidelines for 'palliative' anti-cancer drug use. *Medical Journal of Australia*, 1994; **160**:723–5.
20. Lowenthal RA. A time of change in medical oncology. *Medical Journal of Australia*, 1992; **157**:28–30.
21. Porzsolt F, Tannock I. Goals of palliative cancer therapy. *Journal of Clinical Oncology,* 1993;**11**:378–81.
22. Quill TE. *Death and Dignity: Making Choices and Taking Charge.* New York: WW Norton, 1993.
23. Derogatis LR, *et al.* The prevalence of psychiatric disorders among cancer patients. *Journal of the American Medical Association,* 1983; **249**:751–7.
24. Lancee WJ, Vachon MLS, Ghadirian P, Adair W, Conway B, Dryer D. The impact of pain and impaired role performance on distress in persons with cancer. *Canadian Psychiatric Association Journal*, 1994; **39**(10):617–22.
25. Kaasa S, Malt U, Hagen S, Wist E, Moum T, Kvikstad A. Psychological distress in cancer patients with advanced disease. *Radiotherapy and Oncology,* 1993; **27**:193–7.
26. Miller RD, Walsh D. Psychosocial aspects of palliative care in advanced cancer. *Journal of Pain and Symptom Management*, 1991; **6**:24–9.
27. McCartney CF, *et al.* Effect of psychiatric liason program on consultation rates and on detection of minor psychiatric disorders in cancer patients. *American Journal of Psychiatry,* 1989; **7**:898–901.
28. Pinder KL, Ramirez AJ, Black ME, Richards MA, Gregory WM, Rubens RD. Psychiatric disorder in patients with advanced breast cancer: prevalence and associated factors. *European Journal of Oncology,* 1993; **29A**:524–7.
29. Goldberg D. *Manual of the General Health Questionnaire*: Windsor, Ontario: NFER-Nelson, 1978.
30. Vachon MLS, Fitch M, Greenberg M, Franssen E. *The Needs of Cancer Patients and Their Families Attending Toronto-Sunnybrook Regional Cancer Centre*, in preparation, 1996.
31. Lancee WJ, Vachon MLS. Risk factors and mediators of symptoms of distress in persons with cancer. *Psychosomatic Medicine*, 1995; **57**:57–96:80 (abstract).
32. Kathol RG, Mutgi A, Williams J, Clamon G, Noyes R. Diagnosis of major depression in cancer patients according to four sets of criteria. *American Journal of Psychiatry,* 1990; **147**:1021–4.
33. Chochinov HM, Wilson KG, Enns M, Lander M. Prevalence of depression in the terminally ill: effects of diagnostic criteria and symptom threshold judgements. *American Journal of Psychiatry,* 1994; **151**:537–40.
34. Noyes R, *et al.* Distress associated with cancer as measured by the illness distress scale. *Psychosomatics*, 1990; **31**:321–30.
35. Carroll BT, Kathol RG, Noyes R, Wald TG, Clamon GH. Screening for depression and anxiety in cancer patients using the hospital anxiety and depression scale. *General Hospital Psychiatry,* 1993; **15**:69–74.
36. Given CW, Stommel M, Given B, Osuch J, Kurtz ME, Kurtz JC. The influence of cancer patients' symptoms and functional states on patients' depression and family caregivers' reaction and depression. *Health Psychology,* 1993; **12**:277–85.
37. Spiegel D, Sands S, Koopman C. Pain and depression in patients with cancer. *Cancer,* 1994; **74**:2570–8.
38. Hughson AVM, Cooper AF, McArdles CS, Smith DC. Psychological consequences of mastectomy: levels of morbidity and associated factors. *Journal of Psychosomatic Research*, 1988; **32**:383–91.
39. Goldberg RJ, Cullan LO. Depression in geriatric cancer patients: guide to assessment and treatment. *Hospice Journal*, 1986; **2**:79–98.
40. Hinton J. Comparison of places and policies for terminal care. *Lancet,* 1979; **6 January**:29–32.
41. Mor V. Assessing patient outcomes in hospice: what to measure. *Hospice Journal,* 1986; **2**:17–35.
42. Brown JH, Henteleff P, Barakat S, Rowe CJ. Is it normal for terminally ill patients to desire death? *American Journal of Psychiatry,* 1986; **143**:208–11.
43. Massie MJ. Depression. In: Holland JC, Rowland JH, eds. *Handbook of Psychooncology.* New York: Oxford University Press, 1989:283–90.
44. Rodin G, Voshart K. Depressive symptoms and functional impairment in the medically ill. *General Hospital Psychiatry,* 1987; **9**:251–8.
45. Stolbach LL, Brandt UC. Psychosocial factors in the development and progression of breast cancer. In: Cooper CL, ed. *Stress and Breast Cancer.* Chichester: Wiley, 1988:3–24.
46. Evans E. *A Psychological Study of Cancer.* New York: Dodd-Mead, 1926.
47. LeShan L. Psychological states as factors in the development of malignant disease: a critical review. *Journal of the National Cancer Institute,* 1959; **22**:1–18.
48. LeShan L. An emotional life history pattern associated with neoplastic disease. *Annals of the New York Academy of Sciences*, 1966; **125**:780–93.
49. LeShan L, Worthington RE. Personality as a factor in the pathogenesis of cancer: a review of the literature. *British Journal of Medical Psychology,* 1956; **29**:49–56.
50. Blumberg EM, West PM, Ellis FW. A possible relationship between psychological factors and human cancer. *Psychosomatic Medicine,* 1956; **16**:277–86.
51. Bacon CL, Renneker R, Cutler M. A psychosomatic survey of cancer of the breast. *Psychosomatic Medicine,* 1952; **14**:453–60.
52. Greer S, Morris T. Psychological attributes of women who develop breast cancer: a controlled study. *Journal of Psychosomatic Research*, 1975; **19**:147–53.
53. Cassileth BR, Lusk EJ, Miller DS, Brown LL, Miller C. Psychosocial correlates of survival in advanced malignant disease. *New England Journal of Medicine*, 1985; **312**:1551–5.
54. Derogatis LR, Abeloff MD, Melisaratos N. Psychological coping mechanisms and survival time in metastatic breast cancer. *Journal of the American Medical Association*, 1979; **242**:1504–8.
55. Temoshok L. (1987). Personality, coping style, emotion and cancer: towards an integrative model. *Imperial Cancer Research Fund 1987,* 1987; **6**:545–567.
56. Weisman AD, Worden JW. Psychosocial analysis of cancer deaths. *Omega,* 1975; **6**:61–75.
57. Worden JW, Johnston LC, Harrison RH. Survival quotient as a method for investigating psychosocial aspects of cancer survival. *Psychological Reports,* 1974; **35**:719–26.
58. Greer S, Watson M. Towards a psychobiological model of cancer: psychological considerations. *Social Science and Medicine,* 1985; **20**:773–7.
59. Greer S, Morris T, Pettingale KW. Psychological response to breast cancer: effect on outcome. *Lancet*, 1979; **2**:785–7.
60. Spiegel D. *Living Beyond Limits.* New York: Fawcett Columbine, 1993.
61. Jamison RN, Burish TG, Walston KA. Psychogenic factors in predicting survival of breast cancer patients. *Journal of Clinical Oncology,* 1987; **5**:768–92.
62. Kneier AW, Temoshok L. Repressive coping reactions in patients with malignant melanoma as compared to cardiovascular disease patients. *Journal of Psychosomatic Research*, 1984; **28**:145–55.
63. Morris TA. Type C for cancer: low trait anxiety and the pathogenesis of breast cancer. *Cancer Detection and Prevention*, 1980; **3**:102.
64. Pettingale KW. Towards a psychobiological model of cancer: biological considerations. *Social Science in Medicine*, 1985; **20**:779–87.
65. Cunningham AJ. From neglect to support to coping: the evolution of psychosocial intervention for cancer patients. In: Cooper CL, ed. *Stress and Breast Cancer.* Chichester: Wiley, 1988:135–54.
66. Cunningham AJ *et al.* A group psychoeducational program to help cancer patients cope with and combat their disease. *Advances,* 1991; **7**:41–56.
67. Grossarth-Maticek R, Schmidt P, Vetter H, Arndt, S. Psychotherapy research in oncology. In: Steptoe A, Matthews A, eds. *Health Care and Human Behaviour.* London: Academic Press, 1984:325–41.
68. Siegel BS. *Love, Medicine and Miracles.* New York: Harper and Row, 1988.
69. Simonton OC, Simonton SM, Creighton JL. *Getting Well Again.* New York: Bantam, 1978.

70. Spiegel D, Bloom JR, Kraemer HC, Gottheil E. Effect of psychosocial treatment on survival of patients with metastatic breast cancer. *Lancet*, 1989; **14 October**:888–91.
71. Fawzy FI, *et al.* Malignant melanoma: effects of an early structured psychiatric intervention, coping, and affective state on recurrence and survival six years later. *Archives of General Psychiatry*, 1993; **50**:681–689.
72. Fawzy FI, Fawzy NW. A structured psychoeducational intervention for cancer patients. *General Hospital Psychiatry*, 1994; **16**:149–92.
73. Morgenstern H, Gellert GA, Walter D, Ostfeld AM, Siegel BS. The impact of a psychosocial support program on survival with breast cancer: the importance of selection bias in program evaluation. *Journal of Chronic Diseases*, 1984; **37**:273–82.
74. Anderson BL, Kiecolt-Glaser JK, Glaser R. A biobehavioral model of cancer stress and disease course. *American Psychologist*, 1994; **49**:389–404.
75. Hu D, Silberfarb PM. Psychological factors: do they influence breast cancer? In: Cooper CL, ed. *Stress and Breast Cancer*. Chichester: Wiley, 1988:27–62.
76. Anonymous. Prostate cancer: should you get a PSA test? *University of California Berkeley Wellness Letter*, 1995; **11**:10.
77. Baltrusch HF, Waltz ME. Early family attitudes and the stress process—a life-span and personological model of host–tumour relationships: biopsychosocial research on cancer and stress in Central Europe. In: Day SB, ed. *Cancer, Stress and Death*. 2nd edn. New York: Plenum, 1986:241–83.
78. Vachon MLS. Unresolved grief in persons with cancer referred for psychotherapy. *Psychiatric Clinics of North America*, 1987; **10**:467–86.
79. Thomas CB, Duszynski K, Schaffer J. Family attitudes reported in youth as potential predictors of cancer. *Psychosomatic Medicine*, 1979; **41**:287–302.
80. Thomas CB, Greenstreet RL. Psychobiological characteristics in youth as predictors of five disease states: suicide, mental illness, hypertension, coronary heart disease and tumour. *Johns Hopkins Medical Journal*, 1973; **132**:16–43.
81. Vachon MLS. Psychotherapy and the person with cancer: one nurse's experience. *Oncology Nursing Forum*, 1985;**12**:33–40.
82. Osterweis M, Solomon F, Green M. *Bereavement: Reactions, Consequences and Care*. Washington, DC: National Academy Press, 1984.
83. Temoshok L, Fox BH. Coping styles and other psychosocial factors related to medical status and to prognosis in patients with cutaneous malignant melanoma. In: Fox BH, Newberry BH, eds. *Impact of Psychoendocrine Systems in Cancer and Immunity*, Toronto: Hogrefe, 1984:86–146.
84. Temoshok L, Heller BW. On comparing apples, oranges and fruit salad: a methodological overview of medical outcome studies in psychosocial oncology. In: Cooper CL, ed. *Psychosocial Stress and Cancer*. Chichester: Wiley, 1984:231–60.
85. Morris T, Greer S. A 'Type C' for cancer? Low trait anxiety in the pathogenesis of breast cancer (abstract). *Cancer Detection and Prevention* 1980;**3**:102.
86. Greer S, Watson M. Towards a psychobiological model of cancer: psychological considerations. *Social Science and Medicine*, 1985; **20**:773–7.
87. Levy SM, Wise BD. Psychosocial risk factors and cancer progression. In: Cooper CL, ed. *Stress and Breast Cancer*. Chichester: Wiley, 1988:77–96.
88. Ramirez AJ, Craig TK, Watson JP, Fentiman IS, North WR, Rubens RD. Stress and relapse of breast cancer. *British Medical Journal*, 1989; **298**:291–3.
89. Greer S, Morris T, Pettingale KW, Hybittle JL. Psychological response to breast cancer and 15-year outcome. *Lancet*, 1990; **355**:49–50.
90. Marshall JR, Funch DP. Social environment and breast cancer: a cohort analysis of patient survival. *Cancer*, 1983; **52**:1546–50.
91. Goodwin JS, Hunt WC, Key CR, Samet JM. The effect of marital status on stage, treatment, and survival of cancer patients. *Journal of the American Medical Association*, 1987; **258**:3125–30.
92. Blumenthal SJ, Matthews K, Weiss SM. *New Research Findings in Behavioral Medicine: Proceedings of a National Conference*.Washigton, DC: National Institutes of Health, 1994.
93. Chorot P, Sandin B. Life events and stress reactivity as predictors of cancer, coronary heart disease and anxiety disorders. *International Journal of Psychosomatics*, 1994; **41**(1–4):34–40.
94. Sontag S. *Illness As Metaphor*. New York: Farrar, Strauss and Giroux, 1977.
95. Stein S, Linn MW, Stein EM. Psychological correlates of survival in nursing home cancer patients. *Gerontologist*, 1989; **29**:224–8.
96. Stein S, Linn MW, Stein EM. Patients' anticipation of stress in nursing home care. *Gerontologist*, 1985; **25**:88–94.
97. Ganz PA, Lee JJ, Siau J. Quality of life assessment: an independent prognostic variable for survival in lung cancer. *Cancer*, 1991; **67**:3131–5.
98. Coates A, *et al.* Improving the quality of life during chemotherapy for advanced breast cancer. *New England Journal of Medicine*, 1987; **317**:1490–5.
99. Barinaga M. Can psychotherapy delay cancer deaths? *Science*, 1989; **246**:448–9.
100. Fawzy FI, Cousins N, Fawzy NW, Kemeny ME, Elashf R, Morton D. A structured psychiatric intervention for cancer patients: I changes over time in methods coping and affective disturbance. *Archives of General Psychiatry*, 1990; **47**:720–5.
101. Fawzy FI, *et al.* A structured psychiatric intervention for cancer patients: II , changes over time in immunologic measures. *Archives of General Psychiatry*, 1990; **47**:729–35.
102. *Canada Year Book 1990*. Ottawa: Ministry of Regional Industrial Expansion.
103. Statistics Canada, *1991 Census*, Part A93337 and 93338. Ottawa: Statistics Canada, 1992.
104. Wingo PA, Tong T, Bolden S. Cancer statistics, 1995. *CA: Cancer Journal for Clinicians*, 1995; **45**:8–30.
105. Pearce NE, Howard JK. Occupation, social class and male cancer mortality in New Zealand 1974–1978. *International Journal of Epidemiology*, 1986; **15**:456–62.
106. Levi F, Negri E, La Vecchia C, Cong Te V. Socioeconomic groups and cancer risk at death in the Swiss Canton at Vaud. *International Journal of Epidemiology*, 1988;**17**: 711–17.
107. *Canadian Cancer Statistics 1990*. Ottawa: Health and Welfare Canada, 1990.
108. Barker DJP, Coggon D, Osmond C, Wickham C. Poor housing in childhood and high rates of stomach cancer in England and Wales. *British Journal of Cancer*, 1990; **61**:575–8.
109. Panel on Cancer and the Disadvantaged. *Inequalities in Cancer Control in Canada*. Toronto: Canadian Cancer Society, 1991.
110. D'Arcy C. Prevalence and correlates of nonpsychotic psychiatric symptoms in the general population. *Canadian Journal of Psychiatry*, 1982;**27**:316–24.
111. Addington-Hall JM, MacDonald LD, Anderson HR, Chamberlain J, Freeling P, Bland JMM. Randomized controlled trial of effects of coordinating care for terminally ill cancer patients. *British Medical Journal*, 1992; **305**:1317–22.
112. Coyle N, Adelhardt J, Foley KM, Portenoy RK. Character of terminal illness in the advanced cancer patient: pain and other symptoms during the last four weeks of life. *Journal of Pain and Symptom Management*, 1990; **5**(2):83–93.
113. Hinton J. Can home care maintain an acceptable quality of life for patients with terminal cancer and their relatives? *Palliative Medicine*, 1994; **8**:183–96.
114. Fife BL. The conceptualization of meaning in illness. *Social Science and Medicine*, 1994: **38**:309–16.
115. Barkwell DP. Ascribed meaning: a critical factor in coping and pain attenuation in patients with cancer-related pain. *Journal of Palliative Care*, 1991; **7**(3):5–14.
116. Hinton J. Which patients with terminal cancer are admitted from home care? *Palliative Medicine*, 1994; **8**:197–210.
117. Weisman A. *Coping with Cancer*. New York: McGraw-Hill, 1979.

118. Wool MS. Understanding denial in cancer patients. *Advances in Psychosomatic Medicine*, 1988; **18**:37–53.
119. Glaser BG, Strauss AL. *Awareness of Dying*. Chicago, IL: Aldine, 1965.
120. Freud A. *The Ego and the Mechanisms of Defence*. London: Hogarth, 1966.
121. Stedeford A. *Facing Death: Patients, Families and Professionals*. London: Heinemann Medical, 1984.
122. Shepherd R. *Living with Terminal Cancer*. Toronto: Maclean Hunter, 1991.
123. Weisman AD. Vulnerability and the psychological disturbances of cancer patients. *Psychosomatics*, 1989; **30**:80–5.
124. Heim E. Coping and adaptation in cancer. In: Cooper CL, Watson M, eds. *Cancer and Stress: Psychological, Biological and Coping Studies*. New York: Wiley, 1991:197–235.
125. Houts PS *et al.* Unmet needs of persons with cancer in Pennsylvania during the period of terminal care. *Cancer*, 1988; **62**:627–34.
126. Holland JC. Progress in the psychosocial management of cancer. *Proceedings of the 4th National Conference on Human Values and Cancer*. New York: American Cancer Society, 1984:7–11.
127. Razavi D, Stiefel F. Common psychiatric disorders in cancer patients. 1.Adjustment disorders and depressive disorders. *Supportive Care in Cancer*, 1994; **2**:223–32.
128. Stiefel F, Volkenandt M, Breitbart W. Suizid und Krebserkrankung. *Schweizerische Medizinische Wochenschrift*, 1989; **119**:891–5.
129. Stiefel F, Kornblith A, Holland JH. Changes in the prescription patterns of psychotropic drugs for cancer patients during a 10-year period. *Cancer*, 1990; **65**:1048–53.
130. Horowitz MJ, Wilner N, Marmar C, Krupick J. Pathological grief and the activation of latent self-images. *American Journal of Psychiatry*, 1980; **137**:1157–62.
131. Wellisch DK, Wolcott DL, Pasnau RO, Fawzy FI, Landsverk J. An evaluation of the psychosocial problems of the homebound cancer patient: relationship of patient adjustment to family problems. *Journal of Psychosocial Oncology*, 1989; **7**:55–76.
132. McDaniel JS, Musselman DL, Porter MR, Reed DA, Nemeroff CB. Depression in patients with cancer: diagnosis, biology, and treatment. *Archives of General Psychiatry*, 1995; **52**:89–99.
133. Mor V. Cancer patients' quality of life over the disease course: lessons from the real world. *Journal of Chronic Diseases*, 1987; **40**:535–44.
134. American Psychiatric Association. *Quick Reference to the Diagnostic Criteria from DSM-IV*. Washington, DC: American Psychiatric Association, 1994.
135. Mermelstein HT, Lesko L. Depression in patients with cancer. *Psycho-Oncology*, 1992; **1**:199–215.
136. Vachon MLS. Counselling and psychotherapy in palliative/hospice care: a review. *Palliative Medicine*, 1988; **2**:36–50.
137. Godding PR, McAnulty RD, Wittrock DA, Britt DM, Khansur T. Predictors of depression among male cancer patients. *Journal of Nervous and Mental Disease*, 1995; **183**:95–8.
138. Baile WF, Gibertini M, Scott L, Endicott J. Depression and tumor stage in cancer of the head and neck. *Psycho-Oncology*, 1992; **1**:15–24.
139. Holland JC, *et al.* Comparative disturbance in patients with pancreatic and gastric cancer, *American Journal of Psychiatry*, 1986; **143**:982–6.
140. Pomara NP, Gershon S. Treatment-resistant depression in an elderly patient with pancreatic carcinoma. *Journal of Clinical Psychiatry*, 1984; **45**:439–40.
141. Leibenluft E, Goldberg RL. The suicidal, terminally ill patient with depression. *Psychosomatics*, 1988; **4**:386–97.
142. Allebeck P, Boland C, Ringback G. Increased suicide rate in cancer patients: a cohort study based on the Swedish Cancer-Environment Register. *Journal of Clinical Epidemiology*, 1989; **42**:611–16.
143. Massie MJ, Gagnon P, Holland J. Depression and suicide in patients with cancer. *Journal of Pain and Symptom Management*, 1994; **9**:325–40.
144. Chochinov HM, *et al.* Desire for death in the terminally ill. *American Journal of Psychiatry*, 1995; **152**: 1185–91.
145. Cassileth BR *et al.* Concordance of depression and anxiety in patients with cancer. *Psychological Reports*, 1984; **54**:588–90.
146. Stiefel F, Razavi D. Common psychiatric disorders in cancer patients. II Anxiety and acute confusional states. *Supportive Care in Cancer*, 1994; **2**:233–7.
147. Spiegel D. Health caring: psychosocial support for patients with cancer. *Cancer*, 1994; **74**(Supplement):1453–7.
148. Snaith RP. The concepts and assessment of depression in oncology. *Journal of Psychosocial Oncology*, 1987; **5**:133–9.
149. Silberfarb PM. *Psychiatric Treatment of the Patient during Cancer Treatment. Psychosocial Issues and Cancer*. New York: American Cancer Society, 1988:5–9.
150. Northouse PG, Northouse LL. Communication and cancer: issues confronting patients, health professionals, and family members. *Journal of Psychosocial Oncology*, 1987; **5**:17–46.
151. Cassileth BR *et al.* Survival and quality of life among patients receiving unproven as compared with conventional cancer therapy. *New England Journal of Medicine*, 1991; **324**:1180–5.
152. Silver RL, Wortman CB. Coping with undesirable life events. In: Garber J, Seligman M, eds. *Human Helplessness*. New York: Academic Press, 1980;279–375.
153. Blanchard CG, Labrecque MS, Ruckdeschel JC, Blanchard EB. Information and decision-making preferences of hospitalized adult cancer patients. *Social Science and Medicine*, 1988; **11**:1139–45.
154. Newall DJ, Gadd EM, Priestman TJ. Presentation of information to cancer patients: a comparison of two centres in the UK and USA. *British Journal of Medical Psychology*, 1987; **60**:127–31.
155. Gilhooly MLM, Berkeley JS, McCann K, Gibling F, Murray K. Truth telling with dying cancer patients. *Palliative Medicine*, 1988; **2**:64–71.
156. Lewis FM, Haberman MR, Wallhagen MI. How adults with late stage cancer experience personal control. *Jounal of Psychosocial Oncology*, 1986; **4**:27–42.
157. Cassileth BR, Zupkis RV, Sutton-Smith K, March V. Information and participation preferences among cancer patients. *Annals of Internal Medicine*, 1980; **92**:832–6.
158. Faulkner A, Maguire P, Regnard C. Breaking bad news. *Palliative Medicine*, 1994; 8:145–51.
159. Shinn M, Lehmann S, Wong NW. Social interaction and social support. *Journal of Social Issues*, 1984; **40**:55–76.
160. Heller K, Swindle RW. Social networks, perceived social support, and coping with stress. In: Heller K, Swindle R, eds. *Preventive Psychology: Theory, Research and Practice*. New York: Pergamon Press, 1983:87–103.
161. House JS. *Work, Stress and Social Support*. Reading, MA: Addison-Wesley, 1981.
162. Dunkel-Schetter C. Social support and cancer: findigs based on patient interviews and their implications. *Journal of Social Issues*, 1984; **40**:77–98.
163. Kaczorowski JM. Spiritual well-being and anxiety in adults diagnosed with cancer. *Hospice Journal*, 1989; **5**:105–16.
164. McCrae RR. Situational determinants of coping responses: loss, threat, and challenge. *Journal of Personality and Social Psychology*, 1984; **46**:919–28.
165. Cassel E. The nature of suffering and the goals of medicine. *New England Journal of Medicine*, 1982; **306**:639–45.
166. Cassel EJ. Recognizing suffering. *Hastings Centre Report*, 1991; **21**:24–31.

14.2 The family

Betty R. Ferrell

Introduction

Definition of the family

Cancer has often been described as a family illness and recognized for the impact on all of the individuals surrounding the one family member with the cancer diagnosis. Changing demographics of our society and an aggressive shift of health care into the living room makes the role of family caregivers in chronic and terminal illness even more significant. While the family was traditionally defined as an individual of blood relationship, a broad definition of family is most appropriate and best defined as those individuals considered as family by the patient. Studies in oncology related to family caregiving have generally found that approximately 70 per cent of primary family caregivers are spouses, approximately 20 per cent are children (of which daughters or daughters-in-law are most predominant), and approximately 10 per cent are friends or more distant relatives.[1,2] A review of the literature on the topic of family and palliative care reveals that most of this research has focused on pain management with the second predominant area identified as family bereavement.

While family caregivers confront many patient symptoms, the experience of pain perhaps serves as a model case for exploring the differences between the individual patient's experience as compared to that of the family caregiver. Fig. 1 identifies the experience of pain from the patient's perspective beginning with nociception or the cause of the pain. However, pain is greatly influenced by many factors including prior painful experiences, meaning of pain, culture, and other factors. Pain is an extremely subjective experience and, thus, it is expressed in not only intensity, or the amount of pain, but also in the degree of distress from the pain. This perception results, then, in the global experience of physical pain, associated symptoms and emotions, and the dimension of suffering.

Similarly, Fig. 2 describes the family caregiver's experience of pain as a model symptom of advanced illness. Family caregivers' experience of pain begins with their perceptions of the patient's suffering. However, family caregivers' perspectives of pain vary dramatically and are influenced by many factors including their own personal encounters with pain, the relationship to the patient, culture, and interpretation of cause and meaning. The burden of care giving and observing a family member's pain can lead to severe emotional distress in the caregiver.

These models illustrate the similarities in the shared experience of pain but also the unique experience of the individual with advanced illness versus those who experience it from their vision as caregivers. It is often stated that while the patient experiences greater physical symptoms, family caregivers often experience a greater degree of suffering as they observe the patient.[3,4] Table 1 includes excerpts from some of our prior research related to family caregivers' perceptions of pain. The table includes descriptions by family caregivers of the symptom of pain. Included are family perceptions of pain as an anatomic entity as well as the communication issues that result when patients or families hide the reality of pain to avoid distress. Also included are family caregiver comments regarding the fear and suffering associated with anticipation of future pain and the overwhelming nature of assuming the care of a loved one in pain.[3,4] These same models could be applied to many other patient symptoms to illustrate the shared experiences between patient and family.

Family care giving takes on distinct meaning in situations such as AIDS in which care is shifted to non-blood relatives and often to other individuals experiencing the same illness. Future trends in health care will also shift care from professionals to unlicensed caregivers as our society becomes increasingly dependent upon significant others such as an elderly spouse, whose ability to provide the intensive care of advanced disease is limited.[5,6] Appreciation for the caregivers' perspective is critical to the care of the patient. Decades of work in hospice and palliative care have demonstrated

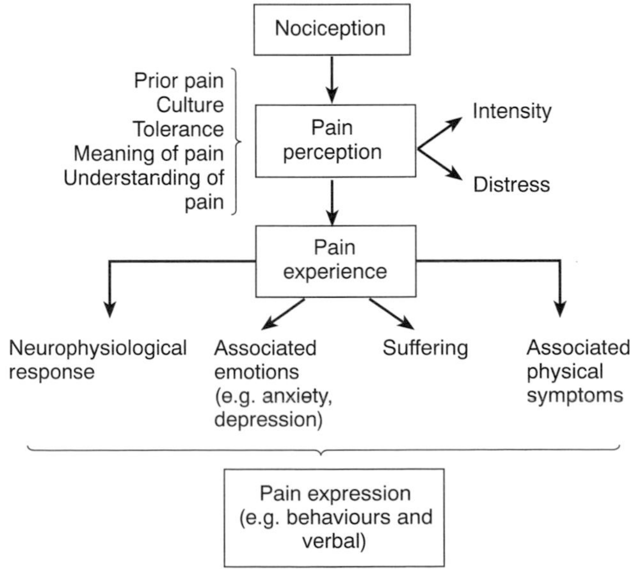

Fig. 1 Patient's experience of pain.[3]

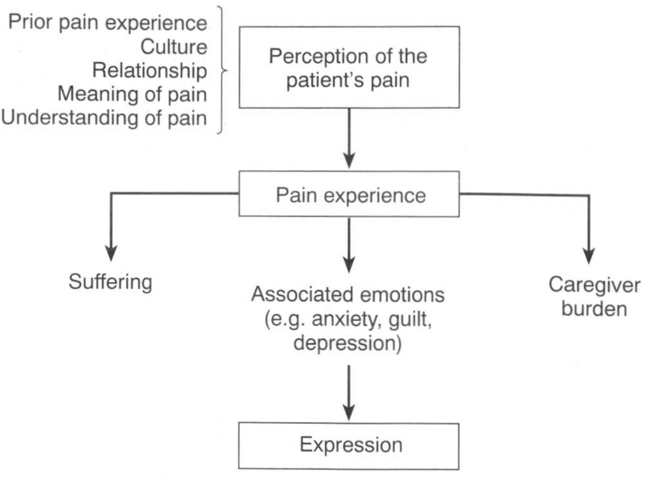

Fig. 2 Caregiver's experience of pain.[3]

that support of family caregivers is an essential feature of quality care for patients with chronic advanced illness.

Terminal illness as a family experience

Families are profoundly influenced by acute and chronic illness. Day-to-day family activities, roles and relationships, and the meaning of life itself becomes altered once life shifts from health to illness. Terminal illness adds an entire dimension, even for those who have faced years or decades of chronic illness. During terminal illness, patients and families struggle not only with the present and all that is included with terminal illness care but with the overwhelming issues associated with death and transcendence beyond death.[7-10]

In a recent study of parents of children with cancer, a mother described having a child diagnosed with cancer as an experience in which the family actually came closer together. Grandparents became supportive in the care of the child. The parents worked together to provide the most comfort to the child and siblings also became co-operative and concerned about their brother with cancer. However, the mother described the experience of having the child suffering pain by saying, 'It was as if someone threw a hand grenade in our living room'.[11] This mother described how having a child with uncontrolled symptoms created an opposite environment in which the grandparents became critical of the parents' care and the parents' became critical of each other. The siblings were frightened of their brother's pain and thus isolated themselves from him.

This is an excellent example of how palliative care has the ability to prevent family crisis and create cohesion in the light of, even, a life-threatening illness. Family intervention is needed to confront the many physical and emotional issues associated with palliative care. This intervention is dependent upon assessment of family functioning and use of an interdisciplinary team to meet the diverse needs of the family.

Role of family caregivers in palliative care

In a review of 7657 citations in *Index Medicus* during 1992 which included 'pain' as a title or index term, only 314 citations (4 per cent) included 'family', 'home', or 'caregivers' as indexing terms. Thus, while the focus on pain has increased in professional literature, many areas, such as family perspectives of pain, remain in need of attention in both clinical care and research.[12] Similar findings are apparent in other topics of palliative care, as descriptive studies as well as interventions have focused on the patient rather than on the family as a unit of care.

Family caregivers are involved with not only the emotional experiences and perceptions of illness but largely involved in the

Table 1 Families' descriptions of pain

Anatomic

'She has pain throughout her sternum—pressure pain; pain in the shoulder blades. Her back is essentially broken—spinal compression.'

'It's in different spots at different times. It travels around and is not so much where the mets to hip was found but is now in the ribs.'

Hidden pain

'A lot of the time I can sense what she is going through, but she doesn't want to burden others, so she minimizes.'

'She pretends she doesn't have any, but when it really gets bad she says, "I just can't stand it." She doesn't want anyone to know it hurts, but since her hospitalization we've made a pact that she'll tell me when she's hurting. She doesn't express her feelings loudly, so when she said she was hurting, you knew it was bad.'

Family fear and suffering

'He was in very severe pain before his surgery, and I'm just waiting for it to start again. I'm so afraid.'

'It's scary. It came on so fast, and now it seems to be constant. Sometimes it's worse than others, but it always seems to be there.'

'She's hurting, and it makes me cry. It's like a knife twisting in her.'

'It was awful watching him being in pain, knowing surely there was something to help him.'

'Intense, terrible—I can't take it any more. The last couple of weeks I thought she was gone because of the pain.'

'It is very, very difficult. It is so hard to watch someone you love suffer.'

'It is the closest thing to hell I can imagine.'

'I don't think I can find the words. Only a mother that has gone through it can describe it.'

'It was awful. It was the most awful thing that you can imagine.'

Overwhelming/unendurable pain

'Horrible pain. Burning with fever inside. Aching, like turning a hot knife. Horrible.'

'It's an unbearable pain. He said he just couldn't take it.'

'Completely overwhelming. Radiates throughout her body, causing tremors. Sharp pain.'

'Really painful; never really goes away. So painful—swollen tongue with sores down his neck. He says it's worse than childbirth.'

'A burning sensation like a branding iron. Within the last month, she has been in agonizing pain, with wild eyes. She felt like she was being stabbed with a knife. She felt like her insides were blowing up.'

'The pain was unbearable, like a bulldozer was going all through her.'

'It is exasperating. She shouts. It is terrrible, sharp pain.'

direct care provided to patients. Our research in the area of family caregivers' involvement in pain management has revealed the direct acts of care giving in pain management as well as the intense ethical dilemmas faced by family caregivers. This research revealed that family caregivers were involved with decisions regarding what medication to take, for example whether they should give only a mild analgesic such as codeine rather than giving morphine.[3] Family caregivers often decided when to give medications and in fact often decided to withhold medications ordered on a 3 to 4 h basis until approximately 5 or 6 h duration.

We have also found that family caregivers are commonly involved in 'night duty,' assuming total care; making decisions at night for patients who perhaps are more independent during the day hours. The family's decisions in pain management seem to range from giving pain medications aggressively (while often being quite concerned about their decisions in medicating) to restricting and withholding medications because of concern that they would be criticized for over-medicating the patient or using too much of the restricted medications.

Barriers to effective symptom management by family caregivers

Frequently cited barriers to effective pain management by family caregivers of patients with cancer include fear of respiratory depression, fear of drug tolerance, fear of drug addiction, and lack of knowledge regarding chronic pain. Investigators have documented that family members play an important role in pain management.[2,13–15] This is increasingly true as family members assume the role of caregivers for patients in the home. Advances in pain technology now require that families manage complex medication regimens, parenteral infusion devices, and even parenteral and intraspinal medications in the home.[12,16–18] Because patients are increasingly being cared for at home, family members are assuming the responsibility for pain relief despite the frequent need to understand basic pain management principles. Family members often deny that the patient is in pain to avoid the realization that the disease is progressing.[19–23]

The caregiver's burden can be described as the emotional and physical demands and responsibilities of one's illness that are placed on family members, friends, or other individuals involved with the patient outside of the health-care system. A study by Grobe, Ilstrup, and Ahmann[22] revealed that family members of terminally ill patients with cancer needed to learn new skills such as assisting with ambulation, comfort care, and pain management in order to provide effective care in the home. These family members reported that specific caregiving skills were not taught by their health-care providers, and they were left with a 'trial and error' method of skill acquisition. The authors concluded that family members may be more receptive to learning new skills from health-care providers while the patient was in the home setting.

Tringali[24] reinforced this conclusion by observing family members of patients with cancer at three different phases of illness including initial treatment, recurrent disease, and follow-up treatment. Family caregivers were evaluated regarding their cognitive, emotional, and physical needs. Regardless of the phase of illness, informational needs were identified as most important. The results suggest that the provision of information prepares family members to support the patient, reinforces the treatment goals, and assists in managing the side-effects of therapy and disease. It is apparent from the reports of these investigators,[22,24] and others,[5,6,25–30] that the needs of family members are not being met, and that understanding needs and assisting families in meeting those needs will contribute to improved care (see Section 16).

Our study of 'Family factors influencing pain management'[1] identified the critical role of family caregivers in pain management. On a scale of 0 = none to 100 = severe, caregivers' mean rating of the patients' pain was 70 while the patients themselves rated the pain at a mean of 45. Caregivers rated their distress with the pain on the same scale at 78. The data revealed mood disruption for caregivers as most severe in the areas of anxiety, depression, and fatigue. Caregivers reported extreme fears of the patient becoming addicted to pain medications and they feared respiratory depression and drug tolerance. Caregivers expressed feelings of helplessness in being unable to provide the patient comfort. The caregivers also had virtually no instruction in the use of non-pharmacological pain management.

Ethical dilemmas encountered by family caregivers

An additional area of study is the ethical dilemmas associated with palliative care. A recent study identified both decisions and conflicts for patients, primary family caregivers, and nurses, as well as this triad's search for the meaning of the pain experience. The impact of major decisions and conflicts encountered while managing pain were described by each group of the triad. Patients reported decisions and conflicts related to: medications; the future in relation to pain, death, suicide, or euthanasia; and spiritual issues. Family caregivers also reported: decisions and conflicts related to medications as well as balancing dichotomies related to control, personal needs, and accepting imminent death; decisions and conflicts related to treatments and interventions; spiritual and existential conflicts; and conflicts related to assessment (see Section 3).[19,20]

There are many decisions and conflicts encountered by families beyond pain management including: those related to other medications, physician relations, patient assessment, personal decisions, religious issues, balancing career and personal life, professional limitations, and nutrition and hydration.[19,20]

Studies to date have identified the important role of family caregivers and their educational needs in assuming care for the person with cancer. Research has also begun to describe conflicts and burdens faced by caregivers. The impact of cancer care on caregivers, their ethical dilemmas and resultant distress, and their knowledge of pain management principles and techniques are areas for additional study.[31–34]

General fears and concerns of family members

A review of the research on the impact of cancer on the family[33] identified 11 separate issues of concern for family members. These included:

(1) emotional strain;

(2) physical demands;

(3) uncertainty;

(4) fear of the patient dying;

(5) altered roles and lifestyles;

(6) finances;

(7) ways to comfort the patient;

(8) perceived inadequacies of services;

(9) existential concern;

(10) sexuality;

(11) non-convergent needs among household members.

Studies of family members caring for persons with advanced cancer have shown that most experience stress in the caregiver role and significant stress in observing patient suffering. Family caregivers report distress from uncertainty about the course of the disease as well as feelings about their inability to provide care (such as effective symptom relief) and also to manage the patient's psychological symptoms such as depression and anxiety.[23]

Hampe[28] identified eight needs of family members of dying persons including:

(1) to be with the dying person;

(2) to be helpful to the dying person;

(3) to receive assurance of the dying person's comfort;

(4) to be informed of the dying person's condition;

(5) to be informed of impending death;

(6) to ventilate emotions;

(7) to receive comfort and support from family members;

(8) to receive acceptance, support, and comfort from health-care professionals.

Family communication

The above discussion emphasizes how frequently issues of communication influence family care giving in palliative care. Family communication begins by assessing needs for information and means of sharing these needs. Understanding family information needs is central to providing the care necessary to maintain patients in the home care setting. The emotional and psychosocial needs, of both patient and family, reinforce the importance of interdisciplinary care in advanced illness.

Three patterns of restricted communication among couples coping with the terminal phase of cancer were identified by Hinton:[29]

(1) consciously avoiding any discussion of the illness as a self-protective way of preventing one's distress level from rising;

(2) avoiding discussion of the illness in order to maintain the positive attitude felt to be essential to coping with the disease, thereby avoiding discussing any pessimistic feelings;

(3) those who had rarely spoken openly about emotional events in the past and maintained this pattern during the terminal illness.

Vachon described many issues related to family communication during advanced illness. Family members, like patients, experience significant distress during the patient's illness. Three major problematic issues can be summarized from the research literature related to family communication and cancer:

(1) concealing feelings

(2) acquiring information

(3) coping with helplessness.

Family communication can become restricted as family members withhold information to protect one another from difficult issues.[32,35-36] Patients often underreport symptoms to avoid distressing family caregivers.

In one study,[8] poor communication between couples in a hospice setting was found to have caused more problems than any other difficulty, with the exception of pain. Families needed help either with the fact that the patient was withdrawing or else that the patient was wanting constant contact.

Dar and colleagues studied 40 married patients with metastatic cancer, who were receiving opioid medication for cancer pain. These patients were asked about their pain and its treatment, their beliefs regarding cancer pain, their concerns about opioid analgesics, their mood state, and the nature of their interaction with their spouse in relation to these issues. The spouses of these cancer patients were interviewed separately about the same issues. The results indicate that patients underestimate the distress their pain causes to their spouses and that spouses tend to downgrade their own support to the patients. These findings are likely to be applicable to other symptoms. An important intervention by

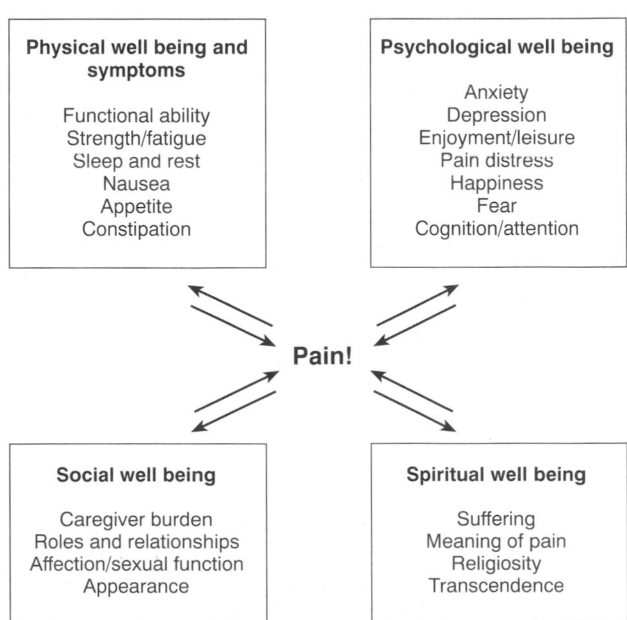

Fig. 3 Pain affects the dimensions of quality of life.

Table 2 Items of the Family Pain Questionnaire (FPQ)

1. Cancer pain can be effectively relieved
2. Pain medicines should be given only when pain is severe
3. Most cancer patients on pain medicines will become addicted to the medicines over time
4. It is important to give the lowest amount of medicine possible to save larger doses for later when the pain is worse
5. It is better to give pain medications around the clock (on a schedule) rather than only when needed
6. Treatments other than medications (such as massage, heat, relaxation) can be effective for relieving pain
7. Pain medicines can be dangerous and can often interfere with breathing
8. Patients are often given too much pain medicine
9. If pain is worse, the cancer must be getting worse.

Experience

10. Over the past week, how much pain do you feel your family member has had?
11. How much pain is your family member having now?
12. How much pain relief is your family member currently receiving?
13. How distressing do you think the pain is to your family member?
14. How distressing is your family member's pain to you?
15. To what extent do you feel you are able to control the patient's pain?
16. What do you expect will happen with your family member's pain in the future?

All items are assessed on as scale of 0–10 to indicate degree of agreement (items 1–9) or extent of pain experience (10–16).

health-care providers is to validate the family caregiver's contributions to the patient's comfort and reinforce their commitment.

There is a need to extend family research beyond a single caregiver or beyond spouses alone. Clinical experience documents the impact of terminal care on all family members yet the entire family unit, and particular individuals such as children, are seldom studied.[37]

Health-care providers play an important role in enhancing communication between various family members, with the patient, and with health-care professionals. In the terminal phase of illness, families often require greater support to overcome barriers to communication which greatly affect patient care. Psychosocial services such as the care provided by a clinical psychologist or psychiatrist are important but all team members can assist in improved family communication. Encouraging expression of concerns, facilitating discussions, active listening, and providing information are all important components of this care.

Clinical issues in supporting family caregivers

What family caregivers need most is information and support. Family caregivers increasingly assume 24-h care that in recent years was provided in acute, inpatient settings with 24-h professional nursing care. In many instances, family caregivers are now assuming procedures and treatments that in recent years were confined to intensive care units. Families assume these responsibilities with little or no education and, perhaps even more importantly, little emotional support. Health-care professionals provide this care with the support of colleagues and with the assurance that the 'next shift' will relieve them soon. Family caregivers seldom have such assurance. There is much to be provided in the way of home care and hospice services and yet even for those individuals with access to optimum care provided by these agencies, the majority of the responsibility rests on the family members themselves.

In recent research, conducted at the City of Hope National Medical Center, we evaluated a structured pain education programme in both elderly patients and family caregivers. The educational programme was quite successful in improving knowledge and attitudes about pain, as well as direct outcomes such as improved pain intensity and overall quality of life. However, the study also revealed the unmet emotional needs of family caregivers arising from the perceived burden of responsibility for the relief of a loved one's suffering.[18] This study, and other literature, demonstrates that providing information alone is not sufficient, but that family caregivers desperately need support for the intense roles they assume and the burdens they shoulder associated with assuming responsibility for patient comfort.

Family members often feel very helpless, despite their best attempts, if symptoms persist. Family caregivers also may deny the presence of symptoms as a means of coping with the situation. Our previous decade of research has also revealed the ever present metaphor of pain as a symbol of death. In this sense, pain is unlike treatment of other symptoms, such as nausea or constipation, in that it carries with it the existential issues of suffering and death.

Alternative therapies

Family caregivers often seek alternative therapies. Family caregivers often seek alternative therapies either as curative treatments to avoid the possibility of terminal illness or as palliative treatments for symptom management.

Montbriand[38] reviewed alternative therapies in cancer care and categorized these as spiritual, psychological, or physical modalities. Spiritual methods include faith healing, psychic surgery, and similar modalities. Psychological therapies include visualization or other cognitive therapies. The most common alternative treatment is use of physical methods such as herbs, vitamins, health foods, and healers.

These methods may be a valuable component of the patient's care, enhancing the effects of traditional methods. Their use may also benefit family caregivers by enhancing their sense of helpfulness and control. However, health-care providers should assess the use of these modalities to determine the potential for misuse or to identify areas of fraud or financial burden too often associated with their use. Work by Montbriand[38] and others[39–42] serves as a useful guide to direct health-care providers in this important aspect of care.

Bereavement issues

Care provided to families during the course of a terminal illness has a profound influence on bereavement following death of the patient. All of the above cited suggestions for family support during illness will also influence subsequent bereavement. Positive bereavement

Table 3 Quality of life scale/CANCER PAIN-FAMILY

Directions: We are interested in knowing how your experience of having a family member with cancer affects your Quality of Life. Please answer all of the following questions based on **your** life at this time.

Please circle the number from 0–10 that best describes your experiences:

Physical well being

To what extent are the following a problem for you:

1. Fatigue
   no problem 0 1 2 3 4 5 6 7 8 9 10 **severe problem**
2. Appetite changes
   no problem 0 1 2 3 4 5 6 7 8 9 10 **severe problem**
3. Pain
   no problem 0 1 2 3 4 5 6 7 8 9 10 **severe problem**
4. Sleep changes
   no problem 0 1 2 3 4 5 6 7 8 9 10 **severe problem**
5. Rate your overall physical health
   excellent 0 1 2 3 4 5 6 7 8 9 10 **extremely poor**

Psychological well being items

6. How difficult is it for you to cope as a result of having a family member with cancer?
   not at all 0 1 2 3 4 5 6 7 8 9 10 **very difficult**
7. How good is your quality of life?
   excellent 0 1 2 3 4 5 6 7 8 9 10 **extremely poor**
8. How much happiness do you feel?
   a great deal 0 1 2 3 4 5 6 7 8 9 10 **none at all**
9. Do you feel like you are in control of things in your life?
   completely 0 1 2 3 4 5 6 7 8 9 10 **not at all**
10. How satisfying is your life?
    completely 0 1 2 3 4 5 6 7 8 9 10 **not at all**
11. How is your present ability to concentrate or to remember things?
    excellent 0 1 2 3 4 5 6 7 8 9 10 **extremely poor**
12. How useful do you feel?
    extremely 0 1 2 3 4 5 6 7 8 9 10 **not at all**
13. How much anxiety do you have?
    none at all 0 1 2 3 4 5 6 7 8 9 10 **a great deal**
14. How much depression do you have?
    none at all 0 1 2 3 4 5 6 7 8 9 10 **a great deal**

Social concerns

15. How distressing has your family member's illness been for you?
    not at all 0 1 2 3 4 5 6 7 8 9 10 **extremely**
16. Is the amount of support you receive from others sufficient to meet your needs?
    a great deal 0 1 2 3 4 5 6 7 8 9 10 **not at all**
17. To what degree has your family member's illness and treatment interfered with your employment?
    not at all 0 1 2 3 4 5 6 7 8 9 10 **a great deal**
18. To what degree has your family member's illness and treatment interfered with your activities at home?
    not at all 0 1 2 3 4 5 6 7 8 9 10 **a great deal**
19. How much isolation do you feel is caused by you family member's illness and treatment?
    none 0 1 2 3 4 5 6 7 8 9 10 **a great deal**
20. How much financial burden have you incurred as a result of your family member's illness and treatment?
    none 0 1 2 3 4 5 6 7 8 9 10 **a great deal**

Spiritual well being

21. How important to you is your participation in religious activities such as praying, going to church, or temple?
very important 0 1 2 3 4 5 6 7 8 9 10 **not at all important**

22. How important to you are other spiritual activities such as meditation?
very important 0 1 2 3 4 5 6 7 8 9 10 **not at all important**

23. How much has your spiritual life changed as a result of your family member's cancer diagnosis?
a great deal 0 1 2 3 4 5 6 7 8 9 10 **not at all**

24. How much uncertainty do you feel about the future?
not at all uncertain 0 1 2 3 4 5 6 7 8 9 10 **very uncertain**

25. To what extent has your family member's illness made positive changes in your life?
a great deal 0 1 2 3 4 5 6 7 8 9 10 **none at all**

26. Do you sense a purpose/mission for your life or a reason for being alive?
a great deal 0 1 2 3 4 5 6 7 8 9 10 **none at all**

27. How hopeful do you feel?
very hopeful 0 1 2 3 4 5 6 7 8 9 10 **not at all hopeful**

outcomes result from a sense by family caregivers of having provided optimum care and relieved symptoms. The physical and psychological burdens of care giving are relieved when family members feel that they were able to minimize the patient's distress and that the patient received appropriate professional care.[7,10]

Implications for future research

As care shifts into the home and family caregivers provide a greater extent of palliative care, research should also expand to understudied areas. It is important to evaluate outcomes of palliative care to include both patient and family caregivers. Outcomes should incorporate all aspects of quality of life including physical, psychological, social, and spiritual well being (Fig. 3).

Examples of family caregiver outcomes are included as Tables 2 and 3. Table 3 is the 'Family Pain Questionnaire' which we have used extensively in both descriptive and experimental studies to evaluate family caregivers' knowledge and experiences of pain management.[43] This questionnaire also provides information useful for directing patient care and family support.

Table 3 is a questionnaire developed for family caregivers. It is analogous to the questionnaire used to assess patients' quality of life.[44] This is an example of methodology which assesses the family caregiver's needs as distinct from those of the patient.

Future research should incorporate cost-benefit outcomes and include direct as well as indirect costs and the costs assumed by patients and families.[45–46] Cost measures are essential in the future restructuring of health care, to establish the benefits of palliative care.

Sexuality and terminal illness

Sexuality is a critical issue to patients and their partners and yet it is often ignored within the context of palliative care. Sexuality encompasses not only sexual intercourse but also dimensions of intimacy, self-concept, and the expression of love which is critical at this phase of life transition. Previous research has documented sexuality as a priority need of patients and family caregivers and that this need is often ignored.[47–49] A patient in our recent research related to breast cancer commented that although many people had given great attention to the loss of her breast not a single health-care provider had acknowledged or addressed the issues of her sexuality as related to vaginal symptoms and ability to have intercourse. Acts of intimacy and/or sexual intercourse have significant meaning during terminal illness. Ability to express intimacy and express sexuality are often acts of important communication during terminal illness. A failure to intervene with this equally important aspect of holistic care creates great distress for patients and their loved ones.

Sexuality can be addressed by first exploring with the patients their needs and assessment of physical or psychological issues associated with sexuality. Issues of sexuality are often examples of divergent needs between patients and family caregivers. Patients may have a continued or even stronger desire for sexual activity yet partners may be reluctant to reciprocate due to either fear of physical harm or avoidance of the intimacy with their loved one given the prognosis. Tension is best addressed by allowing both partners to express their feelings or concerns associated with illness or intimacy. Often there are also basic considerations such as a lack of privacy within institutional settings or physical changes such as altering the hospital bed so that both patient and partner can sleep together.

The first challenge is to facilitate communication with patient or partner regarding issues of sexuality and intimacy. We have found it useful within our quality of life questionnaire (Table 3) to ask questions regarding distress from illness and interference with relationships as ways to begin communication and lead on to more specific aspects of intimacy. This important need is also an example of where co-ordination of the palliative care team is important, to ensure that sexuality is assessed and services are routinely offered by a member of the team and that additional services by a sexual counsellor are available as needed.

Summary

While the emotional problems facing patients and families are significant, there is much to be done to minimize the suffering of

Table 4 Suggested interventions to facilitate family coping with advanced illness

1. Assess family communication patterns prior to and over the course of the illness
2. Acknowledge the specific relationship of the family member to the patient. Family caregiving is significantly influenced by the distinct relationship (i.e. spouse, parent, child) between patient and family caregiver
3. Identify families at risk for dysfunctional coping with terminal illness. Risk factors include families with poor communication patterns, prior history of family stress, and those with prior issues of non-compliance
4. Establish mechanisms for conducting family conferences to facilitate shared communication between patient, family, and health care providers
5. Provide counselling for the direct and indirect financial burdens associated with chronic illness
6. Recognize the family's developmental level and its relationship to their coping with the illness. Family developmental crisis, such as recent retirement, 'empty nest' syndromes, births, marriages, etc., influence coping with illness
7. Recognize areas of concurrent stress which may be unrelated to the patient or illness (i.e. job loss, stress in the extended family, coping by children)
8. Provide opportunities for family caregivers to express their emotions through individual or group support away from the patient
9. Diminish family caregiver's sense of helplessness by empowering them with knowledge and skills to enhance patient comfort (i.e. pain management, use of drug and non-drug modalities)
10. Provide structured pain education to diffuse anxiety regarding issues such as drug addiction and opioid tolerance
11. Provide opportunities for family caregivers to verbalize the emotional strain inherent in care giving during terminal illness
12. Develop family education regarding the basic physical aspects of care giving (e.g. lifting, bathing, toileting)
13. Address the issue of uncertainty. Provide information regarding anticipated symptoms and discuss the distress associated with uncertainty
14. Provide information to family caregivers regarding the actual death event
15. Evaluate and co-ordinate available sources of family support, i.e. social workers, clinical psychologists, psychiatrists, family counselling, peer support groups

terminal illness. Palliative care programmes have demonstrated successful interventions to reduce the physical and emotional burdens of patients and families. Table 4 is a list of suggested interventions derived from the literature. This list can serve as a guide to evaluate the adequacy of support in existing programmes as well as to guide interventions for individual families.

In summary, family aspects are an integral aspect of palliative care. Family care has been a cornerstone of the hospice philosophy and will remain so but such care demands professional support. A mother in our family research recently described having a child with cancer as 'being forced to watch your child dangled over a river'. She went on to say that having a child in pain, however, was like 'watching the child dropped into the river and drown'. Again, while experiencing terminal illness is a terrible event, and observing it perhaps even more so, the important lessons of palliative care demonstrate that much can be done to alleviate the suffering of both the patient and their family.

References

1. Ferrell BR, Ferrell BA, Rhiner M, Grant MM. Family factors influencing cancer pain management. *Post Graduate Medical Journal*, 1991; **67** (Suppl. 2): S64–9.
2. Given B, Given W. Cancer nursing for the elderly. *Cancer Nursing*, 1989; **12**: 71–7.
3. Ferrell BR, Cohen MZ, Rhiner M, Rozek A. Pain as a metaphor for illness Part II: Family caregivers' management of pain. *Oncology Nursing Forum*, 1991; **18**: 1315–21.
4. Ferrell BR, Rhiner M, Cohen MZ, Grant M. Pain as a metaphor for illness. Part I: Impact of cancer pain on family caregivers. *Oncology Nursing Forum*, 1991; **18**:1303–9.
5. Horowitz A. Family caregiving to the frail elderly. *Annual Review of Gerontology and Geriatrics*, 1985; **5**: 194–246.
6. Matthews SH. Provision of care to old patients: Division of responsibility among adult children. *Research in Aging*, 1987; **9**: 45–60.
7. Vachon MLS, Freedman K, Formo A, Rogers J, Lyall WAL, Freeman SJJ. The final illness in cancer: the widow's perspective. *Canadian Medical Association Journal*, 1977; **177**: 1151–4.
8. Stedeford A. Psychological aspects of the management of terminal cancer. *Comprehensive Therapy*, 1984; **10**: 35–40.
9. Bergen A. Nurses caring for the terminally ill in the community: a review of the literature. *International Journal of Nursing Studies*, 1991; **28**: 89–101.
10. Bowen M. Family reaction to death. In: Guerin P, ed. *Family Therapy*. New York: Gardner Press, 1976: 335–348.
11. Ferrell BR, Rhiner M, Shapiro B, Dierkes M. The experience of pediatric cancer pain, Part I: Impact of pain on the family. *Journal of Pediatric Nursing*, 1994; **9**: 368–79.
12. Ferrell BA, Ferrell BR. Pain management at home. *Clinics in Geriatric Medicine*, 1991; **7**: 765–76.
13. Cleeland C. Barriers to the management of cancer pain. *Oncology*, 1987; **1**(2 Suppl.):19–26.
14. Ferrell BR, Schneider C. Experience and management of cancer pain at home. *Cancer Nursing*, 1988; **11**: 84–90.
15. Woods NF, Lewis FM, Ellison ES. Living with cancer: family experiences. *Cancer Nursing*, 1989; **12**: 28–33.
16. Spross J, McGuire D, Schmitt R. Oncology Nursing Society position paper on cancer pain. *Oncology Nursing Forum*, 1991; **17**: 595–614, 751–60, 943–4.
17. Whedon M, Ferrell BR. Ethical issues and high tech pain management. *Oncology Nursing Forum*, 1991; **18**: 1135–43.
18. Ferrell BR, Ferrell BA, Ahn C, Tran K. Pain management for elderly patients with cancer at home. *Cancer*, 1994; **74**: 2139–46.
19. Ferrell BR, Johnston Taylor E, Grant M, Fowler M, Corbisiero RM. Pain management at home: struggle, comfort and mission. *Cancer Nursing*, 1993; **16**: 169–78.
20. Ferrell BR, Johnston Taylor E, Sattler GR, Fowler M, Cheyney BL. Searching for the meaning of pain: cancer patients', caregivers', and nurses' perspectives. *Cancer Practice*, 1993; **1**: 185–94.
21. Dar R, Beach CM, Barden PL, Cleeland CS. Cancer pain in the marital system: a study of patients and their spouses. *Journal of Pain and Symptom Management*, 1992; **7**: 87–93.
22. Grobe ME, Ilstrup EM, Ahmann DL. Skills needed by family members to maintain the care of an advanced cancer patient. *Cancer Nursing*, 1990; **4**: 371–5.
23. Hinds C. The needs of families who care for patients with cancer at home: are we meeting them? *Journal of Advanced Nursing*, 1985; **10**: 575–81.
24. Tringali CA. The needs of family members of cancer patients. *Oncology Nursing Forum*, 1986; **13**: 65–9.

25. Stommel M, Given CW, Given BA. The cost of cancer home care to families. *Cancer,* 1993; **71**: 4–11.
26. Block AR, Boyer SL. The spouse's adjustment to chronic pain: cognitive and emotional factors. *Social Science and Medicine,* 1984; **19**: 1313–7.
27. Flor H, Turk DC, Scholz OB. Impact of chronic pain on the spouse: marital, emotional and physical consequences. *Journal of Psychosomatic Research,* 1987; **31**: 63–71.
28. Hampe SO. Needs of the grieving spouse in a hospital setting. *Nursing Research,* 1975; **24**: 113–9.
29. Hinton J. Sharing or withholding awareness of dying between husband and wife. *Journal of Psychosomatic Research*, 1981; **25**: 337–43.
30. Hull MM. Coping strategies of family caregivers in hospice home care. *Caring,* 1993; **12**: 78–88.
31. Davies B, Reimer JC, Martens N. Family functioning and its implications for palliative care. *Journal of Palliative Care,* 1994; **10**: 29–36.
32. Keitel MS, Zevon MA, Rounds JB, Petrelli NJ, Karakousis C. Spouse adjustment to cancer surgery: distress and coping responses. *Journal of Surgical Oncology,* 1990; **43**: 148–53.
33. Lewis FM. The impact of cancer on the family: a critical analysis of the research literature. *Patient Education and Counselling,* 1986:269–89.
34. Reimer JC, Davies G, Martens N. Palliative care: the nurse's role in helping families through the transition of 'fading away'. *Cancer Nursing,* 1991; **14**: 321–7.
35. Vachon MLS. Emotional problems in palliative medicine: patient, family, and professional. In D Doyle, GWC Hanks, N MacDonald (Eds.) *Oxford Textbook of Palliative Medicine.* Oxford, England:Oxford University Press, 1993:575–605.
36. Oberst MT, Scott DW. Postdischarge distress in surgically treated cancer patients and their spouses. *Research in Nursing and Health,* 1988; **11**: 223–33.
37. Rhiner M, Ferrell BR, Shapiro B, Dierkes M. The experience of pediatric cancer pain, Part II: management of pain. *Journal of Pediatric Nursing,* 1994; **9**: 380–7.
38. Montbriand MJ. An overview of alternate therapies chosen by patients with cancer. *Oncology Nursing Forum,* 1994; **21**: 1547–54.
39. American Cancer Society. Unproven methods of cancer treatment: Macrobiotic diets for the treatment of cancer. *CA: A Cancer Journal for Clinicians,* 1989; **39**: 248–51.
40. American Cancer Society. Unproven methods of cancer treatment: Psychic surgery. *CA: A Cancer Journal for Clinicians,* 1990; **40**: 184–8.
41. American Cancer Society. Questionable methods of cancer management: 'nutritional' therapics. *CA: A Cancer Journal for Clinicians,* 1993; **43**: 309–17.
42. Cassileth BR. Unorthodox cancer medicine. *Cancer Investigation*, 1986; **4**: 591–8.
43. Ferrell BR, Rhiner M, Rivera LM. Development and evaluation of the family pain questionnaire. *Journal of Psychosocial Oncology,* 1993; **10**: 21–35.
44. Ferrell BR, Grant M, Chan J, Ahn C. The impact of cancer pain education on family caregivers of elderly patients. *Oncology Nursing Forum.* In press.
45. Ferrell BR, Griffith H. Cost issues related to pain management: report from the cancer pain panel of the agency for health care policy and research. *Journal of Pain and Symptom Management,* 1994; **9**: 221–34.
46. Ferrell BR. How patients and families pay the price. *Proceedings of the Bristol Pain Symposium*—Johns Hopkins University, 1995, IASP Press.
47. Leiber L. The communication of affection between cancer patients and their spouse. *Psychomatic Medicine,* 1979; **38**: 379–81.
48. MacElveen-Hoehn P, McCorkle R. Understanding sexuality in progressive cancer. *Seminars in Oncology Nursing,* 1985; **1**: 56–62.
49. Vachon MLS. Psychotherapy and the person with cancer: one nurse's experience. *Oncology Nursing Forum,* 1985; **12**: 33–40.

14.3 The stress of professional caregivers

Mary L.S. Vachon

The stress of professional caregivers

Not only do patients and their families suffer distress when confronting terminal illness, so too do those who care for them. The professional caregiver can experience significant stress in response to working with dying persons as well as in response to the death of particular patients. The stress may come from a variety of sources: within the person him/herself as a result of previous or current life experiences; because of a particular death experience with a patient/family; 'death overload' from too many patients dying too close together; or from too much investment in patients over too long a time. Stress may result from the work environment in which there are unrealistic expectations of the amount of work that can be accomplished. There may also be a lack of resources to carry out the work that needs to be done.

Epidemiology of caregiver distress

In an early study in the field of palliative care, nurses starting a palliative care unit were found to have distress scores equal to those of newly widowed women and higher than those of women undergoing radiation treatment for newly diagnosed breast cancer.[1] A later, much larger, international study compared caregivers from all professional groups working in a variety of specialty areas where there was significant exposure to life-threatening illness and death. In that study, caregivers working in palliative care were found to have fewer stressors, fewer manifestations of stress, and more coping mechanisms than those in most other specialties.[2] A recent review of much of the literature of stress in palliative care over the past quarter century found that many studies reported that staff working in palliative care had either less burnout and stress than other professionals or that they experienced no more stress than other health-care professionals working with seriously ill and/or dying persons.[3]

The use of drugs, alcohol, and suicidal ideation by hospice medical directors and matrons was a concern.[4] Hospice nurses were more anxious, with associated psychosomatic complaints, than hospital nurses, although the latter had more job dissatisfaction. High levels of mental ill health were predicted by a lack of social support and involvement in work and high workload.[5] Hospice nurses were found to be higher on the death and dying dimension of the Nursing Stress Scale[6] and were slightly more depressed than medical,surgical, or intensive care unit nurses.

The review concluded that while stress exists in palliative care, it is by no means a universal phenomenon. This finding may well be related to the fact that from the early days of the hospice movement, staff support and team development programmes were felt to be integral to effective palliative care. Undergraduate educational programmes and most postgraduate medical and radiation oncology programmes do not prepare staff to deal with the terminally ill and their grieving relatives.[7] Therefore, much of the preparation for palliative care must take place at the postgraduate level.

This chapter will identify the personal and organizational variables associated with stress in palliative care, identify the manifestations of stress and coping mechanisms, and suggest research questions for the future.

The person–environment model of occupational stress

Occupational stress is viewed within the person–environment fit framework.[8,9] The underlying principle of this model is that adaptation is a function of the 'goodness of fit' between the characteristics of the person and the work environment. 'Fit' is the mesh between the needs of the individual and the supplies or resources available within the environment and/or the abilities of the individual and the demands made by the work environment. In part, fit is determined by the extent to which environmental supplies are available to meet individual needs and values; it is also determined by the ability of the person to manage the environment.[10]

In assessing one's own 'goodness of fit' within the work environment it is important to be able to assess both one's self and the work environment. Individuals need to have an accurate understanding of their personal resources, values, and limitations. They must also be aware of the resources available within the environment to meet their needs and to facilitate their being able to perform in their professional role.[10]

A model of occupational stress

Through interviews with a multidisciplinary, international sample of close to 600 caregivers caring for the critically ill, dying, and bereaved, the author developed the model of occupational stress in Fig. 1.[2] In that study, Antonovsky's[11] definition of stress was used: 'stress is a demand made by the internal or external environment of the organism that upsets its homeostasis, restoration of which depends upon a non-automatic and not readily available energy-expending action' (p. 72). Stress evolves from exposure to stressors

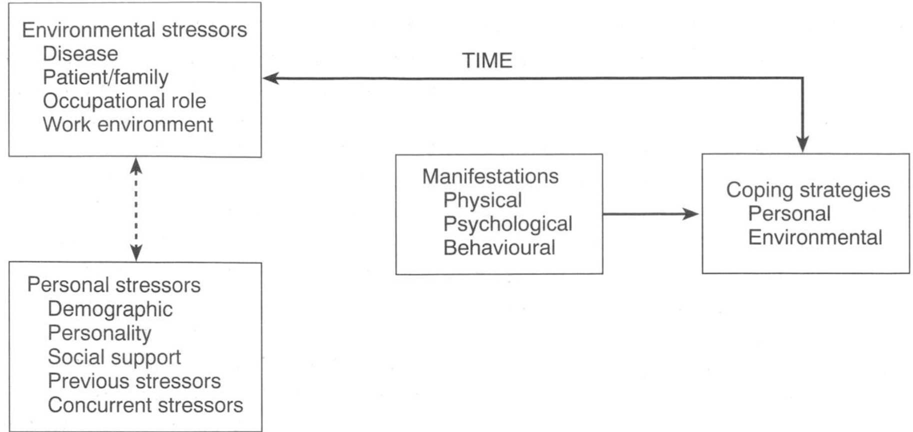

Fig. 1 Occupational stress in caregivers.

that are differentiated from routine stimuli. A routine stimulus might become a stressor under certain circumstances. It is not always possible to determine when and why this is happening. In addition, one person's stressor may be another person's routine stimulus. Whether a given situation is perceived as being a stressor or not is dependent upon the meaning of that stimulus to the person at that point in time and on the person's repertoire of coping mechanisms that are readily available.[2,9]

In the model of stress shown in Fig. 1, job stress is seen as being the result of the interaction between the person and the environment. Personal variables that affect one's perception of a situation as stressful or not include demographic variables, social support, personality, previous stressful life events, and the stressful life events one might currently be experiencing. Work stressors derive from the patients and families with whom we work, illnesses, one's occupational role, and the work environment.

Personal variables

Demographic variables

Age

Younger staff working in hospices have been found to: perceive more stress,[12] to be more prone to burnout,[13,14] and to report more stressors, manifestations of stress, and fewer coping strategies than older caregivers (45 years and over).[2] The age at which a physician had a first encounter with death was found to be associated with communication patterns with terminally ill patients. The later in life a respondent's first exposure to death took place, the more likely it was that he or she would avoid confronting a patient with a terminal prognosis.[15] The older age of caregivers in a hospital-based home care team working with severely ill cancer patients accounted, in part, for the fact that they experienced more job satisfaction than hospital ward caregivers working with similar patients.[16]

Gender

Female physicians experience more role strain than their male counterparts.[17] In a Canadian study of 3352 physicians, women were more likely to report having had suicidal ideation. Sixteen per cent of Quebec female physicians recently studied admitted to thoughts of self-annihilation.[18]

In a study of almost 2000 British family practitioners,[19] female general practitioners had greater job satisfaction and showed greater well-being than matched controls. Male physicians had higher anxiety scores than the norms, had less job satisfaction, and drank more alcohol than their female counterparts. Dealing with death and dying was not a major source of stress; however, it was associated with excess alcohol use—particularly for women physicians. While the authors do not speculate on why this correlation might exist, it might reflect distress from work–home interface and social life experienced by women physicians. Perhaps they felt torn as they tried to balance their home lives with the legitimate needs of dying patients and their families for increased attention.

The contradictory findings that women physicians have both more role strain and more role satisfaction and greater job satisfaction and more suicidal ideation may reflect the fact that if women physicians are satisfied with their careers they are very satisfied. However, if they are not satisfied, and are having difficulty with role strain, then they are at significantly increased risk of problems with alcohol, perhaps because of a tendency to try to self-medicate away their depression, which if untreated is associated with the higher risk of suicidal ideation.

Place of residence

In a Spanish study of physician attitudes towards death and terminal patients,[15] the place where one spent one's adolescence reflected the process of assimilation of cultural patterns and the adoption of certain attitudes. The attitudes of the 153 physicians studied were similar to those of medical students, nurses, and practising physicians previously studied by members of the research team.[20-22] Urban environments, as opposed to rural settings, were associated with greater aversion towards death and its outward manifestations (grieving, funeral, etc.). The rural environment was associated with the acquisition of a more flexible attitude towards death, in part because of having had more frequent exposure to death and funerals during adolescence. Physicians who spent their adolescence in urban areas expressed a greater fear of and anguish over their own death.

Personality

Motivation

Motivation is composed of both conscious and unconscious elements. Job stress may result when there is a discrepancy between the individual's motivation for seeking a particular job and the supplies for meeting that need existing within the job environment.

Studies have found that volunteers entered hospice work to pursue a professional interest in counselling[23] or for the opportunity to experience self-growth, become involved in one's community and a chance for further education in the health field.[24] Volunteer counsellors joined hospice organizations for intellectual, self-centred, and humanitarian reasons; they continued to volunteer in a hospice setting because of the emotional rewards they received from contact with peers and clients.[23]

Previous experience with death is a motive in choosing to work in palliative care.[23,25] In a group of volunteers who choose to work in a hospice programme to have some professional training, over half had experienced one to three deaths in their personal lives in the past 2 years. Experience with fewer deaths prior to hospice experience was associated with higher initial job stress.[23]

Motivation for working in hospices in the initial phases of the movement evolved from: a desire to do the 'in thing' or to affiliate with a charismatic leader; an intellectual appeal and a desire for mastery over death; a sense of calling; and previous personal experience.[26] More recently, staff have chosen to enter hospices as a part of their career development and because of their commitment to a particular quality of care, rather than with the driving conviction of those who initially felt 'called' to hospice work.[27]

Personal value systems

The initial hospice movement had significant spiritual underpinning and organized religions, particularly Christianity, gave impetus to the movement.[3,27] Leaders in the British hospice movement, including Drs Cicely Saunders, Derek Doyle, and Sheila Cassidy, have written of the strong spiritual elements which underpin their work. They have a 'single-minded spiritual devotion to what they are doing' (James and Field, p. 1366).[27]

Hospice workers are more religious than caregivers from other settings.[28] Competency in spiritual aspects of care was studied in 32 nurse hospice experts working with people nearing death. Spiritual care was grounded in self-awareness and a clear personal philosophy.[29] In a group of 181 oncology nurses, self-reported spirituality and religiosity were positively associated with attitudes about spiritual care. However, the more spiritual and religious the nurse was, the more likely was the nurse to perceive the 'unbelieving patient ' as spiritually unhealthy. Furthermore, the more frequently the nurse attended religious services the more likely was the nurse to share personal spiritual beliefs and discuss spiritual issues. The authors suggested that a high degree of religiosity could lead to the nurse having difficulty appreciating the spiritual well-being of a patient who believed differently and to inappropriate proselytizing.[30]

Cassidy, a hospice physician, has reflected on her personal values, personality characteristics, and hospice work. She states: '. . . there emerges a picture of conflicting gifts: of a powerful creativity only partially fulfilled in caring for the sick; and a terrible urge to succeed, to be better than other people, to climb every mountain, that has driven me far in my profession but leaves me still restless and hungry for more. Perhaps because I am a religious person, I understand this hunger in part as a longing for God.'[31]

Personality and coping style

The most commonly studied personality characteristics of hospice care providers are attitude towards death and death anxiety. Working with dying patients has been found to shape one's attitude towards death and dying.[25] Those who coped adequately with death lived in the present, rather than the past or future. They scored higher on inner-directedness, self-actualizing value, existentiality, spontaneity, self-regard, self-acceptance, acceptance of aggression, and capacity for intimate contact.[32]

The death anxiety of hospice workers was within the norm for the general population and those who exhibited a 'higher sense of purpose in life' tended to score lower on death anxiety.[33] Death anxiety was found to correlate significantly with the severity of job stress for medical-surgical but not hospice nurses[6] and was negatively correlated with time competence, inner-directedness, self-regard, self acceptance, and the Personal Orientation Inventory.[32]

A relationship has been found between physician's fear of death and their attitudes towards informing terminally ill patients. Physicians who believe that patients 'should never be made aware that they are dying are likely to have a greater fear of their own death, to avoid references to their own death, and to express more rigid attitudes towards the problems surrounding terminal patients' (Barroso *et al*, p. 530).[15]

Physicians' difficulty in dealing with their own death was also reflected in a study in which physicians were asked about living wills.[34] Almost all the physicians surveyed approved of living wills and 90 per cent would feel bound by the terms of a patient's living will (albeit with many caveats). However, although 81 per cent of the 3400 Canadian physicians surveyed said they would personally consider having a living will for themselves, none of the physicians selected for follow-up telephone calls (N not given but sample 'from 30 something to 65') had personally made a living will.

The Hardy Personality is effective in combating work stress.[35,36] The Hardy Personality involves: a sense of commitment (as opposed to alienation) to oneself and the various areas in one's life, including work, which reflects the Hardy person's curiosity about and a sense of meaningfulness of life; control (as opposed to powerlessness), reflecting the belief that one has the power to influence the course of events; and challenge (as opposed to threat), epitomizing the expectation that it is normal for life to change and for development to be stimulated. Hardiness is associated with fewer mental and physical symptoms of stress. 'Hardiness is said to lead to a perception, interpretation, and handling of stressful events that prevents excessive activation of arousal and therefore results in fewer symptoms of stress' (Kash and Holland, p. 652).[37]

Although a Hardy Personality is effective in combating stress in oncology settings,[37] problems can follow if both the patient and caregiver have a strong need to control the current situation and are working at cross purposes or get into rivalry. Physicians (and other caregivers) often assume that they are the one 'in control' and should be the decision-maker. However, self-care advice usually exhorts patients to adopt a 'take-charge' attitude.[38]

Caregivers may be caught in an ambiguous role—balancing their own previously unchallenged role as an authority figure with the current ethical recognition of the increased role of the patient in decision making.[39] It may be helpful to caregivers in these situations to understand their own need for control and to try to work toward shared control and decision making. If this does not work intermediaries, such as the patient's family member or hospital personnel such as chaplains, social workers, other physicians, or ethics committees, can be used.[39]

In understanding the need for control in either one's self or another it is helpful to recognize that believing that one is in control can, in certain instances, augment feelings of threat.[40,41]

Antonovsky contrasts coherence with control.[11] Coherence emphasizes the importance of predictability in both internal and external environments, coupled with the likelihood of things working out as well as can be expected. He distinguishes between a sense of coherence and control; coherence implies that one can shape one's destiny, not that one is in control. A sense of coherence is partly personality related and partly developed through experience. Those who are personality resourceful and flexible are better able to adjust to most life challenges than those with poor repertoires.[42] For the caregiver and patient alike, a sense of coherence can be helpful in dealing with the cancer experience.

Social support

Social support is crucial to survival in palliative care and the existence of a good support system is one of the qualities of the ideal palliative care nurse.[43] 'Although social support has many facets, a core dimension of it involves participating in a network of caring and reciprocal relationships with others and creating a sense of belonging and a reason for living that transcends one's individual self'.[44] Hospice nurses do not differ significantly in social support from critical care nurses.[45] High levels of mental ill health in hospice nurses correlates with a lack of social support.[5] In addition, a correlation exists between reporting that one's friends were a source of distress and reporting that one's work environment was a source of distress.[23] This may reflect a personality trait, as opposed to the reality of the hospice environment.

One's social support system can be a source of stress, as well as a buffer against life stressors. A professional caregiver's social support system may change. While initially family members and friends may be useful in helping the neophyte practitioner to debrief, over time caregivers turn more to colleagues who are more able to understand the specific stressors to which one is exposed.[46]

Caregivers who use their family and friends as the major source of a professional support system may have difficulty over time. Research on physicians and their social support system has found that as the physician grows and matures, so too will the members of his or her support system. They may no longer want to play the support role.[46,47] Physicians who rely primarily on their personal support system to deal with professional stressors might find that this support system might withdraw under particularly stressful situations leaving the physician open to psychological problems and even to suicide.[48]

Stressful life events

Stressful life events may serve as a source of strength as well as a stressor. For example, many female physicians that were interviewed reported that they had chosen to enter medicine because of having had a sister with a chronic illness. At other times unresolved previous stressful life events such as the death of a parent, a history of sexual abuse, or family alcoholism might leave the caregiver vulnerable to stress reactions in one's professional practice.

Previous experience with death may be a motive in choosing to work in palliative care, as stated above.[23,25] Other studies have shown a more negative impact of previous death experiences, particularly if the grief is unresolved. Recent personal bereavement and unresolved grief from deaths prior to coming into a children's hospice were associated with high distress on the General Health Questionnaire.[49] In a study of palliative care nurses and administrators a significant correlation was found between job satisfaction and absence of loss in the past year.[12]

Concurrent stressors that the caregivers reported included: illness or bereavement in one's personal support system; problems within one's marriage or relationships; personal concerns such as divorce, health problems, and family problems. Caregivers reported that sometimes these personal stressors interfered with their ability to perform their work. At other times they felt that the work situation allowed them to avoid thinking about their personal problems.

Occupational stressors

Stress in a hospice has been found to derive from the work environment, occupational role, patients and families, and illnesses. Most studies do not differentiate the amount of stress derived from various aspects of one's work life. However, in one study[2] 48 per cent of the stressors reported by hospice caregivers derived from the work environment; 29 per cent came from their occupational role; 17 per cent from patients and families; and 7 per cent from illness related variables. In a study of burnout,[13] demographic variables accounted for 15 per cent of the variance in the burnout variable; occupational characteristics added another 6 per cent. In that study no hospice organizational factors tested were significantly related to burnout.

The framework for the discussion of work-related stressors will be those identified in the physicians (N=79) interviewed in an international study of occupational stress in the care of the dying.[2] Table 1 shows a synopsis of the stressors, manifestations of stress, and coping mechanisms of physicians. For purposes of comparison, Table 2 shows a synopsis of the same variables for the 60 people from a variety of professional (including physicians) and volunteer groups who worked in hospice/palliative care.

Communication problems with others in the system

Physicians were the most likely to report problems with dealing with 'others in the system.' This included professional rivalry with and lack of support from colleagues, problems dealing with those in other specialties as well problems with other professional groups, and from the hesitancy of those in other specialties to refer to hospice/palliative care.[2,50]

The problems encountered with 'others in the system' vary with different countries. In the United Kingdom, Australia, and New Zealand, palliative care is now a specialty (see Chapter 2.4). Education and training in the principles of palliation for those with 'advanced mortal illness' is probably little different in content and emphasis in the nursing and medical undergraduate programmes in the United Kingdom from other countries, although more time may be allotted to such training. However, specialist palliative care education is now available for both nurses and physicians at the postgraduate level (see Chapter 21.2). Specialist palliative care is provided in specialist palliative care units. In the United Kingdom, a distinction is made between palliative care as practised by every doctor and nurse (hopefully to an increasingly high standard) and the specialist palliative care provided in specialist palliative care units where all senior staff are accredited as specialists in palliative care (D. Doyle, personal communication, 1995).

Research is not yet available about the stressors encountered dealing with 'others in the system' in the United Kingdom now that palliative care is seen as a 'full specialty' that is seen as being integral and supportive within the system (D. Doyle, personal communication, 1995). However, a recent study comparing United Kingdom palliative care specialists with medical and clinical (formerly known as radiotherapist) oncologists has found that palliative care specialists are least likely to report feeling stressed by factors including 'having organizational responsibilities/conflicts'.[51]

Nevertheless, in the author's international travels during 1995, hospice caregivers in both the United Kingdom and the United States spoke of problems encountered trying to position their hospice/palliative care programmes within the changing health-care environment. Rivalries are encountered as programmes try to determine with which agencies, if any, they will have preferred partner arrangements. The aggressive marketing techniques of some hospice programmes have resulted in conflicts amongst the programmes existing in and/or developing within some communities. This problem is undoubtedly more pronounced in the United States.

Another problem being experienced in the United States is the change to managed health care. Palliative care is still seen as a subdiscipline and health-care providers are feeling threatened by managed care which is changing the traditional roles of many health-care providers, particularly physicians. This scenario has resulted in communication problems with 'others in the system' being somewhat more prevalent as specialists vie to ensure their continued viability.

Some of the difficulties hospice staff have in receiving referrals and some of the ambivalent regard colleagues have for those in palliative care in the United States were reflected by a surgeon in a presidential address. He spoke of the fact that he and his colleagues have become so expert at thwarting death that they have come to regard death as a personal failure, rather than the logical and inevitable outcome of life: 'None of us enjoys failure, and rather than deal with it, we have not only allowed nurses or hospice teams to assume responsibility for that patient and family, we have also turned over responsibility to a seemingly endless array of intruders who make it almost impossible for the physician to have control over the care of the dying patient' (Fletcher, p. 460).[52]

There is also friction within members of the palliative care community. While the position of palliative care as a specialty has been established in the United Kingdom, Australia, and New Zealand, the position of palliative care in the United States and Canada is still in the stages of negotiation. In the United States, palliative care may develop as a subdiscipline within medical oncology.[7] In Canada, negotiations as to the role of palliative care as a specialty or subspecialty are still in progress. This time of uncertainty has, not unexpectedly, led to friction between those with different training and experience. Fear has been expressed that in the move to create the subspecialty of palliative care some

Table 2 Palliative care workers' stressors and coping mechanisms in palliative care

Stressors
Communication problems with others
Role ambiguity
Team communication problems
Administrative communication problems
Role conflict
Nature of the system
Unrealistic expectations
Patient/family communication
Inadequate resources
Patient/family coping/personality problems
Manifestations of stress
Staff conflict
Feelings of depression, grief, and guilt
Job–home interaction
Feelings of helplessness and hopelessness
Coping mechanisms
Team philosophy, support, and team building
Sense of competence, control, and pleasure in work
Develop control over practice
Personal philosophy
Increased education

Table 1 Physicians' stressors and coping mechanisms in the care of the dying

Stressors
Communication problems with others in the system
Role overload
Role strain
Patient/family communication problems
Team communication problems
Inadequate resources/staffing
Role ambiguity
Role conflict
Manifestations of stress
Job–home interaction
Staff conflict
Depression, grief, and guilt
Anger, irritability, and frustration
Helplessness, inadequacy, and insecurity
Distancing, depersonalization, and intellectualization
Errors in judgement
Avoidance of patients
Coping mechanisms
Sense of competence, control, and pleasure in work
Develop control over practice
Personal philosophy of illness, death, and one's role
Team philosophy, support, and team building
Formalized ways of handling decision-making
Staffing policies
Colleagues at work
Leave the work situation

physicians, particularly those with a family practice background, who have been practising palliative care will not be recognized as palliative care specialists in the future.

The anticipated changes in the health-care structure and financing in the United States will continue to influence hospice care[7] and tensions will result. Estimates are that in 1993, the 2600 existing hospice programmes in the United States cared for approximately 30 per cent of patients who died of cancer (J. Magno, personal communication to D. Doyle, 1995). These programmes are significantly affected by Medicare regulations. Tension results from the impact of the lack of reimbursement for physician involvement, per diem reimbursement, and an aggregate cap on reimbursement.[7] Patients may also be forced to enter a hospice programme because of bureaucratic regulations. Serving these 'ambivalent clients' may prove to be a considerable challenge.[53]

Other communication problems in the United States involved issues related to what one hospice administrator referred to as 'The Gates of Heaven' model, reflecting a narrow and inflexibly defined mission. 'Patients must be just right, families in place, the disease one that the programme is comfortable with, etc. Such programmes do not grow and over time they find themselves threatened by other providers whom they identify as somehow taking unfair advantage' (Mount, p. 34).[54]

Role overload

Role overload, or the feeling that there is too much to do in one's job, was a major stressor particularly for those working in oncology and emergency rooms. General practitioners have also been found to experience stress from work overload.[19] When palliative care specialists were compared with clinical and radiation oncologists, problems with 'feeling overloaded and its effects on home life' were found to be significantly greater for the medical and clinical oncologists than for the palliative care specialists.[51]

Physicians in one study acknowledged that at least some of their professional work overload was self-induced. One physician said 'Lots of us feeling overloaded and overworked create it ourselves. We start dancing to a tune that you're called to play by yourself.' Nevertheless, there is a real problem with the work overload that can occur when professionals try to juggle patient care, research, and publication while preserving some time for self and family.[2]

Role strain

Role strain, or having difficulty performing various aspects of one's professional role, for the most part involved difficulty in decision-making and was more often mentioned by physicians than by other professional groups. Physicians mentioned the stress involved in decision making, particularly when they felt isolated with the decisions they had to make. They also had problems with the feeling that 'the buck stops here.' Oncologists reported significantly more difficulty with two elements of role strain 'dealing with patients' suffering' and 'being involved with treatment toxicity and errors' than did palliative care specialists.[51] Such problems are documented elsewhere as well.[19,46]

Role strain in palliative care can also evolve from constant exposure to the terminally ill and the need to be open to developing intimate relationships with dying persons and their families (Vachon, in press).[1,2] Dr David Barnard has spoken of the tension between the promise of intimacy and the fear of our own undoing in the care of the terminally ill. He speaks of the need to give full weight to both the promise and the fear of intimacy in palliative care and refers to palliative care as challenging caregivers to leap into the confrontation with the forces of chaos and disintegration. 'We live in the tension between the promise of intimacy and the fear of our own undoing . . . The fear that accompanies moments of intimacy in palliative care—fear of entering intimately into another person's agony and the fear of being overwhelmed by suffering, chaos and disintegration.'[55] This fear can lead to significant role strain.

Role strain can also derive from difficulty in living up to one's own performance expectations,[56] struggling to narrow the gap between the 'real and the ideal,' the challenge of being both a professional and a friend,[57] and feeling inadequately prepared for one's role.[25,58] Feeling inadequately prepared to deal with the emotional needs of patients and families and feeling that the nursing care offered was purposeless were associated with high stress scores.[59] Further role strain may occur as palliative care becomes more of an academic discipline. There are concerns that this will result in priority being given to research into physical symptoms as opposed to the aspiration of total patient care.[27]

Patient and family communication problems

Communication problems with patients and families can occur with those who have a different cultural or social background as well as with those who are similar to one's own background. Shepard, a psychiatrist who wrote of his experience with terminal cancer, spoke of the difficulty that other physicians had in caring for him—difficulty that was no doubt complicated by their recognition that they could be in Dr Shepherd's shoes.[60,61]

A recent article noted that patients and family members are 'much more demanding than they used to be and, not unreasonably, expect more time and explanation of their doctors'(Weatherall, p. 1671).[62] The author noted that many criticisms levelled at physicians are not about their clinical competence but '. . .seem to reflect a deficiency of the basic skills of handling sick people as humans, poor communication, lack of kindness, thoughtlessness, and in short, all the facets of good interpersonal relationships that society has a right to demand of its doctors. Can such attitudes be taught? And even if they can, given our poor track record who is to teach them?'(Weatherall, p. 1671–2).[63]

A journalist wrote of her anger when she felt that she and her family were being prematurely approached about transferring her newly diagnosed mother to a hospice programme. She felt the nurse meant no harm but felt the question was premature. ' We needed time, and the last thing we wanted was a meeting to discuss Mom's death. We had not yet given up hope, even if the doctors had. This time I was angry. I told the nurse not to dare mention the word hospice to my father at this time and under no circumstances to call our home. Despite this, the hospital did call our home the next day to see if Dad was interested in attending a meeting' (Davis-Barron, p. 562).[63]

Identification with patients and families

Identifying strongly with the patient and or family member can cause the caregiver to become wrapped up in the patient's illness and distress and to experience what Weisman calls 'caregiver plight'.[64] In this situation the caregiver is so overwhelmed by what is happening to the patient that he or she is no longer able to be objective. Caregivers will often identify with patients who remind them of themselves or of people from their past or present life. For example oncologists with young children will often find it difficult to deal with dying children.

Team communication problems

An extensive review of the palliative care literature showed that team communication problems were identified initially and continue to be an ongoing concern.[1-5,16] The problems included a lack of support from one's team members,[65,66] are associated with high levels of depression,[5] and are a major problem for volunteers.[24] Team communication problems involve such factors as dealing with a lack of team stability, intergroup conflict, and intragroup conflict.[2] Colleagues are a major source of stress as well as a major stress reducer.[12,13,57,65,66] Organizational factors such as personality issues and team conflict[16,27,49,57] were more commonly reported stressors than were problems in dealing with patients and families and issues related to death and dying.[2,3,12,13,24,43,57]

Inadequate resources and staffing

Inadequate resources and staffing can result from fiscal restraints within the system. In the current economic climate, the lack of an adequate number of caregivers or of adequately prepared caregivers and limited resources are problems. While caregivers want to be able to deliver the highest quality of care, understaffing and the absence of critical staff members may necessitate compromises and the psychosocial aspects of care are often the first to be sacrificed.[67] Concerns have been expressed that because inpatient hospice care is expensive and labour-intensive, financial constraints have led to the development of a diversity of organizational forms, particularly in the United States. Where costs are shared by 'other health providers, their demands and expectations may constrain work practices in ways which compromise the initial hospice ideals'.[68]

James found[69] that in the hospice she studied, a shift from holistic to physical care occurred as the hospice lost its 'specialness' and became integrated into its host National Health Service hospital.[68] With limited resources hospices may no longer provide as high a level of support as initially and increasing problems with stress and burnout may result.[68] There is already evidence that with increasing workloads in oncology the job satisfaction of oncology nurses is decreasing.[70] 'Finally, the hospices are vulnerable to the processes of institutionalization and rationalization once the dedicated and 'charismatic' idealists who were responsible for their foundation and the first cadre of highly selected staff leave.[69-72] Concerns such as these have led to calls for evaluation of hospices and their organizational functioning'.[68,73]

Mount did an informal survey of New York State hospice directors and asked them to comment on 'the barriers to keeping a balance of mission and management; to keeping the mission uppermost; to meeting mission objectives' (Mount, p. 33).[54] All responses started with inadequate funding. In addition, concerns have been expressed that changes and the increasing bureaucratization of hospice programmes may shift the emphasis of providing high quality services for a few people to providing lesser services for a greater number.[27]

Role ambiguity (see Chapter 2.2)

To perform adequately in one's role, an individual must understand the expectations others have of that role. One must understand the rights, duties, and responsibilities of the office. What activities of the individual will fulfil these responsibilities? How can these activities can best be done? When there is a lack of clear, consistent information about what is expected of a person in a role, or when an individual does not understand what others expect of someone in that role, then role ambiguity exists.[2,74] The more ambiguity one experiences in one's role, the more tension and anxiety are felt. Furthermore, most people want less role ambiguity than they have.[2,3,75]

Role ambiguity was a more common stressor in the early days of the movement[1,2,24,50] when the roles of team members and volunteers were not clearly defined. Early hospices deliberately blurred traditional role definitions and hierarchies, but more recently there has been a move towards clearer job demarcation and specialization within the hospice field. There is now specialist training offered for those working within hospices, reflecting a move away from the 'generalist' hospice worker to the specialization of staff in different aspects of 'holistic' care within hospices.[27]

Role conflict (see Chapter 2.2)

Role conflict follows when several aspects of one's roles in life—professional and personal; researcher and clinician—conflict. Role conflict was one of the biggest stressors identified in a study of general practitioners.[19] Conflicts between hospice work and family life occurred, particularly in the early days of hospices.[2,5,12,25,50,76] For many caregivers the attempt to balance their work and home lives have led to limiting the extensive over involvement in hospice work that often marked the early pioneers in the field. This has then led to the complaints that administrators made to Mount[54] that caregivers were no longer as dedicated and selfless as they once were.

Manifestations of stress

Job–home interaction

Bringing the stressors of one's work life into one's home life occurred when physicians were constantly on call. They returned home exhausted at the end of each professional day. Families came to resent the demands that the physician's work made on their lives. Physicians sometimes came to feel that they were better liked and enjoyed life more at work than at home and thus they increased their work life accordingly. This problem is greater for female physicians than for males.[2] In a Canadian study, 61 per cent of female physicians versus 46 per cent of males said that balancing work and family is the area that has caused the greatest change in stress levels.[77] One quarter of hospice nurses (26 per cent) reported that work had a negative effect on their family life.[25]

Staff conflict

Staff conflict occurred within one's own team and within one's professional group. It often involved power struggles and rivalry, issues of who was in control, and scapegoating of colleagues. The process of scapegoating is common to dysfunctional families.[78] Caregivers who come from alcoholic backgrounds or families that were dysfunctional can easily find themselves unconsciously replicating some of these early family dynamics in the work situation.

Staff conflicts may also result from the fact that individual professionals have an urgent need to be in control of serving patients in the immediate present. Such staff feel that those in palliative care do not have the time to wait to have their needs met.[56] The interpersonal conflicts in hospice nursing are one of the four impediments to preserving one's integrity found in hospice nursing (limitations of the system, intrapersonal conflict, interpersonal conflict, characteristics of palliative care). Handling these conflicts is a part of the secondary work effort of palliative care nurses (role adaptation, intrapersonal conflict management, interpersonal conflict management) as compared with the primary work of hospice nursing (including supportive care to patients and families and facilitating the work of other professionals).[56]

Depression, grief, and guilt

Depression, grief, and guilt can come from the loss of a patient through death but can also occur through the loss of self esteem that occurs when one has not lived up to expected ideals or one has lost previously valued relationships with colleagues. In a study of 49 hospice medical directors and 36 hospice matrons, depressive symptoms were found in many caregivers studied. Of particular concern in that study was the fact that 16 per cent of the physicians reported suicidal thoughts of more than 2 weeks duration and 11 per cent of the matrons and 8 per cent of the physicians acknowledged suicidal thoughts of 2 weeks or less duration.[3]

In a Canadian study of 3352 physicians more than 36 per cent suspected they had suffered from clinical depression at some point and 15 per cent were quite sure they had. Nine per cent reported having had suicidal ideation. This was more common in females.[18]

Feelings of grief in caregivers can be manifest in:

(1) anticipatory grief when it is clear that patients will die and the caregiver begins to withdraw emotionally;

(2) denial of grief when caregivers can never let themselves show any grief over the death of patients;

(3) masked or distorted grief involving caregivers developing physical illness or engaging in acting out or risk taking behaviour;

(4) exaggerated grief involving inappropriate manifestations of grief for all or most patients who die;

(5) chronic grief in which caregivers become lost in the manifestations of grief;

(6) group grief in which most or all team members grieve for a particular patient or group of patients.

Anger, irritability, and frustration

Anger, irritability, and frustration can occur openly or in a more subtle way through put-downs or gossip about colleagues. The 'medical temper tantrum' of high achieving physicians is behaviour that becomes a norm in some settings.

Helplessness, inadequacy, and insecurity

Feelings of helplessness and insecurity may occur because of caregivers' unrealistic expectations of themselves—the need to try to be all things to all people and the often unconscious idea that death represents a medical failure. In palliative care, this latter thought may not be that death is failure, as much as it is the idea that the inability of professionals to be able to handle all physical and emotional symptoms represents a failure—a really good palliative care physician would have been able to handle these symptoms.

Symptoms and situations that left nurses feeling helpless and useless were most stressful.[25] Staff in a children's hospice experienced a sense of impotence when unable to relieve perceived needs or distress.[49] These feelings can begin to eat away at caregivers, seriously interfering with their inability to perform effectively professionally and to maintain and enjoy an outside life.

Distancing, depersonalization, and intellectualization

When caregivers are uncomfortable with the fact that patients are dying, they may find themselves avoiding the patient and family, coming in on rounds at times when patients are sleeping, and avoiding the pain of the situation by using intellectual defences. Direct observation has shown that the distancing behaviour of physicians and nurses can prevent caregivers from getting close to their patients' emotional suffering. This technique may be used to ensure the emotional survival of caregivers, but appropriate coping strategies will keep caregivers from needing to use this strategy.[79]

Errors in judgement

Errors in judgement were more frequent in younger caregivers and surprisingly were mentioned only by nurses and physicians. Such errors were often associated with fatigue or with having ambivalent feelings about the patient.

Avoidance of patients

Caregivers may also choose simply to avoid being available when patients begin to die. Patients often understand the difficulty that death involves for professionals, but they can still feel abandoned. One patient said 'Will my doctor be able to stick by me when I am dying or will he run away?'

Coping mechanisms

The introduction to this section is adapted from Vachon.[9]

Coping comprises both behavioural and cognitive strategies aimed at managing the internal and external demands of stressful transactions.[41] These efforts, directed toward mastering, reducing, or tolerating demands, may be problem-focused or emotion-focused. Problem-focused mechanisms target the environment or self for direct intervention, whereas emotion-focused strategies target negative feelings arising from stressful episodes. Rarely will one coping mode be the answer; mostly, it is a pattern that expresses a person–situation fit.

Coping can be either adaptive or maladaptive. Adaptive coping is task-oriented or goal-directed and deals with the problem or the affect (feeling) associated with the problem. Adaptive coping is an attempt to maintain an emotional and/or physiological balance called health. Maladaptive coping is more defence-oriented and focused on protection, and using these techniques predominantly can be harmful and can result in psychological or somatic disease. Maladaptive coping may include strategies such as use of drugs and alcohol, social isolation, or overuse of strategies that are normally adaptive.[17,80]

The research on coping with job stress is still limited. There have been few long-term longitudinal studies of coping. Studies have found that individual coping is repetitive regarding certain kinds of fixed stimuli but is flexible in the face of new challenges.[17] The effectiveness of strategies for handling stress and burnout have not been studied with reference to impact on performance, productivity, or client outcome.[80,81]

A sense of competence, control, and pleasure from one's work

This was the most common coping mechanism for physicians and the second most common for the group as a whole. When asked what it was that motivated them to be able to continue in their stressful jobs, caregivers would often say 'The bottom line is that I know what I am doing and I am good at it.' This sense of competence developed through a series of stages in which caregivers developed their professional skills, set goals for themselves, had frequent tests of their competence, proved their competence in many situations, learned that because they were secure in their own competence that they could share their competence with others, and eventually were able to report being comfortable living with a sense that they were competent in their work situation. Along with this sense of competence came the realization that one had a certain degree of control in one's work situation and that one could derive pleasure from work. This sense of competence, control, and pleasure in one's work is very similar to Kobasa's Hardy Personality.[35,36]

Develop control over practice

Physicians were more apt to use the coping mechanism of developing control over their clinical practice than were other health professionals. This often came with professional competence and allowed the professional to focus on a personal interest area of specialization or research. Physicians also spoke of organizing their professional day to be able to derive some pleasure for themselves. One family physician said that if he were going to see a patient with whom he had difficulty then he would book someone he enjoyed seeing as the next appointment.

Personal philosophy

A personal philosophy of illness, death, and one's role in life is essential for many caregivers. A philosophy that the author has found helpful[2] was derived from the work of Weisman. He said that when working with young medical students who were having difficulty in their role with dying patients he would tell them they should realize 'Your turn will come and it may be sooner than you think. What can you do today when it's not your turn that you hope that someone will do for you tomorrow when it may be.'

For some, a religious philosophy, centred on a commitment to serve others, may be both helpful and a key to deriving a sense of meaning in difficult times. Religion has been found helpful for a certain group of nurses.[17] However, when caregivers use their personal religious beliefs to reach out to patients this may or may not be helpful.[9,82] One's personal philosophy should be shared with patients only when it is clear that the patient wants this to occur.

Team philosophy, team support, and team building

A sense of team philosophy, team support, and team building was more important to professionals other than physicians than it was to physicians. However, it can be quite helpful when a team is clear on what it is doing, how they will do it and can support one another through personal and professional difficult times.

Regular team meetings have been found important.[49,57] Such meetings serve to set goals to accomplish the work of the team, provide a time of evaluation and reflection on the work being accomplished, and allow for shared decision making.[3] Involvement in decision making has been of greater consequence to hospice nurses than to nurses in other specialties, possibly because they needed more emotional support due to the nature of their work.[5]

Formalized ways of handling decision making

For physicians in particular, the ability to have clearly delineated team or institutional norms to give guidance when there are difficult decisions can be quite helpful. These may include protocol around discussions of 'do not resuscitate' orders with patients and families, the use of ethics committees, the fact that a physician who is caring for a dying person may not be the one to ask the family about organ donation, etc.

Staffing policies

Staffing policies that allow for adequate time off are essential. So too are policies that allow for some flexibility of movement between departments and within the organization. There should be reasonable workloads and on-calls, and avoidance of overwork.[5,12,49] There should be a work environment to stimulate the staff's own initiative,[16] which allows for shared decision-making,[5] and provides sufficient supplies, equipment,[80] and staff to do the work assigned.

Colleagues at work

Talking with colleagues at work was particularly important for those working in emergency rooms and those in oncology. To some extent it implied a sense of isolation from the team as a whole but also reflected the personal relationship that could develop between and among colleagues who trusted one another. This relationship was often with members of one's own discipline but could also involve caregivers making a special effort to develop relationships with those in other disciplines.

Support from colleagues was very important for hospice caregivers.[12,43,57,83] Support from colleagues has been found effective in dealing with work-related stress. Sixty-seven per cent of palliative care nurses used 'talking things over with a colleague' as a coping mechanism compared with 18 per cent who talked with people at home.[25] The overall mental health of hospice nurses was, in part, predicted by staff support.[5] In addition, an association has been found between support from colleagues and low burnout scores for hospice nurses, showing the value of providing staff support within the work setting.[79,84]

Leave work situation

When other coping mechanisms failed, caregivers sometimes chose to leave the work situation—either to change jobs or even, occasionally, leave the profession entirely.

Lifestyle management

Although physicians did not mention lifestyle management, this was an effective coping strategy for many other professionals. This included having outside interests,[2,80] engaging in physical activities and diversions,[2,23,57] organizing non-job-related social interaction,[43] taking time off,[24] attending to one's needs for nutrition and adequate sleep,[12] and meditation and relaxation techniques.[2]

Future research agenda

Future research questions in palliative care might include the following:

1. Does it make a difference to effective patient care whether caregivers are experiencing distress because of their work situation or home life?
2. Which types of programmes serve most effectively to buffer stress for which individuals or which types of hospice organizations?
3. What is the impact of the changing hospice environment on patients and caregivers?
4. Given the sensitivity of some hospice caregivers to work overload, how can these caregivers cope effectively with the changing hospice environment?
5. Does extra support for staff new to palliative care influence their ability to practice effectively and for a longer period?
6. What is the impact of specialist education on patient and family care and caregiver job satisfaction?

References

1. Lyall A, Vachon M, Rogers J. A study of the degree of stress experienced by professionals caring for dying patients. In: Ajemian I, Mount BM, eds. *The RVH Manual on Palliative/Hospice Care*. New York: ARNO Press, 1980: 498–508.
2. Vachon MLS. *Occupational Stress in the Care of the Critically Ill, the Dying and the Bereaved*. New York: Hemisphere Press, 1987.
3. Vachon MLS. Staff stress in hospice/palliative care: a review. *Palliative Medicine*, 1995; **9**: 91–122.
4. Finlay IG. Sources of stress in hospice medical directors and matrons. *Palliative Medicine*, 1990; **4**: 5–9.
5. Cooper CL, Mitchell S. Nursing the critically ill and dying. *Human Relations*, 1990; **43**: 297–311.
6. Bene' B, Foxall MJ. Death anxiety and job stress in hospice and medical-surgical nurses. *The Hospice Journal*, 1991; **7**: 25–41.
7. Walsh D. Palliative care: management of the patient with advanced cancer. *Seminars in Oncology*, 1994; **21** (4 Suppl 7):100–6.
8. French JRP, Rodgers W, Cobb S. Adjustment as person-environment fit. In: Coelho GV, Hamburg DA, Adams E, eds. *Coping and Adaptation*. New York: Basic Books, 1974: 316–33.
9. Vachon MLS, Stylianos SK. Caring for the caregiver: a person-centered framework. In: Baird SB, McCorkle R, Grant M, eds. *Cancer Nursing: A Comprehensive Textbook*. Philadelphia: WB Saunders Co., 1991: 1084–93.
10. Harrison RV. Person-environment fit and job stress. In: Cooper CL, Payne R, eds. *Stress at Work*. Chichester: Wiley, 1979: 175–205.
11. Antonovsky A. *Health, Stress and Coping*. San Francisco: Jossey-Bass, 1979.
12. Krikorian DA, Moser DH. Satisfactions and stresses experienced by professional nurses in hospice programs. *American Journal of Hospice Care*, 1985; **2**: 25–33.
13. Masterson-Allen S, Mor V, Laliberte L, Monteiro L. Staff burnout in a hospice setting. *The Hospice Journal*, 1985; **1**: 1–15.
14. Mor V, Laliberte L. Burnout among hospice staff. *Health and Social Work*, 1984; **9**: 274–83.
15. Barroso P, Osuna E, Luna A. Doctors' death experience and attitudes towards death, euthanasia and informing terminal patients. *Medicine and Law*, 1992; **11**: 527–33.
16. Beck-Friis B, Strang P, Sjoden P-O. Caring for severely ill cancer patients: a comparison of working conditions in hospital-based home care and in hospital. *Supportive Care in Cancer*, 1993; **1**: 145–51.
17. Heim E. Job stressors and coping in health professions. *Psychotherapy and Psychosomatics*, 1991; **55**: 90–9.
18. Cassels D. Tarnished images. *Survey 1993: The Medical Post National Survey of Canadian Doctors*. Toronto: Maclean Hunter, 1993: 8–12.
19. Cooper CL, Rout U, Faragher B. Mental health, job satisfaction, and job stress among general practitioners. *British Medical Journal*, 1989; **298**: 366–70.
20. Luna A. El consentimiento para las actuaciones medicas en los enfermos terminales. In: Luna A, ed. *El Derecho en las Fronteras de la Medicina*, 1985: 53–60.
21. Pacheco R, Osuna E, Gomez-Zapata M, Luna A. Attitudes of medical personnel (doctors and nurses) toward informing the terminal patient. *Medicine and Law*, 1989; **8**: 243–8.
22. Luna A, Caracuel MA, Valenzuela A, Osuna E. Estudio de la ansiedad 334 y de las actitudes ante la muerte y los enfermos terminales en estudiantes de enfermeria. *Folia Neuropsiquiatrica del sur y Este de Espana*, 1987; **22**: 313–20.
23. Garfield CA, Jenkins GJ. Stress and coping of volunteers counseling the dying and bereaved. *Omega*, 1981–2; **12**: 1–13.
24. Paradis LF, Miller B, Runnion VM. Volunteer stress and burnout: issues for administrators. *Hospice Journal*, 1987; **3**: 165–83.
25. Alexander DA, Ritchie E. 'Stressors' and difficulties in dealing with the terminal patient. *Journal of Palliative Care*, 1990; **6**: 28–33.
26. Vachon MLS. Motivation and stress experienced by staff working with the terminally ill. In: Davidson G, ed. *The Hospice: Development and Administration*. New York: Hemisphere, 1978: 113–22.
27. James N, Field D. The routinization of hospice: charisma and bureaucratization. *Social Science and Medicine*, 1992; **34**: 1363–75.
28. Amenta MM. Traits of hospice nurses compared with those who work in traditional settings. *Journal of Clinical Psychology*, 1984; **40**: 414–19.
29. Zerwekh J. Transcending life: the practice wisdom of nursing hospice experts. *The American Journal of Hospice and Palliative Care*, 1993; **5**: 26–31.
30. Taylor EJ, Highfield M, Amenta M. Attitudes and beliefs regarding spiritual care: a survey of cancer nurses. *Cancer Nursing*, 1994; **17**: 479–87.
31. Cassidy S. *Sharing the Darkness*. Maryknoll, NY: Orbis Books, 1991: 79.
32. Robbins RA. Death anxiety, death competency and self-actualization in hospice volunteers. *Hospice Journal*, 1991; **7**: 29–35.
33. Amenta MM, Weiner AW. Death anxiety and purpose in life and duration of service in hospice volunteers. *Psychological Report*, 1984; **54**: 979–84.
34. Murray T. The right to choose death. *The Medical Post National Survey of Canadian Doctors*. Toronto: Maclean Hunter, 1992: 103, 145.
35. Kobasa SC. Stressful life events, personality and health: an inquiry into hardiness. *Journal of Personality and Social Psychology*, 1979; **37**: 1–11.
36. Kobasa SC, Maddi SR, Courington S. Hardiness and health: a prospective study. *Journal of Parsonality and Social Psychology*, 1982; **42**: 168–77.
37. Kash KM, Holland JC. Special problems of physicians and house staff in oncology. In: Holland JC, Roland JH, eds. *Handbook of Psychooncology*. New York: Oxford University Press, 1989: 647–57.
38. Spiegel D. *Living Beyond Limits*. New York: Fawcett Columbine, 1993.
39. Gregory DR, Cotler MP. The problem of futility: III. the importance of physician-patient communication and a suggested guide through the minefield. *Cambridge Quarterly of Healthcare Ethics*, 1994; **3**: 257–69.
40. Folkman F. Personal control and stress and coping processes: a theoretical analysis. *Journal of Personality and Social Psychology*, 1984; **6**: 839–52.
41. Lazarus RS, Folkman S. *Stress, Appraisal and Coping*. New York: Springer Publishing, 1984.
42. Antonovsky A. *Unraveling the Mystery of Health*. San Francisco: Jossey-Bass, 1987.
43. Gotay CC, Crockett S, West C. Palliative home care nursing: nurses' perceptions of roles and stress. *Canada's Mental Health*, 1985; **33**: 6–9.
44. Larson DG. *The Helper's Journey*. Champaign, Ill: Research Press, 1993: 22.
45. Mallett K, Price JH, Jurs SG, Slenker S. Relationships among burnout, death anxiety, and social support in hospice and critical care nursing. *Psychological Report*, 1991; **68**: 1347–59.
46. Hayden WR. Support systems for caregivers: the physician. In: Marshall RE, Kasman C, Cape LS, eds. *Caring for Sick Newborns*. Philadelphia: Saunders, 1982: 66–81.

47. McCue JD. The effects of stress on physicians and their medical practice. *New England Journal of Medicine*, 1982; **306**: 458–63.
48. Sargent DA, Jenson VW, Petty TA, Raskin H. Preventing physician suicide. *Journal of the American Medical Association*, 1977; **237**: 143–5.
49. Woolley H, Stein A, Forrest GC, Baum JD. Staff stress and job satisfaction at a children's hospice. *Archives of Disease in Childhood*, 1989; **64**: 114–18.
50. Vachon MLS. Battle fatigue in hospice/palliative care. In: Gilmore A, Gilmore S, eds. *A Safer Death*. New York: Plenum, 1988: 149–60.
51. Ramirez AJ, Graham J, Richards MA, Cull A, Gregory WM, Leaning MS, Snashall DC, Timothy AR. Burnout and psychiatric disorder among cancer clinicians. *British Journal of Cancer*, 1995; **71**: 1263–9.
52. Fletcher WS. Doctor, am I terminal? *The American Journal of Surgery*, 1992; **163**: 460–2.
53. Hamilton CL, Neubauer BJ. Hospice nursing: serving ambivalent clients. *Nursing and Health Care*, 1989; **10**: 321–2.
54. Mount BM. Keeping the mission. *The American Journal of Hospice and Palliative Care*, 1992; **9**: 32–7.
55. Barnard D. Closing plenary session. *The Tenth International Terminal Care Conference*, Montreal, Quebec, September, 1994.
56. McWilliam CL, Burdock J, Wamsley J. The challenging experience of palliative care support-team nursing. *Oncology Nursing Forum* 1993; **20**: 770–85.
57. Munley A. Sources of hospice staff stress and how to cope with it. *Nursing Clinics of North America*, 1985; **20**: 343–55.
58. Paradis LF, Usui WM. Hospice staff and volunteers: issues for management. *Journal of Psychosocial Oncology*, 1989; 7: 121–39.
59. Power KG, Sharp GR. A comparison of sources of nursing stress and job satisfaction among mental handicap and hospice nursing staff. *Journal of Advanced Nursing*, 1988; **13**: 726–32.
60. Shepherd R. *Living with Terminal Cancer*. Toronto: Maclean Hunter, 1991.
61. Mandell H, Spiro H, eds. *When Doctors Get Sick*. New York: Plenum, 1987.
62. Weatherall DJ. The inhumanity of medicine. *British Medical Journal*, 1994; **308**: 1671–2.
63. Davis-Barron S. Cold hard death, cold hard doctors. *Canadian Medical Association Journal*, 1992; **146**: 560–3.
64. Weisman AD. Understanding the cancer patient: the syndrome of caregiver plight. *Psychiatry*, 1981; **44**: 161–8.
65. Yancik R. Sources of work stress for hospice staff. *Journal of Psychosocial Oncology*, 1984; **2**: 21–31.
66. Yancik R. Coping with hospice work stress. *J ournal of Psychosocial Oncology*, 1984; **2**: 19–35.
67. Slaby AE. Cancer's impact on caregivers. *Advances in Psychosomatic Medicine*, 1988; **18**: 135–53.
68. Field D. *Nursing the Dying*. London: Tavistock/Routledge, 1989: 30–1.
69. James N. *Care and Work in Nursing the Dying*. Ph.D. thesis. University of Aberdeen, 1986.
70. Wilkinson SM. The changing pressures for oncology nurses 1986–93. *European Journal of Cancer Care*, 1995; **4**: 69–74.
71. Weber M. *The Theory of Social and Economic Organization*. London: William Hodge, 1947.
72. Abel EK. The hospice movement: institutionalizing innovation. *International Journal of Health Services*, 1986; **16**: 71–85.
73. Seale CF. What happens in hospices: a review of research evidence. *Social Science and Medicine*, 1989; **28**: 551–9.
74. Kahn RL, Wolfe DM, Quinn RP, Snoek JD. *Organizational Stress: Studies in Role Conflict and Ambiguity*. New York: Wiley, 1981; Malabar, FL.:Kreiger, 1964.
75. French JRP. Person role fit. *Occupational Mental Health*, 1973; **3**, 15–20.
76. Mount BM, Voyer J. Staff stress in palliative/hospice care. In: Ajemian I, Mount BM, eds. *The RVH Manual on Hospice/Palliative Care*. New York: ARNO Press, 1980: 457–8.
77. Skinulus R. Change = stress. *The Medical Post National Survey of Canadian Doctors*. Toronto: Maclean Hunter, 1993: 52–5.
78. Kritsberg W. *The Adult Child of Alcoholics*. Deerfield Beach, FL.:Health Communications, 1985.
79. Maguire P. Barriers to psychological care of the dying. *British Medical Journal*, 1985; **291**: 1711–13.
80. Cohen MZ, Haberman MR, Steeves R, Deatrick JA. Rewards and difficulties of of oncology nursing. *Oncology Nursing Forum*, 1994; **21** Suppl: 9–17.
81. Delvaux N, Razavi D, Farvacques C. Cancer care—a stress for health professionals. *Social Science and Medicine*, 1988; **27**: 159–66.
82. Steeves R, Cohen, MZ, Wise CT. An analysis of critical incidents describing the essence of oncology nursing. *Oncology Nursing Forum*, 1994: **21** Suppl: 19–26.
83. Barstowe J. Stress variance in hospice nursing. *Nursing Outlook*, 1980; **28**: 751–4.
84. Bram PJ, Katz LF. Study of burnout in nurses working in hospice and hospital oncology settings. *Oncology Nursing Forum*, 1989; **16**: 555–60.

15

Psychiatric aspects of palliative care

15 Psychiatric aspects of palliative care

William Breitbart, Harvey Max Chochinov, and Steven Passik

But when the lights are out, the darkness swarms over us and talk between bed and bed is extinguished. Each of us lives in our own light, a drugged semi-sleep in which we darkly swim, sometimes floating up to the surface where the voices are . . . I can't sleep. I'm blurred, but the pain won't let me sleep.

The Stone Angel, Margaret Lawrence.

Introduction

Often, it is not death that is feared but rather the process that leads to death. Images of suffering, or dying in isolation, can be foremost on the minds of those with terminal illness. Unaddressed physical and psychiatric symptoms often interact and impact negatively on quality of life. Therefore, the prompt recognition and effective treatment of both psychiatric and physical symptoms becomes critically important to the well being of the patient with advanced disease. In general, palliative care specialists are quite expert at managing a broad spectrum of difficult and complex physical symptoms. Managing psychiatric complications (such as organic mental disorders, depression, suicide, anxiety) and difficult psychosocial issues (such as bereavement, loss, family dysfunction) facing patients with terminal illness and their families, however, can test the limits of even the most skilled and experienced palliative medicine practitioner. It is for this reason that a multidisciplinary approach to the management of the patient with advanced disease has gained broad acceptance. A psychiatrist or psychologist can play a vital role as a member of such a treatment team. This role includes the assessment and treatment of the psychiatric complications of terminal illness and the application of psychological and psychiatric techniques to the management of physical symptoms. This chapter is designed to both provide psychiatric consultants with a knowledge base specific to terminal illness, and to give the palliative medicine practitioner a framework for approaching psychiatric issues in palliative care.

Prevalence of psychiatric disorders in the terminally ill

The patient with advanced disease faces many stressors during the course of his illness, including fears of a painful death, disability, disfigurement, and dependency. While such concerns are universal, the level of psychological distress is quite variable depending on personality, coping ability, social support, and medical factors. The Psychosocial Collaborative Oncology Group determined the prevalence of psychiatric disorders seen in 215 cancer patients (ambulatory or hospitalized, with a wide range of cancer diagnoses and stages of disease) in three cancer centres utilizing the criteria from the *Diagnostic and Statistical Manual III* classification of disorders.[1] About half (53 per cent) of the patients evaluated were adjusting normally to the stresses of cancer with no diagnosable psychiatric disorder; however, 47 per cent had clinically apparent psychiatric disorders. Of the 47 per cent who had psychiatric disorders, 68 per cent had reactive anxiety and depression (adjustment disorders with depressed or anxious mood); 13 per cent had major depression; 8 per cent had an organic mental disorder (delirium).

Cancer patients with advanced disease are a particularly vulnerable group.[2–5] The incidence of pain, depression, and delirium all increase with higher levels of physical debilitation and advanced illness.[6–8] Approximately 25 per cent of all cancer patients experience severe depressive symptoms, with the prevalence increasing to 77 per cent in those with advanced illness.[7] The prevalence of organic mental disorders (delirium) among cancer patients requiring psychiatric consultation has been found to range from 25 per cent to 40 per cent and as high as 85 per cent during the terminal stages of illness.[8] Opioid analgesics such as pethidine (meperidine), levorphanol, and morphine sulphate commonly cause confusional states, particularly in the elderly and terminally ill.[9,10] Cancer patients with pain are twice as likely to develop a psychiatric complication of cancer than patients without pain. Of the patients who received a psychiatric diagnosis, 39 per cent reported significant pain. In contrast, only 19 per cent of patients without a psychiatric diagnosis had significant pain.[1] The psychiatric diagnoses of these patients with pain were predominantly adjustment disorder with depressed or mixed mood (69 per cent) and major depression in 15 per cent. This finding, of increased frequency of psychiatric disturbance in cancer patients with pain, has been reported by others including Ahles *et al.* and Woodforde.[11,]

Tross and her colleagues[13] reported the prevalence of psychiatric disorders in an ambulatory sample of 279 patients with AIDS spectrum disorders. The study included asymptomatic gay men, gay men with AIDS-related complex, and gay men with AIDS. All patients with organic mental disorders or obvious neurological impairment were excluded. Men with AIDS-related complex showed the greatest distress and frequency of psychiatric disorder. Three-quarters of the men with AIDS-related complex, one-half of the AIDS patients, and two-fifths of the asymptomatic gay men were diagnosed as having a psychiatric disorder. The most common psychiatric diagnosis was adjustment disorder, seen in two-thirds of AIDS patients and more than half of patients with AIDS-related complex. Depression was present in one-quarter of the entire study population. Patients with AIDS thus have quite comparable, if not higher, levels of psychiatric distress than cancer patients. What is striking is that levels of distress are quite high in asymptomatic gay men, and highest in those with AIDS-related complex. Presumably, these are the 'worried well' for whom waiting for a diagnosis of AIDS is more distressing than finally knowing. There is a higher prevalence of psychiatric disorders seen in homosexual men (with or without HIV infection) as compared to the heterosexual men or the general population.[14] Atkinson *et al.*[14] found that homosexual men had higher lifetime rates of substance abuse and affective and anxiety disorders than the general population that may have predated their HIV infection.

There have been several reports of psychiatric diagnoses seen in AIDS patients who were hospitalized and more seriously ill. Karina *et al.* reported that of 357 patients hospitalized with AIDS, 49 (14 per cent) had at least one psychiatric diagnosis.[15] These patients were hospitalized an average 60 days longer than AIDS patients without such psychiatric illnesses. Differences in medical morbidity could not account for the longer length of stay. Barbuto and Fleishman[16] reviewed the psychiatric consultation data collected on 65 hospital inpatients with AIDS. Psychiatric consultations were most frequently requested to evaluate depressive symptoms, suicidal risk, and behaviour related to central nervous system impairment by delirium or dementia. In this study, organic mental disorders, adjustment disorders, anxiety disorders, and affective disorders ranked in order of decreasing prevalence. Eighty per cent of AIDS patients given a functional psychiatric diagnosis had the diagnosis changed to an organic mental disorder as illness progressed and cognitive impairment became more obvious. Perry and Tross[17] reported on the prevalence of psychiatric disorders seen in medically hospitalized AIDS patients at New York Hospital. Sixty five per cent of patients were diagnosed with an organic mental disorder, and 17 per cent were diagnosed with major depression. The organic mental disorders seen were predominantly AIDS dementia complex and delirium, often in combination.

Controlling psychiatric symptoms

Anxiety in the patient with advanced illness

The terminally ill patient presents with a complex mixture of physical and psychological symptoms in the context of a frightening reality. Thus, the recognition of anxious symptoms requiring treatment can be challenging. Patients with anxiety complain of tension or restlessness, or they exhibit jitteriness, autonomic hyperactivity, vigilance, insomnia, distractibility, shortness of breath, numbness, apprehension, worry, or rumination. Often the physical or somatic manifestations of anxiety overshadow the psychological or cognitive ones, and are the symptoms that the patient most often presents.[18] The consultant must use these symptoms as a cue to inquire about the patient's psychological state, which is commonly one of fear, worry, or apprehension. The assumption that a high level of anxiety is inevitably encountered during the terminal phase of illness is neither helpful nor accurate for diagnostic and treatment purposes. In deciding whether to treat anxiety during the terminal phase of illness, the patient's subjective level of distress is the primary impetus for the initiation of treatment. Other considerations include problematic patient behaviour such as non-compliance due to anxiety, family and staff reactions to the patient's distress, and the balancing of the risks and benefits of treatment.[19]

Anxiety, like fever, is a symptom in this population that can have many aetiologies. Anxiety may be encountered as a component of an adjustment disorder, panic disorder, generalized anxiety disorder, phobia, or agitated depression. Additionally, in the terminally ill cancer patient, symptoms of anxiety are most likely to arise from some medical complication of the illness or treatment such as organic anxiety disorder, delirium, or other organic mental disorders.[6,18,19] Hypoxia, sepsis, poorly controlled pain, and adverse drug reactions such as akathisia or withdrawal states are specific entities which often present as anxiety. Patients who have been managed for long periods of time with relatively high doses of benzodiazepines or opioid analgesics for the control of anxiety or pain often become tolerant or physically dependent upon these drugs. During the terminal phase of illness, when patients become less alert, there is a tendency to minimize the use of sedating medications. It is important to consider the need to slowly taper benzodiazepines and opioid analgesics in order to prevent acute withdrawal states. Withdrawal states in terminally ill patients often present first as agitation or anxiety and become clinically evident days later than might be expected in younger, healthier patients due to impaired metabolism. Benzodiazepine withdrawal, for example, can present first as agitation or anxiety, though the diagnosis is often missed in terminally ill patients, and especially the elderly, where physiological dependence on these medications is often unrecognized.[20] In the dying patient, anxiety can represent impending cardiac or respiratory arrest, pulmonary embolism, electrolyte imbalance, or dehydration.[21]

Despite the fact that anxiety in terminal illness commonly results from medical complications, it is important not to forget that psychological factors related to death and dying or existential issues play a role in anxiety, particularly in patients who are alert and not confused.[18] Patients frequently fear the isolation and separation of death. Claustrophobic patients may be afraid of the idea of being confined and buried in a coffin. These issues can be disconcerting to consultants who may find themselves at a loss for words that are consoling to the patient. Nonetheless, one should not avoid eliciting these concerns, listening empathically to them, and enlisting pastoral involvement where appropriate.

The specific treatment of anxiety in the terminally ill often depends on aetiology, presentation, and setting. An example of how the specific aetiology of the anxious symptom is important is the case of hypoxia. Anxiety associated with hypoxia and dyspnoea in a patient with diffuse lung metastases is most responsive to treatment with oxygen and opioid analgesics. If the same patient's presentation included hallucinations and agitation, a neuroleptic would be added to the regimen. In the hospital setting, an arterial blood gas can confirm the diagnosis of hypoxia. However, the good clinician caring for the terminally ill patient at home may conclude, on clinical grounds, that hypoxia is present and therefore would treat anxiety associated with it in an identical fashion to that in the hospital. An arterial blood gas provides confirmatory information but is not essential to considering and treating hypoxia and so may be unnecessary when attempting to maximize the patient's comfort.

Table 1 Anxiolytic medications used in patients with advanced disease

	Generic name	Approximate daily dosage range (mg)	Route[a]
Benzodiazepines			
	Very short-acting		
	midazolam	10–60 per 24 h	IV, SC
	Short-acting		
	alprazolam	0.25–2.0 t.i.d.–q.i.d.	PO, SL
	oxazepam	10–15 t.i.d.–q.i.d.	PO
	lorazepam	0.5–2.0 t.i.d.–q.i.d.	PO, SL, IV, IM
	Intermediate acting		
	chlordiazepoxide	10–50 t.i.d.–q.i.d.	PO, IM
	Long acting		
	diazepam	5–10 bid–q.i.d.	PO, IM, IV, PR
	clorazepate	7.5–15 bid–q.i.d.	PO
	clonazepam	0.5–2 bid–q.i.d.	PO
Non-benzodiazepines			
	buspirone	5–20 t.i.d.	PO
Neuroleptics			
	haloperidol	0.5–5 q.2–12 h	PO, IV, SC, IM
	methotrimeprazine	10–20 q.4–8 h	IV, SC, PO
	thioridazine	10–75 t.i.d.–q.i.d.	PO
	chlorpromazine	12.5–50 q.4–12 h	PO, IM, IV
Antihistamine			
	hydroxyzine	25–50 q4–6 h	PO, IV, SC
Tricyclic antidepressants			
	imipramine	12.5–150 h	PO, IM
	clomipramine	10–150 h	PO

[a] PO, peroral; IM, intramuscular; PR, per rectum; IV, intravenous; SC, subcutaneous; SL, sublingual; b.i.d., two times a day; t.i.d., three times a day; q.i.d., four times a day. Parenteral doses are generally twice as potent as oral doses, intravenous bolus injections or infusions should be administered slowly.

Pharmacological treatment of anxiety in the terminally ill

The pharmacotherapy of anxiety in terminal illness (see Table 1) involves the judicious use of the following classes of medications: benzodiazepines, neuroleptics, antihistamines, antidepressants, and opioid analgesics.[6,18,19,22]

Benzodiazepines

Benzodiazepines are the mainstay of the pharmacological treatment of anxiety in the terminally ill cancer patient. The shorter acting benzodiazepines, such as lorazepam, alprazolam, and oxazepam, are safest in this population. The selection of these drugs avoids toxic accumulation due to impaired metabolism in debilitated individuals.[23]

Lorazepam, oxazepam, and temazepam are metabolized by conjugation in the liver and are therefore safest in patients with hepatic disease. This is in contrast to alprazolam and other benzodiazepines which are metabolized through oxidative pathways in the liver that are more vulnerable to interference resulting from hepatic damage. The disadvantage of using short-acting benzodiazepines is that patients often experience breakthrough anxiety or end-of-dose failure. Such patients benefit from switching to longer-acting benzodiazepines such as diazepam or clonazepam. Dying patients often benefit from parenteral administration of these drugs. Common dosage regimens include: lorazepam 0.5 to 2.0 mg, sublingual peroral, intravenous, intramuscular, or subcutaneous administration, every 3 to 6 h; alprazolam 0.25 to 1.0 mg, administered perorally, three to four times a day; diazepam 2.5 to 10 mg, peroral, per rectum, or intravenous administration every 3 to 6 h; clonazepam 0.5 to 2 mg, administered perorally, two to three times a day. Dying patients can be administered diazepam rectally when no other route is available, with dosages equivalent to oral regimens. Rectal diazepam[24] has been used widely in the palliative care field to control anxiety, restlessness, and agitation associated with the final days of life.

Midazolam, a very short-acting, water-soluble benzodiazepine, is usually administered as an intravenous infusion in critical care settings where sedation is the goal in an agitated or anxious patient on a respirator. Midazolam may also prove useful in controlling anxiety and agitation in the terminal phases of illness.[25, 26]Unlike diazepam, midazolam has a short duration of action and seems to be less irritating to subcutaneous tissues when given by subcutaneous infusion. Since it is several times as potent as diazepam, starting doses should be low and careful monitoring of effects should be initiated. Doses ranging from 10 to 60 mg/day have been found to be safe and effective for most patients. However, doses as high as 125 mg/day have been reported.[27] Clonazepam, a longer-acting benzodiazepine, has been found to be extremely useful in the palliative care setting for the treatment of anxiety, depersonalization, or derealization in patients with seizure disorders, brain tumours, and mild organic mental disorders. Patients who experience end of dose failure with recurrence of anxiety on shorter-acting drugs also find clonazepam helpful. It is not uncommon to switch patients from alprazolam to clonazepam when attempting to taper off alprazolam. Clonazepam is also useful in patients with organic mood disorders who have symptoms of mania, and as an adjuvant analgesic in patients with neuropathic pain.[28–30]

Fears of causing respiratory depression should not prevent the clinician from using adequate dosages of benzodiazepines to control anxiety. The likelihood of respiratory depression is minimized when one utilizes shorter-acting drugs, increases the dosages in small increments, and ultimately switches to longer-acting drugs.

Non-benzodiazepine anxiolytics

Neuroleptics, such as thioridazine and haloperidol, are useful in the treatment of anxiety when benzodiazepines are not sufficient for symptom control.[19] They are also indicated when an organic aetiology is suspected or when psychotic symptoms such as delusions or hallucinations accompany the anxiety. Typically, haloperidol (0.5–5 mg peroral, intravenous, or subcutaneous administration, every 2–12 h) is sufficient to control anxious symptoms and avoid excessive sedation. Low potency neuroleptics such as thioridazine (10–75 mg, peroral administration, three times a day) are effective anxiolytics and can help with insomnia and agitation. Neuroleptics are perhaps the safest class of anxiolytics in patients where there is legitimate concern regarding respiratory depression or compromise. Methotrimeprazine (10–20 mg, every 4–8 h, intramuscular, intravenous, or subcutaneous administration) is a phenothiazine with unique analgesic and anxiolytic properties that is often used for the treatment of pain and anxiety in the dying patient.[31, 32]Its side-effects include sedation, anticholinergic symptoms, and hypotension. Intravenous administration by slow infusion is preferable to avoid problems with hypotension. Chlorpromazine (12.5–50 mg, peroral, intramuscular, or intravenous administration, every 4–12 h) has similar side-effects that limit its application in this setting. However, it can be useful in patients where sedation is desirable. With this class of drugs in general, one must be aware of extrapyramidal side-effects (particularly when patients are taking additional neuroleptics for antiemetic purposes) and the remote possibility of neuroleptic malignant syndrome. Tardive dyskinesia is rarely a concern given the generally short-term usage and low dosages of these medications in this population.[33]

Hydroxyzine is an antihistamine with mild anxiolytic, sedative and analgesic properties. It is particularly useful when treating anxious, terminally ill cancer patients with pain. A dose of 100 mg of hydroxyzine given parenterally has analgesic potency equivalent to 8 mg of morphine and potentiates the analgesic effects of morphine.[34] As an anxiolytic, 25 to 50 mg of hydroxyzine every 4 to 6 h peroral, intravenous, or subcutaneous administration is effective.

Tricyclic, heterocyclic, and second generation antidepressants are the most effective treatment for anxiety accompanying depression and are helpful in treating panic disorder.[35,36,37] Guidelines for their use are discussed in the section on depression below. Their usefulness is often limited in the dying patient due to anticholinergic and sedative side-effects. Very often the consultant is faced with the task of relieving symptoms in a short period of time and so drugs that require a period of weeks to achieve therapeutic effect are unsatisfactory.

Opioid analgesics are primarily indicated for the control of pain. However, these drugs are also effective in the relief of dyspnoea due to cardiopulmonary processes and the anxiety associated with them.[38] Opioid drugs are particularly useful in the treatment of dying patients who are in respiratory distress. Continuous intravenous or subcutaneous infusions of morphine or other opioid analgesics allow for careful titration and control of respiratory distress, anxiety, pain, and agitation.[39] Occasionally, one must maintain the patient in a state of unresponsiveness in order to maximize comfort. When respiratory distress is not a major problem, it is preferable to use the opioid drugs solely for analgesic purposes and to add more specific anxiolytics (such as the benzodiazepines) to control concomitant anxiety.

Buspirone, is a non-benzodiazepine anxiolytic that is useful along with psychotherapy in patients with chronic anxiety or anxiety related to adjustment disorders. The onset of anxiolytic action is delayed in comparison to the benzodiazepines, taking 5 to 10 days for relief of anxiety to begin. Since buspirone is not a benzodiazepine, it will not block benzodiazepine withdrawal, and so one must be cautious when switching from a benzodiazepine to buspirone. The effective dose of buspirone is 10 mg orally, three times a day.[40] Because of its delayed onset of action and indication for use in chronic anxiety states, buspirone may be of limited usefulness to the clinician treating anxiety and agitation in the terminally ill.

Non-pharmacological treatment of anxiety in terminally ill patients

Non-pharmacological interventions for anxiety and distress include supportive psychotherapy and behavioural interventions which are used alone or in combination. Brief supportive psychotherapy is often useful in dealing with both crisis-related issues as well as existential issues confronted by the terminally ill.[41] Psychotherapeutic interventions should include both the patient and family, particularly as the patient with advanced illness becomes increasingly debilitated and less able to interact. Mental health professionals can assist in seeing that the emotional needs of patients and families are met during the terminal phase of illness. Such needs include continuous, updated information regarding the disease status and treatment options available. This information must be delivered repeatedly and with sensitivity as to what they are currently prepared and able to hear and absorb. Families, especially, require a great deal of reassurance that they and the medical staff have done everything possible for the patient. The goals of psychotherapy with the patient are to establish a bond that decreases the sense of isolation experienced with terminal illness; to help the patient face death with a sense of self-worth; to correct misconceptions about the past and present; to integrate the present illness into a continuum of life experiences; and to explore issues of separation, loss, and the unknown that lies ahead. The therapist should emphasize past strengths and support previously successful ways of coping. This helps the patient mobilize inner resources, modify plans for the future, and perhaps even accept the inevitability of death.

It is during the terminal phase of illness that we have the

greatest opportunity to affect the process of adaptation to loss. Mental health professionals must extend their supportive stance to include both the patient and family. Anticipatory bereavement is a common experience which allows patients, loved ones, and health-care providers the opportunity to mentally prepare for the impending death. Patients and family members should be encouraged to use this period to reconcile differences, extend important final communications, and reaffirm feelings and wishes. It is a time of vital importance that can often set the tone for the subsequent bereavement course.[42]

Relaxation, guided imagery, and hypnosis may help reduce anxiety and thereby increase the patient's sense of control. Most patients with advanced illness are still appropriate candidates for useful application of behavioural techniques despite physical debilitation. In assessing the utility of such interventions for a terminally ill patient, the clinician should, however, take into account the mental clarity of the patient. Confusional states interfere dramatically with a patient's ability to focus attention and thus limit the usefulness of these techniques.[2] Occasionally these techniques can be modified so as to include even mildly cognitive-impaired patients. This often involves the therapist taking a more active role by orienting the patient, creating a safe and secure environment, and evoking a conditioned response to the therapist's voice or presence. A typical behavioural intervention for anxiety in a terminally ill patient would include a relaxation exercise combined with some distraction or imagery technique. Typically, the patient is first taught to relax with passive breathing accompanied by either passive or active muscle relaxation. Once in such a relaxed state, the patient is taught a pleasant, distracting imagery exercise. In a randomized study comparing a relaxation technique with alprazolam in the treatment of anxiety and distress in non-terminally ill cancer patients, both treatments were demonstrated to be quite effective for mild to moderate degrees of anxiety or distress. The drug intervention (alprazolam) was more effective for greater levels of distress or anxiety and had a more rapid onset of beneficial effect.[43] Relaxation techniques can be prescribed concurrently with anxiolytic medications in highly anxious cancer patients.

Depression in patients with advanced illness

The incidence of depression in cancer patients ranges from 10 to 25 per cent and increases with higher levels of disability, advanced illness, and pain.[7,44,45] Certain types of cancer are associated with an increased incidence of depression. Patients with pancreatic cancer, for example, are more likely to develop depression than patients with other types of intra-abdominal malignancies.[46,47] The somatic symptoms of depression, for example anorexia, insomnia, fatigue, and weight loss, can be unreliable and lack specificity in the cancer patient.[48] Thus, the psychological symptoms of depression take on greater diagnostic value and include the following: dysphoric mood, hopelessness, worthlessness, guilt, and suicidal ideation.[7,44,45,48] Chochinov *et al.*[5] studied the prevalence of depression in a cohort of 130 terminally ill patients in a palliative care facility. They reported that 9.2 per cent met research diagnostic criteria for major depression when using high-severity thresholds for research diagnostic criteria A symptoms (equivalent to the symptom threshold judgements specified in the *Diagnostic and Statistical Manual* IV).

Table 2 Endicott substitution criteria[48]

Physical/somatic symptom	Psychological symptom substitute
1. Change in appetite, weight	1. Tearfulness, depressed appearance
2. Sleep disturbance	2. Social withdrawal, decreased talkativeness
3. Fatigue, loss of energy	3. Brooding, self-pity, pessimism
4. Diminished ability to think or concentrate, indecisiveness	4. Lack of reactivity

This approach yielded the identical prevalence of major depression whether or not one included somatic symptoms in the diagnostic criteria or used Endicott revised criteria[48] (involving replacement of somatic symptoms with non-somatic alternatives—see Table 2). While concern has been raised about the non-specificity of somatic symptoms in the medically ill, these results—along with those of other recent investigations[49,50]—indicate that their inclusion may not overly influence the diagnostic classification of major depression.

Family history of depression and history of previous depressive episodes further suggest the reliability of a diagnosis. Evaluation of cancer-related organic factors, such as corticosteroids,[51] chemotherapeutic agents [52–55] (vincristine, vinblastine, asparaginase, intrathecal methotrexate, interferon, interleukin), amphotericin,[56] whole brain radiation,[57] central nervous system metabolic-endocrine complications,[58] and paraneoplastic syndromes [59,60] that can present as depression must precede initiation of treatment.

Assessment of depression in the terminally ill

Depressed mood and sadness can be appropriate responses as the terminally ill patient faces death. These emotions can be manifestations of anticipatory grief over the impending loss of one's life, health, loved ones, and autonomy. The diagnosis of a major depressive syndrome in a terminally ill patient often relies more on the psychological or cognitive symptoms of major depression (worthlessness, hopelessness, excessive guilt, and suicidal ideation), rather than the neurovegetative or somatic signs and symptoms of major depression.[44,45,48] The presence of neurovegetative signs and symptoms of depression, such as fatigue, loss of energy, and other somatic symptoms, is often not helpful in establishing a diagnosis of depression in the terminally ill. Terminal illness itself can produce many of these physical symptoms so characteristic of major depression in the physically healthy. The strategy of relying on the psychological or cognitive signs and symptoms of depression for diagnostic specificity is itself not without problems. How is the clinician to interpret feelings of hopelessness in the dying patient when there is no hope for cure or recovery? Feelings of hopelessness, worthlessness, or suicidal ideation must be explored in detail. While many dying patients lose hope of a cure, they are able to maintain hope for better symptom control. For many patients hope is contingent on the ability to find continued meaning in their day-to-day existence. Hopelessness that is pervasive, and accompanied by a sense of despair or despondency, is more likely to represent a symptom of a depressive disorder.[44] Similarly, patients often state that they feel they are burdening their families unfairly, causing them great pain and inconvenience. Those beliefs are less likely to represent a symptom of depression than if the patient feels that their life has never had any worth, or that they are being punished for evil things they have done. Suicidal ideation, even rather mild and passive forms, is very likely to be associated with significant degrees of depression in terminally ill cancer patients.[61,62]

Management of depression in the terminally ill

Depression in cancer patients with advanced disease is optimally managed by utilizing a combination of supportive psychotherapy, cognitive-behavioural techniques, and antidepressant medications.[44] Psychotherapy and cognitive behavioural techniques are useful in the management of psychological distress in cancer patients, and have been applied to the treatment of depressive and anxious symptoms related to cancer and cancer pain. Psychotherapeutic interventions, either in the form of individual or group counselling, have been shown to reduce effectively psychological distress and depressive symptoms in cancer patients.[63,64,41] Cognitive-behavioural interventions, such as relaxation and distraction with pleasant imagery, have also been shown to decrease depressive symptoms in patients with mild to moderate levels of depression.[43] Psychopharmacological interventions (i.e., antidepressant medications, see Table 3), however, are the mainstay of management in the treatment of cancer patients with severe depressive symptoms who meet criteria for a major depressive episode.[44] The efficacy of antidepressants in the treatment of depression in cancer patients has been well established.[36,44,65–67]

Table 3 Antidepressant medications used in patients with advanced disease (adopted from reference 44)

	Generic name	Approximate daily dosage range (mg)	Route[a]
Tricyclic antidepressants			
	amitriptyline	10–150	PO, IM, PR
	doxepin	12.5–150	PO, IM
	imipramine	12.5–150	PO, IM
	desipramine	12.5–150	PO, IM
	nortriptyline	10–125	PO
	clomipramine	10–150	PO
Second generation antidepressants			
	bupropion	200–450	PO
	fluoxetine	10–60	PO
	paroxetine	10–60	PO
	fluvoxamine	50–300	PO
	sertraline	50–200	PO
	nefazodone	100–500	PO
	venlafaxine	37.5–225	PO
	trazodone	25–300	PO
Heterocyclic antidepressants			
	maprotiline	50–75	PO
	amoxapine	100–150	PO
Monoamine oxidase inhibitors			
	isocarboxazid	20–40	PO
	phenelzine	30–60	PO
	tranylcypromine	20–40	PO
	meclobomide	150–600	PO
Psychostimulants			
	dextroamphetamine	2.5–20 b.i.d.	PO
	methylphenidate	2.5–20 b.i.d.	PO
	pemoline	37.5–75 b.i.d.	PO, SL[b]
Benzodiazepines			
	alprazolam	0.25–2.0 t.i.d.	PO
Lithium carbonate		600–1200	PO

[a] PO, peroral; IM, intramuscular; PR, per rectum; b.i.d., two times a day; t.i.d., three times a day; intravenous infusions of a number of tricyclic antidepressants are utilized outside of the United States. This route is, however, not FDA approved.

[b] Comes in chewable tablet form that can be absorbed without swallowing.

Pharmacological treatment of depression in the terminally ill

Any treatment for major depression in the terminally ill will be less effective if given in a context devoid of psychotherapeutic support. Although both psychotherapy and cognitive behavioural therapy have proven effective in reducing psychological distress and mild to moderate depressive symptomatology in the cancer setting, pharmacotherapy is the mainstay for treating terminally ill patients meeting diagnosis criteria for major depression.[44] Factors such as prognosis and the time-frame for treatment may play an important role in determining the type of pharmacotherapy for depression. A depressed patient with several months of life expectancy can afford to wait the 2–4 weeks it may take to respond to a tricyclic antidepressant. The depressed dying patient with less than 3 weeks to live may do best with a rapid acting psychostimulant.[9] Patients who are within hours to days of death and in distress are likely to benefit most from the use of sedatives or opioid analgesic infusions.

Tricyclic antidepressants

Tricyclic antidepressants have been the cornerstone for treating depression in the general cancer setting since the early 1960s. Their application specifically to the terminally ill, however, requires a careful risk–benefit ratio analysis. Although nearly 70 per cent of patients treated with a tricyclic for non-psychotic depression can anticipate a positive response, these medications are associated with a side-effect profile which can be particularly troublesome for terminally ill patients.[68] They have multiple pharmacodynamic actions accounting for these side effects including blockade of muscarinic cholinergic receptors, alpha-adrenoceptor blockade, and H_1 histamine receptor blockade. The tertiary amines (amitriptyline, doxepin, imipramine) have a greater propensity to cause side-effects than do secondary amines (nortriptyline, desipramine).[69] The secondary amines are, thus, often a preferable choice for the terminally ill.

The anticholinergic side-effects can include constipation, dry mouth, and urinary retention. To avoid exacerbating symptoms associated with genitourinary outlet obstruction, decreased gastric motility, or stomatitis a relatively non-anticholinergic tricyclic, such as desipramine or nortriptyline, is a reasonable choice. Those patients who are receiving medication with anticholinergic properties (such as pethidine, atropine, diphenhydramine, or phenothiazines) are at risk of developing an anticholinergic delirium, and thus antidepressants which are potently anticholinergic should be avoided.[70] The anticholinergic actions of tricyclic antidepressants can also cause serious tachycardia which can be problematic for terminally ill patients with cardiac insufficiency. The quinidine like effects of tricyclic antidepressants can also lead to arrhythmias by virtue of their ability to delay conduction via the His–Purkinje system [71] (associated with non-specific ST–T changes and T waves on the electrocardiograph). These effects are particularly concerning for those terminally ill patients with pre-existing conduction defects, especially second or third degree heart block.

Alpha$_1$-blockade is associated with postural hypotension and dizziness. This can be of particular concern for the frail, volume depleted patient who, because of these side-effects, is at risk for falls and possible fractures. Nortriptyline and protriptyline are the tricyclic antidepressants least associated with alpha$_1$-blockade. H$_1$ histamine receptor blockage is associated with sedation and drowsiness.

For dying patients already exposed to a variety of sedating agents (e.g. opioid analgesics, antiemetics, anxiolytics, and neuroleptics) tricyclic antidepressants such as amitriptyline and doxepin are the most likely to accentuate the overall cumulative sedating effects of these medications.

Tricyclic antidepressants should be started at low doses (10–25 mg at bed time) and increased in 10 to 25 mg increments every 2 to 4 days, until a therapeutic dose is attained or side-effects become a dose limiting factor. Depressed cancer patients often achieve a therapeutic response at significantly lower doses of tricyclic antidepressants (25–125 mg) than are necessary in the physically well (150–300 mg).[44] There is also evidence to suggest that patients with advanced cancer achieve higher serum tricyclic levels at modest doses.[72] In order to minimize drug toxicity and more carefully guide the process of drug titration, prescribing tricyclics (desipramine, nortriptyline, amitriptyline, imipramine) with well established therapeutic plasma levels may be advantageous.[73] Desipramine and nortriptyline are generally better tolerated in this population than amitriptyline or imipramine.

The choice of which specific tricyclic antidepressant to use depends on a variety of factors including the nature of the underlying terminal medical condition, the characteristics of the depressive episode, past responses to antidepressant therapy, and the specific drug side-effect profile. Those patients who present with agitation and insomnia may respond favourably to more sedating tricyclics (amitriptyline, doxepin). For the terminally ill depressed patient, the choice of tricyclic antidepressant is made on the basis of a side-effect profile which will be least incompatible with the patient's overall medical condition. Most tricyclics are available as rectal suppositories for patients who are no longer able to take medication orally. Outside of the United States, certain tricyclics are given as intravenous infusion.[74] Although not very practical, amitriptyline, imipramine, and doxepin can also be given intramuscularly.[9,44]

It must be borne in mind that a therapeutic response to tricyclic antidepressants (as with all antidepressants) has a latency time of 2–4 weeks. For the terminally ill, depressed patient whose life expectancy is anticipated to be less than this, psychostimulants may offer a more viable, rapid response alternative.

Second generation antidepressants[75]

Newer antidepressant agents, often with fewer side-effects and simplified dosage regimens have become available and may have important applications in the treatment of depression in patients with advanced disease. Among these agents are the selective serotonin reuptake inhibitors (SSRIs) and serotonin-noradrenaline reuptake inhibitors.

Selective serotonin reuptake inhibitors (SSRIs) The SSRIs are a recent important addition to the available antidepressant medications. They have been found to be as effective in the treatment of depression as the tricyclics[76] and have a number of features which may be particularly advantageous for the terminally ill. The SSRIs have a very low affinity for adrenergic, cholinergic, and histamine receptors and this accounts for negligible orthostatic hypotension, urinary retention, memory impairment, sedation, or reduced awareness.[77] They have not been found to cause clinically significant alterations in cardiac conduction and are, in general, favourably tolerated along with a wider margin of safety than the tricyclic antidepressants in the event of an overdose. They do not, therefore, require therapeutic drug level monitoring.

Most of the side-effects of SSRIs result from their selective central and peripheral serotonin reuptake. These include increased intestinal motility (loose stools, nausea, vomiting, insomnia, headaches, and sexual dysfunction). Some patients may experience anxiety, tremor, restlessness, and akathisia (the latter is relatively rare but it can be problematic for the terminally ill patient with Parkinson's disease).[78] These side-effects tend to be dose related and may be problematic for patients with advanced disease.

There are five SSRIs currently being marketed including sertraline, fluoxetine, paroxetine, nefazodone, and fluvoxamine. With the exception of fluoxetine, whose elimination half-life is 2 to 4 days, the SSRIs have an elimination half-life of about 24 h. Fluoxetine is the only SSRI with a potent active metabolite—norfluoxetine—whose elimination half-life is 7 to 14 days. Fluoxetine can cause mild nausea and a brief period of increased anxiety as well as appetite suppression that usually lasts for a period of several weeks. Some patients can experience transient weight loss but weight usually returns to baseline level. The anorectic properties of fluoxetine has not been a limiting factor in the use of this drug in cancer patients. Fluoxetine and norfluoxetine do not reach a steady state for 5 to 6 weeks, compared with 4 to 14 days for paroxetine, fluvoxamine, and sertraline. These difference are important, especially for the terminally patient in whom a switch from an SSRI to another antidepressant is being considered. If a switch to a monamine oxidase inhibitor is required, the washout period for fluoxetine will be at least 5 weeks given the potential drug interactions between these two agents. Since fluoxetine has entered the market, there have been several reports of significant drug-drug interactions.[79,80] Until it has been studied further in the medically ill, it should be used cautiously in the debilitated dying patient. Paroxetine, fluvoxamine and sertraline on the other hand require considerably shorter washout periods (10–14 days) under similar circumstances.

All the SSRIs have the ability to inhibit the hepatic isoenzyme P450 11D6, with sertraline (and according to some sources, fluvoxamine) being least potent in this regard. This is important with respect to dose/plasma level ratios and drug interactions, since the SSRIs are dependent upon hepatic metabolism. For the elderly patient with advanced disease, the dose response curve for sertraline appears to be relatively linear. On the other hand, particularly for paroxetine (which appears to most potently inhibit the hepatic isoenzyme of cytochrome P450 11D6), small dosage increases can result in dramatic elevations in plasma levels. Paroxetine, and to a somewhat lesser extent fluoxetine, appear to inhibit the hepatic enzymes responsible for their own clearance.[81] The coadministration of these medications with other drugs that are dependent on this enzyme system for their catabolism (e.g., tricyclics, phenothiazines, type IC antiarrhythmics, and quinidine) should be done cautiously. Luvox has been shown, in some instances, to elevate the blood levels of propranolol and warfarin by as much as two fold and, thus, should not be prescribed together with these agents.

SSRIs can generally be started at their minimally effective doses. For the terminally ill, this usually means initiating therapy at approximately half the usual starting dose used in an otherwise healthy patient. For fluoxetine, patients can begin on 5 mg (available in liquid form) given once daily (preferably in the morning) with a range of 10 to 40 mg/day; given its long half-life, some patients may only require this drug every second day. Paroxetine can be started at 10 mg once daily (either morning or evening) for the patient with advanced disease, and has a therapeutic range of 10 to 40 mg/day. Fluvoxamine, which tends to be somewhat more sedating, can be started at 25 mg (in the evenings) and has a therapeutic range of 50 to 300 mg. Sertraline can be initiated at 50 mg, morning or evening, and titrated within a range of 50 to 200 mg/day. Nefazodone can be started at 50 mg twice per day and titrated within a range of 100 to 500 mg/day. If patients experience activating effects on SSRIs, they should not be given at bedtime but rather moved earlier into the day. Gastrointestinal upset can be reduced by ensuring the patient does not take medication on an empty stomach.

Serotonin-noradrenaline reuptake inhibitor (SNRI) Venlaflaxine (Effexor) is the only antidepressant in this class and was just recently released on the market. It is a potent inhibitor of neuronal serotonin and noradrenaline reuptake and appears to have no significant affinity for muscarinic, histamine, or alpha1-adrenergic receptors. Some patients may experience a modest, sustained increase in blood pressure, especially at doses above the recommended initiating dose. Compared with the SSRIs, its protein binding (<35 per cent) is very low. Few drug interactions induced by protein binding are, thus, expected. Like other antidepressants, venlaflaxine should not be used in patients receiving monoamine oxidase inhibitors. Its side-effect profile tends to generally be well tolerated with few discontinuations. While there is currently no data addressing its use in the terminally ill depressed patient, its pharmacokinetic properties and side-effect profile suggest it may have a role to play.

Trazodone If given in sufficient doses (100–300 mg/day), trazodone can be an effective antidepressant. Although its anticholinergic profile is almost negligible, it has considerable affinity for alpha1-adrenoceptors and may thus predispose patients to orthostatic hypotension and its problematic sequelae (i.e. falls, fractures, and head injuries). Trazodone is very sedating and in low doses (100 mg at bedtime) it is helpful in the treatment of the depressed cancer patient with insomnia. It is highly serotonergic and its use should be considered when the patient requires an adjuvant effect in addition to antidepressant effects. Trazodone has little effect on cardiac conduction but can cause arrhythmias in patients with premorbid cardiac disease.[82] Trazodone has also been associated with priapism and should thus be used with caution in male patients.[83] It is highly sedating with drowsiness being its most common adverse side-effect. In smaller doses it can, thus, be used as an effective sedative hypnotic.

Bupropion Bupropion is a relatively new drug in the United States and there has not been much experience with its use in the medically ill. At present, it is not the first drug of choice for depressed patients with cancer. However, one might consider prescribing bupropion if patients have a poor response to a reasonable trial of other antidepressants. Bupropion may have a role in the treatment of the psychomotor retarded, depressed, terminally ill patient as it has energizing effects similar to the stimulant drugs.[84,85] However, because of the increased incidence of seizures in patients with central nervous system disorders, bupropion has a limited role in the oncology population.

Heterocyclic antidepressants

The heterocyclic antidepressants have side-effect profiles that are similar to the tricyclic antidepressants. Maprotiline should be avoided in patients with brain tumours and in those who are at risk for seizures since the incidence of seizures is increased with this medication.[86] Amoxapine has mild dopamine-blocking activity. Hence, patients who are taking other dopamine blockers (e.g. antiemetics) have an increased risk of developing extrapyramidal symptoms and dyskinesias.[87] Mianserin (not available in the United States) is a serotonergic antidepressant with adjuvant analgesic properties that is used widely in Europe and Latin America. Costa and colleagues [67] showed mianserin to be a safe and effective drug for the treatment of depression in cancer.

Psychostimulants

The psychostimulants (dextroamphetamine, methylphenidate, and pemoline) offer an alternative and effective pharmacological approach to the treatment of depression in the terminally ill.[88–95] These drugs have a more rapid onset of action than the tricyclics and are often energizing. They are most helpful in the treatment of depression in cancer patients with advanced disease and those where dysphoric mood is associated with severe psychomotor slowing and even mild cognitive impairment. While psychostimulants have been demonstrated to be effective antidepressants in the medically ill as single-agent therapies, many clinicians occasionally employ combination therapy (e.g. psychostimulants in combination with a more traditional antidepressant such as one of the SSRI agents). One common clinical practice is to start a psychostimulant and an SSRI (in low dose) simultaneously, and then begin to withdraw the stimulant as one titrates the dose of the SSRI. The rationale of such a strategy is to obtain immediate antidepressant effects from the psychostimulant, allowing for a period of 1 to 2 weeks for the SSRI to begin to work. Also, occasionally psychostimulants may be used to augment the antidepressant effects of more traditional antidepressants such as the SSRIs. Such combination therapies must be used with caution and frequent monitoring for cumulative or synergistic side-effects related to elevated levels of serotonin or noradrenaline (e.g. anxiety, palpitations, hypertension, tremor, flushing). Psychostimulants have been shown to improve attention, concentration, and overall performance on neuropsychological testing in the medically ill.[96] In relatively low dose, psychostimulants stimulate appetite, promote a sense of well being, and improve feelings of weakness and fatigue in cancer patients. Treatment with dextroamphetamine or methylphenidate usually begins with a dose of 2.5 mg at 8:00 a.m. and at noon. The dosage is slowly increased over several days until a desired effect is achieved or side-effects (overstimulation, anxiety, insomnia, paranoia, confusion) intervene. Typically a dose greater than 30 mg/day is not necessary, although occasionally patients require up to 60 mg/day. Patients usually are maintained on methylphenidate for 1 to 2 months, and approximately two-thirds will be able to be withdrawn from methylphenidate without a recurrence of depressive symptoms. Those who do recur can be maintained on a psychostimulant for up to 1 year without significant abuse problems. Tolerance will develop and adjustment of dose may be necessary. An additional benefit of such stimulants as methylphenidate and dextroamphetamine are that they have been shown to reduce sedation secondary to opioid analgesics and provide adjuvant analgesia in cancer patients.[97] Common side-effects of stimulants include nervousness, overstimulation, mild increase in blood pressure and pulse rate, and tremor. More rare side-effects include dyskinesias or motor tics as well as a paranoid psychosis or exacerbation of an underlying and unrecognized confusional state.

Pemoline is a unique psychostimulant chemically unrelated to amphetamine. It is a less potent stimulant with little abuse potential.[92] Advantages of pemoline as a psychostimulant in cancer patients include the lack of abuse potential, the lack of federal regulation through special triplicate prescriptions, the mild sympathomimetic effects, and the fact that it comes in a chewable tablet form that can be absorbed through the buccal mucosa and be used by cancer patients who have difficulty swallowing or have intestinal obstruction. Pemoline appears to be as effective as methylphenidate or dextroamphetamine in the treatment of depressive symptoms in terminally ill cancer patients (Breitbart and Mermelstein, in press). Pemoline can be started at a dose of 18.75 mg in the morning and at noon, and increased gradually over days. Typically patients require 75 mg/day or less. Pemoline should be used with caution in patients with liver impairment, and liver function tests should be monitored periodically with longer-term treatment.[98]

Monamine oxidase inhibitors

In general, monamine oxidase inhibitors have been considered a less desirable alternative for treating depression in the terminally ill. Patients who receive monamine oxidase inhibitors must avoid foods rich in tyramine, sympathomimetic drugs (amphetamines, methylphenidate), and medications containing phenylpropanolamine and pseudoephedrine.[78] The combination of these agents with monamine oxidase inhibitors may cause hypertensive crisis, leading to strokes and fatalities. Monamine oxidase inhibitors in combination with opioid analgesics have also been reported to be associated with myoclonus and delirium, and must therefore be used together cautiously.[9] The use of pethidine while on monamine oxidase inhibitors is absolutely contraindicated and can lead to hyperpyrexia, cardiovascular collapses, and death. Monamine oxidase inhibitors can also cause considerable orthostatic hypotension. Avoiding this minefield of adverse interactions can be particularly problematic for the terminally ill. It is not surprising that monamine oxidase inhibitors tend to be reserved in this patient population for those who have shown past preferential responses to them for treatment of their depression.

The new reversible inhibitors of monoamine oxidase-A may reduce some of the problems associated with the older monamine oxidase inhibitors(tranylcypromine, isocarboxazide). There are no studies on the role of reversible inhibitors of monoamine oxidase in the depressed terminally ill but there are interesting theoretical reasons to suggest they may eventually have a larger role to play than the non-selective monamine oxidase inhibitors. Reversible inhibitors of monoamine oxidase-A selectively inhibit monoamine oxidase-A enzyme, therefore leaving monoamine oxidase-B enzyme available to deal with any tyramine challenge. Moclobemide, a reversible inhibitor of monoamine oxidase-A recently introduced onto the Canadian market, appears to be loosely bound to the monoamine oxidase-A receptor and is relatively easily displaced by tyramine from its binding sight. It has a very short half-life, which further reduces the possibility of any prolonged adverse effects such as hypertensive crisis. Dietary restrictions avoidant of tyramine-containing foods are not required. The side-effect profile of moclobemide is far more favourable than non-selective monamine oxidase inhibitors and tends to be well tolerated. Although the risk of hypertensive crisis is significantly reduced, it is not however entirely eliminated. Agents such as pethidine, procarbazine, dextromethorphan, or other ephedrine-containing agents are still best avoided. Its short half-life requires that moclobemide be administered two times daily, with a total dosage range of 150 to 600 mg daily. Coadministration with cimetidine will increase its plasma concentration, thus requiring appropriate dosage adjustments. While reversible inhibitors of monoamine oxidase-A may offer some advantages in the terminally ill depressed patient over tranylcypromine and isocarboxazid, they will likely remain a second line choice to other available non-monamine oxidase inhibitor antidepressants.

Lithium carbonate

Patients who have been receiving lithium carbonate prior to a cancer illness should be maintained on it throughout their cancer treatment, although close monitoring is necessary in the preoperative and postoperative periods when fluids and salt may be restricted.[99] Maintenance doses of lithium may need reduction in seriously ill patients. Lithium should be prescribed with caution for patients receiving cisplatinum because of the potential nephrotoxicity of both drugs. Several authors have reported possible beneficial effects from the use of lithium in neutropenic cancer patients. However, the functional capabilities of these leucocytes have not been determined. The stimulation effect appears to be transient; no mood changes have been noted in these patients.[100]

Benzodiazepines

The triazolobenzodiazepine, alprazolam, has been shown to be a mildly effective antidepressant as well as an anxiolytic. Alprazolam is particularly useful in cancer patients who have mixed symptoms of anxiety and depression. Starting dose is 0.25 mg three times a day, effective doses are usually in the range of 4 to 6 mg daily.[43]

Table 4 Suicide vulnerability factors in patients with advanced disease (adapted from reference 61)

Pain; suffering aspects
Advanced illness; poor prognosis
Depression; hopelessness
Delirium; disinhibition
Control; helplessness
Pre-existing psychopathology
Substance/alcohol abuse
Suicide history; family history
Fatigue; exhaustion
Lack of social support; social isolation

Electroconvulsive therapy

Occasionally, it is necessary to consider electroconvulsive therapy for depressed cancer patients who have depression with psychotic features or in whom treatment with antidepressants pose unacceptable side-effects. The safe, effective use of electroconvulsive therapy in the medically ill has been reviewed by others.[44]

Non-pharmacological treatment of depression in terminally ill patients

Supportive psychotherapy is a useful treatment approach to depression in the terminally ill patient. Psychotherapy with the dying patient consists of active listening with supportive verbal interventions and the occasional interpretation.[101] Despite the seriousness of the patient's plight, it is not necessary for the psychiatrist or psychologist to appear overly solemn or emotionally restrained. Often it is only the psychotherapist, of all the patient's caregivers, who is comfortable enough to converse light-heartedly and allow the patient to talk about their life and experiences, rather than focus solely on impending death. The dying patient who wishes to talk or ask questions about death should be allowed to do so freely, with the therapist maintaining an interested, interactive stance. It is not uncommon for the dying patient to benefit from pastoral counselling. If a chaplaincy service is available, it should be offered to the patient and family.

Suicide and the terminally ill

Cancer patients are at increased risk of suicide relative to the general population, particularly in the terminal stage of illness. Factors associated with increased risk of suicide in patients with advanced disease [61,62] are listed in Table 4. Patients with advanced illness are at highest risk, perhaps because they are most likely to have such cancer complications as pain, depression, delirium, and deficit symptoms. Psychiatric disorders are frequently present in hospitalized cancer patients who are suicidal. A recent review of the psychiatric consultation data from Memorial Sloan-Kettering Cancer Center showed that one-third of suicidal cancer patients had a major depression, about 20 per cent suffered from a delirium, and 50 per cent were diagnosed with an adjustment disorder with both anxious and depressed features at the time of evaluation.[61,62]

Cancer patients commit suicide most frequently in the advanced stages of disease.[102–105] Eighty-six per cent of suicides studied by Farberow *et al.*[103] occurred in the preterminal or terminal stages of illness, despite greatly reduced physical capacity. Poor prognosis and advanced illness usually go hand-in-hand. It is, thus, not surprising that in Sweden, those who were expected to die within a matter of months were the most likely to commit suicide. Of 88 cancer suicides, 14 had an uncertain prognosis and 45 had a poor prognosis.[102] With advancing disease, the incidence of significant cancer pain increases. Uncontrolled pain in cancer patients is a dramatically important risk factor for suicide. The vast majority of cancer suicides in several studies showed that these patients had severe pain which was often inadequately controlled and poorly tolerated.[102,106]

Depression is a factor in 50 per cent of all suicides. Those suffering from depression are at 25 times greater risk of suicide than the general population.[107,108] The role depression plays in cancer suicide is equally significant. Approximately 25 per cent of all cancer patients experience severe depressive symptoms, with about 6 per cent fulfilling *Diagnostic and Statistical Manual* III criteria for the diagnosis of major depression.[1,7,45] Among those with advanced illness and progressively impaired physical function, symptoms of severe depression rise to 77 per cent.[7] Depression also appears to be important in terms of patient preferences for life-sustaining medical therapy. Ganzini *et al.* reported that among elderly depressed patients an increase in desire for life-sustaining medical therapies followed treatment of depression in those subjects who had been initially more severely depressed, more hopeless, and more likely to overestimate the risks and to underestimate the benefits of treatment.[109] They concluded that while patients with mild to moderate depression are unlikely to alter their decisions regarding life-sustaining medical treatment in spite of treatment for their depression, severely depressed patients—particularly those who are hopeless—should be encouraged to defer advance treatment directives. In these patients, decisions about life-sustaining therapy should be discouraged until after treatment of their depression.

Hopelessness is the key variable that links depression and suicide in the general population. Further, hopelessness is a significantly better predictor of completed suicide than is depression alone.[110,111] With the typical cancer suicide being characterized by advanced illness and poor prognosis, hopelessness is commonly experienced. In Scandinavia, the highest incidence of suicide was found in cancer patients who were offered no further treatment and no further contact with the health-care system.[105,102] Being left to face illness alone creates a sense of isolation and abandonment that is critical to the development of hopelessness. The prevalence of organic mental disorders among cancer patients requiring psychiatric consultation has been found to range from 25 per cent to 40 per cent [8,112] and as high as 85 per cent during the terminal stages of illness.[8] While earlier work suggested that delirium was a protective factor in regard to cancer suicide,[103] clinical experience has found these confusional states to be a major contributing factor in impulsive suicide attempts, especially in the hospital setting.

Loss of control and a sense of helplessness in the face of cancer are important factors in suicide vulnerability. Control refers to both the helplessness induced by symptoms or deficits due to cancer or its treatments, as well as the excessive need on the part of some patients to be in control of all aspects of living or dying. Farberow noted that patients who were accepting and adaptable were much less likely to commit suicide than cancer patients who exhibited a need to be in control of even the most minute details of their care.[103] This need to control may be prominent in some patients and cause distress with little provocation. However, it is not uncommon for cancer-related events to induce a great sense of helplessness even in those who are not typically controlling individuals. Impairments or deficits induced by cancer or cancer treatments include loss of mobility, paraplegia, loss of bowel and bladder function, amputation, aphonia, sensory loss, and inability to eat or swallow. Most distressing to patients is the sense that they are losing control of their minds, especially when they are confused or sedated by medications. The risk of suicide is increased in cancer patients with such physical impairments, especially when accompanied by psychological distress and disturbed interpersonal relationships due to these deficit factors.[106]

Fatigue, in the form of exhaustion of emotional, spiritual, financial, familial, communal, and other resources, increases risk of suicide in the cancer patient.[62] Cancer is now often a chronic illness. Increased survival is accompanied by increased numbers of hospitalizations, complications, and expenses. Symptom control thus becomes a prolonged process with frequent advances and setbacks. The dying process also can become extremely long and arduous for all concerned. It is not uncommon for both family members and health-care providers to withdraw prematurely from the cancer patient under these circumstances. A suicidal patient can thus feel even more isolated and abandoned. The presence of a strong support system for the patient that may act as an external control of suicidal behaviour reduces risk of cancer suicide significantly.

Holland[113] advises that it is extremely rare for a cancer patient to commit suicide without some degree of premorbid psychopathology that places them at increased risk. Farberow[103] described a large group of cancer suicides as the 'dependent dissatisfied.' These patients were immature, demanding, complaining, irritable, hostile, and difficult ward management problems. Staff often felt manipulated by these patients and became irritable due to what they saw as excessive demands for attention. Suicide attempts or threats were often seen as 'hysterical' or manipulative. Consultation data from Memorial Sloan Kettering Cancer Center on suicidal cancer patients showed that half had a diagnosable personality disorder.[62]

The frequency of suicide attempts in cancer patients has not been well studied. While the frequency of suicidal thinking in the cancer setting may be in question, its relationship to suicide attempts or completions is clearer. Bolund[102] reports that fully half of all Swedish cancer suicides had previously conveyed suicidal thoughts or plans to their relatives. In addition, many of the completed cancer suicides had been preceded by an attempted suicide. This is consistent with the statistics of suicide in general, which show that a previous suicide attempt greatly increases the risk of completed suicide.[114–116] A family history of suicide is also of relevance in assessing suicide risk.

Frequency of suicidal ideation

Thoughts of suicide probably occur quite frequently, particularly in the setting of advanced cancer, and seem to act as a steam valve for feelings often expressed by patients as 'if it gets too bad, I always have a way out'. Once they develop a trusting and safe relationship, patients almost universally reveal occasional, persistent thoughts of suicide as a means of escaping the threat of being overwhelmed by cancer. Recent published reports, however, suggest that suicidal ideation is relatively infrequent in cancer and is limited to those who are significantly depressed. Silberfarb, *et al.*[117] found that only three of 146 breast cancer patients had suicidal thoughts, while none of the 100 cancer patients interviewed in a Finnish study expressed suicidal thoughts.[118] A study conducted at St. Boniface Hospice in Winnipeg, Canada demonstrated that only 10 of 44 terminally ill cancer patients were suicidal or desired an early death, and all 10 were suffering from clinical depression.[119] Chochinov *et al.* found that of 200 terminally ill patients in a palliative care facility, 44.5 per cent acknowledged at least a fleeting desire to die—these episodes were brief and did not reflect a sustained or committed desire to die (Chochinov, *et al.*, in press). However, 17 patients (8.5 per cent) reported an unequivocal desire for death to come soon and indicated that they held this desire consistently over time. Among this group, 10 (58.8 per cent) received a diagnosis of depression, compared to a prevalence of this diagnosis for 7.7 per cent in patients who did not endorse a genuine, consistent desire for death. Patients with a desire for death were also found to have significantly more pain and less social support than those patients without a desire for death.

At Memorial Hospital, suicide risk evaluation accounted for 8.6 per cent of psychiatric consultations, usually requested by staff in response to a patient verbalizing suicidal wishes.[62] Among 185 cancer patients with pain studied at Memorial Hospital, suicidal ideation was found in 17 per cent of the study population.[61] The actual prevalence of suicidal ideation may be considerably higher in that patients often disclose these thoughts only after a stable, ongoing physician–patient relationship has been established.

Management of the suicidal, terminally ill patient

Assessment of suicide risk and appropriate intervention are critical. Early and comprehensive psychiatric involvement with high risk individuals can often avert suicide in the cancer setting.[115] A careful evaluation includes a search for the meaning of suicidal thoughts, as well as an exploration of the seriousness of the risk. The clinician's ability to establish rapport and elicit a patient's thoughts are essential as he or she assesses history, degree of intent, and quality of internal and external controls. One must listen sympathetically, not appearing critical or stating that such thoughts are inappropriate. Allowing the patient to discuss suicidal thoughts often decreases the risk of suicide. The myth that asking about suicidal thoughts 'puts the idea into their head,' is one that should be dispelled, especially in cancer.[120] Patients often reconsider and reject the idea of suicide when the physician acknowledges the legitimacy of their option and the need to retain a sense of control over aspects of their death.

The suicide vulnerability factors (Table 4) should be utilized as a guide to evaluation and management. Once the setting has been made secure, assessment of the relevant mental status and adequacy of pain control can begin. Analgesics, neuroleptics, or antidepressant drugs should be utilized when appropriate to treat agitation, psychosis, major depression, or pain. Underlying causes of delirium or pain should be addressed specifically, when possible.

Initiation of a crisis-intervention-oriented psychotherapeutic approach, mobilizing as much of the patient's support system as possible, is important. A close family member or friend should be involved in order to support the patient, provide information, and assist in treatment planning. Psychiatric hospitalization can sometimes be helpful but is usually not desirable in the terminally ill patient. Thus, the medical hospital or home is the setting in which management most often takes place. While it is appropriate to intervene when medical or psychiatric factors are clearly the driving force in a cancer suicide, there are circumstances when usurping control from the patient and family with overly aggressive intervention may be less helpful. This is most evident in those with advanced illness where comfort and symptom control are the primary concerns.

The goal of the intervention should not be to prevent suicide at all cost, but to prevent suicide that is driven by desperation. Prolonged suffering due to poorly controlled symptoms leads to such desperation, and it is the consultant's role to provide effective management of such problems as an alternative to suicide in the cancer patient.

AIDS and suicide

There is increased risk of suicide in persons with AIDS.[121,122] A study of the rate of suicide in 1985 in New York City residents diagnosed with AIDS revealed that the relative risk of suicide in men with AIDS aged 20 to 59 years was 36 times that of men without AIDS in the same age range, and 66 times that of the general population.[121] By comparison, the relative risk of suicide in cancer patients is only twice that of the general population. AIDS patients who commit suicide generally do so within 9 months of diagnosis and usually die as a result of falling from heights or hanging. About 25 per cent had made a previous suicide attempt, half were reportedly severely depressed, and 40 per cent saw a psychiatrist within 4 days before committing suicide.[121] At the time of this study, AIDS was primarily seen in the homosexual population and so it is not surprising that all suicides occurred in males. A 1986 review of the psychiatric consultation data at Memorial Sloan Kettering Cancer Center [62] revealed that AIDS with Kaposi's sarcoma was the single most common medical diagnosis amongst suicidal patients. Patients with AIDS and Kaposi's sarcoma who were suicidal frequently had prominent signs of delirium often superimposed on AIDS dementia. Poor prognosis, delirium, depression, hopelessness, loss of control, helplessness, pre-existing psychopathology, and prior suicide attempts are all factors that help identify and seem to contribute to increased risk of suicide. Rundell, *et al.*[123] report a 16 to 24 times higher rate of suicide attempts in HIV infected Air Force personnel than in the Air Force in general. Risk factors for suicide attempts in this group of HIV-seropositive individuals included social isolation, perceived lack of social support, adjustment disorder, personality disorder, substance/alcohol abuse, past history of depression, and HIV-related interpersonal or occupational problems.

Suicidal ideation, either lifetime prevalence or current ideation, is also dramatically higher in HIV-infected individuals than in the general population or even in the cancer population.[124–128] In HIV seropositive populations of homosexual males, alcohol or substance abusers, and psychiatric outpatients, prevalence rates of lifetime suicidal thoughts ranged from 50 per cent to 82 per cent.[124–127,129] Interestingly, HIV-negative individuals in the same at risk populations had similar rates of suicidal ideation, thus suggesting that it is not HIV status *per se* that accounts for such high rates of suicidal ideation, but rather the psychiatric morbidity found in the at risk groups. In addition, stage of HIV illness and the presence of physical and psychiatric symptoms, such as pain and depression, increase rates of current suicidal ideation. Sison *et al.*[130] found that the presence of pain, depressed mood, low T4 lymphocyte counts, and a diagnosis of AIDS increased rates of suicidal ideation. For instance, over 40 per cent of those with pain reported suicidal ideation while 20 per cent of ambulatory HIV infected patients without pain reported suicidal ideation. Clinicians must be alert to this increased risk of suicide in AIDS patients and promote early intervention for such psychiatric complications as delirium and depression and social isolation.

Cognitive disorders in the terminally ill

Cognitive failure is unfortunately all too common in patients with advanced illness. *The Diagnostic and Statistical Manual of Mental Disorders* (4th edn)[131] divides cognitive disorders into the subcategories of:

(1) delirium, dementia, amnesic, and other cognitive disorders;

(2) mental disorders due to a general medical condition (including mood disorder, anxiety disorder, and personality change due to a general medical condition);

(3) substance-related disorders.

While virtually all of these mental syndromes can be seen in the patient with advanced cancer, the most common include delirium, dementia, and mood and anxiety disorders due to a general medical condition. Lipowski[132] categorized organic mental disorders into those that were characterized by general cognitive impairment (i.e. delirium and dementia) and those where cognitive impairment was rather selective or limited (i.e. amnesic disorder, organic hallucinosis, organic mood disorder, etc.). With organic mental disorders where cognitive impairment is selective, limited, or relatively intact, the more prominent symptoms tend to consist of either anxiety, mood disturbance, delusions, hallucinations, or personality change. For instance, the patient with mood disturbance meeting criteria for major depression, who is severely hypothyroid or on high-dose corticosteroids, is most accurately diagnosed as having a mood disorder due to a general medical condition or substance-induced mood disorder respectively (particularly if organic factors are judged to be the primary aetiology related to the mood disturbance). Similarly, the patient with hyponatremia or the patient on acyclovir for central nervous system herpes who is experiencing visual hallucinations but has an intact sensorium with minimal cognitive deficits, is more accurately diagnosed as having a psychotic disorder due to a general medical condition or a substance-induced psychotic disorder respectively.

Delirium and dementia

In spite of very little being known about the neuropathogenesis of delirium, its symptoms suggest that it is a dysfunction of multiple regions of the brain.[133] Delirium has been defined as an aetiologically non-specific, global, cerebral dysfunction characterized by concurrent disturbances of level of consciousness, attention, thinking, perception, memory, psychomotor behaviour, emotion, and the sleep–wake cycle. Disorientation, fluctuation, or waxing and waning of these symptoms, as well as acute or abrupt onset of such disturbances, are other critical features of delirium. Delirium, in contrast with dementia, is conceptualized as a reversible process. Reversibility of the process of delirium is often possible even in the patient with advanced illness; however, it may not be reversible in the last 24 to 48 h of life. This is most likely due to the fact that irreversible processes such as multiple organ failure are occurring in the final hours of life. Delirium occurring in these last days of life is often referred to as terminal restlessness or terminal agitation in the palliative care literature.

At times, it is difficult to differentiate delirium from dementia since they frequently share such common clinical features as impaired memory, thinking, judgement, and disorientation. Dementia appears in relatively alert individuals with little or no clouding of consciousness. The temporal onset of symptoms in dementia is more subacute or chronically progressive, and one's sleep–wake cycle seems less impaired. Most prominent in dementia are difficulties in short and long-term memory, impaired judgement and abstract thinking as well as disturbed higher cortical functions (such as aphasia and apraxia). Occasionally, one will encounter delirium superimposed on an underlying dementia such as in the case of an elderly patient, an AIDS patient, or a patient with a paraneoplastic syndrome. Clinically, we often utilize a number of scales or instruments that aid us in the diagnosis of delirium, dementia, or cognitive failure.

The Delirium Rating Scale, developed by Trzepacz, *et al.*[134] is a ten-item, clinician-rated, symptom rating scale for delirium (Table 5). The scale is based on *Diagnostic and Statistical Manual* III, revised, diagnostic criteria for delirium and is designed to be used by the clinician to identify delirium, and distinguish it reliably from dementia or other neuropsychiatric disorders. Each item is scored by choosing one best rating and carries a numerical weight chosen to distinguish the phenomenological characteristic of delirium. A score of 12 or greater is diagnostic of delirium. The Mini-Mental State Examination[135] is also useful in screening for cognitive failure but does not distinguish between delirium or dementia. The Mini-Mental State Examination provides a quantitative assessment of the cognitive performance and capacity of a patient, and is a measure of severity of cognitive impairment. It is also most sensitive to cortical dementias, such as Alzheimer's disease, and is less sensitive in detecting subcortical deficits such as those found in AIDS dementia. The Mini-Mental State Examination assesses five general cognitive areas including orientation, registration, attention and calculation, recall, and language.

Table 5 Items from the delirium rating scale (adapted from reference 134)

1. Temporal onset of symptoms
2. Perceptual disturbances
3. Hallucination type
4. Delusions
5. Psychomotor behaviour
6. Cognitive status during formal testing
7. Physical disorder
8. Sleep–wake cycle disturbance
9. Lability of mood
10. Variability of symptoms

Table 6 Causes of delirium in patients with advanced disease (adapted from reference 136)

- Direct central nervous system causes
  - primary brain tumour
  - metastatic spread to central nervous system
  - seizures
- Indirect causes
  - metabolic encephalopathy due to organ failure
  - electrolyte imbalance
  - treatment side-effects from
    - chemotherapeutic agents
    - steroids
    - radiation
    - narcotics
    - anticholinergics
    - antiemetics
    - antivirals
  - infection
  - haematological abnormalities
  - nutritional deficiencies
  - paraneoplastic syndromes

Delirium is common in patients with far advanced cancer. Between 15 and 20 per cent of hospitalized cancer patients have organic mental disorders.[136,137] Massie *et al.*[8] found delirium in more than 75 per cent of terminally ill cancer patients they studied. Delirium can be due either to the direct effects of cancer on the central nervous system, or to indirect central nervous system effects of the disease or treatments such as medications, electrolyte imbalance, failure of a vital organ or system, infection, vascular complications, and pre-existing cognitive impairment or dementia (Table 6). Early symptoms of delirium can be misdiagnosed as anxiety, anger, depression, or psychosis. In any patient showing acute onset of agitation, impaired cognitive function, altered attention span, or a fluctuating level of consciousness a diagnosis of delirium should be considered.[132] A common error among medical and nursing staff is to conclude that a new psychological symptom is functional without completely ruling out all possible organic aetiologies. Given the large numbers of drugs cancer patients require, and the fragile state of their physiologic functioning, even routinely ordered hypnotics are enough to tip patients over into a delirium. Opioid analgesics, such as levorphanol, morphine sulphate, and pethidine, are common causes of confusional states, particularly in the elderly and terminally ill.[10] Chemotherapeutic agents known to cause delirium include methotrexate, fluorouracil, vincristine, vinblastine, bleomycin, BCNU, cisplatinum, asparaginase, procarbazine, and the glucocorticosteroids.[51-56] Except for steroids, most patients receiving these agents will not develop prominent central nervous system effects. The spectrum of mental disturbances related to steroids includes minor mood lability, affective disorders (mania or depression), cognitive impairment (reversible dementia), and delirium (steroid psychosis). The incidence of these disorders range from 3 to 57 per cent in non-cancer populations, and they occur most commonly on higher doses. Symptoms usually develop within the first 2 weeks on steroids, but in fact can occur at any time, on any dose, even during the tapering phase.[51] Prior psychiatric illness, or prior disturbance on steroids, is not a good predictor of susceptibility to, or the nature of, mental disturbance with steroids. These disorders are often rapidly reversible upon dose reduction or discontinuation.[51]

Management of delirium in the terminally ill

A standard approach for managing delirium in the cancer patient includes a search for underlying causes, correction of those factors, and management of the symptoms of delirium. The treatment of delirium in the dying cancer patient is unique, however, because:

(1) most often the aetiology of terminal delirium is multifactorial or may not be found;

(2) when a distinct cause is found, it is often irreversible (such as hepatic failure or brain metastases);

(3) work-up may be limited by the setting (home, hospice);

(4) the consultant's focus is usually on the patient's comfort and ordinarily helpful diagnostic procedures that are unpleasant or painful (i.e. CT scan, lumbar puncture) may be avoided.

When confronted with a delirium in the terminally ill or dying cancer patient, a differential diagnosis should always be formulated; however, studies should be pursued only when a suspected factor can be identified easily and treated effectively. Interestingly, Bruera[138] reported that an aetiology was discovered in less than 50 per cent of terminally ill patients with cognitive failure.

In addition to seeking out and correcting the underlying cause for delirium, symptomatic, and supportive therapies are important.[132] In fact, in the dying patient they may be the only steps taken. Fluid and electrolyte balance, nutrition, and vitamins may be helpful. Measures to help reduce anxiety and disorientation (i.e. structure and familiarity) may include a quiet, well-lit room with familiar objects, a visible clock or calendar, and the presence of family. Judicious use of physical restraints, along with one-to-one nursing observation, may also be necessary and useful. Often, these supportive techniques alone are not effective and symptomatic treatment with neuroleptic or sedative medications are necessary (Table 7). Sedation may be necessary to relieve severe agitation or insomnia.[132]

Haloperidol, a neuroleptic agent that is a potent dopamine blocker, is the drug of choice in the treatment of delirium in the medically ill.[132,139-141] Haloperidol in low doses, 1 to 3 mg, is usually effective in targeting agitation, paranoia, and fear. Typically 0.5 to 1.0 mg haloperidol (peroral, intravenous, intramuscular, or subcutaneous) is administered, with repeat doses every 45 to 60 min titrated against target symptoms.[2,8,9] An intravenous route can facilitate rapid onset of medication effects. If intravenous access is unavailable, one can start with intramuscular or subcutaneous administration and switch to the oral route when possible. The majority of delirious patients can be managed with oral haloperidol. Parenteral doses are approximately twice as potent as oral doses. Delivery of haloperidol by the subcutaneous route is utilized by many palliative care practitioners.[4,142] In general, doses need not exceed 20 mg of haloperidol in a 24 h period; however, there are those that advocate high doses (up to 250 mg/24 h of haloperidol, usually intravenously) in selected cases.[139,140,143] A common strategy in the management of symptoms related to delirium is to add parenteral lorazepam to a regimen of haloperidol.[139,140,143] Lorazepam (0.5–1.0 mg every 1–2 h, peroral or intravenous) along with haloperidol may be more effective in rapidly sedating the agitated delirious patient. In a double blind, randomized comparison trial of haloperidol versus chlorpromazine versus lorazepam, Breitbart *et al.* demonstrated that lorazepam alone, in doses up to 8 mg in a 12 h period, was ineffective in the treatment of delirium and in fact contributed to worsening delirium and cognitive impairment.[144] Both neuroleptic drugs, however, in low doses (approximately 2 mg of haloperidol equivalent/per 24 h) were highly effective in controlling the symptoms of delirium (dramatic improvement in Delirium Rating Scale scores) and improving cognitive function (dramatic improvement in Mini-Mental Status Examination scores).

Table 7 Medications useful in managing delirium in patients with advanced disease

	Generic name	Approximate daily dosage range (mg)	Route[a]
Neuroleptics			
	haloperidol	0.5–5 q.2–12 h	PO, IV, SC, IM
	thioridazine	10–75 q.4–8 h	PO
	chlorpromazine	12.5–50 q.4–12 h	PO, IV, IM
	methotrimeprazine	12.5–50 q.4–8 h	IV, SC, PO
Benzodiazepines			
	lorazepam	0.5–2.0 q.1–4 h	PO, IV, IM
	midazolam	30–100 per 24 h	IV, SC

[a] Parenteral doses are generally twice as potent as oral doses; IV, intravenous infusions or bolus injections should be administered slowly; IM, intramuscular injections should be avoided if repeated use becomes necessary; PO, oral forms of medication are preferred, or; SC, subcutaneous infusions are generally accepted modes of drug administration in the terminally ill.

Methotrimeprazine (intravenous or subcutaneous) is often utilized to control confusion and agitation in terminal delirium.[32] Dosages range from 12.5 mg to 50 mg every 4 to 8 h up to 300 mg/24 h for most patients. Hypotension and excessive sedation are problematic limitations of this drug. Midazolam, given by subcutaneous or intravenous infusion in doses ranging from 30 to 100 mg/24 h are also used to control agitation related to delirium in the terminal stages.[25,27] The goal of treatment with midazolam, and to some extent with methotrimeprazine, is quiet sedation only. As opposed to neuroleptic drugs like haloperidol, a midazolam infusion does not clear a delirious patient's sensorium or improve cognition. These clinical differences may be due to the underlying pathophysiology of delirium. One hypothesis postulates that an imbalance of central cholinergic and adrenergic mechanisms underlies delirium, and so a dopamine blocking drug may initiate a rebalancing of these systems.[145] While neuroleptic drugs such as haloperidol are most effective in diminishing agitation, clearing the sensorium, and improving cognition in the delirious patient, this is not always possible in the last days of life. Processes causing delirium may be ongoing and irreversible during the active dying phase. Ventafridda *et al.*[146] and Fainsinger *et al.*[147] have reported that a significant group (10–20 per cent) of terminally ill patients experience delirium that can only be controlled by sedation to the point of a significantly decreased level of consciousness.

Several new antipsychotic agents with less dopamine-blocking effects at low dose are now available (including risperidone and clozapine) and may eventually be shown to have a role in the management of delirium or agitated demented patients. There are no studies on the use of these agents in the treatment of delirium; however, we have begun to use low doses of risperidone (e.g. 0.5–1.0 mg, per oral, twice a day) in the management of delirium in patients with cancer or AIDS who have demonstrated intolerance to the extrapyramidal side-effects of the classic neuroleptics.

The use of neuroleptics in the management of delirium in the dying patient remains controversial in some circles. Some have argued that pharmacological interventions with neuroleptics or benzodiazepines are inappropriate in the dying patient. Delirium is viewed as a natural part of the dying process that should not be altered. Another rationale that is often raised is that these patients are so close to death that aggressive treatment is unnecessary. Parenteral neuroleptics or sedatives may be mistakenly avoided because of exaggerated fears that they might hasten death through hypotension or respiratory depression. Many are unnecessarily pessimistic about the possible results of neuroleptic treatment for delirium. They argue that since the underlying pathophysiological process often continues unabated (such as hepatic or renal failure), no improvement can be expected in the patient's mental status. There is concern that neuroleptics or sedatives may worsen a delirium by making the patient more confused or sedated. Clinical experience in managing delirium in dying cancer patients suggests that the use of neuroleptics in the management of agitation, paranoia, hallucinations, and altered sensorium is safe, effective, and quite appropriate. Management of delirium on a case by case basis seems wisest. The agitated, delirious dying patient should probably be given neuroleptics to help restore calm. A 'wait and see' approach, prior to using neuroleptics, may be most appropriate with patients who have a lethargic or somnolent presentation of delirium. The consultant must educate staff and patients and weigh each of these issues in making the decision of whether to use pharmacological interventions for the dying patient who presents with delirium.

Organic mental disorders in AIDS

The spectrum of organic mental disorders seen in AIDS is similar to that seen in other terminally ill patients (with the exception of AIDS dementia) and includes: delirium, dementia (AIDS dementia complex), organic mood disorder, organic personality disorder, organic hallucinosis, and organic delusional disorders.[148] Several factors make organic mental disorders somewhat unique in the AIDS patient. Concomitant substance abuse, as well as neuropsychiatric side-effects of antiviral or chemotherapeutic agents, can cause organic mental disorders such as organic mood disorder-manic type.[148] Most important is the fact that the HIV virus is neurotropic and thus invades the central nervous system early in infection and can result in AIDS dementia complex.

AIDS dementia complex (dementia due to HIV in *Diagnostic and Statistical Manual* IV) is the most common neurological complication of AIDS.[149] The syndrome of AIDS dementia complex is characterized by disturbances in motor performance, cognition, and behaviour. It is estimated that two-thirds of AIDS patients will develop clinical dementia during the course of their illness. Patients with AIDS dementia complex clinically exhibit a triad of cognitive, motor, and behavioural disturbances. Cognitive and intellectual impairment is typically subtle in onset and progressive. Progression can be rapid or gradual and is quite variable. Initially, the presentation is one of memory impairment, mental slowing, and impaired concentration. This can progress to global cognitive impairment with disorientation, confusion, psychosis, and mutism. Motor disturbances can begin with clumsiness, unsteady gait, tremor, and impaired handwriting, and lead to ataxia, paraplegia, myoclonus, incontinence, and seizures. Early behavioural symptoms included apathy, withdrawal, depression, and anxiety. Late behavioural changes include paranoia, agitation, confusion, psychosis, hallucinations, and affective disturbances, that is mania or depression.[149]

The earliest symptoms of AIDS dementia are often mistaken for functional psychiatric disturbance such as reactive depression or anxiety. As dementia progresses, the organic nature of psychiatric symptoms becomes more obvious. Many of the psychiatric symptoms that develop after a diagnosis of AIDS or AIDS related complex are similar to those reported in patients with cancer.[131,140,150] Patients often react with disbelief, denial, numbness, anxiety, depression, feelings of hopelessness, and, occasionally, suicidal ideation. Differentiating early AIDS dementia complex from a functional psychiatric disorder can be quite difficult. Early behavioural changes seen in AIDS dementia include irritability, anxiety, and depression. These symptoms are common in major depression, anxiety disorders, and adjustment disorders and are easily misconstrued as an understandable reaction to the diagnosis of a life-threatening illness rather than signs of early encephalopathy.[131,148] Formal, neuropsychological testing can be quite helpful in accurately documenting AIDS dementia complex and distinguishing it from depression or adjustment disorder (Table 8). The pattern of neuropsychological abnormalities conforms to what has been termed a 'subcortical dementia.' Characteristic abnormalities include impaired fine and rapid motor movement, difficulty with complex sequencing, reduced verbal fluency, impaired short term memory, diminished visual-motor and visual-spatial abilities, and impaired integrated sequential problem solving. Patients typically have the greatest difficulty, and deficits are most obvious, when tasks are timed and require rapid processing and reaction.[13] Notably, in many patients there is a discrepancy between their complaints of frequent forgetfulness and their relatively preserved performance on formal memory testing. Although depression may mimic AIDS dementia clinically, the pattern of impaired performance on neuropsychological tests that is seen with AIDS dementia complex is somewhat distinctive and not reproduced in depression.

The use of pharmacotherapy in AIDS patients must be prudent and cautious because it is becoming more clear that patients with neurological complications of AIDS are quite sensitive to the adverse side-effects of psychoactive medications. Non-pharmacological treatments such as relaxation techniques, hypnosis, and cognitive coping techniques should be utilized whenever possible to

Table 8 Neuropsychological tests found sensitive to cognitive impairment in HIV-1 infection (adapted from reference 13)

	Domain	Test
I	Attention/concentration	Trail making A
II	Speed of processing information	Trail making A and B Digit symbol substitution (WAISR)
III	Motor functioning	Finger tapping Grooved pegboard Thumb–finger sequential touching
IV	Abstraction/reasoning	Wisconsin card sorting test Halstead category test
V	Visuospatial skills	Block design
VI	Meaning/learning	Rey auditory verbal learning test Visual reproduction (WMS)
VII	Speech/language	Verbal fluency Vocabulary Boston naming Animal naming

help limit medication use to lower dosages. Patients with AIDS dementia complex who present primarily with symptoms of depression, psychomotor retardation, and mild cognitive impairment respond quite well to pharmacotherapy. Barbuto *et al.*[16] have found that AIDS patients respond to relatively low doses of tricyclic antidepressants and may be increasingly sensitive to the anticholinergic effects of these drugs. Fernandez[96] recently reported on the efficacy of psychostimulants in improving both mood as well as cognitive impairment in patients with AIDS dementia. He advocates early use of psychostimulants such as methylphenidate or dextroamphetamine. Psychostimulants can frequently be used to improve mood, energy, and higher cortical functioning.

Neuroleptic drugs are often necessary and effective in the control of confusion and psychosis (delirium) in patients with AIDS dementia.[143,144] There is reason to believe that patients with AIDS dementia have a high degree of sensitivity to the extrapyramidal side-effects of potent neuroleptic drugs.[149,151,152] Supporting this concern are the following points:

(1) AIDS dementia complex is a subcortical process affecting such structures as the basal ganglia;[153]

(2) 11 per cent of AIDS patients with neurological complications have movement disorders such as dystonia, chorea, and parkinsonism even without exposure to neuroleptics indicating a basal ganglia disturbance;[154]

(3) several reports in the literature indicate severe extrapyramidal symptoms in AIDS patients receiving low-dose neuroleptic drugs.[149,151]

Clinical experience indicates that AIDS patients with neurological impairment may be prohibitively sensitive to high potency neuroleptics. Lower-potency neuroleptics, such as thioridazine, or very low doses of high-potency neuroleptics, such as haloperidol, are the most appropriate strategies to manage delirium or confusional states in this population.

Behavioural interventions for the control of selected physical symptoms

While the diagnosis and treatment of psychiatric disorders in the patient with advanced illness is of importance, pain and other troublesome physical symptoms must also be aggressively treated in efforts aimed at the enhancement of the patient's quality of life.[155] The deleterious influence of uncontrolled pain on a patient's psychological state is often intuitively understood and recognized. However, physical symptoms other than pain can go undetected and cause significant emotional distress. This distress often dissipates when effective management is instituted. In a recent study, Coyle *et al.*[156] reported that 70 per cent of terminally ill patients have three or more physical symptoms other than pain. This finding replicates those of earlier papers that elucidate the multiple problems facing the terminally ill patient.[157] These symptoms must be assessed by the psychologist or psychiatrist concerned with the assessment and treatment of affective and other syndromes in the terminally ill population. In other chapters of this text, the management of a variety of physical symptoms experienced in terminal illness (including pain, dyspnoea, nausea, vomiting, asthenia, cachexia, and anorexia) are discussed. In the following section, we will briefly review psychological interventions that may be useful in the management of some selected distressing symptoms.

Pain

The reader is directed to Chapter 9.2.9 for a detailed discussion of the use of behavioural, psychotherapeutic, and psychopharmacological interventions in pain control. In brief, behavioural interventions are effective in the management of acute procedure-related cancer pain, and as an adjunct in the management of chronic cancer pain.[64,158,159] Hypnosis, biofeedback, and multicomponent cognitive behavioural interventions have been used to provide comfort and minimize pain in adults, children, and adolescents undergoing bone marrow aspirations, spinal taps, and other painful procedures.[160–162] Typically, behavioural interventions utilized in the management of acute procedure-related pain employ the basic elements of relaxation and distraction or diversion of attention. In chronic cancer pain, cognitive behavioural techniques are most effective when they are employed as part of a multimodal, multidisciplinary approach.[2] Adequate medical assessment and management of cancer pain is essential. Mild to moderate levels of residual pain can be effectively managed with behavioural techniques that are quite similar to those used for anxiety, phobias, and anticipatory nausea and vomiting. Relaxation techniques are utilized to help the patient achieve a relaxed state. Once in a relaxed state, the cancer patient with pain can use a variety of imagery techniques including pleasant distracting imagery, transformational imagery, and dissociative imagery.[2] Transformational imagery involves the imaginative transformation of either the painful sensation itself, or the context of pain, or both. Patients can imaginatively transform a sensation of pain in their arm, for instance, into a sensation of warmth or cold. They can use such imagery as 'dipping their arm into a bucket of cold spring water', or 'into a vat of warm honey'. Such techniques can also be used to alter the context of the pain. Dissociative imagery or dissociated somatization refers to the use of one's imagination to disconnect or dissociate from the pain experience. Specifically, patients can sometimes imagine that they leave their pain racked body in bed and walk about for 5 or 10 minutes, pain free. Patients can also imagine that a particularly painful part of their body becomes disconnected or dissociated from the rest of them, resulting in a period of freedom from pain. These techniques can provide much needed respite from pain. Even short periods of relief from pain can break the vicious pain cycle that entraps many cancer patients.

Anorexia and weight loss

Cancer patients and their families find weight loss demoralizing, perplexing, and distressing. Weight loss and anorexia in the terminally ill patient are complex problems that can arise from a number of sources. While most often a variety of medical factors account for the anorexia and cachexia associated with terminal illness, psychological and psychiatric factors may also play a role in the aetiology of anorexia and weight loss. Among the most frequent of such causes are anxiety, depression, and conditioned food aversions.[163]

The treatment of anorexia and weight loss begins with the identification and correction of its reversible causes. For example when uncontrolled opioid-induced nausea is identified as a key factor in a patient's inability to eat, adding an antiemetic may completely control the subsequent anorexia. Once specific causes have been ruled out or corrected, subsequent treatment relies upon environmental manipulations.[157] Frequent administration of favourite foods, nutritional supplements, and fluids can reverse weight loss.

When poor appetite is a symptom of underlying major depression or significant anxiety, psychopharmacological interventions with antidepressants and anxiolytics are indicated. Conditioned nausea and vomiting is often quite responsive to relaxation training and other behavioural techniques.[164] These interventions can be employed even by patients with advanced disease if their sensorium is clear and they are capable of concentrating.

Behavioural interventions are commonly used to treat a variety of eating disorders in cancer patients, including conditioned anorexia, swallowing difficulties, and nausea and vomiting. Dixon[165] reported on a study of 55 nutritionally at-risk cancer patients who were randomized to four intervention groups. One group received nutritional support alone; another received relaxation training only; a third group received both supplementation and relaxation; and the fourth group was a no intervention control. Weight gain was greatest for the relaxation groups who were taught deep abdominal breathing, autosuggestion, progressive relaxation, and imagery. Campbell[166] and colleagues showed that a relaxation and imagery exercise programme was associated with weight gain and improvement in performance status. Conditioned difficulties with eating, swallowing, and nausea have been managed successfully with systematic desensitization.[167,168] Hypnosis has been utilized in children with cancer[169] resulting in improved appetite and weight gain.

Asthenia

Asthenia is defined as generalized weakness, and physical or mental fatigue (see Chapter 9.4). Studies suggest that as many as two-thirds of advanced cancer patients complain of weakness. Unfortunately, a treatable cause of asthenia will be identified and corrected in only a minority of cases. The role of psychiatric factors in the presentation of asthenia in the dying cancer patient is small in comparison to that of physical factors. However, psychiatric factors are probably enlisted too often by frustrated house staff who have seen a number of treatments fail, and then view the patient's continuing malaise as a sign of depression. More likely the cause of asthenia arises from some of the following aetiologies: malnutrition, infection, profound anaemia, metabolic abnormalities, and reactions to medication. Chemotherapeutic agents and radiotherapy are frequently employed as palliative therapies in patients with advanced cancer. Both can cause significant weakness that may resolve after treatment is completed.

The psychological and psychiatric treatment of asthenic patients includes patient and family education (especially to address the non-psychological nature of the problem in many cases). An ongoing supportive relationship which permits the patient to express fears and concerns about the meaning of continued weakness, and to address distorted ideas that they may have about its prognostic significance, is critically important.[170] Some patients who suffer with temporary asthenia from chemotherapy or radiotherapy feel that their weakness is a sign of imminent death. The literature in support of the pharmacotherapy of asthenia in cancer patients is largely anecdotal. Some patients respond to steroids (methylprednisone, 15 to 30 mg daily) with improvement in mood, appetite, and physical well-being. Unfortunately, this response tends to be fleeting. Also problematic is the fact that prolonged use of steroids can exacerbate weakness by causing proximal myopathy. Steroids have several other potentially distressing, adverse effects including severe psychiatric syndromes such as organic mood syndromes and delirium. Psychostimulants have been used in the treatment of asthenia with mixed results. However, certain patients do respond well to amphetamine, methylphenidate, or pemoline and it is, thus, appropriate to use stimulants not only for depressive syndromes but for the asthenia/weakness syndrome as well. Despite the appetite suppressing effects of amphetamine-like drugs, stimulants often improve energy and appetite in asthenic terminally ill patients.

Nausea and vomiting

Approximately 50 per cent of patients with advanced cancer experience nausea and vomiting during the course of their illness[157,171] (see Chapter 9.3.1). Common causes of nausea and vomiting in cancer patients include radiation, medications, toxins, metabolic derangements, obstruction of the gastrointestinal tract, and chemotherapy. During the course of chemotherapy, many patients become sensitized to the treatment, develop phobic-like reactions, and even develop conditioned responses to stimuli in the hospital setting. As a result of being conditioned by the experience of profound nausea and vomiting secondary to highly emetic chemotherapy agents, patients report being nauseated in anticipation of treatment. A conservative estimate of the prevalence of anticipatory nausea and vomiting is at least 33 per cent.[172] The factors that increase the likelihood of developing anticipatory nausea and vomiting are as follows:

(1) severity of post-treatment nausea and vomiting (high density, duration, and frequency);

(2) a pattern of increasing nausea and vomiting;

(3) receiving highly emetic drugs (cisplatinum) or combinations of chemotherapies.[173]

Given the relationship between intensity of post-chemotherapy nausea and vomiting and the development of anticipatory nausea and vomiting, the efficacy of antiemetic regimens in the management of these symptoms becomes increasingly important. Antiemetic drugs are the mainstay of managing chemotherapy-induced nausea and vomiting in patients with advanced disease. Several antiemetic drugs have dopamine-blocking properties and so can cause a variety of extrapyramidal side-effects. Akathisia is a common extrapyramidal symptom experienced by the patient as an intense inner sense of restlessness, often accompanied by outward manifestations of agitation. This is often confused with anxiety related to illness by physicians and nurses. Patients can often differentiate feelings of anxiety and nervousness from a sense of motor restlessness. Additionally, akathisia is often accompanied by other extrapyramidal symptoms such as mild tremor or cogwheel rigidity. Treatment of akathisia secondary to antiemetics may involve lowering the dose of the antiemetic, switching to a non-dopamine blocking agent such as ondansetron, or the addition of a benzodiazepine or an anticholinergic agent.

Rapid onset, short-acting benzodiazepines are helpful in controlling anticipatory nausea and vomiting once it has developed. Alprazolam has been shown to be clinically effective in reducing anticipatory nausea and vomiting in doses of 0.25 to 0.5 mg three to four times a day, given for 1 to 2 days prior to chemotherapy.[174] Behavioural control of anticipatory nausea and vomiting has been shown to be highly effective.[171] The techniques that have been studied include relaxation training with guided imagery, video game distraction (in children), and systematic desensitization. It is unclear whether muscular relaxation or cognitive-attentional distraction is the key element in the efficacy of some of these techniques. Chemotherapy nurses trained in these techniques can remarkably improve the quality of life in chemotherapy patients.

Insomnia

Behavioural interventions have been successfully applied to the treatment of insomnia in cancer patients (see Table 5). Cannici and colleagues[175] studied fifteen patients suffering from secondary insomnia due to cancer, and showed a marked reduction in mean sleep onset latency after progressive muscle relaxation training. Stam and Bultz[176] showed an increase in duration of sleep utilizing relaxation and imagery techniques. Such techniques are useful non-pharmacological interventions that help keep medication use to a minimum. Occasionally, sleep disturbance in cancer patients may be due to a concomitant psychiatric disorder such as depression or delirium. Obviously in these cases specific treatment for the underlying disorder is a preferred approach. Pharmacotherapy utilizing benzodiazepines, neuroleptics, or antidepressants may also be indicated when sleep disturbance is due to medication side-effects or to some other organic aetiology.

Conclusion

As the possibility of cure or prolongation of life becomes remote in the care of the patient with advanced cancer or AIDS, the focus of treatment shifts to symptom control and enhancement of quality of life. Such patients are uniquely vulnerable to both physical and psychiatric complications. The high prevalence of distressing physical symptoms, such as pain, make the assessment of psychiatric symptoms difficult. It is critical that physicians and nurses working in the palliative care setting recognize the unique knowledge and skills of psychiatrists and psychologists and the contributions they can make to the care of the terminally ill patient. The role of the psychiatrist, or other mental health professional, in the care of the terminally ill or dying patient is critical to both adequate symptom control and integration of the physical, psychological, and spiritual dimensions of human experience in the last weeks of life. To be most effective in this role, the psychiatrist must not only have specialized knowledge of the psychiatric complications of terminal illness, but must also be familiar with the common physical symptoms that plague the patient with advanced cancer and contribute so dramatically to suffering.

References

1. Derogatis LR, Marrow GR, Fetting J, *et al.* The prevalence of psychiatic disorders among cancer patients. *Journal of the American Medical Association*, 1983; **249**: 751–7.
2. Breitbart W. Psychiatric management of cancer pain. *Cancer*, 1989; **63**: 2336–42.
3. Massie MJ, Holland JC. The cancer patient with pain: psychiatric complications and their management. *Medical Clinics of North America*, 1987; **71**: 243–58.
4. Twycross RG, Lack SA. *Symptom Control in far Advanced Cancer: Pain Relief.* London: Pitman Brooks, 1983.
5. Chochinov HMC, Wilson K, Enns M, Lander S. Prevalence of depression in the terminally ill: effects of diagnostic criteria and symptom threshold judgments. *American Journal of Psychiatry*, 1994; **151**: 537–40.
6. Foley KM. The treatment of cancer pain. *New England Journal of Medicine*, 1985; **313**: 84–95.
7. Bukberg J, Penman D, Holland J.Depression in hospitalized cancer patients. *Psychosomatic Medicine*, 1984; **43**: 199–212.
8. Massie MJ, Holland JC, Glass E. Delirium in terminally ill cancer patients. *American Journal of Psychiatry*, 1983; **140**: 1048–50.
9. Breitbart W. Psychiatric complications of cancer. In: Brain MC, Carbone PP, eds. *Current Therapy in Hematology Oncology-3*. Toronto and Philadelphia: B.C. Decker Inc. 1988: 268–74.
10. Bruera E, MacMillan K, Kuchn N, *et al.* The cognitive effects of the administration of narcotics. *Pain*, 1989; **39**: 13–16.
11. Ahles TA, Blanchard EB, Ruckdeschel JC. The multidimensional nature of cancer realted pain. *Pain*, 1983; **17**: 277–88.
12. Woodforde JM, Fielding JR. Pain and cancer. *Journal of Psychosomatic Research*, 1970; **14**: 365–70.
13. Tross S, Hirsch DA. Psychological distress and neuropsychological complications of HIV infection and AIDS. *American Psychologist*, 1988; **43**: 929–34.
14. Atkinson JH, Grant I, Kennedy CJ. Prevalence of psychiatric disorders among men infected with human immunodeficiency virus. *Archives of General Psychiatry*, 1988; **45**: 859–64.
15. Karina K, Koutsky l, Bradshaw D, Hopkins S, Katon W, Lafferty W. Psychiatriac comorbidity and length of stay in hospitalized AIDS patients. *American Journal of Psychiatry*, 1994; **151**: 1475–8.
16. Barbuto J, Fleishman S, Holland J. Prevalence of psychiatric disorders in AIDS patients. *Current Concepts in Psycho-Oncology and AIDS*. Memorial Sloan-Kettering Cancer Center. September 17–19, 1987.

17. Perry JSW, Tross S. Psychiatric problems of AIDS inpatients at the New York Hospital: A preliminary report. *Public Health Reports*, 1984; **99**: 200–5.
18. Holland JC. Anxiety and cancer: the patient and family. *Journal of Clinical Psychiatry*, 1989; **50**: 20–5.
19. Massie MJ. Anxiety, panic and phobias. In: Holland JC, Rowland J, eds. *Handbook of Psychooncology: Psychological Care of the Patient with Cancer.* New York: Oxford University Press, 1989: 300–9.
20. Whitcup SM, Miller F. Unrecognized drug dependence in psychiatrically hospitalized elderly patients. *Journal of the American Geriatric Society*, 1987; **35**: 297–301.
21. Strain JJ, Liebowitz MR, Klein DF. Anxiety and panic attacks in the medically ill. *Psychiatry Clinics of North America*, 1981; **4**: 333–48.
22. Wald T, Kathol R, Noyes R, Carroll B, Clamon G. Rapid relief of anxiety in cancer patients with both alprazolam and placebo. *Psychosomatics*, 1993; **34(4)**: 324–33
23. Hollister LE. Pharmacotherapeutic considerations in anxiety disorders. *Journal of Clinical Psychiatry*, 1986; **47**: 33–6.
24. Twycross RG, Lack SA. *Therapeutics in Terminal Disease.* London: Pitman, 1984: 99–103.
25. Bottomley DM, Hanks GW. Subcutaneous midazolam infusion in palliative care. *Journal of Pain and Symptom Management*, 1990; **5**: 259–61.
26. Mendoza R, Djenderedjian Att, Adams J *et al.* Midazolam in acute psychotic patients with hyperarousal. *Journal of Clinical Psychiatry*, 1987; **48**: 291–3.
27. De Sousa E, Jepson A. Midazolam in terminal care. *Lancet*, 1988; **i**: 67–8.
28. Chouinard G, Young SN, Annable L. Antimanic effect of clonazepam. *Biological Psychiatry*, 1983; **18**: 451–66.
29. Keck P, McElroy S, Nemeroff, C. Anticonvulsants in the treatment of bipolar disorder. *Journal of Neuropsychiatry and Clinical Neurosciences*; 1992; **4**: 395–405.
30. Walsh TD. Adjuvant analgesic therapy in cancer pain. In: Foley KM, Bonica JJ, Ventafridda V, eds. *Advances in Pain Research and Therapy*, Vol. 16, Second International Congress on Cancer Pain. New York; Raven Press, 1990: 155–66.
31. Beaver WT, Wallenstein SL, Houde RW, *et al.* A comparison of the analgesic effect of methotrimeprazine and morphine in patients with cancer. *Clinical Pharmacology and Therapeutics*, 1966; **7**: 436–46.
32. Oliver DJ. The use of methotrimeprazine in terminal care. *British Journal of Clinical Practice*, 1985; **39**: 339–40.
33. Breitbart W. Tardive dyskinesia associated with high dose intravenous metaclopramide. *New England Journal of Medicine*, 1986; **315**: 518.
34. Beaver WT, Feise G. Comparison of the analgesic effects of morphine, hydroxyzine and their combination in patients with post-operative pain. In: Bonica JJ, Albe-Fessard D, eds. *Advances in Pain Research and Therapy*,. New York; Raven Press, 1976: 553–7.
35. Liebowtiz MR. Imipramine in the treatment of panic disorder and it's complications. *Psychiatry Clinics of North America*, 1985; **8**: 37–47.
36. Popkin MK, Callies AL, Mackenzie TB. The outcome of antidepressant use in the medically ill. *Archives of General Psychiatry*, 1985; **42**: 1160–3.
37. Mavissakalian, MR. Combined behavioral and pharmacological treatment of anxiety disorders. In: Oldham JM, Riba MB, Tasman A, eds. *American Psychiatric Press Review of Psychiatry*; Vol. 12, Washington DC; American Psychiatric Press Inc., 1993.
38. Bruera E, MacMillan K, Pither J, MacDonald RN. Effects of morphine on the dyspnea of terminal cancer patients. *Journal of Pain and Symptom Management*, 1990; **5**: 341–4.
39. Portenoy RK, Moulin DE, Rogers A, Inturrisi Cc, Foley KM. Intravenous infusions of opioids in cancer pain: clinical review and guidelines for use. *Cancer Treatment Reports*, 1986; **70**: 575–81.
40. Robinson D, Napoliello MJ, Schenk J. The safety and usefulness of buspirone as an anxiolytic drug in elderly versus young patients. *Clinical Therapy*, 1988; **10**: 740–6.
41. Massie MJ, Holland JC, Straker N. Psychotherapeutic interventions. In: Holland JC, Rowland JH, eds. *Handbook of Psychooncology: Psychological care of the Patient with Cancer.* New York: Oxford University Press, 1989; 455–69.
42. Chochinov HM, Holland JC. Bereavement. In: Holland JC, Rowland JH, eds. *Handbook of Psychooncology: Psychological Care of the Patient with Cancer.* New York, NY: Oxford University Press 1989; 612–27.
43. Holland JC, Morrow G, Schmale A, *et al.* Reducation of anxiety and depression in cancer patients by alprazolam or by a behavioral technique. (abstract). *Proceedings of the American Society of Clinical Oncology*, 1988; **6**: 258.
44. Massie MJ, Holland JC. Depression and the cancer patient. *Journal of Clinical Psychiatry*, 1990; **51**: 12–17.
45. Plumb MM, Holland JC. Comparative studies of psychological functionin patients with advanced cancer. *Psychosomatic Medicine*, 1977; **39**: 264–76.
46. Holland JC, Hughes Korzun A, Tross S, *et al.* Comparative psychological disturbance in pancreatic and gastric cancer. *American Journal of Psychiatry*, 1986; **143**: 982–6.
47. Green A, Austin, C. Psychopathology of pancreatic cancer. *Psychosomatics*, 1993; **34(3)**: 208–21.
48. Endicott J. Measurement of depression patients with cancer. *Cancer*, 1983; **53**: 2243–8.
49. Kathol RG, Mutgi A, Williams J, Clamon G, Noyes R Jr. Diagnosis of major depression in cancer patients according to four sets of criteria. *American Journal of Psychiatry*, 1990; **147**: 1021–4.
50. Zimmerman M, Coryell WH, Black DW. Variability in the application of contemporary diagnstic criteria: endogenous depression as an example. *American Journal of Psychiatry*, 1990: **147**: 1173–9.
51. Stiefel FC, Breitbart W, Holland JC. Corticosteroids in cancer: neuropsychiatric complications. *Cancer Investigation*, 1989; **7**: 479 91.
52. Young DF. Neurological complications of cancer chemotherapy. In: Silverstein A, ed. *Neurological Complications of Therapy: Selected Topics.* New York, NY: Futura Publishing, 1982: 57–113.
53. Holland JC, Fassanellos, Ohnuma T. Psychiatric symptoms associated with L-asparaginase administration. *Journal of Psychiatric Research*, 1974; **10**: 165.
54. Adams F, Quesada JR, Gutterman JU. Neuropsychiatric manifestations of human leukocyte interferon therapy in patients with cancer. *Journal of the American Medical Association*, 1984; **252**: 938–41.
55. Denicoff KD, RUbinow DR, Papa MZ, *et al.* The neuropsychiatric effects of treatment with interleukin-w and lymphokine-activated killer cells. *Annals of Internal Medicine*, 1987; **107**: 293–300.
56. Weddington WW. Delirium and depression associated with amphotericin B. *Psychosomatics*, 1982; **23**:1076–8.
57. DeAngelis LM, Delattre J, Posner JB. Radiation-induced dementia in patients cured of brain metastases. *Neurology*, 1989; **39**: 789–96.
58. Breitbart WB. Endocrine-related psychiatric disorders. In: Holland J, Rowland J, eds. *The Handbook of Psychooncology: The Psychological Care of the Cancer Patient.* New York: Oxford University Press, 1989: 356–66.
59. Posner JB. Nonmetastatic effects of cancer on the nervous system. In: Wyngaarden JB, Smith LH, eds. *Cecil's Textbook of Medicine.* Philadelphia: WB Saunders, 1988: 1104–7.
60. Patchell RA, Posner JB. Cancer and the nervous system. In: Holland J, Rowland J, eds. *The Handbook of Psychooncology: The Psychological Care of the Cancer Patient.* New York: Oxford University Press, 1989: 327–41.
61. Breitbart W. Cancer pain and suicide. In: K. Foley, *et al.* eds. *Advances in Pain Research and Therapy.* Vol. 16, New York: Raven Press, 1990: 399–412.
62. Breitbart W. Sucide in cancer patients. *Oncology*, 1987; **1**: 49–53.
63. Spiegel D, Bloom JR, Yalom ID. Group support for patients with metastatic cancer: A randomized prospective outcome study. *Archives of General Psychiatry*, 1981; **38**: 527–33.
64. Spiegel D, Bloom JR. Group therapy and hypnosis reduce metastatic breast carcinoma pain. *Psychosomatic Medicine*, 1983; **4**: 333–9.
65. Rifkin A, Reardon G, Siris S, *et al.* Trimipramine in physical illness with depression. *Journal of Clinical Psychiatry*, 1985; **46**: 4–8.

66. Purohit DR, Navlakha PL, Modi RS, *et al.* The role of antidepressants in hospitalized cancer patients. *Journal of the Association of Physicians, India*, 1978; **26**: 245–8.
67. Costa D, Mogos I, Toma T. Efficacy and safety of mianserin in the treatment of depression of women with cancer. *Acta Psychiatrica Scandinavica*, 1985; **72**: 85–92.
68. Davis JM, Glassman AH. Anti-depressant drugs. In: Kaplan HI, Sadock BJ, eds. *Comprehensive Textbook of Psychiatry*, 5th edn. Baltimore: Williams and Wilkins, 1989.
69. Stroudemire A, Fogel BS, Gulley LR. Psychopharmacology in the medically ill. *Medical Psychiatric Practice.* Vol. 1. Washington DC: American Psychiatric Press Inc., 1991: 29–98.
70. Breitbart W, Passik SD. Psychiatric aspects of palliative care. In Doyle D, Hanks GW, MacDonald, eds. *Oxford Texbook of Palliative Medicine.* New York: Oxford University Press, 1993.
71. Glassman AH, Roose SP, Bigger JT. The safety of tricyclic antidepressants in cardiac patients. *Journal of the American Medical Association*, 1993; **269**: 2673–5.
72. Stoudemire A, Fogel BS. Psychopharmacology in the medically ill. In: Stoudemire A, Fogel BS, eds. *Principles of Medical Psychiatry.* Orlando FL: Grune and Stratton, 1987: 79–112.
73. Preskorn SH, Jerkovich GS. Central nervous system toxicity of tricyclic antidepressants: Phenomenology, course, risk factors, and role of therapeutic drug monitoring. *Journal of Clinical Psychopharmacology*, 1990; **10**: 88–95.
74. Massie MJ, Holland JC. Diagnosis and treatment of depression in the cancer patient. *Journal of Clinical Psychiatry*, 1984; **42**: 25–8.
75. Glassman AH. The newer antidepressant drugs and their cardiovascular effects. *Psychopharmacology Bullitin*, 1984; **20**: 272–9.
76. Mendels J. Clinical experience with serotonin reuptake inhibiting antidepressants. *Journal of Clinical Psychiatry*, 1987; **48** (Supp): 26–30
77. Cooper GL: The safety of fluoxetine—an update. *British Journal of Psychiatry*, 1988; **153**: 77–86.
78. Preskorn S, Burke M. Somatic therapy for major depressive disorder: selection of an antidepressant. *Journal of Clinical Psychiatry*, 1992; **53**(suppl): 1–14.
79. Ciraulo DA, Shader RI. Fluoxetine drug-drug interactions: I. Antidepressants and antipsychotics. *Journal of Clinical Psychopharmacology*, 1990; **10**: 48–50.
80. Pearson HJ. Interaction of fluoxetine with carbamazepine. *Journal of Clinical Psychiatry*, 1990; **51**: 126.
81. Preskorn SH. Recent pharmacologic advances in antidepressant therapy for the elderly. *American Journal of Medicine*, 1993; **94** (suppl 5A).
82. Rudorfer MV, Potter WZ. Anti-Depressants. A comparative review of the clinical pharmacology and therapeutic use of the 'newer' versus the 'older' drugs. *Drugs*, 1989; **37**: 713–38.
83. Sher M, Krieger JN, Juergen S. Trazodone and priapism. *American Journal of Psychiatry*, 1983; **140**: 1362–4.
84. Shopsin B: Buproprion: a new clinical profile in the psychobiology of depression. *Journal of Clinical Psychiatry*, 1983; **44**: 140–2.
85. Peck AW, Stern WC, Watkinson C. Incidence of seizures during treatment with tricyclic antidepressant drugs and buproprion. *Journal of Clinical Psychiatry*, 1983; **44**: 197–201.
86. Lloyd AH. Practical consideration in the use of maprotiline (ludiomil) in general practice. *Journal of International Medical Research*, 1977; **5**: 122–5.
87. Ayd F. Amoxapine: a new tricyclic antidepressant. *International Drug Therapy Newsletter*, 1979; **14**: 33–40.
88. Fernandez F, Adams F, Holmes VF, *et al.*. Methylphenidate for depressive disorders in cancer patietns. *Psychosomatics*, 1987; **28**: 455–61.
89. Katon W, Raskind M. Treatment of depressionin the medically ill elderly with methylphenidate. *American Journal of Psychiatry*, 1980; **137**: 963–5.
90. Kaufmann MW, Muarray GB, Cassem NH. Use of psychostimulants in medically ill depressed patients. *Psychosomatics*, 1982; **23**: 817–9.
91. Fisch R. Metylphenidate for medical inpatients. *International Journal of Psychiatry in Medicine*, 1985–1986; **15**: 75–9.
92. Chiarillo RJ, Cole JO. The use of psychostimulants in general psychiatry. A reconsideration. *Archives of General Psychiatry*, 1987; **44**: 286–95.
93. Satel SL, Nelson CJ. Stimulants in the treatment of depression: a critical overview. *Journal of Clinical Psychiatry*, 1989; **50**: 241–9.
94. Woods SW, Tesar GE, Murray GB, Cessem NH. Psychostimulant treatment of depressive disorders secondary to medical illness. *Journal of Clinical Psychiatry*, 1986; **47**: 12–15.
95. Burns MM, Eisendrath SJ. Dextroamphetamine treatment for depression in terminally ill patients. *Psychosomatics*, 1994; **35**: 80–2.
96. Fernandez F, Adams F, Levy J, *et al.* Cognitive impairment due to AIDS related complex and its response to psychostimulants. *Psychosomatics*, 1988; **29**: 38–46.
97. Bruera E. Chadwick S, Brennels C, *et al.*.Methylphenidate associated with narcotics for the treatment of cancer pain. *Cancer Treatment Reports*, 1987; **71**: 67–70.
98. Nehra A, *et al.*. Pemoline associated hepatic injury. *Gastroenterology*, 1990; **99**: 1517–9.
99. Greenberg DB, Younger J, Kaufman SD. Management of lithium in patients with cancer. *Psychosomatics*, 1993; **34**: 388–94.
100. Stein RS, Flexner JH, Graber SE. Lithium and granulocytopenia during induction therapy of acute myelogenous leukemia: update of an ongoing trial. *Advances in Experimental Medical Biology*, 1980; **127**: 187–98.
101. Cassem NH. The dying patient. In: Hackett TP, Cassem NH, eds. *Massachusetts General Hospital Handbook of General Hospital Psychiatry*, 2nd edn. Littleton, Mass: PSG Publishing, 1987: 332–52.
102. Bolund C. Suicide and cancer: II. Medical and care factors in suicide by cancer patients in Sweden. 1973–1976. *Journal of Psychosocial Oncology*, 1985; **3**: 17–30.
103. Farberow NL, Schneidman ES, Leonard CV. *Suicide Among General Medical and Surgical Hospital Patients with Malignant Neoplasms.* Medical Bulletin 9, Washington D.C: U.S. Veterans Administration, 1963.
104. Fox BH, Stanek EJ, Boyd SC, Flannery JT. Suicide rates among cancer patients in Connecticut. *Journal of Chronic Diseases*, 1982; **35**: 85–100.
105. Louhivuori KA, Hakama J. Risk of suicide among cancer patients. *American Journal of Epidemiology*, 1979; **109**: 59–65.
106. Farberow NL, Ganzler S, Cuter F, Reynolds D. An eight year survey of hospital suicides. *Suicide and Life-Threatening Behavior*, 1971; **1**: 194–201.
107. Robins E, Murphy G, Wilkinson Jr RH, Gassner S, Kayes J. Some clinical considerations in the prevention of suicide based on 134 successful suicides. *American Journal of Public Health*, 1950; **49**: 888–9.
108. Guze S, Robins E. Suicide and primary affective disorders. *British Journal of Psychiatry*, 1970; **117**: 437–8.
109. Ganzini L. Lee MA, Heintz RT, Bloom JD, Fenn DS. The effect of depression treatment on elderly patients' preferences for life-sustaining medical therapy. *American Journal of Psychiatry*, 1994; **151**: 1613–6.
110. Beck AT, Kovacs M, Weissman A. Hopelessness and suicidal behavior: an overview. *Journal of the American Medical Association*, 1975; **234**: 1146–9.
111. Kovacs M, Beck AT, Weissman A. Hopelessness: an indication of suicidal risk. *Suicide*, 1975; **5**: 98–103.
112. Levine PM, Silberfarb PM, Lipowski ZJ. Mental disorders in cancer patients. *Cancer*, 1978; **42**:1385–90.
113. Holland JC. Psychological aspects of cancer. In: Holland JF, Frei E, eds. *Cancer Medicine*, 2nd edn. Philadelphia: Lea and Febiger, 1982.
114. Zweig R, Hinrichsen G. Factors associated with suicide attempts by depressed older adults: a prospective study. *American Journal of Psychiatry*, 1993; **150**: 1687–92.
115. Dubovsky SL. Averting suicide in terminally ill patients. *Psychosomatics*, 1978; **19**: 113–5.
116. Murphy GE. Suicide and attempted suicide. *Hospital Practice*, 1977; **12**: 78–81.
117. Silberfarb PM, Maurer LH, Cronthamel CS. Psychosocial aspects of breast cancer patients during different treatment regimens. *American Journal of Psychiatry*, 1980; **137**: 450–5.
118. Achte KA, Vanhkouen ML. Cancer and the psyche. *Omega*, 1971; **2**: 46–56.

119. Brown JH, Henteleff P, Barakat S, Rowe JR. Is it normal for terminally ill patients to desire death? *American Journal of Psychiatry*, 1986; **143**: 208–11.

120. McKegney PP, Lange P. The decision to no longer live on chronic hemodialysis. *American Journal of Psychiatry*, 1971; **128**: 47–55.

121. Marzuk PM, Tierney H, Tardiff K, *et al.* Increased risk of suicide in persons with AIDS. *Journal of the American Medical Association*, 1988; **259**: 1333–7.

122. Cote TR, Biggar RJ, Dannenbert AL. Risk of suicide among persons with AIDS—a national assessment. *Journal of the American Medical Association*, 1992; **208**: 2066–8.

123. Rundell JR, Kyle KM, Brown GR, Thomason JL. Risk factors for suicide attempts in a human immunodeficiency virus screening program. *Psychosomatics*, 1992; **33**: 24–7.

124. Atkinson H, Gutierrez R, Cotter L, Grant I, Pace P, Brown S, Weinrich J, McCutchan J. Suicide ideation and atempts in HIV illness (Abstract) *VI International Conference on AIDS*, June 21–24, 1990, San Francisco, California.

125. Drexler K, Rundell J, Brown C, *et al.*. Suicidal thoughts, suicidal behaviors, and suicde risk of factors in HIV-seropositives and alcoholic controls. (Abstract) *VI International Conference on AIDS*, June 21–24, 1990, San Francisco, California.

126. Gutierrez R, Atkinson H, Velin R, Patterson T, Heaton R, Grant J, Smith K, Pace P, Weinrich J. Coping and neuropsychological correlates of suicidality in HIV. (Abstract) *VI International Conference on AIDS*, June 21–24, 1990, San Francisco, California.

127. Orr D, O'Dowd MA, McKegney FP, Natali C. A comparison of self reported suicidal behaviors in different stages of HIV infection. (Abstract) *VI International AIDS Conference*, June 21–24, 1990, San Francisco, California.

128. McKegney FP, O'Dowd MA. Suicidality and HIV status. *American Journal of Psychiatry*, 1992; **149**: 396–8.

129. Alfonso C, Cohen MA, Aladjem AD , *et al.* HIV seropositivity as a major risk factor for suicide in the general hospital. *Psychosomatics*, 1994; **(35)4**: 368–73.

130. Sison A, Keller K, Segal J, Passik S, Breitbart W. Suicidal ideation in ambulatory HIV infected patients: The roles of pain, mood, and disease status. (Abstract) *Current Concepts in Psycho-oncology IV*, New York, October 10–12, 1991.

131. *American Psychiatric Association Diagnostic and Statistical Manual of Mental Disorders*, 4th edn. Washington, DC: American Psychiatric Association, 1994.

132. Lipowski ZJ. Delirium (acute confusional states). *Journal of the American Medical Association*, 1987; **285**: 1789–92.

133. Trzepacz, P. The neuropathogenesis of delirium. *Psychosomatics*, 1994; **35**: 374–91.

134. Trzepacz PT, Baker RW, Greenhouse J. A symptom rating scale for delirium. *Psychological Research*, 1988; **23**: 89–97.

135. Folstein MF, Folstein SE, McHugh PR. Mini-Mental State. *Journal of Psychiatric Research*, 1975; **12**:189–98.

136. Fleishman SB, Lesko LM. Delirium and dementia. In: Holland J, Rowland J, eds. *Handbook of Psychooncology: Psychological Care of the Patient with Cancer.* New York: Oxford University Press, 1989.

137. Levine PM, Silverfarb PM, Lipowski ZJ. Mental disorders in cancer patients: A study of 100 psychiatric referrals. *Cancer*, 1978; **42**:1385–91.

138. Bruera E, Miller L, McCalion S. Cognitive failure in patients with terminal cancer: A prospective longitudinal study. *Psychosocial Aspects of Cancer*, 1990; **9**: 308–10.

139. Adams F, Fernandez F, Andersson BS. Emergency pharmacotherapy of delirium in the critically ill cancer patient. *Psychosomatics*, 1986; **27**: 33–7.

140. Murray GB. Confusion, delirium, and dementia, In: Hackett TP, Cassem NH, eds. *Massachusetts General Hospital Handbook of General Hospital Psychiatry*, 2nd edn. Littleton, Mass: PSG Publishing, 1987: 84–115.

141. Fernandez F, Holmes VF, Adams F, Kavanaugh JJ. Treatment of severe refactory agitation with a haloperidol drip. *Journal of Clinical Psychiatry*, 1988; **49**: 239–41.

142. Fainsinger R, Bruera E. Treatment of delirium in a terminally ill patient. *Journal of Pain and Symptom Management*, 1992; **7**: 54–6.

143. Fernandez F, Levy JK, Mansell PWA. Management of delirium in terminally ill AIDS patients. *International Journal of Psychiatry in Medicine*, 1989; **19**: 165–72.

144. Breitbart, Platt M, Marotta R, *et al.* Low-dose neuroleptic treatment for AIDS delirium (Abstract). *144th Annual Meeting, American Psychiatric Association*, May 11–16, 1991.

145. Itil T, Fink M. Anticholinergic drug-induced delirium: Experimental modifaction, quantitative EEG and behavioral correlations. *Journal of Nervous and Mental Disease*, 1966; **143**: 492–507.

146. Ventafridda V, Ripamonti C, DeConno F, *et al.* Symptom prevalence and control during cancer patients last days of life. *Journal of Palliative Care*, 1990; **6**: 7–11.

147. Fainsinger R, MacEachern T, Hanson J, *et al.* Symptom control during the last week of life in a palliative care unit. *Journal of Palliative Care*, 1991; **7**: 5–11.

148. Perry SW. Organic mental disorders caused by HIV: Update on early diagnosis and treatment. *American Journal of Psychiatry*, 1990; **147**: 696–712.

149. Brew BJ, Sidtis JJ, Petito CK, Price RW. The neurologic complications of AIDS and human immunodeficiency virus infection. In: Plum F, ed. *Advances in Contemporary Neurology.* New York: P.A. Davis and Co., 1988: 1–49.

150. Treisman GJ, Lyketsos CG, Fishman M, Hanson AL, Rosenblatt A, McHugh PR. Psychiatric care for patients with HIV infection. The varying perspectives. *Psychosomatics*, 1993; **34**: 432–9.

151. Breitbart W, Marotta RF, Call P. AIDS and neuroleptic malignant syndrome. *Lancet*, 1988; **ii**: 1488–9.

152. Edelstein H, Knight RT. Severe parkinsonism in two AIDS patients taking prochlorperazine. *Lancet*, 1987; **2**: 341–2.

153. Rottenberg DA, Moeller JR, Strother SC, *et al.* The metabolic pathology of the AIDS dementia complex. *Annals of Neurology*, 1987; **22**: 700–6.

154. Elder GA, Sever JL. AIDS and neurological disorders: An overview. *Annals of Neurology*, 1988; **23**: 54–6.

155. Bruera E. Symptom control in patients with cancer: *Journal of Psychosocial Oncology*, 1990; **8**: 47–73.

156. Coyle N, Adelhardt J, Foley KM, Portenoy RK. Character of terminal illness in the advanced cancer patient: Pain and other symptoms during the last four weeks of life. *Journal of Pain and Symptom Management*, 1990; **5**: 83–93.

157. Levy M, Catalano R. Control of common physical symptoms other than pain in patients with terminal disease. *Seminars in Oncology*, 1985; **12**: 411–30.

158. Fotopoulos SS, Graham C, Cook MR. Psychophysiologic control of cancer pain. In:Bonica JJ, Ventafridda, V, eds. *Advances in Pain Research and Therapy.* Vol 2. New York: Raven Press, 1979: 231–44.

159. Turk D, Rennert K. Pain and the terminally ill cancer patient: A cognitive-social learning perspective. In: Sobel, ed. Behavior Therapy In Terminal Care. Cambridge: Ballinger, 1981.

160. Hilgard E, LeBaron S. Relief of anxiety and pain in children and adolescents with cancer: Quantitative measures and clinical observations. *International Journal of Clinical and Experimental Hypnosis*, 1982; **30**: 417–42.

161. Jay S, Elliott C, Varni J. Acute and chronic pain in adults and children with cancer. *Journal of Consulting and Clinical Psychology*, 1986; **54**: 601–7.

162. Kellerman J, Zeltzer L, Ellenberg L, Dash J. Adolescents with cancer: Hypnosis for the reduction of acute pain and anxiety associated with medical procedures. *Journal of Adolescent Health Care*, 1983; **4**: 85–90.

163. Lesko L. Anorexia. In: Holland JC, Rowland J, eds. *Handbook of Psychooncology: Psychological Care of the Patient with Cancer.* New York: Oxford University Press, 1989: 434–43.

164. Redd WH, Andresen GV, Minagawa RY. Hypnotic control of anticipatory emesis in patients receiving cancer chemotherapy. *Journal of Consulting and Clinical Psychology*, 1982; **50**: 14–19.
165. Dixon J. Effect of nursing interventions on nutritional and performance status in cancer patients. Nursing Research, 1984; **33**: 330–5.
166. Campbell D, Dixon J, Sanderford L, Denicola M. Relaxation: Its effect on the nutritional status and performance status of clients with cancer. *Journal of the American Dietetic Association*, 1984; **84**: 201–4.
167. Redd WH. Invivo desensitization in the treatment of chronic emesis following gastrorutestinal surgery. *Behavior Therapy*, 1980; **11**: 421–7.
168. West B, Piccionne C. Cognitive-behavioral techniques in treating anorexia and depression in a cancer patient. *The Behavioral Therapist*, 1982; **5**: 115–17.
169. LeBaw W, Holton C, Tewell K, *et al.* The use of self hypnosis by children with cancer. *American Journal of Clinical Hypnosis*, 1975; **17**: 233–8.
170. Bruera E, MacDonald N. Asthenia in patients with advanced cancer. *Journal of Pain and Symptom Management*, 1988; **3**: 9–14.
171. Barnes M. Nausea and vomiting in the patient with advanced cancer. *Journal of Pain and Symptom Management*, 1988; **3**: 81–5.
172. Morrow GR, Morrell BS. Behavioral treatment for the anticipatory nausea and vomiting induced by cancer chemotherapy. *New England Journal of Medicine*, 1982; **307**: 1476–80.
173. Jacobsen PB, Andrykowski MA, Redd WH, *et al.* Non pharmacologic factors in the development of post treatment nausea with adjuvant chemotherapy for breast cancer. *Cancer*, 1988; **61**: 379–85.
174. Greenberg DB, Surman OS, Clarke J, *et al.* Alprazolam for phobic nausea and vomiting related to cancer chemotherapy. *Cancer Treatment Reports*, 1987; **71**: 549–50.
175. Cannici J, Malcolm R, Peck LA. Treatment of insomnia in cancer patients using musele relaxant training. *Journal of Behavior Therapy and Experimental Psychiatry*, 1983; **14**: 251–6.
176. Stamm H, Bultz B, Pittman C. Psychosocial problems and interventions in a referred sample of cancer patients. *Psychosomatic Medicine*, 1986; **48**: 539–48.

16

Domicilliary palliative care

16 Domiciliary palliative care

Derek Doyle

Introduction

This section will deal with the provision of palliative care to the patient in his home and, inseparably, with the care and support of the immediate relatives. The task of providing such care is a difficult and daunting one but uniquely rewarding for all concerned.

What follows is based on the assumption that every terminally ill patient has a fundamental right to receive good palliative care wherever he is, that it is the professional responsibility of all doctors and nurses caring for patients at home to provide such care, and that almost all patients would prefer to be cared for at home as long as possible. These assumptions appear to be increasingly accepted in most parts of the world. What must be questioned is why the quality of such care is so often below the standard the patient has a right to expect and how this deficiency can be corrected.

Those familiar only with hospital practice may be forgiven for thinking that domiciliary care is identical with hospital care in all respects except the place where the patient is resident. This is emphatically not the case. The principles may be very similar but many details of the practice are very different. A more informed and sympathetic understanding of these differences on the part of hospital staff might go some way to improving domiciliary care, if coupled with enhanced skills in family doctors and community nurses. This section will address these and other issues.

The challenge of domiciliary care

Those familiar with the British tradition of general practice may be forgiven for thinking that it is, to a greater or lesser extent, a universal pattern. That is not so. Somewhat similar patterns certainly exist in Canada, Australia, New Zealand, South Africa, United States, and many Scandinavian and mainland European countries but in most parts of the world the concept of a doctor responsible for a patient 'from birth to death' is unfamiliar. Even in some of the countries just named, the family doctor is not always regarded as the doctor of first contact whose responsibility it would be to refer the patient to hospital or specialist services; many patients would often bypass this doctor for a specialist of their own choice. Millions of the world's population have no doctor they can call their own and must attend medical centres and clinics often miles from their homes, with no possibility that any doctor (or a nurse) is ever likely to visit them for any reason in their homes. Even in some countries famed for their ultra-modern hospitals equipped with the latest and most extensive treatment facilities and technical equipment, there is nothing that could conceivably be called domiciliary care. A patient whose condition now merits palliative care must often travel vast distances to see a doctor or nurse skilled and interested in their condition and procure the necessary medications, not from a local pharmacy but from this distant hospital or clinic.

At first sight it might appear that the only common factor is that most dying people would prefer to die at home. This may be the case but it is increasingly apparent, particularly in the more sophisticated Western world, that the chances of achieving this aim are modest.[1] In the United Kingdom, for example, a study of 300 Scottish nurses, half of whom worked in hospitals and half in the community, found that 80 per cent of them would elect to die at home if it were possible.[2] Yet other figures for the United Kingdom, where only a few decades ago 70 per cent of people died at home, show that only 30 per cent currently do so and that the figure is dropping steadily except in areas served by specialist domiciliary palliative care services which have no back-up beds in palliative care units.[3] In North America, the figure for those dying at home is nearer 15 per cent, in Scandinavia only 10 per cent,[4] while in Japan only 8.2 per cent of cancer patients, but 29 per cent of all deaths, are at home.[5] In spite of critical reports of hospital care for the dying in Italy, very few die at home.[6,7] Somewhat similar pictures are described for Germany, France, Australia, and New Zealand.[8]

The reasons for this dramatic change over the last few decades are complex. Though Illich[9] has described the situation as 'The medicalizing of dying and the institutionalizing of death', the responsibility for these changes cannot be laid at the door of the medical and nursing professions. One reason is the disproportionate funding and development of hospital services[6] compared with community care or general practice, exemplified by Finland[10] where, in the 1970s, 90 per cent of health care resources went to specialized hospital services, leaving only 10 per cent for primary health care. Even in the United Kingdom, where primary health care is well developed and reasonably well funded and declared government policy that of encouraging more care in the community, it is clear that deaths at home will become increasingly uncommon. This, however, in no way diminishes the imperative to provide the highest quality of palliative care for whatever time these patients are at home, even if they are subsequently readmitted to hospital or palliative care unit.

It is more than simply a question of funding and allocation of resources. Hospitals are understandably seen by patients and their relatives as centres of hope and health-care excellence, where they undergo sophisticated investigations and treatment, encounter skilled round-the-clock medical and nursing care, and often obtain their first substantial relief of pain. Furthermore, in many countries, as we have seen, hospitals are sometimes the only places where doctors are available, and are often the only places where necessary analgesics of the opioid family are either prescribable or stocked. This latter fact may be the result of legislation based on the mistaken belief that medically-prescribable opioids in the community will inevitably lead to widespread drug abuse, limited supply of the necessary range of opioids for a variety of other reasons, and sometimes a reluctance on the part of community pharmacists to stock drugs so much in demand by drug-abusers.

Increasing evidence suggests that many dying patients agree to return to hospital, or even request it, not for their own sakes but out of selfless consideration for their stressed relatives. They describe how upset and guilty they feel to see carers tired and strained as a result of looking after them, and offer to leave home to assist them.[33,34] Clearly one major challenge to doctors, therefore, is to find the means of reducing avoidable, family strain.

It must, however, be asked if there are other, medical reasons why more die in hospital than are said to want to. Is the quality of domiciliary care offered both to them and their relatives of sufficiently high quality? Do the doctors and nurses caring for patients at home feel sufficiently competent and confident to do so properly? Are community resources for them adequate in terms of staff, equipment, financial assistance, etc? The answers to all these questions would seem to be no. This is another challenge that this present section will seek to address.

The present state of domiciliary care

Allusion has been made to the widely differing patterns of domiciliary care provision world-wide.[3-8,10] It is tempting, writing from the British perspective, to assume that the pattern in this country is the preferable one but such is not the case. Increasing evidence suggests that comprehensive, domiciliary palliative care can be provided in the absence of a traditional 'family doctor system' by appropriately staffed and skilled specialist teams working in the community.[5,8,11-17] These will be described later in this section and in considerable detail in Chapter 2.4. The British experience is described in some detail here because of its long history, well-established training programmes, and the fact that it has been emulated in so many other countries. Lessons from this experience may be helpful, particularly when the shortcomings are studied.

In Britain, each general practitioner, the doctor of first contact for each patient, has a group who have chosen to be cared for by him; the number varying between 1500 to close on 3000, the average being 2400 (although, obviously, those working in remote rural areas may have as few as 600 patients). The general practitioner is totally responsible for these patients at home: for diagnosing, investigating, and treating; for making all referrals for specialist help; for the inviting into the home of any nursing or specialist medical service; and for day and night care except when a patient is discharged from hospital, in which case the hospital nurses liaise directly with their community colleagues. He usually works with colleagues in partnerships of anything of two to fourteen, all sharing practice/office premises. They share out-of-hours work between them, or may employ deputies for these times. Each doctor has, on average, 12 500 consultations a year. They have access to all but the most exclusive drugs (used in, for example, chemotherapy) and have full and free access to almost all diagnostic facilities in local hospitals. A small number may be able to admit patients to 'general practitioner beds' in local hospitals but more usually when a patient enters hospital he temporarily leaves the care of the general practitioner and comes under the clinical care of a hospital consultant/specialist.

Increasingly, community nurses are attached to group practices to provide nursing care and support to patients under the general practitioners; they, too, work exclusively in the community.

General practice is a popular career choice for young doctors who must undertake a period of specialist training after completing their first postgraduate year in hospital work. Increasingly, general practitioners study for higher qualifications, and to qualify for special salary increments they must undertake a prescribed amount of regular postgraduate training pertinent to their work in the community.

In theory, therefore, such 'primary health care teams' of doctors and nurses should be able to offer excellent domiciliary palliative care and, indeed, very many do, but closer study reveals serious deficiencies which must now be addressed.

Reported deficiencies in domiciliary care

Hospital doctors may feel that most of the final year of a cancer patient's life is spent in hospital under their care, but in fact 90 per cent of that period is spent at home,[18] hence the responsibility that falls on the general practitioner and community nurse. Having said that, it must be recognized that those who do most of the caring are not the professionals but the family members.[19] Failure to recognize this fact accounts for many of the problems in palliative care.[20-26]

In spite of the resources already described, which are very similar in many of the countries of the Western world, large studies have shown that many patients feel they are not visited frequently enough.[6-8,27-29] They rate the quality of domiciliary palliative care in terms of their doctor's home-visiting pattern rather than his skills in symptom relief. The more visits, and the more ready he is to listen, the better is their perception of the care.[30] Nevertheless, the number of home visits by doctors, even for the dying, continues to fall, particularly for non-cancer patients and the elderly, who most need such visits. Recent studies have shown that the dying elderly and non-cancer patients are neglected and disadvantaged groups.[27-29,31] However, Higginson[32] has shown that the actual place of death is related to socio-economic class with only 5 per cent of the under-privileged and up to 46 per cent of the more privileged dying at home in the United Kingdom. Hinton[33,34] has shown that the longer home care continues, the fewer patients and families want it, falling from 100 per cent to 54 per cent of patients and 45 per cent of relatives.

Suffering at home is not universally well-relieved.[6,7,19,29,35-40] A report from Sicily, comparing care in 1990 with 1988, found few signs of improvement.[8] Fewer patients were being visited and only one in five of family doctors were prescribing opioids. A seminal British study found that home care was associated with considerable suffering.[41] Six per cent of those at home and one in five in hospital before the terminal phase had severe, unrelieved pain. Although most at home were mobile, 40 per cent had pain severe enough to justify their transfer to hospital for terminal care; but, even there, almost the same percentage were left in unrelieved pain. The principal factor for the discontinuance of home care has been identified as poor pain control, unrelieved emotional distress, and family strain—for a multitude of reasons. Another study[42] has shown that the possibility of dying at home increases with age and is even more likely in females and the married, and is less likely in the young, unmarried, those with higher levels of education and having carcinoma of lung, breast, or prostate.

Pain is certainly not the only problem. A British study of carers found two-thirds reporting inadequate symptom control and was highly critical of communications with and between the professionals involved.[38] Interestingly, before they were questioned as part of the study none had complained or aired this dissatisfaction.

Even when no complaints have been expressed, consumer satisfaction is often low. A study in Sheffield, England, found one-quarter of patients grateful to their general practitioner but 34 per cent critical.[38] The foci of complaints are often the quality of communication or the provision of resources, whether they are nursing, equipment, financial benefits, or simply adequate information.[6,23,24,38,43–48] Some examples will illustrate this.

The director of Britain's first hospice for children found that parents had wanted better control of symptoms in their dying children, better mobilization of resources, and, above all else, wanted to be listened to and to be acknowledged as experts in the care of their own children.[109] Inadequacies of care for a dying child, happily a rare challenge in the life of a general practitioner or nurse, are not surprising and are reflected in the finding that only one-quarter of Scottish nurses feel either confident or competent in this area.[2]

Many reports show that nurses are called in too late, equipment not provided in time, and family support felt to be inadequate;[19,49–54] yet only 26 per cent of general practitioners in one major study felt that family care (as distinct from patient care) was a very important part of their work, and the same percentage declared that this was relatively unimportant, in spite of the fact that 'family medicine' prides itself in care of the whole family, one of whose members is the principal focus of attention.[19] Not surprisingly, the relatives have been identified as the chief carers in 90 per cent of cases.[19] They are usually women, often so elderly that they are physically poorly equipped for the physical and emotional demands of terminal-care nursing.[35,55]

Many studies of community nursing have found deficiencies in the sharing of information between doctors and nurses, a need for improved teamwork, and a need for a lesser controlling role for the general practitioners/family doctors.[56] Community nurses continue to complain that analgesia is inadequate and plead for earlier invitations to become involved in care.[36] One study of a specialist advisory home care service found that one in five of patients were faecally incontinent yet no nurse had been called in to help and no mention had been made to relatives of a special laundry service readily available for just such a problem.[45] The nursing input for a dying patient may be very considerable yet sufficient nurses are not always made available to meet these needs. Even when a nurse is already visiting, the number of visits will increase as death approaches, by almost half for men and 117 per cent for women.[45]

Family stress is inevitable and predictable but often is not dealt with well. As Stedeford points out, families need to discuss their fears—of being alone in the house when a loved one dies, what to do when it happens, how they might cope—all simple and reasonable questions which could be encouraged and answered by the family doctor.[57,58] As has been said, the quality of intimacy of relationships (and not merely sexual) can affect the final phase and how a spouse will cope but how often do professionals recognize this and capitalize on it to facilitate better care?[59]

Families at such a time wonder if they will cope, and their sense of doubt creates either disengagement or enmeshment.[60] Such a crisis, often unlike anything they have ever experienced before, makes it difficult for them to perform the very roles for which they are relied upon. The effects are felt not only by the relatives but, in some cases, by the patients. Work with patients suffering chronic pain (both malignant and non-malignant) shows that there is a tendency for such patients to come from families which include another member with pain or a similar pattern of suffering, and such stressed spouses may reinforce pain behaviour.[61]

It might be asked if this dismal picture is exclusive to domiciliary care in densely populated inner cities where (world-wide) health care resources are often inadequate, or is it also seen in rural areas?

Certainly, a higher percentage die at home in country areas and one has the impression that certain communities remain more closely knit and supportive than many city families, but the picture is not much different from that described for the cities. A semirural British practice recorded 53 per cent of deaths occurring at home. One-third of those who had to be admitted to hospital were there less than a week before they died. The reason for admission in 74 per cent of cases was the emotional strain on the family carers and much avoidable suffering of the patients was found, leaving the doctor to conclude that expert advice in palliative care needed to be made available, something increasingly recognized in other studies.[17,62]

Workers in Israel reported 29 per cent of terminally ill patients dying at home, 40 per cent in general hospitals, and 31 per cent in chronic care institutions but claimed, as others have done, that with better palliative care services and skills two-thirds could have been spared hospitalization.[1,4,8,42,47,48,62,63–70]

In the face of such evidence it is tempting, both in Britain where some doctors have access to hospital beds and in North America where they have extensive admitting rights to general hospitals, to transfer the patient from home to hospital but still continue care under the family doctor.[3,16,71,72] Alternatives are for specialist teams to be available to provide the additional care and support which might enable more to remain at home longer.[1,3,48,50,55,56,62,65,66,69,73–84] Yet another solution is to establish specialist teams capable of providing total care at home without the involvement of family doctors;[4,63,64] both are described in detail in Chapter 2.4. We must be careful, however, not to see these as the only solutions, but to look for ways of capitalizing on the undoubted commitment and developed skills of doctors and nurses already working in the community and the well-documented evidence that properly supported relatives can achieve more than most professionals would ever believe possible.

Factors contributing to inadequate domiciliary care

Insufficiently experienced doctors

It follows that if an ever-diminishing number of people die at home, doctors will have less opportunity to gain experience in providing palliative (and, in particular, terminal) care, and will lose both expertise and confidence. This vicious circle is often forgotten by the critics of general practice. One study of a two-man partnership responsible for 3800 patients had 31 deaths in a year, with only six occurring at home.[85] Another group of five doctors reviewed 85 deaths—35 sudden and unexpected, 25 from malignant disease, and 25 from non-malignant causes, but all anticipated. Thirty-nine of the expected deaths occurred in hospital and 11 at home. Of 34 bereaved relatives interviewed, six were dissatisfied with the medical care or communications, and in eight cases the doctors themselves were dissatisfied with communications and what they regarded as poor pain and symptom control.[43] Clearly, family doctors look after many terminally ill patients at home, though few die at home. Debate continues on whether family doctors care for enough such patients, particularly in the final phase, to maintain clinical expertise.

Improved professional education at both undergraduate and postgraduate levels may go some way to addressing the problem, (see Chapter 21.2), but nothing replaces practical clinical experience in the home; yet it is said that many trainee general practitioners (undergoing three-year training, one year of which is in general practice), had never been involved in the care of a dying patient during their practice attachment, either because there were no such patients or because their trainer did not see fit to entrust the care of such a patient to an inexperienced young colleague. Coupled with this is the problem that many doctors are poor communicators,[43,86] and the disconcerting evidence that some young doctors are reluctant to call in specialist help.[76,79]

Poor skills in pain and symptom control

Even good experience and training in hospital work scarcely prepares a young doctor for similar work at home.[87] The two scenes are very different:[26]

1. The doctor no longer has nurses observing and reporting on patients 24 hours a day. This, however, should not be an obstacle to good palliation. There is abundant evidence that the use of pain charts, whether visual analogue scales (VAS) or numerical scales, can demonstrate the patient's suffering over 24 h,[88,89,90] both for the professionals and the caring relatives. This latter group of care-givers being particularly important in this respect because many studies have now confirmed that relatives perceive the dying patient as having more pain and anxiety than is actually the case.[91,92]

2. There are no nurses to give the medication, monitor its effects, and interpret the doctor's advice and comments to the patient. This, too, should not prove an insurmountable obstacle if pain and symptom charts are used in the home, adequate time spent with patients and relatives explaining the details of medication and possible adverse effects, and a system of shared records employed enabling visiting nurses, doctors, and other professionals to record essential details. Planned, cohesive teamwork with defined guidelines has been shown to be effective.[67,93]

3. Senior medical colleagues with more experience are no longer around as they would be in hospital to advise the young doctor; there are no social workers readily available to deal with psychosocial problems.

4. The doctor no longer sees a patient several times a day, but must learn to plan visits, anticipate problems, and plan care regimens for days and weeks ahead.

5. He is now in sole charge, seeing problems presenting in forms very different from those in hospital wards, hearing of symptoms vaguely and hesitatingly expressed, yet unsure whether to investigate further, to play for time, or to deal with the problems as they present.

6. The doctor is no longer shielded from anxious, grieving relatives, but must cope with their needs, face their anger or questions, and often has to do so on their territory rather than in the safer, sheltered environment of the hospital ward. This is not the problem that it appears to be. There is good evidence that relatives are often happy with the quality of care given to the patient in a hospital but dissatisfied with the quality of support given to them, the relatives, in hospital.[41] In a patient's home, the doctor has the opportunity to mobilize the rich, caring skills of the family if he elects to do so, provided it is remembered that their needs are vastly different from those of the patient, their anxiety levels often higher, their grief and sense of inadequacy often expressed as anger and impotence (see Chapter 14.2).

7. He has to do all this while still having to deal with dozens of other patients each day, many with minor ailments but claiming and expecting his attention, his skills, and his time.[90]

8. The doctor has to decide, as McWhinney has pointed out, whether to be pro-active or re-active in his dealing with his patients and their needs.[94] There is no doubt that palliative care needs to be planned and that many problems of the terminally ill can be anticipated. It is doubtful whether the 're-active' doctor can ever be more than a symptomatologist. This section is written unashamedly from the 'pro-active' viewpoint.

Poor communication skills

Like all doctors, the general practitioner is expected to have consummate communication skills, but will very likely have had little or no training in them. Sadly, as has been shown for medical students and qualified doctors, he may not be aware of his deficiencies and may regard himself as a good communicator.[43,86]

The basic skills differ in no way from those of hospital doctors except that he will have to communicate with more relatives on their territory, often in their time. He must be able to make himself understood and, equally important, be able both to listen and to understand what others are saying to him. Neither is easy, but in domiciliary care there are additional problems not always encountered in hospital practice.

1. The general practitioner may not be fully aware of what a partner or nurse has said or what a hospital doctor has said or done. In domiciliary care, few detailed, written records are usually kept of consultation conversations. There is much to be said for the use of tape-recordings, both in the doctor's consulting room and in

patients' homes, enabling the patient and relatives to replay the tape at their leisure; something found increasingly useful in hospital oncology practice.[97]

2. He may fail to keep either patients or relatives up-to-date with what is happening—investigations, treatment goals, changing objectives, the significance of new symptoms are all areas frequently reported as bewildering to relatives who feel that more explanations are often given to patients than to them, the family care-givers.[19,21,25]

3. He may fail to keep the nurses and his partners and hospital colleagues up-to-date with relevant clinical details, information to and from the patient, details of changed treatments and goals, and how the relatives are coping.[95,96]

4. He may fail to listen to vital information from the nurses who, even in the community, usually spend much longer with the patient than the doctor has time to give. This paucity of communication between the two professional groups is repeatedly alluded to in nursing literature.[93]

Poor co-operation with colleagues

This need not imply an unhappy partnership, or even a bad doctor, but more usually a poorly developed awareness of other colleagues' roles and possible contributions.

1. A partner can only help if he is fully informed and his advice and support invited and welcomed. There are few things more confusing for professionals and family caregivers than to have different professionals giving differing advice or initiating new treatment without explaining the rationale behind it and communicating that to colleagues.

2. A hospital colleague can be of more help if his role in the case is defined with the general practitioner and his possible contribution discussed in advance rather than during an emergency or in a busy outpatient (ambulatory) clinic. It is both feasible and permissible for a general practitioner to enquire of his oncology colleague whether there are any further chemotherapy options and whether he would consider using them, or of his neurosurgical, orthopaedic, respiratory medicine, or cardiology colleague whether they see themselves as having a role in future care. In many countries, home-based patients are being given blood transfusions at home rather than in hospital[98] or benefiting from spinal opioids using epidural cannulas and reservoirs.[90,99] Much more can be done at home than was once thought.

3. A community nurse has a rich spectrum of skills, but may not be able to employ them if he or she is invited to share them too late in the patient's illness, or if his or her contribution is belittled in any way. One of the commonest complaints of community nurses in all the countries where they are to be found is that they were invited to share in care so late that their contribution could not make as big an improvement in the patient's care as would otherwise have been possible.

4. A deputy providing out-of-hours cover cannot ever be expected to replace a competent general practitioner at the bedside of a dying patient, whom he has known for a long time, unless the means are found for making all necessary information about the patient readily available, preferably in the home. This applies particularly to cancer patients whose history may go back years, with complex details of surgery, radiotherapy, chemotherapy, frequently-changing medication regimens, and a plethora of emotional, social, and even spiritual problems. Once again the benefit of shared records which can be kept in the patient's home is obvious.

5. An unnecessarily late involvement (if, indeed, there is any at all) of such colleagues as palliative medicine specialists, physiotherapists, stoma therapists, psychologists, pain specialists, and others, may deprive the patient of better care, the doctor of a chance to share and to learn, and the colleagues of a chance to help as they would wish.

Inadequate support of the family

Care of the relatives is inextricably bound-up with the care of the dying patient and should be a central feature of all good family medicine. Unfortunately, however, an increasing number of reports from many countries suggest that family caregivers are not supported as they need to be. The result is poorer quality care for the patient, increased family strain, premature and sometimes unnecessary admission of the patient to hospital, and long-term disappointment, sometimes anger, and prolonged regret and blame in the bereavement that follows.

It bears repeating that the needs of the family are not the same as the needs of the patient. The latter may be comfortable in all respects, a tribute to the doctor's palliative skills. The family in the adjacent room are grieving his dying, fearful of what lies ahead and how they will have to cope before and after his death, reluctant to express some feelings less they sound selfish or uncaring, understandably hesitant about criticizing the doctor, and needing to have all their needs met—not once, but every day their loved one is still with them, and beyond.

Carers describe how satisfied they were with the doctor's care of the patient and how ignored they, themselves, felt. One widow said of her doctor, 'I almost came to hate him. He would come in every day, spend about half-an-hour upstairs with John, and I could hear them laughing together because he always managed to keep John so comfortable. Then he would come downstairs, put his arm round my shoulder and tell me what a wonderful job I was doing and that I must never hesitate to call him. My friends all said how lucky I was to have such a doctor but never once did he ask how I was. I was so angry that John was leaving me alone in the world, so upset at not understanding what the specialist had said, and nobody seemed to be interested in what I was going through'.

The next most common complaint is that families were not told of the non-medical resources which were available for them—aids to help in the nursing care, special laundry facilities, dietary advice, domiciliary physiotherapy, sitters to stay with the patient for a few hours whilst the relative had a rest, the provision of communication aids, financial assistance, respite admissions, etc.[33,34]

The general practitioner is uniquely able to offer all that is needed:

(1) a sympathetic ear to the questions, needs, and fears of the main carers, recognizing that they are all legitimate, but different from those of the patient. (Obvious as it may be, in our modern society where so much care is institutionalized, few relatives have ever been with a dying person or seen a body, and fewer still have ever provided terminal care for someone so close to them.);

(2) a simple explanation of exactly what is happening, what is likely to happen, what is planned, and what their role is. (Many relatives have the most horrific vision of dying and death, gleaned from television or films, and need to have every detail explained to them in the most reassuring manner.);

(3) an offer to speak to those, for example young children, who may be watching and fearful in the background as their lives undergo an irrevocable and painful change;

(4) a sense of continuity and meaning when nothing seems to make any sense and every day is different;

(5) friendship and shared humanity, a bridge between the past, the present; and the future—a reminder of his continuing interest and caring which will not be diminished by their loved one's death.

As Cartwright found, general practitioners who felt at ease coping with the dying and every aspect of fatal illness were usually the easiest to relate to.[28] The stress on a family can scarcely be measured.[22] Perhaps the highest tribute that can be accorded to the general practitioner is the succinct observation by a relative, 'The general practitioner knows and understands you'.[30] Most families really do not want automatic referral to hospital when things become difficult but, as Rossel has observed, 'good general practice' has often come to mean quick referral to a hospital, a knee-jerk reaction by the general practitioner but often a cause of life-long guilt for the one left behind.[100] Not only that, unexpected moves against the patient's wishes have a serious impact on relatives' bereavements.[101]

Inadequate planning of palliative care

Good palliative care should be an exercise in anticipation rather than in crisis intervention.

1. Many problems can be anticipated. The possibility of hypercalcaemia can be remembered for the patient with a squamous cell carcinoma or multiple bone metastases. The patient with mid-dorsal spine metastases is a candidate for spinal cord compression. Every patient on opioids can be expected to be constipated and will need regular examinations with appropriate bowel treatment rather than urgent admission to relieve faecal impaction. The patient with cerebral metastases should clearly not be burdened with the information that he may suffer personality change or convulsions, but skilled advanced warning of the family may be possible, delicate as such a task is. It is preferable to a middle-of-the-night call for his first acute paranoid episode or grand mal convulsion. The patient who is becoming increasingly weak and frail can be provided with walking aids or a commode in time to prevent a crisis. Plans for more frequent visits can be made as pain becomes a greater problem necessitating more frequent reviews of the analgesic regimen.

The patient who, for some reason, may not be able to remain at home can often be prepared in a skilled and sensitive way for the day when he has to be readmitted to hospital or a palliative care unit. He may understandably be disappointed, but not nearly as upset as he would be if the move were to come unexpectedly, leaving him bewildered and the relatives wondering if it was all their fault or their failure. Research shows that unexpected moves against a patient's wishes have a serious impact on relatives during their subsequent bereavement.[101]

2. Anticipating increasing nursing needs, community/home nurses can be involved as early as possible and certainly before there is a nursing crisis. Similarly, other community resources, if they exist, can be tapped or alerted—linen and laundry services, equipment suppliers, physiotherapy, dietitian, and many others.

3. Specialist services can be reviewed in case they are needed. Some may be seldom used by family doctors and they may need to enquire how to refer patients or invite into the home for advice: pain service, specialist palliative care service, neurosurgery for possible spinal cord compression, direct access radiation oncology for pain or superior vena caval obstruction—and many more.

The role of the doctor in palliative care

The general practitioner/family doctor should regard himself as being responsible for:

(1) comprehensive 24-h care of the dying patient and family members living with that patient (unless they have chosen to come under the care of another local doctor). This will involve the planning and co-ordination of all care and liaison with specialists and nurses.

(2) the emotional and social needs of the patient and immediate relatives at home;

(3) bereavement support of relatives under his care.

These will now be addressed in detail.

Comprehensive palliative care at home

All the principles and many of the details of palliation as described in this textbook apply equally to home care and to hospital/hospice care. What differs is the prevalence of some suffering, the importance of support for the carers, and the different resources available to the family doctor:

(1) fear and apprehensions may be more frequently expressed to the family doctor who has become a friend over many years;

(2) the needs of the relatives will be more evident and pressing, particularly when they must provide most of the nursing;

(3) crises and emergencies require different professional skills at home when the doctor is not so close at hand as in a hospital with all its staff and resources.

It has always to be remembered, as Cartwright points out, that most dying patients have on average ten problems requiring attention at any one time, only 50 per cent of which will be reported as symptoms, the others being equally important to the patient but not reported because the patient suspects they are too trivial for the doctor's attention.[35] Each may reflect a deep fear not recognized even by the family doctor.

The task of the doctor is to identify each symptom and appreciate its significance for the patient rather than its diagnostic value for the doctor. Each must be defined, explained, treated appropriately—and then kept under regular review. Some illustrations may help here:

1. The patient who is sweating copiously may not appreciate that this is due to his cancer or that it can be successfully palliated. He may need to be reassured that he is not, in addition to his malignancy, suffering from an infectious condition such as tuberculosis or AIDS.

2. The patient who is mildly confused but has witnessed many delirious or demented people in hospital needs skilled assessment and reassurance.

3. The patient with steatorrhoea from a pancreatic malignancy needs to be reassured that any faecal matter left adhering to the toilet pan does not contain cancer cells which can endanger family members using the same lavatory.

4. The patient troubled by dyspnoea, whatever its cause, is not asking that further diagnostic tests be done every time he mentions it to his doctor, but needs reassurance that he will not, as he suspects, die of asphyxia. In the same way the patient who knows he has an oesophageal carcinoma, which required an oesophageal stent, needs constant reassurance that he will not starve to death or die from aspiration of food matter.

This obligation to probe deeply, palliate where possible, and explain skilfully at all times applies to all doctors but at home the responsibility to do so falls unequivocally on the family doctor; he is no longer part of a hospital medical team to share the responsibility.

Fears and apprehensions, crises and emergencies do not respect office hours, hence the doctor's undeniable responsibility to make himself, or one of his partners, available throughout twenty-four hours. It can never be acceptable for such a patient and his family to have to depend on medical deputies on call out-of-hours but that is increasingly the practice in many countries. It is grossly unfair for the patient and for a deputy who cannot be expected to know the patient, his past and present medical history, or the complexities of his complicated treatment regimens. The British experience, echoed in other countries, is that pain control and confidence are soon lost when a deputy gives an inappropriate analgesic dose or when the patient is unnecessarily readmitted to hospital at night. Even worse is the situation when no doctor is available to make out-of-hours home visits and the patient has to be taken to an emergency department for palliation which could easily have been provided at home.

Particularly difficult problems in the home

Every doctor caring for a dying patient at home must be prepared to deal skilfully with:

1. *Faecal incontinence*, unlike urinary incontinence, soon leads to requests for hospital admission yet often its cause is obvious and its management simple.

2. *Haemorrhage* is so alarming to patient and carers. Massive haemorrhage, though rare, may be fatal and a doctor must ensure that the family knows what to do and that appropriate tranquillizers are readily available in the home or his emergency bag. Minor bleeding can so easily be controlled topically with haemostatic dressings, 1:5000 silver nitrate, or adrenaline soaks, or, if less urgent, ethamsylate or tranexamic acid; but the patient and family will need much confidence-building.

3. *Unproductive cough,* trivial as it sounds, will exhaust the patient and disturb the most caring family. The doctor will be prepared for this and have available nebulized bupivacaine 0.25 per cent (see Chapter 9.5).

4. *Convulsions,* experienced by 10 per cent of the terminally ill, are much easier to manage at home than often thought but only if the family members are prepared and some taught how to give rectal diazepam solution or even subcutaneous injections of midazolam.[102,103] (See Chapter 9.12.)

5. *Malodorous lesions,* can so distress a family and isolate the patient that, unless well dealt with, admission is soon sought. It is imperative that care is provided by the team of doctor, nurse, and stoma therapist, whether or not it is decided to use activated charcoal dressings, topical metronidazole, or commercial deodorizers (see Chapter 9.6.3).

6. *Paranoid confusional states* can only occasionally be managed at home. The management is described in Section 15 but at home particular care is needed to reassure relatives that it is not 'mental illness' on top of all else or that the cruel allegations and accusations made against loved ones are not the real feelings of the disturbed patient.

7. *Severe incident/breakthrough pain* is dealt with in Chapter 9.2.10 but, even more at home than in hospital, it can be alarming, particularly when most other pains have been brought under control. It is essential for the doctor to identify the patient most likely to have it and to leave adequate supplies of the necessary drugs and instructions for their use in the house. Vague advice or an inadequate analgesic are counter-productive, leaving the patient frightened and the family feeling inadequate in all respects.

Useful emergency drugs are listed in Table 1.

Table 1 Useful drugs for the doctor's bag

Injection morphine (or diamorphine if available)*
Injection dexamethasone
Injection midazolam
Injection hyoscine hydrobromide
Injection metoclopramide
Injection diazepam (for intravenous use)
Injection lignocaine, 2%
Injection frusemide
Rectal diazepam solution
Lignocaine gel
0.25% bupivacaine or 2% lignocaine (for nebulizer use)

* The amount carried should be proportional to the dose any patient is currently on. It is clearly useless to carry 15 mg morphine if a patient is on 100 mg every 4 h, by mouth.

Planning and co-ordinating care

Knowing the clinical pattern and course of the major life-threatening illnesses, the doctor is in a position of being able to plan and participate in many problems. Even better he can, and should, do so with nursing colleagues.

Contrary to what many believe, most patients and relatives do want to know what to expect and, equally important, what is not likely to happen, frightening as have been the forecasts of friends and neighbours. They can, and must, have explained to them:

1. *Progressive weakness*, which few expect, is much commoner than any other symptom (see Chapter 9.4).

2. *Dietary and feeding problems*, often of little importance to the patient, is often worrying to the carers who see his failure to eat as they would wish as the reason for his decline. Seldom is the expert help of a dietitian needed. The simpler the advice, the better—'little and often', 'what he wants, when he wants', 'forget normal meal times and traditional invalid foods', 'plenty to drink even if he doesn't want to eat'— no one is better equipped to give such homely advice than the family doctor and home nurse.

3. *Nursing procedures* can be carried out by relatives who have been taught the basic principles by the nurse: lifting, turning, transferring, bathing and showering, oral hygiene, toileting, etc.

4. *Medications and how to administer them* are basically simple but are daunting or even bewildering to lay carers. The doctor will recognize what a large number of preparations he may need to prescribe (on average 5.7 drugs for each terminally ill patient at any one time), how the number must be kept as low as possible, and how regularly and frequently they need to be reviewed. Medicating in the home is much more difficult than in hospital. Every detail needs to be explained—the exact timing, the way to measure and administer, the rationale and any expected adverse effects, and any storage and security requirements. Some illustrations may help here:

   (a) The instruction '3 times a day' (tid) is understood by doctors and nurses usually to mean 'every 8 h' but to most patients it means simply 3 doses in a day, e.g. after breakfast, around lunch time; and in the evening; with the result that plasma levels are therapeutically unsatisfactory and, in the case of analgesics, pain control is never established or is soon lost.

   (b) Likewise, morphine solution prescribed 'every 4 h' is found to be given '4 times in a day' with pain frequently breaking through.

   (c) Unless the mode of action is explained in a way which is rarely done in hospital, sustained-release morphine preparations are not taken at 12-hourly intervals or else are taken 'as required' for incident pain as if they were immediate-release preparations.

In domiciliary care the focus of attention is the family as much as the patient. The family carers soon lose what little confidence they ever had and the patient still suffers in spite of their efforts when something unexpected happens and they suspect it was their fault, the last dose they gave or something they omitted to report to the doctor. To assist them, it is essential to furnish them with a medication chart (Fig. 1), every detail of which is regularly explained.

Hospital admissions and discharges

The general practitioner/family doctor is responsible for appropriate referral to a hospital service and all the necessary passing on of essential information, and for the care of the patient on return from hospital. It is sad, but true, that doctors caring for the dying often blame their opposite numbers for failing to keep the other fully informed.

NAME JOHN SMITH HOME CARE SERVICE SISTER M. BROWN

	am	am	pm	pm	pm	am	
NAME OF DRUG	6	10	2	6	10	2	
Metoclopramide 10 mg	✓		✓		✓		
Dexamethasone 2 mg		✓					
Morphine solution 10 ml	✓	✓	✓	✓	✓	✓	
Temazepam 10 mg					✓		
Piroxicam 10 mg		✓					

HOME CARE SERVICE (ST ELSEWHERE'S HOSPICE) Tel.

Fig. 1 Suggested chart for recording medication.

On each occasion the patient goes to hospital, whether for an outpatient (ambulatory care) consultation, or admission, the family doctor should endeavour to provide the hospital specialist with details about:

(1) current medication and any recent changes, with reasons for them;

(2) all new symptoms;

(3) what the patient has asked;

(4) what the patient has been told and how it was explained;

(5) how much the patient appears to have understood;

(6) the expressed and apparent needs of the carers;

(7) what the family doctor expects/needs to hear from the hospital specialist;

(8) what plans there are for further hospital consultations, therapy, and investigations.

It is important that such patients are not followed up unnecessarily by hospital colleagues who no longer have a central role, no matter how important their previous role. It is the general practitioner's responsibility to take the initiative in discontinuing such inappropriate continuing care, with a promise to send copies of all relevant correspondence and reports in case the patient should ever again have to consult that specialist. If this is not done, the patient may find himself attending a general physician, an oncologist, and even the surgeon who carried out the original operation, an exhausting exercise and one liable to lead to confusing explanations or even inappropriate changes in therapy.

When the patient returns from hospital, he should be visited as soon as possible, even when it is known that he is mobile and reasonably well. The visit or office consultation serves to remind the patient of the continuing interest and commitment to his care by the family doctor, something often much appreciated if the hospital has felt impersonal and threatening, as can be the case.

The doctor, seeing the patient after discharge, should:

(1) ensure that the patient has a supply of drugs, knows exactly how to take them, and what they are for;

(2) ascertain what the patient has been told and how much the patient understands;

(3) give guidance about daily activities, diet, sex, and visitors;

(4) ascertain what questions or problems the relatives have and deal with them;

(5) explain when he will return and how he may be contacted.

All this may seem very obvious. Experience suggests, however, that many patients return home from hospital unsure of what has happened, even less sure of what has been advised, and needing very confident management by the primary care team.[104]

Emotional and practical support

Dealing with the emotional and social needs of the patient

In addition to the well-recognized fears of the patient that are often expressed in hospital, the patient at home has others:

(1) he fears for the health of his family whom he sees many times each day showing tiredness and stress;

(2) he fears readmission, yet knows it might be better for his family if not necessarily for him;

(3) he fears crises occurring at home when there is no trained person present, and wonders what the indications should be for calling the doctor;

(4) he feels even more embarrassed at home than he might have done in hospital when he is incontinent, sick, sleepless, or confused;

(5) he feels increasingly excluded from decision-making in the home and resents the whispered conversations about him downstairs or with the doctor on the doorstep;

(6) he fears the impact of his illness on his children and grandchildren, yet wants to see them more than ever.

There are no simple solutions. The doctor and nurse must exercise all their skills and become supersensitive to the patient's every spoken and unspoken fear. No one is in a better position to help the patient than the family doctor and nurse. Patients must be enabled to maintain some degree of 'control' as has been demonstrated with patients dying at home with ALS/MND.[105]

Dealing with the emotional and social needs of the carers

It cannot be stated strongly enough that the emotional needs of the carers are often very different from those of the patient, and are often much more difficult to deal with. Explaining the details of the patient's care and the treatment regimen will only go some way to allaying their fears and apprehensions, many of which are related to their own attitude to illness, loss and death, and, in particular, to their own coping and future bereavement. It has also to be remembered that research has clearly demonstrated that relatives perceive the dying patient as having more pain and anxiety than is actually the case.[91]

In Western countries, we seem to have created not only a 'death-denying' society but one often unwilling to suffer or accept loss in any form.[108] It has been aptly described as a 'fix-it' society—one which seems to assume that there is someone, somewhere, if he can be found, who can put everything right, even mortal illness! For some relatives, this may be the promise of a new drug regimen or an operation; for others, a different faith or cult. The result is that family doctors may find themselves caring for a patient who sadly but realistically accepts the inevitability of his decline and death, attended by relatives who insist on exploring new avenues, the possibility of energetic feeding and rehydration regimens, or even taking their loved one to distant medical centres, all in the hope of keeping him alive for a little longer.

When confronted by relatives who wish to try alternative remedies, it is the responsibility of the family doctor not only to explain the pros and cons of alternatives, any hazards which may be involved, and every other implication for the patient but also to remind them that he understands their feelings and will remain available whenever they need him, welcoming back the patient and not condemning their action.

Evidence suggests that the more family carers are kept fully informed, not only of the diagnosis, prognosis, and details of treatment regimen, but also of what may lie ahead, they are less distressed, more co-operative, and feel more confident in their own caring with fewer requests for urgent hospital readmission.

It is essential for the relatives, as well as the patient, to understand what is meant by palliative care. When it is explained to them that it is the relief of suffering, rehabilitation within the limits of the patient's ability, and a constant focus on quality of life rather than preparation for dying, they less frequently talk about 'removing all hope'. The time to begin this regular explanatory process is when evidence shows inexorable disease progression, possibly years before the final phase. There may still be much 'active palliation' possible, months or years of happy, useful living, but the theme for the relatives is that the family doctor is seen as the professional link between the carers and the specialists, a visible reminder of continuing care and concern for everybody involved.

It is sometimes forgotten that, particularly in Western countries, dying has been institutionalized, and relatives may never have seen a dying patient or been present at a death. They feel ill-equipped to cope and have come to regard caring for the dying as a medical/nursing responsibility, something which requires high professional skills of which they have none. This is often at the root of their emotional and social difficulties when a loved one is dying at home. Self-evident as it may appear, the doctor should:

Explain what they can expect to happen day-by-day

Carers need to be prepared for the patient's weakness and increasing dependency; to be forewarned about his eating and dietary difficulties, his changing sleep pattern, his changing moods, his swinging between hope and despair, his sense of being a 'burden' or 'nuisance'. This last feature, that of feeling a burden, is particularly important as research has shown. No matter how effective the pain control and palliation of other symptoms, many dying people feel that they are an unnecessary burden on their carers and on society. They are not comforted by being told that this is untrue. One of the many challenges in palliative care is to give patients a sense of worth, of value, of self-esteem, in spite of their increasing dependency.

Table 2 Nursing aids and equipment for domiciliary care

Very useful	Useful
Additional pillows	Electric fan
Back-rest	Portable suction machine
Commode/urinal	Room-to-room intercom
Walking aid	Deodorizer
Special mattresses	Bed/back elevator
Syringe pump	Angled table lamp
Vacuum flask	Ice-cream/sorbet maker
Special crockery/cutlery	Liquidizer/blender

Carers, in particular, expect death to be painful. Whether this is likely to be a symptom needs to be explained and the strongest reassurance given that pain can usually be controlled. Few carers expect the dying patient to suffer confusion, far less paranoid symptoms, and where appropriate this must be dealt with or even anticipated. No one expects a loved one to suffer a personality change and have no idea how to cope with it.

Explain simple caring techniques

Palliative care nursing does not demand high technical skills or specialized equipment. The doctor or, more usually, the nurse can easily demonstrate how to feed, bath, and how to change a patient; how to make him comfortable in spite of pain or dyspnoea; how to bring down temperature and keep him cool; how to give medications and, so important and often overlooked, how to sit quietly by the bedside creating an aura of love and peace in spite of all that is happening.

Advice on the sickroom and its furnishings

Relatives need to be reassured that their loved one does not necessarily need a special bed or the range of equipment associated with a hospital room, although certainly a few items may be useful and can be made ready[63] (Table 2).

The layout of the sickroom is more important. The bed should be moved to the centre of the room if possible to make it easier to attend to his needs from both sides, and so placed that he can look out of the window to the world outside. A small table should be sited by the bedside within his reach, with a light behind his head, and a bell or call system nearby to call his carers. Chairs should be placed so that when he gets up and walks around he has something substantial to lean on, with all rugs removed in case they slip under his unsteady feet.

Prepare for their own feelings

Often to their surprise, the emotions of the carers change from day to day. They fluctuate between selfless love and resentment that they are to be left alone in the world; between sympathy for the patient and anger that he failed to take their advice and consult the doctor early enough; between gratitude to the medical profession and bitterness about his care and what they perceive as medical apathy or ineptitude.

The doctor must cope with all these feelings—never defensive, or critical, always sensitive, always objective. The carers need to be advised in advance that they will experience this kaleidoscope of reactions, so many of which are painfully, almost alarmingly, new to them.

Building on his unique knowledge of their past lives and how they have coped with other, lesser crises ('small deaths' as they have been termed), the family doctor can help them develop their coping strategies for this supreme test.

Anticipate family tensions

It has been said with some truth, that 'dying brings out the best in a patient and the worst in a family'. The doctor may be able to anticipate some difficulties and help when they occur.

One relative may be confident in their caring, another paralysed by fear. One sadly accepts the inevitable, another argues for immediate hospitalization or a second opinion. One is willing to do anything to help, another only criticizes the first but protests that he and his family are too busy to help in any way. The permutations are endless. The sickroom may be a haven of peace and love, while downstairs there is friction and feuding.

Unless all members of the family are brought together, whether they want to or not, and their roles, their reactions, and their joint responsibilities outlined by the doctor, such a situation soon deteriorates. The doctor is met on the doorstep one day with the request that the patient return to hospital. To make matters worse, the principal carers have to cope with the pressures of the community in which they live. Life and work must go on. Well-meaning friends and neighbours express surprise that they are trying to cope at home. It is frequently put to them that they would actually be showing their love more effectively if they allowed the patient to return to hospital.

Some times only a few sleepless nights, an occasional family disagreement, or an episode of unnecessary, uncontrolled suffering by the patient, brings domiciliary care to an end. Much of this can be avoided. The value of a family conference 'chaired' by the doctor cannot be overstated.[21]

Bereavement support of carers

This is dealt with in detail in Section 18 of this textbook. Here it only remains to state the obvious. Grieving starts when it is first apparent to the carers that they are to lose their loved one—long, long before the death itself.

The loss begins to be felt when the patient is first diagnosed, or even before that when something sinister is suspected by the loved one. Each relapse (and there are so many with most chronic conditions) brings about another sense of loss and each remission a modest return of hope but tinged with doubts and uncertainties made more difficult by the patient's slowly diminishing ability to lead a normal life, to be the breadwinner, or the fulcrum of the family. Fears of the future are very real to the carer but can seldom be mentioned in the presence of the patient. The role of the family doctor at this time can hardly be exaggerated. By giving excellent palliative care to the patient, and personalized care to the relatives, he can do much to ease their sense of loss and, at the same time, show them how they can and will cope in the future, whatever is to happen.

The family doctor must have a plan for care in the subsequent bereavement, no matter if he feels, as so many doctors seem to do, that grief is a physiological process. It has to be remembered that, with his nursing colleagues, he will probably be the only professional involved in the care of the relatives both before and long after the death of the loved one. Here is another role he did not have in hospital practice.

At the time of death

The doctor will visit to complete the legal formalities and spend a few minutes with the family. Experience shows that little or nothing of what he says then may be remembered but, interestingly, relatives may 'remember' comforting words that were in fact never said. What is certainly remembered is how he conducted himself, and this will be recounted for years. At all costs he must avoid such platitudes as, 'He is at peace at last', or 'He has had a good innings' (a peculiarly English allusion to cricket) or, in the case of the elderly person, 'Well, he had a long life, much longer than many people get'. Such expressions are rarely comforting as bereaved relatives readily explain.

At 3 weeks or so after the death

Most family members have had to return to their own homes and the spouse is alone with his or her grief. At this time he or she will want to re-live recent events, recount things that were said, be reassured that they made the right decisions, and speak of the family. This is the time when carers speak in glowing terms of the wonderful professional care their loved one received, often in stark contrast to the criticisms that they voice later on.

At 6 weeks after the death

Life around them has returned to normal but they are feeling more loneliness each day, they are having to pay accounts, and put on a good appearance of coping. This is the time when outsiders stop speaking of the one who has died, make complimentary remarks about how the bereaved is looking, and expect the spouse to have returned to normal activities, Church, clubs, and social events. Very rarely do they feel as composed and brave as they appear to be. To make it worse, about 12 per cent of people experience 'hallucinations', hearing the dead one making familiar remarks, or smelling a wife's perfume. They are not mentally ill but begin to wonder and dread being referred for psychiatric advice.

At 6 months after the death

According to Parkes, this is the time when surviving partners are at most risk.[106] Frequently, they are experiencing some of the symptoms the patient had, and they secretly fear for their own health and life. The doctor may want to visit them at home, but it is probably preferable for them to be invited to visit him for a chat and a complete clinical examination and, hopefully, reassurance. It comes as a surprise to many professionals to realize that, coping satisfactorily as they appear to be, this is the time of most attempted suicides.

On the anniversary of the death

This is a date likely to have been forgotten by most friends and perhaps deliberately 'overlooked' by some of the family. It can be an intensely sad and lonely time for the bereaved one. Some doctors are now following the practice of many palliative care units and sending a simple card for the anniversary, saying something such as, 'Your friends in the surgery (practice/medical centre etc.) are remembering you at this time'. Others are thoughtful enough to take a few minutes to drop in for a chat over coffee. The gratitude of these carers is usually overwhelming. Bearing in mind that the average family doctor has 20 deaths per annum amongst his patients, many of them leaving no close relatives or relatives for whom he, the GP, is responsible, it follows that he will have remarkably few who will need this thoughtful gesture.

Community nurses

In most countries of the world, such professionals are a rare breed, though happily not an endangered species. In some they do not even exist. Even in countries reasonably well supplied with doctors, there may be few trained nurses except in the major hospitals, and even there the senior ones may be expatriates, with none working in patients' homes.

It is recognized, therefore, that this section describes a group of highly-trained professionals found mainly in Western countries but a brief description of their work, particularly with the dying, may still be helpful and hopefully an inspiration to developing health care systems.

In countries where there are community nurses, they have usually completed formal training and gained official recognition after which they have had several years in hospital nursing, probably gained further qualifications in such specialties as oncology, paediatrics, geriatrics, or psychiatric nursing, and then taken an academic year to qualify as a community nurse. In Britain, as in many other countries, such nurses may either take on all nursing responsibilities in the community or confine themselves to public health medicine, disease prevention, and health promotion—the 'health visitors' as they are described in the United Kingdom.

In many countries, community nurses are employed by the National Health Service and are accountable to senior managers in that service but may either be attached to a practice of doctors or work in a designated geographical area. In other countries, they may be employed by a hospital or be based there, or employed by a private agency, or by a local authority.

By and large, the responsibilities of the community nurse can be summarized as:

1. To provide practical nursing care for patients in their own homes. This will include general nursing care, dressings, routine injections, the giving of enemas, catheterization and routine catheter care, and the follow-up of patients after inpatient care or day care surgery.

2. Giving dietary advice. The nurse will offer this when required, liaising with health visitor or dietician if such a colleague exists.

3. Giving emotional support. This is an inseparable part of the nurse's work as he or she encounters psychological problems in patients and carers, related to the patient's underlying organic condition.[58]

4. Ordering essential nursing equipment and aids. The nurse will usually have access to special beds, mattresses, commodes, urinals, sputum mugs, deodorizers, syringe-pumps, electric fans, liquidizers/blenders (many of which can be loaned to patients under his/her care), and a large range of surgical dressings and appliances.

5. Liaising with hospital colleagues. Ideally, no patient with any serious pathology should be discharged home without arrangements having been made for the nurse to visit and continue to provide at home the same quality of care as in the hospital, albeit without some of the high technology equipment there taken for

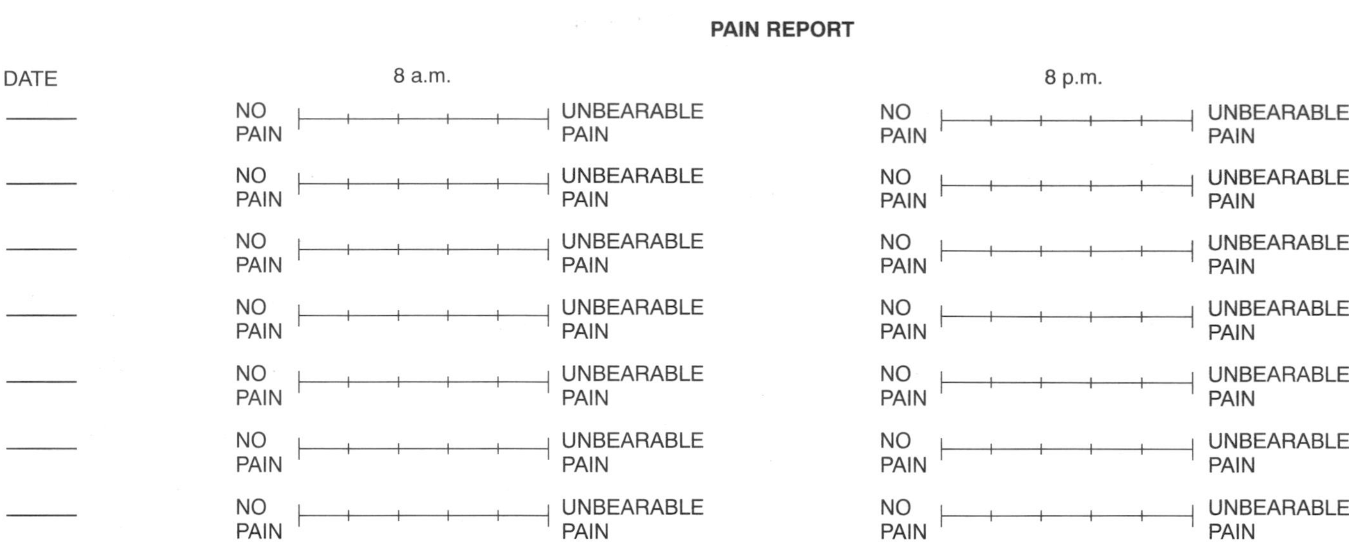

Patient's name: ____________________

Reference number/Date of birth: ____________________

PAIN REPORT

DATE	8 a.m.	8 p.m.
______	NO PAIN |—+—+—+—+—| UNBEARABLE PAIN	NO PAIN |—+—+—+—+—| UNBEARABLE PAIN
______	NO PAIN |—+—+—+—+—| UNBEARABLE PAIN	NO PAIN |—+—+—+—+—| UNBEARABLE PAIN
______	NO PAIN |—+—+—+—+—| UNBEARABLE PAIN	NO PAIN |—+—+—+—+—| UNBEARABLE PAIN
______	NO PAIN |—+—+—+—+—| UNBEARABLE PAIN	NO PAIN |—+—+—+—+—| UNBEARABLE PAIN
______	NO PAIN |—+—+—+—+—| UNBEARABLE PAIN	NO PAIN |—+—+—+—+—| UNBEARABLE PAIN
______	NO PAIN |—+—+—+—+—| UNBEARABLE PAIN	NO PAIN |—+—+—+—+—| UNBEARABLE PAIN
______	NO PAIN |—+—+—+—+—| UNBEARABLE PAIN	NO PAIN |—+—+—+—+—| UNBEARABLE PAIN

NOTE: 1. This record should be completed by the patient, not the family.
2. The report should be left out for doctor and sister to see.

Fig. 2 Pain chart using a visual analogue scale.

granted. Likewise, it is the nurse's responsibility to be in touch with his or her opposite number in hospital about all relevant information when a patient is admitted and prior to his discharge. Optimally, time and workload permitting, he or she will try to visit patients in hospital to maintain contact.

6. Liaising with specialist colleagues. Details of specialist palliative care nurses are given below. Others with whom he or she may be required to work include stoma therapists, community psychiatric nurses, community paediatric nurses, and community occupational therapists and physiotherapists.

7. Assisting in the education of patients and carers. An important but ill-defined responsibility is the education of lay people in simple nursing techniques and procedures: the lifting, handling and transferring of patients, feeding techniques, the preparation and care of the sickroom, the avoidance of infection, and the provision of mutual support.

It should not need to be said that nurses working in the community must work closely with general practitioners and their trainees. Sadly, this sometimes becomes an area of tension and mutual recrimination but need not be so. The reasons for poor working relationships are legion and complex.[54] Some doctors are possessive of 'their' patients and resent what they choose to regard as intrusion in their domain by their nursing colleagues.[93] Some have little appreciation of how comprehensive the nurse's training and experience are, and put insufficient trust in his/her judgement and advice. The nurse, like his or her hospital colleagues, may see a different side of the patient than the general practitioner and is often made privy to important clinical information which the patient is reluctant to share with the doctor. They see pain that could be better controlled and predictably become upset when the doctor shows either less than optimal skill in relieving it, or appears apathetic. There is abundant evidence of this.[19,36,49,51,80]

The fault does not always lie with the doctor. When a nurse has been called in to a patient's care, it then becomes his or her responsibility to decide on the frequency of visits, every detail of nursing needed, and adequate continuity of care when visits are to be done by deputies in his or her absence. There are many reports of this not happening in the care of the dying and the elderly.[31] If the nurse feels that a patient has not described his pain well enough for the doctor to help him, it becomes the nurse's responsibility to elicit a clearer history and report it to the doctor.

It is increasingly recognized that the use of pain or symptom charts can make all the difference to the quality of pain and symptom control in the home (Fig. 2, Fig. 3, and Fig. 4). Such a pain chart can show, for example, the fluctuation of pain at different times of day, the response to medication, and can be used as objective evidence, if needs be, to convince an otherwise sceptical doctor of the pain (or any other symptom) that the patient is suffering.[88,89,90] Just as the doctor has a responsibility to identify each pain, and to treat each specifically, so the attending nurse has a responsibility likewise to know of each pain and its cause, understand the specific treatment regimen being offered for each, and to report on each pain in consultation with the doctor. It is worse than useless for a patient to be reported as having 'pain' without the nurse identifying it, giving the necessary description which will enable the doctor to identify the offending organ or system, and giving precise details of response to medication.

One study of 118 dying patients at home found that 75 per cent had visiting nurses, making an average of 120 visits per patient—a considerable professional input.[52] In spite of this, many relatives said they were largely unaware of any other possible sources of help, such as night sitters and voluntary agencies, yet the nurses could have advised them. A study of the elderly discharged from hospital found that their most common complaints related to insufficient

Patient's name: ____________

Reference number/Date of birth: ____________

NAUSEA REPORT

DATE	8 a.m.			8 p.m.		
______	NO NAUSEA	├──┼──┼──┼──┼──┤	UNBEARABLE NAUSEA	NO NAUSEA	├──┼──┼──┼──┼──┤	UNBEARABLE NAUSEA
______	NO NAUSEA	├──┼──┼──┼──┼──┤	UNBEARABLE NAUSEA	NO NAUSEA	├──┼──┼──┼──┼──┤	UNBEARABLE NAUSEA
______	NO NAUSEA	├──┼──┼──┼──┼──┤	UNBEARABLE NAUSEA	NO NAUSEA	├──┼──┼──┼──┼──┤	UNBEARABLE NAUSEA
______	NO NAUSEA	├──┼──┼──┼──┼──┤	UNBEARABLE NAUSEA	NO NAUSEA	├──┼──┼──┼──┼──┤	UNBEARABLE NAUSEA
______	NO NAUSEA	├──┼──┼──┼──┼──┤	UNBEARABLE NAUSEA	NO NAUSEA	├──┼──┼──┼──┼──┤	UNBEARABLE NAUSEA
______	NO NAUSEA	├──┼──┼──┼──┼──┤	UNBEARABLE NAUSEA	NO NAUSEA	├──┼──┼──┼──┼──┤	UNBEARABLE NAUSEA
______	NO NAUSEA	├──┼──┼──┼──┼──┤	UNBEARABLE NAUSEA	NO NAUSEA	├──┼──┼──┼──┼──┤	UNBEARABLE NAUSEA

NOTE: 1. This record should be completed by the patient, not the family.
2. The report should be left out for doctor and sister to see.

Fig. 3 Recording nausea using a visual analogue scale.

home visits and nursing. Other studies have shown that the disadvantaged ill are those with chronic illnesses and the elderly, two of the groups who form the focus of attention of this textbook.[31]

The picture is not all bleak. Community nurses are very ready to admit to a sense of low confidence and competence with such groups as dying children and terminally ill adults. Surprisingly, 95 per cent expressed confidence in caring for the elderly, making one wonder why the elderly appear to have fewer visits and lesser quality care than other groups.[2] Experience in Britain shows that community nurses are eager to learn and develop their skills, particularly in palliative care. In many centres in the United Kingdom it has been found that nurses unable to obtain funding to go on extended full-time courses are very ready to attend day-

Patient's name: ____________

Reference number/Date of birth: ____________

BREATHLESSNESS REPORT

DATE	8 a.m.			8 p.m.		
______	NO BREATHLESSNESS	├──┼──┼──┼──┼──┤	UNBEARABLE BREATHLESSNESS	NO BREATHLESSNESS	├──┼──┼──┼──┼──┤	UNBEARABLE BREATHLESSNESS
______	NO BREATHLESSNESS	├──┼──┼──┼──┼──┤	UNBEARABLE BREATHLESSNESS	NO BREATHLESSNESS	├──┼──┼──┼──┼──┤	UNBEARABLE BREATHLESSNESS
______	NO BREATHLESSNESS	├──┼──┼──┼──┼──┤	UNBEARABLE BREATHLESSNESS	NO BREATHLESSNESS	├──┼──┼──┼──┼──┤	UNBEARABLE BREATHLESSNESS
______	NO BREATHLESSNESS	├──┼──┼──┼──┼──┤	UNBEARABLE BREATHLESSNESS	NO BREATHLESSNESS	├──┼──┼──┼──┼──┤	UNBEARABLE BREATHLESSNESS
______	NO BREATHLESSNESS	├──┼──┼──┼──┼──┤	UNBEARABLE BREATHLESSNESS	NO BREATHLESSNESS	├──┼──┼──┼──┼──┤	UNBEARABLE BREATHLESSNESS
______	NO BREATHLESSNESS	├──┼──┼──┼──┼──┤	UNBEARABLE BREATHLESSNESS	NO BREATHLESSNESS	├──┼──┼──┼──┼──┤	UNBEARABLE BREATHLESSNESS
______	NO BREATHLESSNESS	├──┼──┼──┼──┼──┤	UNBEARABLE BREATHLESSNESS	NO BREATHLESSNESS	├──┼──┼──┼──┼──┤	UNBEARABLE BREATHLESSNESS

NOTE: 1. This record should be completed by the patient, not the family.
2. The report should be left out for doctor and sister to see.

Fig. 4 Recording breathlessness using a visual analogue scale.

release and evening courses, often at their own expense, and the demand for such training greatly exceeds the number of places.

The community nurse in palliative care

In most respects, the role of the community nurse in palliative care does not differ from that of her colleagues in hospital/hospice. The same principles apply, the same drugs are used, the same equipment is needed, and the same close interdependent relationship with other professional colleagues and, in particular the doctor, is essential.

The principal difference between palliative care in hospital and in the community, so far as nurses are concerned, is that in the community they have a longer term, continuing relationship with the patient and family, must make the family (including the patient) the focus of care, and must be ready to accept the inevitability of inexorable decline and final death. Probably the only feature which radically differs from hospital nursing is that the community nurse may often be the only professional in frequent contact with the family, the one to whom they will turn with more questions than to the doctor, the one who is supposed to know all the answers, the one with whom they will share their grief and their anger, and yet the community nurse will usually be working alone and often feeling isolated, threatened and poorly supported.

Experience shows that even the best general practitioner/family doctor cannot offer optimal, comprehensive palliative care on his own but requires the professional input and support of a nurse colleague. It is equally apparent that a community nurse cannot do this alone and must have the support and respect of a medical colleague. This area of work is fraught with problems and challenges. There is no place for professional competition and certainly not for suspicion, criticism, or defensive distancing.

Specialist advice and support

The following specialist services and colleagues will at some time be found useful or even indispensable in the care of the terminally ill patient at home:

(1) specialist home care service (Chapter 2.4)

(2) stoma therapist (Chapter 12.4)

(3) psychologist, particularly for the children (Chapter 19.4)

(4) physiotherapist (Chapter 12.2)

(5) occupational therapist, able to assess the needs of the patient and to provide such special equipment as bathroom fittings, high chairs, invalid cutlery and crockery, etc. (Chapter 12.3)

Specialist home care services are described in detail in Chapter 2.4. Here it only needs to be emphasized that such a service should never be invited in by the general practitioner/family doctor without prior discussion with the nurse, but apparently this happens in 50 per cent of cases. It is insulting to the nurse, does not permit the best preparation of patient and family, often makes the work of the home care service more difficult, and understandably gives a poor impression to the family of the level of professional co-operation and communication upon which they rightly depend.

Ethical issues in domiciliary care

The subject of ethical issues in palliative care is comprehensively dealt with in Section 3.[107] Reference is here made only to those issues which come into sharper focus in domiciliary care.

Confidentiality and communication with relatives

Every patient has a right to know his diagnosis, prognosis, and what treatment and care are proposed for him. A relative may feel the need for the same information but also may feel that he has a right to veto the patient being told. In western culture he has no right to put such an embargo on communication with the patient, even though his motive may be based on love and the wish to protect the patient, but in many other parts of the world this does not hold true (see Section 10). Another reason is that he fears the emotions that will be unleashed in the patient and his own ability to cope with them.

It has to be remembered that even patients who have not explicitly been told the diagnosis usually suspect it or have come to deduce it for themselves. This comes as a considerable surprise to most relatives who have convinced themselves that their protection has been adequate and the patient is still ignorant of the true facts and the awesome prognosis.

No doctor should accept any embargo on 'truth telling', no matter how well intentioned the carers. As detailed elsewhere in this textbook, he must find ways of communicating honestly yet delicately with his patient, and only with the patient's permission may he then give the same (and no more) information to the relatives. In the safety and sanctity of their own homes, many relatives will feel unusually confident in trying to influence the family doctor to do otherwise but this must be resisted. This responsible task is, however, made easier by the fact that the family doctor has often been known to all parties and indeed become a family friend over many years. He can speak not only with clinical authority but with long-standing and well-established respect for all concerned, knowing their coping strategies, their strengths, and their weaknesses.

Confidentiality and the clergy

The general practitioner, unlike most hospital doctors, may know of his patient's faith and Church affiliations. He may often be aware of spiritual needs and want to help in some way. He has no right to disclose confidential information to a priest or minister of religion, but he can broach the subject with the patient and suggest how helpful it might be if he could bring it to the attention of the priest if he is not already involved. His hands are then untied, and just as he is seen working as a team with a nursing colleague, so he can sometimes offer to be with the patient and spiritual adviser when they get together for the initial discussions on spiritual issues.

It must be admitted that some clergymen, like some doctors, feel uneasy at the bedside of a dying patient, but nevertheless it has been reported that nearly 30 per cent of patients had the help of a spiritual adviser, a clergyman, in the final weeks. There is also substantial evidence that the training of clergy has much improved in the last few decades, many of them having now well-trained insights and sensitivity in this area, though clergy still admit that it is not always easy to co-operate with the medical profession.

Treating the patient for the sake of the relatives

There are a few occasions when the general practitioner finds himself doing something to the patient more for the sake of the relatives than the patient. This is ethically acceptable provided the doctor recognizes what he is doing, does not harm the patient, and does so only until the relatives can, with his help, cope without this form of help.

Some illustrations may help. The unconscious, dying patient is presumably unaware of his death rattle but the relatives may be distressed by it, seeing it as respiratory distress or impending asphyxia. The administration of hyoscine or glycopyrrolate will reduce the offending secretions and so comfort the relatives. A man recently diagnosed as having a disseminated bronchogenic carcinoma with cerebral metastases goes into status epilepticus from which he may die. The relatives, only so recently told of his diagnosis, have not yet come to terms with it and are unprepared for his imminent death. The doctor may, on such an occasion, decide to give high doses of dexamethasone so that in the following weeks as the dose is gradually reduced, the family may enjoy the patient's final days with him.

What is not acceptable is agreeing with the relatives' assessment of the patient's pain and anxiety when the conscious patient would disagree with that perception. As has already been pointed out, research shows that relatives perceive higher levels of pain and anxiety than actually exist.[91] The result is that they can very readily pressurize the doctor into giving larger and larger doses of opioids or other analgesics which the patient does not need and which can, clearly, produce unacceptable side-effects.

Sedation of the patient for the sake of the relatives

If the patient neither wants nor needs to be sedated, it is ethically wrong to do so, no matter how pressing and persuasive the relatives. This is a frequent request at home where their tiredness and strain are so clearly recognized by, and a concern to, the general practitioner.

It has been said that 'sedation' (to the point of deep unconsciousness) is demanded by relatives, reluctantly acceded to by doctors, and usually not wanted by the dying patient. This is probably true. To the grief-stricken carers, the unrousable patient is clearly free of what they perceived as unbearable pain and is now unaware of his impending death. They, the relatives, have seen enough and feel they cannot face any more of his questions or see any more of what they perceive as intolerable suffering. Their needs must clearly be met in other ways but to sedate the patient solely for their sake is wrong.

Maintaining life at any cost

Palliative medicine has as its focus the quality, rather than the quantity, of life. To attempt to prolong it with intravenous hydration, total parenteral nutrition, or other 'life support systems' when they are not wanted by the patient who is aware he is dying, is unethical, no matter how grave the pressure from relatives. As has already been stated, it is often much more difficult for the relatives at home to come to terms with what is happening than it is for the patient himself. Unless consummate skills are employed by the attending family doctor and nurse, many families will continue to feel that their loved one is dying of malnutrition to the point of starvation, or dehydration. It must also be admitted that there are doctors who are only comfortable with the dying when they are 'active'—energetically intervening as they were taught to do in hospital, without due regard for the true state of the patient, his wishes, and his needs. This is one of those many occasions when the work of a family doctor can be eased by calling in a palliative medicine specialist who is able to view the situation objectively and then devote his skill and time to speaking to the relatives on behalf of the family doctor, endorsing his actions and reassuring the family.

Domiciliary care worldwide

It is tempting to think that good domiciliary palliative care can only be provided if there are not only highly-trained general practitioners/family doctors and all the specialist services and other resources described here, but also if the patient lives in a home typical of those in the affluent Western world. This is quite untrue.

Most of the prerequisites for good domiciliary care cost little and are freely available worldwide. They are a loving family, prepared to give unstintingly for the one who has loved them, the commitment of all the available professionals to do as much as possible for the dying as they enjoy doing for the living, and for all concerned to put the patient's needs and dignity at the forefront of all their thinking and doing.

It is quite possible to care for someone in a house which some would describe as poor or even squalid, because that house is a man's home, the creation of his labours and his love. It is certainly possible to keep him comfortable without modern nursing aids if there is the will to do so.

However, one prerequisite, namely the supply of adequate analgesia, coupled with the professional skill to use the necessary drugs, is not yet universally available, and no one can rest until it is. As is graphically illustrated in the final section of this book, most of the world's population has little or no access to strong opioids and must die in unnecessary pain. This must remain a challenge to us all. For those in the West who do have the necessary drugs, but not necessarily everything else which has been described in this section, the challenge is to ensure universal skills in using these drugs and universal willingness to do so.

Perhaps the final challenge is to stem the worldwide swing to hospitalization, the benefits of which have clearly been shown to be much more apparent to doctors than to their patients. Death is a part of life and everyone should have their right to die at home respected. Perhaps Illich was right. We have indeed medicalized and institutionalized death.

References

1. Doyle D. A home care service for terminally ill patients in Edinburgh. *Health Bulletin* (Edinb), 1991; **49**: 14–23.
2. Doyle D. Nursing education in terminal care. *Nurse Education Today*, 1982; **2**(4): 4–6.

3. Ward AWM. *Home Care Services for the Terminally Ill*. Sheffield: Medical Care Research Unit, University of Sheffield, 1985.
4. Palleson AE. Care for the dying in Denmark. *Danish Medical Bulletin*, 1992; **39**: 265–8.
5. Kashiwagi T. Hospice care in Japan. *Postgraduate Medical Journal*, 1991; **67** (suppl 2): S95–9.
6. Toscani F, Mancini C. Inadequacies of care in far advanced cancer patients. *Palliative Medicine*, 1989; **4**: 31–6.
7. Terzoli E, *et al*. Medical oncology and home care in Italy. *Tumori*, 1993; **79**: 30–3.
8. Mercadente S. Family doctor and palliative care team: 1988 versus 1990. *Journal of Palliative Care*, 1991; **7**: 38–9.
9. Illich I. *Limits to Medicine. Medical Nemesis: the Expropriation of Health*. London: Pelican Books, 1977.
10. Vainio A. Palliative care in Finland. *Palliative Medicine*, 1990; **4**: 225–7.
11. Margalit D. The first two years of a palliative home care programme—Jerusalem. *European Journal of Cancer*, 1993; 29a (suppl 6): S268.
12. Tsao SY, Leung A. Palliative care in Hong Kong. *Palliative Medicine* 1991; **5**: 262–6.
13. De Lima L, Bruera E. Palliative care in Columbia: program in 'La Viga'. *Journal of Palliative Care* 1994; **10**: 42–3.
14. Christopoulou I. Factors affecting the decision of cancer patients to be cared for at home or in hospital. *European Journal of Cancer Care*, 1993; **2**(4): 157–60.
15. Walsh TD. Continuing care in a medical center: the Cleveland Clinic Foundation Palliative Care Service. *Journal of Pain and Symptom Management*, 1990; **5**: 273–8.
16. Magno J. USA hospice care in the 1990's. *Palliative Medicine*, 1992; **6**: 158–65.
17. Curtiss CP. Trends and issues for cancer care in rural communities. *Nursing Clinics of North America*, 1993; **28**: 241–51.
18. Levy B, Selare AB. Fatal illness in general practice. *Journal of Royal College of General Practitioners*, 1976; **26**: 303–7.
19. Cartwright N. Changes in life and care in the year before death. *Journal of Public Health Medicine*, 1981; **13**: 81–7.
20. Dar R, *et al*. Cancer pain in the merital system: a study of patients and their spouses. *Journal of Pain and Symptom Management*, 1992; **7**: 87–93.
21. Faulkner A. Helping relatives to cope with a diagnosis of cancer in a loved one. *Journal of Cancer Care*, 1993; **2**(3): 132–6.
22. Grieco AJ, Kowalski W. The 'care partner'. In: Bernstein LH, Grieco Aj, Dete MK, eds. *Primary Care in the Home*. Philadelphia: J.B. Lippincott, 1987: 71–82.
23. Hileman JW, Lackey NR. Self-identified needs of patients with cancer at home and their home caregivers: a descriptive study. *Oncology Nursing Forum*, 1990; **17**: 907–13.
24. Jones RV, Hansford J, Fiske J. Death from cancer at home: the carer's perspective. *British Medical Journal*, 1993; **306**: 249–51.
25. Kissane DW, *et al*. Psychological morbidity in the families of patients with cancer. *Psycho-Oncology*, 1994; **3**: 47–56.
26. Reddall C. People with cancer have the right to expect the best possible treatment and care. *European Journal of Cancer Care*, 1994; **3**: 39–43.
27. Bradshaw PJ. Characteristics of clients referred to home, hospice and hospital palliative care services in Western Australia. *Palliative Medicine*, 1993; **7**: 101–7.
28. Cartwright A. *The Role of the General Practitioners in Caring for People in the Last Year of their Lives*. King Edward's Hospital Fund Report, 1990.
29. Cartwright A. Dying when you're old. *Age and Ageing*, 1993; **22**: 425–30.
30. March G, Kaim-Caudle P. *Terminal Care in General Practice*. London: Croom-Helm. 1976.
31. Williams EL, Fitton F. General practitioner response to elderly patients discharged from hospital. *British Medical Journal*, 1990; **300**: 159–61.
32. Higginson I, Webb D, Lessof L. Reducing hospital beds for patients with advanced cancer. *Lancet*, 1994; **344**: 409.
33. Hinton J. Can home care maintain an acceptable quality of life for patients with terminal cancer and their relatives? *Palliative Medicine*, 1994; **8**: 183–96.
34. Hinton J. Which patients with terminal cancer are admitted from home care? *Palliative Medicine*, 1994; **8**: 197–210.
35. Cartwright A, Hockey L, Anderson R. *Life Before Death*. London: Kegan Paul, 1973.
36. Cartwright A. Balance of care for the dying between hospital and the community; perceptions of general practitioners, hospital consultants, community nurses and relatives. *British Journal of General Practice*, 1991: **41**: 271–4.
37. Mercadente S. Prevalence, causes and mechanisms of pain in home-care patients with advanced cancer. *Pain Clinic*, 1994; **7**: 131–6.
38. Sykes NP, Pearson SE, Chell S. Quality of care of the terminally ill: the carer's perspective. *Palliative Medicine*, 1992; **6**: 227–36.
39. Thorpe G. Enabling more dying people to remain at home. *British Medical Journal*, 1993; **307**: 915–8.
40. Walker J. When self-help begins at home. Pain control in cancer care. *Professional Nurse*, 1992; **7**: 662–3.
41. Parkes CM. Home or hospital? Terminal care as seen by surviving spouses. *Journal of the Royal College of General Practitioners*, 1978; **28**: 19–30.
42. Constantini M, *et al*. Palliative home care and place of death among cancer patients: a population-based study. *Palliative Medicine*, 1993; **7**: 323–31.
43. Blyth AC. Audit of terminal care in a general practice. *British Medical Journal*, 1991; **330**: 983–6.
44. Brivio E, Gamba A. Home care for advanced cancer patients: the efficacy of domiciliary assistance. *European Journal of Cancer Care*, 1992; **1**(2): 24–8.
45. Doyle D. Domiciliary terminal care—demands on statutory services. *Journal of the Royal College of General Practitioners*, 1982; **32**: 285–91.
46. Hileman JW, Lackey NR, Hassanein RS. Identifying the needs of home caregivers of patients with cancer. *Oncology Nursing Forum*, 1992; **19**: 771–7.
47. Norum J, Wist E. When a cancer patient dies at home—experience of the relatives. Kreftavdelingen Regionsykehuset; *Tromso Tidsskr Nor Laegeforen*, 1993; **113**(9): 1107–9.
48. Sanz-Ortiz J, Llamazares Gonzales A. Home care in a palliative care unit. *Medicina Clinica*(Barcelona), 1993; **101**: 446–9.
49. Boyd KJ. Palliative care in the community: views of general practitioners and district nurses in East London. *Journal of Palliative Care*, 1993; **9**: 33–7.
50. Doyle D. Domiciliary terminal care. *Practitioner*, 1980; **224**: 575–82.
51. Dunphy KP, Amesbury BDW. A comparison of hospice and home care patients: patterns of referral, patient characteristics and predictors of place of death. *Palliative Medicine*, 1990; **4**: 105–11.
52. Reilly PM, Patten MP. Terminal care in the home. *Journal of the Royal College of General Practitioners*, 1981; **31**: 531–7.
53. Seale C. Community nurses and the care of the dying. *Social Science and Medicine*, 1992; **34**: 375–82.
54. Seamark DA, *et al*. Knowledge and perceptions of a domiciliary hospice service among general practitioners and community nurses. *British Journal of General Practice*, 1993; **43**: 57–9.
55. Nikkonen M, Siikanen E. Home care nurses' support of the relative caregiver of the patient dying at home. *Sairaanhoitaja* 1993; **8**: 14–15.
56. Kindlen M. Hospice home care services: a Scottish perspective. *Palliative Medicine*, 1988; **2**: 115–21.
57. Stedeford A. Couples facing death II—unsatisfactory communication. *British Medical Journal*, 1981; **283**: 1098–101.
58. Stedeford A. 1994. *Facing Death: Patients, Families and Professionals*, 2nd edition. Oxford: Sobell Publications.
59. Gilley J. Intimacy and terminal care. *Journal of the Royal College of General Practitioners*, 1988; **38**: 121–2.
60. Smith N. The impact of terminal illness on the family. *Palliative Medicine*, 1990; **4**: 127–35.
61. Snelling J. The role of the family in relation to chronic pain: review of the literature. *Journal of Advanced Nursing*, 1990; **15**: 771–6.
62. Herd EB. Terminal care in a semi-rural area. *Journal of the Royal College of General Practitioners*, 1990; **40**: 248–51.

63. Beck-Friis B, Strang P. The organization of hospital-based home care for terminally ill cancer patients: the Motala model. *Palliative Medicine*, 1993; 7: 93–100.
64. Beck-Friis B, Strang P. The family in hospice-based home care with special reference to terminally-ill cancer patients. *Journal of Palliative Care*, 1993; **9**: 5–13.
65. Gomas JM. Palliativecare at home; a reality or 'mission impossible'? *Palliative Medicine*, 1993; **7**(2suppl): 45–59.
66. Gomez-Batiste X. Catalonia's five year plan: basic principles. *European Journal of Palliative Care*, 1994; **1**: 45–9.
67. Jones R. Primary health care: what should we do for people dying at home with cancer? *Eur.J. Cancer Care*. 1992; **1**: 9–11.
68. Lubin S. Palliative care—could your patient have been managed at home? *Journal of Palliative Care*, 1992; **8**: 18–22.
69. MacAdam DB. A review of 715 terminal patients cared for at home by a hospice palliative care service. *Cancer Forum*, 1985; **9**: 101–4.
70. Spencer J. Caring for a terminally ill person with pain, at home: An Australian perspective. *Cancer Nursing*, 1991; **14**: 55–8.
71. Lyon A, Love DR. Terminal care: The role of the general practitioner hospital. *Journal of the Royal College of General Practitioners*, 1984; **34**: 331–3.
72. Thorn CP, *et al.* The influence of general practitioner community hospitals on the place of death of cancer patients. *Palliative Medicine*, 1994; **8**: 122–8.
73. Bennett IJ, Danczak AF. Terminal care: improving teamwork in primary care using significant event analysis (SEA). *European Journal of Cancer Care*, 1994; **3**: 54–7.
74. Berenthal JA. A welcome back for carers? The role of voluntary services in caring for dying people. *Professional Nurse*, 1994; **9**: 267–70.
75. Cavenagh JD, Gunz FW. Palliative hospice care in Australia. *Palliative Medicine*, 1988; **2**: 51–7.
76. Copperman H. Hospice home care service (letter). *Palliative Medicine*, 1992; **6**: 260.
77. Dawson NJ. Need satisfaction in terminal care settings. *Social Science and Medicine*, 1991; **32**: 83–7.
78. Dessloch A, *et al.* Hospital care versus home nursing; on the quality of life of terminal tumor patients. *Psychotherapeutic and Psychosomatic Medicine and Psychology*, 1992; **42**(12): 424–9.
79. Haines A, Booroff A. Terminal care at home: perspective from general practice. *British Medical Journal*, 1986; **292**: 1051–3.
80. Hockey L. St. Columba's Hospice Home Care Service: an evaluation study. *Palliative Medicine*, 1991; **5**: 315–22.
81. McWhinney IR, Stewart MA. Home care of dying patients. Family physicians' experience with a palliative care team. *Canadian Family Physician*, 1994; **40**: 240–6.
82. Maltoni M, *et al.* Description of a home care service for cancer patients through quantitative indexes of evaluation. *Tumori*, 1991; **77**: 453–9.
83. Mercadente S, *et al.* Home palliative care: results of 1991 versus 1988. *Journal of Pain and Symptom Management*, 1992; **7**: 414–8.
84. Roe DJ. Palliative care 2000—home care. *Journal of Palliative Care*, 1992; **8**: 28–32.
85. Barritt PW. Care of the dying in one practice. *Journal of the Royal College of General Practitioners*, 1984; **34**: 446–8.
86. Simpson M, *et al.* Doctor-patient communication: The Toronto Consensus Statement. *British Medical Journal*, 1991; **303**: 1385–7.
87. Hunt RW, *et al.* The community care of terminal ill patients. *Australian Family Physician* 1990; **19**: 1835–41.
88. Raiman J. Monitoring pain at home. *Journal of District Nursing*, 1986; **4**: 4–6.
89. Lloyd-Williams M. Depression among cancer patients (letter). *British Journal of General Practice*, 1994, **44**: 223.
90. Sanders J. Palliative Care—the general practice challenge. *Journal of Cancer Care*, 1993; **2**(1): 2–5.
91. Spiller JA, Alexander DA. Domiciliary care: a comparison of the views of terminally ill patients and their family caregivers. *Palliative Medicine*, 1993; **7**: 109–15.
92. Grossman SA, *et al.* Correlation of patient and caregiver ratings of cancer pain. *Journal of Pain and Symptom Management*, 1991; **6**: 53–7.
93. Robinson L, Stacy R. Palliative Care in the community: setting practice guidelines for primary care teams. *British Journal of General Practice*, 1994; **44**: 461–4.
94. McWhinney IR. *A Textbook of Family Medicine*. London: Oxford University Press. 1989.
95. Johnston TE, *et al.* Managing cancer pain at home: the decisions and ethical conflicts of patients, family caregivers and homecare nurses. *Oncology Nursing Forum*, 1993; **20**: 919–27.
96. Lopez de Maturana A, *et al.* Attitudes of general practitioners in Bizkaia, Spain, towards the terminally ill patient. *Palliative Medicine*, 1993; **7**: 39–45.
97. Saunders J, Rosenthal S. Improving domiciliary terminal care. *Nursing Times*, 1992; **88**: 32–4.
98. Sciortino AD, *et al.* The efficacy of administering blood transfusions at home to terminally ill cancer patients. *Journal of Palliative Care*, 1993; **9**: 14–17.
99. Mercadente S. Intrathecal morphine and bupivicaine in advanced cancer patients implanted at home. *Journal of Pain and Symptom Management*, 1994; **9**: 201–7.
100. Rosser JE, Maguire P. Dilemmas in general practice: the care of the cancer patient. *Social Science and Medicine*, 1982; **16**: 315–22.
101. Dunlop RJ, Hockley J. The distress of inappropriate hospice transfer. *Palliative Medicine*, 1991; **5**: 61–2.
102. Amesbury BDW, Dunphy KP. The use of subcutaneous midazolam in the home care setting. *Palliative Medicine*, 1989; **3**: 299–310.
103. McNamara P, Minton M, Twycross, RG. Use of midazolam in palliative care. *Palliative Medicine*, 1991; **5**: 244–9.
104. McNulty B. Discharge of the terminally ill patient. *Nursing Times*, 1970; **66**: 1160–2.
105. Moore MK. Dying at home: a way of maintaining control for the person with ALS/MND. *Palliative Medicine*, 1993; **7**(4 suppl.2): 65–8.
106. Parkes CM. The effects of bereavement on physical and mental health: a study of the care records of widows. *British Medical Journal*, 1984; **2**: 274.
107. National Council for Hospice and Specialist Palliative Care Services. *Key Ethical Issues in Palliative Care: Evidence to House of Lords Select Committee on Medical Ethics*. Occasional Paper 3, July 1993.
108. Isaacs B. The concept of pre-death. *Lancet*, 1971; **1**: 1115–19.
109. Burne R. The dying child at home. *Journal of the Royal College of General Practitioners*, 1987; **37**: 291.

17

The terminal phase

17 The terminal phase

Robert Twycross and Ivan Lichter

The practical and ethical issues surrounding the care of patients who are close to death are discussed in this section. The patient's condition leaves no room for doubt that death is likely to occur within a matter of days. He or she is:

- profoundly weak
- essentially bedbound
- drowsy for extended periods
- disoriented with respect to time with a severely limited attention span
- increasingly uninterested in food and fluid
- finding it difficult to swallow medication.

The terminal phase is a period when goals must be redefined and when it is appropriate to discontinue certain treatments. Existing symptoms may worsen or new symptoms arise, necessitating modification of management or the initiation of new measures to ensure the comfort of the patient. Good relief of symptoms can be achieved so that the large majority of patients die peacefully.[1] To achieve this, there needs to be a balance between death sooner than is technologically possible and death later than is compatible with a peaceful end.[2]

Management at this stage is the same whatever the cause of the terminal illness. What is offered will depend on the resources available. In developing countries facilities for care are often limited, while in the United States of America methods of medical practice and Medicare regulations for reimbursement can create difficulties.

Telling the patient

The patient sometimes appears to be unaware that the end is near. However, if he or she is already aware that the illness is terminal, there is seldom need to draw attention to the imminence of death. Some patients ask 'When will it be over?', and reassurance that it will not be long is often welcome. Others do not ask even when life no longer holds any pleasure or when the ravages of disease have exhausted them and they long for an end. For them, it is a comfort to be told that release is close at hand. Patients should be assured that they will be kept comfortable and will not suffer pain. They should be told that nothing will be done to prolong dying, that death will be peaceful, and that someone will be with them. This does much to alleviate fears that they may have about dying.[3] Those patients who feel a need to fight to the end and who struggle to keep going, may find it a relief to be told that 'it is all right to let go now'. In this way a difficult death may be transformed into a peaceful one.

Telling the relatives

Even when it appears certain to health care professionals that the patient has very little time left, relatives may be unprepared for the death and are upset because they have not been warned. Opportunity for farewells may have been missed, and this can cause considerable grief, leading to a more difficult bereavement. Therefore care must be taken to ensure that all close relatives are informed that time is short.

However, a patient who appears to have only a matter of hours to live may sometimes survive for many days. Because of the uncertainty of prognostication, relatively wide limits should be given when informing relatives about the imminence of death.

Psychological needs of the patient

What the patient needs is 'safe conduct' at a time when he or she must surrender autonomy and yield control to someone else. It is important to do nothing that infringes a person's individuality or damages self-esteem. An awareness by the carers of factors which influence hope in the terminally ill is important (Table 1). When close to death, hope becomes refocused on 'being' rather than 'doing', and emphasizes relationships—with others and with God

Table 1 Factors that influence hope in the terminally ill

Decrease	Increase
Feeling devalued	Feeling valued
Abandonment and isolation 'conspiracy of silence' 'there is nothing more which can be done'	Meaningful relationship(s) reminiscence humour
Lack of direction/goals	Realistic goals
Unrelieved pain and discomfort	Pain and symptom relief

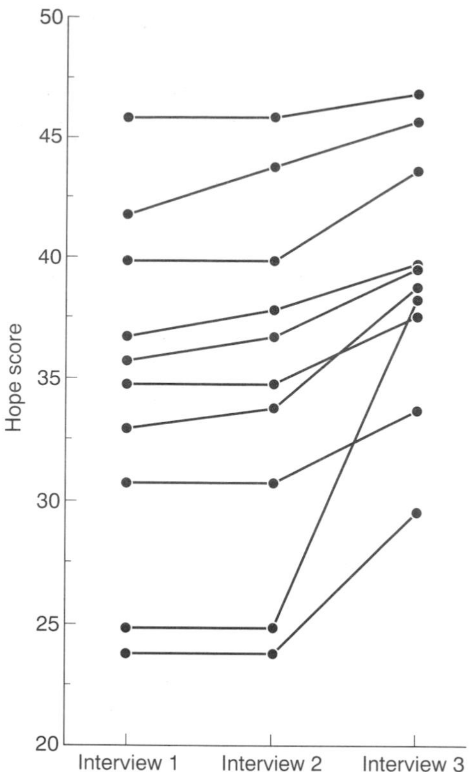

Fig. 1 Hope scores in 10 home-care patients shortly after referral to a hospice programme (interview 1), when ability to complete activities of daily living became severely impaired (interview 2), and when death was thought likely to occur within 2 weeks (interview 3). (Reproduced with permission from ref. 4.)

(or a 'higher being').[4] In consequence, it is possible for hope to increase as death approaches, provided that the standard of care and comfort are good enough (Fig. 1).

Religion, faith, and dying

When religion has been a central dimension in life it is likely to play an important role in the approach to death. However, people for whom religion has not been significant do not often turn to it when they are dying.[5]

Roman Catholic priests have observed that sacramental anointing sometimes results in a patient's accepting death, and dying more easily and quickly.[6] There may be release from anxiety, apprehension, and feelings of guilt which often produces physical relaxation, with relief of pain and other symptoms. Religious rites serve deep psychospiritual needs, comparable with confession in the non-religious setting.

Patients with strong religious beliefs or none at all are usually much less apprehensive about dying than those with weakly held beliefs.[7] However, some patients with strong beliefs may be terrified of punishment for past misdeeds. Others, having led a blameless life, may question a faith which has not protected them from their present suffering. Everybody has spiritual needs, even those without a formal faith. Therefore a clergyman should be available to listen to the patient without pressing any particular doctrine.[8] The clergyman must seek to respond to the patient's questions and help him to examine his fears without the use of religious language and dogma.[9]

Supporting the family

Much of the support which the dying person needs can only be given by the family. Their love and attention are of paramount importance to the well being and psychological comfort of the dying patient. They in turn need support at this critical time, and should have easy access to those providing care for the patient. They need recognition of the strain which they are bearing, and to be told how important their contribution is to the care of the patient.

A major fear of families looking after a loved one at home is that they will not provide the right care or will not know what to do in the event of an emergency. As far as possible, they need to be relieved of the uncertainty as to what may happen, and feel prepared to meet those emergencies that can be anticipated. They must be told how symptoms will be relieved and above all they must be assured of constant and speedy professional support.

Family members need to feel that they are being helpful to the patient and contributing to his comfort. In the terminal stage, they should not be discouraged from any self-sacrifice that they wish to make as their last gift to the dying patient. They should not be made to feel inadequate if they are no longer able to care for the patient at home or to feel intruders at the hospital bedside.[10] They should be encouraged to stay close so that they will learn from the example of nurses who talk to the patient even when he is unconscious and hold his hand, and will develop the confidence to do the same.[3] They may need an opportunity to say their last words to the dying patient in private and to be assured that this is helpful even if the patient is unable to show any response. Reassurance will need to be given to those who find it too painful to be present at the death so that they do not suffer feelings of remorse or guilt. They will be helped by the knowledge that the caring team will not leave their loved one unattended.

What the family is most likely to remember for a long time after the patient's death are the events of the last days. For the sake of both the family and the patient, care must be given to maintain identity and dignity. Patients must not be left exposed or in a soiled condition. Privacy must be ensured and the patient treated with respect even when confused or disordered behaviour occurs. Unrelieved pain or other distressing symptoms are incompatible with full dignity and demand vigorous and speedy relief.

The family will recall details of the patient's symptoms and emotional status as they perceived them. Explanation at the time by staff can prevent distress from lack of understanding or misinterpretation. Reassurance that noisy breathing does not indicate difficulty in breathing, that grunting does not imply distress, and that the patient is indeed comfortable will prevent later doubts. Knowledge that the dying person is aware of their presence and is comforted by it, even when comatose, helps to sustain the relatives in their vigil. They will welcome assurance that they have done all that could be done and have made the best decisions in matters such as placement.

At the time of death, staff need to provide a supporting presence for the family and will subsequently give guidance about making necessary arrangements. There should be an opportunity to talk with a staff member and to weep and express emotion. The presence of a clergyman at this time may bring great comfort.

At an early date, the family should be invited to meet with staff who cared for their relative for discussion and explanation of events surrounding the illness and the death. At this time they can be prepared for some of the experiences of bereavement.

Supporting the team

Patients who do not seem to be near to death may decline very rapidly even when death is not caused by a sudden catastrophe such as major haemorrhage. Staff may find this disconcerting, and they should be reminded from time to time that this does occur and be supported when distressed by an unexpected death.

Health-care professionals also need to recognize their own emotions. This is particularly important when dealing with children and young adults. Younger staff members identify with such patients and experience something of their own fear of suffering and death. Unless provision is made for them to express their feelings, their anxieties and fears may reflect back onto their patients.[11]

Suffering

Suffering is not directly related to the severity of unrelieved symptoms.[12,13] Even mild symptoms may cause considerable suffering if the patient has not come to terms with the prospect of imminent death, and relatives and friends suffer when forced helplessly to witness the physical deterioration of a loved one. Suffering stems from conditions or events which threaten the integrity of a person as a complex psychological and social entity.[14] Suffering is experienced by persons, not by bodies. It can occur in relation to any aspect of the person—physical, psychological, social, or spiritual. A sense of loss of meaning and purpose,[15] helplessness,[16] hopelessness, endlessness, and lack of control[17] are major causes of suffering.

Suffering is influenced by psychological factors which may be rooted in personality traits and attitudes, or may result from disturbed interpersonal dynamics.[18] Personality traits which tend to increase distress and suffering include a negative outlook on life or the need to maintain control. The dying person suffers not only loss of control over external events but also loss of bodily control and mental functions. Those who have been most independent are particularly affected and may refuse help which could make them comfortable.[19] Rigid, controlling, and domineering individuals may be overwhelmed when faced with physical helplessness.[20]

For many people, sorting out unfinished interpersonal business is important in achieving a sense of completeness which promotes tranquillity and inner peace. There is often a need for forgiveness and reconciliation with others.[21] If left unresolved, broken relationships may cause continued suffering, although it is the patient's perception of the situation which ultimately determines the degree of distress.

In addition to physical symptoms and psychological distress, existential concerns are a potent source of suffering. Common existential issues include hopelessness, disappointment, remorse, death anxiety, disruption of personal identity, and the meaninglessness of continued life. There may be distress about the distress of the family, friends, and carers, which may lead to the patient's concluding that ongoing existence only constitutes a perpetuation of the burden to others.[17]

The importance of distinguishing between suffering and symptoms is particularly relevant in the days before death. At this stage most patients are profoundly weak and probably bedbound. It is not possible to alleviate the weakness, but continuing vigilance is needed in the relief of pain and other symptoms. People frequently report suffering when they do not believe that their pain can be relieved, when the pain (although not overwhelming) continues for a long time, when the source of the pain is unknown, or when the meaning of the pain is dire. Suffering is eased by making the source of the pain known, changing its meaning, and demonstrating that it can be relieved and that an end is in sight.[14] The patient must also be sustained spiritually during this time of almost total physical dependence. This task is helped by an appreciation of the factors that provide the basis for a supportive relationship, the so-called 'therapeutic triad':[22]

- empathy, i.e. the ability to imagine what someone else is feeling but not necessarily expressing (e.g. anger or anxiety);
- warmth, i.e. a warm feeling towards others with a non-judgemental acceptance of all that they reveal themselves to be;
- genuineness, i.e. trustworthiness, openness, and a wholeness of character which is real and not a professional facade.

The task of confronting suffering requires both humility and courage. Suffering can always be approached; transformation of suffering often occurs. Those who obtain relief from suffering have surrendered 'who they were' to a new reality of 'who they are'. Interventions must be consonant with the personal matrix of the individual patient, and help him or her regain a sense of integration by discovering a renewed sense of meaning and purpose within his or her personal experience of discomfort and dying.[23]

Suffering is not amenable to relief by others. Ultimately, it is the patient and the family who work through and make sense of their suffering, not the professional carer. Others may provide the conditions which assist patients in working through and coming to terms with their suffering, beginning by recognizing and validating it.

Ethical considerations

The statement of the Council on Ethical and Judicial Affairs of the American Medical Association on withholding or withdrawing life-prolonging medical treatment provides a good summary of the doctor's responsibility to patients at the end of life (see Appendix). The statement stresses that the ethical standards of professional conduct and responsibility may exceed but are never less than, or contrary to, those required by law.[24] The caring team will normally strive to preserve the life of the patient until this is essentially futile and will balance the potential benefits of treatment against potential burdens. The primary aim is no longer to prolong life but to make what life remains as comfortable as possible. In these circumstances, treatment to relieve pain and suffering which coincidentally brings forward the moment of death by a few hours or days is acceptable.[25]

The report from the Hastings Center is recommended for further reading,[26] as is the shorter account in the World Health Organization (WHO) Expert Committee Report.[27]

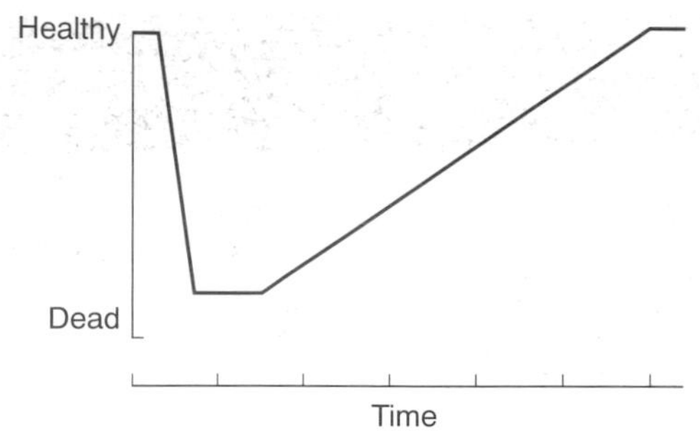

Fig. 2 A graphical representation of acute illness. Biological prospects are generally good. Acute resuscitative measures are important and enable the patient to survive the initial crisis. Recovery is aided by the natural forces of healing; rehabilitation is completed by the patient alone, without continued medical support.

Appropriate treatment

When a patient is close to death, the overriding aim of treatment is to make the person as comfortable as possible. What may be an appropriate treatment in an acutely ill patient could well be inappropriate in someone close to death. Cardiac resuscitation, artificial respiration, intravenous infusion, nasogastric tubes, and antibiotics are all primarily supportive measures for use in acute or acute-on-chronic illnesses to assist a patient through the initial period towards recovery of health (Fig. 2). To use such measures in patients who are clearly close to death and have no expectancy of a return to health is inappropriate, and therefore is bad medicine (Fig. 3). We have no right or duty, legal or ethical, to prescribe a lingering death.[24]

However, treatment remains active; 'passive care' is a contradiction in terms. Efficient good-quality care is what is called for, not just 'tender loving care'—a term sometimes used to justify neglect.[28] The following key points should be borne in mind:

- the patient's biological prospects
- the therapeutic aim and benefits of each treatment
- the adverse effects of treatment
- the need to avoid prescription of a lingering death.

In patients who are close to death it is often appropriate to 'give death a chance'. All patients must die eventually; ultimately nature will take its course. In this respect, the art of medicine is to decide

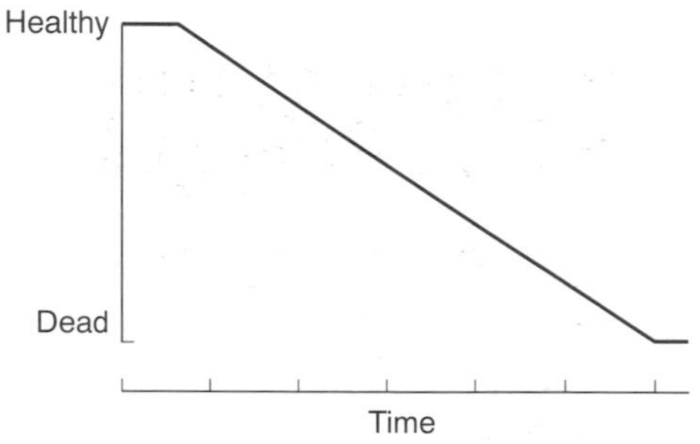

Fig. 3 A graphical representation of acute illness. Biological prospects are generally good. Acute resuscitative measures are important and enable the patient to survive the initial crisis. Recovery is aided by the natural forces of healing; rehabilitation is completed by the patient alone, without continued medical support.

when life sustenance is essentially futile and therefore when to allow death to occur without further impediment. For example, although antibiotics are generally appropriate for the patient with advanced cancer who develops a chest infection while still relatively active and independent, pneumonia should still be 'the old man's friend' in those who have deteriorated and are close to death. It is generally appropriate not to prescribe antibiotics.

If it is difficult to make a decision, the '2-day rule' should be invoked, i.e. if after 2 to 3 days of straightforward symptom management the patient is clearly holding his own, prescribe an antibiotic, but if the patient is clearly much worse, do not.[25] However, not all terminally ill patients who develop a chest infection die from it. Some patients progress only to a 'grumbling pneumonia' but no further. A continuing wet cough may cause much distress and, possibly, loss of sleep. In circumstances when the patient is neither better nor worse after 3 to 4 days, an antibiotic is indicated in order to relieve symptoms.

When death is close it is sensible to simplify medication. Iron, multivitamins, and potassium are usually medium-term supportive treatments and become irrelevant when the patient is close to death. Antihypertensives can often be gradually discontinued. Continued diuretic therapy may cause postural hypotension unless the dose is reduced or stopped in the face of a poor fluid intake or repeated vomiting. In the last days it is generally appropriate to discontinue laxatives and antidepressants. Insulin dose should be reduced as oral intake diminishes. Reductions can be made on the basis of finger-prick blood glucose estimations or by guesswork. When the patient is unconscious, insulin can be discontinued. There is no longer any biological justification for the continued palliation of the diabetic state.

Similarly, some nursing procedures which are normally regarded as essential may be discontinued in the last days. For example, care of pressure areas may be perceived as an unwelcome disturbance and may be reduced or stopped.

Terminal dehydration

Food and fluid intake generally diminish in the terminal stage of illness. It is at this time that the question is raised whether to administer fluids by artificial means.[29] The traditional hospice view is that when interest in food and fluid becomes minimal, the patient should not be forced to receive them. Indeed, eating and drinking may no longer be relevant to the patient who has already withdrawn and whose attention is now inward or 'beyond'.[30] None the less, many dying patients automatically receive intravenous fluids when they are no longer able to maintain a normal fluid balance.[31,32] The main reason for this appears to be a belief that dehydration in a person close to death is distressing. However, hospice staff have generally taken the view that dehydration may well be beneficial, and hydration detrimental. It is claimed that with dehydration there is decreased urine output and less need for the urinal, the bedpan, the commode, or catheterization, and fewer bed-wetting episodes. A reduction in pulmonary secretions is said to result in less coughing and congestion, and a decrease in choking and drowning sensations with less need for suctioning. Likewise, decreased gastrointestinal secretions result in fewer bouts of vomiting in obstructed patients. Pain may also be diminished owing to reduction in tumour oedema.[33]

It is now claimed that hypodermoclysis (e.g. 500–1500 ml/24 h) circumvents many of the objections to other artificial methods of hydration.[34,35] However, there is no evidence to date that rehydration generally makes patients more comfortable.[36] Hypodermoclysis has also been reported to relieve delirium in some dying patients. This suggests that improvement in renal function may promote the excretion of toxic drug metabolites.[37] However, improved cognition has also been reported after withdrawal of hydration.[33]

A possible indication for rehydration is that the patient feels dry despite good mouth care. Dry mouth is a common problem in cancer patients and is related not only to dehydration but to other causes such as drugs (e.g. phenothiazines, tricyclic antidepressants, opioids), candidiasis, local radiotherapy, oxygen therapy, and mouth breathing.[38,39] Thus artificial hydration alone is unlikely to resolve the symptom of dry mouth in most patients.[40] Further, poor fluid intake and laboratory tests do not provide a sound basis for predicting whether a patient will experience dry mouth and thirst or other dehydration-related symptoms.[41] However, dry mouth can be satisfactorily relieved by conscientious mouth care and small amounts of fluid,[42] for example 1 to 2 ml of water delivered by pipette or syringe into the dependent side of the mouth every 30 to 60 min. Small ice chips can also be used.[43]

Intravenous hydration may have negative psychosocial effects in that the infusion acts as a barrier between the patient and the family. It is more difficult to embrace a spouse who is attached to a plastic tube, and doctors and nurses tend to become diverted from the more human aspects of care to the control of fluid balance and electrolytes.[44]

Families are often distressed as patients near death decrease their oral intake. Their feelings on intravenous therapy and its significance to them should be established, and the rationale for discontinuing it should be explained.[45] The decision regarding rehydration should focus on the comfort of the patient, rather than on the goal of providing optimal nutrition and hydration.[33]

Studies of dying

At the beginning of the present century, Sir William Osler stated that:[46]

> I have careful records of about 500 deathbeds, studied particularly with reference to the modes of death and the sensations of the dying. The latter alone concerns us here. Ninety suffered bodily pain or distress of one sort or another, eleven showed mental apprehension, two positive terror, one expressed spiritual exaltation, one bitter remorse. The great majority gave no signs one way or the other; like their birth, their death was a sleep and a forgetting.

Presumably, Osler was talking about a wide range of causes of death including infection. He gives no information about the use of medication to relieve pain or distress. Even so, his conclusion that for the great majority 'death was a sleep and a forgetting' is noteworthy.

Some more recent studies also cover a range of causes of death,[47-50] while others have been limited to cancer patients associated with palliative care services in inpatient[51] and community settings.[52-54] The picture portrayed by these reports is similar to a great extent. Each highlights symptoms which require diligent attention during the final 48 h: pain, dyspnoea, restlessness, and agitation (Table 2).

Table 2 Last 48 h of life: symptoms in a series of 200 patients

Symptom		Frequency (percentage of patients)
Noisy and moist breathing		56
Urinary dysfunction		53
Incontinence	32	
Retention	21	
Pain		51
Restlessness and agitation		42
Dyspnoea		22
Nausea and vomiting		14
Sweating		14
Jerking, twitching, plucking		12
Confusion		9

Source: ref. 54.

The report from Milan[53] is exceptional in that 63 of 120 patients dying at home had one or more unendurable symptoms which necessitated sedating the patient until death (Table 3). The fact that dyspnoea, for example, may worsen as death approaches has been noted by others.[52,55] What is disturbing in the Milan study is the apparent need to sedate more than 25 per cent of dying patients because it became unendurable. These figures contrast strongly with the experience at St Christopher's Hospice, London, where only one patient in a consecutive series of 100 died with uncontrolled dyspnoea.[51] The patient in question had been in the hospice for only 1 day and steps were actively being taken to ease his distress at the time of death.

Data from patients in New Zealand being cared for either at home or as hospice inpatients also demonstrated that death was not always peaceful.[54] Here again, the incidence of respiratory distress and pain was much lower (Table 4). It is possible that cultural factors account for the differences between the data from Italy and those from the United Kingdom and New Zealand. Because several factors could be involved,[56] an international multicentre study would be required to ascertain the reason for the differences.

Level of consciousness immediately before death

Data concerning the level of consciousness in the hours or days before death are given in several studies.[6,48,51,54] Because measures

Table 3 Unendurable symptoms in 63 patients dying of cancer

Symptoms	Number of patients
Dyspnoea	33
Pain	31
Delirium	11
Vomiting	5
Total	80*

* Fifteen patients had two symptoms and one patient had three symptoms.
Source: ref. 53.

Table 4 Factors that prevented a peaceful death in a series of 200 patients

Symptom	Frequency (percentage of patients)
Haemorrhage and haemoptysis	2
Respiratory distress	2
Restlessness	1.5
Pain	1
Myocardial infarction	1
Regurgitation	1
Total	8.5

Source: ref. 54.

of level of consciousness and the time intervals used differ, it is not possible to compare the data from different centres directly. However, all the studies state that some patients were conscious until death or less than 15 min before death. Excluding those who died suddenly and unexpectedly, the proportion of patients coming into this category varied from 6 to 30 per cent. The number stated to be unconscious for more than 24 h varied inversely from 34 to 8 per cent.

Planning and coordinating care

Planning for the last days calls for an understanding of the changes which may take place at this time and a knowledge of the options which are available. While the best physical comfort may be more readily achieved with inpatient care, the wishes of the patient and family (which may be conflicting) are paramount. They must have information about the increasing demands of care which may arise, and of the degree and sources of support which can be offered if they choose home care.

Relatives may be upset and feel guilty if the patient dies very shortly after leaving their care, feeling that they could have 'seen it through' if they had had better information. Others are glad to provide every care during the illness, but are afraid or unwilling to have the patient die at home.

Coping at home

As long as my mother was taking drugs orally that was all right—I could cope. But when it got to the stage that she could not keep anything down and we had to have injections it was a terrifying situation. I could not phone my family practitioner at all hours of the night. There was no 24 hour service as far as I knew. In fact, I was left alone in the middle of the night with my mother in absolute agony not knowing where to turn.[57]

In this situation no advanced technology or new research was needed to relieve the patient's vomiting and pain. The issues were doctor availability, information about community resources, 24-h cover, and instructions about how to administer analgesics by an alternative route to a vomiting patient.

Doctor availability

Doctor availability is a crucial element in symptom management at home. It is vital for the psychological and physical well being of the terminally ill patient that the doctor remains a key figure throughout. A doctor is needed to make routine and emergency home visits for on-the-spot assessments and to decide on appropriate therapeutic measures. In a survey of home-based terminal cancer care,[58] doctors themselves rated medical (as distinct from nursing) needs as heavy in 12 per cent, moderate in 59 per cent, and minimal in 27 per cent. Whereas minimal requirements may be satisfied over the telephone, it is difficult to justify not seeing a patient with heavy or moderate needs.

A doctor whose clinical experience has been in the protective security of the well-staffed medical centre may feel insecure and uncertain when alone with a housebound patient with uncontrolled symptoms. However, people will put up with a great deal of inconvenience and discomfort if they remain confident that their doctor respects them as individuals and is concerned for their comfort. An emergency home visit in the early hours of the morning may do much to reinforce the reality of this concern regardless of what is done in relation to symptom relief (see Section 16).

Drug administration

When swallowing becomes difficult, it is helpful to convert from tablets to oral solutions. Morphine may be given in a concentrated solution as a lingual, sublingual, or buccal administration. Sublingual tablets are the best sublingual preparations because they are less likely to be swallowed. Diamorphine is available in sublingual form in the United Kingdom. Sublingual buprenorphine, which is a partial agonist, can be used in doses of up to 4 to 5 mg per 24 h, equivalent to 240 to 300 mg of morphine by mouth (see Chapter 9.2.3). Several other drugs which may be required in the terminal phase are available in sublingual formulations (Table 5). It may be easier to place tablets or solution in the dependent cheek rather than under the tongue. With most drugs at the end of life, a 1:1 dose conversion ratio is used initially when converting from oral to sublingual and is adjusted according to outcome.[25]

Antiemetic, psychotropic, and analgesic suppositories have a special place in home care as an alternative to parenteral medication when the patient is unable to swallow (Table 6). The carer must be taught to place the suppository against the rectal mucosa. The drug will not be absorbed if pushed into a faecal mass or placed in the anal canal. The widespread availability of portable syringe drivers has considerably simplified the administration of medication to moribund patients wherever they are cared for.[59–61] The use of a syringe driver is less disturbing to the patient than repeated injections or the insertion of suppositories, and relieves the burden on patients and carers when swallowing becomes difficult. Most drugs given by syringe driver are miscible;[62] some must be given separately.

Planning for crises

The situation often changes quickly for the dying patient. With each visit one must expect the situation to have changed. Common problems must be discussed with the relatives because they need to be prepared psychologically and practically. Unless a syringe driver is available, a supply of essential drugs in suppository or parenteral form should be kept in the home. Eventualities should be antici-

Table 5 Sublingual formulations of relevance to palliative care available in the United Kingdom

Drug	Preparation	Strength	Comment
Analgesics			
Aspirin-glycine*	Tablet	500 mg	The glycine enhances the solubility of aspirin. For some patients it is too gritty
Buprenorphine	Tablet	0.2 mg 0.4 mg	
Dextromoramide*	Tablet	5 mg, 10 mg	Rapid onset of action; relatively short-acting and may need to be used every 3 h
Diamorphine	Tablet	10 mg	
Morphine	Liquid	20 mg/ml	Supplied with calibrated dropper. Sublingual administration feasible because of small volume; probably absorbed mainly from stomach. Particularly useful for moribund patients at home
Phenazocine*	Tablet	5 mg	Bitter tasting like other opioids
Antiemetics and psychotropics			
Hyoscine	Tablet	0.3 mg	An over-the-counter preparation (Quick Kwells®)
Lorazepam[a]	Tablet	1 mg, 2.5 mg	Five times more potent than diazepam. Tablets are scored, permitting use of 0.5 mg

* Oral tablets that can be taken sublingually.

pated as far as possible, and drugs charted to be given by the nurse without further consultation with the doctor in the event of an emergency (e.g. haemorrhage or fit).

Most situations are manageable in the home, but poor planning can precipitate inpatient admission. Although even the best laid plans may prove inadequate, families can often manage to cope if they can talk to somebody who knows the patient at any time of the day or night. Families occasionally test out 24-h availability and call for help at an unusual hour for some trivial reason. Once they discover that somebody really is there, most stop testing and do not abuse the service.

'I can't stand seeing her suffer'

It is usually possible to achieve as much at home as in a hospital or hospice. Sometimes, however, family and staff know that symptom relief could be improved by inpatient admission, but the patient prefers to put up with the pain or vomiting in order to stay at home. In this situation it may be harder for those who watch than it is for the patient. There may need to be much discussion with the family (with and without the patient) to prevent their insistence on admission. For example, it helps them to know that a willingness to be less comfortable but at home is not unusual. In one study, mean anxiety and depression ratings were found to be significantly higher among hospice outpatients than hospice inpatients, yet only one in 20 desired inpatient care.[63] However, in a few patients the pain becomes so severe or the vomiting so distressing that it is impossible to cope at home. In these cases, inpatient admission is necessary.

Inpatient admission

Despite initially expressing a wish for care to be at home, many patients and families change their minds as the disease progresses. In a group of patients receiving specialist palliative care at home, preference for home care fell over time from 100 to about 50 per cent.[63] Ultimately, less than one-third died at home, about the same proportion were admitted 1 to 3 days before death, and the rest for longer periods.[63]

A person living alone or with an unfit relative generally needs to be admitted at the terminal stage.[63] Severe dyspnoea is easier to cope with on an inpatient basis. A more prolonged terminal illness is also associated with eventual inpatient admission.[63] Home care until death requires a fit relative who can cope with serious illness, nurses who can visit at least once a day, an attentive doctor, and a capability by the caring team to respond quickly to new problems. A guarantee of rapid admission in the event of a major crisis is also essential.

The inpatient environment

Most hospices have rooms with three to six beds. This arrangement allows mutual support between several patients and their families, and reduces fear by allowing families and patients to observe that death is peaceful. However, death may not be perceived as peaceful if it is associated with noisy breathing for example.

One study showed that most patients and relatives prefer the privacy of a single room, particularly in the terminal phase;[64] at one centre, when inpatient accommodation was changed from multi-bedded to single rooms, this did not appear to be detrimental.[65]

Table 6 Analgesic, anti-emetic, and psychotropic suppositories

Drug	Available strengths
United Kingdom and United States	
Aspirin	120/130, 195/200, 300, 600/650, 1200 mg (USA) 300, 600 mg (UK)
Indomethacin	50 mg (USA) 100 mg (UK)
Morphine	5, 10, 20, 30 mg (USA) 15, 30 mg (UK)
Domperidone	30 mg
Paracetamol (acetaminophen)	120/125, 325, 650 mg (USA) 125, 500 mg (UK)
Prochlorperazine	2.5 mg (USA) 5, 25mg
United Kingdom only	
Flurbiprofen	100 mg
Naproxen	500 mg
Diclofenac	100 mg
Oxycodone pectinate	30 mg[a]
Cyclizine	50 mg
Diazepam	10 mg[b]
United States only	
Opium and belladonna (15 mg) B & O supprettes No., 15A, 16A	30, 60 mg
Oxymorphone	5 mg
Hydromorphone	3 mg
Thiethylperazine	10 mg
Trimethobenzamide	100, 200 mg
Chlorpromazine	25, 100 mg

[a] Available on a named-patient basis, i.e. supplied by manufacturers on receipt of a special order.
[b] Also available as a rectal solution.

Thus, where a choice is available, account should be taken of patients' and families' preferences.

Symptom relief

In many ways, symptom relief in the last days of a patient's life is a continuation of what is already being done. However, new problems do emerge in the terminal phase, and it is these which will be addressed here.

Pain

Even when the patient is close to death careful evaluation is still necessary if he or she appears to be in pain. Temporary relief from a painful bedsore can be obtained by the application of a local anaesthetic gel. A distended bladder can be relieved by catheterization.

Most dying cancer patients receive a strong opioid.[51,66,67] Generally, pain will not be troublesome at the very end if control has previously been good. In one series the analgesic requirements in those receiving strong opioids in the last 48 h were decreased in 13 per cent, increased in 44 per cent, and unchanged in 43 per cent.[54] In more than half the patients with pain in the last 48 h, the pain was a new type that had not previously been present. This would account for most of those receiving an increased dose of opioid.

In two-thirds of these patients pain can be relieved with the first dose or first increase of dose of analgesic administered, sometimes together with a coanalgesic. In the remainder, further adjustments of the dose of analgesic or other treatment may be necessary to control the pain. Pain relief may not be complete in about 10 per cent, but persisting severe pain is very rare.

Patients who have been taking a non-steroidal anti-inflammatory drug for metastatic bone pain occasionally suffer a recurrence of pain if the drug is discontinued because of difficulty with swallowing. Several drugs of this type are now available in liquid and/or suppository forms, and in some countries preparations are available for parenteral use and therefore can be given by continuous subcutaneous infusion.[68-70] It should be noted that acute renal failure has been reported with ketorolac, and contraindications to its use should be observed.[71,72]

Patients may be disturbed by pain even when unconscious. They may also be physically dependent on opioids, and withdrawal restlessness will occur if analgesic medication is stopped suddenly when they can no longer swallow. Therefore continuation of analgesia by suppository, sublingually, by injection, or by subcutaneous infusion is recommended. Data from one hospice indicate that 60 per cent of patients were able to swallow until a few hours before death and needed no change of route for drug administration. Another 25 per cent required one or two doses of opioid by suppository; only 15 per cent needed an injection.[73]

In the terminal phase, patients may appear to suffer pain on movement. They may show signs of discomfort even when apparently deeply unconscious, and may moan or cry out when moved. Such disturbance pain may be due to the development of joint stiffness when little spontaneous movement takes place.[51] Signs of discomfort may also be a form of 'alarm response' to disturbance, and may be particularly evident in the blind, the deaf, and the confused. Dying patients may call out to check whether someone is with them or when they are aware that they are unattended.[51,74] These cries may be misinterpreted as pain and be a source of concern to family and carers.

Disturbance pain is minimized by keeping the patient informed of intended interventions, by describing any procedure that is to be undertaken, and by gentle slow handling. At some centres, activity-related pain is managed by administration of a short-acting strong opioid (e.g. dextromoramide) for major disturbances such as sponging. Increasing the maintenance dose of analgesics leads to sedation for the major part of the day when the patient is undisturbed, although this may not always be undesirable.

Once the patient has become stuporose, it is often possible to convert to a 5- or 6-hourly regimen by increasing the former 4-hourly dose proportionately. However, if for any reason it is decided to reduce the total daily dose, this will not precipitate physical withdrawal since only a quarter of the original daily dose is needed to prevent withdrawal symptoms.[73] Rigid adherence to the previous schedule is unnecessary.

The doctor should warn the family that, at this late stage, any injection may be the last and allay in advance any lingering fears about 'killing the patient'.

She is very ill . . . she could die just five minutes after you give the six o'clock injection. How will you feel if that happens? The important thing to remember is that we are using injections only to keep her free of pain and, whatever we do, she is going to die . . . Because she needs injections every four hours she is bound to die less than four hours after the last one—maybe after three hours but maybe after just five or ten minutes. . . .'

When a syringe driver is available, its use is less disturbing to the patient than repeated injections or the insertion of suppositories. The use of the syringe driver also eliminates the fear associated with administering the injection after which the patient dies. In one series, opioids were administered by syringe driver in 64 per cent of patients in the terminal phase.[64]

Respiratory symptoms

Dyspnoea

Terminal dyspnoea is usually multifactorial and it may not be possible to relieve it completely. In these circumstances the emphasis is on containment.[75] Causes of dyspnoea amenable to specific measures for relief will already have been treated. At this stage the aim of treatment is to relieve the perception of breathlessness. Dyspnoea causing distress is usually associated with tachypnoea and accompanied by anxiety. A comforting hand and soothing voice help to relieve anxiety and, if relaxation techniques and controlled breathing have already been instituted, the distressing tachypnoea may be adequately controlled. A cool draught of air is helpful and can be achieved by opening a window or by the use of a fan.[76] A fan often provides as much relief as nasal oxygen and does not impede bedside companionship. However, oxygen has a place in management if the patient is cyanosed.

Results of studies of the effects on dyspnoea of oxygen[77–79] and of morphine[77,80–84] differ, partly because of differences in the populations studied and the measures used. Hypoxic and hypercapniac patients cannot be compared, nor can the effects of a single dose with repeated or continuous morphine administration. There are few reports and no scientific evaluation of individual titration of morphine.[85]

None the less, common hospice experience is that the perception of breathlessness can be relieved by reducing the rate of breathing to a comfortable level with morphine. The dose of morphine is titrated against the rate of respiration to achieve a resting rate of about 15 to 20 breaths/min. Patients already receiving morphine for pain usually require an increase in dose of about 50 per cent to achieve a suitable reduction in respiratory rate. Anxiety is a concomitant of dyspnoea at rest, and an anxiolytic should also be administered in this circumstance, for example diazepam 5 to 10 mg immediately and 5 to 20 mg at night, but less for those over 70 (e.g. 2–5 mg).

Nebulized morphine is reported to relieve breathlessness with little change in arterial blood gases and vital signs (see Chapter 9.5). Patients with a past history or signs of asthma should be excluded to avoid possibly fatal respiratory arrest.[86] Chlorpromazine is also reported to be effective for the relief of dyspnoea in advanced cancer.[87]

Increased inspired oxygen concentration relieves breathlessness in chronic heart failure.[88] However, for most patients the value of oxygen in relieving dyspnoea remains undecided. The effects of supplemental oxygen on the subjective sensation of dyspnoea in patients with chronic obstructive pulmonary disease have been controversial.[83,89,90] There is some evidence that oxygen is useful in relieving dyspnoea in hypoxaemic terminal cancer patients who do not have chronic obstructive pulmonary disease.[79] The effects of oxygen on subjective dyspnoea in terminal cancer patients with normal oxygen saturation needs to be studied and the above study on hypoxaemic terminal cancer patients needs to be replicated. Evaluation using both nasally administered air and oxygen will help to determine whether oxygen is helpful.

Respiratory panic attacks

Respiratory panic attacks are sudden episodes of acute dyspnoea in patients already experiencing effort dyspnoea. The episodes generally occur on activity, such as climbing stairs. The emphasis in management is on alleviation of the acute anxiety. The patient is urged to breathe slowly and deeply; and a rapidly acting anxiolytic may be administered (lorazepam 0.5 mg sublingually). Advice from a physiotherapist and the introduction of relaxation techniques are important preventive measures.

Severe acute stridor

Severe acute stridor may be caused by haemorrhage into a tumour pressing on the trachea. Measures which can be adopted include intravenous administration of diazepam or midazolam until the patient is asleep (5–20 mg), or diazepam solution 10–20 mg per rectum or midazolam 10–20 mg subcutaneously if intravenous administration is not possible.

'Death rattle'

Inability to clear secretions from the oropharynx and trachea often results in noisy ('rattling') respiration as the secretions oscillate up and down in conjunction with expiration and inspiration. The usual approach to management is as follows:

- explain to the family;
- if the patient is stuporose, place in the 'coma position';
- administer an anticholinergic drug to reduce pharyngeal secretions.

Anticholinergic drugs do not dry up secretions already present. Therefore it is important to act at the first sign of rattling.[91] If secretions have already accumulated, gentle aspiration may be needed. In the home, it may be advisable to act prophylactically in the stuporose patient. Hyoscine (scopolamine) hydrobromide is often used because it also has a sedative effect in most patients (0.4 mg.

Hyoscine butylbromide (Buscopan) and glycopyrronium are being increasingly used as cheaper alternatives.[92] Regimens vary, but most centres administer a dose of a standard ampoule at once, followed by repeated doses as needed and/or at intervals of 4 h, or by a continuous subcutaneous infusion. The latter is easiest and more economical. For example, most patients are well controlled with hyoscine butylbromide 20 mg at once and 20 to 40 mg over 24 h. Atropine or hyoscyamine (L-atropine) can also be used. However, they tend to be excitatory and should be combined with an anxiolytic such as midazolam.

Table 7 Drugs given by subcutaneous infusion at more than one-third of 97 palliative care units in the United Kingdom[94]

	Percentage of units using drug	Range of mean maximum dose (mg/24 h)	Median dose (mg/24 h)
Diamorphine	99	300–10 000	2200
Haloperidol	95	5–100	12.5
Methotrimeprazine	93	25–400	150
Cyclizine	85	50–150	150
Midazolam	64	10–160	40
Metoclopramide	64	10–200	30
Dexamethasone	39	4–30	15.5
Hyoscine hydrobromide	39	0.4–4	1.2

Occasionally, very elderly dying patients may develop a death rattle while still conscious and able to sit up in bed. A smaller dose of hyoscine may be adequate in these patients and can be given transdermally.[93] Each patch contains a reservoir of 1.5 mg, of which 0.5 mg is delivered over the course of 3 days. Intravenous furosemide (20 mg) or bumetanide (0.5 mg) is of benefit if there is concomitant left ventricular failure.

Noisy tachypnoea in a moribund patient

Noisy tachypnoea manifests in a number of forms but basically comprises rapid (30–50 breaths/min) snorting respirations which are very noisy. Muscular movements of the abdomen and chest may be prominent, and the two phenomena give the impression of severe terminal distress. The noise pervades the patient's home or the whole of the ward.

Although the patient is unconscious and therefore unaware, the family and, in hospital, neighbouring patients and visitors are very disturbed. In these circumstances, parenteral morphine or diamorphine (ideally intravenously) is the drug of choice and it should be used without delay to slow the respiratory rate to between 10 and 15 breaths/min. If the patient is not receiving a strong opioid, morphine 20 to 30 mg (diamorphine 10 to15 mg) may be needed. In patients already receiving morphine or diamorphine or hydromorphone, it may be necessary to double or treble the previously satisfactory analgesic dose to contain this form of tachypnoea.

The aim is to reduce the noise by decreasing the respiratory rate and the depth of respiration. If muscular heaving persists, midazolam (10–20 mg injections) or diazepam (20–30 mg per rectum) may be required.

Dysphagia

In patients unable to swallow because of weakness or impaired consciousness medication is given by suppository or injection. When it seems likely that several injections will be needed, a syringe driver will avoid the need for multiple injections (Table 7) (see also Section 7).

Most drugs required can be delivered by a syringe driver and most can be mixed together.[62] The British National Formulary advises that the following can be mixed with diamorphine:[95]

cyclizine

dexamethasone

haloperidol

hyoscine butylbromide

hyoscine hydrobromide

levomepromazine

metoclopramide

midazolam

Experience in other countries has demonstrated that these drugs are also miscible with morphine. The following limitations should be noted.

- Cyclizine may precipitate at concentrations above 20 mg/ml or in physiological saline or as the concentration of diamorphine relative to cyclizine increases.[96] Mixtures of diamorphine and cyclizine are also liable to precipitate after 24 h.
- Special care is needed to avoid precipitation of dexamethasone, i.e. warm the syringe by holding it in the closed hand before adding dexamethasone.
- Midazolam does not mix with dexamethasone, betamethasone, or methylprednisolone.
- Mixtures of haloperidol and diamorphine are liable to precipitate after 24 h if the haloperidol concentration is above 2 mg/ml.
- Under some conditions metoclopramide may become discoloured; such solutions should be discarded.
- Cyclizine usually precipitates if mixed with metoclopramide, but these should not be used together because anticholinergic drugs block the intestinal action of metoclopramide.
- Diclofenac and ketorolac mix with diamorphine provided that the drugs are drawn up in saline; they do not mix with other drugs.
- Chlorpromazine can be given subcutaneously but tends to cause local subcutaneous inflammation.
- Prochlorperazine and diazepam are too irritant for subcutaneous infusion.
- Phenobarbitone is made up in 90 per cent propylene glycol and does not mix with other drugs, except diamorphine and hyoscine.
- Phenytoin is oil based and does not mix with other drugs.

Immiscible drugs should be given in a separate syringe driver or as injections once or twice a day if they have a long duration of action. Skin reactions may occur; the number of drugs used is important in this respect. When four drugs are combined the incidence is almost 50 per cent.[62] Cyclizine is frequently associated with skin reactions. Adding hydrocortisone sodium succinate 25–50 mg reduces inflammation.[97] Hyaluronidase 1500 units/24 h has also been found to prevent inflammatory reactions, presumably by facilitating the dispersion and absorption of the infused drugs (D. Doyle, personal communication).

The use of a syringe driver is less disturbing to the patient than the administration of drugs per rectum. If the patient is only able to swallow with difficulty, a continuous subcutaneous infusion relieves the relatives and the patient of the struggle associated with the administration of oral medications.

Nausea and vomiting

When nausea and vomiting occur in the terminal stage of the disease, suitable antiemetics are best administered by suppository or syringe driver. At this time the cause of vomiting is often multifactorial and a combination of antiemetics may be required.

Intractable vomiting due to intestinal obstruction may be relieved by the continuous subcutaneous infusion of octreotide (0.3–0.6 mg/24 h).[98] Octreotide is a somatostatin analogue which reduces the volume of gastrointestinal secretions by decreasing the secretion of water, sodium, and chloride, and stimulating intestinal absorption of water and electrolytes. It also inhibits peristalsis (see Chapter 9.3.4). If octreotide is not available, hyoscine butylbromide (60–120 mg/24 h) can be used as an alternative antisecretory drug.[99] A nasogastric tube is another option for giving relief for the persistent vomiting of high intestinal obstruction.

Delirium

Delirium has been discussed elsewhere (see Section 15). It is often a prelude to coma and death.[100] In one series,[101] 85 per cent of patients dying of cancer developed delirium; in another,[102] 77 per cent developed serious mental impairment more than a week before death. Delirium may relate to direct malignant involvement of the brain or be a manifestation of a paraneoplastic syndrome.[103] It commonly relates to metabolic encephalopathy resulting from organ failure, electrolyte imbalance, nutritional abnormalities, or sepsis. The condition is generally worse in the evening and at night, and disruptive behaviour increases at these times.

Delirium in the dying is generally multifactorial. Some causes can be avoided, corrected, or modified,[104] but this is not often feasible or appropriate in the terminal phase. The drug regimen should be reviewed. All medications which are not absolutely necessary should be discontinued. Symptoms may be exacerbated by sedation, and consideration should be given to a reduction in medication. Delirium may be caused or exacerbated by toxic opioid metabolites.[105] Changing to another opioid may be helpful in these circumstances. Patients with renal failure have benefited from a change from subcutaneous diamorphine to subcutaneous alfentenil.[106] If the patient is cyanosed, oxygen may bring about improvement.

Delirium is generally best treated with haloperidol which can be given as needed or by continuous infusion in an individually optimized dose. If delirium is not controlled on a haloperidol dose of 20 to 30 mg/24 h, it should be discontinued and more sedating treatment administered, for example subcutaneous midazolam (see below).

Agitated delirium

Up to 50 per cent of elderly patients presenting with delirium experience distressing hallucinations with or without nightmares, and a similar number have paranoid ideas.[107,108] In patients close to death the following approach is recommended for agitated delirium:

- haloperidol (5–10 mg) orally, subcutaneously, or intravenously (depending on weight and previous exposure to psychotropic medication);
- repeat after 30 min if necessary;
- give a double dose after a further 30 min if necessary, with midazolam 10 mg subcutaneously.

Occasionally it is necessary to keep the patient sedated until death ensues. In this circumstance, give midazolam 60 mg/24 h by continuous subcutaneous infusion (or diazepam 10–20 mg per rectum every 6–8 h) and haloperidol 20 mg/24 h, and increase further if necessary. If the patient fails to settle after increasing the dose of midazolam to 100 mg/24 h and haloperidol to 30 to 40 mg/24 h, phenobarbitone should be considered, for example 200 mg subcutaneously or intramuscularly at once and 600 to 1200 mg/24 h by continuous subcutaneous infusion.

Alternatives include chlormethiazole (particularly in the elderly or if alcohol withdrawal is suspected), thioridazine, and chlorpromazine. The dose depends on the response; very agitated patients may require very large doses. Guidelines for the use of intravenous chlormethiazole are included in the British National Formulary in the section on status epilepticus. Some centres use levomepromazine up to 200 mg/24 h. This can be regarded as double-strength chlorpromazine. There is no objective evidence to support the view that it is better than an equisedative dose of chlorpromazine but, because it is less irritant to tissues, it can be administered subcutaneously. If these measures fail, intravenous thiopentone or intravenous propofol should be used as the sole agent.[109,110]

Terminal anguish

Terminal anguish is a tormented state of mind which relates to long-standing unresolved emotional problems and/or interpersonal conflicts, or to long hidden unhappy memories often with guilty content. These problems have festered in the mind but have never been brought into the open.

As long as the patient is well enough to control his or her thoughts and as long as denial can function, all appears to be well. With increasing weakness, the onset of drowsiness, and inability to control thoughts, hidden matter in the unconscious mind is able to surface. The mental anguish manifests with restlessness, thrashing about, moaning, groaning, and even crying out. Inadequate sedation only makes matters worse, and nothing short of deep unconsciousness, natural or induced, provides relief. In this tormented state, when recovery is impossible and death is near, heavy sedation (as for severe agitated delirium) is the only method of relief.[109,111,112]

The possibility of such an outcome highlights the need to make every effort to deal with psychological 'skeletons in the cupboard' before the patient becomes too weak to be able to address them. However, a few resist every attempt to explore what has been suppressed.

Restlessness

Restlessness is commonly observed in the last hours of life. It may have multiple causes, none of which may be obvious, and specific treatment is often not possible. This symptom overlaps but is not necessarily identical with agitated delirium and terminal anguish. Treatable causes include physical discomfort such as unrelieved pain, distended bladder or rectum, dyspnoea, nausea, pruritus, and inability to move because of weakness. Cerebral anoxia may be responsible.

Restlessness is also a feature of delirium. Psychomotor agitation or hyperactivity may occur in the presence of anxiety when there is loss of inhibition. It is also seen in akathisia due to neuroleptic drugs, in benzodiazepine withdrawal, and with corticosteroids.[113] Phenothiazines, butyrophenones, opioids, and tricyclic antidepressants lower the seizure threshold and may exacerbate neuromuscular excitation.[114] Restlessness is a symptom and not a diagnosis. The cause should be identified if possible and treated appropriately. Pain should be excluded as a cause; this may require a trial of an appropriate dose of analgesic.

The presence of a family member or carer, holding a hand and speaking gently, may have a significant calming effect even on the unconscious patient. Drug treatment is similar to that used in agitated delirium. However, midazolam is the drug of choice for patients without delirium[114] and for those in whom more specific measures, for example catheterization or pain relief, are not indicated.

Multifocal myoclonus

Multifocal myoclonus is a central pre-epileptiform phenomenon (see Chapters 9.2.3 and 9.2.10). It is exacerbated by hypoglycaemia and, in the moribund, may be caused or exacerbated by dopamine antagonists (neuroleptics, metoclopramide) and opioids (particularly at higher doses) or as a result of drug withdrawal (benzodiazepines, barbiturates, anticonvulsants, alcohol). It is a feature in cancer patients dying with encephalopathy resulting from multi-organ failure and is seen more specifically in those with renal failure, hepatic failure, and hyponatraemia. It occurs with cerebral oedema and hypoxia.

Management should begin with a review of drug withdrawals and drug doses in the light of failing kidney and liver function. Diazepam, midazolam, and clonazepam are the drugs of choice for myoclonus:

- diazepam 5 to 10 mg solution per rectum every hour until settled and 10 mg per rectum once or twice a day
- midazolam 5 to 10 mg subcutaneously every hour until settled and 10 to 30 mg/24 h by subcutaneous infusion
- clonazepam 0.5 mg subcutaneously every hour until settled and 1 to 2 mg/24 h by subcutaneous infusion.

The dose should be adjusted upwards if two or more 'as-needed' doses are given. Flunitrazepam and phenobarbitone are other alternatives which can also be given by syringe driver.

Grand mal convulsions

Grand mal convulsions have been discussed elsewhere (see Chapter 9.12) but the following points should be made.

Prophylaxis

Patients who are already on anticonvulsants but can no longer swallow need continuing prophylaxis by another route. Phenytoin and sodium valproate have long plasma half-lives and will remain at therapeutically significant concentrations for some time after cessation of oral therapy. If several hours have elapsed since the last oral dose, it may be wise to give an immediate dose of diazepam 10 mg per rectum or midazolam 10 mg subcutaneously, followed by one of the following:

- diazepam 20 mg per rectum at night or twice daily
- midazolam 30 to 60 mg/24 h by continuous subcutaneous infusion.
- phenobarbitone 200 to 600 mg/24 h by continuous subcutaneous infusion.

Higher doses should be used if necessary. Phenobarbitone sodium for injection is made up with 90 per cent propylene glycol (200 mg/1 ml). If given by subcutaneous infusion, it should be diluted 1:10 with water. Of the drugs commonly given by subcutaneous infusion, phenobarbitone is miscible only with diamorphine and hyoscine.

Emergency management

If a moribund patient has a grand mal convulsion, one of the following should be given as emergency treatment:

- diazepam 10 mg per rectum repeated after 15 min and 30 min if not settled
- midazolam 10 mg subcutaneously or intravenously repeated after 15 min if not settled.

If the above fail, consider doubling the dose of diazepam or midazolam or give phenobarbitone 100 mg subcutaneously or 100 mg in 100 ml of saline intravenously over 30 min.

Stopping dexamethasone in patients with intracranial malignancy

Most patients stop taking dexamethasone automatically when they become moribund and can no longer swallow. They may need diamorphine or morphine by subcutaneous infusion to prevent distressing headaches, and diazepam per rectum or midazolam subcutaneously to prevent convulsions.

Occasionally the patient requests that the dexamethasone is stopped because of deterioration despite its continued use and an unacceptable quality of life. This is a situation which tends to cause considerable distress to staff. It is probably best to reduce the dexamethasone gradually on a daily basis, because this gives the patient time to reconsider. At the same time the following steps should be taken.

- Increase the oral anticonvulsant medication.
- Prescribe additional analgesics for breakthrough headache:

if on paracetamol, prescribe coproxamol as needed.

if on coproxamol, prescribe morphine 10 to 20 mg orally, or diamorphine or morphine 5 to 10 mg subcutaneously as needed.

- Review twice a day, preferably personally.
- Consider changing the regular analgesic if two or more 'as needed' doses have been given in the previous 24 h.
- Consider changing anticonvulsants to diazepam per rectum or midazolam subcutaneously if the patient becomes drowsy or finds swallowing difficult.
- Consider changing to diamorphine and midazolam by continuous subcutaneous infusion.

If the morphine or diamorphine causes significant respiratory depression, the elevated $p\text{CO}_2$ induces intracranial vasodilatation which leads to an increase in intracranial pressure and exacerbation of headache. If this is suspected because of restlessness, grimacing, or other physical expressions of pain, it may be necessary to increase the morphine or diamorphine rapidly (possibly double or treble the dose) in order to overcome medication-exacerbated headache. This is rarely necessary in practice.

Incontinence and retention of urine

Retention of urine may be caused by enlargement of the prostate, anticholinergic drugs, weakness, disinterest due to depression, lack of awareness due to delirium or drowsiness, or a combination of factors. A common cause in the terminal phase is a loaded rectum which can be dealt with by a laxative suppository, enema, or manual removal. An indwelling catheter will be needed in most patients, although a male external catheter sometimes suffices.

Incontinence of urine, whether related to tumour, infection, or other cause, will seldom be reversible at this time. Therefore management will be by padding, male external catheter, or indwelling catheter.[115] An indwelling catheter often provides most comfort with least ongoing disturbance.

Haemorrhage

If one or more significant warning haemorrhages have occurred, it may be sensible to draw up a syringe of midazolam 10 mg and a syringe containing morphine or diamorphine so that they are immediately available in the event of a major terminal haemorrhage. The dose of opioid will be equivalent to the four-hourly injection dose if the patient is already receiving morphine or diamorphine; otherwise 10 mg will be appropriate. It is helpful to have green surgical towels available to lessen the frightening sight of blood on white sheets.

Massive haemorrhage from the carotid artery in recurrent neck cancer results in death within minutes. The only sensible response is to stay with the patient and hold his or her hand. If a major artery is eroded by a malignant ulcer (e.g. in the axilla, face, neck, or groin), midazolam 10 mg subcutaneously or diazepam 10 mg (or more if the patient is already receiving anxiolytics) as a rectal solution or suppository should be administered.

A comparable approach can be adopted with severe acute haematemesis, fresh melaena, and vaginal bleeding in a patient already close to death.

At the end of the day

Palliative care developed as a reaction to the attitude, spoken or unspoken, that 'there is nothing more that we can do for you' with the inevitable consequence for the patient and family of a sense of abandonment, hopelessness, and despair. It was stressed that this is never true—there is always something that can be done. Yet, while this is generally the case, there are times when a nurse or doctor has nothing specific to do for a patient and, in consequence, feels that he or she has nothing to offer. In such a situation, we are thrown back on who we are as individuals:

> Slowly, I learn about the importance of powerlessness. I experience it in my own life and I live with it in my work. The secret is not to be afraid of it—not to run away. The dying know we are not God.... All they ask is that we do not desert them.[116]

Therefore there are circumstances in which it is necessary to relinquish the 'Dr. Fix-it' and 'Nurse Fix-it' attitudes imbued during training. When there is nothing to offer except ourselves, a belief that life has meaning and purpose helps to sustain the carer. However, to speak glibly of this to a patient who is in despair is cruel. At such a time actions are better than words. By what we do, we seek to convey the essential message:

> You matter because you are you.
>
> You matter to the last moment of your life,
>
> and we will do all we can
>
> not only to help you die peacefully,
>
> but to live until you die. (Cicely Saunders)

Appendix

Statement on Withholding or Withdrawing Life-prolonging Medical Treatment, Council on Ethical and Judicial Affairs, American Medical Association

The social commitment of the physician is to sustain life and relieve suffering. Where the performance of one duty conflicts with the other, the choice of the patient, or his family or legal representative if the patient is incompetent to act in his own behalf, should prevail. In the absence of the patient's choice or an authorized proxy, the physician must act in the best interest of the patient.

For humane reasons, with informed consent, a physician may do what is medically necessary to alleviate severe pain, or cease or omit treatment to permit a terminally ill patient whose death is imminent to die. However, he should not intentionally cause death. In deciding whether the administration of potentially life-prolonging medical treatment is in the best interest of the patient who is incompetent to act on his own behalf, the physician should determine what the possibility is for extending life under humane and comfortable conditions and what are the prior expressed wishes of the patient and attitudes of the family or those who have responsibility for the custody of the patient.

Even if death is not imminent but a patient's coma is beyond doubt irreversible and there are adequate safeguards to confirm the accuracy of the diagnosis and with the concurrence of those who have responsibility for the care of the patient, it is not unethical to discontinue all means of life-prolonging medical treatment.

Life-prolonging medical treatment includes medication and artificially or technologically supplied respiration, nutrition, or hydration. In treating a terminally ill or irreversibly comatose patient, the physician should determine whether the benefits of treatment outweigh its burdens. At all times, the dignity of the patient should be maintained.[24]

References

1. Fainsinger R, Miller MJ, Bruera E. Symptom control during the last week of life on a palliative care unit. *Journal of Palliative Care*, 1991; **7(1)**:5–11.
2. Callahan D. *The troubled dream of life: living with mortality*. Indianapolis: Hastings Center, Indiana University, 1993: chapter 6.
3. Charles-Edwards A. *The Nursing Care of the Dying Patient*. Beaconsfield: Beaconsfield Publishers, 1993.
4. Herth K. Fostering hope in terminally ill people. *Journal of Advanced Nursing*, 1990; **15**:1250–9.
5. Lichter I. *Communication in Cancer Care*. Edinburgh: Churchill Livingstone, 1987.
6. Saunders C. The care of the dying patient and his family. *Contact*, 1972; **Supplement 38**:12–18.
7. Hinton J. The physical and mental distress of the dying. *Quarterly Journal of Medicine*, 1963; **32**:1–21.
8. Mauritzen J. Pastoral care for the dying and bereaved. *Death Studies*, 1988; **12**:111–22.
9. Lamerton R. Religion and the care of the dying. *Nursing Times*, 1973; **69**:88–9.
10. Parkes CM. Psychological aspects. In: C.M. Saunders, ed. *The Management of Terminal Malignant Disease*. Edward Arnold : London, 1978: 44–64.
11. Bennett MB. Care of the dying. *South African Medical Journal*, 1973; **47**:1558–60.
12. Fishman B. The treatment of suffering in patients with cancer pain: cognitive–behavioural approaches. In: K. Foley, J. Bonica, and V. Ventafridda, eds. *Advances in Pain Research and Therapy*. Raven Press: New York, 1990: 301–16.
13. Portenoy RK. Pain and quality of life. *Oncology*, 1990; **4**:172–8.
14. Cassell E. *The Nature of Suffering and the Goals of Medicine*. Oxford University Press, 1991.
15. Frankl VE. *Man's Search for Meaning*. New York: Washington Square Press, 1984.
16. Chapman CR, Gavrin J. Suffering and its relationship to pain. *Journal of Palliative Care*, 1993; **9(1)**: 5–13.
17. Cherny NI, Coyle N, Foley KM. Suffering in the advanced cancer patient: a definition and taxonomy. *Journal of Palliative Care*, 1994; **10**:57–70.
18. Lichter I. Some psychological causes of distress in the terminally ill. *Palliative Medicine*, 1991; **5**:138–46.
19. Stedeford A. *Facing Death: Patients, Families and Professionals*. London: Heinemann Medical, 1984.
20. Bakhtiar JAH. Care of the dying patient. *International Journal of Social Psychiatry*, 1980; **26**:167–77.
21. Clark R. Forgiveness in the hospice setting. *Palliative Medicine*, 1990; **4**:305–10.
22. Traux C, Carkhuff F. *Towards Effective Counselling*. Chicago, IL: Aldine, 1967.
23. Byock I. When suffering persists. *Journal of Palliative Care*, 1994; **10(2)**: 8–13.
24. Dickey NW. Withholding or withdrawing life-prolonging medical treatment. *Journal of the American Medical Association*, 1986; **256**:471.
25. Twycross R. *Pain Relief in Advanced Cancer*. Edinburgh: Churchill Livingstone, 1994.
26. Hastings Center. *Guidelines on the Termination of Life-sustaining Treatment and the Care of the Dying*. Indianapolis, Hastings Center, Indiana University, 1987.
27. World Health Organization. *Cancer Pain Relief and Palliative Care*. Technical Series No 804. Geneva: World Health Organization, 1990.
28. Saunders C. Principles of symptom control in terminal care. In: M. Reidenberg, ed. *The Medical Clinics of North America. Clinical Pharmacology of Symptom Control*. Philadelphia, PA: WB Saunders, 1982:1169–83.
29. Dunphy K, Finlay I, Rathbone G, Gilbert J, Hicks F. Rehydration in palliative and terminal care: if not—why not? *Palliative Medicine*, 1995; **9**:221–8.
30. Byock I. Patient refusal of nutrition and hydration: walking the ever-fine line. *American Journal of Hospice and Palliative Care*, 1995; **12(2)**:8–13
31. Micetich KC, Steinecker PH, Thomasma DC. Are intravenous fluids morally required for a dying patient? *Archives of Internal Medicine*, 1983; **143**:975–8.
32. Seigler M, Shiedermayer DL. Should fluid and nutritional support be withheld from terminally ill patients? *American Journal of Hospital Care*, 1984; **2**:32–5.
33. Andrews M, Bell E, Smith S, Tischler T, Veglia J. Dehydration in terminally ill patients. *Postgraduate Medicine*, 1993; **93**:201–8.
34. Fainsinger R, Bruera E. The management of dehydration in terminally ill patients. *Journal of Palliative Care* 1994; **10(3)**: 55–9.
35. Fainsinger R *et al.* The use of hypodermoclysis for rehydration in terminally ill cancer patients. *Journal of Pain and Symptom Management*, 1994; **9**:298–302.
36. Waller A, Hershkowitz M, Adunsky A. The effect of intravenous fluid infusion on blood and urine parameters of hydration and on state of consciousness in terminal cancer patients. *American Journal of Hospice and Palliative Care*, 1994; **11(6)**:22–7.
37. Bruera E, Franco JJ, Maltoni M, Watanabe S, Suarez-Almazor M. Changing pattern of agitated impaired mental status in patients with advanced cancer: association with cognitive monitoring, hydration, and opioid rotation. *Journal of Pain and Symptom Management*, 1995; **10**:287–91.
38. Hanks GW. Management of symptoms in advanced cancer. *Update*, 1983; **26**:1961.
39. Holmes S. The oral complications of specific anticancer therapy. *International Journal of Nursing Studies*, 1991; **28**:343–60.
40. Ellershaw JE, Sutcliffe JM, Saunders CM. Dehydration and the dying patient. *Journal of Pain and Symptom Management*, 1995; **10**:192–7.
41. Burge F. Dehydration symptoms of palliative care cancer patients. *Journal of Pain and Symptom Management*, 1993; 8(7):454–64.
42. McCann RM, Hall WJ, Groth-Juncker A. Comfort care for terminally ill patients: the appropriate use of nutrition and hydration. *Journal of the American Medical Association*, 1994; **272**:179–81.
43. Billings J. Comfort measures for the terminally ill: is dehydration painful? *Journal of the American Geriatrics Society*, 1985; **November**:808–10.
44. Editorial. Terminal dehydration. *Lancet*, 1986; **i**:306.
45. Brooker S. Dehydration before death. *Nursing Times*, 1992; **88**:59–62.
46. Osler W. *Science and Immortality*. London: Constable, 1906.
47. Exton-Smith AN. Terminal illness in the aged. *Lancet*, 1961; **ii**:305–8.
48. Witzel L. Behaviour of the dying patient. *British Medical Journal*, 1975; **ii**:81–2.
49. Wilkes E. Dying now. *Lancet*, 1984; **i**:950–2.
50. Wilson JA, Lawson PM, Smith RG. The treatment of terminally ill geriatric patients. *Palliative Medicine*, 1987; **1**:149–53.

51. Saunders C. Pain and impending death. In: P.D. Wall and R. Melzack, eds. *Textbook of Pain*. London:Churchill Livingstone, 1989: 624–31.
52. Higginson I, McCarthy M. Measuring symptoms in terminal cancer: are pain and dyspnoea controlled? *Journal of the Royal Society of Medicine*, 1989; **82**:264–7.
53. Ventafridda V, Ripamonti C, DeConno F, Tamburini M, Cassileth BR. Symptom prevalence and control during cancer patients' last days of life. *Journal of Palliative Care*, 1990; **6(3)**:7–11.
54. Lichter I, Hunt E. The last 48 hours of life. *Journal of Palliative Care*, 1990; **6(4)**:7–15.
55. Reuben DB, Mor V. Dyspnoea in terminally ill cancer patients. *Chest*, 1986; **89**:234–6.
56. Mount B. A final crescendo of pain? *Journal of Palliative Care*, 1990; **6(3)**:5–6.
57. Hancock S. A death in the family. *British Medical Journal*, 1973; **i**:29–30.
58. Wilkes E. Terminal care at home. *Lancet*, 1965; **ii**:799–801.
59. Oliver D. Syringe drivers in the community. *Practitioner*, 1991; **235**:78–80.
60. Moulin D, Kreeft J, Murray-Parson N, Bouquillon A. Comparisons of continuous subcutaneous and intravenous hydromorphone infusion for management of cancer pain. *Lancet*, 1991; **337**:465–8.
61. Venning M, Rogers J. Continuous subcutaneous infusion: flexible option in symptom control. *Australian Nurses Journal*, 1988; **17**:34–7.
62. Lichter I, Hunt E. Drug combinations in syringe drivers. *New Zealand Medical Journal*, 1995; **108**:224–6.
63. Hinton J. Can home care maintain an acceptable quality of life for patients with terminal cancer and their relatives? *Palliative Medicine*, 1994; **8**: 183–96.
64. Lichter I. Unpublished data.
65. Mount BM. Personal communication.
66. Lombard DJ, Oliver DJ. The use of opioid analgesics in the last 24 hours of life of patients with advanced cancer. *Palliative Medicine*, 1989; **3**:27–9.
67. McIllmurray MB, Warreb MR. Evaluation of a new hospice: the relief of symptoms in cancer patients in the first year. *Palliative Medicine*, 1989; **3**:135–40.
68. Myers K, Trotman I. Use of ketorolac by continuous subcutaneous infusion for the control of cancer-related pain. *Postgraduate Medical Journal*, 1994; **70**:359–62.
69. Blackwell N, Bangham N, Hughes L, Hughes M, Melzack D, Trotman I. Subcutaneous ketorolac—a new development in pain control. *Palliative Medicine*, 1993; **7**:63–5.
70. Hall E. Subcutaneous diclofenac: an effective alternative. *Palliative Medicine*, 1993; **7**:339–40.
71. Smith K, Halliwell R, Lawrence S, Kineberg P, O'Connell P. Acute renal failure associated with intramuscular ketorolac. *Anaesthesia and Intensive Care*. 1993; **21**:700–3.
72. Pearce C, Gonzalez F, Wallin D. Renal failure and hyperkalaemia associated with ketorolac tromethamine. *Archives of Internal Medicine*, 1993; **153**:1000–2.
73. Twycross R, Lack S. Symptom control in far advanced cancer: pain relief. 1983, London: Pitman.
74. Livesley B. The management of the dying. In: Pathy MSJ, ed.. *Principles and Practice of Geriatric Medicine*. London: John Wiley, 1985;1287–95.
75. Twycross R. Symptom control: the problem areas. *Palliative Medicine*, 1993; **7**:1–8.
76. Schwartzstein R, Lahive K, Pope A, Weinberger S, Weiss J. Cold facial stimulation reduces breathlessness induced in normal subjects. *American Review of Respiratory Disease*, 1987; **136**:58–61.
77. Cowcher K, Hanks G. Long-term management of respiratory symptoms in advanced cancer. *Journal of Pain and Symptom Management*, 1990; **5**:230–330.
78. Woodcock A, Gross E, Geddes D. Oxygen relieves breathlessness in pink puffers. *Lancet*, 1981; **i**:907–9.
79. Bruera E, de Stoutz ND, Velasco-Leiva A, Schoeller T, Hanson J. Effects of oxygen on dyspnoea in hypoxaemic terminal cancer patients. *Lancet*, 1993; **342**:13–14.
80. Cohen M *et al.* Continuous intravenous infusion of morphine for severe dyspnoea. *Southern Medical Journal*, 1991; **84**:229–34.
81. Walsh T. Opiates and respiratory function in advanced cancer. *Recent Results in Cancer Care*, 1984; **89**:115–17.
82. Gray J, Henry D, Paice B, Gettinby G, Moran F, Lawson D. Acute respiratory failure and CNS-depressing drugs. *Postgraduate Medical Journal*, 1981; **57**:279–82.
83. Bruera E, Macmillan K, MacDonald RN. Effects of morphine on the dyspnea of terminal cancer patients. *Journal of Pain and Symptom Management*, 1990; **5**:341–4.
84. Bruera E, MacEachern RN, Ripamonti C, Hanson J. Subcutaneous morphine for dyspnoea in cancer patients. *Annals of Internal Medicine*, 1993; **119**:906–7.
85. Henteleff P. Dyspnea management. Paper presented at First International Conference on Palliative Care for the Elderly,Toronto, 1989.
86. Farncombe M, Chater S. Case studies outlining use of nebulized morphine for patients with end-stage chronic lung and cardiac disease. *Journal of Pain and Symptom Management*, 1993; **8**:221–5.
87. McIver B, Walsh D, Nelson K. The use of chlorpromazine for symptom control in dying cancer patients. *Journal of Pain and Symptom Management*, 1994; **9**:341–5.
88. Moore D, Weston A, Hughes J, Oakley C, Cleland J. Effects of increased inspired oxygen concentrations on exercise performance in chronic heart failure. *Lancet*, 1992; **339**:850–3.
89. Swinburn C, Mould H, Stone T, Corris P, Gibson G. Symptomatic benefit of supplemental oxygen in hypoxemic patients with chronic lung disease. *American Review of Respiratory Disease*, 1991; **143**:913–15.
90. Liss H, Grant B. The effect of nasal flow on breathlessness in patients with chronic obstructive pulmonary disease. *American Review of Respiratory Disease*, 1988; **137**:1285–8.
91. Power D, Kearney M. Management of the final 24 hours. *Irish Medical Journal*, 1992; **85**:93–5.
92. Bausewein C, Twycross R. Comparative cost of hyoscine injections. *Palliative Medicine* 1995; **9**:256.
93. Dawson HR. The use of transdermal scopolamine in the control of the death rattle. *Journal of Palliative Care*, 1989; **5(1)**:31–3.
94. Johnson I, Patterson S. Drugs used in combination in the syringe driver: a survey of hospice practice. *Palliative Medicine*, 1992; **6**:125–30.
95. Anonymous. Prescribing in terminal care. *British National Formulary*, 1995; **29**:12–15.
96. Regnard CFB. Antiemetics/diamorphine mixture compatibility in infusion pumps. *British Journal of Pharmaceutical Practice*, 1986; **8**:218–20.
97. Shvartzman P, Bonnehn D. Local skin irritation in the course of subcutaneous morphine infusion: a challenge. *Journal of Palliative Care*, 1994; **10(1)**:44–5.
98. Khoo D, Hall E, Motson R, Riley J, Denman K, Waxman J. Palliation of malignant intestinal obstruction using octreotide. *European Journal of Cancer*, 1994; **30**:28–30.
99. De Conno F, Caraceni A, Zecca E, Spoldi E, Ventafridda V. Continuous subcutaneous infusion of hyoscine butylbromide reduces secretions in patients with gastrointestinal obstruction. *Journal of Pain and Symptom Management*, 1991; **6**:484–6.
100. Adams F. Neuropsychiatric evaluation and treatment of delirium in cancer patients. In: T.N. Wise, ed. *Advances in Psychosomatic Medicine*, Basel: Karger, 1988: 26–36.
101. Massie MJ, Holland J, Glass E. Delirium in terminally ill cancer patients. *American Journal of Psychiatry* 1983; **140**:1048–50.
102. Bruera E, Chadwick S, Weinlick A, MacDonald N. Delirium and severe sedation in patients with terminal cancer. *Cancer Treatment Reports*, 1987; **71**:787–8.
103. Posner JB. Neurological complications of systemic cancer. *Medical Clinics of North America*, 1979; **63**:783–800.
104. de Stoutz ND, Tapper M, Fainsinger R. Reversible delirium in terminally ill patients. *Journal of Pain and Symptom Management*, 1995; **10**:249–53.

105. de Stoutz ND, Bruera E, Suarez-Almazor M. Opioid rotation for toxicity reduction in terminal cancer patients. *Journal of Pain and Symptom Control*, 1995; **10**:378–84.
106. Kirkham SR, Pugh R. Opioid analgesia in uraemic patients. *Lancet*, 1995; **345**:1185.
107. Steinhart MJ. The use of haloperidol in geriatric patients with organic mental disorder. *Current Therapeutic Research*, 1983; **33**:132–43.
108. Lipowski ZJ. Delirium in the elderly patient. *New England Journal of Medicine*, 1989; **320**:578–82.
109. Green W, Davis W. Titrated intravenous barbiturates in the control of symptoms in patients with terminal cancer. *Southern Medical Journal*, 1991; **84**:332–7.
110. Moyle J. The use of propofol in palliative medicine. *Journal of Pain and Symptom Management*, 1995; **10**: 643–6.
111. McNamara P, Minton M, Twycross R. Use of midazolam in palliative care. *Palliative Medicine*, 1991; **5**:244–9.
112. Truog R, Berde C, Mitchell C, Grier H. Barbiturates in the care of the terminally ill. *New England Journal of Medicine*, 1992; **327**:1672–82.
113. Back I. Terminal restlessness in patients with advanced malignant disease. *Palliative Medicine*, 1992; **6**:293–8.
114. Burke A, Diamond P, Hulbert J, Yeatman J, Farr E. Terminal restlessness—its management and the role of midazolam. *Medical Journal of Australia*, 1991; **155**:485–7.
115. Fainsinger RL, MacEachern T, Hanson J, Bruera E. The use of urinary catheters in terminally ill cancer patients. *Journal of Pain and Symptom Management*, 1992; **7**:333–8.
116. Cassidy S. *Sharing the Darkness*. London: Darton, Longman and Todd, 1988.

18

Bereavement

18 Bereavement

Colin Murray Parkes

Definitions

Bereavement: the situation of anyone who has lost a person to whom they are attached.

Grief: the psychological and emotional reactions to bereavement.

Mourning: the social face of grief.

Attachment: a strong tendency to remain close to or, from time to time, to return to another individual.

Anticipatory grief: psychological and emotional reaction to anticipation of bereavement.

Normal grief

The anticipation of bereavement

It is inevitable that as long as patients are alive their needs will take precedence over those of the family. This assumption is so obvious that family members who ask for help while a patient is still alive are often made to feel that they are being selfish or unreasonable. Yet the moment the patient is dead they become the focus of attention and may even be expected to 'break down'.

Aware of such attitudes relatives often tend to deny or play down their own needs during the patient's life. 'Don't worry about me' they seem to be saying, 'He (or she) is the one we must care for'. Anticipatory grief cannot be expressed because of their fears that if they don't keep a tight rein on their emotions they will be unable to continue to care for the dying person or because they fear that by getting upset themselves they will upset the patient ('If I start to cry I may not be able to stop'). This collusive denial of emotional needs may lead caring staff to underestimate such needs and it may obstruct any attempt that is made by carers to support the family prior to the patient's death.

Psychological research[1] suggests that the denial or avoidance of distressing thoughts may indeed enable people to get through periods of crisis and that we should not bring undue pressure to bear on them to relinquish such defences. At the same time we also need to recognize that denial is an unstable defence which cannot always be maintained, particularly if it has to be continued over a long period of time. Given proper support most people who choose to express their anticipatory grief do come through it, tears die down, and they cope better than they had feared. As time passes they find themselves better able to think and talk about the distressing facts associated with the illness and this may enable them to communicate more effectively with the patient than they would if they felt it necessary to avoid potentially distressing topics about which the patient is ready to talk. Several research projects have shown that deaths which are expected and timely are less likely to give rise to lasting psychological problems in the bereaved than those which are unexpected and untimely.[2]

It follows that accurate information and emotional support given before a death will reduce the risk of such problems afterwards. The ways in which this support can be given have been discussed in Section 4 and Section 16. In this section we turn our attention to the period of time which follows bereavement.

It is a sad paradox that, just when the family are most aware of their need for help and most likely to accept it, help is usually withdrawn. Doctors, nurses, and others who may have befriended the family while the patient was in hospital say goodbye and the family is left with nothing but a death certificate to take away. There is, however, good reason to regard bereavement as a potential threat to physical and mental health and there is also evidence that that threat can be reduced by support given to the right people in the right way. Bereavement provides us with an opportunity to prevent ill health and to help people to find the new directions which may lead to psychological, social, and spiritual growth.

The nature of grief

The reaction to bereavement is complex and can be viewed from many different perspectives. Three major components are present from the outset although their respective influence is most obvious at different times after the loss.

The urge to cry and to search for the lost person

Human beings share with other social animals a strong tendency to pine for those who are lost. The emotion of pining is accompanied by the impulse to cry aloud and to search restlessly for the lost person. It tends to recur in episodes ('pangs of grief') which are triggered by any reminders of the lost person or of the events associated with the loss.

The urge to avoid or repress crying or searching

Unlike other species human beings are aware that it is illogical to search and to cry for someone who is dead. From early childhood we have been urged not to cry and in most 'Western' countries strong social pressures are brought to bear to limit the overt expressing of negative emotions. Mourning customs which in the past provided social sanction for the expression of grief, have changed and 'civilized' behaviour dictates that the 'stiff upper lip' is to be maintained on all public occasions. Consequently, funerals and the social gatherings which follow them are often an ordeal rather than a support to the bereaved.

There is a great deal of variation in the extent to which individuals resolve the conflict between these competing urges with some crying in private but not in public, some inhibiting all tears, and a few crying openly. Both clinical experience and research[3] suggest that those who repress their grief most fully at the time of bereavement are likely to become more disturbed later.

The urge to review and revise internal models

The death of a loved person invalidates a large number of assumptions about the world, habits of thought, and behaviour which formerly involved or relied upon the existence of that person. Old roles must be relinquished and new roles adopted; plans must change, status, power, and control are often lost and one's very identity alters. For example a widow is very different from a married woman, and a childless woman is very different from a mother.

The psychosocial transition which follows bereavement is usually unwelcome and, like other unwelcome transitions, will tend to be resisted. People do not readily abandon assumptions about the world which have stood them in good stead for a long time or which represent habits of thought or of long-established expectations. They tend to go over in their minds, again and again, the events associated with the loss as if some alternative explanation could be found for what has happened and they continue to think and behave in ways which are often discrepant with their current life situation. The dead person is often felt to be near at hand and the bereaved may speak to them as if they were alive, minimal sights and sounds are misinterpreted as indicating the return of the dead, and in states of drowsiness, vivid hypnagogic hallucinations may occur in which the dead are perceived briefly as if they were present. Transient hallucinations of this kind are reported by up to 50 per cent of widows and may be misinterpreted as signs of incipient mental illness.

Despite this most people recognize the illusory nature of these phenomena and are all too aware of their tendency to operate on a model of the world which is now obsolete. Each mistake in thought or behaviour catches the bereaved unawares and undermines their sense of security, for, however unsatisfactory the world may be, the provision of an accurate internal model of it enables each one of us to 'know where we stand' and to plan our behaviour accordingly. When the accuracy of that model is in question every thought must be checked and a great deal of time devoted to identifying obsolete patterns of thought and updating them. As one widow put it 'It's as if the familiar world has suddenly become unfamiliar'.

Phases of grief

Although these three components of grief are present from the start each is more or less prominent at different times after bereavement. This has given rise to the notion of phases of grief, a model of grief which has some value but which tends to ignore the great variation which exists between people and the fact that people move back and forth between the phases.

Numbness and blunting

Many people find it hard to take in the full reality of a loss, particularly if they were unprepared for that event. An immediate reaction of numbness with feelings of unreality 'I can't take it in, it doesn't seem true' is very common and may last for a few hours or a few days.

Pining and yearning—the pangs of grief

Before long episodes of intense pining for the lost person occur with a tendency to cry aloud interspersed with relatively quiet periods of anxiety and tension. Anger, self-reproach, and bewilderment often add to the emotional turmoil which is associated with a general loss of security and self-esteem such that the bereaved seem to be waiting for another disaster to take place. Physiological accompaniments of anxiety are often misinterpreted and taken as evidence of illness or incipient madness. Anxiety may then escalate to panic attacks and/or hyperventilation.

Disorganization and despair

As time passes the intensity and frequency of the pangs of grief diminish and there are longer and longer periods of apathy and despair. All the appetites are diminished and people live from day to day preferring not to look to the future. Many people remain disengaged from social involvement, and feel and behave as if physically mutilated.

Reorganization and recovery

The first appetite to recover is usually the appetite for food. Weight lost in the first month or two of bereavement is soon regained and by the end of the first year too much weight may have been acquired. Anniversaries are often times of renewed grieving but once they are past there may be a lightening of mood and a renewal of energy. At this time holidays may enable people to escape from the constant reminders of loss; morale improves and on return they may be motivated to clear cupboards, redecorate, or engage in activities directed to the future rather than the past. In this way a new internal model of the world, as it now is, is constructed alongside the old.

There is no end-point to grief. Years after a bereavement an unexpected reminder of the past will trigger another pang of grief and memories of the dead may remain as clear or clearer than they were in the early weeks of bereavement. Many people report that the pain of yearning has diminished to the point where it is outweighed by the pleasure of remembering the good times that are past. Nostalgic recollections in tranquillity can then become one of the joys of advancing years.

Demographic and cultural factors

The above account of the pattern of grieving comes from research which has mainly focused on widows in middle life in the United Kingdom, the United States, and Australia. Even within this nominally Christian population there is great variation in reaction and the differences become greater still when other types of bereavement, other ages and sexes, and other racial and religious populations are studied (see Section 10).

Systematic comparisons are only now beginning to be carried out and shortage of space forbids all but a cursory summary of the current state of our knowledge regarding these factors. More detailed consideration of some of the more important causes of pathology will be given under 'prediction of risk'.

Conjugal bereavement and the death of a child are generally regarded as the most severe types of loss, with conjugal losses giving rise to more protracted disorganization of the world model and loss of a child evoking the most intense and lasting pining and anger. This reaction is more pronounced in mothers than in fathers and bereaved women in general tend to show more overt emotional disturbance and to seek help for emotional problems more frequently than bereaved men. On the other hand, one study[3] showed that the levels of anxiety or depression shown by women during the first year of bereavement return to levels comparable to those of married women more quickly than do those of widowers and there is evidence that the increased risk of death from heart disease which follows conjugal bereavement is greater in men than in women.[4] The social pressures on men to repress or inhibit grieving may well explain these findings.

Age is another important factor influencing the expression and course of grief. In very young children the difference between temporary and permanent separations is not clear. All separations evoke distress, but this soon passes provided adequate substitutes are provided for the lost person. In older children the pattern of grief approaches that of the adult but is likely to be complicated by failure of communication. Adults often attempt to protect children from the impact of a loss by concealing the fact, telling 'fairy stories' in the guise of religious myth and blocking the child's attempts to talk or play about the death. Inversion of parenting may occur with older children finding themselves expected to care for a grief-stricken parent. Such events may complicate and/or delay the process of maturation and the establishment of autonomy.

In old age bereavements are less often unexpected and untimely than in youth. This may account for the less intense emotional disturbance that is often (but not always) found in this age group. The disengagement which follows the many losses of old age is so common that it has been supposed by some to be a normal feature of ageing;[5] however, this phenomenon, in common with other features of grief, will pass if it is not aggravated by physical frailty and loss of mobility.

Cultural and religious influences are described in Section 10. Suffice it to say at this point that, although all known societies allow for the expression of tears in the course of mourning, there is great variation in the degree to which such emotional expression is expected and in the taboos on and privileges of the mourner.[6]

Risks to physical and mental health

Various studies suggest that, after the death of a husband or wife, about one-third of the surviving spouses will suffer a decline in physical or mental health of sufficient magnitude to justify them in seeking help.[7]

Minor problems are a reflection of the disturbance in psychophysiological function which is associated with continuing anxiety and tension. Disturbance of sleep, appetite, concentration, and mood are so common in the first month that they can be regarded as 'normal'. Only if these symptoms persist for several months are they likely to be regarded as abnormal. *In-vitro* studies of the immune response system suggest some reduction in the response to pathogens by β lymphocytes during the first month of bereavement,[8,9] but direct evidence is lacking for any effect on resistance to infection, although some authorities suggest that major losses can contribute to the onset of certain types of cancer.[10] Changes in endocrine function have also been reported[11] but again the implications for clinical practice are unclear. More impressive is the evidence for a significant increase in deaths from heart disease, particularly among men over the age of 55 who have lost their wives.[4] This has given rise to the suggestion that people with known ischaemic heart disease who suffer a major loss should be given a prophylactic β-blocker in order to reduce the influence of strong emotions on the heart.

An increase in consultations with general practitioners in widows and widowers over the age of 60 is largely attributed to muscle and joint conditions (particularly osteoarthritis) but it is unclear whether the bereavement causes the arthritis or simply makes it less tolerable.[12] A wide variety of psychosomatic disorders have been attributed to bereavement and the reader is referred to the review of the scientific literature by Osterweis for a more full account of these.[4]

Almost any psychiatric illness can be triggered by bereavement in those who are already vulnerable. Clinical depression has been found in 47 per cent of older widows during the first year[13] and there is some increase in the risk of suicide[14] among single men losing a parent. Hypochondriacal disorders sometimes resemble the illness of the person who has died (identification symptoms). An interesting and distinctive group are the pathological grief reactions in which the normal course of grief is distorted. Since these are associated with particular types of risk factor they will be discussed separately.

Prediction of risk

The study of risk factors has contributed to our understanding of the causes of psychiatric problems after bereavement; it has also proved useful in helping us to identify people at the time of a bereavement who need help and to guide counsellors towards likely problems.

The assessment of risk factors in those family members who are most affected by a patient's death should be routine and can be a part of the family assessment which is made by a primary care nurse or other caregiver whenever it is clear that a patient is entering the terminal phase of care. In the field of palliative care a genogram is more useful than a stethoscope, yet costs nothing and can be used by professionals and volunteers to good effect. It is the basic tool or starting point of family care. Without it the idea that the family (which includes the patient) is the unit of palliative care is no more than a slogan.

A genogram is a conventional code for recording a family. It employs simple symbols (most often a square for men and a circle for women) to indicate members and joins them by horizontal lines (to indicate ties within generations) and vertical lines (to indicate ties between generations). Further information is then added to the genogram as indicated in the following example (Fig. 1).

The following questions immediately come to mind when considering this genogram.

1. How did Mary's mother die? Mary's preconceptions of her illness are likely to be coloured by that event.

2. How did she and her husband cope with the deaths of their first two babies? Did this influence their attitude to the two who were born alive (overprotection is very likely, particularly of the daughter with Down's syndrome)?

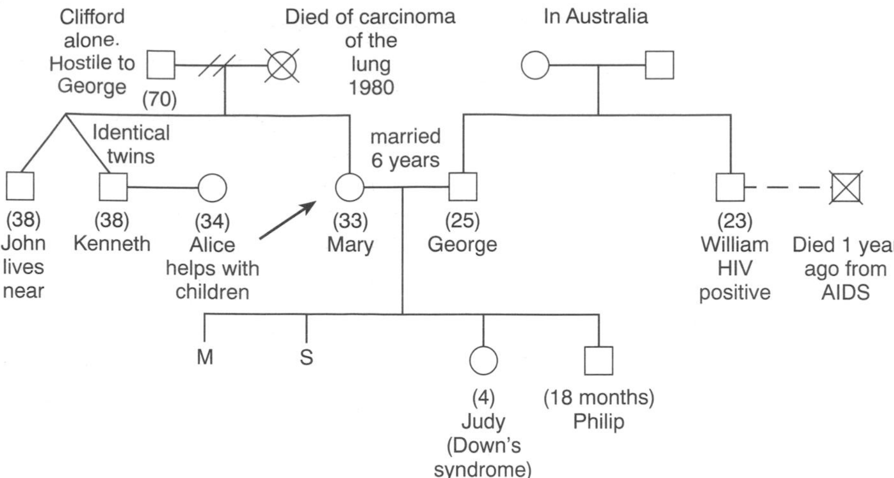

Fig. 1 An example of a genogram. indicates a married couple, a separated couple, a divorced couple, and a cohabiting couple. Siblings are shown or if they are twins. Individuals who are dead are symbolized by a cross superimposed: S= Stillbirth, M= Miscarriage. The patient is indicated by an arrow below and to the left or right of his/her symbol.

3. How is George going to cope with so little support from his own family? His brother is newly bereaved and has a life-threatening illness, his parents are in Australia, Mary's father is antagonistic, and he has to work for a living, cope with his grief, and meet the needs of two children, one of whom has Down's syndrome. A lot will depend on Mary's siblings and sister-in-law but it would not be surprising if George decided to emigrate after his wife's death.

4. Is Clifford in need of counselling? He will have lost his wife and his only daughter. At 70 he may well have difficulties in continuing to live on his own and his needs may conflict with those of Judy and Philip if Alice decides to continue to care for the children. The fact that he was divorced from their mother may well have affected his relationship with his children and adversely affect his reaction to her death.

5. How are the children to be prepared for their mother's death? The fact that Judy has Down's syndrome does not mean that she will not grieve but her intellectual development will influence the ease of communication. Both children are psychologically vulnerable and need consistent parenting with as few changes as possible.

6. How is William coping? He too has few family supports and Mary's illness may well have preoccupied George so that he cannot give William the support and understanding which he needs.

These questions will be most apparent to the person who draws the genogram and, for this reason alone, this act often gives rise to a fruitful discussion of the important issues. It brings home, as nothing else can, the importance of the family and summarizes a great deal of information in a small space. Doctors and others will often need to refer to the genogram which can be located on the front page of the section of the case notes which deals with family problems and can be passed to the bereavement service at the time of the patient's death. Genograms are also invaluable at case conferences and for teaching purposes when they can be drawn on a flip chart or the transparency of an overhead projector.

Predictors of poor outcome

Several factors have emerged from a variety of research projects as predictors of poor outcome after bereavement.[15] Different studies have not always attached the same weight to the same variables but close scrutiny usually explains any differences that exist. Thus, although several studies have inculpated sudden, unexpected deaths as a major determinant of poor outcome,[2] others have found no such association.[16] In this instance it seems that the age of the dead person is important. We seem to cope quite well with the sudden death of elderly people, perhaps because no death in this age group is entirely unexpected; by contrast, the death of a young person is an outrage which is compounded if it happens suddenly and unexpectedly. Deaths which have been anticipated are less traumatic but there are exceptions if the survivors have previously centred their lives on caring for the sick patient.

Vulnerability to bereavement is greatest in those whose trust in themselves and/or others is low.[17] It is also associated with a previous history of psychiatric illness, intolerance of stress, or threats of suicide. The relationship with the dying patient both reflects personal vulnerability and itself influences the outcome of bereavement. Relationships characterized by clinging or ambivalence are particularly important; the former is easily recognized by nursing staff who witness the intensity with which a family member clings to the dying patient.[3] The existence of a caring family who provide support to those of their members who are most affected by bereavement is a predictor of good outcome—it is the survivor's perception of the family that is important and this may not become clear until after the patient's death, when concealed conflicts may emerge or the bereaved may find that family members try to block or divert their attempts to express their grief. Raphael's study[18] suggests that it is this group of high-risk bereaved who will benefit most from the help of a counsellor.

Some hospices make use of formal questionnaires giving a numerical measure of risk. These were used as a means of selecting bereaved people for counselling in two studies which demonstrated the effectiveness of counselling.[18] Other studies which offered counselling to bereaved people regardless of risk showed no such benefits.[19] Despite these findings, formal questionnaires cannot be relied on to give an accurate prediction of risk and the factors described above may prove to be an equally useful way of guiding the assessor to ask questions which will enable a considered judgement to be made. There is, however, no justification for uneducated guesswork or leaving it to bereaved people who may be far too depressed to take the initiative in asking for help.

Abnormal grief

Although the relationship between risk factors and outcome is complex and it would be simplistic to suggest that particular risk factors inevitably give rise to particular types of reactions, correlational studies do reveal some overall patterns of reaction which are, to some extent, explicable in terms of the emotional circumstance which precedes them. Some of these are not specific to bereavements. Thus, general tendencies to anxiety, depression, and alcohol abuse are predictors of grief which will be complicated by these reactions. About half the people who are referred for psychiatric treatment after a bereavement fall into these non-specific categories.[3] The other half are suffering pathological types of grieving which themselves reflect the particular relationships and types of bereavement that precede them. They represent the tip of an iceberg. The group who seek psychiatric help are only a small proportion of the many people with similar problems, most of whom do not seek psychiatric help. Only a proactive, preventive programme aimed at providing counselling to these people early on in the bereavement process is likely to mitigate the suffering to which these disorders give rise.

The classification of pathological grief which follows derives from a prospective study of American widows and widowers in middle life to which reference should be made for further details.[20]

Traumatic loss

Deaths which are sudden, unexpected, and untimely or associated with multiple losses, hideous mutilation, or situations in which the survivor's life is also threatened, commonly give rise to a pattern of grieving in which attempts to avoid, repress, and delay grief continue for many months (or even years) but do not prevent high levels of anxiety and tension. These reactions can be viewed as a type of post-traumatic stress disorder. The events leading up to and including the death are usually recalled with great clarity and may be experienced again and again in the form of panoramic memories or nightmares. Acute anxiety (and even panic) may be triggered by sights and sounds associated with the death and the survivor may go to great lengths to avoid situations in which these will impinge.

Following events of this kind the numbness and blunting which were described above as a normal reaction to loss may persist for abnormal lengths of time. The process of grieving is delayed and the bereaved often attempt to maintain a fantasy relationship with the dead person who is seen as ever present and watching over the living. The bereaved withdraw from society and are less likely to make new relationships or to cope effectively with the challenges and opportunities which they meet. When these reactions follow a man-made event they give good grounds for compensation.

Conflicted grief

Another type of delayed grief tends to follow the loss of a person (usually a spouse or partner) to whom the bereaved had an ambivalent attachment. Here the immediate reaction is often one of relief. The bereaved experience neither the acute anxiety nor the numbness which follow traumatic bereavements and they may not expect to miss the dead person at all. With time, however, it becomes clear that there is unfinished business to be done. People find themselves 'haunted' by memories of the lost person. Feelings of anger and guilt complicate the situation and the bereaved may begin to feel that they have no right to happiness. 'Why should I be happy if he (or she) is dead?', as if they are buying happiness at the cost of the other person's death. A year after bereavement, people whose relationship was complicated by ambivalence are likely to be missing the dead person more than people whose attachment was relatively untrammelled and identification symptoms are not uncommon.

The ambivalence may not be confined to the relationship with the lost person. Stormy relationships with parents may be reflected in stormy relationships with partners and with siblings. Whether it is the parent or the partner who dies, the resulting grief is likely to be complicated by conflicts with the dead person and with the family who survive.

Chronic grief

The term 'dependent' has often been used of relationships which give rise to intense or prolonged grief when they come to an end, but studies of people who seek psychiatric help suggest that this type of reaction also often occurs after the death of the partner who was formerly regarded as dependent on the survivor.[17] It seems that there are some relationships in which the self-esteem and confidence of one person is repeatedly reinforced by a partner who is cast in the role of 'weak'. When the 'weak' one dies the mutually supportive system is disrupted and it is the 'strong' partner who collapses.

It is easy to understand why symbiotic relationships of this kind give rise to severe grief. Having done so the grief may be perpetuated because of the everyday gains which arise from it. Not only does overt mourning elicit sanction for withdrawal from social and other responsibilities but it often dignifies the mourner in the eyes of children and others. Grief being a sign of love and love a virtue in our society, mourning is a way of esteeming both the mourned and the dead person; as such it is tempting for those who feel a need to boost their esteem, or to make restitution to the dead, to persist in endless grieving.

The three categories of abnormal grief described above are not mutually exclusive and mixed pictures are not uncommon. This is hardly surprising when we recognize that relationships can be ambivalent and symbiotic and that any type of relationship may precede a traumatic bereavement. Clearly the greater the concatenation of risk factors the greater the risk.

Provision of care

It will be evident from what has been said that the care of the bereaved should start before the bereavement and that the prevention of psychiatric and physical disorders resulting from bereavement is more important than cure.

The care of the family before the patient's death has been discussed in Section 9. Suffice it to say at this point that this needs to be planned after a genogram has been drawn and assessment of the family needs made. Far from attempting to relieve families of the whole burden of care on the 'Don't worry, we'll look after him' principle, the care which is offered to families needs to recognize that this may be their last chance to make restitution to the dying person for any failure or other psychological debt which the family feel they owe, and to prepare themselves for bereavement by facing up to the realities of the illness, however painful this may be. It follows that we do not serve families best by taking away from them the whole care of the patient or by pretending that the prognosis is better than it really is.

Regular discussions of family problems in which the key nurses and doctors present their views for discussion by the team as a whole are a good way of ensuring that the family remains the focus of care and encourages nurses and doctors to develop the interest and psychological sophistication which makes for a high level of expert care.

Social workers, psychologists, and psychiatrists have important roles to play in support of the front line of care givers but it is as inappropriate to expect that they will look after all the psychological problems as it is to expect the chaplain to look after all the spiritual problems. In fact, the interface between psychological and spiritual care is so unclear that it is unwise to attempt to force people into these procrustean beds. Thus, the statement 'Everybody and everything is against me' could be taken as an example of projection (psychological), paranoia (psychiatric), alienation (social), or spiritual isolation (theological). There is no one of these viewpoints that is 'right'; all are valid ways of viewing a complex situation and each adds something to our understanding. The most effective carers are likely to be those who can move comfortably and flexibly between these various points of view without feeling constrained by any of them. Referral to one of the above professionals is only needed when it is appropriate to make use of their special knowledge. Sophisticated understanding is needed if we are to avoid inappropriate referrals. It would be as inappropriate to refer a widow to a psychiatrist because she has an illusion of the presence of her dead husband as it would be to ask the chaplain to provide absolution for delusions of guilt.

Part of the difficulty is the temptation to find simple solutions to complex problems. All of the theoretical models employed in psychology, or other human sciences, attempt to increase our understanding by dissecting out parts of a complex picture and focusing attention on them in the hope that they will simplify our ability to plan. The danger is that the plan will turn out to be as simplistic as the theory. Thus, depressed people may be given antidepressants on the assumption that depression is a kind of illness, newly bereaved people may be urged to cry on the assumption that everyone needs to grieve, and lonely old people may be bullied into old people's institutions on the grounds that proximity to others will dispel loneliness. Each of these plans may be appropriate in some cases. The danger is in applying them to all without due consideration of other possible factors; depression may be a transient unhappiness, the bereaved may not yet have had time or need to grieve, or loneliness may itself be a reflection of grief which will only be aggravated if the old person is uprooted.

The damage done by simplistic theories is such that some are tempted to eschew all theory. Counsellors are enjoined never to give advice and become a passive channel reflecting the client's perception back to the client in the hope that the clients will develop their own plans. This policy itself implies a whole set of theoretical assumptions which, like all the others, will only help some people.

In youth it is fitting that we embrace with enthusiasm the ideas and insights which help to explain the mysteries of the world we meet. (There is even one school of thought which believes that it is the enthusiasm of the therapist which matters more than the school of thought!) With increasing years we learn the limits of our knowledge and may lose some of our blinkered enthusiasm but we also, if we are patient, build up a repertoire of ideas which can prove useful in a widening range of circumstances.

The foregoing sections have presented ideas about the world of the bereaved, some of which will prove useful in enabling us to understand the problems they face. Flexibility, tact, and discretion are needed when we come to apply this understanding to the creation of support services to the bereaved. Many different models of care have been introduced but few have been submitted to the rigours of scientific evaluation (see below for a review of the research in this field). In the section which follows some widely used services will be described and the arguments for and against them reviewed, although this is a developing field in which there are few certainties. Local conditions will often dictate what is possible and the 'ideal' models which have been set up in some places are not necessarily appropriate to all circumstances.

In the long run no doubt a consensus of good practice will be reached, and some organizations (such as Cruse) are already laying down minimum standards that they expect all of their branches to achieve. The range of practice in hospices is enormous and although funding agencies sometimes demand the provision of bereavement services (for example, in the United States) these may mean no more than an occasional telephone call to the bereaved by a hospice volunteer.

There are large differences between the services which can be provided by a local hospice in an urban area where most of the bereaved clients live within a short distance, those provided by a rural team whose clients are more widely dispersed, and by a large oncology unit whose patients may have travelled hundreds of miles for treatment. The urban hospice may well opt for setting up its own bereavement service to provide individual counselling in the client's home, while the oncology unit is more likely to rely on telephone contact, referring those who are thought to need more intensive counselling to any local resources which happen to exist in their own area. Rural teams will be constrained by the distances which clients and counsellor are able to travel but may choose to support a number of small services scattered throughout the catchment area.

Whatever model is selected, it is important that it maintains an active and effective liaison with other services available to bereaved people in the area. If the area is large, this implies the creation and regular updating of a databank containing basic information about local services for the bereaved. Of course, specialized bereavement services are only one of several possible sources of help to the bereaved; others include social workers, general practitioners, and clergy, all of whom should receive training which prepares them for the problems they will meet. Local bereavement services are often in a position to provide this training.

Types of service

These vary according to the method of selection of clients (proactive/reactive), time of intervention (pre- or post-bereavement), identity of helper (professional, volunteer, or mutual support), location of base (hospital, hospice, or community), affiliation (local or national), location of intervention (home, office, or telephone), unit of care (individual, family, or group), type of support (befriending, counselling, pastoral, social, psychotherapy, psychiatric, or other psychological), and duration of intervention (long or short-term).

Selection of clients

The following choices are available.

(1) proactive services which reach out to clients who are thought to be at special risk;

(2) reactive services which respond to requests for help from any client;

(3) secondary care services which rely on referral from a primary caregiver.

At the time of writing the only bereavement services which have passed the test of scientific evaluation by random allocation (see below) are all proactive, i.e. they rely on a systematic assessment of risk factors made before or shortly after bereavement to identify individuals at special risk. Clients are then offered the service by personal or telephone contact with the counsellor who will provide the care.

Reactive services are much more common. Bereaved people are provided with information about the service (usually in the form of a printed leaflet) and it is left to them to decide whether to contact the service. While this probably increases the chances that those clients who respond are motivated to accept the help that is offered and reduces the counsellor's fear of intruding, it requires an act of courage on the part of the newly bereaved person, who may well be too depressed, too insecure, or too suspicious to take this initiative.

Secondary care services are typified by the traditional psychiatric service, most of whose referrals come from members of a primary care team. Since there may well have been a lapse of time before the client achieved the courage to ask for help, a further delay before he or she is seen by the primary caregiver, more delay before the referral is made, and even more delay before the first visit is made, several months may well have elapsed between the recognition of a problem and the provision of care. Psychiatric services all carry a stigma and should preferably be reserved for the very small minority of bereaved people who become mentally ill or who are thought to be a suicidal risk. In the latter case every possible step should be taken to avoid the delays described above. It is, of course, possible and appropriate for a service to be proactive, reactive, and to accept referrals.

In the United States, where insurance schemes currently provide funding for hospice service conditional on the provision of bereavement follow-up, a telephone call is usually made after bereavement to assess bereavement risk and to offer further support. It remains to be seen whether or not assessments made in this way are more reliable predictors of need than those made by professional staff. Home-care teams often make routine visits to families after bereavement in order to assess bereavement risk and to express their condolences; some routinely attend funerals. Whether the behaviour of newly bereaved persons at funerals, when they are often on their best behaviour and surrounded by their family, is any indication of their future adjustment is doubtful.

The main conclusion to be drawn from this section is that, regardless of who makes a risk assessment, or when and where it is made, it should be structured in such a way that valid conclusions can be drawn regarding the need for follow-up. All staff involved in this work should have a basic knowledge of risk factors and be trained to make assessments without offence to the family. If counselling is offered because of an assumption of high risk the would-be counsellor should not be alarmist in explaining the need: this would only add to the risk. On the other hand the client has a right to know of the concern which is felt for their welfare.

Timing of intervention

There is currently some disagreement regarding the best time to initiate bereavement support to those who need and want it. Some home-care teams see this as starting before bereavement and argue that a stranger coming in for the first time after a death is likely to be seen as an intruder, whereas a person who is already known to the family is more acceptable. Other teams prefer to introduce a new person after the bereavement on the grounds that bereavement counselling requires different skills from those needed to support families before bereavement (when the focus of care is on the patient), and the advent of a new person requires the bereaved to 'tell the story'; in doing so they are not only informing the counsellor, they are also clarifying in their own minds the reality of what has happened. They are setting up a pattern of interaction with the counsellor which is thought to facilitate the work of grieving.

Among those who wait until after bereavement to make a visit there is a general consensus that the best time to start is between 3 and 8 weeks after the event. Before this time the bereaved are often too 'wrapped up' in their families whereas after 8 weeks some will already have stopped crying, sealed off their feelings, and become reluctant to 'start all that again'. Between 3 and 8 weeks the family have often withdrawn, the bereaved are on their own, and grief is at a peak. This is usually a time when the bereaved are glad to talk and when a counsellor is most welcome.

There are, of course, exceptions to this rule. Some people are in urgent need of help after a bereavement and need to be seen the same day. Others will not accept help until many months have passed. It follows that an organized response should be flexible and sensitively aware of the needs and wishes of the bereaved.

Identity of helper

Having undergone the rigours and tests of a professional training it is not surprising that doctors, nurses, and social workers are often sceptical of the ability of lay people to provide help which requires 'professional' levels of knowledge, reliability, and confidentiality. Yet there is evidence from research that, with proper selection, training, and supervision, volunteer counsellors can achieve as much if not more than professionals. The way in which this can be carried out will be considered below but it is worth noting at this point that volunteer counsellors often have certain advantages over professionals. They often have more time to spare, and they are perceived as less distant and threatening. By devoting themselves to one type of service they soon become more experienced and 'expert' at bereavement care than most doctors and others for whom this is only a minor aspect of their work. Finally, they are considerably cheaper and can often provide a service which would not otherwise be economically viable.

Since many of those who offer themselves as volunteer counsellors to the bereaved have themselves been bereaved this type of service provides them with an opportunity to turn their most painful experience to good use. There is something appealing about an organization in which people who come for help can stay on to help others and this philosophy has given rise to the idea of widow-to-widow and other mutual help groups for bereaved people.[21] These groups usually adopt the extreme position that only those who have suffered a major loss are qualified to help the bereaved and that this is the only qualification that is needed. They are often deliberately unselective and provide little or no supervision of the 'befrienders' who offer help to the newly bereaved.

While there is no doubt that many of those who come for help to such organizations are satisfied with what they get there are certain dangers which must cause us to pause. Without proper selection of helpers there is always a danger that the group will become dominated by its most discontented or angry members. There is a danger that members will over-generalize from their own personal experience of bereavement, to that of others ('I know what you're feeling, I've been through it all myself' may be intrusive and a block to further communication). Ignorance of the special problems which sometimes arise may lead to failure to diagnose illnesses for which psychiatric treatment is needed and naïve management of other complex issues. The fact that the 'aggrievement' of grief is sometimes directed against doctors, nurses, and other professionals may lead to the development of antiprofessional attitudes within the group and a species of group paranoia which discourages its members from seeking help which they may need. At the time of writing, no satisfactory scientific evidence has been published indicating that mutual help groups without professional support are effective in reducing the risks to health of the bereaved.

For these reasons unqualified endorsement cannot be given to those mutual help groups which lack effective links with professional caring agencies and which do not provide proper selection, training, and supervision for those individuals who offer help to the newly bereaved. Further consideration of the roles open to professional and trained volunteer counsellors will be given below.

Location of base

There is no doubt that the base from which a service operates will colour the attitude of potential clients to that service. Thus, a bereavement service based around a church is likely to be favoured by the adherents of that church but distrusted by those who lack this affiliation. Since a well-run bereavement service brings credit to the institution to which it belongs there may even be competition between caring agencies to provide such services.

Effective risk assessment and liaison between those who care for the family before and after bereavement can best be achieved if a bereavement service is based in a local hospital or hospice, but this will only be able to provide face-to-face help to the families of patients living within a limited catchment area.

Affiliation

All services need to be part of a responsible and respected organization which is acceptable to the majority of those who might need help. A hospital or hospice can often provide that type of respectability, as can membership of a national body which sets minimum standards. In Britain, the organization Cruse does this and many hospices have developed close working links with their local branch. (The name 'Cruse' comes from the widow's cruse or jar of oil which was blessed by the prophet Elijah with a promise that it would not run out until famine was gone from the land (*Kings I,* Chapter 8:8–16)). Cruse has a national headquarters in London, a network of area organizers in each part of the United Kingdom, and 190 local branches. Smaller rural branches are based in the homes of particular members but larger urban branches usually have an office in the community.

This model has much to recommend it. Cruse provides a corporate identity which has become widely approved, accepts self-referrals as well as referrals from professional agencies, and, through its links with local hospitals and hospices, is capable of proactive involvement (although this is not widespread at the present time).[22] Multiple affiliation is, of course, quite possible with services benefiting from working links with local and national organizations.

Location of intervention

For most people their home is the place in which they feel most secure and many will not accept an offer of help in the early stages of bereavement unless the counsellor is willing to visit them at home. Places such as hospitals and hospices are particularly hard to face because of their association with the death which took place there and there are many bereaved people who are too insecure to attend open meetings or visit strange places. Most will answer the telephone and a few prefer the anonymity of a lengthy telephone conversation to admitting a counsellor to their homes, but most clients and counsellors feel more comfortable in face-to-face contact with each other and non-verbal communication adds an important dimension to all counselling. It follows that bereavement services are best advised to offer support in the home of the client in the first instance. At later stages it may benefit the client to return to the hospital or to other places in order to foster social integration.

The unit of care

For the same reasons many bereaved people will refuse to join groups but will be grateful for personal care for themselves and their families. The decision whether to include more than one member of the family is not always easy. When a spouse has died the surviving widow or widower will often prefer to be seen alone but following other bereavements, especially the death of children, couples may prefer to be seen conjointly.

Children are seldom invited to participate in counselling unless they are seen as having a major problem, but there may well be good grounds for including them in at least some sessions. As in our work with families before bereavement it is always best to regard the entire family as the unit of care and to maintain an active interest in members who have not been seen.

Group counselling and social meetings may well be of value once the bereaved are through the early stages of grieving. Groups may be set up to meet the special needs of particular segments of the population (e.g. parents' circles for widows and widowers with children under 16 years of age) or they may be heterogeneous groups aiming to draw people from a variety of backgrounds together. Open groups whose membership changes from week to week, or closed groups meeting for a set period of time and with a membership that is expected to remain constant, provide other alternatives. The former suit people who like to be able to 'drop in' to a group when they feel in need of help, the latter provide the opportunity for the group to reach a level of mutual contact and trust which enables them to share emotionally distressing problems and to achieve a greater depth of understanding than is possible in an open group.

Type of support

'Befriending' is a term which is used to refer to offers of friendship by untrained persons who may or may not have been bereaved. 'Mutual help' (or self help) is reserved for people whose qualification for offering help is their own experience of bereavement; they are usually untrained and sometimes unselected. Thus, mutual help groups are often leaderless open groups who rely entirely on their members to support each other. The term 'counselling' is best reserved for help given by people who have been selected and trained for the purpose. They may or may not have been bereaved. In the United Kingdom, most bereavement counsellors are volunteers, but there are also increasing numbers of professionals (such as doctors, social workers, or nurses) who have received training in counselling the bereaved.

'Psychotherapy' refers to the treatment of psychiatric illness by interaction with a therapist who has undergone a recognized course of training. It is expensive, time-consuming, and only appropriate for bereaved people who are also psychiatrically disordered. Since physical methods of treatment such as drugs may be required as well as, or instead of, this form of treatment it is advisable for referral to a non-medical psychotherapist to be made only after a proper diagnostic assessment has been made by a psychiatrist. Other psychological treatments have been developed by psychologists for the treatment of post-traumatic stress disorders, phobias, depression, and avoided grief reactions, all of which can occur following bereavements.

Duration of intervention

No hard and fast rules can be laid down since needs very so much. It is, however, reasonable to state at the outset that intervention and therapies should usually be brief, consonant with movement towards a satisfactory adjustment. Grief, as we have seen, lasts a long time but there is no need for us to assume that counselling or therapy should continue until the bereaved have come through their grief. Sometimes a single visit is sufficient to reassure people about the normality of the symptoms from which they are suffering. More often five or six visits at increasing intervals will ensure that the bereaved are on course to achieve recovery. Even patients with overt mental disorders seldom need prolonged therapy.

It is in the nature of human attachments that those people whose security has not been satisfactorily established in childhood and who grew up with little basic trust in themselves or others, often have difficulties in forming secure attachments in adult life. When insecure attachments are severed by death their precarious adjustment is thrown off course and the bereaved may well seek or be referred for help. It is hardly surprising if they then form an equally tenacious attachment to any friend, counsellor, or therapist who reaches out to them. The handling of these insecure attachments requires great tact and sensitivity and it is not surprising that some carers have difficulty in detaching themselves from clients whose insecurity causes them to cling immoderately. Like good parents, they must convince the clients of their own strength and autonomy without hostility or rejection. The relationship between client and carer is further complicated by financial considerations and there are some clients who will attempt to buy the attention (love) of a professional carer and there are some carers whose time is for sale regardless of the real needs of the client.

The withdrawal of support is as important as its initiation and can be hard for the carer as well as the client. This emphasizes the need for the carer to have the guidance and supervision of a third party who is capable of helping them to cope with the complex nuances of such relationships. These considerations also emphasize the importance of selecting carers who are not motivated by greed or the desire to satisfy their own insecure needs for attachment.

Choice of a bereavement support service

The foregoing catalogue may leave the reader somewhat bemused. Is there such a thing as an 'ideal' service, and even if there is, how can it be achieved with the limited constraints of time, money, and staff which most of us face? The answer must be that, in the present state of our knowledge, there can be no such thing and the main purpose of drawing attention to these issues is to help people to make the best possible use of the resources available to them in their particular area. This applies whether we are trying to decide how to advise a particular bereaved person to choose between existing services or whether we are tying to plan services at local, regional, or national levels.

The best known, large-scale services for the bereaved are probably the Widow-to-Widow services in the United States,[21] Cruse in the United Kingdom, and the Compassionate Friends[23] who cover both countries. In addition, hospices have developed patterns of service which, although they lack central organization, do follow particular patterns in each country.

The Widow-to-Widow programmes were introduced by Phyllis Silverman in the United States and have had a wide influence in other countries. They are limited to widows and rely on the assumption that the best person to help a widow is another widow. Individual counselling in the home and mutual help groups are both offered and, although no scientific evaluation has been undertaken at the time of writing, most people who seek their help are said to be satisfied. Unfortunately, they are not always well supported by professionals and some, indeed, have antiprofessional attitudes which might make liaison difficult.

Cruse provides a range of services to all who are bereaved by death, including individual counselling by volunteer counsellors who have been selected and trained for the purpose, group counselling, social groups, and information on a wide range of issues relevant to the bereaved. Introduced by Margaret Torrie in 1958, Cruse now has over 3000 counsellors across the United Kingdom.[22] Links with hospices are encouraged. The organization draws on the (voluntary) support of members of the caring professions to provide training and supervision of its counsellors. In return it is able to relieve these professionals of some of the burden of care and to provide training and information to student social workers and others who work with the bereaved. It produces three journals: the *Cruse Chronicle*, for bereaved clients; the *Cruse Bulletin*, an in-house news bulletin for Cruse staff and volunteers; and *Bereavement Care,* a quarterly journal for all who work with the bereaved (this has an international readership).

The Compassionate Friends is a mutual help organization run by and for parents who have lost a child. Started in 1969 by the Reverend Simon Stephens,[23] this organization has numerous branches in the United States and the United Kingdom. It produces a journal for its members and supporters. Closely associated is the mutual support group Support after Murder and Manslaughter.

Most hospices (but very few hospitals) provide some kind of bereavement follow-up. There is no uniform model, but the family service provided at St Christopher's Hospice provides an example which has been widely followed. Although initiated by the writer in 1970,[20] this service is now the responsibility of the social work department whose staff are closely involved in the selection, training, and support of volunteer counsellors. These are assigned to clients on the basis of a risk assessment made by the nurses and other staff of the hospice. Further details are given below.

Social support, pastoral care, and the place of ritual

Social support, spiritual support, and the rituals associated with death all play an important part in ensuring psychological recovery after bereavement. Together they contribute to providing a meaning to death and to the life that the bereaved must now lead. Social support does this by reassuring people that they are not alone, by providing succour and relief from responsibilities during the early stages of grief, and opportunities for social reintegration as grief subsides; pastoral care provides answers to the questions that science cannot answer about ultimate meaning and the support of a loving God. Rituals of the funeral and memorial services articulate these in ways which make the dead person both more incontrovertibly dead and more mystically sacred. By making death grand the funeral invests it with meaning, beautifies the ugliness of death, accredits the special status of the mourners, and articulates in poetic form ideas which defy rational explanation. In many societies, the spirits of the dead are believed to remain earthbound during the period of mourning.[6] A second ceremony then releases the dead to go to their final resting place and relieves the bereaved of the obligation to mourn them. This is thought to help mourners to move out of their special status and to enter the society which now awaits them.

Western Christianity has no such second ceremony but the social and religious events that have been introduced in some hospices can have similar psychological effects. Thus, at St Christopher's Hospice the relatives of patients who have died 9 to 15 months previously are invited to return to the hospice, to attend a service of remembrance in the chapel and to meet each other and the staff at a social gathering. For many it is an ordeal to return to the place where the death occurred but it is one worth suffering. Bereaved people often feel they have taken an important step towards accepting the full reality of the death and subsequently find it easier to take further steps towards a new social identity.

The rituals of bereavement have traditionally been organized and performed by funeral directors and clergy. In recent years, however, psychologists such as Rando,[24] recognizing the great value of these ways of helping people, have begun to make use of them as an aid to counselling. While this may seem a logical development it should still be regarded as experimental and it may be that, in the long run, its greatest value will be to stimulate a closer collaboration between the 'ritual experts' and the 'psychological experts'. Rituals are significant social events that may influence a lot of people and it is, perhaps, naïve for psychologists to assume that, simply because a ritual such as a funeral is of benefit to the bereaved, this is its only function. Tony Walter[25] points out that we are in danger of forgetting that the funeral belongs to the dead as much as the living.

These issues are discussed in more detail in Section 11.

Roles, training, and supervision of professional and volunteer staff

Bereavement care is too important to be left to chance and should be organized as efficiently as is the care of patients. Many different members of staff have a role to play and these are summarized below. Flexibility is needed and there are many ways in which roles can be allocated to suit the particular circumstances of large or small organizations with various types of catchment area (or none at all).

Records

Records need to be kept of all visits and these must be treated with the same, if not greater, confidentiality than patient's records. Such records serve several functions.

1. They enable basic information to be recorded regarding the identity, location, and accessibility of all family members who may need or give help.
2. They impose on carers the discipline of thinking about each interaction with the client and help them to clarify their aims.
3. They remind carers of what has been discussed in previous visits and enable them to hand over to others if the need arises.
4. They enable supervisors and counsellors to check on progress.
5. They facilitate the preparation of reports and referrals when needed.
6. They can be shown to the client to provide reassurances of progress and to allay any suspicions.
7. They form a valuable source of research data and can be used, with the client's permission, to teach others and to develop our knowledge of a developing field of care.

All records should be kept under lock and key when not in use and should be accessible only to the caring team (and, with permission, to authorized researchers). Clients should be informed of the existence of all records that are kept and reassured of their confidentiality. They should also be informed of their right of access to personal records (though not to those of other family members). This information can be provided as part of the basic information leaflet which explains the service.

Some services have adopted formal methods of record keeping which include problem lists organized under particular headings. These have particular value while a counsellor is under training and may help to focus attention on likely areas of concern. The danger of such forms is that they may encourage the counsellor to adopt an equally rigid approach to the interview as if the purpose was to fill in the questionnaire rather than to help the client.

Roles of nursing staff in bereavement care

The role of the nursing staff is summarized below:

1. Pre-bereavement support for families (see Section 13)
2. Assessment of bereavement risk
3. Support for the family at the time of death (see Section 16)
4. Home care nurses sometimes carry out visits to bereaved people in their homes. These are usually single visits to express sympathy, assess the need for further support, and provide 'one-off' counselling. Those bereaved people who need further support will normally be referred on to other sources of help but there are some hospice services in which the nurse is expected to provide all the bereavement counselling that is needed. In such cases the same training, supervision, and accreditation as other counsellors will be required.
5. Ward nurses often have an opportunity to meet families who are returning to a ward to collect items such as a patient's belongings or the death certificate. They too have the opportunity to provide 'one-off' counselling at this time.

One-off counselling is often helpful. It enables newly bereaved people to take stock of what has happened, and to ask questions about the causes and circumstances of the death. It also helps them to make real the fact of death, to share grief, and to obtain reassurance regarding the normality of the painful symptoms which are often present at this stage of bereavement. Training in such counselling can best be provided by role play in the presence of an experienced nurse counsellor. This should be an essential element in the training of nurses.

Roles of medical staff in bereavement care

These are listed below.

1. Anticipatory guidance to patient and family, including methods to break bad news and other communication with and support for, the family before bereavement.

2. Meeting the family after bereavement when they come to collect the death certificate provides doctors with a chance to answer questions about any aspect of the death that is of concern to them and provide reassurance and emotional support. Doctors, more than nurses, are expected to understand the medical causes of the death and can often provide positive reassurance that everything was done that could have been done and that the survivors were in no way to blame for the death or for any suffering which led up to it.

If permission is required for postmortem examination or organ donation it is essential to take time and trouble explaining the reasons for the request and the possible benefits that will result. Newly bereaved people will often find it difficult to make an immediate decision and emotional pressure will only increase their anxiety and indecisiveness.

3. General practitioners are sometimes able to follow up bereaved people by visiting them in their homes a week or two after bereavement. Others may be seen in the surgery. This is a time when many bereaved people are worried about their health and there may indeed be some increased risk. A careful history and examination, however, will usually disclose that most of the symptoms of newly bereaved people are due to the psychophysiological effects of grief. For these, explanation and reassurance, in language which the patient can understand, is all that is needed. If tranquillizers or sedatives are prescribed they should be in the form of a few single doses and not for regular consumption.

The general practitioner may also be in a position to reassure people that to 'break down' and show grief is not a sign of 'nervous breakdown'. He or she may also be able to give people permission to grieve, and provide them with the emotional support which makes that possible. It will be for the general practitioner to decide whether and how to provide further counselling for those who need it. The relationship between the doctor and patient may well be such that he or she will want to continue to provide counselling for some patients. It follows that general practitioners require the same kind of training and support as others who provide this type of counselling (see Section 16).

4. Medical practitioners in many specialties and in general practice will often come across patients whose medical problems are attributable to bereavements of one sort or another. A good knowledge of these problems is, therefore, an essential requirement for every doctor and is increasingly imparted in medical schools. Much of the therapy for these conditions can be provided by these doctors and only a minority require referral to psychiatrists and psychologists. Regardless of the need for referral, doctors have many opportunities to reassure their patients of the need to grieve and, in due time, to reassure them that their duty to the dead has been done and to foster their reintegration in society. Above all they should beware of the temptation to see normal life crises in medical terms and to label people who are suffering from normal grief as 'sick'.

Roles of social workers in bereavement care

The training of social workers in family care fits them well to take a lead in supporting families before and after bereavement.

1. Social work departments should initiate and organize services for families which continue or are introduced after bereavement. They should take prime responsibility with the volunteer organizer for the recruitment, selection, training, and support of volunteer counsellors (as described below), and they also have important roles to play in the training of other professionals in this field. Their own basic training should prepare them for these responsibilities but

they should also make full use of the help of psychiatrists and psychologists who are available to them.

2. Social workers often have the opportunity to work with families before and after bereavement. At these times they are in a position to contribute to the assessment of bereavement risk as well as providing counselling.

3. Like doctors, social workers are often asked for help as a consequence of a wide range of bereavements. A good knowledge of the nature of grief and the management of the problems resulting from bereavement is essential.

Roles of clergy and chaplains in bereavement care

Traditionally it was the clergyman who was expected to provide counselling and support to the bereaved and there are still many bereaved people who turn to their church for help. Sadly the training of clergy in pastoral care often leaves them poorly prepared for their role.

1. Hospital and hospice chaplains have opportunities to meet families before and at the time of bereavement and to help them to grapple with the problems of meaning alluded to in the foregoing section.

2. Funeral and memorial services also provide clergy with opportunities to work with families to plan and perform rituals of great psychological and spiritual significance. Time spent in discovering the family's 'religious language' and involving them as fully as possible in the service can change an horrific ordeal into a moving and elevating experience. It can also build a relationship of trust which will facilitate later pastoral care and counselling.

3. For those with a religious faith bereavement counselling by a pastor of similar faith has an added dimension which other counsellors may lack. This is less obvious when the bereaved person has little or no faith, but even here the clergyman or minister who is not bent on proselytizing may still have a pastoral role.

Role of volunteers in bereavement care

Before bereavement takes place volunteers working on hospice wards or home-care teams may get to know and befriend families who will share with them thoughts and feelings that they will never share with a doctor or nurse. At that time they may develop the kind of supportive relationships which make them the best person to support a family member after bereavement. If this is to be encouraged and to happen on a regular basis it is important that they be selected and trained with this in mind. Even when this is not the case some basic training should be given to alert volunteers to the problems they are likely to meet and to the sources of help available (see Chapter 21.6).

Volunteers who have been selected and trained as bereavement counsellors as indicated below should have the following skills:

1. They should be able to assess bereavement risk and the need for counselling or other forms of help.
2. They should be able to recognize, explain, and reassure bereaved people about the normality of many of the physical and emotional concomitants of bereavement.
3. They should be able to give emotional support and facilitate the expression of grief.
4. They should recognize the limits of their own skills; in particular they should know when to refer people for psychiatric or other medical help.
5. They should provide sanction and encouragement for both the expression of grief and, in due time, the ending of mourning. They should be able to reassure the bereaved that they have a right to life and the pursuit of happiness for themselves and their families.
6. They should know how to help bereaved people to review their assumptions about themselves and their world in the expectation that they will find new meanings, roles, and directions in life.
7. They should be able to recognize their own needs for help and accept the supervision and support which they need.

Roles of psychologists and psychiatrists in bereavement

Although grief is not a mental illness and should not be treated as such there is a minority of bereaved people who do become psychiatrically ill and a greater number whose degree or duration of emotional disturbance comes close to justifying such a diagnosis.[26] Since there is no sharp dividing line between mental health and mental illness it makes sense for psychologists and psychiatrists to work in close collaboration with palliative care and bereavement services to insure that problems are appropriately dealt with. Their roles include reassuring people that they are not mentally ill more often than assigning diagnoses but it is important that they be readily available whenever a counsellor or other member of staff feels that their attempts to help are not succeeding, that a person is so disturbed as to represent a suicidal risk, or that they are showing some evidence of pathology.

Psychologists and psychiatrists have useful roles to play in the training and selection of counsellors. It is important for counsellors to be aware of the psychiatric problems that may arise and to have the benefit of the depth of knowledge of the dynamics of family and individual psychology which is the stock in trade of these professions. Psychiatrists have the advantage of a medical training which makes them the best people to assess and treat any health problems. Psychologists, on the other hand, have special skills in the management of anxiety and other manifestations of stress. In recent years, many of them have become skilled in staff support (both individual and in groups) and in some parts of the world they are playing a major role in the provision of bereavement care.

Because there is a considerable overlap between the roles of psychiatrists and psychologists, local conditions will often decide who is available and interested in providing the support that is needed. Their training also fits them well to carry out the research which is needed if the care of the bereaved is to develop on a proper scientific footing.

Recruitment and selection of counsellors

The staff of hospices and other palliative care units have discovered repeatedly the goodwill that exists towards their work and the large numbers of people who offer to help. Only a small proportion of hospice volunteers are likely to be suitable or interested in bereavement counselling, but there are many ways in which volunteers can be of service and it should rarely be necessary to reject help out of hand. People who are unsuited to one set of roles can usually be steered towards others.

As indicated above, the roles of the bereavement counsellor are demanding and require a major commitment. It may, therefore, be necessary to seek out suitable persons by advertising widely and by drawing on the help of local clergy and other community leaders. Public meetings at which interested persons can learn about the service are a good way to start. On the whole, most of those who express an interest in undergoing the necessary training are well motivated and it is not usually necessary to reject many of those who apply. Some will withdraw their offer of help once they realize what is expected of them and no attempts should be made to dissuade them. The rest should be subjected to a thorough selection process. This also applies to professionals who wish to add bereavement counselling to their other caring skills and who often assume that their prior experience or training makes further instruction unnecessary. Sadly, experience teaches that there are some doctors, nurses, social workers, clergy, and other members of caring professions who are too vulnerable or busy to cope with the rigours of training let alone the regular counselling of the bereaved.

The selection process should, at a minimum, include taking up references from people who can vouch for the character, resilience, and suitability of the applicants and one-to-one interviews in which they are asked to talk about the worst losses and other distressing events which they have experienced and to explain their reasons for choosing this type of service. Most applicants will be found to have suffered a major loss of some kind and the interviewer needs to assess the extent to which they can now share thoughts and feelings about the loss, not without emotion, but without being overwhelmed with grief. In the end it is the interviewer's feeling that he or she could cry on this person's shoulder that is probably the best indication that they would make a bereavement counsellor. Previous experience, training, or paper qualifications, though welcome, are not necessary.

All applicants need to be able to make a firm commitment to attend the training course and to complete the approved number of counselling visits under supervision. It is an interesting side-light on volunteering that the more that is demanded of volunteers the more seriously they tend to take their commitment to the service. Expect little and you will get little.

Training and supervision

The aims of training are to impart skills as well as information. Information can be provided by guided reading, backed by seminar/discussions, and should cover the main topics in this section along with a more detailed exposition of the management of grief and its variants than is possible here. Skills are more difficult to teach and require the use of experiential methods such as role play. Trainees will also benefit from talking, in the training group, about their own experiences of loss, such as what they felt or what was helpful. Role play is usually evaluated as the most painful and the most worthwhile part of the course. Just as the counsellor will eventually provide the emotional support which will enable clients to share disturbing thoughts and feelings, so the group leader must provide the trainees with a secure base from which to explore the frightening world of the bereaved. Time should be spent in getting to know trainees before embarking on role play. The more extrovert members of the group may lead the way but all should be expected to play the roles of both clients and counsellors.

The aim of role play is to give the trainees opportunities to meet, in advance, the kinds of situations they are likely to meet when counselling the bereaved and to understand them from the point of view of the bereaved as well as the counsellor. The leader selects a range of likely scenarios and as many of the group as are needed play the parts of family members and counsellors. The 'family' will need to spend some time drawing genograms and discussing their life situation but the 'counsellors' should be told no more about them than they would be likely to know in real life. If a role play gets 'stuck' (e.g. the counsellor cannot think of what to say or do and/or tension is rising, despite counselling) it is important for the leader to interrupt the play, to invite the participants to report back what they are feeling and ask the group to make suggestions. It is sometimes useful to ask a non-participating member of the group to take over a role.

Role play is different to theatrical acting in that the players are expected to identify with the part and to feel as if they were undergoing the trials and tribulations of the people they represent. As well as being emotionally taxing it can be hard for some players to put aside the part they have been playing and resume their former identities. The group leader has important roles to play in maintaining the security of the group and ensuring that the roles of the players are properly discarded after the play. At the conclusion of the play the actors should move out of the acting area and indicate their awareness that they are no longer in their roles by talking in the past tense about their parts. If necessary the leader should point out that 'you are no longer a widow, you are Mary Jones again', and obtain the assent of the trainee. The group leader should be available after role play sessions to discuss any problems that persist and to provide appropriate counselling.

Cruse expects trainee counsellors to spend a minimum of 20 hours in seminar/discussion groups and 12 hours in experiential learning. The timing of the training sessions is determined by local circumstances but each session should be long enough to allow the participation of all trainees. Some trainees will drop out in the course of training when they realize the problems that face them. Others may need to be redirected to more suitable work. For this reason a formal review of progress should be made at the end of the period of basic training to decide whether or not each trainee should continue in the programme. Those who clear this hurdle begin a period during which they carry out bereavement counselling under supervision. They must attend supervision meetings at which they will report on the work they are doing and discuss any problems that emerge. Some services use report forms as a means of focusing on likely problem areas. Subject to satisfactory completion of an agreed number (Cruse say 60) of supervised counselling sessions, a certificate or letter of accreditation can be issued. Thereafter the amount of supervision is reduced, but counsellors should continue to attend group discussions and occasional advanced level training (for example in group work). In due course they may become sufficiently experienced to take on the supervision of others.

In this way, a bereavement service eventually becomes more independent of the professionals who initiated it although their skills will always be needed in training courses and to provide back-up when special problems arise.

Principles of counselling the bereaved

It would take us beyond the scope of this volume to attempt anything but the briefest exposition of the principles which underlie counselling for the bereaved and, once again, the reader is warned against simplistic or mechanistic techniques. Every counselling situation is different; there are no rules of thumb and we are venturing into uncharted territory whenever we reach out to a bereaved person.

The first and most important principle is to take time. Counselling cannot be hurried and we shall get nowhere if we try to force the pace. The first visit, which may be the longest, may well last for as long as 2 hours.

The counsellor must not talk too much. A brief introduction, explaining his or her presence in a relaxed and friendly way will soon put the client at ease. A cup of tea is the traditional British way of breaking the ice and establishes the counsellor as a guest if the interview is taking place in the client's home. It is better to say too little than too much, and to listen attentively to everything the client has to say.

Since grief is a way of making real inside oneself an event which is already an established reality outside, the best way to facilitate grief is to ask bereaved people to tell their own story. While they are explaining themselves to us they are explaining themselves to themselves. The events they describe are becoming more real and the implications clearer. The counsellor can facilitate feelings by asking about them: 'What do you feel about that?', and by echoing them 'That makes me feel very sad (angry, etc.)'. Such statements about one's own feelings must come from the heart. We should never pretend to feelings we lack.

Non-verbal communication is as important as speech and the counsellor must become sensitively aware of the client's, as well as his own, unspoken messages. Showing interest is a powerful message, so is sharing grief. At times there is no harm in the counsellor shedding a tear, but it must be the counsellor's shoulder on which the client is crying, not vice versa. If anxiety or tension is becoming unbearable, the best way of reducing it is usually to move closer to the bereaved, and to smile and touch or hold them in a comforting manner (much as a mother can quiet a frightened child). Again we must allow time for tears to subside before expecting the bereaved to go on talking, and not block off tears by changing the topic or rushing in too quickly with a tissue (the non-verbal message here being 'dry your eyes and stop crying'!). Some clients cannot tolerate closeness and the counsellor must watch carefully how they react to any movement and respect their need for distance.

Positive reassurances about the normality of grief and simple explanations of any symptoms that are frightening or bothering the client are often necessary. If referral or examination is needed this should be explained as a reasonable precaution rather than an indication of danger. Counsellors should never blame, criticize, denigrate, tease, or talk down to clients, even when they are being most unreasonable; we must understand and tolerate their anger. By the same token they should avoid agreeing with points of view that may be distorted and should not be in a hurry to counteract the client's feelings of guilt. It may be more appropriate to say 'If that's the way you feel, what can you do about it?' than to say 'Oh you shouldn't feel like that, it's not your fault'. Confronting people with their feelings and asking them to consider what to do implies that there is always something useful to be done with feelings—a positive attitude that can lead to some very creative actions.

If the conversation should dry up, become trivial, or show other evidence of being blocked it is important to work out the reason. The client may be tired, in which case the meeting should be brought to an end and resumed some other time; feelings that are just too intense may have arisen, in which case the client may need time to calm down before continuing; or anger or mistrust may have been evoked. This will need time to be examined if the relationship is to get on the right wavelength. It is often useful to repeat back to the client the last sentence uttered since this is often the key to the block.

Counsellors can implicitly and explicitly give people permission and encouragement to grieve. In due time, they can also give them permission and encouragement to stop grieving and get on with living. Grief is not only a reaction to bereavement, it is also a duty to the dead and mourners may need reassurance that their duty has been done. Sensitive counsellors will not push people to make plans for the future too soon; in fact they are more likely to find themselves warning them not to sell up and move out or to adopt other means of escaping from a situation from which there is no escape. But the time will come when the social sanction for mourning, and the special protection that goes with it, can be withdrawn; it is time for the bereaved to re-enter the world, to discover what can be carried forward from the past and what must be left behind. It is not the counsellor's job to direct or advise but to have faith in the client's strengths and to encourage them to make their own plans.

Because, in general, men have more problems than women in the expression of emotion they are likely to benefit most from an approach that focuses on helping them to do this. Women, on the other hand, are more likely to need help in thinking through the implications of their bereavement and reorganizing their lives (Schut *et al.*).[27]

Research: psychological and social

Because bereavement often constitutes a major stress which occurs at a clearly identifiable time and is the subject of medical census records it has been the subject of much research in recent years (see Osterweis[4] and Rando[24] for reviews). Retrospective and prospective studies have demonstrated the effects of major losses (especially the death of a spouse) on the physical and mental health of the survivors, while short longitudinal studies have provided detailed accounts of the course and range of variation of grief and have enabled risk factors to be identified. Random allocation studies have enabled the effects of counselling and other types of intervention to be evaluated. Between them these studies have provided a firm foundation for much of the knowledge which is summarized in Section 13.

Retrospective studies of the incidence of losses in sick populations have been bedevilled by the usual biases of such studies. Losses by death of a spouse, parent, or child is unlikely to be misremembered and studies, such as the examination by Parkes of the case records of 3245 psychiatric patients[28] and the study by Bunch *et al.* of the precursors of suicide,[29] provide convincing data for an association between bereavement and clinical depression or suicide.

Prospective studies of the health of bereaved people have ranged from studies of the incidence of minor disorders, prescription of medication, and health-care utilization in small samples of bereaved people[12] to studies of the mortality rates in very large populations of widowers[30,31] followed-up over 10 years.

Methodological issues need to be addressed in such studies.

1. What is the range of normality of the psychophysiological reaction to bereavement. What is the distinction between 'grief' and 'clinical depression'? By what criteria is 'ill health' defined?

2. Given that traumatic life events occur repeatedly in all our lives, how soon after a bereavement must an illness occur for a causal relationship to be established and how long should it persist for it to be seen as more than transient? These issues are important in determining the timing and duration of follow-up.

3. Few of the symptoms and other psychological consequences of bereavement are capable of objective measurement. How can sensitive and reliable measures of subjective phenomena be developed which will ensure that the findings of one study can be verified in another and that the words used have a consistent and communicable meaning?

4. The psychological meaning of a life event can only be understood from its context. Thus, a bereavement which, to one person, might be a disaster, to another may be an unmitigated blessing. Even an event as clear-cut as the death of a spouse cannot be regarded as of equal significance to all who suffer it; nor can it be assumed that all who experience this event are equally in need of help. It follows that appraisal of the circumstances of a death and the meaning which it has for the bereaved must be taken into account in planning and interpreting research in this field.

5. However great the damage which can result from a life event the provision of help on more than an experimental scale can only be justified if it can be demonstrated that such help is effective in reducing or preventing such damage. To evaluate effectiveness both the help and the damage which it is intended to mitigate must be clearly measured and a group of people who receive the help be compared with another who do not. The two groups should resemble each other in all relevant criteria (such as age, sex, socio-economic status, or life circumstances) and account should be taken of the possibility that those who do not receive help from one source will seek it from another.

Examples

Research in the field of bereavement has now developed to the point where it is possible to cite examples of good research which take account of these methodological problems.

1. Clayton *et al.* have used clear operational definitions of 'clinical depression' which meet established psychiatric criteria to investigate the incidence and prevalence of depression after conjugal bereavement.[13]

2. Repeated observation of widows and widowers at intervals after bereavement have provided a picture of the changes which occur over time and comparison with non-bereaved control groups has enabled the bereavement effect to be measured. Thus, the study by Young *et al.* of the mortality during the first year of bereavement[27] has been extended to 10 years and compared with the mortality in age-matched controls.[28]

3. Operational definitions of the subjective phenomena under study and reproducible questionnaires such as the Texas grief inventory[32] have provided us with instruments which enable one sample to be compared with another.

4. A number of longitudinal studies have not only revealed a wide range of variation in the response to bereavement such that the model of grief as a series of fixed stages which the bereaved must pass on the way to recovery has been called into question, but has enabled many of the contextual circumstances which explain this variation to be identified and related to the consequent patterns of grieving (grief syndromes) which result.

A spin-off of this type of research has been the identification of 'risk factors' which enable people who are likely to need counselling to be identified before or at the time of bereavement and provide the counsellor with guidance regarding the kind of help likely to be needed. A good example of the application of this approach to the study of conjugal bereavement in young to middle-aged adults is the Harvard bereavement study.[20]

5. Evidence for the effectiveness of bereavement counselling comes from two random-allocation studies focused on high-risk bereaved.[18,19] Both studies used questionnaires to identify widows (in Parkes' study also widowers) at special risk and provided counselling during the first year of bereavement to one group while offering no proactive help to the other. Follow-up interviews during the second year of bereavement showed statistically significant differences in psychophysical adjustment favouring the counselled groups. The main difference between these studies was that the counselling in Raphael's Australian study was provided by herself (an experienced psychiatrist) whereas that in Parkes' London study was provided by volunteers who had been selected and trained for the purpose.

Problems

Several other studies have shown little or no differences between counselled and non-counselled groups of unselected bereaved people but problems of sample size, insensitive outcome measures (health change being a more sensitive indicator than health status), and inexperienced or poorly trained counsellors probably account for most of the negative findings. The possibility must also be considered that counselling may even do harm to some of those who would otherwise do well, perhaps by evoking anxiety and introspective doubts or by displacing the support of a caring family.

At the time of writing, no satisfactory evaluations of mutual help groups without professional backing are known to the writer, perhaps because of the difficulty of randomizing the people who seek help from these organizations. Likewise difficulty in obtaining access to bereaved children accounts for the paucity of information about this age group. The inadequacy of much of the research which has been published on the effects on parents of intrauterine deaths and the death of children is less easily explained. Much of this remains at an anecdotal level.

Studies of bereavement in the elderly has given rise to much controversy mainly because of the complicating effects of the multiple losses which often occur in this age group and the high prevalence of health problems in non-bereaved controls.

Conclusion

Hospices and other organizations providing care for families before and after bereavement are in a unique position to carry out the longitudinal studies which are needed to fill in the many gaps which exist in our knowledge of bereavement. As in the case of research with patients, the implications of this research extend beyond the field of palliative care.

References

1. Lararus RS, Averill JR, Opton EM. Towards a cognitive theory of emotion. In: Magda A, ed. *Feelings and Emotions.* New York: Basic Books, 1974.
2. Lundin T. Morbidity following sudden and unexpected bereavement. *British Journal of Psychiatry,* 1984; **144**: 84–8.
3. Parkes, CM. *Bereavement: Studies of Grief in Adult Life.* 3rd edn. London: Routledge, 1996.
4. Osterweis M, Solomon F, Green M. *Bereavement: Reactions, Consequences and Care.* Washington DC: National Academy Press, 1984.
5. Cumming E, Henry WE. *Growing Old.* New York: Basic Books, 1961.
6. Rosenblatt PC, Walsh RP, Jackson DA. *Grief and Mourning in Cross-cultural Perspective.* New York: H R A F Press, 1976.
7. Raphael B. *The Anatomy of Bereavement: a Handbook for the Caring Professions.* London: Hutchinson, 1984.
8. Bartrop RW, Lazarus L, Luckhurse E, Kiloh LG, Pennoy R. Depressed lymphocyte function after bereavement. *Lancet*, 1977; **ii**: 834–6.
9. Schleiffer SJ, Keller SE, Camerino N, Thornton JC, Stein M. Supression of lymphocyte stimulation following bereavement. *Journal of the American Medical Association*, 1983; **250**: 374–7.
10. Schmale AHJ, Iker HP. The affect of hopelessness and the development of cancer. I, Identification of uterine cervical cancer in women with atypical cytology. *Psychosomatic Medicine*, 1966; **28**: 714.
11. Hofer M, Wolff C, Friedman S, Mason PW. A psycho-endocrine study of bereavement. *Psychosomatic Medicine*, 1977; **39**: 481–504.
12. Parkes CM. The effects of bereavement on physical and mental health: a study of the case records of widows. *British Medical Journal*, 1984; **2**: 274.
13. Clayton PJ, Halikas IA, Maurice WL. The depression of widowhood. *British Journal of Psychiatry,* 1972; **120**: 71–8.
14. Bunch J, Barraclough B, Nelson B, Sainsbury P. Suicide following the death of parents. *Social Psychiatry,* 1971; **6**: 193–9.
15. Parkes CM. Risk factors in bereavement: implications for the prevention and treatment of pathologic grief. *Psychiatric Annals*, 1990; **20**: 308–13.
16. Helsing KJ, Szklo M. Mortality after bereavement. *American Journal of Epidemiology,* 1981; **114**: 41.
17. Parkes CM. Attachment, bonding and psychiatric problems after bereavement in adulthood. In: Parkes CM, Stevenson-Hinde J, Marris P, eds. *Attachment Across the Life Cycle.* London: Routledge, 1991.
18. Raphael B. Preventive intervention with the recently bereaved. *Archives of General Psychiatry,* 1977; **34**: 1450–4.
19. Parkes CM. Evaluation of a bereavement service. *Journal of Preventive Psychiatry,* 1981; **1**: 179–88.
20. Parkes CM, Weiss RS. *Recovery from Bereavement.* New York: Basic Books, 1983.
21. Silverman P. Services for the widowed: first steps in a program of preventive intervention. *Community Mental Health Journal*, 1967; **3**: 37.
22. Parkes CM. Models of bereavement care. *Death Studies*, 1987; **11**: 257–301.
23. Stephens S. *Death Comes Home.* London: Mowbray, 1972.
24. Rando TA. *Treatment of Complicated Mourning.* Champaign, Illinois: Research Press, 1993.
25. Walter T. *Funerals and How to Improve Them.* London, Sydney, Auckland and Toronto: Hodder & Stoughton, 1990.
26. Jacobs S. *Pathologic Grief: Maladaptation to Loss.* Washington, DC and London, England: American Psychiatric Press, 1993.
27. Schut HAW, de Keijser J, van den Bout J. Short-term inpatient therapy in groups. *Proceedings of the Fourth International Conference on Grief and Bereavement in Contemporary Society.* Swedish Association for Mental Health, 1994.
28. Parkes CM. Recent bereavement as a cause of mental illness. *British Journal of Psychiatry,* 1964; **110**: 198.
29. Bunch J, Barraclough B, Nelson B, Sainsbury P. Suicide following the death of parents. *Social Psychiatry,* 1991; **6**: 193–9.
30. Young M, Benjamin B, Wallis C. Mortality of widowers. *Lancet*, 1963; **ii**: 454.
31. Parkes CM, Benjamin B, Fitzgerald RG. Broken heart: a statistical study of increased mortality among widowers. *British Medical Journal*, 1969; **i**: 740–3.
32. Fashingbauer TR. *Texas Inventory of Grief* (test manual). Houston: Honeycomb, 1981.

19

Paediatric palliative care

19.1 Pain control

Patricia A. McGrath

Introduction

The topic of pain control in paediatric palliative care is receiving increasing attention from health-care professionals.[1-7] During the past decade, unprecedented interest has focused on the special pain problems of infants, children, and adolescents, so that there have been enormous advances in our understanding of children's pain perception and in our ability to alleviate their suffering.[8-16] Many of the myths underlying our past treatment of children's pain have been refuted. We recognize that infants can experience pain at birth and that failing to alleviate their pain causes adverse physiological consequences, in addition to needless suffering. We now know that children, like adults, can experience many different types of acute, recurrent, and persistent pain. We know that children can describe their pain and that we should assess their pain regularly to monitor the effectiveness of the interventions we provide. We know that children do suffer prolonged pain due to disease, trauma, and psychological factors. We know that children in severe pain require potent analgesics for pain relief, and that appropriate opioid administration does not lead to addiction. Furthermore, we know that pain control for infants and children receiving palliative care (as for adults) should include regular pain assessments, appropriate analgesics administered at regular dosing intervals, adjunctive drug therapy for symptom and side-effects control, and non-pharmacological interventions to modify the situational factors that can exacerbate pain and suffering.

This chapter focuses on the special challenge of caring for children with pain, particularly children who may or will die with pain. A practical approach for treating children's pain from a multidimensional perspective, consistent with the neural and psychological mechanisms that mediate their pain is presented. Since much specific information on pain control (presented in Section 9.2) is also relevant for children, basic information on pathophysiology, pharmacology, and physical interventions is not repeated in this chapter. Instead, this chapter provides a complementary focus to the other contributions in this textbook by describing the unique nature of children's pain and presenting guidelines for selecting and administering analgesics to control their pain.

The nature of children's pain

One of the most remarkable advances in our understanding of children's pain—due to its important implications for pain management—has been our gradual realization that the system that mediates children's pain perceptions is a marvel of subtlety and complexity. Like adults, children can experience pain without tissue injury or apparent injury. They can also sustain injury without experiencing pain, and can experience very different pains from the same type of tissue damage. Children's nociceptive systems are plastic, in that they have the capacity to respond differently to the same amount of tissue damage. Impulses generated by tissue damage can be modified by impulses in other ascending systems activated by innocuous stimuli (e.g. touch) and by impulses in descending pain-suppressing systems activated by various factors (e.g. expectations about what will happen).[11,17,18] Since a child's pain is not simply and directly related to the extent of physical injury or to disease severity, we cannot completely control a child's pain by gearing our interventions solely to the source of tissue damage. Instead, we must also modify the factors that affect his or her nociceptive processing. Controlling children's pain requires a dual emphasis on administering appropriate analgesics and on selectively modifying the factors that exacerbate their pain.

The factors that modify children's pain perception are shown in the model in Fig. 1. Some factors are relatively stable for a child, such as age, gender, cognitive level, previous pain experience, family learning, and cultural background (listed in the clear box). These child characteristics shape how children generally interpret and experience the various sensations caused by tissue damage. In contrast, the cognitive, behavioural, and emotional factors (listed in the shaded boxes) can vary dynamically, depending on the specific circumstances in which children experience pain. These situational factors represent a unique interaction between the child experiencing pain and the context in which the pain is experienced.[11,14] Differences in situational factors may account for why the same tissue damage can evoke pains that differ in strength and may partially explain why proven analgesics can vary in effectiveness for different children and for the same child at different times. Even though the pain source may remain constant, the particular set of situational factors is unique for each occurrence of pain. Moreover, unlike the child characteristics listed in Fig. 1, health professionals can modify situational factors and dramatically lessen children's pain.

The impact of situational factors on children's pain

What children understand, what they do, and how they feel have a profound impact on their pain experience. Cognitive factors

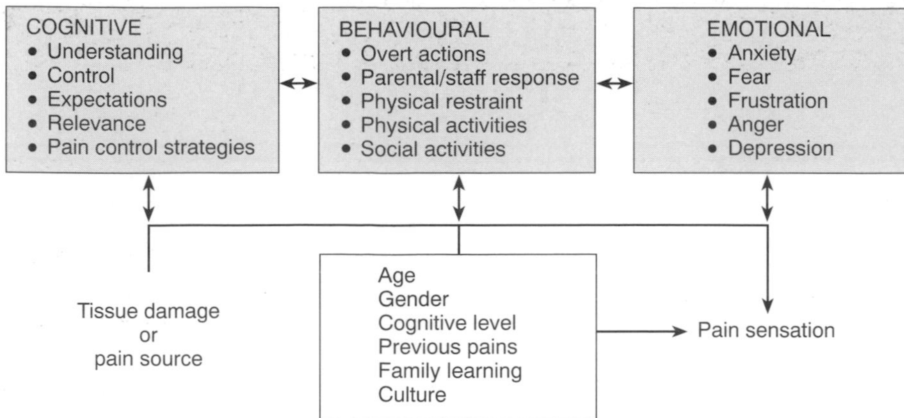

Fig. 1 A model depicting the situational factors that modify children's pain perception. (Reproduced with permission from PA McGrath and LM Hillier. Controlling children's pain. In: *Psychological Treatments for Pain: A Practitioner's Handbook*, RJ Gatchel and DC Turk, editors. Guilford Publications Inc., 1996: 333.)

include children's understanding about the pain source, their ability to control what will happen, their expectations regarding the quality and strength of pain sensations that they will experience, their primary focus of attention (that is distracted away from the pain or focused on what is happening), the relevance or meaning of the pain—particularly it's life-threatening potential, and their knowledge of pain control strategies. In general, children's pain can be lessened by providing accurate age-appropriate information about pain, for example emphasizing the specific sensations that children will experience (such as the stinging quality of an injection, rather than the general hurting aspects), by increasing their control and choices, by explaining the rationale for what can be done to reduce pain, and by teaching them some independent pain reducing strategies.[19–25]

Behavioural factors include children's overt physical behaviours (e.g., crying, withdrawal, using a pain control strategy) and parent's and health staff's behavioural responses to them (e.g., displaying frustration, calmly providing encouragement for children to use pain control strategies). They also include the extent to which children are physically restrained during treatments and the broader physical and social restrictions on children's lives. Distress behaviours and some altered behavioural patterns may initiate, exacerbate, or maintain children's pain. In general, as children's physical activity increases, as children use coping and pain control methods, as their distress and disability behaviours decrease, and as staff and parental responses become more consistent in encouraging them to use pain control methods, their pain should lessen.[11,12,26–28]

Children's emotions affect their ability to understand what is happening, their ability to cope positively, their behaviours, and ultimately their pain. Children's immediate emotional reactions to pain may vary from a relatively neutral acceptance to annoyance, anxiety, fear, frustration, anger, or sadness. The specific emotions depend on the nature of the pain—type, cause, intensity, and duration—and its impact on their lives. In general, the more emotionally distressed children are the stronger or more unpleasant their pain. When children do not understand what is happening, when they lack control and do not know independent pain control strategies, their emotional distress increases and their pain intensifies. Similarly, when children's behaviours are restricted, when they are physically restrained during medical procedures, or when their usual sports and peer activities are disrupted, their emotional distress and pain can intensify.[11]

There are dynamic interactions among cognitive, behavioural, and emotional factors. Health staff can significantly lessen children's pain, not only by administering potent analgesics but also by increasing children's understanding and control, by decreasing their emotional distress, and by teaching children some simple physical, behavioural, and cognitive methods to complement analgesic medications and further reduce their pain.[11,29]

Situational factors in paediatric palliative care

Cognitive and emotional factors are the most salient situational factors that affect pain for children receiving palliative care. Children probably have already endured a prolonged period of physical disability, intermittent pain, and multiple aversive treatments. Children who were receiving curative therapies become more focused on the future consequences of their disease. Their thoughts, behaviours, and feelings change as they begin to understand that they are dying. Naturally, the type of support, information, and guidance children require also changes. While the impact is profound for all children and families, each child and family is unique with respect to their specific psychological, medical, social, and spiritual needs. All families experience anguish and grief, but they may also experience denial, anxiety, anger, guilt, frustration, and depression. It is essential that health professionals listen attentively and observe carefully not only to ensure that all the needs of both the child and family are met but also to resolve the myriad factors that can exacerbate children's pain and suffering. The primary situational factors in paediatric palliative care are listed in Table 1. This summary has evolved from our treatment of children referred to the pain clinic. Child and family factors are listed in italics; the factors that are relevant for health staff, as well as families, are listed in roman print.

The shift in care from curative to palliative therapies may signify to some children and families that health professionals are giving up on the child. Children and families must understand that stopping ineffective therapies is not giving up, but represents a

Table 1 Situational factors in paediatric palliative care

Cognitive	Behavioural	Emotional
Meaning of death	Physical inactivity	Anxiety about dying and death
Inaccurate understanding: course of disease	Social withdrawal	Fear of separation
palliation	Passive approach to pain control	Anxiety regarding meaning of life
Little independent control over pain	Secondary gains from stress reduction and parental/staff attention	Distress and suffering from pain and aversive symptoms
Limited choices		
Expectation for continuing pain	Inappropriate choice or mode of drug administration	Fear of inadequate pain control
		Fear for family
Misunderstanding of opioids	Failure to evaluate and document pain	
		Anger
Misunderstanding of drug prescription and administration (dosing etc.)	Failure to aggressively treat opioid-related side-effects	Sadness and depression
Misunderstanding of criteria for pain/drug efficacy	Failure to use effective non-drug therapies	Distancing by staff

rational decision based on children's best interests. Pain control is an essential component of palliative care. Children and parents should not fear that health professionals have given up on controlling pain and aversive symptoms. Pain and all symptoms must be treated aggressively from the dual perspective of targeting the primary source of tissue damage and modifying the secondary contributing factors. Although most children receive accurate information about their disease and required treatments, few children or their parents receive concrete information about their pain, the factors that can attenuate or exacerbate it, a rationale for the interventions they receive, and training in effective non-pharmacological pain control techniques. The latter may be particularly important for children in palliative care, who have diminishing control in their lives. Children and their parents do not know that prescribed pain control treatments may vary in efficacy at different times throughout their treatment due to variations in disease activity or situational factors. Without this knowledge, their confidence in certain therapies can decrease, even though these therapies would effectively alleviate pain at another time. The fear of inadequate pain control places an enormous emotional burden on an already distressed child and family and can create a situation in which their pain and disability intensifies.

Generally, children's physical activity has been progressively restricted due to the disability caused by their condition. Parents who encourage children to adopt passive patient roles, to behave differently than other children, and to depend primarily on others for pain control will undoubtedly create a situation wherein children's pain is maximized. Even when children are somnolent, it is possible to create some 'normal environment' in which children can participate and actively involve themselves during their alert periods. Children should live as fully as possible, even as they are dying. Parents who encourage children to engage in as many normal activities as possible create a situation wherein their children's pain should be lessened.

Children who experienced adverse physical effects from medication, such as hair loss and weight gain, may become acutely self conscious about their appearance. They become ill at ease with their peers and may progressively withdraw because they anticipate negative reactions from their friends. Increased withdrawal and social isolation can exacerbate their pain. Their withdrawal may increase when treatment emphasis shifts from cure and palliation to palliation alone. Parents may 'close-in', spending even more exclusive time with the dying child as a closed family unit. While important for children and families, the exclusive focus on the family increases a child's social isolation and may cause more anxiety for some children—particularly when the family does not openly address children's concerns about death and dying. Inadvertently, the family may prevent children from interacting both with peers who can lessen their anxiety through play and conversation and also with health professionals who can help them to resolve their anxiety and fears about dying. Children seem to know intuitively, even when dying has not been discussed directly with them. They fear separation and abandonment; some children may fear that their illness is a punishment. Dying children may feel frightened, isolated, and guilty unless they are able to openly express and resolve their concerns.

Many observers have noted that children who are dying have a level of maturity 'far beyond their years'.[3] It is essential to acknowledge and resolve their fears. Children should receive accurate information, consistent with their religious beliefs, presented in a calm reassuring manner. They may need concrete reassurance that they will not suffer when they die, that they will not be alone, and that their families will remember them. Unresolved emotions add anguish and may intensify their pain as shown by the following case study.

Mary, an 11-year-old girl with leukaemia, was referred to the pain clinic for treatment of severe pain caused by the effects of chemotherapy.[29] The therapist reviewed her medical chart and interviewed her to determine the sensory characteristics of her pain, to evaluate her analgesic regimen, to assess the impact of

Table 2 Primary components of pain assessment

Sensory characteristics: Onset Location Intensity Quality Duration Spread to other sites (consistent with neurological pattern) Temporal pattern Accompanying symptoms	**Cognitive factors:** Understanding of pain source Understanding of diagnosis, treatment, and prognosis Expectations Perceived control Relevance of disease or pain-inducing stimuli Knowledge of pain control
Medical/surgical: Investigations conducted Consult results Analgesic and adjuvant medications (type, dose, frequency, route)	**Behavioural factors:** General coping style Learned pain behaviours Overt distress Parent's behaviours Physical activities and limitations Social activities and limitations
Clinical factors: Environment features Roles of medical and health staff Nature of interventions Documentation of pain Criteria for determining analgesic efficacy	**Emotional factors:** Frustration Anger Sadness Fear Anxiety

situational factors, and to recommend additional pain interventions. At the time of her assessment, medical staff had already discussed with her parents that Mary's care should shift from curative to palliative therapies. Mary was a hospital inpatient and receiving morphine (3.3 mg/h) by continuous infusion, plus bolus morphine (2.5 mg every 20 min) for pain control. During the 24-h period preceding the assessment, she had complained about pain frequently and received 26 boluses. When the therapist entered the room, Mary seemed depressed and barely acknowledged the therapist's presence. She was lying in a darkened room, in which there were none of the personal mementoes that children often bring with them to the hospital, even though Mary had been in hospital for a few weeks. Mary's mother was in the room with her and had been with her at all times during the previous weeks. She regularly indicated to nursing staff that her daughter was in a lot of pain. Nurses reported that Mary had refused to participate when Child Life specialists entered the room and had not attempted to attend any of the hospital activities available for children, even before her pain had increased to its current level. The pain consultation was requested by nursing staff, who were concerned about the morphine dose Mary was receiving and wondered whether she was demanding boluses when she primarily needed attention.

Therapists begin inpatient consultations by obtaining the information listed in Table 2 through a chart review and brief interviews with children, parents, and relevant health staff. Mary described her pain as a severe burning sensation arising from her enlarged haemorrhoids and spreading diffusely as a moderate pain sensation throughout her body. After explaining her role, the therapist described pain systems and gates to Mary (general teaching explanations are described later in the section on non-pharmacological interventions). She then used the television set in Mary's room and the three attached coloured wires to explain that morphine controlled pain via one pathway, but there were other pathways—a physical set activated by sensory stimulation and a cognitive set activated by mental concentration. The therapist explained that Mary was receiving partial pain control, because she was relying exclusively on only one of these systems. Mary showed much interest and easily understood that if each of the three cables attached to the television were necessary for it to work well, then two other methods of pain control should complement her morphine so that she would have even less pain.

Mary's mother also listened very attentively to the therapist's explanation. Nurses had informed the therapist that Mary's mother asked Mary repeatedly whether she was in pain. She did not seem to have any other interactions with Mary beyond comforting and holding her when Mary said 'yes' that she did have pain. (Note: Some parents may focus on children's pain or other physical signs because they wish to help and comfort their children, but do not know how to best assist them. Some parents may be more frightened by the pain, because they interpret it as a tangible sign of the child's impending death, while other parents may focus excessively on the physical pain because they cannot address the emotional pain that they or their children are experiencing. Thus, a pain assessment must include information on both what parents are doing for their children and why they are doing it.)

In order to assist Mary's mother, the therapist used another analogy to explain why Mary should not monitor her pain too closely. 'Imagine that you are going to see a movie and people are sitting near you; they have popcorn and many candies wrapped in crinkly paper. Suppose I ask you to ignore the sounds of people unwrapping and eating their candies, and just pay attention to the movie. But, what if every two minutes I ask you if you can still hear the crinkling?'. Mary smiled and said that the more she paid attention to the noise, the less she would be able to truly ignore it and watch the movie. The therapist then explained that people should not ask her too often about whether she had pain; otherwise, they might accidentally interfere with how well the morphine worked. Instead, the nurses and doctors would ensure that she had enough drug and non-drug techniques to lessen her pain, and the therapist would help her to set up a plan to ensure that all three systems were working to relieve her pain. Her mother's role would change from checking on Mary's pain to actively massaging her at specified times during the day and encouraging Mary to participate in Child Life activities (to the extent that it was possible). Mary was asked to remind people entering her room to talk with her about other aspects of her life and not constantly ask about her pain. She was also asked to have her dad bring some pictures from home to display, so that she could let people know about other things in her life and they could talk about more interesting topics. In order to assist her mother, the therapist further explained why regular periods of massage, combined with increased and varied physical stimulation, would be beneficial for Mary. Nurses began to assess and chart Mary's pain level regularly, rather than relying on Mary's mother to constantly monitor the level.

In addition, the therapist designed a simple behavioural management programme. Mary would earn stickers on a calendar for following the previous recommendations as her 'get rid of pain' plan. Six hours later, when the therapist returned with the calendar and some stickers, Mary was remarkably different. She was sitting up and her affect was quite positive, she had participated in Child Life activities for approximately 2 h, and she had not requested any morphine boluses since the therapist met with her earlier. She and her mother received stars for the day because they had worked as a team. She was gradually weaned off morphine, as her haemorrhoidal inflammation subsided. (Note: local anaesthesia for pain control was contraindicated; morphine was the appropriate analgesic.) Mary was painfree at discharge but required opioids at subsequent readmissions and during the period prior to her death.

Mary's inadequate pain control was due to dramatically changing situational factors as her family began to adjust to the change in her condition, not to an inadequate analgesic or dosing regimen. The presence of situational factors that can exacerbate pain led the therapist to recommend modifying those factors as practically and immediately as possible, while maintaining the same dosing schedule. If those factors had not been present or if there had not been concurrent reductions in Mary's pain, the therapist would have recommended an increase in Mary's continuous infusion dose as described later in Analgesic selection and administration.

Optimal pain control for children

A sixteenth-century aphorism, penned by an anonymous author to define the role of a physician, defines the essence of paediatric palliative care 'To cure sometimes, to relieve often, to comfort always'. The comprehensive care of children includes curative therapies when available, pain and symptom management, and compassionate support for children and their families. It is essential to focus not only on the medical management of children's disease but also on the psychosocial and spiritual factors that affect children's pain and suffering.

The optimal relief of pain in paediatric palliative care begins with the recognition that you are assessing and treating an individual child with pain, not managing pain as a symptom apart from the child. The assessment must be conducted from a dual perspective—an objective appraisal of the sources of nociceptive stimulation and a thorough evaluation of the factors that modify nociceptive processing for that child. The characteristics of the pain, the chronology of the disease, previous therapy, and the child's individual characteristics must be carefully considered. After a careful and thorough assessment to determine the causative and contributing factors, an effective treatment plan can be designed to adequately alleviate children's pain. The most appropriate pharmacological and non-pharmacological interventions are selected to address all the responsible factors, as outlined by the treatment algorithm in Fig. 2.[30] A primary pharmacological intervention, either analgesics or anaesthetics, is usually selected to attenuate nociceptive activity. However, cognitive, physical, and behavioural interventions must also be used to mitigate the pain-exacerbating impact of situational factors. Controlling children's pain requires an integrated approach because many factors are responsible, no matter how seemingly clear cut the aetiology. Adequate analgesic prescriptions, administered at regular dosing intervals, must be complemented by a practical cognitive-behavioural approach to ensure optimal pain relief.

Children receiving palliative care are often at risk for higher pain levels due to the unique constellation of factors associated with a life-threatening disease. Since space limitations preclude an adequate review of the primary sources of pain and mediating factors for each disease, the remainder of this chapter focuses on children dying from cancer. Cancer pain provides a model for understanding the myriad issues that must be addressed to ensure optimal pain control for children in palliative care. The principles of analgesic therapy, the guidelines for drug administration, and the guidelines for a supportive cognitive-behavioural approach are those that should be followed in all paediatric palliative care, including the care of children with AIDS. These guidelines are not restricted to children with cancer pain.

Children with cancer pain

Although cancer is a relatively rare disease in children, with an approximate incidence of 1 per 600, cancer ranks second to accidents as the leading cause of death in children from 1 to 14 years old.[31,32] Approximately two-thirds of children can be cured when they are diagnosed early and receive curative therapies. Unfortunately, though, most children with cancer do not receive curative therapies because the majority of children with cancer are in developing countries.[33] These children will die either because their disease is too far advanced by the time they are diagnosed or because curative therapies are not available due to a lack of trained medical and health personnel, unavailability of drugs, and limited resources. Thus, the care of many children must shift from an equal emphasis on cure and palliation, including pain relief, to a primary emphasis on palliation.

Almost all children with cancer will experience some pain during the course of their illness—due to active disease, effects of therapy, invasive procedures, and psychological factors. Children can experience persistent pain when the disease process activates nociceptors by invading bone, compressing nerves, infiltrating blood vessels, and injuring healthy tissue. Pain arises from the tissue damage produced by blood sampling procedures, lumbar punctures, bone marrow aspirations, intramuscular and intravenous injections, surgery, chemotherapy, and radiation therapy. In addition, children with cancer can develop pain due to the psychological stress of living with a potentially fatal disease. (Reviews of the nociceptive mechanisms associated with different types of cancer are listed in the references.)[31,34–39]

Children with cancer generally do not experience the same chronic debilitating pain from disease as do adults with cancer, presumably due to the different types of cancer that they experience.[40–42] One-third of all childhood cancers are leukaemias, while approximately 20 per cent are brain and spinal tumours—in contrast to the lung, breast, and gastrointestinal cancers common in adults. Leukaemias and lymphomas can cause diffuse bone and joint pain. Children can experience headaches from meningeal irritation and obstruction with increased intracranial pressure. There are no accurate estimates on the world-wide prevalence of different types of cancer pain in children because countries differ widely in their diagnostic capabilities and reporting systems. We do know that children's cancer pain may recur intermittently in different sites and at different strengths, predictably reflecting

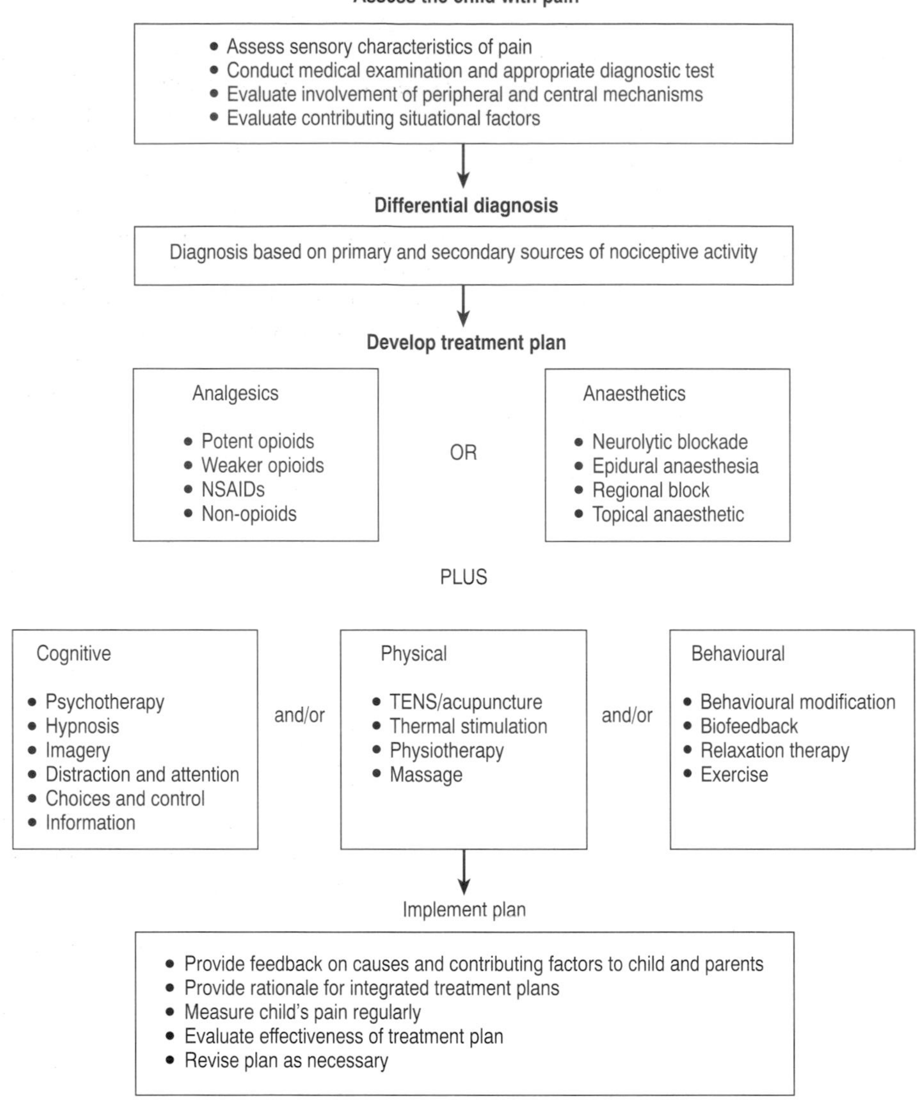

Fig. 2 A model of an integrated pharmacological and non-pharmacological approach for controlling children's pain. (Adapted with permission from PA McGrath. Pain control in children. In: *Innovations in Pain Management; A Practical Guide for Clinicians*, RS Weiner, editor. Paul M. Deutsch, 1992: 32–43.)

disease progression, or pain may recur in an unpredictable manner with no clear relationship to advancing disease. In some conditions little pain arises from the disease, but invasive treatments cause intense pain seemingly out of proportion to the extent of tissue damage. In other cases, pain may increase steadily throughout an illness so that children experience severe pain in the terminal phase. Additional pain can arise during the course of an illness if children suppress their emotional reactions to the disease and treatment. Children who are dying are more susceptible to increased pain due to the emotional impact of the situation.

Misconceptions regarding pain control in children with cancer

Several misconceptions have led to inadequate pain control in children with cancer as described in the following (revised from McGrath, 1990 and McGrath, 1993).[11,23]

Misconceptions about children's pain systems

Many individuals who treat children with cancer have lacked information about the plasticity and complexity of children's nociceptive systems. As a consequence, they treated pain from an erroneous perspective that tissue damage was synonymous with pain. They focused on the primary source of noxious stimulation but not on all the causative and contributing factors that affected nociceptive processing.

Misconceptions about the pharmacodynamics and pharmacokinetics of opioid analgesics

As a result of misconceptions about the pharmacodynamics and pharmacokinetics of opioid analgesics, health professionals have not always selected the most appropriate drugs, doses, dosing intervals, or administration routes.

Misconceptions about the risk of addiction

Some health professionals and parents believe that opioid analgesics should be administered only as a last resort, to avoid drug addiction. They have not understood that TOLERANCE + PHYSICAL DEPENDENCE ≠ ADDICTION. As a result, children have not always received the potent analgesics required to relieve severe pain.

Misconceptions about the efficacy of non-drug therapies

Many health professionals have not known that simple cognitive, physical, and behavioural strategies can lessen children's pain. As a result, they have not taught children practical strategies that are effective for reducing their acute and persistent pain. Similarly, they have not taught parents the importance of evaluating and modifying situational and familial factors to lessen children's pain.

Misconceptions about comprehensive pain control

Many health professionals have believed that pharmacological interventions are both necessary and sufficient to control children's cancer pain. They have not prescribed non-pharmacological interventions to supplement or complement analgesics, even when situational factors are impeding analgesic efficacy.

Misconceptions about pain assessment

Most health professionals have not routinely assessed and documented children's pain levels. As a result, children's pain and need for pain-relief were dismissed as irrelevant in clinical practice.

Misconceptions about who is in charge of pain control

Usually, one individual has not assumed primary responsibility for ensuring that a child's pain is controlled adequately, so that the diffusion of responsibility among various health professionals has led to suboptimal pain control.

Misconceptions about the importance of pain control

Oncology services have not always adopted a consistent approach to pain assessment and pain control, similar to their consistent approach to diagnosis and medical treatment.

Controlling cancer pain: guidelines for assessment, analgesic selection and administration, and non-pharmacological interventions

Evaluating children's pain

A comprehensive pain assessment is necessary initially to establish a correct clinical diagnosis. Subsequent assessments of pain intensity enable us to evaluate which treatments are most effective for reducing different types of pain and which treatments are most beneficial for which children. However, even though pain assessment should be an intrinsic component of paediatric practice, few clinicians regularly use validated measures to evaluate and monitor children's pain. Anecdotal reports suggest that physicians lack information about convenient age-appropriate pain measures that they could readily incorporate into their practices. In view of the diverse array of pain measures now available for infants and children, it is understandable that there is some uncertainty about which measures are best for clinical use (reviews are given in the reference list).[43-47]

Like adult pain measures, children's pain measures are classified as behavioural, physiological, or self-report, depending on the nature of the response that is measured—that is children's overt distress behaviours (e.g. grimaces, cries, protective guarding gestures), children's physical parameters (e.g. heart rate, sweat index, blood pressure, cortisol level), or children's direct self-reports (e.g. their words or numerical ratings). The criteria for an accurate pain measure are similar to those required for any measuring instrument—validity, reliability, and minimal bias. A pain measure must be valid, in that it measures a specific aspect of pain, for example intensity, so that changes in children's pain ratings accurately reflect a meaningful and proportional change in their pain experience. The measure must be reliable, in that it provides trustworthy and consistent pain ratings, that do not change over time. The measure must be relatively free from response bias, in that children use it similarly regardless of how they may wish to please adults or how adults administer it. In addition, pain measures should be practical and versatile for assessing different types of pain (e.g. disease-related, procedural pain) with many different children (according to age, cognitive level, cultural background) in both clinical and home settings.

Behavioural and physiological signs provide indirect pain measures for infants and for children who are unable to communicate verbally. We can only infer the presence or strength of pain from the type and magnitude of children's behaviours or physical states. In contrast, self-report measures can provide direct information about many aspects of a child's pain—the sensory characteristics, the aversive component, and contributing cognitive, behavioural, and emotional factors. At present, self-report measures represent the gold standard for assessing children's pain. Children can express what they feel, describe what they do, use diaries to record prospectively how often pain occurs, and rate pain intensity on quantitative scales.

Many thermometer, facial, and visual analogue rating scales are available as reliable and valid measures of pain intensity for children above 5 years of age.[44] The poker chip method may be the best pain measure for younger children, who choose the number of poker chips (from 0–4, designated as pieces of hurt) to show how much they hurt.[48]. Four pain scales are shown in Figs 3 and 4. A common rating scale is a 100 cm thermometer, graded in 10 cm intervals. The 0 level represents no pain and the 100 level usually represents 'intense' pain. Children point to the level on the thermometer that matches their pain severity. However, when numbers are clearly visible on a scale, some children may judge their pain by making numerical ratings while others may judge their pain by evaluating the level on the thermometer. Thus, there is a potential risk that children use the same scale differently. To avoid this risk, children could rate their pain on a scale in which the numbers are mounted on the back, visible to health staff. A coloured analogue scale (a 10 cm wedge shaped visual analogue scale) is a convenient tool for children to use to measure pain intensity; its psychometric properties are equivalent to those of the visual analogue scale (McGrath *et al*, in press). As shown in Fig. 4, the bottom of the scale is a light pink narrow wedge, designated as 'no pain'. The wedge increases progressively in hue and thickness to a deep red, wide wedge at the top of the scale, designated as 'most pain'. Children adjust the position of a slider along the scale to match their pain intensity. Numbers corresponding to the different scale positions are mounted on the back of the scale, so that health professionals and parents can read and record children's pain levels.

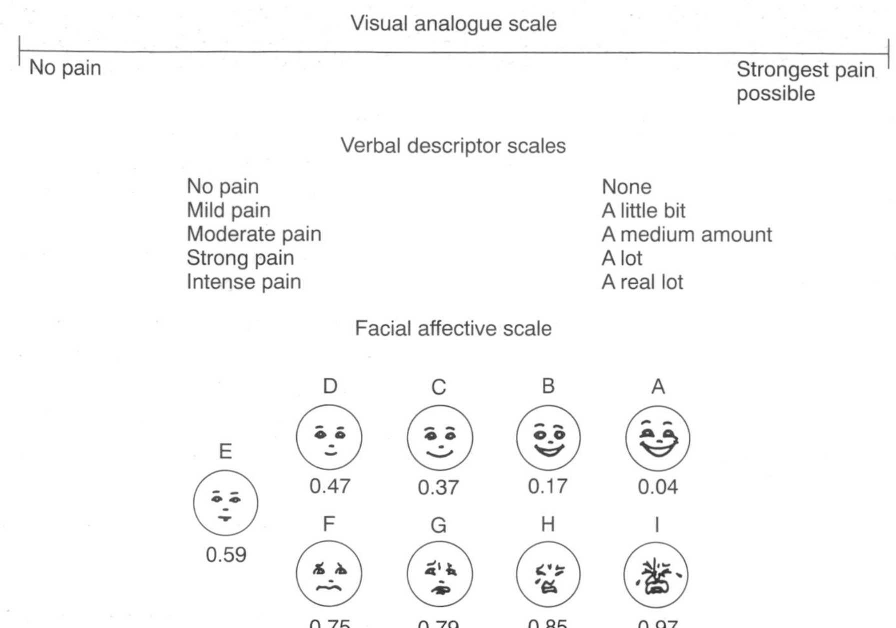

Fig. 3 Pain measures used for children: visual analogue scale to assess pain intensity, verbal descriptor scales to assess pain intensity for children above 7 (list on left) and for children younger than 7 (list on right), and facial scale to assess pain affect.

Physicians should always ask children directly about their pain to determine its sensory characteristics and facilitate an accurate diagnosis. They should also assess relevant situational factors in order to modify their pain-exacerbating impact, especially the factors listed in Table 1. When possible, children should rate their pain intensity on a standardized scale. Then, physicians should select the most appropriate pharmacological and non-pharmacological interventions and regularly measure children's pain-intensity to monitor the efficacy of those interventions.

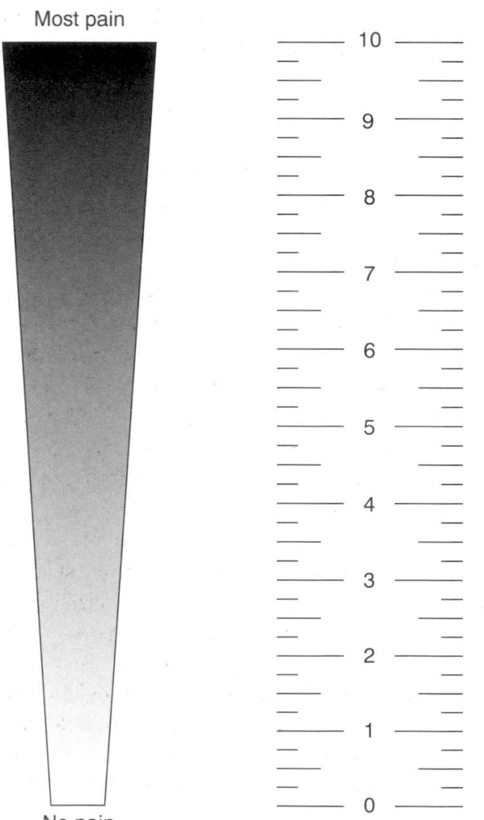

Fig. 4 A coloured analogue scale (CAS) to assess pain intensity. (Left) Front of the CAS as seen by children. (Right) Back of the CAS which shows the numerical value of the intensity rating shown of the CAS.

Analgesic selection and administration

The control of pain due to advanced cancer consists of three main approaches: anticancer modalities to decrease or eliminate the neoplasm (through chemotherapy, endocrine therapy, radiation therapy, radioisotope therapy); interventions to control the pain without affecting the neoplasm (through systemic drugs, therapeutic nerve blocks, neurosurgical operations, and psychological methods); and a combination of the two approaches. We have achieved enormous progress in controlling children's pain since Swafford and Allan's survey on postoperative pain management in which they state 'paediatric patients seldom need medication for relief of pain. They tolerate discomfort well.'[49] All health professionals who treat children with cancer should have a working knowledge of the main categories of analgesic and adjuvant drugs administered to children and the major types of anaesthetic techniques available for children. Information about what type, how much, and how often children receive drugs is an essential component of their pain assessment, particularly for children who are in hospital. Health professionals must ensure that the general principles of analgesic administration—'by the ladder', 'by the clock', 'by the child', and 'by the mouth'—are followed.[7]

'By the ladder' refers to a three step approach for selecting progressively stronger analgesic drugs—paracetamol, codeine, and morphine—based on the child's pain level—mild, moderate, strong. If pain persists despite using the appropriate drug, recommended dose, and dosing schedule, children should receive the

Table 3 Non-opioid drugs for relieving cancer pain in children

Drug	Dosage	Comments
Paracetamol (acetaminophen)	10–15 mg/kg PO, every 4–6 h	Lacks gastrointestinal and haematological side-effects; lacks anti-inflammatory effects (may mask infection-associated fever)
Choline magnesium trisalicylate	10-15 mg/kg PO, every 8–12 h	May have minimal antiplatelet effect; lacks gastrointestinal effects
Ibuprofen	10 mg/kg every 6–8 h	Anti-inflammatory activity, but may have gastrointestinal and haematological effects
Naproxen	~5 mg/kg every 12 h	Anti-inflammatory effects, but may have gastrointestinal and haematological effects

Note: Increasing the dose of non-opioids beyond the recommended therapeutic level produces a 'ceiling effect', in that there is no additional analgesia but there are major increases in toxicity and side-effects.
PO, by mouth.
Adapted with permission, from World Health Organization monograph, *Cancer Pain Relief and Palliative Care in Children*, in press.

next more potent analgesic. This ladder approach was initially developed by the World Health Organization.[50] Even when children require opioid analgesics, they should continue to receive paracetamol (and non-steroidal anti-inflammatory drugs if appropriate) as supplemental analgesics. More extensive reviews of analgesic and anaesthetic interventions for children are given in the reference list.[36,51–58] The analgesic ladder approach is based on the premise that paracetamol, codeine, and morphine should be available in all countries and that doctors and health-care professionals can relieve cancer pain in the majority of children with a few drugs.

Non-steroidal anti-inflammatory drugs, typically similar in potency to aspirin, are used primarily to treat inflammatory disorders and to relieve mild to moderate acute pain. Until relatively recently, most non-steroidal anti-inflammatory drugs were not approved for children. Since concern for bleeding problems is common for children with cancer, indications for aspirin and non-steroidal anti-inflammatory drugs are much narrower than for other painful conditions in children. Although paracetamol should be considered the routine non-opioid analgesic for children with cancer, non-steroidal anti-inflammatory drugs are effective for patients with bony metastases, who have adequate platelet counts.

Although the specific drugs and doses are determined by the needs of each child, general guidelines for pharmacological pain management have been developed through a Consensus Conference on the Management of Pain in Childhood Cancer, published as a supplement to *Pediatrics*,[59] in a monograph, *Cancer Pain Relief and Palliative Care for Children*,[7] and through the Agency for Health Care Policy and Research.[36] Recommended starting doses for analgesic medications to control children's disease-related pain are listed in Tables 3 and 4; starting doses for adjunctive medications to control side-effects and other symptoms are listed in Table 5.

'By the clock' refers to the timing for administering analgesic medications. Analgesics should be administered on a regular schedule (e.g. every 4 or 6 h, based on the drug's duration of action and the child's pain severity), not on a *pro re nata* basis, unless children's pain episodes are truly intermittent and unpredictable. On a *pro re nata* basis, children must first experience pain before they can obtain pain relief. Moreover, the doses of opioids that are required to relieve existing or breakthrough pain are higher than those required to prevent the recurrence of pain. Children should receive analgesics at regular times, 'by the clock', to provide consistent pain relief and prevent breakthrough pain. Although breakthrough pain episodes have been recognized as a problem in adult pain control, they may represent an even more serious problem for children. Unlike adults, who generally realize that they can demand more potent analgesic medications or demand more frequent dosing intervals, children have little control, little awareness of alternatives, and fear that their pain cannot be controlled. They become progressively frightened, upset, and preoccupied with their symptoms. Thus, it is essential to establish and maintain a therapeutic window of pain relief for children.

'By the child' refers to the need to adjust analgesic doses based on the individual child. There is no one final dose that will be appropriate for all children with pain. The goal is to select a dose which prevents children from experiencing pain before they receive the next dose. It is essential to monitor the child's pain regularly and adjust analgesic doses as necessary to control the pain. The effective opioid dose to relieve pain varies widely among different children or in the same child at different times. Some children require massive opioid doses at frequent intervals to control their pain. If such large doses are necessary for effective pain control, and the side-effects can be managed by adjunctive medication so that children are comfortable, then the doses are appropriate. Children receiving opioids may develop altered sleep patterns so that they are awake at night, fearful and complaining about pain, and they sleep intermittently throughout the day. They should receive adequate analgesics at night with hypnotics or antidepressants as necessary to enable them to sleep throughout the night. To relieve severe ongoing pain, opioid doses should be increased steadily until comfort is achieved, unless the child experiences unacceptable side-effects such as somnolence and respiratory depression.

'By the mouth' refers to the route of drug administration. Medication should be administered to children by the simplest and most effective route, usually by mouth. Since children are afraid of

Table 4 Opioid analgesic dosing*

Drug	Equianalgesic dose (Parenteral)	Usual starting dose IV/SC		IV/SC: PO ratio	Usual starting dose PO		Biological half-life
		< 50 kg	≥ 50 kg		< 50 kg	≥ 50kg	
Short half-life opioids							
Morphine	10 mg	Bolus dose = 0.1 mg/kg every 2–3 h Continuous infusion = 0.03–0.05 mg/kg/h	5–10 mg every 2–4 h	3:1	0.3 mg/kg every 3–4 h	30 mg every 3–4 h	2.5–3 h
Hydromorphone	1.5 mg	0.015 mg/kg every 3–4 h	1–1.5 mg every 3–4 h	5:1	0.06 mg/kg every 3–4 h	4–8 mg every 3–4 h	2–3 h
Codeine	130 mg				0.5–1 mg/kg every 3–4 h	60 mg every 3–4 h	2.5–3 h
Oxycodone					0.2 mg/kg every 3–4 h	10 mg every 3–4 h	1.5 h
Pethidine[a]	75 mg	0.75 mg/kg every 2–3 h	75–100 mg every 3 h	4:1	1–1.5 mg/kg every 3–4 h	50–75 mg every 3–4 h[b]	3 h[a]
Fentanyl	100 µg	0.5–2 µg/kg/h as continuous infusion	25–75 µg every 1 h				
Long half-life opioids							
Controlled release morphine					0.6 mg/kg every 8 h or 0.9 mg/kg every 12 h	30–60 mg every 12 h	
Methadone	10 mg	0.1 mg/kg every 4–8 h	5–10 mg every 4–8 h	2:1	0.2 mg/kg every 4–8 h	10 mg every 4–8 h	12–50h

Doses are for opioid naïve patients. For infants under 6 months, start at one-quarter to one-third the suggested dose and titrate to effect.

Principles of opioid administration:
1. If inadequate pain relief and no toxicity at peak onset of opioid action, increase dose in 50% increments.
2. IV and SC are essentially equivalent. Avoid IM administration.
3. Whenever using continuous infusion, hourly *pro re nata* rescue doses with short onset opioids should be available. Rescue dose is usually 50–200% of continuous hourly dose. If greater than 6 rescues are necessary in 24-h period, increase daily infusion total by the total amount of rescues for previous 24 h ÷ 24. An alternative is to increase infusion by 50%.
4. To change opioids—Because of incomplete cross tolerance, if changing between short half-life opioids, start new opioid at 50% of equianalgesic dose. Titrate to effect. If changing from short to long half-life opioid (i.e. morphine to methadone), start at 25% of equianalgesic dose and titrate to effect.
5. To taper opioids—Anyone on opioids over 1 week must be tapered to avoid withdrawal symptoms. Taper by 50% for 2 days, then decrease by 25% every 2 days. When dose is equianalgesic to an oral morphine dose of 0.6 mg/kg/day if less than 50 kg or 30 mg day if greater than 50 kg, it may be stopped.

[a] Pethidine not recommended in chronic use as toxic long half-life metabolite norpethidine may accumulate.
[b] 'Usual' starting doses are often empiric, not always dosed according to equianalgesic principles (i.e. starting dose of pethidine IV/PO of 75 mg even though IV:PO ratio is 1:4).

Abbreviations: PO, by mouth; IV, intravenous; SC, subcutaneous; IM, intramuscular.
Adapted with permission, from World Health Organization monograph. *Cancer Pain Relief and Palliative Care in Children*, in press.

painful injections they may deny that they have pain or they may not request medication. When possible children should receive medications through routes that do not cause additional pain. Although optimal analgesic administration for children requires flexibility in selecting routes according to children's needs, parenteral administration is often the most efficient route for providing direct and rapid pain relief. Since intravenous, intramuscular, and subcutaneous routes cause additional pain for children, serious efforts have been expended on developing more pain-free modes of administration that still provide relatively direct and rapid analgesia. Attention has focused on improving the effectiveness of oral routes. As an example, a 'fentanyl lollipop', oral transmucosal fentanyl citrate, provides rapid onset and safe analgesia via a pleasant route for children with cancer receiving painful medical procedures.[60] Some hospitals have already restricted the use of intramuscular injections because they are painful and drug absorption is not reliable; they advocate the use of intravenous lines into which drugs can be administered directly without further hurting children. Topical anaesthetic creams should be applied before inserting these needles into children. The use of portacatheters has increased in paediatrics, particularly for children with cancer who require administration of multiple drugs at weekly intervals.

Continuous infusion has several advantages over intermittent subcutaneous, intramuscular, or intravenous routes. This method

Table 5 Adjuvant analgesic drugs

Drug category	Drug, dosage	Indications	Comments
Antidepressants	Amitriptyline, 0.2–0.5 mg/kg. Escalate by 25% every 2–3 days up to 1–2 mg/kg if needed. Alternatives: doxepin, imipramine, nortriptyline	Neuropathic pain (i.e. vincristine-induced, radiation plexopathy, tumour invasion) Insomnia	Usually, improved sleep and pain relief within 3–5 days. Anticholinergic side-effects are dose-limiting. Use with caution for children with increased risk for cardiac dysfunction
Anticonvulsants	Carbamazepine, 2 mg/kg PO every 12 h Phenytoin, 2.5–2 mg/kg PO every 12 h Clonazepam, 0.01 mg/kg every 12 h	Neuropathic pain, especially shooting, stabbing pain	Monitor for haematological, hepatic, and allergic reactions. Side-effects: gastrointestinal upset, ataxia, disorientation, somnolence
Neuroleptics	Chlorpromazine. 0.5 mg/kg IV/PO every 4–6 h Promethazine, 0.5–1 mg/kg IV/PO every 4–6 h Haloperidol, 0.01–0.1 mg/kg IV/PO every 8 h	Nausea, confused child, psychosis, acute agitation, Enhancement of opioid analgesia	Consider concurrent use of antihistamine (i.e. diphenhydramine) to avoid dystonic reaction if high doses or prolonged course is used
Sedatives, hypnotics, anxiolytics	Diazepam, 0.05–0.1 mg/kg PO every 4–6 h Lorazepam, 0.02–0.04 mg/kg PO/IV every 4–6 h Midazolam, 0.05 mg/kg IV every 5 min prior to procedure; 0.3–0.5 mg/kg PO every 30–°45 min prior to procedure	Acute anxiety, muscle spasm. Premedication for painful procedures	Sedative effect may limit opioid use. Other side-effects include depression and dependence with prolonged use
Antihistamines	Hydroxyzine, 0.5–1 mg/kg every 4–6 h Diphenhydramine, 0.5–1 mg/kg every 4–6 h	Opioid-induced pruritus, anxiety, nausea	Sedative side-effects may be helpful.
Psychostimulants	Dextroamphetamine, methylphenidate, 0.1–0.2 mg/kg twice a day. Escalate to 0.3–0.5 as needed	Opioid-induced somnolence, potentiation of opioid analgesia	Side-effects include agitation, sleep disturbance, and anorexia. Administer second dose in early afternoon to avoid sleep disturbances
Corticosteroids	Prednisone, prednisolone, and dexamethasone dosage depends on clinical situation (i.e. dexamethasone 6–12 mg/m^2/day	Headache from raised intracranial pressure, spinal, or nerve compression; widespread metastases	Side-effects include oedema, dyspeptic symptoms, and occasional gastrointestinal bleeding

Abbreviations: PO, by mouth; IV, intravenous.
Adapted with permission, from World Health Organization monograph. *Cancer Pain Relief and Palliative Care in Children*, in press.

circumvents repetitive injections, prevents delays in analgesic drug administration, and provides continuous levels of pain control without children experiencing increased side-effects at peak level and pain breakthroughs at trough level.[51,54,57,61–71] Continuous infusion should be considered when children have strong pain for which oral and intermittent parenteral opioids do not provide satisfactory pain control, when intractable vomiting prevents oral medications, when intravenous lines are not desirable, and when children would like to remain at home despite severe pain.[55] However, children receiving a continuous infusion should still receive 'rescue doses' to control breakthrough pain, as necessary. As outlined in Table 4, the rescue doses should be 50 to 200 per cent of the continuous infusion hourly dose. If children experience repeated breakthrough pain, the basal rate can be increased by 50 per cent or by the total amount of morphine administered through the rescue doses over a 24-h period (divided by 24 h).

Patient-controlled analgesia provides patients with the ability to administer small bolus doses against a background infusion rate (for review see Gaukroger).[72] A fixed dose (based on child's pain severity) is programmed into the pump, so that children can deliver additional doses to control breakthrough pain. (Note: there is a safety lock-out feature to prevent over-doses.) Children from 6 to 18 years old have obtained excellent pain relief with patient-controlled analgesia pumps.[73–89] Initial fears that children would be unable to responsibly control their analgesia were unfounded. But the issue of a lower age limit and the extent to which patient-controlled analgesia should become 'parent controlled analgesia' remain controversial. Gaukroger[72] reports that the majority of 5 and 6-year-olds can use patient-controlled analgesia successfully. Clearly, patient-controlled analgesia offers special advantages to children who have little control and who are extremely frightened about uncontrolled pain.

The use of spinal administration routes (epidural and intrathecal) for opioids and local anaesthetics for children is increasing.[15,51,90–104] Epidural administration of opioids and/or local anaesthetics are feasible techniques for managing cancer pain in children of all ages. Experience from many centres suggests that these techniques can be extremely useful for children with advanced cancer.[105] It is often feasible for children to receive epidural and subarachnoid infusions at home on an extended basis. Although infection is possible, the reported infection rates in several series of cancer patients have been quite low.[105]

Dosing considerations for neonates and infants

Recent research on controlling pain in neonates, concurrent with neurobiological studies of the development of the nociceptive system, has led to improved rational therapeutic regimens which provide safe and effective analgesia with a minimum of side-effects.[106] (Note: please see the reference list for a detailed discussion of neonatal pain control[107,108] and for a detailed discussion of developmental neuroanatomy and neurophysiology.[109,110])

Neonates and infants require the same three categories of analgesic drugs as older children. However, the differences in pharmacokinetics and pharmacodynamics among neonates, preterm infants, and full-term infants, warrant special dosing considerations for infants and close monitoring when they receive opioids. Paracetamol can be safely administered to neonates and infants without concern for hepatotoxicity, when given for short courses at the recommended dose (10–15 mg/kg). The rate of absorption is slower in neonates and its plasma half-life prolonged, so peak serum concentrations are reached at approximately 60 min after an oral dose, and subsequent doses may be required after 6 h rather than 4 h.[106,111] Paracetamol does not cause respiratory depression and does not produce tolerance.

Opioid analgesics are the mainstay of treatment for controlling severe pain in neonates. As shown in Table 4, the starting doses for opioid analgesics in infants under 6 months of age are one-quarter to one-half the suggested doses. As for children, the dosage and mode of administration of opioids needs to be titrated between the degree of analgesia required and a reasonable level of sedation. (Note: theoretically postulated long-term effects of opioid administration include the alteration of endogenous opioid receptor development but these effects are irrelevant in neonatal palliative care.) The drug clearance and the analgesic effects of morphine, fentanyl, sufentanil, and methadone for infants above the age of 6 months and children resemble those for young adults.[106] Thus, the general clinical impression is that morphine and other opioids have a reasonable margin of safety and excellent efficacy for most children over 6 months of age with cancer pain. However, premature and term new-borns show reduced clearance of most opioids.[112] The widely observed sensitivity of new-borns to morphine is probably due to kinetic factors, including smaller volume of distribution, diminished clearance, possible increased entry into the brain, and increased sensitivity on a pharmacodynamic basis associated with the immaturity of ventilatory responses to hypoxaemia and hypercarbia. Therefore, opioids must be used more cautiously with infants under the age of 6 months; infants must be monitored extremely carefully. Respiratory depression can be controlled by judicious dosing and careful monitoring, while tolerance has significance only as a signal of receptor function or a potential indicator of withdrawal when therapy is discontinued.

Neonates who have pain severe enough to require opioids usually have an intravenous line in place. If a limited number of doses is needed and if intravenous access is not available, intramuscular or subcutaneous routes may be used occasionally in full term neonates. However, these routes are painful and not suitable for preterm neonates because of their sparse muscle mass and delicate skin. They are also not suitable for long-term pain management in term neonates because plasma levels and clinical effects are less controlled and difficult to titrate from intramuscular administrations. Similarly, intravenous doses may produce peak levels resulting in coma and respiratory depression with rapid decline in plasma levels, causing alternate periods of pain and analgesia. Thus, continuous intravenous infusion of opioids, producing constant blood levels and minimal fluctuations in analgesia, is the most effective route. Anand, Shapiro, and Berde,[106] recommend a loading dose of 50 μg/kg followed by a continuous infusion of morphine at 10 to 20 μg/kg per h. Further increases in the infusion rate may be required to titrate to clinical effect or with the development of tolerance. However, infants must be monitored carefully because most opioids have prolonged half lives in neonates, so that continuous infusions can result in slow accumulation of the drug over time with high blood levels that may not be detected immediately.

The principal and potentially life threatening side-effect of all opioid drugs is the dose-dependent respiratory depression leading to apnoea, which may be observed in infants and neonates at relatively low doses. This is advantageous in the incubated and ventilated patients, but poses considerable challenges when using opioids for spontaneously breathing new-borns. Opioid-induced respiratory depression can be reversed with naloxone, but the effect of the drug diminishes within 30 min so that repeated naloxone dosing may be required. If apnoea does occur, stimulation of the baby will usually elicit some respiratory effort temporarily while emergency arrangements are made to inject naloxone or provide respiratory support. Naloxone should be titrated to effect in increments of 10 μg/kg until a desired effect is obtained, or up to a total dose of 100 μg/kg.[106] High doses of naloxone may produce a massive stress response from sudden nociception and withdrawal, or may result in undesirable fluid shifts. Following an effective dose of naloxone, the neonate should be monitored closely for at least 24 h. In fact, because plasma concentrations of morphine can increase in some neonates, even after an opioid infusion is discontinued, neonates require close monitoring for at least 24 h after morphine administration is discontinued.[112]

Young infants, especially premature babies or those who have neurological abnormalities or pulmonary disease, are susceptible to apnoea and respiratory depression when systemic opioids are used.[113] The infants' metabolism is altered so that the elimination half life is longer and the blood–brain barrier is more permeable.[114,115] Both factors result in young infants having higher concentrations of opioids in the brain for a given dose than mature infants or adults. Thus, non-ventilated infants who are less then 1 year of age should be monitored intensively when they receive opioids because extreme sedation and decreased respiratory effort may be difficult to assess. Institutions where neonates and infants are treated for cancer should train personnel in the safe and effective administration of analgesia and provide appropriate technologies for monitoring. Aggressive monitoring should include frequent assessments of heart and respiratory rates, respiratory effort, blood pressure, level of alertness, and arterial oxygen saturation.

Epidural analgesia is now widely used for infants with post-operative pain. The haemodynamic effects of major regional analgesia in infants with postoperative pain appear minimal.[116] For paediatric epidural infusion rates, the maximal recommended local anaesthetic rates per hour are roughly 0.4 mg/kg for bupivacaine and 2 mg/kg for lignocaine. Epidural infusions that exceed those recommended rates may lead to convulsions.[117] Epidural morphine has been used successfully, even for very young infants with cancer.[118] The proper use of infusions or intermittent doses of epidural opioids or local anaesthetics requires expertise and close monitoring.

Physical dependence + tolerance ≠ addiction

The fear of opioid addiction in children has been greatly exaggerated. While physical dependence, the body's gradual and routine adjustment to the drug so that the body requires the drug on some regular basis, is common, the dependence can be controlled easily by gradually tapering medication. Similarly, tolerance is common in that progressively higher levels of the drug are required to achieve the same physiological effect. Nevertheless, the terms 'physical dependence' and 'tolerance' are not synonyms for 'addiction'. Addiction represents a pattern of drug use in which an individual is wholly absorbed in the compulsive use and procurement of a drug and has a tendency to relapse after withdrawal.[119] There is no empirical evidence that children receiving opioid analgesics for pain control are at risk for addiction. In contrast, children who do not receive appropriate analgesic medications are probably more at risk for 'pseudoaddiction' by becoming excessively concerned about receiving their next medication dose in the hope that they might eventually relieve their suffering.

Parents, and occasionally staff, may have misconceptions about the use of potent opioids. Although the sensory characteristics of children's pain should be consistent with the known pattern from the presumed source of tissue injury, the source is not easily identified for all children. This is particularly true for children who have cancer, since there may be multiple sources of noxious stimulation due to disease and the effects of curative therapies. Yet, children's pain must be controlled, even when the specific aetiology is not yet determined. Otherwise children become increasingly anxious, fearful, and distressed—beginning a cycle of increasing pain that will be more difficult to alleviate.

Parents are often anxious about opioids for their children, particularly when children require dose increments. Staff must assist parents to understand that physical dependence and tolerance are very different from addiction. Physical dependence and tolerance are normal drug effects; they do not mean that their children with pain have become addicted. Physical drug dependence is well recognized. When opioids are suddenly withdrawn, children suffer irritability, anxiety, insomnia, diaphoresis, rhinorrhoea, nausea, vomiting, abdominal cramps, and diarrhoea. These withdrawal symptoms are prevented by gradually tapering doses for all children who have been on opioid therapy for longer than a week. Even though children with severe pain may require progressively higher and more frequent opioid doses due to drug tolerance, they should receive the doses they need to relieve their pain. However, children who require increased opioids to relieve previously controlled pain should also be assessed carefully to determine whether the disease has progressed, since pain may be the first sign of advancing disease.

Therapists can use familiar analogies to explain dependence, tolerance, and addiction. For example parents are often accustomed to drinking coffee in the morning. They know that they will experience some noticeable effects without their usual caffeine intake, but they also know that they can withdraw from coffee by gradually lowering their daily consumption. The fact that their body is used to a certain amount of caffeine at certain times of the day means that they are dependent. Similarly, many people become accustomed to a certain level of salt for a food to taste 'salty'. After a while they may need to increase their salt intake if they want foods to taste the same, because their bodies have adjusted to or now tolerate the previous amount of salt so that it no longer has the same effect. In the same way, their children can become tolerant to a morphine dose so that they require a slightly higher dose to achieve the same pain reduction. These benign examples of a body's normal responses to substances often help parents understand that when opioids are prescribed for their children the effects of those drugs are well-known, well-understood, and will not lead to adverse effects, including addiction.

Opioid-related side-effects

The safe, rational use of opioid analgesics requires an understanding of their clinical pharmacology. Unlike weak opioids, strong opioids have no fixed upper dosage limit. Instead, the dose can be increased as necessary to relieve a child's pain, as long as children do not experience dose-limiting side effects (i.e. toxicity, respiratory depression). Opioid analgesic doses should be titrated to clinical effect. Side-effects must be anticipated and treated aggressively. Since opioids produce physical dependence and tolerance, doses must be increased over time to control severe pain. Doses must be adjusted according to the child's need depending on pain severity, prior analgesic medication, and the distribution and availability of the drug in the body.

All opioid drugs cause similar side-effects. These well-known problems should be anticipated and treated whenever opioids are administered, so that children can receive pain control without suffering from intolerable side-effects. Children may not report all side-effects (e.g. constipation, dysphoria, and pruritus) voluntarily, so they should be asked specific questions about these problems. Some side-effects may resolve within the first week of initiating therapy as the child develops tolerance to them (e.g. nausea, vomiting, and somnolence). Other side-effects require aggressive treatment. If these persist despite appropriate interventions, change to a different opioid because a child may be able to better tolerate the specific side-effects of another opioid. There is generally incomplete cross-tolerance between opioids, so that the guidelines for switching from one opioid to another is to begin at the lower dosing range, considering the presence or absence of central nervous system side-effects, and titrate up accordingly. The treatment of opioid side-effects is summarized in Table 6.

Non-pharmacological interventions: pain control strategies for children

Cognitive interventions are the most powerful and versatile non-pharmacological pain therapies for children. When health professionals provide age-appropriate information about a pain source to children, or teach them to use a simple coping strategy, they are administering a basic cognitive intervention. Accurate information about what will happen and what children may feel can improve children's understanding, increase their control, lessen their distress, and reduce their pain. Additional information about pain gates—that is how thoughts, actions, and feelings can modify their pain—and the simple strategies children can use to close these gates, can further reduce their pain. The extent of detailed information that children receive should be based on the child's individual needs, interest, and developmental level. There has been a renewed interest in the use of these therapies for children, concurrent with our improved understanding of the plasticity of nociceptive processing.

Table 6 Opioid side-effects

Side-effect	Management
Respiratory depression	Reduction in opioid dose by 50%, titrate to maintain pain relief without respiratory depression.
Respiratory arrest	Naloxone 0.5–2 mg/kg or by 20 μg IV every 1–2 min. Small frequent doses of diluted naloxone or naloxone drip preferable for patients on chronic opioid therapy to avoid severe, painful withdrawal syndrome. Repeated doses often required until opioid effect subsides.
Drowsiness/sedation	Frequently subsides after a few days without dosage reduction; methylphenidate or dextroamphetamine (0.1 mg/kg administered twice daily, in the morning and mid-day so as not to interfere with night-time sleep). The dose can be escalated in increments of 0.05–0.1 mg/kg to a maximum of 0.5 mg/kg/day (WHO Guidelines, in press).
Constipation	Increased fluids and bulk, prophylactic laxatives indicated.
Nausea/vomiting	Administer an antiemetic (e.g. metoclopramide, 0.1–0.2 mg/kg IV or PO every 6 h to a maximum dose of 15 mg per dose) or a phenothiazine (e.g. prochlorperazine, 0.1–0.2 mg/kg PO or IV every 6 h to a maximum of 10 mg dose). Antihistamines such as diphenhydramine or hydroxyzine (0.5–1 mg/kg PO or (IV hydroxyzine slowly) every 6 h to a maximum 50 mg per dose) can also be used.
Confusion, nightmares, hallucinations	Reassurance only, if symptoms mild; change to a different opioid or add neuroleptic (e.g. haloperidol 0.01–0.1 mg/kg PO or IV every 8 h to a maximum of 30 mg per day).
Multifocal myoclonus; seizures	Generally occur only during extremely high dose therapy; reduction in opioid dose indicated if possible. Add a benzodiazepine (e.g. clonazepam 0.01 mg/kg PO every 12 h to a maximum dose of 0.5 mg per dose).
Urinary retention	Rule out bladder outlet obstruction, neurogenic bladder, and other precipitating drugs (e.g. tricyclic antidepressant). Particularly common with epidural opioids. Change of opioid, route of administration, and dose may relieve symptom. Bethanechol, crede, or catheter may be required.

Abbreviations: IV, intravenous; PO, by mouth.

Non-pharmacological interventions are categorized primarily as physical, behavioural, and cognitive, depending on whether they influence children's thoughts, change children's behaviours, or modify children's sensory systems. As shown in Fig. 2, non-pharmacological therapies should be used to relieve children's cancer pain because treatments must be directed at all the causes of children's pain and suffering. The specific cognitive, physical, and behavioural interventions listed in Fig. 2 are ranked in an order similar to the analgesic ladder, in which the different methods required to control progressively stronger or more prolonged pain are listed in an ascending order. Although each method is listed within a main category, most methods vary in the particular combination of cognitive, physical, and behavioural modulation involved. For example hypnosis is considered primarily a cognitive intervention because children learn to reduce pain by their intense mental concentration, even though a hypnotic induction process often includes a behavioural component of progressive muscle relaxation.

Distraction and attention as well as guided imagery are practical tools that health professionals and parents can routinely use when children experience pain. Unfortunately, distraction is often not used appropriately because it has been incorrectly perceived as a simple diversionary tactic in which a child's attention is passively diverted away from pain. The implication is that the pain is still there but the child is momentarily focused elsewhere. However, when the child's attention is fully absorbed by an activity or topic other than his or her pain, is a very active process that can lessen the neuronal responses evoked by tissue damage. Children do not simply ignore their pain, they are actually reducing it. Parents and staff can assist children to concentrate fully on something else besides their pain. Music, lights, coloured objects, tactile toys, sweet tastes, and other children are effective attention grabbing stimuli for infants and young children. Conversation, games, computers, and interesting movies are effective distracters for older children and adolescents.

Guided imagery is a specific method of distraction and attention. Health professionals and parents guide children to remember and vividly describe some previous positive experience, a story they have seen, read or written, or relaxing pain-free sensations associated with pleasurable experience. The more vividly they imagine their positive experiences, the less pain they experience. Guided imagery and story telling provide useful techniques for assisting children to undergo potentially aversive treatments, such as magnetic resonance imaging scans. Children can incorporate the features of the procedures, such as the tunnel shape or loud banging of the magnetic resonance imaging, as features in the story, so when children encounter those stimuli they will not be as frightened.

Many cognitive and behavioural interventions, including relaxation training, operant conditioning, desensitization, and hypnosis, have been used to reduce anticipatory anxiety, nausea, emesis, pain, and behavioural distress for children undergoing cancer therapy.[120-131] Hypnosis has been the most widely used intervention for controlling children's therapy related cancer pain (see reference list for reviews).[122,132] Children can easily learn self-hypnotic techniques to reduce pain during medical treatments and can use hypnosis to supplement analgesic therapy for the control of disease related pain.

Most parents have successfully used a variety of non-pharmacological interventions to relieve their child's typical aches and pains. They reassure children that they will be okay, teach them how to cope, distract their attention away from pain, provide a special hug or kiss, rub a sore body site, or encourage children to continue playing. Children already know that these methods can relieve the pain, so that health-care providers can then teach children new methods to use for the types of cancer pain that they experience. In our pain clinic, we use Fig. 1 to teach children and parents about pain and pain gates. We begin by informing them that the traditional belief, that pain was directly proportional to tissue damage, is wrong. We explain about plasticity, that the same tissue damage or pain source can produce very different pains, depending on the factors listed in the figure. We ask them about whether pain would be stronger or weaker if they were frightened, restrained, had choices, etc. so that they recognize that there are many factors that influence their pain.

Health professionals and parents can relieve children's pain, not only by administering analgesic drugs, but also by increasing their understanding and control, decreasing their emotional distress, and teaching them some simple methods to reduce their pain and anxiety. In addition to providing support and reassurance, parents can help children to understand what will happen, make choices, gain whatever control is possible within the setting, and independently use plain reducing methods. Thus the family, as well as health professionals, share a fundamental role in managing their children's cancer pain. The key concept underlying the use of all analgesic and non-analgesic therapies for children is 'by the child', as described above. Specific pain control methods that require the child to concentrate and focus attention should always be used for children with cancer pain. Beales[133] noted critical differences between adults and children in their perceptions of pain, especially cancer pain. Children's cancer pain seemed even less positively correlated with pathology than adults' cancer pain. Beales suggested that some of the psychological mechanisms involved in pain perception may be manipulated more easily in children than in adults, consistent with our clinical observations that children's cancer pain is more plastic than that of adults. Children seem to possess an enhanced ability to absorb themselves completely in a task, game, or imagined event and, thus, might be more able than adults to trigger endogenous pain-inhibitory mechanisms. Even very young children can easily learn to use a variety of practical pain control methods. The goals of therapy are to enable children to understand what is happening and to have something that they can actively do to lessen their anxiety, distress, and pain.

The specific methods selected depend on the age of the child, the type of pain experienced, and the resources available. Simple methods such as deep breathing, blowing bubbles, alternately tightening and relaxing their fists, squeezing their mother's hand, listening to stories or music, and imagining that they are in a pleasant setting can be very effective for reducing procedural-related pain, when used with appropriate analgesics. When possible, children should learn a few basic methods to reduce their pain and distress. They should not be encouraged to develop a false reliance on the magical benefits of any one method. Instead, they should understand that these practical methods relieve pain because they change the factors that usually increase pain and they help to restore normal sensory input.

All children should learn that pain from some procedures is generally less when they are able to choose the site and rub the area before and after the injection or finger prick. They should learn that pain is less when they are very relaxed. Progressive muscle relaxation with simple exercises in which they tense and relax their body limbs, and biofeedback can help to show them that any type of pain can be intensified if the muscles are always tightened. Children should learn that fear and anxiety can make them tense and increase pain. Then they need practical tools to alleviate their fear about the cancer or their anxiety towards necessary treatments. Children and families must learn that what they think, how they behave, and how they feel affect their children's cancer pain. Then they can begin to work independently and with staff to create additional non-drug pain control methods based on the child's interest, the cultural setting, and the availability of resources. The most important aspect of cognitive therapies is that children concentrate fully on something else.

Although much more research is needed to determine the comparative efficacy of hypnosis, hypnotic-like suggestions for analgesia, distraction, relaxation, and visual imagery for reducing children's cancer pain, all these interventions can provide valuable assistance to children in palliative care. Non-pharmacological interventions can alter many relevant situational factors, such as improving a child's control, and can directly activate endogenous pain-inhibitory systems. Specific interventions should be selected and administered to children as part of a comprehensive pain programme, in the same manner as the most appropriate analgesics are selected and administered in adequate doses, at regular dosing intervals, through the most efficient routes.

Summary

Optimal pain control for children in palliative care includes a judicious blend of pharmacological and non-pharmacological interventions. However, specific interventions must be selected after determination of the primary and secondary sources of noxious stimulation and after a thorough assessment of the unique situational, behavioural, emotional, and familial factors which affect a child's pain. It is impossible to adequately relieve children's pain from a unidimensional perspective, in which pain is considered as synonymous with the nature and extent of tissue damage. Childhood pain must be viewed from a multidimensional perspective because multiple sensory, environmental, and emotional factors are responsible for the pain—no matter how seemingly clear cut an aetiology. Treatment begins with a thorough assessment of these multiple factors, using structured interviews and standardized measures. Pharmacological, physical, and psychological strategies must be incorporated into a flexible intervention programme for children, in which parents and siblings form an essential component of treatment.

All analgesics should be selected 'by the ladder' and administered 'by the clock', 'by the child', and in an effective and painless route. Dosing intervals should be frequent enough to adequately control pain, so that children do not experience an alternating cycle of pain, drowsy analgesia, pain, etc. Children should also learn some simple pain control strategies so that they can reduce acute pain caused by invasive treatments and disease or therapy related pain. Adjuvant medications should be administered to control aversive symptoms and side-effects. Non-pharmacological interventions should be used to control pain.

Special problems in pain control may arise when children die at home, unless parents and medical and nursing teams communicate openly about the availability of potent analgesics and the flexibility of dosing routes and regimens. Parents may be unduly anxious because even small children, like adults with cancer, require larger opioid doses at frequent intervals. Parents' fears can lead them to deny the extent to which their children are in pain or children may fail to report pain because they do not want to further distress parents or because they fear injections.

Multiple sources of noxious stimulation are usually responsible for pain in dying children, as the disease progressively affects many systems. Increased disability, toxic side-effects of medication, physical impairment, and the emotional adjustment of children and their families can intensify pain and suffering. Like adults, children's pain affects the entire family and must be viewed within a broader context. Effective pain control is possible when the goals are to reduce or block nociceptive activity by attenuating responses in peripheral afferents and central pathways, activate endogenous pain inhibitory systems, and modify situational factors that exacerbate pain. Thus, the choice for pain control is not merely 'drug versus non-drug therapy', but rather a therapy that mitigates both the causative and contributing factors for pain. Pain management is a continuous dynamic process, since the disease state and factors that influence pain are not static. Different combinations of drug and non-drug therapies will be required at different times. Thus, health professionals must continually assume as much responsibility for monitoring and relieving children's pain as for medically managing their diseases. Children should not suffer. We have the knowledge to ensure that children receive adequate pain control, from the time they are diagnosed to their death. Parents' memories of their children should not be marred by memories that they experienced unrelieved pain.

References

1. Goldman A, Feret J, Bartolotta C, Weisman SJ. Pain in terminal illness (home care). In: Schechter NL, Berde CB, Yaster M, eds. *Pain in Infants, Children and Adolescents.* Baltimore, MD: Williams and Wilkins, 1993: 425–34.
2. Howell DA. Special services for children. In: Doyle D, Hanks GWC, MacDonald N, eds. *Oxford Textbook of Palliative Medicine,* 1st edn. Oxford: Oxford University Press, 1993: 718–24.
3. Howell DA, Martinson IM. Management of the dying child. In: Pizzo PA, Poplack DG, eds. *Principles and Practice of Pediatric Oncology,* 2nd edn. Philadelphia: J.B. Lippincott, 1993: 1115–24.
4. Davies B, Eng BWS. Special issues in bereavement and staff support. In: Doyle D, Hanks GWC, MacDonald N, eds. *Oxford Textbook of Palliative Medicine,* 1st edn. Oxford: Oxford University Press, 1993: 725–34.
5. Stevens MM. Psychological adaptation of the dying. In: Doyle D, Hanks GWC, MacDonald N, eds. *Oxford Textbook of Palliative Medicine,* 1st edn. Oxford: Oxford University Press, 1993: 699–706.
6. Stevens MM. Family adjustment and support. In: Doyle D, Hanks GWC, MacDonald N, eds. *Oxford Textbook of Palliative Medicine,* 1st edn. Oxford: Oxford University Press, 1993: 707–17.
7. World Health Organization. *Cancer Pain Relief and Palliative Care in Children.* Geneva: World Health Organization, in press.
8. Barr RG. Pain experience in children: developmental and clinical characteristics. In: Wall PD, Melzack R, eds. *Textbook of Pain.* 3rd edn. London: Churchill Livingstone, 1994: 739–65.
9. Bush JP, Harkins SW, eds. *Children in Pain: Clinical and Research Issues from a Developmental Perspective.* New York: Springer-Verlag, 1991.
10. Pichard-Leandri E, Gauvain-Piquard A, eds. *La Douleur Chez l'Enfant.* Paris: Medsi/McGraw-Hill, 1989.
11. McGrath PA. *Pain in Children: Nature, Assessment and Treatment.* New York: Guilford Publications, 1990.
12. McGrath PA. Alleviating children's pain: a cognitive–behavioural approach. In: Wall PD, Melzack R, eds. *Textbook of Pain,* 3rd ed. London: Churchill Livingstone, 1994: 1403–18.
13. McGrath PJ, Unruh A. *Pain in Children and Adolescents.* Amsterdam: Elsevier, 1987.
14. Ross DM, Ross SA. *Childhood Pain: Current Issues, Research, and Management.* Baltimore: Urban and Schwarzenberg, 1988.
15. Schechter NL, Berde CB, Yaster M, eds. *Pain in Infants, Children and Adolescents.* Baltimore: Williams and Wilkins, 1993.
16. Tyler DC, Krane EJ, eds. *Advances in Pain Research and Therapy.* New York: Raven Press, 1990.
17. Price DD. *Psychological and Neural Mechanisms of Pain.* New York: Raven Press, 1988.
18. Wall PD, Melzack R, eds. *Textbook of Pain,* 3rd edn. London: Churchill Livingstone, 1994.
19. Anderson CTM, Zeltzer LK, Fanurik D. Procedural pain. In: Schechter NL, Berde CB, Yaster M, eds. Pain in Infants, Children and Adolescents. Baltimore: Williams and Wilkins, 1993: 435–57.
20. Beales JG. Factors influencing the expectation of pain among patients in a children's burn unit. *Burns,* 1983; **9**: 187–92.
21. Beales JG, Keen JH, Holt PJL. The child's perception of the disease and the experience of pain in juvenile chronic arthritis. *Journal of Rheumatology,* 1983; **10**: 61–5.
22. Kavanagh CK, Lasoff E, Eide Y, *et al.* Learned helplessness and the pediatric burn patient: dressing change behavior and serum cortisol and beta-endorphin. In: Barness L, ed. *Advances in Pediatrics,* vol. 38. St. Louis: Mosby-Year Book, 1991: 335–63.
23. McGrath PA. Psychological aspects of pain perception. In: Schechter NL, Berde CB, Yaster M, eds. *Pain in Infants, Children and Adolescents.* Baltimore: Williams and Wilkins, 1993: 39–63.
24. Peterson L, Shigetomi C. The use of coping techniques to minimize anxiety in hospitalized children. *Behavioral Therapy,* 1981; **12**: 1–14.
25. Ross DM, Ross SA. *A Study of the Pain Experience in Children* (final report, ref. no. 1 RO1 HD13672–01). Bethesda, Maryland: National Institute of Child Health and Human Development, 1982.
26. Cataldo MR, Jacobs HE, Rogers MC. Behavioral/environmental considerations in pediatric inpatient care. In: Russo DC, Varni JW, eds. *Behavioral Pediatrics: Research and Practice.* New York: Plenum Press, 1982: 271–98.
27. Melamed BG, Robbins RL, Graves S. Preparation for surgery and medical procedures. In: Russo DC, Varni JW, eds. *Behavioral Pediatrics: Research and Practice.* New York: Plenum Press, 1982: 225–67.

28. Varni JW, Katz ER, Dash J. Behavioral and neurochemical aspects of pediatric pain. In: Russo DC, Varni JW, eds. *Behavioral Pediatrics: Research and Practice.* New York: Plenum Press, 1982: 177–224.
29. McGrath PA, Hillier LM. Controlling children's pain. In: Gatchel R, Turk D, eds. *Psychological Treatment for Pain: A Practitioner's Handbook.* New York: Guilford Press, 1996:331–70.
30. McGrath PA. Pain control in children. In: Weiner RS, ed. *Innovations in Pain Management: A practical guide for clinicians.* Orlando, Florida: Paul M. Deutsch Press, 1992:32.1–32.79.
31. Pizzo PA, Poplack DG, eds. *Principles and Practice of Pediatric Oncology,* 2nd edn. Philadelphia: J.P. Lippincott, 1993.
32. Stiller CA. Malignancies. In: Pless IB, ed. *The Epidemiology of Childhood Disorders.* New York: Oxford University Press, 1994: 439–72.
33. Robison LL. General principles of the epidemiology of childhood cancer. In: Pizzo PA, Poplack DG, eds. *Principles and Practice of Pediatric Oncology,* 2nd edn. Philadelphia: J.B. Lippincott, 1993: 3–10.
34. Chapman CR, Foley KM, eds. *Current and Emerging Issues in Cancer Pain: Research and Practice.* New York: Raven Press, 1993.
35. Foley K. Pain syndromes in patients with cancer. In: Bonica JJ, Ventafridda V, eds. *Advances in Pain Research and Therapy.* New York: Raven Press, 1979: 59–75.
36. Jacox A, Carr DB, Payne R, *et al. Management of Cancer Pain. Clinical Practice Guideline.* Rockville, MD: Agency for Health Care Policy and Research, U.S. Department of Health and Human Services, Public Health Service, 1994.
37. Bonica JJ. Introduction to management of pain of advanced cancer. In: Bonica JJ, Ventafridda V, eds. *Advances in Pain Research and Therapy.* New York: Raven Press, 1979: 115–30.
38. Janig W. Neurophysiological mechanisms of cancer pain. *Recent Results in Cancer Research,* 1984; **89**: 45–58.
39. Twycross R. *Pain Relief in Advanced Cancer.* New York: Churchill Livingstone, 1994.
40. Altman AJ, Schwartz AD. *Malignant Diseases of Infancy, Childhood and Adolescence,* 2nd edn. Philadelphia: W.B Saunders Company, 1983: 1–149.
41. Kellerman J, Varni JW. Pediatric hematology/oncology. In: Russo DC, Varni JW, eds. *Behavioral Pediatrics: Research and Practice.* New York: Plenum Press, 1982: 67–100.
42. Schechter NL. Pain and pain control in children. *Current Problems in Pediatrics,* 1985;**15**: 1–67.
43. McGrath PA. Pain assessment in children—a practical approach. In: Tyler DC, Krane EJ, eds. *Advances in Pain Research and Therapy.* New York: Raven Press, 1990: 5–30.
44. McGrath PA. Pain in the pediatric patient: practical aspects of assessment. *Pediatric Annals,* 1995; **24**: 126–38.
45. Beyer JE, Wells N. The assessment of pain in children. *Pediatric Clinics of North America,* 1989; **36**: 837–54.
46. Craig KD, Grunau RVE. Neonatal pain perception and behavioral measurement. In: Anand KJS, McGrath PJ, eds. *Pain in Neonates.* Amsterdam: Elsevier Science, 1993: 67–105.
47. Porter F. Pain assessment in children: infants. In: Schechter NL, Berde CB, Yaster M, eds. *Pain in Infants, Children, and Adolescents.* Baltimore: Williams and Wilkins, 1993: 87–96.
48. Hester NO, Foster R, Kristensen K. Measurement of pain in children: generalizability and validity of the pain ladder and the poker chip tool. In: Tyler DC, Krane EJ, eds. *Advances in Pain Research and Therapy: Pediatric Pain.* New York: Raven Press, 1990: 79–84.
49. Swafford LI, Allan D. Pain relief in the pediatric patient. *Medical Clinics of North America,* 1968; **52**: 131–6.
50. World Health Organization. *Cancer Pain Relief and Palliative Care.* Geneva, Switzerland, 1990.
51. Cohen DE. Management of postoperative pain in children. In: Schechter NL, Berde CB, Yaster M, eds. *Pain in Infants, Children, and Adolescents.* Baltimore: Williams and Wilkins, 1993: 357–84.
52. Houck CS, Troshynski T, Berde CB. Treatment of pain in children. In: Wall PD, Melzack R, eds. *Textbook of Pain,* 3rd edn. London: Churchill Livingstone, 1994: 1419–34.
53. Maunuksela EL. Nonsteroidal anti-inflammatory drugs in pediatric pain management. In: Schechter NL, Berde CB, Yaster M, eds. *Pain in Infants, Children, and Adolescents.* Baltimore: Williams and Wilkins, 1993: 135–44.
54. Miser AW. Management of pain associated with childhood cancer. In: Schechter NL, Berde CB, Yaster M, eds. *Pain in Infants, Children, and Adolescents.* Baltimore: Williams and Wilkins, 1993: 411–24.
55. Miser AW, Miser JS. Management of childhood cancer pain. In: Pizzo PA, Poplack DG, eds. *Principles and Practice of Pediatric Oncology,* 2nd edn. Philadelphia: J.B. Lippincott Company, 1993: 1039–50.
56. Schechter NL. Management of pain associated with acute medical illness. In: Schechter NL, Berde CB, Yaster M, eds. *Pain in Infants, Children, and Adolescents.* Baltimore: Williams and Wilkins, 1993: 537–46.
57. Yaster M, Maxwell LG. Opioid agonists and antagonists. In: Schechter NL, Berde CB, Yaster M, eds. *Pain in Infants, Children, and Adolescents.* Baltimore: Williams and Wilkins, 1993: 145–72.
58. Yaster M, Tobin JR, Maxwell LG. Local anesthetics. In: Schechter NL, Berde CB, Yaster M, eds. *Pain in Infants, Children, and Adolescents.* Baltimore: Williams and Wilkins, 1993: 179–94.
59. Schechter NL, Altman A, Weisman S. Report of the consensus conference on the management of pain in childhood cancer. *Pediatrics,* 1990; **86** (suppl.).
60. Schechter NL, Weisman SJ, Rosenblum M, *et al.* Oral transmucosal fentanyl citrate for pediatric procedures: a randomized clinical trial. *Journal of Pain and Symptom Management,* 1991; **6**: 178.
61. Bray RJ. Postoperative analgesia provided by morphine infusion in children. *Anaesthesia,* 1983; **38**: 1075–8.
62. Bray RJ, Beeton C, Hinton W, Seviour JA. Plasma morphine levels produced by continuous infusion in children. *Anaesthesia,* 1986; **41**: 753–5.
63. Cousins MM, Mather LE. Intrathecal and epidural administration of opioids. *Anesthesiology,* 1984; **61**: 276–310.
64. Hendrickson M, Myre L, Johnson DG, Matlak ME, Black RE, Sullivan JJ. Postoperative analgesia in children: a prospective study of intermittent intramuscular injections vs. continuous intravenous infusion of morphine. *Journal of Pediatric Surgery,* 1990; **25**: 185–91.
65. Lynn A, Opheim KE. Morphine intravenous infusions and effects of PaCO2 in infants and toddlers following cardiac surgery. *Journal of Pain and Symptom Management,* 1991; **6**: 207.
66. Robieux IC, Kellner J, Coppes M, *et al.* Continuous intravenous infusion of morphine for the treatment of severe vaso-occlusive painful crises in children with sickle cell anemia. *Journal of Pain and Symptom Management,* 1991; **6**: 176.
67. Ure LM, Ward Platt MP. Tolerance to continuous morphine infusion in children. *Journal of Pain and Symptom Management,* 1991; **6**: 207.
68. Weisman SJ, Driscoll L, Schechter NL, Blanchard D, Bernstein B. Continuous infusion morphine sulfate for pain management in children. *Journal of Pain and Symptom Management,* 1991; **6**: 208.
69. Coyle N, Mauskop A, Maggard J, Foley KM. Continuous subcutaneous infusions of opiates in cancer patients with pain. *Oncology Nursing Forum,* 1986; **13**: 53–7.
70. Miser AW, Davis DM, Hughes CS, Mulne AF, Miser JS. Continuous subcutaneous infusion of morphine in children with cancer. *American Journal of Diseases of Children,* 1983; **137**: 383–5.
71. Ventafridda V, Spoldi E, Caraceni A, Tamburini M, DeConno F. The importance of continuous subcutaneous morphine administration for cancer pain control. *Pain Clinic,* 1986; **1**: 47–55.
72. Gaukroger PB. Patient-controlled analgesia in children. In: Schechter NL, Berde CB, Yaster M, eds. *Pain in Infants, Children, and Adolescents.* Baltimore: Williams and Wilkins, 1993: 203–12.
73. Berde CB, Lehn BM, Yee JD, Sethna NF, Russo D. Patient-controlled analgesia in children and adolescents: a randomized, prospective comparison with intramuscular administration of morphine for postoperative for postoperative analgesia. *Journal of Pediatrics,* 1991; **118**: 460–6.

74. Hill HF, Chapman CR, Kornell JA, Sullivan KM, Saeger LC, Bendetti C. Self-administration of morphine in bone marrow transplant patients reduces drug requirement. *Pain*, 1990; **40**: 121–9.
75. Brown REJr, Broadman LM. Patient-controlled analgesia (PCA) for postoperative pain control in adolescents. *Anesthesia and Analgesia*, 1987; **66**: S22.
76. Cahill C, Gondek E, Strafford M, Sethna N, Berde C. Implementation of PCA program. *Journal of Pain and Symptom Management*, 1991; **6**: 187.
77. Dodd E, Wang JM, Rauck RL. Patient controlled analgesia for post-surgical pediatric patients ages 6–16 years. *Anesthesiology*, 1988; **69**: A372.
78. Gaukroger PB, Chapman M. PCA for children with burns. *Journal of Pain and Symptom Management*, 1991; **6**: 143.
79. Lewe D, Ryan C. Medication use and frequency of side effects in children using patient-controlled analgesia. *Journal of Pain and Symptom Management*, 1991; **6**: 186.
80. Means LJ, Allen HM, Lookabill SJ, Krishna G. Recovery room initiation of patient-controlled analgesia in pediatric patients. *Anesthesiology*, 1988; **69**: A772.
81. Meretoja OA, Korpela R, Dunkel P. Critical evaluation of PCA in children. *Journal of Pain and Symptom Management*, 1991; **6**: 143.
82. Morton NS, Gillespie A. Safety of PCA in children: The role of pulse oximetry. *Journal of Pain and Symptom Management*, 1991; **6**: 142.
83. Reichenback MAB, Bender LH, Stodghill P. Children's use of analgesia under two administration methods. *Journal of Pain and Symptom Management*, 1991; **6**: 161.
84. Rodgers BM, Webb CJ, Stergios D, Newman BM. Patient-controlled analgesia in pediatric surgery. *Journal of Pediatric Surgery*, 1988; **23**: 259–62.
85. Shapiro B, Cohen D, Howe C. Use of patient-controlled analgesia for patients with sickle cell disease. *Journal of Pain and Symptom Management*, 1991; **6**: 176.
86. Tahmooressi J, Schmalzle S, Tobin J. Patient-controlled analgesia in the adolescent undergoing Cotrel-Dubosset Rod. *Journal of Pain and Symptom Management*, 1991; **6**: 160.
87. Tyler DC. Patient controlled analgesia in adolescents. *Pain*, 1987; **4** (suppl): S236.
88. Webb CJ, Paarlberg JM, Sussman M. The use of a PCA device by parents or nurses for postoperative pain in children with cerebral palsy. *Journal of Pain and Symptom Management*, 1991; **6**: 160.
89. Barkas G, Duafala ME. Advances in cancer pain management: A review of patient controlled analgesia. *Journal of Pain and Symptom Management*, 1988; **3**: 150–60.
90. Arora MK, Rajeshwari R, Kaul HL. Comparison of caudal morphine and bupivacaine for postoperative analgesia in children. *Journal of Pain and Symptom Management*, 1991; **6**: 165.
91. Attia J, Ecoffey C, Sandouk P, Gross JB, Samii K. Epidural morphine in children: pharmacokinetics and CO2 sensitivity. *Anesthesiology*, 1986; **65**: 590–4.
92. Finholt DA, Stirt JA, DiFazio CA. Epidural morphine for postoperative analgesia in pediatric patients. *Anesthesia and Analgesia*, 1985; **64**: 211.
93. Glenski JA, Warner MA, Dawson B, Kaufman B. Postoperative use of epidurally administered morphine in children and adolescents. *Mayo Clinic Proceedings*, 1984; **59**: 530–3.
94. Goresky GV, Klassen K, Kuwahara B, Neil SG. Bupivacaine serum concentrations during continuous epidural infusion in children are high. *Journal of Pain and Symptom Management*, 1991; **6**: 166.
95. Henneberg SW, Hole P. Epidural morphine in children for postoperative pain relief. *Journal of Pain and Symptom Management*, 1991; **6**: 165.
96. Jacobson LE, Krane EJ, Pomietto M. Continuous epidural sufentanil for postoperative pain relief. *Journal of Pain and Symptom Management*, 1991; **6**: 208.
97. Klein AS. Comparison of epidural fentanyl versus fentanyl plus bupivacaine continuous infusions for control of postoperative pain after selective dorsal rhizotomy in children. *Journal of Pain and Symptom Management*, 1991; **6**: 163.
98. McNeely JK. Epidural analgesia versus parental analgesia in pediatric postoperative patients. *Journal of Pain and Symptom Management*, 1991; **6**: 166.
99. Pruden PB, Israels SJ. Use of intrathecal narcotics in adolescents with relapsed CNS lymphoma. *Journal of Pain and Symptom Management*, 1991; **6**: 165.
100. Bosenberg AT, Hadley GP, Murray WB. Epidural analgesia reduces postoperative ventilation requirements following esophageal atresia repair. *Journal of Pain and Symptom Management*, 1991; 6: 209.
101. Sethna N, Strafford M, Berde C. Experience with 852 epidural infusions in a children's hospital. *Journal of Pain and Symptom Management*, 1991; **6**: 164.
102. Shapiro LA, Jedeikin RJ, Shalev D, Hoffman S. Epidural morphine analgesia in children. *Anesthesiology*, 1984; **61**: 210–2.
103. Taylor GC, Boswell MV. Continuous epidural infusion of low-dose morphine for postoperative analgesia in children. *Journal of Pain and Symptom Management*, 1991; **6**: 209.
104. Yaster M, Nichols DG, Lynner AM. Respiratory effects and disposition of intrathecal morphine in children. *Journal of Pain and Symptom Management*, 1991; **6**: 181.
105. Berde C, Ablin A, Glazer J, *et al*. Report of the subcommittee on disease-related pain in childhood cancer. *Pediatrics*, 1990; **86**: S818–25.
106. Anand KJS, Shapiro BS, Berde CB. Pharmacotherapy with systemic analgesics. In: Anand KJS, McGrath PJ, eds. *Pain in Neonates*. New York: Elsevier, 1993: 155–98.
107. Anand KJS, McGrath PJ, eds. *Pain in Neonates*. New York: Elsevier, 1993.
108. Franck LS, Gregory GA. Clinical evaluation and treatment of infant pain in the neonatal intensive care unit. In: Schechter NL, Berde CB, Yaster M, eds. *Pain in Infants, Children, and Adolescents*. Baltimre: Williams and Wilkins, 1993: 519–36.
109. Fitzgerald M, Anand KJS. Developmental neuroanatomy and neurophysiology of pain. In: Schechter NL, Berde CB, Yaster M, eds. *Pain in Infants, Children and Adolescents*. Baltimore: Williams and Wilkins, 1993: 11–31.
110. Fitzgerald M. Development of pain pathways and mechanisms. In: Anand KJS, McGrath PJ, eds. *Pain in Neonates*. Amsterdam: Elsevier, 1993: 19–38.
111. Greeley WJ, Boyd JLI, Kern FH. Pharmacokinetics of analgesic drugs. In: Anand KJS, McGrath PJ, eds. *Pain in Neonates*. Amsterdam: Elsevier, 1993: 107–54.
112. Koren G, Butt W, Chinyanga H, Soldin S, Tan YK, Pape K. Postoperative morphine infusion in newborn infants: assessment of disposition characteristics and safety. *Journal of Pediatrics*, 1985; **107**: 963–7.
113. Purcell-Jones G, Dormon F, Sumner E. Paediatric anaesthetists' perceptions of neonatal and infant pain. *Pain*, 1988; **33**: 181–7.
114. Collins C, Koren G, Crean P, Klein J, Roy WL, MacLeod SM. Fentanyl pharmacokinetics and hemodynamic effects in preterm infants during ligation of patent ductus arteriosus. *Anesthesia and Analgesia*, 1985; **64**: 1078–80.
115. Lynn SM, Slattery JT. Morphine pharmacokinetics in early infancy. *Anesthesiology*, 1987; **66**: 136–9.
116. Meignier M, Souron R, Le Neel J-C. Postoperative dorsal epidural analgesia in the child with respiratory disabilities. *Anesthesiology*, 1983; **59**: 473–5.
117. Berde CB. Convulsions associated with pediatric regional anesthesia. *Anesthesia and Analgesia*, 1992; **75**: 164–6.
118. Berde CB, Fischel N, Filardi JP, Coe CS, Grier HE, Bernstein SC. Caudal epidural morphine analgesia for an infant with advanced neuroblastoma: report of a case. *Pain*, 1989; **36**: 219–23.
119. Yaffe SJ, ed. *Pediatric Pharmacology: Therapeutic Principles in Practice*. New York: Grune and Stratton, 1980.
120. Dahlquist LM, Gil KM, Armstrong FD, Ginsberg A, Jones B. Behavioral management of children's distress during chemotherapy. *Journal of Behavioral Therapy and Experimental Psychiatry*, 1985; **16**: 325–9.
121. Dash J. Hypnosis for symptom amelioration. In: Kellerman J, ed.

Psychological Aspects of Childhood Cancer. Springfield: Charles C. Thomas, 1980: 215–30.

122. Hartman GA. Hypnosis as an adjuvant in the treatment of childhood cancer. In: Spinetta JJ, Deasy-Spinetta P, eds. *Living with Childhood Cancer.* Toronto: C.V. Mosby Co, 1981: 143–52.
123. Hilgard JR, LeBaron S. Relief of anxiety and pain in children and adolescents with cancer: quantitative measures and clinical observations. *International Journal of Clinical Experimental Hypnosis*, 1982; **30**: 417–42.
124. Hilgard JR, LeBaron S. *Hypnotherapy of Pain in Children with Cancer.* Los Altos,CA: William Kaufman, 1984.
125. Jay SM, Elliott CH, Ozolins M, Olson RA, Pruitt SD. Behavioural management of children's distress during painful medical procedures. *Behaviour Research and Therapy*, 1985; **23**: 513–52.
126. Katz ER, Kellerman J, Ellenberg L. Hypnosis in the reduction of acute pain and distress in children with cancer. *Journal of Pediatric Psychology*, 1987; **12**: 379–94.
127. LaBaw WL, Holton C, Tewell K, Eccles D. The use of self-hypnosis by children with cancer. *American Journal of Clinical Hypnosis*, 1975; **17**: 233–8.
128. McGrath PA, deVeber LL. The management of acute pain evoked by medical procedures in children with cancer. *Journal of Pain and Symptom Management*, 1986; **1**: 145–50.
129. Olness K. Imagery (self-hypnosis) as adjunct therapy in childhood cancer: clinical experience with 25 patients. *American Journal of Pediatric Hematology/Oncology*, 1981; **3**: 313–21.
130. Olness K. Hypnosis in pediatric practice. *Current Problems in Pediatrics*, 1981; **12**: 1–47.
131. Zeltzer L, LeBaron S. Hypnosis and nonhypnotic techniques for reduction of pain and anxiety during painful procedures in children and adolescents with cancer. *Journal of Pediatrics*, 1982; **101**: 1032–5.
132. Spinetta JJ, Deasy-Spinetta P, eds. *Living with Childhood Cancer.* St. Louis: C.V. Mosby, 1981.
133. Beales JG. Pain in children with cancer. In: Bonica JJ, Ventafridda V, eds. *Advances in Pain Research and Therapy.* New York: Raven Press, 1979: 89–98.

19.2 Life threatening illnesses and symptom control in children

Ann Goldman

Introduction

Relatively few children die from an illness and the spectrum of life threatening illnesses in children is different from that in adults. Most children who are dying are cared for either by general paediatricians or by paediatric specialists in a child's particular disease. Since training in the care of dying children is still not commonly available, this chapter hopes to help those who encounter this situation infrequently. It will consider common symptoms, other than pain, which are associated with a variety of life threatening illnesses.

One of the challenges of paediatrics comes from looking after patients across a wide age range, from neonates through childhood to adolescence. Each child's care must be appropriate for his or her physical, cognitive, and emotional status. It is also impossible to care for children without considering them within the context of their family unit. Parents need to be seen not only as part of the family unit requiring support but also as an integral part of the team looking after the sick child. The needs of siblings and grandparents must also be considered.

Symptom care needs to be incorporated into an holistic plan of care for the child and family. This has been summarized in a charter (Fig. 1) that was developed in the United Kingdom through the Association for Children with Life Threatening and Terminal Conditions and their Families (ACT). ACT serves as an advocate for families and links the work of statutory services and voluntary organizations.

Symptom management

Systematic collection of data and trials specific to symptom care in children are still sparse. Much of the literature reflects personal practice. Some of the symptoms encountered frequently in children are discussed below. Others can be managed by reference to experience in general paediatrics and adult palliative care.

Symptoms and signs tend to develop more quickly in children than adults and are often less clearly localized, especially in the very young. The general approach to management of all symptoms is similar (Fig. 2). The initial step is to take a careful history and make a thorough assessment. In contrast with pain, formal assessment tools for other symptoms in children are not available. The picture developed is often a synthesis of the child's own description, which depends on the child's age and level of understanding, and the parents' observations and opinion. Particular issues to consider are how much distress the symptom causes the child himself, and how much it interferes with the child's and family's daily living. If the cause can be identified it may help in planning treatment, although often at this stage it will not be reversible. Approaches to management need to include drug treatments, practical nursing care, and psychological support both for the child and the family. Regular reassessment will help maintain optimal symptom relief.

Pharmacological considerations

The choice of drugs for children, particularly in palliative care, can be difficult as many of the products are not recommended by the manufacturers either for the particular age range or use. In some cases this is due to proven problems, but more often it is due to a lack of information and paediatric trials. Reasons contributing to this lack include the difficulty of establishing reliable data in small numbers of patients of wide age ranges, the practical and ethical problems of arranging trials when children are terminally ill, and the limited market for drug companies for their products. In practice, physicians often take the responsibility of using unlicensed drugs, and a body of clinical experience develops in the absence of formal trials or pharmacokinetic data.

Children differ from adults in their ability to absorb, distribute, metabolize, and eliminate drugs.[1,2,3] Details are shown in Table 1. These differences are most marked in neonates and alter as the child gets older. Although the many variables affecting how drugs are handled in children make it difficult to generalize, neonates tend to have a low renal and hepatic clearance and a high volume of distribution, resulting in a longer elimination half-life for many drugs. However, in infancy and childhood a relatively high clearance with a 'normal' volume of distribution leads to shorter drug half-lives compared with adults. The clinical implications are that neonates tend to need reduced doses relative to their overall size, though a loading dose may be important to prevent delayed onset of therapeutic effect, whilst infants and young children may need comparatively higher doses and at shorter intervals.

The most common approach to calculating doses for children is to estimate in milligrams of drug per kilogram of body weight. For drugs with a low therapeutic index, and therefore a high risk of adverse effects (for example cytotoxics) dose calculations may be

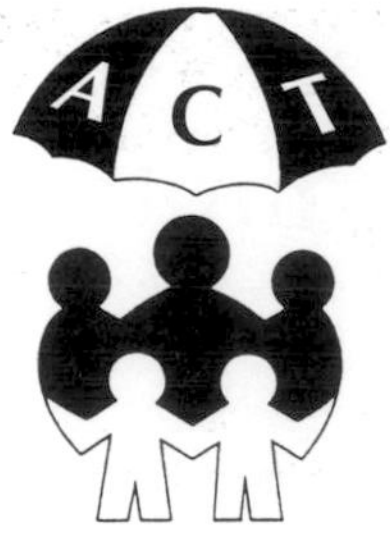

ACT Charter

for Children with Life-threatening Conditions and their Families

1. Every child shall be treated with dignity and respect and shall be afforded privacy whatever the child's physical or intellectual ability.
2. Parents shall be acknowledged as the primary carers and shall be centrally involved as partners in all care and decisions involving their child.
3. Every child shall be given the opportunity to participate in decisions affecting his or her care, according to age and understanding.
4. Every family shall be given the opportunity of a consultation with a paediatric specialist who has particular knowledge of the child's condition.
5. Information shall be provided for the parents, and for the child and the siblings according to age and understanding. The needs of other relatives shall also be addressed.
6. An honest and open approach shall be the basis of all communication which shall be sensitive and appropriate to age and understanding.
7. The family home shall remain the centre of caring whenever possible. All other care shall be provided by paediatric trained staff in a child-centred environment.
8. Every child shall have access to education. Efforts shall be made to enable the child to engage in other childhood activities.
9. Every family shall be entitled to a named key worker who will enable the family to build up and maintain an appropriate support system.
10. Every family shall have access to flexible respite care in their own home and in a home-from-home setting for the whole family, with appropriate paediatric nursing and medical support.
11. Every family shall have access to paediatric nursing support in the home when required.
12. Every family shall have access to expert, sensitive advice in procuring practical aids and financial support.
13. Every family shall have access to domestic help at times of stress at home.
14. Bereavement support shall be offered to the whole family and be available for as long as required.

Fig. 1 ACT charter, developed in 1992 and available from ACT, 65 St. Michael's Hill, Bristol BS2 8D7, United Kingdom.

made according to surface area. For drugs with a higher therapeutic index, the dose may be given according to age range.

Children may also react differently from adults to individual drugs. Dystonic reactions with metoclopramide and phenothiazines are more common in children. With opioids, the side-effect of itching seems more frequent whilst nausea and vomiting are less of a problem. In neonates, the greater permeability of the blood–brain barrier contributes to their greater sensitivity to morphine. Children taking steroids appear to develop a cushingoid appearance relatively quickly, they also often suffer marked mood and behaviour changes.

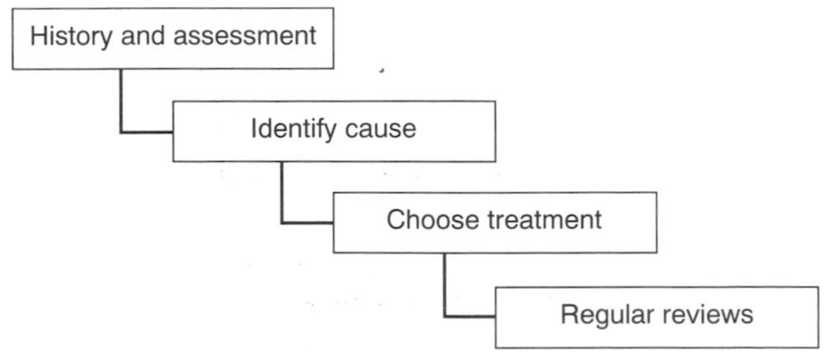

Fig. 2 Systematic plan for symptom management.

Administering drugs

Many seriously ill children will have been taking a variety of medicines for a long time; however, as they become more sick, they may find taking them more difficult and distressing. Planning a drug regimen which is both practical and acceptable to the child

Table 1

Physiological	Variable factor	Effect
Absorption		
Gastric pH	Birth — neutral Adult values by 3 years	↑ Absorption of acid labile drugs ↓ Absorption of acidic drugs
Gastric emptying	Neonates — prolonged Adult values by 6–8 months	↓ Drug absorption
Pancreatic enzymes	Decreased in cystic fibrosis	↓ Absorption of drugs requiring hydrolysis
Splanchnic blood flow	Decreased in cardiac failure	↓ Absorption of drugs
Skin	Thin in neonates and infants	↑ Absorption
Muscle	Smaller mass, more variable blood flow in neonates, infants, and seriously ill	↓ Absorption after intramuscular injection
Distribution		
Plasma albumin	Low levels up to 1 year, lower binding affinity in neonatal albumin	↓ Protein binding acidic drugs
Displacement by bilirubin	Free fatty acids and other substances in cord blood	↑ Fraction absorbed
Plasma globulin	Reduced, adult values 7–12 years	↓ Protein binding of basic drugs
Body fluids	Neonates — 75% total body weight, extracellular fluid 40% 1 year — 60% total body weight, extracellular fluid 25% Adult — 55% total body weight, extracellular fluid 20%	Higher volumes for distribution of water soluble drugs
Metabolism		
Cytochrome oxidases, hydroxylation	Reduced in neonates	Slow clearance of diazepam, phenytoin, phenobarbitone, lignocaine, theophylline
Dealkylation	Efficient from birth	e.g. diazepam
Glucuronidation	Absent in neonates, adult values at 3 years	↑ Risk of respiratory depression with opioids up to 6 months ↓ Clearance of chloramphenicol, altered pathway for paracetamol
Sulphate and glycine conjugation	Efficient from birth	Preferred pathway in neonates
Protein binding	Reduced for many drugs in neonates	Enhanced metabolism of total drug
Excretion		
Glomerular filtration rate (GFR)	2–4 ml/min birth 8–20 ml/min day 3 adult values 5 months	Prolonged half-life of renally excreted drugs
Renal blood flow	Increase over neonatal period	↑ Clearance of above drugs
Active secretion	Low in neonates adult values 7–10 months	↓ Clearance for some drugs
Urinary pH	Lower than adults	↑ Reabsorption weak acids ↓ Reabsorption bases
Protein binding	Increased free fractions in neonates	↑ Filtration efficiency

and family is essential. Sometimes this can only be achieved by giving priority to the most important drugs, particularly as the illness progresses.

As in adults the oral route is the first choice for drugs. Children can be offered either liquid or tablet formulations. Young children often prefer crushed tablets to elixir and the taste can be disguised with juice, yoghurt, or other food. Long-acting preparations, whenever they are available, are helpful in reducing the inconvenience of frequent doses thus making the illness seem less intrusive. If the oral route is not possible, because of vomiting or decreased level of consciousness for example, then another must be used. Rectal preparations are available for many drugs and may be acceptable. Some children prefer this route to any needles, even subcutaneous, and it can also be useful if the child has become unconscious, or in the final stages of life. Otherwise a subcutaneous infusion can be established or drugs given through a central intravenous line if one is already *in situ*. A simple syringe pump is effective and straightforward for parents to manage. Complex and expensive systems with patient controlled analgesia, often appropriate for postoperative pain management in children, are not necessary for terminal care, especially at home.

Gastrointestinal problems

Eating and drinking

Concerns and problems with feeding often assume great importance in paediatrics, and may be equally so when a child is receiving palliative care. Providing food and nourishment for their child is at the core of being parents, often symbolizing their love. Being unable to provide this essential need can cause intense distress and anxiety, and represents, on an emotional level, their failure as parents. Children, especially those who are ill, have relatively little influence over their own lives and their eating habits may be one area where they can retain some control. This can lead to conflict within the family and further distress. Eating, chewing, and sucking are an important part of all children's lives and development, providing comfort, pleasure, and stimulation. When children are ill, or brain damaged, they may regress in their behaviour and adopt patterns usually associated with a younger child.

These issues need to be considered and addressed, alongside the child's medical and practical problems with eating, when planning care. Attitudes to food and drink need to be adjusted in accordance with the child's prognosis and condition, so that invasive procedures are not used to prolong the process or distress of dying.

Feeding problems are particularly prominent for children with progressive degenerative conditions when they affect the neurological and neuromuscular mechanisms of swallowing. Realistic eating goals need to be set for pleasure and comfort, whilst nutritional goals aimed at restoring or maintaining health may be of secondary importance. Discussion, support, and training with families can help them provide for the child's practical needs and also reduce tension and enable eating to be more enjoyable.

For children with neuromuscular problems, careful attention to the child's position and surroundings is helpful. This may include stabilizing the head with the chin tilted downwards, helping the swallowing reflex by stroking the child's neck, and providing the right aids or appliances to assist the child. Often frequent, small meals are more acceptable. Depending on the child's abilities, solids may need to be cut into small pieces and moistened with gravy or sauce. Purees may be easier to swallow than liquids. Hard or dry feeds should be avoided and uncooked dairy foods may thicken mucus and be troublesome. Consideration of details may prolong a child's ability to feed independently or help parents who are feeding a totally dependent child.

Assisted feeding

Whether assisted feeding is appropriate must be considered individually for each child and family. It can be considered where significant stress would be relieved or where it may extend a child's useful or enjoyable life. For children with slowly progressive diseases, when feeding becomes impossible but death is not imminent assisted feeding may be entirely appropriate. Some children may have had assisted feeding from an early stage of their disease, for example to maintain blood sugar levels in a metabolic disorder, and discontinuing feeding at a later stage of the illness would be more distressing for the family than maintaining it. In contrast, starting assisted feeding in an anorexic child with a metastatic and rapidly progressive tumour would seem inappropriate.

Assisted feeding can be through a nasogastric tube. Small-bore silk tubes are usually well tolerated although they can sometimes aggravate the problems caused by excess secretions. If tube feeding is likely to be necessary for a long time a gastrostomy is often preferable.

Anorexia and dehydration

Severely ill children, nearing death, naturally become less interested in food and may survive many weeks with surprisingly little nutrition and without discomfort. The severe cachexia seen in adults with cancer seems less common in children but no data are available about its incidence or accompanying metabolic changes. Reversible causes such as nausea, fear of vomiting, constipation, sore mouth, depression, or the presentation of too much or unappetizing food should be considered. If none of these is present, attention should focus on other family members, helping them to acknowledge anorexia as part of the child's progressing disease. Steroids, as an appetite stimulant, are generally not recommended in children. They may result in unpleasant mood changes and a rapid onset of a Cushingoid appearance, which both the children and the families find disturbing.

Failure to maintain an oral fluid intake tends to occur at a very late stage. The main discomfort from dehydration appears to be a dry mouth, which can be helped by mouth care and moistening.

Nausea and vomiting

Nausea and vomiting are relatively common and unpleasant symptoms for children. Causes which may be identified include raised intracranial pressure, metabolic disturbance, drug side-effects, gastric irritation, constipation, and external pressure on the bowel from tumours. Frank intestinal obstruction from tumours is uncommon in children. Often no single cause can be found.

The control and neurophysiology of nausea and vomiting are complex and not fully understood (Chapter 9.3.1). The act of vomiting appears to be co-ordinated by the vomiting centre in the medulla, and can be induced by a variety of stimuli. Antiemetics may work at one or a number of sites and can be selected rationally, according to the presumed cause. If vomiting is persistent, then combining a number of drugs which act in different ways may be successful (Fig. 3). Drugs are given orally if possible, but the rectal

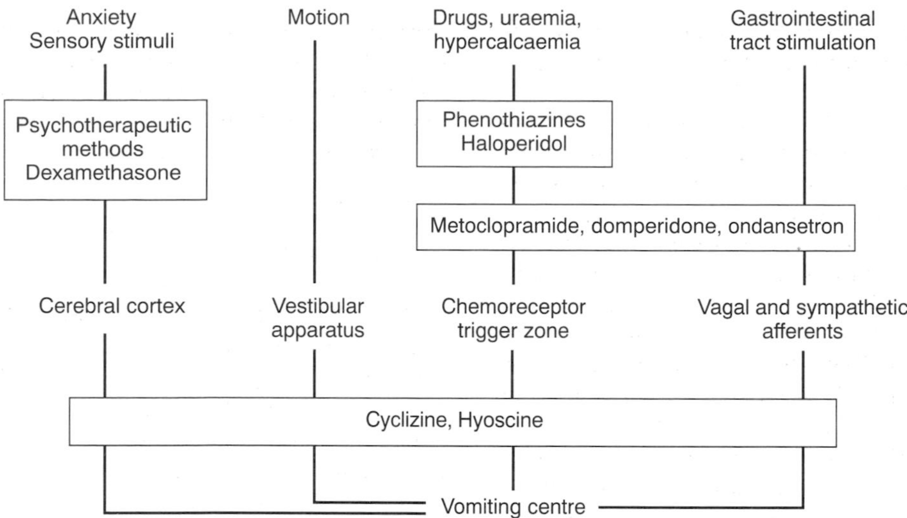

Fig. 3 Selection of antiemetics in relation to the causes of nausea and vomiting.

or subcutaneous routes can be used if necessary. Haloperidol or cyclizine are usually the first choice for administration by subcutaneous infusion. Metoclopramide may also be used, and methotrimeprazine if sedation is also required.

Cyclizine, a drug available in the United Kingdom but not in many other countries, appears to be particularly effective for vomiting due to raised intracranial pressure. Although the role of ondansetron in palliative care, even in adults, has not been defined and only one case report appears in the literature,[4] clinical experience in children suggests it can be very helpful when the vomiting is severe and resistant to other antiemetics. It can also be a useful addition with cyclizine in the vomiting of raised intracranial pressure when it is preferable to using increasing doses of corticosteroids. Short courses of corticosteroids may, however, be helpful to cover special short-term situations such as holidays. Dystonic reactions with metoclopramide and occasionally haloperidol and domperidone are more frequent in children than adults, but can be treated effectively with benztropine.

Constipation

Terminally ill children, like adults, have many problems which can contribute towards constipation. These include poor fluid and dietary intake, lack of mobility, weakness and wasting, and the use of drugs, particularly opioids but also phenothiazines and anticholinergic drugs. Fortunately in children this is balanced, to some extent, by their younger and fitter bowels. If parents are aware of the possibility of constipation developing and keep a note of bowel actions, then simple measures and mild laxatives can be instituted quickly and severe problems avoided.

Children taking opioids should always be prescribed regular laxatives. A mild osmotic laxative such as lactulose may be sufficient, and is well tolerated by children, although those with neurodegenerative diseases can find it difficult to swallow. If this is not effective, gastrointestinal stimulants (such as bisacodyl or senna) and drugs which combine stool softening and stimulant activity (such as co-danthrusate) can be substituted. Adequate doses and combinations of oral drugs should be tried before resorting to suppositories (bisacodyl) or enemas (sodium citrate or docusate sodium).

Diarrhoea

Chronic and severe diarrhoea is a particular problem for children with HIV/AIDS infection. It can be very distressing to families and cause considerable practical problems. Pharmacological approaches to relieve the symptoms need to be given alongside investigations to identify the cause. Oral loperamide is often effective in reducing the diarrhoea; if not, oral morphine may be introduced. If the diarrhoea is so severe that oral absorption is prevented, morphine, diamorphine, or hydromorphone can be given subcutaneously. Octreotide, the synthetic somatostatin analogue, has been used successfully to help severe secretory diarrhoea in adults and may also have a role in children. Consideration of practical issues such as skin hygiene, laundry services, and preplanning journeys are also particularly appreciated by families.

Mouth care

Terminally ill children with general debility and lowered immunity often develop mouth problems, but they are frequently reluctant to undertake regular or intensive mouth care. Persuasion and compromise may be called for. The mouth can be cleansed with povidone-iodine, chlorhexidine, or hexetidine using mouth washes or gentle cleaning and moistening with a foam stick. Candida infections should be looked for regularly and treated with nystatin or ketoconazole. During chemotherapy, painful ulceration is common and may be relieved with benzydamine hydrochloride mouthwash or local anaesthetic lozenges. Hydrocortisone pellets may also be helpful in palliative care. Children can be given some choice to allow for individual preferences.

Neurological symptoms

Convulsions

Seizures may have been a significant symptom throughout the illness for some children, such as those with neurodegenerative diseases. For others, for example some of those with malignant diseases, they may only develop terminally. Watching a child having a seizure is extremely frightening for parents, particularly if it is totally unexpected. They should always be warned and prepared if it is a risk. As with all symptoms in palliative care, the need for drug intervention should be balanced against the distress the seizure causes the child. Occasional short fits may not warrant drug treatment.

Children with a history of recurrent seizures may be taking long-term anticonvulsants. Doses and combinations of drugs will have been adjusted to give optimum control with minimal side-effects. An overall deterioration in the illness may require the regular medication to be readjusted. Often children with satisfactory seizure control have occasional, prolonged fits and need drugs for this acute situation, although their regular anticonvulsants may not need to be changed.

For acute management of seizures diazepam is valuable, although it needs to be given rectally or intravenously. Families looking after a child for whom fits are a possibility should have a supply of rectal diazepam available and be taught how to use it. Although it is helpful for terminating fits acutely it does not have an extended anticonvulsant effect. Regular oral anticonvulsants such as carbamazepine or phenytoin can be introduced if the seizures are frequent and the child still has a life expectancy of several months.

If severe, repeated seizures develop towards the end of life, alternative drugs which are helpful include midazolam, paraldehyde, or phenobarbitone. Midazolam can be given by subcutaneous infusion and is both a sedative and anticonvulsant. It is also compatible with a subcutaneous infusion of opioids. Although intramuscular paraldehyde is inappropriate and painful, it can be given rectally diluted in an equal volume of arachis oil. Traditionally it is given with a glass syringe but problems are not encountered using modern plastic syringes if it is given promptly. Phenobarbitone is often avoided as a regular anticonvulsant in childhood because of sedation and behaviour problems but this may not be applicable in the case of a terminally ill child. For severe, prolonged seizures it can be given subcutaneously as an aqueous solution through a syringe driver, and the dose increased as necessary. It is not compatible with morphine or diamorphine and must be given separately.

Anxiety and agitation

Anxiety as the disease progresses may reflect children's need to express their fears and distress. It may be helped by discussion or, particularly in younger children, by age appropriate play, stories, or art work. Low-dose oral diazepam may also be valuable.

Drugs may be helpful when a child is very close to death and agitation and confusion result from irreversible organ failure. Benzodiazepines are often the first choice, either oral diazepam or midazolam given subcutaneously via a syringe pump. Haloperidol, which also has antiemetic activities, is useful and methotrimeprazine, with antiemetic and analgesic effects, is a helpful sedative. All of these can be given either subcutaneously and are compatible with morphine and diamorphine.

Respiratory symptoms

The incidence and severity of respiratory symptoms as a problem in paediatric palliative care is uncertain. For those with cystic fibrosis and muscular dystrophy they are a major feature of the final illness. For children with cancer, the clinical impression is that it is less of a problem than in adults but very little data are available. A retrospective review of the case notes of children with cancer identified some respiratory symptoms in 40 per cent of children in the last 3 months of their life.[5] In children dying from neurodegenerative diseases in a children's hospice, 17 of 45 (38 per cent) children experienced dyspnoea and 31 per cent had difficulties from excess secretions.[10]

Dyspnoea, cough, and excess secretions can all cause distress to children and anxiety for their parents. Haemoptysis is, fortunately, rare but the possibility is particularly frightening. The degree of the child's distress often depends not only on the severity of the underlying disease but also on the speed of onset of the problems and the child's level of anxiety. As well as pulmonary disease from lung damage, infection, malignant infiltration, or pleural effusion difficulty in breathing can also result from cardiac failure, superior vena caval obstruction, or extrathoracic problems such as anaemia, ascites, or chest wall pain. If treatment can be directed at relieving the cause, even temporarily, this may be worthwhile.

If the underlying cause is not amenable to treatment, relief can be achieved by combining drugs with practical and supportive approaches. Fear is often a powerful element in dyspnoea and the confidence of staff to manage the situation is readily conveyed to families. Simple practical measures, according to what seems to help each individual child, can be employed. Finding the optimum position with pillows or a table to lean on, open windows, using a fan, and relaxation exercises may all help.

The sensation of breathlessness can be relieved with opioid drugs. These are usually given orally, or if necessary, subcutaneously. The role of nebulized morphine in children has not been established. Systemic opioids and nebulized local anaesthetic agents can be helpful for cough which may cause distress by aggravating chest wall pain and headache and disturbing sleep. Small doses of sedatives such as diazepam can be helpful in relieving anxiety associated with dyspnoea.

Children with gradually increasing hypoxemia from chronic chest diseases may suffer from headaches, nausea, drowsiness during the day, and poor quality sleep. Intermittent or eventually continuous oxygen therapy may help relieve these symptoms and can be given at home via nasal prongs. Children with dyspnoea in the later stages of malignant disease do not usually find oxygen helpful and often dislike the use of facial masks or prongs.

Excess secretions are often a prominent problem for children with chronic neurodegenerative diseases as their illness progresses and they are less able to cough and swallow. They may also occur in other terminally ill children as they near death. Portable suction equipment for use at home may be helpful for children with chronic problems but is less appropriate for those nearing death. Hyoscine hydrobromide can reduce secretions, and can be given conveniently transdermally or subcutaneously. Glycopyrrolate can also be used in oral form in the United States and as an injection elsewhere.

Anaemia and bleeding

Anaemia

Treatment of anaemia in the latter stages of a child's life should be directed towards relief of symptoms, rather than in response to the level of haemoglobin. Each situation needs to be judged individually and in consultation with the family. If the child has been enjoying a good quality of life and becomes limited or distressed by symptoms attributable to the anaemia, most often tiredness but also dyspnoea, headaches, or palpitations, then red cell transfusions are justified. Parents should understand the purpose of transfusions and appreciate that as the illness progresses there is likely to come a point when transfusions no longer relieve symptoms and are therefore inappropriate.

Transfusions are usually given as packed cells, and should aim to restore the haemoglobin to around 12 g/dL. The total quantity of blood needed can be estimated according the child's current haemoglobin (Hb) and weight.[6]

Volume of packed cells in millilitres = (desired - observed Hb concentration) × body weight in kilograms × 3

Children cared for at home can receive the blood there, if staff are available to be with them, otherwise they need to be admitted to hospital for as brief a time as possible.

Bleeding

Although an internal or intracerebral bleed may seem a relatively peaceful way to die, florid external bleeding, haemoptysis, or haematemesis are frightening for the child, distressing for the carers, and may leave the family with unforgettable, painful memories. If there is a risk of serious bleeding an appropriate analgesic and sedative, for example an opioid and midazolam, should be prescribed and available. The correct dose should be calculated ahead of time and the drugs and syringes immediately accessible at home or in hospital.

Children with liver disease and portal hypertension may develop serious bleeding from oesophageal varices. Endoscopic sclerosis of the varices with injections of ethanolamine can help this. Children with liver disease may also have low levels of clotting factors (which may be helped by regular vitamin K) and low platelets from hypersplenism.

Many children with malignant disease have widespread bone marrow infiltration and consequently low platelets. Petechiae and minor nasal and gum bleeding are common but fortunately serious bleeding is not usual. During chemotherapy, families become familiar with receiving platelet transfusions whenever the platelet levels are low. They may find it difficult adjusting to the pattern in palliative care where routine transfusion is confined to bleeding which is severe or interferes with the quality of life. Children with acute promyelocytic leukaemia or a strong history of bleeding throughout their illness may require regular platelets. Platelet transfusions can often be given at home, with antihistamine and steroid cover. Haemostatics, such as tranexamic acid and ethamsylate, can help reduce spontaneous bleeding, even when platelets are low. They can be taken orally, or for bleeding gums the intravenous solution can be used as a mouthwash.

Common illnesses from which children die

Every child who is dying and his or her family are unique. However, knowledge of and experience with the child's illness can help staff anticipate likely symptoms and prepare for them.

Cancer

Cancer in children is uncommon. In the United Kingdom, with a childhood population of 12 million, about 1200 new cases are diagnosed each year.[7] The incidence in other countries world-wide has been published by the World Health Organization.[8] The range of tumours differs from adults as carcinomas are unusual while leukaemias, brain tumours, and soft tissue sarcomas are common. In the United Kingdom, cure can be anticipated in about two-thirds of all children diagnosed. However, there are still some tumours, particularly those which are widespread at diagnosis, where cure rates are low.[7] In developing countries where less aggressive therapy is available, survival is correspondingly lower.

In developed countries, the majority of children are treated at specialist paediatric oncology centres where they enter formal therapeutic trials. Care is provided by a multidisciplinary team with a strong emphasis on psychosocial support throughout treatment. Treatment for symptoms related to the therapy, such as pain from procedures and nausea and vomiting from chemotherapy, should run alongside treatment directed against the cancer. It is essential to give such symptoms a high priority. For those children who will be cured, symptoms will form their lasting memory of the illness and can affect the ability of long-term survivors to cope.[9]

Acknowledging that treatment has failed and a child's cancer cannot be cured is always a difficult time. Decisions about the value of further anticancer treatment against the cancer must be taken by the family and medical team together. Many factors, including whether it will be possible to induce temporary remission, the role of new phase I and II agents, and how the child has tolerated therapy so far, are taken into consideration. During this period of transition, palliative care gradually assumes a more prominent role and for most children eventually becomes the focus of management.

When a child has progressive cancer the spectrum of symptoms which he or she develops depends on the sites of the primary tumour and metastatic disease. Common sites of spread include bone and bone marrow, the lymphatic system, and lungs. Many childhood tumours spread very widely and aggressively, so that compared with adults the length of the final illness is often relatively short, although children with brain tumours may have a more prolonged illness.

Pain is a great fear for families and its management forms a major part of the care for a child dying from progressive cancer (see Chapter 19.1). Other symptoms are also likely to develop and should be addressed equally vigorously. Symptoms from bone marrow failure, with anaemia and thrombocytopenia, are frequent. Gastrointestinal problems of nausea and vomiting are also common and may be difficult to eradicate entirely. Dyspnoea may develop either in association with lung metastases or anaemia, although many younger children appear to have less severe symptoms than might be expected from their X-rays or level of haemoglobin. Children with brain tumours often have distressing, progressive neurological deficits with paralysis, loss of vision, loss of speech, and difficulty in swallowing. In the case of brainstem tumours these problems may develop without loss of consciousness or understanding. Convulsions may also occur in children with brain tumours or central nervous system leukaemia.

Although parents often fear the moment of death they can be reassured that for almost all children it is peaceful. Terminal fits or bleeding are uncommon. Terminal restlessness and agitation and excess secretions may develop in the late stages of the illness but these respond well to treatment. Parents are also helped by knowing

Table 2

Disease group	Examples	Inheritance	Some typical features
Neuronal storage diseases	Nieman–Pick Battens	Recessive Recessive	Damage to grey matter. Progressive mental deterioration, seizures, blindness
Mucopolysaccharidoses	Hurlers Hunters	Recessive Sex linked	Typical facies, skeletal abnormalities, progressive mental deterioration, corneal clouding, behavioural difficulties
Leucodystrophies	Metachromatic Krabbes	Recessive Recessive	Damage to white matter. Gait disorders, ataxia, paralysis, progressive mental deterioration
Primary neuronal degenerative diseases	Leigh's encephalopathy	Recessive	Psychomotor delay and deterioration, blindness, spasticity, vomiting, respiratory irregularity
	Ataxia telangiectasia	Recessive	Ataxia, telangiectasia, growth retardation, increased risk of infection and malignancy

that death is rarely sudden and there will be enough time for them to know that the end is approaching.

Neurodegenerative and metabolic diseases

As more children with cancer are cured, the relative importance of these diseases as a cause of death in childhood increases. A large number of conditions with a diverse range of neuromuscular, metabolic, and other features can be included under this broad heading. Individually, many are extremely rare but as a group they are united by their progressive nature, the inevitability of death, and, in the majority, an inherited cause. Some examples are given in Table 2. For families of an affected child, their grief often begins at birth or soon after, and since no cure is available all the child's treatment is palliative.

Many of the children become profoundly mentally and physically disabled and some have difficult behaviour problems. Some of the illnesses progress over a relatively long time, with periods where the disease seems almost static. Assessment of symptoms is a particular problem in these children and parents and carers must often rely on observation, experience, and trials of therapy. Pain does not appear to be a major feature though it may be underestimated; muscle spasm, joint pain, gastro-oesophageal reflux, constipation, and routine childhood conditions such as otitis media may be underlying causes. Convulsions are often a problem, particularly in degenerative diseases involving the grey matter of the brain. The nature, frequency, and severity of the fits may vary during the course of the illness and status epilepticus can sometimes occur. Problems from declining mobility, difficulty feeding, incontinence, deteriorating vision and speech, and respiratory symptoms occur frequently.[10]

As these illnesses are so uncommon, families often feel isolated and find it difficult to obtain information. They may need help to access the financial benefits and practical help to which they are entitled, and any charitable support which is available. Social workers and specific disease-related support groups may provide this help. The burden of care for families is prolonged and is both physically and emotionally exhausting. Strain within the parents' marriage, for siblings, and across the wider family is common. Respite care is a vital and underprovided aspect of palliative care. It may be offered by volunteer families who take children for short periods, by carers who take over from the parents at the child's home for a limited period, or less appropriately, by admission to acute paediatric hospital wards. In some countries, children's hospices now offer this type of help (see Chapter 19.5). The needs are currently greater than the services available.

Particular problems are associated with inherited conditions. Most commonly, the inheritance is autosomal or sex linked recessive. Families need genetic counselling and information about the possibility of prenatal diagnosis. Unfortunately, some diseases do not present until some years after birth and so several affected children may be born in the same family, compounding the grief, stress, and practical problems involved. Feelings of guilt and blame are common in families whose children have inherited disorders.

Cystic fibrosis

The estimated world-wide incidence of cystic fibrosis varies from 1:620 to 1:90 000 and is generally most prevalent in northern and central Europeans.[11] Prognosis has gradually been improving and three-quarters of those suffering are still alive in their teens, with increasing numbers surviving into young adult life.[12] Identification of the cystic fibrosis gene in 1989 offers the potential for gene therapy. Heart and lung transplant has also become available recently, offering a dramatic treatment for terminal disease for some patients.

Cystic fibrosis is a systemic disease which can affect almost every organ in the body. Problems in the respiratory and digestive systems dominate and are progressive. Comprehensive and lifelong care is essential to maintain good quality life for as long as possible. Specialist care by a multidisciplinary team has been shown to improve survival.[13]

Chest management to delay the onset of problems involves regular physiotherapy, exercise, and aggressive antibiotic therapy.

However, in time, lung damage develops inevitably and infections become increasingly difficult to eradicate. Symptoms which invariably become troublesome include cough, dyspnoea, headaches, exhaustion, insomnia, and back and chest pain; eventually hypoxia and cor pulmonale develop. Severe lung disease may be complicated by pneumothoraces. If small these may reabsorb spontaneously, otherwise intercostal drainage is needed, and if this fails, thoracic surgery is required. Unfortunately this may prejudice future transplantation. Small haemoptyses are also common with progressive lung disease. These are usually self limiting but, when more severe, they may be helped temporarily with vasopressin. Bronchial artery embolization is required for permanent relief.

Nutritional status is maintained by pancreatic enzyme replacement and good dietary intake. Oral supplements and more aggressive enteric feeding, via a gastrostomy, may also be used. Glucose intolerance increases with age and insulin dependent diabetes may develop.

After chest disease, the main cause of mortality is hepatobiliary disease. Cirrhosis with portal hypertension, hypersplenism, oesophageal varices, and jaundice occur in over 10 per cent of adolescents and adults. Haematemesis may develop and, although the varices may be treated with sclerotherapy, this is made more difficult by the increased risk of anaesthesia due to pulmonary disease.

The time consuming and unremitting care places a heavy emotional and practical burden on families. From the time of diagnosis, cystic fibrosis families live with the knowledge that the child's death will be premature. The children themselves develop an increasing insight into their own prognosis as they get older. They anticipate and experience the death of siblings and friends and see themselves moving inexorably in the same direction.

In the past, eventually, the imminence of death was obvious and acknowledged and the focus of care changed to symptom relief. There was an opportunity to make plans about the death and for the family to grieve together. This has changed in recent years with the possibility of heart and lung transplant. Families can now postpone the need to face death and continue to fight actively against the illness. For those who do receive a transplant, considerable improvement in quality of life occurs but survival is only 70 per cent at 2 years and the possibility of graft rejection and complications of immunosuppressive drugs continue.

Transplants are not available for all patients. Physical contraindications include previous major thoracic surgery, invasive Aspergillus infection, severe malnutrition, and liver disease. Patients also need a positive psychological approach and a history of good compliance with past treatments. Even after selection, a transplant cannot be guaranteed as insufficient donor organs are available. Many patients die on the waiting list. The pressure is great for those awaiting transplant, hoping desperately that they will be called but gradually becoming more and more ill. Managing symptoms and addressing the emotional support for patients under these ambivalent circumstances can be particularly difficult.

Muscle disorders

The majority of muscle disorders in children are genetically determined and, since none can be cured, treatment for the children is palliative from the time of diagnosis. Problems can range from mild disability to those which are life-threatening. Some, such as severe spinal muscular atrophy, cause death during infancy; others, such as Duchenne muscular dystrophy, develop and progress through childhood with death in adolescence anticipated. The practical needs, problems of symptom management, and psychosocial issues are closely linked and change and increase as the disease progresses.

Problems in infancy

Infants with major problems are characterized by those with spinal muscular atrophy (Werdnig–Hoffman). From their child's birth, parents are faced with both emotional distress and with immediate and progressive physical disability. Babies with spinal muscular atrophy are not intellectually impaired. Since they have the curiosity of a normal baby but the inability to be satisfied, due to their severe weakness, they can be demanding to care for. Initially they are able to swallow and suck but later assisted feeding is usually required. Secretions, which become an increasing problem, can be reduced with transdermal hyoscine and portable suction machines are needed at home from an early stage. Many families prefer to care for their child at home as much as possible, treating recurrent chest infections as they arise. Most children die by the age of two years, usually from pneumonia.

Problems in older children

Duchenne is the most common form of muscular dystrophy. There are about 1500 boys living with the disorder in the United Kingdom at any one time, and there are about 100 boys born with it each year.[14] It is a genetically determined (sex linked recessive), progressive, degenerative disorder, resulting from a defect in the protein dystrophin in muscle. The boys may also have an associated cardiomyopathy and about one-third are intellectually impaired.

The onset of symptoms is within the first 5 years of life, and from then, the course of the disease is relentlessly downhill. Early management focuses on maintaining optimum mobility, with exercise and physiotherapy and efforts to prevent and treat contractures and spinal deformity. The ability to walk is usually lost between the ages of 8 and 11, although it may be delayed for a short time by the use of leg callipers. Eventually an electric wheel chair will be needed. Later, as the shoulder girdle muscles weaken, arm rests can be fitted to the wheelchair to allow the boys to retain as much use of their hands as possible. Electric beds, with hand controlled switches, may help discomfort at night. Eventually unable to feed themselves, chewing and swallowing also become increasingly difficult and weight loss is common over the last months.

Respiratory failure is the major cause of death. Deterioration in respiratory function parallels the decline in overall muscle strength. Problems with chest infections become more frequent and more serious, and recurrent admissions to hospital for treatment of pneumonia are usual. Hypoventilation, especially at night, can cause headaches, nausea, drowsiness during the day, and restlessness at night. Oxygen through nasal prongs, initially at night and later also during the day, may help relieve these symptoms. Cardiac disease also accounts for a number of deaths. Occasionally these are sudden but often cardiomyopathy and lung damage result in increasing cardiac failure. End-of-life care for boys with Duchenne muscular dystrophy has become increasingly complex in recent years, as the potential of long-term ventilation and home ventilator programmes have been developed.[15] Decisions in this area remain controversial and vary with different cultures and resources.

Cardiac diseases

Life threatening cardiac problems commonly result from congenital abnormalities affecting the structure of the heart, major blood vessels, or pulmonary circulation. They may also develop through cardiomyopathy or in association with other diseases such as cystic fibrosis or muscular dystrophy.

Sophisticated, corrective cardiac surgery and the possibility of heart and heart and lung transplants have altered the outlook for families and staff. This aggressive approach to treatment means that the majority of sick children who die from cardiac disease do so in an acute perioperative or intensive care unit setting. A small group of children with chronic heart disease die suddenly and unexpectedly, and this is probably related to arrhythmias. There are only a few situations where everyone involved agrees that aggressive treatment is not appropriate and the focus moves to symptom management and palliative care.

The symptoms children develop are the result of heart failure and hypoxia. Initially, symptoms may be related to increased demands such as exercise, emotion, or intercurrent illness but then they progress to occur with minimal exertion or temperature change and eventually at rest. Fatigue and exhaustion are very frequent complaints and are related to the poor blood supply to the skeletal muscles. Dyspnoea is also common as the heart is unable to meet demands for oxygenated blood and the ensuing oxygen debt results in an increased respiratory rate. This may be exacerbated by fluid accumulating in the lungs. Progressive hepatomegaly can cause abdominal discomfort, nausea, and vomiting with increased pressure on the stomach and compromised blood supply to the bowel. Eventually this can result in reduced absorption of food, reduced bowel motility, and progressive weight loss. Peripheral oedema may also develop in the legs, face, and abdomen. Dizziness and fainting may occur as the heart fails to meet the demands of the cerebral blood supply, as well as through sudden arrhythmias. Pain is not common but some children suffer from angina-like chest pain.

General advice and support may help family members adapt their lifestyle to reduce the demands on the heart, increase their understanding of the situation, and allow them to express their feelings about the progressing disease. Short-term goals, appropriate to the child's level of activity, and aids to mobility may be helpful. Adequate rest is important and comfort at night may be improved with extra pillows and night sedation. Nutrition may be enhanced by eating frequent, small-volume meals; a lower fat diet, which allows stomach emptying, may help alleviate nausea.

Specific therapy may help delay the onset or severity of symptoms. Captopril or vasodilators can reduce the blood pressure and muscle work and nifedipine may help by increasing the blood flow through the lungs. The role of digoxin, to increase the force of contraction of the heart muscle, is debatable. Diuretics help relieve symptoms, though they should be used gently to avoid compromising the heart's need for good filling pressure. Nausea and vomiting may be helped with antiemetics and opioids may reduce dyspnoea. A low dose of diazepam for anxiety may also be valuable. Headaches and drowsiness from hypoxia may be improved by oxygen. At home, this is usually supplied via nasal prongs using an oxygen concentrator or a portable oxygen cylinder for mobility.

Hepatic and renal disease

For children with irreversible hepatic or renal disease, the development of transplantation programmes has altered the pattern of care and the expectations of families. Although families are aware that the illness is life-threatening, and that much of the treatment is palliative, they are always aware of the possibility of transplant in the future. Virtually all deaths occur in hospital whilst staff are striving to deal with situations they hope and believe can be altered, such as awaiting a transplant, during a crisis after surgery, or because of infection or complications of treatment. Occasionally a decision is taken not to enter a child into a transplant programme or after many years of intensive treatment children may themselves elect to discontinue. In developing countries, transplant programmes are not universally available. In these situations palliative care becomes the main focus for treatment.

Liver disease

The signs and symptoms of progressive liver disease reflect the liver's importance and range of functions. These include its role in digestion and carbohydrate metabolism, production of blood clotting factors, its role in metabolism and detoxifying substances, and its importance in the immune process. Damage to other organs, particularly the brain and kidneys, can also result from a failing liver.

Jaundice may develop, and be particularly severe if there is hypoplasia of the bile ducts. Itching associated with cholestasis can be severe. Ascites and oedema are common as liver disease progresses. Fluid restriction, spironolactone, and albumin infusions may help; paracentesis is only a very temporary measure. If hypoglycaemia is a problem it can usually be controlled by giving the child small and regular feeds either orally or nasogastrically. Many of these children also have anorexia, nausea, anaemia, fatigue, and growth failure.

Serious bleeding may be associated with the presence of portal hypertension and oesophageal varices. It is exacerbated by the low levels of clotting factors and low platelets from hypersplenism. Haematemesis can be life threatening and unpredictable. Sclerosis of the abnormal vessels with injection of ethanolamine via an endoscope is helpful treatment. It may need to be undertaken regularly and can eventually result in oesophageal narrowing and reflux. Some children with liver failure develop chronic neurological problems and progressive loss of skills. This can be particularly distressing for families and also for some of the children who retain insight into their situation. Low protein diets and lactulose may be recommended. Acute hepatic encephalopathy with confusion, agitation, fits, and coma may develop suddenly or be precipitated by a gastrointestinal bleed. Benzodiazepines (for example diazepam or midazolam) may be helpful but chlorpromazine and haloperidol, which can precipitate coma, should be avoided.

Renal disease

It can be difficult to predict how long a child will live with progressive renal disease. Death may be very rapid and sudden, possibly from cardiac arrhythmias due to electrolyte imbalance or the children may decline very gradually over many months and even years. Many of the treatments for chronic renal failure can continue as part of palliative care. These may include dietary manipulation, correction of acidosis and salt wasting, prevention of renal osteodystrophy, erythropoietin, and antihypertensive agents. How tolerable these are for the child, which are important for symptom relief, and which might be appropriately discontinued needs careful consideration.

As the disease progresses, pain is unusual but anaemia, with tiredness and weakness, is common. Nausea and vomiting often result from uraemia. A high carbohydrate diet can reduce the uraemia, and the symptoms resulting from it, and this may need to be given by a nasogastric tube. Antiemetics may also help. Platelet dysfunction may result in bleeding into the skin and gut. As renal function declines, fluid overload with oedema and dyspnoea may develop; associated with this, pericardial infusion and tamponade may be a terminal event. Other children may develop convulsions and coma before death.

Conclusions

Careful attention to all symptoms and their management is vital for children dying from any illness. It can improve the child's quality of life and help relieve distress for them and their families. This can contribute to a more peaceful and dignified death for the child and leave the family with easier memories of the final illness. As health-care providers in palliative care, we face the challenge of increasing the quality and quantity of information available about symptom relief in children so that future care can be improved on the basis of sound data as well as good clinical practice.

References

1. Bryson S, McGovern L. Dosing decisions in paediatrics. *Current Views in Pharmacy and Therapeutics*, 1987; **9**: 6–8.
2. Reed MD. Developmental Pharmacology: relationship to drug use. *DICP, The Annals of Pharmacotherapy*, 1989; **23**: 521–6.
3. Timmins JG. Pharmaceutical problems in children. *British Journal of Pharmaceutical Practice*, 1985; **7**: 242–6.
4. Cole RM, Robinson F, Harvey L, Trethowen K, Murdoch V. Succcessful control of intractable nausea and vomiting requiring ondansetron and haloperidol in a patient with advanced cancer. *Journal of Pain and Symptom Management*, 1994; **9**: 48–50.
5. Hain R, Patel N, Crabtree S, Pinkerton R. Respiratory symptoms in children dying from malignant disease. *Palliative Medicine*, 1995; **9**: 203–5.
6. DePalma L, Ness P, Luban N. Red blood cell transfusion. In: Luban N, ed. *Transfusion Therapy in Infants and Children*. Baltimore: Johns Hopkins University Press, 1991: 12.
7. Stiller CA. Aetiology and epidemiology. In: Plowman P, Pinkerton C, eds. *Paediatric Oncology Clinical Practice and Controversies*. Chapman and Hall, 1992: 1–20.
8. Parkin DM, Stiller CA, Draper GS, Bieber CA, Terracini B, Young JL, eds. *International Incidence of Childhood Cancer*. World Health Organization, International Agency for Research on Cancer, 1988.
9. Stuber ML, Meeske K, Gonzalez S, Houskamp B, Pynoos R. Post traumatic stress after childhood cancer. *Psycho-oncology*, 1994: **3**: 302–12.
10. Hunt A, Burne R. Medical and nursing problems of children with neurodegenerative disease. *Palliative Medicine*, 1995; **9**: 19–26.
11. Doershuk CF, Boat TF. Cystic fibrosis. In: Berhman RE, Vaughan VC, eds. *Nelson Textbook of Pediatrics*. WB Saunders. 1987: 926–36.
12. British Paediatric Association Working Party on Cystic Fibrosis. Cystic Fibrosis in the United Kingdom 1977–85: an improving picture. *British Medical Journal*, 1988; **297**: 1599–602.
13. Webb AK, David TJ. Clinical management of children and adults with cystic fibrosis. *British Medical Journal*, 1994; **308**: 459–62.
14. Baum D. The magnitude of the problem. In: Goldman A, ed. *Care of the Dying Child*. Oxford: Oxford University Press, 1994: 1–14.
15. Hilton T, Orr R, Perkin R, Ashwal S. End of life care in Duchenne Muscular Dystrophy. *Paediatric Neurology*, 1993; **9**: 165–77.

19.3 Psychological adaptation of the dying child

Michael M. Stevens

What do children think and fear about death—particularly their own death? Do children who are dying develop insight to adjust and cope? These questions, currently amongst the most topical in psychosocial paediatrics, are clearly relevant to paediatric palliative medicine and are discussed in this chapter.

Psychological development of the normal child

An understanding of what sick children think and fear about death and how they adjust requires a brief discussion of how healthy children begin to think and form concepts including a concept of death.

Jean Piaget is regarded as this century's leading developmental psychologist. His stage theory of child development[1,2] describes the development of the child's intellect (thoughts, perceptions, judgement, reasoning) as an orderly hierarchical sequence of three major periods, each integrating and extending the previous one. This theory is widely used as a model in experimental child psychology (Table 1).

In the first period (sensorimotor intelligence, birth to 2 years), intellectual development begins with motor and sensory actions which, by being repeated, become behavioural sequences. These form the basis for later intellectual structure. Piaget believed that infants in this period are still unable to think or form concepts.

The second period (preparation and organization of concrete operations, early childhood to adolescence) consists of two stages, referred to as preoperational thought and concrete operations. During the stage of preoperational thought (age 2–7) the child is still unable to differentiate between the internal and external worlds (egocentricity), and has thoughts which do not follow logical rules. The child will attribute life and consciousness to inanimate objects (animistic thinking) and believes that inanimate objects can be commanded to obey actions or thoughts (magical thinking). This assists the child in making order out of the world and ascribing causes to events. The child will ascribe magical prelogical explanations in discovering what differentiates life from death. The child will also believe that all objects and events in the world are manufactured to serve people (artificialism) .

During the stage of concrete operations (age 7–12), the child gradually becomes less egocentrically orientated. Animistic, magical, and artificialistic thinking decrease and gradually disappear, and the child comes to realize the personal nature of his or her views. Language and communications skills increase dramatically, and the child acquires the concepts of conservation, space, time, and rate. The child's thinking becomes logical and influenced by the rules of disciplines such as arithmetic and mechanics. The child is concerned with the actual rather than the hypothetical, and his or her reasoning will be connected as much as possible to beliefs based on direct observation. The child confronted by death will now know that animals and people do not die because a magic spell was put upon them that can be lifted, and will seek to discover what differentiates life from death.

During formal operations (adolescence to adulthood) previous cognitive structures and functions are integrated to achieve full intellectual capacities, including the ability to deal effectively with the world of abstract ideas.

The sequence of these periods will be orderly in all children, but children may differ widely in the ages at which they move through the sequence. Occasional reversions to a less-developed mode of thought will occur.

The well child's concept of death and its development

The development of an understanding of death in the well child parallels Piaget's sequence of periods of cognitive development.

Specific cognitive achievements suggested as essential for understanding the various components of a concept of death include classification abilities (ability to categorize in hierarchies and to attend to multiple classifications simultaneously, for example a banana is yellow and long and belongs to the fruit family), the ability to focus on transformations as well as states, a linear notion of time, the ability to perform reversible operations (ability to follow a process from beginning to end and retrace steps back to the starting point), reciprocity skills (recognition that others may feel and/or think differently to oneself) that enable children to learn from the experience of others, increased objectivity, decreased egocentrism, and the universal application of rules. A child's concept of death will vary according to his or her level of cognitive development.

Maria Nagy conducted 484 assessments on 378 Hungarian children aged between 3 and 10 in Budapest and its environs, using compositions written by those aged 7 to 10 years on the subject of death, drawings by those aged 6 to 10 years, and discussions with those aged 3 to 10 years. Her results were published in English in 1948,[5] although much of the work was done as early as 1936. Nagy found three stages of development of a concept of death.

Table 1 The child's cognitive development and development of death concepts: recommendations for caregivers

Period/stage of cognitive development (Piaget)*	Life period†	Some major characteristics	Predominant death concepts	Recommendations for caregivers‡
I Period of sensorimotor intelligence	Infancy (0–2)	'Intelligence' consists of sensory and motor actions. No conscious thinking. Limited language§ no concept of reality	No concept of death	Provide maximum physical relief and comfort
II Period of preparation and organization of concrete operations				
1. Stage of pre-operational thought	Early childhood (2–7)	Egocentric orientation. Magical, animistic, and artificialistic thinking. Thinking is irreversible. Reality is subjective	Death is reversible: a temporary restriction, departure, or sleep	Minimize child's separation from parents. If parents unavailable, provide reliable and consistent substitute. Correct misperception of illness as punishment for bad thoughts or actions. Evaluate for feelings of guilt, rejection, anger, resentment of self or others
2. Stage of concrete operations	Middle childhood/ preadolescence (7–11/12)	Orientation ego-decentred. Thinking is limited to actual (although possibly absent) features of a situation rather than exploring abstract relationships and hypotheses. More adaptive thinking but confined to objects. No abstract reasoning. Understands conservation, reversibility. Multiple classification ability	Death is irreversible but capricious: external –internal physiological explanations	Evaluate for fears of abandonment, destruction, or body mutilation. Be truthful and open. Provide details about treatments. Reassure treatments are not punishments. Maintain access to peers. Foster child's sense of control, mastery
III Period of formal operations	Adolescence and adulthood (12 +)	Propositional and hypodeductive thinking. Generality of thinking. Reality is objective	Death is irreversible, universal, personal, but distant: natural, physiological, and theological explanations	Reinforce comfortable body image, self-esteem. Allow ventilation of anger. Provide privacy. Support reasonable measures for independence. Be clear, honest, and direct. Maintain access to peers. Consider mutual support groups

* Each stage includes an initial period of preparation and a final period of attainment; thus whatever characterizes a stage is in the process of formation.
† There are individual differences in chronological ages.
‡ Adapted from ref. 3.
§ By the end of their second year children have attained a vocabulary of approximately 250–300 words on average.
Adapted with permission from ref. 4.

1. Age 3–5: death seen as temporary and reversible, and not distinguished completely from life.
2. Age 5–9: death is personified and imagined as a separate person.
3. Age 9 years and upwards: death is seen as the cessation of corporal activities, and is universal and inevitable.

Sylvia Anthony studied definitions of the word 'dead' by 128 children.[6] Their responses fell into five categories:

(1) apparent ignorance of the meaning of the word 'dead';

(2) limited or erroneous concept;

(3) no evidence of non-comprehension of the meaning of 'dead' but definition by reference to (a) associated phenomena that were not biologically or logically essential or (b) humans specifically but not other living things;

(4) correct, essential, but limited reference;

(5) general, logical, or biological definition or description.

As the child grew older, his or her concept of 'dead' changed in the order of the classification from (1) to (5). Anthony noted that

Table 2 Concepts of death and implications of incomplete understanding for adjustment to loss

Component of death concept	Definition	Example of incomplete understanding	Implication of incomplete understanding
Irreversibility	The understanding that once a living thing dies, its physical body cannot be made alive again. Death as final, as irrevocable, as permanent	The child expects the deceased to return, as if from a trip	Failure to comprehend this concept prevents the child from detaching personal ties to the deceased, a necessary first step in mourning
Finality: non-functionality, dysfunctionality, cessation	The understanding that all life-defining functions cease completely at death	The child worries about a buried relative being cold or in pain; the child wishes to bury food with the deceased	May lead to preoccupation with the physical suffering of the deceased and impair adjustment
Universality (inevitability)	The understanding that all living things die. Death as a natural phenomenon that no living being can escape indefinitely	The child views significant individuals (i.e. self, parents) as immortal	If the child does not view death as inevitable, he or she is likely to view death as punishment (either for actions or thoughts of the deceased, or the child) leading to excessive guilt and shame
Causality	A realistic understanding of the causes of death	Child who relies on magical thinking is apt to assume responsibility for death of a loved one by assuming that bad thoughts or unrelated actions were causative	Tends to lead to excessive guilt that is difficult for the child to resolve

Reproduced from ref. 10 with permission; additional data taken from refs. 8 and 11.

immature death concepts take the form of oral fantasy. She also observed that fairy tales are full of such oral fantasy about death of a kind which is not death: Red Riding Hood's grandmother is eaten by the wolf and is later recovered from the beast's belly; Hansel and Gretel eat part of the witch's house, and she welcomes them inside but plans to cook and eat them.

Components of the child's concept of death: the current view

Although earlier studies have been valuable, it now appears that the child's concept of death is virtually complete by the age of 8 years. Studies have confirmed that different components of the child's concept of death are acquired at differing ages. In one study, 3-year-olds were often found to have some realization of death, but only at the age of 12 years would a child be likely to have an accurate idea of what a dead body would look like.[7]

In a more recent review of three key components of a death concept,[8] it was concluded that, under at least some circumstances, young children think that death is reversible, attribute various life-defining functions to dead things, and think that certain individuals (often including themselves) will not die. Irreversibility, non-functionality, and universality are understood at roughly the same time (for most children between 5 and 7 years). In a second recent study[9] of the age of acquisition of seven of Kane's[7] components of the concept (separation, universality, causality, irrevocability, appearance of the body, insensitivity, and cessation of body function) in well children, about 60 per cent of the 5-year-olds, 70 per cent of the 6-year-olds and 66 per cent of the 7-year-olds had complete or almost complete concepts. By the age of 8 and 9 years the figures were almost 100 per cent.

Some caution is required in comparing various studies of age of acquisition.

1. Differing statistical criteria are used by various investigators (e.g. a varying percentage of positive responses are defined to consider a concept acquired).
2. There are variations in the socio-economic and educational standards of the children tested.
3. There are other influences related to the date of the particular study (e.g. the opportunity for the child to encounter death more commonly in the modern media).

The currently accepted components of the concept of death as summarized recently by Schonfeld[10] are presented in Table 2, with examples of incomplete understanding and implications of incomplete understanding for adjustment to loss.

Development in well children of fears and anxieties concerning death

There are at least three views on how children acquire fears and anxieties about death.[12]

1. The psychoanalytic view suggests that death anxieties and fears in children and adults are derivatives of other anxieties and fears that develop in early life, principally separation anxiety, fear of object loss, fear of castration, fear of abandonment, and fears of physical immobility and the dark. Anthony[13] suggests that risk-taking behaviour such as 'dares' is one type of defence against such anxieties.

2. The cognitive view relates children's fears and anxieties about death to the stage of development of their concept of death. The young child may fear waking up after death and being trapped in the grave. After the child develops the concept of the irreversibility of death, there will be a fear of its permanence.

3. The social learning view puts forward the idea that children's ideas and feelings are influenced by their experiences and by the observations of others. Thus death fears and anxieties in children will be influenced by their parents, as well as by siblings, peers, teachers, and relatives. Siblings and peers can provide 'information' about death that can be truly frightening. The media (particularly television), children's books, and fairy tales have also been noted to be significant influences.

Death education

Educating children about death has recently been advocated on the basis that it is desirable to promote conceptual development related to death, and that death should be introduced as a general concept prior to the child's exposure to personal loss in order to lessen anxiety about it and to assist more successful adjustment to loss.[11,14]

The sick child's perception of death

Although the survival rates for a variety of chronic illnesses have dramatically improved over the last 30 years, many children still do not survive. Thus the issue of their concept of death is still pertinent. Anxiety about death is an issue for all chronically ill children, particularly those with leukaemia or other malignancies, whether or not they eventually survive.

Prior to 1970, most caregivers believed that unless a child was aged over 10, he or she was incapable of understanding death and therefore did not experience anxiety about it. It was felt that children did not need information about their disease and that they would be incapable of coping with the distress and anxiety of knowing that they were dying. A closed protective approach was advocated.[15–18]

Revised concepts of illness and death in children with leukaemia

In the late 1960s and early 1970s, pioneering work by Vernick and Karon,[19,20] Waechter,[21] and Bluebond-Langner[22] prompted a complete revision of this perspective.

The views of those advocating a closed protective approach were challenged bluntly for the first time in 1971 by the late Eugenia Waechter. In a key article[21] published in mid-1971, which was prepared from research on anxiety about death in terminally ill children conducted for her doctoral dissertation, Waechter reported on 64 children between the ages of 6 and 10 divided into four groups of equal size: those with a fatal disorder, those with a chronic non-fatal disease, those with a brief illness, and a group of well elementary school children who were not in hospital. A General Anxiety Scale for Children,[23] measuring concerns in many areas of living, was administered to each child. A set of eight pictures was also shown individually to each child, and stories were requested in order to elicit fantasy expression of the child's concern regarding present and future body integrity and functioning. Four pictures were selected from the Thermatic Apperception Test.[24] Four other pictures which were designed specifically for the study are reproduced in Fig. 1.

Parents of the children in the first three groups were interviewed to assess how the quality and quantity of the fatally ill children's concerns about death were influenced by their previous experience with death, the religious devoutness within the family, the quality of maternal warmth towards them, and the opportunities that they had had to discuss their concerns or the nature of their illness with their parents, professional personnel, or other meaningful adults.

Although only two of the 16 fatally ill children had been told their prognoses, the generalized anxiety was extremely high in all 16 cases, almost double that of the two comparison groups of children in hospital and three times that of healthy children. The children threatened with death discussed loneliness, separation, and death much more frequently in their fantasy stories. Waechter's most striking finding was the dichotomy between the children's degree of awareness of their prognosis, as inferred from their imaginative stories, and the parents' beliefs about their child's awareness. Only two of the 16 fatally ill children had discussed their concerns about death with their parents, but 63 per cent of stories told by these children related to death. The children often gave the characters in the stories their own diagnoses and symptoms; they frequently depicted death in their drawings and occasionally they would express awareness of their prognoses to persons outside their immediate family. Waechter concluded that denial and protectiveness by adults may not be entirely effective in preventing these children from experiencing anxiety or in keeping their diagnosis and probable prognosis from them. She recommended that the child's questions and concerns should be dealt with in a way that did not further alienate and isolate the child from the parents and other meaningful adults.

In the early 1970s, Myra Bluebond-Langner, an anthropologist, confirmed and extended Waechter's research by conducting detailed long-term observations of leukaemic children, their parents, and the various health professionals caring for them in the haematology–oncology clinic and ward of an American hospital. Her observations and conclusions, published in 1978,[22] together with those of Waechter, have been pivotal in changing the views of the establishment on how to work most effectively with dying children.

Stages of acquisition of factual information about the disease (Bluebond-Langner)

Although parents and staff provided little or no information to the child about any aspect of the illness in the hope of lessening his or her anxiety, it was found that over time such children acquired information about their disease in five stages and that particular experiences were critical to passage through these stages. As the children passed through these stages, they also passed through five different definitions of themselves (Table 3).

The children's personal experiences were a much more significant determinant than age or intellectual ability in determining concepts of their sickness. Thus a 3- or 4-year-old might know more about his or her prognosis than a very intelligent 9-year-old.

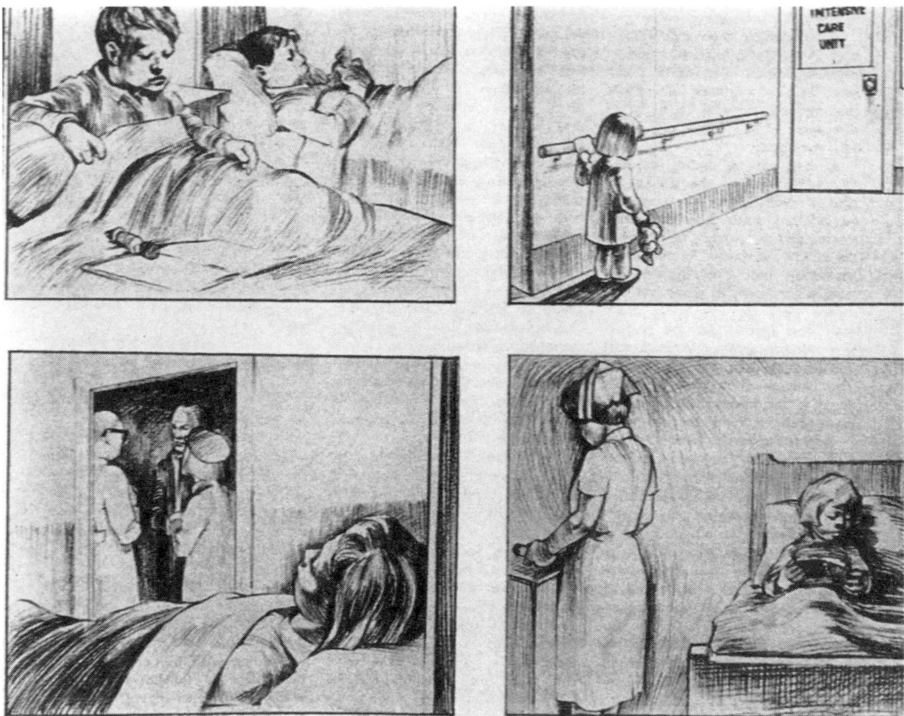

Fig. 1 Four specifically designed pictures used by Waechter[21] to elicit fantasy expressions of concerns related to present and future body integrity from dying children aged 6 to 10. The children were asked to tell stories about the pictures. They often gave the characters their own diagnosis and symptoms and 63 per cent related their stories to death. (Reproduced from ref. 21 with permission.)

Mutual pretence

Bluebond-Langner's research confirmed that not only did terminally ill children know that they were dying before death became imminent, but they also kept such knowledge a secret, mainly to avoid upsetting their parents and to lessen the probability of being abandoned by loved ones or caregivers because of the anxieties that such disclosures might cause in the latter. Instead, the children, together with their parents and the caregivers, practised an elaborate ritual of mutual pretence, in which all parties defined the patient as dying but acted as if the patient was going to live (Table

Table 3 Stages in a sick child's acquisition of information about illness, and critical experiences required for passage through stages

Stage of acquisition of information	Child's information	Experience required for passage to this stage	Child's self-concept at this stage
First stage	'It' is a serious illness (not all know the name of the disease)	Parents being informed of diagnosis	I was previously well but am now seriously ill
Second stage	The names of the drugs used in treatment, how they are given, and their side-effects	Parents being informed that child is in remission; child speaking to other children at clinic	I am seriously ill and will get better
Third stage	Purposes of special procedures and additional treatments consequent to the side-effects of therapy, and the relationship between particular symptoms and procedures	The first relapse	I am always ill and will get better
Fourth stage	A larger perspective of the disease as an endless series of relapses and remission	Several further relapses and remissions	I am always ill and will never get better
Fifth stage	The disease as a series of relapses and remissions, ending in death	Child learns of the death of an ill peer	I am dying

Adapted from ref. 22.

Table 4 Rules for practice of mutual pretence*

1. All parties to the interaction should avoid dangerous topics
2. Talk about dangerous topics is permissible as long as neither party breaks down
3. All parties to the interaction should focus on safe topics and activities
4. Props should be used to sustain the 'crucial illusion'
5. When something happens or is said which tends to expose the fiction that both parties are attempting to sustain, then each must pretend that nothing has gone awry
6. All parties to the interaction must strive to keep the interaction normal
7. All parties must strive to keep the interaction brief
8. When the rules become impossible to follow and the breakdown of mutual pretence appears imminent, avoid or terminate the interaction

* Dying children, their parents, and their caregivers are observed to adhere to these rules when practising mutual pretence.
Data from refs. 22 and 25.

4). Interestingly, in the children studied by Bluebond-Langner, breaches in these rules did not lead to open awareness. Mutual pretence remained the dominant mode of interaction in all children studied, who practised it to the end.

Many patients practise mutual pretence because they find it the most comfortable way to relate to many staff members in the treatment team. The important thing is to be aware that it exists and that it is not a suitable medium for honest communication.

Other research on sick children's concepts of death, illness, and isolation

An evaluation of anxiety and withdrawal in children aged between 6 and 10 years who were terminally ill with leukaemia was conducted in 1974.[26,27] It was found that they appeared to be aware of the seriousness of their illness (even though they might not be yet capable of talking about this awareness in adult terms), expressed more anxiety than controls, and, of greater concern, perceived a growing psychological distance from those around them.

A contemporary study[28] of concepts of death, illness, and isolation in 21 children with leukaemia aged between 4 and 9 years, conducted in the United Kingdom, found no indications that the sick children interviewed had radically different concepts of death from those shown by healthy children. Some of the perceptions of the sick children about themselves in hospital were worrying. The children's feelings of being alone, even with ample company, suggested deprivation of another sort. There was a large variation in the concept of death between individual children, particularly in those younger than 8 years.

The family's culture and environment and the child's concept of death

Little research is yet available to indicate how a child's concept of death will be affected by the family's culture and environment. However, there is a recurrent theme in the death literature that the way in which parents and others discuss death within the family will have a significant effect on the child's developing concept. Virtually all the literature encourages openness and honesty, and opportunity for the child to talk about the subject. Some predictions that could be tested by research can be attempted based on knowledge already available about how various cultures handle serious illness, dying, death, and mourning (see Table 4 in Chapter 19.4). For instance, the Buddhist regards illness and death as a natural part of life, whereas the Aboriginal regards death as punishment or resulting from evil magic. It is likely that the Buddhist child would have a different concept of death from that of the Aboriginal child, and would be less afraid of it and accept it more as a part of life. Some cultures, for example that of the Lebanese, are rich in mourning rituals but have a closed attitude to discussion of death. It is not yet known how Lebanese children who attend a relative's funeral or who are seriously ill themselves deal with the sudden massive displays of emotion that they witness without the benefit of discussion with other members of the family.

Guidelines for working with the dying child

Clearly, seriously ill and dying children are much more aware of their illness and prognosis than it is comfortable to acknowledge. They are known to harbour anxiety about their situation and are helped by the provision of age-appropriate information. Equipped with this knowledge, the caregiver can certainly be more attentive to the child's verbal and non-verbal communications and seek, where possible, to lessen the child's anxiety.

The emotional needs of the dying child are as follows:

- those of all children regardless of health;
- those arising from the child's reaction to illness and admission to hospital;
- those arising from the child's concept of death.

The following guidelines[29] can be used to help seriously ill children to communicate the inner experiences related to their illness.

1. Before proceeding with communication, ascertain the child's own perception of the situation, taking into account his or her developmental level and experience.
2. Understand the child's symbolic language. Children often experience emotions without being able to put them into concepts or words, and young children can use symbolic language to communicate their worries.
3. Clarify reality and dispel fantasy. Children often have difficulty distinguishing between reality and fantasy and between actions and thoughts. A common fantasy of sick children is that of being responsible for the illness. Thus admission to hospital and medical procedures are interpreted as punishment.
4. Encourage the expression of feelings. When children are allowed to express their anger, sadness, and anxiety, they are able to examine these feelings, place them in perspective, and gain control over them.

5. Promote self-esteem through mastery. The self-esteem of the child with cancer is threatened by pain, frustration, deprivation, changes in body image, and the possibility of death. As a result, his or her school attendance and peer relationships may both suffer. School is the ideal setting in which to encourage the child to communicate about his or her illness in a way that will promote self-esteem through mastery.

6. When approaching the child with cancer, make no assumptions about what the situation will entail. Be open to what each encounter can teach. Do not underestimate the child's ability to master life's challenges creatively and with humour and dignity.

A child who asks 'Am I going to die?' has already picked the person to ask. The wisest and best response is to be honest and confirm that such is the case. How one replies and the words one uses will vary greatly because the details of each child's situation and management, and the relationship with the caregiver asked the question, make every case unique. The important thing is to be honest, confirm that the answer to the question is 'yes', and stay with the child to deal with whatever specific concerns he or she may mention next. Like adults, children are concerned that they will be comfortable, safe, and not alone.

Recommendations for caregivers working with a terminally ill child are referred to in Table 1 and are also discussed in Chapter 19.4.

Methods of assessing children's psychological adaptation

Art therapy and music therapy are both forms of expressive therapy that can be used for effective communication by the child. Both can also be used as effective measures of the child's psychological adaptation.

Art therapy

Children are natural artists and can express themselves with few inhibitions. The child's art may communicate what words cannot. While the therapist needs to understand the images produced by children, interpretations of their work are most reliable when provided by the children themselves.

Art therapy can be used to rechannel acting-out behaviour and aggression, provide periods of normality in the midst of frequent examinations, tests, and treatments, and provide opportunity for the children's expressions of creativity. Group art therapy provides opportunities for socializing and communication with peers and for countering feelings of withdrawal or isolation.

The art work of terminally ill children has been found to share common features and to follow particular trends. Objects and forms tend to move towards the upper left quadrant of a page as death approaches. An unusual treatment of a body area has corresponded to new areas of disease unsuspected by the medical staff. Pictures depicting extreme weather conditions have been noted frequently in the art work of terminally ill children: clouds, heavy rain, or snow (often with a brightly shining sun nearby) are said to indicate feelings of anxiety or of being overwhelmed. There may also be a decreased selection of bright colours as the disease progresses, reflecting decreased physical stamina and emotional energy. The reader is referred to a recent report[30] for a more detailed account of this useful medium for communication and assessment.

Music therapy

Music therapy is also effective in uncovering and working through fears and anxieties related to death and mourning, and it offers the opportunity for creative acts. As illustrated by the case histories of one therapist working with children terminally ill with cancer,[31] music therapy may energize or relax, promote thought or distract, and provide an opportunity for expression. A variety of music therapy techniques, including song writing and selection, lyric substitution, improvisation, and guided imagery, can all be used to encourage the child to release his or her fears through a creative act. Music may facilitate a therapeutic relationship, which in turn may supply the security and trust that enables the child to let go of his or her fears. Concerns that are too threatening to be talked about openly can be indirectly expressed during music therapy activities.

The use of music therapy in paediatric settings is currently confined largely to the United States but, with the continuing encouragement of a small but growing number of advocates in other countries,[32] its application and acceptance in this field will extend elsewhere (see Chapter 12.6).

Books about death for adults and children

There are a wide variety of books dealing with death in both fiction and non-fiction for children and parents, including such well-known works as *Litle Women* by L.M. Alcott and *Charlotte's Web* by E.B. White. There is some difference of opinion about the usefulness of such material for working with children.[33-36] Such books are useful when they assist parents or health professionals in explaining aspects of death to a questioning child, particularly when they allow a dialogue on the subject to develop between parent and child. Lists of recommended titles for adults and children appear in Tables 5 and 6.

The terminally ill child at school

As a result of their illness, children with cancer will have acquired concepts and experiences of pain, loss, and grief which will have changed them and distinguish them from their peers. Children who receive treatment for cancer encounter a loss of self-esteem. Their unusual situation requires them to deal with new and significant issues, occasionally with some anxiety, so that they may have less attention and energy for the day-to-day matters of school. They will be less assertive. They will be more reluctant than their healthy peers to attempt new concepts in which failure is possible because of the risk of losing more self-esteem through failure. Schooling for these children should always start out from areas and levels of competence in which they feel absolutely comfortable.[37]

Children who are terminally ill with cancer may be continuing with further treatment, and in many cases will remain well enough to attend school for many months. Even though they may be in an advanced stage of their disease, it is very important for their self-esteem and sense of mastery over a deteriorating situation to continue to attend school when they wish to, if only for a few hours a day.

An explanation to the class about the child's illness will have been given by a member of the treatment team earlier in the course of the illness, usually soon after the diagnosis. At the outset,

Table 5 Books for adults about death

Adams DW. *Childhood Malignancy: The Psychosocial Care of the Child and his Family.* Springfield, IL: C.C. Thomas, 1979

Adams DW, Deveau EJ. *Coping with Childhood Cancer—Where Do We Go From Here?* 3rd edn. Hamilton, Ont: Kinbridge, 1993

Deitrick R, Armstrong-Dailey A. *Approaching Grief* (pamphlet). Children's Hospice International, 1850 M Street, NW, Suite 900, Washington, DC 20036 USA

Grollman EA. *Talking About Death: A Dialogue between Parent and Child*. Boston, MA: Beacon Press, 1976

Martinson IM. *Home Care for the Dying Child: Professional and Family Perspectives*. New York: Appleton-Century-Crofts, 1976

McKissock M. *Coping with Grief*. Australian Broadcasting Corporation Box 8888, Crows Nest, NSW, 2065, Australia

Miles MS. *The Grief of Parents*. Privately printed, 1978. Available from Compassionate Friends Inc., PO Box 1347, Oak Brook, IL 60521, USA

Schiff HS. *The Bereaved Parent*. New York: Crown Publishers, 1977

Schulman JL. *Coping with Tragedy: Successfully Facing the Problem of a Seriously Ill Child*. Chicago: Follett, 1976.

Sherman M. *The Leukemic Child.* Publication NIH 76–863. Washington DC: US Department of Health, Education & Welfare, 1976

Stephens S. *Death Comes Home*. New York: Morehouse-Barlow, 1973.

Wass H, Corr CA, eds. *Helping Children Cope with Death: Guidelines and Resources*. 2nd edn. Washington, DC: Hemisphere, 1984

Wells R. *Helping Children Cope with Grief—Facing a Death in the Family*. London: Sheldon Press, 1988

Zagdanski D. *Something I've Never Felt Before—How Teenagers Cope with Grief*. Melbourne: Hill of Content Press, 1990

classmates are most frequently concerned about whether or not they can catch the disease from the patient.

In the event of the child becoming terminally ill, the child's teacher will have to confront and deal with the impending death of the child and the resulting effects on the classmates, other teachers, and students at the school. Under these circumstances, it is wise to have made some preparation beforehand. Discussion at a staff meeting might take place involving other teachers and the principal to examine their attitudes to death and dying. This would enable staff to formulate an appropriate plan which the child's teacher could then implement with the class. The teacher should also confer with the child's parents, who need to be involved in these plans.

The child's treatment team, particularly the hospital school teacher, will liaise with the school and the child's school teachers to maximize his or her educational opportunities. Terminally ill children may wish to be included and need to be treated as normally as possible. A bean chair or similar comfortable support in the corner of the classroom close to the focus of interest may enable such children to enjoy many hours of satisfaction, even though they may not be able to participate actively in all lessons.

Deterioration is usually gradual and death is not expected to occur suddenly or unexpectedly, for example during class. If the terminally ill student deteriorated rapidly or unexpectedly collapsed, there would still be sufficient time to take him or her home or to hospital with the parents and family.

Table 6 Books for children about death

Alcott LM. *Little Women.* Boston: Little, Brown, 1968

Alex M, Alex B. *Grandpa and Me.* Hertford: Lion, 1981

Bernstein JE, Gullo SV. *When People Die.* New York: Dutton, 1977

Fassler J. *My Grandpa Died Today.* New York: Human Sciences Press, 1971

Grollman EA. *Talking About Death—A Dialogue Between Parent and Child*. Boston, MA: Beacon Press, 1976

White EB. *Charlotte's Web*. New York: Harper & Row, 1952

Zim H, Bleeker S. *Life and Death*. New York: Morrow, 1970

Saying goodbye: the child's preparation for death

Children who are seriously or terminally ill will usually take steps to put their affairs in order. During her preparation for a mismatched bone marrow transplant, one of the author's patients completed tapestries bearing personal notes of thanks for the author and another doctor. These were presented after her death by her parents, who reported that she had discussed her funeral with her friends, requesting that her two closest girlfriends sing a favoured hymn.

Another patient, a teenage boy dying of progressive non-Hodgkin's lymphoma, summoned all the ward staff to his room to say goodbye to each. Later, with many of his friends present, he bequeathed one of his possessions to each, including his most cherished possession, a CB radio.

The following example from the author's department provides even more striking evidence of preparation for and acceptance of imminent death.

Case history

Patient A had acute myeloid leukaemia which was diagnosed in 1982 when she was aged 13. Following relapse in January 1984, she proceeded to a mismatched bone marrow transplant in April 1984, with her mother as the donor. She died 5 weeks after the transplant. A's mother reported that, during her last few months, A spoke more about the possibility of death and of the need to plan for the disposal of her material possessions. After her relapse she frequently spoke of not wanting to die, mainly confiding her thoughts to her mother. She attended three healing masses and was noted to have fewer periods of depression afterwards. One of the pages from her notebook on which she recorded her observations of what she thought death would be like, is reproduced with the family's permission in Fig. 2.A's mother reported A's great self-control as she planned for the possibility of not surviving the transplant. She asked that the family have a holiday together before the transplant. She asked if she owned her bedroom furniture and her piano, and about her right to make a will. Those attending her funeral were to wear bright colours. The service was to be held in her school chapel and the madrigal group of which she was a member was to

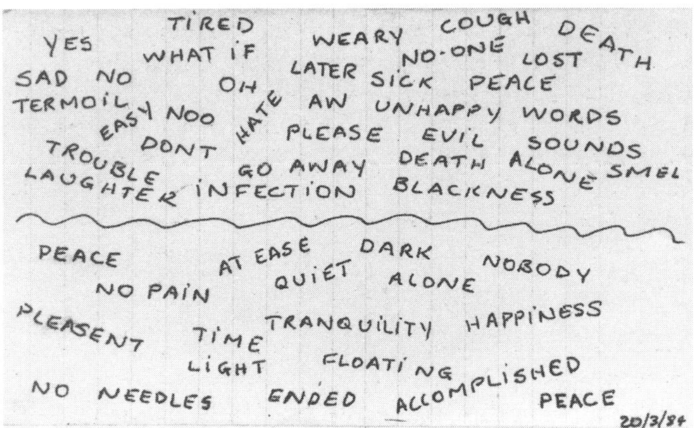

Fig. 2 A page from A's notebook recording her own observations of what she thought death would be like (reproduced with her parents' permission).

sing a favourite hymn. A nominated a white coffin, named the clothing for her burial ('not a nightie, under any circumstances'), and asked that a family photograph, a Bible, and her rosary beads be placed in her coffin. She purchased a remembrance gift for her parents and wrote them a personal letter. She recorded herself playing a special piece of music on the piano. She asked her parents not to remain sad, to be kind and loving to each other, and always to stay together.

These examples show that dying children may respond in a manner well beyond their years.

The dying child's premonition of imminent death

Terminally ill children often know when they are about to die and may even share this information with their parents.

One of the author's patients, a 9-year-old boy, died suddenly shortly after the abrupt onset of severe interstitial pneumonitis 8 months after bone marrow transplant. His family owned one of a number of shops clustered in a marina, and their son was well known to the other tenants. After he had died, the parents learnt that he had spent time chatting with each and every tenant in the marina on the day before his death.

Another of the author's patients, a 5-year-old boy with terminal acute lymphoblastic leukaemia, died at home. On the night that he died, he came into his parents' bedroom. He explained that he did not quite know what to say to them and, instead, sang a familiar children's song *I can sing a rainbow*.[38]

Needing permission to die

Young people who are dying may linger close to death for prolonged periods. They may simply need permission from their loved ones to die and will often die promptly when such permission is given. One of the author's patients, an 11-year-old boy with osteogenic sarcoma, was dying at home after a 5-year illness. Throughout his illness, he had demonstrated a notable tenacity to survive and willingness to endure continuing and painful treatment as long as it entailed some hope for further quality survival. After his death, his father reported that as the boy's death drew close, he lingered on in a coma for more than 7 days. An Aboriginal community nurse who was caring for the patient spoke with his father, informing him that the boy needed his parents' permission to die. The father and mother ushered the boy's grandmother and other relatives out of his room, sat down alone by the boy's bed, spoke to him of their love for him, and gave him their permission to die. The boy died peacefully a few hours later.

Future prospects in paediatric palliative care

One can anticipate further studies in the near future on the psychological aspects of death and dying in both well and sick children. The challenge for the caregiver will be to keep abreast of current thought and to respond to new principles of care as they become validated.

An area of current research that may become of increasing relevance to paediatrics concerns a relatively new field known as psychoneuroimmunology.

Psychoneuroimmunology: the physiological effects of wish-granting

Severe psychological stress can produce a measurable abnormality in immune function.[39] A recent review of the effects of stress on the immune system illustrates the variety of currently understood mechanisms by which stress affects most, if not all, neuroendocrine functions.[40] An inaugural international congress was held in mid-1990.[41]

In related developments, many children who are chronically or terminally ill have now participated in a wish-granting experience with the assistance of benevolent wish-granting organizations such as the Starlight Foundation. Children enrolled in such programmes are granted one of three wishes that they have settled on in advance. Common wishes are to meet someone famous, to visit a special place, or to receive a sought-after gift. It is not known whether this is simply palliative or has a therapeutic effect. It seems relevant that a dying child may 'set a date' and look forward to a significant event such as a birthday or special trip, with a slowing of deterioration during that time.

Psychoneuroimmunology seeks to evaluate possible physiological effects of participating in such an experience. One hypothesis is that the wish-granting experience may influence the patient's immune system and possibly even favourably influence the course of the patient's disease. Clearly, evaluation of well-controlled and relevant studies will be required to establish this new and intriguing field. Diseases with immunological implications, such as cancer, and autoimmune processes, such as rheumatoid arthritis, asthma, and certain kidney diseases, would be the obvious target for psychoneuroimmunology research.[42]

Conclusion: implications for staff

Staff caring for terminally ill children face similar stresses to those confronted by the family. Because the family's outlook is greatly influenced by the personality and reactions of the staff, a special degree of maturity and caring is required. Staff need to recognize their own limitations and the importance of the support which an interdisciplinary team approach can offer. Staff need to be realistic in the goals that they set and use supports available to them. Regular periods of leave, and interests and commitments outside the workplace, will all help to ensure a continuing effective level of care to those in need.

It is often asked how one could work in such an emotionally charged field, and the response (as most who work in this field will know) is that one enjoys the work and finds working with children such as these and their families rewarding, fascinating, frequently unpredictable, never boring, and always a privilege.

References

1. Piaget J, Inhelder B. *The Psychology of the Child*. Translated from the French by Helen Weaver. New York: Basic Books, 1969.
2. Singer D, Revenson T. *A Piaget Primer: How a Child Thinks*. New York: Universities Press, 1978.
3. Rando TA. *Grief, Dying and Death: Clinical Interventions for Caregivers*. Champaign, IL: Research Press, 1984:385–91.
4. Wass H. Concepts of death: a developmental perspective. In: Wass H, Corr CA, eds. *Childhood and Death*. Washington, DC, DC: Hemisphere, 1984:4,18.
5. Nagy M. The child's theories concerning death. *Journal of Genetic Psychology*, 1948; **73**:3–27.
6. Anthony S. *The Discovery of Death in Childhood and After*. New York: Basic Books, 1972.
7. Kane B. Children's concepts of death. *Journal of Genetic Psychology*, 1979; **134**:141–53.
8. Speece MW, Brent SB. Children's understanding of death: a review of three components of a death concept. *Child Development*, 1984; **55**:1671–86.
9. Lansdown R, Benjamin G. The development of the concept of death in children aged 5–9 years. *Child: Care, Health and Development*, 1985; **11**:13–20.
10. Schonfeld D. Crisis intervention for bereavement support: a model of intervention in the children's school. *Clinical Pediatrics*, 1989; **28**:29.
11. Schonfeld DJ, Kappelman M. The impact of school-based education on the young child's understanding of death. *Developmental and Behavioural Pediatrics*, 1990; **11**:247–52.
12. Wass H, Cason L. Fears and anxieties about death. In: Wass H, Corr CA, eds. *Childhood and Death*. Washington, DC, DC: Hemisphere, 1984:25–45.
13. Anthony S. *The Discovery of Death in Childhood and After*. New York: Basic Books, 1972:163–5.
14. McNeil J. Young mothers' communication about death with their children. *Death Education*, 1983; **6**:323–39.
15. Knudson AG, Natterson JM. Participation of parents in the hospital care of their fatally ill children. *Pediatrics*, 1960; **26**:482–90.
16. Morrissey JR. Death anxiety in children with a fatal illness. In Parad HJ, ed. *Crisis Intervention*. New York: Family Service Association of America, 1965:324–38.
17. Natterson JM, Knudson AG. Observations concerning fear of death in fatally ill children and their mothers. *Psychosomatic Medicine*, 1960; **22**:456–65.
18. Richmond JB, Waisman HA. Psychologic aspects of management of children with malignant diseases. *American Journal of Diseases of Children*, 1955; **89**:42–7.
19. Vernick J and Karon M. Who's afraid of death on a leukemia ward? *American Journal of Diseases of Children*, 1965; **109**:393–7.
20. Karon M, Vernick J. An approach to the emotional support of fatally ill children. *Clinical Pediatrics*, 1968; **7**:274–80.
21. Waechter EH. Children's awareness of fatal illness. *American Journal of Nursing*, 1971; **71**:1168–72.
22. Bluebond-Langner, M. *The Private Worlds of Dying Children*. Princeton, NJ:Princeton University Press, 1978.
23. Sarason SB *et al*. *Anxiety in Elementary School Children*. New York: Wiley, 1960.
24. Murray, HA. *Thematic Apperception Test*. Cambridge, MA: Harvard University Press, 1943.
25. Glaser B, Strauss A. *Awareness of Dying: A Study of Social Interaction*. Chicago: Aldine, 1965.
26. Spinetta JJ, Rigler D, Karon M. Personal space as a measure of a dying child's sense of isolation. *Journal of Consulting and Clinical Psychology*, 1974; **42**:751–6.
27. Spinetta JJ, Rigler D, Karon M. Anxiety in the dying child. *Pediatrics*, 1973; **52**:841–5.
28. Clunies-Ross C, Lansdown R. Concepts of death, illness and isolation found in children with leukaemia. *Child: Care, Health and Development*, 1988; **14**:373–86.
29. Adams-Greenly M. Helping children communicate about serious illness and death. *Journal of Psychosocial Oncology*, 1984; **2**(2):61–72.
30. Schmitt BB, Guzzino MH. Expressive therapy with children in crisis: a new avenue of communication. In: Corr CA, Corr DM, eds. *Hospice Approaches to Pediatric Care*. New York: Springer, 1985:155–77.
31. Fagen TS. Music therapy in the treatment of anxiety and fear in terminal pediatric patients. *Music Therapy: Journal of the Atnerican Association for Music Therapy*, 1982; **2**:13–23.
32. Bright R. *Grieving: A Handbook for Those who Care*. St. Louis MO: MMB Music, 1986.
33. Corr CA: Books for adults. In: Wass H, Corr CA, eds. *Childhood and Death*. Washington, DC: Hemisphere, 1984:367–71.
34. Wass H. Books for children. In: Wass H, Corr CA, eds. *Childhood and Death*. Washington, DC: Hemisphere, 1984:373–6.
35. Lamers E. Books for adolescents. In: Corr CA, McNeil JN, eds. *Adolescence and Death*. New York: Springer, 1986:233–42.
36. Aradire C. Books for children about death. *Pediatrics*, 1976; **57**:372.
37. Stevens MM. Cancer in childhood. In Stevens MM, Rayner J, Turnell R, Smith T, Piper D, Graham B, eds. *Physical as Anything: Collaborative Support for Students with Physical Disabilities and Medical Conditions*. Sydney: New South Wales Department of School Education, 1996.
38. Stevens M. Palliative care in paediatrics. *Cancer Forum*, 1989; **13**:21–5.
39. Bartrop RW, Luckhurst E, Lazarus L, Kiloh LG, Penny R. Depressed lymphocyte function after bereavement. *Lancet*, 1977; **i**:834–6.
40. Khansari DN, Anthony JM, Faith RE. Effects of stress on the immune system. *Immunology Today*, 1990; **11**:170–5.
41. Spector NH. Neuroimmunomodulation takes off. *Immunology Today*, 1990; **11**:381–3.
42. Weiner LP, personal communication.

Bibliography

Anthony S. *The Discovery of Death in Childhood and After*. New York: Basic Books, 1972.

Bluebond-Langner M. *The Private Worlds of Dying Children*. Princeton, NJ: Princeton University Press, 1978.

Binger CM, Ablin AR *et al*. Childhood leukemia: emotional impact on patient and family. *New England Journal of Medicine*, 1969;**280**:414–18.

Brent D. A death in the family: the pediatrician's role. *Pediatrics*, 1983; **72**:645–51.

Bright R. *Grieving: A Handbook for Those Who Care*. St. Louis, MO: MMB Music, 1986.

Clunies-Ross C, Lansdown R. Concepts of death, illness and isolation found in children with leukaemia. *Child: Care, Health and Development,* 1988; **14**:373–86.

Corr CA, Corr DM, eds. *Hospice Approaches to Pediatric Care.* New York: Springer, 1985:219–40.

Foley GV, Whittam EH. Care of the child dying of cancer: Part I. *CA–A Cancer Journal for Clinicians,* 1990; **40**:327–54.

Lansdown R, Benjamin G. The development of the concept of death in children aged 5–9 years. *Child: Care, Health and Development,* 1985; **11**:13–20.

Nagy M. The child's theories concerning death. *Journal of Genetic Psychology,* 1948; **73**:3–27.

Parkes CM. *Bereavement: Studies of Grief in Adult Life.* London: Tavistock, 1972.

Pettle MSA, Lansdown RG. Adjustment to the death of a sibling. *Archives of Disease in Childhood,* 1986; **61**:278–83.

Piaget J, Inhelder B. *The Psychology of the Child.* Translated from the French by Helen Weaver. New York: Basic Books, 1969.

Raphael B. *The Anatomy qf Bereavement.* New York: Basic Books, 1983.

Rando TA. *Grief,Dying and Death: Clinical Interventions for Caregivers.* Champaign, IL: Research Press, 1984:179.

Vernick J, Karon M. Who's afraid of death on a leukemia ward? *American Journal of Diseases of Children,* 1965; **109**:393–97.

Wass H, Corr CA, eds. *Childhood and Death.* Washington, DC: Hemisphere, 1984:25–45.

19.4 Care of the dying child and adolescent: family adjustment and support

Michael M. Stevens

This chapter discusses the family's adjustment during the experience of coping with the child's illness and impending death, and provides some suggestions for support by caregivers.

Phases of the child's illness and the family's adjustment

There are various phases in the child's illness. For a child who develops cancer, the first begins at diagnosis and extends through the phase of treatment, which is almost always curative in intent. This phase ends either with completion of therapy and follow-up of the presumably cured survivor, or with the passage through one or more relapses. If relapse occurs, therapy may be intensified with cure still the goal. If the disease progresses despite further therapy, a decision will become necessary to cease curative therapy and alter the emphasis of therapy from cure to palliation. The family then experiences a passage into palliative care which extends on to the child's death and beyond.

The family's successful transition to palliative care is strongly affected by its experiences earlier in the child's management. The caregiver's attention to earlier aspects of the family's management does much to help the family cope with the child's palliative care and death. Hence, an evaluation of the family's experience will be given, along with suggestions for support in each phase.

The family can be regarded as a system of parts or components. Like any system, the family attempts to maintain a degree of balance and equilibrium, and each will have distinct patterns of communication, behaviour, roles, rules, and expectations. A family may be seen as an open system if family members have full freedom to communicate, boundaries between family members are flexible, and family rules are up to date and promote growth. In contrast, a family may be seen as a closed system if communication is restricted or indirect, boundaries are enmeshed, members are overly involved with and dependent on one another, and rules are too inflexible to allow change or permit growth.[1] Clearly, the experiences that each family encounters and the challenges generated will vary considerably.

Foundations for effective palliative care: the family's early experience

The quality of the family's experience in the earliest phase of the child's illness, in the first few weeks after diagnosis, is particularly important in determining later adjustment to palliative care, should that become necessary.

The initial treatment goals set for a child with cancer are almost always curative in intent. Considerable advances in surgery, radiotherapy, and particularly chemotherapy have occurred over the last 40 years. The advent of multi-institutional randomized trials of therapy for paediatric cancer in the United Kingdom, the United States, and elsewhere has led to encouraging improvements in the cure rate for many types of childhood cancer. About 60 per cent of children who develop the most common type of childhood cancer, acute lymphoblastic leukaemia, will be cured with current conventional therapy. Over 80 per cent of children who develop some of the most common paediatric solid tumours, including localized Wilms' tumour, localized non-Hodgkin's lymphoma, and Hodgkin's disease, will also be cured with current therapy. The outlook for others with less common types of leukaemia, certain cerebral tumours, disseminated neuroblastoma, and other solid tumours where detectable spread has occurred prior to diagnosis remains less favourable. Overall, about 75 per cent of today's young patients with malignant disease will be cured. The remainder will ultimately die of their disease and need palliative care.

At diagnosis the child should be referred to a paediatric institution offering skilled multimodal cancer therapy. Occasionally children may be very ill at the time of diagnosis and may almost immediately enter the terminal phase. However, for most children the emphasis of initial therapy will be strongly directed towards cure.

Communicating with the child's parents at diagnosis: foundation for successful palliative care

On receiving the diagnosis the child's parents always assume the worst, that their child is certainly going to die and soon. One of the goals of the initial consultations with the child's paediatrician and other significant caregivers is to readjust the parents' expectations to a more hopeful level in keeping with the child's actual prognosis.

However, there are other equally important goals in these initial consultations. Effective communication with the child's parents in the days after diagnosis is vital in laying the foundation for effective palliative care later, should that become necessary. If information, friendly encouragement, practical support, and hope have been made freely available to the family by the treatment team from the time of diagnosis, parents will be much more likely to cope successfully with palliative care than if they feel uninformed, misunderstood, and unsupported.

In interviews of 20 families of children who died of leukaemia in the mid-1960s, many of the parents described the events at diagnosis as the hardest blow they had to bear throughout the course of the child's illness. All families expressed appreciation for the frankness and honesty of the initial discussions with the treatment team, and eight specifically singled them out as one of the major sources of help.[2] Disagreements and misunderstandings arising from poor communication between paediatric patients with leukaemia, their parents, and physicians may be responsible for seemingly unusual or maladaptive coping by patients or families.[3]

The diagnosis of cancer in a child is a crisis for the child and the family. The parents will usually be stunned and disbelieving at the outset, and there will be an initial period of shock, confusion, and numbness. The parents will describe a feeling of being overwhelmed by the situation, or of feeling unable to function. There may be denial of the diagnosis, or intellectual acceptance of the diagnosis without any emotional release.

As the initial shock declines, a progressive testing of reality occurs. This is usually accompanied by feelings of anger, guilt, sadness, and depression. With no explanation of the cause of the child's cancer forthcoming, the parents may blame themselves or each other for a failure of some sort. They may hold themselves responsible by having 'passed the disease on' to the child. This will not be so except in cases of hereditary retinoblastoma or other rare family cancer syndromes. There is often guilt over a perceived delay in diagnosis and a sentiment that the illness would not have occurred had they sought attention earlier. They may also fear for the child's siblings or even themselves, lest they develop the same illness. There is a definite similarity between these early reactions at diagnosis and those experienced in the early phases of bereavement.

Effective communication with parents under these circumstances is always difficult and may fail even in skilled hands. Pointers to good communication early in therapy are provided in Table 1. As the child's therapy progresses and the parents meet more caregivers and other families who corroborate what the family has been told, parents develop trust in the treatment team and willingly co-operate. Longer-term pointers for good communication with parents are also provided in Table 1. Pointers for good communication with adolescents with cancer are provided later in this chapter.

Rarely, an assessment of the child's initial outlook (e.g. the presence of irreversible paralysis due to spinal metastases from disseminated rhabdomyosarcoma involving additional distant sites) may indicate that therapy is best not undertaken and a programme of palliative care adopted immediately. This requires that the treatment team not only develop an effective relationship with the child's family immediately but also move directly to the transition phase to palliative care.

Occasionally, a child may have a favourable prognosis, but the family will steadfastly refuse consent for potentially curative therapy. One has the option of adopting legal means to displace the parents' right to withhold consent. A decision about such action cannot be taken until the motives for the parents' actions have been discussed fully with them and an objective appraisal made of the child's prognosis and anticipated quality of life during therapy. One may decide that the treatment is in the child's best interests,

Table 1 Pointers to good communication with parents of children with cancer[4]

Ensure that both parents are present for the initial consultation. This recognizes the importance of both parents and makes it less likely that one partner will misinterpret information.

Interview parents in a quiet, comfortable room, with everyone seated.

During important discussions, allow the parents to include a close friend or relative, who may recall information that parents forget.

Have another member of the caregiving team, e.g. the nurse, present to help identify areas for discussion.

Give parents a clear description of their child's illness; identify the illness as cancer; use plain English.

Emphasize that the parents did not cause the disease and could not have prevented it; that the disease is not hereditary (if that is so); that the diagnosis has been made without undue delay; and that effective therapy is available that has cured other children.

Provide enough time so that parents can ask questions and not feel rushed. Encourage them to write down any points of concern as they occur for discussion at the next consultation. Seek feedback about what parents have understood from each consultation.

On receiving the diagnosis, parents always assume that their child is going to die, and soon. Aim to readjust their expectations to a hopeful level, in keeping with the child's actual outlook.

A written summary or tape-recording of the discussion may be helpful.

With parental approval, involve the child in some of the early discussions to lessen his or her anxiety.

Parents will be shocked initially and even disbelieving, then angry, guilty, and depressed. This limits their ability to absorb and retain information. Repeat information patiently over several consultations.

In the beginning, do not provide detailed technical information that the family may misunderstand or forget.

At an early stage, spend time with the patient's siblings and grandparents and liaise with the child's school to help allay anxiety and reduce family members' stress.

Have the family meet a child with a similar diagnosis who has done well.

Longer-term pointers

Be easy to contact by parents.

A patient-held medical record[5] provides the family with readily accessible information about their child's progress.

Regular seminars, support meetings, and newsletters for parents of surviving and deceased patients improve parents' knowledge and help them feel supported.

Have parents attending the treatment centre elect a liaison committee to assist in optimal patient management. The liaison committee is a group of elected members of the parent body who act as conductors of information between the oncology staff and the patients' families. This is achieved through a quarterly magazine, an annual parents' seminar day, casual wine and cheese nights in different parts of the city, and meetings with the oncology staff during which the committee can act as parent advocates.

Always allow parents hope, no matter how poor the outlook. Support the family in their current hope and help them maintain a realistic focus on what their child can still do.

although the consequences of such action on the family's relationship with the treatment team may be adverse (see Chapter 19.8).

Grandparents, siblings, and the child's school at diagnosis

The child's grandparents, brothers and sisters, family friends, and school will all be deeply disturbed by the diagnosis.

In one study of families' adaptation to a child's final illness, half the families studied considered that one or both sets of grandparents had become a burden or hindrance, but in many other families the grandparents offered considerable support. Negative interactions reflected to a considerable extent past relations between parents and grandparents.[2]

Grandparents benefit considerably from an early consultation with the child's physician, undertaken with the parents' consent, soon after diagnosis. This allows any misconceptions or irrational guilt to be dealt with. The grandparents may subsequently become closely involved in the day-to-day care of their grandchild and thus provide support and practical assistance to the parents. Those grandparents who have coped well during the child's illness will also cope more successfully with bereavement after the child's death.

The caregiving team must pay special attention to the welfare of the sick child's siblings. A number of studies have documented that brothers and sisters of a seriously ill child undergo significant anxieties and stresses during the child's illness. Not only do they face the potential loss of their sibling, but also the loss of their family as they have known it and the loss of their parents' attention. This may engender feelings of being rejected by the parents and also resentment towards the dying child.

A study[6] of school-aged patients from 71 families attending a paediatric oncology clinic and their healthy siblings aged 6 to 16 years revealed that siblings of children with cancer have the same significant anxieties, fears for their own health, social isolation, and other stresses once thought to be peculiar to the patients themselves. The siblings' anxiety about their own health frequently found expression in physical symptoms. The siblings felt very isolated from their parents, from other family members, and from friends. Divisions in the family were caused by the patient's hospital admissions accompanied by the mother, while the father attempted to cope at home and with job responsibilities. The siblings were frequently found to be left at home, alone, worried, and cut off from reassurance and support. Despite the siblings' isolation and relative neglect, they were reluctant to express anger or negative feelings towards other family members.

Healthy adaptation for siblings would be encouraged by allowing them to participate in conferences with the physician, by directing parents' attention to their needs, and by encouraging them to visit the ward whenever the patient is in hospital.

The welfare of siblings of the dying child is discussed again later in this chapter.

Liaison with the child's school soon after diagnosis assists the family in re-establishing some degree of equilibrium during therapy. Ideally, with the parents' permission, a member of the treatment team should visit the school and provide the school's staff with relevant information about the child's illness and treatment. Precautions helpful to the child's therapy can be emphasized, such as the importance of minimizing exposure to varicella or morbilli, which may be lethal to the immunocompromised patient on chemotherapy. The child's classmates can be reassured, and arrangements can be made with the hospital's school for work to be sent to the hospital or home and for selected classmates to visit the child in hospital. Educational resources providing information about the child's illness and its treatment should be available to the parents[7] and the school.[8]

These measures will help to alleviate the anxiety of the child and family and assist their attempts to regain control and some degree of normality in their day-to-day life.

Recognizing the family at risk

Families will be encountered that for one reason or another experience significant difficulties during the child's illness, for example families already coping with physically or intellectually handicapped children, single-parent families, families where parents are separating at the time of the child's diagnosis, and families struggling because of financial difficulties, unemployment, or cultural or language difficulties.

Such families require extra help at diagnosis and during therapy to lessen the likelihood of additional crises other than those unavoidably linked to the child's diagnosis and treatment. Excessive criticism of health professionals already encountered earlier in the child's management indicates poor adjustment and the need for additional support. The family that places unreasonable demands on the treatment team needs to be recognized since compliance with all the family's requests may lead to conflict later. Some early agreement about level of service should be tactfully negotiated with such families in order to avoid problems.

Parent support groups in the early phases of the child's illness

Convincing documentation that parents of other leukaemic children are a source of support to parents was provided at least 25 years ago[2] and has been confirmed by others.[9,10] The author's team strongly believes in the value of parent support and has fostered the development of parent support groups both for families of children attending for treatment and bereaved families. Families with newly diagnosed children are encouraged to contact these groups and to meet other members at periodic conferences or luncheons held at the hospital specifically for this purpose. Most families find the groups a valuable source of support, information, and practical assistance.

Transition to palliative care

The recognition that a child's leukaemia or cancer is entering a terminal phase after one or more unsuccessfully treated relapses heralds the onset of renewed stress for all concerned. Prior to this, the child will have been receiving chemotherapy and supportive treatment in a planned and methodical attempt at cure. During this time the child's cancer will have been under control and the child will have been reasonably or completely well. The family's shock, grief, and depression present at the time of diagnosis will have eased, although anxiety about the implications of relapse is constantly present in both parents and patients, even in those very long-term survivors already declared cured. Relapse and the eventual advent of palliative care plunges the family into renewed crisis.

All the reactions present at the original diagnosis resurface with heightened intensity, now overshadowed by the loss of hope implicit in relapse. The parents experience feelings of hopelessness and helplessness, coupled with grief, fear, depression, anger, and denial. Parents who constantly dread relapse and terminal care may express some sentiments of relief that the worst has at last occurred.

There is no easy way to convey bad news. All aids to communication employed at diagnosis and discussed previously become more important now. The paediatrician responsible for the child's cancer therapy should accept the responsibility of these painful consultations. One must be honest, frank, gentle, and sympathetic. The last requires a certain degree of empathy and therefore pain for the caregiving team.

Investigational or palliative therapy?

There are several paths to follow for the child who is fatally ill at diagnosis or who has failed curative therapy and is entering a terminal phase.[11]

One basic treatment plan is to give no medical or nursing treatment at all other than to enhance the physical, personal, and social comfort of the dying child. This plan may be very difficult for the treatment team to accept because it implies that the caregivers as well as their treatments have failed. Comfort measures, such as a manageable diet, pain control, and prevention or treatment of skin breakdown, are the only form of medical or nursing treatment provided.

A second plan is for palliative care which places the highest priority on the control of pain in its broadest sense. Certain medications, chemotherapy protocols, irradiation, and even surgery may eventually result in a higher quality of remaining life for the child even though extension of life is not the goal of palliative care. The treatment team must consider carefully the enhanced quality of life after such palliative procedures when measured against their inherent discomfort. Recovery time must not use up long portions of the child's remaining life.

The third and most controversial plan is to administer investigational treatments which offer only a slight chance of cure and very frequently cause a significant increase in the pain and morbidity suffered by the child. This option is the only one that offers any chance at all of cure.

In explaining the implications of the terminal nature of the child's illness, the paediatrician will already have made a judgement that further therapy directed against the underlying cancer is not appropriate. This places a responsibility on the doctor to be fully informed of all recent advances in treatment, particularly those involving investigational agents or techniques of unproven activity against the disease involved. A decision by the child's paediatrician to change to palliative care should only be taken after full discussion of possible treatment options with the other team members. Occasional conflict will arise within the team over whether to proceed with investigational therapy or change to palliative care. While the need for trials of investigational therapy is not disputed, foremost consideration must be given to the anticipated benefits and disadvantages of the proposed therapy for the particular child. The need for a sensible advocate for the child within the treatment team is vital.

Making the transition to palliative care

Surprisingly, most families make the transition from curative to palliative therapy smoothly and effectively, even though it is an extremely demanding time for them. The time taken in earlier phases of the child's management to establish a trusting relationship between the child and family and the staff will be invaluable in helping them through this crisis. The caregiving team can help make this transition more successfully by providing the necessary information and support to assist the family's decisions. Most families are able to retain sufficient equilibrium to deal with the situation effectively. Information is most commonly relayed from the treatment team to the parents, who then convey it to the other members of the family. Maintenance of confidentiality at this stage is even more important than at diagnosis in order to allow the family to retain some control over how widely information is disseminated.

Parents need a careful and sympathetic explanation of the situation including available options for further therapy, so they can participate in the decisions being made. It is necessary that parents, and ultimately the patient and family, adjust to a shift in emphasis from cure to relief of symptoms. In acknowledging that the underlying disease will not be successfully eradicated, the goal of further treatment becomes that of ensuring optimal comfort and quality for each remaining day of the child's life.

The parents must be reassured that treatment failure is not their fault as there will be considerable guilt about previous minor and insignificant non-compliance with medication schedules. An estimate of how long the child is expected to live will be sought and should be provided. This may be only a matter of days when there is rapidly progressing infection or metabolic disturbance, or several months in a well child with a slowly growing tumour. A summary of the plan for the child's management during the terminal phase should be presented to the family and subsequently discussed with them by other members of the treatment team, all of whom play a role in the child's palliative care. Such a plan requires personal knowledge of the individual child.

It is best to inform the parents first without the child and give them time to adjust to the new situation before consulting directly with the child. The patient's brothers and sisters, grandparents, other relatives, and friends are also involved in the crisis. A brother or sister of the patient who has acted as a donor for a bone marrow transplant will face special difficulties, as will single parents and families hampered by cultural or language barriers. Allowance must be made for a wide range of reactions from families of different cultural backgrounds. Such reactions should not be allowed to prejudice the caregiving team's treatment of the child.

Occasionally a family will refuse to accept the transition to palliative care. Such families will continue to insist that 'everything possible be done' and may seek alternative sources of therapy which may be of unproven benefit or even potentially harmful. The best approach is to continue discussing the issues objectively and patiently, emphasizing what is best for the child. The parents in such families may need to confront and acknowledge fears and other negative emotions relating to the potential loss of the child that may have been denied at diagnosis or in earlier phases of treatment.

Communicating with the child

As discussed in the previous section, ill and dying children know a great deal more about their situation than might otherwise be thought. Furthermore, attempts to conceal the situation from them have been proved ineffective and damaging. Dying children invariably know the true situation from their past experiences in the treatment unit. Their own bodies provide strong additional clues that death may be imminent.

Consequently, it is essential to involve the child in at least some of the discussions about further management. With the consent of the parents one should consult directly with children over 5 or 6 years of age at this important phase of their management. A tactful but honest explanation as to why specific therapy is being discontinued should be given and ample opportunity for discussion of the implications provided. Children older than 6 or 7 are often very matter-of-fact in their approach to their own situation.

The child's questions should be answered truthfully. The most difficult questions asked by the child may be directed to the parents or to a trusted member of the team other than the doctor and may be asked at a later time. Again, truthful answers are best. A child who asks a difficult question almost always knows the answer beforehand and is merely seeking confirmation to assess if it is permissible to discuss the subject with the person to whom the question has been directed. Failure to respond openly to such a question because of a fear of not coping deprives the child of a valuable opportunity for communication.

The child's perception and understanding of death will be influenced by chronological age, developmental level, individual personality, past experiences with death and loss, and the family's religious beliefs. It may be difficult for young children to express their fears. In particular they fear separation from parents and loved ones, and sense and respond strongly to the level of anxiety surrounding them. Expressive play with art or music will assist them in working through and expressing their concerns, and they have a continuing need for reassurance and security. In not wishing to discuss painful matters and seemingly putting on a brave front, the child may in fact be seeking to protect the parents from further emotional turmoil for which he or she may feel responsible.

Additional suggestions for helping seriously ill children communicate the inner experiences relating to their illness are given in Chapter 19.3.

Communicating with the siblings

The young patient's brothers and sisters also face emotional difficulties during the terminal period. While grieving for the sick child, they may resent the lack of attention they receive because of the parents' preoccupation with him or her. This may lead to hostility towards the sick child and even a wish for his or her death. Later there may be guilt over these feelings. As with the parents, an opportunity for counselling by the child's doctor or other members of the treatment team to deal with some of these issues prior to the child's death will help to reduce disturbance afterwards.

The adolescent with a life-threatening illness

In times of crisis most adolescents require support to some extent from their parents, but also sufficient freedom to be able to experiment with coping with the challenge by themselves. Their response, typically, is that they want to be loved and supported, but not 'wrapped in cotton wool'.

Adolescents with a life-threatening illness may welcome the support from parents that may have developed during the crisis, yet will feel confused as to how best to be a 'normal adolescent' when an opportunity arises to spend time away from their parents. Rather than confide in their parents, they may prefer to confide in their peer group, particularly with peers who are in a similar situation, about their needs to experiment and for discussion of personal issues.

Much of the usual stress experienced by well adolescents is related to an inevitable struggle with developmental tasks, social changes, and relationships with family and peers. Adolescents with a life-threatening illness must deal not only with these challenges, but also with additional stresses associated with their illness, its treatment, and side-effects of therapy. How those around them react will have a significant effect on how successfully adolescents with a life-threatening illness cope and on their freedom to make their own choices.

Adolescents with a life-threatening illness react to crises occasioned by the normal process of growing up in a similar manner to their well peers. By remembering to consider the reactions and needs of adolescents with a life-threatening illness in the context of normal adolescence, a practical view may be gained of the problems they encounter and of potential solutions. Most terminally ill adolescents are more concerned about how their family and friends will be affected by their death than about themselves. Further, they are not so much afraid of death as of the process of dying. With patient and attentive listening, an accurate understanding is acquired of young persons' perceptions of death and of their own prognosis.

Phases of adolescence: implications of life-threatening illness

Adolescence is arbitrarily divided into early, middle, and late phases. Although in practice the boundaries between these phases may be blurred, some differences between phases are evident in key issues, behaviour, and relationships with peers and in the impact of a life-threatening illness. The characteristics of adolescence and implications of a life-threatening illness in adolescence are summarized in Table 2.

Life-threatening illness and the early adolescent

Early adolescence generally occurs between the ages of 12 and 14 years in girls and 13 and 15 years in boys. This is a time of rapid physical growth and the onset of puberty. Early adolescents focus strongly on the development of their bodies. Membership of a peer group is very important.

Early adolescents with a life-threatening illness are most concerned about the effects of the illness on their physical appearance and mobility. Significant distress is common in adolescents with cancer if treatment results in weight gain, hair loss, scarring, or

Table 2 Characteristics of adolescence and implications of a life-threatening illness in adolescence[a]

Age	Early adolescence	Middle adolescence	Late adolescence
	12–14 years (female) 13–15 years (male)	14–16 years	17–24 years
Key issues and characteristics, focus	Focus on development of body Most pubertal changes occur Rapid physical growth Acceptance by peers Idealism Mood swings, contrariness, stubbornness, temper tantrums Day dreaming	Sexual awakening Emancipation from parents and authority figures Discovery of identity by testing limitations, boundaries Role of peer group increases	Defining and understanding functional roles in life in terms of: Careers Relationships Lifestyles
Social/relationships, behaviour	Skills in abstract thinking improve Foreseeing of consequences, planning for future Physical mobility prominent Energy levels high Appetite increased Social interaction mostly in groups Membership of a peer group very important	Relationships very narcissistic Risk-taking behaviour increases Intense peer interaction Most vulnerable to psychological problems	Increasing financial independence Planning for the future Establishment of permanent relationships Increasing time away from family
Relationships with adults	Parents and other authority figures still mostly respected As part of adjustment to new 'adult' bodies, may assert themselves as adults while still dependent on parents and caregivers Some testing out e.g. with time away from home	Parental relationships strained Separation from family begins Some hero worship	Culmination of separation from family Increasing financial independence Sense of being equal to adults
Relationships with peers	Peers used as standards for measurement of developmental progress and assessment of 'normality' Comparisons of strength and prowess Friendships with same sex generally more important	Interaction with peers increases Questioning increases concerning who are one's friends and one's own identity and value Sexuality and sexual preference of more concern	Increasing experimentation with intimacy outside family
Impact of life-threatening illness	Concerns about physical appearance and mobility Privacy all-important Possible interference with normal cognitive development and learning (school absence, medication, pain, depression, fatigue) Comparison with peers hindered, making self-assessment of normality more difficult Possible lack of acceptance by peers Reliance on parents and other authorities in decision-making Hospitals perceived as very disturbing	Illness particularly threatening and least well tolerated at this stage Compromised sense of autonomy Emancipation from parents and authority figures impeded Interference with attraction of partner Fear of rejection by peers Limited interaction with peers may lead to social withdrawal Dependence on family for companionship and social support Hospitalization, school absences interfere with social relationships and acquisition of social skills Non-compliance with treatment	Absences from work, study Interference with plans for vocation and relationship Difficulties in securing employment and promotion at work Unemployment hinders achieving separation from family and financial independence Discrimination in employment, health cover, and life insurance Loss of financial independence and self-esteem Concerns about fertility and health of offspring

[a]Reprinted from Stevens MM, Dunsmore JC. Adolescents who are living with (a) life-threatening illness. In: Corr CA, Balk DE, eds. *Handbook of Adolescent Death and Bereavement*. New York: Springer Publishing Co. 1996, with permission from the publisher.

similar alterations to their physical appearance, which are perceived as drawing attention to their disability. Because privacy is all-important to early adolescents, large ward rounds are often excruciatingly embarrassing. Being less assertive than older adolescents, their concerns about such issues may go unrecognized.

Most early adolescents are still reliant on authority figures and are content to let parents act on their behalf. They do, however, wish to be involved in decisions and to have opportunities to talk with their doctor on their own. Because many early adolescents are very disturbed by hospitals, the presence of familiar, friendly staff is all-important. Younger adolescents tend to rely on nursing or social work staff and parents to be their advocates, particularly with doctors.

The use of symbolic language is very common in this age group. Frequently, just giving voice to their thoughts reduces their anxiety. Encouraging them to do so will often be beneficial by helping them regain some control over their situation and to feel less overwhelmed. There is no need to force young people to confront their situation. If a carer listens to what is said, a gentle easing into the truth of the situation is possible.

Life-threatening illness and the middle adolescent

This period is defined as approximately 14 to 16 years of age for both females and males. Middle adolescents most commonly focus on attracting a boyfriend or girlfriend, emancipation from parents and authority figures, and increasing interaction with peers.

Middle adolescents with a life-threatening illness are most concerned about the effects the illness will have on their ability to attract a girlfriend or boyfriend, on their emancipation from parents and authority figures, and about being rejected by their peers. Time in hospital, and away from school, can severely interfere with social relationships and the acquisition of social skills. Social standing within a peer group can be threatened. The ability to attract a boyfriend or girlfriend can be reduced if illness or treatment affects the way a young person looks. Being different within a peer group can signal disaster for that adolescent. Fear of rejection by peers can lead to a number of adjustment problems, including a lowering of self-esteem, withdrawal, depression, and acting-out behaviours.

Non-compliance with medical treatments and lifestyle changes is highest in this age group. To young people in this age group, side-effects of treatment may be much more alarming than the threat of death. They understand the threat of death but appear to make choices based on an unrealistic view of their invincibility.

With a life-threatening illness, middle adolescents often find themselves totally dependent on family again. This dependence and accompanying regression reduce self-esteem. A sense of personal autonomy is often compromised by admissions to hospital and frequent trips to clinics and specialists involved in routine treatment. As control issues are so important in middle adolescence, informed consent and open communication with authority figures involved in management is vital.

Life-threatening illness and the late adolescent

This period is defined as approximately 17 to 24 years for both females and males. Significant issues for the late adolescent include defining of careers, permanent relationships and lifestyles, increasing financial independence where this is possible, and separation from family.

Late adolescents with a life-threatening illness are most concerned about the effects of the illness on their plans for career and relationships, and on their lifestyle. Time off work or away from study can interfere with work promotion and academic achievement. This in turn can have ramifications on economic independence and self esteem. Job discrimination, and life insurance and health insurance rejection are also common. Illness and treatment can cause major social disruptions and increase dependence on parents, and thus interfere with the formation of intimate relationships. Some adolescents have to return home after having lived independently for a number of years.

Reproductive capabilities are reduced in some conditions, causing concern in this age group about intimate relationships and having children. Low energy or weakened physical capabilities can interfere with independence, economic security, and social flexibility. Questions from ill adolescents about fertility are common, even in the terminal stages of their illness. Sadness about possible loss of fertility, and loss, therefore, of the chance to live on through their children, can displace sadness over the prospect of death.

Significant losses mourned by adolescents with cancer

Being an adolescent and living with a life-threatening illness involves significant grieving, both at the onset of the illness, during its course, and in its terminal phase. Not all of the losses are related to death or dying. Many are related to the process of having a chronic or debilitating illness. For example, some significant losses mourned by adolescents with cancer are as follows.

Prediagnosis person

Adolescents with a serious illness often find themselves grieving for their former healthy selves. The onset of their illness prevents them from living in the style they enjoyed while well. The sick role makes them different because of feelings of weakness, lack of energy, and physical changes to their bodies. This can lower their standing within their peer group. One young person remarked, 'People don't treat me like the person I used to be.' Spontaneity is reduced and many young people, after diagnosis, question their place in the world, as in 'I wish it could just go back to the way it was.'

Body image

Amputation, hair loss, weight gain, weight loss, and other side-effects of treatment alter the young person's body image at a time when concerns about physical attractiveness and prowess are greatest. Compared with other age groups, the adolescent feels most the unpleasant and upsetting side-effects of radiotherapy and chemotherapy. Adolescents report how upset they felt when their hair fell out. This upset may not be evident to a casual observer at the time because many patients put on a brave front, but the pain of that experience is often expressed for many years. Loss of hair and related side-effects may have an isolating effect on the adolescent, because of the resultant self-imposed restriction on socializing and in some cases, rejection by peers. Use of cosmetic aids such as artificial limbs and wigs only superficially restores the adolescent's composure and confidence; the insult to his or her body image is internal and cannot be restored properly by an external prosthesis.

Health

Young people with a serious illness describe losing the perception by others that as a healthy person one is independent, in control, and not unreasonably vulnerable to physical harm or emotional upset. This altered perception results instead in their being regarded as 'precious'. As one young person said, 'It's the 'wrapped up in cotton wool' syndrome. My parents are paranoid about me catching infections and relapsing. "Don't be too late", they say,

"You'll get sick".' Some continue to experience avoidance by others, including friends and parents of friends, long after treatment is completed because of fears of contagion.

School life

Young people with a life-threatening illness are upset by missing out on developmentally important milestones associated with day-to-day life at school, such as sitting for exams, dating, poking fun at authority figures, and participation in group experimentation with risk behaviour (e.g. smoking, playing truant from school). Young men report the most disturbing losses as being associated with loss of prowess, loss of energy, not being able to take part in sports, and being seen as wimps. Girls experience losses resulting from school absence most strongly in a social context, for example, isolation from their 'group', missing out on the latest gossip, and activities with best friends.

Independence

Most adolescents test out and establish their independence between the ages of 12 and 18 years and attempt to identify their capabilities. The onset of a life-threatening illness during this stage makes it difficult for adolescents to become independent of parents and other authority figures. Ill adolescents are ambivalent about having to depend on parents for even their most basic care (e.g. changing of beds, toileting, washing, dressing, feeding). Considerable anger may be generated by the helplessness they experience over the loss of their independence. Matters are made worse if adolescents are treated unwittingly by staff of paediatric units in the same way as younger children. The dying adolescent's frustration may be taken out on a parent, usually the one that has been constantly at the bedside, by attempting to drive the parent away. If the attempt succeeds, or even seems likely to succeed, there is often an immediate plea for the parent to return.

A young man aged 21 who was dying said, 'I hate to see the sadness in my mother's eyes. She is also not well and yet she tries to do everything for me and fusses over everything like I'm 5 years old again. I want to scream at her but then I get scared she will leave me and no one will care for me then.'

Pre-diagnosis family

Following diagnosis of a life-threatening illness in a young person, family relationships may deteriorate or improve. Life in the family is no longer the same as it used to be. There is often a plea for life to return to the way it was.

Relationships with parents

Adolescent patients are often attempting to deal with feelings of anger and ambivalence about their parents. There is now doubt that eventual independence from the parents will be achieved. There are often concerns about the commitment of time and expense required by their parents, and about the demands placed on their own relationship. Roles within the family are often threatened.

Relationships with siblings

The patient's siblings may experience feelings of hostility and guilt. They may become angry because of all the attention given to their brother or sister and the various secondary gains that this can bring. They may be afraid of developing a similar illness. They may feel guilty, believing they have caused their brother's or sister's cancer because of some crisis which might have occurred at an earlier phase in their family life.

Relationships with girlfriends/boyfriends

Deterioration of the young person's appearance causes embarrassment. Ill adolescents frequently prefer to break off friendships, rather than risk causing their friends embarrassment or being abandoned by them. Their interest in sex appears to be similar to others their age, although those in relapse have commented on missing out on sexual experiences because of their physical appearance and low energy levels. Lack of opportunity for sexual intimacy is often not addressed by parents or caregivers of adolescents with a terminal illness.

Uncertainty about the future may adversely influence the development of a new relationship. The terminally ill young person may choose to break off a relationship with a partner to try and protect the partner from the pain of separation associated with death. Young people with a life-threatening illness do not want to be pitied. Their biggest fear is that someone may stay with them only because of pity.

Certainty about the future

The adolescent has a more mature concept of death and dying than does the younger child, being able to see the permanence of death and the finality of separation which it involves. The terminally ill adolescent mourns the loss of the future as well as of the past. It is in adolescence that life goals are becoming more strongly established in the mind. The adolescent senses this loss when confronting the possibility of death. It is difficult to predict with certainty which patients will be cured of their disease. The adolescent with cancer is left in a limbo of uncertainty about the results of treatment, often for many years after diagnosis and commencement of therapy. 'Living one day at a time' is a common dictum of adolescents with cancer.

Indicators of the future

A sense of worth in adolescence is linked to experiencing milestones along the journey to adulthood. If milestones such as examinations are missed due to illness, the young person's sense of worth may deteriorate. Adolescents who have been given a poor prognosis may experience difficulty in resuming studies after completion of treatment, if they perceive the likely duration of their survival to be limited. Other milestones include planning what one will do after leaving school, planning to have a family, planning for travel, and the attainment of increasing economic independence.

Hope

Young people living with a life-threatening illness have the same developmental needs as well adolescents. Young people facing death require opportunities to develop peer relationships, to experiment with different sides of their personalities, and to interact in the manner of their well peers. Frequently, young people who have been told that they may die soon report that people start to treat them as if they are already dead. As one 18-year-old said, 'They treat me like a non-person. It is as though I am in the coffin already and they are waiting to hammer in the final nails.' Hope becomes an essential ingredient for living successfully for these young people. Their hopes may not necessarily be for a cure or magical recovery, but more often for joy and for success with the challenges of living. One can be very clear about the implications of one's life-threatening illness and still maintain hope. One adolescent had on her bedroom wall, 'Be realistic. Plan for a miracle.'

Implications of life-threatening illnesses other than cancer in adolescence

Many of the implications for management of young people with cancer also apply to the management of young people with life-threatening illnesses other than cancer. However, the need for some modification is evident when specific diseases are discussed.

HIV/AIDS (see Chapter 20.2)

Young people may acquire HIV/AIDS because of sexual activity or, in a relatively much smaller group, by drug misuse or medically acquired HIV/AIDS. Specific factors that further complicate the experience of young people with HIV/AIDS, as compared to other life-threatening illnesses, include the following.

Stigma—community fear and ignorance

The stigma associated with this diagnosis, which is related to community fear and ignorance, adversely colours many of the contacts that the young person has with others who are aware of the diagnosis.

Disclosure

Young gay men often need to disclose their homosexuality, as well as their antibody status, to their parents, siblings, peers, and health-care workers when symptoms of AIDS develop and medical attention is required. There is also a legal requirement to disclose their status to intending sexual partners. This disclosure is frequently met with a very negative response, causes distress to all, and is described by young gay people as 'the double whammy'.[12] Similar distress is also experienced by young people with medically acquired HIV/AIDS.

Communication issues

Young people ill with HIV/AIDS express a fear that they will be treated differently or will be discriminated against by health-care workers because of the diagnosis. This concern commonly arises in the context of communication with the patient about the illness and plans for management.

Appearance and self-esteem

A healthy appearance ('healthiness, looking good, having a healthy body, going to the gym') is considered crucial for self-esteem by young gay people, especially in organized gay communities in urban areas. The adverse effect on appearance both of HIV/AIDS-related illnesses such as Kaposi's sarcoma, and of treatment devices such as central venous catheters and subcutaneous injection portals, results in further social isolation, both from the gay community as well as family and friends.

Internalized guilt and blame

The young person with HIV/AIDS internalizes the homophobic thoughts and prejudices of others, manifested by convictions such as that if only one was not gay, the catastrophe of developing HIV/AIDS would not have happened. As one young gay person said, 'I always knew that because I was gay something like this would happen.'

A poorer prognosis than with cancer

There is much less hope of survival for a young person with a diagnosis of HIV/AIDS than with cancer. One young gay person who was HIV-positive said, 'If only I had cancer then there'd be a chance. With HIV, there's no chance.'

Loss of friends within gay community

The young person with HIV/AIDS experiences repeated bereavements as friends within the gay community (not established through hospital-related contact) die from HIV/AIDS.

There is current concern by providers of health care for young people about the likelihood of an imminent and significant increase in the incidence of HIV/AIDS in young people. This concern is based on research such as that reported in North America[13] and Australia[14] which indicates that the majority of university students have engaged in sexual intercourse by the end of their first year at university, that only a minority practise safe sex, and that a small but disturbing proportion are HIV-positive.

Cystic fibrosis

A diagnosis is commonly established early in childhood. Thus, young people with cystic fibrosis learn at an early age that their life-span is expected to be limited. Problems associated with issues of dependency and of attaining goals in adolescence are experienced, as by young people with cancer. Denial is a common reaction in young patients with cystic fibrosis, evidenced, for example, by non-compliance with physiotherapy, diet, and other important components of long-term therapy.

Severe brain damage

Issues affecting the family may be more significant than those affecting the patient. Families of patients who are vegetative, apparently unresponsive, and totally dependent on them, may exhaust their reserves of energy in caring for such young people. These families will benefit from the patient receiving periodic respite care, to assist them in recharging their spiritual batteries. Families of such patients should be encouraged to remember that the patient may still be able to hear despite being unable to respond, and to continue talking to the patient at the bedside, even if about simple matters, such as what one is doing at that moment. These families may describe being in a dilemma of wanting the patient to die in order to be released, yet experiencing guilt over such feelings. Opportunities are required for these families to work through their anticipatory grieving. Just being able to discuss their feelings will assist them in the grieving process. Others will remain adamant that miracles do happen.

Catastrophic illness with short life-expectancy

When a catastrophic illness (e.g. motor vehicle accident, acute cardiomyopathy, viral meningitis, overwhelming sepsis) occurs in a previously well young patient and death is imminent, issues of honesty with the young patient become important. Young people in this situation are very likely to suspect that they are about to die and deserve honesty from their caregivers to ensure, for example, that something they want to say or have done can be accomplished. Families in this situation are often required to make urgent and painful decisions about treatment or organ donation. Additional support may be required in such a death and also in removal of the deceased patient's body to the mortuary. The after-care of such families is as important as would have been the ongoing care of the young patient, had he or she survived.[15]

The family in palliative care: guidelines for support

As the child's palliative care commences, liaison must occur both with the treatment team and between it and the available support in the community. All members of the treatment team should be informed of the child's continuing condition and the plans for palliative care. Community resources must be mobilized to ensure that much of the child's care can be based at home. This is particularly important for families in isolated areas, where considerable distances exist between the family's home and local caregiving agencies and the palliative treatment team's hospital. As the programme of care commences, the parents will require further education about the ill child, particularly in practical matters such as maintenance of central lines and the nursing and biomedical equipment used in symptom control.

Home care versus hospital care—making the decision

As the emphasis of treatment shifts from cure to palliation and making the best of what time remains, care of the child at home becomes a priority for the family. Returning a terminally ill child to the home will support the family by keeping all its members together and allowing everyone to share in the child's care and provide mutual support. The home care programme needs to be flexible to meet the needs of the individual family. Parents will need reassurance to help them cope with fears of having the child at home. Careful preparation and planning and securing lines of communication usually help allay these fears. The parents and older brothers and sisters will become primary caregivers in the home and will need much support and encouragement from the treatment team.

With the change in emphasis from complex therapy to supportive care, the family's general practitioner may be pleased to become more closely involved in management and to provide much of the emotional support needed. Where possible, regular home visits by members of the treatment team (e.g. the community nurse consultant, the social worker, and the child's oncologist) will help to ensure that care is optimal. Regular telephone contact to discuss day-to-day difficulties also assists the parents in coping. Even with the best planning, care of the child at home may become too difficult because of parental exhaustion, stress, or development of symptoms requiring hospital admission (e.g. bleeding or recurrent seizures). The child may express a desire to return to the security of the hospital and the closer support of the medical team. Under these circumstances a return to the treatment team's inpatient facility for respite care is preferable. A few days only may be required to allow the parents to rest. Longer periods may be necessary according to the wishes of the child and the family.

From a family's perspective, it is not easy to care for a terminally ill child. The strain and loneliness can be great. The advent of free-standing children's hospices, initially in the United Kingdom and more recently in Canada and Australia, provide a welcome alternative to hospitals for respite care for children and their families. A home-like atmosphere can be maintained more successfully in a children's hospice than in a hospital, while the burden of responsibility for the child's care can be temporarily transferred to hospice staff.

Benefits and disadvantages of home care

Care in the home offers the family the advantage of being together with the child in a secure, familiar, and comfortable environment. There is less disruption to family life. Nursing the child at home is perceived by parents as a positive experience. Siblings can participate in the child's care and their needs can be met more easily. The child's food preferences can be catered to more readily. There is greater privacy and freedom from the hospital environment which holds unpleasant associations for the child. There is ready access to parents, brothers and sisters, friends, possessions, and pets. The parents will feel more in control since all the family can participate in the child's care. By witnessing the child's gradual deterioration they will be able to face the approaching death more realistically. Family members are more likely to be present at the time of death and to grieve afterwards in an unhurried manner.

From the parents' perspective, the commonest difficulties of home care are watching the child's physical decline, coping with nights, handling fears of what will happen at the time of death, dealing with medical complications such as haemorrhage and seizures, and coping with domestic difficulties, including care of siblings.

Care in the hospital offers a greater degree of security for management of potentially frightening complications such as seizures or haemorrhage. However, the hospital may not be able to provide the same degree of privacy and informality that is available in the home.

An inquiry into the management of dying children and their families was recently conducted by the patient care review committee of a large Australian paediatric teaching hospital.[16] A 12-month sample of deaths of the hospital's patients was analysed, examining age at death, place of death, and cause of death. Fifteen hospital staff members and four parents were interviewed, and written submissions were received from ten staff members and two parents. No anonymous contributions were received. During the 12-month period (July 1988–June 1989) there were 80 deaths, 66 in hospital and 14 at home. Of 22 cancer patients, 13 died in hospital and nine at home. Parents whose children had died and clinical staff were able to offer the committee many valuable and practical suggestions (Table 3).

Evaluation of home-based care

Those working in paediatric palliative care commonly advocate the advantages of home care over hospital care for dying children. However, to date, there is little published information about how parents themselves actually perceive the care and support that they receive in this situation. A recent Australian study provides information obtained from parents whose children died after receiving care at home (Collins, Stevens, and Cousens, in press). Recommendations for improved care of such children based on the parents' suggestions are as follows:

1. Families need to be able to opt for home-based, hospital-based, or hospice-based care for their child and receive adequate professional support to validate their choice. If circumstances

Table 3 Suggestions from parents and staff on improving management of dying children and their families: results of a recent enquiry by a patient care review committee of a large Australian paediatric teaching hospital[16]

Provide better facilities including quiet rooms for communication, private grieving, rest, reflection, and privacy
Provide more sensitive body viewing, mortuary, autopsy, and funeral arrangements
Provide a more accessible chapel
Relocate telephones so that calls cannot be overheard
Provide better accommodation facilities for parents, better facilities for siblings, hot food available out of working hours, car parking
Provide facilities appropriate to the age of adolescent patients
Provide better in-service education for staff and information for families
Deal with issues well in advance to avoid crises
Ensure good communication and preparation over a period of time to allow smooth transition from curative to palliative to terminal management
Develop stronger links with palliative and hospice care teams, general practitioners, and community nurses

change, the family needs to be able to change freely from one option to another. An integrated, co-ordinated programme of palliative care is required that offers these options.

2. Professional support needs to be available on a 24 hours a day, seven days a week basis, so that medical and nursing needs of children receiving palliative care at home can be met at all times.

3. Parents providing care at home need to receive sufficient information about drug treatment and about what to expect. Adequate opportunities for communication with, and feedback from, parents must be provided prospectively during home visits by members of the caregiving team.

4. Parents often benefit from speaking to another parent who has had a similar experience. Opportunities for such contact should be offered.

5. Parents require assistance with routine home duties to enable them to spend more time with their dying child. A co-ordinated volunteer service will fulfil this requirement.

6. Relief for parents at night is required to ensure adequate sleep. The presence of a non-professional volunteer may suffice but in some cases professional nursing skills will be required. Relief for parents by provision of respite care in hospital or hospice should also be available.

7. Readmission to hospital, when necessary, should be expedited. Parents, if they desire, should be permitted to remain the primary caregivers while their child is in hospital.

8. Local doctors and community nurses assisting families may need additional information about aspects of symptom control or nursing that are essential for successful management. This information can be provided via a case conference for all involved, by written instructions, and by ongoing contact between caregivers.

Each family needs to make its own decision about where care will be centred, without pressure one way or the other from the treatment team. The child's personal wishes should play a significant role in making this decision. Some parents and patients who initially feel that they will not be able to cope with death at home given good support will change their minds and subsequently manage successfully.

It is important to preserve hope at all stages during the terminal illness. To take away all hope will destroy a child's ability to live on from day to day and will foster feelings of hopelessness and helplessness. No matter how grim the situation, one should always strive to deal with matters with a positive attitude. The focus of hope changes over time, for example from hope for cure to hope for a longer remission than last time, to hope that the child can be cared for at home, to hope that the child will die without pain. It is necessary to acknowledge the gradual accumulation of losses and the change in the focus of hope. The family should be supported in their current hope and helped to maintain a realistic focus on what the child can still do (EMB Davies, personal communication, February 1991).

Guidelines for working with the dying child

The reader is encouraged to review the psychological adaptation of the dying child as outlined in Chapter 19.3.

For the infant too young to have a concept of death, one should aim to provide maximum physical relief and comfort. The child of 2 to 7 years of age will fear the separation from parents and other loved ones that death entails. Such separations should be minimized during the phase of palliative care. The child aged between 7 and 12 years will fear abandonment, destruction, and body mutilation. One should be open and honest and provide truthful explanations of symptoms and their management. Access to peers should be maintained, and the child's sense of control over his or her deteriorating body should be fostered.

Some members of the treatment team may feel less equipped to work directly with the dying child. Such members can direct their skills to working with the child's parents, helping them to cope more effectively with the situation. If one is uncomfortable working directly with the child, another caregiver that the child trusts should be involved.

Honesty and compassion must somehow be combined to alleviate the child's anxiety and preserve hope, as in the response of a colleague of the author during their haematology-oncology fellowship. One of his colleague's patients, a boy with non-Hodgkin's lymphoma who had experienced multiple relapses and was dying, arrived at the clinic with his mother. Despite receiving ample supportive care from the treatment team, in the middle of the reception area, he asked his mother tearfully whether he was going to die. The mother was unable to respond and looked to the author's colleague for assistance. She in turn promptly hugged him and said laughingly, 'Well, it looks like that might be the case, but you're certainly not going to die today.' In the midst of a busy clinic where no one was expecting such a question and no one else could respond, this doctor had the necessary presence of mind to respond quickly and honestly, establishing a beneficial conversation with the child.

To summarize, the emotional needs of the dying child include those of all children regardless of health, those arising from the child's reaction to illness and admission to hospital, and those arising from the child's concept of death.

Guidelines for working with the dying adolescent

The dying adolescent represents the greatest challenge to the caregiver.[17,18] It is necessary to reinforce the adolescent's self-esteem and body image, and allow adequate opportunity for ventilation of anger. The adolescent needs privacy and his or her sense of independence should be preserved as much as possible. Access to peers should be maintained and contact with mutual support groups may be helpful.

Pointers for improved communication with parents of children with cancer at diagnosis provided in Table 1 apply equally as well to adolescents with cancer. During interviews, young people may be intimidated by close eye to eye contact ('being eye-balled'); a side by side arrangement may be preferred. Interviews may be held effectively in settings other than a room, for example a hospital coffee shop or garden. At an early stage, and with the patient's consent, spend time with the patient's partner as well as parents, siblings, and grandparents and liaise with the patient's school or employer, to help allay anxiety. Encourage the young person to meet another young person who has or has had cancer and is doing well. In the longer term, another member of the caregiving team approved by the patient can be appointed as the patient's 'buddy', to be available for discussion and to act as an advocate for the patient with the rest of the team. The patient and siblings should be encouraged to join a peer support organization.

How attentive listening and improved communication help

Much of the tension these adolescents experience can be released to assist them in successfully coping with their predicament, by simply permitting them to discuss their thoughts and feelings and share their dreams and frustrations. All too often, an issue of importance to the patient is ignored in the hope that it will go away. Denial is a coping strategy used by patients and carers alike. Health professionals and patients alike may not discuss important issues, fearing that doing so may 'open the flood-gates' and precipitate unacceptable levels of emotion. As one young person said, 'I thought if I started crying, I'd never stop!'

In order to be able to listen to adolescents and discuss death and dying with them without putting up barriers, caregivers need to be aware of their own beliefs and fears about death. It is quite normal to have uncomfortable feelings surface when working with a young person who is facing death. But if one becomes overwhelmed by these feelings one will have little energy left to assist one's patients. Time out, and occasionally supervision, assist the caregiver to deal with a range of feelings, including sadness and anger, that emerge when dealing with the death of a young person and with past experiences of one's own that are brought to the surface at such times.

Negotiation and being offered choices

Adolescents value opportunities for negotiations concerning their treatment, whether early in the course of their illness, in follow-up, and for those who are dying, in palliative care. Being offered choices affords them a sense of control over their situation. In early phases of treatment, better compliance with therapy is likely. For those in palliative care, adverse emotions such as anger, frustration, depression, and anxiety will be lessened. Choices in even apparently mundane matters such as what to eat, wear, or watch on television can boost morale effectively.

Recognition of small achievements

When one is required to redefine one's hopes from hope for cure to hope for prolonged survival with good quality, the positive value of small achievements becomes significant. Hope is better preserved if the ill adolescent's small achievements, from day to day, are acknowledged and respected.

Hospital and health-care team issues

Adolescents prefer to be nursed in the company of their peers in an adolescent ward, rather than in a paediatric or adult ward. Hospital rules concerning visiting hours, rooming in, decoration of the patient's room, and related issues may need to be relaxed during hospital-based care of terminally ill patients, in order to foster a more home-like atmosphere.

Those caring for terminally ill adolescents must face the prospect of repeated losses and will frequently experience painful emotions including sadness, anger, frustration, and guilt. Caregivers must recognize their own limitations and use appropriate support within their institution or treatment team.

Jealousy and resentment may occur in staff who feel threatened by perceived intrusions into their area of responsibility by other health-care professionals who are involved in the patient's care, or who feel displaced in the patient's affections. The patient's wishes and preferences should be respected and dialogue should occur between carers so that any conflict between carers may be lessened.

Occasional conflict will arise within the treatment team over whether to proceed with further attempts at curative therapy or change to palliative care. Foremost consideration must be given to the anticipated benefits and disadvantages of the proposed therapy for the patient. The need for a sensible advocate for the patient within the treatment team is vital.

Certain health professionals evoke striking affection, respect, and loyalty from their adolescent patients and develop close 'professional friendships'. These friendships are valued highly by patients. One adolescent said, 'It makes me feel that I'm alive that I affect someone else, it's not all one-sided.'

Leisure activities

Participation in activities such as camps affords chronically and terminally ill adolescents a valuable opportunity to escape from the tedium and concerns of their day to day routine. Recreational camps provide an ideal opportunity to mix socially with other teenagers and to have fun and take risks in a safe environment. Group discussions are easily arranged at camps. One to one discussions also are facilitated, because the teenagers are able to choose when, and with whom, they will talk. Camps afford a good opportunity for teenagers to talk informally amongst themselves and to become better acquainted with those who care for them, often seeing their health professionals in a different light for the first time. Self-esteem can be effectively built up by success with simple accomplishments.

Peer support and its value

Just as parents of other children with leukaemia or cancer are a source of support to parents, so too can young people with cancer or leukaemia offer helpful support and encouragement to each other. A young person with cancer should be encouraged to meet other young people who have or have had cancer and are doing well. Such contact helps to lessen feelings of social isolation and to maintain participation in social and leisure activities. Research currently being undertaken is beginning to demonstrate the benefits for young people with cancer. However, further research is required into the value of peer support for young people with a life-threatening illness, and into the reasons why some young people prefer not to avail themselves of peer support.

Aids to the adolescent's communication with health professionals

Adolescents often benefit from having a focus other than the health professional, when discussing difficult issues. The use of photographs or photo albums which enable the adolescent to talk about his or her family and friends has been found to be very productive. Encouraging the writing of poems, letters (which may or may not be posted), or a journal can all assist in the release of pent-up emotions, and help clarify issues and decisions that may need to be made.

Drawing as an aid to expression

Drawing is a creative activity which may be very therapeutic by facilitating non-verbal communication and enabling the release of emotions. Drawing assists adolescents in telling their stories.

Leaving behind a permanent record

When discussing their death and the effect their death may have on those that they love, many adolescents mention the importance of leaving behind some permanent record. Although painful for some, many adolescents who were dying have made a tape-recording of messages for their friends and family and some have made a video. Composing these messages in the company of a friend or counsellor may be less threatening, because a two-way conversation or interview is less artificial and often results in much more of the real personality of the young person being displayed. There may be much laughter, as well as more serious messages.

Because hope is so important to these adolescents, preparations such as these are often best completed while putting these tasks in the 'just in case' category. Discussion usually centres around all the energy that is required to suppress feelings of fear and anxiety associated with the possibility of dying. Nightmares are reported as common. Often when adolescents have 'put their house in order', they find they can invest additional energy into living.

Guidelines for working with the parents

Sources of distress that parents face include the following.

The parental role

The parent must face not only the child's imminent death but also the perceived loss of part of himself or herself and must cope with the feeling of having failed as a parent. Feelings of loss of self-esteem are common.

The unnaturalness of a child predeceasing a parent

There may be strong feelings of guilt associated with surviving where one perceived as 'more worthy of life' is dying prematurely.

Societal reactions to the child's death

The approaching death is unnatural and threatening to the parents of other children. They fear the loss of their own child and withdraw, leaving the parents with little of the social support that is helpful in coping with the stresses of palliative care.

Loss of support of spouse

The threat of impending death strikes both parents simultaneously. Each is preoccupied with his or her own grief and is unavailable for support to the other. Each becomes vulnerable to feelings of anger or blame displaced by the other. One spouse may misinterpret the other's withdrawal and depression as rejection.

Parenting of remaining children

The parents are obliged to continue in the very role they are attempting to grieve for and relinquish. The surviving children serve as a painful reminder of the dying child. Feelings of hostility may be displaced onto the surviving children, leading to deepening guilt.

Identifying these issues and discussing them will help the parents focus on and talk about their feelings and deal more effectively with the issues confronting them.

The employment of one or both parents may be put at risk during the child's final illness. Simple liaison with the employer by the treatment team may be sufficient to obtain compassionate leave. The family may experience significant financial difficulties at this time because of loss of work and the increasing demands of the child's care. The assistance of supportive agencies and funds can often be obtained to help make ends meet and to have important bills paid on time. The practical difficulties involved in managing other children and the household may be significant. Grandparents or other members of the extended family may be available and willing to assist the parents with the care of other children and management of the household during this time.

The family will need adequate breaks from the stresses of caring for the child. Parents exhausted by care at home may benefit from the child receiving periods of respite care in hospital. The family may simply 'need permission' to take a break.

Occasionally, significant behavioural problems will occur in families attempting to deal with the stresses and threats of a terminal illness. The caregiving team must be alert to early signs of decompensation and make whatever interventions are required.

An example of extremely maladaptive behaviour has been described involving the childhood cancer patient and one parent, almost always the mother.[19] The child becomes so locked into an infantile tight-knit relationship with the mother that the two cannot be separated without panic. In some instances the distress is more severe in the parent than the child. A rigid pattern of extreme mutual dependency develops, and together they withdraw socially. The parent and child may separate completely from the other parent and other children in the family. The patient sleeps with the mother and will usually exhibit classical school phobia. Typically there is progressive social and physical isolation of the parent–child unit until the child dies, and then the parent makes a very poor later adjustment. Identification and intervention can do much to help with this significant problem.

Guidelines for working with the siblings

A recent study[20] documented the following reactions seen in the siblings of paediatric cancer patients.

(1) the sibling may have his or her own private version of the causation of the patient's illness;

(2) there may be misconceptions about the nature of the illness because of the lack of a visible focus of disease (e.g. in leukaemia compared to an amputation);

(3) there may be misconceptions about the hospital clinic and the treatment programme;

(4) there may be a fear of developing the same illness;

(5) there may be guilt and shame relating to relief for not developing the illness, ambivalent feelings about the patient (envy, resentment over family's preoccupation with patient), and shame over the patient's disfigurement as marking the family as different;

(6) there may be compromised academic and social functioning because of preoccupation with the stress of illness.

These emotions may lead the sibling to exhibit irritability, social withdrawal, academic underachievement, enuresis, and acting-out behaviour.

The sibling bone marrow transplant donor

It has been recognized for some time that siblings who act as donors for bone marrow transplantation feel a responsibility for the outcome of the transplant and experience inappropriate feelings of guilt when graft-versus-host disease or other complications arise. At the outset they are required to undergo a bone marrow harvest, a painful procedure not primarily in the donor's interest. The sibling donor may also feel neglected and jealous when coping with the increased family disruption associated with the transplant. Less attention may be given to siblings by parents who are required to spend longer periods at hospital during the patient's admission.[21] If the transplant fails, the surviving donor will feel guilty for playing a seemingly easily identified role in the patient's death, if the death is due to severe graft-versus-host disease.

Donors' attitudes appear to differ in renal and bone marrow transplants. In renal transplants, the donor mourns the lost kidney, expresses concern about whether the patient will appreciate the sacrifice and take proper care of the donated organ, and focuses on anticipating personal gain such as military discharge or praise from the family.[22] The recipient of the kidney initially feels guilty about jeopardizing the life of the donor. In comparison, the bone marrow donor's reaction is of anxiety appropriate for any simple surgical procedure but with little concern for self. The direction of guilt is reversed, with the bone marrow donor usually experiencing significant guilt and the recipient showing either no guilt or expressing only mild concern that the donor had to be briefly admitted to hospital.[21]

These family members require additional counselling and support to reverse and preferably prevent such misapprehensions.

Recommendations for parents

Suggestions which may help parents to assist the siblings of the ill child are given below.[23]

1. Treat the children equally by taking into account each child's special needs.

2. Keep in contact with the siblings during hospital stays with the ill child.

3. Spend even limited time alone with the siblings.

4. Permit the siblings to continue with their lives as normally as possible.

Counselling the sibling

Specific recommendations for the caregiver in counselling the sick child's sibling during the phase of palliative care include the following:

1. Give the sibling a clear and unambiguous concept of the child's illness and its cause.

2. Encourage the sibling to dispense with any erroneous concepts of the cause of the child's illness.

3. Allow the sibling to visit the clinic, meet staff caring for the child, and witness the child's treatment programme.

4. Assign the sibling helpful tasks in the child's home care.

5. Reassure the sibling that he or she will not develop the same illness (this is always slightly difficult, as the physician may have had personal experience of a sibling developing the same illness).

6. Provide the sibling with appropriate opportunities for ventilation (verbal and non-verbal) of feelings of resentment towards parents or the patient.

7. Liaise with the sibling's school.

8. Provide an opportunity for the sibling 'to say good-bye' as the child's death approaches.

9. Allow the sibling to attend the funeral along with the rest of the family if he or she wishes to do so. Children should not be forced to attend such events, and they need the freedom to participate to the degree they feel comfortable.

Support groups or discussion groups for siblings of children with cancer offer another source of support for working through such conflicts.

Many of the emotional reactions of the family of the terminally ill child are manifestations of anticipatory grief. It is well documented that the grieving process may commence prior to the patient's death. Anticipatory grieving is characterized by depression, a heightened concern for the terminally ill person, rehearsal of the death, and attempts to adjust to the consequences of the death. Anticipatory grief is discussed more fully in Section 18 and Chapter 19.6.

Roles of support groups in palliative phase

The parent support groups which are of value in earlier phases of the child's illness may assume special importance during the child's palliative care. Other parents who have already experienced the loss of a child may provide compassionate understanding and support which can help the parents dealing with the approaching death of their own child. These groups may also provide practical assistance with cooking, housekeeping, shopping, child-minding, running errands, and other similar day to day tasks that otherwise may tax the ill child's family.

The child's impending death

Some time should be spent gently discussing with the parents the practical implications of the child's impending death. Members of the family will feel a need to make their final farewells to the child and should be encouraged to do so in whatever way each feels is appropriate. The child's condition usually deteriorates gradually and the parents are often considerably reassured to know that the death, when it occurs, will almost always be peaceful and free of fear and distress for the child. At this time the child will become more withdrawn and detached from those providing care. The family may need reassurance that this detachment is a normal part of the distancing and separation inherent in dying.

Lazarus syndrome

This occurs when the child is expected to die, the child's family have worked through their anticipatory grief and consider themselves fully prepared for the child's death, and the child then goes into remission. The family members may be unable to reinvest emotional attachment to the child and may feel frustration, anger, and resentment that the expected death has not occurred.

Planning for the funeral

As the child's death draws near, the question of an autopsy should also be raised. There is considerable fear of and misconception about autopsies, and parents usually welcome some information to assist them in making a decision. Further, if there are significant and unanswered questions about the child's illness, an autopsy may provide information which will be of assistance to the parents during their bereavement. If an autopsy is planned after a death managed at home, provision must be made for the removal of the child's body from the home to the hospital. Parents should also be encouraged to give some thought to the child's funeral. They will be required to decide whether the child's body is to be buried or cremated, and will need to be in touch with a funeral director who will make the necessary preparations. Although seemingly difficult subjects, a small amount of planning in advance will later be regarded by the parents as valuable.

After the child dies, the family may benefit from a quiet time with the child's body. Hasty attempts to remove the body by well-meaning but uninformed staff or relatives are not to be encouraged. Brothers and sisters should be asked if they wish to see the child's body and allowed to do so. Family members who are excluded may harbour distressing fantasies of how the deceased looked after death and are deprived of the opportunity of 'saying good-bye'. Such issues may lead to considerable additional emotional disturbance during the period of bereavement. In effect, it is necessary to relearn practices which were considered perfectly familiar and desirable in earlier generations.

The family's culture: implications for palliative care

Culture is defined as the sum total of ways of living built up by a group of human beings, which is transmitted from one generation to another and includes language, ideas, beliefs, customs, taboos, and ceremonies.

It is important to note that in any culturally diverse society, customs and expectations surrounding the events of serious illness, dying, death, and mourning will vary. Members of a given culture will often maintain religious beliefs differing from those of the host country's predominant culture. There will usually be a strong overlap between religious and cultural practices, often with no distinction between the two made by the members of the culture themselves. Traditional practices within the culture will have been modified by the effects of mixing with other cultures, by the laws or practices of the host country's culture, and by the requirements of modern society.

The culture's customs and religious beliefs will have been learnt by experience and living rather than by learning *per se*. Thus, people of a given culture may find difficulty in explaining their particular beliefs, though they may still have deep significance to those practising them. Within any culture or religion, people will have their individual interpretations and beliefs. Understanding of the customs of other cultures assists those providing care to avoid causing needless offence or additional stress to patients and their families during palliative care and in the early days after the patient's death. Attitudes to serious illness, dying, death, and mourning in various cultures resident in Australia and New Zealand are summarized in Table 4 .

Staff should ask the family about their particular beliefs and needs. Cultural requirements tend to be modified or relaxed by families in the case of an ill or deceased child in comparison with an adult.

Interestingly, there are striking parallels in the customs of quite disparate cultures with regard to attitudes to visitation of the dying, last rites, funeral and burial rites, and support of the bereaved during mourning. More research is required into the impact of culture on palliative care and bereavement, and into the influence of the family's culture and environment on the child's concept of death.

A potential advance in paediatric palliative care

As further studies unravel the complex psychological reactions of a family to the loss of a child, the ability of caregivers to provide effective support will surely improve. An area of current research that will become increasingly relevant to paediatric palliative care concerns the impact of the palliative care movement on the care of dying children. Despite the widespread acceptance of palliative care for dying adults, there are still relatively very few palliative care services dedicated to children and few reports of the efficacy of palliative care in the paediatric setting.[24]

Free-standing children's hospices are being established in Melbourne and Sydney. Very Special Kids Inc., established in 1985, is a non-profit organization based in Melbourne providing support by trained volunteers to families who have a child with a progressive life-limiting illness. Very Special Kids House opened in November 1996. The Royal Alexandra Hospital for Children, a tertiary level 350-bed paediatric referral hospital in Sydney, is establishing a palliative care service. The service will operate a free-standing children's hospice, Bear Cottage, to be established at a separate site away from the hospital. Bear Cottage will provide respite care and terminal care for children with life limiting illnesses, and their families, and will open during 1998. The palliative care service will also provide consultative advice on pain and symptom relief for the hospital's inpatients, and an outreach programme to support families caring for terminally ill children at home. These programmes are described in more detail in Chapter 19.5. As these and other forward-thinking organizations adopt the principles of palliative care in the management of chronically and terminally ill children and adolescents, it will be important to plan and conduct

Table 4 Serious illness, dying, death, and mourning in various cultures

Culture	Important perspectives	Cultural practices	Religious practices	Funeral practices
Australian Aboriginal[a]	Traditional view that death seen not as end of life but as last ceremony in present life. Urban Aboriginals may have a similar perspective on death and dying to non-Aboriginals. Importance of extended family. Relatives may be slow in coming to terms with reality of impending death. Senior members of extended family involved in decision-making. Deliberate slowness in making arrangements. Cultural/religious overlap and possible conflict between Aboriginal and non-Aboriginal beliefs and practices. Social rules for separation of male and female discourse and activity may require that patient is cared for by member of same sex. Also multiple avoidance rules determined by kin relationships, e.g. son-in-law/mother-in-law. Offence to use name of the deceased. Survivors with same name renamed. Photographs of deceased destroyed. Community involvement in dying process and funeral. Because of variations between communities, and even between families within a community, close and careful consultation is always required.	Traditional belief that spirits of dead return to their places of origin as part of eternal stream of Dreamtime cycle. Disease and death may be seen as unnatural and resulting from evil magic by enemies identifiable by elders' inquests and interpretation of signs. However, contemporary Aboriginals (even remote tribes) known to relate to serious illness, dying, death, and mourning in similar ways to Western society. Relatives travel vast distances to visit sick or dying person or to attend funeral. Large undemanding gatherings at patient's home. Family may seek help of traditional healer. Personal space required. Discomfort in crowded and unfamiliar settings such as hospitals. Avoidance of eye contact by health professionals advisable as respect for personal space. In clinical encounter, Aboriginal people find it easier to talk about medical problems if the health professional first establishes a personal relationship with them.	Spirits of the dead and burial grounds may be held in awe or fear by traditionally orientated Aboriginals. Many Aboriginals may use Christian rites, funeral, and burial services, sometimes in addition to traditional ceremonies. During terminal illness, family may ask healer to treat sufferer. Healer 'somebody spiritual'. Family relate to healer as person rather than to healer's status.	Traditional practices included destroying possessions of the dead, burning of shelters, moving away of whole camp, names of dead not spoken. Essential that burial be in own territory and spirit sung properly to rest, with burial ceremonies lasting months or even years for an important person. Mummification by heat, body placed on platform or in hollow log, or cremation. Mourners painted with white clay, venting of grief in body laceration and wailing, widows observing prolonged food taboos and period of silence. Regional and tribal variations. Autopsy usually not permitted, offence to deceased person's spirit and integrity of body. If death at home, traditional practice of smoking out home after death to free spirit. All residents leave and do not re-enter after deceased's death until home smoked by selected person. May be deferred for months after death. Burial now almost universal. Little available literature or information on practices in urban or rural communities. Traditional ceremonies adapted widely in response to availability of technology, mortuaries, hospitals, Western medical care, and Christian beliefs.

Culture	Important perspectives	Cultural practices	Religious practices	Funeral practices
New Zealand Maori[b]	Events surrounding time of death are among the most sacred and important in Maori life. Traditional grieving and mourning practices affected significantly by influences of modern society. It is essential to acknowledge formally and make legitimate the contribution of traditional healers in the care of Maori patients. Bereaved family receive sustained support from relatives and friends.	*He Kanohi kitea*: 'The seen face'. The Maoris believe it is much better to see a dying person whilst he or she is still alive. Friends relatives and family visit and gather at bedside prior to patient's death to pray. There is an obligation to visit especially for those closely related to patient. This may strain hospital resources.	Reciting and chanting of special prayers at ill patient's bedside led by elders. Traditional belief that deceased person's spirit journeys to the Spirit World.	There is a complex protocol governing commencement of formal mourning, preparation of the body for burial, and ceremonies held between death and interment. The body is not left unaccompanied during this time. Body lies in state on home *marae* (community gathering area). Paying of respects to deceased and bereaved with long speeches over 2 to 3 days after death. Church and graveside ceremony held on day of interment. Burial not cremation, preferably in family's traditional burial grounds. All who attend give gift of money (*koha*) to help with funeral expenses. Tramping of the deceased person's house by an elder after interment. Unveiling of memorial stone 1 to 5 years after burial.
Chinese[c]	Death regarded as one of three great events in life, along with birth and marriage. Extended family valued. Many are superstitious, believing in evil spirits.	Death and dying might not be discussed to avoid invoking bad luck on patient or speaker. Reluctance to visit dying for fear of consequences. Dying child's parents might avoid discussion of subject for fear of accelerating process. Wills not made. If death at home, deceased's remains must have direct and straight access to street, i.e. no corners (does not allow spirit free access to next life), may require temporary structural alterations to building. Acceptance of host country's and hospital's rules. Deceased's eyes not fully closed indicates final message left uncommunicated. Number 4 equated with death; similar phonetic sound.	Multiple religions—Buddhism, Taoism, Confucianism, Christianity. Buddhist view of serious illness as result of past life (karma—fruits of action), emphasis on non-violence, brotherhood, meditation, and doctrine of rebirth. No special rites for dying but patient and family may wish to be visited by Buddhist monk. Important that prayers are said after death.	Autopsy distasteful—usually refused. Buddhist regards soul as remaining in deceased's body for several days after death, thus crying avoided near body. After death, mantra recited to help spirit to be taken to better place. Washing of body with warm water. Food left for deceased 'food for journey'. Body dressed in layered longevity clothes. Usually burial. Funeral generally elaborate to speed spirit on its way. Wailing essential to denote proper mourning. Burning of paper cars, houses, and money to allow spirit a good time. Mourners dress humbly. Diviner often consulted for good aspect burial site. Monetary contributions to family costs of funeral, burial. Money, food given to guests. Mourning for 49 days.
Lebanese/Turkish[d]	Muslim practices and interpretation of beliefs vary from country to country. Turkish Muslims more open to Western practices than	People's expectations of health care influenced by attitude that people with money receive best treatment. Tendency not to	Close mixing of genders restricted by religious regulations. Touching or observation of opposite sex disapproved. Ideally female	Autopsy forbidden unless where suspicious circumstances, e.g. poisoning, murder. After death, eyes to be closed,

Culture	Important perspectives	Cultural practices	Religious practices	Funeral practices
	Lebanese. Muslim culture influences other religions in the country of origin (e.g. Catholicism). Equal proportion Muslim/Christian in Lebanon. Most Turks are Muslims. Strong expectations of gender roles. Strong identification with family mores. Preservation of family heart by women. Grief displayed openly and volubly.	disclose diagnosis of serious illness to patient to prevent anxiety, e.g. one parent may request child's diagnosis withheld from spouse, both parents may request child not informed of deterioration. Cancer classified as male (benign) or female (malignant). Pork, alcohol, blood-based food, gelatin prohibited. Other meat permitted provided that it is killed according to Islamic law.	patient should be attended by female staff and male by male staff. Ritual washing and prayers required at five definite times each day even in debility. Fasting during holy month each year. Presence of religious elder (Imam) or Muslim over 18 years very important at death.	lower jaw bound to head to avoid sagging, washing of body by Muslim with soap and warm water. After cleansing, body wrapped in white, placed in coffin, removed to mosque for burial prayer. Burial, not cremation, preferably in direct contact with ground. Body to be on right-hand side and facing Mecca. Crying during funeral and burial encouraged by most. Can be ritualized. Discouraged at graveside by some who says tears may drown the body. Mourning for 3 days (40 days by some Muslims). Family visited 3rd, 40th day. House open 40 days. Widow indoors 130 days.
Greek[e]	Strong identification with family unit. More pronounced in new country then in Greece because used as a method to 'survive'—people staying together for self-protection. Word 'cancer' not used. Often referred to as 'the disease' or 'the bad illness'. Belief that surgery (e.g. laparotomy) accelerates spread of cancer through the body.	Strong overlap with religious practices. Wearing of black by bereaved: most women wear black, length of time varies (if husband has died, may be for life), men do not wear black, may wear armband. Men may not shave for 40 days. Family does no cooking for 40 days, cooking done by extended family. Some cultural (and religious) beliefs based on superstition (e.g. belief in adverse consequences if 40-day observance broken).	Strong overlap with cultural practices. Strong belief in life after death, concepts of heaven and hell similar to other Christian religions. Important to maintain religious practices when ill. Access to sacraments important. In case of sudden death, last rites should be administered as soon as possible. If a child is sick, need for baptism may become important. Icons common near dying person—the saint after whom the patient is named or of the local church. Most Greeks are Greek Orthodox. A second church (Greek Community Church) has similar beliefs and practices.	When a young girl dies, it is common that she be dressed as a bride for her burial. Services are advertised in the local Greek papers with a picture of the deceased. Poems are often written. Coffins are often open in church. Congregation files past, face of deceased may be kissed. Holy bread or special bread often taken by family to bless soul of deceased. Kolyva (boiled wheat) distributed to mourners leaving church. Burial not cremation. Meal after funeral (lunch or afternoon tea) including fish, dairy products rather than meat, which is regarded as a luxury. Mourners returning to home for meal wash hands at front door 'to wash death away'. Memorial services may be held after 9 and 40 days, 3, 6, 9, and 12 months then annually.

Sources: Dr M Stevens, Head, Oncology Unit and Ms P Jones, Malcolm Sargent Social Worker, Oncology Unit, Royal Alexandra Hospital for Children, Camperdown 1991 and [a]Parbury N. *Survival: a history of aboriginal life in New South Wales*: Sydney: Ministry of Aboriginal Affairs, 1986.
Mobbs, R. In sickness and health: the sociocultural context of Aboriginal well-being, illness and healing. In: Reid J. Trompf P, eds. *The Health of Aboriginal Australia* Marrickville NSW: Harcourt Brace Jovanovich Group (Australia) Pty Ltd, 1991: 292-325. Ms R Williams, Aboriginal Social Worker, Royal Alexandra Hospital for Children, Camperdown September 1991. Dr G Henderson, Visiting Research Fellow, Australian Institute for Aboriginal and Torres Strait Islander Studies, Canberra ACT, September 1991. Mr S Houston, Administrator, Tharawal Aboriginal Health Service, Campbelltown NSW, September 1991. Professor J Reid, Pro-Vice Chancellor (Academic), Queensland University of Technology, Brisbane Qld, October 1991. [b]Na Paratene Ngata. *The undiscovered country: customs of the cultural and ethnic groups of New Zealand concerning death and dying*. NZ Dept Health: 1986, Drs D Mauger and J Skeen, Auckland Hospital, Auckland NZ, 1991. [c]Lee Sio Mong, *Spectrum of Chinese Culture*. Selangor Darul Ehsan, Malaysia: Pelanduk Publications, 1986. Drs M Gett and A Lam, Mr N Lee, Camperdown, Ms B Eng, British Columbia Children's Hospital 1991. [d]Circular, Islamic Funeral Services, 71 Wangee Road Lakemba Sydney April 1991. Mr I Kurdi, Islamic Centre Lakemba Sydney, Sept 1991. Dr M Bashir, Camperdown Nov 1991. [e]Ms K Karatasas, Oncology Social Worker, King George V Hospital, Camperdown, Sydney, April 1991.

as much relevant research as such programmes will reasonably permit.

Conclusion: implications for staff

Those providing care to dying children and their families face the prospect of repeated losses associated with the deaths of many of their patients. Caregivers must recognize their own limitations and use appropriate support within their institution or treatment team. A well-balanced and effective level of care can only be maintained by provision of adequate and regular periods of leave and by fulfilling interests outside the work-place.

Detailed discussion of the implications of paediatric palliative care for staff will be found in Chapter 19.6.

In an excerpt from her novel *George Beneath a Paper Moon*, appearing in an excellent article on the psychological care of children with malignant disease by Lansdown and Goldman,[25] Nina Bawden writes:

> The really unexpected happens so seldom that few of us know how to deal with it. We all move, for most of the time, in a small circle of known possibilities to which we have learned the responses. Outside this circle lies chaos; a dark land without guidelines.

Caring for children with malignant diseases, as Lansdown and Goldman add, involves helping them and their families to find some guidelines through the chaos.

References

1. Rando TA. *Grief, Dying and Death: Clinical Interventions for Caregivers.* Champaign, IL: Research Press, 1984: 327–8.
2. Binger CM, Ablin AR, Feuerstein RC, Kushner JH, Zoger S, Mikkelsen C. Childhood leukemia: emotional impact on patient and family. *New England Journal of Medicine,* 1969; **280**: 414–18.
3. Mulhern RK, Crisco JJ, Camitta BM. Patterns of communication among pediatric patients with leukaemia, parents and physicians: prognostic disagreements and misunderstandings. *Journal of Pediatrics,* 1981; **99**: 480–3.
4. Stevens MM. Palliative care for children dying of cancer: psychosocial issues. In: Adams DW, Deveau EJ, eds. *Beyond the Innocence of Childhood: Helping Children and Adolescents Cope with Threat to their Lives, Death, Dying and Bereavement.* Amityville, New York: Baywood Publishing Company, 1995.
5. Stevens MM. 'Shuttle sheet': a patient-held medical record for pediatric oncology families. *Medical and Pediatric Oncology,* 1992; **200**: 330–5.
6. Cairns NU, Clark GM, Smith SD, Lansky SB. Adaptation of siblings to childhood malignancy. *Journal of Pediatrics,* 1979; **95**: 484–7.
7. Adams DW, Deveau EJ. *Coping with Childhood Cancer: Where Do We Go From Here?* Hamilton Ontario: Kinbridge Publications, 1993.
8. Stevens MM. Cancer in childhood. In: Stevens MM, Rayner J, Turnell R, Graham B, Piper D Smith T, eds. *Physical as Anything: Collaborative Support for Students with Physical Disabilities and Medical Conditions.* Sydney: Special Education Directorate, NSW Dept of School Education, 1996.
9. Heffron WA, Bommelaere K, Masters R. Group discussions with the parents of leukemic children. *Pediatrics,* 1973; **52**: 831–40.
10. Klass D. Self-help groups: grieving parents and community resources. In: Corr CA, Corr DM, eds. *Hospice Approaches to Pediatric Care.* New York: Springer, 1985: 241–60.
11. Snyder CC. Nursing care of the child with cancer. In: Snyder CC, ed. *Oncology Nursing.* Boston: Little, Brown, 1986: 247–97.
12. Schembri AM. The double whammy: social work practice with HIV-positive young gay men. *Proceedings of Social Work and Adolescent Health Care Conference. Prince of Wales Children's Hospital, Sydney NSW, August 1994.*
13. Fulton R. Children at risk because of AIDS. *Proceedings 10th International Conference on Death, Dying and Bereavement, King's College, London Ontario, 11–13 May, 1992.*
14. Schembri AM. '*Heads Down and Tails Up': a report of the 1992 gay mens' welfare survey at the University of New South Wales,* Sydney, New South Wales: University of New South Wales Student Guild, 1992.
15. Stevens MM, Dunsmore JC. Adolescents who are living with a life-threatening illness. In: Corr CA, Balk DE, eds. *Handbook of Adolescent Death and Bereavement.* New York: Springer Publishing, 1996: 107–35.
16. Ashby MA, Kosky RJ, Laver HT, Sims EB. An enquiry into death and dying at the Adelaide Children's Hospital: a useful model? *Medical Journal of Australia,* 1991; **154**: 165–70.
17. Stevens MM, Dunn CJ, Li A, Gulliver D. Adolescent health - 1: coping with cancer. *Australian Family Physician,* 1983; **12**: 107–9.
18. Stevens MM, Dunsmore JC. Helping adolescents who are coping with a life-threatening illness, along with their siblings, parents, and peers. In: Corr CA, Balk DE, eds. *Handbook of Adolescent Death and Bereavement.* New York: Springer Publishing, 1996: 329–53.
19. Lansky S, Gendel M. Symbiotic regressive behavior patterns in childhood malignancy. *Clinical Pediatrics,* 1978; **17**: 133–8.
20. Sourkes BM. Siblings of the pediatric cancer patient. In: Kellerman J, ed. *Psychological Aspects of Childhood Cancer.* Springfield, IL: Charles C Thomas, 1980: 47–69.
21. Gardner GG, August CS, Githens J. Psychological issues in bone marrow transplantation. *Pediatrics,* 1977; **60**: 625–31.
22. Fellner CH, Marshall JR. Twelve kidney donors. *Journal of the American Medical Association,* 1968; **206**: 2703.
23. Davies B, Martinson IM. Care of the family: special emphasis on siblings during and after the death of a child. In: Martin BB, ed. *Pediatric Hospice Care: What Helps.* Los Angeles CA: Children's Hospital of Los Angeles, 1989: 189–90.
24. Corr CA, Corr DM, eds. *Hospice Approaches to Pediatric Care.* New York: Springer, 1985.
25. Lansdown R, Goldman A. The psychological care of children with malignant disease. *Journal of Child Psychology and Psychiatry,* 1988; **29**: 555–67.

Bibliography

Adams DW, Deveau EJ, eds. *Beyond the Innocence of Childhood: Helping Children and Adolescents Cope with Threat to their Lives, Dying, Death, and Bereavement.* Amityville NY: Baywood Publishing, 1995.

Aradine C. Books for children about death. *Pediatrics,* 1976; **57**: 372.

Binger CM, Ablin AR, Feuerstein RC, Kushner JH, Zoger S, Mikkelsen, C. Childhood leukemia: emotional impact on patient and family. *New England Journal of Medicine,* 1969; **280**: 414–18.

Brent D. A death in the family: the pediatrician's role. *Pediatrics,* 1983; **72**: 645–51.

Cairns NU, Clark GM, Smith SD, Lansky SB. Adaptation of siblings to childhood malignancy. *Journal of Pediatrics,* 1979; **95**: 484–7.

Corr CA, Corr DM, eds. *Hospice Approaches to Pediatric Care.* New York: Springer, 1985: 219–40.

Corr CA, Balk DE, eds. *Handbook of Adolescent Death and Bereavement.* New York: Springer Publishing, 1996.

Heffron WA, Bommelaere K, Masters R. Group discussions with the parents of leukemic children. *Pediatrics,* 1973; **52**: 831–40.

Rando TA. *Grief, Dying and Death: Clinical Interventions for Caregivers.* Champaign, IL: Research Press, 1984.

Robbins J. *Caring for the Dying Patient and the Family.* London: Harper and Row, 1989.

Spinetta JJ, Deasy-Spinetta P, eds. *Living with Childhood Cancer.* St. Louis: CV Mosby, 1981.

19.5 Special services for children

Betty Davies and Doris Howell

Differences between care for adult and child

The concept of paediatric palliative care is an extension of palliative care philosophy. Taken broadly, the phrase paediatric palliative care designates a programme or approach to care that seeks to maximize present quality of life by adapting principles of palliative care to children themselves, or their family members, and to other concerned persons who are coping with any of the following as they relate to a child: living with serious or life-threatening illness, the imminent likelihood of dying, or the aftermath of death.[1] Professional staff and volunteers in such programmes provide direct support and co-ordinate assistance from other sources to meet the total needs of this unique population.

Since the late 1960s, the adult palliative care movement has gradually increased in size as a result of a growing awareness of the needs of terminally ill people and their families. Palliative care for adults has evolved to a stage where it is fairly well understood and is perceived as a reasonable option of care for individuals who may be suffering from an incurable illness. Palliative care for children, however, is in much earlier stages of societal acceptance, and is only beginning to receive its rightful place in the spectrum of health-care services. Children require specialized services to meet their unique needs, and they require specialized caregivers in addition to their family.[2] Additionally, family members, especially siblings, require special attention and support. The needs and how they are met will vary greatly according to the characteristics of the child, the family, and caregivers.

The child

Dependent status of child

As the child progresses from birth to adulthood, the degree of his dependency is in constant flux, moving steadily towards total independence. This innate drive is impeded by serious illness, adding to the confusion of the child. Parents, overwhelmed by the fear of impending loss of their child, cling more possessively and seek to be all things to him. The young child, dependent for all things, adjusts accordingly, but the adolescent suffers. At the stage that he experiences his greatest need for independence, privacy, and control, the authority of medicine, the over protectiveness of his parents, and his own apprehension add to his burden.

Diagnosis

Children requiring palliative care have different diagnoses than do most adults receiving palliative care. The common perception is that children's programmes are just for children dying of cancer, as is the case for the majority of adult patients. With children, however, only about 20 per cent of children admitted to palliative care programmes have cancer. Many of them have progressive neurological and metabolic disease, many with associated mental and physical impairments. These diagnoses mean that a major focus of paediatric palliative care is on the provision of respite services. Most adult programmes admit patients close to death. In contrast, children's programmes admit children close to the time of diagnosis and provide services to the children and their families as they progress through the various phases of the illness trajectory and eventual death. Accordingly, the length of stay may be considerably longer than is usual in adult programmes.

Legal and ethical status of children

In adult palliative care programmes, the wishes of the patient are paramount. In caring for children, it is sometimes more difficult to determine whose wishes should be followed. Parents sometimes see the child's needs quite differently than the way the child sees them, or the parents and various staff members may hold differing views. The age and cognitive level of the child must, of course, be taken into account. In addition, the child's legal status must be considered. As minors in the eyes of the law, children are subservient to the will of their parents under usual circumstances. This dictum has been challenged in the past decade as the need for advocacy for the child has become more evident in the light of more sophisticated modalities of care.

Ethical concerns, arising originally around the status of the fetus and, more recently, organ donations and transplantation, recognize the child as an individual deserving of a voice in his own destiny. If the child is unable to speak for himself, the ombudsman may intercede on his behalf to assure that his best interests are met. For further discussion of related ethical issues, see Chapter 19.8.

Family

Family size and experience

The families of young children tend to be more inclusive, and therefore, larger than families of adults. Parents and grandparents are still living, siblings are often present, and school and neighbourhood friends are part of the affected family group. Moreover, most family members will not have faced the death of a child before so the task of meeting family needs requires special attention, skill, and time.

Care provision

Most parents expect to care for their dependent children. Moreover, grief-filled parents, seeking to assuage the anguish and pain of impending loss, may compensate by trying to be all things to their child and tend to resist help from outsiders. The hospital environment, with its wide variety of caregivers, often puts parents in an ambiguous position where they are appreciative of the expert care but resent the control exerted over their child and themselves by busy professionals. Parents, when inadvertently displaced from the bedside by well-meaning staff, have been electing to care for their dying child at home, turning to home care support where available. Such support programmes, as an adjunct to hospital care, are needed to provide timely assistance in a sensitive and responsive manner in accord with the parents' desires. The providers of such support services serve primarily as assistants and teachers to the parents rather than in the classical hands-on role of the professional caregiver. The need for parents to be everything and maintain control of their child's life serves as a major recourse for their anguish and grief.

Bereavement needs

As a rule, families suffer the death of a child more severely than the death of an adult.[3] And, because of the composition of the family group and the differences in age of its members, there is the potential for more disruption following a child's death. Bereavement care must be a major programme component, with family support provided more frequently, to a more diverse group of bereaved members, and for a longer time than in typical adult hospice programmes.

Caregivers

Knowledge

A natural result of the past emphasis on adult palliative care is that there is little available research, experience, and knowledge pertaining to the details of care for paediatric patients. This is particularly apparent in techniques for pain and symptom management. Adapting existing knowledge to the care of children and seeking new approaches to the management of problems should be major programme goals of any children's palliative care programme.

Caregivers also require extensive knowledge of children and their perceptions of illness, death, and dying. Childhood development progresses through an orderly sequence of increasing comprehension, interpretation, and independence (see Chapter 19.2, Table 1). The ill child is delayed in his milestones and with prolonged or serious illness, will regress. This does not mean, however, that the ill child can be ignored, since such children seem mature beyond their years in their perception of death.

Many adults assume that children are not affected to the same degree as are adults by serious illness and death because they are 'too young to understand', or because they 'will forget as time passes by'. Children are less verbal and communicate their thoughts and feelings in different ways than adults, but it is not true that children are not affected by such events.

Caregivers who are knowledgeable and experienced in childhood development are needed to assess the child's status repeatedly and to design care plans appropriate to his functional rather than chronological stage. Allowances have to be made to obtain a match between the child's waning capabilities and his parents' expectations. Communicating with the ill child in accord with the level at which he is functioning will help the child express his feelings, his needs, his wishes, and his fears more freely. A child's understanding of life and death, sickness and health, and self and non-self reflect his level of maturity along the developmental pathway (see Chapter 19.2, Table 3). Understanding the child's functional level permits the caregiver to provide the patient with as much control over his life and circumstances as he is willing and able to handle. Sharing the developmental evaluation with the parents will enlighten them as they seek to cope with the patient's behaviour and reassure them that the regressive pattern is the expected norm.

Team work

Special services for children require a highly skilled team in which the contributions of each discipline must synchronize to attend to the needs of each member of the family, and not only the patient.[2,4,5] Experienced caregivers must be closely tuned to the emotional, mental, and physical stamina of the child's parents. Paediatric personnel must acquire a thorough understanding of the family's lifestyle, personalities, religion, and cultural mores, and the parent–child relationship. The impact of these influences will be seen in the behaviour and coping mechanisms used by the child. The ill child usually wants all care to be rendered by the parents, but most will respond to sensitive caregivers if the parents take the lead in accepting assistance. As the legally responsible persons, all decisions regarding the dependent child rest with the parents. Their ability to function well and remain in charge will benefit from consistent support and guidance by an empathetic staff who incorporate the needs of all family members into the care plan and help the entire family to sustain and cope. The pioneer efforts of Martinson in 1978 and, later, Lauer and coworkers demonstrated the value of the team concept in providing support to families.[6–11] This support permitted parents, even those living at a distance from the patient's hospital base, to be fully involved in the care of their child in the home, even choosing the place for death to occur.

Successful palliation permits the child and family to share each day to the fullest degree possible, defining with their caregivers appropriate care plans. Bonds of trust, communication, and support with the caregivers develop from the time of diagnosis and are essential to sustain child and family—for children, particularly when ill, do not adapt well to changes in caregivers.

Recruitment and retention of competent and sensitive caregivers is often difficult because of the personal pain and sadness associated with the impending death of a child (see Chapter19.6). Staff needs to be protected from burnout, as they must sustain the entire family in their supportive caregiving role.

Location of care for children

In the provision of special services for children, the location of care is a major issue. The child who faces death and his parents reserve the right to select where his final weeks should be spent, and deserve the full endorsement and help of the caregiving staff. Hospitals, the classical site over the past four decades, have become less essential since parents have become more knowledgeable and assertive in their active involvement in care, as pain control and support systems for the patient are now available in the home. However, admission should always be readily available for those families in need of the hospital for its sense of security and availability of sophisticated personnel.[12] The child himself would rarely choose the hospital as his preference except when he senses his parents' inability to cope at home and, to protect them, will subjugate his own wishes to theirs.

The dependent nature of the relationship of child to family makes the isolation of the hospital, with separation from the familiar, undesirable for most children under any circumstance. In terminal illness, the emotional tensions of the despairing family and the subtle withdrawal of discomfited hospital staff confuse and disturb the child, who may already be anxious. Whereas home would be the natural place for a child to want to spend his final days, this decision must be reached within the context of the family with awareness of the impact which the impending death will have on each member. The child's physical condition and possible emergency needs must be anticipated and the parents prepared so that they can cope with a sudden or unexpected change of status. Without the security of love and appropriate bodily care in the home, the child's sense of safety and protection can be lost. The decision for locus of care is weighty and should be made with serious attention to all aspects of family life and the ability of the chosen location to meet the quality of life expectations of the child and the parents.

Home care is generally thought to be the best alternative for care of children with life-limiting illnesses. Despite this emphasis, however, relatively few children in the industrialized world die at home. This may be due, in part, to certain conditions not being met; such conditions are requisite to paediatric home care.

Requirements for home care

Caregiver availability

Paediatric home care is feasible when a mother, father, or other responsible person is in the home and is able and willing to care for the child with some outside help and support. This is not surprising—caregiver availability and ability are major factors in determining feasibility for palliative home care for adult patients.[13] For families with children, it is not always possible for parents to be in the home consistently, especially since the once dominant scene, where father went out to work and mother stayed home with the children, is now more and more a phenomenon of the past.

Educated caregivers and professional staff

Caring for a seriously ill child at home places a heavy responsibility on the parents, as well as on the primary health-care team who rarely encounter dying children and often feel ill equipped to deal with either the medical or emotional needs of the child and family. Moreover, since most health-care professionals' education occurs in the hospital setting, most health-care workers are not comfortable with, nor skilled at, providing care in the home. There is, therefore, a need for teaching both parents and health-care professionals.

Twenty-four-hour nurse availability

A third condition necessary for paediatric palliative home care has been put forward by those who have implemented and evaluated such programmes.[14,15] Both concluded that the effectiveness of the programme depended upon a nurse being available 24 hours a day, 7 days a week for professional consultation and support.

Respite services

Providing home care to a seriously ill child becomes impossible for all families without the support of home care services and some form of respite service. With periodic respite care, families gain a much needed period of rest and revitalization and are better able to resume care, refreshed. Respite care may be needed under other circumstances as well, when for example a sibling or parent is ill, particularly if someone is ill with a contagious disease which could spread to the already debilitated child.

Co-ordination of services

It is critical that a continuum of care exists so that families do not experience fragmented services or feelings of abandonment resulting from a disruptive shifting of care between home and hospital and hospice. The goal of care, regardless of setting, is to normalize living and to optimize quality of life. To meet this goal, inpatient care must always be an option. Families may need assistance with symptom control, or they may become increasingly anxious and need the reassurance of the familiar hospital and/or the quiet support of the hospice environment. Services offered between the various locations must be co-ordinated, with the child and family always remaining the central focus. Families are greatly reassured by the knowledge that an alternative exists if they find themselves unable to care for the child at home. They are further reassured when no guilt is attached to their choice for location of care.

Other supportive environments for children

School

Special services for children need to take into consideration that school plays a vital role in the lives of children. Consequently, although palliative care focuses primarily on the child in the final stage of life, there may be many weeks to months of slow decline during which encouragement of the child to continue to attend school may give him satisfaction and even pleasure through participation in normal activities with his peers. The child should be encouraged to participate, although he should be the final judge of what he is able to do.

Schooling represents a child's life work and by continuing participation in school he can feel that he is assuming his responsibility. Teachers, who in recent years have become more accustomed to 'mainstreaming' children with chronic illnesses, will be co-operative and supportive if well informed. The time in class need not be long but should be rewarding. The child must be an active member in the decision process.

Day care

Day care programmes for daytime activities and companionship, increasingly utilized for adult patients with cancer, have not yet found widespread use in paediatrics, although such programmes are able to offer respite to parents and an opportunity for some freedom from surveillance for the child whose illness and terminal course is prolonged. For the preschool child, day care provides the peer companionship, stimulation, and sense of belonging as does school for the older child. St Mary's Hospital for Children in Bayside, New York, provides a stimulating day care programme for their handicapped children and has extended enrolment to some of the terminally ill children from the hospice unit no longer able to attend school (personal communication, St Mary's Hospital, 1991). Personal communication from several other hospital-based programmes indicates that a variety of day programmes for family respite are being explored but are still experimental. The value of day care is well regarded during the diagnostic and treatment phase of illness when the child feels fairly well and is physically active, but in the palliative stage is of use primarily if both parents are working or caregivers become ill or are in need of respite time.

Play therapy is a recognized modality of care for all children. When utilized in day care, as in the school system, the activities need to be tailored to the child's level of function and endurance. Meaningful play is the ideal way to help the child patient express his feelings and reduce anxiety, anger, and depression.

Multidisciplinary staff

The many needs of the dying child are best met by people who have had previous experience with sick children and their anxious parents. This is not to exclude those who wish to learn to relate to children who are seriously or terminally ill, but, since time is of the essence, the dying child deserves skilled caregivers. The learning curve to becoming such a caregiver is slow for persons starting from no experience, as the process of integrating child development, child psychology, cultural and religious influences, pathophysiology of disease, therapeutics, and pain control is long and difficult. The care of the child receiving palliation demands the same commitment to excellence and the same level of monitoring as does acute care.

Professional health-care workers

The nurse

In palliative care the nurse emerges as the natural leader of the team. Time spent with the child and the ability to read his body language and incorporate pertinent pieces of scientific knowledge into an effective care plan equips the nurse with the ability to co-ordinate the collaborative team efforts which may significantly influence the emotional stress and ease the coming events. The nurse must be mindful not to displace the parents in their need to care for their child and simultaneously not demand of them more than they can handle. In addition, the nurse serves as the gatekeeper, recognizing when to call in the strengths and services of others. In times of limited resources or in areas less well endowed, the nurse may need to fill multiple roles, as well as train volunteers to assist.

The physician

Most seriously ill and dying children have been treated by multiple physician specialists. To optimize communication and facilitate supportive services, the specialists need to work in close collaboration with the child's primary physician. With the acceptance of the transition from curative to palliative care, the parents need to clarify one person who will serve as the primary physician. Close collaboration of physician and nurse is needed to gain complete symptom control and to provide continuity of care to the patient and reassurance to the family. Constancy of the caregivers is essential, for as the child weakens he will relate well to fewer and fewer people, and not at all to strangers.

The social worker

In the care of children with life-threatening diseases or conditions, the social worker plays many roles. As an experienced listener, the social worker prioritizes the problems and concerns of all involved parties and seeks to expedite solutions for them. Resources and pertinent information are provided, as is expert negotiation of management crises and red tape. The social worker's contributions to and support of the family do not end with the death, but continue throughout the bereavement period. A valuable liaison role between parents, nurse, psychologist, clergy, and others is well served by an experienced social worker.

The clergy

The child tends to cleave to and reflect the religious beliefs and commitment of his parents in accord with his age and level of comprehension. Whenever possible, a clergy person of the family's religious conviction should be recruited to the team. Many are well trained as counsellors, and the spiritual support and hope which they convey will be of comfort to patient, family, and caregivers. Clergy provide formal rites, hear concerns, fears, and confessions, offer counselling, serve as a friend, and, most importantly, signify a link to the unknown future. Their presence offers comfort to many patients and families, and sustains the family members after the death.

The psychologist/psychiatrist

The mental health disciplines are not usually involved when the patient has reached the palliative stage, but the family and the staff may well benefit from their continued support, or gain reassurance through clarification of the patterns of behaviour of the dying child. Adolescents, often filled with anger and resentment as well as fear, may benefit from their counsel or role as a sounding board. Having not been directly involved in their care, they may, therefore, help teenagers express their feelings and expend their anger.

Other support persons

Parent groups

The relationship with other parents suffering similar potential loss is ambivalent initially as denial is a major factor in parents' coping skills. Supportive family members are invaluable in rallying round the stricken family. Parent support groups become increasingly effective as the parents adjust to their pain and identify with others who have suffered similarly. Parent groups can be most beneficial if they provide parents with the freedom to move in and out of the group until they find their own level of comfort and choose to participate with the group. Encouragement by the caregivers, and sensitivity on their part to introduce parents likely to be compatible, smooths the adjustment for parents and child and helps to create a supportive ambience for all concerned.

Others

Flexibility and adaptability are key elements of palliative care staffing. To attain the goal of meeting the needs of the patient and his family the team needs to include, on an *ad hoc* basis, whoever is most capable of accomplishing each given task. Classmates, teachers, coaches, scout leaders, etc., may contribute a sense of still belonging to a peer group and should be encouraged to participate in accord with the patient's wishes, emotional state, and physical reserves.

A fine line exists between responding to the child's wishes and exhausting him with excessive activities or ministrations. As the child's fatigue increases and his attention span shortens, brevity becomes the order of the day. As death approaches, physical comfort and freedom from pain will make a peaceful death more bearable for the survivors.

Volunteers have proved to be a valuable asset in staffing home care programmes. The volunteers should be well trained so that they augment the staff, benefit the family, and in no way antagonize or inadvertently do harm to the patient. Volunteers can bring a fresh outlook to the scene, provide beneficial services to the child and family, and relieve parents and staff, providing them with respite from stress.

Ombudsmen are invaluable in ascertaining that the patient's point of view is heard and that decisions are made in his best interest. The parent-child relationship is of such magnitude that bringing in a third party is not common, but time has shown that utilizing an ombudsman as a 'neutral observer' may provide excellent service in prevention of miscommunication.

The multidisciplinary team and spirituality

Palliation to the physical body without concern for the mind and spirit is incomplete and frequently ineffective. The child is inherently a spiritual being not yet fully burdened by the complexities of life. His religious orientation, imitative or parent-directed, has limited meaning for him. The spiritual dimension or life force of the family imprints the child from birth and provides him with a model for developing his own person. The strength of the family spirit becomes his strength, and his trust in the love and protection of his family sustains him.

Holistic care is essential for fulfilment of palliation. Spiritual care is not only appropriate but is an innate need of all persons, religious or not. In offering spiritual care the caregiver goes the extra mile to seek out the inner person of the patient or family member, share their anguish, and provide solace.

Appreciation of the family's values, strengths, beliefs, and fears enhances the ability of the caregiver to encourage uninhibited communication on all matters and to offer constructive coping skills. The goal of spiritual care is to provide non-judgmental love and the promise of non-abandonment.[16] Providing spiritual care transcends the empathic communication used to meet the family's daily psychosocial needs and invokes a sharing of self when needed. Caregivers are challenged to reach beyond their personal religious belief system to help each family probe its own religious ties and nurture them. For parents facing the loss of a child, the search for meaning is painful but inevitable as they struggle through guilt, defiance, anger, and finally acceptance. The unconditional spiritual support of a caring person can be the glue which holds the family together through and beyond the death of their child.

Cost of paediatric palliative care

Palliative care must be quality care—efficient and yet cost effective. In the field of paediatrics, particularly in life-threatening illnesses, no family would let cost deprive their child of life-saving care. Health professionals concerned with the dynamics of the whole family have long been aware of the devastating impact of serious and terminal illness on the needs of other members of the family. As technology has increased in sophistication, with its resultant escalation in costs, families are facing unbearable financial burdens which impact on all the members.

The growth and success of the palliative care movement since the 1960s has been described as a social movement provoked by rising health care costs.[17,18] Certainly, the survival of the hospice philosophy of home care in a highly competitive hospital-dominated environment can be attributed in part to the need to control rising costs recognized by both provider and consumer. It would be inappropriate, however, if the intent of pioneer Dame Cicely Saunders and her associates—to relieve pain, alleviate symptoms, and provide comfort to those suffering in their final days of life—and the contributions of countless numbers of volunteers committed to palliative care were perceived to be driven primarily by money.

The outstanding advances in pain control made through research in pharmacology and neurology have been welcomed, but the price of these gains is to increase the cost of care which will need further evaluation to demonstrate if the benefits gained are truly cost effective. Analysis of the elements of costs, the rightful assignment of charges, and the measurement of out-of-pocket costs must also include the savings in hospital costs, in-kind contributions of family and volunteers, and reduction in physical and mental health costs in survivors.[19,20]

Work in progress by Birenbaum,[21] comparing hospital care and home care costs for children, indicates the importance of a breakdown of subcategories of cost in order to identify the burden of the cost to families using home care who must bear the higher out-of-pocket social costs and direct non-health costs. The literature reports a variety of conflicting observations, but in general seems to favour the position that home care *in toto* is less costly than hospital admission.[22] More definitive studies are needed to analyse actual costs in a prospective manner, since retrospective studies, even with diaries, are limited in their ability to capture many of the important details. In the United States, financial assistance for non-medical expenses is sorely needed as, increasingly, the financial burden can break an already emotionally strained marriage and/or leave the family with an insurmountable debt as well as an irreparable marital relationship. Definitive cost analyses will be essential to move the policy-makers to provide the additional financing needed for the current unacknowledged expenditures.

Children present a particularly poignant problem, especially in the United States where there is no national health insurance. Most young parents are poorly insured, if at all. The most impoverished may be sustained by federal and state programmes for hospital therapeutic care, but little is available for palliative services. Both Bloom *et al.*[23] and Lansky *et al.*[24] have provided data suggesting that, although the family portion of the total costs may be only 5 percent, on a per family basis this will consume approximately 38 per cent of the gross annual family income.

Paediatric palliative care is more costly than adult care, primarily because of the large number of specialized personnel needed to provide definitive paediatric care and support services to entire families. Further studies on cost effectiveness and cost benefits of palliative care will be critical to its continued existence as an integral part of the health-care system. Survival of palliative care hinges on cost wise management and hard evidence that the cost-benefit ratio is favourable.[25]

Research and evaluation of palliative care

The opportunities for research in paediatric palliative care are unlimited, since well-controlled studies with significant data are minimal. At the present time, there are very few paediatric centres or programmes able to conduct large-scale controlled evaluations on either the physical or behavioural aspects of palliative therapy or to provide validated outcome measures.

In palliative care, the quality of remaining life of the patient is primary and is a product of optimal symptom control. Evaluation of quality of life is both complex and multifactorial. For children, most evaluation tools lack validation. One major difficulty has been separation of the child's statements and values from those of the parents. Paediatric patients present a demanding challenge to investigators in questions of design, measurement, analysis, and ethics.[26] The behaviour of a developing infant or child is in constant flux, with continuously changing norms. Children frequently present barriers to communication—limited comprehension, unpredictable behaviour, and capricious co-operation—which may frustrate efforts to evaluate even the most simple actions. In the adolescent age group the natural rebelliousness and need for control are heightened by the teenager's anger at the injustice of a foreshortened life. The more tenuous the child's hold on life, the less inclined will the patient or family be to participate in any but the most necessary activities, and even the most co-operative will become resistant to measurements and evaluations which impinge on their remaining time. The researcher, in turn, feels guilty about adding to the burden of a family under such agonizing stress.

The problems of conducting randomized controlled studies of paediatric palliative care procedures seem overwhelming, given the wide diversity of the existing programmes, services, and personnel.[27] Financial support from health agencies and foundations will continue only if there is hard evidence of the values to be realized by high calibre palliative care. In the United States, there has been growing dissatisfaction with the peer review system of individual cases as the major tool for monitoring outcomes and evaluating patient care. Increasingly, funding sources are demanding more definitive monitoring, audit, and quality assurance. Certification and licensing also require improved methods of documentation. In children, clinical judgement, clouded by emotional overlay, may influence the evaluation and interfere with the orderly collection of comparative data needed for improved quantitative systems of review. The 1990 report of the Institute of Medicine, *Medicare: A Strategy for Quality Assurance*,[28] urged the use of data-driven studies to promote improved patient outcomes and mould clinical decision-making by meaningful feedback to both caregivers and consumers alike.

Within the National Health Service of the United Kingdom, efforts to evaluate care have focused increasingly on cost. Audit tools, particularly performance indicators, used in the National Health Service compare one hospital with another rather than with established standards. For many hospitals these indicators serve the same purpose as the diagnosis-related groups in the United States to encourage early discharge of patients who are incurable, with little concern for the patient's wishes or quality of care.

Such a dangerous trend threatens the care of children, for whom most terminal care continues to be hospital-based despite the growing trend for home as the site of terminal care. For a variety of reasons, not all parents are capable of caring for terminal illness in the home, and in some cases the child's physical condition and needs are of such a magnitude that only hospital care will suffice.

Comparisons of paediatric palliative care benefits in the United Kingdom and the United States have frequently shown different outcome conclusions, particularly when measured by patient satisfaction. These differences may reflect the variations in cultural backgrounds and social mores, despite a common language. Research questions should be addressed to infants, children, and youth across each age and developmental category, with the data analysed accordingly rather than amassed under the single euphemism—children. Although there may be similar responses to research questions, regardless of age, the variations at each developmental milestone are of such a magnitude as to cloud the outcome if not carefully segregated before the fact. Additionally, cultural variations in child-rearing practices and subsequent child behaviour may be so different across countries that data will not be generalizable, but will have to be viewed and interpreted culturally.

Very few paediatric programmes have evaluated critical issues such as staff attitudes towards children dying in a 'do not resuscitate' status, patient-controlled opioid administration, acceptance of the parent as a cocaregiver, or, most basically, how, when, and by whom the decision should be made to move from curative to palliative care. In addition, many of the same questions need to be addressed to the child and his family in each of the different locations where a child might receive palliative care. Children, more than adults, react quite differently in various environments—a hospital, hospice home care, non-hospice home care, or a paediatric hospice facility.

Although Lauer and coworkers have demonstrated successful parental adaptation and psychological adjustment to the child dying at home, there are still many questions to be answered concerning when hospital admission is appropriate, and desired by all parties, and when an alternative is preferable to the patient and the family members.[8] Regardless of location, research is needed on the components and provisions of quality care during a child's final weeks.

If indeed, as earlier studies have shown, the child with terminal illness wants to be in his own home, further definitive research is needed to identify the ideal characteristics of successful home care.[10,11] The coping mechanisms most useful to parents to handle the stress, the influence of various types of support services, the role reversal between parent and nurse caregivers, and the grief work necessary to each member of the family, as well as the patient, are just a few of the issues requiring well-controlled studies.

The need for 'hospice' or specialist palliative care facilities for paediatric patients, a current debate in the United Kingdom, deserves study in the light of criticisms regarding the use of limited resources for such highly specialized low-census centres.[29,30] Demographic research of regions or districts could better define the extent of the need for facilities offering respite care to children with chronic disease and their parents. The marked difference in geography and population distribution in countries such as Canada, the United States, and Australia, compared with the United Kingdom, will require multisite studies of the similarities and disparities of styles, services, and staffing to render the findings applicable across countries. Now that alternative sites of care are available, it is incumbent upon the physician to justify using the precious numbered days of a child's life in hospital if other adequate alternatives, more preferable to the child, are available.

The future of paediatric palliative care

As medicine, with its increasingly sophisticated diagnostic tools and therapies, has grown, the relentless pursuit of cure has riveted attention on disease and away from the patient. The medical graduate of the 1990s is poorly prepared to function competently in the presence of terminal illness, death, or bereavement.

The last half century has seen a dramatic fall in morbidity and mortality in children, with improved survival rates for many diseases. Most families have never experienced the death of a child, and even the demise of elderly parents or relatives has occurred at a distance, in hospital or a nursing home. At a time when families have become less confident in their competence to care for their severely ill, the hospitals, beset with burgeoning costs to sustain the new technology, cannot assign expensive paediatric beds to patients needing non-reimbursable, symptom-directed palliation. Patients in need of palliation are refused admission or are discharged prematurely to fend for themselves in an unprepared community environment or at the hands of their overwhelmed family members.

The community has tried to respond to the needs of such patients with significant improvement in broader services, increased availability of home care nursing, and the development of hospice programmes and facilities. These may prevent those who are not curable from being discarded, but only if financing for their care can be procured and guaranteed. The equally difficult challenge of educating health professionals to recognize that medicine was designed to serve the patient, not the disease, and to perfect the skills necessary to provide compassionate care until death will be much harder to influence.

For children with chronic or prolonged illnesses, care during the final weeks of life should be provided, whenever possible, by the family in the home where the child is most secure. When the hospital must be used to provide special services and complex care, the parents should be incorporated into the care plan and remain with the young or very ill child. As quickly as possible, in keeping with safety, the child whose life is limited needs to be returned to his home environment. During this terminal phase, the family will require physical, emotional, and spiritual support.

For parents, the decision to move their child from a course of curative medicine to palliation is often interpreted as accepting no further therapeutic care. The unfortunate interpretation from early hospice days that palliation replaces all treatment modalities has been a serious drawback to timely and effective symptom control. Successful palliation often requires full utilization of chemotherapy, radiation, antibiotics, and even surgical intervention on occasion.[31] The goal of palliation—to effect the best quality of life for the patient—will be best met by utilizing every means appropriate to alleviate the patient's symptoms. Even the most realistic parents cling to the hope that some event will transpire to prevent the death of their child. Continuance of treatment permits hope to sustain the family until such time as the side-effects or lack of symptom control lead them to embrace palliation.

Palliative care has served an even larger and more diverse group of patients as the public and professional acceptance of home care for irreversible and chronic illness has increased. The paediatric conditions previously excluded from most palliative care services by nature of the unpredictability of the date of death and the long terminal projectory, namely cystic fibrosis, neurodegenerative disorders, brain damage, and, most recently, AIDS, are pressing for much needed support. With the removal of the original restrictive life expectancy limitation imposed by third party payers in the United States, they too can receive care and the help of caregivers throughout their lifespan. The nature of each of these conditions will require special services and collaboration amongst the many disciplines involved in their care to provide them with a better quality of remaining life.

The rapid increase in paediatric AIDS from contaminated blood products and transplacental infection from infected mothers brings new challenges to the delivery of palliative care, requiring a major increase in psychosocial support to serve a blighted population of young families. Although services are being provided by a few programmes, the need for research, education, and testing of services to meet their needs is only beginning.[32,33]

References

1. Corr CA, Corr DM. In our opinion... What is pediatric hospice care? *Children's Health Care*, 1988; **17**: 4–11.
2. Wilson DC. Caring for dying children: General principles. In: Corr CA, Corr DM, eds. *Hospice Approaches to Pediatric Care*. New York: Springer Publishing Company, 1985: 5–30.
3. Fischoff J, O'Brien N. After a child dies. *Journal of Pediatrics*, 1976; **88**: 140–6.
4. Bakke K, Pomietto M. Family care when a child has late stage cancer: a research review. *Oncology Nursing Forum*, 1986; **13**: 71–6.
5. Martin BB. Pediatric hospice care: what does it mean? In: Martin BB, ed. *Pediatric Hospice Care: What Helps*. Los Angeles: Children's Hospital of Los Angeles, 1989: 1–10.
6. Martinson IM, Armstrong GD, Geis DP. Home care for children dying of cancer. *Pediatrics*, 1978; **62**: 106–13.
7. Lauer ME, Mulhern RK, Wallskog JM, Camitta BM. A comparison study of parental adaptation following a child's death at home or in the hospital. *Pediatrics*, 1983; **71**: 107–11.
8. Mulhern, RK, Lauer ME, Hoffmann RG. Death of a child at home or in the hospital: subsequent psychological adjustment of the family. *Pediatrics*, 1983; **71**: 743–7.
9. Corr CA, Corr M. Pediatric hospice care. *Pediatrics*, 1985; **76**: 774–80.
10. Lauer ME, Mulhern RK, Hoffman RG, Camitta BM. Utilization of hospice/home care in pediatric oncology: a national survey. *Cancer Nursing*, 1986; **9**:102–7.
11. Lauer ME, Mulhern RK, Hoffman RG, Schell MJ, Camitta BM. Longterm follow-up of parental adjustment following a child's death at home or hospital. *Cancer*, 1989; **63**: 988–94.
12. Lauer ME, Mulhern RK. Home care referral: parental self selection vs psycho-social predictors of capacity. *American Journal of Hospice Care*, 1984; **1**: 35–8.
13. Brown P, Davies B, Martens N. Families in supportive care, Part II: Palliative care at home—a viable care setting. *Journal of Palliative Care*, 1990; **6**: 21–7.
14. Martinson IM, Enos M. The dying child: At home. In: Corr CA, Corr DM, eds. *Hospice Approaches to Pediatric Care*. New York: Springer Publishing Company, 1985: 31–42.

15. Martin BB. Home care for terminally ill children and their families. In: Corr CA, Corr DM, eds. *Hospice Approaches to Pediatric Care*. New York: Springer Publishing Company, 1985: 65–86.
16. Saunders C. Moment of truth; care of the dying person. In Pearson L, ed. *Death and Dying: Current Issues in Treatment of the Dying Person*. Cleveland, OH: Cleveland Press of Case Western Reserve University, 1969.
17. Mor V, Greer DS, Kastenbaum R, eds. Public policy and the hospice movement. In: *The Hospice Experiment*. Baltimore: Johns Hopkins University Press, 1988: 227–44.
18. Paradis LF. An assessment of sociology's contributions to hospice: priorities for future research. *Hospice Journal*, 1988; **4**: 57–71.
19. Mor V, Kidder D. Cost savings in hospice: final results of the National Hospice Study. *Health Services Research*, 1985; **20**: 407–22.
20. Houts P, *et al.* Non-medical costs to patients and their families associated with outpatient chemotherapy. *Cancer*, 1984; **53**: 2388–92.
21. Birenbaum LK. Cost of terminal care for families of children with cancer. *Phyllis J. Verhonick Nursing Research Conference, Delivering Nursing Care in the 90s: Growing Needs, Shrinking Resources, Charlottesville, VA, 6 April 1990.*
22. Bloom BS. Is hospice care least expensive for the terminally ill? *Hospice Journal*, 1987; **3**: 67–76.
23. Bloom BS, Knorr R, Evans A. The epidemiology of disease expenses. *Journal of the American Medical Association*, 1985; **253**: 2393–7.
24. Lansky SB, Black JL, Cairns NU. Childhood cancer: medical costs. *Cancer*, 1983; **52**:762–6.
25. Hill F, Oliver C. Hospice—an update on the cost of patient care. *Palliative Medicine*, 1989; **3**: 119–24.
26. Moore IM, Ruccione K. Challenges to conducting research with children with cancer. *Oncology Nursing Forum*, 1989; **16**: 587–9.
27. Kohler JA, Radford M. Terminal care for children dying of cancer: quantity and quality of life. *British Medical Journal*, 1985; **291**: 115–16.
28. Institute of Medicine, Division of Health Care Services. In: Lohr KN, ed. *Medicare: A Strategy for Quality Assurance*. Washington, DC: National Academy Press, 1990.
29. Chambers TL. Hospices for children. *British Medical Journal*, 1987; **295**: 1309–10.
30. Wilkinson JM, *et al.* Hospices for children? Correspondence. *British Medical Journal*, 1987; **295**: 210–11.
31. Miller RJ. The role of chemotherapy in the hospice patient: a problem of definition. *American Journal of Hospice Care*, 1989; **6**: 19–26.
32. Boland MG, Mahan RP, Evans P. Special issues in the case of the child with HIV infection/AIDS. In: Martin BB, ed. *Pediatric Hospice Care: What Helps*. Los Angeles: Children's Hospital of Los Angeles, 1989: 116–36.
33. Dailey AA. Terminal care for the child with AIDS. In: Pizzo PA, Wilfert CM, eds. *Pediatric AIDS: The Challenge of HIV Infection in Infants, Children, and Adolescents*. Baltimore: Williams and Wilkins, 1991: 619–29.

19.6 Special issues in bereavement and staff support

Betty Davies and Brenda Eng

Bereavement: significance of the concept

Despite advances in medical technology and delivery of health care, despite our efforts to preserve life, children will continue to die of incurable disease such as cancer, congenital anomalies, and genetic defects. Though sometimes difficult to admit, the end result of the paediatric palliative care experience is the death of a child. A child's death is considered a greater loss because the child has not had the opportunity to live a full life as compared to the adult or aged individual; a child's death confounds our expectation that children will grow into adulthood and live a normal lifespan. A child's death confounds our hope that this child may be the one who recovers. All concerned—the parents, the child, the physician, and the other professionals involved in the care—face difficulties in acknowledging the death of a child. A child's death evokes in each one of us the 'inner bereaved child;' it reawakens those painful and repressed effects of separation and loss from our earliest development and makes for a rapid withdrawal from the pain involved. The purpose of this chapter is to bridge the gap between theory and practice and to offer some practical suggestions for assisting parents and siblings following the death of a child from life-threatening illness, and for assisting health-care professionals with this emotion-filled experience.

Death of a child: impact on the family

The family provides for its members the necessary relationships, both in quality and intensity, out of which normal growth and development occur. Because of these relationships, the system behaves, not as a simple composition of independent elements, but coherently and inseparably as a whole. Following this perspective, illness or death in any family member is a potential assault on the family system. The death of a child, therefore, affects not only individual family members, but also the family unit as a whole.

Empty space

Interviews with 49 families, 7 to 9 years after a death from childhood cancer, suggested that the death of a child creates an empty space for surviving family members, a sense in the family that there is always something missing.[1] Three patterns of grieving characterized family members' responses to this sense of emptiness; getting over it, filling the emptiness, and keeping the connection. Those families who placed emphasis on getting over the grief tended to have a somewhat concrete plan for putting the death of the child behind them. They accepted the death matter of factly as either God's will or as something we all have to face. The second group of families filled the empty space by keeping busy (for example building a new house or performing two jobs) or by substituting other problems or situations to take their mind off their grief. They acknowledged the emptiness, but made an effort to fill up the space with activities. The largest number of families accepted the empty space but tried never to forget or become very busy. They acknowledged the empty space, allowed it to exist, treasured their remaining children more, and valued life in general.

No pattern of grieving is suggested as superior to the others. The patterns only serve to emphasize that grief, for any family or family member, should not be expected to follow a specific path within specified time limits.

Additional findings from this same study reported that the child's death requires individual reorganization and adjustments within the family system.[2] Changes in marital status and or the addition of other children required adjustments in the relationships of family members. Some changes were developmental in nature while others, according to the informants, were directly related to the death of the child. Regardless of the changes, however, a child's death is perceived as a significant event, a reference point to which all subsequent events can be related.

Levels of functioning

Family theorists have attempted to delineate functional and dysfunctional coping strategies used by families following stressful events. In one study, combining data from three groups of families whose child died from cancer between 2 months and 9 years previously, several characteristics of functional and dysfunctional families were delineated.[3]

Open versus closed

The first characteristics of families who coped effectively during bereavement was openness. Such families communicated freely in discussing the child's illness, death, and family members' responses since death. Discussion occurred in the presence of other family members, and all persons were allowed to express their own thoughts and feelings. Closed families did not have this freedom of expression nor was each person's individual grief related to the grief of others in the family.

Process versus content

Functional families focused not only on events, but also on the thoughts and feelings associated with such events. As a result, they were more aware of process; this awareness led to action. The opposite was true for less functional families. They were less able to focus on feelings, to anticipate potentially difficult occasions, such as special holidays, and consequently became stuck in their sadness.

Reality versus illusion

The responses of less functional families reflected escape from the reality of the situation as well as suppression of natural feelings. They remembered only the good aspects of the deceased child, ignoring that the child had been a normal child with both good and bad behaviour. They regretted that they had not done more for their child. Functional families, on the other hand, were more realistic in their recall of their child and in their assessment of their own behaviour.

Flexible versus rigid roles

Functional families were more flexible in assuming new roles, acknowledging that no one could take the place of the child who had died. In less functional grieving families, roles were rigidly maintained. Functional families used a wide range of resources, accepting their vulnerabilities and their need for support. The less functional families withdrew from sources of support, claiming that they were able to manage on their own and sometimes denying the extent of their grief.

Parental grief

The loss of a child through death is quite unlike any other loss known. In comparison with other individuals in different role relationships to the deceased (e.g. spouse, sibling, and child) the grief of parents is more intense, more complex, and longer lasting.[4,5] When a child dies, the parents feel each day as grey, hollow, empty; each day is a burden. Parents feel overwhelmed with feelings of anger, depression, uncontrollable tears, hopelessness, frustration, and fear for their remaining children. Parents can be reassured that the psychosomatic symptoms they experience are not congruent with mental illness. This reassurance is underscored by a study of parents 2 years after their child had died from cancer.[6] These parents presented a profile on a symptom checklist (Symptom Checklist 90-Revised) that was significantly different from the normal non-clinical and psychiatric outpatient group. This suggests that these bereaved mothers and fathers display a psychological pattern that is more symptomatic than normal, but less symptomatic than diagnosed outpatients. Despite the recognition of parental grief as an intensely difficult psychological experience, relatively few researchers have empirically addressed this issue. Study samples vary widely in composition and results have been contradictory. Four types of factors potentially related to bereavement outcome have been identified:

(1) demographic factors;

(2) factors related to parents' premorbid personalities or experiences;

(3) factors related to the child's hospitalization or death;

(4) postdeath factors.[7]

Duration and intensity of grief

It has often been assumed that the pain of grief decreases with the passing of time. However, recent studies[7,8] report that parents who had been grieving for longer than 2 years reported similar patterns to parents who had experienced a loss within the past 3 months to 2 years and that parental grief appears to remain fairly intense for at least 4 years. These findings concur with more recent conceptualizations of grief as an active process which occurs over time[9] rather than as an event from which individuals recover.

Survival guilt

The unique difficulties inherent in the loss of a child stem from the view that the death of a child is not only inappropriate in the context of living, but its tragic and untimely nature is also a basic threat to the function of parenthood. Parents feel victimized by the realistic loss of their child, by the loss of their hopes and dreams, and by their own loss of self-esteem because they failed as parents in protecting their child. This victimization is sometimes referred to as survival guilt.[10] This phenomenon lends evidence as to why the resolution of grief may be a difficult task and why bereaved parents face so many more difficulties than other bereaved individuals. Thoughts of suicide, self-accusations, inconsolable grief, and withdrawal from family and friends are common parental reactions to the loss.

Complicated grief

The experience of parental grief is profound, affected by a myriad of factors which predisposed parents to be exceptionally vulnerable to complicated or unresolved grief. Complicated bereavement is characterized by an inability to adapt to the loss and bring grieving to a satisfactory conclusion.[11] Research into the elements of complicated parental bereavement has been limited. It is inappropriate therefore to evaluate parental bereavement with traditional criteria. A new model of parental mourning must be developed. Until such a model is developed, the following behaviours remain the most useful for the clinician in assessing complicated bereavement. These behaviours, displayed years after the actual death, include, but are not limited to, maintaining the dead child's environment just as it was at the time of death, developing physical symptoms similar to those of the deceased, feeling unacceptable and intense sadness at various anniversary times, and being unable to talk about the deceased child without intense reactivation of the feelings experienced at the time of the death.[12]

The marital dyad

Parents as individuals are affected by the death of their child; the marital dyad is also affected. Mothers and fathers may deal differently with expression of feelings, working and doing daily activities, relating to things that trigger memories of the deceased, and searching for the meaning of what has happened. One of the most difficult aspects of parental bereavement is that the death of a child strikes both partners in the marital dyad simultaneously and confronts them with the same overwhelming loss. Consequently, each partner's primary and most therapeutic source of support is taken away. The person to whom each would turn for support is confronting and working through his or her own grief.

Divorce

A common occurrence is that one spouse may misinterpret the behaviour of the other. The erroneous assumption that because partners suffer the same loss, they will experience the same grief, may set up unrealistic expectations that most likely will not be met. The expectation of going through the entire crisis together is often thwarted for bereaved parents. This in itself constitutes a loss for the couple as they may have been accustomed to pulling together through crises. When combined with other factors, this loss places additional burdens of grief, loss, and demands for adaptation on an already over-burdened individual. Such reactions have led to the assertion that there may be higher divorce rates in bereaved couples. However, the assumption that parental loss of a child invariably destroys the marital relationship is an erroneous interpretation of early research findings; these reports have failed to take into account normal divorce rates and longitudinal designs. Several studies[13-15] suggest that while stresses of childhood illness and subsequent death of the child are exceptionally high, and may exacerbate pre-existing marital discord, family relationships do not automatically have to be disrupted and end in divorce. In one study[2] of 56 families 7 to 9 years following a child's death from cancer, nine couples were divorced. Four of the nine divorced couples stated that the death of the child was a major factor contributing to their divorce. The other five couples did not attribute the divorce to the child's death but viewed it as a result of other problems which existed before the child was diagnosed with cancer.

Intimacy

The lack of synchronicity in grieving styles and grief experiences commonly results in dissimilar expectations and coping strategies. Husbands and wives may deal differently with expression of feelings, working, and doing daily activities, relating to things that trigger memories of the deceased, and searching for the meaning of what has happened. One problem frequently discussed is the inhibition of sexual response and intimacy in bereaved parents. This area of difficulty may be the result of fear related to having and losing other children and/or guilt over experiencing pleasure and/or it may be a symptom of grief and/or depression experienced by one or both partners.[16] It is not uncommon for the couple to sustain some sexual difficulties for up to 2 years following a child's death because of disinterest or grief-related symptomatology in one or both partners. In fact, in one cross-sectional study of 54 bereaved parents,[17] the response pattern was characterized by a decrease in intensity of the grief experience in the second year following the child's death, followed by an increase in intensity in the third year. Mothers tended to exhibit more intense grief experiences and poorer subsequent adjustment than fathers. Parental bereavement may intensify rather than decline, over time.

Search for meaning

The death of a child is so profound that it ultimately sends bereaved parents into a deep and painful existential 'search for meaning' and this search may be a key factor in a positive 'growth' versus negative 'despair' resolution of the grief experience. Of the numerous comments made by 36 parents in one study,[18] 40 responses indicated a positive outlook, whereas only 13 responses were negative. Positive growth responses included: learning to live each day to the fullest; being more understanding of others; having a stronger faith; being aware of the precariousness of life; being a better person in general. Focusing on the potential for growth when a child has died is meant in no way to minimize the deep and long-lasting pain of grief; rather, it is meant to point out the importance of channelling the pain and rage into meaningful endeavours which can contribute to recovery.

Table 1 Sibling responses to the death of a brother or sister from cancer[54]

Psychological
Fearful of own death and parents' death
Tearful
Anxiety (over people leaving, with new situations)
Loneliness
Angry outbursts or temper tantrums
Concerns about getting cancer
Attention-seeking from parents
Withdrawn (guarding feelings and thoughts)
Sadness
Daydreaming
Change in school performance (decreased concentration)
Physiological
Sleep disturbances (reluctant to go to bed, nightmares)
Eating disturbances (loss of appetite, lack of interest in food)
Bodily complaints (e.g. head aches; stomach aches, generalized aches)
Increased incidence of colds and influenza episodes
Frequent infections (urinary tract, respiratory tract)

Sibling grief

If paediatric health-care providers are concerned about the death of children, then these professionals must pay attention to the needs of the siblings of children who die. The responses of children to the death of a sibling have not been extensively examined, yet to lose a brother or sister can have traumatic effects. Most individuals have at least one sibling with whom they share a greater part of life than with any other person. Children spend more time together than any other family subsystem and exert a powerful influence on shaping each others' identity in varying roles, as mentor, supporter, comforter, protector, and socializer. When the sibling dies, an emptiness remains that cannot be filled.

Behaviour problems

A wide range of behaviour problems occurs after the death of a child. Since children often work out their feelings through their behaviours and since behaviour represents a relatively easy way of assessing children's responses to critical events, it is logical that the focus of research in this area has been on behaviour. Many studies, however, define the behaviour changes seen in bereaved children as problematic, if not even pathological, although positive responses also have been identified. Problems have included a range of behaviours, attitudes, emotions, symptoms, cognitions, and diagnoses (Table 1). Reported research has produced contradictory findings on the frequency, severity, and persistence of problems following the death of a child. The most common behaviours to pay attention to include psychophysiological responses such as headaches, general aches and pains, and stomach cramps. Sleeping disturbances are common—children may not want to go to bed at night, especially if they shared a room with the deceased child; they may have bad dreams or nightmares, or walk in their sleep. Eating disturbances may include overeating or a loss of appetite. Anxiety may be evident, and school performance may deteriorate. Children will frequently complain of loneliness. If, over time, children are noted to demonstrate a pattern of behaviour which includes persistent sadness and withdrawal, decreased involvement in activities and hobbies, acting out, diminished self-esteem, and a loss of interest and achievement in school, the child should be given individualized attention through referrals to the school counsellor or to a specialist in children's grief.

Influencing factors

A child's response to the death of a brother or sister can be influenced by several factors. Loss occurring at younger than 5 years of age or during early adolescence, and the presence of pre-existing psychological difficulties are warning signs for children at risk. The contribution of the family environment to sibling bereavement has been noted.[19] The greater the degree of commitment, help, and support family members provide for one another, the fewer withdrawing and acting out behaviour reported for the bereaved children. Furthermore, families with a greater emphasis on social, cultural, recreational, and religious involvement tended to have children with fewer behavioural problems following a sibling's death.

The relationship between the deceased and the bereaved also influences grief resolution among siblings. Siblings who shared close relationships with their brother or sister tend to demonstrate more internalizing behaviour after the death of the child. Emotional closeness between siblings exerts a stronger influence on bereavement outcome than closeness in age, length of illness, or number of surviving children in the family. Health-care professionals therefore need to be particularly sensitive to the needs of the children who shared a close relationship with their brother or sister.

Long-term effects

Most studies of sibling bereavement, and in fact most bereavement studies, focus on the months immediately after the death or up to 1 or 2 years following the death; consequently, the longer-term effects of sibling bereavement are relatively unknown. Several studies[20,21] indicate that symptoms persisted with siblings in the majority of families even 2 to 3 years after the death. At 7 to 9 years after the death, siblings continued to experience effects of the death. Several continued to dream about their deceased brother or sister; such dreams were not disturbing, but rather comforting in that they provided a feeling of closeness to the sibling. Feelings of loneliness and sadness persisted, not always in the forefront of their minds but still identifiable. Many of the siblings still continued to think about their sibling frequently, many as often as once a day. Such thoughts were triggered by internal and external reminders, and were more prevalent at certain times, like when they themselves reached the age at which the sibling had died or when they had children of their own. Long-term outcomes for 12 adults who, in their early adolescence, lost a sibling through death reported psychological growth, a sense of feeling different, and withdrawal from peers.[22] The study presents a theoretical schema relating these outcomes. The sense of personal growth and maturity arouses feelings of being different from peers, and may result in an intolerance of the developmentally appropriate behaviours demonstrated by peers. Some siblings respond to these feelings by withdrawing from their peers at a time when peer relationships are critical to completing developmental tasks. For such siblings, feelings of sadness and loneliness become long-term. Up to 10, 20, or 30 years after the death, siblings perceive that the death had a long-term impact on their lives, often as a constant reminder about the value of life. The long-term effects of sibling bereavement are not necessarily pathological, but they are long-lasting.

Situational variables affecting bereavement

At the time of death

Cause of death

Whenever parents find their child is in a stressful situation, they respond with thoughts of 'What did I do to have caused this?' or 'What could I have done to prevent this from happening?' Such responses are natural for parents whose child dies, especially when the death is sudden, dramatic, or unexpected. When a child dies following a long-term illness, there is reason to believe that parents most often perceive the death as an outcome of the illness rather than of personal action.[23] At the time of diagnosis, however, parents often hold themselves responsible for not producing a healthy child. It is not uncommon for them to search all the way back to the earliest prenatal experiences in an attempt to identify a reason for the untoward condition. If parents have been adequately supported in expressing and handling these feelings during their child's illness, they will be less likely to harbour feelings of responsibility for the child's death. Family reactions at the time of diagnosis are discussed more fully in Chapter 14.2.

Anticipatory grief in childhood cancer

The concept of anticipatory grief has been viewed as a potential coping mechanism for a prospective loss. When death results from a sudden event, the subsequent grief for survivors is more difficult than when the death follows a long-term, life-threatening illness. However, reported findings are inconclusive as to the value and function of anticipatory grief, even though there is consensus that having time to prepare for a death serves an adaptive function in reducing seriousness and frequency of psychological sequelae after a child's death[23–25] and consideration must be given to the idea that there are optimum amounts of anticipatory grief. Further research is needed to clarify what constitutes 'optimum' anticipatory grief and to be able to identify, differentiate, and predict what will be most therapeutic for different parents in differing situations.

One difficulty with the concept of anticipatory grief is that is leads to the assumption that an 'unexpected' death is more difficult than an 'expected' death. It is critical to realize that every child's death is unexpected at the time at which it occurs. After the death, parents and siblings who had accepted the inevitable outcome of the illness, have been heard to comment, 'But I didn't think he would die until after he graduated', 'I didn't think he would die this morning.' Even with preparation time, the actual death is a final surprise. No degree of education or anticipatory grief adequately prepares one for the reality of death until all bodily functions cease permanently. Anticipatory grief does not replace the need to grieve over the death of a child, and to grieve over time. Therefore, health professionals must be prepared to support family members at the time of their child's death and to continue their support for extended periods of time.

Place of death

If given a choice, most ill children prefer to be with their parents, their families, and friends, among familiar belongings at home. When children are dying, their preference for being at home is even stronger. Many parents share this wish. In her pioneering work in providing home care for dying children,[26] Martinson expected that about half the children would die at home; in fact, 80 per cent of them did. The reader is referred to Section 16 for a discussion of home care as an alternative to hospital care.

Some families may not choose home care as an option but for those who do, home care has been remarkably effective from a cost-saving perspective and from the perspective of siblings and parents following the child's death. Studies examining the differential adjustment of siblings and parents have shown that a child's death at home has long-term benefits over that in hospital. First, the behaviour reactions of children 3 to 29 months following a sibling's death at home were within normal limits on a standardized checklist, whereas those children whose sibling had died in hospital had higher scores of fear and neurotic behaviour.[27] Secondly, 1 year after the death, siblings described a significantly different experience depending on the place of death. Those whose siblings had died in hospital generally described themselves as having been inadequately prepared for the death, isolated from the dying child and their parents, unable to use their parents for support information, unclear as to the circumstances of the death, and useless in terms of their own involvement. By contrast. siblings of children who died at home were prepared for their impending death, received consistent information and support from their parents, were involved in most activities concerning the dying child, were present for the death, and viewed their own involvement as the most important aspect of the experience. Open and ongoing communication and involvement in the care of the dying child, and in events after the death, are positively related to optimal bereavement outcomes in children. Thirdly, 6 to 8 years following a child's death at home or in hospital, parental adjustment was related to location of care.[28] Parents who provided home care experienced a relatively efficient and enduring resolution of their grief. While this relationship requires further empirical testing among home care and non-home care sibling populations, these early findings provide more definitive support for the role of home care as a determinant of differential profiles of bereavement.

Following the death

Caring for the child's belongings

Knowing what to do with the belongings of a child after his death usually presents a dilemma for families, and often they share their concerns with those who are caring for the child during the terminal phase or with those who follow the family after the death. To respond to such questions is not an easy task. An exploration of what families actually did with their child's belongings provides some guidelines for health-care professionals whose opinions may be sought.[29] The belongings of the deceased child have the potential of serving as memories, and the meaning associated with a particular belonging determines whether or not the belonging is kept. Therefore, health-care professionals should avoid telling families what to do with their child's belongings and should avoid giving families explicit time lines to follow. Furthermore, memories may vary in meaning for individuals within the family. Memories may have a mutually held meaning for the family as a whole and private meanings for its individual members. Consequently, health-care professionals can encourage families to be aware of the subtle meanings that may be associated with various belongings which serve as memories. For example, most bereaved families keep visible mementoes of their child. When such mementoes (photographs, for example) are displayed within a grouping of photos of all the children in the family, a different message is conveyed than if the photo is the only one displayed. In the first instance, the surviving children perceive that the deceased child was 'one of the family;' in the second instance, they may perceive that the deceased child is the most important child in the family. There is also evidence to suggest that the greater the discrepancy between the family's mutually held meaning of the memory and the individual's private meanings of the memory, the less the integration of the loss by the family and its individual members. It is important, therefore, to encourage family members to share openly their private meanings, and to help them realize that not having the same meanings and memories is acceptable.

Parenting

Parents who have other children must continue to function in the very role that they are trying to grieve for and relinquish. Parenting the remaining children presents what is often a challenge to parents, and is the source of potential problems between bereaved parents and their remaining children. Parents may overprotect their other children, wanting not to risk losing another child. Parents may worry excessively about how the surviving children are dealing with their grief; conversely, parents may be distressed because the surviving children appear not to be grieving enough. Sometimes, parents harbour resentments because their other children continue to live. None of these feelings are abnormal in the context of grief but it is important that such feelings are acknowledged by parents, preferably with the assistance of health-care providers, and that parents are provided with information about what to expect in their other children. It is critical for parents to understand that children may differ from adults in the way they demonstrate their grief. For example, younger children may cope best by continuing with their lives as if nothing had happened. Play is the child's vehicle for learning and for expressing feelings and concerns. So, for a child to resume play activities 'as if nothing had happened' is usually the only means available to the child for dealing with the loss. Parents, and other adults, must not assume to 'know' what the children are thinking and feeling unless they have spoken with them. Parents must also recognize the unique difficulties of surviving siblings as these children will live longer with the loss than anyone else. Knowledge about children's responses to loss, as well about the similarities and differences between childhood and parental bereavement, can better prepare parents to communicate with their children about loss and death and to help them cope.

Replacement child

Parents who are unable to integrate the loss of their child into their lives are at risk for having a 'replacement child'—a substitute for the dead child. A child can be conceived or adopted for the purpose of comforting and alleviating the pain of the parents' loss. Sometimes, a surviving child may become a replacement child. Consequences for the child assigned this role are potentially traumatic; the child never becomes his 'own person,' and continually feels as if he is 'not enough' to satisfy the parents' longings. In some families, the surviving child perceives that the child who died was the parents' favourite child or that the deceased child was perfect, and these children often feel as though they are not enough. Such feelings can negatively affect the child's self-concept.[30]

Physicians and other health-care providers can do much to prevent the phenomenon of replacement children. First, they should refrain from suggesting that parents have another child after the death of one child. Often, parents are told to have another child to give them something else to live for or to take their mind off the child who died. Instead, parents must be made aware of the potential for creating a replacement child; they must be helped to realize that other children will not help them resolve their grief. Moreover, the focus of intervention must be on clarifying expectations for grief and on explaining feelings that are common for bereaved parents and siblings. Parents must be assisted in realizing that their pain will eventually lessen but that their memories will last forever.

Parent–child communication

The importance of effective communication has been recognized as an essential element in facilitating individual and family coping with childhood chronic, life-threatening illness. However, effective communication refers not just to the sharing of information but to the creation of a climate that allows and encourages the expression of feelings. Several studies support that suggestion that parent–sibling communication differs before and after the death. Before the death, talking about the illness and death is related specifically to the events of day-to-day care. After the death, while open expression may pertain to many topics and areas of concern to family members, discussion about the feelings aroused by the death may be excluded. Similarly, the open expression of grief may not be supported, even in the most expressive families. This exclusion may not, and is usually not, conscious. Often, it is communicated implicitly by the lack of willingness to experience and openly express the painful emotions associated with grief. Therefore, it seems that parents, including those who communicated openly with their children before the death, need encouragement in communicating openly with their surviving children after the death so that the sadness and sorrow is shared and expressed.

Health-care professional intervention

In recent years, a limited number of studies have begun to examine the relationship between parental bereavement outcome and health-care professionals' interventions prior to, at the time of, and after the child's death.[8,31] The results of the studies revealed that, in many cases, the actions that were considered helpful or not helpful varied according to each individual's personal perceptions and situations. Due to the uniqueness of every parent's grieving response, health-care professionals' intervention cannot be simply standardized but must be individualized to meet the needs of each bereaved parent. The most consistently helpful action was related to the attitude of the health-care providers—showing a caring, concerned attitude and also demonstrating an ability to be involved with parents.[31]

Summary

The death of a child has a potentially traumatic impact on the family. The death induces profound parental grief which affects parents as individuals and as marital partners; the death alters the behaviour of siblings. From the literature reviewed, it can be concluded that the death of a child is not something to 'get over.' Instead, it is an event that surviving parents and siblings must learn to integrate into the ongoing fabric of their lives. Only by understanding this to be the case can health professionals offer their knowledgeable, sensitive, and long-term support that such families require.

Caregiver response

Helping a child die well, physically comfortable and psychologically at peace; helping parents get through the experience of their child's death as well as they possibly can; helping siblings and other children close to the dying child master the experience to the full potential of their developmental level—each of these is a challenge to health-care professionals personally and professionally. Caregivers absorb much of the same stress experienced by the family members of a dying child and experience similar conflict. This stress, and the associated disruption, pressure, and depletion require significant personal and professional effort at adaptation and balance. Furthermore, the death of a child characteristically leads to a core conflict in persons caring for the child—a tendency to overprotect and become overinvolved with the child and an opposing tendency to move away from the child to protect oneself from painful involvement.

Showing compassion

In order for those in helping professions to function effectively—to 'enjoy' being a good doctor, nurse, clergyman, lawyer, or whatever—professionals must allow themselves to approach, and to a degree share, the distress of those they are attempting to help.[32,33] They must show compassion. Yet, when confronted with a dying child, professionals are sometimes compelled to respond with analysis, clinical judgement, and 'doing' behaviours in an effort to maintain some sense of control and composure.

However, compassion and control seem incompatible. Professionals vary widely in the extent to which they can retain their compassion. Two things are crucial: the magnitude of the distress and the individual's own confidence in his or her ability to cope with it. As long as professionals feel that their participation is worthwhile, they will find themselves able to tolerate high levels of disturbance in others without disengaging. Confidence in one's ability to cope with the distress of others can be, and normally is, obtained by a process of attunement. By repeated, reflective exposure, professionals gradually discover what they can do to alleviate distress and how much of it is inevitable and insurmountable.

Key attributes

Some health-care professionals are more suitable than others for the demanding role of working with dying children and adolescents.[34] Those who are best suited to this role have specific personal attributes, including: a high tolerance for ambiguity, flexibility, and an appreciation for individual differences; good external support networks and a realistic awareness of personal limits; *joie de vivre* and sense of humour; an open communication style and tendency to value self-awareness as assets; empathy and a willingness to continually learn.[35,36] Perhaps the most basic characteristic is one's comfort with death. Becoming a clinical practitioner who can move toward instead of away from children who are dying does not come easily. Only by coming to terms with one's own thoughts and feelings about death and about children, is it possible to adapt philosophically to working with children who might die. Self-awareness is integral to effective care of the dying; caregivers needs to be conscious of their own agendas as they interface with patient, family, team, and institution directions and goals.[37]

Nurse–patient–family relationship

The duration of relationships with patients who have long-term, chronic illness provides nurses with both the opportunity and the obligation to establish relationships as persons as well as professionals. The nurse may become a 'professional friend'. The relationship is a professional one—it is time limited, goal oriented, and patient centred with professional knowledge and skills employed on the patient's behalf.[38] However, the relationship may also assume some of the qualities usually described as part of a socially meaningful relationship. When the patient is a child, the nurse often becomes a professional friend not only of the child but also of the family. As the child enters the terminal phase, the closeness of the relationship may enhance personal and professional distress. A recent study[39] described the 'struggle' nurses experience while caring for children with chronic, life-threatening illness who die. They struggle with grief but their expression of such distress was hampered by a code of conduct either self-imposed or imposed by their profession, their organization, or society in general. Nurses also struggled with moral distress when directives for painful, life-prolonging treatment for children in the dying process challenged their professional ethic to provide for the patient the most comfort they could.

Manifestations of stress: cost of caring

In a study of occupational stress in the care of the critically ill, the dying, and the bereaved, three major categories of stress—physical, psychological, and behavioural—were reported.[37] Of these, physical symptoms of stress were reported less often, and psychological symptoms were reported more often than behavioural ones. Furthermore, younger caregivers reported more symptoms of stress and fewer coping strategies than older caregivers. By being aware of the manifestations of stress, professionals can monitor their own responses, taking appropriate action when they begin to experience such symptoms. Appropriate actions include approaches at both institutional and personal levels.

Much of the literature cites the paediatric ward as a potential source of ultimate frustration, anguish, and personal and professional stress for caregivers; however, there are few studies which describe the stress experienced by staff working with such children.[39,40] In the one published study describing staff stress in a paediatric hospice setting,[40] a small but distinct subgroup of staff who manifested symptoms of psychological distress were characterized in two ways. First, they experienced relatively recent bereavement in their personal lives. Second, they failed to resolve their grief about a bereavement which had occurred some considerable time before. Deep distress can be rekindled when a trigger event echoes back to and resurrects a sense of personal loss. The very nature of the work serves as a constant reminder of their loss and may interfere with their own natural grieving.

Institutional actions

Within agencies, primary consideration must be given to staff selection. Individuals must want to work in paediatric palliative care, and must come with a repertoire of coping abilities developed through previous work and personal experiences. They must be trained in the care of dying children. On the whole, physicians and nurses are inadequately prepared to care for the dying; education has emphasized life-saving activities, maintenance of personal control, and the avoidance of failure. Lack of emphasis on the accountability of psychosocial care has contributed to this lack of education for all health professionals. The need for systematic education for nurses was identified more than 20 years ago;[41] however, in the interim, few such programmes have been described and even fewer programmes have been evaluated.[42] There are similar findings in medical literature pertaining to the education of physicians.[43–46] The need for appropriate training in the care of the dying remains strong.

Recent findings suggest that the milieu of the ward when a child died affects the nurse's grief.[39] When it was acknowledged how difficult it might be for the nurse when her patient died, the nurse felt supported and felt better able to resolve her grief. Another strategy that facilitates nurses' successful moving though the grieving process is clearly establishing the palliative focus of nursing care goals. Being able to make the patient comfortable, free from pain, and the family satisfied made it easier for nurses to cope with the situation. The difficulty in an acute care setting is that not all members of the team may be able to acknowledge that the child will not recover. In spite of these barriers, the opportunity to brief, debrief, review, and analyse the situation in a safe, supportive environment can help nurses cope with current and subsequent stresses in their practice setting.

The necessity of teambuilding and support in interdisciplinary teamwork has been the focus of long-standing debate. There are three primary advantages to allowing staff as a group the time and means to understand and tackle the difficult issues that necessarily arise in any team.[47] First, understanding of interpersonal dynamics and pitfalls amongst the team will further the team's understanding of the families for whom they care. Second, while some may argue that teams are really too busy helping families to waste time on the unnecessary nicety of promoting understanding, the contrary is true in that time is saved. Prolonged and unresolved staff conflict saps and debilitates the individual and undermines his or her self-esteem, commitment, and efficiency. At its worst, it leads to high staff turnover with consequent fragmentation in care and delivery. Third, 'problems and difficulties encountered by those facing great distress have a way of echoing and reverberating in the service set up to help them, with the danger that a service inadvertently mirrors, and therefore remirrors, the very difficulties it aims to ease.'[47] Any group claiming to work as a team should show their battle scars. 'If they don't have them, they haven't worked as a team.'[48]

Personal actions

The person best equipped to deal with the care of the dying child is that person who has developed a wide repertoire of coping skills through exposure to previous life stressors, both personal and professional. Conversely, the professional who deals with feelings of helplessness and passivity by excessive intellectualization, flight into activity, denial, projection, rationalization, or withdrawal is going to experience personal distress as well as finding himself or herself in the middle of considerable staff conflict.[33] Effective coping requires a high degree of self-awareness and personal responsibility. Personal approaches therefore must include developing outlets for physical and emotional expression, creating periods of solitude for reflection and integration, and finding meaning through one's personal philosophy.

Implications for practice

Helping the bereaved

According to the Committee for the Study of Health Consequences of the Stress of Bereavement[49] health-care providers and institutions are professionally and morally obligated to assist the bereaved by offering support and information and by being sensitive to and knowledgeable about grief's impact. To carry out this role responsibly, they should be able to communicate about sensitive issues, to understand the nature of normal and abnormal bereavement reactions, and to be knowledgeable about community resources to which the bereaved can be referred for specialized help if needed. A recent review of models in the field of death, dying, and bereavement suggests the need to shift perspective from passive victimization to an opportunity for active processes (task-based model), whereby one can regain some measure of control and meaning in living with loss.[9,50] Limitations in the attention paid to the bereaved by health-care professionals appear to derive from three factors:

(1) their inadequate training about the nature of bereavement and their own personal feelings toward death;

(2) the failure of health-care institutions to acknowledge their responsibility for bereavement follow-up, the stress that caring for dying and bereaved persons puts on their staff, and the need for sufficient staff time for these activities;

(3) the financial constraints imposed by the current structure of third-party reimbursement arrangements.

Despite these constraints, and despite currently inadequate therapeutic guidelines, it is necessary for health professionals to formulate some approach to the bereaved because, whether they are trained or untrained, those who interact with a bereaved person will have an impact—negative or positive—on that individual.

Although there has been much documentation in the literature addressing assessment and intervention strategies when working with bereaved individuals,[51-53] there is a dearth of coherent, systematic synthesis of this material. While one must always be weary of 'cookbook' approaches to grief counselling, consideration of some general principles for helping individuals may be beneficial.

Bereaved parents

In working with bereaved parents, it is critical to maintain a family systems perspective, recognizing the impact of the death on family members and on their interactions with one another. Interventions by health-care professionals begin by making contact with the parents and letting them know that caregivers are available to meet with them should they desire such contact. Parents often have many questions about the child's death, and the nurses and physicians who are willing to discuss these sensitive issues provide a meaningful service to the family. Parents especially value contact with those care providers who cared directly for their child, and in particular with the nurse who was with the child at the moment of death.

Almost all the evidence recommends professional intervention following the death of a child; the need for a trained professional in the area of bereavement seems evident. Follow-up by the care providers focuses on facilitating communication within the family, allowing parents to vent their anxieties and concerns, assessing the family's grief in order to promote the mental health of the family, and referring the parents to other useful resources. One major resource may be books written for bereaved individuals, particularly bereaved parents. The most potent resources available, however, are specific support groups for bereaved parents, which provide ongoing social support. Options include groups such as The Compassionate Friends, an international self-help group for all types of bereaved parents, Candlelighters, a group for parents of children with cancer, or other local groups devoted to helping bereaved parents. Through mutual sharing, learning, modelling, and support these groups support parents in their grief.[54,55]

Probably the most critical realization for caregivers who are providing bereavement support to parents is that they cannot take away the parents' pain and suffering. Therefore, the follow-up that caregivers offer must be supportive in nature, and provided over time. Caregivers will no doubt feel helpless in such situations, and want to do something more. Instead, they must value the 'gift of presence,' of being there to share the pain. Table 2 provides a synthesis of principles and intervention strategies for working with bereaved parents.[56,57]

Bereaved siblings

Two critical assumptions provide the foundation for interventions with bereaved siblings. First, health-care providers must acknowledge the impact of a child's death on the surviving siblings. Until very recently, the focus of all attention has been the parents of the child who died; siblings have been forgotten. Research into the long-term effects of sibling bereavement continues to validate the significance of this event for siblings. Secondly, health-care providers must understand that the child's parents are the best one to help the siblings; therefore, the focus of interventions for the siblings becomes the parents. This is not to say, however, that direct contact with siblings is not helpful; indeed, direct interventions with caregivers can be particularly advantageous for older children, who need a less emotionally involved adult with whom to discuss their concerns. Such children often avoid discussing their own grief with their parents because they are trying to protect their parents from further distress.

There is considerable similarity between the techniques used to help children cope with a dying sibling and those used to help children adjust to the death of a sibling. In both cases, in order to guide parents in supporting their other children, care providers must understand children's view of death, and must be aware of the normal responses of children to death. This information then serves as the foundation upon which parents' questions and concerns about their surviving children can be discussed. Communication with siblings needs to be open, and must take into account each child's individual needs and developmental level. For all children, however, parents and caregivers need to remember the CHILD when helping him or her to cope with grief (Table 3).

Conclusion

Facing the impending death of a child is an experience like no other. The unnaturalness of a child's death compounds the pain, the sorrow, and the sadness. And yet, children too must face life-threatening illness. It is crucial that we pay attention to this experience, and that we realize that the effects of the experience do not end with the child's death. The loss of a child triggers profound grief in all those who knew and cared for the child—the parents, siblings, grandparents, teachers, and the nurses and doctors and other health providers who, on a daily basis, were witness to the plight of the child and his family. Health-care professionals can do much to facilitate optimal bereavement outcomes in the child's family. Such individuals must realize the child's need to be cared for in a style that promotes comfort and dignity. In addition, such individuals must remember that the experiences of the family during the dying process will significantly

Table 2 Principles and strategies for working with bereaved parents[11,57]

1. Make contact and assess the bereaved parents
2. Provide assurance that they can survive their loss, keeping in mind the parents' unique perspective
3. Provide times to grieve, remembering that grief has its own time
4. Facilitate the identification and expression of feelings, including anger, hostility, sadness, relief, guilt
5. Encourage verbalization of thoughts and recollections of the deceased child; do not be afraid to mention the deceased child's name
6. Interpret 'normal' grieving behaviour and responses
7. Maintain a therapeutic and realistic perspective; do not rush to 'fix' the pain
8. Allow for individual differences relating to gender, age, personality, culture, ethnicity, religion, characteristics of the death
9. Avoid analysing or interrupting parents' repeated stories and tears
10. Help to identify and resolve secondary losses, such as the hopes, dreams, and expectations the parents had for the deceased child
11. Examine defences and coping strategies; carefully examine resistance to the grief process
12. Assist in finding sources of continuing support
13. Identify and refer 'pathology'
14. Interpret 'recovery' for them; correct unrealistic expectations of themselves and of the grief process

Table 3 Helping children cope with grief: Remember the CHILD

C— CONSIDER

Consider the unique situation of the child, his/her developmental capacity to understand, his/her concerns, his/her thoughts, his/her feelings, his/her relationship to his sibling

A child is a child: do not expect a child to be 'the man around the house' or the 'little mother'; it is unfair to the child's future development and often limiting to the grieving process to assign inappropriate role responsibilities to the child

H— HONESTY

Use the 'd' word: death, die, dying

Realize that it is all right to not have all the answers

Avoid euphemisms—words which are confusing or have other meanings for the child

Avoid words such as gone away or went on a trip; expressions such as these can make everyday events—leaving on a vacation, going to work—very frightening for the child

Do not explain to a child that the dead person is sleeping; he/she will be afraid of sleeping

I— INVOLVE

Let the child know what is happening; if possible, before the death occurs

Give the child factual knowledge about the cause of death—especially the school-age child

Involve the child in saying good-bye to the dying and deceased—allow the child the choice to participate in the funeral to the level at which he/she is comfortable

L— LISTEN

Concentrate on discussing the stumbling block of the moment—too often when the subject is sensitive, adults want to rush ahead to explain and reassure in order to finish the conversation; rather, let the child talk through what is on his/her mind

Let the child know that it is all right to not want to talk to anyone anymore about the death for a while

Give the child outlets for expressing his/her grief—art, drawing, play, writing letters, poetry, stories, hammering

Be aware of thoughts and fantasies children may have of being reunited with the person who has died; each child must be considered potentially at risk for suicide and any kind of communication that suggests this possibility should be promptly and fully evaluated; careful attention to any suggestion of suicidal risk, no matter what the age of the child, is essential

Clarify that death is NOT the result of the child's action or thoughts; be attuned to magical thinking involved in the child's explanation of the death and correct it to avoid guilt and inappropriate grief reactions

D— DO IT OVER AND OVER AGAIN

Appropriately share your grief; realize that children cannot do grief work without permission and role models; children need to see an honest expression of emotions from adults accompanied by explanations and reassurance

Keep in mind the developmental capacities of the child and his/her age-related concerns and needs affect their future lives as survivors. Professionals must be aware of the various reactions that comprise 'normal' grief in parents and siblings, recognizing that such reactions may be influenced by a variety of mediating factors, some of which have been identified. Further, health-care professionals must be aware that the intensity of the immediate impact does seem to diminish over time but the long-term effects, though not easily identified or measured, last a life time.

Health-care professionals who choose to care for dying children and their families do not engage in this work without needing support themselves. This is a challenging field, one which demands that professionals struggle with the difficult task of maintaining balance and perspective. In addition, however, working with such children and their families provides meaning to life. Working with these children helps to give a clear perspective on what is really valuable. Working with these children helps us to grow, to develop as both persons and professionals. It has been said that all of us need to learn about our own mortality, limitations, and vulnerabilities. These children and their families teach these lessons well.

References

1. McClowry SG, Davies EB, Kulenkamp ME, Martinson IM. The empty space phenomenon: the process of grief in the bereaved family. *Death Studies*, 1987; **11**: 361–74.
2. Martinson IM, McClowry SG, Davies B, Kulenkamp EJ. Changes over time: a study of family bereavement following childhood cancer. *Journal of Palliative Care*, 1994; **10**: 19–25
3. Davies B, Spinetta J, Martinson I, McClowry S, Kulenkamp E. Manifestations of levels of functioning in grieving families. *Journal of Family Issues*, 1986; **7**: 297–313.
4. Clayton P, Desmarais L, Winokur G. A study of normal bereavement. *American Journal of Psychiatry*, 1968; **125**: 168–78.
5. Sanders CM. A comparison of adult bereavement in the death of a spouse, child, and parent. *Omega*, 1979–80; **10**: 303–22.
6. Moore IM, Gilliss CL, Martinson IM. Psychosomatic symptoms in parents 2 years after the death of a child with cancer. *Nursing Research*, 1988; **37**: 104–6.
7. Hazzard A, Weston J, Gutteres C. After a child's death: Factors related to parental bereavement. *Developmental and Behavioral Pediatrics*, 1992; **13**: 24–30.
8. Neidig JR, Dalgas-Pelish P. Parental grieving and perceptions regarding health care professionals' interventions. *Issues in Comprehensive Nursing*, 1991; **14**: 179–91.
9. Attig TW. The importance of conceiving of grieving as an active process. *Death Studies*, 1991; **15**: 383–93.
10. Miles MS. Helping adults mourn the death of a child. In: Wass H, Corr CA, eds. *Issues in Comprehensive Pediatric Nursing*, Vol. 1. Washington DC: Hemisphere Publishing, 1985: 219–41.
11. Worden JW. *Grief Counselling and Grief Therapy: A Handbook for the Mental Health Practitioner.* New York: Springer, 1982.
12. Foley GV, Whittham EH. Care of the child dying of cancer: Part II. *Ca A Cancer Journal for Clinicians*, 1991; **41**: 52–64.
13. Foster DJ, O'Malley JE, Koocher GP. The parent interviews. In: Koocher GP, O'Malley JE, eds. *The Damocles Syndrome: Psychosocial Consequences of Surviving Childhood Cancer.* New York: McGraw-Hill, 1981: 86–100.
14. Lansky SB, Cairns NU, Hassaneim R, Wehr J, Lowman JT. Childhood cancer: parental discord and divorce. *Pediatrics*, 1978; **62**: 184–8.
15. Spinetta J, Swarner J, Sheoposh J. Effective parental coping following death of a child from cancer. *Journal of Pediatric Psychology*, 1981; **6**: 251–63.
16. Rando TA. The unique issues and impact of the death of a child. In: Rando TA, ed. *Parental Loss of a Child.* Champaign, IL: Research Press, 1986: 5–43.
17. Rando TA. An investigation of grief and adaptation in parents whose children have died from cancer. *Journal of Pediatric Psychology*, 1983; **8**: 3–20.
18. Miles MS, Crandall EK. The search for meaning and its potential for affecting growth in bereaved parents. *Health Values: Achieving High Level Wellness*, 1983; **7**: 19–23.
19. Davies B. The family environment in bereaved families and its relationship to surviving sibling behaviour. *Children's Health Care*, 1988; **17**: 22–30.
20. Davies B. After a sibling dies. In: Morgan MA, ed. *Bereavement: Helping the Survivors. Proceedings of the 1987 King's College Conference.* London: King's College, 1987: 55–65.
21. Rosen H. *Unspoken Grief: Coping with Childhood Sibling Loss.* Lexington, DC: Health and Company, 1986.
22. Davies B. Long-term outcomes of adolescent sibling bereavement. *Journal of Adolescent Research*, 1991; **6**: 83–96.
23. Kupst MJ. Death of a child from a serious illness. In: Rando TA, ed. *Parental Loss of a Child.* Champaign, IL: Research Press, 1986: 191–9.
24. Futterman EH, Hoffman I. Mourning the fatally ill child. In: Schowalter JE, Patterson PR, Tallmer M, Kutscher AH, Gull SV, Peretz D, eds. *The Child and Death.* New York: Columbia University Press, 1983: 366–81.
25. Kemler B. Anticipatory grief and survival. In: Koocher GP, O'Malley JE, eds. *The Damocles Syndrome: Psychosocial Consequences of Survival of Childhood Cancer.* New York: McGraw-Hill, 1981: 131–43.
26. Martinson IM. *Home Care for the Child with Cancer* (Final report grant CA 19490). Washington DC: National Cancer Institute, 1980.
27. Lauer ME, Mulhern RK, Bohne JB, Camitta BM. Children's perceptions of their siblings' death at home or hospital: the precursors of differential adjustment. *Cancer Nursing*, 1985; **8**: 21–7.
28. Lauer ME, Mulhern RK, Schell MJ, Camitta BM. Long-term follow-up of parental adjustment following a child's death at home or hospital. *Cancer*, 1989; **63**: 988–94.
29. Davies B. Family responses to the death of a child: The meaning of memories. *Journal of Palliative Care*, 1987; **3**: 9–15.
30. Martinson I, Davies B, McClowry S. The long-term effects of sibling death on self-concept. *Journal of Pediatric Nursing*, 1987; **2**: 227–35.
31. Jost KE, Hasse JE. At the time of death: Help for the child's parents. *Children's Health Care*, 1989; **18**: 146–52.
32. Parkes CM. *Bereavement: Studies of Grief in Adult Life.* 2nd edn. New York: Tavistock Publications, 1986.
33. Vachon MLS, Pakes E. Staff stress in the care of the critically ill and dying child. *Issues in Comprehensive Pediatric Nursing*, 1985; **8**: 151–82.
34. Davies B, Eng B. Factors influencing nursing care of children who are terminally ill: A selective review. *Pediatric Nursing*, 1993; **19**: 9–14.
35. Benoliel JQ. The cancer patient's right to know and decide: An ethical perspective. In: McCorkle R, Hongladarom G, eds. *Issues and Topics in Cancer Nursing.* Norwalk, CONN: Appleton-Century-Crofts, 1986: 5–17.
36. Zerwekh JY. Professional stress and distress. In: Blues AG, Zerwekh JY, eds. *Hospice and Palliative Nursing Care.* New York: Grune and Stratton, 1984: 347–62.
37. Vachon MLS. *Occupational Stress in the Care of the Critically Ill, the Dying and the Bereaved.* New York: Hemisphere Publishing, 1987.
38. Trygstad L. Professional friends: The inclusion of the personal into the professional. *Cancer Nursing*, 1986; **9**: 326–32.
39. Davies B, Clarke D, Connaughty S, *et al.* The Experience of Nursing Care for Chronically Ill Children Who Die. Final Report. *Pediatric Nursing*, 1996; **22**:500–7.
40. Woolley H, Stein A, Forrest GC, Baum JD. Staff stress and job satisfaction at a children's hospice. *Archives of Disease in Childhood*, 1989; **64**: 114–18.
41. Quint JC. *The Nurse and the Dying Patient.* New York: Macmillan, 1967.

42. Degner LF, Gow CM. Evaluation of death education in nursing: A critical review. *Cancer Nursing*, 1988; **11**: 151–9.
43. Penney JC. The evolution of a medical school curriculum in death and dying. *Journal of Palliative Care*, 1987; **3**: 14–18.
44. Irwin WG. Teaching terminal care at Queen's University of Belfast. I–Course, sessional educational objectives and content. *British Medical Journal*, 1984; **289**: 1509–11.
45. Irwin WG. Teaching terminal care at Queen's University of Belfast. II–Teaching arrangements and assessment of topic. *British Medical Journal*, 1984; **289**: 1604–5.
46. Scofield GR. Terminal care and the continuing need for professional education. *Journal of Palliative Care*, 1989; **5**: 32–6.
47. Stein A, Woolley H. Care for the carers. In Goldman A, ed. *Care of the Dying Child*. Oxford: Oxford University Press, 1994: 164–81.
48. Mount BM, Voyer S. Staff stress in palliative hospice care. In: Ajemaian I, Mount BM, eds. *The Royal Victoria Hospital Manual on Palliative Hospice Care*. New York: Arno Press, 1980: 146.
49. Osterweiss M, Solomon F, Green M, eds. *Bereavement Reactions, Consequences, and Care*. Report by the Committee for the Study of Health Consequences of the Stress of Bereavement, Institute of Medicine, National Academy of Sciences. Washington, DC: National Academy Press, 1984.
50. Corr CA, Doka KJ. Current models of death, dying and bereavement. *Critical Care Nursing Clinics of North America*, 1994; **6**: 545–52.
51. McCollum A. Counselling the grieving parent. In: Burton L, ed. *Care of the Child Facing Death*. London: Routledge and Kegan Paul, 1974: 177–88.
52. Pine YR, Brauer C. Parental grief: A synthesis of theory research, and intervention. In: Rando TA, ed. *Parental Loss of a Child*. Champaign, IL: Research Press, 1986: 59–96.
53. Rando TA. *Grief, Dying, and Death: Interventions for Caregivers*. Champaign, IL: Research Press, 1984.
54. Davies B, Martinson IM. Care of the family: Special emphasis on siblings during and after the death of a child. In: Martin BB, ed. *Pediatric Hospice Care: What Helps*. Los Angeles: Children's Hospital of Los Angeles, 1989: 186–99.
55. Dorsel SJ, Dorsel TN. Helping parents whose child has died: a review of coping strategies and alternatives for support. *American Journal of Hospice Care*, 1986; **3**: 17–20.
56. Rando TA. Individual and couples treatment following the death of a child. In: Rando TA, ed. *Parental Loss of a Child*. Champaign, IL: Research Press, 1986: 341–414.
57. Schmidt L. Working with bereaved parents. In: Krulik T, Holaday B, Martinson IM, eds. *The Child and Family Facing Life-Threatening Illness*. Philadelphia: J.B. Lippincott, 1987: 327–44.

Bibliography

The list of references contains a number of sources of general information in addition to the useful references cited here.

Adams-Greenly M. Helping children communicate about serious illness and death. *Journal of Psychosocial Oncology*, 1984; **2**: 61–72.

Graham-Pole J, Wass H, Eyberg S, Chu L, Olejnik S. Communicating with dying children and their siblings. A retrospective analysis. *Death Studies*, 1989; **13**: 465–83.

Rando TA. *Parental Loss of a Child*. Champaign, IL: Research Press, 1986.

19.7 The development of paediatric palliative care

19.7.1 Introduction

Betty Davies

As recognition of the need for palliative services for children and support for their families has increased, so has the variety of ways in which such care can be provided. A thorough knowledge of the resources available within a geographical area is essential in order to determine how the specific needs of patients and families can be met. The model of palliative care most likely to be successful will evolve from local lay and professional collaborative efforts.[1] Desirable as it may be, it may not be realistic or cost effective to propose separate units for children except in heavily populated areas or in referral centres serving a large area.

The development of palliative care in the United Kingdom in the 1960s created hospital-based, and later free-standing, residential beds for adults with terminal illnesses. In the United States, the hospice concept was not embraced immediately by medical professionals and the hospice movement grew from a grass-roots beginning with most programmes designed as home-care support. In Canada, specialized palliative care units have been established in many hospitals following the lead of Dr Balfour Mount in Montreal. Home-care programmes have developed more recently. Establishment of the modern palliative care movement in Australia began fairly recently when a group of 30 Australian nurses and physicians discovered each others' mutual interests in palliative care while attending the International Congress on the Care of the Terminally Ill in Montreal in the late 1980s (personal communication, Dr M. Stevens, The New Children's Hospital, Sydney, 1995). In all these countries, the development of palliative care services for children has followed adult programmes and is, therefore, very recent.

Standards for paediatric hospice care

Regardless of their setting, it would be wise to assess paediatric palliative programmes against general, uniform standards. A United Kingdom publication, *Care of the Dying: A Guide for Health Authorities*, outlines several criteria for assessing 'terminal care schemes'.[2] These same criteria are relevant to children's hospice services and could be used to begin to develop uniform standards, as in the following.

It is necessary that programmes have flexibility—the capacity to respond to the varying needs of the patient and to respond quickly. Costs are obviously a major consideration. Issues to be addressed should include capital expenditure and revenue consequences, the rate at which services can and should be implemented, and the possibility of shared funding with national or local charities. It is also necessary to allow for the fact that the new service may lead to financial savings elsewhere; or in cases where actual expenditure is increased, a more effective use of the resources may be achieved. Acceptability to patients is also a critical element. Often, parents find the hospital a safe and familiar place, but they also resent the lack of parental control and the 'high-tech', often cramped environment. Other parents may perceive that using palliative care is tantamount to admitting that their child will die. Public education and having current palliative care users share their experiences with other parents often helps to alter such perceptions. Moreover, since we live in a multicultural society, it is important that the services are planned and care is provided in such a way that the diverse needs of the various ethnic, religious, and cultural groups are met appropriately.

Acceptability to colleagues in hospital and in the community is also significant. Co-ordination of services and open communication are critical to successful paediatric hospice programmes. It is important that hospice programmes are developed and maintained in ways that they complement, not duplicate or compete with, existing services. Good communication before the service is started, good management, and a clear operational policy go a long way to ensuring co-operative endeavours. Finally, location is critical. The programme must be easily accessible to families, either by car or public transportation. When an inpatient facility serves a large geographical region, then it must be within relatively easy access from train, bus, or plane terminals.

Locations of paediatric palliative care

A variety of locations where palliation for children is provided has evolved over the last 10 to 12 years. As no universal standards have yet been agreed upon, the location and services reflect the influence of the local professional and lay communities. The pressure for delineated areas for children receiving palliation came originally from those services carrying significant numbers of children with chronic illnesses in their terminal phase, such as oncology and cystic fibrosis services. Some medical school departments of paediatrics and tertiary care paediatric programmes, especially those affiliated with children's hospitals, responded to such models of extended care by establishing palliative care units staffed by specially trained paediatric nurses. Not every hospital can offer such services.

The loci of care available for palliation in children can be loosely categorized into inpatient or domiciliary facilities and outpatient or home-based programmes. In some places, the home-care programmes are co-ordinated through inpatient facilities. The facilities may be hospitals—general in nature or specialized. In turn, within these, children may be cared for in general units, intensive care units, undifferentiated palliative care units, or specific paediatric palliative care units. In addition to the standard hospital, there are free-standing palliative care facilities, commonly referred to as hospices. The first of these, Helen House, was established in England in 1982, and others have since developed. This model of care provides the basis for the first free-standing children's hospice in North America—in Vancouver, Canada, and for Australia's first free-standing hospice in Sydney, Australia.

Following are summaries of the status of paediatric palliative care in four of the industrialized countries: the United Kingdom, Canada, Australia, and the United States. It is acknowledged that we have much to learn about paediatric palliative care in not only other industrialized countries, but in the rest of the world as well.

References

1. Lazarus KH. Developing a pediatric hospice: organizational dynamics. In: Paradis LF, ed. *Hospice Handbook: A Guide for Managers and Planners.* Rockville: Aspen Publications, 1985: 147–71.
2. National Association of Health Authorities. *Care of the Dying—A Guide for Health Authorities.* Birmingham, England, 1987.

19.7.2 Development in the United Kingdom

Frances Dominica

A variety of paediatric hospice care programmes have developed in the United Kingdom.[1] In the late 1970s, Chapman and Goodall drew attention to the needs of dying children and their families for emotional and practical support.[2,3] A need for home-based, as well as hospital-based care was recognized, both for children receiving treatment and for children in the terminal stage of their illness. However, at about the same time another need became apparent: that of non-hospital based respite care for those families caring for children with life-limiting and often long-term disease.

Helen House, the first purpose-built, free-standing facility providing respite and terminal care to children with life-limiting disease was opened in 1982.[4] Helen, after whom the house was named, had been a happy, healthy child who, in 1978 at the age of two, was diagnosed as having a massive cerebral tumour. Surgery successfully removed the tumour but resulted in devastating brain damage. Helen's parents were told that nothing further could be done towards recovery and they determined that they would care for her at home. A friendship between Helen's parents and Sister Frances Dominica, then Mother Superior of All Saints Convent, Oxford, led to the idea of a facility that could offer friendship, respite, and support to families caring for their sick child at home. The facility would aim to complement existing services rather than to be an alternative. From the original concept to completion took less than 3 years, the entire cost of building—and subsequent running costs—coming from voluntary sources.[5,6]

In 1995, at the time of writing, there are eight free-standing children's hospices in the United Kingdom offering respite and terminal care to children with life-limiting illnesses and their families. These are Helen House, Oxford (1982), Martin House, West Yorkshire (1987), Acorns, Birmingham (1988), Cambridge Hospice for the Eastern Region (1989), Francis House, Manchester (1991), Quidenham Children's Hospice, Norfolk (1991), Derian House, Chorley (1993), and Rainbows, Leicestershire (1994). A number of other paediatric hospices are in various stages of planning and development.

Each hospice offers inpatient care. Some also give support to families through care in the home. The children's hospices are designed to be as light and attractive as possible, home rather than hospital being the model. Most have beds available for eight to ten children at any one time and can provide accommodation for members of the families who may wish to stay with them. Parents may choose to care for their child in the hospice themselves, to hand over care to the team, or to share the care. In response, the care teams aim to respond as flexibly as they can to meet the needs of the families. Well brothers and sisters are welcome to stay, too, and it is recognized that their needs, though different, are nevertheless as great as those of the sick child. Grandparents, who play an important role in many families, are also welcome.

Examination of patterns of use at three of the hospices suggests that the average length of stay for children on a visit is from four to six nights and the average number of nights per year per child is from 16 to 21. However, the frequency and duration of visits varies tremendously with the changing needs of each child and family during the course of the illness. Whilst most admissions at Helen House have been for planned respite care, approximately 10 per cent have been for emergency respite, symptom control, or terminal care.[7,8]

As independent establishments, each hospice has developed its own criteria for admission. At Helen House, any child under 17 years with a life-threatening condition may be referred. During the 11 years from opening until the end of 1994, 325 children were admitted. From 60 to 70 per cent of children had a genetic disease and over 10 per cent of families have had more than one child with the same disease. Up to the end of 1994, 206 children had died, 50 per cent of these within 2 years of their first admission. However, reflecting the chronicity of many of the conditions, nearly 20 per cent had lived more than 5 years after their first admission.

The provision of respite care attracts to the children's hospices those families whose need for respite is paramount, that is, where the child's needs are physically and emotionally demanding and time-consuming. However, patterns at each hospice may vary according to local needs and sources of referral. In 1994, at Helen House, the group who used the hospice most were those families whose child had a neurodegenerative condition.[9] At Martin House, the greatest proportion was those children with neuromuscular disease, in particular, those with Duchenne muscular dystrophy (Table 1).

Referrals to Helen House have come from many sources, including 30 per cent from the families themselves (Table 2). Registering authorities for some of the hospices have limited the use so that if a child reaches 19 years of age they may no longer use the facility. However, at Helen House, if children, previously

Table 1 Diagnostic groups of children staying at three UK children's hospices in 1994

	Helen House		Martin House		Cambridge	
	Number	%	Number	%	Number	%
Degenerative central nervous system disease	38	45	41	22	9	10
Non-progressive central nervous system	14	17	24	13	34	36
Mucopolysaccharidoses	12	14	15	8	3	3
Other inborn errors	5	6	10	5	3	3
Neuromuscular disease	8	9	50	28	7	8
Congenital disease	7	8	16	9	24	26
Cancer	1	1	19	10	7	8
Other	0	0	9	5	6	6
Total	85	100	184	100	94	100

accepted, live on in to their late teens and early 20s they may continue to use the facility if it remains the most appropriate one available for the child and family. Some of the hospices have a specific catchment area, whilst others have no regional boundaries. Whilst some have endeavoured to accept all appropriate children who are referred, Helen House found, after about 8 years of operation, that once the number of children currently using the facility exceeded 90 (with six out of eight beds available for respite) flexibility of the service deteriorated and it became difficult to admit children in an emergency. They have aimed to run at an occupancy of from 60 to 65 per cent in order to allow for such flexibility. Hence, a waiting list for respite care exists. Martin House, however (with seven out of nine beds available for respite), aiming to meet the needs of their area in the north of England, in 1994 served over 180 children on an inpatient basis, and had an occupancy of nearly 95 per cent. Both practices, though different, suggest that the need for respite care and support for families whose child has a life-threatening illness is not yet met. Current research programmes, funded by the Department of Health, are attempting to estimate the needs of families in various areas of the country.

Most of the children's hospices have assumed a model by which day-to-day care of the children is provided by a multidisciplinary team. The teams may include registered sick children's nurses, teachers, social workers, nursery nurses, physiotherapists, and others without formal qualifications but wide experience in the care of children and families. Children and families have a member of the team allocated to them for each shift, with greater emphasis on compatibility than on particular qualification. At Helen House, as well as caring for the child and family, the team members look after the housekeeping and catering aspects of the house whilst at others more formal catering and administration arrangements may exist. Staff support is considered vital and each hospice has implemented programmes by which support is available.[10] Medical care is provided by a local general practitioner, who, like other members of the team, does his utmost to work in co-operation with those supporting the family in their home environment. Indeed the hospice is seen as one part of a network of support. At present, all the hospices, modelling themselves on home rather than hospital, are supported medically by general practitioners rather than specialists. The child's own specialist and general practitioner remain responsible for the child's overall medical care.

Table 2 Helen House: sources of referral of 325 children who stayed from 1982–1994

Source of referral	Number of children	%
Parents	98	30
Social worker	65	20
Hospital	54	17
Primary care team	45	14
Other	63	19

Place of death

Every effort should be made to give terminal care in the place chosen by the child and family.[11] Often this will be at home, but a family may feel that they cannot cope at home or that, for instance, if the child dies in the house they will not be able to carry on living there. Not infrequently the death will occur suddenly, either at home or perhaps in hospital following an acute episode of illness. If the family is aware that the child's condition is deteriorating rapidly, they may wish the child to be admitted to the hospice and the family will, unless they live very close, come and stay also. Alternatively, a family staying at the hospice when a child's condition seems imminently terminal may choose to take the child home to die in his own familiar surroundings.

Most of the hospices has a small bedroom, which can be kept cool, for use as a 'chapel of rest'. When a child dies at the hospice, the child's body often remains there for several days, perhaps until the funeral. Here, the family, which may include parents, brothers and sisters, grandparents, and many others, may come and go as they wish. This time saying good-bye to the dead child is seen as very important in adjusting to the death of the child.[12] When the child has died in hospital or at home, some families have brought the child's body to the hospice so that this time is available to them. Alternatively, the hospice has made a cooler available to the family so that they can keep the dead child's body at home for a while. If it is needed, help and support is available to the family in making arrangements for the funeral service and burial or cremation. The place of death in 1994 of children who attended three of the hospices is listed in Table 3.

Table 3 Place of death of children dying in 1994

	Helen House	Martin House	Cambridge	Total	%
	n	*n*	*n*	*n*	
At home	7	12	3	22	39
In hospice	2	10	3	15	27
In hospital	5	8	3	16	29
Other	3			3	5
Total	17	30	9	56	100

Bereavement support

Loneliness is one of the experiences almost all of the families have in common during the illness of their children and this is often even greater during the months and years following the death of the children. Bereavement support is seen as a vital part of the hospice programme. Each of the hospices has developed a programme by which families who have previously used the hospice are supported. At Helen House, bereavement workers continue to visit families and maintain telephone contact after the death of the child. Whilst this level of support may continue as long as thought helpful to each family, the usual length of time is in the region of 2 years. As the hospices have developed, one of the needs that has become most apparent is for support and understanding for the brothers and sisters of the sick child. Play therapists or other specialist workers are now employed at some of the hospices to work specifically with the siblings, to build up a relationship with them during their visits to the hospice and to support them in their bereavement. Each member of the family grieves as an individual and relationships are often strained. It is untrue to suggest that a family 'gets over' the death of their child, although eventually they do normally adjust to a different way of living and very gradually good days begin to outnumber bad ones.

Conclusion

The children's hospice is just a small part in a programme that may be developed to support children with life-limiting disease and their families. The child's home is recognized as the centre of care, the hospice offering an occasional alternative. The parents are the acknowledged experts in the care of their child and their wishes are of paramount importance. What is offered is not so much a relationship of professional to patient and relatives, as that of friendship with the whole family backed up by practical and professional skills. We need to be flexible to respond to the very different needs of each family through the stages of chronic illness, terminal illness, and bereavement.

Whilst each hospice is independent, links are maintained through meetings of head nurses and administrators, through an annual clinical meeting for the hospice doctors, and through occasional exchanges of staff. The children's hospices are represented on the Council of ACT (Association for Children with Life-threatening or Terminal Conditions and their Families), which in turn holds an annual meeting open to all those working in, or interested in, the area of paediatric hospice and palliative care.

Inevitably there are a number of differences in the way in which each hospice programme is implemented. Some offer home care, others share their experience by providing educational programmes which are open to other professionals. Referral and admission policies vary slightly, as does the make up of each team. However, all are united in the fundamental philosophy of offering friendship and practical, emotional, and spiritual help to children with life-limiting illness and their families.

References

1. Goldman A, Baum D. Provision of care. In: Goldman A, ed. *Care of the Dying Child*. Oxford: Oxford University Press, 1994: 107–14.
2. Chapman JA, Goodall J. Dying children need help too. *British Medical Journal*, 1979; **1**: 593–4.
3. Chapman JA, Goodall J. Helping a child live whilst dying. *Lancet*, 1980; **1**: 753–6.
4. Burne R, Dominica F, Baum D. Helen House—a hospice for children: analysis of the first year. *British Medical Journal*, 1984; 289:1655–68.
5. Dominica F, Hunt A. Children's Hospices. In: Glasper EA, Tucker A, eds. *Advances in Child Health Nursing*. London: Scutari Press, 1993.
6. Worswick J. *A House Called Helen*. London: Harper Collins, 1993.
7. Burne R, Hunt A. Use of opiates in terminally ill children. *Palliative Medicine*, 1987; **1**: 27–30.
8. Hunt A. A survey of signs, symptoms and symptom control in 30 terminally ill children. *Developmental Medicine and Child Neurology*, 1990; **32**: 341–6.
9. Hunt A, Burne R. Medical and nursing problems of children with neurodegenerative disease. *Palliative Medicine*, 1995; **9**: 19–26.
10. Woolley H, Stein A, Forrest GC, Baum JD. Staff stress and job satisfaction at a children's hospice. *Archives of Disease in Childhood*, 1989; **64**: 114–8.
11. Hill L. The role of the children's hospice. In: Hill L, ed. *Caring for Dying Children and their Families*. London: Chapman and Hall, 1993.
12. Dominica F. Reflections on death in childhood. *British Medical Journal*, 1987; **294**: 108–10.

19.7.3 Development in Canada

Betty Davies

The status of paediatric palliative care in Canada is in an active stage of development, but to varying degrees across the country. There are pockets of activity, usually related to or connected with children's hospitals or oncology centres, and some home-care programmes.

Informal palliative care programmes

In several provinces, paediatric staff in oncology centres or in children's hospitals offer well organized support to children with cancer and to their families, but have not created formal palliative care programmes. These programmes maintain a constant liaison with families and provide support to health-care providers in the child's home community, particularly regarding symptom control.

In other provinces, children's hospitals have instituted palliative care programmes to provide support and follow-up to children with cancer and their families. Other hospitals are beginning to develop such programmes (personal communications, Dr I. Mitchell, Alberta Children's Hospital, Calgary, Alberta, 1995, and Dr A. Finley, IWK Children's Hospital, Halifax, Nova Scotia, 1995). Some of these programmes now include children with other life-limiting illnesses, not just cancer. And, in some areas, palliative care associations, though not usually providing direct care to dying children, offer emotional, spiritual, or social support to children coping with the terminal illness and death of a family member or classmate (personal communication, Sudbury Regional Palliative Care Association, Sudbury, Ontario, 1995).

Hospital palliative care programmes

One of the longest running hospital-based programmes is the palliative care programme at the Hospital for Sick Children in Toronto which has been in existence since 1986.[1] The programme is headed by a nurse co-ordinator and a doctor from the Division of Clinical Pharmacology, who help co-ordinate the care of the child in the hospital and at home. They prepare parents and child for care at home, and the nurse phones regularly and makes home visits as necessary. Home visiting by community health nurses can also be arranged. In the first 7 years of its operation, approximately 120 children received care in the programme. The majority of these children had neurosurgical (55 per cent) or genetic/metabolic (22 per cent) conditions. The programme is funded through the hospital's global budget as part of Clinical Pharmacology and Toxicology. The programme also receives private donations which are specifically used to help families with a variety of expenses, such as medications that are not covered by insurance or the government or additional nursing respite hours.

Bloorview Children's Hospital, also in Ontario, has a hospital-based palliative care programme which provides care for children (and their families) who have severe birth defects or terminal illness and who are unable to benefit from further curative treatment (personal communicaton, Bloorview Children's Hospital, Willowdale, Ontario, 1995). Children are admitted for short term respite, interim (en route home from an acute centre), or terminal palliative care. The costs of hospital care are covered by the provincial health plan, but the programme welcomes donations to the Bloorview Children's Hospital Foundation which are designated for the palliative care programme.

A Clinical Nurse Specialist and a Child Life Worker laid the groundwork for the palliative care programme at the Montreal Children's Hospital between 1987 and 1991.[2] They were joined by a part-time medical director at the end of 1991. Two years later, the programme was completed as originally envisaged, with 'consultant members' added to the original team of three. The programme is primarily consultative in promoting a hospice approach to the care of all dying children and their families (not just oncology patients) in the setting of a paediatric teaching hospital. The programme averages about 60 consultations per year, and notes the increasing importance of symptom control as a reason prompting requests for consultation. In addition, the programme is beginning to offer a home-care consultation service, and does offer bereavement follow-up.

Community/home-care palliative care programmes

Children's hospitals in Canada are limited in number, and serve as tertiary referral centres for large geographical areas. Therefore, children from distant parts of each region are referred to these centres. This presents challenges for palliative care since these families return to isolated areas, where nearly all health professionals have had limited experience with palliative paediatrics. In these cases, especially in the far northern communities, palliative care programmes work to set up a care team within the child's community and provide education and consultation for the professionals. A variation of this concept characterizes the palliative home-care programme for terminally ill children in Newfoundland and Labrador.[3] This programme began in 1988. When the decision is made to discontinue active treatment, a multidisciplinary team of professionals at the Janeway Child Health Centre combine their expertise and are identified as the Janeway Palliative Care Team. These professionals are normally involved with the child and family (to greater and lesser degrees) from the time of diagnosis.

Each professional involved in the case contacts his/her counterpart in the child's home community. This facilitates the creation of an holistic team approach to be of support to the dying child and family anywhere in the province. In areas served by a regional palliative home care programme (a programme operated by a health care agency to provide services to terminally ill patients in the geographical region), the Janeway Team makes every effort to work with and through that community resource. Thus, as the need arises, there is a palliative care team for the specific patient and family at the Janeway and in the home community. Such a programme allows for co-ordinating a smooth transition from active treatment to home palliative care for any child with a terminal illness in Newfoundland and Labrador.

Saskatchewan offers a similar, province wide, family directed, community based Palliative Care Outreach Program for children terminally ill with cancer.[4] The model consists of a multi-disciplinary hospital palliative care team (consisting of paediatric oncologists, nurses, social worker, and pastoral care person) located in each of the two provincial cancer centres in the cities of Saskatoon and Regina. A 'twin' community palliative care team is identified in each case through contact with the family physician or local community hospital, physician (depending on the child's physical status, distance from home to the nearest hospital/community health-care resources, and ability of the parents or family to care for the child), or the existing network of palliative care providers such as home care and public health nurses. Prior to the child's transfer home, a phone teleconference will be held between the two teams to review the child's clinical status, list of problems, medications, family and psychosocial issues, and support and crisis intervention. The local team will organize personnel and support services in advance of the child's arrival. Once the child is transferred back to the community, the two teams will continue to teleconference at a minimum of once a week until the child dies. A final 'wrap up' teleconference will be held subsequently. Parents will be invited to attend and participate in each teleconference. The benefits of the programme are:

(1) it can be provided in remote areas;

(2) it draws on existing community health-care personnel and resources;

(3) it serves as a model for the care of other children with potentially fatal diseases such as cystic fibrosis and neuro-degenerative disorders.

Free-standing hospice programme

Opened in November, 1995, Canuck Place is the first free-standing children's hospice in North America.[5,6] The idea for a children's hospice for British Columbia arose from the experience of paediatric health-care professionals in collaboration with parents of children who had died from progressive, life-threatening illness. A group of parents and professionals comprised a Steering Committee (March 1989) which a year later, became the first Board of the HUGS (Human Growth, Understanding and Sharing) Children's Hospice Society, the non-profit organization responsible for the development and operation of Canuck Place. In 1991, HUGS entered into a partnership with numerous volunteers and community-based donors, most significantly the Canuck Foundation (the charity arm of the Vancouver Canucks, a team in the National Hockey League) to work together to make the dream of a children's hospice a reality. Founding patrons of Canuck Place also include the Loewen Group, a large funeral home company, and the Vancouver Sun, the local newspaper. Operating costs come from combined sources which include corporations, private donors, the Ministry of Health, and others.

An assessment of the situation in British Columbia[7,8] documented the need for a children's hospice in that province. Canuck Place has a provincial mandate to provide hospice care to children with progressive, life-threatening illness and their families. The Canuck Place Program, through its multidisciplinary team, provides care to children and their families as they experience two transitions:

(1) the transition through the various phases of illness, which require respite, palliative, and bereavement care;

(2) the transition of moving from one location to another; that is, from home, to hospital, to the hospice facility, and back into the community.

Centre-based care is offered to children and their families while they are in Canuck Place at Glen Brae (a renovated, turn-of-the century heritage mansion located close to the provincial children's hospital); community-based care is offered through an Interlink programme of community consultation and resource-sharing.

The Canuck Place Program focuses on maximizing the quality of remaining life for children with progressive, life-threatening illness by providing comprehensive services that meet the combined physical, sociological, emotional, and spiritual needs of the child/family unit. The type and scope of services provided are based upon initial and ongoing assessment of the child and family needs and upon comprehensive care plans that define child/family problems and strengths, goals for intervention, and methods of achieving those goals. The exact combination of services and the level of care (e.g. frequency of visits, numbers of hours of care by various interdisciplinary team members) is unique to each child/family unit and changes as the child/family needs evolve over the course of the involvement with Canuck Place.[9]

As do most other palliative care programmes across the country, Canuck Place offers educational programmes pertaining to paediatric palliative care. In addition, it has an active mandate to incorporate research and evaluation into its programme from its inception. And it offers, under one umbrella, all three components of paediatric hospice care—respite, palliative, and bereavement.

References

1. The Hospital for Sick Children. *Patient Information: The Palliative Care Program*. Toronto, 1994.
2. Hutcheon RA. *MCH Palliative Care Program Medical Director's Final Report* (1992–1995). 1995.
3. Singleton R. *The Palliative Home Care Program for Terminally Ill Children in Newfoundland and Labrador*. St. John's: Janeway Child Health Centre, 1994.
4. Ali K, Krespin H, Goh S. Outreach Palliative Care Program using a teleconference 'twinning' model. *Children's Hospice International 8th Conference, Sydney, Australia, June 1993*.
5. Davies B, Eng B, Arcand R, Collins J, Bhanji N. Canuck Place—A Hospice for Children. *British Columbia Medical Journal*, 1995; **17**: 533–7.
6. Davies B, Eng B. Challenges in developing a children's hospice. In: Adams D, Deveau E, eds. *Helping Children and Adolescents: the Impact of Threat to their Lives—Death, Dying and Bereavement*. Amityville, NY: Baywood Press, in press.
7. Davies B. *Assessment of Need for a Children's Hospice in British Columbia*. HUGS Children's Hospice Society, Vancouver, B.C., June 1992.
8. Davies B. Assessment of need for a children's hospice program. *Death Studies*, 1996; **20**: 247–68.
9. Hospice Care Committee. *Canuck Place Hospice Care Program: Blueprint*. Vancouver, B.C.,1994.

19.7.4 Development in Australia

Michael M. Stevens and Brian Pollard

Historical overview of palliative care services in Australia

A hospice was established by a Catholic order of nuns in 1890 in Sydney and has operated continuously since then. Establishment of the modern palliative care movement in Australia began much more recently. The stimulus to commence palliative care formally in Australia came from a single event. About 30 Australian nurses and doctors, who mostly knew nothing of each other, unexpectedly met at the World Congress in Montreal in 1980. Enthused by the discovery of their common interest in palliative care and by the new knowledge gained and contacts made, they resolved that it was time to establish the new form of care back home. At a national meeting in Adelaide 3 months later, ways and means were discussed, resulting in groups being set up in major centres almost at once, and elsewhere more gradually, the latest only in 1992.

With a land area over 30 times that of Great Britain, Australia has a population only three times that of London. Its geography and demography determined that palliative care services developed not to plan, but randomly, springing up autonomously, shaped by the perceived still unmet needs of the local community.

Now each state has its own professional association, with membership ranging from 50 to over 300, all affiliated to a national association with its headquarters rotating around the states. In one state, separate bodies for nurses and doctors, additional to the common association, have been formed, and some of the more populous states have regional associations also. Membership is mixed, predominantly consisting of nurses, with smaller numbers of doctors, other professionals and community members. In smaller regions, the latter are very valuable in providing funding and support.

In major cities, bed units or ready access to beds exist in most, and generally all, large hospitals, supplemented by hospices, to many of which are attached outreach community services, assisting family doctors to care for patients dying at home. Regional cities and rural areas also have nursing outreach teams which cover variable proportions of the local population, depending on distance. Some of these are supplemented by radio communication and air ambulances.

A directory of hospice and palliative care services in Australia compiled in 1993 and revised in April 1995, is available from the Australian Association for Hospice and Palliative Care Inc., PO Box 7450 Cloisters Square, Perth WA 6850 Australia, tel +61-9-324 1001, fax +61-9-324 1002.

Paediatric malignancy

In Australia, as in other developed countries, childhood cancer remains the commonest cause of death after accidents in children aged between 1 and 14 years. Thus, most children requiring palliative care in Australia have terminal malignancy.

In Australia, treatment of children and teenagers with cancer is supervised by paediatric oncology units within tertiary level children's hospitals in the capital cities of each state. There are two such units in Sydney providing paediatric cancer services for New South Wales—at The New Children's Hospital at Westmead, and at the Sydney Children's Hospital, Randwick. Each unit has a community nurse consultant in paediatric oncology and palliative care.

When palliative care commences for a child or teenager with cancer and the family opt for home-based care, the paediatric community nurse consultant liaises with palliative care services or community nursing services available in the family's district to arrange provision of home care for the child and family. Such services are orientated to the care of terminally ill adults, but may have had some experience in the care of children dying of cancer through earlier referrals. The child's family practitioner or local paediatrician is also contacted and advised of the plan of management. Members of the child's hospital-based treatment team, including the child's oncologist, social worker, and ward nurses, keep in touch with the family and child with regular telephone contact and home visits.[1]

The major children's hospitals have developed a range of services that reinforce the clinical and medical care they provide. The clinical team is likely to develop an extremely close relationship with these families and to offer grief counselling, liaison with community-based support services, and palliative care in hospital or in the home. It is recognized that for many patients no additional services are required. With the development of pain relief techniques, in particular, families are increasingly able to care for children at home up to and including the time of death.

For families residing many hundreds of kilometres from Sydney, home visits by members of the hospital-based treatment team are usually not possible. The care of such children and their families has to be largely handed over to whatever paediatric and palliative nursing services are available locally. Regular contact by telephone after hand-over provides support to the family and to the primary caregivers and offers advice on matters such as symptom control.

If the family chooses to return to the treatment team's hospital for terminal care, such care is provided, whenever possible, in the unit's acute care ward. Ward routines and procedures that would normally impinge on the child are adjusted or relaxed as much as permissible to provide the child and family with privacy and a more home-like atmosphere.

Management of such children at home proceeds most successfully when the family reside close to the treatment team's hospital and home visits by members of the treatment team can be maintained without the routine care of other patients becoming compromised. Quality home-based care is also usually well maintained when the nursing and medical personnel in the community, to whom the referral has been made, are experienced in paediatric palliative care and are comfortable accepting the referral. Successful management of the dying child at home may be more difficult for families who live long distances from the treatment team's hospital or in a district in which palliative care resources are lacking.

Services provided through hospitals are reinforced by the network of community-based support services. These can include clinical care (e.g. Sydney Home Nursing Service in New South Wales), as well as vital support and counselling, and even financial assistance services, provided by a range of organizations such as the Malcolm Sargent Cancer Fund For Children In Australia and the Australian Teenage Cancer Patients Society (CanTeen). Older teenagers may also be treated in an adult hospice or palliative care ward. However, these environments, which may have no provision for teenagers, are considered inappropriate from both the patients' and supervising staff's perspective.

Paediatric terminal illnesses other than malignancy

Few if any hospital-based palliative care services currently exist for children dying of diseases other than cancer. Outreach or consultative services to assist a family caring for a terminally ill child at home may be negotiated on a case by case basis with hospices or palliative care services caring for adults, or provided directly by the paediatrician and associated caregivers managing the child's illness. The nature and chronicity of many non-malignant, life-limiting illnesses of childhood and adolescence mean that, in many cases, the family is no longer under the supervision of physicians with admitting rights to acute care hospital beds which might otherwise have been accessed for palliative and respite care.

Deficiencies in services currently available

There are four striking absences in this range of services:

(1) a facility specializing in the palliative care component for that small portion of terminally ill children who cannot be cared for at home during the last phase of their illness;

(2) a centre providing much-needed respite care, in a supported but non-hospital environment, for terminally ill children and their families;

(3) a facility which acts as the focal point for the provision and co-ordination of non-hospital-based palliative care services for children with progressive life-limiting illnesses and their families;

(4) a facility to meet the special needs of teenagers.

To the authors' knowledge, no tertiary level, Australian children's hospital is providing a formal in-house consultative palliative care service, and there is only one paediatric palliative medicine specialist in training. A residential palliative care service specifically for children (i.e. free-standing children's hospice) has been established in Melbourne, Victoria, by Very Special Kids Inc., to provide respite and palliative care for children with life-limiting and terminal illnesses and their families. A similar initiative is planned for Sydney, New South Wales, by the Royal Alexandra Hospital for Children (The New Children's Hospital at Westmead).

Melbourne, Victoria—Very Special Kids House

Very Special Kids Inc., established in 1985, is a non-profit organization based in Melbourne Victoria, providing support by trained volunteers to families who have a child with a progressive life-limiting illness. Families are referred to Very Special Kids by hospitals, health care, and community agencies. Services provided by Very Special Kids include child and family support provided by trained volunteers; information and advice on available social welfare and community services; bereavement care; opportunities for families to share experiences; and community and professional education. In the period 1986 to 1994, 413 families had been referred to Very Special Kids and 106 children had died after referral. Child and family support services were being provided to 176 families in 1994, by a pool of 100 trained volunteers.[2] Very Special Kids House, Australia's first free-standing children's hospice , was opened in Malvern, Melbourne, in November 1996.

Sydney, New South Wales—Bear Cottage: a children's hospice

The Bear Cottage children's hospice project was launched by The New Children's Hospital at Westmead (Royal Alexandra Hospital for Children) in June 1993, as one component of a proposed palliative care service for the hospital.

A Core Planning Committee for Bear Cottage chaired by one of the authors (MS) was appointed in mid-1993, comprising three nurses (deputy director of nursing, oncology clinical nurse consultant, community nurse consultant in oncology and palliative care), three paediatricians (oncologist, intensive care specialist, advanced trainee in pain and paediatric palliative medicine), a clinical psychologist working with dying adolescents, a social worker, and two couples each of whom had previously received home-based palliative care for their dying child. This committee reports directly to the hospital's chief executive officer. The committee acknowledges the significant support received from colleagues overseas, particularly those associated with Helen House, Children's Hospice for the Eastern Region, Martin House, Acorns, and Little Bridge House in the United Kingdom and Canuck Place in Vancouver.

The Core Planning Committee's initial priority was to draft a philosophy for Bear Cottage, to serve as a mission statement for the project and as the introductory section of more detailed documentation of the project. The second task was to arrange for collection of data to estimate the likely demand for the services of a children's hospice based in Sydney. This information was required to determine an optimal size for the hospice and a schedule of accommodation that would be both efficient and flexible, and to identify specific characteristics of children and families in need of hospice-based palliative care and the implications of those characteristics for the hospice's design.

International experience has already shown, and was confirmed in the needs analysis for Bear Cottage,[3] that, while firmly based in a palliative care model, the majority of clients of a children's hospice are likely to be children not in the terminal phase of an illness but rather children with a long-lasting, albeit progressive and life-limiting condition, who with their families are in need of respite care that can best be provided in a facility rather than their home. The combination of these two groups (terminal care and respite care) has significant implications for the facility's design, as well as education of patients, the community, and health practitioners.

The utilization estimates and bed requirements derived from the needs assessment corroborated an accommodation schedule that includes at least seven to eight beds/rooms (six in regular use and two held for emergencies) plus two family suites. By the time Bear Cottage opens, it is likely that there will have been sufficient gain in understanding and acceptance of its role such that actual utilization exceeds the conservative estimates documented in the analysis. A prevalent belief was noted in those interviewed that a hospice is a place to go to die and that its services are quite detached from previous, ongoing clinical, and other care. The amount of public and professional education required to adjust these professionals' beliefs to an accurate understanding of the services that will be provided by Bear Cottage should not be underestimated.

Some confusion has been encountered in the community about the difference between children's hospices and Ronald McDonald Houses. The mission of the hospice to care for children with terminal illness and their families, and the presence within the hospice of professional staff trained in paediatric palliative care, are two distinguishing features. As occurred in the British Columbia experience, an explanation to the community has also been required about important differences between a hospice for adults and a children's hospice.

Since March 1993, a total of $5.2m has been received in donations and pledges towards the establishment target of $6m. A site for Bear Cottage at Manly, Sydney, was approved by the local council in December 1996. Bear Cottage is scheduled to open in September 1998.

References

1. Stevens M, Luxon R, Jones P. Home care of the child dying of cancer. *New South Wales Cancer Council Professional Information News Sheet*, October 1991.
2. Annual Report, *Very Special Kids* Inc.
3. Australian Health Innovations. *Bear Cottage: Needs Analysis*, May, 1994.

19.7.5 Development in the United States

Kathleen W. Faulkner

The paediatric palliative care movement in the United States has been primarily directed toward supporting the dying child and family in their home environment. Although several paediatric hospice inpatient units exist, the overwhelming majority of children who receive hospice support die at home, or at the hospital in which they have received treatment for their life-threatening illness. Because their care is geographically far-flung, and not concentrated in a few physical inpatient facilities, the statistics on how many children are served by hospice is difficult to determine with certainty.

Historically, Children's Hospice International made its first attempt to determine how accessible hospice care was to children and adolescents in the United States in 1984 (personal comunication, A Armstrong-Dailey, founder Children's Hospice International). At that time, the organization surveyed approximately 1500 hospices and children's hospitals to ascertain if hospice care was provided to children and what constituted that care. At that time, only about 22 per cent of the hospices in the United States admitted and cared for children. In a repeat survey in 1989, this number had increased slightly in both absolute numbers of programmes serving children and in the percentage of hospice programmes that provided care. Of the 1700 hospices and children's hospitals surveyed, 26 per cent admitted and cared for paediatric hospice patients.

In recent years the growth of paediatric hospice programmes has been dramatic, as is reflected by the 1992 National Hospice Organization census.[1] In that year, there were estimated to be 1935 operational hospice programmes in the United States, and 90 per cent of those programmes were willing to admit terminally ill children. The data indicated that in 1992, 2460 children and their families were served by hospice programmes. This represented 1 per cent of the total hospice population.

The National Hospice Organization national hospice profile also confirmed a growth in bereavement services directed specifically towards children and families. In that survey, 35 per cent of all hospices provided specific children's bereavement services. In addition, 50 per cent of hospice programmes indicated that they worked in the community with the school system on bereavement issues. Twenty-seven per cent of hospice programmes also indicated a working relationship with community organizations, such as Compassionate Friends, which serve bereaved families.

In 1995, the interest in providing paediatric hospice care continues to grow. Last year, Kaleidoscope® Kids received over 1500 telephone enquiries from hospices and home-care agencies, requesting information on the implementation or improvement of paediatric hospice/home care programmes (personal comunication, C Byrnes, founder Kaleidoscope® Kids). Kaleidoscope® Kids is a non-profit federally-trademarked paediatric hospice programme which has been available for consultation since 1991.

This new commitment to paediatric palliative care services reflects an overall renaissance in paediatric home care which was stimulated by the former Surgeon General C. Everett Koop, who was responding to children with special needs. The Health Care Financing Administration of the United States Government has described home care for all ages as the fastest-growing component of personal health care spending and has noted that paediatrics is now the fastest growing segment of that industry.[2]

The steady growth of paediatric palliative care in the United States is the culmination of an effort to improve the care for dying children and their families which began over two decades ago. In the late 1970s, there were three pioneering efforts to provide home palliative care for children. The first documentation that good medical care could be provided in a home environment came from Ida M. Martinson, R.N., and her group at the University of Minnesota. In their seminal study of 32 families who had a child dying of cancer and wished to be supported at home, Martinson demonstrated the effectiveness of utilizing local nursing agencies with paediatric consultative back up.[3] In addition to demonstrating the medical effectiveness of terminal home care, this group also documented that home care was less costly than hospitalized care.[4] They also began the ethical and practical discussions of exploring the decision-making process of physicians and parents in choosing between the hospital and home care for children in the terminal phase of cancer.[5,6] The same cohort of families, followed after the deaths of their children, showed improved bereavement adaptation with home death.[7,8,9]

The Midwest Children's Cancer Center corroborated the feasibility and desirability of providing terminal home care for children with cancer. A nursing co-ordinator either provided direct care to the 42 families enrolled in the study or arranged for that care to be delivered by nurses from health agencies in the family's residential area.[10] In addition to confirming that the medical needs of the dying children could be met by a home care team, this group also documented the positive psychological adjustment of the bereaved family and siblings.[11,12] They also looked at the utilization of hospice/home care for children dying of cancer and found that, at that time (1986), there were problems with community agencies, including inexperience with paediatric issues and procedures, inadequate pain management, and the reluctance of families to work with unfamiliar staff.[13] This co-ordination of services between the paediatric cancer centre and the community hospice or home-care agency continues to be a challenging aspect of care.

While paediatric cancer centres were reaching out to the communities to provide care for dying children, one community was developing a model of care which included children dying of non-oncological diseases. In 1978, Edmarc Hospice for Children was created as a ministry of a small church in rural south-east Virginia, by a young couple whose own child was dying.[14] Initially, the hospice was a volunteer agency providing, primarily, nursing support. As the programme grew, ancillary services were added such as physical therapy, occupational therapy, speech therapy, home health aide services, medical social services, bereavement care, and volunteer co-ordination. In addition to pioneering the effort to include children facing life-threatening diseases other than cancer, Edmarc Hospice also recognized and explored the difficulties in labelling a child as 'terminal' based exclusively on the number of days of predicted survival.

Although most of the early efforts in developing paediatric palliative care programmes in the United States were directed toward improving the care of children in their own home environment, it was recognized at an early date that this would not always be feasible. One of the first inpatient units for children's hospice care was developed at St. Mary's Hospital in Bayside, New York. This group has published a comprehensive description of their planning process, and the difficulties faced in bringing this project to reality.[15] Today, the concept of a paediatric inpatient unit is well established and there are several such programmes in existence. The spread of the HIV epidemic has led some hospices to consider 'family-type' inpatient units to serve the needs of their HIV infected families.

In addition to designated hospice units, utilizing a hospice approach to the families of seriously ill children has become more commonplace in all hospitals. More home-like physical surroundings, an involved social work staff, and a commitment to bereavement follow-up are only a few of the innovative approaches that are now incorporated into many hospital programmes.

References

1. National Hospice Organization. 1992 Stats Show Continued Growth in Progress and Patients. *NewsLine*, 1993; **3**: 1–2.
2. Goldberg AI, Gardner HG, Gibson LE. Home care: The next frontier of paediatric practice. *Journal of Pediatrics*, 1994; **125**: 686–90.
3. Martinson IM, Armstrong GD, Geis DP, *et al.* Home care for children dying of cancer. *Pediatrics*, 1978; **62**: 106–13.
4. Maldow DG, Armstrong GD, Henry WF, Martinson IM. The cost of home care for dying children. *Medical Care*, 1982; **20**: 1154–60.
5. Edwardson SR. The choice between hospital and home care for terminally ill children. *Nursing Research*, 1983; **32**: 29–34.
6. Edwardson SR. Physician acceptance of home care for terminally ill children. *Health Services Research*, 1985; **20**: 83–101.
7. Martinson, IM, Nesbitt M, Kersey V. Children's adjustment to the death of a sibling from cancer. *Advances in Thonatology*, 1987; **6**: 1–7.
8. Smith C, Garvis M, Martinson IM. Content analysis of interviews using a nursing model: A look at parents adapting to the impact of childhood cancer. *Cancer Nursing*, 1983; **6**: 269–75.
9. Martinson IM, McClowry SG, Davies B, Kuhlen-kang EV. Changes over time: a study of family bereavement following childhood cancer. *Journal of Palliative Care*, 1994; **10**: 19–25.
10. Lauer MF, Camitta BM. Home care for dying children: A nursing model. *Journal of Pediatrics*, 1980; **97**: 1032–5.
11. Mulhern RK, Lauer ME, Hoffman RG. Death of a child at home or in the hospital: subsequent psychological adjustment of the family. *Pediatrics*, 1983; **71**: 743–7.
12. Lauer ME, Mulhern RK, Bohne JB, Camitta BM. Children's perceptions of their sibling's death at home or hospital: the precursors of differential adjustment. *Cancer Nursing*, 1985; **8**: 21–7.
13. Lauer, ME, Mulhern RK, Hoffman RG, Camitta BM. Utilization of hospice/home care in paediatric oncology. *Cancer Nursing*, 1986; **9**: 102–7.
14. Sligh JS. An early model of care. In: Armstrong-Dailey A, Zarback Gottzer S, eds. *Hospice Care for Children*. New York: Oxford University Press, 1993: 219–30.
15. Wilson DC. Developing a hospice program for children. In: Corr CA, Corr DM, eds. *Hospice Approaches to Paediatric Care*. New York: Springer Publishing Company, 1985: 5–29.

19.8 Child-centred care in terminal illness: an ethical framework

Marcia Levetown and Michele A. Carter

Introduction: towards a child-centred approach

The ethical root of child advocacy is the shared commitment by parents, teachers, health care workers, and society itself to the protection and nurturing of the young. As normal human development proceeds, the child's vulnerability and powerlessness diminish; the child takes on new rights, liberties, and responsibilities as a full member of society.

Children are vulnerable not only because they are dependent on others to provide for them the basic necessities of life, but because they lack the full maturity and the legal authority to make independent decisions. Their inherent vulnerabilities and dependencies are exacerbated by illness, particularly chronic, life-threatening illness. The special mission of paediatric medicine is to help the child compromised by illness to nevertheless develop his or her unique potential as a human being.

Terminal illness deepens a child's need to be nurtured, to belong, to be cared for and about, and to exist in an intimate relationship with others. The ideal of caring is reflected in many cultures and societies; there is a universal expectation that compassion will motivate people to help those who cannot help themselves. Thus the basic premise of this chapter—the practice of paediatric palliative medicine is grounded in an 'ethic of care.' This ethic is rooted in human relationships which, especially in the case of children, involve the human condition in its most fragile state. The ethical ideal of caring is not simply a lofty, abstract, or philosophical ideal, but is a concrete, practical framework for medical decision-making.

This chapter reviews the historical origins of paediatric medical decision-making models, explores the contemporary ethical standards and principles that inform the ethic of care as it applies to children with life-limiting illness, and suggests modifications of the current paradigms that might allow closer alignment to the ideal of the ethic of care.

The ethic of care

The concept of care has been expressed throughout history as a fundamental form of relating to another, with rich cultural, philosophical, religious, and existential meanings.[1] Caring is understood as the human motivation to provide protection, belonging, nourishment, solicitude, and humanistic concern. Caring is not merely a sentimental attitude toward someone or something, but an integral component of human relationships, without which the essence of humanity is lost. According to the psychologist Rollo May,[2] our ethical duties to others arise out of our common humanity, impelling us to act responsibly toward ourselves and others. For Erikson,[3] care is the capacity to take care of another—to have a concern for and a commitment toward another. Mayeroff[4] identifies eight components of the caring process: knowledge, harmony, honesty, trust, humility, hope, courage, and patience.

Caring, whether it be articulated as a theory, an ethic, a framework, or a model of practice, is the moral centrepiece of palliative medicine. It provides the moral context for the relationship between the patient, his family, health professionals, and society.

Ethical obligations of practitioners towards the dying child

The ethic of care incorporates the values and ethical principles that justify the decisions made on behalf of children. One of the most important duties of the paediatric practitioner is to help the child achieve his or her uniqueness and potential as a human being, reflecting the principle of self-determination. Adherence to this principle gives rise to important rights: autonomy of the patient/family, privacy, dignity, and confidentiality. Respecting the developing autonomy of the child recognizes the child's individual worth; this can best be exemplified by assisting the child to make choices regarding the management of his illness based on his own experience.

The child's need for support, affection, understanding, consolation, and comfort requires an individualized framework of care that is centred on the child's perception of his own well being, even if his illness is incurable. The dying child has a deepened need for care and concern. The caregivers' responsibilities are to help the child, to talk with him about what he feels, knows, fears, wishes, and believes about life, as well as about death and dying.

Dying children should have the information they desire about their illnesses, including the relative merits or burdens of any proposed treatments or procedures so that they can exercise some personal choice. This is true regardless of whether they have the full maturity of an adult. For example, choices of the day or time of treatment or the hand or leg in which the intravenous line will be inserted can be offered even to very young children.

Respecting the child also includes taking seriously the child's subjective complaint of pain or discomfort—the best guide to attentive, individualized pain and symptom management strategies. The child, when able to demonstrate the competency presumed of all adults (ability to understand the risks and benefits of proposed interventions; ability to understand personal death and its irreversibility) should also be allowed to refuse any unwanted interventions, including those considered 'life saving'.

Social attitudes regarding the death of the child

The 'unnatural': the child dying before the parent

Prior to the last 50 years, the death of children was commonplace. Improvement in hygiene, development of vaccines and antibiotics, and increasingly sophisticated technological advances have all contributed to decreasing child mortality in developed nations.[5] The death of a child has thus come to be viewed as an anomaly, as a tragic, unnatural, and unacceptable event.[6] In contrast, in developing countries, in which hygiene remains poor and basic medical care is often unavailable, the death of a child, although a loss, is not as unacceptable as it is in the West.[7] Thus, social attitudes towards childhood death are influenced to a large degree by its frequency and social experience. Furthermore, the value and meaning of children has varied over time in the context of changing social, cultural, and economic values.[8,9] Whereas in the past children have been seen as property even in developed countries, current conceptions in Western countries place extremely high value on the life of a child. The personhood of the child is undermined, however, in the all-too-common relentless pursuit of maintaining biological life. The person of the child is thus still undervalued. The implementation of all technological means to preserve life, even in the face of irreversible illness, creates suffering for the child, suffering which often goes unrecognized and thus untreated.

The 'immature' self: the child's own wishes

The concept of the child as property, coupled with the traditional stronghold of paternalistic medical decision-making in paediatrics, has resulted in the neglect of the child as a decision-maker. The Children Act of 1989 in the United Kingdom[10] and the United Nations' convention on the Rights of the Child of 1989[11] exhort those involved in the care of children to inform the child of his situation, to solicit his opinion, and, when appropriate, to regard his opinion as determinative. Children, in their developing maturity, have opinions and desires that may not align with their caretakers' opinions. There is evidence that the experience of illness, in particular, confers a different perspective of its meaning for the child-patient than for the family.[12] These differences must be acknowledged and honoured, particularly for the developmentally mature child and adolescent.

Even very young children should be given developmentally appropriate information, have the opportunity to express an opinion, and have that opinion factored into the ultimate decision.[9,13-16] By not soliciting the child's input, his autonomy is violated, not only showing him disrespect, but neglecting the duty of caregivers to ensure the continued development of the emerging adult.[17]

There have been numerous publications over the last decade giving guidelines for the determination of capacity of the child to give 'assent with parental permission' or to give legally binding consent.[13,16-24] The American Academy of Pediatrics Committee on Bioethics established that parents and physicians should not exclude children and adolescents from decision-making without 'persuasive reasons', citing literature supporting the position that adolescents, especially age 14 and older, may have a similar capacity to make informed health care decisions as adults.[20] William Bartholome,[14] a noted paediatrician and child autonomy advocate, objects to the 'loophole' of 'persuasive reasons' and admonishes that all children should be allowed to participate in decisions governing the care of themselves. Some children are competent at a very early age. The individual child's capacity therefore needs to be investigated in most cases. As we come to understand the developmental capabilities of children more thoroughly,[12,25] perhaps they will be accorded greater respect as individuals in terms of medical decision making.

The 'incompetent' versus the 'knowing' child

That the child's views are not always sought and respected in medical decisions today is illustrated by two cases in the United States. Billy Best[26,27] was a 16-year-old with lymphoma who ran away from home in order to avoid ongoing medical treatment, consented to by his parents, but against his wishes. He returned home only when promised no further coercion and went on to be 'cured' by an unconventional therapy he became aware of through his own research. Benito Agrelo was a 15-year-old liver transplant recipient who faced retransplantation because of rejection of the first organ. Based on his own illness experience, he preferred to forgo a second transplant. He was taken to court in an attempt to override or confirm the validity of his decision, was proven to be competent, and won the right of self determination.[28] Though not of legal majority, Billy and Benito both, through their experience and developmental capacity, were very sophisticated in their understanding of their medical conditions, the proposed treatments, and the risks of non-treatment, including death. The treatment plans arrived at by their physicians and parents failed due to lack of respect for the person most directly affected by those plans.

Children often have insights about their illnesses and prognoses of which others, even parents, are unaware.[29] These realizations must be recognized and accounted for in creating any treatment regimen. In addition, the concept of informed consent also implies the ability to give informed dissent, even in the case of life-sustaining treatment.[17,18,30-32] If a minor has experienced an illness for some time, understands the illness and the benefits and burdens of treatment, has the ability to reason, and has a comprehension of personal death that encompasses its finality, then that person, irrespective of age, is competent from an ethical standpoint to forgo life-sustaining treatment.[33] To state otherwise is to propose to violate the ethical principles of autonomy, privacy, dignity, and self-determination.[34]

Ethical guidelines for providers of paediatric medical care

In a pluralistic society where diverse conceptions of what is good are equally authoritative, ethical guidelines are critical. Some guidelines on the ethical treatment of children are broad and meant to apply in all contexts. For example the United Nations *Declaration of the Rights of the Child*[35] asserts the essential rights and special protections to which all children are entitled. These include rights to freedom, dignity, education, and medical services. The Declaration also asserts that the guiding principle for decisions regarding the welfare of a child is the determination of his or her best interests. In general, this responsibility resides with the child's parents but should be influenced, if not determined, by the child's own opinion.

One of the most influential guidelines affecting the care of children in the United States was developed in 1974. The National Commission for the Protection of Human Subjects of Biomedical and Behavioural Research was created by the United States Congress (P.L. 93–348). The National Commission identified three ethical principles which are applicable to the paediatric clinical and research contexts; respect for persons, beneficence, and justice.[36] Respect for persons was understood to refer to the obligation to provide added protections against undue physical, psychological, or moral harms to which children are vulnerable, especially when they are ill. The principle of beneficence was understood as both the obligation to avoid harm and to maximize the good of children. Finally, justice was understood as the obligation to be fair in the distribution of resources. The Commission understood the importance of human judgment in the careful balancing of these principles and the various ethical duties they invoke. Additionally, their recommendations became an authoritative guideline for many professionals in health care, law, and applied ethics.

Another significant guideline concerning the responsibilities health care professionals in the United States have toward children was the President's Commission for the Study of Ethical Problems in Medicine and Biomedical and Behavioural Research. The President's Commission proposed that decision-making about difficult health matters and policy matters was best accomplished by appeal to a set of ethical principles. These include: the right to autonomy, which asserts that a particular person has the right to have choices about matters affecting himself, implemented in the procedure of obtaining informed consent; the principle of privacy, which protects an individual against unwarranted intrusion by others; the principle of confidentiality, which ensures that information about patients obtained in the course of the therapeutic relationship is to be held in confidence; the principle of trust, which asserts that others can be depended upon to act in honest and truthful ways; and the principle of equity, which the Commission understood as the requirement that people have access to an adequate level of care and that the costs of that care be fairly distributed. In addition, the President's Commission studied the complexities pertaining to life-sustaining therapies. Four guidelines regarding medical care of children with serious illness, summarized from the section 'Deciding to Forgo Life-Sustaining Treatment' are:

1. Health-care professionals serve patients best by maintaining a presumption in favour of sustaining life, unless the state of life is such that 'prolongation would be inhumane and unconscionable.'[12,25]

2. Families, health-care institutions, and professionals should work together to make decisions for patients who lack decision-making capacity.[36]

3. Parents should be surrogates for a seriously ill newborn unless they are disqualified by decision-making incapacity, an unresolvable disagreement between them, or their choice of a course of action that is clearly against the infant's best interests.[37,38]

4. Therapies expected to be futile...need not be provided.[39–41]

Clearly, the principles espoused by these important reports continue to exert a powerful influence on the understanding and resolution of ethical problems in health care and research. Medical decisions involving ethical and/or cultural values should be based on sound principles or standards that have achieved some degree of authority in society, and never simply on emotion, intuition, or local precedent. Ethical problems in paediatric medicine occur as a result of changes in society, advances in technology, conflicts within the roles of practitioners, and conflicts among the duties to patients, families, employers, and the law.

Over the last few years, there has been increasing public awareness of the complexities involved in medical decision-making for children, including seriously ill or damaged newborns. Common ethical problems include disagreement about the sanctity, meaning, or quality of life; relative benefits or burdens of medical interventions; the justifiability of medical paternalism; arguments regarding the existence and understanding of medical futility; resource allocation and distribution of health care; and disagreements about the importance of truth-telling, advocacy, and power. Decision-making about whether and/or how much to treat are, by necessity, laden with cultural, social, political, and philosophical values. Currently, several ethical standards applicable to paediatric medicine are employed in the United States to assist health care providers in making ethically competent decisions with their patients.

Standards of decision-making in the care of a child with a terminal illness

The ethical principles that guide the medical decision-making and care of the paediatric patient are the same as for the adult patient. These include respecting individual liberty (autonomy), promoting self-determination, maximizing good and minimizing unavoidable harm (beneficence and non-maleficence), and acting in ways that promote honesty, fairness, and compassion. Although the principles in both cases are the same, their application to the child require extreme integrity of the involved adults due to the ease with which adults can undermine and usurp the rights of the child.

A discussion of the ethical standards relevant to medical decision-making follows.

Substituted judgment

It is an axiomatic principle of medical ethics that the competent adult patient has the right to consent to or refuse medical interventions, based on the assumption that adults have developed a system of individual preferences or values regarding what matters to them. The substituted judgment standard of decision-making is grounded in the ethical values of autonomy and self-determination. In the paediatric context, it only applies to minors who previously were mature enough to make decisions but who are now no longer able to articulate for themselves decisions based on their own values, wishes, and preferences. Such individuals must have another person substitute in the role of the primary decision-maker. The surrogate decision-maker is required to make those decisions believed to most adequately represent the known preferences of the minor, preserving the ethical value of individual autonomy.

Best interests

Children and other minors who have never been able to formulate a value system typically have this right exercised on their behalf by parents or legal surrogates. In the current social and legal setting, parents are presumed to have the ability to make decisions regarding a child's best interest. The 'best interest' standard is derived from the ethical principle of beneficence, obligating the physician to attempt to do that which promotes the patient's good. In general, the best interests of a child are usually presumed to be life-preserving, but in the face of irreversible illness, this presumption requires careful exploration. Best interests may require a plan of care that focuses on the child's need for comfort and symptom relief, rather than the provision of life-saving medical therapy, to ease the process of dying in a way that promotes the safety, comfort, and dignity of the child.

The Baby Doe regulations

The care and medical decision-making for infants with life-threatening illnesses is often driven by the imperative to sustain life, regardless of the best interests of the person of the infant. In the United States, this was even formalized in regulations implemented briefly by the federal government. The United States federal Baby Doe regulations[39–41] arose after public exposure of a case of involving a baby with Down's syndrome and duodenal atresia whose parents and physicians elected medical non-intervention. Uninvolved parties, including the President of the United States, rapidly intervened to put a stop to such 'medical neglect' of handicapped infants, implementing regulations governing medical decision-making for infants. These regulations were struck down by the Supreme Court but replacement 'antidiscrimination' regulations[42] based on the Rehabilitation Act soon followed. These regulations failed to recognize all the situations in which the best interests of the infant might be served by forgoing life-sustaining intervention. In the United States District Court opinion leading to the eventual overthrow of these regulations, Judge Gerhard Gesell stated that Section 504 of the Rehabilitation Act (upon which the Baby Doe regulations were based) was never meant to be applied so 'blindly and without any consideration of burdens'. He also noted that 'to the extent the regulation is read to eliminate the role of the infant's parents in choosing an appropriate course of medical treatment, its application may, in some cases infringe upon the (right to privacy interests)'. He also characterized the regulations as having an *in terrorum* effect (causing disproportionate fear, expanding and exaggerating the original meaning of the regulations, and thus leading to altered decision-making), and as not facilitating more compassionate decision-making.[43] The 'chilling effect'[37,38] of the Baby Doe regulations, despite their overthrow, nevertheless remains, exerting significant influence on the options provided to families and the decisions made for infants. For example some American physicians believe that the option of forgoing life-sustaining interventions, even in the face of terminal illness, is one they cannot offer to families of infants. The regulations were intended to prevent medical neglect of infants with impairments who, with medical attention, could survive to enjoy a life of value to themselves. However, the regulations are now incorrectly perceived by many physicians to not allow termination of life-sustaining intervention in virtually any case. Inclusion of quality-of-life valuations in medical decision-making for infants under 1 year of age is particularly avoided.[44,45]

Since the initiation of the Baby Doe guidelines, the voices of family and child advocates have been raised. The replacement 'antidiscrimination law' enacted by Congress, allows the withholding of life-sustaining interventions in three instances, namely:

(1) permanent unconsciousness;

(2) provision of treatment would merely prolong dying, not be effective in ameliorating the life-threatening condition(s), or the treatment is otherwise futile in terms of the infant's survival;

(3) the provision of such services would be 'virtually futile' in achieving the infant's survival and the provision of treatment would thus be 'inhumane'.

This has never been legally challenged, however, leaving physicians, families, and infants in an ambiguous position. Recently, a group of prominent ethicists and paediatricians have again spoken out against the abandonment of the family's quality-of-life determination in neonatal decision-making in the United States, proposing new guidelines to assist in rational and ethical decisions for these infants and their families.[46] Additionally, the American Academy of Pediatrics and the American College of Obstetricians and Gynecologists have just issued a statement calling for parents to be given full information regarding the risks involved with the aggressive care of their severely premature infants, though they stopped short of recommending that families' opinions of the benefit/burden ratio be determinative of the goals of ongoing care.[47]

Quality-of-life standard

The quality-of-life standard is notoriously difficult to apply as it rests on subjective judgments that may represent a wide variety of beliefs and attitudes regarding the benefits and burdens of life, disability, and death. It is generally accepted that quality of life judgments ought not be made unilaterally by caregivers but require the collaboration of the child (where possible), his or her parents or surrogates, and paediatric practitioners familiar with the values and wishes of the patient. In the face of terminal illness in particular, quality-of-life assessments require careful, patient-centred discussions. Dying children and their parents may legitimately and appropriately reject medical treatments believed to result only in pain or suffering.

Quality-of-life determinations are acknowledged by nearly everyone as an appropriate and major factor in adult medical decision-making.[48-58] There are numerous guidelines on ethical decision-making for infants and children which cogently argue for anticipated quality of life to be factored in to life-and-death decision-making for them as well.[59,60] The lack of consideration of quality of life in medical decision-making for infants directly contravenes respect for persons and autonomy and constitutes discrimination solely on the basis of age.[61-63] Incompetent adults are able to exercise, through surrogates, the 'reasonable person standard' in medical decision-making, yet infants may not, as interpreted by some physicians in the United States. This approach results in lack of respect for the humanity of the infant, the deprivation of family rights of decision-making in the best interests of their infants, as well as the injudicious use of resources.[64] Even when families plead to stop, some United States physicians caring for incurably ill or neurologically devastated infants, often against their own consciences, refuse to forgo attempts to cure, putting forever out of reach the possibility of a peaceful, natural dying process.

The physician must not only take credit for saving lives, but also must assume responsibility for incurring injury and suffering.[35] The current medical model places low priority on the consequences of unrelenting quests to sustain life. Documentation of the harms done by ignoring the long-standing ramifications of our actions can be found in the essays of Constance Battle, a physician caring for patients in paediatric nursing homes, as well as by William Silverman, a neonatologist looking back on his whole career.[65,66] A paper documenting the poor conditions and services rendered to paediatric patients in the Massachusetts nursing homes reveals that the majority are patients who may have benefited from the option of palliative care.[67] The remainder were children with congenital syndromes and anomalies, who may also have benefited from alternative goals of therapy.

Quality-of-life estimations are routinely factored into decisions for infants in countries other than the United States,[68,69] demonstrating a lack of universal opinion that quality-of-life judgments are inappropriate for those who, by virtue of age alone, cannot speak for themselves.

There is documentation that in The Netherlands,[70,71] Canada,[69,72] New Zealand,[68,73] Australia,[74,75] and England[76] the parents are actively involved in these decisions. In other countries such as Japan,[73,77] India, Nepal, Sri Lanka,[4] and Poland,[78] however, it seems to be less common for the parents to have a say in the decision. Excluding parents from this process endangers their ability to act on their valuations of their infant's or family's best interests and violates their autonomy, and the personhood of their infants. In Japan, autonomy as a principle may be less valued in society[79] but this does not discount the ethical principle of the best-interest standard and respect for personhood. One wonders about the private suffering of families when the authoritarian physician determines the medical treatment of their children. The effects of paternalistic decision-making on bereavement has not been studied, but there are several cases indicating that parents and physicians do not always concur on the best interests of the child.[80-83] Thus, the child and family may be harmed by a perceived 'wrongful life' or, just as greatly, by their perception of a premature and unnecessary death. Just as competent children must have a voice in determining their own care, so must the parents of the imperilled newborn.

Beneficence and non-maleficence; the prevention of suffering

As Cassell and Bluebond-Langner explain,[84,85] suffering involves the loss of social roles and the inability to achieve expectations. Who suffers more than a child with a fatal illness, who will never reap the rewards of completed maturity? Suffering occurs in the knowledge that one will never play on the all-star team, never do the things older siblings have done and that younger siblings will do, never go to the prom, never graduate from high school, never marry or have sexual relations.

In some cases, the suffering of children is more profound than that of adults since their opinions and concerns are rarely solicited due to caregivers' fears of increasing their own pain.[86] Control regarding medical decisions is 'granted' too infrequently to the dying child, leaving him to feel unimportant as well as scared and ill. Children are known to feel responsible for the causes of their illnesses and the burdens imposed on their families as a result.[87] When unaddressed by caregivers, these feelings may cause untold suffering for the child. Children also place the needs of their grieving parents first, often at the expense of their own increased suffering. Children will allow continued futile treatments and hospitalizations for their parents' sake, as well as create situations to allow the parents to be alone if that is their desire, when what the child desires most is continuing demonstrations of parental love and attention.[88]

The terminally ill child: persisting problems and paradoxes

Failure of the acute care medical model

For a variety of reasons, regardless of the age of the patient, the promises of modern medicine have led many to place a high value on hospitalization, even at the end of a terminal illness. The increasing acceptance of the medicalized death, occurring as it too often does in the hospital after futile attempts to resuscitate, contributes to the feeling that death should not occur at home, without the 'benefit' of high technology. This is particularly true for the child, whose medical caregivers may have entered the field of paediatrics, in which death is a rare occurrence, in part because of their own discomfort with death.[29] The unrelenting pursuit of cure is often a result of the rejection of the concept of death as a natural phenomenon, a lack of understanding that making comfort the priority may actually be preferable to the burdens of ongoing attempts to preserve life. This is often the case in spite of the fact that the principle of beneficence is clearly not being served, and that the principle of non-maleficence is being breached.[89] As David Todres, a paediatric intensivist and neonatologist states, 'life is not the ultimate good nor death the ultimate evil.'[90] Ashwal *et al.*, referring to neonates, point out that 'we must resist the urge to institute desperate remedies for desperate patients and families. Unless a reversal or amelioration of the underlying condition can be expected, treatments should be questioned. Physicians should not be slaves to technology, and patients should not be its prisoners.'[33] In our highly technical practise of medicine, the imperative to 'do something' seems to include unrelenting attempts to cure or more rarely 'pull the plug,' but offering palliative care, particularly for children, occurs far too infrequently.

Futile ongoing attempts to cure are related directly to the failure of the acute care medical model. We labour under the misconception that we are the masters of death; that if we spend enough money and use enough technology, we can succeed in fending it off.[91] A death that is not preceded by an intensive care unit stay and an attempt at cardiopulmonary resuscitation is seen as one that might have been prevented. Thus, death can no longer be a peaceful though bittersweet time of last goodbyes, to be cherished by family and friends.

If maintenance of life at all costs is the overriding goal, however, the individual and human elements of care are often neglected. Life as the ultimate good has been rejected by many commentators, including the Catholic Church.[33,89,92-96] The failure to provide holistic, child-centred care, which is sensitive to diverse interpretations regarding the value of life, undermines the importance of self determination and other individual values, and thus overlooks an essential element of care in a pluralistic society.[97] The concept of suffering, as only the affected child[98,99] and family[100-102] can know suffering, is thus often ignored in designing treatment plans.[103]

The role of uncertainty in paediatric care

Neonatal medicine

One of the most difficult decision tasks in neonatal medicine has to do with medical uncertainty. King[104] has noted that parents need information about their seriously ill infants to allow realistic expectations regarding their children's prognoses. As clinicians and parents evaluate specific ways to manage medical uncertainty, it is essential that consideration is made of whether a given treatment or intervention is ethically appropriate for a particular patient. As the likelihood of a good outcome decreases, despite the lack of complete certainty regarding the neonate's prognosis or life course, it is important to discuss and align the overall goals of medical management with the values and preferences of the family. Good decisions result from sensitive balancing of anticipated benefits with the probable immediate or long-term burdens associated with the intervention. Parents are generally the stewards of the values and desires of their non-autonomous children; thus their opinions must be elicited and respected. The ethical value promoted by this respect is autonomy, supporting family integrity and acknowledging the legitimate role parents have in shaping their children's development.[92]

Although it is easily demonstrated that the rights of infants are not always acknowledged, particularly when it comes to refusal of 'life-saving' therapies, the palliative care community has not stepped forward as their advocates. It is difficult to prove the suffering of infants. However, it is not difficult to prove the suffering of the survivors of some of those therapies. As Constance Battle, Medical Director and CEO of The Hospital for Sick Children, a paediatric nursing home in Washington, D.C. elaborates:

> 'I walk the halls every day and see the lives these children lead long after the drama and glamour of treatment decisions have been made. . . . (T)he children whose families have moved onto new chapters in their lives with guilt and recrimination . . . and therapists coming and going, feeding the children, teaching, reteaching and reinforcing the simplest tasks. . . . And I think of the long, lonely Saturday afternoons when . . . the therapists are gone and the children are slowly passing the time, minute by minute. . . . It is time that we acknowledged that the interests being served are not those of the baby and the family but rather of the physician engaged in a great, momentary professional challenge . . . Just as the neonatologists' doors close, the often bleak doors to the survivors' futures open.'[65]

Data regarding the profundity of the grief and loss of infants (and even pregnancy losses) show that these losses are equally painful as the loss of an older child. In the United States alone, there are estimated to be 40 000 infant deaths per year.[105] Most of these children die without the benefits of palliative care interventions, and bereavement follow-up is unusual and of short duration when it is offered.[106-108] Hospice interventions for the critically ill newborn can have great salutary effect for the family.[109-113] The ethic of care may mandate the implementation of palliative care programmes for these families. As Janet Goodall comments, 'dying babies, too, can be helped to live until they die... To ignore the normal reaction to grief and to destroy the opportunity for parents and the child to have even a brief time to enjoy each other is to sow a legacy of chronic emotional pain.'[114] Even the neonatal intensive care unit can be a place where palliative care interventions can be made.

Permanent vegetative state

Permanent unconsciousness, a state which greater than 75 per cent of Americans reject as an acceptable quality of life for themselves,[115] when present in childhood often leads to medical 'treatment'. The causes of this phenomenon include: physician misinterpretation of the law; ignorance of position statements of bodies such as the President's Commission,[48] the Hastings Center,[49,116] and of ethical principles in general; parental guilt caused by being made to feel that their decision, not the disease, is the direct cause of the child's death;[117] and persistent lack of certainty on the part of the medical community about prognosis, sometimes based on single case reports.[118-120] This latter is particularly problematic for the diagnosis of permanent vegetative state, a condition which is often confused with the continuing vegetative state which precedes it.[119]

The permanent vegetative state is a state of irreversible unconsciousness. The prognosis for children in persistent vegetative state of a year's duration is no different than for adults.[120-122] For both adults and children, the prognosis is better with traumatic aetiologies.[123,124] Permanent vegetative state is in fact a terminal illness, even with all means of support being continued.[125,126] Life expectancies vary by age, with younger children generally having a shorter life-expectancy. Ashwal, *et al.* documented life-expectancies ranging from 2.6 years in the infant with permanent vegetative state to 7 years for the patients greater than 19 years of age at onset of persistent vegetative state.[118] The reluctance to forgo life-sustaining treatment for children even in the face of permanent vegetative state[118] may constitute a form of age discrimination, depriving children of the rights afforded to adults for the simple fact that they were never of age to indicate their preferences or construct an advance directive.[62]

Rare diseases

Uncertainty of prognosis of childhood diseases exists not only in the case of permanent vegetative state but for a whole host of other paediatric conditions and diseases as well. The child may suffer from a rare genetic or metabolic abnormality, too rare to allow statistical certainty for a population, let alone an individual. Profound parental guilt in these congenital disorders creates problems in the unbiased application of the principle of best interests. Even the care of paediatric cancer patients is fraught with uncertainty.[127] The resilience of the child's physiology leads to uncertainty of prognosis, causing unduly optimistic predictions in many instances, and leaving the child and family ill-prepared when death makes its inevitable presence known. Finally, emerging technology and the willingness of parents and physicians to subject the child unknowingly to experimental treatments in order to attempt to preserve life conspire to deprive the child and family of the option of a palliative approach.[63] Bone marrow transplantations are more willingly offered than comfort, holding hands, and hugs.

A proposal for humanistic care for children with terminal illnesses

A new paradigm of supportive care

It is known that we fear most that with which we are least familiar. The increasingly rare phenomenon of childhood death in developed nations and the ever-changing spectrum of rare diseases that cause it breed fear; fear of being wrong and thus fear of acknowledging either the terminal nature of the illness or the terminal status of the child. Uncertainty on the part of the medical community has a significant influence on the decision-making of the child and family regarding treatment options in the face of terminal illness. Palliative care options are simply not considered. Some physicians relentlessly pursue cure based on anecdotal reports of one or two child survivors in the same circumstances in 28 years.[128] Others would remind us of the costs incurred by such an approach—'. . . the psychological costs of false hope, the prolongation of the acceptance of death and the initiation of grieving, the last visual memory of one's child invaded by technology'.[129] These factors, too should be part of the decision-making paradigm.

Parents, however, justifiably see themselves as their children's champions; their natural tendency is to want to preserve life and with it their social roles as parents.[130] It is only when the physician offers the information from the beginning of treatment that the burdens of ongoing treatment may at some point outweigh the benefits, that loving parents may, with their child's input when available, decide to forgo further attempts at cure. They must be helped to see that forgoing treatment designed to cure can be an even greater manifestation of love, thus freeing them to spend precious time with their child, enjoying the last days, weeks, or months, unencumbered by medical trappings and overwhelming guilt. There must be simultaneous reassurances that if forgoing curative measures is chosen, that the comfort of the child and family will be maintained at all costs and that the treatment team will stand by them until death and thereafter in bereavement.

The 'admission criterion' for paediatric palliative care interventions is simple: there is a significant possibility of death prior to achieving adulthood. Entering the family dynamic early allows the team to address the grief and loss that occurs at the time of diagnosis and which ebbs and flows thereafter. It allows sharing of the good times and the bad. It allows for respite interventions to be made and for promotion of family unity through the work of the child life specialist and social worker. Attention to symptom management to maximize the ability to enjoy life, and attention to developing social issues can be achieved best by early intervention.

Visits in the early stages can be infrequent, often substituting phone calls just as a lifeline of people who care. Curative interventions may be undertaken as long as the child and family feel they are of benefit. When curative care is seen as not helping, the efforts of the palliative care team will be accelerated, increasing visit frequency and intensity. Inpatient and outpatient options need to be available. The team needs to feel comfortable attending to the family in the intensive care unit setting since some children (particularly neonates) will only be off the ventilator for a short time prior to death.

Home care for these patients is cost-effective for third party payers as well as for hospitals.[127] As it currently stands, home care is not financially cost-effective for families, but it is emotionally cost-effective. The lost wages by at least one adult caregiver needs to be factored into the equation when evaluating the benefits of home care. Supporting the family in attending to their child both by providing respite services as well as by structuring reimbursement methods to make allowances for the caregiving done by the family is a needed change, one reflective of a society that is just and empathic. It will be cost-effective for society, we believe, as the number of unnecessary hospitalizations will decrease and, more importantly, as the effects of a poorly handled and prolonged grieving process will more often be avoided through the provision of effective, family-centred supportive care.

A mandate for educational change

In order for the ethic of care to be utilized in the care of paediatric patients, it must be incorporated in the training of medical personnel. The unavoidability of death for some children needs to be acknowledged. The fears of the caregivers need to be confronted and ameliorated by giving them tools to use. Knowledge of how to approach these children and their families and how to calm their fears and effectively manage their symptoms, both physical and psychological, must be taught and modelled by senior caregivers.

For the same reasons as in adult care, children with the diagnosis of: chronic lung disease (even on the basis of bronchopulmonary dysplasia); profound irreversible dementia (whether based on hypoxic–ischaemic injury, intracranial haemorrhage, neurodegenerative processes, anatomic malformations, trauma, infection, or any other cause, at any age); cancers with poor prognoses (even at the time of diagnosis); malformations incompatible with meaningful life (including chromosomal defects, other anatomical anomalies); or other less common incurable conditions (AIDS, storage diseases, and other metabolic deficiencies) should be given the option of supportive care close to the time of diagnosis. Though it may not be accepted at first, if its availability is made known at the outset, and the physician acknowledges the difficulties ahead, if and when the family needs to avail themselves of additional help, they will feel supported in their decision.

The technological imperative versus the ethic of care

The effects of the technological imperative can be seen most clearly as they affect medical decision-making as well reimbursement strategies. It is far easier for the medical care team to persist in efforts to sustain life than to sit down with the child and family to have an earnest discussion of the goals of therapy. For some medical caregivers, the ability to pursue cure has even taken on a moral imperative.[131] For others, particularly in the United States, continued reimbursement for curative care is attractive, though neither the child nor the family may be benefiting. There are significant financial disincentives to physicians, who still seem to be determinative regarding the goals of care, to implement palliative care and, in particular, to refer to a hospice programme. Only in 1995 did it become possible for a physician in the United States to bill for charges associated with a home visit for a patient on hospice services. Case management at the interdisciplinary team meeting or via phone is not directly reimbursable. As a result, most physicians in the United States volunteer their time to palliative care patients, particularly in the home setting.

Additionally, not only in the context of palliative care, but throughout the United States' medical reimbursement paradigms, the services of social workers, child life therapists, pastoral workers, occupational therapists, and music therapists are not reimbursed. This reinforces the notion that these non-technical services are not of value and are unnecessary 'frills'. Likewise, in the American hospice setting, bereavement services are not reimbursable. The prolonged and more intense bereavement needs of families who lose a child are thus unattractive for hospices to undertake. It also creates an incentive to have non-professional volunteers handle this aspect of hospice services, potentially creating harm for families who need more.

Implications for a just society

One of the reasons that palliative care is not offered to families of dying children with greater frequency is that the prospect of a child dying is accepted neither by the medical community nor the family. This follows in part from the technological imperative discussed above, in part from historic and social constructs as introduced in the first part of the chapter, and, in large measure, from the reimbursement mechanisms available. In Britain, where the cost of most medical care is covered by the comprehensive National Health Service, palliative care is offered for the long term,[132] with some children enrolled in a hospice for years. In contrast, in the United States, where palliative care is an either/or option as opposed to curative care, parents and children who would still like to undergo some forms of curative measures must forgo hospice services, including respite care. Alternatively, hospices can provide the services without reimbursement. The latter tactic is frequently used, but hospices cannot survive long without receiving reimbursement, particularly if long-term involvement with paediatric patients is contemplated.

Conclusion

Ethical principles apply to all individuals, regardless of age or maturity. Children deserve the right to autonomy, whether exercised on their behalf by parents in the case of infants and the very young child, or in partnership with the parents in the young child, or with parental input in the case of the adolescent. Each decision must be mindful not only of emerging technology, but also of the emerging adult. The developing person of the child must be honoured in the creation of all treatment plans, and, with his parents, he must be told of all available options, including palliative care.

Supportive care of the infant and child throughout chronic, life-limiting illness is a concept whose time has come. An understanding of the values, principles, and duties that inform the ethic of care creates the imperative to provide humanistic, holistic, and competent palliative care to the child, honouring the intrinsic value of each individual, regardless of age.

Despite our technical expertise in curing illness, there are still a substantial number of children who will die of irreversible illness every year. These children may be found in neonatal intensive care units, on hospital wards, and at home. None should be excluded from having the benefits of child-oriented supportive care.

Promoting education of the medical community and society at large about the benefits of holistic supportive care, pain and symptom management, as well as ethical principles and their practical applications in paediatric medicine, will perhaps increase the acceptability of the inevitable death of a child and allow it to be a peaceful time. For progress to occur, however, reimbursement structures must stop rewarding non-beneficial uses of biotechnology and start encouraging the humane application of palliative care to children.

References

1. Reich WT, editor-in-chief. Care: history of the notion. In: *Encyclopedia of Bioethics*. New York: Macmillan, 1995: 319–36.
2. May R. *Love and will*. New York: WW Norton, 1969.
3. Erikson E. *Childhood and Society*, 2nd edn. New York: W.W. Norton, 1963.
4. Mayeroff M. *On Caring*. New York: Harper and Row, 1971.
5. Dominica F. Reflections on death in childhood. *British Medical Journal*, 1987; **294**: 108–10.
6. Evans PR. The management of fatal illness in childhood. *Proceedings of the Royal Society of Medicine*, 1969; **62**: 549–50.
7. Subramanian KNS. In India, Nepal, and Sri Lanka, quality of life weighs heavily. *Hastings Center Report*, 1986; **16**: 20–2.
8. Fost N. Parents as decision-makers for children. *Biomedical Ethics*, 1986; **13**: 285–93.
9. Kurtz Z. Do children's rights to health care in the UK ensure their best interests? *Journal of the Royal College of Physicians of London*, 1995; **9**: 508–16.
10. *The Children Act, Great Britain, 1989*. London: Her Majesty's Stationery Office, 1989, 218 pp.
11. General Assembly of the United Nations. *Adoption of a Convention on the Rights of the Child*. New York: United Nations General Assembly, 1989.
12. Susman EJ, Hersh SP, Nannis ED, *et al.* Conceptions of cancer: the perspectives of child and adolescent patients and their families. *Journal of Pediatric Psychiatry*, 1982; **7**: 253–61.
13. Leikin S. The role of adolescents in decisions concerning their cancer therapy. *Cancer* (suppl.), 1993; **71**: 3342–6.
14. Bartholome WG. A new understanding of consent in pediatric practice:

consent, parental permission and child assent. *Pediatric Annals*, 1989; **18**: 262–5.

15. Alderson P. *Children's Consent to Surgery*. Philadelphia: Open University Press, 1993.
16. Freyer DR. Children with cancer: special considerations in the discontinuation of life sustaining treatment. *Journal of Medical and Pediatric Oncology*, 1992; **20**: 136–42.
17. King NMP, Cross AW. Children as decision-makers: Guidelines for pediatricians. *Journal of Pediatrics*, 1989; **115**: 10–16.
18. Doyal L, Henning P. Stopping treatment for end-stage renal failure: the rights of children and adolescents. *Journal of Pediatric Nephrology*, 1994; 8: 768–91.
19. Grant VJ. Consent in pediatrics: a complex teaching assignment. *Journal of Medical Ethics*, 1991; **17**: 199–204.
20. Committee on Bioethics, American Academy of Pediatrics. Informed consent, parental permission and assent in pediatric practice. *Pediatrics*, 1995; **95**: 314–17.
21. Leikin S. A proposal concerning decisions to forgo life-sustaining treatment for young people. *Journal of Pediatrics*, 1989; **115**: 17–22.
22. Robinson RJ. Ethics committees and research in children. *British Medical Journal*, 1987; **294**: 1243–4.
23. Holder AR. Disclosure and consent problems in pediatrics. *Law, Medicine and Healthcare*, 1988; **16**: 219–28.
24. Rothenberg KH. Medical decision making for children. In: Childress JF, King PA, Rothenberg KH, *et al*., eds. *Biolaw: A Legal and Ethical Reporter on Medical, Health Care and Bioengineering*, Vol.1. Frederick, MD: University Publications of America, 1986.
25. Grisso T, Vierling L. Minors' consent to treatment: a developmental perspective. *Professional Psychology*, 1978; **9**: 412–27.
26. Culbert ML. *The Choice*, 1995; **21**:15.
27. Roberts E. Refusal of treatment by 16 year old. *Lancet*, 1992; **340**: 108–9.
28. Feeg VD. Ethics lessons in a teenager's story. *Pediatric Nursing*, 1994: **20**: 436.
29. Bluebond-Langner M. *The Private Worlds of Dying Children*. Princeton, NJ: Princeton University Press, 1978.
30. Landwirth J. Ethical issues in pediatric and neonatal resuscitation. *Annals of Emergency Medicine*, 1993; **22**: 502–7.
31. Elton A, Honig P, Bentovim A, *et al*. Withholding consent to lifesaving treatment: three cases. *British Medical Journal*, 1995; **310**: 373–7.
32. Robb N. Ruling on Jehovah's Witness teen in New Brunswick may have 'settled the law' for MD's. *Canadian Medical Association Journal*, 1994; **151**: 625–8.
33. Ashwal S, Perkin RM, Orr R. When too much is not enough. *Pediatric Annals*, 1992; **21**: 311–14, 316–17.
34. Devereux JA, Jones DPH, Dickenson DL. Can children withhold consent to treatment? *British Medical Journa*l, 1993; **306**: 1459–61.
35. United Nations General Assembly. Resolution 1386(XIV), November 20, 1959. In: *Official Records of the General Assembly, Fourteenth Session*, 1960 (Supplement 16): 19.
36. US National Commission for the Protection of Human Subjects of Biomedical and Behavioral Research. *The Belmont Report. Ethical Principles and Guidelines for the Protection of Human Subjects of Research*. Federal Register, **44** (Apr 18, 1979) 3 volumes. Washington, DC: US Government Printing Office, 1988: 23192–7.
37. Moskop JC, Saldanha RA. The Baby Doe rule: Still a threat. *Hastings Center Report*, 1986; **16**: 2.
38. Lantos J. Baby Doe five years later: implications for child health. *New England Journal of Medicine*, 1987; **317**: 444–7.
39. Department of Health and Human Services, Office of Civil Rights. Notice to health care providers. *Federal Register*, 1982; **47** (May 18): 26027.
40. Department of Health and Human Services. Nondiscrimination on the basis of handicap, interim final rule. *Federal Register*, 1983; **48** (March 7): 9630–2.
41. Department of Health and Human Services. Nondiscrimination on the basis of handicap; procedures and guidelines relating to health care for handicapped infants; final rule. *Federal Register*, 1984; **49** (January 12): 1622–54.
42. US Congress. Public Law 98–457, amending Child Abuse Prevention and Treatment Act: *Federal Register*, 1985; **50** (April 15): 1340.
43. Annas GJ. Disconnecting the Baby Doe hotline. *The Hastings Center Report*, 1983; **13**: 14–16.
44. Kopelman LM, Irons TG, Kopelman AE. Neonatologists judge the 'Baby Doe' regulations. *New England Journal of Medicine*, 1988; **318**: 677–83.
45. Nelson LJ. Forgoing treatment of critically ill newborns and the legal legacy of Baby Doe. *Clinical Ethics Report*, 1992; **6**: 1–6.
46. Lantos JD, Tyson JE, Allen A, *et al*. Withholding and withdrawing life sustaining treatment in neonatal intensive care: issues for the 1990's. *Archives of Disease in Childhood*, 1994; **71**: F218–23.
47. American Academy of Pediatrics Committee on Fetus and Newborn, American College of Obstetricians and Gynecologists Committee on Obstetric Practice. Perinatal care at the threshhold of viability. *Pediatrics*, 1995; **96**: 974–6.
48. President's Commission for the Study of Ethical Problems in Medicine and Biomedical and Behavioral Research. *Deciding to Forgo Life-sustaining Treatment: a Report on the Ethical, Medical and Legal issues in Treatment Decisions*. Washington, DC: Government Printing Office, 1987.
49. Members of the Hastings Center Research Project on the Care of Imperiled Newborns. Standards of judgment for treatment of imperiled newborns. *Hastings Center Report*, 1987; **17**: 13–16.
50. Current Opinions of the Council on Ethical and Judicial Affairs of the American Medical Association. *Withholding or Withdrawing Life-prolonging Treatment*. Chicago: American Medical Association, 1986.
51. Executive Board of the American Academy of Neurology. Position of the AAN on certain aspects of the care and management of the PVS patient. *Neurology*, 1989; **39**: 125–6.
52. Kass LR. Ethical dilemmas in the care of the ill: what is the patient's good? *Journal of the American Medical Association*, 1980; **244**: 1946–9.
53. Wanzer SH, Federman DD, Adelstein SJ, *et al*. The physician's responsibility toward hopelessly ill patients: A second look. *New England Journal of Medicine*, 1989; **320**: 844–9.
54. Howie KE, Gomberg FK. How does the law treat the doctor? *Canadian Medical Association Journal*, 1983; **129**: 1034–8.
55. Council on Scientific Affairs and Council on Ethical and Judicial Affairs, American Medical Association. Persistent vegetative state and the decision to withhold or withdraw life support. *Journal of the American Medical Association*, 1990; **263**: 426–30.
56. Jennett B. Letting vegetative patients die. *British Medical Journal*, 1992; **305**: 1305–6.
57. British Medical Association Medical Ethics Comittee. *Discussion Paper on Treatment of Patients in Persistent Vegetative State*. BMA House, Tavistock Square, London: British Medical Association, 1992.
58. Institute of Medical Ethics Working Party on the Ethics of Prolonging Life and Assisting Death. *Lancet*, 1991; **337**: 96–8.
59. Walters JW. Approaches to ethical decision-making in the neonatal intensive care unit. *American Journal of Diseases in Children*, 1988; **142**: 825–30.
60. Neal BW. Ethical aspects in the care of very low birth weight infants. *Pediatrician*, 1990; **17**: 92–9.
61. Stahlman M. Presidential address, American Pediatric Society: Medical ethics and the law. *Pediatric Research*, 1986; **20**: 913–14.
62. Gustaitis R. Right to refuse life-sustaining treatment. *Pediatrics*, 1988; **81**: 317–21.
63. Tyson J. Evidence-based ethics and the care of premature infants. *The Future of Children*, 1995; **5**: 197–213.
64. Angell M. Handicapped children: Baby Doe and Uncle Sam. *New England Journal of Medicine*, 1983; **309**: 659–61.
65. Battle CU. Beyond the nursery door: The obligation to survivors of technology. *Clinics in Perinatology*, 1987; **14**: 417–27.
66. Silverman WA. Overtreatment of neonates? A personal retrospective. *Pediatrics*, 1992; **90**: 971–6.

67. Glick PS, Guyer B, Burr BH, *et al.* Pediatric nursing homes: implications of the Massachusetts experience for residential care of multiply handicapped children. *New England Journal of Medicine*, 1983; **309**: 640–6.
68. Mitchell DR. Medical treatment of severely impaired infants in New Zealand hospitals. *New Zealand Medical Journal*, 1986; **99**: 364–8.
69. Bioethics Committee, Canadian Pediatric Society. Treatment decisions for infants and children. *Canadian Medical Association Journal*, 1986; **135**: 447–8.
70. Visser HKA. Paediatrics in the Netherlands: challenges for today and tomorrow. *Archives of Disease in Childhood*, 1993; **69**: 251–5.
71. Visser HKA, Aartsen HGM, de Beaufort ID. Medical decisions concerning the end of life in children in the Netherlands. *American Journal of Diseases of Children*, 1992; **146**: 1429–31.
72. Bagwell CE, Goodwin SR. Spinning the wheels: a CAPS survey of ethical issues in pediatric surgery. *Journal of Pediatric Surgery*, 1992; **27**: 1385–90.
73. Charlton R, Dovey S. Attitudes to death and dying in the UK, New Zealand, and Japan. *Journal of Palliative Care*, 1995; **11**: 42–7.
74. Yu VYH. The extremely low birth weight infant: ethical issues in treatment. *Australian Paediatric Journal*, 1987; **23**: 97–103.
75. Working Party, Council of the Australian College of Paediatrics. Non-intervention in children with major handicaps; legal and ethical issues. *Australian Journal of Paediatrics*, 1983; **19**: 217–22.
76. Innes-Williams D. Medical ethics in paediatric surgery. *Irish Journal of Medical Science*, 1990; **159**: 237–40.
77. Kimura R. In Japan, parents participate but doctors decide. *Hastings Center Report*, 1986; **16**: 22–3.
78. Szawarski Z, Tulczynski A. Treatment of defective newborns—a survey of paediatricians in Poland. *Journal of Medical Ethics*, 1988; **14**: 11–17.
79. Hoshino K. Telling the truth and decision making in the context of the family: two issues in Japanese bioethics.
80. Glover JJ, Rushton CH. Introduction: from Baby Doe to Baby K: evolving challenges in pediatric ethics. *Journal of Law, Medicine and Ethics*, 1995; **23**: 5–6.
81. Richmond C. Is the issue the price of a child's life or the futility of heroic measures? *Canadian Medical Association*, 1995; **152**: 2035–6.
82. Capron AM. Baby Ryan and virtual futility. *Hastings Center Report*, 1995; **25**: 20–21.
83. Rolbein S. A matter of life and death. *Boston Magazine*, 1987; **179** Oct: 246–54.
84. Bluebond-Langner M. *The Private Worlds of Dying Children*. Princeton, NJ: Princeton University Press, 1978: 204, 212–15.
85. Cassell E. *The Nature of Suffering and the Goals of Medicine*. New York: Oxford University Press, 1991: Chapter 3.
86. Goldman A. *Care of the Dying Child*. New York: Oxford University Press, 1994: 133.
87. Wheeler PR, Lange NF, Bertolone SJ. Improving care for hospitalized terminally ill children: a practicable model. In: Corr CA, Corr DM, eds. *Hospice Approaches to Pediatric Care*. New York: Springer Publishing, 1983: 43–60.
88. Bluebond-Langner M. *The Private Worlds of Dying Children*. Princeton, NJ: Princeton University Press, 1978: 198–230.
89. Young EWD, Stevenson DK. Limiting treatment for extremely premature, low-birth-weight infants (500–750g). *American Journal of Diseases in Childhood*, 1990; **144**: 549–52.
90. Todres ID. Ethical dilemmas in pediatric critical care. *Critical Care Clinics*, 1992; **8**: 219–27.
91. Landau RL, Gustafson JM. Death is not the enemy. *Journal of the American Medical Association*, 1984; **252**: 2458.
92. Fleischman AR, Nolan K, Dubler NN, *et al.* Caring for gravely ill children. *Pediatrics*, 1994; **94**: 433–9.
93. Huault G. The place of a pediatric intensivist in our society. *Intensive Care Medicine*, 1989; **15**: S1–4.
94. Coulter DL, Murray TH, Cerreto MC. Practical ethics in pediatrics. *Current Problems in Pediatrics*, 1988; **18**: 137–95.
95. Paris JJ, McCormick RA. The Catholic tradition on the use of nutrition and fluids. *America*, 1987; May 2: 356–61.
96. Coggan D. On dying and dying well: spiritual and moral aspects. *Proceedings of the Royal Society of Medicine*, 1977; **70**: 75–81.
97. Englehardt HT. Bioethics in pluralistic societies. *Perspectives in Biology and Medicine*, 1982; **26**: 64–78.
98. Bracegirdle KE. A time to die: withdrawal of pediatric intensive care. *British Journal of Nursing*, 1994; **3**: 513–17.
99. Wikler D. Patient interests: clinical implications of philosophical distinctions. *Journal of the American Gerontological Society*, 1988; **36**: 951–8.
100. Lantos JD. Treatment refusal, noncompliance, and the pediatrician's responsibilities. *Pediatric Annals*, 1989; **18**: 255–60.
101. Lo B, Rouse F, Dornbrand L. Family decision-making on trial; who decides for incompetent patients? *New England Journal of Medicine*, 1990; **322**: 1228–32.
102. Gale R, Armon Y, Stern L, *et al.* Ethical problems in cardiac surgery for a lethal, congenital malformation. *Journal of Perinatology*, 1988; **8**: 137–40.
103. Cassell EJ. The nature of suffering and the goals of medicine. *New England Journal of Medicine*, 1982; **306**; 639–45.
104. King NM. Transparency in the neonatal intensive care. *Hastings Center Report*, 1992; **22**: 18–25.
105. Ashwal S. Are we diagnosing brain death in newborns accurately? *Journal of Heart and Lung Transplantation*, 1991; **10**: 867.
106. Lewis E. Mourning by the family after a stillbirth or neonatal death. *Archives of Disease in Childhood*, 1979; **54**: 303–6.
107. Bourne S, Lewis E. Perinatal bereavement. *British Medical Journal*, 1991; **302**: 1167–8.
108. Rosenfeld JA. Bereavement and grieving after spontaneous abortion. *American Family Physician*, 1991; **43**(5):1679–84.
109. Silverman WA. A hospice setting for humane neonatal death. *Pediatrics*, 1982; **69**: 239–40.
110. Harmon RJ, Glicken AD, Siegel RE. Neonatal loss in the intensive care nursery: Effects of maternal grieving and a program for intervention. *Journal of the American Academy of Child Psychiatry*, 1984; **23**: 68–71.
111. Whitfield JM, Siegel RE, Glicken AD, *et al.* The application of hospice concepts to neonatal care. *American Journal of Diseases of Children*, 1982; **136**: 421–4.
112. Landon KA, Kirkpatrick JM, Stull SP, *et al.* Incorporating hospice care in a community hospital NICU. *Neonatal Network*, 1987; **6**: 13–19.
113. Siegel R. A family-centered program of neonatal care. *Social Work*, 1982; **7**: 50–8.
114. Goodall J. Dutch doctor convicted of murdering disabled infant. *British Medical Journal*, 1995; **310**: 1603.
115. Knox RA. *Americans favor mercy killing*. Boston Globe/Harvard Poll, Oct 18–20, 1991, p.1 of National/foreign section.
116. The American Academy of Pediatrics Committee on Bioethics. Guidelines on forgoing life-sustaining treatment. *Pediatrics*, 1994; **93**: 532–6.
117. Nelson LJ, Nelson RM. Ethics and the provision of futile, harmful or burdensome treatment to children. *Critical Care Medicine*, 1992; **20**: 427–33.
118. Ashwal S, Bale JF, Coulter DL, *et al.* The persistent vegetative state in children: Report of the Child Neurology Society Ethics Committee. *Annals of Neurology*, 1992; **32**: 570–6.
119. Coulter DL. The vegetative state in infants: criteria and prognosis (abstract 78). *Annals of Neurology*, 1991; **30**: 473.
120. Coulter DL. Neurologic uncertainty in newborn intensive care. *New England Journal of Medicine*, 1987; **316**: 840–4.
121. The Multi-Society Task Force on PVS. Medical aspects of the persistent vegetative state, (first of two parts). *New England Journal of Medicine*, 1994; **330**: 1499–508.
122. Ashwal S, Eyman RK, Call TL. Life expectancy of children in a persistent vegetative state. *Pediatric Neurology*, 1994; **10**: 27–33.
123. The Multi-Society Task Force on PVS. Medical aspects of the persistent vegetative state, (second of two parts). *New England Journal of Medicine*, 1994; **330**: 1572–9.
124. Fields AI, Coble DH, Pollack MM, *et al.* Outcomes of children in a persistent vegetative state. *Critical Care Medicine*, 1993; **21**: 1890–4.
125. Kriel RL, Krach LE, Jones-Saete C. Outcome of children with prolonged

unconsciousness and vegetative state. *Pediatric Neurology*, 1993; **9**: 362–8.

126. Jennett B, Plum F. Persistent vegetative state after brain damage. *Lancet*, 1975; **1**: 480–4.
127. Martinson IM. Improving the care of dying children. *Western Journal of Medicine*, 1995; **163**: 258–62.
128. Orlowski JP. How much resuscitation is enough resuscitation? *Pediatrics*, 1992; **90**: 997–8.
129. Quan L. How much resuscitation is enough resuscitation? (Letter to the editor). *Pediatrics*, 1993; **91**: 516–17.
130. Bluebond-Langner M. *The Private Worlds of Dying Children*. Princeton, NJ: Princeton University Press, 1978: 214–17.
131. Fost N. Treatment of seriously ill and handicapped newborns. *Critical Care Clinics*, 1986; **2**: 149–59.
132. Dominica MF. The role of the hospice for the dying child. *British Journal of Hospital Medicine*, 1987; **38**: 334–43.

20

Palliative care aspects of acquired immune deficiency syndrome

20.1 AIDS: aspects in adults

Philip D. Welsby, Alison Richardson, and R.P. Brettle

Introduction

The original description of AIDS, the acquired immune deficiency syndrome, appeared in 1981[1,2] and described 26 patients with Kaposi's sarcoma (a skin tumour which until then had only been seen in elderly men, in African races, and in those with considerable iatrogenic immunosuppression) plus five men with oral thrush and *Pneumocystis carinii* pneumonia (which was usually associated with iatrogenic immunosuppression). The connection between the two groups was that all the men were homosexuals. The causative virus was first isolated in 1983 by Dr Luc Montagnier and was propagated in a cell line by Dr Robert Gallo in 1984. A variety of names were used for the virus but these have all now been replaced by human immunodeficiency virus (**HIV**). The definition of the clinical syndrome was revised in 1987[3] (see Appendix) and 1993.

In essence, AIDS is the occurrence of a reliably diagnosed disease that is at least moderately indicative of a defect in underlying cellular immunity, in an HIV positive person, in the absence of other conditions known to be associated with cellular immunodeficiency. AIDS is now a major, and increasing, cause of mortality throughout the world. Infection with HIV is even more widespread and the extent of the final problem can only be surmised.

The transmission of HIV occurs by three routes—any form of unprotected penetrative sexual intercourse, inoculation of blood or blood products, or mother to child transmission (during pregnancy, childbirth, or breast feeding). The World Health Organization has classified HIV transmission into three patterns. Pattern 1 is characterized mainly by spread through homo- or bisexual intercourse or intravenous drug use, pattern 2 is characterized by transmission by heterosexual intercourse, and pattern 3 is associated with visitors to and from pattern 1 and 2 areas together with infection associated with imported blood products from such areas. The United States, Europe, and Australia initially showed pattern 1 transmission, Africa showed pattern 2 transmission, and the Middle East, Oceania, and Russia pattern 3 transmission. However, such categorizations are becoming less relevant and, for example, transmission in the Far East shows features of all three patterns. In developed countries, injection drug users are an important reservoir of infection and are a critical bridge by which infection spreads via the sexual route into the general heterosexual population.[4] Britain is in a transition period and, although absolute numbers are relatively small, the greatest rate of increase of infection is from heterosexual contacts with high-risk groups.

A variety of social factors combined to produce the HIV and AIDS epidemic including: increased movement of populations around the world, partly as a consequence of cheaper and more available travel; changes in the sexual life-style; the economic drive or move toward urbanization; and the epidemics of injection drug misuse. In developing countries, such as Africa, other factors include: the migration of prostitutes between neighbouring countries (presumably for economic reasons); the influx of travellers from other countries for tourism; the opening of overland trade routes; and mass population migrations, usually as a result of war.

Epidemics of injection drug use seem to have occurred secondary to unemployment combined with widespread availability of cheap heroin. Epidemics of HIV associated with injection drug use were produced by widespread sharing of injecting equipment, possibly caused by a lack of simple hygiene knowledge together with a paucity of injecting equipment. Gathering of injection drug users in so called 'shooting galleries,' where equipment was shared, guaranteed rapid transmission of infection to all involved. The mobility of injection drug users then spread infection nationally and internationally. It is important to realize that the term injection drug user includes a large number of people who, in their youth, experimented only transitorily with drugs in much the same way that some others (the more fortunate) experimented with alcohol. In the United States, at the time of writing, injection drug users are the predominant AIDS sufferers.

From 1970 to 80, there were changes in sexual lifestyle, particularly amongst American homosexuals. The development of the 'gay' movement was partly characterized by an increased frequency of sex, together with increasing commercialization of sex (via bath houses and sex clubs). On average, individuals had two to three sexual contacts per night and epidemics of traditional sexually transmitted diseases and an, initially unnoticed, epidemic of HIV infection followed. The crucial factor in overall sexual transmission is not related to particular sexual practices but rather to the number of sexual partners, although sexual transmission may happen after one episode of heterosexual intercourse. In certain areas of Africa, HIV is a 'general sexually transmitted disease' affecting males and females equally with infection rates of up to 20 per cent in certain urban populations.

Future HIV and AIDS facilities, and in particular the hospice movement, will have to cater for male homosexuals, injection drug users, an increasing number of patients with heterosexually acquired infection, and a smaller group of patients who acquired

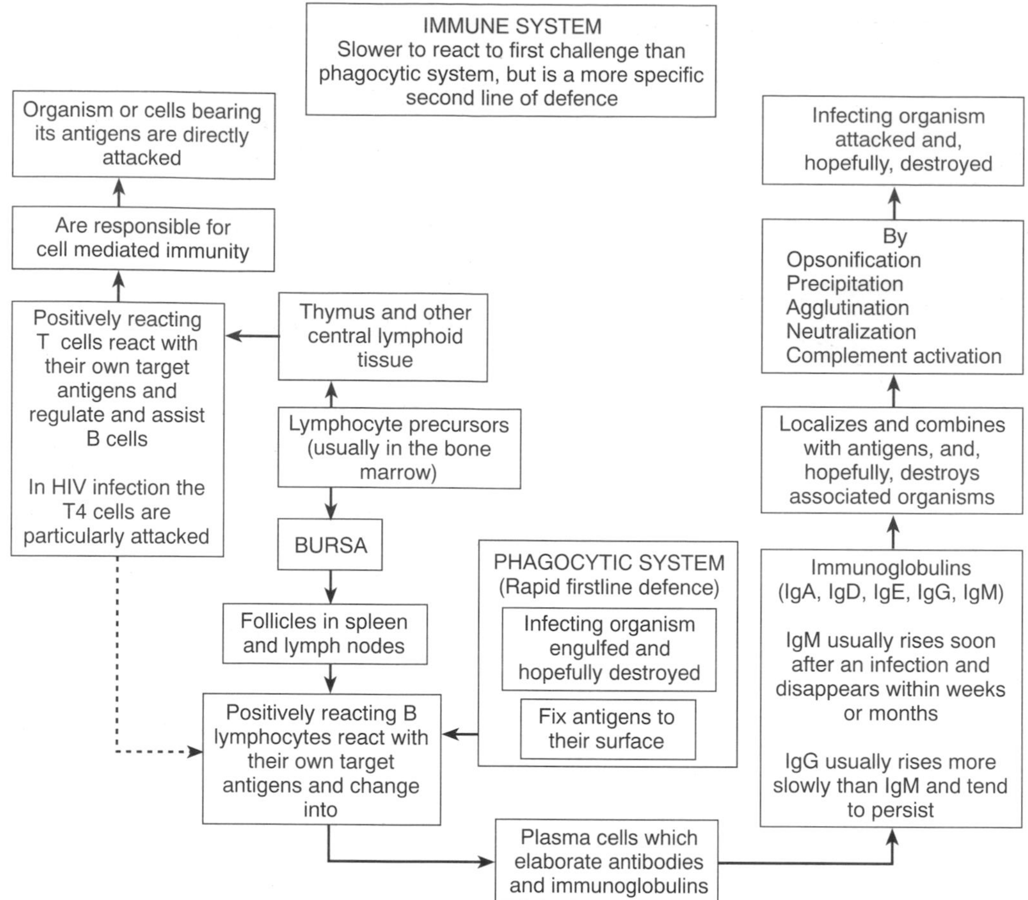

Fig. 1 The host's defences against infection or antigenic challenge: a simplified account.

their infection from medically administered blood or blood products.

Pathogenesis and immunological aspects

An understanding of the immune system is necessary in order to explain the pathogenesis of HIV/AIDS (Fig. 1).

Thymus derived (T) lymphocytes are responsible for cell mediated immunity which deals with host cells containing (intracellular) pathogens. HIV infection affects many host cells but particularly attacks T-lymphocytes so that, in AIDS, infections are often with obligate or facultative intracellular parasites. Certain lymphocytes (T4 or CD4 cells) have a number of surface proteins, including CD4, which act as receptors for HIV; these 'helper' cells are particularly damaged and decline in number and function, contributing to immunodeficiency.

Cell mediated immunity is also partially responsible for containing certain infections which persist after the initial infection. Such infections include all herpes viruses, herpes simplex, cytomegalovirus, and herpes varicella zoster and (of particular relevance in AIDS) mycobacteria and toxoplasmosis. Each may reactivate once immunodeficiency becomes significant. When the T4 or CD4 lymphocyte count falls below 200 cells/mm^3 the risk of developing an AIDS-defining opportunistic infection is high (some individuals with no CD4 cells remain well for several months, demonstrating that other host defence mechanisms must be operating). Malignancies are also a feature of late-stage HIV infection because cell mediated immunity is necessary to recognize and eliminate abnormal or malignant cells.

B-lymphocytes are polyclonally stimulated and produce large quantities of mostly ineffective immunoglobulins and the host may be unable to mount an adequate humoral response to challenge with specific organisms. Two consequences follow in late-stage HIV infection. Firstly, there is an increased incidence of infection with 'usual' organisms which attack opportunistically. Secondly, the production of abnormal immunoglobulins and/or failure of specific immunoglobulin responses interferes with diagnostic tests which depend on detection of organism-specific antibodies produced by the host. Thus, identification of organism-specific antibody in the HIV-positive patient confirms that the patient had been infected with that organism at some time but does not confirm that the patient's current symptoms were caused by that organism; organism specific IgM, if detected, might indicate a recent infection. Ideally, organisms must be seen or grown. Paradoxically, HIV-positive patients with hypergammaglobulinaemia benefit from high-dose intravenous immunoglobulin if they have recurrent infections.[5]

The clinical manifestations of most infections are partially or wholly produced by the host's defence mechanisms; if these are defective the clinical manifestations of infection may be non-specific or atypical. Unless infections can be completely eradicated

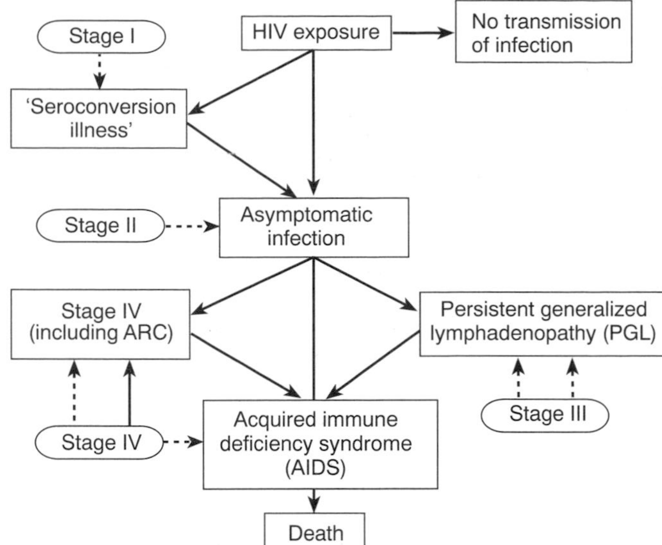

Fig. 2 The natural history of HIV infection and classification.

they will recur. Thus, after successful therapy continued prophylactic treatment may be essential.

Patients in late-stage AIDS often accumulate a variety of prophylactic therapies. To complicate matters further the abnormal immune system causes an increased incidence of drug allergy.[6]

Classification of HIV infection

Classification of HIV infection is essentially clinical and the most widely used system is that of the Center for Disease Control in Atlanta. There are four mutually exclusive stages, as shown in Fig. 2. Individuals do not necessarily ascend sequentially through all stages. Once an individual has ascended, descent is not possible; it is, thus, a hierarchical categorization except in Stage IV disease when it is possible to occupy more than one such stage.

Stage I is an illness developed by a proportion of those infected; at the time of seroconversion (usually about 6 weeks after infection), the illness resembles glandular fever with combinations of fever, lymphadenopathy, sweats, myalgia, rash, sore throat, and possibly meningitic or gastroenteritic features. Patients can be infectious prior to seroconversion and, thus, absence of HIV antibody does not exclude infectivity. Most patients then progress to asymptomatic Stage II; some patients may have asymptomatic low platelet count. Some patients develop Stage III illness (persistent generalized lymphadenopathy). Stage II and III patients are constitutionally well. In the vast majority of HIV-infected patients there is a slow decline in T4 cells. Eventually, patients develop Stage IV infection. Some Stage IV patients are ill but they have not developed relevant, AIDS-defining, opportunistic infections (see Appendix) or neoplasm, and are described clinically as having AIDS related complex (ARC). Stage IV infection is divided into five subsections—IVA (constitutional symptoms), IVB (neurological illness), IVC (secondary infections), IVD (secondary neoplasms), and IVE (certain other HIV-related conditions). Thus Stage IV includes patients with ARC or AIDS.

Stage I infection is marked by high levels of HIV production (and almost certainly high levels of infectivity), Stage II and III by smouldering low levels of HIV expression (and almost certainly lower but not absent infectivity), and Stage IV by an increase of viral replication. There is no stage of infection in which circulating virus is not present. All HIV-positive patients must be presumed to have infectious body fluids.

Progression from HIV infection to AIDS

The mechanisms which cause disease in HIV infection are unknown. Factors involved include genetic susceptibility, coinfection with other viruses, and age. Markers of faster progression including higher age at seroconversion, anaemia, CD4 lymphopenia (a count of less than 200 suggests that 50 per cent of patients will develop AIDS within 2 years), a rapidly falling CD4 count, high levels of serum IgA, immune thrombocytopenic purpura, HIV antigenaemia, and high levels of β_2-microglobulin.[7]

The proportion of HIV-infected patients who develop AIDS is 0 to 2 per cent after 2 years of infection, 5 to 10 per cent after 4 years, 10 to 25 per cent after 6 years, 30 to 40 per cent after 8 years, and 48 to 51 per cent after 10 years.[8,9] The median time for progression from seroconversion to AIDS is 11 years with about 8 per cent of a group of those infected with HIV developing AIDS each year.

Survival after AIDS

Approximately 50 per cent of patients survive 1 year after a diagnosis of AIDS,[10] about 25 per cent survive 2 years, about 5 per cent 3 to 4 years, and a handful survive more than 5 years.

Deciding the prognosis of individual AIDS patients is simultaneously difficult but important in determining the extent of investigatory and therapeutic intervention. An American study of AIDS patients[11] gave one point for each of the following:

severe diarrhoea or albumin level under 2 g/dl;

any neurological deficit;

arterial oxygen tension of 50 mm or less,

haematocrit below 30 per cent;

lymphocyte count below 150/mm^3;

white cell count below 2500/mm^3;

a platelet count below 140 000/mm^3.

Patients with no points had a median survival time of 11.6 months, patients with one point 5.1 months, and patients with two to seven points 2.1 months. No other analysed variable provided additional predictive power. This study covered the years 1981 to 1987 and therapeutic advances will have improved the quoted survival times.

The importance of the level of viral RNA in plasma (viral load) in determining both risk of progression and response to treatment has recently been reported. Blood samples that had been collected from 180 people with HIV in the mid-1980s were tested for viral load. Only 8 per cent of individuals with a viral load of less than 4350 copies progressed to AIDS within 5 years, compared with 62 per cent of people who had a viral load of over 36 270 copies. Also, only 5 per cent of those with a viral load of less than 4350 copies died within 5 years, compared with 49 per cent of people who started with a viral load of over 36 270 copies. A single viral load estimate was also superior to a single CD4 cell count in predicting disease progression; 50 per cent of those with viral loads over 10 900 copies per millilitre but a CD4 count greater than 500 cells/mm^3 died within 6 years compared with only 5 per cent of those with similar CD4 cell counts but viral loads less than 10 900 copies. Viral load also seems better at predicting the response to treatment than the CD4 cell count response. It is likely that this will become a standard virological assay in the near future.

Effect of risk group on presentation

Kaposi's sarcoma is commoner in homosexually acquired infection or from sexual contact with an individual with Kaposi's sarcoma. Cytomegalovirus infection, cryptosporidiosis, and Kaposi's sarcoma are all less common in injection drug users; tuberculosis, *Pneumocystis carinii* pneumonia, oesophageal candidiasis, and extrapulmonary cryptococcosis are more common.[10]

Treatment of HIV infection

There are a number of drugs that have an effect on HIV; none are viricidal. The first to be discovered, and as a consequence the best characterized drug, is zidovudine (also known as AZT, azidothymidine, or Retrovir®). Didanosine and zalcitabine are similar nucleoside analogues.

At present, anti-HIV therapy has, unequivocally, been shown to increase survival time for those with AIDS or near AIDS, to delay the onset of AIDS for those with symptoms or illness due to HIV, and to reduce the chances of HIV being passed to a child born to a mother infected with HIV.[12,13]

Zidovudine

The usual dosage of zidovudine is 250 mg twice daily or 200 mg three times daily. The chances of having a side-effect that prevents an individual from continuing with zidovudine increases with the progression of HIV. Nausea, vomiting, abdominal pain, headache, and muscle pains are common at the start of treatment but often improve or disappear with continued administration.[14,15]

A long-term side-effects of zidovudine, which may necessitate discontinuation and replacement with zalcitabine or didanosine, is myelosuppression, with 1 to 30 per cent of patients requiring transfusion and this increasing with advanced disease. Up to 10 per cent of patients develop neutropenia, myopathy, or myositis (as evidenced by muscle pain, tenderness, or a raised creatinine kinase). Rarely, abdominal pain, rashes, fever, insomnia, blue nail pigmentation, or abnormal liver function tests may occur. The manufacturer's literature recommends that zidovudine be discontinued if the neutrophil count falls to less than 0.7×10^9/l. If a patient has a favourable clinical and CD4 response to zidovudine then repeated blood transfusions (with cytomegalovirus negative blood for patients with no serological evidence of prior cytomegalovirus infection) may be justified rather than changing to zalcitabine or didanosine .

There are a number of important interactions. The use of long-term opioids doubles the effect of zidovudine so that these patients can be maintained on lower doses.[16] Variable phenytoin levels occur and blood levels should be measured. The use of zidovudine with ganciclovir (for cytomegalovirus infection) commonly produces haematological toxicity.[17] Zidovudine given with pyrimethamine, trimethoprim, interferon, cytotoxics, sulphonamides, flucytosine, dapsone, foscarnet, or amphotericin may also result in major myelosuppression. Coadministration of zidovudine and acyclovir has been reported to reduce mortality but the mechanism is uncertain.[18]

Zidovudine has no effect on cell-associated HIV for (at least) 4 weeks after treatment has commenced.[19] It is, therefore, probably not worth starting zidovudine if a patient is likely to die within the following few weeks. In most AIDS patients there comes a time to stop zidovudine when disadvantages outweigh benefits.

Two other drugs similar to zidovudine (didanosine and zalcitabine) have been shown to be of benefit in HIV infection.[20]

Didanosine (ddI, dideoxyinosine, or Videx®)

Didanosine has different side-effects to zidovudine; notably it does not cause anaemia. The recommended dose is 125 mg, 12 hourly, if the patient weighs less than 60 kg, or 200 mg, 12 hourly, if the patient weighs more than 60 kg. Didanosine needs to be chewed and taken on an empty stomach half an hour before eating. Diarrhoea is the commonest side-effect. Other side-effects include painful tingling of the hands or feet (neuropathy) and abdominal pain (which may be due to pancreatitis, especially if the dose is high). Its use with other potential pancreatitis-inducing agents (including intravenous pentamidine, high-dose sulphonamides, frusemide, tetracyclines, steroids, or thiazides) may precipitate pancreatitis. Didanosine should not be used with tetracyclines. Its use with drugs known to cause peripheral neuropathy (such as isoniazid, chloramphenicol, metronidazole, phenytoin, ribavirin, thalidomide, vinblastine, or vincristine) may precipitate neuropathy. Certain drugs (including ketoconazole, dapsone, itraconazole, trimethoprim, rifampicin, ciprofloxacin, or pyrimethamine) should be given 2 h before didanosine, otherwise impaired absorption of didanosine may occur. Didanosine may be given in combination with zidovudine to produce a more sustained CD4 cell count although the result of several studies on combination therapy are awaited.[21]

Zalcitabine (ddC, dideoxycytidine, or Hivid®)

Zalcitabine is effective for those who cannot tolerate zidovudine; it has similar side-effects to didanosine. Patients with ARC or AIDS who had received more than 48 weeks of zidovudine showed no clinical benefit from changing to zalcidabine.[22] The usual dose is 0.375 to 0.75 mg, three times daily. The major side-effects are peripheral neuropathy and pancreatitis. The neuropathy is sensorimotor in 20 to 25 per cent of instances and usually recovers slowly.

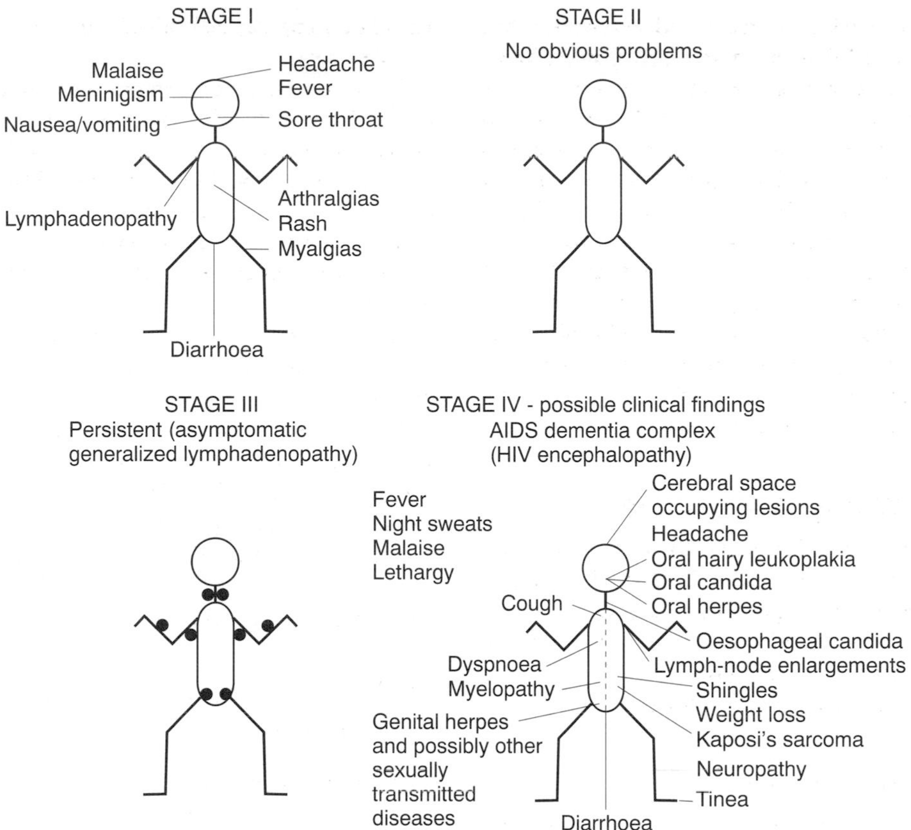

Fig. 3 Possible symptoms and signs of HIV infections.

Pancreatitis occurs in less than 1 per cent of patients. Interactions occur particularly with drugs associated with peripheral neuropathy or drugs associated with pancreatitis (e.g. didanosine). Contraindications include known peripheral neuropathy and abnormal liver function tests may be a relative contraindication.

Combination therapies

Two recent trials, one in Europe and the other in the United States (Delta and ACTG 175) have both shown that, for those who had never taken any zidovudine, taking two drugs (zidovudine/didanosine or zidovudine/zalcitabine) was better than zidovudine alone at slowing the loss of CD4 cells, delaying the onset of AIDS, and reducing further infections after the onset of AIDS, as well as increasing survival. For those already on zidovudine adding didanosine had some additional benefit. At present, for those already on zidovudine, the addition of a second drug or starting a completely new combination seems to be the best option. A number of ongoing clinical trials have shown that combinations of three drugs reduce the viral load for most individuals with HIV at whatever stage of infection.

At the time of writing several new drugs have been licensed which affect different targets in the HIV lifecycle: these include non-nucleoside reverse transcriptase inhibitors (which inhibit the change of HIV RNA into DNA) and protease inhibitors (which interfere with the formation of new viral particles). Each drug has particular indications and side-effects. By using combination therapy there is now the prospect of long-term suppression of HIV and further studies are awaited to reveal which combinations are appropriate at each stage of HIV disease.

Clinical manifestations of HIV and AIDS (Fig. 3 and Table 1)

The causes of HIV-related illnesses are drawn from a much wider spectrum than are the causes of illness in patients with normal immunity but it should not be forgotten that the patient, who may know little of the implications of immunology and opportunistic infection (which are major concerns for the doctors), might well perceive more benefit from simpler caring measures (massage for example) than from any technical intervention.

The three main presentations that enable a diagnosis of AIDS are *Pneumocystis carinii* pneumonia, Kaposi's sarcoma, or candida involving the oesophagus or bronchi. Other less common presentations include cryptococcal infection, tuberculosis, atypical mycobacterial infection, cytomegalovirus infection, recurrent *Herpes simplex* infection, cerebral toxoplasmosis, HIV encephalopathy, or non-Hodgkin's lymphoma. The presenting illnesses vary geographically; for example in the United Kingdom *Pneumocystis carinii* pneumonia is a less common presentation than in the United States but Kaposi's sarcoma is more common. In France, central nervous system toxoplasmosis is a very common presenting complaint. About 10 per cent of AIDS patients present with neurological problems. With advances in treatment and changes in behaviour, the pattern of AIDS defining illnesses will continue to change.

Table 1 The causes of HIV-related illness

Causative condition or organism	Syndrome or site of pathology												
	Skin lesions	Lymph node enlargement	Non-specific severe illness (PUO)	Retinitis	Encephalitis, myelopathy, encephalopathy	Meningitis, fits, cerebral abscess	Pneumonia without effusion	Pneumonia with effusion	Perianal lesions	Diarrhoea with/without malabsorption	Hepatitis, cholestasis	Dysphagia	Sore mouth, oral lesions
Pyogenic bacteria	?	?	P			?	P	P					?
Salmonellae			P							P			
Mycobacteria (typical or atypical)		M	P	?	?	P	P	M		P	?		
Nocardia asteroides							?	?					
CMV	?	?	M	M	?	?	?	?		P	?	P	?
Herpes simplex	P	?			?	?			P	?		P	P
Herpes varicella zoster	P		?		?		?						
HIV		M	P	?	M	?	?			P			
Molluscum contagiosum	P												
Candida albicans	?		?				?		?			M	M
Cryptococcus neoformans	?		P		?	M	?	?					
Cryptosporidiosis										M	?		
Isosporiasis										P			
P. carinii			P				M	?			?		
Toxoplasma gondii		?	?	?	P	M					?		
Kaposi's sarcoma	P	P	?				?	P	?	?		?	P
Lymphoma	?	P	?		?	?				?	?	?	

?, possible causes (not including extremely rare causes).
P, probable causes.
M, major causes.
PUO, pyrexia of unknown origin.
Certain infections (including amoebiasis, chlamydiasis, gonorrhoea, hepatitis B, and syphilis) are associated with various 'HIV at-risk' activities, rather than HIV itself and should be considered in differential diagnosis.

Haematological abnormalities of HIV and AIDS

Haematological abnormalities become more common as HIV progresses. About 93 per cent of AIDS patients are anaemic, about 12 per cent are leucopenic, about 20 per cent are neutropenic, and about 75 per cent are lymphopenic.

Anaemia

Anaemia in AIDS is almost always multifactorial in aetiology with inadequate diet, general debility, malabsorption, or gastrointestinal blood loss (from Kaposi's sarcoma for example) contributing. Drug treatment (notably with zidovudine and ganciclovir given together) may exacerbate HIV-induced anaemia as may treatment with long-term cotrimoxazole (which should be accompanied by folinic acid supplimentation). Transfusion may be required and indeed may be the price to be paid to allow necessary treatment to continue with zidovudine or ganciclovir.

Pancytopenia

Pancytopenia may be caused by bone marrow dysfunction induced by drugs, HIV infection, opportunistic infections (especially atypical mycobacterial infection), or infiltration (especially with lymphoma).

Thrombocytopenia

A form of idiopathic thrombocytopenic purpura, more properly described as HIV-related thrombocytopenia, is not uncommon, particularly early in the course of HIV infection. Patients seldom bleed with platelet counts over $20\times10^9/l$, and major haemorrhage is rare. In the absence of bleeding, non-intervention may be the best policy. Acute life-threatening bleeding is best managed by platelet transfusion and high dose immunoglobulin (0.5 mg/kg) although the latter is less useful when bone marrow failure is the cause. HIV-related thrombocytopenia is a chronic condition; platelet transfusions only provide short-lived protection and patients with recurrent symptoms may respond to steroids, gammaglobulin, danazol, interferon, or splenectomy. Zidovudine seems to have a beneficial effect.[23]

Lymph node enlargement

Uncomplicated and asymptomatic HIV infection may cause lymph node enlargement but other causes include Kaposi's sarcoma, lymphoma, and mycobacterial infections. Less common causes include pyogenic bacteria, cytomegalovirus, nocardia, herpes simplex, or toxoplasmosis. If the patient is plainly preterminal, diagnosis of lymph node enlargement is not essential—providing

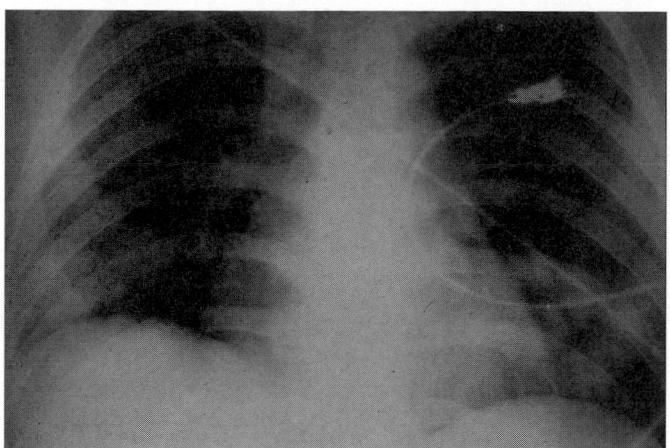

Fig. 4 *Pneumocystis carinii* pneumonia.

that the patient is not also coughing up *Mycobacterium tuberculosis* in his sputum.

Pneumonia

Pneumocystis carinii pneumonia (Fig. 4) is the initial presentation of AIDS in 60 per cent of patients overall and 85 per cent of patients develop *P. carinii* pneumonia at some stage.[24] *P. carinii* is a ubiquitous organism, it is a major cause of pneumonia (without effusion) in patients with AIDS, and may cause significant shortness of breath without any chest radiograph abnormalities.[25] *P. carinii* infection in AIDS is usually confined to the lungs with thickening of the alveolar basement membrane, and gas exchange is compromised. Common symptoms are progressive shortness of breath, weight loss, fever, and dry cough. The diagnosis can be made by taking samples of sputum (obtained by induced sputum, bronchoalveolar lavage, or lung biopsy) in which the organism can be identified by a variety of means.

Mycobacterium tuberculosis infection, although not a major cause of pneumonia, is of major importance because other people might become infected—in particular those who are HIV positive or who have AIDS. It is, thus, essential that *M. tuberculosis* should be excluded in all cases of HIV-related pneumonia.

One of the hidden 'expenses' of HIV is an increased incidence of pneumonia caused by 'standard' bacteria, usually *Haemophilus influenzae* or *Streptococcus pneumoniae*. Other HIV-related causes of pneumonia include cryptococci, cytomegalovirus, or nocardia, and less commonly herpes simplex or varicella zoster. Kaposi's sarcoma may predispose to infective pneumonias by obstructing bronchi or by infiltrating lung parenchyma.

Treatment of acute *Pneumocystis carinii* pneumonia

The mainstay of treatment is cotrimoxazole (sulphamethoxazole 100 mg/kg per day with trimethoprim 20 mg/kg) per day in divided doses intravenously. Usually, 1920 mg are given every 6 h, either orally or intravenously. If $Pa\text{O}_2$ is more than 10 kPa it is reasonable to try oral therapy; when $Pa\text{O}_2$ is less than 8 kPa, initial intravenous treatment is recommended. If $Pa\text{O}_2$ is less than 6 kPa, the addition of steroids (oral prednisolone 40–60 mg/day for 5 days, or equivalent intravenous doses of hydrocortisone/ methyl prednisolone) is recommended.[26–28] If the creatinine clearance is less than 25 ml/min then dose reduction of cotrimoxazole is required. The total treatment time is usually around 3 weeks.

Side-effects from cotrimoxazole occur in up to two-thirds of patients and include nausea, fever, tremor, rashes, diarrhoea, fever, abnormal liver function tests, thrombocytopenia, leucopenia, neutropenia, agranulocytosis, and haemolysis in glucose 6-phosphatase dehydrogenase deficient patients. Problems are more likely in combination with other myelosuppressive drugs (e.g. ganciclovir, zidovudine, and pyrimethamine).

Other possible treatment regimens include: daily continuous infusion of trimethoprim alone (in saline or 5 per cent dextrose) plus dapsone 100 mg, orally; and clindamycin 450 mg four times daily, orally or intravenously, together with primaquine 15 mg/day, orally. Atovaquone 250 mg, 8 hourly, is another option.

Intravenous pentamidine, 2 mg/kg over 6 h daily, for 2 to 3 days, followed by inhaled pentamidine, is another alternative. Side-effects are common, however, and include hypoglycaemia, hyperglycaemia, postural hypotension, neutropenia, nephrotoxicity, rash, hypocalcaemia, thrombophlebitis, cardiac arryhthmias, and pancreatitis. There are potential interactions with nephrotoxic agents.

Nebulized pentamidine isothianate 600 mg dissolved in 6 ml of sterile water (not saline) can be given via a nebulizer but is unsuitable for patients with any degree of hypoxia. Pretreatment with nebulized salbutamol or ipratropium in 4 ml of saline can prevent pentamidine-induced bronchospasm. The common side-effects include cough, bronchospasm, and hypersalivation.

Prophylaxis of *Pneumocystis carinii* pneumonia

Following an acute episode of *P. carinii* pneumonia, secondary prophylaxis is usually given with oral cotrimoxazole (480 mg/day), inhaled pentamidine (300 mg every 2–4 weeks), dapsone (100 mg/day), dapsone (100 mg) with pyrimethamine (25 mg twice per week), or sulphadoxine/ pyrimethamine one to two tablets per week. A number of trials[29–36] confirm the efficacy of prophylaxis and have clearly demonstrated the superiority of oral agents such as cotrimoxazole over inhaled pentamidine. If anti-*P. carinii* pneumonia treatment precipitates thrush, fluconazole can be added which also probably acts as prophylaxis against cryptococcal infection.[37]

Mycobacterial pneumonias

Mycobacterium tuberculosis pneumonias always have to be treated but if atypical mycobacterial organisms (including *Mycobacterium avium intracellulare*—MAI or MAC) are identified the need for treatment should be carefully considered; preterminal patients may not benefit because the response to treatment may be slow. Treatment of pulmonary *M. tuberculosis* is along standard lines but if infection is with an atypical mycobacterium, standard treatment will usually have to be modified depending on local sensitivity patterns, although some atypical infections respond to drugs to which they are insensitive *in vitro*.

Skin lesions

Kaposi's sarcoma

About 15 per cent of patients have Kaposi's sarcoma at diagnosis of AIDS and 8 per cent have Kaposi's sarcoma in addition to an opportunistic infection. Kaposi's sarcoma lesions are unusual in AIDS acquired by injection drug use and they may represent another sexually acquired infection (as outlined below). Kaposi's sarcoma lesions are usually brownish-purple, circular, papular lesions ranging from 0.5 to 1.0 cm in diameter; occasionally lesions may be larger or may become confluent. Kaposi's sarcoma must be assumed to be multiple at presentation, even if only one lesion is apparent, as internal organs (except, curiously, hardly ever the brain) may be involved. Vigorous 'curative' surgical attack on isolated lesions is inappropriate because Kaposi's sarcoma is rarely life-threatening and because most patients with Kaposi's sarcoma die from opportunistic infections. Kaposi's sarcoma on exposed parts of the body may cause severe embarrassment and lesions in the gut, in the bronchi, or blocking lymphatic drainage may cause problems.

Treatment can be given with cosmetic camouflage, radiotherapy, injecting the lesions, or freezing with liquid nitrogen. A number of options are possible for small lesions (less than 1 cm diameter): liquid nitrogen can by applied by cotton wool applicator until a halo of erythema is observed or direct injection of dilute vinblastine (0.2 mg/ml, usually less than 0.5 ml) may be given into the centre of a lesion. Local radiotherapy usually produces a rapid involution of lesions but treatment of intraoral lesions is problematical as the normal oral mucosa is particularly sensitive to radiation.

Systemic drugs may be used for multiple or symptomatic lesions: vincristine 2 mg, intravenously (given slowly); bleomycin 30 mg in 1 litre of normal saline over 12 to 24 h (limit lifetime total dose to less than 150 mg to reduce the risks of pulmonary fibrosis); or adriamycin intravenously, every 2 weeks (15 mg/m^2 or 10–30 mg total dose)

Combination treatment with adriamycin 20 mg/m^2 plus bleomycin 10 mg/m^2 and vincristine 1.4 mg/m^2 is also possible but toxicity is common. If a patient has peripheral neuropathy, it is advisable to replace vincristine with vinblastine. Treatment is given intravenously every 2 weeks with monitoring for cardiac, pulmonary, and neurological toxicities. Interferon treatment for Kaposi's sarcoma is reserved for those patients with well preserved immunity (CD4 count of more than 350 cells/mm^3). Liposomal daunorubicin (Daunoxome®) 40 mg/m^2 intravenously in 5 per cent dextrose every 2 weeks) is a promising new therapy with reduced side-effects. A viral cause for Kaposi's sarcoma has recently been proposed (herpes simplex virus type 8) and this may well have implications for future treatment regimens.

Herpes simplex

Herpes simplex (notably genital herpes) may be a recurrent problem. Herpes in AIDS, unlike the usual herpes in the immunocompetent, may present as areas of mild or severe ulceration.

Acyclovir 200 mg orally, five times daily for 5 days, or intravenously 5 mg/kg eight hourly, is usually effective but if a recurrence occurs, follow-on prophylaxis is required. Usually, the therapeutic dosage can be slowly reduced until a minor breakthrough occurs with subsequent return to the previous dosage. If prophylaxis is required it should be continued until death to prevent recurrences. Topical acyclovir has little or no role to play in HIV-associated herpes.

Shingles

Herpes varicella zoster infection, presenting as shingles, is not common in AIDS (it usually antedates development of the full-blown AIDS syndrome by 18 months or so). Shingles should be treated with acyclovir 800 mg orally, five times daily, for 7 days (or intravenously 10 mg/kg for severe zoster). Shingles may occur early and require treatment similar to that of a non-immunocompromised person, or late when more aggressive therapy is needed. In late-stage HIV infection, shingles may be multidermatomal and may occur on non-contiguous nerve root areas. Follow-on prophylaxis is not usually indicated but persistent or recurrent lesions may occur in late-stage disease.

Eosinophilic pustular folliculitis

Eosinophilic pustular folliculitis comprises sterile pruritic papules and pustules on the face, trunk, and extremities; the lesions may coalesce to form plaques with a tendency to central clearing, they may spontaneously remit, and may be accompanied by leukocytosis, eosinophilia, or both. Treatment is possible with ultraviolet light.[38]

Molluscum contagiosum

Molluscum contagiosum is a poxvirus infection producing umbilicated waxy papules, usually most prominent on the face. Although harmless they may cause much distress. Treatment is either with liquid nitrogen applied with a cotton wool bud, or with phenol applied with the tip of an orange stick.

Scabies

In the immunocompromised extensive scabies may result—so-called Norwegian scabies—in which there is spread outside the classical areas. Such patients are very contagious. Treatment is along standard lines but repeated courses may be necessary. Scabies should be considered as a diagnostic possibility in all itchy rashes as early action is required to prevent potentially rapid spread to other patients.

Seborrhoea

Seborrhoeic dermatitis is very common in AIDS and causes dry, flaky, eventually red, skin. It classically starts around the nose, behind the ears, and in the perineum. Topical agents such as ketoconazole cream and shampoo (plus or minus steroids) are often effective but may need to be given repeatedly. In severe cases, orally administered treatment may be indicated.

Other causes of skin lesions include pyogenic bacteria, cytomegalovirus infection, candida, cryptococci, and lymphoma. Psoriasis may appear to worsen with immunodeficiency.

Retinitis

Blindness is generally worth preventing even in a preterminal state although occasional patients are willing to risk blindness if the treatment becomes particularly difficult. Because the appearances of any infective process are dependent on the host responses (which are always abnormal in AIDS), retinal appearances may not be characteristic of any one disease process and diagnosis may have to rest upon serological tests or organism culture from other sites. An expert ophthalmological opinion is essential in any patient with retinal abnormalities.

'Cotton-wool' spots of uncertain aetiology may appear transiently in AIDS but should be monitored closely. HIV itself may produce small waxy exudates and microaneurysms, and haemorrhages may be seen.

Cytomegalovirus is the commonest cause of visual problems and may cause a 'bushfire, ketchup, and cottage cheese' retinal appearance—perivascular waxy exudates ('cottage cheese'), often with surrounding haemorrhage ('ketchup'), with activity round the edge but less so in the centre ('bush fire'). If untreated, bilateral lesions would develop in about 60 per cent of patients. Probably all patients with cytomegalovirus retinitis should receive urgent therapeutic, and then prophylactic, treatment. Cytomegalovirus retinitis can progress so rapidly that a 'wait and see' approach by doctors may lose the patient his or her ability to see.

Ganciclovir is the traditional treatment for cytomegalovirus, given initially in a dose of 10 mg/kg per day in two divided doses as a 1 h infusion in dextrose or saline, for 2 to 3 weeks, followed by maintenance therapy in a daily dose of 5 mg/kg per day, 7 days a week (or 6 mg/kg per day for 5 days). If the serum creatinine is more than 125 mmol/l, dose reduction is required.

Ganciclovir is myelotoxic and there is a need for frequent full blood counts (especially if the patients is also on zidovudine) to detect neutropenia, thrombocytopenia, or anaemia. Ganciclovir is both mutagenic and teratogenic and thus effective contraception for both men and women should be advised. If myelosuppression occurs, folinic acid can be given but often discontinuation of ganciclovir or drugs being given at the same time (e.g. zidovudine) may be required. Erythropoetin and granulocyte colony stimulating factor may have a role to allow treatment to continue.

Foscarnet (phosphonoformic acid/ Foscavir®) can be used to replace ganciclovir for resistant cytomegalovirus or herpes simplex infections. It is available in 250 ml and 500 ml bottles containing 24 mg/ml of foscarnet and 124 mmol sodium. It should, preferably, be administered undiluted into a central line to avoid peripheral vein thrombophlebitis. Side-effects include hypocalcaemia (the most important clinical problem), hypomagnesaemia, nephrotoxicity, hypercalcaemia, hypokalaemia, hypo- or hyperphosphataemia, headaches, nausea, fatigue, rash, convulsions, genital ulcerations, or anaemia. Drug interactions may occur with other nephrotoxic drugs. Before administration, patients should receive prehydration of at least 1 litre normal saline, infused over 6 h or overnight. The induction course is usually for at least 2 to 3 weeks. The usual treatment dose for those with normal renal function is 180 to 200 mg/kg daily. Usually, a single infusion over 4 to 6 h, with at least 1 litre of fluid, is given either orally or intravenously. An initial test dose of 20 mg/kg over 30 min should be infused. Foscarnet infusions should be discontinued if renal function is deteriorating or creatinine clearance drops below 25 ml/min. The maintenance dose of foscarnet is as a single daily dose of 90 to 120 mg/kg, ensuring adequate hydration as mentioned above.

P. carinii may produce multiple exudates with minimal evidence of inflammation, usually in patients who have underlying *P. carinii* pneumonia. Herpes simplex or zoster may cause retinal necrosis. Toxoplasmosis may produce areas of retinal necrosis but haemorrhages are unusual. Other causes of retinitis include mycobacterial infection and fungi. Candida may produce yellowish-white exudates with indistinct borders; retinal haemorrhages are not a feature and there may be an intense vitreous reaction.

Central nervous system

Meningitis

Cryptococcus neoformans, a fungus, is the most common cause of meningitis in patients with AIDS; the onset may be insidious with vague headache and fever, and meningitic signs then develop. Diagnosis is confirmed by lumbar puncture, with specific staining of the cerebrospinal fluid and detection of cryptococcal antigen. Treatment is with intravenous amphotericin B, either alone or with flucytosine. Fluconazole also has an important role, particularly for mild cases and for continuing prophylaxis after initial treatment of the acute episode.[39]

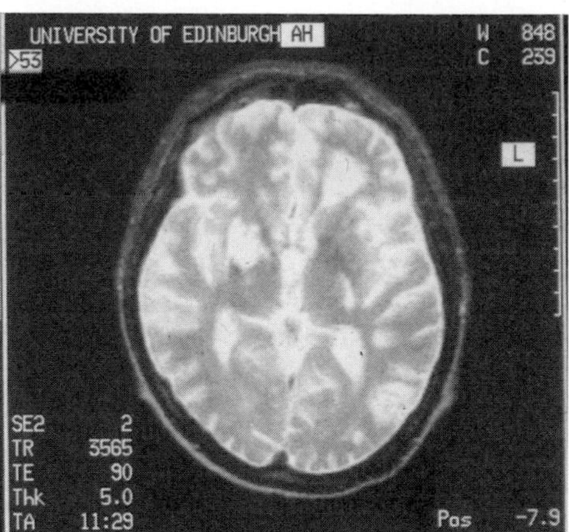

Fig. 5 Cerebral toxoplasmosis.

Space occupying lesions

Toxoplasmosis is a major cause of cerebral space occupying lesions (in some series up to about 30 per cent of AIDS patients have had cerebral toxoplasmosis); there may be suggestive fundal appearances but computerized axial tomography (**CT**) scanning or magnetic resonance imaging (**MRI**) may be required. Cerebral toxoplasmosis (Fig. 5) usually presents with headache, fever, and/or focal neurological symptoms such as stroke or visual disturbance.

The initial treatment is with intravenous sulphadiazine 1 g in 500 ml saline every 6 h, plus pyrimethamine 50 mg orally every 6 h for the first 24 h, followed by pyrimethamine 50 mg/day and folinic acid 15 mg/day orally.[40] Intravenous sulphadiazine can be changed to oral sulphadiazine once the patient feels better and the focal signs disappear. If there is any evidence of cerebral oedema, dexamethasone (usually 4 mg six hourly, initially) should be considered. Alternative therapies include replacing sulphadiazine with dapsone 100 mg/day or clindamycin 600 mg six hourly. Maintenance therapy commences after at least 4 weeks of primary treatment, with pyrimethamine 25 to 50 mg and sulphadiazine 2 to 4 g/day. Alternative maintenance regimens include fansidar one tablet daily or dapsone 100 mg/day plus pyrimethamine 25 mg/day. Side-effects of such regimens are common and include pancytopenia (folinic acid 15 mg/day may be useful), nausea and vomiting, diarrhoea, rash, fever, nephritis, and haemorrhagic cystitis.

Primary central nervous system lymphoma (Fig. 6) is the major non-infective cause of a cerebral space occupying lesion, occurring in about 5 per cent of AIDS patients. Prognosis is poor (usually months) even with therapy. The diagnosis may be suggested by progression of lesions on **CT** scan despite adequate antitoxoplasma therapy. Brain biopsy may be useful, particularly for those patients that wish to avoid toxic drug combinations in the last few months of life.

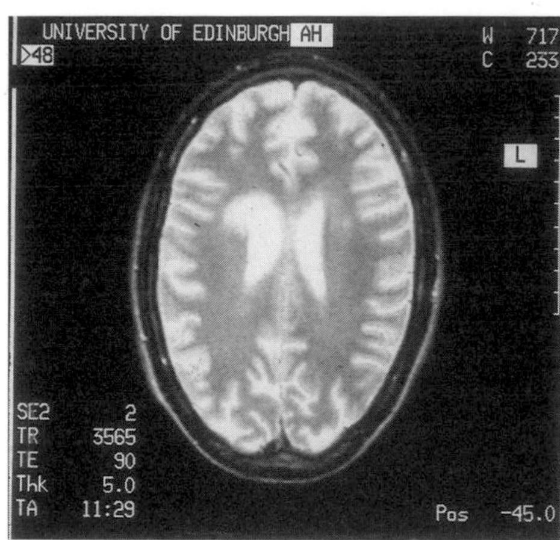

Fig. 6 Cerebral lymphoma.

Seizures

Seizures should be treated along conventional lines. In preterminal patients, further investigations of meningitis, seizures, or cerebral abscess may not be indicated. Seizures, particularly if non-focal, may be drug-related, including the withdrawal of psychoactive drugs. Seizures may be a manifestation of cerebral space occupying lesions. A decision has to be made as to whether to investigate (CT scan first, followed by lumbar puncture) or to treat symptomatically. If a patient has seizures or meningitis with no suspicion of a space occupying lesion, a lumbar puncture is necessary to exclude or confirm meningitis. A counsel of perfection is that a CT scan should precede lumbar puncture to avoid the risk of precipitating coning caused by unsuspected space occupying lesions. Exclusion of syphilis may require lumbar puncture for diagnosis.[41]

HIV encephalopathy and AIDS dementia complex

The price for longer survival conferred by prophylactic treatment for opportunistic infections may be an increased incidence of other manifestations of HIV, including progressive AIDS dementia complex which occurs in around 20 per cent of patients with AIDS and an annual incidence after AIDS diagnosis of 7 per cent.[42] An increasing number of patients will survive to develop dementia with prevention of opportunistic infections.

Cognitive function (memory, attention, visiospacial ability) is impaired. Early symptoms are forgetfulness, poor concentration, clumsiness, ataxia, generalized slowing, problems with sequences, social withdrawal, or disinhibition. AIDS dementia complex patients may be abnormally sensitive to psychoactive drugs. A vacuolar myelopathy may also develop which presents as a progressive spastic paraplegia with bladder dysfunction.

The differential diagnosis of AIDS dementia complex includes treatable infections such as cryptococcal infection, mycobacterial infection, cytomegalovirus, herpes simplex infection, and cerebral lymphoma. In all these situations (with the exception of those with coincidental pulmonary *M. tuberculosis* infection), if the patient is preterminal it may be kinder not to treat but concentrate on symptom relief. Neurophysiological tests for AIDS dementia complex are available which quantify brain function impairment. CT scans may reveal cerebral atrophy but MRI is required to identify early encephalitis. Treatment with zidovudine delays the onset of dementia and in some patients with established dementia there is clinical improvement (Goodwin, *et al.*, in press).[43] Patients whose AIDS dementia complex has responded to zidovudine may wish to continue with treatment until death.

Progressive multifocal leukoencephalopathy

Progressive multifocal leukoencephalopathy is a demyelinating condition due to infection by a papovavirus. Patients may have headache, ataxia, hemiparesis, and mental changes. CT scans and MRI may be suggestive but definitive diagnosis may require a brain biopsy. There is no effective treatment and the prognosis is very poor.

Peripheral nerve problems

HIV may cause peripheral nerve dysfunction in 20 to 40 per cent of patients with AIDS but symptoms may develop at any stage of HIV infection. A distal, mostly sensory, neuropathy is the most common abnormality and persisting pain may be a considerable problem.[44]

Myopathy

HIV may cause a myositis which clinically may overlap with zidovudine-induced myopathy.[45] Other problems include a chronic inflammatory demyelinating polyneuropathy (which may antedate other signs of HIV infection) and Guillain–Barré syndrome. Neuropathy may also be a drug side-effect or related to cytomegalovirus infection.

Gastrointestinal problems

Anal and perianal lesions

Herpes simplex, gonococcal, syphilitic, and chlamydial infections should be excluded, particularly in the homosexual population. Herpes simplex usually presents with ulcerative lesions. Anal warts may be florid but cause relatively few symptoms. Candida and Kaposi's sarcoma are other HIV-related possibilities. Defecation may be painful whatever the aetiology and topical lignocaine and faecal softening agents may be required until specific therapy is effective.

Diarrhoea

Diarrhoea may be a major problem in AIDS and eradication of causative infections may be impossible. Non-AIDS pathogens should be sought but an infective aetiology for diarrhoea may not be found and AIDS-related infections should be excluded. Empirical treatment may have to be given. Salmonella infections may persist despite treatment but an appropriate antibiotic is usually given to protect the patient from extraintestinal spread and in an attempt to reduce their infectivity. Always exclude faecal impaction in patients on opioids or other constipating drugs.

Cryptosporidiosis is found in about one-third of AIDS patients with persistent diarrhoea.[46] Cryptosporidiosis is a water-borne protozoan infection which may cause a profuse, continual watery diarrhoea in AIDS with marked fluid or electrolyte loss or malabsorption. Treatment is disappointing but successes have been reported using paromomycin. Other protozoal organisms have to be excluded including *Isospora belli* (which may respond initially to cotrimoxazole), *Entamoeba histolytica*, or *Giardia lamblia*.

Cytomegalovirus colitis gives rise to classical large bowel type diarrhoea with frequent small amounts of stool. Diagnosis is important because treatment is available which may result in symptomatic improvement. The diagnosis is usually made on the histology of biopsy specimens but positive stool, throat, blood, or urine cultures with supportive serological evidence in a patient with diarrhoea or abdominal pain would provide strong support for a trial of ganciclovir.

Mycobacterial enteritis or colitis is usually caused by *Mycobacterium avium intracellulare*, but *Mycobacterium tuberculosis* is also a possibility. Either may cause diarrhoea, weight loss, abdominal pain, and high fever.

All diarrhoeal stools should be submitted for culture of standard enteropathogenic bacteria, mycobacteria, fungi, and viruses plus microscopy for protozoa. If results are negative, then sigmoidoscopy and biopsy should be performed with microscopy and culture of the biopsy (for cytomegalovirus and *Mycobacterium tuberculosis*) and histological examination of abnormal areas to exclude Kaposi's sarcoma or lymphoma. If all studies are negative then a trial of ciprofloxacin or metronidazole may be appropriate but if symptoms persist consider the possibility that HIV, which might respond to zidovudine, may be the cause.

During investigations of chronic diarrhoea codeine phosphate (initially 30–60 mg four times daily) or loperamide (initially 2–4 mg four times daily) should be tried. In terminal AIDS, intractable diarrhoea may respond to oral morphine or subcutaneous diamorphine. Some success has occurred with octreotide (a somatostatin analogue) but the need for parenteral administration is a disadvantage. In our experience, symptoms in the majority of patients are controlled by oral morphine.

Hepatitis and cholestasis

Many drugs used in AIDS (including zidovudine, ganciclovir, foscarnet, and most antituberculous drugs) have hepatic dysfunction as a possible side-effect. The major infective causes of hepatitis, include hepatitis A, B, or C, cytomegalovirus, or toxoplasmosis. Occasionally *Pneumocystis carinii* or mycobacteria may be responsible and lymphomas may infiltrate the liver. In preterminal AIDS, it may be appropriate not to investigate patients with asymptomatic hepatitis. Interferon therapy for both chronic hepatitis B or C is disappointing in HIV-positive patients. Successful therapy is more likely to occur in those with preserved immunity.

Oral hairy leukoplakia

These are asymptomatic whitish, vertical fissures on the side of the tongue which were thought to be specific to HIV but are now recognized as features of advanced immunosuppression.

Sore mouth or oral lesions (see Chapter 9.10)

Candida albicans is the most common cause of sore mouths or oral lesions in AIDS, but cytomegalovirus or toxoplasmosis may cause a mild sore throat. Trivial oral candida may be treated with nystatin solution (100 000 IU), nystatin pastilles six hourly, or amphotericin lozenges 10 mg six hourly either singularly or alternating. Higher and/or more frequent administration is often required but is often poorly tolerated by patients because of lack of efficacy. If patients are intolerant or efficacy declines, systemic therapy is required with fluconazole 50 to 100 mg/day for 3 to 5 days or 350 to 400 mg as a single dose, which may need to be repeated. It may be necessary to use higher doses. Side-effects of fluconazole include nausea, abdominal discomfort, diarrhoea, and flatulence and rarely rash and urticaria. Important interactions include potentiation of anticoagulants, increase in the half-life of oral hypoglycaemic agents, and increases in phenytoin levels. Alternative therapies include oral ketoconazole, itraconazole, clotrimazole pessaries (given orally), or occasionally intravenous amphotericin (starting at a dose of 0.25 mg/kg per day rising to 0.5 mg/kg per day).

If there is no response to the anticandida therapy the patient may either have resistant candida or have atypical herpes simplex infection. Herpes simplex causes clusters of vesicles but intraoral vesicles invariably break down to leave shallow ulcers, which may be confluent. Kaposi's sarcoma may be found intraorally; most are asymptomatic but occasionally lesions in and around the gums cause dental pain. Aphthous ulcers may be troublesome and usually respond to topical steroids but for persistent or recurrent lesions, provided there is no risk of pregnancy, thalidomide 50 to100 mg can be given at night (to minimize daytime drowsiness). Other causes of sore mouth include severe gum recession or periodontitis and gingivitis; these may respond to metronidazole 400 mg eight hourly or penicillin V 500 mg six hourly, in addition to dental hygiene and antiseptic mouth washes.

Dysphagia (see Chapter 9.3.2)

Dysphagia may be caused by pain (which usually has an inflammatory or infective aetiology and is commonly treatable by simple measures) or by obstruction, which implies a space occupying lesion and may be less easily treated.

Candida albicans is the classical cause of painful dysphagia. Patients with oesophageal candida (an AIDS defining diagnosis) almost always have oral candida. A barium swallow may be diagnostic, showing a lace-like pattern of barium (Fig. 7). Treatment with nystatin pastilles or amphotericin B lozenges is often effective in mild oral candidiasis, but fluconazole or itraconazole are usually required for initial treatment of oesophageal candida. Intravenous amphotericin, (perhaps with flucytosine) may be necessary for severe or resistant candida.

Cytomegalovirus infection, herpes simplex infection, Kaposi's sarcoma, or lymphoma may also cause dysphagia and endoscopy with biopsy and culture may be required for a definitive diagnosis. Investigation must precede treatment even in preterminal AIDS so that effective treatment can be given.

Non-specific severe illness

In preterminal AIDS, a decision has to be made either to pursue a diagnosis (or diagnoses) or to treat symptomatically. In either case the presence of transmissible, opportunistic infections should be excluded. Cytomegalovirus may cause severe illness with few focal manifestations (fundoscopy, even in patients with no ocular symptoms, might provide diagnostic clues). Disseminated opportunistic infections which may present without obvious focal manifestations include 'standard' pyogenic bacteria, salmonella, mycobacteria (typical or atypical), cryptococcal infection, candida, toxoplasmosis, pulmonary *Pneumocystis carinii* infection, and herpes simplex. Other causes of non-specific severe illness include Kaposi's sarcoma in certain anatomical situations and lymphoma.

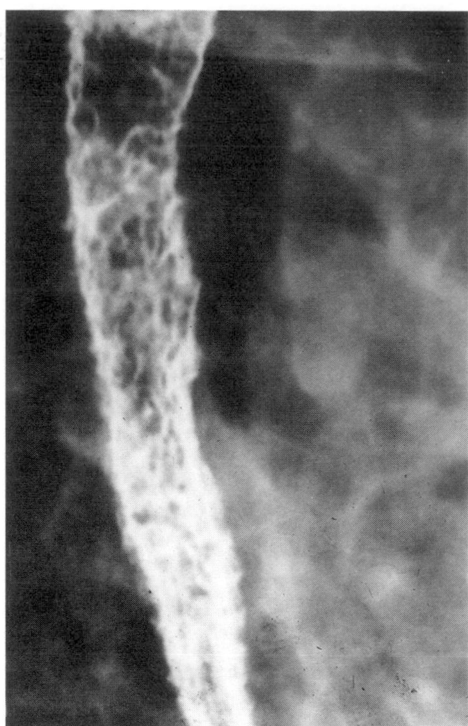

Fig. 7 Oesophageal candida.

Colonization with atypical mycobacteria may occur at sites such as the respiratory and gastrointestinal tracts but isolation from blood or other sterile sites indicates invasive infection. *Mycobacterium avium intracellulare* tends to occur late in AIDS, often when the CD4 count is less than 50 cells/mm^3. Treatment for *Mycobacterium avium intracellulare* is usually difficult because the majority of strains are resistant to conventional chemotherapy. Combination therapy is the rule; drugs to be considered include ethambutol, clarithromycin, ciprofloxacin, rifabutin, pyrazinamide, and amikacin.

Non-specific loss of weight

This is a common manifestation of endstage disease; in Africa, AIDS is known as slim disease. Opportunistic infections or complicating neoplasia should be excluded. Advice from a dietitian is important, especially if nasogastric tube feeding has to be used. Pressure sores must be anticipated and prevented, if weight loss and debility are profound.

If nausea and vomiting are a problem, all drugs that may cause nausea and vomiting should be given after meals and/or antiemetics given 1 h before meals. In terminally ill patients, opioids, cyclizine, haloperiodol, methotrimeprazine, or metoclopramide can be given via a syringe driver. Appetite stimulants, such as megestrol[47] and corticosteroids, may produce a transient increase in appetite, well being, and weight (see Chapter 9.4).

Neoplasms in AIDS

Forty per cent of AIDS patients develop a neoplasm at some stage. Kaposi's sarcoma has been mentioned previously but other neoplasms also occur. Non-Hodgkin's lymphoma develops in up to 10 per cent of patients with AIDS and, unlike classical lymphoma, often develops in sites other than lymph nodes, including the central nervous system, bone marrow, gastrointestinal tract, or liver. Disease is often advanced and disseminated at presentation even if seemingly localized to one site. Treatment, except to relieve symptoms, may be inappropriate as the prognosis is so poor, with or without treatment.

Other neoplasms that may be associated with HIV infection[48] include hepatoma, germ cell tumours, Hodgkin's disease, urinary tract tumours, and acute lymphoblastic leukaemia. Classical treatment rules for tumours—elimination of every malignant cell, toxicity being a reasonable price to pay for cure, the need for complete rather than partial response to treatment, and the need for cure rather than palliation—are not applicable because of the poor prognosis of AIDS patients as a result of the underlying immunosuppression.

Other specific organ failures

Renal impairment, in particular an HIV-related nephropathy with heavy proteinuria, biochemical features of the nephrotic syndrome, and rapid progressive renal failure, is well recognized.[49] Dialysis can be undertaken if clinically indicated.

Treatment and investigations

Tables 2 and 3 detail investigation of illness in HIV infection and Table 4 details the treatment of infection in HIV.

Women and HIV

Pregnancy

The majority of HIV-infected women are of reproductive age and would often have one or two children during the time they are infected. In Scotland, 86 per cent of HIV-infected women are in the 15 to 44 age group. In the Edinburgh cohort there is no evidence that pregnancy in symptomatic women hastens immunological decline.

The chances of having a baby infected *in utero* are probably partially dependent on the stage of the infection in the mother,[50] and ranges from around 13 to 50 per cent of babies. Caesarean section reduces transmission of HIV to the fetus[51] as may administration of zidovudine to mother and child.[52,53] Nearly all babies will have received maternally derived antibody whilst *in utero* and thus will be HIV antibody positive after birth. Parents have to wait 6 months, or occasionally longer, to discover if their baby clears this antibody (and are thus presumably not infected). Specialized methods, other than antibody measurements, including viral culture, exist to determine whether infection has occurred. Some babies are persistently seronegative but HIV can be cultured.[54]

The appropriate use of prophylaxis against opportunistic infections may be necessary. Cotrimoxazole may give rise to problems (particularly kernicterus in the neonate) in late pregnancy. There is little experience of pregnancy with other agents commonly used in the treatment of AIDS related conditions such as cytomegalovirus

Table 2 Investigation of illness in HIV infection

Suggested investigations	Syndrome or site of pathology											
	Sore mouth, oral lesions	Dysphagia	Hepatitis, cholestasis	Diarrhoea with/ without malab-sorption	Perianal lesions	Pneumonia with effusion	Pneumonia without effusion	Meningitis, fits, cerebral abscess	Encephalitis, myelopathy, encephalo-pathy	Retinitis	Non-specific severe illness (PUO)	Lymph node enlarge-ment	Skin lesions
Respiratory													
Chest radiography		Usual				Almost always	Almost always	Usual	Usual	Consider	Almost always	Usual	
Induced sputum						Consider	Consider				Consider		
Blood gases and lung function tests						Usual (first)	Usual (first)				Consider		
Bronchoscopy with bronchoalveolar lavage						Usual (second)	Usual (second)				Consider		
Transbronchial lung biopsy						Consider	Consider				Consider		
Central nervous system													
CT								Almost always (first)	Almost always (first)		Consider	Consider	
Lumbar puncture								Almost always (second)	Almost always (second)		Consider		
EEG								Consider	Consider		Consider		
Gastrointestinal													
Barium contrast studies, ?endoscopy		Almost always		Consider									
General													
Blood culture			Almost always (BMFV)	Consider		Almost always (BMV)	Almost always (BMV)	Almost always (BMFV)	Almost always (BMFV)	Almost always (MV)	Almost always (BMFV)		
Blood for serological testing			Almost always (TV)			Usual	Usual	Usual	Usual	Usual	Usual	Usual	
Bone marrow											Consider	Consider	
Lesion biopsy	Consider	Consider	Consider	Usual	Consider	Consider	Consider	Consider	Consider		Consider	Consider	Almost always
Lesion culture	Almost always (BFV)	Consider (FV)	Consider	Almost always	Usual (V)	Almost always (BFMPV)	Almost always (BFMPV)	Almost always (BFMTV)	Consider (BMTV)		Consider	Almost always (BMTV)	Usual (BMV)
Lymph node biopsy											Consider	Almost always	
Stool			Almost always (MP)	Almost always (BFMPV)	Usual (BMV)								

B, bacteria; M, mycobacteria; F, fungi; V, viruses; P, protozoa; T, toxoplasmosis; PUO, pyrexia of unknown origin.

or atypical mycobacteria. Zidovudine given in the last two trimesters reduces the infection rate of the unborn.[56]

Breast feeding should be discouraged because HIV may be persistently present in breast milk.[55]

Gender

Gender has not emerged as a significant factor in HIV progression.[57] Women are less likely to present with *Pneumocystis carinii* pneumonia as the AIDS defining illness and significantly more women than men suffer from oesophageal candidiasis, atypical mycobacteria, and the wasting syndrome.[58] Most of such reports come from the United States, where clinical presentations may be affected by the time of presentation and access to medical care. In Edinburgh, there does not appear to be a particular spectrum of clinical HIV disease occurring in women. In a retrospective survey of 612 HIV-related admissions, there was no excess of female admissions except for detoxification, investigation of loss of consciousness, or urinary tract infections.[59]

Survival of women after AIDS diagnosis

Following a diagnosis of AIDS about 50 per cent of patients survive 1 year. Early reports suggested that HIV-infected women had a reduced survival but this is most probably related to poorer access to medical services rather than gender.[60–62] Where there is good access to medical care women have a similar prognosis.[63] Genital herpes, candidiasis, and pelvic inflammatory disease are more common, more aggressive, and more often recurrent in HIV-positive women. Women were less likely to present with Kaposi's

Table 3 Investigation of illness in HIV infection

Suggested investigations	Request	Comments
Respiratory		
Chest radiography		Normal chest radiography does not exclude significant pathology, particularly pneumocystis infection
Induced sputum	Microscopy for pneumocystis; microscopy and culture for bacteria, mycobacteria, fungi viruses	Sputum production induced by nebulized hypertonic saline
Blood gases and lung function tests	P_{O_2} and P_{CO_2} (low CO transfer factor may suggest pneumocystis infection)	O_2 desaturation may be an early marker of pneumocystis infection
Bronchoscopy with bronchoalveolor lavage	Microscopy for pneumocystis; microscopy and culture for bacteria, mycobacteria, fungi, viruses	
Transbronchial lung biopsy	Histology, microscopy, and culture for bacteria, mycobacteria, fungi, viruses	Risks increased if patient is very dyspnoeic or has a low platelet count
Central nervous system		
Computed tomography (CT)		Focal ring enhancement suggests toxoplasma or lymphoma; atrophy suggests HIV encephalopathy
Lumbar puncture	Microscopy for cell count; microscopy and culture for bacteria, mycobacteria, fungi, viruses	Also obtain cerebrospinal fluid glucose and protein; do CT scan of brain first; ask for cryptococcal antigen
EEG		
Gastrointestinal		
Barium contrast studies; ? endoscopy		
General		
Blood culture	Bacteria; ? mycobacteria, fungi, viruses	At least two sets initially
Blood for serological testing	'Viral' titres and save serum; ? HIV serology; ? hepatitis B; ? syphilis serology	Anticipated serological responses may be absent in HIV infection; ask for cryptococcal antigen if indicated
Bone marrow	Histology, microscopy, and culture for bacteria, mycobacteria, fungi	
Lesion biopsy	Histology, microscopy, and culture for bacteria, mycobacteria, fungi	
Lesion culture	Microscopy and culture for bacteria, mycobacteria, fungi, viruses; microscopy for protozoa	
Lymph node biopsy	Histology, microscopy, and culture for bacteria, mycobacteria, fungi, viruses	Consider if there is systemic illness, if nodes are painful, change size rapidly, or are asymmetric or hilar
Stool	Microscopy and culture for enteropathogenic bacteria and mycobacteria; microscopy for protozoa	

Always remember that more than one pathogen may be active. Thus identification of a pathogen does not necessarily mean that it is the only one present.

sarcoma than men. In an Italian study of over 10 000 cases of AIDS, 6 per cent had Kaposi's sarcoma[64] but in Africa Kaposi's sarcoma seems to affect women fairly frequently; the male:female ratio of HIV-related Kaposi's sarcoma being 2:1.

Genital neoplasms

Since individuals who acquire HIV may be more sexually active, it is difficult to isolate the effect of HIV on the incidence of genital neoplasms. In a study of HIV-infected women who were clinically well, 18 of 109 had abnormalities of their lower genital tract[65] and HIV-positive women from a variety of sources have an incidence of cervical intraepithelial neoplasia varying between 35 and 80 per cent. The risk of HIV-infected women having cervical neoplasia is 4.9 times that of an HIV-negative women.[66]

Regular (six monthly) screening of HIV-positive women by clinical smear or colposcopy is indicated (HIV counselling and testing should be considered in cases of women receiving palliative care for cervical neoplasia who are at risk of HIV but whose HIV status is not known).

Specific issues in management for women

All HIV infected women should be aware of effective contraception to enable them to avoid unplanned pregnancy.

Pain syndromes in HIV and AIDS

The principles of pain relief for patients with HIV/AIDS are broadly similar to that of other conditions such as carcinoma. However, there are unusual causes of pain which can be improved by treatment.[67] The early stages of infection with HIV are rarely associated with pain. Patients with seroconversion illness may present with symptoms of acute aseptic meningitis, for example headache, fever, photophobia, and neck stiffness. Other painful neurological manifestations include myelopathy, Guillain–Barré

Table 4 Treatment of infection in HIV

Causative condition or organism	Appropriate standard antimicrobials	Acyclovir	Zidovudine (AZT) Didanosine Zalcitabine	Phosphonoformate (Foscarnet)	Ganciclovir (DHPG)	Nystatin	Ketoconazole or fluconazole	Amphotericin B	Flucytosine	Co-trimoxazole	Pentamidine isothionate	Toxoplasmosis therapy	Radiotherapy chemotherapy, or interferon
Bacteria													
Pyogenic bacteria	Valuable												
Salmonellae	Possible												
Mycobacteria (typical or atypical)	Valuable												
Nocardia asteroides	Valuable												
Viruses													
Cytomegalovirus				Valuable	Valuable								
Herpes simplex		Valuable											
Herpes varicella zoster		Valuable											
HIV			Valuable										
Molluscum contagiosum													
Fungi													
Candida albicans						Valuable	Valuable	Valuable	Valuable				
Cryptococcus neoformans							Valuable	Valuable	Valuable				
Protozoa													
Cryptosporidia													
Isosporida										Valuable			
Pneumocystis carinii										Valuable	Valuable		
Toxoplasma gondii												Valuable	
Other													
Kaposi's sarcoma													Valuable
Lymphoma													Valuable

(b) Appropriate dosages in HIV infection

Acyclovir	Herpes zoster 800 mg orally 5 times daily for 7 days (or intravenously 10 mg/kg 8 hourly for severe zoster); herpes simplex 200 mg orally 5 times daily for at least 5 days or intravenously 5 mg/kg 8 hourly (10 mg/kg for encephalitis); suppression of herpes simplex 200 mg 4 times daily
Zidovudine (AZT)	For serious manifestations of HIV infections in patients with AIDS or AIDS-related complex: 250 mg twice daily or 200 mg three-times daily; if haemoglobin falls below 7.5 g/dl or neutrophil count falls below 750/mm^3 consult data sheet; blood transfusion support may be necessary
Didanosine (ddI)	125 mg twice daily if body weight less than 60 kg, 200 mg twice daily if the body weight is more than 60 kg.
Zalcitabine (ddc)	0.375–0.75 mg three times daily
Phosphonoformate (Foscarnet)	Intravenously 0.05–0.16 mg/kg/min for 14–21 days; maintenance regimen not yet defined
Ganciclovir (DHPG)	5 mg/kg in 100 ml of 0.9% saline or 5% dextrose (each dose given over 1 h) for 14–21 days; maintenance therapy may be needed especially for retinitis
Nystatin	For upper gastrointestinal candidiasis: one 100000 IU pastille 6 hourly, suspension 1 ml 6 hourly; in severe candidiasis these doses may have to be exceeded; consider 4 hourly alternation with amphotericin lozenges
Ketoconazole or fluconazole	Ketoconazole 200 mg tablets 200–400 mg orally once daily with meals for 5 days, fluconazole 50 mg 24 hourly for 7–14 days (either may need to be continued longer (perhaps long term)); also consider fluconazole or itraconazole for candida or cryptococcal infections
Amphotericin B	100 mg tablets or 100 mg/ml suspension, one to two tablets or 2 ml suspension 6 hourly or 10 mg lozenges 6 hourly for mucosal involvement; intravenously 0.25 mg/kg daily, increased rapidly to 1.0 mg/kg daily, possibly to 0.6 mg/kg by day 2 (maximum daily dose 1.5 mg/kg) for systemic involvement; consider combining amphotericin with flucytosine
Flucytosine	100–200 mg/kg/day given orally 6 hourly or by intravenous infusion; usually given in addition to amphotericin B; avoid if there is severe bone marrow suppression
Cotrimoxazole	For pneumocystis 16 tablets (1280 mg as trimethoprim content) daily for 21 days, intravenously 20 mg/kg daily (dose as trimethoprim diluted 1:25 in 0.9% saline or 5% dextrose); a brief course of systemic steroids may be useful in severe pneumonia; dapsone + trimethoprim may also have a role; for isosporiasis two tablets 6 hourly long term
Pentamidine isethionate	4 mg/kg/day intramuscularly or by slow intravenous infusion in 5% dextrose for 14–21 days; aerosol administration using special nebulizer possible; prophylactic use is promising, a brief course of systemic steroids may be useful in severe cases
Toxoplasmosis therapy	Sulphadiazine 4 g daily + pyrimethamine 25–50 mg daily + folinic acid 5–10 mg daily for 3–4 weeks, then maintenance therapy; dapsone may also be used

syndrome, and radiculopathy. Bleeding into tissues may be associated with thrombocytopenia, which may cause short-term pain.

Respiratory system

Many HIV positive patients, but especially heavy smokers, suffer from recurrent bacterial chest infections. Shingles may present initially with chest pain and cause diagnostic uncertainty until the rash appears. *Pneumocystis carinii* pneumonia, is associated with pain in only a minority of cases. In our own experience, pain with *Pneumocystis carinii* pneumonia is more common with drug users than other risk groups but this may be because of associated bacterial infection. Even so, it occurs in under 20 per cent of our patients. *Pneumocystis carinii* pneumonia can, however, present with severe pleuritic type chest pain or this may develop during the illness and indicates the development of the complication of pneumothorax. Oesophagitis may present as chest pain if there is minimal pain on swallowing.

Gastrointestinal system

Oral candida is usually asymptomatic but it can cause burning oral discomfort. Severe retrosternal chest pain with burning on swallowing is usually caused by an erosive oesophagitis (a grimace associated with swallowing of hot tea or coffee is diagnostic) which is usually caused by candidiasis. Cytomegalovirus or herpes simplex virus infection are other possible causes. Poor appetite or weight loss may be non-specific accompaniments. Oesophagitis can be a particular problem in the later stages of AIDS if resistance to oral antifungal agents develops. Oesophageal pain may be relived by H_2 blockers until treatment of the causative organism has taken effect. Extensive and painful idiopathic aphthous ulcers may develop in the mouth or oesophagus. Thalidomide may be effective (but is contraindicated in woman at risk of pregnancy).

Abdominal pain in injection drug users on methadone or other opioids is commonly associated with constipation which may be excluded by rectal examination and/or a plain radiograph of the abdomen. Pancreatitis may be secondary to antiretroviral treatment (including didanosine) or it may occur spontaneously in late HIV disease. In injection drug users cholecystitis, appendicitis, or peptic ulceration may be masked by opioids. Infection with atypical mycobacteria or cryptosporidiosis may cause persistent abdominal pain. Cryptosporidiosis, which is usually associated with persistent diarrhoea, may also cause a painful obstructive cholangitis. Cytomegalovirus can also cause intestinal pain and diarrhoea. Definitive diagnosis is by microscopy and culture of rectal or colonic biopsies. A large number of patients with HIV, especially drug users, have also been exposed to agents such as hepatitis B or C. Chronic hepatitis or frank cirrhosis may, therefore, develop and in our experience this is an important cause of non-AIDS morbidity and mortality—nearly 20 per cent of the causes of death in drug users. Pain as a consequence of liver capsule expansion or ascites is certainly a possibility as a terminal event. Another possible explanation for abdominal pain may be enlarging lymph nodes secondary to lymphoma. Other mechanisms of abdominal pain include infiltration of Kaposi's sarcoma, with lymphoma or enlargement of lymph nodes.

Anorectal pain may be severe and disabling. It is usually associated with herpes simplex infection; this infection should be excluded in all instances of rectal pain as it is treatable with acyclovir. Ulceration (rather than vesicle formation) is typical. Lymphoma should always be remembered as a possibility if the symptoms do not settle on acyclovir.

Other systems

Painful neuropathies may occur at any stage of HIV infection and may be caused by HIV, cytomegalovirus, varicella zoster virus, herpes simplex virus, syphilis, or by antiretroviral drugs including didanosine and zalcitabine. A 'burning feet' syndrome is a fairly common complaint. Treatment (in addition to specific antiorganism therapy) usually requires additional antidepressants. Occasionally antiepilepsy drugs are helpful, as is mexiletine or other antiarrythmic drugs.

Headache may be caused by space occupying lesions (including toxoplasmosis or lymphoma) or by meningitis (usually cryptococcal). Headaches also occur with HIV encephalopathy or cerebral atrophy. Sinusitis is very common in late stage AIDS.

Neuropathies secondary to injection drug injury are problematical because they tend to present after the signs of local injury have settled. Development of weakness or wasting suggests an organic rather than a manipulative pain, as discussed below.

Additional diagnostic problems associated with drug use

Continued drug use may interfere with clinical assessment. Lymphadenopathy may be associated with AIDS or injection of foreign materials. Fatigue, lethargy, diarrhoea, and excessive sweating can be caused by opioid withdrawal. Weight loss and sweating may be associated with opioid use or stimulants such as amphetamines or cocaine. Epileptic fits may be caused by benzodiazepine withdrawal. Excessive use of cannabis and benzodiazepines interferes with memory and other cognitive functions. Syncopal attacks may be caused by antidepressant tricyclic drugs (rather than HIV-related autonomic neuropathy or hypoadrenalism). Dyspnoea or a persistent cough can occur with endocarditis, bacterial pneumonia, excessive smoking, recurrent bronchitis, and obstructive airways disease (rather than with *Pneumocystis carinii* pneumonia).

Assessment of pain is a problem in injection drug users who often wish to obtain opioid for reasons other than pain relief. Complaints of pain are a method of increasing opioid prescribing and considerable experience is required in both the investigation and management of the problem to avoid ever larger prescriptions. Injection drug users may not be able to afford their habit and so may wish the medical services to provide for their habit needs. Dental pain is one of the commonest fictional (and genuine) complains. Dental caries are very common in injection drug users and input from a dentist experienced in the treatment of injection drug users is invaluable.

Painful injection-related abscesses may occur in a surprising variety of anatomical situations and drugs such as temazepam cause extensive local tissue destruction when extravasation occurs.

Perhaps the most difficult pains to diagnose are the traumatic neuropathies secondary to injection drug injury. These tend to present some time after the local injury has settled with little in the way of physical signs. They may be difficult to distinguish from manipulation for more drugs and may only be diagnosed with the development of weakness or wasting. Equally, they are difficult to distinguish from HIV-related causes of neuropathies, especially if the patient is not keen on admitting their injection drug injury.

Problems of pain management in HIV related to injection drug use

The advent of HIV has resulted in large numbers of drug users, who previously have not had much contact with health services, requiring help for a variety of problems, including the very difficult problem of pain control. These difficulties occur not only in the every-day management of drug users but also in the terminal phase of HIV. The problems described above with regard to careful investigation of pain need to be reiterated. The commonest problem in the management of new pain in drug users is probably one of insufficient doses as a consequence of existing high levels of opioid use. It is important to involve nursing staff in all discussions about the reality of a patient's pain.

The problems in the management of recent-onset pain in injection drug users may be resolved by rescheduling the pre-existing opioid to an analgesic frequency rather than a frequency to prevent drug withdrawal. For example methadone is usually given in a once daily dose to prevent withdrawal symptoms but for pain relief it should be given initially every 6 to 8 h, after which it can usually be reduced to once or twice daily.

Use of inappropriate drugs such as dipipanone or buprenorphine should be resisted whenever possible because they are highly sought after as recreational drugs. Our current practice is to use increasing frequency and/or doses of drugs such as methadone, slow release morphine, or subcutaneous morphine/diamorphine as subcutaneous infusions. Domiciliary therapy, which entails giving the patient unsupervised access to his medication, may result in over-rapid use of supplied opioid and genuine pain thereafter. If a brief increase of opioid is indicated (for example after operative procedures) we use either a continuous subcutaneous pump or fixed intermittent dose delivery system for opioid delivery (but tampering with infusion pumps can occur). It may take some while to return patients to their previous level of opioid use.

Provision of adequate sedation during necessary procedures is difficult; patients may require unusually large doses of midazolam because tolerance of their regular intake of other benzodiazepines is high. Alternatively, respiratory depression may result in patients because of concurrent therapy (known or unknown) with benzodiazepines, and flumazenil (which reverses symptoms and signs of benzodiazepine overdose) should be available. In an emergency, it is always worth giving naloxone because reversal of opioid action may be sufficient to restore spontaneous respiration. Additionally, some HIV/AIDS patients exhibit an unusual sensitivity to neuroleptics or benzodiazepines, probably because of concomitant HIV encephalopathy. A gradual introduction of such drugs is required.

Drug users may complain of pain to obtain an increased opioid prescription but close and sensitive questioning may reveal that the problem is actually one of psychosocial distress and the difficulty of facing death rather than actual physical pain. In these circumstances prescribe additional drugs for distress rather than pain. In endstage AIDS it may be appropriate to give drug users what they request.

Drug interactions

Drug interactions may be a major problem in HIV/AIDS therapies because patients in endstage AIDS have often accumulated a larger number of drug treatments and, thus, potential drug interactions. Treatment failures may result. Notably, pain control may fail because of lower opioid levels. The most important adverse reactions are caused by induction of hepatic enzymes. Induction of hepatic enzymes occurs with a number of antiepileptics (including phenytoin) and with antibiotics used to treat atypical mycobacteria (including rifampicin or rifabutin). Fluconazole levels may also fall (fluconazole therapy also increases the levels of rifabutin which in turn may cause uveitis).

Withdrawal of therapies

It is very difficult to issue dogmatic guidelines concerning which treatments can be withdrawn as palliative care replaces acute interventions. In general terms, organism-specific prophylactic treatment should continue until death. Depending upon circumstances the following may need to be continued until quite close to death:

(1) prophylaxis for *Pneumocystis carinii* pneumonia;

(2) prophylaxis for herpes simplex infections;

(3) prophylaxis for cytomegalovirus retinitis;

(4) treatment and prophylaxis of oral and oesophageal candidiasis;

(5) treatment to control infections, such as tuberculosis, that are transmissible to others (especially other immunocompromised patients);

(6) treatment of central nervous system toxoplasmosis unless there has been:

    no evidence of treatment efficacy (including slowing of disease progression)

    unacceptable toxicity or side-effects

    severe dementia

    or the patient is plainly near to death.

HIV and AIDS in tropical and developing countries

HIV and AIDS is a medical and social disaster for most developing countries where medical care is limited. The discrepancy between health-care resources in the developed and developing world is stark and has been well illustrated by an AIDS resource index relating the AIDS epidemic to the *per capita* income in various countries.[68]

Affordable diagnostic tests, treatments for HIV itself, and related opportunistic infections are often expensive, and therefore unavailable. The extent of HIV-related problems is difficult to ascertain as surveillance is difficult and the extent of problems is hidden because patients do not die of AIDS itself—they die with AIDS as the underlying cause of opportunistic infections. AIDS in developing countries tends to be a disease of active young people (active both sexually and economically) who, had they lived, would have provided the infrastructure for their country's development.

Patterns of opportunistic infections are different in tropical countries. There are four reasons for this.

1. Prior infection with HIV may facilitate acquisition of endemic tropical diseases.
2. Prior infection with a tropical disease may increase susceptibility to, or transmission of, HIV (or both).
3. HIV may exacerbate latent infections or accelerate the normal course of such infections.
4. Acquisition of a tropical disease might accelerate the progress of the HIV infection.

Most of what follows applies to Africa, which is at the forefront of the world HIV pandemic, but patterns are usually similar, in nature if not in extent, elsewhere in most of the developing world.[69]

In Africa, HIV infection is mostly spread by heterosexual intercourse, from mother to child, and by infected blood transfusions (transfusions were often used for malarial or sickle cell anaemias) and to a lesser extent by repeated medical use of needles or by ritual scarifications. Insect bites do not appear to transmit HIV. Twenty nine per cent of those attending sexually transmitted disease clinics in some central African cities are seropositive; 8 per cent of blood donors and 3 to 11 per cent of pregnant women are seropositive. The male:female ratio approaches 1:1. Such seropositivity rates make the concept of 'at risk' groups unhelpful as nearly all of the population is at risk.

In Africa, AIDS has as its main presentation a (secretory) diarrhoea/wasting syndrome known to local populations as 'slim'. The survival time is reduced (for example in Kinshasa there is about 40 per cent 3 month survival rates from a diagnosis of AIDS until death); late diagnosis and unavailability of treatment no doubt both contribute to this mortality rate. Gastroenterological problems and dermatological manifestations are more common in African AIDS (although Kaposi's sarcoma is less common—the classical African Kaposi's sarcoma is almost a separate disease). The spectrum of AIDS-related opportunistic infections is related to the local background prevalence of potentially pathogenic organisms. Toxoplasmosis, salmonellosis, shigellosis, giardiasis, cryptosporidiosis, cryptococcal infection, hepatosplenomegaly, and diarrhoea of unknown origin are all common. Pre-existing latent infections with syphilis (varying between 5 and 30 per cent of certain populations), cytomegalovirus (100 per cent), toxoplasmosis (50 to 75 per cent), and hepatitis B (15 per cent) may all be reactivated when HIV-related immunosuppression is profound. Tuberculosis is common as it may be reactivated and/or more easily acquired; typically about one-third of patients with tuberculosis are HIV positive and about two-thirds of patients with extrapulmonary tuberculosis are HIV positive. Interestingly, *Pneumocystis carinii* pneumonia is relatively uncommon and worm infections (with the possible exception of *Strongyloides*) seem to cause few problems.

Prophylaxis of opportunistic infections is not practicable, except in rare pockets of high technology medical care, and palliative care must concentrate on relief of symptoms rather than treatment directed at underlying causes. A high degree of palliation can be achieved with antituberculous drugs, where indicated, plus nine relatively inexpensive drugs—cotrimoxazole, metronidazole, ketoconazole, chlorpromazine, chloroquine, aspirin or paracetamol (acetaminophen), codeine, calamine lotion, and petroleum jelly.[70]

Counselling, particularly counselling to reduce at risk behaviour, is difficult, especially if communication networks are poor. Additionally, patients may not wish for complete exposition of their illness and its implications.[71] Control of infection measures may be difficult to implement because of religious, cultural, or financial reasons and significant cultural differences may exist in customs surrounding dying and death.

Psychological and psychiatric aspects of patient care

Psychological problems may be very similar to those which arise in any patient with a life-threatening disease. However, a number of differences are evident—patients are almost all young, they are often extremely well informed about the disease, and lastly, of course, it is an infectious disease.

The psychological responses to illness may vary between the various at risk groups, not because of differences in the presentation of illness but largely because of pre-existing social or psychological circumstances.

For many drug users, HIV is the last in a long line of previous personal disasters, most of which involved rejection and stigmatization. They may have had backgrounds that were subject to multiple deprivations, frequently culminating in neglect or rejection by exasperated care agencies. They frequently receive a psychiatric diagnosis of personality disorder—a diagnosis which may discourage sustained therapeutic endeavours. Drug users may have an history of overdose (accidental or intended) and other suicide attempts. However, it is important to remember that because a patient acquired HIV through intravenous drug use it does not necessarily mean that he or she will continue to use drugs or behave stereotypically.

Many homosexual men are happy about their sexual orientation but others may be chronically unhappy because of their own or others' inability to accept it. Those who were heterosexually infected may or may not have been aware that they were at risk from a sexual partner and many have the burden of being in a continuing relationship with someone who has infected them, often unwittingly.

Haemophiliacs are a more homogeneous group and usually have a common bond of life-long, life-threatening illness. A new medically endorsed treatment which promised them hope, but which unpredictably contained HIV, then devastated their lives and that of their families. This understandably may cause bewilderment, disbelief, and despair; disillusionment and anger have been directed at those who treated their haemophilia and at the government. Many are also angry with homosexuals and drug users who had inadvertently donated the blood which infected them.

Those infected by blood transfusion are vulnerable because there is no sense of identity with any other HIV at-risk group—including others infected by transfusion—because they are such a heterogeneous and small population.

Bewilderment, disbelief, and despair are similar to reactions experienced by most people who develop a life-threatening disease, and with HIV there is the additional stigma which is still often associated with it.

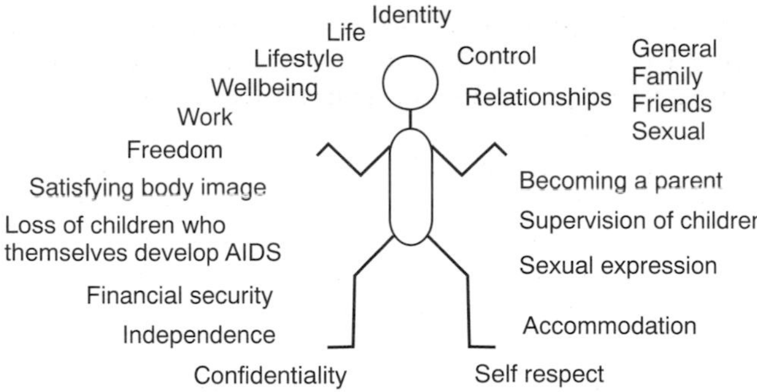

Fig. 8 The real or perceived losses for a patient with HIV infection or AIDS.

Those who give palliative care for HIV positive patients need to be aware of these consequences associated with the mode of acquisition of HIV. However, there are many common problems confronting those with AIDS and carers should be encouraged to see AIDS as 'yet another fatal disease' and to realize, despite any initial prejudices, that the way in which the patient acquired the infection is irrelevant to the care they should receive. The following account emphasizes the shared problems of patients with AIDS and, where indicated, the problems associated with particular groups.

Coping with losses

Any dying person experiences feelings of loss but for those with AIDS there are extra burdens and fears (Fig. 8).

Loss of relationships

Patients with HIV infection may fear the stigma and alienation associated with drug use, the disease itself, or with homosexuality. The diagnosis of HIV may give rise to a fear of loss of family and friends if the existence of a previously hidden lifestyle becomes apparent. Patients also worry that families and friends may fear infection, even if no real risk exists. AIDS patients, their families, and friends are all told that HIV is not infectious except by well-defined means but they may have difficulty in accepting this. In particular, they may have difficulty in believing that children are safe from infection.

Many HIV positive people often have personal experience of others who have fallen ill and died of AIDS. In Edinburgh (where in one cohort it is estimated that about 65 per cent of injection drug users were infected prior to 1986), whole families are infected—parents, brothers and sisters, and the next generation of children.[72]

Loss of identity

Most people have several foundations for their identity; their status in society, their families, their work, their sexual preferences, and their habits or their interests. Those who have HIV often feel that they are losing one or more of these identities to become 'AIDS victims'. This role of victim may be exacerbated by media publicity, the necessarily repeated visits to hospitals, or constant enquiries about the nature of their ill health from others. Networks of support may be helpful at different stages of illness but at other times the patient may need to be encouraged to carry on as normal a life as possible so that he or she is not constantly focused on an infection which may not have any manifestations of illness. Generally, once the patient has developed HIV related illness more support is helpful.

Others may find that their HIV infection or AIDS gives them an identity which is fulfilling. Contribution to self-help and other support groups enables some patients to discover a role, a sense of self value, which may otherwise have been unobtainable.

Loss of control

Patients with AIDS usually need to attend medical clinics on a regular basis; those that do have a better prognosis but this may cause patients to feel that the virus is taking control of their lives. Most treatments (especially antiviral therapies and ganciclovir) need to be monitored so that opportunistic infections and serious side-effects can be detected and treated at an early stage.

Loss of sexual expression

A patient's knowledge that he or she is infected with HIV inevitably implies a change in sexual behaviour with (at least) the use of condoms to protect others. Surveys have shown that condoms are often considered unacceptable as their use is incompatible with spontaneous, uninhibited sex. Informing a partner of your HIV positivity risks the loss of that partner. Many of those infected only have non-penetrative sexual activities or eschew intercourse to protect their loved ones—whose affection may therefore be lost.

Support and counselling must include discussion about the appropriateness of these restrictions and, in particular, explore alternatives to unprotected penetrative sex. Whilst safe sex can be enjoyable it is important to be realistic and acknowledge that it may be less physically fulfilling than previous sexual behaviour. Presentation of safe and safer sex as being as enjoyable as unprotected sex is unrealistic, not generally successful, and may be resented by patients. Having said this, many people do adjust successfully to having safer sex, albeit with a sense of loss.

Loss of body image

Kaposi's sarcoma or severe weight loss may be unmistakable evidence of severe illness and the former is diagnostic of AIDS to anyone with some knowledge of HIV infection. In any event, awkward questions and answers may result which may lead to a conspiracy of isolation between the patient and others. Facial Kaposi's sarcoma can be unsightly and cause distress to patients, although families and acquaintances may be more embarrassed than the patients. Although patients with Kaposi's sarcoma often are relatively healthy and may survive for months or years, they may suffer psychologically. Cosmetic advice and medical treatment may be helpful. It is unhelpful to attempt to minimize problems of obvious lesions—rather, the patient needs sensitively delivered help in coming to terms with the problems. Severe weight loss may also cause a loss of previous self image which may affect general and sexual relationships.

Loss of children

The implications of HIV infection in pregnancy have been mentioned previously. Women with HIV or AIDS who become pregnant need to be confronted with objective information, sensitive counselling, and safe sex advice. The risk of having an infected baby is unacceptably high for many couples to contemplate and they may require help to reconcile themselves to being childless or having no more children. This may be as painful for men as for women. Some homosexual and bisexual men may also feel that they have lost the opportunity to father children; any assumption that homosexuality precludes a desire to have children may be incorrect.

Couples in whom one or both are infected who do initiate a pregnancy have to be assisted to cope with the possibility that their babies may develop AIDS. Since maternally derived HIV antibody may take time to clear, parents may have to cope with the possibility that their baby is infected during this time,[73] though more sophisticated laboratory tests than the HIV antibody test now make it possible to be relatively sure what the baby's HIV status is at an earlier stage.

Not only this, but an infected parent will fear that he or she might well die before the children grow up; if both parents are infected (or in a single-parent family) this fear is accentuated if there are no close relatives who are willing to adopt the children and parents have to face the possibility that children will be taken into care.

A single parent may fear that an unsuitable, estranged partner will have automatic custody of children after their death. Drug users, at the time of writing, are the group most likely to be affected by these problems and may fear that their children will be taken away by social workers, either before or after their own death. Wherever possible, carers should help parents to make arrangements in advance, even if in some cases children will have to be taken into care, fostered, or adopted. In these circumstances, parents should be encouraged to develop a close shared-care relationship with the future carers, prior to or during the terminal illness. Authoritative assurances that children will be cared for, without any tangible evidence, are unlikely to alleviate concerns about the children's future.

Loss of lifestyle

In Europe, unlike the United States, people with AIDS rarely become destitute because of medical bills, but those who become unable to work may find themselves in considerably reduced financial circumstances. Others may lose their accommodation because of adverse reactions of neighbours who discover the diagnosis. Travel abroad may be curtailed since some governments (including the United States) have in the past restricted or forbidden entry to the HIV positive.[74]

Problems associated with particular stages of HIV disease

Whilst psychological problems may arise at any stage there are eight possible landmark events (Table 5) which may initiate severe stress and uncertainty. The initial diagnosis of HIV positivity, development of AIDS itself, and any complicating illnesses are obvious examples.

Other landmark events are less obvious. For example the initiation of opportunistic infection prophylaxis or anti-HIV-therapy. Doctors perceive introduction of such therapy as of positive benefit whereas the patient's perception can be exclusively negative, with the introduction of each new therapy being seen as a marker of disease progression. Other, more ominous landmarks occur when long-term treatments are discontinued because they are no longer indicated or effective or when side-effects become unacceptable. Patients should be encouraged to participate fully in such therapeutic decision-making after discussion about the benefits, possible side-effects, and anticipated duration of efficacy of the treatments. Patients may wish to discuss how they can set their finances and associated matters in order prior to their death. Others will wish to discuss whether an autopsy will be performed, or whether they will be cremated or buried. Especially when there might be a conflict of wishes between relatives and a patient's partner, it is wise to suggest that the patient provides a written account of his wishes. Living wills (advance directives) are often left by patients with AIDS. These may detail whether or not the patient wishes medical interventions in different circumstances.

Table 5 The eight major possible landmark events in HIV disease

1. Initial diagnosis of HIV positivity
2. Initiation of anti-HIV or antiopportunistic infection therapy
3. Development of AIDS
4. Complicating illnesses
5. Discontinuation of therapies
6. Pregnancy in patients (or their partners)
7. Peer group illness and death
8. Dying and death

Through all their illnesses, AIDS patients require extensive support. They and their carers know that something will happen, but not exactly what or exactly when. Throughout the disease progression there is anxiety because of the uncertainties; unpredictability is an essential part of AIDS and prevention of the predictable only postpones other essentially unpredictable events.

Psychological, psychiatric, and neuropsychological problems in HIV infection

There are two categories of problems: those caused by psychological or psychiatric factors and those caused by organic brain dysfunction. These categories may overlap and it is important to attempt to identify and treat the contribution each makes in any one patient.

Psychological problems

Anxiety, depression, or a preoccupation with infection may be a normal response to a life-threatening situation and may be exacerbated in response to any of the significant landmarks. Knowledge of HIV positivity may precipitate or exacerbate pre-existing problems.[75]

In acute anxiety, patients may experience chest pain, sweating, trembling, diarrhoea, and numerous other physical symptoms. These may be interpreted as manifestations of HIV disease. Anxiety induces adrenaline-mediated effects, which in turn exacerbate anxiety, constituting a symptomatic vicious circle. Explanation of this self-perpetuating mechanism may help the patient break out of the vicious circle of symptoms but specific anxiety management techniques (including relaxation training and cognitive therapy) can enable patients to regain control of their somatic symptoms. Anxiolytic medication, using minor or major tranquillizers, may be helpful in symptom relief, particularly at times of crisis, but such drugs should generally only be prescribed for short periods of time, especially if there is a history of drug dependency.

Symptoms of clinical depression include early morning waken-ing, loss of appetite, weight loss, variations or blunting of mood, psychomotor retardation, and loss of libido. Some of these may also be symptoms of progressing HIV disease and definitive diagnosis may be difficult.[76]

Suicidal thoughts are common and patients should be encour-aged to discuss these so that mistaken impressions or misinforma-tion can be corrected and appropriate support, both psychological and physical, provided. Suicidal thoughts may reflect an underlying depressive illness, the treatment of which may allow the patient to make a more realistic assessment of their situation. Drug users may be at particular risk of suicide as they have access to potentially lethal drugs. Although many drug overdoses are regarded as accidental, trivial, attention seeking, or manipulative rather than suicidal in intent, all should be taken seriously. In the United States it has been reported that the risk of suicide is 36 times greater among HIV infected men than non-infected men.[77]

Obsessional thoughts and behaviour and hypochondriacal fears may arise. Obsessional checking of the body for blemishes or rashes, fixation on thoughts of death, repetitive attempts to identify how and from whom they acquired infection, or repeated visits to the doctor for check-ups may dominate a patient's life. In severe forms reassurance is only of transitory help and referral for more formal assessment to appropriate psychological or psychiatric agencies should be made.

Psychotic illness

Psychotic illnesses, with severe abnormalities in thought, feeling, or behaviour, are well recognized in HIV disease; the patient may have thoughts, worries, and suspicions which have no realistic basis. However, there is no strong evidence that psychoses are more common in HIV positive patients.[78]

Psychotic illnesses are more likely when there has been a previous history of such illness. Manic, schizophrenic, or depres-sive psychoses may occur. Mania may present with ideas of grandeur—such as a belief that the individual has found a cure for AIDS or has been miraculously cured. Schizophrenia may cause ideas of reference, auditory or visual hallucinations, thought block, etc. and may cause a patient to believe that he is being persecuted by his carers or family.

Neurological illnesses

HIV dementia

HIV/AIDS is unusual in that it combines immunological, neuro-logical, and psychiatric disorders and as a consequence patients may develop a variety of disabilities ranging from wasting dis-orders, severe pain, neurological dysfunction (such as paralysis or cognitive impairment), and psychological symptoms. These con-stellations of disabilities may result in considerable problems for both patients and carers. A detailed description of the problems of HIV dementia is beyond the scope of this section. However, some mention will be made of the difficulties of management, with particular reference to drug users. HIV-related drug misuse itself causes considerable problems for medical units (Brettle, in press).

The common cause of cognitive impairment is HIV encephalitis and this may occur quite early in the disease process or as a terminal event. It appears that not everyone is at risk—perhaps only 10#per cent of patients. Zidovudine treatment may be protective, and to a certain extent the inability to cope may be more obvious the lower the initial intelligence of the patient. Whilst all risk groups may be affected, management issues are more complex with drug users since the patients may become quite susceptible to neuroleptic and other drugs. The patients find it quite difficult to accept that they can no longer tolerate their 'normal' dose of recreational drugs. The symptoms of cognitive impairment are often worsened by benzodiazepines, marijuana, or stimulants as well as intercurrent infections or fever. Despite severe impairment of short-term memory, the patients often appear quite normal with very good preservation of long-term memories, reflex actions, and repetitive events such as the volume of methadone or the number of tablets of opioid required each day. They are often very good at confabulating and hiding their disabilities.

As ill health develops most patients with HIV suffer a loss of income as a result of possibly both physical and mental deteriora-tion. The disease process also occurs in those engaged in illegal activities and they are far more likely to be apprehended in pursuit of criminal activities. Effectively, this phenomenon could be described as criminal unemployment and it creates considerable difficulties for those funding an illegal drug habit. Consequently, as HIV progresses there may be an increased dependency on the state. This dependency often manifests itself via numerous demands on the health service to prescribe substitute drugs as an attempt to offset a deficiency of illegal funds. This increasing pressure to replace lost income may result in additional difficulties for a national health service; increased theft in and around hospitals, drug dealing in hospital settings, blatant requests for medical help in making fraudulent social security claims (spurious travel expenses, non-existent weight loss, enhanced physical disability), requests for inappropriate hospitalization, or manipulated emer-gency admissions which allow an individual to actually save money which would otherwise have been spent on food and heating, etc.

The physical weakness and mental slowing which may accom-pany injection drug use and HIV also results in other problems for the drug user such as victimization, harassment, and/or exploita-tion. This may in part be related to a prior position of superiority in the drug culture and a desire on the part of others in the community to repay past wrongs or previous harassment. Alter-natively, it may simply be related to the exploitation of weaker individuals. The net result, however, is a gradual inability to cope in the community. When this is combined with a very real difficulty in accepting the discipline of a hospital regimen the scene is set for frequent precipitous admissions and discharges. The unwillingness or inability to adapt to changed circumstances result in 'revolving door' type admissions to hospital with considerable frustration for patients, relatives, and staff. In our experience increasing family anxiety, frequent hospital admissions and self discharges, increasing use of illegal drugs, and harassment often herald the onset of serious HIV encephalopathy or frank dementia.[79]

The diagnosis of HIV encephalopathy requires access to a number of specialized techniques for diagnosis such as psycho-metric testing, neurophysiological testing (e.g. auditory evoked potentials), or magnetic resonance imaging (MRI). An accurate diagnosis is important both for patient and carers since it helps prevent misunderstandings—particularly of difficult behaviour which is often misinterpreted as bad behaviour rather than as a consequence of ill health. An accurate diagnosis is an aid to a management plan which is often based around behavioural therapy. Considerable supervision of the patient is required to prevent wandering or harm to either the patient or others. This is obviously important in wards where patients with infective conditions are located. Considerable resources are required to keep the patient in the community. Much of the care and management is based on that used for older demented patients the only difference being that the patients are often in their twenties or thirties. Other patients with HIV/AIDS are remarkably tolerant of the problems and may be of help in care and supervision. The greatest danger for injection drug use-related HIV dementia is access to illegal drugs from patients or visitors who do not appreciate the sensitivity and dangers for the patient of additional drugs.

Some 30 to 40 per cent of AIDS patients have been reported to have neurological dysfunction at some stage during life and 80 per cent of patients with AIDS show signs of neurological problems post-mortem.[80] Only 3 per cent of patients present with AIDS dementia complex as the first sign of AIDS. However, the incidence is increasing as life-threatening opportunistic infections are prevented; indeed doctors tend not to fully discuss with patients the inevitable increased chance of other disorders consequent upon successful prophylaxis. Thus, there is obviously much clinically undetectable neurological damage of uncertain relevance to the patient's mental state. Many of those infected are highly knowledgeable about the disease and are understandably fearful that they may become demented, blind, or incontinent.

Early manifestations of AIDS dementia complex include forgetfulness, poor concentration, loss of interest, weight loss, loss of libido, blunted affect, and psychomotor retardation. Later manifestations include motor disturbance, which may cause difficulty in walking, seizures, spasticity, and mutism. Early symptoms of AIDS dementia complex may be indistinguishable from those of depression and a combined medical, neuropsychological, and psychiatric assessment is essential. The fear of late stage AIDS dementia complex may present as 'false presentation' of early AIDS dementia complex itself in that patients present with memory and concentration difficulties, which reflect an acute anxiety state or depression rather than early AIDS dementia complex.

Psychological stages of dying

The process of adjustment to an illness which leads to death often starts when the diagnosis of HIV or AIDS is confirmed. It is important to stress four facts to patients:

1. HIV infection itself is mostly asymptomatic; immunodeficiency by itself has no symptoms or signs.
2. Patients feel well providing complications are prevented or controlled.
3. Most patients with AIDS are mostly well for most of the time.
4. People do not usually die of HIV or AIDS but of the complications associated with it.

Although not all patients experience similar progressions the different stages of dying have been described as shock, denial, anger, bargaining, and acceptance.[81]

All the above reactions may be present at different times but some patients may remain angry or remain in a state of denial from diagnosis to death. Skilled counselling is invaluable if it allows patients to come to terms with the inevitable, no matter at what stage they die. Some patients maintain denial throughout their illness; this may be a successful defence mechanism which should be respected.

Anger may be difficult to cope with, particularly if anger is directed towards those who care for the patient. Anger or denial may not be harmful to the patient but can be a successful coping mechanism, which carers should respect. Thus, it is important that carers should try to understand the mechanism of anger and, if possible, assist the patient to express emotions constructively in a way more to the patient's benefit. There is no doubt that anger, sometimes from those with a history of violence, may be difficult and frightening for carers to manage. Do not fail to consider that the patient may have genuine grievances including inadequate symptom relief ('it's just thrush') or other shortcomings in medical or nursing support. Always respond positively to the basis of the patient's grievances.

There are extra problems remaining after the death of a patient with AIDS. Those remaining may not feel they can involve others in their grieving process without full disclosure of the diagnosis of AIDS. This is a particular problem for those who do not wish others to know that the patient was infected. It is important that counselling services, who have supported the patient and family whilst the patient was alive, should be available to give families continued support during their grieving process.

Counselling in AIDS

The spectrum of possible losses as detailed in Fig. 8 would be unusual in any other disease but when occurring in minority groups who may feel themselves outside mainstream society, when illness occurs in disadvantaged circumstances, and when patients may wish to conceal their diagnosis from those who would normally rally round, it is apparent that a particularly wide range of personality, attributes, and skills are required in psychosocial services. Versatility is essential with care being taken not to encourage a dependency role, whilst providing maximum support.

Self-help groups

Self-help groups are invaluable for many reasons too obvious to mention. HIV self-help groups have one feature in common; they are unusually well informed about all aspects of their illness including the numerous media announcements of significant advances in treatment—both genuine and worthless. All carers, but particularly medical carers, have to be up to date with relevant developments and occasionally have to adopt forceful stances against the introduction or discontinuation of therapy suggested by patients if such therapies may be harmful or reduce the patient's quality of life. 'Substance X might be a miracle breakthrough, but there is no evidence that it is'. 'The fact that you have seen others on zidovudine therapy eventually become ill is the effect of their disease, not the zidovudine, and this is no reason for you to discontinue therapy'. 'Visiting such a (alternative medicine) practitioner is unlikely to produce a significant effect on the disease itself, but if you feel it helps, why not?' 'Whatever alternative therapies you try, keep us informed and do not discontinue your current treatments that have been proven to be of benefit.'

Organization of carers

The keynote of caring must be the well publicized, but unobtrusive, availability of a variety of caring agencies and individuals who can respond to each crisis that may arise. No one carer can cope with all the problems associated with the losses that a patient with AIDS may experience (Fig. 8). A team is required with medical and nursing input as the foundation but with counsellors, psychologist, psychiatrist, social workers, health visitors, occupational therapists, physiotherapists, dietitians, drug workers, district nurses, community workers, and others as indicated. The patient, or his or her representative, should have the right to attend the relevant parts of the meeting if they wish. Such a team should meet regularly as in a case conference.

As a general rule all members of the team should know each other and each should know the patients being discussed. Other interested parties who wish to attend should be ascertained to have a legitimate reason. There are six purposes of such conference: identification of problems, pooling of skills and resources, division of labour, stimulation of members' realization of problems faced by other members, and mutual support and encouragement. Such groups should discuss, but not make, important medical decisions; since 1967 it has been known that, contrary to popular opinion, groups arrive at riskier decisions than individuals do alone.[82] In particular, there is a risk that enthusiasts always triumph over sceptics when the addition of another possibly helpful, but probably inappropriate, treatment is being considered.

There are problems of confidentiality when organizing support in the community; provision of certain assistance by certain persons may imply a certain diagnosis to onlookers. Some patients never wish to go to particular hospital departments or AIDS specific hospices because to do so would make their diagnosis immediately obvious. Similarly, the training needs of professionals outside the primary care team may require sensitive management to preserve confidentiality.

The actual diagnosis of HIV infection or AIDS must be restricted to those who need to know—and these are surprisingly few in number. For many carers the only confirmed knowledge necessary is which infection precautions are necessary.

Table 6 Possible contributors to HIV–AIDS caring teams

Medical and nursing staff
Counsellor
Psychologist
General practitioner when indicated
Psychiatrist if relevant
Social worker
Health visitor
Community worker
Occupational therapist
Physiotherapist
Dietitian
Patient or representative when appropriate

Caring for carers

Caring for those with HIV infection and with AIDS provides stresses additional to non-HIV terminal care; the patients are often relatively young adults and there are difficulties associated with some high-risk groups. Patients with AIDS have, over the course of many years, established a relationship with a variety of carers and, whenever possible, those carers should be available to patients throughout the illness, so that if the patient wishes he or she can initiate discussion. Implicit in this is that care should be given by teams that cover both in- and outpatient work. Additionally, carers may have long-term contact with patients, often from when they are first diagnosed HIV positive until death. Inevitably interpersonal associations are more intense than standard patient contacts. The large breadth of a patient's possible needs encourage his dependency, which might not be in a patient's best interest. Carers who allow themselves to become emotionally involved may not be able to provide objective counselling, advice, or medical care.

HIV infection and AIDS should not be allowed to dominate the life of individual carers. This is a risk if conscientious carers (the majority) are exposed to an expanding work load (which may be of their own seeking), especially if facilities are limited. Carers may be unable to cope with the numerous demands or may immerse themselves in caring; both may cause exhaustion—AIDS burnout—with anxiety or depression. Avoidance of this requires regular discussion groups specifically for carers to discuss their individual problems and problems that other members of the group may be having. Feedback and interchange of insights should minimize burnout.

Some carers will know themselves to be HIV positive and will experience the additional stresses of anticipation of the manifestations which their illness might take.

Organization of medical care

The medical care of endstage patients with AIDS requires a teamwork approach (Table 6) comprising, at least, nursing staff, a physiotherapist, a dietitian, appropriate social workers, a psychologist, occupational therapists, counsellors and, where appropriate, a psychiatrist. It would be important to include community carers such as the general practitioner and (with the permission of the patient) relatives, partners of the patient, or any self-help support group worker who may be appropriate. A financial adviser may be another useful member of the team. It is important that the team should be led by a doctor, given the relative importance of medical aspects. It is ideal if such teams cover both in- and outpatient work, as patients often alternate between the two forms of care. Because complicating and essentially unpredictable illnesses occur in AIDS such meetings should be held weekly. Given the appropriate supportive infrastructure and with highly motivated services, in San Francisco 90 per cent of patients with AIDS are now able to die at home.[83]

There is a need to vary the style but not the content of patient care according to their medical condition and life situation. In general, homosexuals have much more organized and reliable self-help support groups in the community, whereas injection drug users tend to have less support and sometimes may actively alienate those who try to help. However, parents of injection drug users, who have previously been exasperated and exhausted by their offspring's behaviour, often show incredible tolerance and forgiveness once the inevitable outcome becomes obvious.

Hospice care for the AIDS patient

Three questions have to be answered. Can hospices deal with the medical problems? Can hospices deal with the relevant patient groups? And, most importantly, should general hospices attempt to deal with patients with AIDS within their current facilities?

Medical problems

Patients with AIDS may have multiple pathology, but so do many hospice patients. There are important differences. Firstly, patients with AIDS may have unusual infections or unusual malignancies, or both. Secondly, the HIV-induced defective immune system causes unusual presentations of illness, that may be different from those in patients with normal immunity, and such patients need to be treated by staff who should have received adequate training in the various aspects of infection and infection control. Thirdly, and perhaps most significantly for maximum effective palliation, it is important that complicating infections or neoplasms are diagnosed rapidly and accurately even at a late stage, and for this to occur general hospital facilities are likely to be required. Most hospices will not have these facilities and nursing care for control of infection might prove difficult to institute. The reason for this is not that nursing staff could not be trained, but rather that it would be difficult to be selective about the control of infection precautions to be employed; in infectious diseases units and AIDS-specific hospices it is easy (and non-discriminatory) to treat all patients as though they were capable of spreading infection, but if a selective policy were employed errors of omission might well occur. Fourthly, patients with AIDS might develop infections that are infectious to others, including tuberculosis,[84] and such illnesses may have to be repeatedly excluded.

Most patients with HIV and AIDS are mostly well for most of the time and may well wish to continue sexual activity and may need specific information and advice regarding safe sex.

Management aspects of certain patient groups

Whilst it would be unrealistic to deny that there is prejudice against homosexuals, malicious prejudice seems rare and probably such prejudice as exists is the misunderstanding that almost all minority groups must expect. However, it may be that non-homosexual patients and their visitors might be more intolerant and it might well be inappropriate to try to educate them in a hospice situation.

Unfortunately, a proportion of injection drug users are truly addicted or vary between abuse, addiction, and abstinence and these patients can provide much disruption. The potential problems are numerous and may be caused by the patients themselves or their visitors. Free floating aggression and antisocial behaviour places a strain on all caring staff. Incessant demands for drugs and unassessable claims to be in severe pain are common. Thefts may occur. Drugs of abuse are smuggled into wards and intravenous lines used for their administration. Security arrangements need to be enhanced, not just for terminal care drugs—an obvious focus of attention—but also for any easily removed, saleable ward property. It is likely that injection drug users, or some of their friends, would alter and dominate the running of a general hospice such that the current achievements of the hospice movement were affected and thereby diminished.

At present, the question of where patients with HIV/AIDS should receive palliative care has not been defined for all situations. Not surprisingly, it is very dependent on local circumstances and there is no generic solution that should be adopted for all situations. In areas with large numbers of patients (such as London or Edinburgh) dedicated hospices are viable. However, since they are dedicated at present they cannot serve all patients since a number of patients require confidentiality which is lost on entering a dedicated hospice. In other areas, care (including palliative care) may be delivered by the local HIV/AIDS unit.

Should current hospice facilities be used?

The answers to this question are controversial, ranging from opinions that any hospice that doesn't accept people with AIDS should not be called a hospice,[85] to opinions that specialized services are required.[86] Perhaps it would be unwise to jeopardize the present achievements by attempting to integrate people with AIDS into the current general hospices. People with AIDS require something different. Perhaps the challenge is either to develop specific AIDS hospices or to integrate hospice facilities and experiences into the existing hospital-based AIDS facilities. In any event, ready access to general hospital diagnostic and treatment facilities would seem essential.

Problems for hospice management

The question of when and where individuals would prefer to die is often a difficult area for an HIV unit that is used to delivering acute and active therapy to broach, since the staff often feel that this may cast a rather too gloomy outlook on the admission. The transition from acute care to palliative care is very difficult for patients with HIV—they may be initially acutely ill with eminently treatable conditions, they may require complex medical treatment such as the treatment of cytomegalovirus retinitis until the last days of life, and not all patients are able to make the decision to opt for palliative care. In those areas where the numbers of HIV patients are low the limited experience of HIV may also make it difficult for carers to determine exactly when it is reasonable to switch from active to palliative care. It is not uncommon for patients to present with what appears to be an easily treatable condition and then it becomes obvious that the problems are insurmountable. It takes considerable experience to know when carers should be discussing quality as much as quantity in terms of a patient's survival and this is perhaps the major reason why HIV units need to be involved in the decisions concerning palliative care. Despite all these problems in our experience it is possible, even with the most difficult patients, to enter into discussions over choices relating to death.

In Edinburgh, where the average patient with HIV/AIDS is aged 33, one-third are female and 60 per cent of the patients have become infected with HIV via injection drug use, to date the majority of patients have died in an acute dedicated unit (37 per cent). The rest have died at home (28 per cent), the local HIV hospice (14 per cent) which only opened in 1991, other locations such as hospices or hospitals (12 per cent), and unknown (8 per cent) (Brettle, in press).

In Edinburgh, unlike other areas dealing with HIV in the United Kingdom, a considerable number of patients (29.5 per cent) died suddenly or unexpectedly (84.5 per cent infected via injection drug use) and planning for death was therefore not possible with all patients. Over an 8 year period, 55 per cent of the expected deaths amongst the patients attending the AIDS unit in an infectious diseases hospital had occurred in the hospital, 19 per cent in the local AIDS hospice, 20 per cent at home, and 5 per cent elsewhere. A preference over place of death had been elicited overall in 55 per cent of the expected deaths, although by 1992 84 per cent of the expected deaths had a documented preference for the place of death compared with only 25 per cent in 1989. The preference of the patients was equally split (32 per cent) between three locations, the AIDS hospital, the local AIDS hospice, and at home with only 4 per cent choosing any other location. Only three expected deaths did not achieve their preference for location of death. All three died in the AIDS hospital rather than at home; one because of a lack of a night sitting service, one because they came from a small community and were concerned over loss of confidentiality, and one who wished for active therapy for cytomegalovirus retinitis until 1 week before death which at that time could not be delivered at home.

Most patients with AIDS are young adults and their present caring team (including doctors, nurses, and counsellors) may only have known them for about 1 year, usually from (at least) the diagnosis of AIDS. All patients, even possibly difficult injection drug users, may develop a strong bond with their hospital team during the necessary repetitive in- and outpatient attendances and it may be unreasonable to expect them to transfer their allegiance to a new team at the endstage of the battle they have fought along with their previous team.

Death

In the United Kingdom, death certificates are public documents yet patients or relatives may wish for confidentiality to be maintained after death. In such circumstances it should be remembered that patients usually die because of complications of their immunodeficiency and that these can be given alone as the cause of death (e.g. skin cancer for Kaposi's sarcoma or severe pneumonia for *Pneumocystis carinii* pneumonia) along with the information that further information may be available later; the death certificate is not amended as a result of further information.

HIV remains infectious for around 1 week after death and a body should be dealt with according to local control of infection protocols, usually ending with the patient being placed in protective coverings (a plastic body bag). This is usually done by the staff on the ward. Those who deal with the patient thereafter have no need to know anything other than that the bag should not be opened. Because viewing of the body after placement in such a bag poses problems, it is important that arrangements are made in advance to allow all those who would wish to say their last farewells to have the opportunity to do so before the deceased patient is placed in the body bag. This may entail keeping the body in bed on the ward for longer than is usually the case. The handling of bodies after death should, of course, observe any religious requirements associated with the patient's beliefs.

There is often a mistaken belief by relatives (and inexperienced carers) that patients dying with HIV or AIDS have to undergo cremation because of the infection risks. It may, therefore, be important to correct this mistaken belief and positively point out to patients or relatives that there is no directive that all patients with HIV have to choose a cremation. In addition, it may be important to emphasize that undertakers are not automatically informed of the diagnosis, simply that the patient died and that there is a danger of infection—however, because of the measures taken to protect the undertakers from any danger of infection they may have a good idea. If the patient comes from a small village or community and dies away from home it certainly may be better to arrange a local cremation and then to transport the ashes back home in order to preserve confidentiality beyond death.

Appendix

The surveillance definitions of AIDS (1987)

The Center for Disease Control, Atlanta, produced a revised definition of AIDS in 1987 which is as follows:

I Without laboratory evidence of HIV infection

If laboratory tests for HIV are not available then provided the following conditions (under 1A) are not present a diagnosis of AIDS can be made provided the disease is diagnosed definitively (under 1B).

IA Causes of immunodeficiency that disqualify diseases as indicators of AIDS in the absence of evidence of HIV infection:

1. high-dose or long-term systemic corticosteroid therapy or other immunosuppressive/cytotoxic therapy for < or = 3 months before the onset of the indicator disease;
2. any of the following diseases diagnosed for < or = 3 months after the diagnosis of the indicator disease: Hodgkin's disease, non-Hodgkin's lymphoma (other than primary brain lymphoma), lymphocytic leukaemia, multiple myeloma, any other cancer of the lymphoreticular or histiocytic tissue, or angioimmunoblastic lymphadenopathy;
3. a genetic (congenital) immunodeficiency syndrome or an acquired immunodeficiency syndrome atypical of HIV infection, such as one involving hypogammaglobulinaemia.

IB Indicator disease diagnosed definitively:

1. candidiasis of the oesophagus, trachea, bronchi, or lungs;
2. cryptococcosis, extrapulmonary;
3. cryptosporidiosis with diarrhoea for > 1 month;
4. cytomegalovirus disease of an organ other than the liver, spleen, or lymph nodes in a patient > or = 1 month of age;

5. herpes simplex virus infection causing a mucocutaneous ulcer that persists for > 1 month; or bronchitis, pneumonitis, or oesophagitis for any duration affecting a patient > or = 1 month of age;
6. Kaposi's sarcoma affecting a patient < or = 60 years of age;
7. lymphoma of the brain (primary) affecting a patient < or = 60 years of age;
8. lymphoid interstitial pneumonia and or pulmonary lymphoid hyperplasia (LIP/PLH) complex affecting a child < or = 12 years of age;
9. *Mycobacterium avium* complex or *M. kansasii* disease, disseminated (at a site other than or in addition to lungs, skin, or cervical or hilar lymph nodes);
10. *Pneumocystis carinii* pneumonia;
11. progressive multifocal leucoencephalopathy;
12. toxoplasmosis of the brain affecting a patient > or = 1 month of age.

II With laboratory evidence of HIV infection

Regardless of the presence of other causes of immunodeficiency outlined above (under IA), in the presence of laboratory evidence of HIV infection, any disease listed above (under IB) or below (under IIA or IIB) indicates a diagnosis of AIDS.

IIA The following conditions, diagnosed definitively:

1. bacterial infections, multiple or recurrent (any combination of at least two within a 2-year period), of the following types affecting a child < 13 years of age: septicaemia, pneumonia, meningitis, bone or joint infection, or abscess of an internal organ or body cavity (excluding otitis media or superficial skin or mucosal abscesses), caused by Haemophilus, Streptococcus (including pneumococcus), or other pyogenic bacteria;
2. coccidioidomycosis, disseminated (at a site other than or in addition to lungs or cervical or hilar lymph nodes);
3. HIV encephalopathy (also called HIV dementia, AIDS dementia, or subacute encephalitis due to HIV);
4. histoplasmosis, disseminated (at a site other than or in addition to lungs or cervical or hilar lymph nodes);
5. isosporiasis with diarrhoea persisting > 1 month;
6. Kaposi's sarcoma at any age;
7. lymphoma of the brain (primary) at any age;
8. other non-Hodgkin's lymphoma of B-cell or unknown immunological phenotype and the following histological types:
   (a) small non-cleaved lymphoma (either Burkitt or non-Burkitt type);
   (b) immunoblastic sarcoma (equivalent to any of the following, although not necessarily in all combinations: immunoblastic lymphoma, large-cell lymphoma, diffuse histiocytic lymphoma, diffuse undifferentiated lymphoma, or a high grade lymphoma).

   Note: lymphomas are not included here if they are of T-cell immunological phenotype or their histological type is not described or is described as lymphocytic, lymphoblastic, small cleaved, or plasmacytoid lymphocytic.
9. any mycobacterial disease caused by mycobacteria other than *M. tuberculosis*, disseminated (at a site other than or in addition to lungs, skin, or cervical or hilar lymph nodes);
10. disease caused by *M. tuberculosis*, extrapulmonary (involving at least one site outside the lungs, regardless of whether there is concurrent pulmonary involvement);
11. salmonella (non-typhoid) septicaemia, recurrent;
12. HIV wasting syndrome (emaciation, slim disease).

IIB The following conditions, diagnosed presumptively:

1. candidiasis of the oesophagus;
2. cytomegalovirus retinitis with loss of vision;
3. Kaposi's sarcoma;
4. lymphoid interstitial pneumonia and or pulmonary lymphoid hyperplasia (LIP/PLH) affecting a child < or = 13 years of age;
5. mycobacterial disease (acid-fast bacilli with species not identified by culture), disseminated (involving at least one site other than or in addition to lungs, skin, or cervical or hilar lymph nodes);
6. *Pneumocystis carinii* pneumonia;
7. toxoplasmosis of the brain affecting a patient > or = 1 month of age.

III With laboratory evidence against HIV infection

With laboratory test results negative for HIV infection, a diagnosis of AIDS for surveillance purposes is ruled out unless:

IIIA all the other causes of immunodeficiency listed above are excluded and

IIIB the patient has had either:

1. *Pneumocystis carinii* pneumonia diagnosed by a definitive method or

2.(a) any of the other diseases indicative of AIDS listed above diagnosed by a definitive method and

2.(b) CD4 count of < or = 400 cells/cm^3.

In 1993, the Center for Disease Control added four AIDS-defining conditions to the 1987 definition of AIDS; these are cervical cancer, two episodes of bacterial pneumonia in a 12 month period, pulmonary tuberculosis, or a CD4 count of less than 200 cells/mm^3. The United Kingdom definition does not include a CD4 count of less than 200 cells/mm^3.

References

1. Centres for Disease Control. Pneumocystis pneumonia—Los Angeles. *Morbidity and Mortality Weekly Report*, 1981; **30**: 250–3.
2. Gottlieb MS, Schroff R, Schanker HM, *et al. Pneumocystis carinii* pneumonia and mucosal candidiasis in previously healthy homosexual men. *New England Journal of Medicine*, 1981; **305**: 1425–31.
3. Revision of the CDC surveillance case definition for acquired immunodeficiency syndrome. *Mortality and Morbidity Weekly Report*, 1987; **36**(Suppl. 1): 1S–15S.
4. Moss AR. AIDS and intravenous drug abuse; the real heterosexual epidemic. *British Medical Journal*, 1987; **294**; 389–90.
5. Schrappe-Bacher M, Rasokat H, Bauer P. High dose intravenous immunoglobulins in HIV-1 infected adults with AIDS-related complex and Walter-Reed 5. *Vox Sanguis*, 1990; **59** (Suppl 1): 3–14.
6. Lee, BL, Safrin S. Drug Interactions and toxicities with patients with AIDS. In: Sande M, Volberding PWB, eds. *Medical Management of AIDS*, 3rd edn. Philadephia: Saunders Co, 1992: 129.
7. Moss AR. Predicting who will progress to AIDS. *British Medical Journal* 1988; **297**: 1067–8.
8. Moss AR, Bacchetti P. Natural history of HIV infection. *AIDS*, 1989; **3**: 55–61.
9. Rutherford GW, Lifson AR, Hessol NA, *et al.* Course of HIV-1 infection in a cohort of homosexual and bisexual men: an 11 year follow up study. *British Medical Journal*, 1990; **301**: 1183–8.
10. Rothenberg R, Woelfel M, Stoneburner R, Milberg J, Parker R, Truman B. Survival with the acquired immunodeficiency syndrome. *New England Journal of Medicine*, 1987; **317**: 1297–302.
11. Justice AC, Feinstein AR, Wells CK. A new prognostic staging system for the acquired immunodeficiency syndrome. *New England Journal of Medicine*, 1989; **320**: 1388–93
12. Fischl MA, Rickman DD, Grieco MH, *et al.* The efficacy of azidothymidine (AZT) in the treatment of patients with AIDS and AIDS-related complex; a double blind controlled trial. *New England Journal of Medicine*, 1987; **317**; 185–91.
13. Fischl MA, Rickman DD, Hansen N, *et al.* The safety and efficacy of Zidovudine (AZT) in the treatment of subjects with mildly symptomatic human immunodeficiency virus—Type 1 (HIV) infection. *Annals of Internal Medicine*, 1990; **112**: 727–37.
14. Anonymous. *Retrovir (Zidovudine)*. Beckenham, Kent: Wellcome Foundation Product Monograph 1988: 1–38.
15. Richman DD, Fischl MA, Greico MH, *et al.* The toxicity of azidothymidine (AZT) in the treatment of patients with AIDS and AIDS-related complex; a double-blind, placebo-controlled trial. *New England Journal of Medicine*, 1987; **317**: 192–6.
16. Schwartz EL, *et al.* Pharmacokinetic interactions of Zidovudine and Methadone in intravenous drug patients. *AIDS*, 1992: **5**: 619–26.
17. Hochster H, Dieterich D, Bozzette S, *et al.* Toxicity of combined ganciclovir and zidovudine for cytomegalovirus disease associated with AIDS. *Annals of Internal Medicine*, 1990; **113**: 111–17.
18. Cooper DA, Pehrson PO, Pederson C, *et al.* The efficacy and safety of zidovudine alone or as cotherapy with acyclovir for the treatment of patients with AIDS and AIDS-related complex: a double-blind, randomized trial. *AIDS*, 1993; **7**: 197–207.
19. Ho DD, Moudgil T, Alam M. Quantitation of human immunodeficiency virus type 1 in the blood of infected persons. *New England Journal of Medicine*, 1989; **321**: 1621–5.
20. Lambert JS, Seidlin M, Reichman RC, *et al.* 2′,3′-dideoxyinosine in patients with the acquired immunodeficiency syndrome or AIDS-related complex. *New England Journal of Medicine*, 1990; **322**: 1333–40.
21. Collier A C, Coombs R W, Fischl M A, *et al.* Combination therapy with zidovudine and didanosine compared with zidovudine alone in HIV-1 infection. *Annals of Internal Medicine*, 1993; **119**: 786–93.
22. Fischl MA, Olson RM, Follansbee SE, *et al.* Zalcitabine compared with zidovudine in patients with advanced HIV-1 infection who received previous zidovudine therapy. *Annals of Internal Medicine*, 1993; **118**: 762–9.
23. Flegg PJ, Jones ME, MacCallum LR, Williams KG, Cook MK, Brettle RP. Effect of Zidovudine on platelet count. *British Medical Journal*, 1989; **298**: 1074–5.
24. Kovacs JA, Masur H. AIDS commentary; Prophylaxis of *Pneumocystis carinii* pneumonia: an update. *Journal of Infectious Diseases*, 1989; **160**: 882–6.
25. Smith DE, McLuckie A, Wyatt J, Gazzard B. Severe exercise hypoxaemia with normal or near normal x-rays: a feature of *Pneumocystis carinii* infection. *Lancet*, 1988; **ii**: 1049–51.
26. National Institutes of Health–University of California Expert Panel for Cortico Steroids as Adjunctive Therapy for Pneumocystis Pneumonia. Consensus Statement. *New England Journal of Medicine*, 1990; **323**: 1500–4.
27. MacFadden DK, Edelson JD, Hyland RH, Rodriguez CH, Inouye T, Rebuck AS. Corticosteroids as an adjunctive therapy in treatment of *Pneumocystis carinii* pneumonia in patients with acquired immunodeficiency syndrome. *Lancet*, 1987; **i**: 1477–9.
28. Miller RF, Semple SJG. Glutocorticoid therapy for severe *Pneumocystitis carinii* pneumonia. *Journal of Infection*, 1990; **21**: 131–7.
29. Fischl MA. Treatment and prophylaxis of *Pneumocystis carinii* pneumonia. *AIDS*, 1988; **2** (Suppl 1): 5143–50.
30. Medina I, Mills J, Leoung G, *et al.* Oral therapy for *Pneumocystis carinii* pneumonia in the acquired immunodeficiency syndrome. *New England Journal of Medicine*, 1990: **323**: 776–82.
31. Toma E, Fournier S, Poisson M, Morrisset R, Phaneut D, Vega C. Clindamycin with Primaquine for *Pneumocystis carinii* pneumonia. *Lancet*, 1989; **i**: 1046–8.
32. Fischl MA, Dickinson GM, LaVoie L. The safety and efficacy of Sulfamethoxazole and trimethoprim chemoprophylaxis for *Pneumocystis carinii* pneumonia in AIDS. *Journal of the American Medical Association*, 1988; **259**: 1185–9.
33. Centres of Disease Control. Guidelines for prophylaxis against *Pneumocystis carinii* pneumonia for persons infected with human immunodeficiency virus. *Journal of the American Medical Association*, 1989; **262**: 335–9.
34. Golden JA, Chernoft D, Hollander H, Feigal D, Conte JE. Prevention of *Pneumocystis carinii* pneumonia by inhaled Pentamidine. *Lancet*, 1989; **i**: 654–7.
35. Leoung GS, Feigal DW, Montgomery AB, *et al.* Aerosolized pentamidine for prophylaxis against *Pneumocystis carinii* pneumonia. *New England Journal of Medicine*, 1990; **323**: 769–75.
36. Thomas S, O'Docherty M, Bateman N. *Pneumocystis carinii* pneumonia (Editorial). *British Medical Journal*, 1990; **300**: 211–2.
37. Stern JJ, Hartman BJ, Sharkey P, *et al.* Oral fluconazole therapy for patients with acquired immunodeficiency syndrome and cryptococcosis: experience with 22 patients. *American Journal of Medicine*, 1988; **85**: 477–89.
38. Buchness MR, Lim HW, Hatcher VA, Sanchez M, Soter NA. Eosinophilic pustular folliculitis in the acquired immunodeficiency syndrome. *New England Journal of Medicine*, 1988; **318**: 1183–6.
39. Esposito R, Foppa Cu, Antinori S. Fluconazole for cryptococcal meningitis. *Annals of Internal Medicine*, 1989; **110**: 170.
40. Leport C, Raffi F, Matheron S, *et al.* Treatment of central nervous system toxoplasmosis with Pyrimethamine/Sulphadiazine combination in thirty-five patients with the Acquired Immunodeficiency Syndrome. *American Journal of Medicine*, 1988; **84**: 94–100.
41. Johns DR, Tierney M, Felsenstein D. Activation of syphilis in AIDS. *New England Journal of Medicine*, 1987; **316**: 1569–72.
42. McArthur JC, Hoover DR, Bacellar H, *et al.* Dementia in AIDS patients: incidence and risk factors. *Neurology*, 1993; **43**: 2245–52.
43. Sidtis JJ, Gatsonis C, Price RW, *et al.*: Zidovudine treatment of the AIDS dementia complex: results of a placebo-controlled trial. *Annals of Neurology*, 1993; **33**: 343–9
44. Cornblath DR, McArthur JC. Predominantly sensory neuropathy in patients with AIDS and AIDS-related complex. *Neurology* (NY), 1988; **38**: 794–96.

45. Simpson DM, Citak KA, Godfrey D, Godbold J, Wolfe DE. Myopathies associated with human immunodeficiency virus and zidovudine. Can their effects be distinguished. *Neurology*, 1993; **43**: 971–6.
46. Whiteside ME, Barkin JS, May RG, *et al.* Enteric coccidiosis in patients with the acquired immunodeficiency syndrome. *American Journal of Tropical Medicine and Hygiene*, 1984; **33**: 1065–72.
47. Von Roenn JH, Murphy RL, Weber KM, Williams LM, Weitzman SA. Megestrol acetate for treatment of cachexia associated with human immunodeficiency virus (HIV) infection. *Annals of Internal Medicine*, 1988; **109**: 840–1.
48. Monfardini S, Vaccher E, Pizzocaro G. Unusual malignant tumours in 49 patients with HIV infection. *AIDS*, 1989; **3**: 447–52.
49. Glassock RJ, Cohen AH, Danovitch G, Parsa KP. Human immunodeficiency virus (HIV) infection and the kidney. *Annals of Internal Medicine*, 1990; **112**: 35–49.
50. Rouzioux C, Costagliola D, Burgard M, Blanche S, Mayaux M-J, Griscelli C, Valleron A-J, the HIV infection in Newborns French Collaborative Study Group. Timing of mother-to-child transmission depends on maternal status. *AIDS*, 1993; **7**(suppl): S49–S52.
51. European Collaborative Study. Caesarean section and risk of vertical transmission of HIV-1 infection. *Lancet*, 1994; **343**: 1464–7.
52. Connor EM, Sperling RS, Gelber RD, *et al.* Reduction of maternal-infant transmission of human immunodeficiency virus type 1 with zidovudine treatment. *New England Journal of Medicine*, 1994; **331**: 1173–80.
53. Bradbeer C. Women and HIV. *British Medical Journal*, 1989; **298**: 342–3.
54. Mok JQ, Giaquinto C, DeRossi A, Grosch-Worner I, Ades AE, Peckham CJ. Infants born to mothers seropositive for human immunodeficiency virus. Preliminary findings from a multicentre European Study. *Lancet*, 1987; **i**: 1164–8.
55. Ruff AL, Coberly J, Halsey NA, *et al.* Prevalence of HIV-1 DNA and p24 antigen in breast mild and correlation with maternal factors. *AIDS*, 1994; **7**: 68–73.
56. Centers for Disease Control: Zidovudine for the prevention of HIV transmission from mother to infant. *Morbidity and Mortality Weekly Report*, 1994; **43**: 285–7.
57. Selwyn PA, Alcabes P, Hartel D, Buono D, *et al.* Clinical manifestations and predictors of disease progression in drug users with HIV infection. *New England Journal of Medicine*, 1992; **327**: 1697–703.
58. Thompson M, Whyte B, Morris A, Rimland D, Thompson S. Gender differences in the spectrum of HIV disease in Atlanta. *VII International Conference on AIDS, June 1991 Florence Italy*; Abstract MC 3115.
59. Willocks L, Cowan FM, Brettle RP, MacCallum LR, McHardy S, Richardson A. Early HIV infection in Scottish women. *VII International Conference on AIDS, June 1991, Florence Italy*; Abstract MB 2433.
60. Rothenberg R, Woelfel M, Stoneburner R, Milberg J, Parker R, Truman B. Survival with the acquired immunodeficiency syndrome. *New England Journal of Medicine*, 1987; **317**: 1297–302.
61. Lemp GF, Payne SF, Neal D, Temelso T, Rutherford GW. Survival trends for patients with AIDS. *Journal of the American Medical Association*, 1990; **263**: 402–6.
62. Lindan CP, Allen S, Serufilira A, *et al.* Predictors of mortality among HIV infected women in Kigali, Rwanda. *Annals of Internal Medicine*, 1992; **116**: 320–8.
63. Areneta MC, Young MA, Pierce P. Natural History of HIV disease in an urban cohort of women. *VIth International Conference on AIDS, June 1990, San Francisco, USA*. Abstract FB 432.
64. Serraino D, Zaccarelli M, Franceschi S, Greco D. The epidemiology of AIDS-associated Kaposi's sarcoma in Italy. *AIDS*, 1992; **6**: 1015–9.
65. Byrne MA, Taylor-Robinson D, Munday PE, Harris JRW. The common occurrence of human papillomavirus infection and intraepithelial neoplasia in women infected by HIV. *AIDS*, 1989; **3**: 379–82.
66. Mandelblatt JS, Fahs M, Garibaldi K, Senie RT, Peterson HB. Association between HIV infection and cervical neoplasia: implications for clinical care of women at risk for both conditions. *AIDS*, 1992; **6**: 173–8.
67. O'Neill WM, Sherrard J. Pain in human immunodeficiency virus disease: a review. *Pain*, 1993; **54**: 3–14.
68. The Panos Institute. *AIDS and the Third World*. London: Panos Publications, 1988: 83.
69. Conlon CP. Clinical aspects of HIV infection in developing countries. *British Medical Bulletin*, 1988; **44**: 104–14.
70. Katabira E, Goodgame RW, eds. *AIDS Care: Diagnostic and Treatment Strategies for Health Workers*. Entebbe, Republic of Uganda: AIDS Control Program, Ministry of Health, 1989.
71. Goodgame RW. AIDS in Uganda—clinical and social features. *New England Journal of Medicine*, 1990; **323**: 383–9.
72. Robertson JR, Skidmore CA. *AIDS in the Family*. Second report by project number k/OPR/2/2/C668(C754). Scottish Home and Health Department, 1989.
73. Mok J. Paediatric HIV infection. In: Green J, McCreaner A, eds. *Counselling in HIV Infection and AIDS*. Oxford: Blackwell Scientific Publications, 1989: 157–66
74. Duckett M, Orkin AJ. AIDS-related migration and travel policies and restrictions: a global survey. *AIDS*, 1989; **3** (suppl 1): S231–S252.
75. Atkinson H, Grant I, Kennedy CJ, *et al.* Prevalence of psychiatric disorder among men infected with human immunodeficiency virus. *Archives of General Psychiatry*, 1988; **45**: 859–64.
76. Richardson AM. Psychiatric and neuropsychological aspects of HIV infection. In: Anderson C, Wilkie P, eds. *Reflective Helping in HIV and AIDS*. Open University Press, 1992.
77. Marzuk PM, Tierney H, Tardiff K, *et al.* Increased risk of suicide in persons with AIDS. *Journal of the American Medical Association*, 1988; **259**: 1333–7.
78. King MB. Psychological aspects of HIV Infection and AIDS. What have we learned? *British Journal of Psychology*, 1990; **156**: 151–6.
79. Maxwell J, Egan V, Chiswick A, *et al.* HIV-1 associated cognitive/motor complex in an injecting drug user. *AIDS Care*, 1991; **3**: 381.
80. Lechtenberg R, Sher JH. *AIDS in the Nervous System*. Edinburgh: Churchill Livingstone, 1988.
81. Kubler-Ross E. *On Death and Dying*. London: Tavistock,1970.
82. Wallach MA, Kogan N, Burt RB. Group risk taking and field dependence–independence of group members. *Sociometry*, 1967; **30**: 323–38.
83. Martin JP. The AIDS home care and hospice programme. *American Journal of Hospice Care*, 1986; **3**: 35–7.
84. Pitchenik AE, Burr J, Laufter M, *et al.* Outbreaks of drug-resistant tuberculosis at AIDS centre. *Lancet*, 1990; **ii**: 440–1.
85. Di Tullio SA. Where can an AIDS patient turn for care? *American Journal of Hospice Care*, 1986; **3**: 4.
86. Saunders C. Sounding board: hospice for AIDS patients. New teams should be developed for AIDS care. *American Journal of Hospice Care*, 1987; **4**: 7–8.

20.2 AIDS: aspects in children

Stephen D.R. Green

Introduction

The World Health Organization (WHO) estimates that almost half of all newly infected HIV adults world-wide are women. In Europe the number of women of childbearing age with AIDS has increased from 11 per cent in 1989 to 19 per cent in 1993.[1] As this figure increases so does the number of infants with HIV infection.

The brunt of paediatric HIV infection falls on countries which have the fewest resources to cope. For many people the illness of the young infant is the first indication that the virus has a foothold in the family. It often destabilizes relationships; affected families are frequently isolated and may lack the support from the extended family and friends normally expected when coping with a chronic disease.

Effective palliative care of children with AIDS requires an understanding of how the disease affects the child and his family, careful clinical assessment, and familiarity with the range of problems that may benefit from physical, social, and spiritual intervention. With increasing scientific knowledge and the development of new treatments, improved social awareness and responsibility, changing systems of health care delivery, and the recognition of the rights and needs of particular groups (e.g. women and adolescents), there is a continuing need to develop imaginative family-based services for people affected by HIV.

Transmission

Children acquire HIV infection from infected blood products, their infected mothers, injecting equipment that has not been properly sterilized, non-sexual contact with infected bodily fluids, or sexual contact, either voluntarily in adolescents or through sexual abuse by an infected perpetrator.

Routine blood testing was introduced in the United Kingdom in 1985 and this procedure has virtually eliminated the risk of infection from blood or its products. However, nearly 300 haemophiliac children were reported HIV positive in the United Kingdom in 1986.[2]

Transmission through infected blood remains an important problem in many countries where testing is not routine. The magnitude of this problem may be underestimated. During 1986 in one large hospital in Kinshasa, 27 000 units of blood were transfused of which 67 per cent were to children. The estimated seroprevalence rate of 6.3 per cent meant that 1114 children would have been infected with HIV (unpublished observation). Following this, strict transfusion guidelines were established to achieve a reduction in unnecessary transfusions.[3]

Household transmission of HIV infection (other than through sexual contact, injecting drug use, or breast feeding) is rare. The risk of transmission is less than 0.1 per cent in a single mucous membrane exposure.[4] Eight cases (five children) have been described and emphasize the importance of proper care and protection in the home when nursing infected persons.[5]

Most children acquire the infection from their mothers. This accounted for 90 per cent of childhood AIDS cases reported to the Center for Disease Control, Atlanta, in 1992. Several factors have been implicated in vertical transmission (Table 1).

Transmission rates vary from 14 to 40 per cent.[17–19] They are higher in developing countries than in Europe or North America. Inadequate facilities for diagnosing infection in young infants and breast feeding have been offered as explanations for these differences. Vertical transmission of HIV-2 is rare.[20,21]

Transmission may be *in utero*, intrapartum, or post partum through breast feeding. The bimodal onset of HIV-related disease in infants and children supports this hypothesis. The detection of HIV in fetal tissue as early as 12 to 15 weeks' gestation,[22] placental abnormalities (chorioamnionitis, funisitis), and detection of the virus within a week of birth in infants subsequently shown to be infected support *in utero* acquisition of HIV.

Intrapartum transmission occurs through contact with infected blood and amniotic fluid during delivery. HIV may enter the circulation through the mucosa, stomach, conjunctiva, or skin abrasions. HIV cannot be cultured for about 6 weeks following

Table-1 Factors which may be implicated in vertical transmission[6–16]

Advanced stage of maternal infection
Impaired maternal immunological status
Maternal virus load
High levels of viral replications
Unprotected sex with multiple partners before and during pregnancy
Low maternal vitamin A levels
Vaginal delivery
Breast feeding
Low gestational age (<34 weeks)
Neonatal skin abrasion
Neutral neonatal stomach pH

Table 2 Sensitivities of early diagnostic tests of HIV infection in infants

Method	Sensitivity (%)				
	1 week	2–4 weeks	1–2 months	3–6 months	>6 months
Culture	30–50	50	70–90	>90	>90
PCR	30–50	50	70–90	>90	>90
p24ag	10–25	20–50	30–60	30–50	20–40
ICDp24ag	63*	85–100	ND	ND	ND
IgA	<10	10–30	20–50	50–80	>90
IVAP			44†	>95	>95
IVAG		80‡	85–100	85–100	85–100

Abbreviations: PCR, polymerase chain reaction; ICDp24ag, immune complex dissociated p24 antigen; IVAP, *in vitro* antibody production; IVAG, *in vitro* antigen.
* From ref. 28.
† From ref. 29.
‡ From ref. 30 (small sample size).

transmission in adults and children, and the inability to demonstrate the virus at birth in infants subsequently shown to be infected suggests the intrapartum timing of infection. Fifty to seventy per cent of infants may be infected in this way.[23]

HIV-1 may be transmitted through breast milk.[24] The additional risk of HIV-1 transmission through breast feeding has been estimated at 14 per cent.[25] Where seroconversion occurs during lactation, the postnatal transmission rate may be as high as 60 per cent.[24] Not all infants breast fed by infected mothers become infected. The presence of HIV-1-infected cells and a defective IgM response in the milk 15 days post partum are strongly predictive of infection in the child. Anti-HIV-1 IgM and IgA may protect against postnatal transmission of the virus.[26]

Therefore there are compelling arguments against breast feeding, but only in countries where there are safe alternative feeding methods. In many poor communities breast feeding is essential for survival, and the risk of death from common infections is two to 14 times higher in non-breast-fed infants.[27]

Diagnosis

The hope of extending survival and improving the quality of life through effective prophylaxis for *Pneumocystis carinii* pneumonia and antiviral therapy depends on the early identification of infected infants before symptoms develop.

Diagnosis in the older child and adult is by the detection of anti-HIV IgG antibodies. Identification of the infected infant is complicated by the placental transfer of maternal IgG antibodies to HIV, the timing of HIV acquisition, and the relative immaturity of the newborn's immune system. The inability to establish the timing of infection leads to difficulties in determining the sensitivity of the various diagnostic tests available (Table 2).

Viral culture is considered to be the gold standard. Both viral culture and polymerase chain reaction are expensive. *In vitro* antibody production and *in vitro* antigen production depend on cultured peripheral blood mononuclear cells and are expensive techniques. Immune complex dissociated p24 antigen has a sensitivity approaching that of culture and polymerase chain reaction and is much cheaper. IgA is very sensitive for infants aged over 6 months and is the most appropriate technique for laboratories unable to perform complex and expensive tests.[31]

The Center for Disease Control, Atlanta, has established the following criteria for the diagnosis of HIV infection (1987 AIDS surveillance case definition).[32]

(1) HIV infected

  (a) child less than 18 months

  - positive results on two separate occasions (not cord blood) for virus culture, polymerase chain reaction, or p24 antigen, or
  - meets criteria for AIDS

  (b) child aged 18 months or more

  - HIV antibody positive by repeatedly reactive enzyme immunoassay and confirmatory test (e.g. Western blot), or
  - meets any criterion in (a)

(2) Seroreverter: child who is born to an HIV-infected mother and who has

- two or more antibody negative tests at 6 to 18 months or one negative antibody test after 18 months, and
- no other laboratory evidence of infection, and
- has not had an AIDS-defining condition

Immunology

An overview of the immunological aspects of HIV infection has been given in the previous chapter. Essentially, the T4 cell controls all levels of immune response: inflammation, antigen processing and presentation, primary immune response, and the development of immune memory.

In immunological terms, HIV infection in children is a different disease from that in adults. HIV infection in adults occurs in the presence of a competent immune system. Immune memory helps to protect the adult against secondary infections after contact with

Table 3 CD4 counts and the revised classification of paediatric HIV infection

Immunological category	CD4 count (μl (%))					
	<12 months		1–5 years		6–12 years	
1. No evidence of suppression	≥1500	(25)	≥1000	(≥25)	≥500	(≥25)
2. Moderate suppression	750–1499	(15–24)	500–999	(15–24)	200–499	(15–24)
3. Severe suppression	<750	(<15)	<500	(<15)	<200	<15

From ref. 34.

HIV, and clinical latency can be prolonged for 8 to10 years. As the defences are gradually overwhelmed, so the disease expresses itself clinically.

HIV infection in infants occurs at a time when the immune system is still naïve but encountering many new antigens. Not only does the infant mount a suboptimal response to infection through a poor inflammatory reaction and inadequate antigen processing, but he or she is unable to develop a repertoire of specific antibodies and sensitized T cells because of damage to the memory cells. Thus the infant becomes very vulnerable to secondary infections. The rate of progression of the disease is much faster, and the period of latency is much briefer (18–24 months). Symptomatic infants usually die by the age of 3 years.

Certain immunological markers are helpful in determining the rate of progression of the disease and the optimum time to instigate preventive or therapeutic measures. In adults the CD4 count has been used for many years. Normal CD4 counts have only recently been established in children[33] and incorporated into the revised classification of paediatric HIV infection (Table 3).[34]

Other useful markers of disease progression include serial IgA measurements and *in vitro* antibody production, but these have not yet been linked to therapeutic interventions.

Classification

The classification of HIV infection in children under 13 years was revised in 1994.[34] Children are classified according to clinical, immunological, and infection status, with the aim of reflecting the stage of the disease and therefore having some prognostic significance.

Infection status is determined by the various tests discussed above (Table 2). Immunological status is determined by CD4 counts (Table 3) and immunosuppression can be rated as severe (3), moderate (2), or none (1). Children are classified into one of four clinical categories (A1–3, B1–3, C1–3, N1–3) based on signs, symptoms, or diagnoses related to HIV infection (Table 4. If a perinatally exposed child's HIV status is undetermined, the prefix E is added before the appropriate code (Fig. 1). Comparison with the 1987 classification is shown in Table 5.[34]

In areas where laboratory information cannot be obtained, the WHO AIDS surveillance case definition (modified 1994)[35] is useful for identifying infected children (Table 6). However, its specificity and sensitivity are not very high, particularly where tuberculosis is prevalent. Its advantages are ease of use and low cost.

Clinical manifestations and their management

There are no significant differences between HIV-infected and uninfected infants at birth. An HIV dysmorphology syndrome has been described, but is more likely to be due to other factors, such as maternal drug abuse during pregnancy and coinfections, than to be an effect of the virus itself.

There are marked differences between adults and children in the clinical expression of HIV infection (Table 7). A small number of infants will present with serious bacterial infections or *Pneumocystis carinii* pneumonia within a few months. However, the majority will present with a slowly progressive course typified by the symptoms and signs listed in Table 4.

Growth and nutrition

Poor nutrition and growth failure increase morbidity and shorten the lifespan of children with HIV infection. The majority of infected children fail to thrive, and this has been shown to be a prognostic marker for progression to AIDS and survival (Fig. 2).[36,37] Nutritional management may be difficult because of anorexia, recurrent fevers and infections, mouth ulceration, chronic diarrhoea, neurological, renal or cardiac complications or neglect. The resulting malnutrition affects the integrity of mucosal barriers, the ability to mount an acute phase response and cellular immune function.

Early nutritional intervention may help to protect the immune system and therefore reduce the susceptibility to disease and improve the quality of life. All children should have their weight, length, and head circumference plotted monthly on standard charts. Any child who fails to gain weight or grow must be fully assessed by both a paediatrician and a dietitian. This assessment will include the following:

(1) history (feeding; fever, diarrhoea or vomiting);

(2) estimation of dietary intake by 24-h recall;

(3) treatment of underlying problems;

(4) estimation of catch-up requirements (this should take into account the increased caloric requirements for stress, e.g. 12 per cent per °C rise in temperature, 25 per cent for diarrhoea);

(5) formulation of altered diet.

Table 4 The 1994 classification of HIV infection in children: clinical categories

Category N: not symptomatic
No symptoms or signs due to HIV infection or only one condition listed in A

Category A: mildly symptomatic
Two or more of the conditions listed below but none of those listed in B or C
- Lymphadenopathy (≥0.5 cm at more than two sites; bilateral = one site)
- Hepatomegaly
- Splenomegaly
- Dermatitis
- Parotitis
- Recurrent or persistent upper respiratory infection, sinusitis, or otitis media

Category B: moderately symptomatic
Symptomatic conditions other than those in A or C, including the following
- Anaemia (<8 g/dl), neutropenia (<1000/mm^3), or thrombocytopenia (<100 000/mm^3) persisting more than 30 days
- Bacterial meningitis, pneumonia, or sepsis (single episode)
- Oropharyngeal candidiasis (thrush), persisting more than 2 months in children aged more than 6 months
- Cardiomyopathy
- Cytomegalovirus infection, onset before 1 month of age
- Diarrhoea, recurrent or chronic
- Hepatitis
- Herpes simplex virus stomatitis, recurrent (more than two episodes in one year)
- Herpes simplex virus bronchitis, pneumonitis, or oesophagitis with onset before 1 month of age
- Herpes zoster (shingles) involving at least two distinct episodes or more than one dermatome
- Leiomyosarcoma
- Lymphoid interstitial pneumonia
- Nephropathy
- Nocardiasis
- Persisting fever (lasting > 1 month)
- Toxoplasmosis, onset before 1 month of age
- Varicella, disseminated (complicated chickenpox)

Category C: severely symptomatic
- Serious bacterial infections*
- Candidiasis, oesophageal or pulmonary
- Coccidioidomycosis, disseminated
- Cryptococcosis, extrapulmonary
- Cryptosporidiosis or isosporiasis with diarrhoea for more than 1 month
- Cytomegalovirus disease with onset of symptoms after 1 month of age (at a site other than liver, spleen, or lymph nodes)
- Encephalopathy†
- Herpes simplex virus infection‡
- Histoplasmosis, disseminated
- Kaposi's sarcoma
- Lymphoma
- *Mycobacterium tuberculosis*, disseminated or extrapulmonary
- *Mycobacterium avium* or *Mycobacterium kansasii* disseminated
- *Pneumocystis carinii* pneumonia
- Progressive multifocal leucoencephalopathy
- Salmonella (non-typhoid) septicaemia, recurrent
- Toxoplasmosis of the brain with onset at more than 1 month of age
- Wasting syndrome§

* Multiple or recurrent infections (i.e. any combination of at least two culture-confirmed infections within a 2-year period) of the following types: septicaemia, pneumonia, meningitis, bone or joint infection, abscess of an internal organ or body cavity.

† At least one of the following progressive findings present for at least 2 months in the absence of a concurrent illness other than HIV which could explain the findings: (a) failure to attain or loss of developmental milestones; (b) impaired brain growth or acquired microcephaly; (c) symmetric motor deficit (paresis, pathological reflexes, ataxia, or gait disturbance).

‡ Causing a mucocutaneous ulcer persisting for more than 1 month, or bronchitis, pneumonitis, or oesophagitis for any duration affecting a child more than 1 month of age.

§ (a) Persistent weight loss more than 10 per cent of baseline, or (b) downward crossing of at least two percentile lines on the weight-for-age chart in a child 1 year of age or more, or (c) less than fifth percentile on weight-for-height chart on two consecutive measurements at least 30 days apart plus (i) chronic diarrhoea (two stools or more per day for at least 30 days) or (ii) documented fever (at least 30 days intermittent or constant).

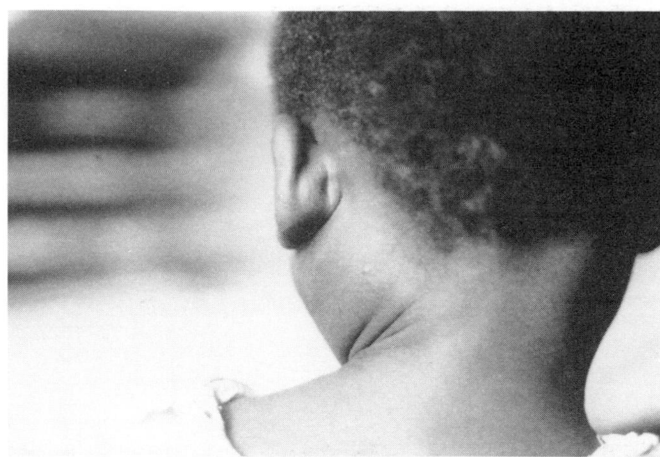

Fig. 1 Parotid enlargement in an African girl with HIV infection.

Table 6 WHO AIDS surveillance case definition (1994)

Major signs	Weight loss at least 10% or abnormally slow growth
	Chronic diarrhoea for more than 1 month
	Prolonged fever for more than 1 month, intermittent or constant
Minor signs	Persistent cough for more than 1 month
	Generalized pruritic dermatitis
	History of herpes zoster
	Oropharyngeal candidiasis
	Chronic progressive or disseminated herpes simplex infection
	Generalized lymphadenopathy
	Confirmed maternal HIV infection

AIDS is suspected when a child presents with two major and two minor signs in the absence of known causes of immunosuppression.
From ref. 35.

Simple interventions such as the use of special teats to reduce the amount of work of sucking (e.g. the Haberman teat), or smaller more frequent feeds and correction of maternal feeding habits, should be considered. Caloric intake can be increased in small children by adding glucose polymers or medium-chain triglyceride oil to the feed. Oral supplements may not be adequate, and recourse to nasogastric feeding (intermittent or continuous overnight), gastrostomy tube, or parenteral hyperalimentation may be required. Oral feeding should be maintained so that children retain the ability to chew, suck, and swallow. This should all be carried out at home; hospital admission is only used in refractory cases to assess growth when optimum intake is provided. Zidovudine therapy has been helpful in improving nutritional status.

Neurological assessment

HIV-associated progressive encephalopathy describes the active primary infection of the brain by HIV.[38] Opportunistic infections and tumours may also affect the central nervous system (see below). Some infants have a 'subacute progressive' syndrome with increasing motor dysfunction, acquired microcephaly, and loss of milestones. A spastic quadriparesis with or without pseudobulbar signs may result.

Table 5 Comparison of the 1987 and 1994 classifications

1987	1994
P–0	Prefix E
P–1	N
P–2A	A,B,C
P–2B	C
P–2C	B
P–2D1	C
P–2D2	C
P–2D3	B
P–2E1	C
P–2E2	B
P–2F	B

From ref. 34.

The rule in most children is a gradual slowing of development. The rate of acquisition of new skills is slow. There is no loss of milestones. Serial head circumference measurements may indicate poor brain growth (Fig. 3). Some children may develop motor signs. In school-age children, loss of interest in school performance, social withdrawal, or increased emotional lability may be early signs of central nervous system impairment.

Brain scans in affected children may show variable degrees of cerebral atrophy and white matter abnormalities. There may be calcification of the basal ganglia.[39] The cerebrospinal fluid is generally normal.

Ideally, children should be followed regularly by a multidisciplinary team in a child development centre. Full neurological examination must be performed on any child found to have developmental delay or neurological symptoms. Children with developmental delay but no other neurological findings should be reassessed in 6 months. Those with focal neurological signs or progressive dysfunction should have further tests which might include the following:

- full blood count and VDRL;
- cerebrospinal fluid examination (protein, cells, VDRL, cultures);
- ophthalmological examination for retinitis;
- CT or MRI scan of brain;
- electroencephalogram in the case of seizures.

Specific infections of the central nervous system will require treatment (see later). Anticonvulsants may be required for seizures.

Prompt recognition of deficits allows the child to be enrolled in an early intervention programme or to have an early nursery placement. Older children with deficits should be assessed by a psychologist to determine any special educational needs.

Table 7 Comparison of the clinical expression of HIV infection in adults and children

Children	Adults
1. Total lymphocyte levels and CD4 counts higher in child <2 years	1. Kaposi's sarcoma more common
2. Hypergammaglobulinaemia common	2. Acute 'mononucleosis-like' onset may occur
3. Recurrent pyogenic infections more common	3. Latency period longer
4. Lymphoid intersitial pneumonia more common	4. *P. carinii* pneumonia and other AIDS-defining opportunistic infections have a better prognosis
5. Encephalopathy more common and more severe	5. Parotid swelling infrequent

Gastrointestinal tract

The gastrointestinal tract is a major site of disease. Enteric infections are common but disaccharide intolerance and an HIV enteropathy leading to malabsorption have been described.[40,41] In cases of diarrhoea stool examination will include the following:

- microscopy for white cells (more than five cells with acute diarrhoea suggests bacterial infection);
- examination for ova, cysts, and parasites;
- culture for bacterial pathogens;
- presence of *Clostridium difficile* toxin;
- viral studies;
- smear for acid-fast bacilli;
- reducing substances.

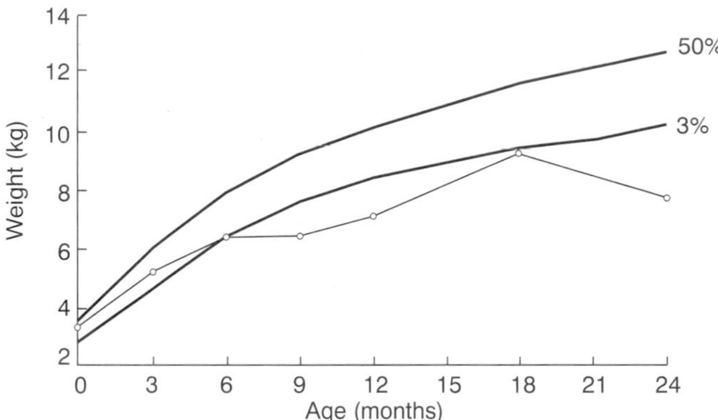

Fig. 2 Failure to thrive in a Zairian child with HIV infection. He died at 26 months.

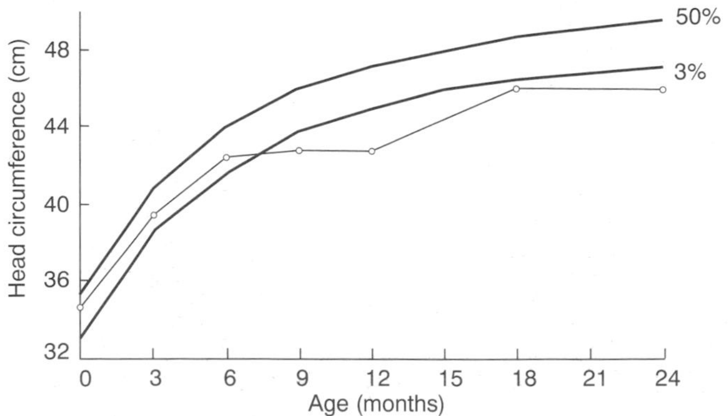

Fig. 3 Head circumference of the child in Fig. 2.

Therapy aimed at treating and preventing dehydration should be given to all children with diarrhoea regardless of aetiology. Ideally, oral rehydration solution should be used. Intravenous treatment may be required in severe cases where there is considerable electrolyte disturbance. Rehydration by nasogastric tube is a cheap and effective alternative in many countries where sterile solutions are expensive and in short supply.[42]

Chronic diarrhoea is a frequent and frustrating problem. It may be due to identifiable pathogens which should be treated. In many cases no obvious cause is found and many mechanisms may be involved, for example bacterial overgrowth, antibiotics, malabsorption, and irritation by bile salts. A small-bowel biopsy may show villous atrophy.

In non-specific chronic diarrhoea metronidazole 25 mg/kg/day three times daily for 7 to 14 days is often effective with or without cholestyramine (to bind bile salts) for 7 days. Antidiarrhoeal agents (loperamide or opioids) should be used cautiously.

Dysphagia is often associated with Candida or herpes simplex infections of the mouth or oesophagus (Fig. 4). The presence of oral thrush and retrosternal pain on swallowing are suggestive. Confirmation may be obtained by the demonstration of mucosal ulceration on barium swallow or endoscopy. A barium swallow will not distinguish between Candida and herpes simplex ulceration. Cytomegalovirus oesophagitis may occur.

Symptomatic relief can be obtained with local topical anaesthetics, for example lignocaine 5 per cent lozenges or benzydamine mouthwash or spray. Nystatin and clotrimazole are useful for oral thrush, but ketoconazole or fluconazole may be required for oesophageal disease. Treatment may be required for 2 to 4 weeks. Acyclovir is indicated for herpes simplex oesophagitis. Ganciclovir suppresses symptoms due to cytomegalovirus. It should not be forgotten that gastro-oesophageal reflux is a common cause of oesophagitis in children.

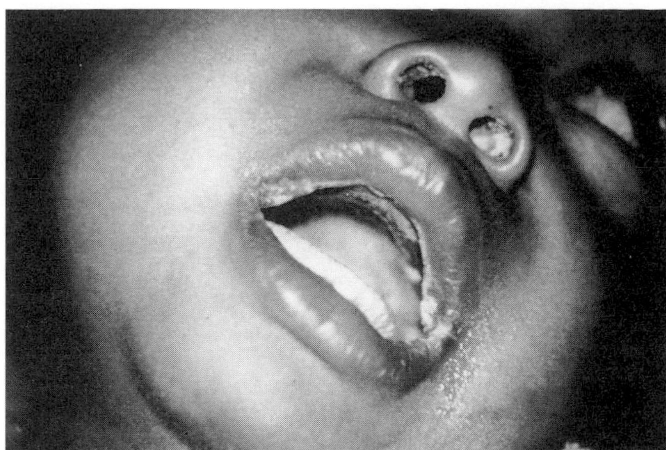

Fig. 4 Severe oral candidiasis in an African infant.

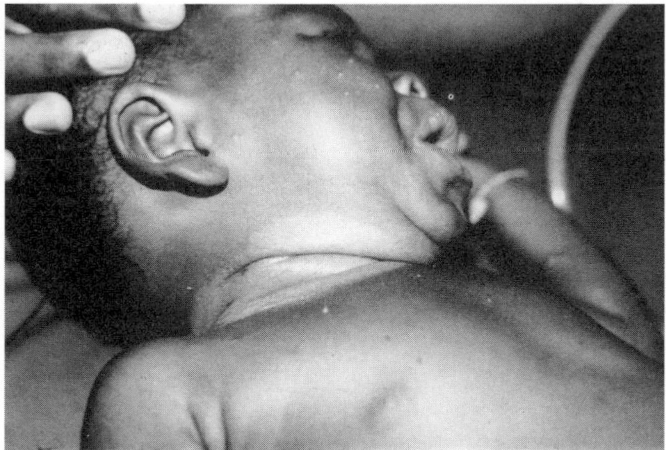

Fig. 6 Candida infection of neck skin fold.

The liver is frequently affected. Hepatomegaly and raised liver enzymes are often noted, but clinical jaundice is rare. Specific pathogens (e.g. cytomegalovirus, *Mycobacterium avium intracellulare*, Epstein–Barr virus) may be implicated, but this is usually as part of a disseminated infection.

Skin

The most common skin manifestations of HIV in children are infections (bacterial, viral, or fungal), exacerbations of childhood dermatoses, or drug reactions. Cutaneous Kaposi sarcoma is rare in children.

Staphylococci and streptococci are the most common bacterial agents causing impetigo, cellulitis, and abscesses. They should be treated with appropriate oral antibiotics. Severe infections may require intravenous therapy.

Recalcitrant napkin candidiasis is one of the most common skin infections (Fig. 5). Candida may also affect the skin folds (neck and axilla) (Fig. 6) and nails (paronychia). Topical nystatin or an imidazole cream are usually effective, but oral therapy may be required in addition to eradicate a gastrointestinal source of infection.

Fungal infections may become severe and widespread in HIV. *Tinea corporis* will respond to an imidazole cream, but Whitfield's ointment is a cheap and effective alternative. Nail and scalp ringworm are best treated with oral griseofulvin for 4 to 6 weeks.

Herpes simplex commonly causes persistent severe erosion of the lips and tongue, but vesicular lesions may occur on the fingers. Severe cases should be treated with intravenous acyclovir (750 mg/m^2/day every 8 h) for 7 to 10 days, whereas milder cases will respond to oral treatment (200 mg five times daily). Herpes zoster infection may be atypical and more severe in HIV, and may cause significant discomfort and scarring. It is treated with intravenous acyclovir 1200 mg/m^2/day every 8 h for 1 to 2 weeks (Fig. 7).

Molluscum contagiosum may be widespread in HIV. Small numbers of lesions can be dealt with by curettage, but this is difficult where they are numerous. Recurrence following removal is common. Human papillomavirus infection may manifest as multiple verruca vulgaris and condylomata acuminata. The presence of the latter may alert the paediatrician to possible sexual abuse. Cryotherapy, podophyllin, and surgical excision are standard treatments, but recurrence is frequent.

Scabies is frequent, and children may develop the severe crusted or Norwegian form. There is a widespread scaling papular eruption harbouring hundreds of mites, and the child is very contagious.

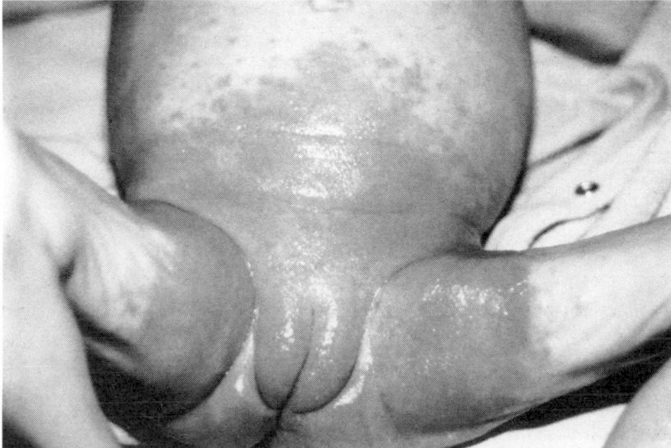

Fig. 5 Severe napkin candidiasis. Note wasting of the thighs. (By courtesy of Dr A Minford.)

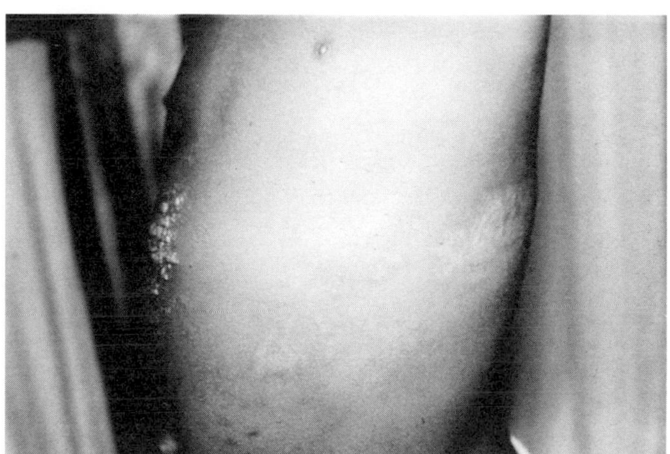

Fig. 7 Recurrent varicella zoster in an African child. Note the scars from previous varicella infection and the vesicles of recent infection.

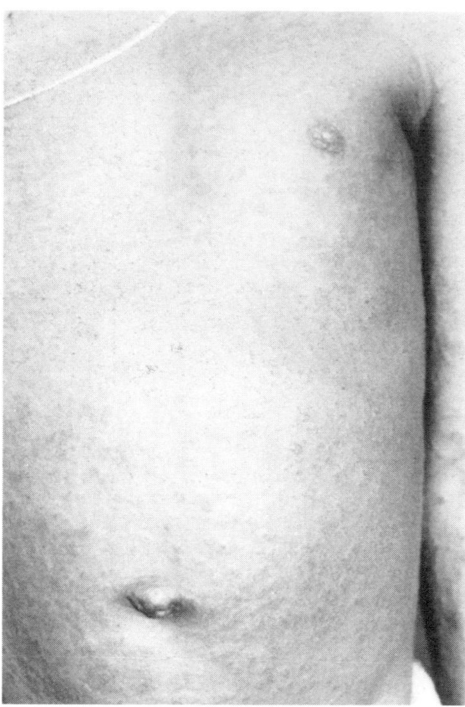

Fig. 8 Drug eruption due to thiacetazone.

The affected child and all household members should be treated by an application of aqueous lindane or permethrin to the whole body. This may need to be repeated. All clothing and bedding should be washed at the time of treatment.

Seborrhoeic dermatitis may be severe in HIV. It should be treated with topical steroids combined with an imidazole. Atopic dermatitis may be exacerbated by HIV infection. It will generally respond to standard treatment with topical steroids, emollients, and antihistamines.

Drug eruptions are common and present most frequently as with a generalized morbilliform eruption (Fig. 8). Occasionally, the Stevens–Johnson syndrome may occur (Fig. 9). This is particularly likely with thiacetazone, an antituberculosis drug widely used in the Third World. Thiacetazone is contraindicated in the presence of HIV infection. Co-trimoxazole is often implicated.

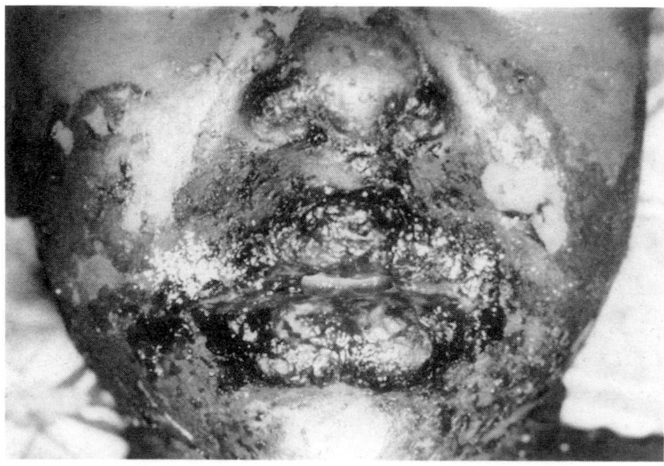

Fig. 9 Stevens–Johnson syndrome due to thiacetazone.

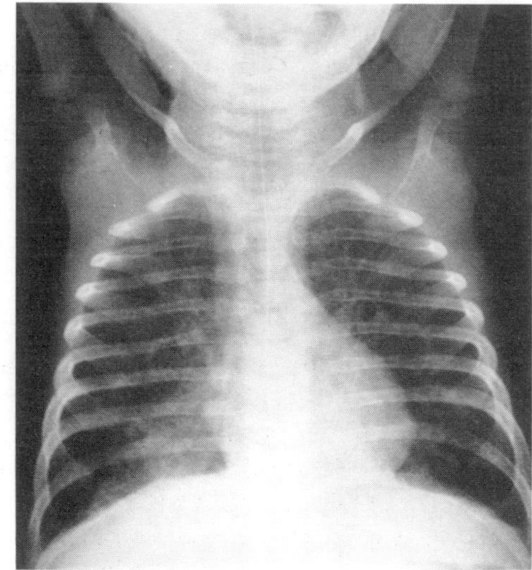

Fig. 10 *Pneumocystis carinii* pneumonia.

Pulmonary complications

The lung is frequently involved in children with HIV infection. Perinatally infected infants will often develop symptoms within the first year of life. Bacterial and viral infections may be more frequent and more severe in HIV-infected children, but a number of conditions are AIDS-defining.

Pneumocystis carinii pneumonia is the most common opportunistic infection in children with HIV infection. It may present within the first year of life as a rapidly progressive respiratory illness with a high mortality, or more insidiously in older immunocompromised children with reduced exercise tolerance. Fever, cough, and tachypnoea are the most frequent presenting signs, with surprisingly few chest signs for the degree of respiratory distress. Chest radiography may also appear normal at the early stage of the illness, but will later show diffuse interstitial infiltrates (Fig. 10). The white count is often normal, but lactic dehydrogenase is frequently elevated (>500 IU/l). There may be a rapid progression characterized by increasing respiratory distress and hypoxia.

Diagnosis should be made by microscopy identification of the organism from secretions (obtained by bronchoalveolar lavage or sputum induction by nebulized saline) or by lung biopsy. Early treatment should be started on presumptive diagnosis based on the following:

- history of acute respiratory decompensation;
- diffuse interstitial infiltrates on chest radiograph;
- oxygen desaturation on oximetry or blood gases;
- raised serum lactic dehydrogenase (>500 IU/l).

Pneumocystis carinii pneumonia is treated with co-trimoxazole (trimethoprim 20 mg/kg/day and sulphamethoxazole 100 mg/kg/day) in four daily doses for 3 weeks. Intravenous pentamidine 4 mg/kg once daily for at least 14 days may be used. There are insufficient data about the use of steroids for *Pneumocystis carinii* pneumonia in children but they reduce morbidity in adults.

Prophylaxis for *Pneumocystis carinii* pneumonia is given according to the level of immune suppression, but should probably be started empirically at the age of 2 months in an infant born to an infected mother where the CD4 count is unknown. Any child with a previous episode of *Pneumocystis carinii* pneumonia should receive prophylaxis (Table 8).

Co-trimoxazole (trimethoprim 150 mg/m^2 and sulphamethoxazole 750 mg/m^2) in two divided doses daily for 3 days a week is most commonly used. Nebulized pentamidine (300 mg/month for a child more than 5 years old), intravenous pentamidine (4 mg/kg every 2–4 weeks), or dapsone (1 mg/kg daily orally, maximum 100 mg/day) can also be used.

Lymphocytic interstitial pneumonitis is the most common respiratory complication in paediatric HIV infection. Early symptoms and signs will typically be mild, but in many cases will progress slowly to chronic hypoxia and finger clubbing. Hepatosplenomegaly, generalized lymphadenopathy, and parotid enlargement are usually associated, emphasizing the lymphoproliferative state. Chest radiography reveals a typical reticulonodular pattern. Lung biopsy shows lymphocytic infiltrates. As immunosuppression increases, the nodules seen radiographically appear to diminish in tandem with decreasing lymphadenopathy and hepatosplenomegaly. This is a poor prognostic sign.

There is no specific treatment. Intercurrent bacterial infections should be treated with antibiotics and immunoglobulin. Where chronic hypoxia becomes a problem, prednisolone 2 mg/kg/day should be given for 2 to 4 weeks until there is improvement. The dose should then be slowly tapered off.

Renal disease

Significant renal disease may occur in up to 30 per cent of HIV-infected children. It is more common in children with perinatally acquired infection than those infected through blood products. Most commonly it is due to an irreversible glomerular lesion. Children may present with the nephrotic syndrome, haematuria, hypertension, acidosis, electrolyte imbalance, or renal failure. Investigations will include full urinalysis, urea, creatinine, and electrolytes. An ultrasound scan and radiological studies may be indicated. A renal biopsy should be performed in cases of non-obstructive renal failure, persistent proteinuria, or haematuria-.Treatment may consist of diuretics, careful nutrition, and fluid balance.

Cardiac disease

Approximately 20 per cent of children will develop an AIDS cardiomyopathy. Baseline evaluation of cardiac status will include a thorough physical examination, an ECG, chest radiography, and an echocardiogram. Six-monthly cardiac assessment should include an ECG, looking for chamber enlargement or hypertrophy, and chest radiography looking for cardiac enlargement. More frequent follow-up will be required once the child develops any signs of cardiomyopathy. Subtle signs may only be unmasked by an intercurrent febrile illness or intolerance to intravenous fluids. The classical signs of failure can often be attributed to non-cardiac causes. Tachypnoea, tachycardia, and a gallop rhythm are the most reliable diagnostic features.

The principles of treatment are to reduce preload and afterload and improve myocardial function. Diuretics, vasodilators, and inotropes are indicated. Arrhythmias and pericardial effusion must be treated in the standard way.

Table 8 Guidelines for prophylaxis for *Pneumocystis carinii* pneumonia

Age	CD4 count
1–12 months	<1500/mm^3
12–24 months	<750/mm^3
2–6 years	<500/mm^3
>6 years	<200/mm^3

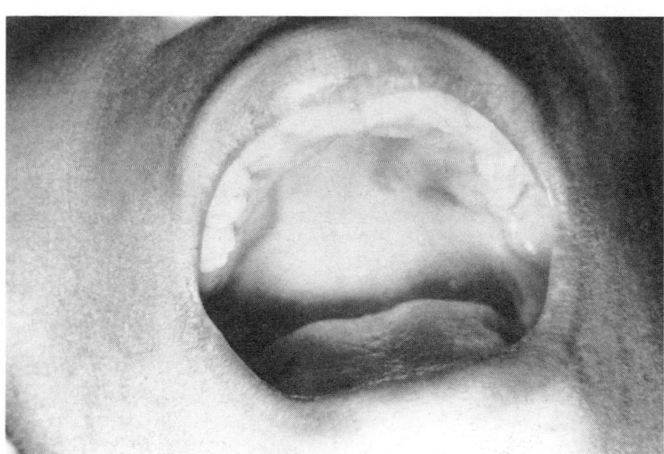

Fig. 11 Kaposi's sarcoma on the palate of a 12-year-old African girl with HIV infection.

Haematological manifestations

HIV affects the haematological system through the direct effect of the virus on stem cells, resulting in the loss of erythroid, myeloid, and megakaryocyte precursors, and also by the production of autoantibodies to stem cells in the peripheral circulation. Thus anaemia, neutropenia, and thrombocytopenia are all common in HIV infection.

Ferrous sulphate and/or transfusions with washed red cells may be required for anaemia. Intravenous immunoglobulin (400 mg/kg/day for 5 days) may be useful in neutropenia if infections become a clinical problem. Intravenous gammaglobulin (1 g/kg per dose for three doses at daily intervals) should be given in thrombocytopenia to achieve platelet levels above 40 000/mm^3. Steroids may be used, but will cause further immunosuppression. Zidovudine has been effective in adults but data for children are scanty. Granulocyte–monocyte colony-stimulating factor and erythropoietin may be effective in treating the cytopenias seen in HIV.

Neoplastic disorders

Neoplasia appears to be relatively rare in children with AIDS. Malignant lymphomas and smooth muscle tumours are the most common manifestations. Kaposi's sarcoma (Fig. 11) is much less frequent in children than adults. Transmitting mothers are most commonly infected through intravenous drug abuse or through a partner who is a drug abuser. Thus the child is infected with the strain that affects drug abusers and not that which affects homosexual males in whom Kaposi's sarcoma predominates.[43]

Infections

Bacterial infections

Defects in humoral and cellular immunity render the child more susceptible to bacterial infections. Agents causing serious invasive disease include *Streptococcus pneumoniae, Haemophilus influenzae, Staphylococcus aureus*, coagulase-negative staphylococci, *Streptococcus viridans*, Salmonella, and *Pseudomonas aeruginosa*. Antibiotic treatment of these infections is similar to that in non-HIV-infected children. However, more broad-spectrum agents may be necessary for empirical therapy. The pneumococcal vaccine should be given to HIV-infected children aged 2 years or older.

Regular intravenous infusions of immunoglobulin (400 mg/kg/month[44] or 300 mg/kg every 2 weeks[45]) reduce bacterial infections where the CD4 count is more than 200 cells/mm^3. This enhances the quality of life but does not increase survival time. Antibiotic prophylaxis alone may be as effective and much cheaper, but comparative trials are awaited.

Mycobacterial infections

Mycobacterial infections are a serious threat to HIV-infected children. The world-wide resurgence of tuberculosis is closely linked to the HIV pandemic. HIV-infected children are more likely to develop clinical disease after primary exposure. Complications of the primary focus and miliary spread are more frequent. A three-drug regimen should be used (four for disseminated disease): isoniazid 10 to 15 mg/kg/day, rifampicin 10 to 20 mg/kg/day; pyrazinamide 20 to 40 mg/kg/day, and ethambutol 15 to 25 mg/kg/day (not advised in very small children because of potential effects on the eye). Annual Mantoux testing is advisable. Children with a positive test but without clinical signs of tuberculosis should receive prophylaxis, preferably with a two-drug regimen (rifampicin and isoniazid), for 6 months.

Mycobacterium avium intracellulare is becoming increasingly common, but only when the CD4 count has fallen to low levels ('50 cells/mm^3). Presenting features include fever, night sweats, diarrhoea, weight loss, neutropenia, hepatomegaly, abdominal pain, anaemia, and lymphadenopathy. Mycobacterium avium intracellulare is usually cultured from blood, bone marrow, or stool in disseminated infection. Mycobacterium avium intracellulare in the sputum is a non-specific finding. A five-drug regimen is usually recommended for initial treatment. This should include clarithromycin (7.5 mg/kg every 12 h), ethambutol (15–25 mg/kg/day), and rifabutin (10–20 mg/kg/day in one or two doses). Other drugs to be considered include amikacin, clofazimine, and ciprofloxacin.

Viral infections

Herpes simplex virus and varicella zoster virus have been discussed above. Cytomegalovirus can cause retinitis, enterocolitis, pneumonitis, hepatitis, and encephalitis. The diagnosis may be difficult to establish. The presence of the virus in bodily secretions does not necessarily imply cause, and antibody levels are variable. Biopsy specimens are more reliable (inclusion bodies) but obtaining them may be more risky than giving empirical treatment. The presence of visual symptoms with fundoscopic evidence of retinitis is sufficient to warrant starting treatment. Intravenous ganciclovir 5 mg/kg twice daily for 14 days may be used. Maintenance therapy will be required for retinitis (5 mg/kg/day 5–7 days per week) to prevent relapses. Foscarnet is equally effective but has not been licensed for children.

Table 9 Immunization schedule

Age	Vaccine
2 months	DTP IPV HIB first dose
3 months	DTP IPV HIB second dose
4 months	DTP IPV HIB third dose
12–18 months	MMR
4–5 years	DT IPV booster

Abbreviations: DPT, diphtheria–pertussis–tetanus; IPV, inactivated poliomyelitis vaccine; HIB, *Haemophilus influenzae* type B vaccine; MMR, measles–mumps–rubella.

Measles carries a significant morbidity and mortality. Measles vaccination should be performed according to the schedule given in Table 9). Exposed children can be given immunoglobulin within 6 days of exposure. Ribavirin may be given intravenously in severe cases (5 mg/kg every 8 h) or by aerosol in measles pneumonitis. Vitamin A should be given to children with measles, particularly if they are malnourished.[46]

Fungal infections

Topical infections have been referred to earlier. Cryptococcal infection most often presents as meningitis and is the most frequent cause of cranial nerve palsy. Amphotericin B with or without 5-flucytosine should be used. Maintenance therapy should be continued with oral fluconazole. Amphotericin B is also effective in treating invasive infections with Histoplasma, Coccidioides, Blastomyces or Aspergillus (Fig. 12)

Parasitic infections

Toxoplasmosis may present as encephalitis or in a disseminated form resulting from intrauterine infection. Treatment is with pyrimethamine (1 mg/kg/day, maximum 25 mg/day) and sulphadiazine (50 mg/kg every 6 h) with folinic acid (5 mg every 3 days)

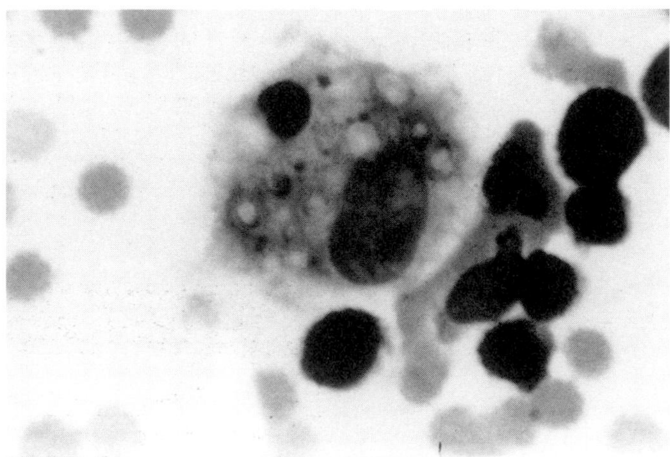

Fig. 12 *Histoplasma duboisii* in a bone marrow specimen from an African child with HIV infection.

for 3 to 6 weeks. Clarithromycin, azithromycin, and atovaquone may also be useful.

Isospora belli may cause intractable diarrhoea and malnutrition. Co-trimoxazole (TMP-SMX) is frequently successful in a dose of 10 mg TMP+50 mg SMX/kg/day in four divided doses for 10 days and then half the daily dose in two divided doses for 3 weeks or longer. Indefinite prophylaxis with sulphadoxine–pyrimethamine (Fansidar) may be the best way of preventing relapse. There are no consistently effective treatment regimens for cryptosporidiosis. Paromycin, azithromycin, and letrazuril may prove helpful. Where antimicrobial agents have failed, octreotide may help in reducing stool output and controlling fluid losses.

Prevention of infections

Infants born to HIV-infected mothers should receive the recommended immunizations against childhood diseases (Table 9). Inactivated poliomyelitis vaccine is used in place of the live strain. In addition, they should receive influenza vaccine annually and pneumococcal vaccine.[47] If the mother has positive hepatitis B serology, the infant should receive hepatitis-B-immune globulin at birth followed by hepatitis B vaccine at 1 month and 6 months of age.

Children with symptomatic HIV infection progressively lose vaccine-associated antibody titres. Therefore immediate appropriate prophylaxis after exposure to measles (immunoglobulin), pertussis (erythromycin), diphtheria (erythromycin), or *Haemophilus influenzae* type B (rifampicin) is recommended even if the child has been previously vaccinated.

BCG is not recommended because there have been reports of disseminated infection following vaccination. However, WHO recommend that BCG should still be given in the newborn period in countries with a high prevalence of tuberculosis (Fig. 13).

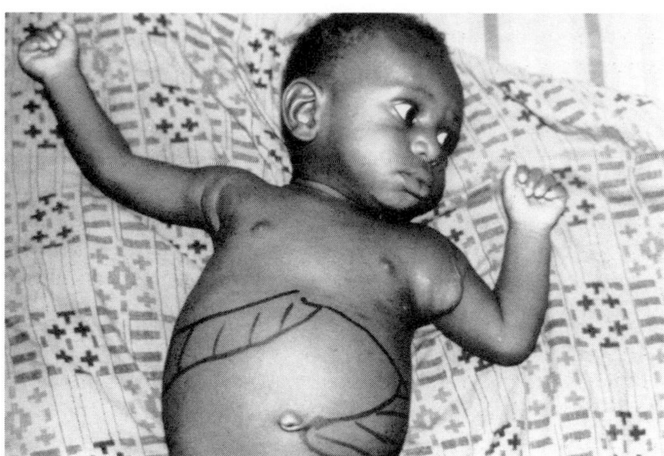

Fig. 13 Miliary tuberculosis from BCG vaccination in an African infant with HIV infection.

Antiretroviral therapy

The current recommendations are that specific therapy should be used in symptomatic children and those showing significant immunosuppression (Table 3). Beneficial effects are seen in terms of weight gain, reduced organomegaly, improved cognitive function, reduced p24 antigen levels, and increased CD4 counts.

The development of resistant strains of HIV is common in prolonged monotherapy. Combination therapy may help to reduce the rate of development of drug resistance and at the same time has the potential advantage of reducing toxicity if lower doses of each drug can be used. Alternating regimens may also be used.

Children receiving treatment should be monitored for signs of toxicity and therapeutic effect. Measures should include full blood count, presence of HIV-related physical signs, growth, neurodevelopmental status, CD4 count, serum immunoglobulins, and p24 antigen levels.

The commonly used drugs and their side-effects are shown in Table 10.

Repeated blood transfusions may be needed for recurrent anaemia in zidovudine treatment. In addition, granulocyte–monocyte colony-stimulating factor and erythropoietin may be of benefit. Future antiretroviral drugs may include newer nucleoside reverse transcriptase inhibitors (stavudine-d4T), non-nucleoside reverse transcriptase inhibitors, *tat* antagonists, and protease inhibitors.

Measures to reduce perinatal transmission include the following:

- Caesarian section[48,49]
- avoidance of breast feeding
- zidovudine during pregnancy and in the neonatal period
- immunization[50]

Zidovudine given in pregnancy reduced transmission to 8.3 per cent from 25.5 per cent in the placebo group:[51]

- zidovudine 100 mg orally five times daily throughout pregnancy from 14 to 34 weeks' gestation;
- zidovudine 2 mg/kg intravenous loading dose over 1 h during labour followed by a continuous infusions of 1 mg/kg/h until delivery;
- zidovudine syrup 2 mg/kg four times daily orally to newborns starting 8 to 12 h after delivery and continuing for 6 weeks.

Zidovudine toxicity was minimal in the women and was well tolerated by the infants. A mild transient anaemia was the only

Table 10 Antiretroviral drugs: doses and toxic effects

Drug	Dose	Toxic effects
Zidovudine	180 mg/m^2 orally every 6 h	Anaemia, neutropenia
Didanosine	90–135 mg/m^2 orally every 12 h	Pancreatitis, diarrhoea
Zalcitabine	0.005–0.01 mg/kg orally every 8 h	Mouth sores, rashes

reported adverse effect in babies. Birth parameters were similar in both groups and there was no increase in birth defects in the treated group.[52,53]

Zidovudine does not completely stop transmission and its efficacy in women with advanced infection or with zidovudine-resistant strains is not known. The long-term effects of zidovudine on children are not known and adverse effects may become more apparent as it is used more widely. A major constraint in the use of zidovudine is that many women present late in pregnancy or are unaware that they are infected.

Caring for the HIV-infected child and family

The majority of children with HIV infection world-wide are born into families where the mother has acquired the infection heterosexually. Serious illness in the child may be the first indication of HIV infection in the family, or the child may be born into a situation where illness and death have already occurred. The presence of a seriously ill child affects the whole family. It brings uncertainties and loss of routine, and it puts a strain on relationships. Planning ahead is difficult. The focus on the sick child may bring out jealousy in a sibling.

In Europe and North America most perinatally infected children are born into single-parent families with a chaotic lifestyle centred around drug abuse. Many are homeless and may be ill themselves.

Most palliative care programmes for children with terminal illness focus around the parents' own instincts of care for their children. Clearly, where parents are ill or under the influence of drugs their caring ability will be affected. For this reason careful planning and co-operation between different agencies is vital.

In the United Kingdom the 1989 Children Act sets out important principles regarding children's rights and choices and parental responsibility. It also makes clear the duties of social services departments to provide services for people who are sick and disabled and to provide support for children 'in need'. The Act makes it clear that parents should be helped as much as possible to look after their children and that children should be helped to understand and have a say in the plans being made for them. However, the range of services available in each area varies depending on how the local authority has decided to spend its funds. For this reason many charitable groups have been set up to support the statutory provision by the social services.

A care programme should attempt to maintain as normal a life as possible for the child, whilst providing adequate care for the physical, emotional, spiritual, and cultural needs of the child and family. There should be good liaison between hospital and community services, particularly the primary health care team. A care programme should include the following:

- multidisciplinary approach
- involving the whole family
- respecting parents' wishes on confidentiality
- providing care at home as much as possible
- giving parents access to back-up professional care
- counselling to parents, grandparents, and siblings
- training in prevention of infection
- providing information about support groups
- identifying special educational needs.

Services available from the social services or voluntary agencies (a list of agencies is given in the Appendix) should include the following:

- special equipment or adaptations to make it easier to manage at home
- assistance with telephone and travel costs
- day care or overnight respite care
- practical help in the house (e.g. babysitting, taking children to school if parent unwell)
- adoption and fostering services
- welfare rights advice
- group meetings with crêche facility
- volunteers to provide practical and emotional support

Confidentiality

HIV is not a notifiable disease. Parents should be allowed to determine who is informed about their child's status. Even if parents or guardians feel the need to disclose in order to obtain appropriate services for their children, further disclosure should only be made with the written consent of the parents.

Community-based care programmes

In Europe and North America the basic care of HIV-infected children is provided by community and health services. However, in many parts of the world there are no government services to provide even basic home care and the traditional extended family is overwhelmed. Charitable agencies play a much greater role and have been able to pioneer the concept of community-based home care services, for example Chikinkata Hospital, Zambia, and TASO, Uganda (see the Appendix for details).

Schooling

Children with HIV should attend normal schools and nurseries. The risk of transmission is negligible under normal circumstances, although special care should be exercised if the child has open wounds or behaviour likely to be risky (e.g. biting). Parents of infected children are often aware of the possibility of social isolation if the child's condition becomes known at school. The number of people who are aware of the situation should be rigorously confined to those who need to know in order to ensure the proper care of the child.

The paediatrician has an important role in initiating early evaluation of special educational needs. This may result in an early nursery placement for preschool children, a special needs teacher in a mainstream school, or even placement in a special school.

Providing emotional and spiritual support

The discovery of HIV infection in the family will raise a mixture of emotions. Different members of the family will react in different ways. There may be guilt (of having inflicted the infection on an innocent child), anger (stemming from frustration), or fear (of illness, rejection, pain, and death). Siblings will need reassurance that they are not responsible for the infection and that they will not catch it. Grandparents often feel guilty, and want to die in the place of their child or grandchild in order to restore the natural cycle of life and death. They need to be reassured that these are normal emotions. Help may be obtained through a counsellor, a trusted friend, or a support group.

After coming to terms with the diagnosis, the family will need to cope with chronic illness and death. Parents will gain help from friends and support groups. Children react in different ways. Below the age of 5 they have no concept of the permanence of death. Often they seem uninterested and may feel 'abandonment' rather than grief or sadness. From 6 to 11 years they begin to understand that death is forever. Their moods change rapidly from happy one moment to sad the next. They often express their feelings through play or pictures. From 11 years onwards they begin to have a more sophisticated understanding of death and will be confused if adults are not honest with them. Answers to their questions will have to be pitched to their level of understanding (see Chapter 19.3).

Most adults with HIV have an inner need to make sense of the experience of living and dying, and to do so with hope and creativity. Children who are dying have a similar need. Frequently parents find it difficult to talk about death with their sick child, but many children are aware of what is happening and confused by a conspiracy of silence. Helping parents know what to say is important and should be in accordance with their own religious beliefs (see Appendix).

Adolescents

The social stigma that has been attached to HIV infection poses special problems for infected adolescents who have just begun the process of defining their identity and sexuality. This is a sensitive area for all teenagers, but is aggravated by HIV infection which may cause delays in growth and sexual maturation and imposes the further burden of a limited future and the prevention of transmission. Sensitive and sympathetic support coupled with adequate knowledge about HIV is required.

Respite care

Psychosocial services should include respite care for parents, foster carers, or adoptive families. Hospital care may be required at times as the disease progresses. Hospice care for children is becoming increasingly available in the United Kingdom. Ten children's hospices are open in the United Kingdom, and there are plans for another 12. The Mildmay Hospital, London, has the first purpose-built family care centre for HIV of its kind in the world; it provides 24-h respite, rehabilitative, and terminal care for children and parents, with nursery facilities for healthy siblings.

Stopping treatment

In contrast with cancer, pain in HIV disease is likely to have an underlying treatable cause.[54] Symptomatic treatments (e.g. for candidiasis) should continue until death. Any benefits have to be considered against side-effects and inconvenience. The treatment of some infections (e.g. Mycobacterium avium intracellulare) may result in drug toxicity without affecting the survival of the child. This may also be true of antiretroviral agents. Withdrawal of these therapies in the terminal stages should be considered in full consultation with the parents and even the child him- or herself. However, parents should be warned that death does not always ensue rapidly following withdrawal.

Appendix: Useful addresses and publications

ACET (AIDS Care, Education and Training). Practical home care services. PO Box 1323, London W5 5TF. Tel: 0181-840 7879.

Barnardo's Positive Options. Information and practical help for parents. 354 Goswell Road, London EC1V 7LQ. Tel: 0171-278 5039.

Childline. A 24-h freephone line for children and young people. Tel: 0800 1111.

Grandma's. A service for children affected by HIV/AIDS. PO Box 1392, London SW6 4EJ. Tel: 0171-610 3904.

Mildmay Mission Hospital. Family Unit for parents and children. Hackney Road, London E2 7NA. Tel: 0171-739 1200.

Milestone House. Hospice and respite centre for people with AIDS. Children can be admitted with their parents. 113 Oxgangs Road, Edinburgh EH14 1EB. Tel: 0131-441 6989.

Paediatric AIDS Resource Centre (PARC). Information service covering all aspects of HIV in children. 20 Sylvan Place, Edinburgh EH9 1UW. Tel: 0131-536 0806.

Strategies for Hope series. Covers Chikinkata and TASO home care programmes. Available from: TALC, PO Box 49, St Albans, AL1 4AX.

AIDS Action. Quarterly newsletter aimed at medical staff and health workers. Free of charge in developing countries. Available from: AHRTAG, 1 London Bridge Street, London SE1 9SG.

Helping Children Cope with Grief by Rosemary Wells. Sheldon Press.

Let's Talk About AIDS by Peter Sanders and Clare Farquhar, Gloucester Press. For older children.

Let's Talk About Death and Dying by Peter Sanders. Gloucester Press. For older children.

Badger's Parting Gifts by Susan Varley, Collins Picture Lions. For younger children.

When Uncle Bob Died by Athea, Dinosaur Publications. For younger children.

References

1. European Centre for the Epidemiological Monitoring of AIDS. Quarterly Report 31 December 1993. *AIDS Surveillance in Europe*, No. 40. Saint-Maurice, France: WHO–EC Collaborating Centre on AIDS, 1994.

2. AIDS Group of the Haemophilia Centre Directors. Prevalence of antibody to HIV in haemophiliacs in the United Kingdom. *Clinical and Laboratory Haematology*, 1988; **10**:187–91.
3. Jager H, *et al.* Prevention of transfusion-associated HIV transmission in Kinshasa, Zaire. HIV screening is not enough. *AIDS*, 1990; **4**:571–4.
4. Ippolito G, Puro V, De Carli G. The risk of occupational human immunodeficiency virus infection in health care workers: Italian Multicenter Study. *Archives of Internal Medicine*, 1993; **153**:1451–8.
5. Center for Disease Control and Prevention. Human immunodeficiency virus transmission in household settings—United States. *Morbidity and Mortality Weekly Reports*, 1994; **43**:347, 353–6.
6. St Louis ME, *et al.* Risk for perinatal HIV-1 transmission according to maternal immunologic, virologic and placental factors. *Journal of the American Medical Association*, 1993; **269**:2853–9.
7. European Collaborative Study. Risk factors for mother to child transmission of human immunodeficiency virus type 1. *Lancet*, 1992; **339**:1007–12.
8. Report of a Consensus Workshop. Maternal factors involved in mother-to-child transmission of HIV-1. *Journal of Acquired Immune Deficiency Syndromes*, 1992; **5**:1019–29.
9. Rouzioux C, *et al.* Timing of mother-to-child HIV-1 transmission depends on maternal status. The HIV in Newborns French Collaborative Study Group. *AIDS*, 1993; **7**(Supplement 2):S49–52.
10. Thomas PA, *et al.* Maternal predictors of perinatal human immunodeficiency virus transmission. The New York City Perinatal HIV Transmission Study Group. *Pediatric Infectious Disease Journal*, 1994; **13**(6):498–95.
11. Yerly S, Chamot E, Hirschel B, Perrin LH. Quantitation of human immunodeficiency virus provirus and circulating virus: relationship with immunologic parameters. *Journal of Infectious Disease*, 1992; **166**:269–76.
12. Kliks SC, Wara DW, Landers DV, Levy JA. Features of HIV-1 that could influence maternal–child transmission. *Journal of the American Medical Association*, 1994; **272**(6):467–74.
13. Bulterys M, *et al.* Multuiple sexual partners and mother-to-child tranmission of HIV-1. *AIDS*, 1993; **7**:1639–45.
14. Semba RD, *et al.* Maternal Vitamin A deficiency and mother-to-child transmission of HIV-1. *Lancet*, 1994; **343**:1593–97.
15. Goedert JJ, *et al.* High risk of HIV-1 infection for first-born twins. *Lancet*, 1992; **338**:1471–5.
16. Wara DW, Luzuriaga K, Martin NL, Sullivan JL, Bryson JB. Maternal transmission and diagnosis of human immunodeficiency virus during infancy. *Annals of the New York Academy of Sciences* 1993; **693**:14–19.
17. European Collaborative Study. Children born to women with HIV-1 infection: natural history and risk of transmission. *Lancet*, 1991; **337**:253–60.
18. Ryder RW, *et al.* Perinatal transmission of the human immunodeficiency virus type 1 to infants of seropositive women in Zaire. *New England Journal of Medicine*, 1989; **320**:1637–42.
19. Lepage P, *et al.* Mother-to-child transmission of human immunodeficiency virus type 1 and its determinants: a cohort study in Kigali, Rwanda. *American Journal of Epidemiology*, 1993; **137**(6):589–99.
20. Adjorlolo-Johnson G, *et al.* Prospective comparison of mother-to-child transmission of HIV-1 and HIV-2 in Abidjan, Ivory Coast. *Journal of the American Medical Association*,1994; **272**(6):462–6.
21. Anonymous. Comparison of vertical HIV-2 and HIV-1 transmission in the French Prospective Cohort. The HIV infection in Newborns French Collaborative Study Group. *Pediatric Infectious Disease Journal*, 1994; **13**:502–6.
22. Sprecher S, Soumenkoff G, Puissant F, De Gueldra M. Vertical transmission of HIV in a 15-week fetus. *Lancet*, 1985; **ii**:288–9
23. Mofenson LM, Wolinsky SM. Vertical transmission of HIV. Part C: Current insights regarding vertical transmission. In: Pizzo PA, Wiffert CM, eds. *Pediatric AIDS: The Challenge of HIV Infection in Infants, Children and Adolescents.*2nd edn. Baltimore, MD: Williams and Wilkins, 1994:179–203.
24. Van de Perre P, *et al.* Postnatal transmission of human immunodeficiency virus type 1 from mother to infant. A prospective cohort study in Kigali, Rwanda. *New England Journal of Medicine*, 1991; **325**:594–8.
25. Dunn DT, Newell ML, Ades AE, Peckham CS. Risk of human immunodeficiency virus type 1 transmission through breastfeeding. *Lancet*, 1992; **340**:585–8.
26. Van de Perre P, *et al.* Infective and anti-infective properties of breastmilk from HIV-1 infected women. *Lancet*, 1993; **341**:914–18.
27. Victoria CG, *et al.*Evidence for protection by breast-feeding against infant deaths from infectious diseases in Brazil. *Lancet*, 1987; **ii**:319–22.
28. Miles S, *et al.* Rapid serologic testing with immune-complex dissociated HIV p24 antigen for early detection of HIV infection in neonates. *New England Journal of Medicine*, 1993; **328**:297–302.
29. Wang X, *et al.* Improved specificity of *in vitro* anti-HIV antibody production: implications for diagnosis and timing of transmission in infants born to HIV-seropositive mothers. *AIDS Research and Human Retroviruses*, 1994; **10**(6):691–9.
30. Pollack H, Zhan MX, Ilmet-Moore T, Tao P, Krasinski K, Borkowsky W. A novel detection assay for the early diagnosis of HIV-1 infected infants. *Journal of Acquired Immune Deficiency Syndromes*, 1993; **6**:582–6.
31. Mokili JLK, Connell JA, Parry JV, Green SDR, Davies AG, Cutting WAM. How valuable are IgA and IgM anti-HIV tests for the diagnosis of mother–child transmission of HIV in an African. *Clinical and Diagnostic Virology*, 1996; **5**:3–12.
32. Center for Disease Control and Prevention. Revision of the CDC surveillance case definition for acquired immune deficiency syndrome. *Morbidity and Mortality Weekly*, 1987; **36**(Supplement):1–15s.
33. The European Collaborative Study. Age-related standards for T lymphocyte subsets based on uninfected children born to human immunodeficiency virus-1-infected women. *Pediatric Infectious Disease Journal*, 1992; **11**:1018–26.
34. Center for Disease Control and Prevention. *Morbidity and Mortality Weekly*, 1994; **43**(RR-12):1–9.
35. World Health Organization. *Weekly Epidemiological Record*, 1994; **69**(37):273–5.
36. Brettler DB, Forsberg A, Bolivar E, Brewster F, Sullivan J. Growth failure as a prognositc indicator for progression to acquired immunodeficiency syndrome in children with hemophilia. *Journal of Pediatrics*, 1990; **117**:584–8.
37. McKinney R, *et al.* Weight growth rates as a prognostic factor in pediatric HIV infections. *Pediatric Research*, 1993; **33**:175A.
38. Janssen RS, *et al.* American Academy of Neurology AIDS Task Force: nomenclature and research case definitions for neurologic manifestations of human immunodeficiency type 1. *Neurology*, 1991; **41**:778–85.
39. Belman AL. Pediatric AIDS. Neurologic syndromes. *Annals of the New York Academy of Sciences*, 1993; **693**:107–22.
40. Yolken RH, Hart W, Oung I, Shiff C, Greenson J, Perman JA. Gastrointestinal dysfunction and disaccharide intolerance in children infected with human immunodeficiency virus. *Journal of Pediatrics*, 1991; **118**:359–63.
41. Ulrich R, *et al.* Small intestinal structure and function in patients infected with human immunodeficiency virus (HIV): evidence for HIV-induced enteropathy. *Annals of Internal Medicine*, 1989;**111**:15–21
42. Green SDR. Treatment of moderate and severe dehydration by nasogastric drip. *Tropical Doctor*, 1987; **17**:86–8.
43. Joshi VV. Pathology of pediatric AIDS. *Annals of the New York Academy of Sciences*, 1993; **693**:71–92.
44. NICHD IVIG Collaborative Group. Efficacy of intravenous immunoglobulin for the prophylaxis of serious bacterial infections in dsymptomatic HIV-infected children. *New England Journal of Medicine*, 1991; **325**:73–80.
45. Rubenstein A, Calvelli T, Rubenstein R. Intravenous gammaglobulin for pediatric HIV-1 infection. *Annals of the New York Academy of Sciences*, 1993; **693**:151–7.
46. American Academy of Pediatrics Committee on Infectious Diseases. Vitamin A treatment of measles. *Pediatrics*, 1993; **91**:1014–15.
47. Gibb D, *et al.* Antibody responses to *Haemophilus influenzae* type B and

Streptococcus pneumoniae vaccines in children with human immunodeficiency virus infection. *Paediatric Infectious Diseases Journal* 1995; **14**:129–35.

48. European Collaborative Study. Caesarian section and the risk of vertical transmission of HIV-1 infection. *Lancet*, 1994; **343**:1464–7.
49. Dunn DT, *et al*. Mode of delivery and vertical transmission of HIV-1: a review of prospective studies. Perinatal AIDS Collaborative Transmission Studies. *Journal of Acquired Immune Deficiency Syndromes*, 1994; **7**(10):1034–9.
50. Cryz SJ, *et al*. Prospects for prevention of vertical transmission of human immunodeficiency virus by immunisation. *Annals of the New York Academy of Sciences*, 1993; **693**:194–201.
51. Center for Disease Control and Prevention. Recommendations of the U.S. Public Health Service Task Force on the use of zidovudine to reduce perinatal transmission of human immunodeficiency virus. *Morbidity and Mortality Weekly*, 1994; **43**:285–7.
52. Center for Disease Control and Prevention. Birth outcomes following zidovudine therapy in pregnant women. *Morbidity and Mortality Weekly*, 1994; **43**(22):409, 415–16.
53. Kumar RM, Hughes PF, Khurrana A. Zidovudine use in pregnant women; a report on 104 cases and the occurrence of birth defects. *Journal of Acquired Immune Deficiency Syndromes*, 1994; **7**(10):1034–9.
54. O'Neill WM, Sherrard JS. Pain in immunodeficiency virus disease: a review. *Pain*, 1993; **54**:3–14

21

Education and training in palliative care

21.1 Multiprofessional education

Gillian Ford

The contributors to this section on education in palliative care are all professionals with experience in education and training. Each was asked to write about one professional group and its needs. Yet, in the practice of palliative care, they are all well aware that people with different professional backgrounds should, and do, collaborate, and thus provide mutual support in their work for, and with, patients.

With the growth of palliative care in recent years, and with both public and professional expectations extending its scope from specialist care for the terminally ill, particularly those with cancer, to much wider patient interests, new questions arise around the concept of teamwork. How far, and in what ways, should professionals who are going to work together, learn together? As Brooking wrote in 1991 (and the point still stands), it is difficult to understand why the divisions between medical and nursing education should still be so sharp, when so much of their education has so much common ground. Whatever may be the historical causes of such differences (which range from differences of status to differences in educational background, styles, and professional objectives) the conclusion from practice is crisp and irrefutable: 'It is self-evident that teams function most effectively when their various members understand and respect each others' ideas and perspectives.'[1]

It takes a regrettably long time to recast medical and nursing curricula, let alone involve members of related professions in the teaching–learning process. Nevertheless, the scale of palliative care, and the teamwork ethos that pervades it, suggest that multiprofessional education is beginning to move from an accepted principle to a necessary practice. How easily the change is made clearly depends upon the social context of each health-care system, on its resources, its challenges, and prevailing attitudes to professional education.

In the United Kingdom, where there has now been quite a long lead-time in palliative care, the development of team working may well be easier than in other countries, where those seeking change have to work back from the evident benefits to, and implications for, the health system generally, where professional prejudices and staff structures may still prevent the idea of teamwork from being fully accepted, and where change may be slow and weakly supported.

Indeed, the critical mass required to achieve change may be long delayed. A Council of Europe study in 1994, for instance, showed that very few centres currently provide any multiprofessional education at the undergraduate level.[2] The commonest argument is that the curriculum is already too crowded and that the professional pressure is towards career specialization and away from generalist ideas, which are seen to operate at lower levels of competence, responsibility and status.

Much the same attitude seems to operate in postgraduate multiprofessional education; moreover, it is customarily offered widely but thinly, in short seminar and workshop courses, occasionally in joint diplomas, or in the degree work which (particularly in Britain) is developing in the field of palliative care. Even in continuing education, to judge from a published report,[3] and anecdotal knowledge, it is evident that there are too few examples of established health-care staff learning together, and that where progress has been made it is usually due to local initiatives, to responses to perceived needs, or to significant departmental or personal initiatives. Certainly, it is not yet a serious issue in the higher reaches of the relevant professions and the Council of Europe report concludes that no member state has yet committed itself to multiprofessional education in its health-care policy.

There is, of course, a significant difference in focus between undergraduate and postgraduate multiprofessional education. A very good case can be made for involving trainees from related but distinct professions in sequences of learning, as a foundation for the interpersonal exchanges which are so vital. However, there are obvious practical difficulties, of which timetabling and location are often the most immediately restrictive. In any case, at this stage, the main objective must be to raise the awareness of problems and lay out the varying approaches to the common goals of patient well-being. The aim, to put it simply, must be a significant shift towards openness in place of a closed view of roles. It will be easier to suggest how this can be done most effectively when there have been more evaluated attempts to do it at all. All the same, this line of thought helps to identify new ways of thinking about the teaching of palliative care and the relationship to other established specialties and subspecialties.

While there must be a continuing search for a common core of knowledge and experience, at all levels, if collaboration is to become a generally accepted style, it is a fair generalization to say that the emphasis in undergraduate multiprofessional education is bound to be on concepts and attitudes, and in postgraduate multiprofessional education it will be on practice and skills. It should, indeed, depend significantly upon the feedback of experience which, in palliative care, will come not only from a variety of staff, but also a variety of settings.

The problems in postgraduate, interactive, multiprofessional education in palliative care are likely to be more organizational than conceptual. But the gain to team working seems worth the effort and suggests that alongside the policy of increasing awareness of palliative care in wider health policy generally there might be specific instructional programmes for those whose daily work with patients with very late stage disease establishes the need to work together.

However, what can be said about instructional programmes? The case for working back from experience is very strong, for three reasons. First, this approach draws upon real working knowledge of the situations in which that knowledge is applied. It can emphasize the differing skills which should be focused on the common goal of patient care and encourage a collaborative spirit which can infuse the more formal teaching and learning process. Secondly, the status and knowledge structures which differing professionals seek to project into a curriculum, even into a nominally common core of work, are unavoidably competitive if the learning design is preconceived and denies opportunity for interaction. The third reason relates to some very real practical difficulties in devising a common core based on a bundle of concepts and practices drawn from different professional training systems. Like will not be matched with like, and that will also be true of the capacities of participants in a joint programme (medical, nurse, and social work education each has its own levels of difficulty, its own framing body of assumptions, and relevant skills). The tendency could be to reduce the training programme to the lowest common denominator, so that it offers generalities with little practical value, which creates a prevailing sense of boredom and frustration. Anyone working in this field has seen this happen time and again at conferences, workshops, seminars, and lectures.

An educational approach which defines and tackles specific tasks and deploys a range of personal skills in concert is clearly the way out of such constraints, not least because it mirrors and anticipates the real-life situation for which the training is being undertaken. In teamwork, after all, the participants take and give differently within a team; and learning how to balance talents and responses within a group is perhaps the most important element in its preparation as well as in its practice. This can only be done properly when task definition and task performance are the central themes in designing a programme and implementing it. Needs have to be defined, challenges faced, resources assessed, interpersonal as well as interprofessional problems solved; in the process, the meaningful participation of all the group members becomes the essential condition of success for the group as a whole—whether it is learning what to do, how to do it, or simply doing it.

There is another argument for this approach to multiprofessional education. In palliative care, it is necessary to take account of factors which are not simply units of professional education. There are ethical issues involved, spiritual, social, cultural, and communication problems to be resolved; the ability of group members to contribute is not directly or necessarily correlated to their formal knowledge, skills, and professional designation. A nurse or a counsellor may well have much more to contribute about the moment of death than an oncology consultant; a social worker may prove to be a natural communicator or facilitator; but without group experience in training, and enhanced awareness of lines of collaboration and support in the hospital or hospice ward, such potential contributions may lie dormant or be disregarded.

The research literature on multiprofessional education is still sparse, although not completely missing. Evaluation and long-term follow-up do indicate value,[4,5] but the final virtue of task-directed education is that it provides a basis for the task-orientated research on which the further development of palliative care in part depends.

Meanwhile, a pragmatic approach to the challenge of interactive multiprofessional education is essential.[6] Progress, even by small steps, will enhance teamwork in practice; new learning materials and technology will overcome some difficulties of scheduling and the act of participating will promote the individual professional's own obligation to develop personal and organizational expertise and quality.[7]

References

1. Brooking J. Doctors and nurses: a personal view. *Nursing Standard*, 1991; **6**: 24–8.
2. Goble R. Multi-professional education: European network for development of MPE in health services. *Journal of Inter-professional Care*, 1994; **8**: 85–92.
3. Storrie J. Mastering interprofessionalism—an enquiry into the development of masters programmes with an interprofessional focus. *Journal of Interprofessional Care*, 1992; **6**: 253–9.
4. Bolden KJ, Lewis AP. A joint course for general practitioners and practice nurse trainers. *British Journal of General Practice*, 1990; **40**: 386–7.
5. Jones R. Working together: a description of residential multi-professional workshops. *Postgraduate Education for General Practice*, 1990; **1**: 154–9.
6. National Council for Hospice and Specialist Palliative Care Services. *Education in Palliative Care*. Occasional Paper 9, 1996: 7.
7. Eraut M. *Training, Quality and Accountability*. University of Sussex, Professorial lecture, 1992.

21.2 Palliative medicine education

John F. Scott, Neil MacDonald, and Balfour M. Mount, with contributions from Anthony M. Smith, J. Andrew Billings, J. Norelle Lickiss, Franco DeConno, and Luigi Saita

Introduction

The World Health Organization has challenged training institutions to ensure that palliative care is:

compulsory in courses leading to a basic professional qualification;

accepted as a suitable subject for testing by examination boards;

recognized by universities and professional bodies as an appropriate subject for study, dissertations, certificates, diplomas, and advanced degrees;

included in postgraduate programmes of continuing professional education;

recognized as an appropriate subject for scholarships, fellowships, and grants by academic institutions and research-funding bodies.[1]

Expert Committee on Palliative Care, World Health Organization, 1989.

In the last decade, we have witnessed exciting developments in palliative medicine education. Nonetheless, the challenge of the next decade will demand far greater and more creative responses. The factors which drive educational development are multiple and their interaction is complex.

Growth factors

The burden of suffering

The most important factor underlying the demand for palliative medicine training is the existence of a large and rapidly expanding population of patients who are dying with unrelieved suffering. In the developed world, this increase is largely due to the ageing of a relatively stable population but in the developing world there continues to be rapid population growth and radical shifts in disease patterns, such that cancer and AIDS will become major problems for all parts of the world.

Programme expansion

Training opportunities must parallel the growth of palliative care services. In many countries, driven by community interest, a variety of programmes bearing the label 'palliative care' or 'hospice' have developed. Many of these include volunteers and health professionals, often working in a part-time capacity, who identify the need for a programme but who may not have had the opportunity to train for their tasks. The well being of patients and families in these programmes, and the overall credibility of the palliative care movement, depend upon ensuring that educational experience matches responsibility.

A number of national organizations have established a set of standards which will assist palliative care programmes in the assessment of their current activities and in planning for the future.[2,3,4] Uniformly, these standards include statements on adequacy of education.

Economics

The last year of life for patients with chronic illness accounts for a large proportion of their total lifetime health-care costs.[5,6] In developed countries, much of this expense originates in acute care institutions and is often related to aggressive, costly, and futile therapeutic initiatives. Palliative care educational initiatives can improve both the clinical and the economic climate for patients, their families, and the society which supports them. Training health professionals in the art of caring for dying patients may result in:

(1) limitation in the use of expensive investigations when the results would not change therapy;

(2) limitation of ineffective, costly, and potentially harmful therapies;

(3) facilitating a shift in the focus of care away from hospitals and into the community.

Patients can do more to care for themselves if they have access to first rate counselling and education. Similarly, with appropriate training and backup from health professionals, caregivers can be prepared to take on levels of care now restricted to institutions.

Medical education philosophy

In the past, the dominant philosophy of medical education has been antithetical to the thrust of palliative medicine. The focus on diagnosis, investigation, and cure left little room or respect for a focus on relief of symptoms and suffering. Superspecialization often gives undue prominence to rare diseases as a focus of clinical interest. The integration of knowledge with the clinical and personal skills and attitudes that nurture patient–doctor relationships has lagged behind technological instruction.

However, in the last decade we have witnessed a shift in the philosophy of medical schools. The old curricula of lectures transmitting knowledge are being replaced by small-group, learner-centred, problem-based strategies. Increasingly, the site of learning is shifting into the community as high technology, tertiary care is de-emphasized. Medical schools are becoming more aware of societal demands, seeking alliances with the people whom they serve. The patient is viewed as the teacher, and the professor and the hospital as only adjuncts to learning. Communication skills, ethics, interdisciplinary collaboration, and the psychosocial needs of the physician are becoming prominent topics. These shifts mean that palliative medicine should become crucial to a medical school's ability to meet its objectives. This represents a major opportunity and danger for palliative medicine, since we seek and may be offered a major role in tutoring whole-person attitudes and communication skills in both undergraduate and postgraduate programmes. While at first glance this is an exciting opportunity, we must examine our scarce faculty resources and decide how we can collaborate with other faculty members so that we do not become overwhelmed by the tasks of general medical education.

A new reflective literature is arising on the role of medicine in society. For example the Royal College of Physicians and Surgeons of Canada seeks to prepare trainees to be competent in six essential roles:[7]

medical expert

communicator

collaborator

manager

health advocate

professional.

This new medical education literature calls for a social contract with the communities we serve and espouses a philosophy attuned to palliative medicine. The literature of diffusion theory, and its focus on changing physicians' behaviour and practice patterns, provides a helpful framework for our postgraduate and continuing medical education efforts.[8,9] The strategies derived from evidence-based medicine and technology transfer studies can be adapted for palliative medicine.

Specialists in medical education can provide us with an increasingly rich menu of innovative learning methods. However, their greatest impact is felt when we adopt their systematic and systemic educational planning framework. Figure 1 illustrates one such planning loop which urges us to initiate programme development with a careful assessment of learning needs.[10]

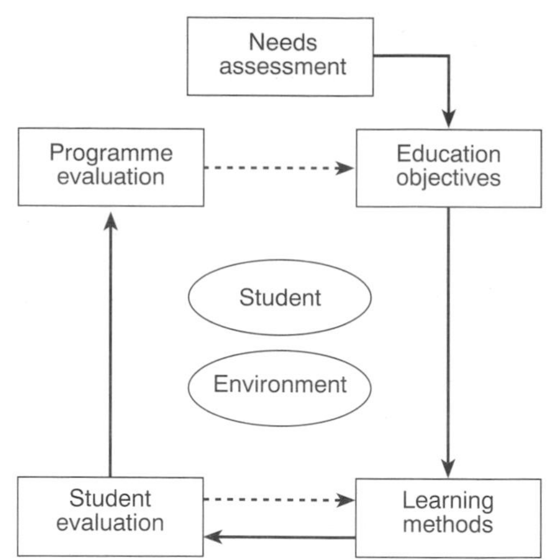

Fig. 1 An illustration of the systematic educational planning loop (adapted from reference 10).

Politics of medicine

Palliative medicine is a small player in the academic political world, particularly vulnerable to suppression by more powerful and long-standing academic disciplines as budgets for both clinical and educational programmes shrink. This risk is balanced by the current ferment for change in medical education.

In the United Kingdom and Australia, academic palliative medicine has found a home within internal medicine. In other settings, departments of family and community medicine, oncology, paediatrics, geriatrics, or anaesthesia may also provide a nurturing environment. Because the interests of palliative medicine cut across traditional departmental lines, novel approaches such as interdepartmental programmes and independent divisions of palliative medicine are being explored. The ideal administrative home for palliative medicine will vary from country to country, and from faculty to faculty. The most important principle influencing the organizational arrangements for palliative care must be its placement within a department which cherishes it, facilitates early access to the majority of patients who will be involved in the palliative care programme, and provides it with a secure academic base. From this position of relative strength, palliative care can reach out to collaborate with colleagues. A 'neutral' arrangement, where no one regards it as a priority issue, is far less likely to enable a palliative care programme to meet its educational obligations to patients with cancer and other disorders, and their professional caregivers.

Public attitude

Overarching many of the changes in the philosophy of medical education and the growth of hospice programmes is a shift in public expectation. In many developed countries, health-care costs are consuming an unprecedented proportion of total government expenditure. While the public is demanding fiscal restraints, paradoxically they continue to expect increasing sophistication and effectiveness in medical therapy. They also expect the health-care system to be more personal and more responsive to personal choices and societal issues. Society demands that we teach physicians to be more effective in communicating information and more sensitive in eliciting and managing the emotional and social components of patients' problems. Despite the continuing importance of denial in both the individual and societal reaction to death, there is increasing public demand for 'dignified' care of the dying.

Community attitudes must be matched by the availability of training opportunities enabling physicians to respond to the patient's agenda. The public's fear that suffering will not be adequately addressed may drive society to some form of sanctioned euthanasia unless medicine can develop a covenant of trust with the public, and demonstrate uniform competence in relieving suffering. Current public interest in end-of-life issues can strengthen support for palliative care; conversely, if academic medicine is not responsive, the public support for euthanasia and physician-assisted suicide may grow. At the present time, public expectation certainly adds to the demand for more training opportunities in palliative medicine.

Scope

The definition and description of 'palliative medicine education' is not clearly demarcated, reflecting its relevance to a wide spectrum of medical education issues. Nonetheless, there is a growing consensus about its core content and objectives.

Palliative medicine as philosophy

Palliative medicine seeks to relieve suffering and increase the meaning and quality of life in the face of terminal illness. Several concepts (including rigorous symptom analysis and treatment, care for the whole person, patient-centred communication, ethical decision-making, interdisciplinary team work, dealing with patients and families as a whole unit of care, and creation of therapeutic environments) have found a secure home in palliative medicine. As a philosophy, palliative medicine has relevance to much of health care beyond the context of terminal disease. Indeed, its lessons in humane care find relevance in most clinical settings. It may well be that palliative medicine's largest impact will be at this macro level. Our education programmes must meet the needs of this wider vision while keeping it in balance with more specific mandates.

Palliative medicine as a programme

In order to address specific needs in a specific population, a wide variety of palliative medicine programmes have developed around the world. These can be entirely new services or co-ordination networks that link existing services in order to optimize care. While all claim to be multidisciplinary, there are radical differences in the role of physicians in these programmes. In each local community, palliative medicine training will be defined largely by the scope and depth of services provided by the local hospice programmes. At a philosophical level, palliative medicine seeks to emphasize the need to care for patients in the setting of their choice—home, hospital, office, clinic, or specialized palliative care unit. However, the training may often be incomplete because the full range of settings is not available in every community. Scarce resources may lead programmes to restrict their admissions to a subpopulation of patients or limit their services to provide only some components of palliative care. Subsequently, the scope of these local programmes can become entrenched in government policies. Restricted definitions of palliative medicine result in anaemic educational models.

Palliative medicine as a discipline

The scope of palliative medicine education is increasingly defined by the growing number of career physicians who view palliative medicine as their professional home. As a discipline, palliative medicine defines its scope of practice, sets training and programme standards, and establishes a research base. Its core body of knowledge is being stated with increasing clarity—a major objective of this textbook.

The demarcation of the academic limits of palliative medicine remains in flux. Palliative medicine teaches the principles of care for the dying and the bereaved, particularly, to date, in the settings of cancer and AIDS. It presumes that many of these principles also apply to patients with other chronic progressive illnesses. It also stresses that its principles, applied early in the trajectory of illness, will reduce the pain and suffering that is experienced later in the illness.

A discipline that serves not only the needs of the dying, but also has application across the total trajectory of chronic illness, clearly has a demarcation dilemma. This issue should not be addressed using traditional 'turf defining' methods. Rather, the attitude whereby palliative medicine is regarded as a discipline, where principles serve as a model for clinical medical teaching, will enable schools to consider practically which topics are addressed in which courses.

Palliative medicine as a vocation

As a vocation palliative medicine is a publicly sanctioned 'call' to serve a particular population and set of needs. The starting point is the recognition of need and a personal/societal commitment to address that need. In this sense, the vocation of palliative medicine issues from the patients themselves. The characteristics of their suffering and the therapies required to relieve their suffering must define the content of palliative medicine education. We cannot fully understand the growth of palliative medicine if we ignore the emotional urgency and spiritual dimension of the 'call' to serve the dying. In fact, much of the power of palliative medicine as a training experience for physicians is derived from the emotional and relational demands placed on a learner in an arena that challenges one to confront issues concerning meaning, freedom, our essential aloneness, and death. Palliative medicine education must seek to utilize this strong vocational flavour and preserve palliative medicine's covenant with vulnerable, fearful, and suffering patients.

Learning needs and objectives

The need for improved educational programmes relating to palliative care has never been more evident; it is suggested by the numerous studies that continue to document inadequate end-of-life treatment in the international community. A quarter century has passed since Saunders showed that there was a better way[11] and Hinton observed that professional caregivers emerge deserving of little credit, 'We, who are capable of ignoring the conditions which make muted people suffer. The dissatisfied dead cannot noise abroad the negligence they have experienced.'[12]

A 2-year prospective observational study in five American teaching hospitals, involving 4301 seriously ill adults with an overall 6-month mortality of 47 per cent, demonstrated shortcomings in communication, frequency of aggressive treatment, and the characteristics of death. Only 47 per cent of physicians knew when their patients preferred to avoid cardiopulmonary resuscitation; 46 per cent of do-not-resuscitate orders were written within 2 days of death; 38 per cent of patients who died spent at least 10 days in an intensive care unit; and for 50 per cent of conscious patients dying in hospital, family members reported moderate to severe pain at least half the time.[13] Suffering associated with poor pain control and resultant impairment in functional status has been noted in cancer patients, in both outpatient[14,15] and inpatient[16] settings. Zenz describes an endemic 'opiophobia' in Europe;[17] physician surveys in Canada and the United States suggest a high prevalence of poor pain assessment skills and an inadequate knowledge base concerning the use of opioids and other therapeutic strategies (MacDonald, in press).[18]

The cost of palliative care incompetence may be reflected in the findings of Chochinov *et al.* who showed that the desire for death among 200 terminally ill patients correlated with ratings of pain, low levels of family support, and depression.[19] At a time when over 60 per cent of the population now favour the legalization of voluntary euthanasia for patients with terminal illness,[20,21] the demonstrated link between desire for death among the dying and factors that are potentially remediable through medical or social intervention stands as both indictment and motivator of those responsible for palliative care education.

The deficiencies in palliative care knowledge that are consistently noted in the literature may not be seen as personal areas of knowledge deficit by medical practitioners. Goldberg *et al.* surveyed 173 internal medicine and surgical residents concerning their perceived terminal care education needs.[22] While respondents recognized their need for improved skills in the psychosocial domain, they felt more secure with respect to symptom control. Only 35 per cent of the sample indicated the need for more training in pain management and only 27 per cent in the treatment of dyspnoea. A similar tendency to acknowledge personal lack of comfort in meeting psychological needs but greater confidence in personal ability to control physical symptoms was found in Ahmedzai's survey of 78 junior house officers in Glasgow.[23] On the other hand, inadequacy of personal ability to provide terminal care may be recognized but rationalized as being irrelevant to one's mandate as a physician. Herman reported on a sample of 50 housestaff and faculty at a New York teaching hospital. While 58 per cent rated their palliative care giving skills as poor, all the physicians felt that having to care for terminally ill patients interfered with learning and the majority expressed the view that patients with a terminal illness had no place in a teaching hospital.[24]

In the Goldberg survey, the lack of confidence concerning psychological support and communication skill was particularly evident among first year residents and was less evident among senior residents, though there is little evidence to confirm that senior residents are more skilled in terminal care. The Goldberg sample indicated that the preferred method of learning terminal care was to observe others doing this work (83 per cent of respondents). However two-thirds of the sample indicated that they did not have a palliative care role model. Likewise, the house officers in Ahmedzai's survey indicated that ward nursing staff contributed much more than their senior medical colleagues in both the psychological and medical aspects of terminal care.

The findings of the Goldberg study paralleled a survey of clinical medical students in the United Kingdom, New Zealand, and Japan which suggested that improved medical education in palliative care is needed. The students preferred multidisciplinary teaching that included specialists, family physicians, psychiatrists, clergy, and patients.[25]

There is wide agreement that the learning objectives in palliative care medical education include the exploration of:

(1) death as part of life and transcultural issues concerning death;

(2) issues defining the decision for palliative care in a variety of clinical settings and the impact of that decision on both the patient's quality of life and health-care costs;

(3) the physical, psychological, social, and spiritual impact of dying on patients and their families;

(4) the control of pain and other symptoms;

(5) psychosocial and existential support of patients and their families;

(6) one's own attitude toward death;

(7) communication skills;

(8) strategies enabling a continuum of care across a variety of inpatient and outpatient settings, particularly care in the home.[26-28]

The American Board of Internal Medicine has identified core competencies expected of board-certified internists in the care of dying patients.[29] These are listed along with their specific components in Table 1.

In order to develop and validate educational objectives in the care of the terminally ill for inclusion in the various levels of medical training, Schonwetter and Robinson[27] asked randomly selected members of the Academy of Hospice Physicians to evaluate 39 educational objectives as -1 (inappropriate), 0 (unsure), or 1 (appropriate). Of the 200 physicians surveyed, 127 (64 per cent) responded. The participants included internists (54 per cent) and family practitioners (23 per cent). Thirty per cent had subspecialties in haematology or oncology, 12 per cent in geriatric medicine, and 7 per cent in palliative medicine. Eighty-eight per cent were primarily involved in patient care, 85 per cent were hospice physicians, and 44 per cent were involved in physician training. Thirty-four of the objectives were validated, all with the mean scores of ≥.8. The 39 educational objectives and their mean ratings are tabulated in Table 2.

Undergraduate training

Objectives

The World Health Organization report *Cancer Pain Relief and Palliative Care*[1] described the scope and task of palliative medicine education:

Education is concerned with the following three interrelated aspects of palliative care:

1. Attitudes, beliefs, and values—minimum learning in this area should include the following topics:

    the philosophy and ethics of palliative care;

    personal attitudes towards cancer, pain, dying, death, and bereavement;

    illness as a complex state with physical, psychological, social, and spiritual dimensions;

    multiprofessional team-work;

    the family as the unit of care.

2. Knowledge base—as a minimum, learning in this area should include the following topics:

Table 1 Physician competencies and definitive components

Components	Core competencies
Medical knowledge	Palliative care Assessment and treatment of psychological distress Pharmacological and non-pharmacological treatment of pain and other symptoms
Interviewing and counselling skills	Listening Truth telling Discussing dying as a process Giving bad news Dealing with families of dying patients
Team approach	Understanding the multidisciplinary nature of end-of-life care—physician, nursing staff, social services, palliative care or hospice team, pharmacist, chaplain, patient, patient's family, patient advocate Promoting collegiality Enhancing ability of team members to fulfill professional responsibilities
Symptom and pain control assessment and management	Communication skills Comfort Use of opioids, sedation, or adjuvant analgesics NSAIDs Control of dyspnoea, anxiety AHCPR and WHO guidelines
Professionalism	Altruism Non-abandonment Respect for colleagues Accountability Honouring patient's wishes Confidentiality Transference and countertransference
Humanistic qualities	Integrity Respect Compassion Courtesy Sensitivity to patients' needs for comfort and dignity
Medical ethics	Advance directives Do-not-resuscitate or do-not-intubate orders Nutrition and hydration Conflicts of interest Futility Double effect Surrogate decision making Physician-assisted suicide

AHCPR = Agency for Health Care Policy and Research, NSAIDs = nonsteroidal anti-inflammatory drugs, WHO = World Health Organization

principles of effective communication;

pathophysiology of the common symptoms of advanced cancer;

assessment and management of pain and other symptoms;

psychological and spiritual needs of seriously ill and dying patients;

treatment of emotional and spiritual distress;

psychological needs of the family and other key people;

availability of community resources to assist patients and their families;

physiological and psychological responses to bereavement.

3. Skills—opportunities should be provided for the application of learned knowledge through practice in the classroom, making use of role-play and discussion of real case-histories. Important areas for practice include:

Table 2 Physicians' mean ratings of educational objectives for medical training in the care of the terminally ill, Academy of Hospice Physicians*

Educational objectives	Mean rating
At the completion of the training period, the physician will:	
Attitude	
1. Propose care for patients when cure is no longer a rational goal, and health services are most appropriately directed at comfort.	0.99
2. Defend the provision of comfort care to the dying as an active, desirable, and important service.	0.98
3. Discuss death as a natural part of the lifecycle.	0.94
4. Discuss the skills necessary to communicate about death and dying with the terminally ill patient and the family (or caregiver).	0.93
5. Honour medical decisions that are guided by the philosophy and values of the patient.	0.92
6. Describe the multiple determinants of suffering; physical, psychological, social, and spiritual.	0.91
7. Identify when disease-specific approaches may be the most appropriate techniques to control symptoms in the terminally-ill patient (e.g., radiotherapy, surgery, chemotherapy, pharmacotherapy).	0.90
8. Identify his or her role as a member and leader of an interdisciplinary team in evaluating and managing a patient's suffering.	0.84
9. Explain the unit of care for the terminally-ill patient as the patient and family (or caregiver).	0.80
10. Identify his or her own conflicts and anxieties about death and dying that may interfere with physician comfort in caring for the dying.	0.76
11. Discuss different approaches to medical care, death, and burial rituals among various cultures and religions.	0.53
12. Explain a patient's and/or family's need to utilize unorthodox or non-conventional therapies available to treat the terminally ill patient.	0.42
Knowledge	
13. Appraise various routes of administration of medication, with advantages and disadvantages of each, used for control of the following symptoms in the terminally ill patient: A. Pain B. Nausea and/or vomiting C. Dyspnoea D. Constipation E. Depression F. Anxiety G. Confusion H. Pruritus I. Anorexia J. Weakness/fatigue K. Other.	1.00
14. Identify and quantify the above symptoms along with the evaluation necessary for their control in the terminally-ill patient.	0.98
15. Discuss the concepts and philosophies of palliative care.	0.98
16. Discuss uncertainties in prognostication when managing the terminally-ill patient.	0.97
17. Identify the potential adverse effects of common medications used for control of the above symptoms in the terminally-ill patient.	0.97
18. Discuss various adjuvant medications used for control of the above symptoms in the terminally-ill patient.	0.97
19. Compare advantages and disadvantages of the various settings that are available for the terminally-ill patient. (In particular, gain an understanding of the patient in the context of the home environment.)	0.96
20. Describe the pharmacology of common oral medications with appropriate dosages for effective control of the above symptoms in the terminally-ill patient.	0.94
21. Explain the classification system of analgesic medications and associated principles for pain control in the terminally-ill patient.	0.94
22. Summarize the signs and symptoms of approaching death in a terminally-ill patient.	0.94
23. Discuss the different non-pharmacological (psychological and physical) approaches to control of the above symptoms in the terminally-ill patient.	0.94
24. Differentiate addiction, physical dependence, psychological dependence, and tolerance.	0.90
25. Contrast the appropriate management for the terminally-ill patient with acute versus chronic symptoms.	0.90
26. Describe the principles of biomedical ethics, including beneficence, non-maleficence, autonomy, competence, informed consent, advance directives, and guidelines for medical decision making for people near the end of life.	0.85
27. Describe the common disorders causing terminal illness, along with their usual disease courses, presentations, and progression.	0.83
28. Distinguish normal and complicated bereavement in order to make appropriate referrals.	0.83
29. Discuss specific regional laws that impact decisions near the end of life as well as opioid prescription requirements.	0.81
30. Explain the importance of the pastoral approach to assist patients and families with the psychospiritual issues that face the terminally-ill patient and family.	0.77
31. Discuss issues of access to and financing of health care for terminally-ill patients in various settings.	0.71
Skills	
32. Collaborate with the interdisciplinary team and provide specific information about diseases, diagnostic processes, prognoses, medical management, and symptom control.	0.99
33. Utilize the interdisciplinary team to manage the patient or family with the common psychosocial issues or problems that face the terminally-ill patient and his or her family (or caregiver).	0.98
34. Treat the dying patient in various settings, showing sensitivity and skill in organizing care responsive to the advantages and disadvantages of the particular environment.	0.97
35. Communicate with the patient and family (or caregiver).	0.96
36. Balance the values of the dying patient, medical factors, and environmental factors in medical decision making.	0.96
37. Control the above symptoms and other gastrointestinal, respiratory, urinary, cutaneous, central nervous system, musculoskeletal, and systemic symptoms in the terminally-ill patient.	0.94
38. Encourage patient control of as many aspects of life as possible with terminal illness.	0.91
39. Assess a terminally-ill patient in multiple relevant dimensions, describing current physical and psychosocial problems, as well as obtaining appropriate information, including social support systems and functional status.	0.92

* Of the 200 academy members who were randomly selected to rate objectives, 127 (64%) responded. The respondents rated each of the 39 objectives as −1 (inappropriate), 0 (unsure), or 1 (appropriate). Thirty-four objectives had mean ratings of ≥8 and were included in the authors' final version of valid educational objectives.

goal-setting in physical, psychological, social, and spiritual dimensions;

development of a family care plan;

monitoring of pain and symptom management.'[1]

These topics are not unique to palliative medicine as they are the foundation for humane medical practice in all of its dimensions. Some of them are already taught in medical schools, although the contact and emphasis are modest in comparison to their subjects.

It is essential that the material outlined within the World Health Organization report is emphasized in medical training to enhance the care of the dying and to improve the general quality of medical care. The realization of this objective depends on the introduction of palliative medicine as a formal designated subject within the medical school curriculum and, of equal importance, the integration of palliative medicine principles within other parts of the curriculum.

Palliative medicine enters the competition for curriculum space at a time when most medical schools are already concerned about information overload. Recognizing the changing relevance of today's facts for students practising medicine tomorrow, pure vocational training is contained, with increased emphasis placed on teaching students the art of medical practice and the value of continuing education. These currents in medical education will create a problem for palliative care groups who wish to carve out large designated blocks of teaching time. They may provide an opportunity for those who wish to integrate palliative medicine into the modern curriculum with emphasis on the fundamental tenets of good practice such as communication skills, cultural empathy, symptom assessment, and family studies.

The medical school curriculum has been in constant ferment for 35 years with no sign of abatement. A study of American faculties revealed that, with the exception of basic science faculties, all groups currently engaged in medical student teaching believe that there is a need for 'fundamental changes'.[30] The recommended reforms, which should be broadly supported within palliative medicine circles, include better integration of the basic and clinical sciences, a change from an institutional to a community teaching base, and a greater emphasis on general medical education and independent learning. American educators strongly support a reduction in formalized teaching blocks, particularly of the set-piece lecture type.

In another section, we have commented on the adoption of a biological model of disease by physicians, with consequent failure to recognize illness as a family and community problem with broad-ranging psychosocial and spiritual dimensions. In part this has occurred as a continuing reaction to the polyglot medical education system of the early part of the century when standards were not uniform and scientific teaching often incredibly bad. The placement of medical training on a scientific base appears to have overshot the mark with a resultant default of the 'social responsibility to train physicians for society's most basic health-care needs.'[31]

The academic base of palliative medicine is drawn from many other disciplines, some of whom may state that 'this topic is our purview' or 'we already teach how to care for dying people'. As discussed in the section on specialized training, a new discipline which intends to influence training practices must clearly identify the tenets of the discipline and itemize instructional objectives which are not addressed in the current curriculum. Otherwise a fruitless wrestling match for curriculum influence may occur with the new discipline usually losing in the final process. While palliative medicine is a discipline, it must be clearly recognized that its principles should imbue all of medical practice. Skill in communications and an emphasis on psychosocial aspects and team development are needed in obstetrics, ophthalmology, and orthopaedics, among many other medical fields. Thus, it is important that palliative medicine be integrated rather than isolated in a curriculum.

A problem could be presented to most palliative care groups if they indeed got what they desired and were granted a large bloc of curriculum time. Almost every programme is understaffed and may not be prepared for major new educational commitments. The lack of resources within any single programme provides a major impetus for co-ordinating palliative medicine instruction with colleagues in other disciplines, other professions (nurses, psychologists, etc.), and sharing teaching resources between faculties.

Guidelines for co-ordination include:

1. Spend less effort on expanding designated curriculum time and more effort on defining and integrating palliative care principles into the current programme. As curriculum time is scarce and the time of palliative care physicians is limited, infuse the concepts of palliative care throughout the curriculum recognizing that colleagues from other disciplines will often be teaching those concepts.

2. In keeping with current trends in medical education, designated time is best devoted to small-group teaching with experience in palliative-care units or clinics. 'Hands on' experience and guided contact with palliative care patients, families, and staff is essential.

3. Following on the above point, role models remain important in medical education. 'The acquisition of new knowledge requires the experience of positive exemplars.'[32] The prominent Canadian neurosurgeon, Wilder Penfield, at the peak of his career would remind McGill medical undergraduates in the course of his Osler Lecture that he continued to look up to his 'medical heroes'; teachers whom he continued to revere and who continued to influence his practice and standards. Role models are more clearly identified by their acts than their words.

4. Good palliative medicine depends on interdisciplinary teams. Teaching must reflect this approach—include nurses and other team members as instructors. In turn, if the nursing school welcomes physician instructors, offer to participate in nursing and other professional instruction.

5. Learning occurs when behaviour changes based on experience; this does not necessarily require a teacher. Use the wealth of education manuals, videos, computer programmes, and other information aids which are now available.

6. Ensure that principles of palliative medicine are included in student evaluation.

7. Offer the best elective in the faculty.

Organizational models—curriculum design

The palliative medicine groups in the Canadian medical schools have approached undergraduate teaching through a process which may be usefully considered in other countries. The deans of 16 Canadian medical schools were asked to name representatives to a Canadian Undergraduate Palliative Care Education Group in 1988. Representatives from 12 schools (out of 16) worked together over the ensuing 2 years to write a palliative medicine curriculum.

Initial discussion focused on the need for designated curriculum time for palliative medicine. In view, however, of the disparate structure of medical school curricula and the general cut back in formalized teaching blocks, the final report stated that palliative medicine needed a defined segment of each school's curriculum but that the size and content of the palliative medicine block was dependent upon each school's unique educational pattern. The committee decided that it was more important to define the content base of palliative medicine teaching.

This report, carrying the support of 12 school representatives and containing specific itemized instructional objectives, can be used to both plan the integration of palliative medicine tenets into the existing curriculum and to provide the foundation for a designated palliative medicine block where topic integration was judged not to be possible or desirable. An important principle of integration holds that palliative medicine physicians should actually take part in the integrated teaching exercise; it is not sufficient to simply identify, for example, that 'the anaesthetists teach how to manage pain'. As stated earlier, it is not possible for the palliative medicine team to cover all topics but they should be included in programme planning and, as time allows, co-ordinated teaching exercises.

The Canadian curriculum, completed in 1990, is divided into symptom control, psychosocial, and organizational sections. Within each subsection, specific objectives are stated which call for the student to learn available skills, adopt available attitudes, and possess an evaluable knowledge base.[28] The Canadian palliative care curriculum was revised and expanded in 1996, now with the input of 15 of the 16 Canadian medical schools. The new edition matches curriculum goals with case studies illustrating these goals. The manual will be published by Oxford University Press as *Palliative Medicine: A Case-Based Manual*. Although it reflects Canadian practice, it has been carefully reviewed by an international contributing editor and should find use in other countries.

When palliative medicine asks for a stronger place in the curriculum, the request may be more readily granted when the proposal is not based on generalities but is backed up by a specific educational plan with clearly outlined objectives and case examples illustrating these objectives. As in other countries, a case-based approach to teaching is in vogue in Canadian schools.[33] The principles of palliative care are readily taught through this process. The Canadian Committee presumes that the development of case-based educational material will not only find favour with students but also with faculties of medicine who need soundly established, case-based material in order to meet their mandates. Early experience suggests that our colleagues in other disciplines welcome our expanded involvement in case-based teaching. One hopes that their response in part is a favourable comment on the quality of the teaching material; it probably also relates to their relief in finding readily applied case-based teaching models at a time when they are overloaded with new demands for small-group teaching and might otherwise be required to fashion case-based material themselves.

In 1992, the Association for Palliative Medicine of Great Britain and Ireland published the *Palliative Medicine Curriculum for Medical Students, General Professional Training, and Higher Specialist Training*.[34] Notable features of this curriculum include designation of curriculum goals by level of training. This curriculum serves as the basic text employed by the European Association for Palliative Care for development of a master palliative care curriculum for Europe. A *Core Curriculum for a Post Basic Course in Palliative Nursing* was published by the International Society for Nurses in Cancer Care in 1991.[35] Recently, under the aegis of the Singapore Hospice Association, Asian and Western educators are developing a palliative care curriculum for Asian nations.

Specialty curricula concentrating on a specific topic, pain, have been published by the American Society of Clinical Oncology[36] and by the International Association for the Study of Pain.[37] These detailed outlines are aimed primarily at postgraduate trainees but serve as excellent reference sources for course planners. The work of Schonwetter and Robinson, formulating specific training objectives, was cited earlier in this chapter.[27]

Formulating curriculum goals is an important first step for palliative care educational groups. Paraphrasing Marshall McLuhan, 'the medium can become the message'—that is the process draws colleagues together in common purpose and leads to the establishment of formalized educational committees who, maintaining contact with each other, may take on other educational pursuits. These may include regular national surveys, sharing educational material, publishing teaching manuals, and using their collective strengths to influence medical schools. A curriculum can also be used by instructors to define expected competencies and to state clearly the goals of a specific educational exercise. In turn, these goals should be used to set examinations and to assess educational programmes. While the above outcomes of curriculum design are useful, the ultimate test of the process depends upon demonstration that curriculum principles are included in medical school teaching, and successfully influence the behaviour of graduates.

Evaluation

Evaluation—educational process

What are the baseline palliative care competencies of physicians—is palliative care teaching improving in quality and quantity, and is patient care improving? Few studies on these issues have been published. An Australian survey on this topic provides both a model for following up on student knowledge after graduation and information on their acquired skills and perceived weaknesses.[38] Smith, Tattersall *et al.* carried out a self-administered questionnaire study involving a sample of graduates of Australian schools who began internship in January 1990 (a total of 389 physicians). The study concluded that both radiotherapeutic and palliative care aspects of oncology teaching were inadequate. Approximately half the respondents had no exposure to a palliative care unit or clinic and more than 70 per cent felt that they were not sufficiently competent to discuss skilfully death with a dying patient. Palliative radiotherapy was not recognized as a principal analgesic technique, reflecting the lack of exposure to both palliative medicine and radiation oncology.

In view of the relative prominence of palliative medicine in Australia, one expects that similar or worse results would emerge from studies in most countries. Subsequent surveys of the views of oncologists and a mix of physicians in Canada also show that North American doctors view their undergraduate training in pain management with a jaundiced eye. A range of studies from various parts of the world (see section on Physician Competence—Chapter on Ethics) have demonstrated that many physicians do not competently address pain and their patients suffer inordinately as a result. Indeed, the authors are not aware of any general pain survey with a positive conclusion. While most surveys concentrate on pain, some have studied other educational outcomes. The concern of students that they cannot discuss emotive issues with patients is worthy of further comment. Repeated studies demonstrate that physicians possess inadequate communication skills. This includes both basic skills in history taking, where two studies demonstrated that nurse practitioners are superior to American physicians in eliciting a good history of gastritis and sleep disturbances[39,40] and skills in eliciting psychosocial information. Recent quality-of-life studies have provided further evidence that physicians are poor assessors of another's symptoms, limitations, and concerns.[41,42]

The failure of doctors to pick up physical and psychosocial problems is not simply placed on the doctors' shoulders. Patients do not like to give their physicians bad news. When they do, they probably fear at a subliminal level that the doctor will then interpret their problems and return even worse prognostic news to them. They also may not wish to disappoint their doctor whose disease controlling efforts may be going for naught.

Content surveys

Numerous surveys have recently been conducted in many countries to determine palliative medicine involvement in undergraduate teaching. As often happens in questionnaire surveys gathering information from different school models, the information is extremely difficult to interpret. Recognizing the distaste with which physicians view extraneous questionnaires, the accuracy of information is always suspect. Moreover, while designated 'palliative medicine' lectures and seminars can be identified, the number of bedside teaching hours devoted to the care of dying patients is difficult to define, and surely fluctuates with patient availability and instructor interest. The quality of these clinical teaching exercises is usually not defined in published surveys. Currently, an in-depth analysis of palliative care teaching in 10 American schools is under way (Greenwell Foundation, Dartmouth study, personal communication). This study is linked to an evaluation of the programmes and a critique of educational approaches. Detailed surveys of this type may create models for both review and implementation of palliative care initiatives.

With these caveats, a few useful points of information can be gleaned from survey data contained in the section on national reports below.

Evaluation—student knowledge

The examination process establishes crude, negative, but very influential priorities for students. Examinations reflect views of the faculty or licensing body on the importance of a subject. Therefore it is imperative that positive educational moves, such as curriculum design, should be accompanied by concomitant changes in student evaluation.

Each country should endeavour to monitor its national or principal examination system to determine the palliative medicine contents. When judged to be inadequate (which is probably the case in every nation today), a campaign to bring about evaluation change should ensue.

Teaching resources

Palliative medicine is replete with 'how to do it' books, manuals, audiotapes, videos, and published highlights of meeting. There are a number of scholarly journals which include reviews and symptom flow charts of generally high quality.

The World Health Organization has been a leader in this field. Their 1986 manual on cancer pain relief was the World Health Organization 'best-seller' at time of publication, and has been translated into 16 languages. This manual has been completely re-edited by a World Health Organization Expert Committee, with publication in 1996. The same Committee commissioned a companion manual on symptom control which, at time of printing, is caught up in the backlog of the World Health Organization publication process. These manuals are primarily directed at health professionals in developing countries although they can complement the many existing treatment manuals prepared by national committees and individual palliative care physicians and nurses.

Several countries have prepared practice guidelines on pain management.[43,44] Guidelines may not influence practice in the absence of other reinforcements.[8] Relevant to undergraduate training, endorsement by faculty leaders who are observed to put these guidelines to practical use could strongly influence medical students currently influenced by otherwise exemplary physicians who may not prioritize pain and palliative care.

Integration with the humanities

It is difficult to get news from poems, yet men die miserably every day for lack of what is found there.

William Carlos Williams

The teaching of medical students remains rooted in the acute care hospital. These institutions have not, over the centuries, given a priority to the humane care of dying patients; their tradition was one of excellence in disease investigation and management, not in whole-person care. Recent trends in medical education may ameliorate this situation, although educators must face the paradox whereby their efforts to humanize institutional care come at a time when administrative and economic forces call for increasing hospital 'efficiency'. A government authority in one of the Canadian provinces characterized this attitude recently when she stated 'Canadians love the concept of the hospital as a hotel. We have to give them the feeling the hospital is a muffler shop where you drive in and drive out.'[45] Her view, shared by many government apparatchiks, managed care technocrats, and some hospital administrators, makes the role of home care in education all the more important.

An emphasis on home care will assist in balancing medical education. A sense of history and familiarity with the humanities will also enhance student appreciation of whole-patient care and will assist them in placing end-of-life care in proper perspective.

Medical events and the characters involved in these events provide the narrative focus for much of literature in every culture. Few physicians, after reflecting upon their experiences, would have any difficulty in sketching the plot for a compelling story. And yet, until recently, the medical curriculum did not use the humanities to assist students to appreciate fully the depth of their experiences and, through literature, to encourage them to 'change places' with their patients in order to see life from a patient perspective. As so much of the literature which touches on medicine concerns human drama at the end of life, an infusion of the humanities into the curriculum should enhance and reinforce the teaching of palliative care. A recent issue of *Academic Medicine* and a *Lancet* editorial set out in greater detail the reasons for welcoming the humanities into our medical schools.[46–48]

Aside from teaching students to encompass a broader vision of human illness, studies in the humanities may also influence the language we use in our case accounts. Perhaps inducing students to use warmer language in describing human events may break the protective carapace tending to distance them from their patients. Rita Charon of Columbia University has analysed hospital chart language. An example from the record of a patient with a carcinoma of the bladder: 'He was noted to have Cheyne-Stokes respirations. He was seen acutely by neurology—an EEG was scheduled following their recommendations. A family conference went over all the complications that had occurred over the past few months, and it was elected not to pursue heroic treatment. The patient was found pulseless and unresponsive, with no blood pressure, at 6:50 a.m.'.[49] Dr Charon notes '..the extensive and bizarre use of the passive voice to explain human events'. The common use of the third person singular with reference to patients in clinical accounts, which may reinforce remoteness and distance, stands in contrast to the more animated use of first person present and future tenses in literature. Perhaps we not only 'are what we eat', but also 'act as we write'.

The *Academic Medicine* series[47] provides a number of examples of approaches to teaching the humanities in American medical schools. Pennsylvania State University College of Medicine (Hershey) was probably the first medical faculty to offer an appointment in literature. Subsequently, this school has continued to develop exemplary programmes. The first year outline of their course on 'The humanities and medicine' illustrates this point. Throughout the course, in addition to lectures and patient interviews, film and literacy readings are used to illustrate:

the patient's experience of illness;

ethical issues in medicine;

ethics and care near the end of life;

medicine and culture;

medicine and gender;

medicine and religion;

social and ethical issues in genetics.

(Personal communication from Dr David Barnard, Pennsylvania State University College of Medicine.)

Other new instructional approaches

'Medical education must foster self-directed learning and lifelong learning skills' and 'medical students...must be given a strong grounding in the use of computer technology to manage information, support patient care decisions, select treatments, and develop their abilities as lifelong learners.'[50]

The current generation of medical students and residents represents the first computer literate cohort of medical trainees. The dual recognition that today's information is often transient in accuracy and importance and that information needed to practice is increasing at a near logarithmic rate, leads inescapably to the conclusion that today's medical students must possess upon graduation the skills to manage information in a highly sophisticated fashion, a task which will require the student to have a friendly relationship with a computer. A variety of forms of computer-assisted instruction suitable for palliative care teaching have been developed but, to date, as in other areas of medical teaching, this material is usually available only as an option 'at the periphery of the curriculum'.[51] Also at the periphery are palliative care educators. It would seem that mastering the new technologies of information transfer and demonstrating their use in innovative programmes could provide an educational leadership role for palliative care.

Postgraduate training

Apart from specialized training for physicians who plan to make palliative medicine their career, we can identify three major target populations in palliative medicine postgraduate education:

(1) family medicine and general practice;

(2) oncology (including medical, radiation, haematological, surgical, and gynaecological oncology);

(3) junior hospital doctors (early, relatively undifferentiated, postgraduate trainees).

Other training programmes in which palliative medicine is extremely relevant include infectious diseases, geriatrics, paediatrics, psychiatry, cardiology, respirology, neurology, nephrology, anaesthesia, general internal medicine, and gastroenterology.

Family medicine

The training programmes for family medicine and general practice are faced with a task of staggering proportions—to enable large numbers of residents and registrars to handle a massive and diverse set of curriculum objectives in a short training period (2 years in many countries). Acquiring the skills of palliative medicine is now considered to be among the important objectives in almost all training programmes in the United Kingdom, the United States, Canada, and Australia. However, these objectives often focus on generic communication skills with less explicit attention to symptom management. Many programmes lack faculty members with specialized expertise in palliative medicine. To fit the objectives of family medicine training programmes, palliative medicine should be taught longitudinally over the 2 year programme with exposure to dying patients in the normal settings of primary care, office, and home. However, many argue that the low prevalence of terminal illness in a typical academic unit fails to provide adequate levels of tutored experience to develop competent and autonomous practice in the community. Many universities lack specialized palliative care teaching units where trainees could experience a telescoped, supervised experience in the care of the dying. None the less, palliative medicine, where available, is recognized by most training programmes as an ideal setting to teach family medicine. The severity of both physical and psychosocial problems and the emotional demands on the trainee act as powerful motivators for learning. Palliative medicine offers a compact opportunity to face difficult clinical, communication, and ethical issues in home, hospital, and office settings.

Elective rotations are widely available and Doyle's 1988 study[52] of 110 palliative care services in the British Isles revealed that 46 per cent were giving clinical instruction to trainee general practitioners and 63 per cent were giving lectures to such trainees. A number of jurisdictions make palliative medicine a compulsory rotation for trainee general practitioners. These rotations usually include responsibility on a specialized unit for 2 to 4 weeks and opportunities to observe palliative medicine in the home, office, and general hospital ward setting. Such an intensive rotation is supplemented by a longitudinal approach over the entire programme with seminars, self-learning programmes, and accessibility of palliative medicine consultants to advise residents on the management of their patients. In parallel to obstetrics, a minimum case requirement for dying patients, in combination with a clear evaluation strategy, will signal to all trainees that learning palliative medicine is an important goal of their programme.

Oncology

In many countries, oncology specialties or subspecialties have emerged in the last four decades. These disciplines have been treatment, rather than system, oriented with the treatment aspects focusing on tumour removal or destruction rather than on symptom control. Medical oncology exemplifies this skew more than radiation oncology where the palliative use of radiotherapy is more clearly recognized.

The fourth phase of cancer control is the control of suffering.[53] Few oncology training programmes have accepted this concept in practice as reflected in the research output of the major oncology centres and in their stated training objectives or examination content. Using cancer pain as a index, recent studies suggest that oncologists in various parts of the world have deficient training in symptom management.[15,18,54,55]

In 1991, the American Society of Clinical Oncology (**ASCO**) was concerned by the modest quantity of submitted cancer pain abstracts and by evidence that cancer pain was not always well handled by American oncologists. An ASCO Committee was formed which developed the following resolutions which were accepted by the ASCO Board:

ASCO recognizes that the treatment of cancer pain is an integral part of an oncologist's responsibilities.

ASCO recognizes that patients with cancer have a right to expect prompt and effective treatment of pain.

ASCO will do all it can to ensure that oncologists are well equipped to treat cancer pain patients who will receive prompt and effective treatment of cancer pain.

Following up on these resolutions, ASCO took the following initiatives:

An oncology pain curriculum was published and distributed to oncology training programmes.[36]

Discussions ensued with the American Board of Internal Medicine and other certifying bodies in an effort to reflect the content of this curriculum in board examinations.

An educational manual, accompanied by illustrative slides, was prepared and presented at a workshop to which all oncology training directors were invited.

The success of these initiatives is not as yet reflected in the clinical research presentations at ASCO's annual meetings. For example in 1996, presentation abstracts include 14 pain studies (out of a total of 1819) in contrast to over 100 reports on a single chemotherapeutic agent, paclitaxel. In oncological training, the thrust of clinical research heavily influences educational experience, as the formulation of clinical trials and the conduct of protocol work occupy a large part of a fellow's or resident's time. Therefore, while a systematic analysis of the exposure of resident to end-of-life care education has not been published, one suspects that, to the present time, the ASCO initiative is in abeyance. The excellent educational manual has been widely distributed throughout the world but its major influence on the training of American oncologists is problematic.

Studies on initiatives to expand the teaching of palliative care in the oncology programmes of other nations have not come to the authors' attention.

Elsewhere in this chapter, factors influencing the introduction of palliative medicine into clinical practice have been commented upon. In essence, these initiatives must be regarded as important by credible leaders in the field who are seen to apply related principles in their daily practice. The leaders are noted to expect others to give these principles a priority, as demonstrated by the emphasis on palliative medicine in evaluation and accreditation examinations.

The oncology training culture centres on the conduct of clinical trials and therapy by protocol. Reflecting what one hopes is progress, the therapy '*du jour*' for the most common forms of adult advanced cancer constantly changes based upon analysis of the latest major clinical trials and the introduction of new chemotherapeutic or biologic agents. These trials usually do not assess patient symptoms, although some phase III trials now gather data on quality of life. Unfortunately, the quality-of-life process is often a psychometric exercise whose assessment instruments are judged too complex for day-to-day clinical care. For example the 1996 American Society of Clinical Oncology abstract booklet contained 17 phase II–phase III studies on stage 3B–stage 4 non-small cell lung cancer which were judged of sufficient merit to be selected for presentation. Only one of these 17 abstracts contains any information on symptoms or quality of life. Despite evidence of tumour regression following therapy in a proportion of these patients, only modest increases in median survival are reported. Nevertheless, as reported elsewhere in this textbook (see Chapter 9.1.1), certain chemotherapeutic regimens have a highly favourable effect on the symptoms of patients with lung cancer.

How to interest oncology training directors in the principles of symptom management and palliative medicine? As oncologists are constantly involved in protocol work which involves careful assessments, one technique may be to recognize this trait and to work with oncology colleagues to convince them that their exemplary approach to analysis should be extended to include scales for symptom relief and psychosocial functioning. Once patient suffering is clearly recognized, it is likely that the compassionate nature of most oncologists will lead them to emphasize further relief of suffering as a component of an oncologist's role, even beyond the point when a patient may qualify for a protocol.

Junior housestaff

Between 70 and 85 per cent of deaths in the developed nations occur in hospitals, and most junior members of the hospital medical staff are often responsible for the care of these dying patients. In many cases the burden of terminal care falls 'by default on the shoulders of the most newly qualified and inexperienced doctor'.[56] Junior hospital doctors have the most physical contact with dying patients and are the ones summoned to certify death and then request an autopsy from grieving relatives. Often these experiences occur with patients or families who are unknown to them or at night when senior medical colleagues are not available. The survey by Goldberg *et al.*[22] indicates that first year house staff were more acutely aware of their deficiencies, confirming the opportunity to introduce teaching at an early stage when the junior doctor still feels the need for it. Doyle[52] believes that palliative medicine's teaching in undergraduate years either can be consolidated or wiped out by negative, unsupported experiences as junior doctors.

The task of palliative medicine education for the junior hospital doctor is formidable. The schedules of these doctors are extremely busy with a high service commitment. There is often little if any formal teaching time, with fierce competition for whatever exists. The junior house doctor is faced with the highest levels of stress that will be experienced at any time in his career. Fatigue, sleep deprivation, heavy professional responsibility, fear of making mistakes, and stresses of building a new family life will all lead to emotional vulnerability and at times to depression and anxiety. Some junior doctors will cope with this stress by avoiding care of the dying or discussions that would increase emotional stress. For others, the professional emotional strains will act as motivators for learning.

Teaching strategies for this group of physicians will require special attention. Calman[56] has suggested a very simple method of a log book which is maintained and then discussed with a supervisor. Where a general hospital palliative medicine consultation team exists, the accessibility to specialized advice on a case-by-case basis would appear to have tremendous educational benefit. However, we must continue to develop the competence and confidence of the senior faculty and ensure that junior hospital doctors are not left unprepared and unsupported. While didactic sessions on the specifics of palliative medicine will rarely be feasible at this stage of training, the use of informal small-group sessions has been introduced in a number of programmes. While serving an educational function, the main agenda for such small groups would be mutual support through discussion of cases and physicians' reactions to those cases.

Learning strategies

Jones *et al.*[57] provides a set of adult education principles (see Table 3) which should be integrated into postgraduate education.

Table 3 Principles of adult education

An adult education programme should:

- Meet the needs of learners
- Be relevant
- Be directly related to daily work
- Be problem-based
- Build on learner's experience
- Challenge learners to commit themselves
- Provide feedback
- Provide a consistent logical approach
- Lead to further study
- Be learner centred
- Be learner controlled
- Use visual as well as intellectual input
- Involve emotions and behaviour as well as fact
- Involve a holistic approach

Adapted from Jones *et al.* [57]

When these principles are used, there will be fewer lectures and more small-group formats and self-directed learning techniques. Ingram, Jones, *et al.*[58] have authored an interactive videodisc (computer-assisted learning with a laserdisc and a resource book) embodying these principles which has been used successfully in postgraduate medical and nursing education around the United Kingdom as well as Europe and India; produced by Marie Curie Cancer Care, it has been translated into Danish and Dutch. This technique is of great importance for learners who have schedules that make large-group teaching difficult. Interactive seminar designs such as the one described by Von Roenn *et al.*[59] has met with marked learner enthusiasm.

The survey of attitudes in 173 residents by Goldberg *et al.*[22] revealed the tremendous variability in the content and teaching methods preferred by residents. When asked to list the most effective methods of learning, 83 per cent indicated observation of others doing the work, 80 per cent supervised practice, 80 per cent discussion, 45 per cent videotape feedback, and 35 per cent included reading and lectures. These results underscore the need for faculty development in order to increase the competence and sensitivity of senior staff so that they can function as role models.

A number of American centres have emphasized the importance of psychiatry for assisting postgraduate trainees as they face the emotional impact of terminal care. There have been reports on the use of a psychiatric supervisor, the participation of liaison psychiatry in case management, and individualized psychotherapy sessions.

However, the optimal methodology of palliative medicine education at the postgraduate level is far from resolved. Some educators argue for a clinical rotation on a model palliative care unit.[60] Others believe that general ward experience supplemented by adequate levels of instruction, supervision, emotional support, and consultation advice is the superior model. Many programmes believe that the use of a mobile consultation team of specialists participating in individual case management is the most effective teaching method. The use of the home setting for postgraduate teaching is an exciting development which should be pursued vigorously despite logistical problems.[61] It is unfortunate that very little has been published on the use of the doctor's office or other outpatient settings for teaching palliative medicine.

Using the physician behaviour check list, an instrument to rate physician supportive behaviours, Blanchard *et al.*[62] compared internal medicine residents assigned to specially designated oncology units and similar residents assigned to general medicine floors. Patients seen by oncology teams were sicker and physicians engaged in less support behaviour than did their general medicine colleagues. The authors proposed that the concentration of very sick cancer patients in a unit diminishes the ability of house staff to engage in supportive behaviour and to address the needs of patients during morning rounds. While these results cannot be extrapolated to a hospice or a palliative care unit, they underline the fact that clinical exposure to dying patients will not in itself lead to learning and altered behaviour. The dying patient can be an effective teacher of palliative medicine only when this interaction occurs in a supportive milieu, with role models who can demonstrate optimal care, with supervisors who can motivate, steer, and support, and with sufficient protected time to allow learning to occur.

Postgraduate diplomas/degrees

Another form of higher academic training is the postgraduate degree or diploma. The appendices to this chapter from the United Kingdom and Australia describe a number of choices. Some, like the University of Wales diploma course, are specifically designed for physicians with a clinical focus. Most are more conceptual and methodological in nature, offering physicians the opportunity to study for an advanced degree alongside other health-care professionals and non-clinicians (Flinders University, Australia; Trent, Glasgow, and Dundee Universities, United Kingdom).

Continuing medical education

Far and away the largest effort in palliative medicine education has been aimed at practising physicians and not undergraduate or postgraduate students. The initial and continuing demand for assistance and information comes from physicians who are struggling to control suffering in their own patients and who are seeking to enhance their own ' zone of mastery'.[63] Solving a management problem in a patient is the most important stimulus to learning for a physician. Other stimuli include

(1) reflecting on the management of a series of patients or problems;

(2) completing an audit of practice for a self-assessment programme;

(3) reading journals or discussing issues with peers and experts;

(4) attending group continuing medical education activities including rounds and conferences;

(5) undertaking scholarly activities such as teaching, writing, and research.

In large part, the goal of continuing medical education is to eliminate ineffective, old practices and to replace them with new ones that have been shown to be more efficacious. The goal of continuing medical education is not so much to increase theoretical knowledge or specific skills but to bring about appropriate behavioural changes in the practitioner so that palliative care learning is integrated into practice. An extensive review of continuing medical education research[64] documents the power of combining several educational strategies. Usually most effort goes into the design and implementation of a specific programme which communicates or disseminates new information or skills. However, for learning to be consolidated and to result in practice changes, it must be combined with 'enabling' strategies (facilitating changes in practice environment) and 'reinforcing' strategies (performance feedback and practice reminders).

Major challenges face palliative medicine continuing medical education. There are huge numbers of generalists and specialists who are gatekeepers or primary care physicians for terminally ill patients. Each of them may only have a very small number of palliative care patients per year which limits the stimuli and weakens the facility to change practice patterns through repetition of newly acquired information. The number of faculty or tutors is small. The learning needs of practitioners are varied, requiring very individualized approaches to continuing medical education. There is also a major problem of access to community physicians in busy isolated practices.

Figure 2 illustrates the need for continuing medical education to be evidence based, patient centred, and sensitive to the context of medicine, if learning is to occur and be integrated into practice. The practitioner lives in an environment in which multiple influences compete and interact on his or her behaviour. The pharmaceutical industry is well aware of these factors in designing marketing strategies. Most of our attention in planning continuing medical education goes into manipulating the educational environment through rounds and other group events. However, administrations, licensing bodies, specialty colleges, etc. can alter regulations by creating maintenance of competence programmes or a mandatory peer review system. Palliative care dramatically illustrates the impact of the economic environment on learning. In many jurisdictions the labour intensive 'cognitive' style of practice required by dying patients is not reimbursed at the same rate as a 'procedural' or high volume practice pattern. Media and public education mechanisms can generate community pressure on physicians. A sociological analysis of the palliative care movement would demonstrate the power of this strategy in shifting what physicians learn. We must not forget the critical importance of personal circumstances on the learner's receptivity. The present and past experience of death in the physician's family and the psychological denial of death present major hurdles or palliative care education, that is there may be complex emotional reasons to avoid learning in this field. Figure 2 also advocates for the dissemination of new information in synthesized, packaged forms. The growth of practice guidelines and care maps is an important part of the continuing medical education strategy for the next decade.

Consultation as continuing medical education

The way in which we organize our clinical care can either encourage or block the education of colleagues. If the delivery system invites a primary care physician to transfer responsibility of all complex cases to a palliative medicine specialist in a different facility, learning will be minimal. However, if the model of

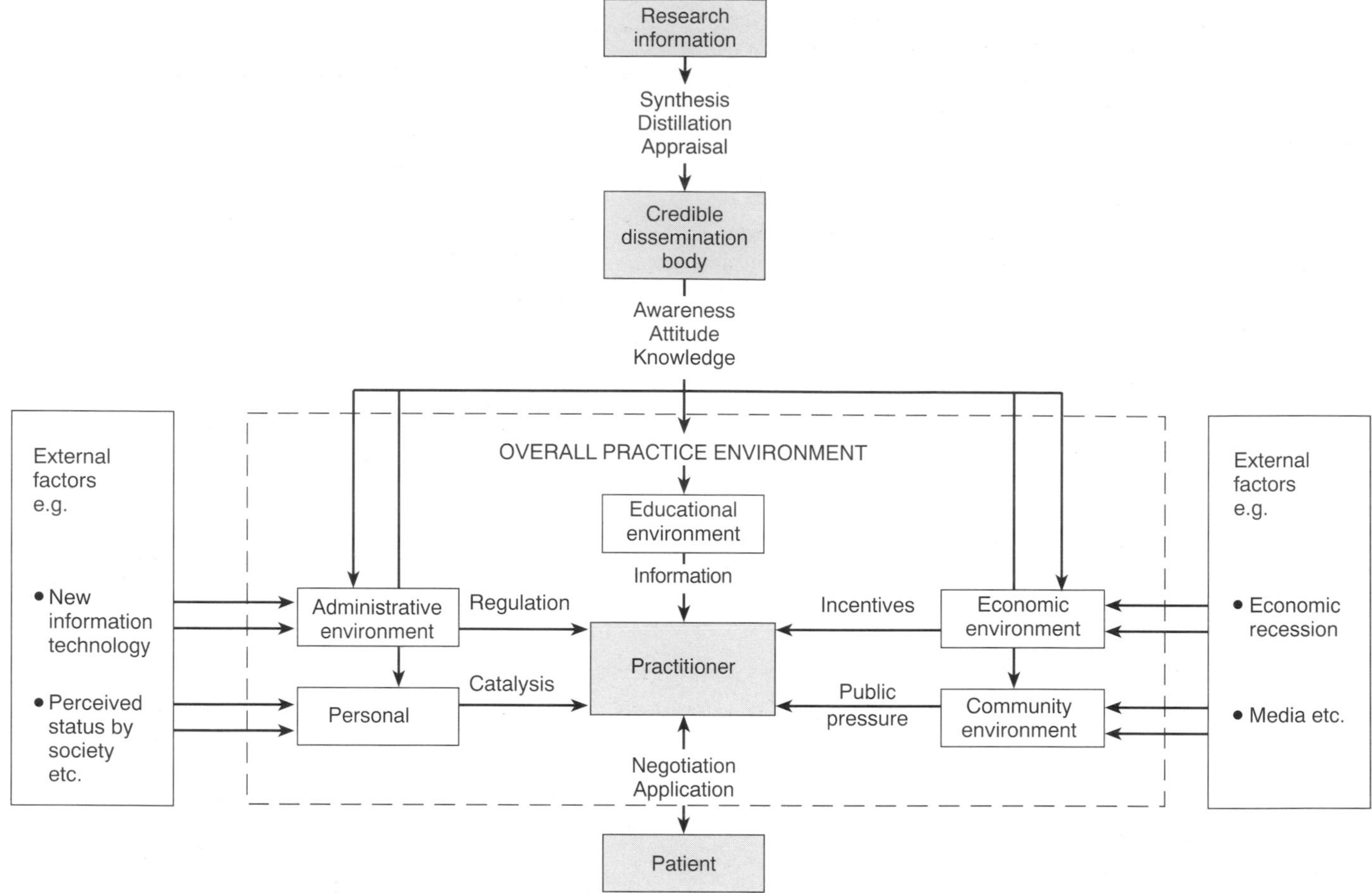

Fig. 2 The co-ordinated implementation model (adapted from reference 8).

consultation provides the primary physician with a thorough analysis of symptoms and issues and a detailed management strategy (including its rationale), the consultation may be more effective than any other method of learning. This style of consultation can occur in hospital, home, clinic, or office settings but should also form the ultimate goal of admissions to hospices or palliative care units. The admission to such units should be a special form of consultation in which patients with complex or intense symptoms are provided with a rapid, thorough, multidisciplinary assessment and monitored following a set of new interventions in a more controlled milieu. Through research, this specialized unit also designs and tests new management techniques, feeding these back to primary care.

All forms of consultation must be intended to teach, enable, and encourage our colleagues who have referred the patient. While assessment requires a relationship of trust between patient and consultant, this must never undermine the key relationship with the primary care physician. The consultation note on hospital charts, the letter and telephone call to the referring family physician, and the discussion of a case during rounds or in the corridor are among the most effective learning tools at our disposal.

Clinical practicums

It is difficult to teach palliative medicine without adequate clinical settings in which to demonstrate methods of assessment and treatment. While transfer of factual knowledge can occur through lectures, journals, computers, and videos most physicians will not have sufficient motivation or confidence to shift practice patterns until they can observe and participate in patient care that utilized this new knowledge.

The specialized palliative care unit or hospice provides an ideal environment for palliative medicine education for the following reasons:

(1) learning can be telescoped by participation in the care of large numbers of patients in a relatively short time;

(2) the emotional context of high intensity suffering and frequent death can force some students to recognize areas of weakness and motivate the learning of new strategies;

(3) high staffing levels, specially trained staff, and treatment protocols allow the learner to observe care that is consistent with the standards being taught by the faculty;

(4) a large multidisciplinary team can provide a safe supportive home base in which learners can shift attitudes and try out new skills that may still be at an awkward stage.

However, the specialized unit has weaknesses in fulfilling the educational mandate. The population tends to be admitted late in the course of disease and my fail to assist learners in dealing with problems of palliation when attempts to prolong life may coexist with the symptom control agenda. The resources of the unit are relatively rich so that learners may feel lost when faced with the task of palliative care in the 'real' world of home, office, or general hospital.

Palliative medicine must utilize the other consultation models of outpatient clinic, hospital consultation team, and home assessment to allow demonstration of care for learners in continuing medical education. However, these settings pose major challenges for faculty members. The advice of consultants is not always fully welcomed or implemented, and therefore consultants often focus on one or two of the most urgent problems. In some cases, students may learn more about the skills of consultation (diplomacy, negotiation, and public relations) than the specifics of palliative medicine. Consultants cannot afford to allow junior learners to try out new skills if this might endanger the reputation of a fragile programme.

Palliative medicine was founded on the belief that the patient is our teacher, and we shall require innovative designs to ensure that this can continue to occur.

Lectures and rounds

In many countries, nurses and other health-care professionals have welcomed palliative care more enthusiastically than physicians and therefore lectures have often been organized as multidisciplinary events. Since these were generally poorly attended by physicians, organizers were frustrated and the assumption was made that physicians were uninterested in, threatened by, or hostile towards palliative medicine. However, a major factor may be the physician's traditional distrust of multidisciplinary education. Most physicians are conditioned to value tightly structured lectures by physician colleagues on topics that can be immediately implemented in practice. To be attractive, a continuing medical education event must be packaged and advertised in ways that ensure that the physician feels safe, in terms both of being among his peers and of predicted benefit. The sponsor of the lecture must have a track record in delivering continuing medical education and be able to provide credits for medical societies and colleges. Special single lectures can be effective, but often must be presented by charismatic well-known speakers and advertised as a medical lecture, even if other professionals are invited. However, this still tends to draw the converted. Perhaps the most effective method of providing basic information for physicians naive to palliative medicine is through participation in the existing system of continuing medical education; that is adding palliative medicine cases to the regular hospital rounds of various disciplines and inserting palliative medicine topics into the continuing medical education lectures of universities or regional medical societies. This should also be the strategy for introducing palliative medicine topics into the conferences of national medical organizations and annual meetings of related disciplines, for example the International Association for the Study of Pain and World Cancer Congress. However, these scientific congresses are unlikely to include palliative medicine in plenary or discussion sessions until there is a substantial increase in the number of research abstracts arising from our discipline and palliative medicine may fail to gain access to some major meetings until it is recognized as a specialty.

Courses and conferences

The International Congress on Care of the Terminally Ill began in 1976 and has subsequently drawn up to 1000 delegates to Montreal every 2 years. Acclaimed as among the most creative and eclectic health-care conferences, this single event has spurred the development of many programmes around the globe and encouraged the diversion of many careers into palliative medicine. Now several national or continental conferences have developed, including the Annual Meetings of the National Hospice Organization (United States), the European Association for Palliative Care, and the Canadian Palliative Care Association. While the large scientific conferences of other disciplines generally focus on the dissemination of new research data, palliative care, until recently, has had relatively few presentations of original research. Almost all conferences are aimed at the full interdisciplinary team including volunteers, and are not structured to attract scholars or scientists. The content of plenary sessions are often philosophical and conceptual in nature. A few conferences, such as those organized by the Association for Palliative Medicine of Great Britain and Ireland and the American Academy of Hospice and Palliative Medicine, have been more clearly targeted to physicians. During this pioneer phase of development, palliative medicine conferences have attracted a combination of veterans and new recruits, leaving organizers faced with the dilemma of presenting the basics once again while simultaneously challenging senior delegates to go deeper.

Most palliative care programmes have developed a method of providing basic and advanced information on medical management to practising physicians, usually in the form of an intensive course of lectures and workshops. The length may vary from 1 to 10 days or more, depending on the course goal and the needs of the target group. Some programmes offer a longer experience of several weeks in which regular lectures are combined with apprentice participation in clinical care. Because the needs and preferences of learners in continuing medical education vary so widely, a wide spectrum of choices is required.

Journals and self-learning programmes

The major medical journals and the journals of our sister disciplines, such as oncology, have largely failed to provide space for palliative medicine. Part of this stems from the dearth of research results sent for publication but it also reflects the underlying philosophy that palliative medicine and the control of suffering is a soft subject and not an essential component of medical science.

More recently, this relative vacuum has been filled by a set of journals aimed at a multidisciplinary care audience. These journals include *Palliative Medicine* (United Kingdom), the *Journal of Palliative Care* (Canada), the *Journal of Pain and Symptom Management* (United States), the *American Journal of Hospice and Palliative Care* (United States), *Progress in Palliative Care* (United Kingdom), and the *European Journal of Palliative Care* (United Kingdom). Much of the content is review material or general discussion of political and programme development issues although the quantity of original research is increasing rapidly. However, the majority of medical publications relevant to palliative medicine are spread throughout the scientific literature. Scholarship has been aided by the more frequent presence of computer hardware and the introduction of more user-friendly software for literature searching. The

World Health Organization and other governmental and pharmaceutical sponsors have published a variety of monographs and newsletters and annotated abstract services. Very few palliative care centres are on the World Wide Web of the internet but we expect this to change rapidly in the next few years.

A wide selection of books, audiotapes, and videotapes are available to the continuing medical education audience, although orderly access can be difficult for the new learner. Perhaps more effective will be interactive self-learning continuing medical education programmes using computers and/or video discs and feedbacks from distance-based faculty members. As training accreditation becomes mandatory and as the research base of palliative medicine expands, we shall require methods of ongoing continuing medical education which include a form of self-evaluation followed by the provision of learning strategies for correcting deficiencies, as are presently provided by a number of national family medicine and paediatric continuing medical education programmes.

Reflective practice

The literature of academic nursing challenges us to utilize the concept of reflective practice in our continuing medical education strategy.[65] New programmes aimed at maintenance of competence in physicians are becoming less focused on the accumulation of credits from lectures and tapes. Instead they encourage colleagues to learn through reflection—either using individual patients (evidence-based management or interactive approach to consultation) or reflect on their practice patterns (chart reviews or practice audits). Palliative medicine, which espouses a client-centred and community-oriented care, must seek innovative ways of integrating patient feedback into learning strategies.

Specialized training

History

In November 1987, the United Kingdom became the first country in the world to recognize palliative medicine as a medical specialty. The Royal Colleges of Physicians of the United Kingdom and Ireland recognized palliative medicine as a new specialty and shortly thereafter the Joint Committee on Higher Medical Training approved a 4-year training programme for senior registrars in this new discipline.[66,67]

Long before this landmark decision, however, we can trace the concept of specialized training back to the 1940s and 1950s when a few physicians focused their career on the care of terminally ill patients. These first pioneers, especially Dame Cicely Saunders, have had enormous impact on developments. What could be achieved when a physician devoted an entire career to this population of patients was demonstrated to the world. With a few notable exceptions, hospice and palliative medicine has only flourished where there have been full-time, career physicians. Historical accounts of hospice and palliative medicine often focus on the disparate training and backgrounds of these early physician pioneers. They were largely 'self-trained' in the specific elements of this new field and most of them did not have formal links with an academic community. None the less they became the first 'specialists' in palliative medicine. The lack of university affiliation did not stop them from using academic methods to revolutionize care. Through careful assessment and documentation of clinical data, through the introduction of innovative therapies, through publication and dissemination of their experience at international conferences, and through the development of education programmes at their hospices they captured the imagination of the world and initiated a global shift in practice and philosophy.

The growth of palliative medicine follows the spiralling demand for health services for the dying. There was an explosion of hospice programmes in the United Kingdom in the 1970s and 1980s to meet this demand. While the rapid ageing of the population speeded development, the major factor underlying this change was a dramatic shift in public philosophy concerning technology and communication. With the growth in hospice programmes, so came a demand for physicians to provide services. By the mid 1980s a serious lack of qualified physicians to direct hospices and National Health Service hospice teams was looming.

Many of the early palliative care programmes developed short and long-term training opportunities to meet the spiralling demand for training. These lacked accreditation standards or any form of certification. Funding bodies and students began demanding increased uniformity and some form of recognition that would assist in later career development.

Universities and scholarly societies began to see the academic opportunities within palliative medicine and new journals and several conferences became available to report on palliative medicine research and programme development. Hospices began to control a substantial number of beds in the health-care system and therefore were increasingly viewed with interest by training programmes. Yet there was no recognized way of developing academic faculty that could make full use of these new academic opportunities.

The relatively rapid growth of palliative medicine in the United Kingdom reflects the recognition by the National Health Service that the proper development of palliative medicine had the potential to decrease the cost of health care in the last year of life. They recognized that shifting attitudes and the provision of skills to enable patients to stay in the community longer and to prevent costly, futile attempts at prolongation would require the development of a small set of specialists in this field. Governments in other parts of the world have been much more ambivalent towards specialty development in this field.

Two other essential components were present in the United Kingdom. First, there was a cancer charity which assisted in the funding of specialized training in palliative medicine. The Cancer Relief Macmillan Fund catalysed the development of palliative medicine by providing funds at a critical time. Secondly, in 1985, The Association of Hospice and Palliative Care Doctors of the United Kingdom and Ireland (now called the Association for Palliative Medicine of Great Britain and Ireland) was formed. This association developed a clear consensus which supported the development of specialty training while continuing to support general practitioners who would provide palliative medicine services in many parts of the country.

Palliative medicine in Australia and New Zealand has followed a path similar to that in the United Kingdom, with a subspecialty programme approved in 1988. In many parts of the world, including Canada and the United States, a firm consensus on specialty development among physicians now practising palliative medicine has not developed, nor is there a governmental or charitable funding body willing to underwrite this development.

Canada provides a case in point. In 1994, The Canadian Society of Palliative Care Physicians applied to the Royal College of Physicians and Surgeons of Canada for subspecialty recognition. Initially, the application was very well received and both Internal Medicine and General Surgery agreed to be base specialties. However, in 1996 the application was rejected for apparently economic and political reasons. The current economic environment has led to massive downsizing in postgraduate training and a new subspecialty was viewed with suspicion as creating yet another slice in a shrinking pie. The structures of medical politics are seldom designed to make rapid shifts to meet changes in the needs of our patients. Governments may also fail to analyse this issue from a population health perspective. Despite the rapid increase in the population of terminally ill patients, governments may focus on cutting costs and reject all new specialization in favour of espousing enhanced generalism and primary care. Palliative medicine must learn to argue more effectively that limited and focused specialization to provide teachers and consultants for the primary care system is critical if we are to meet the huge shift in the burden of illness. Specialization is the most effective strategy to ensure basic palliative competency in a primary care system. In fact the options are not specialization or generalism. The true choice is between standardized, controlled specialization which focuses on consultation and education versus haphazard pseudospecialization in which a set of generalist physicians without training or accountability develop an isolated primary care system for the dying.

Rationale

In 1988, the *Journal of Palliative Care* published six articles centred on the question 'Is palliative care a well-defined discipline or specialty'? While the majority of authors supported the development of specialty, this was not unanimous. Scott[68] defined a discipline as 'a body of knowledge which can be defined, organized, analysed, administered and taught, which requires mental and moral training to be mastered, and which entails a system of principles and standards'. Calman[69] and Levy[70] both examined the historical development of the 45 to 100 recognized specialities and subspecialties of medicine. Most specialties are focused upon specific organ systems (cardiology, nephrology, neurology) or disease categories (infectious diseases, oncology, rheumatology). Other specialties focus upon the more general, yet unique, needs of particular patient populations (paediatrics, obstetrics, geriatrics, physical medicine and rehabilitation). Levy points out that palliative medicine fits most closely into this last category.

A variety of authors have examined the following essential elements of a medical specialty or discipline.

Population

A specialty requires a clearly defined patient population of sufficient size to justify development of a discipline. Palliative medicine arose as a response to the unique needs of the terminally ill, who form a large and rapidly growing segment of the population of both developed and developing countries. The health-care needs of this population are severe, complex, and urgent. The boundaries of this patient population remain somewhat unclear—especially those not suffering from cancer or AIDS and those with advanced disease for whom therapy aimed at prolongation is continuing. None the less there exists a consensus on the core population towards whom this discipline has been directed.

Body of knowledge and skills

A specialty requires a clearly defined body of knowledge. While this is linked with specialties, this body of knowledge must be seen as forming a coherent cohesive whole. In palliative medicine, the presence of journals, textbooks, educational materials, professional societies, congresses, and government commissions attests to the development of this body of knowledge. Several authors point, with concern, to the relative lack of a research base underpinning this body of knowledge. Most of the theoretical base of palliative care has been derived from the research of other disciplines but this is beginning to change. The journals of the discipline document the rapid growth in scholarship and the formation of clinical research programmes. A discipline is also associated with a set of skills and/or technical procedures. The specialist is usually able to provide care which the generalist is unable or unwilling to provide. In palliative medicine, the physician is the source of expertise on the assessment, analysis, and management of the symptoms of advanced disease. At the present time, there is no equivalent to cardiac catheterization or chemotherapy. Palliative medicine skills should be more closely compared with those of paediatrics or geriatrics.

Philosophy and mission

The development of a specialty requires that a group of physicians recognize a shared set of principles and desire to form a 'community' with a common unique mission in health care. This has been one of the strongest factors holding palliative medicine together since the beginnings of hospice care in the 1960s.

Careers

A specialty can develop only when a group of physicians are already working full time with patients who require the specialized body of knowledge mentioned above. These early pioneers must be able to demonstrate the successful application of knowledge and skills in such a way that care is improved. There must be evidence that attractive and effective full-time careers are available.

Public acceptance

Calman[69] points to the need for a well-defined specialty to have value in the eyes of patients, the public, and other professionals. He views this as an important barrier that palliative medicine must break. The natural resistance to the removal of a group of patients from other medical specialties can only be overcome if there is strong public demand for the growth of specialized services.

Shared service with generalists

The spectrum of shared versus unique services varies from specialty to specialty. In all areas of health care, generalists provide the majority of medical care using the information largely developed by specialists. Patients who fail to respond to usual therapies or who have complex or rare problems are those most commonly referred to specialists. Palliative medicine cannot develop as a discipline unless generalists recognize the need to refer. In most countries, the process of referral and negotiation of shared service has been speeded by the fact that palliative medicine has control over the admission policy of a relatively large number of beds in the health-care system.

Calman,[69] Levy,[70] and Librach[71] all explore the relationship between the specialty of palliative medicine and the generalist physician. Levy is confident that general practitioners need palliative medicine specialists to develop the safest and most effective care for dying patients and their families, while Librach is opposed to this development, fearing that palliative medicine would compete with general practitioners in the care of the dying. Care for the dying poses several obstacles for the generalist, including disruption of office and hospital practice patterns and unfair reimbursement for time spent. Despite this, generalists often view this care as central to their vocation. While emotionally draining, it is usually viewed as rewarding and affirming. Calman supports the development of palliative medicine as a distinct discipline, but believes that we have an important responsibility to teach and support the many other doctors, both generalists and specialists, who will be delivering the bulk of palliative care in our society.

The dynamic that exists between generalist and specialist is not unique to palliative medicine. However, since continuity of care is at the core of our mandate, elitism in palliative medicine is particularly destructive.

Standards

A specialty must have a clearly defined training programme, usually with peer accreditation leading to some type of training certification. This is clearly occurring in palliative medicine in a number of countries, although it is far from complete in most.

A specialty includes the formation of clearly defined programmes that are directed by 'specialists'. Palliative medicine, as a body of knowledge, must be able to be administered in a systematic, multidisciplinary programme encompassing a number of clinical settings including inpatient beds, home care, and outpatient and acute care consultations. Here again, the control of beds and other resources is often the key to the development of a distinct discipline. Unlike coronary care units, one cannot go to a hospice or a palliative care unit and assume that it is delivering comparable services to those delivered in other units in the same country. While the nature of palliative medicine will require ongoing diversity, the standardization of programmes will need to increase if specialization occurs. With increasing uniformity, accreditation and quality assurance programmes can be designed.

Learning objectives

The primary goal of a specialized training programme is to provide the resources in which a physician can learn to function as a specialist in palliative medicine. The United Kingdom Senior (Specialist) Registrar Programme aims 'to equip individuals to carry the responsibility of a consultant working full time in a hospice or in a hospital unit or team with the responsibility for a substantial number of patients (with malignant or non-malignant disease such as ALS and AIDS) in the end-stages of illness'. A survey of international fellowships reveal a broad range of objectives (Hall PG, Hobbs N, Scott JF. Postgraduate medical education programs in palliative care: a survey, in press). The longer programmes seek to enable a physician to become a clinician, consultant, team leader, manager, teacher, and researcher in palliative medicine, in order to develop and/or direct palliative care programmes or function as a regional or hospital consultant in pain and symptom control. A secondary goal of these programmes is to provide a structured training experience for those intending a career in another specialty (medical or radiation oncology, general and family medicine, infectious diseases, geriatrics, haematology, neurology, paediatrics, etc.) where a substantial proportion of patients will have end-stage disease.

The appendices to this chapter describe the curriculum models that have developed in the United Kingdom, Australia, New Zealand, and elsewhere.

Politics and careers

Despite the enormous increase in the number of palliative care patients, programmes, teams, and beds, physicians in training might well ask whether a career in palliative medicine is a wise choice. In most countries, funding of hospices and palliative care programmes has been short term and precarious, with unclear methods of physician reimbursement. Will there be a job waiting for those who undertake specialized training in palliative medicine? The United Kingdom is the only country that has undertaken to estimate future career opportunities. In 1986, the Hospice Information Service (based at St Christopher's Hospice, London), undertook a survey at the request of the Association of Palliative Care and Hospice Doctors of Great Britain and Ireland.[72] Based on the 75 per cent response rate from National Health Service and independent hospice units and supplemented by information available from other sources, the survey estimated that there were 68 career posts in the United Kingdom (46 in independent hospices and 22 in the National Health Service). These were all senior positions classified at the consultant level and included both medical directors of hospice units and university appointments in palliative medicine. Based on stated plans, the survey estimated 10 new career posts in hospices during the period 1989 to 94, not including possible expansion of National Health Service programmes. During a 2-year period (1986–7), 22 posts (13 new) at the consultant level were advertised in the United Kingdom, several of which were not captured by the survey described above. Many had to be readvertised since applicants did not have the necessary experience and training.

The same survey examined the ages of those presently holding career posts at the consultant grade and estimated a retirement rate of 3.6 per year for 1990 to 94 (18 vacancies) and 2.4 per year for 1995 to 99 (12 vacancies). Based on these data, the Association of Palliative Medicine estimated that at least 10 new posts per year would be advertised over the decade following the survey. However, this is probably a conservative estimate since the establishment of palliative medicine as a specialty is likely to fuel an upward spiral of demand.

In projecting demands and targeting for the optimal number of trainees, each country must examine a number of service, academic, and funding indicators. Projections for the United Kingdom are complicated by the fact that two-thirds of the career posts and training slots are in independent hospices who rely on charitable sources of funding. In 1996, only 38 per cent of the income in 167 independent units derived from the National Health Service. The demand for specialized physicians will increase as service needs increase. Important variables include the total number of deaths (especially cancer and AIDS), the total number of distinct palliative care programmes, the total number of beds devoted to palliative care, and the total number of patients seen in consultation by hospital palliative care teams. Changes concerning funding will have a major impact on the availability of career posts. Career opportunities for palliative medicine will also be determined by the number of medical schools and regional cancer centres who assign a priority to palliative medicine.

The successful development of specialty training programmes in palliative medicine depends on a careful balance of political elements. The total number of training slots, the allocation of those positions across the country, and the length and character of the training programme is determined by a number of players, many of whom are far removed from palliative medicine itself. Each nation will have a distinct pattern of health care services and medical training and therefore will develop a unique method of providing specialty training in palliative medicine. For example in the United Kingdom there are clear distinctions between specialists and general practitioners and between hospital and community care which do not exist in some other countries. The United Kingdom also has a very long period of training for most specialists. There are relatively few consultant grade posts and all expansion is under firm National Health Service control. The palliative medicine specialty that is now developing in the United Kingdom conforms to the medical manpower principles which applies within all National Health Services universities, including the definition of consultant. These principles were agreed upon by the Association for Palliative Medicine during their negotiations with the Government and the Royal Colleges. At the time of writing there are 112 Specialist Registrar training posts in palliative medicine in the United Kingdom.

Future directions

In the twenty-first century, a staggering increase in the demand for palliative medicine education is anticipated. This demand will be impossible to meet unless a major shift in resources and attitudes can be negotiated. The increased demand will be generated largely by the rapid growth in the patient population requiring palliative care in both developed and developing nations fuelled by radical changes in societal attitudes. This burden of suffering will drive governments to seek more effective and efficient methods of delivering care during the last year of life for patients with cancer, AIDS, and other chronic illness. If the growth of rigorous education programmes aimed at symptom analysis and management cannot keep pace with this rise in suffering, we envisage the proliferation of bastardized forms of palliative care and/or sanctioned euthanasia programmes. While we have witnessed remarkable advances in the last decade, such that most medical graduates of the English-speaking world have had some exposure to palliative medicine, we shall need strong prophetic voices if we are to fight for the public mind and the public purse.

Obstacles and opportunities

As palliative medicine approaches the year 2000, a number of factors may impact on its development. Government reliance on cost analysis will be a double-edged sword. While cost–utility analysis should lead to increased funding for palliative medicine education, attempts to portray palliative care as a cheap way to die may lead to anaemic models of care. The anticipated explosion in the patient population requiring palliative care may appear to be an important impetus to educational development. However, if this increase is too rapid, existing resources will be overwhelmed. In such a milieu, service may take precedence over education.

With the notable exception of the United Kingdom, palliative doctors have not developed a common policy on pivotal issues such as specialization. Until the community itself can develop more cohesion and consensus, its educational effectiveness will be diminished. The demand for training and programme standards will force palliative medicine to define more carefully the scope of the patient population. As palliative medicine becomes more closely tied to researchers and scholarship in sister fields, we shall observe more rigorous documentation, more investigational techniques, and more complex management strategies. Some will be concerned that such high technology interventions may lead to a reversion into aggressive, impersonal models of care.

Palliative medicine has tended to develop in small, isolated, and poorly funded programmes. Effective teaching programmes will demand the creation of centres of palliative medicine in which there is a critical mass of academic physicians working together. There must be a firm academic home base and a clear faculty recruitment strategy.

Palliative medicine must brace for a major assault from the euthanasia/assisted suicide controversy. This debate has the potential to split and destroy palliative medicine. Yet it also provides an opportunity to teach the public and politicians about pain control while vigorously standing against the confusion and distortion which portrays palliative care as a form of passive euthanasia.

Recommendations

International standards

A set of standards and recommendations should be developed at the international level in the arena of palliative medicine education. These should include the essential learning objectives for curricula, faculty standards, and the core components of clinical experience. Such a set of guidelines could be the work of a consensus process organized by the World Health Organization and multinational palliative care organizations. As demonstrated by the remarkable success of the World Health Organization Cancer Pain Relief Programme, such an international consensus will enable and empower national and local programmes to fulfil their specific mandates.

Educational methodology

The international community requires several academic centres of palliative medicine where attention can be focused on the methodology of palliative medicine education. New learning resources must be developed including multimedia self-learning packages, distance-based or computerized continuing medical education techniques, and inexpensive simple resources for the developing world. Improved techniques for evaluating the learner, the teacher, and the training programme must be developed with careful attention to measuring the full scope of essential outcomes—for example not only an understanding of opioid pharmacology but also the skill of communicating and assessing bereaved persons.

Practice orientation

We must focus our attention on community patterns of practice and practitioner behaviours. Practice guidelines, decision trees, and care maps must be developed and used as the framework for educational programmes. We must ensure palliative medicine is a core component of the maintenance of competence and recertification programmes being undertaken by licensing and accreditation bodies.

Target selection

In the face of limited resources, training programmes must select the most appropriate learners who will have the largest impact on the burden of suffering in a population. This will require a dynamic balance between our need to train specialists and our need to educate generalists. The latter objective will require broad programmes to teach basic knowledge, skills, and attitudes at both the undergraduate and the junior house officer level, while developing more focused programmes in selected postgraduate fields—most particularly oncology and family medicine.

Faculty

We shall fail to meet the challenge unless we can produce a cadre of full-time career physicians with extensive training in palliative medicine who hold faculty posts in the major medical schools of the world. These academic positions must allow for adequate protection from service demands in order for scholarship, research, and education to flourish. However, we can never hope to develop enough specialists to teach all the objectives of a palliative medicine curriculum—nor should we. Palliative medicine must develop coalitions and co-ordinate instruction with medical colleagues from other disciplines as well as with other members of the multi/interdisciplinary team. Nurses, social workers, clergy, and other professionals must be recognized as important faculty resources.

Research

It is essential that palliative medicine develop a strong research base in order to fulfil its educational mandate. Palliative medicine cannot attract excellence in learners or faculty members without this strength, and the content of its curriculum will rapidly become stale and anaemic. With scarce faculty and financial resources, this will require innovative alliances with sister disciplines and private industry. We must excite researchers in related fields and woo them into recognizing the academic and economic potential of palliative medicine research. We must learn the skills of critical appraisal and systematic reviews to ensure that training is evidence-based.

Funding

Financing palliative medicine education will require a coalition of funding bodies including governments, universities, private industry, and national charities for cancer and other palliative care issues. This will only develop if we can shift public attitudes and exert political pressure on the process of health-care rationing. We must alert governments to the economic benefit of controlling suffering and, even more importantly, demonstrate the political potential of controlling the pain and fear of dying. We must ensure that palliative care is not judged on the basis of cost saving but on cost–utility analysis including the outcomes of symptoms, suffering, quality of life, and satisfaction.

Appendices

United Kingdom

Anthony M. Smith

Introduction

Palliative medicine in the United Kingdom is a recognized specialty, a branch of general internal medicine. From 1987 it has had its own 4-year specialty training programme leading to accreditation. It is also a recognized subject for academic study. A chair of palliative medicine was established in London in 1991 and by 1996 a further six chairs had been established in Bristol, Sheffield, London, Wales, Sunderland, and Glasgow Universities with professors appointed to each. A clinical readership in palliative medicine was established in Oxford University in 1988. Senior lectureships in palliative medicine were established in university medical schools in six cities as well as in five London medical schools, largely with initial funding from the Cancer Relief Macmillan Fund, a very important independent charity.

The Association for Palliative Medicine of Great Britain and Ireland appointed, in 1991, a regional educational representative in each of the British health regions. They are responsible for encouraging the teaching of palliative medicine at undergraduate and postgraduate levels and its incorporation into continuing medical education. A working party of these educational representatives developed a curriculum for the teaching of palliative medicine at all grades, published by the Association for Palliative Medicine in 1992, and subsequently adopted by the European Association for Palliative Care as basic to teaching of palliative care throughout the European Community.

Undergraduate teaching

Palliative medicine now forms part of the curriculum for medical students in most of the British medical schools. A survey at the end of 1992 showed that:

1. In at least 22 of 28 medical schools students received specific education in palliative medicine.
2. Six to 11 schools recognized palliative medicine sessions as appropriate to teach analgesia for chronic non-cancer pain, communication with patients and relatives, grief and bereavement, and multiprofessional team working.
3. Such sessions are used to teach analgesia for cancer pain and symptom relief in advanced terminal disease in 17 and 18 schools respectively.
4. A majority of schools taught all these subjects in sessions within other specialties as well.
5. In 22 out of 26 medical schools students had an opportunity to visit a hospice or palliative care unit during the student years—at Oxford this was a compulsory 5-day visit and included systematic teaching.
6. Sixteen schools reported that a palliative medicine question featured regularly or occasionally in final examinations.[73]

A report was circulated to deans of medical education faculties in which it was pointed out that medical students study most thoroughly those subjects which are examined in finals and it was urged that palliative medicine should so feature. Much change is currently occurring in the British medical student curriculum and there is evidence that palliative care is being given a higher profile. A further study by Field (in 1995) indicated the rapidity of this development.[74]

In 1993, the Open University's Department of Health and Social Welfare instituted a half-credit distance learning course in Death, Dying, and Bereavement. This has appealed to a very wide studentship including doctors, nurses, social workers, chaplains, police and fire service staff, housewives, and carers—even patients themselves. It includes study of ethical issues such as autonomy, disclosure of information, advance directives, and euthanasia as well as giving a sound introduction to communication skills and palliative care.

Postgraduate training

In 1991, a Diploma in Palliative Medicine course was started at the University of Wales and the Holme Tower Marie Curie Centre in Penarth. By 1995, 110 doctors had completed the course and obtained their diplomas and a further 65 were studying the course. This is a course by correspondence (distance learning) but requiring three weekend attendances at Penarth. Study for the diploma can be completed in 1 year, although some students take longer to complete the course. The students are hospital and hospice doctors, general medical practitioners, and overseas palliative physicians in about equal numbers.

Multidisciplinary diplomata in palliative care are being taught at Trent and Glasgow Universities (since 1994) and Dundee University (from April 1995). These are being studied by doctors, nurses, and professionals allied to medicine, in proportion of about two nurses to one doctor.

Masters courses in palliative care nursing had been established in four schools by 1995 for a Master of Science degree, and Trent University was starting a similar course on a multiprofessional basis leading to a Masters in Medical Science degree. Southampton University started a Diploma in Psychosocial Palliative Care in 1992 and in 1994 the first diplomates were admitted to a further year for a Masters of Science in Psychosocial Palliative Care.

It is obvious that academic postgraduate training in the specialty is expanding and deepening in the United Kingdom.

Continuing medical education

A wide variety of 1 to 10-day seminars and courses are available for continuing education in palliative medicine in the United Kingdom.

Vocational trainees for general medical practice in one health region are offered a day's intensive exposure to clinical, communication, and bereavement aspects of palliative care every 6 months at St Christopher's Hospice. Six palliative care facilitators have been appointed by the Royal College of General Practitioners, who are encouraging this aspect of continuing medical education for general practitioners in other parts of the country.

'Choices', a six-weekly publication listing conferences and courses on offer, shows some of the many events available in Britain. In a 3-month period in 1994:

(1) 40 1-day educational events were available in 26 sites for multidisciplinary palliative care education appropriate to doctors and nurses;

(2) 16 multidisciplinary courses lasting between 2 and 10 days were offered;

(3) 6 courses lasting 2 to 4 days, specifically for doctors, occurred;

(4) 2 1-day events were run for doctors by the Association for Palliative Medicine.

Seven of these events had been approved under the general practitioners' continuing medical education scheme, and a further four would have met criteria then being developed for hospital consultants' continuing medical education.

Many other events are arranged in postgraduate medical centres throughout the country, using palliative care specialists to speak to physicians and other colleagues, often including hospital and community nurses, during regular weekly programmes of education for general practitioners and hospital doctors, and these meetings are accredited for continuing medical education.

Specialized training

In Britain and Ireland the student years and the first year of medical practice are basic medical training. Then follows a period of general professional training at senior house officer level during which the doctor generally aims to achieve a postgraduate Membership or Fellowship of a Royal Professional College which acts as an entry examination for higher specialist training. This requires a further 4 years of study and practice as a specialist registrar culminating in the acquisition of a Certificate of Completion of Specialist Training (**CCST**).

Since 1987, a recognized course of higher specialist training for palliative medicine has been identified. During this 4-year period, experience is gained in inpatient palliative care (in a hospice or palliative care unit), in hospital support team work, and domiciliary care; many patients with cancers, AIDS, and neurological conditions such as motor neurone disease (amyotrophic lateral sclerosis) are seen and opportunity is taken to remedy deficiencies in training in various specialties. Special placements are arranged for the specialist-in-training in, for example, oncology, radiotherapy, ear, nose and throat medicine, neurology, pain clinics, and anaesthetics. Often the doctor takes a special course of study, such as the Palliative Medicine Diploma. Such training and experience, regularly appraised, leads to accreditation or the CCST, followed by appointment to a consultant or medical director post. There are now about 112 of these programmes in the United Kingdom.

Conclusion

The Standing Medical Advisory Committee/ Standing Nursing and Midwifery Advisory Committee recommended that all patients needing palliative care services should have access to them, and that the principles and good practice of palliative care which had been stimulated by the voluntary sector should be incorporated at all levels in the National Health Service.[75],[76] It also recommended that there should be an expansion of education programmes in palliative care to ensure continued support for higher medical training programmes and advanced nursing studies.

It is generally encouraging to see the impact on medical practice that has been made by the example of the hospice movement and by education emanating from this movement in Britain. However, we cannot be complacent for too many examples of poor practice in the care of the dying continue to be reported.

United States

J. Andrew Billings

Introduction

In the United States, hospice developed as a 'grass roots' movement, growing up largely outside academic medicine and often conveying an antiestablishment, antiphysician sentiment. Over the past decade, however, hospice has become a familiar, established feature of the country's health-care system, widely accepted by physicians and other health personnel. Hospice programmes serve about a third of the nation's dying cancer patients, and provide end-of-life care for many other patients and families. However, only now are hospice systems becoming better integrated with the academic health centres where medical students, house officers, and fellows learn clinical practice. Departments or divisions or academic positions in palliative medicine have yet to be developed.

In the United States, 'palliative care' and 'palliative medicine' are not commonly recognized terms but 'hospice' is widely used in both professional and popular circles to describe specialized services for terminally ill patients and their families. Although derived from British and Canadian models, hospice programmes in the United States primarily provide comprehensive, co-ordinated, interdisciplinary home care—specialized inpatient units are uncommon.

In the past few years, 'palliative care,' 'supportive care,' and similar terms have emerged in the United States to describe clinical programmes that may differ from hospice care insofar as they try to address a broader range of patients and clinical problems (sometimes including comfort measures for non-terminal patients). Such programmes often represent a more physician-centred, academic, specialty-oriented, institution-based style of care, perhaps with less emphasis than in hospice on interdisciplinary team management, home care, and broad, family-oriented psychosocial and spiritual care. The role of this form of palliative medicine in medical education and in clinical care remains ill defined.

Undergraduate medical education

While courses or teaching modules on 'death and dying' have become standard offerings in most United States medical schools over the past 25 years, few undergraduate students receive systematic training in this area. No national standards for undergraduate medical training in end-of-life care have been proposed by accrediting organizations or groups concerned with medical education. In a recent proposal about reforming undergraduate medical education that was adopted by many schools, hospice is mentioned prominently as a desirable new site for teaching.[77]

Periodic surveys of medical school deans[78,79,80,81] indicate that 89 per cent of institutions now offer formal teaching on 'death and dying,' and that in roughly three-quarters of these schools at least half of medical students take such a course. Courses are primarily elective. Only 11 per cent of schools offer a full term course and only 18 per cent offer a separate course on death and dying; 30 per cent offer one or two lectures as part of another course; and 52 per cent offer a module as part of a required, larger course. Training is predominantly preclinical, although many educators have stressed the importance of clinical exposure and the availability of clinical role models for learning good end-of-life care. Additional disappointing observations about the state of undergraduate palliative medicine education include: curriculum offerings are scattered throughout the curriculum, rather than consciously integrated; the major teaching format is the lecture; patient contact is limited (generally consisting, at best, of a presentation before a large class); and opportunities for students to reflect on their personal attitudes about death and terminal care are rarely mentioned. Moreover, non-psychiatric physicians have played a decreasing role in teaching over the past decade, participating now in only 58 per cent of courses. No data are available on such key issues as whether students actually learn about or participate in a hospice programme, make home visits, get supervision in talking to dying patients, study symptom control, partake in interdisciplinary team work, or address fundamental attitudes about the role of the physician in terminal care.

In reviewing evaluations of palliative care training, a discrepancy between educators and students is noteworthy; whereas cancer centre directors and directors of oncology nursing reported high levels (91–100 per cent) of satisfaction with instruction in supportive care, students at one such institution expressed a low level (27 per cent) of satisfaction.[82] When medical class presidents were surveyed about death education curricula, less than half reported greater than 3 hours of required class time in medical school, only about a third took a course with required reading on some aspect of the dying process, and over a third rated training to be ineffective.[83]

Systematic course evaluation is relatively uncommon in the medical literature and similarly in the literature about palliative care education. A number of reports of enthusiastically received elective and selective courses have been published.[84] One study relied on nurse ratings of clinician behaviours.[60] A few additional observations are worth noting:

A hospice course[85] or rotation[86] has been well received.

Communication skills have been taught effectively.[87,88,89]

Teaching reduced excessive hopelessness about cancer.[90,91]

A 7-week, 1.3-hour per week course lowered student death anxiety.[92]

Postgraduate medical education

While some training programmes in family practice, internal medicine, oncology, geriatrics, and pain medicine have included substantial exposure to hospices, most physicians-in-training have very limited and haphazard training in palliative medicine.[93] The lack of standards in undergraduate teaching is mirrored in a lack of standards for postgraduate education or practice. Young physicians regularly cite end-of-life care as an area that was inadequately covered in their training.[94]

Happily, the American Board of Internal Medicine Subcommittee on Clinical Competence in End-of-Life Care is proposing to identify core skills and knowledge in this area, including social, legal, and ethical issues, underscoring the role of professionalism in terminal care.[95] This group is notable for its emphasis on establishing valid assessment methods. Elsewhere, a curriculum has been developed for an internal medicine housestaff rotation in palliative care.[96] A set of educational objectives have been proposed, based on evaluations of hospice medical directors.[27] In oncology, pain management has received increasing attention, and the inclusion on the oncology board examination of a substantial number of questions about pain control has been viewed as a significant boost to palliative care training.[43]

Additional efforts are noteworthy. The publication of national standards for cancer pain management[22] and the development of detailed curricula for pain specialists[97] should help with a central issue in palliative care education. A number of states have developed initiatives to improve pain management, following the model of the Wisconsin Cancer Pain Initiative.[98] The Catholic Health Association has published guidelines for end-of-life care.[99]

Opportunities for licensed physicians to obtain supervision and intensive exposure to palliative care are rare in the United States. Most hospice clinicians 'learn on the job,' perhaps assisted by textbooks and journals and by attending courses that last 1 to 5 days. Indeed, anyone with a medical degree can serve as a hospice medical director in the United States, even if they have limited clinical training, let alone specialized knowledge about palliative care. No standards or certification procedure for assessing competence in palliative medicine has been established. A few palliative care programmes now offer brief visiting fellowships and even 1 or 2-year training programmes. The National Hospice Organization, a 'trade organization' for hospice programmes, provides a number of courses and conferences, some addressed to physicians, and has developed a physician interest group, but has made no attempt to set standards for training or practice. The Academy of Hospice Physicians has offered courses for new hospice medical directors, and, along with the International Hospice Institute and College, sponsors an annual conference on the management of terminal illness, including a research symposium.

Conclusion

While the current state of education in palliative medicine in the United States leaves much to be desired, increasing attention to this field is evident, and further expansion and development can be anticipated. The foremost factor promoting change is the growth of hospice/palliative care programmes, their increasing integration into conventional care and academic medicine, and greater recognition of the essential role of the medical director in such programmes. National debates on legalizing assisted suicide and voluntary euthanasia have brought further attention to the importance of good palliative care. The current, dramatic changes in United States health care organization will have uncertain effects on medical training, but seems to be focusing increased attention on primary care and ambulatory care disciplines generally hospitable to palliative care concerns. The growing emphasis on 'managed care' may also be favourable to hospice programmes, which have functioned largely under a *per diem* capitated reimbursement system for the past decade, and which can claim to provide better care and improved satisfaction at lesser costs than conventional care, reducing the 'high cost of dying'.[100,101] Finally, two major initiatives to improve palliative care education are noteworthy: the National Cancer Institute has, for the first time, funded proposals for Hospice and Palliative Care Education Programmes, while the Open Society Institute's Project on Death in America has committed substantial resources to 'changing the culture of dying' in this country.

Acknowledgements

Earlier versions of this paper were presented at the 1995 Annual Meeting of the Association of Canadian Medical Colleges, Association of Canadian Teaching Hospitals, and Canadian Association for Medical Education, Quebec City, Canada, 2 May 1995, sponsored in part by the Canadian Society of Palliative Care Physicians, and at the Project on Death in America Faculty Scholar's Retreat, Snoqualamie, WA, 9 July 1995. I am grateful to the recipients of the National Cancer Institute grants on Hospice and Palliative Care Education Programs who furnished their research proposals for review.

Australia and New Zealand

J. Norelle Lickiss

Australia and New Zealand have traditionally been profoundly influenced by British medicine. Medical schools and specialist colleges were initially founded, on the whole, by British graduates or doctors with specialist training in British institutions. Palliative medicine as a discipline in the Antipodes owes much to personal encounters of Australasian doctors with British leaders in the hospice movement in the 1970s and 1980s, and by visits to the antipodes of British and Canadian pioneers in palliative medicine. Increasing links with Asia, including academic links with major centres, are a feature of the present.

Palliative care, as distinct from palliative medicine, has taken on the diversity of the local social, professional, and political environments in the various states of Australia and New Zealand—and there are very considerable differences in concept as well as practice.[102] In some areas, palliative care is based within inpatient units, in other areas community palliative care has been the leading feature. Elsewhere (notably in Sydney) teaching hospitals have been the catalyst and major sites of activity but in most areas all these elements are beginning to emerge with varying forms of linkage. In Australia, the vast majority of palliative care resources in community, palliative care units, and in acute hospitals are government funded as part of the health system—health policy, at national and state level, consistently supports palliative care as a core element in health care. Government support is less prominent in New Zealand with more input from the non-government sector.

The diversity of concept and practice in palliative care throughout Australia and New Zealand has influenced the evolution of educational approaches in palliative medicine—at all levels. However, most involved in education, either in formal structures or in the myriad one-to-one encounters which are the stuff of professional life, recognize the fields in which growth and development needs to occur with reference to a definable body of knowledge and competence, but also in the personal capacity to share pain and tragedy.

Undergraduate medical education

Undergraduate medical education in virtually every medical school in Australia and New Zealand includes explicit teaching in the various aspects palliative medicine. This includes: communication skills, medical decision making, counselling, understanding and treatment of symptoms, care of the dying patient, care of the family, bereavement care, and so on, but it is sufficient that the teaching may be given under the aegis of several departments, especially in larger medical schools. Teaching is given at different stages of the medical course in most schools, with usually some teaching based in a palliative care unit associated with the medical school wherever possible. Some schools have community experience, with students visiting patients in their homes. The role of other disciplines is well recognized.

Formal enquiries into undergraduate medical education in Australia have included comments concerning the need for improvement in the teaching of palliative care within most undergraduate courses in Australia—with more emphasis in general, more attention to experience in patient and family care, and more integration of teaching in palliative care within the curriculum.[103] The Australia and New Zealand Society of Palliative Medicine (ANZSPM) is now developing an undergraduate curriculum.

Schools in the process of change to graduate medical schools (for example the University of Sydney, Queensland University, and Flinders University in South Australia) have particular challenges to ensure opportunities for learning palliative medicine within the 4-year course, capitalizing on the greater maturity of the incoming students, and the intensity of interaction in the course of problem-based learning.

Postgraduate and specialized training

In Australia and New Zealand, graduates from medical schools undertake a brief period of hospital experience (usually 1 year) before registration; they subsequently differentiate into various postgraduate or specialist streams—surgery, internal medicine, obstetrics and gynaecology, medicine, pathology etc., each with its fairly well defined training track. Within each major stream there is opportunity for subspecialization with the need to fulfil further training requirements.

Whilst palliative care involves a wide range of doctors and other professionals, and some palliative medicine is therefore practised in many contexts, palliative medicine as a subspecialty finds its place within internal medicine with a training pathway supervised by the Royal Australasian College of Physicians, with separate supervising committees in Australia and New Zealand. In order to enter the palliative medicine pathway (3 years) as an advanced trainee, the would-be specialist in palliative medicine must pass first the written and clinical Royal Australasian College of Physicians examination, thereafter the candidate undertakes supervised training but no exit examination. In Australia, specific requirements include: 18 months medicine associated with a teaching hospital; 6 months medical oncology; and an elective period involving further experience in palliative medicine or a cognate field. In New Zealand, experience as an advanced trainee must include: 1 year in oncology training (including 6 months of radiotherapy); 18 months in a specialized unit with direct experience for patient care; and 6 months may be spent in a discipline related to palliative care. Post-FRACP supervised training may be arranged.

In addition to the Royal Australasian College of Physicians training track, other training and academic programmes do exist in Australasia, and specialist status may well be conferred on the graduates of some of these programmes.

In Adelaide, South Australia, the Masters programme developed in Flinders Medical School offers interdisciplinary learning in comprehensive palliative care, with a short period of clinical training as a basis for skill enhancement.[104] There is provision for distance learning to assist isolated doctors and nurses unable to commit time in Adelaide. This educational programme has undergone further evolution, with provision for a Graduate Certificate, within the International Institute of Hospice Studies, Flinders University of South Australia. Analogous developments are occurring in other capital cites such as at the University of Melbourne, Monash University (Melbourne), and Edith Cowan University (Perth).

The Sydney Institute of Palliative Medicine, based first in Royal Prince Alfred Hospital with subsequent involvement with three other Sydney teaching hospitals (involving both the University of Sydney and the University of New South Wales) offers clinical training in various contexts (inpatient units, hospital consultancy, community consultancy) with training tailored to the educational needs of the trainee, such as advanced trainees (Royal Australian College of Physicians), trainees preparing for the Certificate of the Institute, family medicine trainees, and international fellows.[105]

Junior doctors preparing for the Royal Australasian College of Physicians barrier examination or for a career in family medicine may undertake a rotation in palliative medicine as part of basic internal medicine training in some teaching hospitals where there is an in house palliative care service. Family medicine trainees elect to undertake clinical training posts in palliative care services in capital cities and academic centres such as Newcastle, New South Wales.

Continuing medical education

Continuing medical education is a feature of Australasian medical practice although participation varies. Various forms of recertification requirements are beginning to influence participation. The Royal Australian College of General Practitioners has been active in fostering general practitioner education in palliative medicine. There continues to be a perceived need for education in palliative medicine for general practitioners.[106]

In general, in most states of Australia and in New Zealand interested doctors (even in country areas) can find opportunities for enhancing knowledge in palliative medicine either by attending short courses, by distance education, by brief clinical attachment, or participation in a formal training programme.

Although an excellent level of health care is available to the vast majority of the people in Australia and New Zealand, poor communication, poor decision making in marginal situations, poor symptom relief, and inadequate family and bereavement care still occur despite efforts of clinicians, health administrators, and political leaders to take steps to improve the quality of care for all the people. Educational deficiencies contribute significantly to some of this and there is a long way to go, especially in Australia, to meet the challenges of distance, multiculturalism, and a complex society in the course of rapid change with high expectations of both health and comfort. Education in palliative medicine as a whole offers the opportunity for medicine to regain focus in the Antipodes.

Continental Europe

Franco DeConno and Luigi Saita

Since the first edition of this textbook there has been an explosion of interest and opportunities in palliative care in Europe, although in most countries palliative care/medicine initiatives are not co-ordinated at a national or governmental level. A grant and support from the programme Europe against Cancer enabled the European Association for Palliative Care to run a workshop in

Brussels attended by 32 experts from the 12 European Union member states and observers from Sweden, the outcome of which was the production and adoption of the report and recommendations for medical education already referred to in this section. Since then, copies have been distributed to all medical schools in Europe by the European Association for Palliative Care under the aegis of the 'Europe against Cancer' programme and workshops have been held entitled 'Teaching for the Teachers'.

The biennial European Association for Palliative Care conferences are hugely successful and well attended by close on 2000 delegates. Equally successful have been the journals, in particularly the European Journal of Palliative Care, and smaller national ones.

Belgium

Presently there is no structured programmes for undergraduates. Some individual non-standardized initiatives have been taken to address this issue in courses on medical psychology and a course on medicine and society. The second year of the doctorate programme includes a couple of hours devoted to the study of pain and in the fourth year there is a course on palliative care (primarily for future general practitioners) as well as a course on bioethics. In the undergraduate course, 2 hours are devoted to palliative care, one of which is on pain control. Each year, four to six students spend a certain period in a Brussels palliative care unit. Training in pain therapy is available at postgraduate levels. Many physicians work full time in palliative units although palliative medicine is still not a recognized and approved medical specialty. Basic teaching of palliative care is done in the fourth or fifth year at the Faculty of Medicine. An introduction to palliative care is given in every medical specialty in the sixth and seventh year, particularly for cancer, AIDS, and neurological diseases. A course organized by nursing instructors is open to all health professionals but is mainly attended by nurses.

Denmark

A group called the Danish Association for the Care of People at the End of Life has been formed to promote better professional education. There is also:

a project on physician–cancer patient communication;

an educational project 'Teaching cancer care in general practice';

an annual ESO course on palliative care, held in Copenhagen each October, with leading experts from the European Association for Palliative Care.

France

The Joseph-Fourier University (Grenoble) offers a diploma course in palliative care open to medical students, doctors, nurses, physiotherapists, psychologists, social workers, and midwives. The course extends over an academic year (124 hours) with 85 hours of general and directed learning and 40 hours of clinical attachment with a written examination at the end. It is a comprehensive course, covering every aspect of palliative care (physical, emotional, social, and spiritual) emphasizing teamwork, the multidisciplinary approach, and the organization of such care.

In other areas of France there is not much emphasis on the training of palliative care and this is usually left to the various institutions and professionals without any definite outline.

Germany

Several palliative care wards have recently opened as part of the Federal programme which finances one ward in every State. Palliative Medicine is not a recognized specialty and few doctors work in it full time. There is some teaching on death and dying in medical schools, with some limited experience in palliative care units where they are available.

Greece, Crete

Courses for doctors and nurses on symptomatic treatment of cancer patients at the palliative care centre of Areteion Hospital is supported financially by the Tzeni Karezi Foundation. The course extends over 500 hours, 250 hours of which are theoretical and 250 hours practical. Instruction covers every aspect of cancer prevention, treatment, and palliative care as well as physical, psychological, and spiritual issues. This same centre is also responsible for undergraduate education, the production of a book on palliative care, the updating of qualified doctors, and intends establishing institutions for pain relief and palliative care in all Greek provinces.

Ireland (Eire)

Palliative Medicine is now an integral part of the undergraduate medical curriculum in all of the medical schools in the Republic of Ireland. There is no standard curriculum and teaching is very much dependent on local factors. However, there has been considerable improvement in this area. The Irish College of General Practitioners has designed a weekend course which takes place throughout the whole country in its twelve faculties, and within 3 years all general practitioners will have had the opportunity to attend it.

Italy

There are no formalized national training policies in palliative care for undergraduates or postgraduates. In a few universities, lectures on palliative care are included, some in the specialties of anaesthesia and oncology. However, these are dependent on the initiative of lecturers and the good will of the directors. Practical training at the existing palliative care units is common, but again this is based on personal initiatives. Most of the attending doctors are specialists. There are many doctors involved full time in palliative care units and home care, although palliative care is not a recognized specialty.

The Italian School of Palliative Medicine, founded and supported by the Floriani Foundation in Milan, organizes two residential courses (15 days each) for physicians and nurses. The Italian Society of Palliative Care, in addition to a national congress every other year, has set up 14 regional committees which organize annual meetings, scientific seminars, etc. Furthermore, the Floriani Foundation has created the most important library on palliative care in the country which is connected with nine international data banks and open to all those interested in the field.

The Netherlands

The specialty of palliative care is not recognized and the very first hospice only opened in 1992. Medical students learn about pain control but otherwise there is no formal teaching on other aspects of palliative care at undergraduate or postgraduate levels.

Poland

Medical students are being trained in Poznan in aspects of palliative care. Seminars, workshops, and practical instruction are also included. In Gdansk, medical students receive instruction on psycho-oncology and palliative medicine. Symposia are organized for a great number of participants and the various hospices plan their own programmes of education for the different disciplines. Advanced postgraduate courses for general practitioners and hospital doctors are organized every 6 months. Foundation courses are being organized every year for nurses by the palliative care service in Poznan together with Sir Michael Sobell House, Oxford. Nursing students in their fouth year attend the University of Medical Science and spend 5 days on theoretical instruction with workshops on skills in communication, terminal care, symptom control, family education, and the care of the bereaved. There is also a specialist course for district nurses. Six hours of lectures on palliative care are being given to fourth year seminarians on such topics as psychothanatology, hospice philosophy, communication, care of the dying and their families, and bereavement.

Spain

Universities in Bilbao and Madrid have recently organized postgraduate courses on medical care open to all professionals in the field as well as two courses on social and family aspects. The Training Faculty of Family Doctors has a course in palliative care and the Spanish Academy of Family Doctors has been developing educational research activities in palliative care, working closely with the Spanish Association for Palliative Care, to develop curricula and educational standards. Furthermore, in Granada there is a 350-hour course for physicians. In January 1993, the Spanish Health Department published its *Guide to Palliative Care* and has a committee of palliative care experts defining standards. The two scientific societies for palliative care have between them more than 700 members. In Spain, there are 11 palliative care centres with 150 beds, six support teams in district general hospitals, and 34 support teams working alongside primary care workers. All are involved in palliative care education.

Sweden

In Sweden there are many conferences on palliative care for doctors, nurses, and others but no formal input in medical student curriculum, nor any formal recognition of palliative medicine as a specialty with its own training programme. However, in May 1992, a Society for Palliative Medicine was inaugurated to set standards and initiate appropriate professional training and there are plans to start a Masters Degree course in pain management at the University of Umea; such a degree course already exists in Stockholm. In the southern health region the 'Oncology Centre' has produced a comprehensive list of all educational activities in palliative care for doctors and nurses. A programme for education in pain for nurses has recently been introduced at the University of Umea and in Stockholm there is now a specialist course in palliative care for nurses as well as a university level course in pain.

Switzerland

A comprehensive course covering every aspect of palliative care is offered by the University Institute Kurt Boesch, the University of Geneva, and the Swiss Society for Palliative Medicine. It is a multidisciplinary course for 25 to 30 participants. The teaching on death and dying and the bereavement process is part of pastoral counselling training. The general tendency in seminaries is to increase education on death and dying, both on theoretical and practical aspects.

Canada

Neil MacDonald

The first Canadian palliative care programmes were organized in teaching hospitals. In 1975, within 2 months of each other, the St Boniface General Hospital (a teaching hospital of the University of Manitoba) and the Royal Victoria Hospital (affiliated with McGill University) opened palliative care units, with associated consult and home-care teams. At the Royal Victoria Hospital, support for the programme was generated following completion of a research programme, sponsored by the Department of Surgery, which demonstrated the need for palliative care within a sophisticated tertiary care facility. Perhaps because of the early support of two academic centres and the charismatic efforts of the first Canadian leaders in the field, palliative medicine has established academic links within the majority of Canadian schools. However, 21 years is not sufficient time to anchor secure academic roots; Canada is facing budgetary cuts in health and education far beyond any experienced before. 'Everything is on the table' and not every Canadian school offers the long-term stability required for cementing the successes achieved by current programmes and allowing palliative care academic leaders to plan for the future and recruit new colleagues. Ironically, while several programmes are threatened, the Canadian community, both formally through a number of political bodies and informally through expressed media views of public interest, understands and supports the need to provide special services for patients with advanced chronic illness.

The Canadian Senate Subcommittee on Euthanasia and Assisted Suicide tabled its final report in 1995. By majority vote, the Senate Committee rejected the changing of Canadian law to allow legally sanctioned euthanasia. In the course of reaching its decision, the Committee travelled across the land hearing testimony and receiving many briefs on these topics. Consistently, regardless of one's views on euthanasia, the testimony strongly supported the introduction and expansion of palliative care programmes. Even organized medicine, as represented by the Canadian Medical Association and the Royal College of Physicians and Surgeons of Canada, previously not noted for their initiatives in this field, indicated support for palliative care.

Thus, at the time of writing, Canadian leaders in palliative care, cognizant of the community's appreciation of the need for palliative care services, must convince their colleagues in academia and organized medicine to convert their expressions of general support to tangible programme development. These programmes will not flower unless a recognized, funded role for palliative care physicians is established, thus allowing career development and the attraction of excellent young colleagues to establish firmly the educational and research foundation on which quality service programmes can develop. While currently threatened in many schools, palliative medicine does have an academic tradition in Canada. Consequently, Canadian palliative care leaders are in a position to profit from the wisdom of those who launched their programmes within medical schools.

Undergraduate teaching

The 1996 national survey of palliative care education clearly demonstrated that the principles of palliative care are offered only modest curriculum time in the majority of Canadian schools. Some survey highlights are:

1. Specific palliative care teaching within other courses was offered at 16 out of 16 schools while six schools also have a formal palliative care course.
2. Teaching hours ranged from 20 h at McGill and Memorial (Newfoundland) to four schools which could identify less than 5 designated palliative care hours.
3. Eleven schools had recently increased teaching hours.
4. Ten schools provided university salaries for palliative care physicians, with the University of Ottawa and University of Alberta funding six positions.
5. On the familiar score of 1 (best)–10 (worst), palliative care colleagues averaged 6 on a scale of satisfaction with the current status of palliative care teaching in their schools. McGill and Memorial colleagues were most satisfied (a score of 2); six schools expressed their level of satisfaction as 10.

Our 1994 survey (presenting a bleaker scenario than the 1996 review) was presented to the Canadian Senate. We posited that questions on euthanasia and physician-assisted suicide could be ethically and logically discussed only when Canadian physicians were reasonably trained in the principles of palliative care and Canadian patients had access to excellent palliative care programmes.

The Canadian Society of Palliative Care Physicians was formed in 1994. Subsequently, the Society assumed responsibility for the Canadian Palliative Care Education Group which now serves as a committee of the Society. All 16 Canadian medical schools have representatives in the Group which continues to take on specific joint educational programmes. In addition to the above survey, work was completed in 1996 on an update of the Canadian Palliative Care Curriculum, which will be published by Oxford University Press as a component of a case-based Manual on palliative care. Funding is on hand allowing the purchase and distribution of the Manual to a graduating class of every Canadian medical school.

Postgraduate training

Palliative medicine as a discipline

Under the aegis of the Canadian Society of Palliative Care Physicians, planning commenced in 1994 for the establishment of palliative medicine as a recognized, formal specialty in Canada. While the specialty training group in Canada, the Royal College of Physicians and Surgeons, expressed early support, at present the specialty proposal is tabled. Part of the problem in establishing an academic graduate base for palliative medicine may lie with the current misunderstanding which appears to exist between organized family medicine, which feels threatened by the development of a palliative care specialty, and academic palliative care physicians who are advancing this idea. The latter group do not believe that they threaten their family practice colleagues; rather, they believe that palliative medicine, which holds a rightful place of prominence within family practice, will only flourish with the creation of a core of fully dedicated palliative care physicians which can continue to produce the educational materials and generate the research studies required to sustain their colleagues in medical practice. At the time of writing, this issue is not resolved. Although the community may be mildly sympathetic to the angst of organized medicine which must adapt to new funding and organizational realities, it may be less tolerant if what it perceives as arcane and self-interested medical politics impedes the community will. The influence of broad-based public concern on medical training policies remains to be determined.

Through private support, fellowship positions in palliative care are available at the University of Ottawa and the University of Alberta. The graduates of these programmes cannot fill the Canadian need. Urgent consideration of publicly-funded training and staff positions for each Canadian province is needed.

General residency posts

Many family practice programmes now include palliative care rotations, ranging from a week to 6 months in length. In some, palliative care is a required rotation; others include it as an elective. Required rotations for oncology residents are a sensible idea but are not a compulsory feature of all Canadian training programmes to date. For the present, oncology trainees may opt to take a rotation in palliative medicine as part of their elective training options. Palliative care electives remain as unusual elective choices for other specialty trainees.

To date, only medical oncology has made a measured effort to include questions relevant to palliative care on professional examinations.

Continuing education

One province, Ontario, is funding a programme allowing family physicians to take short (normally 1–2 weeks) intensive palliative care courses. It is anticipated that these physicians will serve as local mentors and maintain an ongoing liaison with the core palliative care group providing their training.

World Health Organization

Neil MacDonald

The case for the primacy of palliative care in the health programmes of developing countries is eloquently put forward by Dr Stjernswärd in Section 22. For some years to come, over 80 per cent of cancer patients will present with advanced, incurable disease in the developing world. The incidence of cancer is rising in these countries; a devastating problem compounded by the parallel rise in the incidence of AIDS in many nations.

The World Health Organization (WHO) recognizes the skewed balance between overwhelming need and the minimal resources available to help patients with advanced cancer, AIDS, and other chronic disorders that progress to death. Palliative care espouses principles which are simple to teach and will not burden impoverished health systems. Therefore it must be given a priority in developing countries. As Dr Stjernswärd states, 'Nothing would have more immediate effect on quality of life and relief from suffering, not only for the cancer patients but also for their families, than implementing the knowledge accumulated in the field of palliative care.'

In most developed countries, AIDS programmes and the AIDS education of health professionals are distinct from cancer control programmes. Developing countries cannot afford the duplication of educational effort and care implicit in this scenario. A co-ordinated approach addressing the needs of both AIDS and advanced cancer patients must be introduced in countries where both disorders are common.

The WHO espouses a two-phase approach to palliative care education in developing countries, as described below.

Phase I

Phase I is a basic educational programme in palliative care that can be introduced in any country. Ideally, the programme is blended with a parallel initiative to ensure that morphine and other inexpensive agents are available for import and distribution. Teaching palliative care, however, includes many elements aside from opioid use. Their introduction should not be held up pending resolution of opioid bureaucratic snarls. The elements of a phase I programme include:

1. Distribution of teaching resources—the second edition of the World Health Organization manual on cancer pain relief was published in 1996. It may be complemented by the World Health Organization symptom manual. Many excellent monographs on pain and symptom control, particularly relevant to the country of origin, have also been published in several countries. WHO manuals on paediatric pain and home care will be published with private support in 1997–8.

2. Training workshops—using the teaching materials mentioned above as the basic tools for instruction the WHO workshop format teaches the WHO approach to palliative care to national leaders who, in turn, are expected to organize regional workshops in their countries.

3. Curriculum review—a review of the palliative curriculum content should be conducted at the regional university and appropriate changes introduced. The teaching of health professionals in a country should reflect the burden of illness within that land and should not simply follow the established teaching priorities of developed countries. Recently, a curriculum for Asian medical students and physicians was published (1997) by an Asian curriculum group who met in Singapore in March 1996. The curriculum is in preparation at the time of writing.

4. Local training courses—removing palliative care professionals from their home environment is expensive, and deprives, for a time, the local population of needed professional help. Correspondence courses (primarily in the United Kingdom, with a few in Australia at the time of writing) are available, but the cost is often prohibitive. There is a need for affordable programmes which may be linked with short-term fellowships abroad (see below).

5. International fellowships—although almost all palliative care training should be carried out in the country of origin, fellowships enabling students or faculty members to complete short-term training assignments in palliative care in centres of excellence are helpful. If these are not available in the region (see below), opportunities for external training in developed countries will be necessary. Ideally, these should be linked to 'learning at a distance' programmes.

6. Family teaching—the burden of care increasingly falls upon family members in developing countries. Excellent instruction manuals for patients and families are available in most developed countries. The WHO home care manual includes a teaching module for both patients and families, together with a section aimed at village health workers or volunteers. Recognizing different cultural patterns around the world, the home care manual serves as a template which countries can edit, reflecting their culture and family needs.

7. National educational networks have successfully developed curricula and teaching materials. Similar networking on a regional international level would be fruitful.

Information on access to these manuals or other World Health Organization teaching materials can be obtained from one of the authors, from Global Cancer Concern (Britain), or from the World Health Organization Collaborating Centres in Palliative Care.

A Phase I educational programme is not expensive and should be within the capabilities of any country whose government has given the development of palliative care programmes a reasonable priority. External aid in the form of teaching materials and personal commitments by educators in developed countries is necessary.

Phase II

Ideally, training in palliative care should be organized within each region. The World Health Organization had hoped to establish palliative care training centres in core developing countries, but this goal remains to be reached. Countries establishing these centres will have established a palliative care national policy as part of their national cancer control plan and assigned a top priority to palliative care as demonstrated by the introduction of a successful plan for Phase I palliative care educational projects.

The regional university will have similarly assigned a top priority to palliative care education. Tangible expressions of priority setting will include an agreement to appoint full-time academics in palliative care and the provision of appropriate beds, hospital appointments, outpatient arrangements, office space, etc. Responsibilities for a palliative care training centre will include:

(1) establishment of symptom control consult teams in the principal teaching hospitals—these teams will provide 'hands-on teaching';

(2) establishment of a liaison with local palliative care services and introduction of an institution–community interface providing teaching in the home;

(3) establishment of a continuing education programme at the community level;

(4) further development and implementation of curriculum decisions;

(5) training of colleagues in the country of origin and training of colleagues in adjacent countries with a similar culture;

(6) liaison with palliative care colleagues throughout the world with the co-ordination of the World Health Organization.

The World Health Organization palliative care initiative was conceived and advanced by the then Director of the WHO Cancer and Palliative Care Unit, Dr Jan Stjernswärd. At the time of publication, Dr Stjernswärd heads a non-governmental organization (NGO), and the leadership role of the WHO in palliative care has shifted from Geneva to the regional WHO offices. A cooperative thrust involving NGOs, WHO Collaborative Centres, and the Regional WHO programmes can maintain momentum, pending reinstitution of a core WHO leadership group.

References

1. World Health Organization. *Cancer Pain Relief and Palliative Care*. WHO Techinical Report Series 804. Geneva: World Health Organization, 1990.
2. Canadian Palliative Care Association. *Palliative care: Towards a Consensus in Standardized Principles of Practice*. Ottawa: Canadian Palliative Care Association, 1995.
3. Trent Hospice Audit Group. *Palliative Care Core Standards*. Derby UK: Trent Hospice Audit Group, 1992.
4. National Hospice Organization. *Standards of a Hospice Programme of Care*. Arlington, Virginia: National Hospice Organization, 1993.
5. Fries JF. Reduction of national morbidity. In: Lewis SJ, ed. *Aging and Health: Linking Research and Public Policy*. Chelsea, Michigan: Lewis Publishers, 1989.
6. Emanuel EJ, Emanuel LL. The economics of dying. *New England Journal of Medicine*, 1994; **330**: 540–4.
7. Societal Working Needs Group, CanMEDS 2000 Project. Skills for the new millennium. *Annals of the Royal College of Physicians and Surgeons of Canada*, 1996; **29**: 206–16.
8. Lomas J. Retailing research: increasing the role of evidence in clinical services for childbirth. *Milbank Quarterly*, 1993; **7**: 439–75.
9. Hagen N, Young J, MacDonald N. Diffusion of standards of care for cancer pain. *Canadian Medical Association Journal*, 1995; **152**: 1205–9.
10. DesMarchais JE, Pierre J, Delorme P. Basic training program in medical pedagogy: a 1-year program for medical faculty. *Canadian Medical Association Journal*, 1990; **142**: 734–40.
11. Saunders CM. (ed). *The Management of Terminal Illness*. London: Edward Arnold, 1978.
12. Hinton J. *Dying*, 2nd edn. Harmondsworth, UK: Penguin Books, 1972: 159.
13. Support Principal Investigators. A controlled trial to improve care for seriously ill hospitalized patients. The study to understand prognoses and preferences for outcomes and risks of treatments. *Journal of the American Medical Assocation*, 1995; **274**: 274.
14. Cleeland CS, Gonin R, Hatfield AK, Edmonson JH, Blum RH, Stewart JA, Pandya KJ N. Pain and its treatment in outpatients with metastatic cancer. *New England Journal of Medicine*, 1994; **330**: 592–6.
15. Portenoy RK, Miransky J, Thaler HT, Hornung J, Bianchi C, Cibas-Kong I, Feldhamer E, Lewis F, Matamoros I, Sugar MZ, *et al.* Pain in ambulatory patients with lung or colon cancer: prevalence, characteristics and effect. *Cancer*, 1992; **70**: 1616–24.
16. Larue F, Colleau SM, Brasseur L, Cleeland CS. Multicentre study of cancer pain and its treatment in France. *British Medical Journal*, 1995; **310**: 1034–7.
17. Zenz M, Willweber-Strumpf A. Opiophobia and cancer pain in Europe. *Lancet*, 1993; **341**: 1075–6.
18. Von-Roenn JH, Cleeland CS, Gonin R, Hatfield AK, Pandya KJ. Physician attitudes and practice in cancer pain management. A survey from the Eastern Cooperative Oncology Group. *Annals of Internal Medicine*, 1993; **119**: 121–6.
19. Chochinov HM, Wilson KG, Enns M, Mowchun N, Lander S, Levitt M, Clinch JJ. Desire for death in the terminally ill. *American Journal of Psychiatry*, 1995; **152**: 1185–91.
20. Blendon RJ, Szalay US, Knox RA. Should physicians aid their patients in dying? The public perspective. *Journal of the American Medical Assocation*, 1992; **267**: 2658–62.
21. Genuis SJ, Genuis SK, Chang WC. Public attitudes toward the right to die. *Canadian Medical Association Journal*, 1994; **150**: 701–8.
22. Goldberg R, Guadagnoli E, LaFarge S. A survey of housestaff attitudes towards terminal care education. *Journal of Cancer Education*, 1987; **2**: 159–63.
23. Ahmedzai S. Dying in hospital: the resident's viewpoint. *British Medical Journal*, 1982; **285**: 712–14.
24. Herman TA. Terminally-ill patients: assessment of physician attitudes within a teaching instruction. *New York State Journal of Medicine*, 1980; **80**: 200–7.
25. Charlton R, Dovey S, Mizushima Y. Attitudes to death and dying in the U.K., New Zealand and Japan. *Journal of Palliative Care*, 1995; **11**: 42–7.
26. Charlton R, Ford E. Medical education in palliative care. *Academic Medicine*, 1995; **70**: 258–9.
27. Schonwetter RS, Robinson BE. Educational objectives for medical training in the care of the terminally ill. *Academic Medicine*, 1994; **69**: 688–90.
28. MacDonald N, Mount B, Boston W, Scott JF. The Canadian Palliative Care Undergraduate Curriculum. *Journal of Cancer Education*, 1993; **8**: 197–201.
29. Blank LL. Defining and evaluating physician competence in end-of-life patient care. A matter of awareness and emphasis. *Western Journal of Medicine*, 1995; **163**: 297–301.
30. Cantor JC, Cohen AB, Barker DC, *et al.* Medical educators views on medical education reform. *Journal of the American Medical Association*, 1991; **265**: 1002–6.
31. Bloom SW. Structure and ideology in medical education: an analysis of resistance to change. *Journal of Health and Social Behaviour*, 1988; **29**: 294–306.
32. Calman KC. New methods of teaching and the evaluation of teaching. In: Twycross RG, ed. *The Edinburgh Symposium on Pain Control and Medical Education*. Royal Society of Medicine, 1989: 175–80.
33. Mandin H, Harasym P, Eagle C, Watanabe M. Developing a 'clinical presentation' curriculum at the University of Calgary. *Academic Medicine*, 1995; **70**: 186–93.
34. Association for Palliative Medicine and the Royal College of General Practitioners. *Palliative Medicine Curriculum*. Southampton: Association for Palliative Medicine for Great Britain and Ireland, 1993.
35. International Society of Nurses in Cancer Care. *A Core Curriculum for a Post Basic Course in Palliative Nursing Care*. Manchester: Haigh and Hochland, 1991.
36. Ad Hoc Committee on Cancer Pain. Cancer pain assessment and treatment curriculum guidelines. *American Society of Clinical Oncology*, 1992; **10**: 1976–82.
37. Fields HL (ed). *Core Curriculum for Professional Education in Pain: A Report of the Task Force on Professional Education of the International Association for the Study of Pain*. 2nd edn. Seattle: IASP press, 1995.
38. Smith WT. Tattersall MHN, Irwig LM, Langlands AO. Undergraduate education about cancer. *European Journal of Medicine*, 1991; **27**: 1448–53.
39. Everitt DE, Avorn K. Clinician decision-making in the evaluation and treatment of insomnia. *American Journal of Medicine*, 1990; **89**: 357–62.
40. Everitt DE, Avorn K. The neglected medical history and therapeutic choices for abdominal pain. A nationwide study of 799 physicians and nurses. *Archives of Internal Medicine*, 1991; **151**: 694–8.
41. Fosså SD, Aaronson NK, Newling D, *et al.* Quality of life and treatment of hormone resistant metastatic prostatic cancer. *European Journal of Cancer*, 1990; **26**: 11–12, 1133–6.
42. Slevin ML, Plant H, Lynch D, Drinkwater J, *et al.* Who should measure quality of life, the doctor or the patient? *British Journal of Cancer*, 1988; **57**: 109–12.
43. Jacox A, Carr DB, Payne R, *et al. Management of Cancer Pain*. Clinical Practice Guideline No. 9 AHCPR Publication No. 94-0592. Rockville, MD: Agency for Health Care Policy and Research, U.S. Department of Health and Human Services, Public Health Service, March 1994.
44. MacDonald N. *Clinical Practice Guidelines for the Care and Treatment of Breast Cancer. Topic 4. Pain Management for Breast Cancer Patients*. Canadian Breast Cancer Initiative, 1996.
45. Fulton J. As quoted in *The Gazette* (Montreal, Canada), June 4, 1995.

46. Montgomery Hunter K, Charon R, Colehan JL. The study of literature in medical education. *Academic Medicine*, 1995; **70**: 787–91.
47. Charon R, Williams P. Introduction: the humanities and medical education. *Academic Medicine*, 1995; **70**: 758–60.
48. Calman K, Downie R. Why arts courses for medical curricula. *Lancet*, 1996; **347**: 1499–500.
49. Charon R. *Examining the Language of Death*. Working paper: Project on Death in America. Sponsored by Open Society Institute. Soros Foundation, January 1995.
50. Swanson AG, Anderson MB. Educating medical students: assessing change in medical education—the road to implementation (ACME-TRI report). *Academic Medicine*, 1993; **68** (Suppl.): 31–46.
51. Koschmann T. Medical education and computer literacy: learning about, through and with computers. *Academic Medicine*, 1995; **70**: 818–21.
52. Doyle D. Education in palliative medicine and pain therapy: an overview. In: Twycross RG, ed. *Edinburgh Symposium of Pain Control and Medical Education*. Royal Society of Medicine, 1989: 165–74.
53. MacDonald N. Palliative care—the fourth phase of cancer prevention. *Cancer Detection and Prevention*, 1991; **15**: 253–5.
54. Cleeland CS, Gonin R. Hatfield AK, *et al.* Pain and its treatment in outpatients with metastatic cancer. *New England Journal of Medicine*, 1994; **330**: 392–6.
55. Vainio A. Treatment of terminal cancer pain in France: a questionnaire study. *Pain*, 1995; **62**: 155–62.
56. Calman KC. Medical training—the early postgraduate years. *Palliative Medicine*, 1988; **2**: 143–6.
57. Jones RVH, Ingram D, Finlay I, Lant A. CAL in cancer nursing: an adult learning approach. *Information Technology in Nursing*, 1990; **2**: 34–5.
58. Ingram D, Jones RVH, Lant AF, Finlay IG. Carer patients and their families at home. An interative videodisc for doctors and district nurses. *Computers Education*, 1991; **16**: 211–16.
59. Von Roenn JH, Neely KJ, Curry RH, Weitzman SH. A curriculum in palliative care for internal medicine housestaff: a pilot project. *Journal of Cancer Education*, 1988; **3**: 259–63.
60. Glickman EF, Greene HL Jr. Assessment of resident performance in a hospital-based palliative care unit. *Death Education*, 1984; **8**: 99–111.
61. Sankar A, Becker SL. The home as a site for teaching gerontology and chronic illness. *Journal of Medical Education*, 1985; **60**: 308–13.
62. Blanchard CG, Ruckdeschel JC, Labrecque MS, Frisch S, Blanchard EB. The impact of a designated cancer unit on house staff behaviours towards patients. *Cancer*, 1987; **60**: 2348–54.
63. Schon DA. *Educating the Reflective Practitioner Toward a New Design for Teaching and Learning in the Professions*. San Francisco: Jossey Bass Publications, 1987.
64. Davis DA, Thomson MA, Oxman AD, Haynes RB. Evidence for the effectiveness of CME: a review of 50 randomized controlled trials. *Journal of the American Medical Assocation*, 1992; **268**: 1111–17.
65. Atkins S, Murphy K. Reflection: a review of the literature. *Journal of Advanced Nursing*, 1993; **18**: 1188–92.
66. Hillier R. Editorial: palliative medicine—a new specialty. *British Medical Journal*, 1988; **297**: 874–5.
67. Ford G. Specialist medical training in the U.K. *Palliative Medicine*, 1988; **2**: 147–52.
68. Scott DH. Is palliative care a discipline. *Journal of Palliative Care*, 1988; **4**: 10–11.
69. Calman KC. Palliative medicine: on the way to becoming a recognized discipline. *Journal of Palliative Care*, 1988; **4**: 12–14.
70. Levy MH. Palliative care: special and deserving of specialty status. *Journal of Palliative Care*, 1988; **4**: 19–22.
71. Librach SL. Defining palliative care as a specialty could do more harm than good. *Journal of Palliative Care*, 1988; **4**: 23–4.
72. Hospice Information Service. *Hospice Manpower Study*. London: St Christopher's Hospice, 1986.
73. Smith AM. Palliative medicine education for medical students: a survey of British medical schools, 1992. *Medical Education*, 1994; **28**: 197–9.
74. Field D. Education for palliative care; formal education about death, dying, and bereavement in U.K. medical schools in 1983 and 1994. *Medical Education*, 1995; **29**: 414–19.
75. *House of Lords Report of the Select Committee on Medical Ethics*. London: Her Majesty's Stationery Office, 1994.
76. Standing Medical Advisory Committee and Standing Nursing and Midwifery Advisory Committee. *The Principles and Provisions of Palliative Care*. London: Her Majesty's Stationery Office, 1992: 17–28.
77. UK Department of Health. *Government Response to the Report of the Select Committee on Medical Ethics*. Command Paper 2553. London: Her Majesty's Stationery Office, 1994: 2, Para. 288.
78. Marston RQ, Bloom SW, Estabrook RW, Fletcher SW, Haggerty RI, Mechanic D, *et al.* Medical education in transition: report of the Robert Wood Johnson Foundation Commission on Medical Education: The Sciences of Medical Practice. In: Marston RQ, Jones RM, ed. *Medical Education in Transition*. Commission on Medical Education: The Sciences of Medical Practice. Princeton, NJ: Robert Wood Johnson Foundation, 1992: 6–7.
79. Liston EH. Education on death and dying: a survey of American medical schools. *Journal of Medical Education*, 1973; **48**: 577–8.
80. Dickinson G. Death education in U.S. medical schools. *Journal of Medical Education*, 1976; **51**: 34–6.
81. Dickinson G. Changes in death education in U.S. medical schools during 1975–1985. *Journal of Medical Education*, 1985; **60**: 942–3.
82. Merman AC, Gunn DB, Dickinson GE. Learning to care for the dying: A survey of medical schools and a model course. *Academic Medicine*, 1991; **66**: 35–8.
83. Belani CP, Belcher AE, Sridhara R, Schimpff SC. Instruction in the techniques and concept of supportive care in oncology. *Support Care Cancer*, 1994; **2**: 50–5.
84. Holleman WL, Holleman MC, Gershenhorn S. Death education curricula in U.S. medical schools. *Teaching and Learning in Medicine*, 1994; **6**: 260–3.
85. Martin RW, Wylie N. Teaching third-year medical students how to care for terminally ill patients. *Academic Medicine*, 1989; **64**: 413–14.
86. Cassileth BR, Brown C, Liberatore C, Lovejoy J, Parry SA, Streeto C, Watkins K, Berlyne D. Medical students' reactions to a hospice preceptorship. *Journal of Cancer Education*, 1989; **4**: 261–3.
87. Knight CF, Knight PF, Gellula MH, Holman GH. Training our future physicians: A hospice rotation for medical students. *American Journal of Hospice and Palliative Care*, 1992; **9**: 23–8.
88. Anderson JL. Evaluation of a practical approach to teaching about communication with terminal cancer patients. *Medical Education*, 1982; **16**: 202–7.
89. Irwin WB, McClelland R, Love AHG. Communication skills training for medical students: an integrated approach. *Medical Education*, 1989; **23**: 387–94.
90. Evans BJ, Stanley RO, Mestrovic P, Rose L. Effects of communications skills training on students' diagnostic efficiency. *Medical Education*, 1991; **25**: 517–26.
91. Blanchard CG, Ruckdeschel JC, Cohen RE, Shaw E, McSharry J, Horton J. Attitudes toward cancer: 1. The impact of a comprehensive oncology course on second-year medical students. *Cancer*, 1981; **47**: 2756–62.
92. Cassileth BR, Egan TA. Modification of medical student perceptions of the cancer experience. *Journal of Medical Education*, 1979; **54**: 797–802.
93. Kaye JM. Will a course on death and dying lower students' death and dying anxiety? *Journal of Cancer Education*, 1991; **6**: 21–4.
94. Plumb JD, Segraves M. Terminal care in primary care postgraduate medical education programs: a national survey. *American Journal of Hospice Palliative Care*, 1992; **9**: 32–5.
95. Cantor JC, Baker LC, Hughes RG. Preparedness for practice: young physicians' views of their profesional education. *Journal of the American Medical Assocation*, 1993; **270**: 1035–40.
96. ABIM End-of-Life Patient Care Project on the Identification and Promotion of Physician Competency. *Phase I: Resource Document Pilot*, American Board of Internal Medicine, 1995.

97. Von Roenn JH, Neely KJ, Curry RH, Weigzman SA. A curriculum in palliative care for internal medicine housestaff: A pilot project. *Journal of Cancer Education*, 1988; **3**: 259–63.
98. International Association for the Study of Pain Task Force on Professional Education. *Core Curriculum for Professional Education in Pain*. Seattle, WA: International Association for the Study of Pain, 1989.
99. Weissman DE, Dahl JL. Update on the cancer pain role model education program. *Journal of Pain and Symptom Management*, 1995; **10**: 292–7.
100. *Care of the Dying: A Catholic Perspective*. St. Louis, MO: Catholic Health Association of the United States, 1993.
101. Scitovsky AA. 'The high cost of dying' revisited. *Milbank Quarterly*, 1994; **72**: 561–91.
102. Lickiss JN. Australia: statistics of cancer pain and palliative care. *Journal of Pain and Symptom Management*, 1993, **8**: 388–94.
103. Committee of Inquiry into Medical Education and Medical Workforce (Chair: R.L. Doherty). *Australian Medical Education and Workforce into the 21st Century*. Australian Government Publishing Service, 1988.
104. Maddocks I. A master's degree and graduate diploma in palliative care. *Palliative Medicine*, 1992; **6**: 317–20.
105. Turner KS, Lickiss JN. *Post-graduate Training in Palliative Medicine; the Experience of the Sydney Institute of Palliative Medicine, Occasional Paper*. Sydney Institute of Palliative Medicine, 1996.
106. Ashby MA, Wakefield MA, Beilby J. General practitioners and palliative care. *Palliative Medicine*, 1993; **7**: 117–26.

21.3 Nurse education

Nora Jodrell

Introduction

Palliative care, it could be argued, is the single biggest challenge facing health-care professionals today. The delivery of palliative care poses many challenges, not only in the complexity of care that is required but also because it calls into question our belief that cure is our most important aim, that health care means the absence of illness, and that if we do not achieve cure in our patients then somehow we have failed. It is only through education that we are likely to dispel this concept and instil in those caring for patients in a palliative care setting that the delivery of palliative care is active care and should be scientifically, clinically, and educationally sound.

Palliative care is a global but neglected public-health problem.[1] The development of palliative care as a specialty has led to considerable advances in palliative-care knowledge. However, to date, little of this knowledge is being applied generally in the clinical setting. It is likely that a major reason for this is the deficiency in the education of health-care workers and it is probable that the integration of palliative care into health care generally will not happen until it becomes an integral aspect of the basic training of health-care personnel.

During the past three decades, numerous studies have illustrated the need for palliative care and death education to be explicit in nursing programmes.[2,3,4] Traditionally, in nurse education palliative care has been equated with death and dying, and in most curricula the term 'palliative care' is not utilized. Whilst not disputing the importance of education in relation to death and dying, palliative-care education must surely incorporate the broader aspects of whole-patient care. Perhaps we should be more specific in stating the rationale of palliative care in nurse education in an attempt to ensure that rehabilitation and symptom management, as well as death and dying, are seen as identifiable concepts of palliative care, as a continuum of care threaded throughout educational programmes as distinct from being independently taught subjects. In addition, the delivery of nursing care, in the sense of palliative care, is not disease specific. Education, therefore, must ensure that the principles of palliative care are recognized as transferable skills which can be utilized in different clinical environments.

Current trends in palliative-care delivery

The number of individuals requiring palliative care worldwide is increasing, largely due to advances in treatment, scientific knowledge of chronic illnesses such as cancer, and an ageing population. Consequently, there is a greater demand on health-care professionals to deliver palliative care in a variety of settings. In each of these settings it is likely that it will be nurses who carry the burden of care.

Whilst the concept of palliative care originated from the developing hospice movement, the philosophy which underpins it is by no means modern. Hippocrates stated that medicine was intended 'to do away with the sufferings of the sick, to lessen the violence of disease'. With the ever-increasing technology of medical practice, nursing has allowed itself to become task oriented and reductionist.[5] This reductionist ethic still pervades hospitals despite attempts by some nurses to redefine nursing in a patient-oriented way.[6] The philosophy of palliative care, however, provides an opportunity to lead nursing back to the principles of nursing and emphasize care as the essential element[7] as palliative care is more than alleviating the physical suffering of disease—it is the provision of care to sustain a meaningful life for the individual and their carers.

It has been stated that care of the dying is essentially a nursing, and not a medical, problem.[8,9] As patients shift from a 'sick' to a dying role, it is the nurse who assumes the dominant role. As economics drives health care out of the hospital and towards community care, the supportive care required by patients and their carers will largely be the responsibility of the nurse. It is essential, therefore, that nurses are aware of the meaning of palliative care and are appropriately educated in aspects of physical, psychological, and social care. Education is important to ensure that care delivered in the hospice or specialist setting can be as effectively delivered in the community or non-specialist setting. If the trend towards home care continues, there is an urgent need to address the educational needs of the nurses who will provide the bulk of care. Across Europe and at an international level, the delivery of health care is changing to reflect the changing health-care needs of the population. Nurse education must also reflect these changes to ensure the provision of quality care. The changing face of nursing, in a professional sense, should incorporate clear standards for the delivery of care and not allow economic constraints to undermine the importance of an educated work force.

Trends in nursing education

In recent years considerable progress has been made in developing rigorous education programmes for nurses which are patient focused, practice led, and responsive to service goals. The intention is to prepare practitioners with the appropriate knowledge, skills, and attitudes, together with the commitment to ongoing personal and professional development. Quint's work on the education of nurses dealing with dying patients highlighted the inadequacy of educational provision for nurses in this area.[2] In the United Kingdom, Field and Kitson[6] found, however, that death education appeared to receive serious attention in curricula. Despite this, numerous authors uphold the concerns of Quint and have identified nurses' lack of knowledge and concern when caring for individuals who are dying.[10,11,12,13]

The notion that palliative care is synonymous with death education is still apparent in many curricula and tends to focus on two perspectives—on teaching about death and dying and on exploring nurses' experiences with dying patients. As stated previously, however, palliative care encompasses much more than care of the dying or nurses' attitudes towards death. The regulatory and awarding bodies of individual countries are responsible for assuring that curricula design, development, and implementation address appropriate and relevant issues at all stages of education. It is also their responsibility to ensure that teachers of nursing, midwifery, and health visiting are adequately prepared to undertake effective educational approaches to palliative care. Burocoa[14] argues that palliative care is not an exact science and cannot be taken as a purely intellectual discipline. Rather, it is an approach—'palliative care is more a re-discovery of ideas, more adaptation than creation. The whole socio–medico profession should be concerned'. There is a widespread need to develop, through education, palliative 'attitudes' in health-care professionals, to ensure a palliative approach to care when and where it is appropriate for patients.

Although nursing has developed its own window on the world, as have other professions, it recognizes that palliative care crosses all care boundaries and that its success, at the point of delivery, depends upon a team approach. Therefore, all professions, including nursing, must be assured that their teachers are competent in palliative-care education and, particularly, that the selection of teaching methods are appropriate in formulating student learning.

Nurse education for palliative care

The term palliative care now includes specialist practice as well as the principles and approaches which were developed within the hospice movement and defined by the World Health Organization in 1990. The majority of patients requiring palliative care may not be cared for by a recognized specialist but will benefit from the key elements and principles which can be taught to all nurses whatever their field of practice. A recent paper by Mills *et al.*[15] highlighted the need to improve the education of non-specialists, that care of many of the dying patients ($n = 50$) observed in four large teaching hospitals in the west of Scotland received poor care. The authors go on to say that basic interventions to maintain patient comfort were not provided and that nurses, along with their medical colleagues, distanced themselves from the patients requiring care. The physical aspects of caring for dying patients have been identified by others[10,16] as being areas where nurses feel their knowledge is lacking and that their basic education is not sufficient to allow them to feel confident in providing care.

Internationally, there is a wide variation in the provision of education for nurses in palliative care. In the Americas, Australia, the United Kingdom, and elsewhere in northern Europe, there are established educational programmes alongside seminar programmes and conferences specifically relating to palliative care. However, this is not reflected worldwide. For example in Botswana there are no educational programmes in palliative care for nurses and in Thailand and Japan palliative care is taught within cancer nursing courses. That there is a need to address education in palliative care for nurses is evident from the development of short courses in a number of countries in the last few years. The Nairobi Hospice in Kenya has, since 1990, been providing palliative-care courses for nurses and other health-care professionals and, indeed, they have extended this programme to various nursing schools throughout Kenya, with work ongoing to incorporate palliative care into the curriculum of all nursing schools. Relatively small communities are also developing palliative-care services and therefore require education for their nurses. In Bermuda, with 22 registered nurses who are directly involved with the delivery of palliative care, it is believed that it is more cost effective to educate these nurses outside their own country, supplementing this with seminar programmes on specific issues. Eastern Europe also has seen an increase in the availability of education in palliative care, largely due to charitable sources who have supported palliative care development in Russia and the Czech Republic.

Developing education

There has been relatively little research and academic scrutiny in palliative care and the fact that palliative care is an emerging field has many implications. The educator is faced with the challenge of educating care givers about 'a domain of practice of which the limits, objectives, and nature are neither clearly defined nor unequivocally agreed upon'.[17] A number of researchers have addressed this issue,[3,5,13] highlighting areas of concern and thereby offering useful data for the development of course content.

Given that all nurses, whatever their setting, will deliver palliative care to patients, education in palliative care must extend beyond their basic training and continue throughout their career. Education for specialist practice in palliative-care nursing is available at diploma, degree, and postgraduate level. Programmes in the United Kingdom are required by the regulatory bodies to be modular in their approach and flexible in their mode of study. Nursing diplomas, undergraduate, and postgraduate degrees specifically in palliative care or including options for palliative care are becoming more readily available. Increasingly, these are being developed in tandem with clinical specialists in palliative care, together with users and carers; thus acknowledging that competent palliative-care provision, at the point of delivery, is a team responsibility.

It is vital that nurses have the opportunity to develop both educationally and clinically as a result of an educational programme. Professional socialization studies indicate that nursing students are often confused between what they learn in schools and what is expected of them in practice.[18] This may result in rejection of the knowledge they have gained.[19]

The ideal must be that students themselves (at all levels) should experience real contact with a palliative-care environment in which all professionals involved demonstrate appropriate levels of care and acknowledge the importance of the multidisciplinary team; a team which frequently consists of professionals, patients, families, and carers. The notion of education in palliative care then extends far beyond the profession. Patients, families, and carers also require adequate knowledge and skills to facilitate living with illness.[20] It is imperative that nurses, together with their professional colleagues, are suitably prepared to facilitate such learning and thus are able to contribute to a more comprehensive provision of quality care for patients. To some extent palliative care has already accepted this challenge through the context and focus of current provision and its commitment to multiprofessional training.

Preregistration education

That there is a need for a systematic approach to the inclusion of palliative care education in student nurse programmes is a long standing argument probably initiated by Quint 30 years ago.[2] Despite the findings of Field and Kitson[6] that death education appears to be given serious attention in curricula, newly-registered nurses continue to experience feelings of inadequacy when caring for dying patients.[10,21] In many countries, palliative care is a recent development and specialists everywhere are agreed that its integration into health schemes will not happen until it becomes an integral part of the basic training of every student nurse.[22] It should be remembered that in many cases the training received by students will last for life and it is therefore important to bear in mind that education must extend beyond the initial preparation.[23]

Undoubtedly the practice of palliative care is not easy for students, who almost always adhere intellectually to procedures taught in the classroom but do not know what to do with it when they are confronted with a different scenario in practice.[19,22] The ideal must surely be for the students themselves to experience real contact with a palliative care environment, in which they can observe the behaviour of all professionals involved in palliative care.

As has been argued previously, no amount of role play can replace the effects, positive or negative, of actual experience.[24] Wouters[22] argues that student nurses early in their training have not yet learnt to be afraid of the dying or see dying patients as a failure of science. She goes on to state that educators involved in teaching palliative care at this level have a responsibility to equip student nurses with theoretical and practical knowledge which will allow them to function, and initiate change, in the clinical environments in which they will find themselves.

These arguments are supported by the aims of Paillot-Schmidt:[25]

(1) to prevent young professionals resolving their difficulties and insecurity, in the face of patients who are dying, by escapist behaviour;

(2) to enable these nurses to experience palliative care not as a failure but as a natural dimension, a normal and inevitable part of nursing care;

(3) to integrate with nursing care the idea of accompanying the dying patient like a state of mind, an attitude of heart, allowing the nurse to offer both the dying and to their families responses suited to their needs and personality.

A recent report from a European Oncology Nursing Society initiative, which was funded by the European Commission's Europe Against Cancer programme and the Cancer Relief Macmillan Fund (a United Kingdom based cancer charity), highlights some of the difficulties in educational development at a European level. Educational provision varies in terms of the level and length of courses. In addition, the way in which a life-threatening diagnosis (such as cancer) is dealt with varies across Europe from open discussion with patients and relatives to no information being given to patients.[26] Despite these difficulties, however, a workshop of 14 nurses representing different European countries developed guidelines for curriculum content in basic nurse education for Europe.

Areas for inclusion of palliative nursing in basic nursing courses includes a number of themes:

(1) The principles of palliative care:

- attitudes to death in society;
- definitions of palliative care;
- principles and philosophy of palliative care;
- settings for palliative care;
- interdisciplinary perspectives.

(2) Communication:

- self awareness;
- professional vulnerability;
- recognizing personal limitations;
- characteristics of the therapeutic relationship;
- creating a supportive environment;
- foundational communication skills;
- understanding and dealing with communication issues;
- assessing communication needs;
- talking to families;
- issues of confidentiality;
- communication within the multiprofessional team.

(3) Management of nursing problems related to pain and other symptoms:

- definition of pain;
- subjective nature of pain and other symptoms;
- incidence of pain;
- review of pain theories;
- concept of total pain;
- pain assessment tools;
- principles of pain management;

common patterns of spread of advanced disease;

common symptoms of advanced disease;

impact of symptoms on the individual and the family;

review of nursing assessment;

patient and family education.

(4) Facing loss and death:

impact of loss on the patient;

impact of loss on the family;

overview of relevant theories;

uncomplicated grief reaction;

tasks of mourning;

resources available to the individual and family.

(5) Ethical and legal issues:

impact of personal values;

ethical issues encountered in palliative care;

ethical decision-making;

areas of potential conflict;

professional codes of conduct;

legal requirements relating to illness and health.

The working group members recommend that a minimum of 12 hours be set aside in basic education to address palliative nursing and that the framework be piloted in each country represented, with evaluation fed back to the group for possible further development. Perhaps through such a co-ordinated approach to curriculum development the palliative care content of preregistration educational programmes will be both more obvious and more beneficial.

Postregistration education

As stated previously, all nurses provide palliative care with only a small minority doing so within the realm of a specialist palliative care team. The majority of patients receiving palliative care, therefore, do so in a non-specialist health-care setting. There is undoubtedly then a need to ensure education for these nurses, as Hockley's study indicates that nurses' difficulty in caring for terminally ill patients relates to inadequate teaching.[10] Numerous authors have detailed the lack of knowledge,[2,21] increased anxiety,[2,27,28], and concern regarding physical care[10,12,13] of nurses when caring for patients who are dying. In support of this, a number of studies have evaluated the effect of educational interventions in palliative care.[3,5,29,30,31] The majority of these studies explored the change in nurses attitudes towards death or life-threatening illness following the educational intervention. Some researchers have attempted to explore the effect of educational programmes on the problems nurses have identified when caring for patients who are dying[3,5,32] and have shown that educational programmes were effective in reducing some of the problems experienced by nurses. Despite this evidence, educational programmes in palliative care are relatively new, especially outside the United Kingdom, and have largely been initiated by those working within the hospice movement. Such initiatives include study days, short courses, and, more recently, degree programmes and have been developed in response to the needs of nurses providing palliative care outside the hospice setting. There is no doubt that there is an enormous amount of knowledge and expertise amongst nurses and nurse educators in the field of palliative care: the question is, how best can we utilize this expertise and incorporate it into educational programmes? It could be argued that nothing would have more immediate effect on quality of life and relief of suffering for patients and their families than implementing the knowledge accumulated in specialist palliative care areas.

Education offered at postregistration level is varied and there appears little conformity at either a European or international level as to course content, predicted outcomes, or approach. In the United Kingdom, the United Kingdom Central Council for Nursing Midwifery and Health Visiting[33] has stated that programmes leading to specialist qualification should be at a minimum of degree level.

The confusion over the lack of uniformity in palliative care education led the International Society of Nurses in Cancer Care, supported by the World Health Organization, to produce a core curriculum in palliative care nursing.[34] Core areas of curriculum content are:

(1) the politics of health care:

death society and palliative care;

(2) nursing theory:

the nurse in palliative care;

(3) counselling theory and practice:

communication and counselling;

(4) interdisciplinary teamwork;

(5) pain and symptom management:

management of pain;

management of symptoms other than pain;

(6) loss and grief;

(7) spirituality;

(8) legal and ethical issues.

It is recommended that the minimum course length should be 2 weeks. Whilst this falls short of other recommendations, it provides a basis to develop a co-ordinated approach to international palliative care education for nurses. The course content identified by the International Society of Nurses in Cancer Care builds upon basic knowledge and has the potential to develop both cognitive and affective skills through the utilization of theoretical concepts. Underpinning the delivery of palliative care in such a way is vital if we are to enhance its delivery.

In a recent survey of 100 Canadian nurses[35] it was demonstrated that nurses had two main areas of concern:

(1) the education needs of palliative care nurses;

(2) the need to develop standards of practice in palliative care.

This would support the argument made by Copp[4] that there is a need for researchers and educators in palliative care to work more closely together as the issues relating to education, nurses, and patients in palliative care are not mutually exclusive. Only through this co-operation can we ensure that the curriculum content will reflect the needs of those requiring care.

As the specialty of palliative care has developed so too has the recognition that advanced practice demands high levels of clinical, research, management, and leadership skills. Education to address these areas is being developed in many countries. The move in the United Kingdom of nurse education into institutions of higher education is reflected in a number of other European countries and has been evident in the United States, Canada, and Australia for some time. Internationally, there remains confusion however as to what advanced practice is, and therefore the level of educational preparation required for advanced practice is diverse and specific to each country. Indeed, in many countries, of which the United Kingdom is one, there is currently an absence of clear national guidelines as to what education should be undertaken by nurses functioning at an advanced level. In the United States, Bachelor's, Master's, and Doctoral studies are available to nurses working as clinical nurse specialists and in the United Kingdom a similar situation is developing, focusing upon numerous specialisms, one of which is palliative care. Elsewhere in Europe, and in the Middle and Far East, the situation is very patchy and many nurses will leave their own country to undertake further education if they wish to specialize in palliative care.

Multiprofessional education

By definition the delivery of palliative care in specialist settings is, in the majority of situations, a multiprofessional activity. Nurses working in this environment are often highly skilled in palliative care and it is perhaps in this situation where multiprofessional education would be of most benefit. Multiprofessional education in palliative care is still a relatively new concept and one which appears to face a number of difficulties. Whilst the idea of multiprofessional education may be educationally sound, there are intradisciplinary issues which appear to limit its potential.[36]

Nurses functioning at what may be considered an advanced level will, along with clinical experience, be expected to have acquired leadership and management skills and are therefore perhaps more capable of learning in a multiprofessional environment. However, multiprofessional courses in palliative care continue to experience difficulty in attracting a professionally balanced group of students. This may be a consequence of the perception by potential students of the diversity of their educational needs and abilities. It has been argued that the introduction of multiprofessional education would help to raise the awareness of the different approaches of various professions and would create an awareness of the skills of those other professions with whom each will work in the clinical setting, thus enhancing collaboration and mutual respect.[37] In a recent evaluation of the current needs of general practitioners and community nurses, Jeffrey identified that the majority of doctors (88 per cent) and nurses (95 per cent) in his study felt that multidisciplinary learning would be helpful.[16] He contends that there is a need to develop multidisciplinary educational initiatives in palliative care and argues that whilst palliative care in the community depends on team work, doctors and nurses have few opportunities to learn together.

A significant problem in postgraduate education is that a large number of nurses within the profession do not possess a first degree. This is equally valid in the specialty of palliative care. There is a move towards assessment of prior learning, flexible learning, and modular approaches to learning which would facilitate entry into higher education for a greater number of nurses. Also, within the United Kingdom, some institutions acknowledge previous clinical and life experience when considering students for their higher awards.[38] As stated by Davis and Burnard[38] the problem with this approach is whether professional experience can be quantified and equated with academic ability. Despite these concerns, many nurses have successfully accessed higher education via this route and indeed professional profiling is now an important aspect of professional development.

Perhaps to be of most benefit interdisciplinary education should begin at undergraduate level in preparation for more effective team working in clinical practice. Learning together at an early stage in their career may facilitate mutual understanding between health-care professionals before they become socialized into distinct roles. The success of palliative care in specialist settings may be a result of multiprofessional team working. It could be argued, therefore, that an important aspect of education in palliative care for all health-care professionals should be access to an environment which demonstrates collaborative care of patients and their relatives.

Evaluation of educational programmes

The paucity of systematic evaluations of educational programmes in palliative care has not improved since the first edition of this Textbook. As noted by several authors, this lack of evaluation is characteristic of education in this area and is not confined to nurse education.[31,39,40] It is argued that the contribution of education for nurses in palliative care is unknown,[8,40] with conflicting information being presented in the literature. Some studies have shown that nurses' levels of anxiety are reduced following educational intervention[8,41] whilst other authors have not shown this effect.[29,42] While measurement scales are available, there are difficulties in measuring attitudes as highlighted by Hurtig and Stewin.[43] Yet to date, measuring nurses attitudes remains the focus for evaluation of educational programmes. Few studies have evaluated the effects of educational programmes on clinical care and the effect, if any, on patient outcomes. In a review of the literature Webber[40] noted that the influence of variables such as teaching strategies, the length of the course, or characteristics of the trainers have not systematically been researched. The narrow focus of evaluation in palliative care education offers little to educators developing curricula for nurses in palliative care. There is a need for evaluation of education to have a broader focus than that which predominates currently.

There is also a need to look more closely at the process of education, who delivers it, identification of individual educational needs, and whether education in this area is resulting in enhanced patient care.

Education in response to health-care policies

As has been demonstrated, the delivery of palliative care and the availability of education in this area varies greatly throughout the world. The recommendations of the World Health Organisation which have appeared over recent years in relation to palliative care are to be applauded. However, their implementation has been slow and it is often not evaluated, resulting in the fragmented service which exists today. In Europe, the Commission of the European Communities through its Europe Against Cancer programme is addressing some of these variations with a number of recommendations. In their second action plan the Commission acknowledges that palliative care provides extremely valuable support for patients for whom treatment has failed. It also recommends exchange of experience between member states for health professionals in the area of palliative care to improve training.[44] This is reiterated in their third action plan for 1995 to 1999.[45] Such recommendations allow policy makers, as well as individual nurses, access to funds which would assist in the development of care for individuals requiring palliative care. The Europe Against Cancer programme, however, is only one aspect of the European Commissions remit. The ratification of the Treaty on the European Union (Maastricht Treaty) offers the European Union the potential to play a leading role in shaping health-care policy on a European and a national level.[46] An important aspect of this responsibility includes promoting education. Educators in palliative care therefore have an opportunity to argue, within a legal structure, for the development of palliative care through education.

In order to improve the quality of health-care provision, the Health Service within the United Kingdom has undergone unprecedented changes and development. The new service is seeking to achieve greater response to individual needs, better value for money, and an improvement in the quality of patient/client care. Nurses are clearly a major resource and the quality of their care will depend on the quality of their education.[47] The newly structured Health Service expects that purchasers of health care will assess the total needs of the population they serve and in so doing will highlight the needs of palliative care provision. In order to meet those needs, an appropriately prepared and qualified work force is required to be in place. Legislation within the United Kingdom is insistent that future education and training for nurses must reflect the Regional Heath Authorities' manpower planning.[48]

Therefore, in the future, the education of nurses will be based upon regional needs analysis, demographic trends, skill mix, and financial resources. To date, reports on palliative-care provision within the United Kingdom and elsewhere have highlighted an uneven and unco-ordinated service.[49,50]

The Barcelona Declaration from the World Health Organization and others[51] states that 'families and other informal carers are essential contributors to the delivery of effective palliative care. They should be recognized and empowered by government policy'. The declaration also recommends that governments should utilize knowledge of palliative care in a rational way by:

(1) establishing clear and informed policies;

(2) implementing specific services;

(3) educating health professionals;

(4) making necessary drugs available;

(5) systematic assessment of needs in palliative care.

Assessing the needs of communities and populations is likely to result in an increasing demand for appropriate palliative care and the provision of adequate and appropriately prepared staff. Currently in Britain, as in other European countries, a significant percentage of individuals die in hospital.[52] It is therefore essential that all levels of nursing staff can access relevant information and education regarding the care of dying patients and their significant others. However, the current shift of patient care from hospitals into the community requires that all nurses are prepared to be competent practitioners whatever the health-care setting. This has implications for nursing education. It is essential that palliative care education prepares its students to be versatile and to practice competently in a variety of environments.

It is not essential nor desirable, particularly in today's economic climate, that all nurses should be specialists in palliative care. What is important is the availability of palliative care education at various professional and academic levels and that those interested can access modules and programmes of study so that the public can expect a quality service irrespective of the setting and by whom it is delivered. In a number of developing countries, active care of chronic illnesses, such as cancer, is limited. Often care in this situation is, from the outset, palliative. We need therefore to ensure that through education we can address this phenomenon.

Future directions

The quality of palliative-care delivery, as in all nursing care, is dependent upon continuing research. There has been notable progress in highlighting the needs of patients and families.[53] Such research continues to raise the awareness of the need to look critically at the ways in which dying patients and their families are cared for. Research into practice has enabled, and continues to enable, advances to be made in identifying a body of knowledge in palliative care with which to educate health-care professionals. However, questions remain in relation to how we can best enable nurses to learn specific knowledge and skills; for instance handling difficult questions, knowledge of therapeutics, responding sensitively to choices made by patients that may challenge the inherent values and beliefs of the individual nurse, and the ability to continue to support the patient and their carers during those occasions when dying is difficult. It has been stated that structuring the thinking of nurses by utilizing tools (such as care theories, the scientific process of nursing, and, more recently, nursing diagnosis) have advanced the quality of nursing care.[22] Nurse educators involved in teaching palliative care have a responsibility to ensure that such theoretical knowledge underpins the content of their curriculum.

Providing nurses with knowledge is only part of the solution to improving palliative care. Nurses must also learn the skills of negotiation and management if they are to function as an equal member of the health-care team responsible for the delivery of care to patients. The developing role of specialist nurses in palliative care has largely evolved in a piecemeal fashion in response to local need and the availability of resource. Yet in 1989 the World Health Organization recommended that national governments should institute palliative (cancer) care programmes. However, despite this recommendation the need for a co-ordinated, strategic approach to nurse education remains, along with ensuring accessibility to education in palliative care for nurses worldwide. There are undoubtedly moves towards improving nurse education in a number of developing areas, such as Eastern Europe, India, and parts of Africa. Evaluation of these programmes will be important to ensure that they are addressing the needs of the local population, nurses, and patients. Work needs to be undertaken to identify the specific aims and objectives of educational programmes in relation to the skills and knowledge that such programmes aim to produce. There is an urgent need to identify what constitutes competent practice in palliative nursing and the educational input necessary to provide this. There is a growing awareness that palliative care is much more than care of the dying and bereaved. This awareness needs to be reflected in educational programmes at all levels in nursing. The concept of rehabilitation and enhancement of quality of life for individuals with a chronic illness should be integral components of any programme.

Education needs to be more accessible than it is at the moment with consideration given to those who are remote from educational centres. The developments in computer technology should be exploited in nurse education. There is almost unlimited potential to utilize information technology in education, by for example tutorials, teleconferencing, and computer simulation.

Nurse education in palliative care needs to look forward to the changing trends in epidemiology and population requirements to ensure that what is being offered will be relevant in a changing health-care environment. The need for palliative care is likely to increase and nurses along with other health-care professionals need to be prepared to accept the responsibility of providing expert care. Only through education will this be possible.

References

1. World Health Organization. *Palliative Cancer Care.* Regional Office for Europe, WHO, 1989.
2. Quint JC. *The Nurse and the Dying Patient.* New York, Macmillan, 1967.
3. Webber J. The Effects of an Educational Course on Problems Identified by Nurses Caring for Patients with Advanced Cancer. Unpublished MSc dissertation, Kings College, University of London, 1989.
4. Copp G. Palliative care nursing education: a review of research findings. *Journal of Advanced Nursing,* 1994; **19**: 552–7.
5. Nebaur M, Prior D, Berggren L, Haberect J, Ku M, Mitchell A, and Davies E. Nurses' perceptions of palliative care nursing. *International Journal of Palliative Nursing,* 1996; **2**: 26–34.
6. Field D and Kitson C. Formal teaching about death and dying in UK nursing schools. *Nurse Education Today,* 1986; **6**: 270–6.
7. Williams G. Role consideration in the care of the dying patient. *Image,* 1982; **14**: 8–11.
8. Benoliel JQ. Nursing research on death, dying and terminal illness: development, present state and prospects. *Annual Review of Nursing Research,* 1983; **1**: 101–30.
9. Jeffrey D. Appropriate palliative care: when does it begin. *European Journal of Cancer Care,* 1995; **4**: 122–6.
10. Hockley J. Caring for the dying in acute hospitals. *Nursing Times,* 1989; **85**: 47–50.
11. Bramwell L. Cancer nursing—a problem finding survey. *Cancer Nursing,* 1989; **12**: 320–8.
12. Field D. *Nursing the Dying.* Tavistock, Routledge, 1989
13. Copp G and Dunn V. Frequent and difficult problems perceived by nurses caring for the dying in the community, hospice and acute care settings. *Palliative Medicine,* 1993; **7**: 19–25.
14. Burocoa B. Pitfalls of palliative care. *Journal of Palliative Care,* 1993, **9**, 29–32.
15. Mills M, Davies HT, and MacRae WA. Care of dying patients in hospital. *British Medical Journal,* 1994; **309**: 583–6.
16. Jeffrey D. Education in palliative care: a qualitative evaluation of the present state and the needs of general practitioners and community nurses. *European Journal of Cancer Care,* 1994; **3**: 67–74.
17. James C and Macleod R. The problematic nature of education in palliative care. *Journal of Palliative Care,* 1993; **9**: 5–10.
18. Kelly B. The professional values of English nursing undergraduates. *Journal of Advanced Nursing,* 1991; **16**: 867–72.
19. Sneddon M. Continuing Education in Palliative Care Nursing: an exploration of perceived outcome and factors influencing application of learning. Unpublished MSc Thesis, University of Glasgow, 1992.
20. Grahn G. Learning to cope—an intervention in cancer care. *Supportive Care in Cancer,* 1993; **1**: 266–71.
21. Corner J and Wilson-Barnett J. The newly registered nurse and the cancer patient: an educational evaluation. *International Journal of Nursing Studies,* 1992; **29**: 177–90.
22. Wouters B. Teaching palliative care: a challenge to nursing trainers. *European Journal of Palliative Care,* 1994; **1**: 178–83.
23. Uzel P. Soins palliatifs et accompagnement des personnes en fin de vie et de leurs proches. *Infirmirière enseignante,* 1991; **21**: 7–12.
24. Corner J. The nursing perspective. In: Doyle D, Hanks GWC, and MacDonald N, eds. *Oxford Textbook of Palliative Medicine.* Oxford University Press, 1993.
25. Paillot-Schmidt M. Pout une sensibilisation des élèves infirmières à l'approche des malades mourants dans l'exercise des soins palliatifs. *Infirmière-enseignante,* 1987; **6**: 27–9.
26. European Oncology Nursing Society. *Report and Recommendations of a Workshop to Study the Feasibility of Educational Programmes in Palliative Care for Nurses in Europe.* London: Good News Press, 1994.
27. Whitfield S. A Descriptive Study of Student Nurses' Ward Experiences with Dying Patients and their Attitudes Towards Them. Unpublished MSc. thesis, University of Manchester, 1979.
28. Birch JA. Anxiety and conflict in nurse education. In: Davis DB, ed. *Research in Nurse Education.* Kent, Croom-Helm, 1983.
29. Chodil J and Dulaney P. Outcome evaluation. Continuing education on dying and death. *Journal of Continuing Education in Nursing,* 1984; **15**: 5–8.
30. Caty S and Tamlyn D. Positive effects of education on nursing students attitudes towards death and dying. *Nursing Papers,* 1985; **16**: 41–55.
31. Corner J. The Newly Registered Nurse and the Cancer Patient. Unpublished PhD thesis, Kings College, University of London, 1990.
32. Duke S. The Effect of an Educational Course (ENB 931) on the Perceived Problems of Nurses Caring for the Dying. Unpublished BSc dissertation, University of Surrey, 1991.
33. United Kingdom Central Council for Nursing, Midwifery and Health Visiting. *The Future of Professional Practice—the councils standards for education and practice following registration.* London, United Kingdom Central Council, 1994.
34. International Society for Nurses in Cancer Care. *A Core Curriculum for a Post-basic Course in Palliative Nursing.* Manchester, Haigh and Hochland, 1991.
35. Kristjanson L and Balneaves L. Directions for palliative care nursing in Canada: report of a national survey. *Journal of Palliative Care,* 1995; **11**: 5–8.
36. National Council for Hospice and Specialist Palliative Care Services. *Education in Palliative Care.* Occasional Paper 9, 1996.

37. Macleod RD. Teaching hospice medicine to medical students, house staff and other care-givers in the United Kingdom. *Hospice Journal,* 1993; **9**: 55–67.
38. Davis B and Burnard P. Academic levels in nursing. *Journal of Advanced Nursing,* 1992; **17**: 1395–400.
39. Degner LF, Chekryn J, Deegan M, Gow C, Koop P, Mills J, and Reid J. An undergraduate course in palliative care. In: Quint Benoliel J, ed. *Death Education for the Health Professional.* Washington, Hemisphere, 1982.
40. Webber J. New directions in palliative care education. *Support Cancer Care,* 1994; **2**: 16–20.
41. Degner LF and Gow CM. Evaluation of death education in nursing. *Cancer Nursing,* 1988; **11**: 151–9.
42. Yarbel WL, Gobel P, and Rublee DA. Effects of death education on nursing students' anxiety and locus of control. *Journal of School Health,* 1981; **51**: 367–72.
43. Hurtig W and Stewin L. The effect of death education and experience on nursing students' attitudes towards death. *Journal of Advanced Nursing,* 1990; **15**: 29–34.
44. Europe Against Cancer Programme. Adopting a 1990–1994 Action Plan in the Context of the Europe Against Cancer Programme. *Official Journal of the European Communities* No. L 137/31, 1990.
45. Commission of the European Communities. *Adopting an Action Plan 1995–1999 to Combat Cancer within the Framework for Action in the Field of Public Health.* Official Publication of the European Communities Cat. No. CB-CO-95–138-EN-C, 1995.
46. Pritchard P. The Maastricht Treaty: setting a health care agenda for Europe. *European Journal of Cancer Care,* 1994; **3**: 6–11.
47. Department of Health. *Nursing Midwifery and Health Visiting Statement of Strategic Intent.* HMSO, 1994.
48. Department of Health. *Challenges for Nursing and Midwifery in the 21st century; The Heathrow Debate.* HMSO, 1993.
49. Clark D. Whither the hospices. In: Clark D, ed. *The Future of Palliative Care.* Milton Keynes, UK: Open University Press, 1993.
50. Douglas C. For all the saints. *British Medical Journal,* 1992; **304**: 579.
51. Ministry of Health, Government of Catalonia, WHO, EAPC, SECPAL. The Barcelona declaration on palliative care. *European Journal of Palliative Care*, 1996; **3**: 15.
52. Field D and James N. Where and how people die. In: Clark D, ed. *The Future for Palliative Care.* Milton Keynes, UK: Open University Press, 1993.
53. Addington-Hall JM, MacDonald LD, Anderson HR, and Freeling P. Dying from cancer: the views of bereaved family and friends about the experiences of terminally ill cancer patients. *Palliative Medicine,* 1991; **5**: 207–15.

21.4 Education for social workers

F.M. Sheldon

Introduction

Palliative care recognizes the interdependence of physical, psychosocial, and spiritual care. Difficult relationships within a family or anxieties about money or housing can exacerbate or even produce physical symptoms. Therefore attention to the emotional and social needs of patient and family must go alongside control of pain and vomiting. However, the psychosocial aspects of care are not just handmaidens to help with the control of physical symptoms. Any system of care which concerns itself with the whole quality of life of patient and family must recognize that social and emotional needs are equally important.

Where there is a social worker in the team, he or she will be concerned with these aspects of care. Patients needing palliative care may be in specialist hospice inpatient units, or in their own homes supported by specialist palliative care teams. They will often be present in the wards of large general hospitals, in oncology and radiotherapy units, in children's wards, in units for those with mental illness or learning disabilities, and in specialist services for those with chronic disabilities. People who are dying are likely to spend most of the last year of their life at home, wherever they die.[1] Primary health care teams are increasingly supporting the dying in their own homes and calling on local social work organizations for help. Therefore social workers may meet patients needing palliative care or their families if they work in any of the above services. A firm grounding in palliative care at qualifying level is needed together with opportunities for postqualifying study for more specialist workers in the hospice, oncology, or radiotherapy services.

The knowledge, attitudes, and skills needed by social workers in palliative care at generalist and specialist levels are described in this chapter, and ways of delivering such an education are discussed. Finally, we consider how social work education in palliative care has developed and what the future might hold.

Content of educational programmes

Theory of loss and bereavement

Working with loss is an inescapable task for social workers. The loss may involve a child going into foster care, an elderly man going into residential care, or a young mother dying. An understanding of how human beings form emotional attachments to others, how the quality of these attachments may influence development, and how disruption of attachment may affect the individual is basic to all social work. In palliative care the focus is frequently on the effects of loss of attachment as members of a family experience the death of a loved one. Allied to this is the need for an understanding of the way in which individuals build up for themselves a sense of meaning in life and a sense of self-worth. Faced with the crisis of death, both the dying person and those attached to him or her may find their deepest beliefs about themselves and the world challenged and undermined. A number of writers have contributed to our knowledge and understanding in this field, among them Bowlby[2] and his critics,[3] who have shown how human beings develop attachments and the factors that may affect this development.

Erikson[4] has postulated eight crisis periods in the human lifecycle whose resolution influences the mature adjustment of the individual. Parkes[5] has been particularly influential in building on the work on attachment to describe the process of bereavement. His paper on psychosocial transitions[6] is important as it sets out some general principles which underlie all loss experiences. Marris's[7] work on loss and change in a range of life experiences and Caplan's[8] theory of crisis intervention also contribute to the understanding that social workers need to have when working with the dying and their families in any setting. A discriminating approach to Kübler-Ross,[9] which values her clinical insights without treating them as a prescription for action, is an important component of qualifying study.

This appreciation of the varieties of loss experience needs to be deeper for those in specialist palliative care settings. A knowledge of the development of theories of bereavement, encompassing Freud[10] and Lindemann[11] as well as Parkes,[5,6] and including the recent challenges to accepted theories from Wortman and Silver[12] and Stroebe,[13] is essential. Part of this is a broader consideration of the factors which contribute to complicating the grief process and the therapies that have been developed to address particular complications by workers like Liebermann[14] and Ramsay.[15]

Historical and sociological perspectives

Social workers working with the dying and their families form part of a team of professional and non-professional carers. Specific contributions that social workers can make to that team are an understanding of social interaction and family dynamics and an ability to work in a positive way with these elements of the situation. This has to be grounded in both history and sociology. Many professionals in health care have a sadly pessimistic view of contemporary family life which harks back to a 'golden age' when families cared for and valued their elderly members and no one coped with the crisis of death alone. Laslett[16] and the Cambridge Group for the History of Population and Social Structure provide evidence to challenge these popular misconceptions about family life in the past. Current changes in the age structure of the population, the position of women, and changing views of family life form part of the social climate in which the dying, their families, and their professional helpers operate. These changes need to be grappled with rather than simply viewed with abhorrence. These issues are part of the basic training of all social workers and areas relevant to palliative care as any other form of social and health care.

Of more particular application to palliative care is a knowledge of how and why attitudes to death and bereavement have changed over time. Added to this is an appreciation of a variety of responses to death and bereavement found in different cultures. Only if professionals appreciate this will they cease to be prisoners of a particular cultural or social approach to the crisis of death. Their new freedom should enable them to help the dying and their families from any social or cultural background to feel more in control of this experience, and to understand that there is a range of choices about behaviour and ritual. A recent study,[17] shows that equal access to palliative care services in the United Kingdom for those from ethnic minorities has not always been achieved. Training for specialist social workers in palliative care should enable them to assist their teams in developing an organization and work style which allows patients and families to be comfortable using the service, whatever their cultural background.

Ethical issues

A basic training in ethics should be part of all training courses for professionals in health care. In palliative care the issues with which staff most often grapple are those concerning the right of the patient and his or her relatives to determine the treatment and to control information, confidentiality, conflicts of conscience and professional duty, interprofessional conflicts, euthanasia, and the medicalization of bereavement. Edge[18] identifies awareness of the sociological factors which help to determine attitudes as an important component of education in ethics. Social workers in general settings need to have clear ethical principles and an ability to apply them constructively. In specialist palliative care settings, social workers, as members of a team outside the medical and nursing hierarchies, can be helpful in identifying issues and fostering debate. Therefore their training needs to include not only the basics of ethical principles and their application to palliative care issues, but also ways in which teams can be helped to generate debate and resolve issues.

Communication skills

Individual

Good communication skills underlie sensitive palliative care. Although medical and nurse training is catching up fast, social work training is still the most rigorous in preparing students to communicate. The vast majority of social work courses now have some input on counselling skills, often using the popular Egan[19] model and drawing on the work of Rogers.[20] Techniques of opening up discussion about sensitive topics in a non-judgemental way and enabling clients to make decisions for themselves are basic to all social work. The skills can be applied equally well to work in palliative care and bereavement counselling. However, if workers are to be able to mobilize the techniques skilfully, they need the knowledge and attitudes which will help them both to be unafraid of discussing death and dying and to give a positive approach to this type of care. A knowledge of Gestalt techniques such as 'the empty chair' can also be particularly useful to the specialist worker with bereaved clients.[21]

Group work

The social worker is the member of the palliative care team who is likely to have received the most preparation for working in groups, whether these are family groups, groups of patients or relatives, or groups of staff. There are two important aspects of working with families: the understanding of the sociology of a family and its changing nature, which have been alluded to already, and the techniques of family therapy. Writers such as Minuchin[22] and members of the Milan School have been influential in developing a variety of methods which workers can use in partnership with troubled families who wish to change the way that they relate to each other or to mobilize family resources to deal with a life crisis such as the death of a family member. While the sociological aspects of family work are likely to be part of basic social work training, formal training in family therapy will usually only be part of a particular placement for a few students. Family therapy will form part of postqualifying training for most social workers. Its techniques can be adapted for use in palliative care, and practical guidance on this is available.[23-25] Social workers in specialist services need to be prepared to work both with families for whom the death of a family member is the major stress and with families who have already had difficulties in family relationships which the threat of loss or actual bereavement has intensified. Since such work should be done with a coworker, training at postqualifying levels should be multidisciplinary to give the opportunity for different professionals in the palliative care team to work together. Group work with patients or relatives is a valuable therapeutic tool. Opportunities to meet others facing the same crisis, to learn from them, and to give to them add a dimension which the professional–client relationship cannot provide. Qualifying training courses vary in the extent to which group work is included. Again there are two components: an understanding of group dynamics and the use of group work techniques and skills. Groups for patients are most likely to be found in the specialist setting, but groups for relatives, particularly bereaved relatives, are also becoming much more common in community settings. Social workers may develop these as part of their role in social work agencies or in conjunction with voluntary bereavement support organizations such as Cruse in the United Kingdom. Work with groups of bereaved children is a rapidly developing aspect of group work. Kitchener and Smith[26] have developed this technique in a child guidance clinic in the United Kingdom. As yet, there is little formal training for specialist workers in group work with patients or the bereaved. Social workers with a general grounding have built on knowledge and skills, and often develop these by joining an experienced group worker who runs a group for the bereaved. Any specialist training programme for social workers in palliative care should have applications of group work in this field as part of its programme.

Another area of training yet to be developed is the use of creative methods to enable the dying and their families to explore the experience. Work with dying[27] and bereaved children has shown the value of drawing and music in helping children to express their feelings. Hospice arts programmes and the use of music and art therapy are all opening up a variety of ways for adults to understand and express emotional pain. Social workers should be ready to enable clients to tap these sources of help. Again, little training has been directed specifically at social workers in developing these methods of work, and they should form part of the education of specialist workers.

Practical issues

The skills of social workers in obtaining resources for their clients are greatly valued by both the clients themselves and other professionals. Understanding the social welfare and income maintenance systems of the society in which they work forms a part of the basic training of all social workers. The skills of advocating for clients and their families to obtain resources, either financial or practical, are generally learnt during the practical placements that are a part of every social work training course. Anxieties about paying bills and securing help in caring for a sick and dependent partner are as much a concern for the dying and their families as for any disabled person. Since social workers in any setting may come across life-threatening conditions, they all need to be aware of the range of resources available to the seriously ill and disabled. Specialists need to develop a more detailed database and close working relationships with any state or voluntary body particularly concerned with those areas. The specialist knowledge that they develop may sometimes be appropriately mobilized for change on a national scale. A successful campaign in the United Kingdom, led by the Association of Hospice Social Workers, to enable dying people to benefit more fully from a particular benefit for the disabled (the Attendance Allowance) grew out of the practical experience of client need reported by individual social workers at training days on welfare benefits. Lobbying of political parties and ministers cannot be a standard part of social work training but it can improve the quality of life for clients.

Delivery of education for social work in palliative care

Methods of teaching

Good palliative care is not just an intellectual exercise relying on knowledge alone. Since it challenges every part of the professional providing it, the attitude of that professional to death and dying and the ability to work close to deep emotional pain are key areas to be addressed in education in palliative care. The formal lecture is one appropriate medium for developing knowledge of theories of loss and bereavement, sociological and social welfare issues, and information about resources. Other ways of acquiring knowledge are by guided reading and increasingly by the use of interactive computer programs. Attitudes and skills cannot be taught in the lecture theatre, although the lecturer's own attitude to the topic may influence those listening—for good or ill. Small-group teaching with opportunities for students to share views and fears, for instance about the questions that dying people may ask them, provides a far better arena for developing confidence in opening up sensitive topics with a client and engendering an open approach to death. With the development of distance learning programmes in palliative care, some thought needs to be given to how students may learn from each other in this way despite seldom meeting together as a group.

Small groups not only provide a safer setting for discussion than the formal lecture, but also provide the opportunity for using a variety of experiential methods which assist in both attitude change and learning skills. The most commonly used experiential method is role play. Maguire[28] and his colleagues have particularly developed this form of training in palliative care in the United Kingdom. By mimicking the actual interview situation, it can offer increased mastery of the skills of listening, clarifying, and exploring problems, and setting goals. However, role play is not universally popular with students. Moreover, its emphasis on the verbal aspects of the interaction may undervalue the significance of non-verbal communication. The use of role play must be underpinned by a broad approach to communication skills, work on attitudes, and an understanding of the importance of the context in which communication takes place.

A number of videotapes have been developed which model good practice in communication. Another type of videotape offers a 'trigger'—a brief interaction between client and worker—which students can use to develop role play interviews. Videotaping role play interviews by students and playing them back is another potent method of learning communication skills. All these methods require careful preparation by the tutor. Students often feel vulnerable and exposed performing for others or on video, and they will only be able to use these learning methods if they feel encouraged and valued by the tutor and student group.

Another experiential method useful in teaching palliative care is sculpting. This provides a unique way of examining family dynamics and helping to understand death and bereavement from a family-centred rather than an individual point of view. Sculpting first developed as a therapeutic method in family therapy. Very little has been written on this method. In the teaching session, one member of the group will choose a family that they have worked with and place each family member in a particular bodily position and in a spatial relationship to other family members which symbolize the relationships within their family. Discussion can develop in a number of ways, looking at how family relationships change as death approaches, or how family members might go about changing relationships. Participants usually perceive this method as less stressful than role play, and it produces a deeper understanding of the intensity of feeling experienced by all family members when one of them is dying. Students from a range of cultural groups can use it successfully.

Another type of experiential method uses exercises to develop empathy and deepen the students' understanding of their own attitudes and feelings.[29] These may involve paper and pencil exercises such as completing a questionnaire on the students' attitudes to their own death or may use drawing to express feeling. Enabling each student to bring to a small group an object which symbolizes death or bereavement to them is another way of exploring feelings. It must be a cardinal principle in the use of any experiential method that all participants should be clear about what a session will entail, that no student should be compelled to participate, and that students may withdraw even after a session has started.

Case discussion is a well-tried method in social work teaching. The cases may be provided by experienced students from their own practice or by the tutor. Videos of bereaved or dying people talking about their own experience are increasingly being used to stimulate discussion of issues in psychosocial care. Case discussion provides a particularly useful base for discussion of ethical issues. All may agree about general ethical principles, but disagree about their application.

Clients are often the best teachers. Supervised placements with a palliative care team give an opportunity to work with dying people and their families in depth and over time, and to test skills and attitudes. The possibility of such placements is increasing rapidly as social workers become integral members of the palliative care team[30] and can provide the experience and supervision necessary. No classroom experience can match this provided that it is properly supported. The learning is not just about clients but is also about the pleasures and pitfalls of working with a multidisciplinary team.

Collaborative teaching and learning must play a part in social work education in palliative care. Working with other professionals is often perceived as a greater challenge than working with the dying. For example, Lunt and Yardley[31] found that 52 per cent of the Macmillan nurses that they surveyed expected contacts with other professionals to be stressful. Although each profession in palliative care has core skills and knowledge, there is a considerable overlap, particularly in the emotional aspect of care. This overlap will only be fruitful if all professionals have a clear idea of their own role and an appreciation of what other professions can offer. There are two ways of contributing to this in the training process. First, multidisciplinary groups of pre- or postqualifying students can learn together. Second, teachers from different professions can combine to offer a model of co-operation and may help students to confront issues of scapegoating and stereotyping other professions. Palliative care topics such as loss and bereavement, ethical issues, family work, and communication lend themselves particularly well to multidisciplinary learning and teaching.

The current scene

Some components of education for social workers in palliative care have been in place for a long time. In 1987 Mark[32] surveyed field work teachers in health and community settings in the United Kingdom and found that virtually all saw the topic of loss and change as essential for all social work students. A follow-up study of community-based social workers by Cullen and Millard,[33] who looked at the training that community-based social workers had received and its relevance for their work, found that loss and change were highly rated for relevance by all workers and were well covered in training. Care of the dying was not seen as so important, but some training had been available at pre- or postqualifying levels for those who saw it as relevant.

A series of surveys for the European Association for Palliative Care[34–36] record an increasing number of opportunities for social workers in Europe to acquire training in palliative care. In Denmark, Poland, and Switzerland palliative care topics are well covered in the qualifying courses, and such teaching is developing in France too. Where specialist palliative care services exist, students are often able to visit them as part of their course. In some countries in Europe training opportunities arise at postqualifying rather than qualifying level, and such opportunities may be available for multidisciplinary groups rather than for social workers alone. Spain and Belgium are examples of countries which now have short courses at postqualifying level on aspects of palliative care which are open to all professionals. There are well-established Diplomas in Palliative Care at a number of French universities which have a multiprofessional intake.

Social work education in palliative care is perhaps best developed in the United Kingdom following the funding of six Macmillan lectureships in social work, five at universities and one at an Institute of Higher Education, by a national charity, the Cancer Relief Macmillan Fund. All the lecturers contribute specialist palliative care teaching to the qualifying courses run in their departments and are developing modules on Masters courses. In 1992 a postgraduate diploma and Masters degree in psychosocial palliative care was established at Southampton University by one of the Macmillan lecturers, providing one of the first opportunities for advanced level education for social workers in palliative care. The United Kingdom, with its network of specialist palliative care services in hospices, hospitals, and the community, provides many opportunities for social work students on qualifying courses to undertake practice placements in those settings.

Future trends

Two trends, one in health care generally and one in palliative care itself, will ensure that more social workers will require training in this field. In most health-care provision in the developed countries the emphasis is now on reducing the length of time spent in hospital and supporting those who are ill in their own homes or in home-like settings. Therefore those who are dying and are spending more of the last year of their life at home will increasingly require the co-ordination of specialist palliative care services and local community-based services. Social workers in those more general services will be brought into closer contact with the dying and the bereaved, and will need to develop their knowledge and skills. The trend within palliative care itself is to move beyond the needs of people with cancer and their families to consider the needs of anyone who is dying. There is still a debate about the extent to which the principles and practice developed in cancer palliative care apply to any dying person. However, any extension of palliative care will necessarily involve social workers in other health settings, such as geriatrics and disability, and they will require palliative care education.

Advanced level education to meet the needs of experienced specialist social workers is beginning to be developed. The possibility of undertaking diploma and Masters courses with a research element is increasing, and the results of such research are beginning to feed back into both practice and the more basic levels of education. A much more critical approach to current practice is starting to appear. As the specialty develops, experienced palliative care social workers are facing increasing demands that they become teachers of members of their own profession, of other health care professionals, and of the numerous voluntary groups who are concerned about the care of the dying and bereaved. Any education programme for the specialist must prepare its students to be educators in their turn.

The future is exciting for social work education in palliative care. A fruitful interaction of practice, teaching, and research is beginning to emerge which can only improve the quality of education for practitioners in the field.

References

1. Hinton J. Which patients with terminal cancer are admitted from home care? *Palliative Medicine*, 1994; 8:197–210.
2. Bowlby J. *Attachment and Loss: I. Attachment*. London: Hogarth Press, 1969.
3. Rutter M. *Maternal Deprivation Reassessed*. Harmondsworth: Penguin, 1972.
4. Erikson E. *Childhood and Society*. London: Hogarth Press, 1965.
5. Parkes CM. *Bereavement—Studies of Grief in Adult Life*. 2nd edn. Harmondsworth: Penguin, 1986.
6. Parkes CM. Psychosocial transitions: a field for study. *Social Science and Medicine*, 1971; 5(2):101–5.
7. Marris P. *Loss and Change*. Revised edn. London: Routledge and Kegan Paul, 1986.
8. Caplan G. *An Approach to Community Mental Health*. London: Tavistock, 1961.
9. Kübler-Ross E. *On Death and Dying*. London: Tavistock, 1970.
10. Freud S. *Mourning and Melancholia*. Strachey J, ed. Standard Edition. London: Hogarth Press, 1974, vol. 14.
11. Lindemann E. The symptomatology and management of acute grief. *American Journal of Psychiatry*, 1944; **101**: 41.
12. Wortman C, Silver RS. The myths of coping with loss. *Journal of Consulting and Clinical Psychology*, 1989; **57**(3):349–57.
13. Stroebe M. Coping with bereavement—a review of the griefwork hypothesis. *Omega*, 1992–1993; **26**(1):19–42.
14. Liebermann S. Nineteen cases of morbid grief. *British Journal of Psychiatry*, 1978; **132**:159–63.
15. Ramsay RW. Bereavement: a behavioral treatment for pathological grief. In Sioden PO, Bates S, Darkens WS, III, eds. *Trends in Behaviour Therapy*. New York: Academic Press, 1979.
16. Laslett P. *The World We Have Lost*. 2nd edn. London: Methuen, 1971.
17. National Council for Hospice and Specialist Palliative Care Services. *Opening Doors—Improving Access to Hospice and Specialist Palliative Care Services by Members of the Black and Ethnic Minority Communities*. London: National Council for Hospice and Specialist Palliative Care Services, 1995.
18. Edge D. The education of attitudes to death and bereavement. In Thompson I, ed. *Dilemmas of Dying: A Study in the Ethics of Terminal Care*. Edinburgh: Edinburgh University Press, 1979.
19. Egan G. *The Skilled Helper*. 4th edn. California: Brooks/Cole, 1990.
20. Rogers RC. *On Becoming a Person*. London: Constable, 1961.
21. Clarkson P. *Gestalt Counselling in Action*. London: Sage, 1989.
22. Minuchin S. *Families and Family Therapy*. London: Tavistock, 1974.
23. Hildebrand J. Working with a bereaved family: focusing on prevention not pathology. *Palliative Medicine*, 1989; **3**:105–11.
24. Smith N. The impact of terminal illness on the family. *Palliative Medicine*, 1990; **4**:127–36.
25. Bruggen P, Acworth A. Family therapy when one member is on the deathbed. *Journal of Family Therapy* 1985; **7**:379–85.
26. Kitchener M, Smith S. *The Forgotten Mourners: Guidelines for Working with Bereaved Children*. London: Jessica Kingsley, 1994.
27. Judd D. *Give Sorrow Words: Working with a Dying Child*. London: Free Association, 1989
28. Maguire P. Barriers to psychological care of the dying. *British Medical Journal*, 1985; **291**:1711–13.
29. The Open University Coping with Crisis Research Group. *Running Workshops—A Guide for Trainers in the Helping Professions*. London: Croom Helm, 1987.
30. WHO Expert Committee on Cancer Pain Relief and Active Support Care. *Cancer Pain Relief and Palliative Care. World Health Organisation Technical Report, Series 804*. Geneva: World Health Organization, 1990.
31. Lunt B, Yardley J. *Home Care Teams and Hospital Support Teams for the Terminally ill*. London: Cancer Relief Macmillan Fund, 1988.
32. Mark S. *The Training Needs of Social Workers in Health Care*. Report for the Inter-County Workshop, Oxford, 1987.
33. Cullen R, Millard D. Health related and medical information as a tool of social work. A study among area-based social workers. Private communication, 1990.
34. European Association of Palliative Care. *Professional Education in Palliative Care*. Report of the Education Sub-Committee of the European Association for Palliative Care, Infokara, October 1990.
35. European Association of Palliative Care. *Survey of the Current Status of Professional Education in Palliative Care*. Report of the Education Committee of the European Association for Palliative Care,. Infokara, October 1992.
36. European Association of Palliative Care. *New Developments and Initiatives in Palliative Care Education*. Third Report of the European Association for Palliative Care Education Committee. EAPC, June 1994.

21.5 Education and training of clergy

Derek B. Murray

The historic role of clergy in care of the dying

The content of this chapter is deliberately confined to the work and training of clergy of the various branches of the Christian church, but much that is said may be applied to the leaders of the other world religions, and also to lay pastoral workers.

In the faith of the Old Testament the dying and the dead were treated with great honour. With the coming of the Christian religion, with its emphasis both on the necessity to treat each individual life with care, and on the hope of a new life after death, dying and death continued to be subjects of great importance. The priest was expected to prepare people for the fact of death, to elicit and hear confessions, and to administer the sacramental aid which the church prescribed. He had the skill to conduct the funeral rites, to comfort the bereaved, and to ensure that the dead were at rest. The dead, and especially the martyred dead in the days of persecution, were given great honour, and prayers were said at tombs.

When the church emerged from the dark days of persecution and became free to develop within the Roman world, orders of men and women were instituted, many of which had special responsibility for the very sick. Care for the dying was a holy work. In some sense this idea persists, even in the Western secularized world. The great majority of funerals are conducted by clergy, even if families have only a very remote connection with the church, and it is only recently, in Australia, Holland, and to a very limited extent in the United Kingdom and other countries, that secular celebrants of funerals, on the analogy of celebrants of non-religious weddings, have emerged.[1] The role of conductor of this particular rite of passage, and of comforter of the bereaved, is one that has remained the preserve of the clergy, and no active ordained person is likely to avoid contact with palliative care, or to escape the demand for pastoral support for the dying and the bereaved. Mauritzen, writing from a Norwegian perspective, says 'some have concluded that the nurse is the logical person to take on the spiritual aspect of care [of the dying patient]. It sounds exciting . . . First of all comes the question whether the patient is in favour of such integration. My 15 years of experience at the bedside of hospital patients do not lend [credence] to the idea. Seldom have patients opened up for questions and needs of that kind to the nurse'. He concludes that trained chaplains must be available for this care.[2] This seems an extreme point of view. Co-operation among the disciplines and mutual support in the giving of spiritual care should be the aim in teamwork. Often the chaplain's role is to affirm the spiritual care given by the doctor or the nurse.

This being so, the paucity of written discussion about the role of the clergy in palliative care is the more remarkable. There has been very little published, until recently, about the methods of training of clergy in this particular area, and it would appear that most learning was from older practitioners until recent decades. There has also existed the superstition that ordination conveyed the ability and skill to minister to the dying, without further instruction. There is no doubt that some clergy have cared for the dying with an instinctive skill, which can be communicated without books and articles, but as expectations are high such an important area dare not be neglected, and there are signs that much good work is now being carried out.

The current situation in training

The persistence of the apprenticeship model

Clergymen who are at work now have probably learnt most of what they know about the care of the dying from experience, and from the teaching of more experienced practitioners. A survey of Scottish clergy showed that many had learnt more in their years as curates or assistants, or outside the clerical profession in social work or nursing, than in seminary.[3] Only the most traditional denominations teach totally by the apprenticeship model, thus ensuring no change in the tradition, but such an important area as palliative care is often, and quite effectively, learnt in this way. Different churches have different expectations. The older Scottish tradition taught ministers to help parishioners come to terms with mortality, to make peace with neighbours, and to set out a valid will. Roman Catholics have sometimes suggested that the aim of all teaching is preparation for dying and certainly in earlier days there has been a strong emphasis on seriousness in facing mortality. More recent emphasis has shifted to teaching about life in this world, and preaching about death has sometimes been seen as morbid. Rumbold points out that 'current religious attitudes towards death seem to be a curious mixture of fragments of their historical precursors and our contemporary denial or isolation of death . . . this fragmentation is reflected in the cursory treatment given to death in most contemporary theological writing'.[4] This ambivalence is also reflected in training of clergy. There is an acknowledgement that there can be a 'good death', but the pastoral preparation for such an event is lacking. All clergy have received some instruction about the conduct of funerary rites, yet then can feel helpless in the face of spiritual pain and even offended by the anger against God often expressed by dying people and their relatives. More theological exploration needs to be done in these areas.

Changes in pastoral education

Since the 1960s, great changes have been made in the teaching of pastoral and practical theology. No longer does the imparting of 'hints and tips' seem enough, and practical theology has fought for its place alongside other theological disciplines. In the United States, the concept of clinical pastoral education has taken root since the 1920s and spread to many parts of the developed and developing world. The basic elements of this are 'some didactic instruction in the field of pastoral care and theology, the undertaking of a limited amount of pastoral work in the institution, an interpersonal group experience and supervision, either individually or in a group situation'.[5] In the United Kingdom, there has been much writing about the refinement of practical theological training. Basically the shift has been from a course of lectures to field experience, mainly in hospital settings, and to a rigorous examination of attitudes, reactions, and responses. In the 1989 study of the training and education received by a sample of Scottish clergy it is evident that from the early 1960s a new form of pastoral training was offered, taking far more account of the life sciences and counselling as it had developed in the secular world, and of the contributions of other caring professionals. Specifically, in both Protestant and Roman Catholic training, internal lecturers began to share with visiting experts in such fields as psychology and ethics.[6] Those trained in the earlier manner regretted the lack of expert teaching, and were often eager for opportunities to learn.

Clinical pastoral education

In the United States and in other cultures influenced by American models, clinical pastoral education has become a requirement for chaplaincy work. The supervisor, often a hospital chaplain, helps students to confront and explore psychological, emotional, and spiritual issues in pastoral care, and, in specific instances, care of the dying. Presentations, often in the form of a verbatim report, are analysed, and the student is led to confront his and the patient's situation. Alongside this has been the development of interdisciplinary case conferences such as those recorded by Kubler-Ross in *On Death and Dying* (see Bibliography below). In the United States and other English-speaking parts of the world, but not in the United Kingdom, clinical pastoral education is a recognized component of training. Indeed it is a requirement for ordination in most churches.

While clinical pastoral education covers the whole of chaplaincy work, there is still little evidence of specialized training for work with the dying. A description of an experiment in death education in the medical curriculum where medical students and clergy were 'on call' together has been published. Most perceived this as an opportunity to share skills and knowledge, and to demonstrate to future clinicians the value of clergy in health care.[7] Certainly the subject of death cannot be avoided, and there is evidence in recent publications that much more attention is being given to the clergy's part in palliative care. But such books are not in themselves evidence that training needs are being met.

The needs of different types of clergy

When examining the practice and development of the training of clergy in palliative care several factors need to be taken into account. The majority of priests and ministers will be working in parishes, responsible for a wide variety of functions, of which caring for the dying and bereaved will be one among others, although, in the nature of parochial life, a large area of concern. In such care clergy will encounter loss amongst parishioners well known to them and may themselves experience quite profound grief when friends and helpers die. There is a need to learn how to balance experiences, how to share grief, and how to avoid imagining that ordination conveys an ability to avoid pain and loss. They will also, especially in countries with a Christian tradition, find themselves asked to officiate at the funeral of persons who are strangers, and they will have to face grief in people they have met only for this purpose. Quick sympathy is required and a wide comprehension of the varieties of belief, unbelief, and response.

In most churches there are a number of clergy set apart as part-time or whole-time hospital chaplains. Such clergy will meet many dying patients, victims of accidents, chronically sick people, and patients who are expected to recover and do not, as well as those conventionally known as terminally ill. It is such chaplains who meet the widest spectrum of death, and who need some training in both immediate aid and long-term care.

The specialty of hospice chaplaincy is comparatively recent. Such chaplains deal in the main with prolonged, expected death and work in interdisciplinary teams. In the United Kingdom, they are organized in an association for mutual support and learning, and particular needs and pressures are being identified. As in all disciplines working in hospices, chaplains must adjust to living with constant encounter and loss. Until recently there has been no specific training for such work, and clergy are still appointed without reference to the difficulties and special needs, which might be identified as the stress of constant exposure to death and a never-ending series of losses. Hospice chaplains need not only a mature attitude to death but also the ability to make friendships quickly, and to let go just as swiftly. There seem to be as yet no specific training courses offered to certify clergy as hospice chaplains, but in the United Kingdom a start is being made and courses are offered. There are also opportunities for interdisciplinary experience for theological students, and a pastoral studies unit for theological students only has been offered for the past 9 years in one hospice. Students are confronted with the need for close co-operation among the caring professions, and receive some insights into the way in which other professionals work and think.

The theological basis for palliative care

Enough has already been said to indicate that this is no straightforward matter. Belief in an afterlife appears to have receded in many parts of the modern world, and this has influenced thinking and practice. A minister or priest must come to terms with the fact that many folk have a private understanding of the meaning of death, either as an end, or as the beginning of something unknown, which is at variance with traditional Christianity. Caring for the dying requires clergy to learn tolerance for folk religion, as well as to develop firm beliefs of their own. Dying people are not usually fit for theological argument, but they are open to acceptance and love.

This poses problems for belief systems. In the Catholic tradition there are recognized sacramental ways of reconciliation with the church and with God, and many dying patients, who have lapsed from the practice of their religion, are able to return to the trust of their childhood. In the Protestant tradition lines are less clear, and the variety of individual belief and unbelief is wider. Here too clergy must be prepared to build on what is there, to affirm and not to threaten.

Teaching about the meaning of death is generally given in systematic or dogmatic theology courses. It is essential that the subject is taken seriously by trainers and students, and it is also essential that an understanding of what people really believe is conveyed . The balance between personal assurance and tolerance is a fine one. From personal observation it would appear that clergy share the fears, doubts, and spiritual sufferings of other people when they are confronted with their own death and that of their loved ones. In training there should be time for reflection, both on the nature of human mortality and on pastoral interaction with dying people, remembering always the important insight that the dying are still the living, open to new discoveries about themselves and God. Active spiritual care will emphasize and enhance quality of life for the terminally ill.

An area of concern for many clergy is the appropriate approach to ethnic communities representing the other world religions. Co-operation with leaders of these communities is essential, and most Christian clergy would agree that the time of death is not the occasion for proselytization.

The needs of the pastor

Pastoral education is not given in a vacuum. Recent study in the field of death education has isolated several important needs of the student for ministry. Both instruction and practical experience are necessary. Certain skills may be passed on by observation, by group and individual training, and by textbook study. Facts about death and dying are freely available, and different cultural situations pose different problems. A general, if somewhat idealized, statement of intent is found in a booklet issued by the Baptist Union of Great Britain's health and healing advisory group. 'During the course of his training, the pastor will have had the preparation necessary for this important part of the Christian ministry.

1. He or she will have been encouraged to develop a right self-attitude to death.

2. He or she will have developed a theology of death. His (or her) clear if infrequent teaching on death will have shown something of the breadth of his or her understanding.

3. He or she will undoubtedly have some experience of death and dying, probably having spent some time with a hospital or hospice chaplain during which he or she will have experienced the presence of death.

4. He or she will have learnt how to bring comfort to the dying and their relatives.

5. He or she will have been taught the relevant cultural and traditional attitudes to death, and traditions relating to funerals.

6. He or she will have been instructed in the emotional battles involved in coming to terms with the reality of death'.[8]

Research has shown that few clergy would feel confident enough to claim such training and such expertise.[9] Indeed it is doubtful whether confidence to deal with death and dying can be conveyed during a course of training. Certainly the ideal is stated. Natural abilities and sympathies can be encouraged and developed, and the emotional and spiritual questions and problems connected with death can be explored. A good foundation can be laid for future learning through experience.

In one field in particular clergy are assumed to be experts. The preparation for, and conduct of, funerals is still in most Christian societies, their domain. Liturgical requirements vary, and the mode of disposal shapes the approach to the service. Until the beginning of this century burial was all but universal. In British cities today the great majority of funerals are concluded at a crematorium. In most Christian cultures a previous service may have been held in a church. In others, such as Protestant churches in Scotland, a house service was customary until quite recently, and is still expected in rural areas. Mourning customs vary even in such a small country as Scotland, and although the same elements are usually present, a wide variety of rites may be found throughout the Christian world. The pastor will therefore require instruction, not only in the immediate expectations of his region and denomination, but in a wider area, and will need to be aware of changing customs, and the possibility of adapting liturgies to the requirements of individuals, both religious and non-religious. Some interesting research has been done recently and useful suggestions made.[10] Research into the needs of the bereaved is widely available, and the secular exploration of bereavement is of great use to the pastor. A knowledge of the course of reactions to bereavement and an ability to recognize and distinguish good and pathological grief is possible if the pastor is made aware of such research.

It is also important that pastors recognize the need for real and trusting interdisciplinary co-operation in palliative care. In the survey of Scottish clergy it emerged that there are continuing difficulties in this area. Few clergy find it easy to consult doctors and nurses in charge of the care of parishioners, and they are as likely to consult textbooks or medical or nursing friends as to go to those involved in the immediate care of the patient. Too often the picture is of mutual suspicion, clergy fearing a brusque dismissal by doctors, and doctors suspicious of a lack of confidentiality in the clergy.[11]

Methods of training

Recent research suggests that training received even by quite newly ordained clergy has been minimal. A German Lutheran pastor reports that as training is very academic there is no special course on death, dying, and bereavement, and only one week's course on funerals and counselling bereaved people. While care of the dying has a part in clinical pastoral education courses, there seem to be no specific training opportunities in the United States for work in hospices. In Poland and other countries where the hospice movement is largely church based, clergy have been able to share in the general training given to other professions in palliative care. From 1993, a student from the Metropolitan Seminary in Cracow, Poland, has shared in the Pastoral Studies Unit at a specialist palliative care unit in Scotland, with a view to working eventually in hospice care (personal communications from Rev. B. Marloth-Claas, Mainz, Germany; Rev. J. Backe, New York, USA; and Fr J. Luczak, Poznan, Poland). The overall picture is of a new specialism developing and of the churches gradually beginning to recognize a need.

Lectures in seminaries and theological colleges

Short questionnaires issued to theological colleges and seminaries within the United Kingdom in 1990 produced 27 replies (60 per cent response rate). This has been supplemented by a further enquiry in 1996. All who replied had a course of some sort teaching death, dying, and bereavement; in almost all, the subject was taught within practical/pastoral theology. In the two Roman Catholic seminaries replying, it was also taught in dogmatic theology, and in one Anglican college also in liturgics. In all of the colleges, some of the lectures were given by resident staff; 20 (74 per cent) held lectures by visiting professionals (doctors, psychologists, and others). From the other perspective, it was reported in 1985 that 10 per cent of hospices in the United Kingdom offer lectures by their doctors to theological colleges.[12]

Visits to hospitals, hospices, and other institutions caring for the dying

Twenty of the colleges (74 per cent) reported that such visits were arranged, ranging from a day spent visiting a hospice, with videos, lectures, and discussion, and no patient contact, to a hospitals week, in which a wider view of dying in different contexts is offered within a general introduction to the work of general and psychiatric hospitals. In 1985, 11 (22 per cent) hospice units in the United Kingdom offered study days for theological students and 12 (24 per cent) offered study days for ordained clergy.

Thirteen (48 per cent) colleges regularly sent students on attachments to hospices, and 5 (19 per cent) occasionally did so. Such attachments may be weekly, or for a three-week period. Students 'shadow' the chaplain, have the opportunity to talk with other staff, and to meet regularly with selected patients. Eight (30 per cent) offered postgraduate courses incorporating teaching about death and dying. Diplomas in ministry and certificate courses were available to those who seek such qualifications.

Specially designed courses

In 1996, one Anglican college, in Oxford, held a course on death, dying, and bereavement, aiming to combine understanding of the dying and bereavement process with practical knowledge about funeral liturgies. It is based on lectures, the BBC video series *Living with Dying*, and personal reading and reflection. It includes a session on perinatal death. This is one of several similar syllabuses submitted and suggests that in most colleges more and more imaginative attention is being paid to death and dying.

Multidisciplinary courses

Only five (19 per cent) of the colleges replying offered any training in multidisciplinary teamwork in caring for the terminally ill, and this is clearly a difficult area. The recent (1996) publication of the National Council for Hospice and Specialist Palliative Care Services on *Education in Palliative Care* seeks to give guidance in this area and will reach theological colleges and Church Headquarters.

Pastoral studies' units

Some units for pastoral studies are now established for theological colleges in hospices, and these give a longer and more sustained opportunity for students to absorb atmosphere and to face the emotional, spiritual, and, to some extent, the physical problems of caring for the dying. There are openings for theological students to do ward work in some places. At St Christopher's Hospice in London ordained clergy may join practitioners of other disciplines (medical, nursing, and social work) in an extended course, sharing in lectures and multidisciplinary discussions. At St Columba's Hospice in Edinburgh there has been for the past decade a unit for six or seven senior theological students from Anglican, Presbyterian, Baptist, and Roman Catholic colleges. Lectures, seminars, and daily meetings with patients, under supervision, have led to a good response, a lessening of fear and, it is hoped, to a more effective ministry. It has been considered important to listen to specialists in the death of children and the care of geriatric patients, to examine the place of the clergy in the wider community, and to discover what is offered by other professionals. Some theological rigour is expected and a case study is produced by each student from his or her own experience, reflecting on a particular patient and the student's reactions. General reaction to this course has been positive, from patients, other staff, and the students themselves.

Placements

Other forms of training available in several parts of the world are attachments, for a period of a semester or longer, to the chaplaincy of a general hospital or to a specialist palliative care unit. Supervised placements in a parish with an experienced pastor are also inevitably concerned with wide issues of death and bereavement. Occasionally, a student has been placed with a funeral director. At Countess Mountbatten House, a specialist palliative care unit in Southampton, United Kingdom, the chaplain has led weekly sessions for local clergy on various aspects of death and dying, and St Christopher's Hospice, London, and St Columba's Hospice, Edinburgh, offer day courses for clergy to discuss issues and update knowledge. Sabbatical leave has been used for investigating palliative care, and increasingly students from continental Europe have been studying in British hospices, and Britons have studied in the United States. Hospice chaplains are hoping soon to visit Russia and Zaire to lecture to local clergy (personal communication).

Availability of training

It is very difficult to assess the proportion of clergy who receive special training in palliative care. Certainly, there are more now than in earlier decades. Many more possibilities are available to those who seek them but it is still possible to enter ministry with minimal instruction, and it is the student, or the trainer with the desire to pursue the subject, who gains most. Limited availability of time in all seminary and college courses means that space for practical theology is often curtailed, and within that discipline experience and instruction in care of the dying is too often, with honourable exceptions, not yet adequately represented.

Research

At St Christopher's Hospice, London, a research assistant is completing a PhD on spiritual pain, an MTh is in progress in Edinburgh on feminist theology and palliative care, and in Scotland and Canada there are several projects in progress concerning the measurement of spiritual pain and the efficacy of pastoral care.

Literature (see Bibliography below)

Beginning with Kubler Ross, *On Death and Dying,* a specialist literature in English on terminal care has gradually accumulated. Such books as Ainsworth Smith and Speck, *Letting Go,* and Rumbold, *Helplessness and Hope,* have been widely used in theological seminaries. Translations and original work in other European languages have recently become more available.

Conclusion

Clergy have always, by the nature of their calling, been deeply concerned in caring for the dying and the bereaved. For many centuries this was simply an accepted task, taught, if at all, on the apprenticeship model. In recent decades, and especially since the 1960s, increasingly sophisticated methods of training have gradually been introduced for an increasing proportion of clergy in training. The greatest change has been from the purely academic, supplemented by experience, to supervised placements, reflective and self-conscious investigation of particular problems, and fieldwork within the developing hospice movement.

Questions for discussion

1. How can clergy be better instructed in multidisciplinary teamwork?
2. How can a greater proportion of trainee clergy be given the opportunity to work with dying people?
3. How can spiritual insights be shared with other members of the caring team, whether Christian or not?
4. How can the spiritual concerns of patients be met by clergy, lay workers, and others?

References

1. Walter T. *Funerals.* London: Hodder and Stoughton, 1990.
2. Mauritzen J. Pastoral care for the dying and bereaved. *Death Studies,* 1988; **12**: 114–15.
3. Murray DB. The education and training of Scottish clergy in the care of the dying. *Palliative Medicine,* 1989; **4**: 17–23.
4. Rumbold B. *Helplessness and Hope.* London: SCM Press, 1986: 85.
5. Lyall D. Clinical pastoral education. In: Campbell AV, ed. *A Dictionary of Pastoral Care.* London: SPCK, 1990: 37.
6. Murray DB. The education and training of Scottish clergy in the care of the dying. *Palliative Medicine,* 1989; **4**: 19.
7. Davis G, Jensen A. An experiment in death education in the medical curriculum. *Omega,* 1980–81; **11**: 157.
8. Hart J, ed. *Care of the Dying.* London: Baptist Union health and healing advisory group, 1987: 25–6.
9. Murray DB. The education and training of Scottish clergy in the care of the dying. *Palliative Medicine,* 1989; **4**: 21.
10. Walter T. *Funerals.* London: Hodder and Stoughton, 1990.
11. Murray DB. Attitudes and perceptions affecting Scottish clergy in their care of the dying. *Palliative Medicine,* 1991; **5**: 233–6.
12. Doyle D. *Education in Terminal Care—Burden or Bonus.* Paper presented to the Association of Hospice Administrators, Manchester 17 April 1985, Edinburgh: St Columba's Hospice, 1985: 8.

Bibliography

Kubler-Ross E. *On Death and Dying.* London: Tavistock, 1973.
Rumbold E. *Helplessness and Hope.* London: SCM Press, 1986.
Ainsworth-Smith I, Speck P. *Letting Go.* London: SPCK, 1982.
Campbell AV. *The Gospel of Anger.* London: SPCK, 1986.
Anderson RS. *Theology, Death and Dying.* Oxford: Blackwell, 1986.
Walter T. *Funerals.* London: Hodder and Stoughton, 1990.
Aries P. *The Hour of our Death.* Harmondsworth: Penguin, 1981.
Riem R. *Stronger than Death.* London: DLT, 1993.
National Council for Hospice and Specialist Palliative Care Sources. *Education in Palliative Care.* Occasional Paper No. 9. London, 1996.

21.6 Training of volunteers

Ina Cummings

Palliative care has as its central focus the well-being of patients and close family members as individuals, each with their unique gifts and strengths, and unique problems and stresses. By its very nature, palliative care is labour intensive, taxing the limits of time and creativity of any health-care team. Incorporating volunteers in the palliative care team assists the team to meet the many and diverse needs of those they serve.

Three characteristics distinguish volunteer workers generally: commitment, enthusiasm, and caring. A survey of volunteer activity carried out by Statistics Canada indicated that nine out of ten volunteers come forward for the following four reasons; to help others, to help a cause that they believe in, to do something that they like to do, and to feel that they have accomplished something.[1] The goal of any training programme will be to help the volunteer achieve these goals as they apply to palliative care.

Roles of the volunteer

The possible volunteer roles are extremely varied. Many programmes begin with only volunteers who come together, organize themselves, do fund raising to develop some resources, and begin to have patient/family contact. With time, many of these programmes will become larger and more developed, with health professionals giving most of the care, and volunteers playing a role that supports, supplements, and enhances that of the health professionals. In a larger programme, volunteers may have a choice of one of the supporting roles, such as working in a fund raising shop, tending the hospice garden, or driving patients, or a role that is more immediately involved with the health professional team. Most roles fall into one of the following categories:

(1) direct service to patient and family; volunteering in one's professional role, serving as a volunteer in the home or inpatient facility;

(2) administrative support; clerical or office support, fund raising, board of directors, other administrative areas;

(3) public relations and community education; speaker's bureau, newsletter;

(4) special interest volunteers; spiritual care, bereavement, music, puppets, pets, art;

(5) volunteers as consultants.

Volunteers who have been recruited and selected for work in one of these areas will need to be prepared for the tasks that they will face. Training programmes that are overly ambitious, and raise expectations that are not met by the reality of the task will be as inappropriate as those that fail to give the volunteer enough information to feel confident in the required tasks.

Volunteer selection

The qualities of volunteers that do well with a palliative care programme are often paradoxical.[2] They must be self-directed, yet respond to appropriate directives. They need to think independently, and yet work well as a team member. They should be good at problem solving, knowing that many times solutions do not exist. They must be aware of their own beliefs and values, while at the same time being open to those of others. They must be aware of their own limitations and know when and where to ask for help. The selection process must identify those volunteers who are ready immediately, those who can develop the skills required, and those who are inappropriate for this time of endeavour.

Volunteer selection will begin with an interview to assess: motivation; special needs; special abilities; experience with serious illness, death, and dying; potential for working in a role which is predominantly supportive to paid staff; and personal expectations.[3,4] Volunteers who have overriding personal agendas, who are not team players, who lack the personal qualities of empathy, sensitivity, and maturity may be steered into a supporting role removed from direct patient/family contact. Those who are still grieving for a personal loss may be advised to wait a while before offering their services. The training programme will act as a further screening mechanism, during which candidates have a chance to see if their personal expectations are congruent with those of the programme.

Volunteer training programmes

All volunteers will need some level of orientation and training, the extent of which will be proportional to the roles and responsibilities that they will be undertaking. The possible exception would be professionals who are volunteering as consultants in a limited way. General principles for educational programmes for volunteers and non-professionals have been developed and serve as the foundation.[5] Each programme will develop its own educational goals and objectives to reflect the particular functions required. Most programmes will include a theoretical component and some supervised experiential training.

The training programme can be divided into four components:

(1) an introduction and orientation that is appropriate for all volunteers regardless of function and includes practicalities such as payment of expenses;

(2) a more extensive programme of preparation for all volunteers who will work directly with patients/families;

(3) additional specialized content for volunteers who will be focusing in a special interest area;

(4) continuing education programmes, which serve to correct deficiencies in knowledge and to further interest and commitment in volunteers who have been involved for some time.

Training course content

Introduction and orientation, confidentiality

Volunteers need an overview of what hospice/palliative care is, how it has evolved historically, and how the particular programme has developed both its service provision and its ethos since its inception. Volunteers will identify with the programme whatever their role may be, and this is the opportunity to start to build this loyalty and commitment. Volunteers who are working in supporting roles in the community may not need any further training although their own needs for support should be remembered.

Confidentiality needs to be stressed with all volunteers, particularly in small towns where many hospices are located. Even those volunteers indirectly involved with patients may be asked questions about individuals, and they need to know how to respond.

Volunteer training for direct service to patients and families

Most palliative care programmes will require potential volunteers to take the training course prior to beginning any work with patients and families. Basic knowledge is important, particularly in a community setting where volunteers will be functioning independently much of the time.[6] Programmes with an inpatient facility may allow new volunteers to begin working in a 'buddy system' under supervision from a senior volunteer and subsequently enter the training programme. This has the advantage of giving the volunteer an immediate context of experience and allows the training sessions to be more focused and of greater depth.

The training programme may draw on the resources of a number of people: the volunteer co-ordinator; other members of the interdisciplinary team; consultants; and local community resource persons. The experience of learning together in the presence of other members of the palliative care team fosters team cohesion. Involving local community resource people encourages community involvement and ownership. The facilitators of the programme serve as role models for palliative care workers, and thus should exhibit the qualities of caring, listening, openness, and competence. A variety of learning methods may be utilized: didactic lectures, discussion groups, use of audiovisual material, planned interactive exercises, use of reading materials, and site visits. An average of 15 to 30 h is devoted to this basic training programme, usually in periods of 2 to 3 h over a period of 6 to 12 weeks.

Many examples of course curricula are now available with varying emphasis and content.[7,8] The following topic areas are among those frequently covered:

1. Palliative care philosophy: this session focuses on the history of hospice care and the local programme and presents the essential principles—an emphasis on quality of life, a view of the patient as a whole person with physical, psychological, social, and spiritual needs, a focus on the family as the unit of care, and the introduction of the multiprofessional team as the best response to these varied needs.
2. Attitudes toward death and dying in society: volunteers have an opportunity to look at their own view of death and how this has been moulded by the attitudes of the society in which they live.
3. Coping with cancer: a basic presentation of the common types of cancer, the common treatment modalities, cure versus palliation, and current unorthodox or alternative therapies.
4. HIV disease and other terminal illness: depending on the admission criteria of the programme, a brief introduction to other disease states that the volunteers may encounter.
5. Pain and symptom management: an overview of how symptoms can be controlled, with particular emphasis on how the care and comfort measures of the volunteer augment the interventions of other team members.
6. Psychosocial dynamics: the many losses of progressive disease and common responses; ways in which the volunteer can support the patient/family.
7. Spiritual dynamics: spiritual dimensions of death and dying, respect for rituals and beliefs of different faiths and cultures.
8. Families facing a death: family dynamics, changing roles in the family with progressive illness of a family member, symptoms of family dysfunction, and ways in which the volunteer can be supportive.
9. The role of the volunteer: establishing a relationship, verbal and non-verbal communication, active listening skills, confidentiality, and comfort measures; accountability, reporting, and documentation in the programme.[9]
10. Introduction to specialized volunteer roles in the programme.
11. Understanding the bereavement process: influence of past losses, anticipatory grieving, grief process, tasks of bereavement, and introduction to local bereavement programme.
12. Personal stress: understanding common life stressors and those related to palliative care; how to prevent when possible and cope with stress; local programme volunteer support activities.

Evaluation of the training programme is essential if subsequent programmes are to benefit from present experience. Cognitive learning can be measured, but more important, and more difficult to assess, is attitudinal change. Parameters that may be evaluated include the following:

(1) participant satisfaction;

(2) degree to which learning objectives were met;

(3) assessment of presenter performance;

(4) perceived applicability of material to the work setting.

Specialized direct service volunteer roles

Over time many programmes will add on one or more new dimensions to possible volunteer direct service roles. It is assumed that such volunteers will have already had training and experience as palliative care volunteers, and be familiar with the impact of progressive illness and anticipatory loss. Examples of such roles are given below.

Pastoral volunteers

It is seldom possible for a chaplain to visit a patient as often as may be desirable. Volunteers with an interest in the spiritual dimension working under the supervision of a chaplain can extend this pastoral availability. Such volunteers are screened for personal, emotional, and spiritual maturity, and any theological or religious training they may have already received. They are given additional training in pastoral care of the sick, including discussions of the following:

(1) pastoral identity and the theology of pastoral care;

(2) pastoral care in the non-confessional setting;

(3) use of the person's spiritual resources;

(4) making a spiritual diagnosis;

(5) pastoral role at the time of death.

Music/art/recreation volunteers

Volunteers may choose to work with a therapist, taking selected taped music to a bedside, assisting a counselling psychologist with relaxation exercises, or introducing a hobby to a patient whose status is stable and whose days are long. Such volunteers will usually be individually trained and supervised by the therapist.

Bereavement volunteers

Bereavement care has been accepted as an integral part of palliative care, and most programmes will rely on volunteers to assist, if not totally constitute, a bereavement support service. It is essential that programmes totally staffed by volunteers have professional supervision if the standard of care is to be assured. The goal of the bereavement volunteer is to act as a friendly helper to the bereaved individual, remaining available until the grief is resolving and he/she can once again pick up normal activities and relationships. Emotional problems predating and unrelated to the bereavement are not the domain of the volunteer. Appropriate limits must be identified in each case. The volunteers are unlikely to have had extensive training as counsellors, and so it is essential that the programme ensures that the interventions offered by these volunteers are safe and hopefully helpful to those in grief. As one client put it, 'volunteers were the splint that enabled my family's fractures to heal.'[10]

Features of a training programme include the following:

(1) a knowledge of the process of normal grief, the tasks of grief work, and how to recognize abnormal grief;

(2) a knowledge of the professional resources available in the programme and community—when and how to refer for professional help;

(3) a knowledge of the role of volunteer helper versus the role of friend, and of appropriate interventions available to the untrained counsellor:[11]

   (a) support—acceptance, empathy, active listening, facilitating the expression of feelings;

   (b) review—facilitating the telling and retelling of stories of the past relationships;

   (c) problem-solving—how to be a sounding board, to clarify possible options, to evaluate options, and to minimize advice.

Training on the job

Volunteers armed with theoretical knowledge will still be uncertain when faced with situations that seem different to those described in the training course. A probationary period should be established, during which time the volunteer works as a 'buddy' to an experienced volunteer or with other team members who are quickly available. At the end of this time, most volunteers will have gained confidence and be ready to function in assigned roles as full team members. Other volunteers will have found that the work is not what they anticipated, and the interim evaluation will give an opportunity to recognize this and withdraw.

Reporting and documentation

If direct service volunteers are to work as integral team members, they must be aware of the goals of other staff, so that their efforts are complementary and not conflicting. Volunteers will not usually have direct access to the confidential information in the medical record and must obtain their information by some other route. Reporting to the volunteer can take a number of forms. The volunteer co-ordinator may sit in on the interdisciplinary team conferences and transmit the information to the volunteers. The primary nurse may prepare a brief written report to orient the volunteer and periodically meet with him/her to update information. In an inpatient setting, the nurse in charge may give a verbal report to the volunteers early each day, and an audio tape of this report be made available to volunteers coming on duty later.

There needs to be a mechanism for volunteers to report back to the professional team any information that may be important in understanding more fully the concerns or needs of the patient and family. In the community, or when beds are dispersed in an institution, this will require the volunteer to document each intervention (date, time involved, nature of the intervention, any key observations) and make the report available in some systematic way to the professional staff. If the volunteer is working closely with nurses in an inpatient unit, a verbal report to the nurse allows the observations to be documented as part of the notes. Each programme must develop policies outlining the expectations for systematic reporting and documentation on the part of the volunteer.

Supervision, support, and continuing education

Recognition and appreciation of the efforts of volunteers are important in developing a strong volunteer programme. Appreciation begins in preparing volunteers for the problems that they will encounter, listening and supporting them in their activities, and recognizing the commitment that they have made. Volunteers will not feel appreciated if they are given little to do, or if they are thrown into activities for which they are poorly equipped and where there is little supervision.

Volunteer supervision is the responsibility of the volunteer co-ordinator, with the understanding that volunteers working on special tasks may report to the team member whom they are assisting. The goals of supervision, support, and continuing education are often best carried out by a regular team meeting, which can use a case review format. As volunteers share their experience, there is ample opportunity to identify whether the volunteer is aware of programme policies, to review compliance, to support and encourage the volunteers involved, and to identify areas that need further education. Seriously considering the needs of the volunteer in this way validates the importance of his/her role in the total team effort.

References

1. *Survey of Volunteer Activity*, Department of the Secretary of State, Statistics Canada, 1987.
2. Dubik-Unruh S. Group activities: their role as screening and placement indicators in hospice volunteer training. *Journal of Palliative Care*, 1988; **4**: 33–7.
3. Caldwell J, Scott JP. Effective hospice volunteers: demographic and personality characteristics. *American Journal of Hospice and Palliative Care*, 1994; **11**:40–5.
4. Fusco-Karmann C, Tamburini M. Training volunteer trainers. *European Journal of Palliative Care*, 1994; **1**: 50–1.
5. International Work Group on Death, Dying and Bereavement. A statement of assumptions and principles concerning education about life-threatening illness, death, dying and bereavement for volunteers and non-professionals *American Journal of Hospice and Palliative Care*, 1991; **8**: 26–7.
6. Leete EB. Becoming a hospice volunteer. *American Journal of Hospice and Palliative Care*, 1994; **11**: 27–32.
7. Bates IJ, Brandt KE, eds. *Volunteer Training Curriculum recommended by National Hospice Organization.* Arlington: National Hospice Organization, 1990.
8. Brenner PR. The Volunteer Component. In: Armstrong-Dailey A, Goltzer SZ, eds. *Hospice Care for Children*. Oxford: Oxford University Press, 1993.
9. Stephany TM. Identifying the roles of hospice volunteers. *American Journal of Hospice Care*,1984; **1**: 6–7.
10. Craig M. Volunteer services. *American Journal of Hospice and Palliative Care*,1994; **11**:33–5.
11. Dush DM. Balance and boundaries in grief counseling: an intervention framework for volunteer training. *Hospice Journal*, 1988; **4**: 79–93.

22

Palliative medicine—a global perspective

22 Palliative medicine—a global perspective

Jan Stjernswärd and Sandro Pampallona

Introduction

We are all born to die. At present, 50 million people die yearly.[1,2] We ought to give those who are to leave life the same care and attention that we give to those who enter life—the newborns. By enabling the implementation of the vast amount of knowledge available in the field of palliative care both the quality of life and the quality of death of the terminally ill can be significantly improved.

Application of existing knowledge in a rational way is paramount if we are to reach the majority of those in need of palliative care and to achieve maximum coverage. Palliative medicine has the advantage of being a new and emerging speciality without too much vested interest. Therefore the mistakes sometimes made in other areas of medicine, such as achieving a lot for a few or not reaching or covering the great majority who should benefit, can be avoided. For such an approach it is important that we have a worldwide perspective and identify where the 'consumers' are.

Palliative medicine must, from the outset, encompass a global perspective with the aim of reaching the greatest number of people who can benefit from it, namely those in the developing countries. There cannot be one ideal future for the developed nations and another future for the developing nations. It is either one joint future or none. Within any country most must be covered, whether they are the 'haves' or the 'have nots'.

In this chapter we address the following issues:

- the size of the problem now and in the future;
- evaluation and costs;
- priorities and strategies to achieve optimal coverage of patients in need of palliative care;
- cross-cultural aspects;
- recommendations for the implementation of existing knowledge, which are realistic with respect to the available resources, using the relief of cancer pain as a model.

Data describing the pattern of mortality in the world will be presented, pointing out how the incidence of diseases like cancer will increase in the next few decades in the developing countries as a consequence of the extension of life expectancy. Until primary prevention and availability of standard therapies become the norm in all parts of the world, palliative care will represent the only pragmatic and humane answer to the millions affected annually by such diseases. A comprehensive approach to the achievement of freedom from cancer pain, based on implementing existing knowledge in a rational public health manner, by establishing clear policies, drug availability, and education of caregivers will be presented.

Cancer pain relief is used as the model for what can be done, although total palliative care is the goal. The knowledge achieved in cancer palliative care should be applied to as many as possible of the terminally ill, including the elderly, individuals with chronic diseases, and AIDS patients.

The strategies outlined are relevant for both developed and developing countries; in this chapter we shall stress the developing countries, which are often forgotten and which contain the majority of people in need of palliative care worldwide.

Experience shows that implementation of the knowledge already accumulated in palliative care, including symptom control and pain relief, improves the quality of life for the terminally ill and their families. However, even in many resource-rich countries application of available knowledge is inadequate. There is often a lack of clear policies and adequate training of health professionals, and a lack of access to, or unavailability of, palliative care services. Furthermore, both health professionals and the public have unrealistic expectations regarding the limits of modern high-technology medicine and its applications to improving and prolonging life in patients with chronic diseases. When this is combined with a frequent inability in modern Western cultures to accept the unavoidable, namely death, a maldistribution of dwindling health care resources results.

Quality of life and comfort before death could be considerably improved by palliative care, but all too often it is ignored or seen as a last resort— a type of 'waste-paper basket' alternative. Rather, palliative care needs to be projected as an integral part of management which should be applied earlier in the course of illnesses.[3]

A multidisciplinary approach is needed for the implementation of effective palliative care. Political vision and leadership are also necessary, as the problems are not only medical but also socio-economic, social, and ethical. Input is required from sectors of society other than the medical sector, and the role of family members needs to be re-evaluated and their resources utilized, if an acceptable coverage worldwide is ever to be achieved.[4]

'Doing better and feeling worse' is a chapter heading in a textbook which bears the same title.[5] The point it made was that 'according to the Great Equation, Medical Care Equals Health'. But the Great Equation is wrong. More available medical care does not equal better health. The best estimates are that medicine can

Table 1 Causes of death: estimates for 1990

Cause of death	Number of deaths (thousands)			Percentage of deaths from each cause
	Developing countries	Developed countries	Total	
Cardiovascular	9017	5328	14 345	28.7
Infectious and parasitic	13 285	483	13 768	27.5
Neoplasms	3698	2431	6129	12.3
Injuries	3420	807	4227	8.4
Maternal and perinatal	2830	92	2922	6.0
Respiratory	2336	509	2845	5.7
Other causes	4502	1233	5735	11.4
All causes	39 088	10 883	49 971	100.0

From ref. 8.

increase the values of the usual indices by which health is measured (whether you live at all (infant mortality), how well you live (days lost due to sickness), and how long you live (adult mortality)) by only 10 per cent. Thus health is only marginally affected by medical care.[4] This has been brilliantly analysed and demonstrated[6] by the observation that the remarkable decline in infectious diseases, such as tuberculosis, was due largely to socio-economic progress and not to specific medical interventions, a point reinforced by a new way of measuring progress in living standards.[7] Income statistics give a highly inaccurate picture of living standards in subsistence communities. The quality of life can be estimated more accurately by measurement of infant mortality, days lost because of sickness, and adult mortality. The situation will probably be the same for palliative medicine. The behaviour of the individual and the attitudes and habits of society will probably have a greater impact than purely technical medical advances and efforts on the implementation of palliative care.

It is important that providers of palliative care realize this. It means that a broader approach is needed from the outset and that institutionalization should be avoided, scientifically valid methods that are acceptable and maintainable at family and community level should be established, research into practical health services will be required, priorities must be established for the use of available resources, and governments should formulate clear palliative care policies. Emphasis on health systems and not just biomedical development will be a priority in palliative care research.

Ultimately, palliative care should be able to provide good standards of bodily comfort and emotional, psychological, and spiritual support to terminally ill patients and those close to them.

Size of the problem

Causes of death

The total number of deaths estimated to have occurred in 1990 was approximately 50 million,[8] of which 39 million occurred in developing countries and 11 million in developed countries (Table 1). World-wide, cardiovascular disease accounted for 28.7 per cent of deaths, infectious and parasitic diseases for 27.5 per cent, and cancer for 12.3 per cent.[8] Infections and parasitic diseases are by far the most frequent causes of death in the developing world, accounting for almost 34 per cent of deaths compared with 23 per cent for cardiovascular disease and 9.5 per cent for cancer. The same figures for the developed countries are 4.5 per cent, 49 per cent, and 22 per cent. However, this relative distribution is expected to change dramatically as the population structure shifts toward older ages in developing countries. Projected figures for 2015 estimate the total number of deaths at over 62 million;[9] today's percentages of selected causes of death[10] are compared with the projections for 2015 in Table 2. Today, worldwide, for every death due to cancer there are just over two deaths due to infectious and parasitic diseases; by 2015 this ratio will be reduced to almost one-to-one. In 2015, with 15 million new cancer cases yearly, cancer will account for almost nine million deaths, six million of which will occur in the developing world.

Mortality patterns are closely related to lifestyles. Table 3

Table 2 Percentage of selected causes of deaths in 1990 and 2015

	Developing countries		Developed countries		Total	
	1990	2015	1990	2015	1990	2015
Cardiovascular	23.1	35.4	48.9	52.9	28.7	39.4
Infectious and parasitic	33.9	19.4	4.4	6.9	27.5	16.5
Neoplasms	9.5	13.6	22.3	28.1	12.3	14.6

Data from refs. 9 and 10.

Table 3 Changes in the percentage of total mortality due to chronic diseases in five subregions of the Americas between 1970 and 1980

Subregion	Percentage mortality attributed to chronic diseases (1980)	Relative percentage increase (1970–1980)
North America (USA and Canada)	75	0.4
Temperate South America (Southern Cone countries)	60	11
Caribbean area	57	21
Tropical South America	45	105
Continental Middle America (Central America, Mexico, and Panama)	28	56

Adapted from refs. 9 and 11.

illustrates the spread of such changes. The changes in the percentage of total mortality due to chronic diseases between 1970 and 1980 show a 100 per cent relative increase for tropical South American countries.[11] A similar rapid change was seen in Shanghai county, where within a mere 20 years (from 1960 to 1980) cancer shifted from being the sixth most common to the leading cause of death.[12]

Future scene

The need for palliative care will certainly increase. At present, there are proportionally limited resources for palliative care and the future will demand more because of the rapid ageing of the world population, the increase of deaths related to tobacco use, and the increase of AIDS.

Ageing

In 1990 the world population reached 5.3 billion, and it is expected to increase to 6.2 billion by the year 2000 and to 8.9 billion by 2030. The size of the population aged 60 years and over is also increasing: it represented 8.4 per cent of the world population in 1980 and 9.3 per cent in 1990; this proportion is expected to be 10.6 per cent by the year 2000 and to increase to 15.2 per cent by 2030. Developing countries will show the fastest increase in the proportion of elderly: the current 6.9 per cent of the population aged 60 years or more will jump to 13 per cent by 2030, thus almost doubling in 40 years.[13] In absolute terms, these proportions represent 286 million today compared with just over a billion in 2030. In the same time period, the proportion of elderly in developed countries will increase from 18 to 28 per cent, corresponding to 203 million and 358 million respectively.[14] A graphical representation of demographic trends for the population aged 60 or over is given in Fig. 1. By 2030, 73 per cent of people aged 60 or older will be living in developing countries. At present, 1.2 million people celebrate their 55th birthday every month, and 80 per cent of them live in the developing countries.[15] With regard to the oldest old, i.e. that section of the population aged 80 or over, there are 53 million today; in 2025 they will represent 1.6 per cent of the population, i.e. about 135 million, of whom 80 million will be living in the developing countries.[16]

All this will result in an increased need for social and economic support, including palliative care of the elderly, and this will have to be provided by a proportionally decreased working-age population of caregivers. The ratio of tax payers/caregivers to care receivers, which is now 4:1, will soon change to 2:1 in many developed countries.

In developed countries, for example the United Kingdom, the curse of a long life may soon be that the average cost of residential care from admission to death might be about £60 000, coincidentally the value of the average house.[17] Thus children could be robbed of their legacy when a lifetime's wealth assets are required to pay for long-term care. The amount spent on residential and nursing home care could more than double in real terms over the next four decades. With present social trends, changes in family structure, such as geographical dispersion of the three-generation family, increased female participation in the workforce, and high divorce rates, it is unlikely that the amount of care now provided by the family free of charge can continue. In contrast, in the developing countries empowerment of family members as effective caregivers in palliative care is the most realistic approach to achieving a meaningful coverage. However, in view of the intensive urbanization and social changes taking place in these countries, it is

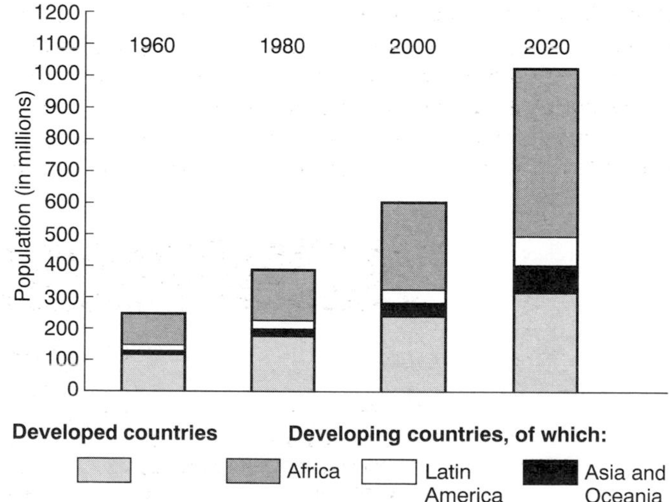

Fig. 1 Population aged 60 years and over, by major world regions, 1960–2020. (Reproduced with permission from ref. 14.)

not certain whether it will be possible to rely on the three-generation family for care of the elderly in the future.

Cancers

What will be the common diseases of the twenty-first century? As a group, the non-communicable diseases will increase, and infections and tropical and parasitic diseases will decrease. Among individual diseases, lung cancer and AIDS are already major causes of death and it is likely that these two diseases will be two of the most common killers in the early part of the twenty-first century.[1]

It is interesting to consider the similarities between lung cancer and AIDS. While neither disease was known at the beginning of this century, both are rapidly increasing worldwide as the century draws to a close. They are among the few diseases to show substantial increases in industrialized countries over the past decade, and they are emerging as major health problems in many developing countries, particularly Africa. Both are virtually preventable because the primary causes—lifestyle factors—are known. However, the health sector is finding it extremely difficult, in practical terms, to bring about the changes in human behaviour necessary for their prevention. On the contrary, high mortality rates appear to be spreading from industrialized countries to the rest of the world, particularly with regard to tobacco-related diseases. Both lung cancer and AIDS are essentially incurable—the overall survival curves are quite similar.[18] While considerable resources are spent on treating advanced cases, the curative effort is usually fruitless and the main role of the health care services will be to provide palliative care.

Lung cancer can be singled out as an example of the increase in cancers mentioned earlier. It is already the most frequent cancer worldwide,[19] and by the year 2000 there are likely to be about a million cases each year. This is a result of increasing tobacco use. Of these lung cancers, 90 per cent will be incurable and most patients will need palliative care. Currently, tobacco use is estimated to account for three million deaths per year, with slightly more than half of these occurring in the developed world where the cumulative exposure (primarily smoking) has been higher than in the developing world. At the global level, the annual number of tobacco-related deaths is expected to rise dramatically, from three million to about 10 million, by the year 2025.[20,21]

Of the estimated 10 million tobacco-related deaths occurring in the year 2025, about three million are expected to occur in China alone. Almost a million of these will be exclusively from lung cancer. Moreover, with current trends, about 200 million children and teenagers living in China today will become regular smokers. Of these, about 50 million or one-quarter will die prematurely of smoking-related illnesses.[20]

AIDS

The cumulative global number of AIDS cases reported to the World Health Organization (WHO) as of 1 July 1995 was 1 169 811. However, it has been estimated that, when underdiagnosis, under-reporting, and delays in reporting are taken into account, there may have been more than 4.5 million cases of AIDS in adults to date.[22] Up to 1990, an estimated nine million persons in the world had been infected with HIV.[23] About 50 per cent of HIV-infected adults will develop AIDS within 10 years of infection, and 78 to 100 per cent of HIV-infected persons will develop AIDS within 15 years. The projected cumulative total of adult AIDS cases by the year 2000 is close to 10 million, of which almost 90 per cent will be in the developing countries.[17] An estimated 26 million adults will be infected with HIV by the year 2000.[23] The WHO also predicts that at least 10 million children will be born with HIV during the 1990s, the majority of them in sub-Saharan Africa and South and Southeast Asia where HIV infection continues. In addition, 10 to 15 million children, mainly in Africa, will be orphaned by the year 2000 because their parents will have died of AIDS.[24]

It is estimated that a high proportion of HIV patients will develop tumours. The earlier estimated increase in cancer (Table 2) does not include these tumours. Apart from the true therapeutic issues that offer their own novel challenges in immunodepressed patients, there are important quality-of-life issues to be addressed regarding the balance between curative and symptomatic/palliative approaches in these patients.

It has become standard practice in the AIDS literature to use cumulative date, starting from the epidemic in the late 1970s. However, this may be misleading. For comparison, if we used the same advocacy strategy for cancer for the next 5 years at the current incidence of nine million cases per year, this would lead to a cumulative number of 45 million cases by the year 2000, of which the cumulative total of deaths would be 30 million.

Priorities, strategies, approaches

Priorities

Globally, palliative care is a neglected area. The need today is enormous and will increase dramatically in the near future. The size of the problem must be made clear to both individuals and society, particularly policy-makers and the medical profession. They must recognize that something really can be done.

A public assessment of the priorities required of health services was recently completed in Oregon. Out of more than 700 services, palliative therapy for patients in whom death is imminent was ranked as a priority and identified as an essential service.[25] However, the professionals often consider other services, often their own, as a priority. This can be shown by taking cancer control as an example. Although at least one-third of cancers can be prevented and major symptom control could be offered to six million cancer patients who die each year, this knowledge is not applied to a sufficient extent. Cancer incidence and mortality continues to increase,[26] and no efficient palliative care is offered to the eight or nine out of ten cancer patients in developing countries who are already incurable at the time of diagnosis. These patients represent 55 to 60 per cent of the world's cancer patients.[27]

Table 4 summarizes the state of the art in cancer control—priorities and strategies for the eight most common cancers. It shows the importance of prevention and palliative care. Unfortunately most resources go to therapy, with proportionally few going to primary prevention and palliative care. Of the eight most common cancers worldwide, five are more prevalent in developing countries. Even if diagnosis is made at an early stage of the disease, treatment is curative in only three of these cancers but palliative care is needed in all eight.[28]

Much progress has been made in cancer therapy over the past

Table 4 Cancer control—priorities and strategies for the eight most common cancers

Tumour[a]	Primary prevention	Early diagnosis	Curative therapy[b]	Pain relief and palliative care
Lung	++	—	—	++
Stomach	+	—	—	++
Breast	—	++	++	++
Colon/rectum	+	+	+	++
Cervix	+	++	++	++
Mouth/pharynx	++	++	++	++
Oesophagus	+	—	—	++
Liver	++	—	—	++

++ effective; +, partly effective; —, not effective.
[a] Listed in the order of the eight most common tumours globally.
[b] Curative for the majority of cases with a realistic opportunity of finding them early.

20 years. The high cure rate of childhood cancers demonstrates this. However, developed countries also need to place greater emphasis on palliative care: 'When you have a hammer (therapy), everything (the patient and the tumour) looks like a nail'. Some important recent data illustrate this. When 40 therapists (20 head and neck surgeons and 20 radiotherapists) were asked how to take care of three patients with incurable disease of the head and neck, 75 per cent estimated that the patients had less than a 20 per cent chance of a cure. However, they were reluctant to withhold therapy, even when 95 per cent of them expected the incurable patients to be dead within a year. The 40 specialists came up with 119 treatment plans, of which less than 10 per cent were palliative only (Table 5).[29,30] Between countries, there are great variations among specialists as to when to treat. Thus American radiotherapists are four times more likely than their British colleagues to give radiotherapy to lung cancer patients.[31]

With almost 60 per cent of the world's new cancer patients presenting in developing countries, at least 80 per cent of whom are incurable at the time of diagnosis, with only 5 per cent of the world's total resources for cancer control in these countries, and with the knowledge that relatively inexpensive, effective, and scientifically valid methods exist for palliative care,[3,32] it is tragic to see how almost all efforts and resources in the developing countries are concentrated on therapeutic approaches, with very limited effect. Frequently, there is an almost complete lack of effort and resources for palliative care in these countries. For years to come, until early referral is common and enough therapists have been trained, palliative care will be the only pragmatic and humane solution.

Table 5 Three advanced ENT patients—overtreatment?

- 40 therapists (20 ENT surgeons + 20 radiotherapists)
- 75% estimated < 20% chance of cure
- Reluctant to withhold therapy even when 95% expected incurable patients to be dead within 1 year
- 119 plans of intervention of which < 10% palliation only

From ref. 30.

About 70 to 80 per cent of total health-care spending, both public and private, in developing countries goes to curative efforts. Within the curative sector, hospitals often account for more than 80 per cent of the total health care costs. Most of these hospitals are located in urban areas, whereas most of the population still lives in rural areas.[33] However, mega-cities and global urbanization are rapidly increasing.

Considerable resources are spent on treating the advanced cases. The curative effort is frequently unsuccessful, and the main role of the health care services should have been to provide palliative care. Technically and in principle, the same guidelines that have been used for cancer patients could be employed for much of the palliative care of the elderly terminally ill and AIDS patients.

The provision of palliative care requires attention at the top decision-making and political levels. There is a need for a comprehensive approach to the development of a coherent prevention, treatment, and care policy for application to the problems of AIDS, cancer, and the elderly terminally ill which can be implemented worldwide.

The WHO has made palliative care a priority in its Global Cancer Control Programme and has made support available to countries that want to implement existing knowledge in cancer control by setting up national cancer control programmes.[34] In addition, in a number of countries the WHO has made several non-governmental organizations, the policy-makers, and the public aware of palliative care.

Search for priorities—coverage

A principle of the public health approaches that we have used has been that, in order to achieve coverage, a search must be made for scientifically valid methods that are acceptable and maintainable at the community level. This is exemplified by the consensus, established in 1982 by WHO and a group of international experts, that drugs are the mainstay of cancer pain relief and that a relatively inexpensive and easily applicable approach exists.[32] This approach, which is known as the three-step pain ladder, has become accepted worldwide and, following a period of field-testing, is being implemented in several countries.

Table 6 summarizes reports in the literature that have explicitly referred to the use of the WHO three-step ladder for pain relief in

Table 6 Studies which have explicitly used the WHO guidelines for cancer pain control

Reference Year	Country	Cancer site	Type of study	No. of patients	Outcome
35	Switzerland	Mixed	Retrospective	63	97% of patients had appropriate pain control
36	Japan	Mixed	Prospective	156	87% of patients with total pain control
37	Italy	Mixed	Retrospective	1229	Over 70% of cases were appropriately treated without any other approach than the 3-step ladder
38	Italy	Mixed	Prospective	45	93% of patients obtained total control or had mild pain
39	India	Mixed	Prospective	88	86% of patients had satisfactory pain control
40	United Kingdom	Mixed	Prospective	20	Good relief was achieved in 100% of the patients
41	Germany	Mixed	Prospective	174	More than 80% of patients rated pain between none or moderate
42	Germany	Mixed	Retrospective	1070	70% of patients had no pain or mild pain
43	Germany	Mixed, dying patients	Prospective	401	No to moderate pain in 76% of patients at time of death
44	Italy	Mixed, last 2 months	Prospective	98	Over 70% achieved good pain relief
45	Germany	Breast	Prospective	106	In 92% of 6767 treatment days pain was at most moderate
46	Netherlands	Head and neck	Prospective	25	Adequate pain relief was achieved in 72% of patients
47	Germany	Head and neck	Prospective	167	Highly effective; severe pain experienced only in 5% of 8106 treatment days

advanced cancer patients.[35-47] A total of 13 reports have been identified in which strict adherence to WHO guidelines had been observed. A total of 3642 patients with different primary pathologies were treated in various European countries as well as in India and Japan. The results invariably suggest that pain control was adequate in about 80 per cent of patients, and often even more. A very low frequency of side-effects was reported, and the management of almost all patients was successful with standard approaches. Relief of cancer pain has served as the spearhead in the search for a comprehensive palliative care programme. Such a programme must be structured in a way that it can be adopted worldwide and will provide coverage for the majority of the 50 million terminally ill patients that require treatment every year.[3]

In view of the demographic data—the need to know where the individuals in need of palliative care are, and who and where they will be in the future—and taking into account the available resources, it is clear that the principles of the above approach, aimed at achieving coverage, must be followed rather than the conventional institutionalized approach alone.

It will be necessary to involve family members to achieve coverage. Fortunately, the developing countries still have an actively functioning three-generation family, which is often absent in the developed countries where families have to compensate with more institutionalized care[48] or new socio-economic health policies that allow them economic compensation so that they can care for their dying relatives.[49] In most developed countries it is widely recognized that families have a serious duty to provide care, but families often have to set limits on the care that they can give.[49] A major aspect of policy will be to identify a proper balance between family and government assistance, so that the family can continue to respond to the needs of elderly family members, knowing that outside care is available when, and if, required. The provision of community and home-based care for the elderly will be essential for effective palliative care and to achieve coverage. Home care should avoid becoming a version of acute care delivery at home, as this will only be a domestic version of institutionalized care.[50] It should encompass personal care, personal services, social companionship, and applied medical care.

In developing countries, the involvement of family members in achieving effective coverage is essential. For example, in sub-Saharan Africa (with the exception of South Africa) there are fewer than 75 cancer specialists of any description (radiotherapists, chemotherapists, cytologists, cancer nurses, etc.) for a population of more than 300 million. Policies and training in palliative care are non-existent in most African countries. With a few exceptions (e.g. Zimbabwe and South Africa), no essential drugs, such as oral morphine, are available. This is despite the fact that Africa has a cancer incidence of over 100 per 100 000 and that 80 to 90 per cent of cancer patients are incurable. Pain, the most common symptom in palliative care, cannot be controlled adequately without access to opioids. There are still 51 countries in which there is no registered morphine consumption.[3] Twenty-seven of these countries are in Africa, nine in the Americas, four in south-east Asia, eight in the eastern Mediterranean region, and three in the western Pacific. In many countries, such as Pakistan, even weak opioids such as codeine are unavailable.

India, with one-sixth of the world's population, has 10 comprehensive cancer centres. They account for the major part of the cancer care and control resources available, and most of these resources are allotted to therapy. However, these centres deal with fewer than 10 per cent of an estimated 700 000 new cancer patients every year. Recently, several Indian states, in collaboration with the WHO, have set rational priorities and strategies through the establishment of national cancer control programmes, in which cancer pain relief and palliative care are always included.[3,34,51,52] Figure 2 shows the situation that existed before this plan was adopted and the need for implementing policies that achieve coverage. Only 16 000 patients are covered annually by all hospitals having expertise in cancer pain in India,[33] although an estimated 350 000 patients suffer daily from moderate to severe cancer pain. Total pain relief is attempted for the 16 000 patients treated in hospital, often using sophisticated approaches from developed countries. Application of the WHO cancer pain relief method should enable coverage to be achieved relatively simply in 80 per cent of all the 350 000 sufferers.[53]

The great majority of Indian cancer patients are encountered at the district level. India has nearly 500 districts, each with a population of one to four million. To increase the impact of cancer control strategies at this level, 20 districts have been selected for joint Indian Ministry of Health–WHO demonstration projects. If these strategies are found to be effective, the programme can be extended on a national scale. A successful extension throughout India, with one-sixth of the world's population, over a 10-year period would have a worldwide impact in palliative care.

The strategies, which are common to those of most national cancer control programmes, include anti-tobacco measures, health education, promotion of early detection and referral to curative treatment, and establishment of cobalt-60 units. Radiotherapy also has an important role in palliation. The district demonstration projects will strongly emphasize palliative care.

Search for priorities—cost considerations

Significant developments in health care provision during the latter part of the twentieth century include the following:

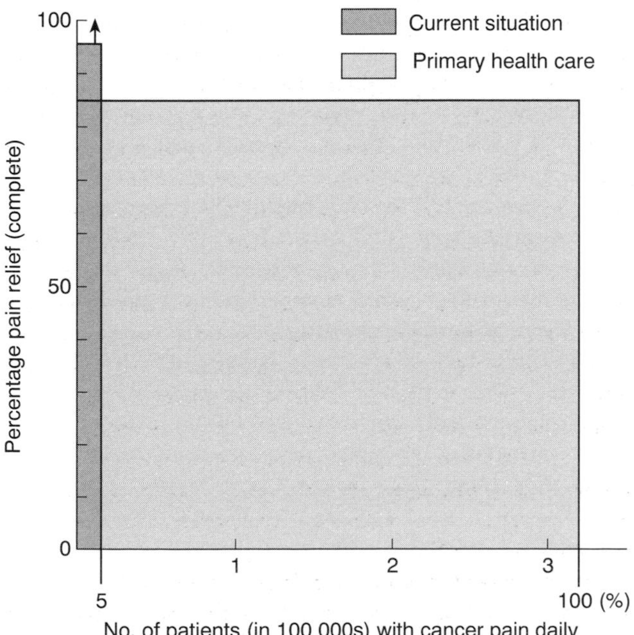

Fig. 2 Patient coverage by strategy. (Reproduced with permission from ref. 28.)

Table 7 Comparative world views

European	**African**
Values and customs	
Competition	Co-operation
Individual rights	Collective responsibility
Separateness	Co-operativeness
Independence	Interdependence
Psychobehavioural modalities	
Individuality	Groupness
Uniqueness	Sameness
Differences	Community
Ethos	
Survival of the fittest	Survival of the tribe
Control over nature	One with nature

From ref. 82.

- the enormous increase in the number and proportion of the elderly (there will be over a billion elderly people by 2020, of whom 70 to 80 per cent will live in developing countries);
- the number of patients needing palliative care, including those with lung cancer and AIDS;
- the decreasing proportion of caregivers to care receivers, and of tax providers to utilizers.

Society and/or governments must improve the overall quality of life of the population while acting within the limits of available financial and human resources.[54] It seems unrealistic for the developing world to adopt the system of delivering terminal/palliative care existing in the developed countries, particularly the United States, rather than adapting existing knowledge in palliative medicine, establishing their own methods at a lower cost to society.

The exorbitant health expenditures in some Western countries are partially driven by an unrealistic belief in what can be achieved by the application of life-prolonging efforts and modern high technology to chronic non-communicable diseases. Figure 3 shows the cumulative expenditures for medical services during the last year of life of terminal cancer patients.

Costs

Despite the diversity of approaches used to quantify the costs of caring for the terminally ill, there is a convergence of results indicating a dramatic increase in health expenditure during the last period of life. North American studies suggest that 18 per cent of lifetime costs for medical care are likely to be incurred in the last year of life;[56] similarly, almost 30 per cent of Medicare and Medicaid payments for individuals aged 65 or older are made during their last year of life.[57] It has been suggested that costs for terminal cancer patients escalate exponentially during the last year of life,[58] Figure 3, with 80 per cent of the expenditure occurring during the final 6 months. Expensive and unnecessary cancer therapies, not palliative care, are the cause of most of these high

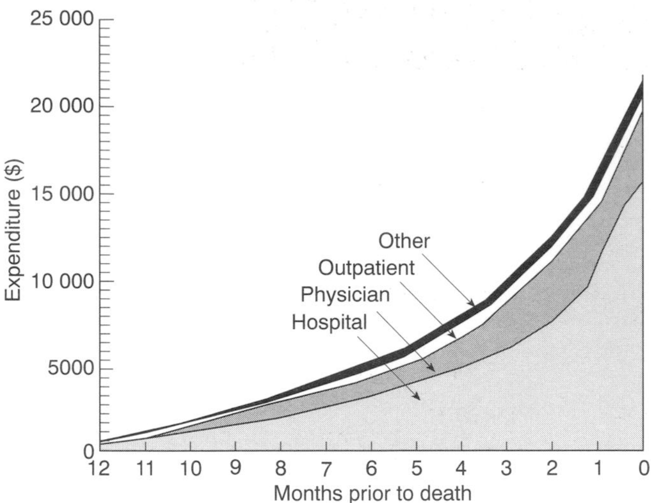

Fig. 3 Cumulative expenditures for medical services during the last year of life. (Reproduced with permission from ref. 55.)

costs. The projected increase in the number of elderly people in the coming decades will inflate the share of health-care costs allocated to this section of the population.[59] One approach to containing the problem is to achieve a reduction of morbidity (compression of morbidity) among the elderly through appropriate prevention programmes[60–62] and thus reduce the demands of the elderly on the medical structure.[63] However, there is controversy as to whether the knowledge that is available today concerning risk factors for mortality also extends to morbidity, and therefore whether the preventive measures suggested would be effective in reducing chronic disability as well as shortening the time interval between its appearance and eventual death.[64] However, it will be several decades before it is established whether or not compression of morbidity can be attained, during which time the problem of costs associated with ageing will have to be addressed. There is evidence that when patients are given the choice and are presented with adequate information, older people request less of the expensive medical technology used to palliate their terminal illnesses.[65,66] However, there is also evidence that advance directives, less aggressive care, and hospice care do not have a substantial impact on eventual costs.[67,68] It has been suggested that the classical methods of evaluating relative costs and benefits of alternative strategies of care are not appropriate in this setting, since they inevitably penalize the elderly, necessarily in their least productive years, without duly considering their pain and suffering or giving them a dignified role in society.[69]

The results available need to be considered in a global perspective, as they only are representative of developed countries. Their extension of findings about costs, their determinants, and ways to contain them may not apply to the developing world; local societal structures and values as well as the comprehensiveness and co-ordination of future geriatric services in these countries will need to be taken into consideration.

The attitude of the state and the family towards the elderly needs to be considered with respect to cultural differences.[70] Ultimately cultural values will have to soften the dry and rational economic considerations which alone cannot provide satisfactory guidance in the choice of what to offer to those who leave life in pain and suffering.

It is up to practitioners of palliative medicine to prove that value for money and improved quality of life can be achieved in the treatment of the terminally ill, despite the sometimes frightening economic figures for medical costs at end of life in the West. It is doubtful that the high costs discussed above were spent on effective palliative care. It is more likely that they were for high-technology approaches with marginal effects. For example, at a leading centre in the United States, a terminally ill patient with pancreatic cancer developed gastric intestinal bleeding, which is a relatively good way to die. Rather than being allowed to die, he was rushed to laser surgery and ended up in an intensive care unit. Whether such approaches are 'life-saving' or a 'prolongation of the act of dying' is open to debate; however, it is clear that this approach is very expensive. Another example, again from the United States, is that patients with solid lung cancer were mandatorily placed in a respirator at the end of their disease, provided that they had not made a 'living will' withholding permission for this.

Assessment and accountability will be critical in medical care, and have even been called the 'third revolution' in care,[71] the first being the scientific achievements in diagnosis and therapy, and the second being society's financing of medical care in many countries. At the present time the elderly, the main consumers of palliative care, use about 40 per cent of the care resources and a 25 per cent increase over the next 10 years has been estimated.[72] Priorities in care, paid for by increasingly limited resources, must be established.[73]

Methodological aspects

Care for the terminally ill consists not only of drug prescriptions but also of a composite set of interventions, including pharmacological and medical, psychological, and spiritual support, hospital care, home care, etc. Quantification of the efficacy of these varied interventions is difficult and requires several measures including quality of life, control of symptoms, containment of costs, place of death, and family distress. Thus the comparative study of alternative palliative care strategies must be classified under health services evaluation. Application of appropriate methodology in this area has been rare.[74] Two endpoints will be considered here: evaluation of efficacy and costs of alternative palliative care strategies.

Even in recent years, very few attempts have been made to use adequate research methods to assess efficacy.[75,76,77] Studies in this area face ethical problems, relating to possible denial of support to a group of dying patients when randomization is applied, as well as methodological difficulties. The latter include the setting and study inclusion criteria, both of which may hamper the extrapolation of the observed results to the more general population of terminally ill patients, patient refusal, which may also result in reduced external validity of the studies, incomplete data because of the difficulty in eliciting information from patients in a rapidly deteriorating condition or their death, and the need for additional specialized care that is not allowed for by the study protocol, resulting in potentially biased results. A higher standard of research and alternative methodologies have been advocated, although these are difficult to achieve.[78] When cost containment is the endpoint, despite warnings that such issues are complex in this setting,[79] the

Table 8 Comparison of traditional (south and southeast Asia) and modern (Western) cultures

	Traditional	Modern
Religion, philosophy, folk beliefs	Hinduism, Buddhism, Islam, Filipino Catholicism, animism, spirit possession, casting spells, astrology, ancestor worship, acceptance/fatalism	Judeao-Christian beliefs, determinism, scientism, pragmatism, materialism, innovation, 'maker of one's fate'
Social relations	Groupism, collectivism, familism, conformity, interdependeence, hierarchical, status, rigidity, holistic (whole person)	Individualism, autonomy, competition, independence, status, flexibility, fragmented roles
Environmental relations	Harmony with nature, dependence on nature, close to nature	Dominance over nature, exploitation, technical, distant from nature
Orientation to time	Cyclical, relaxed about clocks and appointments	Linear, clock awareness, fast paced, concern for future, 'time is money'
Cognitive approach	Synthetic, multilectic, harmony seking (both . . . and)	Analytical, dialectic, critical (either . . . or)
Communication	Passive, indirect, control of emotions	Active, direct, expression of emotions
Coals	Harmony with family and environment, enlightenment (Hinduism, Buddhism), gaining merit by giving submission to authorities	Self-reliance, salvation/ adjustment, material 'success', equality, doubting authority
Self	Defined by relation to others, particularly in family relations	Defined by self, identified in accomplishments
Causes of mental illness	Physical and mental closely related, caused by karma, spells and charms, spirits, cosmic imbalance, etc.	Compartmentalization, genetics, socialization, unconscious motives, etc.
Expectations	Rapid cure, physical/medical treatment, authoritative prescription	Talking cure, joint participation
Disorders of thought and emotion	Organic connection, so organic treatment	Mental causes, so talking helps
Responsibilities of change	Family centred	Person centred
Self-disclosure	Low to non-family	Higher to helper
Relation with helper	Distant	Intimate
Acceptance of problems	Suffering expected, exercise will-power	Pain can be helped
Mode of treatment	Physical or meditation	Verbal, 'talking cure'

From ref. 83.

approaches adopted have been so disparate, although novel, that the data obtained are often conflicting.[57,59,67]

An additional difficulty encountered in this area of research is the importance of local culture and structure, unlike most other medical issues where the functioning of the body can be taken as a cross-cultural constant. Cultural and socio-economic differences in family support to the elderly[70] and attitudes to ageing and death[80,81] do not allow indiscriminate generalization of approaches.

Cross-cultural aspects

Cultural traditions and differences should be respected and will affect the implementation of effective palliative care programmes. Tables 7 and 8 give a simplified indication of the problems that may be worth considering in the search for scientifically valid and cross-culturally robust programmes.[82,83]

Differences in values, religious beliefs, customs, psychobehavioural patterns, and ethos, as well as the ethics of care of the

Table 9 Examples of process measures for cancer pain relief*

- Over 80% of oncologists and cancer professionals must receive training in the WHO method for relief of cancer pain
- More than 50% of general practitioners must be aware of the WHO analgesic ladder
- More than 50% of cancer patients and their families must know that cancer pain can be relieved

* Similar measures should be applied to palliative care.

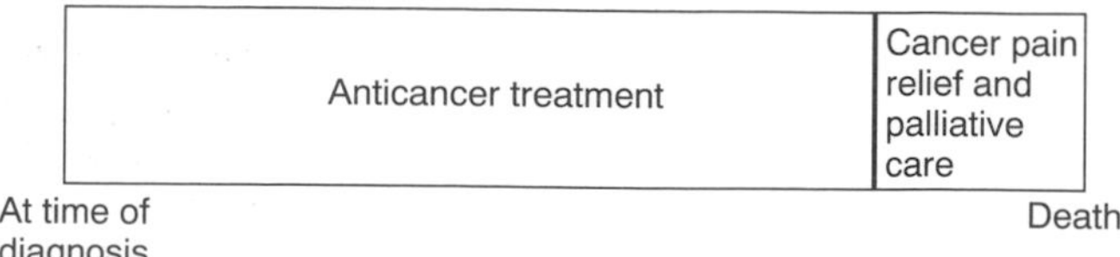

Fig. 4 Present allocation of cancer resources. (Reproduced with permission from ref. 3.)

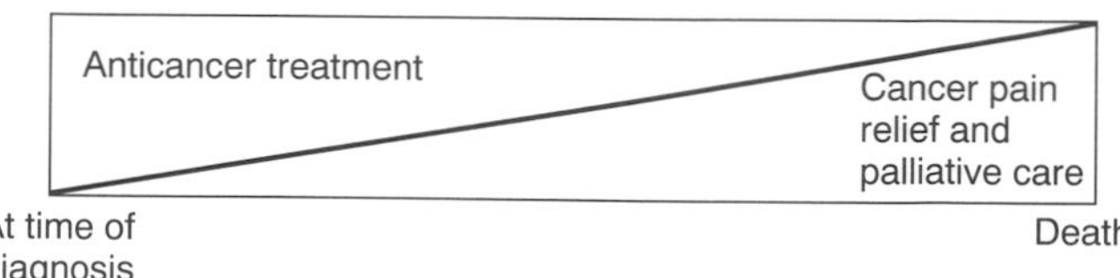

Fig. 5 Proposed allocation of cancer resources in developed countries. (Reproduced with permission from ref. 3).

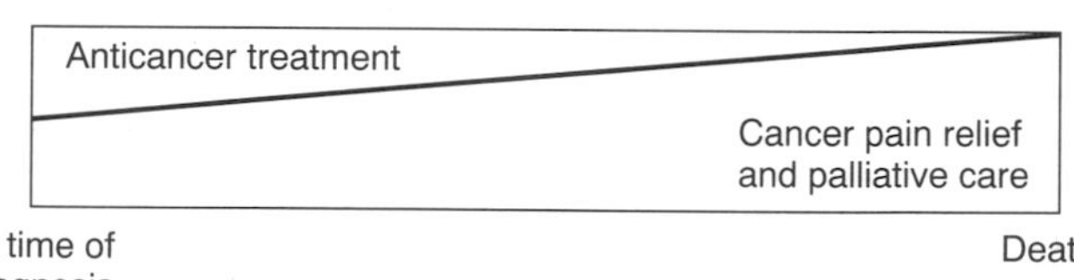

Fig. 6 Proposed allocation of cancer resources in developing countries. (Reproduced with permission from ref. 3.)

elderly and sharing of limited resources, must be taken into account when addressing the attitudes of various societies to pain, suffering, terminal care, and death, as well as when considering the problem of euthanasia. A knowledge of the diversity of cultures, as outlined in Tables 7 and 8, could be helpful when planning the specifics of palliative care programmes around the world.

The different religions both overlap and vary in their attitudes to illness and death. In animism man and nature share the same spiritual essence, and spiritis exists. Illness and unbalance could be caused by breaking taboos, and counter-sorcery is used. Death means a return to nature, often via a second journey in which rituals ensure the success of the passage.

Eastern religions, such as Hinduism and Buddhism, envisage the cosmos/universe and man as one; humans are expected finally to be absorbed in the ultimate energy that is the reality. Illness is often cured by ‘restoring energy flows’. Death leads to a change of living state, perhaps via numerous reincarnations on earth, until ultimately merging with energy, reality, atma.

In Judaeo-Christianity man and nature are often in opposition. God should be obeyed, and in the past illness was seen as the result of sin and disobedience to God’s will. Death led to eternal life in heaven or hell.

According to modern Existentialism, the only world we know is the one mediated by our senses. Illness is defeated by science and the individual is totally responsible. Death is final. Thus life, that’s it— nothing thereafter.

Strategies

With limited resources worldwide for palliative care, rational approaches are essential. Even limited resources may have an impact, provided that the relevant priorities are set and strategies are implemented.

Palliative care should attract more of the available cancer control resources. It is an option that is all too often ignored and not offered to the patient until it is too late in the course of the disease (Fig. 4). In both developed and developing countries, palliative care should be seen as an integral part of cancer care from the outset (Figs. 5 and 6). Curative care and palliative care are not mutually exclusive. The present allocation of cancer care resources (Fig. 4) should be changed in future strategies in both developed (Fig. 5) and developing countries (Fig. 6).

The three figures also show the policies. Palliative care should be an alternative at the time of diagnosis and not seen as a ‘waste basket’ alternative as in Fig. 4. Thus planning of the multidisciplinary clinical team should include adequate personnel resources for palliative care.

Model: implementation of a cancer pain relief programme

In advocating ‘Why not freedom from cancer pain’?, the WHO recommends that countries first establish the three specific measures of governmental policy, education, and drug availability, as symbolized by the triangle in Fig. 7. These could be called foundation measures. They cost comparatively little, but can have large effects. However, they need people with vision, commitment, and leadership to establish them. All three measures are necessary—achieving two without the third will severely limit the effect. For example, developing a national policy on relieving cancer pain and successfully educating the public, health care professionals, and policy-makers will be inadequate if the necessary drugs, particularly opioid analgesics, are not available for patients.

Specific outcomes, as well as indicators for monitoring and evaluation, should be formulated in each area, and target dates should be set. The principles are the same for palliative care. The implementation of palliative care should be continually monitored and evaluated at national level. A rational stepwise approach includes the establishment of process measures (Table 9) and outcome measures (Table 10). The two tables give some examples, but each country must specify its own, depending on its level of palliative care and its health care system. Thus some countries will

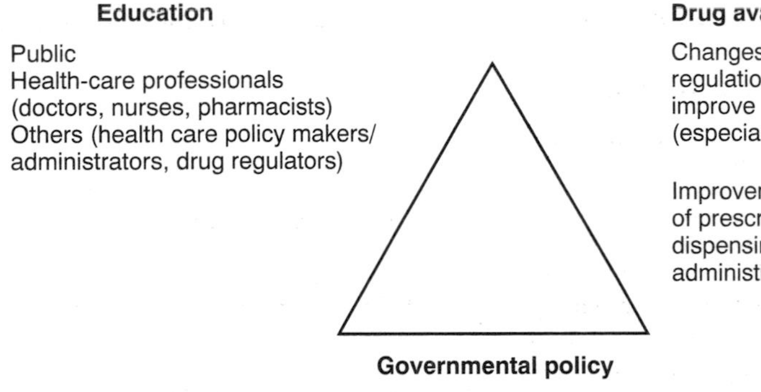

Fig. 7 Foundation measures necessary for an effective national programme.

be monitoring percentages of control of major symptoms, changes in quality of life, and degree of coverage, whereas others will have to start with foundation and process measures, and then proceed to outcome measures in a stepwise fashion.

National policy

During the past few years, evidence has been accumulating that national governments are beginning to recognize the importance of pain relief and terminal care, and to declare them part of their health priorities. The first countries to do so and examples of their policies are listed in Table 11. In addition, palliative care and/or pain relief have been declared as part of the establishment and implementation of national cancer control policies and programmes. Today over 60 countries have established or are planning to establish national palliative care programmes, either separately or as part of their national cancer control programmes. They include Argentina, Cameroon, Colombia, Chile, Cuba, Greece, Indonesia, Jordan, Lebanon, Malaysia, Morocco, Oman, Portugal, Spain, South Africa, Tunisia, Zimbabwe, and the United States. Within larger countries, individual states or provincial governments have also proclaimed or established guidelines on cancer pain relief.[51,52,95–99]

The pioneering efforts of the Wisconsin Pain Initiative, which also serves as a WHO demonstration project, have led over 37 states in the United States to adopt their own state pain initiatives.[100] A federal policy has also been established in the United States,[101] together with excellent reference guides for clinicians covering management of cancer pain in adults[102] and children[103] and a patient's guide.[104]

The three South Indian states of Karnataka, Kerala, and Tamil Nadu introduced their own policies after the federal government made cancer pain relief a priority within their National Cancer Control Programme in 1986.

In Spain, the province of Catalonia has rapidly extended palliative care to over 40 per cent of their terminal cases by establishing clear policies and rational approaches.[105,106] They created 51 palliative care teams, comprising 34 community teams, eight hospital teams, and nine referral units. The aim of the visionary Catalan leadership is to extend such care to at least 80 per cent of their population of six million within the next 5 years by using a multidisease approach encompassing not only cancer patients but also the elderly terminally ill and AIDS patients. In the first 3 years total consumption of morphine for pain release, which is used as an indicator for evaluation, has increased from less than 1 to over 36 kg. The province of Las Palmas has achieved its aim of allowing 80 per cent of their terminally ill patients to die where they choose. In the population of 350 000 people, morphine consumption increased from 37 g to 4 kg. Las Palmas has an effective coverage by home care teams. Moreover, the economic savings have been considerable, with hospital costs reduced and hospital beds released for other patients.[107]

The WHO demonstration projects in Wisconsin, Catalonia, and Las Palmas discussed above show that, with the right leadership,

Table 10 Examples of outcome measures for cancer pain relief*

- Reduction by 30% in the prevalence of pain among cancer patients
- Administration of oral morphine to 50% of cancer patients with pain
- Adoption of the WHO method for relief of cancer pain by more than 50% of general hospitals.

* Similar measures should be applied to palliative care.

Table 11 National policies on pain, cancer pain, and terminal care

Year	Country	Title of document	Issued by	Reference
1984	Canada	*Douleurs Cancereuses Cancer Pain*	Ministry of Health and Welfare, Canada	84
1986	France	*Soigner et Accompagner jusqu au Bout. Soulager la Souffrance* (Caring and Accompanying until the End. Alleviate the Suffering)	Ministry of Social Affairs and Employment, Ministry of Health and the Family, France	85
1988	Australia	*Management of Severe Pain*	National Health and Medical Research Council, Australia	86
1989	Japan	*Manual of Care for Terminally Ill Cancer Patients*	Ministry of Health and Japan Medical Association, Japan	87
1989	Sweden	*The Management of Pain in the Terminal Stage of Life*	National Board of Health and Welfare, Sweden	88
1989	Finland	*Syopapotilaan Kivun Hotto* (Treatment of Pain in Cancer Patients)	National Board of Health, Finland	89
1989	Italy	*Decreta Art. 1 Gazzetta Uffictale della Repubblica Italiana* (Decree on Prescription of Opioid Drugs)	Ministry of Health, Italy	90
1990	Mexico	*Health Policy for Cancer Pain Relief*	Ministry of Health, Mexico	91
1999	Netherlands	*Pijn en Pijnbehandeling bij de Patient met Kanker* (Pain and Pain Treatment for Patients with Cancer)	Dutch chapter of IASP subsidized by the Ministry of Health, Welfare, and Cultural Affairs, The Netherlands	92
1990	Vietnam	*Cancer Pain Policy Statement*	Ministry of Health, Socialist Republic of Vietnam	93
1991	Philippines	*Guidelines on Cancer Pain Relief*	Department of Health, Republic of the Philippines	94

meaningful coverage and effective pain relief can be achieved at reasonable cost and within a relatively short time period.

Drug availability

Some drugs, particularly oral morphine, are essential for the effective control of moderate to severe pain in most patients. On the international level, the International Narcotics Control Board (INCB),[108] in collaboration with the WHO, called on governments to re-evaluate their needs for opioids in the treatment of pain, particularly cancer pain. The INCB, which is a component of the United Nations Drug Control Programme, is responsible for preventing the illicit cultivation, manufacture, and use of controlled drugs, and for ensuring that adequate quantities are available for medical and scientific purposes worldwide. Its duties are established by treaties, including the Single Convention on Narcotic Drugs,[109] the Convention on Psychotropic Substances,[110] and the 1988 Convention on Precursors.

In the past few years, there has been increasing evidence that vague and ambiguous laws and regulations, at both state and national levels, are being revised to accommodate the legitimate use of opioids, particularly for patients with chronic intractable pain.[84–107] Methods of assessing and monitoring the medical need for opioids are being improved. This is reflected in the substantial increase in the estimated annual requirements for morphine reported by various countries to the INCB.

Morphine consumption has increased rapidly (Fig. 8) since the inception of the WHO cancer pain relief programme in 1984. Global medical morphine consumption was relatively constant between 1972 and 1984 at around 2 tons. In 1984 it started to increase and by 1992 it had reached 10 tons. Today it is estimated to be 12 tons, and within two decades it is likely to be 25 tons. However, between 1984 and 1993 most morphine use was concentrated in the 10 industrialized countries that have consistently ranked highest in *per capita* consumption: Australia, Canada, Denmark, Iceland, Ireland, New Zealand, Norway, Sweden, the United Kingdom, and the United States.[111] During this period morphine consumption in the top 10 countries increased by 450 per cent, while in the remainder of the world it increased by 150 per cent. Although the top 10 consuming countries represent

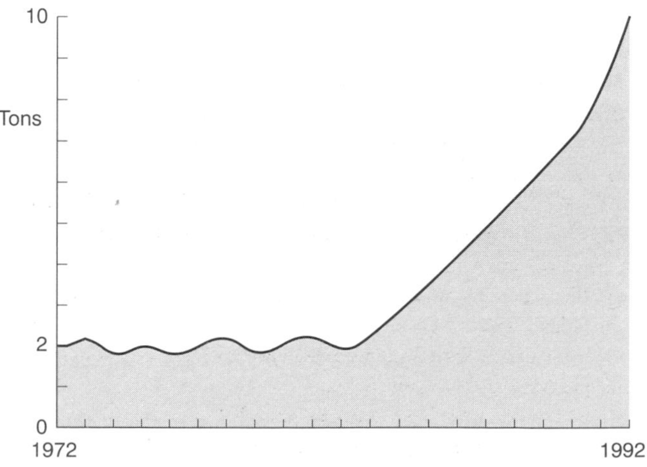

Fig. 8 Global consumption of morphine.

only 7 per cent of the world's population, in 1993 they accounted for approximately 77 per cent of the total morphine used![112]

Morphine consumption for the period 1972 to 1993 broken down by country is shown in Fig. 9.[113] In 1993, approximately 120 countries representing more than 80 per cent of the world's population consumed only 23 per cent of the total morphine used (Fig. 10).[114] These are mainly, but not exclusively, developing countries in Asia, all of South America, Africa, Eastern Europe, and the Mediterranean region. There may be small quantities of opioids in some hospitals in these countries, but most cancer patients have extremely limited access to them, if any. There are still about 50 countries where no oral morphine is available. In these countries most cancer patients are incurable and symptom control is at present the only pragmatic and realistic approach that can be offered.

Under the Single Convention on Narcotic Drugs,[109] to which most governments are party, governments are responsible for assuring the availability of opioid analgesics for medical purposes in their country. Medical organizations have a parallel duty to relieve pain and suffering. To date, over 60 national health ministries have initiated actions to develop policy, education, and drug availability.

However, if there is no co-operative medical and government leadership, there will be little improvement in opioid availability and relief of cancer pain. During 1995, the WHO Cancer and Palliative Care Unit assisted the INCB in a study to ascertain whether governments have fully implemented the recommendations to improve opioid availability made by the INCB in 1989.[108] The INCB sent a questionnaire to governments in 1995 and plans to propose new measures to improve the situation. Fortunately, the supply of opioids in the world is not fixed, and can rise on request from countries to meet increasing medical demand if it is anticipated. WHO has advocated the establishment of clear palliative care policies over the years and this includes opioid availability.[115]

Regional workshops involving national drug regulators, pharmacists, palliative care doctors and nurses, and representatives from the industry offer a rational approach to speeding up the implementation of adequate pain programmes. A recent workshop held in Florianopólis, Brazil, made recommendations for opioid availability in Latin America, after having analysed the situation and identified the impediments.[116] It could serve as a good example for other parts of the world.

Education

Governments and professional organizations should ensure that cancer pain relief and palliative care programmes are incorporated in existing health care systems; separate care systems are neither necessary nor desirable.[3]

There are numerous barriers to the use of available information, one of which is lack of education of health professionals.[117] Education is a priority for ensuring the effective implementation of a palliative care and cancer pain relief programme. The following examples demonstrate how both government and the medical profession have started to address education, and how education of the public is being approached.

Several reports have emphasized that doctors and nurses lack education in the management of cancer pain, and this is also true of palliative care in general.[3,48,118-121] Therefore education is a priority

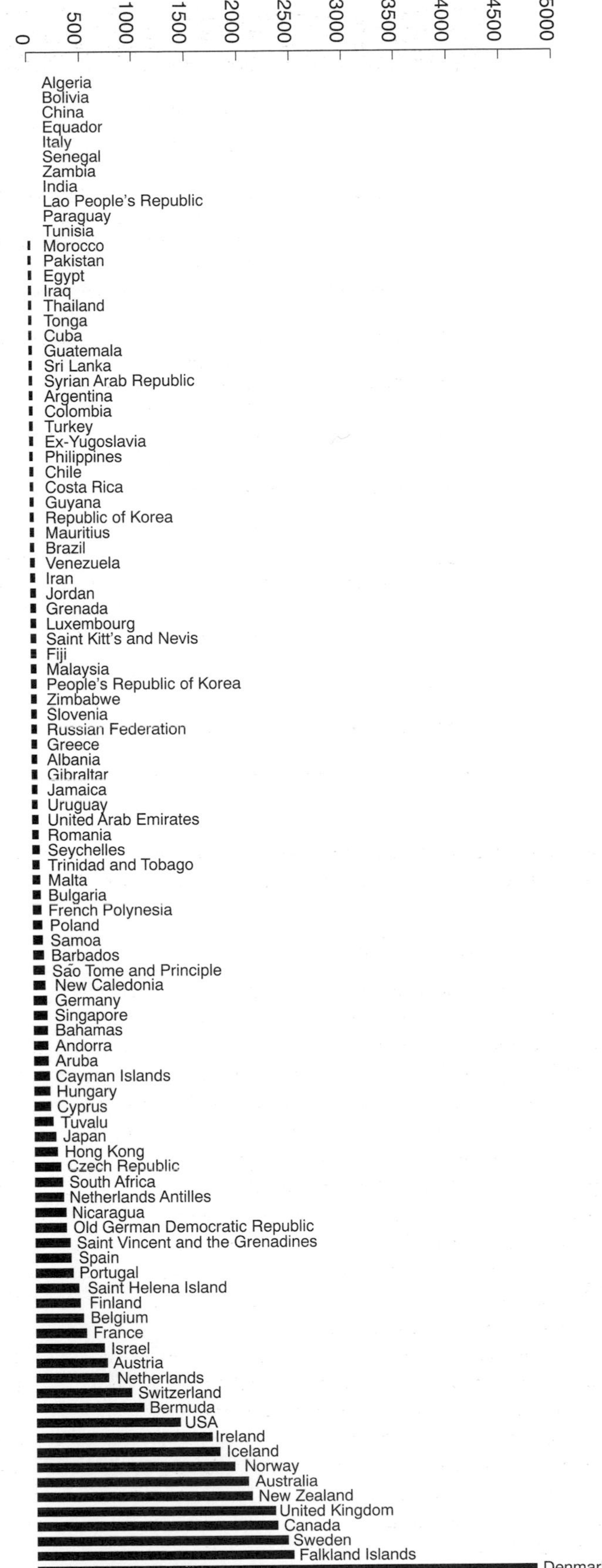

Fig. 9 Average daily consumption of defined daily doses of morphine per million inhabitants.

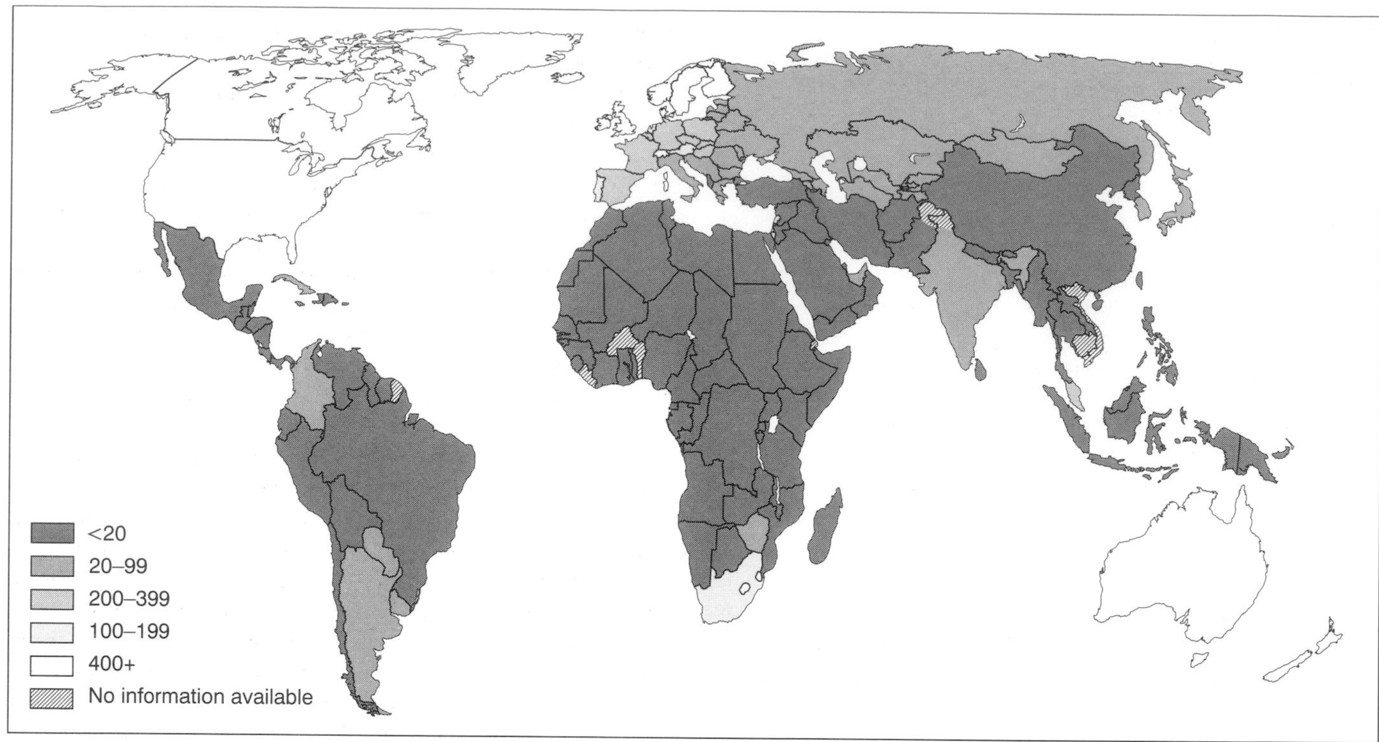

Fig. 10 Global morphine consumption, 1985–1989 (number of daily defined doses per million population per day).

for ensuring the effective implementation of a palliative care programme. The success of palliative care in a number of countries indicates that education in palliative care can be transferred to, and incorporated into, existing health care systems.[3]

The Australian government recently issued regulations making the review of pain assessment and analgesic outcome mandatory in all hospitals.[86] This will certainly influence the future education of health professionals. The body accrediting health facilities in Canada recently issued accreditation standards for palliative care.[122] In the United Kingdom, the Royal College of Physicians recognized palliative medicine as a new subspecialty of general internal medicine in 1987. (It is now recognized as a full specialty.) This was followed by approval of a training programme for senior registrars in palliative medicine by the Joint Committee on Higher Medical Training.[123] In the United States, the American Pain Society is collaborating with the Joint Commission of the Accreditation of Health Care Organizations in field testing quality assurance guidelines for analgesic treatment.[124]

The International Society of Nurses in Cancer Care has outlined a core curriculum in palliative nursing care,[125] and the Oncology Nursing Society of the United States has recommended pragmatic strategies for nurses, including familiarization with the basic principles of the WHO's three-step pain ladder and development of expertise with at least one drug in each class of pharmacological agent identified in the ladder.[126] The International Association for the Study of Pain has also published a core curriculum for professional education in pain.[127]

Concise guides to analgesics should be made available and should be easily accessible to the health professional when the information is needed.[48,128–131]

It is important to monitor and evaluate the effect of education. Thus it was shown that 3 years after Sweden had introduced an official policy for management of pain in the terminally ill, the great majority of chief nurses and doctors responsible for pain management (86 to 100 per cent, depending on specialty, of the 456 asked) were familiar with the WHO three-step pain ladder.[132] Similar surveys were performed in Finland,[133] Norway,[134] Denmark,[135] France,[136] and the United States.[137,138] Even though there has been excellent progress in improving cancer pain relief in the above countries, these studies and two carried out more recently in the United States[139] and France[140] show that cancer pain is still inadequately treated when compared with WHO analgesic standards.

After having achieved the first international consensus that drugs are the mainstay of cancer pain relief and established the three-step pain ladder,[37] allowing a public health dissemination of the enormous amount of knowledge pioneered by the hospice movement, the WHO has established policies for implementing existing knowledge[3] and continued its educational efforts. Thus a second updated version of cancer pain relief,[141] guidelines for opioid availability[142] and symptom relief in terminal illness,[143] policies and managerial guidelines for national cancer control programmes, and, in conjunction with the International Association for the Study of Pain (IASP), recommendations for cancer pain relief and palliative care in children[144] have been produced.

A manual for home caregivers, which is essential for achieving coverage in developing countries, is in preparation, and the Philippines have already produced their own culture-specific version.[145] The quarterly journal *Cancer Pain Release* is an important tool in international networking, and the collaborating centres, demonstration projects, and focal points around the world are crucial for carrying out the mission.[146]

Public education

It is essential that the public are made aware of the following:

- palliative care will improve a patient's quality of life, even if the cancer is incurable;
- cancer is not always painful;
- treatments exist that can relieve pain in many of the symptoms of advanced cancer;
- drug therapy is the mainstay of cancer pain management;
- there is no need for patients to suffer prolonged intolerable pain or other distressing symptoms;
- drugs for the relief of pain can be taken indefinitely without losing their effectiveness;
- psychological dependence (addiction) does not occur when morphine is taken to relieve cancer pain;
- the medical use of morphine does not lead to abuse.

An article in *Reader's Digest* exemplifies what can be done in public education. This article, entitled 'We can win the war against pain',[147] is estimated to have reached over 20 million readers worldwide in 12 different versions. In some editions, leading national figures commented on the article, giving practical information on where services were available. Patients and families need to know how to obtain support from a palliative care service, where and whether home care support is available, and what they can do themselves.[148-151]

The Wisconsin initiative, which is a WHO demonstration project, shows comprehensively how coverage in education is being achieved. Wisconsin was the first state to organize a cancer pain initiative covering the whole state and including educational efforts directed towards doctors, nurses, pharmacists, and cancer patients and their families. The initiative is noted for its success in initiating cancer pain management as part of the curricula of the state's medical and pharmacy schools. Some nursing schools provide courses on the assessment and management of cancer pain[152-154] Inspired by the Wisconsin initiative, professionals in more than 37 states in the United States are now organizing similar state-wide programmes.[155]

In many developing countries, the implementation must be carried out in a stepwise fashion as there is no critical mass of professionals to educate from the beginning. Therefore we recommend the stepwise approach which addresses the implementation for monitoring outcome, starting with a centrally located high-level centre.

Continued advocacy of palliative care, particularly the public health approach and pragmatic approach for developing countries, is important. Numerous international workshops and large congresses are being addressed, as well as the health profession through editorials in journals[156-159] and the general public through press releases. Several informative and emotionally engaging video films are available that ought to be shown more often on public television.

Networks

Institutions, organizations, and countries are not excellent in themselves. However, excellent individuals make excellent institutions, organizations, and countries. The individuals and their initiatives remain essential.[160,161]

Over the years, leaders in the field have demonstrated that major negative symptoms can be controlled and efficient terminal care can be given.[162-173] Large organizations, such as the WHO, have reacted to this and produced state-of-the-art consensus reports and practical field-tested guidelines,[3,32,141-144] as well as policies on how best to implement knowledge gained in palliative care. Some national policies are becoming established, directives for professional education in palliative care are emerging, and vital drugs are becoming available. Excellent journals, associations, and regular forums for palliative care have been established over the past few years, allowing a rapid exchange of information and ideas.

Nothing can stop an idea once its time has come. Palliative medicine is here to stay, and will increase in importance over the years. However, if we are to achieve coverage, reaching all those who are in need of palliative care, it is important to remember that compassion that is not combined with wisdom is inefficient in relieving suffering.[174] A rational method, stressing a public health rather than an institutionalized approach, should be a priority for the individuals, organizations, and countries in the worldwide network involved in implementing existing knowledge in palliative care. Of course, this should not exclude continued academic research. We should never lose sight of the fact that there is a time to be born, and a time to die: 'No death is evil, but a shameful death'.[175] Palliative medicine will be of great importance in avoiding the latter.

Conclusions

Implementation of the following recommendations, which could have a major impact on the quality of life of cancer patients, will require strong political motivation and leadership and can be undertaken without excessive expenditure. A WHO Expert Committee on the relief of cancer pain and palliative care has made the following recommendations to countries for achieving effective palliative care.

1. Governments should establish national policies and programmes for palliative care.
2. Governments of member states should ensure that palliative care programmes are incorporated into their existing health care systems; separate systems of care are neither necessary nor desirable.
3. Governments should ensure that health-care workers (physicians, nurses, pharmacists, or other categories appropriate to local needs) are adequately trained in palliative care.
4. Governments should review their national health policies to ensure that equitable support is provided for programmes of palliative care in the home.
5. In the light of the financial, emotional, physical, and social burdens carried by family members who are willing to care for cancer patients in the home, governments should consider establishing formal systems of recompense for the principal family caregivers.
6. Governments should recognize the singular importance of home care for patients with advanced cancer and should

ensure that hospitals are able to offer appropriate back-up and support for home care.

7. Governments should ensure the availability of both non-opioid and opioid analgesics, particularly morphine for oral administration. Further, they should make realistic determinations of their opioid requirements and ensure that annual estimates submitted to the INCB reflect actual needs.

8. Governments should ensure that their drug legislation makes full provision for the following:

   (a) regular review, with the aim of permitting importation, manufacture, prescribing, stocking, dispensing, and administration of opioids for medical reasons;

   (b) legally empowering physicians, nurses, pharmacists, and where necessary, other categories of health-care worker to prescribe, stock, dispense, and administer opioids;

   (c) review of the controls governing opioid use, with a view to simplification, so that drugs are available in the necessary quantities for legitimate use.

9. With pressure for the legalization of euthanasia likely to increase, governments should make strenuous efforts to keep fully informed of all developments in the field of cancer pain relief, palliative care, and management of terminal cancer.

References

1. Lopez AD. Causes of death: an assessment of global patterns of mortality around 1985. *World Health Statistics Quarterly*, 1990; **43**:91–104.
2. WHO. *World Health Statistics Annual 1990*. Geneva: WHO, 1991.
3. WHO. *Cancer Pain Relief and Palliative Care*. Technical Report Series No. 804. Geneva: WHO, 1990.
4. Stjernswärd J. Editorial. *Newsletter. European Association for Palliative Care*, No.2, Winter 1989–1990.
5. Wildawsky A. Doing better and feeling worse: the political pathology of health policy. In: Knowles JH, ed. *Doing Better and Feeling Worse: Health in the United States*. New York: Norton, 1977: 105–23.
6. McKeown T. *The Role of Medicine: Mirage or Nemesis*. London: Nuffield Provincial Hospital Trust, 1976.
7. Grant J. A new way of measuring progress in living standards. *World Health Forum*, 1981; **2**:373–84.
8. Murray CJL, Lopez A. Global and regional cause-of-death patterns in 1990. *Bulletin of the WHO*, 1994; **72**:447–80.
9. Bulatao RA, Stephens PW. Estimates and projections of mortality by cause: a global overview 1970–2015. In: Jamison DT, Mosley HW, eds. *The World Bank Health Sector Priorities Review*. Washington, DC: World Bank, 1991.
10. Lopez A, Murray CJL. To be published.
11. WHO. *Diet, Nutrition and the Prevention of Chronic Diseases*. Technical Report Series No. 797. Geneva: WHO, 1990.
12. Gu LY, Chen ML. Vital statistics: health services in Shanghai county. *American Journal of Public Health*, 1982; **72**:19–23.
13. WHO. *Health of the Elderly*. Technical Report Series No. 779. Geneva: WHO, 1989.
14. World Bank. *World Development Report 1993*. Oxford University Press, New York, 1993.
15. Macfayden D. International demographic trends. In: Kane RL, Evans JG, Macfayden D, eds. *Improving the Health of Older People: A World View*. Oxford University Press, 1990.
16. *World Population Prospects: 1992 Revision*. Quoted in: *World Economic and Social Survey*. New York: United Nations, 1994.
17. Stephen P. The curse of longlife. *Financial Times*, 1995 **Aug 4**:18.
18. Stanley K, Stjernswärd J. Lung cancer—a world wide health problem. *Chest*, 1989; **96**(Supplement 1):115–55.
19. Parkin DM. Läära E, Muir CS. Estimates of the world wide frequency of sixteen major cancers. *International Journal of Cancer*, 1988; **41**:184–97.
20. Peto R, Lopez AD. Worldwide mortality from current smoking patterns. In Durston B, Jamrozik K, eds. *The Global War. Proceedings of the 7th World Conference on Tobacco and Health*. Perth: Health Department of Western Australia, 1991:66–8.
21. WHO. Tobacco—attributable mortality: global estimates and projections. *Tobacco Alert*, January 1991. Geneva: WHO, 1991.
22. WHO. Current and future dimensions of the HIV/AIDS pandemic: a capsule summary. *Global Programme on AIDS*, April 1991. Geneva: WHO, 1991.
23. World Bank. *World Development Report 1993*. Oxford University Press, New York, 1993.
24. WHO. *Global Strategy for the Prevention and Control of AIDS*. (Report of the Director General, 44th World Health Assembly.) Geneva: WHO, 1991.
25. Dougherty CJ. Setting health care priorities: Oregon's next step. A conference report. *Hastings Center Report*, 1991; **May–June**:1–11.
26. WHO. Cancer in developed countries: assessing the trends. *WHO Chronicle*, 1985; **39**:109–10.
27. Stjernswärd J. Cancer pain relief: an important global public health issue. In: Field HL, *et al*., eds. *Advances in Pain Research and Therapy*, Vol. 9. New York: Raven Press, 1985: 555–8.
28. Stjernswärd J. WHO Cancer Pain Relief Programme. *Cancer Surveys*, 1988; **7**:196–208.
29. Maher EJ. Decision making in the management of advanced cance of the head and neck: Difference in perspective between doctors and patients: future avenues for research. *Palliative Medicine*, 1990; **4**:185–9.
30. Maher EJ, Jefferis A. Decision-making in the management of advanced cancer of the head and neck: variations in the views of medical specialists. *Journal of the Royal Society of Medicine*, 1990; **83**:356–9
31. Lawton PA, Maher EJ, in association with ESTRO. Treatment strategies for advanced and metabolic cancer in Europe. *Radiotherapy and Oncology*, 1991; **22**:1–6.
32. WHO. *Cancer Pain Relief.* Geneva: WHO, 1986.
33. WHO. *Cities and the Population Issue*. (44th World Health Assembly, Technical Discussion 7, Background Document.) Geneva: WHO, 1991.
34. WHO. *National Cancer Control Programmes: Priorities and Managerial Guidelines*. WHO, Geneva, 1995.
35. Rappaz O, Tripiana J, Rapin Ch-H, Stjernswärd J, Junod JP. Soins palliatifs et traitement de la douleur cancereuse en gériatrie. *Therapeutische Umschau*, 1985; **42**:843–8.
36. Takeda F. Results of field testing in Japan of the WHO draft interim guideline on relief of cancer pain. *Pain Clinic*, 1986; **2**:83–9.
37. Ventafridda V, Tamburini M. Caraceri A, De Conno F, Naldi F. A validation study of the WHO method for cancer pain relief. *Cancer* 1987; **59**:850–6.
38. Goisis A, Gorini M, Ratti R, Luliri P. Application of a WHO protocol on medical therapy for oncologic pain in an internal medicine hospital. *Tumori* 1989; **75**:470–2.
39. Vijayaram S, *et al*. Experience with oral morphine for cancer pain relief. *Journal of Pain and Symptom Management*, 1988; **3**:145–9.
40. Walker VA, Hoskin PJ, Hanks GW, White ID. Evaluation of WHO analgesic guidelines. *Journal of Pain and Symptom Management*, 1988; **3**:145–9.
41. Schug SA, Zech D, Dorr U. Cancer pain management according to WHO analgesic guidelines. *Journal of Pain and Symptom Management*, 1990; **5**:27–32.
42. Grond S, Zech D, Schug SA, Lynch J, Lehman KA. The importance of non-opioid analgesics for cancer pain relief according to the guidelines of the WHO. *International Journal of Clinical Pharmacology Research*, 1991; **11**:253–60.
43. Grond S, Zech D, Schug SA, Lunch J, Lehmann KA. Validation of WHO guidelines for cancer pain relief during the last days and hours of life. *Journal of Pain and Symptom Management*, 1991; **6**:411–22.

44. Mercadente S, Maddaloni S, Roccella S, Salvaggio L. Predictive factors in advanced cancer pain treated only by analgesics. *Pain*, 1992; **50**:151–5.
45. Radbruch L, Zech D, Grond S, Jung H. Therapy for somatic pain in advanced breast cancer. *Geburtshilfe und Frauenheildkunde*, 1992; **52**:404–11.
46. Vecht CJ, Hoff AM, Kansen PJ, de-Boer MF, Bosch DA. Types and causes of pain in cancer of the head and neck. *Cancer*, 1992;**70**:178–84.
47. Grond S, Zech D, Lunch J, Diefenbach C, Schug SA, Lehman KA. Validation of WHO guidelines for pain relief in head and neck cancer. *Annals of Otology, Rhinology and Laryngology*, 1993; **102**:342–8.
48. Collopy B, Boyle P, Jennings B. New directions in nursing home ethics. *Hastings Center Report*, 1991; **March–April**:1–16.
49. Swedish National Board of Health and Welfare. *Sweden: Social Styrelsens Allmänna Rad (SOSFS 1989:14) om Bedömningen inom Hälso—och Sjukvarden av Rätt Till Ersättning och Ledighet for Närstaende*. Stockholm: Socialstyrelsen, 1989.
50. Collopy B, Dubler N, Zuckerman C. The ethics of home care: autonomy and accommodation. *Hastings Center Report*, 1991; **March–April**:1–16.
51. Nair MK. *Ten Year Action Plan for Cancer Control in Kerala*. Trivandrum Regional Cancer Centre, 1988.
52. Bhargava MK. *Karnataka State Cancer Control Programme*. Bangalore: Kidwai Memorial Institute of Oncology, 1989.
53. Stjernswärd J, Stanley K, Tsechkovski M. Cancer pain relief: an urgent public health problem in India. *Indian Journal of Pain*, 1986; **1**:8–17.
54. Hadorn DC. The Oregon priority-setting exercise: quality of life and public policy. *Hastings Center Report*, 1991; **May–June**:11–16.
55. Long SH, Gibbs JO, Grozier JP, Cooper DI, Newman JF, Larsen AM. Medical expenditure of terminal cancer patients during the last year of life. *Inquiry*, 1984; **21**:315–27.
56. Fuchs VR. Though much is taken: reflections on ageing, health and medical care. *Milbank Memorial Fund Quarterly: Health and Society*, 1984; **62**:143–66.
57. Temkin-Greener H, Meiners MR, Petty EA, Szydlowski JS. The use and costs of health services prior to death: a comparison of the Medicare-only and the Medicare–Medicaid elderly populations. *Milbank Memorial Fund Quarterly: Health and Society*, 1992; **70**:679–701.
58. Long SH, Gibbs JO, Crozier JP, Cooper DI, Jr, Newman JF, Jr, Larsen AM. Medical expenditures of terminal cancer patients during the last year of life. *Inquiry*, 1984; **21**:315–27.
59. Schneider EL, Guralnick JM. The ageing of America. Impact on health care costs. *Journal of the American Medical Association*, 1990; **263**:2335–40.
60. Fries JF. Ageing, natural death, and the compression of morbidity. *New England Journal of Medicine* 1980; **303**:130–6.
61. Fries JF. The compression of morbidity: near or far? *Milbank Memorial Fund Quarterly: Health and Society*, 1990; **67**:208–32.
62. Patterson C, Chambers LW. Preventive health care. *Lancet*, 1995;**345**: 1611–15.
63. Fries JF, *et al.* Reducing health care costs by reducing the need and demand for medical services. *New England Journal of Medicine*, 1993;**329**:321–5.
64. Kane RL, Radosevich DM, Vaupel JW. Compression of morbidity: issues and irrelevancies. In: Kane RL, Evans JG, Macfayden D, eds. *Improving the Health of Older People: A World View*. Oxford University Press, 1990.
65. Fried TR, Gillick MR. Medical decision-making in the last six months of life: choices about limitation of care. *Journal of the American Geriatric Society*, 1994; **42**:303–7.
66. Murphy DJ, *et al.* The influence of the probability of survival on patients' preferences regarding cardiopulmonary resuscitation. *New England Journal of Medicine* 1994; **330**:545–9.
67. Schneiderman LJ, Kronick R, Kaplan RM, Anderson JP, Langer RD. Effects of offering advance directives on medical treatment and costs. *Annals of Internal Medicine*, 1992; **117**:599–606.
68. Emanuel EJ, Emanuel LL. The economics of dying. The illusion of cost savings at the end of life. *New England Journal of Medicine*, 1994; **330(8)**:540–4.
69. Avorn J. Benefit and cost analysis in geriatric care. *New England Journal of Medicine*, 1984; **310**:1294–1301.
70. Bass SA, Morris R, eds. *International Perspectives on State and Family Support for the Elderly*. Binghamton, NY: Haworth Press, 1994.
71. Relman AS. Assessment and accountability. The third revolution in medical care. *New England Journal of Medicine*, 1988; **317**:1220–2.
72. Calltrop J. *Prioritering och Beslutsprocess i Sjukvardsfragor. Nogra Drag i de Nenaste Decenniernas Svenska Hälsopolitik*. Academic Dissertation, Uppsala University, 1989.
73. Callahan D. *What Kind of Life: The Limits of Medical Progress*. New York: Simon and Schuster, 1990.
74. Bloom BS, Super KA. Health and medical care for the elderly and aged population: the state of the evidence. *Journal of the American Geriatric Society*, 1980; **28**:451–5.
75. Kane LR, Wales J, Bernstein L, Leibowitz A, Kaplan S. A randomized controlled trial of hospice care. *Lancet*, 1984; 890–4.
76. Addington-Hall JM, *et al.* Randomized controlled trial of effects of coordinating care for terminally ill cancer patients. *British Medical Journal*, 1992; **305**:1317–22.
77. McWinney IR, Bass MJ, Donner A. Evaluation of palliative care services: problems and pitfalls. *British Medical Journal*, 1994; **309**:1340–42.
78. McQuay H, Moore A. Need for rigorous assessment of palliative care. *British Medical Journal*,1994; **309**:1315–16.
79. Avorn J. Benefit and cost analysis in geriatric care. *New England Journal of Medicine*, 1984; **310**:1294–1301.
80. Clements WM, ed. *Religion, Ageing and Health: A Global Perspective*. New York, NY: Haworth Press, 1988.
81. Fulton R. The contemporary funeral: functional or dysfunctional? In: Wass H, Niemeyer RA, eds. *Dying. Facing the Facts*. Washington, DC: Taylor and Francis, 1995.
82. Osborne T, Noble CE, Weyl N. *Human Variations: The Biopsychology of Age, Race and Sex*. New York: Academic Press, 1978:1–392.
83. Sundberg ND, Hadiyono JP, Latkin LA, Padilla J. Cross-cultural prevention programme transfer: questions regarding developing countries. *Journal of Primary Prevention*, 1995; **15**(4):361–76.
84. Ministry of Health and Welfare, Canada. *Cancer Pain. A Monograph on the Management of Pain*. Ottawa: Department of Supply and Services, 1984.
85. Ministry of Social Affairs and Employment, Ministry of Health and the Family, France. *Soigner et Accompagner jusqu'au Bout. Soulager la Souffrance*. Paris: Ministry of Social Affairs and Employment, Ministry of Health and the Family, 1986.
86. National Health and Medical Research Council, Australia. *Management of Severe Pain*. Canberra: Australian Government Publishing Service, 1988.
87. Ministry of Health, Japan, and Japanese Medical Association. *Manual of Care for Terminally Ill Cancer Patients*. Tokyo: Ministry of Health and Japanese Medical Association, 1989.
88. Swedish National Board of Health and Welfare. *The Management of Pain in the Terminal Stage of Life*. Stockholm: Swedish National Board of Health and Welfare, 1989.
89. Vainio A, ed. *Syöpäpotilaan kivun Hoito, Lääkintöhallituksen Oppissarja*, No. 5. Helsinki: National Board of Health, 1989.
90. Ministry of Health, Italy. *Decreta Art. 1 Gazzetta Ufficiale della Repubblica Italiana*. Rome: Ministry of Health, 1989.
91. Ministry of Health, Mexico. *Health Policy for Cancer Pain Relief*. (Book No 1 of Laws, Decrees, Agreements and Various Documents that Regulate the Administrative Activities of the Health Secretariat and the Health Sector.) Mexico City: Ministry of Health, 1990:121.
92. Nederlandse Vereniging ter Bestudering van Pijn (NVBP). *Pijn en Pijnbehandeling bij de Patient met Kanker*. Groningen: Academisch Ziekenhuis, 1991.
93. Ministry of Health, Vietnam. *Cancer Pain Policy Statement*. Ministry of Health: Ho Chi Minh City, Socialist Republic of Vietnam, 1990.
94. Philippine Cancer Control Program. *Guidelines on Cancer Pain Relief*. Manila: Department of Health, Republic of the Philippines, 1991.
95. State of Wisconsin Legislature. *Resolution on Cancer Pain*. Madison, WI: State of Wisconsin Legislature, 1987.

96. Office of the Governor, State of Ohio. *Proclamation on the Ohio Cancer Pain Initiative*. Columbus, OH: Office of the Governor, 1990.
97. Hill CS, Jr. *Guidelines for Treatment of Cancer Pain. Final Report of the Texas Cancer Council's Workgroup on Pain Control in Cancer Patients*. Texas Cancer Council, 1990.
98. Generalitat de Catalunya, Departament de Sanitat i Seguretat Social, Direccio General d'Ordenacio i Planifacacio Sanitaria. *Catalan Cancer Control Programme*. Barcelona: Generalitat de Catalunya, 1991.
99. WHO and IASP. Progress in cancer pain relief and palliative care. *Journal of Pain and Symptom Management* (Special Issue), 1993; **8**(6):335–443.
100. Dahl JL. State cancer pain initiatives. *Journal of Pain and Symptom Management*, 1993; **8**(6):372–5.
101. Jacox AK, *et al. Management of Cancer Pain. Clinical Practice Guideline No. 9*. AHCPR Publication No. 94–0592. Rockville, MD.: Agency for Health Care Policy and Research, 1994.
102. Jacox AK, *et al. Management of Cancer Pain. Adults. Quick Reference Guide for Clinicians No. 9*. AHCPR Publication No. 94–0593. Rockville, MD: Agency for Health Care Policy and Research, 1994.
103. Jacox AK, *et al. Management of Cancer Pain. Pediatric. Quick Reference Guide for Clinicians No. 9*. AHCPR Publication No. 94–0594. Rockville, MD: Agency for Health Care Policy and Research, 1994.
104. Jacox AK, *et al. Management of Cancer Pain: A Patient's Guide. Clinical Practice Guideline No. 9* (Adult version—English). AHCPR Publication No. 94–0595. Rockville, MD: Agency for Health Care Policy and Research, 1994.
105. Gomez-Batiste X. Catalonia's five year plan: basic principles. *European Journal of Palliative Care*, 1994, **1**(1):45–9.
106. Gomez-Batiste X, *et al.* Catalonia's five year plan: preliminary results. *European Journal of Palliative Care*, 1994, **1**(2):98–101.
107. Gomez M. Personal communication, Las Palmas, 1995.
108. International Narcotics Control Board. *Demand for and Supply of Opiates for Medical and Scientific Needs*. New York: United Nations, 1989.
109. United Nations. *Single Convention on Narcotic Drugs 1961* (as amended by the 1972 protocol). New York: United Nations, 1977.
110. United Nations. *Convention on Psychotropic Substances 1971*. New York: United Nations, 1977.
111. Joranson D. Availability of opioids for cancer pain: recent trends, assessment of system barriers. New WHO Guidelines, the rise for diversion. *Journal of Pain Symptom Management*, 1993; 8:353–60.
112. Stjernswärd J, Joranson D. Opioid availability and cancer pain—an unnecessary tragedy. *Support Care in Cancer*, 1995, **3**:157–8.
113. International Narcotics Control Board. Table IX: Average daily consumption of defined daily doses per million inhibitants during the years 1989 to 1993. *International Narcotics Control Board Report*. Vienna: United Nations, 1995:152–6.
114. International Narcotics Control Board. *Estimated World Requirements for 1995. Statistics for 1993*. Vienna: United Nations, 1995.
115. WHO. *Cancer Pain Relief: A Guide to Opioid Availability*. WHO/CAN/ 92.3. Geneva: WHO, 1992.
116. Bruera E, Schoeller MT, Stjernswärd J. Opioid Availability in Latin America. The Declaration of Florianopolis. *Support Care Cancer*, 1995; 3:164–7.
117. McCaffery M. Pain control. Barriers to the use of available information. *Cancer*, 1992; **70**:1438–49.
118. Bonica JJ. Cancer pain. In: Bonica JJ, ed. *Pain*. New York: Raven Press, 1980:335–62.
119. American College of Physicians Health and Public Policy Committee. Drug therapy for severe chronic pain in terminal illness. *Annals of Internal Medicine*, 1983; **99**:870–3.
120. Marks RM, Sachar EJ. Undertreatment of medical inpatients with narcotic analgesics. *Annals of Internal Medicine*, 1973; **78**:173–81.
121. Foley KM. Pharmacologic approaches to cancer pain management. In: Fields HL, ed. *Advances in Pain Research and Therapy*, Vol. 9, New York: Raven Press, 1985:629–53.
122. Canadian Council on Health Facilities Accreditation. *Accreditation Standards for Palliative Care Programme*. Ottawa: Canadian Council on Health Facilities Accreditation, 1991.
123. Hillier R. Palliative medicine: a new specialty. *British Medical Journal*, 1988; **297**:874–5.
124. Max M. Improving outcomes of analgesic treatment: is education enough? *Annals of Internal Medicine*, 1990; 885–9.
125. International Society of Nurses in Cancer Care. A core curriculum for a post basic course in palliative nursing care. *Palliative Medicine*, 1990; 4:261–70.
126. Spross JA, McGuire DB, Schmitt RM. *Oncology Nursing Society Position Paper on Cancer Pain*. Oncology Nursing Press, 1991. Also published as three parts in *Oncology Nursing Forum*. 1991; **17**(4–6).
127. Fields HL, ed. *Task Force on Professional Education in Pain. Core Curriculum for Professional Education in Pain*. Seattle, WA: International Association for the Study of Pain Publications, 1991.
128. American Pain Society. *Principles of Analgesic Use in the Treatment of Acute Pain and Chronic Cancer Pain: a Concise Guide to Medical Practice*. Washington, DC: American Pain Society, 1987.
129. Weissman DE, Burchman SL, Dinndorf PA, Dahl JL. *Handbook of Cancer Pain Management*. Madison, WI: Wisconsin Cancer Pain Initiative, 1988.
130. Ligue Suisse Contre le Cancer. *Vivre avec le Cancer, sans Douleur*. Geneva: Ligue Suisse Contre le Cancer, 1990. (Also available in German and Italian.)
131. Librach LS. *The Pain Manual, Canadian Cancer Society*. Montreal: Pegasus Health Care, 1991.
132. Rawal N, Hylander J, Arner S. Management of cancer pain in Sweden: a nationwide survey. *Pain*, 1993; **54**(2):169–79.
133. Vainio A. Treatment of terminal cancer pain in Finland: a second look. *Acta Anaesthesiologica Scandinavica*, 1992, **36**:89–95.
134. Warncke T, Breivik H, Vainio A. Treatment of cancer pain in Norway. A questionnaire study. *Pain*, 1994; **57**(1):109–16.
135. Sjögren P, Banning AM, Jensen N-H, Jensen M, Klee M, Vainio A. Management of cancer pain in Denmark. A nationwide questionnaire study. *Pain*, 1995.
136. Vainio A. Treatment of terminal cancer pain in France: a questionnaire study. *Pain*, 1995.
137. Diekmann JM, Wassem RA. A survey of nursing students' knowledge of cancer pain control. *Cancer Nursing*, 1991, **14**(6):314–20.
138. Schmidt K, Eland J, Weiler K. Pediatric cancer pain management: a survey of nurses' knowledge. *Journal of Pediatric Oncology Nursing*, 1994; **11**(1):4–12.
139. Cleeland CS, *et al.* Pain and its treatment in outpatients with metastatic cancer. *New England Journal of Medicine*, 1994; **330**(9):592–6.
140. Larue F, Colleau SM, Brasseur L, Cleeland CS. Multicenter study of cancer pain and its treatment in France. *British Medical Journal*, 1995; **310**:1034–7.
141. WHO. *Cancer Pain Relief*. 2nd edn. Geneva: WHO, 1995.
142. WHO. Guide to opioid availability: Annex to *Cancer Pain Relief*. 2nd edn. Geneva: WHO, 1995.
143. WHO. *Symptom Relief in the Terminally Ill*. Geneva: WHO, 1995.
144. WHO. *Cancer Pain Relief and Palliative Care in Children*. Joint IASP/ WHO Monograph. Geneva: WHO, 1995.
145. Department of Health, The Philippines. *Caring at Home—Hospice Care, Philippine Cancer Control Programme*. Manila: Department of Health and Philippine Cancer Society, 1995:1–32.
146. Anonymous. Cancer pain, palliative care and the WHO priorities; 1995–99. *Cancer Pain Release*, 1995; 8(1).
147. Englebardt L. We can win the war against pain. *Reader's Digest*, 1991; **February**: 17–21. (Also published in Spanish (Mexico), Portuguese (Portugal, Brazil), Swedish, Norwegian, German, Dutch, Italian, and Chinese between September 1990 and February 1991.)
148. Wisconsin Cancer Pain Initiative. *Cancer Pain Can be Relieved: A Guide for Patients and Families*. Madison, WI: Wisconsin Cancer Pain Initiative, 1988.
149. Wisconsin Cancer Pain Initiative. *Children's Cancer Pain Can be Relieved: A Guide for Parents and Families*. Madison, WI: Wisconsin Cancer Pain Initiative, 1989.

150. Wisconsin Cancer Pain Initiative. *Jeff Asks About Cancer Pain: A Booklet for Teens About Cancer Pain*. Madison, WI: Wisconsin Cancer Pain Initiative, 1990.
151. American Cancer Society. *Questions and Answers About Pain control. A Guide for People with Cancer and their Families*. New York: American Cancer Society, 1983.
152. Dahl J. The Wisconsin Pain Initiative. *Journal of Psychosocial Oncology*, 1990; 8:125–37.
153. Cleeland CS. (1987). Barriers to the management of cancer pain. *Oncology*, 1987; **Special Supplement**:19–26.
154. Dahl JL, Joranson DE, Engber D, Dosch J. The cancer pain problem: Wisconsin's response. *Journal of Pain and Symptom Management*, 1988; 3:S1–20.
155. WHO Collaborating Center for Symptom Evaluation. State cancer pain initiatives. Networking to relieve cancer pain. *Cancer Pain Release*, 1991; **5**:1–4.
156. Stjernswärd J. Point of view. *Asian Hospital*, 1994; **March–April**:2.
157. Stjernswärd J. The case for palliative care: a global problem addressed. *European Journal of Palliative Care*, 1994; **1**(1):6–7.
158. Stjernswärd J. Future trends in palliative care. *European Journal of Palliative Care*, 1994; **1**(2):69.
159. Stjernswärd J. Nurses in the front lines of palliative care. *International Journal of Palliative Nursing*, 1995, **1**(3):124–5.
160. MacDonald N. The WHO volunteer network. *Palliative Medicine*, **5**:93–5.
161. Burn G. A personal initiative to improve palliative care in India. *Palliative Medicine*, 1990; **4**:257–9.
162. Saunders C, Baines M. *Living with Dying: The Management of Terminal Disease*. 2nd edn. Oxford University Press, 1989.
163. Saunders C. *Hospice and Palliative Care: An Interdisciplinary Approach*. London: Edward Arnold, 1990.
164. Bonica J. Treatment of cancer pain: Current status and future needs. In: Fields HL, Dubner R, Cervero F, eds. *Advances in Pain Research and Therapy*, Vol. 9. New York: Raven Press, 1985: 589–616.
165. Ventafridda V. Providing continuity of care for cancer patients. *Journal of Psychosocial Oncology*, 1990; **8**:3–10.
166. Twycross RG, Lack SA. *Symptom Control in Far Advanced Cancer: Pain Relief*. London: Pitman, 1983.
167. Twycross RG, Lack SA. *Therapeutics in Terminal Cancer*, 2nd edn. London: Churchill Livingstone, 1990.
168. Doyle D. *Palliative Care: The Management of the Far Advanced Illness*. London: Croom Helm, 1984.
169. Foley KM. The treatment of cancer pain. *New England Journal of Medicine*, 1985; **313**:84–95
170. Portenoy RK. Pharmacologic approaches to the control of cancer pain. *Journal of Psychosocial Oncology*, 1990; **8**:75–107.
171. Wilkes E, ed. *A Source Book of Terminal Care*. University of Sheffield Printing Unit, 1986.
172. Kübler-Ross E. *On Death and Dying*. London: Tavistock, 1970.
173. Wilson-Barnett J, Raiman J, eds. Nursing issues and research in terminal care. *Developments in Nursing Research*, Vol. 6. Chichester: Wiley, 1988.
174. Rinpoche TT. High resolve: an interview with the venerable Tara Talku Rinpoche. *Parabola*, 1986; **11**(3).
175. Epictetus. *Discourses*, Book II, AD 60–138, quoting *Euripides' Fragments* 480–906 BC.

Index

Note: Since the main subjects of this book are palliative medicine and palliative care, index entries under these keywords have been kept to a minimum, and readers are advised to seek more specific entries.

Page numbers in **bold** refer to major discussions in the text; those in *italics* indicate tables. The alphabetical order of the index is letter-by-letter, so that hyphens, en-rules and spaces within index headings are ignored. *vs* denotes differential diagnosis or comparisons.

Abbreviations used in subentries (without explanation):

AIDS acquired immune deficiency syndrome
CNS central nervous system
GPs general practitioners
HIV human immunodeficiency virus
MAOIs monoamine oxidase inhibitors
NSAIDs non-steroidal anti-inflammatory drugs
TENS transcutaneous electrical nerve stimulation

E

F

G

I

O